YAQUTA PATNI MD
FAMILY PRACTICE

YAQUTA PATNI MD
FAMILY PRACTICE

The
5 Minute
Pediatric
Consult

Second Edition

ASSOCIATE EDITORS

LOUIS M. BELL, JR., M.D.
ASSOCIATE PROFESSOR OF PEDIATRICS
ATTENDING PHYSICIAN, INFECTIOUS DISEASES AND EMERGENCY MEDICINE

PETER M. BINGHAM, M.D.
ASSISTANT PROFESSOR OF NEUROLOGY IN PEDIATRICS
ASSISTANT PHYSICIAN

ESTHER K. CHUNG, M.D.
CLINICAL ASSISTANT PROFESSOR OF PEDIATRICS

DAVID F. FRIEDMAN, M.D.
ASSISTANT PROFESSOR OF PEDIATRICS
ASSISTANT PHYSICIAN, DEPARTMENT OF HEMATOLOGY

ANDREW E. MULBERG, M.D.
DIRECTOR, GASTROENTEROLOGY FELLOWSHIP PROGRAM
DEPARTMENTS OF PEDIATRICS, GASTROENTEROLOGY AND NUTRITION

ASSISTANT EDITORS
MITCHEL I. COHEN, M.D.
CHARLES I. SCHWARTZ, M.D.

MANAGING EDITOR
CHERYL KOSMOWSKI

UNIVERSITY OF PENNSYLVANIA
SCHOOL OF MEDICINE

CHILDREN'S HOSPITAL OF PHILADELPHIA
PHILADELPHIA, PENNSYLVANIA

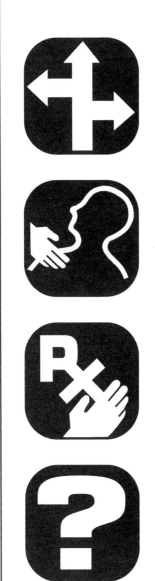

The
5 Minute
Pediatric
Consult

Second Edition

EDITOR

M. WILLIAM SCHWARTZ, M.D.

PROFESSOR OF PEDIATRICS

UNIVERSITY OF PENNSYLVANIA SCHOOL OF MEDICINE

CHILDREN'S HOSPITAL OF PHILADELPHIA

PHILADELPHIA, PENNSYLVANIA

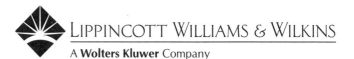

LIPPINCOTT WILLIAMS & WILKINS

A **Wolters Kluwer** Company

Philadelphia • Baltimore • New York • London
Buenos Aires • Hong Kong • Sydney • Tokyo

Editor: Timothy Y. Hiscock
Developmental Editor: Joyce A. Murphy
Manufacturing Manager: Tim Reynolds
Supervising Editor: Mary Ann McLaughlin
Production Service: Colophon
Compositor: The PRD Group, Inc.
Printer: R.R. Donnelley Crawfordsville

© 2000 by LIPPINCOTT WILLIAMS & WILKINS
227 East Washington Square
Philadelphia, PA 19106-3780
lww.com

First edition, 1997

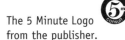 The 5 Minute Logo is a registered trademark of Lippincott Williams & Wilkins. This mark may not be used without written permission from the publisher.

Printed in the USA

Library of Congress Cataloging-in-Publication Data

The 5 minute pediatric consult / editor, M. William Schwartz — 2nd
  ed.
     p.   cm.
  Includes bibliographical references and index.
  ISBN 0-683-30744-4 (alk. paper)
  1. Pediatrics Handbooks, manuals, etc. I. Schwartz, M. William,
1935– . II. Title: Five minute pediatric consult.
  [DNLM: 1. Pediatrics Handbooks.   WS 39 Z99 2000]
RJ48.A15 2000
618.92—dc21
DNLM/DLC
for Library of Congress   99–34055
                               CIP

Care has been taken to confirm the accuracy of the information presented and to describe generally accepted practices. However, the authors, editors, and publisher are not responsible for errors or omissions or for any consequences from application of the information in this book and make no warranty, expressed or implied, with respect to the currency, completeness, or accuracy of the contents of the publication. Application of this information in a particular situation remains the professional responsibility of the practitioner.

The authors, editors, and publisher have exerted every effort to ensure that drug selection and dosage set forth in this text are in accordance with current recommendations and practice at the time of publication. However, in view of ongoing research, changes in government regulations, and the constant flow of information relating to drug therapy and drug reactions, the reader is urged to check the package insert for each drug for any change in indications and dosage and for added warnings and precautions. This is particularly important when the recommended agent is a new or infrequently employed drug.

Some drugs and medical devices presented in this publication have Food and Drug Administration (FDA) clearance for limited use in restricted research settings. It is the responsibility of health care providers to ascertain the FDA status of each drug or device planned for use in their clinical practice.

10 9 8 7 6 5 4 3 2 1

TO

Susan, David, Charlie and memory of Burte and Sloan

MWS

Barbara, Sue, Amy, Chris, Sarak

LMB

Nishan, Tikki, and Aram

PMB

Dennis and Marissa

EKC

Marisa, Elias, Henry, and Isabel, and to Sidney and Adele

DFF

Elyse, Nathaniel and Rebecca

AEM

Brandie and my parents

CS

This second edition is dedicated to the life and memory of Barbara Wei Bell, M.D.
1954–1998

Preface

"The second edition should be the best effort" advised a former book editor. She said that the first edition is the product of a vision about the book tempered by the human elements of writing, missed deadlines, and compromises made while getting the book ready for the publisher. The second edition, she told me, is better, because the staff has had time to see what was successful, what was missing, and how the book was useful to the readers. Hence the challenge we faced in preparing this second edition.

Assembling the content, deciding on a format, and finding authors to write constituted the initial effort for the first edition. The first edition of *The 5 Minute Pediatric Consult*, with its distinctive pink cover, was a big success. Doctors and nurses taking care of children found that the book's easy-to-read format fulfilled their need for rapid retrieval of information about children's diseases and problems. The nurses in the emergency department (Children's Hospital of Philadelphia) wore out the book because they used it as it was designed to be used: to find out information quickly as they were busy caring for patients. Former residents who seldom agreed with anything that came from a faculty member were quite complimentary. At last! Traveling from Kiev, Ukraine to Gallup, New Mexico, I saw the familiar pink book in use. It was even recommended on Amazon.com's web site. The Five Minute Consult format proved to be a success. There are now a series of 5 Minute Consult books available for a variety of medical and veterinary specialties.

Comments from users of the first edition helped shape the second edition. Users appreciated the two-page format concerning each topic and the placement of like components of similar positions in the columns. Users asked for more tables and facts as well as more topics. In the second edition, the first section, Chief Complaints, has been expanded and redesigned. There are more topics in Section II: Specific Diseases, and more tables, and the additional information on surgical procedures, cardiac laboratory information, and laboratory values that add to the use of the book as a reference tool. A section on herbal treatments introduces the topic and includes a table of common herbs that patients either take or accidentally ingest.

This edition could not have been done without the expertise and assistance of many people. Kudos to Cheryl Kosmowski who kept track of all the files and lists of authors, and who maintained communications with Lippincott Williams & Wilkins throughout the publishing process. Thanks to her competence and skills, and exceptional ability to function in the deadline driven activity, the book was delivered on time. Once again, the associate editors did their job of recruiting writers and editing their material. Without the help of Lou Bell, Peter Bingham, Esther Chung, David Friedman, Andy Mulburg, and Charlie Schwartz, the book would not have been completed. I value their friendships and thank them for another excellent effort. Thanks also to Rich Kravitz, Mitch Cohen, and Greg Kennan for managing the pulmonary, cardiology, and collagen disease sections.

During work on this revision, the Williams & Wilkins company merged with Lippincott to become Lippincott Williams & Wilkins. Through this transition, we were fortunate to work with the excellent members of the LWW staff, specifically Joyce Murphy, our developmental editor, Tim Hiscock, acquisition editor, and the production staff. It was a pleasure to work with Joyce as she readied the book for publication; the variety of authors and their expressions of individuality did not faze her. My thanks for her help. We were pleased to see the return to LWW of Katey Millet who helped so significantly in the first edition. She reminds us to cherish each day and work through problems with smiles and positivity. Lastly, the many associations with new and former writers remain an invaluable experience for me.

As always, these efforts to revise the book followed our principles of finding fun in the work, and remembering that our group goal is to improve the health of children by helping others to make good decisions using facts and experience of experts. I hope we met the challenge of making this second edition our best effort.

Since publication of the first edition, we lost an invaluable member of our extended family. We miss Barbara Wei Bell, wife of Lou Bell. Although no longer with us, her charm, special smile, courage, and positivity remain an inspiration to all of us. Her bravery during her illness was a model for everyone, and reminds us to remember what is truly important and that we should not become sidetracked in mundane and insignificant details. This book is dedicated to Barb.

Contributing Authors

Unless otherwise indicated, faculty appointments are at the University of Pennsylvania School of Medicine, and hospital appointments are at Children's Hospital of Philadelphia, Pennsylvania.

WILLIAM J. ALMS, M.D.,Ph.D.
Department of Dermatology

RAANAN ARENS, M.D.
Director
Sleep Disorders Laboratory
Division of Pulmonary Medicine

PHILIPPE F. BACKELJAUW, M.D.
Associate Professor of Pediatrics
Division of Endocrinology
Children's Medical Center
Cincinnati, Ohio 45229

MARK L. BAGARAZZI, M.D.
Assistant Professor of Pediatrics
MCP/Hahnemann School of Medicine
Allegheny University of the Health Sciences
St. Christopher's Hospital for Children
Philadelphia, Pennsylvania 19104

ROBERT N. BALDASSANO, M.D.
Assistant Professor of Pediatrics
Division of Gastroenterology and Nutrition

MEENA SCAVENA BALDI, M.D.
Division of Neurology

LOUIS M. BELL, M.D.
Associate Professor of Pediatrics
Attending Physician
Section of Infectious Diseases
Division of Emergency Medicine

A.G. CHRISTINA BERGQVIST, M.D.
Fellow
EEG and Epilepsy
Division of Neurology

LISA M. BIGGS, M.D.
Clinical Assistant Professor
Department of Pediatrics

PETER M. BINGHAM, M.D.
Assistant Professor of Neurology in Pediatrics
Assistant Physician
Department of Pediatrics

NATHAN J. BLUM, M.D.
Assistant Professor of Pediatrics
Division of Developmental and Behavioral Pediatrics
The Children's Seashore House

JULIE A. BOOM, M.D.
Assistant Professor
Department of Pediatrics
Baylor College of Medicine
Houston, Texas 77030

DEBRA BOYER, M.D.

AMY R. BROOKS-KAYAL, M.D.
Assistant Professor
Departments of Neurology and Pediatrics

KURT A. BROWN, M.D.
Assistant Professor of Pediatrics
Department of Pediatrics
Attending Physician
Division of Gastroenterology and Nutrition

DAVID M. BUSH, M.D.
Division of Cardiology

MAYRA BUSTILLO, M.D.
Division of Pulmonary Medicine

JAMES M. CALLAHAN, M.D.
Assistant Professor and Clinical Investigator
Departments of Emergency Medicine and Pediatrics
SUNY Health Science Center at Syracuse
Attending Physician
Departments of Emergency Medicine and Pediatrics
University Hospital
Syracuse, New York 13210

CARLA CAMPBELL, M.D., M.D.
Clinical Assistant Professor of Pediatrics
Department of Pediatrics
CoMedical Director
Lead Poisoning and Toxicology Clinic

WILLIAM B. CAREY, M.D.
Clinical Professor of Pediatrics
Director
Section on Behavioral Pediatrics
Division of General Pediatrics

CHRISTINE A. CARMAN-DILLON, M.D.
Department of Plastic Surgery

AARON E. CARROLL, M.D.

ROSEMARY CASEY, M.D.
Assistant Professor of Pediatrics

SUZETTE SURRATT CAUDLE, M.D.
Clinical Associate Professor of Pediatrics
University of North Carolina
Chapel Hill, North Carolina
Attending Physician
Division of General Pediatrics
Carolinas Medical Center
Charlotte, North Carolina 28232

ELIZABETH CANDELL CHALOM, M.D.
Director
Pediatric Lyme Disease Program
Section Head
Pediatric Rheumatology
St. Barnabas Medical Center
Director
Pediatric Rheumatology
Children's Hospital of New Jersey
Livington, New Jersey 07039

CINDY W. CHRISTIAN, M.D.
Assistant Professor of Pediatrics
Director
Child Abuse Services

THOMAS H. CHUN, M.D.
Fellow
Division of Emergency Medicine

ESTHER K. CHUNG, M.D., M.P.H.
Clinical Assistant Professor
Department of General Pediatrics
Pediatric Consultant
Office of Maternal and Child Health
City of Philadelphia Department of Public Health
Philadelphia, Pennsylvania 19132

MICHAEL D. CIRIGLIANO, M.D.

LIANA R. CLARK, M.D.
Clinical Assistant Professor
Department of General Pediatrics
Section of Adolescent Medicine

SUSAN E. COFFIN, M.D.
Assistant Professor
Section of Infectious Diseases
Department of Pediatrics

ADAM COHEN, B.A.
Medical Student

MERYL S. COHEN, M.D.
Assistant Professor of Pediatrics
Department of Pediatric Cardiology

MITCHELL I. COHEN, M.D.
Assistant Professor of Pediatrics
Division of Cardiology

ROBERT M. COHN , M.D.
Deputy Director
Clinical Laboratories

PAULO F. COLLETT-SOLBERG, M.D.
Fellow
Division of Endocrinology

DANIEL H. CONWAY, M.D.
Fellow
Section of Neonatology
Department of Pediatrics
St. Christopher's Hospital
Philadelphia, Pennsylvania 19132

PETER B. CRINO, M.D., Ph.D.
Howard Hughes Medical Institute Research Fellow
Department of Pharmacology

GERD CROPP, M.D., Ph.D.
Professor of Clinical Pediatrics
Chief of Pediatric Pulmonary
Department of Pediatrics
University of California San Francisco
San Francisco, California 94143

MONICA DARBY

RICHARD S. DAVIDSON, M.D.
Associate Professor of Orthopaedic Surgery
Attending Surgeon
Division of Orthopaedic Surgery

SUSAN DIBS, M.D.
Instructor in Pediatrics
Division of Emergency Medicine

MARK F. DITMAR, M.D.
Assistant Clinical Professor of Pediatrics
Yale University School of Medicine
New Haven, Connecticut
Chief
Section of General Pediatrics
Norwalk Hospital
Norwalk, Connecticut 06856

DENNIS J. DLUGOS, M.D.
Instructor in Neurology

JOHN P. DORMANS, M.D.
Associate Professor of Orthopaedic Surgery
Chief of Orthopaedic Surgery

HENRY R. DROTT, Ph.D.
Director
Clinical Chemistry Laboratory

DENNIS R. DURBIN, M.D.
Assistant Professor of Pediatrics and Epidemiology
Department of Pediatrics

KAREN D. FAIRCHILD, M.D.
Associate Professor of Pediatrics
Division of Neonatology
University of Maryland Hospital
Baltimore, Maryland 21201

JOEL A. FEIN, M.D.
Assistant Professor of Pediatrics
Attending Physician
Emergency Department

ROBERT J. FERRY, JR., M.D.
Fellow
Division of Endocrinology and Diabetes

HECTOR L. FLORES-ARROYO, M.D.
Assistant Professor of Pediatrics
University of Illinois College of Medicine
Director
Pediatric Pulmonary Medicine
Swedish American Children's Medical Center
Rockford, Illinois 61104

JILL A. FOSTER, M.D.
Assistant Professor of Pediatrics
Allegheny University of the Health Sciences
Attending Physician
St. Christopher's Hospital for Children
Philadelphia, Pennsylvania 19134

JANET H. FRIDAY, M.D.
Assistant Professor
Department of Pediatrics
University of Connecticut
Farmington, Connecticut
Attending Physician
Department of Pediatric Emergency Medicine
Connecticut Children's Medical Center
Hartford, Connecticut 06030

DAVID F. FRIEDMAN, M.D.
Assistant Professor of Pediatrics
Division of Pediatric Hematology

DEBRA L. FRIEDMAN, M.D.
Assistant Professor
Department of Pediatrics
University of Washington School of Medicine
Children's Hospital and Regional Medical Center
Seattle, Washington 98105

KENNETH R. GINSBURG, M.D., MS ED.
Assistant Professor of Pediatrics
Department of Pediatrics

SHMUEL GOLDBERG, M.D.
Fellow
Division of Pulmonary Medicine

JOHN M. GOOD, M.D.

MARC H. GORELICK, M.D.
Assistant Professor of Pediatrics and Epidemiology
Attending Physician
Division of Pediatric Emergency Medicine

JANE M. GOULD, M.D.
Fellow
Department of Pediatric Infectious Diseases

WILLIAM R. GRAESSLE, M.D.

ERNEST M. GRAHAM, M.D.
Assistant Professor
Department of Obstetrics and Gynecology
Allegheny University of the Health Sciences
Philadelphia, Pennsylvani 19130

KATHLEEN GRAHAM

ROBERTA S. GRAY, M.D.
Clinical Professor of Pediatrics
Chief
Pediatric Nephrology
Carolinas Medical Center
Charlotte, North Carolina 28232

ADDA GRIMBERG, M.D.
Instructor
Department of Pediatrics
Fellow
Department of Pediatric Endocrinology and Diabetes

BLAZE ROBERT GUSIC, M.D.
Instructor in Pediatrics
Department of Pediatrics
Attending Physician

CYNTHIA GUZZO, M.D.
Associate Professor
Department of Dermatology

BARBARA HABER, M.D.
Assistant Professor of Pediatrics
Division of Gastroenterology and Nutrition

J. NATHAN HAGSTROM, M.D.
Assistant Professor
Department of Pediatrics
University of Connecticut
Farmington, Connecticut
Director
Hemostasis Program
Connecticut Children's Medical Center
Hartford, Connecticut 06106

HAKON HAKONARSON, M.D.
Assistant Professor
Department of Pediatrics

CHERYL L. HAUSMAN, M.D.
Medical Director
Pediatric and Adolescent Ambulatory Center
Department of Pediatrics
Albert Einstein Medical Center
Philadelphia, Pennsylvania 19141

KATRINKA L. HEHER, M.D.
Assistant Professor of Ophthalmology
Division of Ophthalmology

RICHARD W. HERTLE, M.D., F.A.C.S.
Clinical Scientist
National Eye Institute and Laboratory of Sensory Motor Research
National Institutes of Health
Bethesda, Maryland 20892

TIMOTHY M. HOFFMAN, M.D.
Fellow
Division of Cardiology
Department of Pediatrics

ALEXA N. HOGARTY, M.D.
Fellow
Pediatric Cardiology Division

MICHAEL D. HOGARTY, M.D.
Division of Oncology

DOUGLAS HYDER, M.D.

CYNTHIA R. JACOBSTEIN, M.D.
Instructor
Department of Pediatrics
Fellow
Division of Pediataric Emergency Medicine

STEPHANIE D. JAMES, M.D.
Primary Care

ROBERT KAMEI, M.D.
Director
Pediatric Residency Training Program
Associate Professor of Clinical Pediatrics
University of California San Francisco
San Francisco, California 94143

PETER B. KANG
Fellow
Department of Neurology

LORRAINE KATZ, M.D.
Assistant Professor
Division of Endocrinology and Diabetes

GREGORY F. KEENAN, M.D.
Assistant Professor of Pediatrics
Section of Rheumatology

KARA M. KELLY, M.D.
Assistant Professor of Pediatrics
College of Physicians and Surgeons of Columbia University
Assistant Attending Physician
Division of Pediatric Oncology
The New York Presbyterian Hospital
New York, New York 10032

HELEN ANITA JOHN-KELLY, M.D.
Pediatric Gastroenterologist
Raymond Blank Children's Hospital
Des Moines, Iowa 50321

THOMAS L. KENNEDY III, M.D.
Professor of Clinical Pediatrics
The Yale University School of Medicine
New Haven, Connecticut
Chairman
Department of Pediatrics
Bridgeport Hospital
Bridgeport, Connecticut 06601

HO JIN KIM

MICHELLE M. KLINEK, M.D.
Family Center for Allergy and Asthma
York, Pennsylvania 17403

LAZAROS KOCHILAS, M.D., Ph.D.
Fellow
Pediatric Cardiology
Division of Cardiology

DEBORAH L. KRAMER, M.D.
Assistant Professor of Pediatrics
Department of Pediatric Hematology and Oncology
University of Miami School of Medicine
Miami, Florida 33101

RICHARD MARK KRAVITZ, M.D.
Assistant Professor of Pediatrics
Department of Pediatrics
Division of Pediatric Pulmonary Diseases
Duke University Medical Center
Durham, North Carolina 27710

JANE LAVELLE, M.D.
Assistant Professor
Department of Pediatrics
Assistant Director
Pediatric Emergency Medicine
Department of Emergency Medicine

ANN MARIE LEAHEY, M.D.
Assistant Professor of Pediatrics
Division of Oncology

HAE-RHI LEE, M.D.
Cardiology Fellow
Department of Pediatric Cardiology

MARY B. LEONARD, M.D.
Assistant Professor of Pediatrics and Epidemiology

CHRIS A. LIACOURAS, M.D.
Assistant Professor in Pediatrics
Attending Pediatric Gastroenterologist
Division of Gastroenterology and Nutrition

KAREN LIQUORNIK, M.D.
Fellow
Division of Gastroenterology

KATHLEEN M. LOOMES, M.D.
Fellow
Department of Gastroenterology and Nutrition

JEFFREY P. LOUIE, M.D.
Fellow
Department of Emergency Medicine
Clinical Instructor

DAVID W. LOW, M.D.
Assistant Professor of Surgery
Division of Plastic Surgery

KRISTINE K. MACARTNEY, M.B.B.S.
Fellow
Infectious Disease
Instructor in Pediatrics
Immunologic and Infectious Diseases

ERIC S. MALLER, M.D.
Assistant Professor of Pediatrics
Medical Director
Liver Transplant Program
Division of Gastroenterology and Nutrition

BRADLEY S. MARINO, M.D., M.P.P.
Fellow
Division of Cardiology

MARIA R. MASCARENHAS, M.D.
Assistant Professor of Pediatrics
Division of Gastroenterology and Nutrition
Department of Pediatrics
Director
Nutrition Support Services

CHRISTINA LIN MASTER, M.D.
Attending Physician
Department of Pediatrics
Division of General Pediatrics and Primary Care

ANDREA McGEARY, M.D.
Attending Physician
Primary Care, Cobbs Creek

MARGARET McNAMARA, M.D.
Assistant Clinical Professor
Department of Pediatrics
University of California San Francisco
San Francisco, California 94143

D. ELIZABETH McNEIL, M.D.
Division of Neurology

KEVIN E.C. MEYERS, M.D.
Pediatric Nephrologist
Department of Pediatrics

NAHUSH A. MOKADAM, M.D.

PATRICIA T. MOLLOY, M.D.
Division of Neurology

CHRISTEN MOWAD, M.D.
Associate
Department of Dermatology
Geisinger Medical Center
Danville, Pennsylvania 17821

ANDREW E. MULBERG, M.D., F.A.A.P.
Director
Gastroenterology Fellowship Program
Department of Pediatrics, Gastroenterology and Nutrition

ROBERTO V. NACHAJON, M.D.
Attending Pediatric Pulmonologist
Division of Pediatric Pulmonology
St. Joseph's Children's Hospital
Paterson, New Jersey 07503

FRANCES M. NADEL, M.D.
Assistant Professor
Department of Pediatric Emergency Medicine

MICHAEL E. NORMAN, M.D.
Clinical Professor
Department of Pediatrics
University of North Carolina
Chapel Hill, North Carolina
Chairman and Residency Program Director
Department of Pediatrics
Carolinas Medical Center
Charlotte, North Carolina 28232

CYNTHIA F. NORRIS, M.D.
Clinical Associate in Pediatrics
Division of Hematology
Department of Pediatrics

BRUCE ORIEL, M.D.
Assistant Physician
Primary Care Center, Cobbs Creek

KEVIN C. OSTERHOUDT, M.D.
Assistant Professor of Pediatrics
Division of Emergency Medicine

RITA PANOSCHA, M.D.
Clinical Assistant Professor
Department of Developmental Pediatrics
Children's Seashore House
Philadelphia, Pennsylvania 19104

CARMEN M. PARROTT, M.D.
Fellow
Department of Dermatology

LOUIS PELLIGRINO, M.D.

SHANNON CONNOR PHILLIPS, M.D.
Clinical Assistant Professor
Department of Pediatrics
Indiana University School of Medicine
Indianapolis, Indiana 46202

JONATHAN R. PLETCHER, M.D.
Fellow
Division of Adolescent Medicine

BRENDA PORTER, M.D.

GRAHAM E. QUINN, M.D.
Professor of Ophthalmology
Assistant Surgeon
Division of Ophthalmology

VENKAT RAMESH, M.D., M.R.C.P. (EDIN)
Cardiology Fellow
Division of Cardiology

SUSAN R. RHEINGOLD, M.D.
Fellow
Department of Hematology and Oncology

PAMELA S. RO, M.D.
Cardiology Fellow
Pediatric Cardiology

BRET J. RUDY, M.D.
Assistant Professor of Pediatrics
Attending Physician
General Pediatrics

RICHARD M. RUTSTEIN, M.D.
Associate Professor of Pediatrics
Division of General Pediatrics
Medical Director
Special Immunology Service

DENISE SALERNO, M.D.

MARTA SATIN-SMITH, M.D.
Fellow
Department of Pediatrics
Division of Endocrinology and Diabetes

DAVID B. SCHAFFER, M.D.
Professor of Ophthalmology
Chairman
Division of Opthalmology

SETH L. SCHULMAN, M.D.
Attending Physician
Department of Pediatric Nephrology

CHARLES I. SCHWARTZ, M.D.

M. WILLIAM SCHWARTZ, M.D.
Professor of Pediatrics
Associate Dean
Primary Care Education

PHILIP V. SCRIBANO, D.O.
Assistant Professor
Department of Pediatrics
University of Connecticut School of Medicine
Farmington, Connecticut
Attending Physician
Division of Emergency Medicine
Connecticut Children's Medical Center
Hartford, Connecticut 06106

STEVEN M. SELBST, M.D.
Professor and Vice Chairman
Director
Pediatric Residency Program
Jefferson Medical College of Thomas Jefferson University
Philadelphia, Pennsylvania
Attending Physician
Division of Emergency Medicine
A.I.Dupont Hospital for Children
Wilmington, Delaware 19899

EDISIO SEMEAO, M.D.
Assistant Professor of Pediatrics
Division of Gastroenterology
Saint Christopher's Hospital for Children
Philadelphia, Pennsylvania 19134

TIMOTHY A.S. SENTONGO, M.D.
Fellow
Division of Gastroenterology and Nutrition

MAULLY SHAH, M.B.B.S.
Cardiology Fellow
Department of Pediatric Cardiology

SADHNA C. SHAPIRO, M.D.
Assistant Professor of Pediatrics
Division of Pediatric Hematology and Oncology
Vanderbilt University Medical Center
Nashville, Tennessee 37232

STEVEN C. SHAPIRO, M.D.
Clinical Associate Professor
Department of Pediatrics

KATHY N. SHAW, M.D., M.S.C.E.
Associate Professor of Pediatrics
Director
Emergency Medical Services
Chief
Division of Emergency Medicine

JENNIFER C. SHORES, M.D.
Cardiology Fellow
Cardiac Center

SUZANNE SHUSTERMAN, M.D.
Fellow
Department of Hematology and Oncology

DEBORAH L. SILVER, M.D.
Clinical Assistant Professor
Division of General Pediatrics
Medical Director
CHOP Connection at Abington Memorial Hospital
Abington, Pennsylvania 19001

LAURA N. SINAI, M.D.
Pediatrician
Erdenheim Pediatrics
Abington Memorial Hospital
Abington, Pennsylvania 19001

CHRISTOPHER A. SMITH, M.D.
Allergist and Immunologist
Asthma and Allergy Associates
Ithaca, New York 14850

KIM SMITH-WHITLEY, M.D.
Assistant Professor of Pediatrics
Assistant Physician
Division of Hematology

PHILIP R. SPANDORFER, M.D.
Chief Resident
Department of Pediatrics

H. LYNN STARR, M.D.
Clinical Affiliate
Department of General Pediatrics

JULIE W. STERN, M.D.
Fellow
Department of Hematology and Oncology

MOLLY (MARTHA) W. STEVENS, M.D.
Assistant Professor of Pediatrics
Division of Emergency Medicine

CATHERINE B. SULLIVAN, M.D.
Clinical Staff Associate
Department of Pediatrics

RONN E. TANEL, M.D.
Assistant Professor
Department of Pediatrics
Arrhythmia Service
Division of Cardiology

JAMES W. TEENER, M.D.
Assistant Professor
Department of Neurology

GREGORZ TELEGA, M.D.
Fellow
Department of Gastroenterology

BRUCE TEMPEST, M.D.
Consultant
Gallup Indian Medical Center
Indian Health Service (USPHS)
Gallup, New Mexico 87301

OLAFUR THORARENSON, M.D.
Department of Neurology

NICHOLAS TSAROUHAS, M.D.
Assistant Professor of Clinical Pediatrics and Surgery
Robert Wood Johnson Medical School
Director
Pediatric Emergency Medicine
Department of Emergency Medicine
Cooper Hospital/University Medical Center
Camden, New Jersey 08103

JOHN TUNG, M.B.B.S., M.R.C.P.
Fellow
Division of Pediatric Gastroenterology

ALAN UBA, M.D.
Assistant Clinical Professor
Department of Pediatrics
Division of General Pediatrics
University of California San Francisco
San Francisco, California 94143

ELIZABETH C. UONG, M.D.
Fellow
Instructor of Pediatrics
Department of Pulmonary Medicine

SHEILA VAUGHAN, R.N., B.S.N.
Division of Neurology

EMILY VON SCHEVEN, M.D.
Assistant Professor of Pediatrics
Section of Pediatric Rheumatology
University of California San Francisco
San Francisco, California 94143

SAMEER WAGLE, M.D.
Attending Physician
Department of Pediatrics
Family Health Center and South Regional Medical Center
Laurel, Mississippi 39440

PAUL P. WANG, M.D.
Assistant Professor of Pediatrics
Divisions of Child Development and Neurology
Attending Physician

DROR WASSERMAN, M.D.
Assistant Professor of Clinical Pediatrics, Gastroenterology and Clinical Nutrition
State University of New York
Stony Brook Health Sciences Center
Stony Brook, New York 11794

BARBARA WATSON, M.D.
Director of Vaccine Evaluation
Department of Pediatrics
Albert Einstein Medical Center
Associate Director
Tuberculosis Control Program
Philadelphia Department of Public Health
Philadelphia, Pennsylvania 19132

STUART A. WEINZIMER, M.D.
Assistant Professor of Pediatrics
Division of Endocrinology and Diabetes

MARTIN C. WILSON, M.D.
Assistant Professor of Ophthalmology
Attending Surgeon
Department of Pediatric Opthalmology

GEORGE ANTHONY WOODWARD, M.D.
Director
Emergency Transport Service
Attending Physician
Department of Pediatrics

SONG-GUI YANG, M.D., Ph.D.
Clinic Fellow
Division of Cardiology

ALEX G. YIP, M.D.
Clinical Allergy and Immunology
Southeastern Asthma and Allergy Associates
Wilmington, North Carolina 28403

DONNA ZEITER, M.D.
Assistant Professor
Department of Pediatrics
Connecticut Children's Medical Center
Hartford, Connecticut 06106

KATHY WHOLEY ZSOLWAY, D.O.
Assistant Professor of Pediatrics

Contents

SECTION III: SYNDROMES / 885

SECTION IV: CARDIOLOGY LABORATORY / 891

Timothy M. Hoffman

SECTION V: SURGICAL GLOSSARY / 899

Aaron E. Carroll, Nahush A. Mokadam

SECTION VI: LABORATORY VALUES / 903

Henry R. Drott

SECTION VII: HERBAL TREATMENTS IN PRACTICE / 907

Michael D. Cirigliano

SECTION VIII: TABLES / 917

Monica Darby

DEVELOPMENT

IMMUNIZATION

FEEDING AND NUTRITION

INFECTIOUS DISEASES

GASTROINTESTINAL

SECTION I
Chief Complaints

Abdominal Mass

Database

DEFINITION

An abdominal mass is defined as either an un-usually enlarged abdominal organ (i.e., hepato-megaly, splenomegaly, or an enlarged kidney) or a defined fullness in the abdominal cavity not directly associated with an abdominal organ.

Differential Diagnosis

STOMACH

- Gastroparesis
- Duplication
- Foreign body/bezoar
- Gastric torsion

SPLEEN

- Infiltrative disease (Gaucher, Niemann-Pick)
- Histiocytosis X
- Leukemia
- Hematologic (hemolytic disease, sickle cell disease, hereditary spherocytosis/ellipto-cytosis)

INTESTINE

- Feces (constipation)
- Duplication
- Volvulus
- Intussusception
- Inflammatory bowel disease complications (abscess, phlegmon)
- Toxic megacolon
- Mesenteric/omental cyst
- Lymphoma
- Foreign body
- Appendiceal abscess

PANCREAS

- Pseudocyst (trauma)

LIVER

- Endocrinologic (glycogen storage disease)
- Infectious (hepatitis A, B, C)
- Congenital hepatic fibrosis
- Tumor (neuroblastoma, Wilms, leukemia)
- Vascular (hemangioma, hemangioendo-thelioma)

BLADDER

- Urethral valves
- Neurogenic bladder

OVARY

- Dermoid
- Follicular cyst
- Torsion
- Gonadal tumor

KIDNEY

- Hydronephrosis/ureteropelvic obstruction
- Polycystic/multicystic disease[1]
- Wilms tumor
- Renal vein thrombosis
- Nephroblastomatosis

PERITONEAL

- Ascites
- Teratoma

UTERUS

- Pregnancy
- Hydrometrocolpos

ADRENAL

- Neuroblastoma
- Adrenal hemorrhage
- Pheochromocytoma

GALLBLADDER

- Choledochal cyst
- Hydrops
- Obstruction (stone, stricture, trauma)

ABDOMINAL WALL

- Umbilical/inguinal/ventral hernia
- Omphalocele/gastroschisis
- Trauma (rectus hematoma)
- Tumor (fibroma, lipoma, rhabdomyosarcoma)

OTHER

- Mesenteric cyst
- Omental cyst
- Lymphangioma

Approach to the Patient

GENERAL GOALS

Often, abdominal masses in children are found by an unsuspecting parent or by a physician during a routine physical examination. Most masses have no specific signs or symptoms. In children, abdominal masses require immediate attention. When evaluating a pediatric abdomi-nal mass, an organized approach is paramount in determining its etiology.

Phase 1: Determine the location of the ab-dominal mass and its association with intra-abdominal organs.

Phase 2: Perform diagnostic tests, the abdom-inal ultrasound is the most efficient way to start the evaluation.

Phase 3: Treatment (see Laboratory Aids)

Data Gathering

HISTORY

Question: Frequency and quality of bowel move-ments?
Significance: Constipation, intussusception

Question: History of abdominal trauma?
Significance: Pancreatic pseudocyst

Question: History of weight loss?
Significance: Tumor, posterior urethral valves, inflammatory bowel disease

Question: Presence of jaundice?
Significance: Liver/biliary disease

Question: Hematuria or dysuria?
Significance: Renal disease

Question: Sexual activity?
Significance: Pregnancy

Question: Fever?
Significance: Abscess

Question: What is the age of the patient?
Significance: The age of the patient is often a helpful clue in investigating the cause of the abdominal mass. The most common types of ab-dominal mass in newborns include renal dis-ease (cystic kidney disease, renal vein thrombo-sis, hydronephrosis), adrenal hemorrhage, congenital anomalies, and teratoma. In pre-school-aged children and adolescents, approxi-mately 20% of abdominal masses arise from the gastrointestinal tract, while 5% have their ori-gin in the liver or biliary tree. Wilms tumor typ-ically occurs in preschool-aged children, while ovarian disorders present in adolescents.

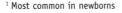

[1] Most common in newborns

Physical Examination

Finding: Location of the mass
Significance:

- Left upper quadrant mass typically involves the kidney or spleen
- Right upper quadrant mass involves the liver or gallbladder or indicates a choledochal cyst
- Right lower quadrant mass indicates an abscess (inflammatory bowel disease), intestinal phlegmon, intussusception, or ovarian process
- Left lower quadrant mass indicates constipation

Finding: Epigastric mass
Significance: Commonly arises from an abnormality of the stomach (bezoar, torsion) or the pancreas (pseudocyst)

Finding: Flank masses
Significance: Often represent renal disease

Finding: Hard and immobile
Significance: Palpable tumors

Finding: Large, extends across the midline
Significance: Teratomas

The abdomen of a normal infant and child should be completely soft and non-tender. As a child ages, an increase in abdominal wall musculature may give greater resistance on examination, but the abdomen should continue to be soft to deep palpation.

 ## Laboratory Aids

Test: CBC
Significance: Anemia or hemolysis

Test: Chemistry panel
Significance: Renal disease (BUN, creatinine), liver disease (ALT, AST, alkaline phosphatase), gallbladder disease (bilirubin, GGTP), pancreatic disease (amylase), or intestinal disease (hypoalbuminemia)

Test: Abdominal ultrasound
Significance: Most useful pediatric diagnostic test for the evaluation of abdominal masses because the paucity of fat in children enhances its diagnostic detail; the disadvantage of ultrasound is its operator variability and its limitations when bowel gas obscures underlying abdominal tissues.

Test: Computed tomography scan
Significance: Can provide more detail when there is overlying gas or bone

Test: Plain abdominal x-ray studies
Significance: Presence of calcifications, extension into the chest

Test: Magnetic resonance imaging
Significance: Vascular lesions of liver, major vessels, and tumors

Test: Radioisotope HIDA scan
Significance: Liver, gallbladder, and intravenous urography (Wilms tumor, cystic kidney disease)

Test: Upper gastrointestinal, barium enema
Significance: Can be of benefit when the mass involves the intestine

Test: Laparoscopy
Significance: Can be useful for direct intraperitoneal visualization and biopsy of abdominal masses

 ## Emergency Care

Of all the diseases listed in the differential diagnosis, patients who present with an abdominal mass and signs and/or symptoms of intestinal obstruction (intussusception, volvulus, gastric torsion, bezoar, foreign body), toxic megacolon, ovarian torsion, biliary obstruction (stone, hydrops), fever, or pancreatitis (pseudocyst) require immediate hospitalization. Initial diagnostic studies should include an abdominal ultrasound, plain abdominal x-ray studies, and a surgical consultation. The remaining causes of abdominal masses require urgent care and timely evaluation.

Issues for Referral

Except for the diagnosis of constipation, the presence of an abdominal mass requires immediate attention. For all masses in children, diagnostic studies should be performed expeditiously at a facility capable of diagnosing pediatric disorders. Once the abnormality is identified, the appropriate pediatric subspecialist should be consulted.

Clinical Pearls

In infants, a full bladder is often mistaken for an abdominal mass, while in neonates, a palpable liver edge can be normal and is often appreciated. Severe constipation in older children and adolescents can present as a large, hard mass extending from the pubis past the umbilicus. Finally, gastric distention should be considered in all children who present with a tympanitic epigastric mass.

BIBLIOGRAPHY

Mahaffey SM, Rychman RC, Martin LW. Clinical aspects of abdominal masses in children. *Semin Roentgenol* 1988;23:161–174.

Merten DF, Kirks DR. Diagnostic imaging of pediatric abdominal masses. *Pediatr Clin North Am* 1985;32:1397–1426.

Schwartz MW. Abdominal masses. In: Schwartz MW, Curry TA, Charney ED, Ludwig S, eds. *Principle and practice of clinical pediatrics*. Chicago: Yearbook, 1987, 139–144.

Swischuk LE, Hayden CK Jr. Abdominal masses in children. *Pediatr Clin North Am* 1985;32:1281–1298.

Taylor LA, Ross AJ III. Abdominal masses. In: Walker WA, Durie PR, Hamilton JR, Walker-Smith JA, Watkins JB, eds. *Pediatric gastrointestinal disease*. Philadelphia: BC Decker, 1991, 132–146.

Author: Chris A. Liacouras

Abdominal Pain

 Database

DEFINITION

Abdominal pain is a frequent complaint in the pediatric age group (see table More Common Causes of Abdominal Pain by Age, below). Pain may be acute or chronic, focal or non-specific. A child's complaint of abdominal pain can originate from gastrointestinal and non-gastrointestinal sources within the abdomen, or can be the manifestation of referred pain from extra-abdominal sites. A careful, complete history and physical examination are required to elucidate the origins of this chief complaint.

 Differential Diagnosis

CONGENITAL/ANATOMIC

- Incarcerated hernia
- Intestinal adhesions
- Intussusception
- Malrotation with volvulus
- Ovarian torsion
- Testicular torsion
- Uteropelvic junction obstruction

INFECTIOUS

- Cystitis and urinary tract infections
- Fitz-Hugh-Curtis syndrome
- Gastroenteritis (bacterial, viral or parasitic)
- *Helicobacter pylori* gastritis
- Mononucleosis with splenic enlargement/rupture
- Otitis media
- Pharyngitis
- Pelvic inflammatory disease
- Peritonitis
- Pneumonia
- Psoas abscess
- Sepsis
- Tubo-ovarian abscess
- Varicella

TOXIC, ENVIRONMENTAL, DRUGS

- Anticholinergic drugs
- Caustic ingestions
- Intestinal foreign body
- Heavy metal (i.e., lead) ingestion
- Mushroom poisoning
- Sympathomimetic drugs

TRAUMA

- Child abuse
- Duodenal hematoma
- Perforated viscus
- Splenic hematoma/rupture

TUMOR

- Any tumor, benign or malignant, leading to viscous obstruction
- Leukemia
- Lymphoma
- Nephroblastoma
- Wilms tumor

METABOLIC

- Diabetic ketoacidosis

ALLERGIC/INFLAMMATORY

- Appendicitis
- Cholecystitis
- Eosinophilic gastroenteritis
- Hemolytic-uremic syndrome
- Henoch-Schöein purpura
- Hepatitis
- Inflammatory bowel disease
- Mesenteric adenitis
- Necrotizing enterocolitis
- Pancreatitis
- Peptic ulcer or gastritis
- Esophagitis or duodenitis

FUNCTIONAL

- Depression
- Functional abdominal pain
- Malingering
- Munchausen syndrome (±by proxy)

MISCELLANEOUS

- Abdominal migraine
- Cholelithiasis
- Colic
- Constipation
- Dysmenorrhea
- Ectopic pregnancy
- Endometriosis
- Ileus
- Intestinal pseudo-obstruction
- Irritable bowel syndrome
- Lactose intolerance
- Mittelschmerz
- Nephrolithiasis
- Ovarian cyst
- Pregnancy
- Porphyria
- Sickle-cell disease
- Typhlitis (in the presence of an immunocompromised host)

Approach to the Patient
GENERAL GOALS

Decide if abdominal pain complaints require emergent, urgent or non-immediate intervention.

Phase 1: Careful and complete history and physical examination to narrow this extensive differential diagnosis.

Phase 2: Directed laboratory evaluations should be made to support more likely portions of the differential diagnosis. If a narrowed differential is difficult to formulate, every effort should be made to assure that the patient is clinically stable. A limited blood and/or radiographic evaluation screening with a CBC, ESR, comprehensive metabolic panel (i.e., Na+, K+, Cl−, CO_2, BUN, creatinine, glucose, total protein, albumin, ALT, uric acid, LDH) and/or abdominal x-ray for significant abnormalities could be made to ensure there are no significant abnormalities above one's clinical suspicion.

Phase 3: Institute appropriate therapy related to diagnosis.

More Common Causes of Abdominal Pain by Age

INFANTS	TODDLERS TO PRETEENS	ADOLESCENTS
Colic	Appendicitis	Appendicitis
Child abuse	Child abuse	Constipation
Infectious gastroenteritis	Constipation	Dysmenorrhea
Intestinal obstruction	Infectious gastroenteritis	Infectious gastroenteritis
Intussusception	Ingestions	Inflammatory bowel disease
Incarcerated hernia	Otitis media	Irritable bowel disease
Necrotizing enterocolitis	Pancreatitis	Lactose intolerance
Pneumonia	Pharyngitis	Mittelschmerz
Pancreatitis	Pneumonia	Ovarian cyst
Sepsis	Trauma	Pancreatitis
Testicular torsion	Urinary tract infections	Pelvic inflammatory disease
Urinary tract infections		Sickle cell disease
		Trauma
		Urinary tract infections

Data Gathering

HISTORY

Question: Location of pain?
Significance: Pain etiology (see table below)

Question: Duration of pain?
Significance: Acute versus chronic illness

Question: Onset and progression of symptoms?
Significance: Evolution of painful process to help discriminate the exact pathological process

Question: Frank hematochezia?
Significance: Colonic bleeding or massive upper gastrointestinal bleeding

Question: Abdominal distension?
Significance: Distension of an abdominal viscus by air, stool, or fluid

Question: Radiation of pain?
Significance: Certain entities characteristically have radiation of pain (i.e., pancreatitis to the back, appendicitis to the right lower quadrant, gallstones to the shoulder).

Question: Pain relieved by bowel movements?
Significance: Etiology may be related to colonic distension (by air or stool) or inflammation (colitis).

Question: Bowel movement pattern?
Significance: Constipation

Question: Relationship to emesis?
Significance: Usually upper intestinal tract disorders

 ## Physical Examination

Finding: Location of pain
Significance: See table Etiology of Abdominal Pain Based on Most Common Symptom Location, below

Finding: Re-examinations by the same health care provider for changing characteristics
Significance: Evolution of abdominal process

Finding: Rebound tenderness
Significance: Peritonitis and the potential need for surgical intervention

Finding: Rectal examination
Significance: Peritoneal irritation, additional localization of pain, masses, presence and consistency of stool, and/or heme positive stools

 ## Laboratory Aids

Test: CBC with differential
Significance: Total white count is non-specific and may be a poor indicator of intestinal inflammation.

Test: Erythrocyte sedimentation rate (ESR)
Significance: Non-specific indicator of systemic inflammation

Test: Urinalysis
Significance: General screen for urinary tract abnormalities

Test: Two position abdominal x-ray
Significance: Possible clue to ileus, intussusception, intestinal obstruction, retained feces, or gas.

 ## Emergency Care

Every effort should be made to ensure that the patient is clinically stable. Frequent evaluation of vital signs and physical examination are a means of assessing evolving pain and ensure the patient is well enough for potential discharge.

Common Questions and Answers

Q: What is the most common cause of abdominal pain in children?
A: Constipation is probably still the most common presentation of abdominal pain. It can easily imitate the presentation of any organic disease, with localization of pain to any quadrant with any symptoms, including vomiting, diarrhea, or reflux.

Q: What are some of the physical findings associated with various abdominal pain syndromes?
A: In the presence of acute pancreatitis, there may be discoloration of the umbilicus (Cullen sign) and/or flank area (Grey Turner) sign. These are seen only in severe hemorrhagic pancreatitis. The presence of Murphy's sign is associated with gallbladder pathology. Tenderness over McBurney's point could suggest a process in the appendix.

Q: What is Rovsing sign?
A: This is tenderness over the left lower quadrant, which also causes pain in the right lower quadrant. This is highly suspicious for appendicitis.

Issues for Referral

Persistent abdominal pain without clear etiology or chronic gastrointestinal diseases should be referred to a pediatric gastroenterologist.

Clinical Pearls

• The farther the complaint of pain is away from the periumbilical region, the more likely the pain etiology represents organic disease.
• True nighttime waking with pain is more often correlated with organic disease than functional pain.

BIBLIOGRAPHY

Apley J. Psychosomatic aspects of gastrointestinal problems in children. *Clin Gastroenterol* 1977;6:311–320.

Hatch EI. The acute abdomen in children. *Pediatr Clin North Am* 1985;32:1151–1164.

Mason JD. The evaluation of acute abdominal pain in children. *Emerg Med Clin North Am* 1996;14:629–643.

Pearigen PD. Unusual causes of abdominal pain. *Emerg Med Clin North Am* 1996;14:593–613.

Author: Kurt A. Brown

Etiology of Abdominal Pain Based on Most Common Symptom Location*

LEFT UPPER QUADRANT	EPIGASTRIC	RIGHT UPPER QUADRANT
Splenic trauma	Esophagitis	Cholecystitis
	Gastritis	Cholelithiasis
	Gastroesophageal reflux disease	Fitz-Hugh-
	Pancreatitis	Curtis syndrome
	Peptic disease	Pneumonia
	SUPRAPUBIC	*RIGHT LOWER QUADRANT*
	Cystitis	Appendicitis
	Dysmenorrhea	Crohn disease
	Pelvic inflammatory disease	Mesenteric adenitis

*Non-lateralizing symptoms are not listed.

Abnormal Bleeding

 Database

DEFINITION

Abnormal bleeding may present as (1) an increase in severity or frequency of nose bleeds, bruising, or menstrual bleeding; (2) as bleeding in unusual sites such as joints or internal organs; or (3) as excessive bleeding for the degree of trauma experienced (see table Common Causes of Abnormal Bleeding).

 Differential Diagnosis

Abnormal bleeding can be the result of an acquired or congenital disorder of the procoagulant factors, platelets, or the vessel wall; disorders of procoagulant factors may be singular or multiple, disorders of platelets may be quantitative or qualitative, and disorders of the vessel wall may be inflammatory or structural. Consider child abuse in children with unusual bruising.

THROMBOCYTOPENIA RESULTING FROM DEFECTIVE PRODUCTION

Congenital/Genetic

- Thrombocytopenia with absent radii (TAR) syndrome
- Amegakaryocytic thrombocytopenia
- Wiskott-Aldrich syndrome
- May-Hegglin anomaly
- Chédiak-Higashi anomaly
- Fanconi anemia
- Metabolic disorders

Acquired

- Aplastic anemia
- Drug-induced marrow suppression
- Virus-induced marrow suppression
- Chemotherapy
- Radiation injury

Marrow Infiltration

- Neoplasia (leukemia, neuroblastoma)
- Histiocytosis
- Osteopetrosis
- Myelofibrosis
- Storage diseases

THROMBOCYTOPENIA RESULTING FROM INCREASED DESTRUCTION

Immune Thrombocytopenia

- Idiopathic thrombocytopenic purpura (ITP)
- Neonatal alloimmune thrombocytopenia
- Maternal autoimmune [e.g., maternal ITP and systemic lupus erythematosus (SLE)]
- Drug-induced (heparin, sulfonamides, digoxin, chloroquine)
- Infection
- Viral, bacterial, fungal, rickettsial

PLATELET FUNCTION DISORDERS

Congenital

- von Willebrand disease (vWD)

Drug

- Aspirin, NSAIDs, guaifenesin, antihistamines, phenothiazines, anticonvulsants

Other

- Uremia
- Paraproteinemia

COAGULATION DISORDERS

Prolongation of aPTT

- Deficiency of factor VIII, IX, XI, or XII
- Acquired inhibitor or lupus anticoagulant
- vWD (often normal)

Prolongation of PT

- Mild vitamin K deficiency
- Liver disease, mild to moderate
- Deficiency of factor VII
- Factor VII inhibitor

Prolongation of PT and aPTT

- Liver disease, severe
- DIC
- Severe vitamin K deficiency
- Hemorrhagic disease of the newborn
- Deficiency of factors II, V, or X or fibrinogen
- Dysfibrinogenemia
- Hypoprothrombinemia associated with a lupus anticoagulant

Normal Screening Laboratory Tests

- vWD
- Factor XIII deficiency

VESSEL WALL DISORDERS

Congenital

- Hereditary hemorrhagic telangiectasia
- Ehlers-Danlos syndrome
- Osteogenesis imperfecta
- Marfan syndrome

Acquired

- Vasculitis (SLE, HSP, etc.)
- Scurvy

Approach to the Patient

Phase 1: Includes a thorough history and physical examination as well as standard screening laboratory tests: PT/aPTT and platelet count. A familial history is an important component of this phase.

Phase 2: If a bleeding disorder is suspected but the initial screening tests are negative then testing for vWD, factor XIII deficiency, and dysfibrinogenemia is warranted. A bleeding time should be performed at this phase if a platelet dysfunction is suspected.

Phase 3: Any abnormal screening tests need further evaluation with additional testing to define the specific disorder (e.g., factor assays, platelet aggregations).

 Data Gathering

HISTORY

Questions that help confirm presence of a bleeding disorder and assist in determining severity:

- Spontaneous bleeding?
- Bleeding in unusual places without significant trauma (intracranial, joints, etc.)?
- Bruising and bleeding disproportionate to injury? Large or palpable bruising?
- Poorly controlled epistaxis? [localized trauma (nosepicking) can exacerbate epistaxis, or be the sole cause of it, unilateral epistaxis may indicate local vascular problems, rather than bleeding disorder]
- Excessive bleeding with tooth extraction?
- Abnormal bleeding at or after circumcision or surgical procedure?
- Prolonged bleeding from minor cuts?
- Excessive bleeding following a fracture?
- Familial history of bleeding disorder?

Questions that help target the defective component of hemostasis.

Question: Mucosal bleeding (gum bleeding, epistaxis)?
Significance: Platelet disorder, vWD, hereditary hemorrhagic telangiectasia, dysfibrinogenemia)

Question: Petechiae?
Significance: Platelet disorders, vWD

Question: Menorrhagia?
Significance: Common in vWD and platelet disorders

Question: Recent medications?
Significance: Aspirin and other drugs affect platelet function

---

Common Causes of Abnormal Bleeding

	COAGULATION FACTORS	PLATELET DISORDERS	VASCULAR DEFECTS
Congenital/Genetic	• Hemophilia (factors VIII, IX, or XI) • von Willebrand disease	• Neonatal alloimmune thrombocytopenia • Storage pool disease	• Hereditary hemorrhagic telangiectasias
Acquired	• Liver disease	• ITP • Leukemia	• Vasculitis: HSP

Question: Presence of renal or liver disease?
Significance: Azoturia contributes to bleeding. Liver disease reduces clotting factors.

Question: Severe malnutrition?
Significance: Scurvy, decreased hepatic synthesis

 ## Physical Examination

Finding: Petechiae in skin and mucous membranes
Significance: Disorder of platelet number or function, vWD

Finding: Small bruises in unusual places (trunk)
Significance: Possible platelet disorder, vWD

Finding: Large bruises or palpable bruises
Significance: Coagulation deficiencies, severe platelet disorders, or vWD

Finding: Delayed wound healing
Significance: Factor XIII deficiency and dysfibrinogenemia

Finding: Purpura localized to lower body (buttocks, legs, ankles)
Significance: Henoch-Schönlein purpura (HSP)

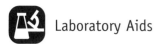 ## Laboratory Aids

Phase 1: Initial Laboratory Screening

- Platelet count
- PT and aPTT
- Bleeding time to screen for qualitative platelet disorders and may also help identify vWD (may be delayed until phase 2)

Phase 2

- Qualitative platelet defect suspected

—Platelet aggregation studies with ristocetin, collagen, thrombin, and ADP
—vWD suspected
—Factor VIII:C
—von Willebrand factor (vWF; VIIIR:Ag)
—Ristocetin cofactor activity
—vWF multimeric analysis

- Thrombin time or fibrinogen assay to screen for hypo- or dysfibrinogenemia

Phase 3: Discriminating Laboratory Studies for Abnormal Phase 1 Tests

When thrombocytopenia is present:

- Inspection of blood smear (screening for bone marrow diseases)
- Mean platelet volume (elevated in destructive causes, low in Wiskott-Aldrich)
- Bone marrow aspiration (rarely necessary)

—When DIC is suspected (infection, liver disease, massive trauma, PT/aPTT prolonged, etc.):

- Fibrinogen
- D-dimer or fibrin split products
- Peripheral smear inspection for RBC fragments

—Prolonged aPTT

- Inhibitor screen (50:50 mixing study of patient's and normal plasma)
- aPTT fully corrects

—Specific factor assays in the following order: VIII, IX, XI, X

- Partial or no correction after mixing study

—Inhibitor present
—Confirmatory test for the presence of a lupus anticoagulant with a platelet neutralizing procedure

Prolonged PT

- Inhibitor screen should also be considered for prolonged PT
- Specific factor levels (II, VII, X)
- Prolonged PT and aPTT

—Test for DIC, liver disease, and fibrinogen disorders, as described previously
—Vitamin K deficiency, moderate to severe
—Factor assays: X and II (prothrombin)

PITFALLS OF TESTING

Bleeding Time

- May be prolonged when platelet count below 100,000/mm³
- Affected when aspirin is ingested within 7 days
- Other drugs taken within 8 to 12 hours may also effect result (NSAIDs, antihistamines)
- Prolongation does not correlate with bleeding risk
- Result depends on method and on experience of technician

PT and aPTT

- Clotting times are longer and standard deviation wider in neonates than in adult controls
- Polycythemia (Hct.65%) or too little blood collected will result in a spuriously high result
- Consider heparin contamination in samples from arterial or central venous catheters

vWD Studies

- Normal reference ranges depend on patient's ABO blood group type
- Values fluctuate over time and may periodically be normal in affected individuals
- May require repeated testing to make diagnosis

 ## Emergency Care

- Pressure, elevation, and ice are generally helpful for most bleeding disorders when active bleeding is present.
- Monitoring for complications of significant blood loss in the acute setting is important.
- More definitive care is dictated by the nature of the underlying hemostatic defect. Platelet transfusions are useful in disorders of thrombocytopenia due to decreased production and for intrinsic qualitative platelet disorders but not for immune platelet disorders. Frozen plasma should only be used in severe cases when the exact diagnosis is not readily available but a defect in coagulation is suspected.
- Head injuries in patients with thrombocytopenia or hemophilia require immediate medical attention.

Common Questions and Answers

Q: What are the proper preoperative screening tests for bleeding disorders prior to elective surgery such as tonsillectomy?
A: A thorough personal history, familial history, and physical examination are by far the most important screening tests. The bleeding time is not recommended. A CBC and PT/aPTT are often requested by the surgeon but normal results do not assure that a bleeding complication will not occur. Overall the sensitivity and specificity of these screening tests is poor.

Q: Bruising is a normal part of childhood. How does one know when bruising is "too much"?
A: There is no proven set of clinical criteria that can reliably predict who should undergo an evaluation and who should not.

Issues for Referral

Indications

- If the history and physical examination strongly suggest the presence of a bleeding disorder or if the screening tests are abnormal the patient should be referred to a pediatric hematologist.
- If von Willebrand disease is suspected, referral to a pediatric hematologist is usually necessary to determine the exact type and for testing that will assess the patient's response to ddAVP therapy.
- Patients with hemophilia should have regular visits to a hemophilia treatment center for follow-up and coordination of care.
- Consultation with a hematologist is recommended prior to invasive procedures, surgery, or dental work.

Screening Tests

Most clinical laboratories can do PT/aPTT and CBC, but may not be able to do bleeding times in young children.

Clinical Pearls

Children with bleeding disorders are more likely to have large bruises (greater than 5 cm), hematomas (palpable bruises), and have bruises on more than one body part.

BIBLIOGRAPHY

Bell B, Canty D, Audet M. Hemophilia: an updated review. *Pediatr Rev* 1995;16(8):290–298.

Laposata M, Connor AM, Hicks DG, Phillips DK. *The clinical hemostasis handbook.* Chicago: Year Book, 1989.

Manno CS. Difficult pediatric diagnoses—bruising and bleeding. *Pediatr Clin North Am* 1991;38:637–655.

Pramanik AK. Bleeding disorders in neonates. *Pediatr Rev* 1992;13(5):163–173.

Author: J. Nathan Hagstrom

Allergic Child

Database

DEFINITION

The allergic child has the tendency toward IgE mediated reactions in response to pollens, molds, environmental allergens, drugs, or foods. These reactions may manifest as any of the following: eczema, allergic rhinitis, asthma, angioedema, hives, or anaphylaxis. These children may have dark circles under their eyes (allergic shiners), a nasal crease, or the child may give you an allergic salute (upward rubbing of nose to relieve a nasal itch). A careful environmental history is essential. The history may reveal seasonal or year round symptoms.

Differential Diagnosis

EYES
- Physical and chemical irritants
- Viral or bacterial infection

NOSE
- Recurrent upper respiratory tract infections
- Rhinitis medicamentosum
- Drugs that cause nasal congestion

—Oral contraceptives
—Reserpine
—Guanethidine
—Propranolol
—Thioridazine
—Tricyclic antidepressants
—Aspirin

- Airway irritants

—Smoke
—Environmental pollution
—Cold air

- Kartagener syndrome
- Cystic fibrosis
- Sinusitis

LUNGS
- Intrinsic asthma
- Airway irritants

—Smoke
—Environmental pollution
—Cold air

- Gastroesophageal reflux
- Foreign body aspiration
- Anatomic defect in airway
- Cystic Fibrosis
- Kartagener syndrome
- Immune deficiency

SKIN
- Viral exanthams
- Autoimmune disorders
- Physical and chemical irritants

Data Gathering

HISTORY

Specific questions are best asked systematically in a review of systems format.

Ears
- Otitis
- Myringotomy Tubes
- Hearing Loss

Nasal
- Frequent URIs
- Sinusitis
- Polyps
- Epistaxis
- Snoring
- Sneezing
- Rhinitis
- Deviated septum
- Obstruction
- Itch
- Mouth breathing
- Nasal discharge

Throat
- Sore throat
- Throat clearing
- Postnasal drip
- Palate itch
- Tonsillitis
- Tonsillectomy
- Croup

Chest
- Day cough
- Night cough
- Sputum production
- Pain
- Wheeze
- Shortness of breath
- Cyanosis

Eyes
- Itching
- Tearing
- Discharge
- Swelling
- Redness
- Rubbing

Gastrointestinal
- Anorexia
- Nausea
- Vomiting
- Diarrhea
- Constipation
- Gas
- Belching
- Abdominal pain
- Fatty or foul-smelling stools

Skin
- Eczema
- Hives
- Angioedema
- Contact dermatitis
- Seborrheic dermatitis
- Skin infections
- Pruritis

Genitourinary
- Dysuria
- Burning
- Polyuria
- Hematuria
- Enuresis

Headache
- Location
- Character
- Frequency
- Duration
- Nausea
- Vomiting
- Scotomata

Other important questions include:

Question: Does your child have food or drug allergies?
Significance: Be sure to ask what type of reaction the child had (many types of intolerances are called allergies by parents). Generally, allergies are IgE mediated reactions resulting in wheezing, allergic rhinitis, hives, angioedema, eczema, or anaphylaxis. Intolerances generally include a non-specific rash, diarrhea, gas, headache, or hyperactivity. Specifically ask about peanut, nut, and shellfish allergy (allergy to any of these is an indication for an EpiPen (Center Labs, Port Washington, NY), and lifelong avoidance).

Question: Has your child ever been stung by a bee, and, if so, what was the reaction?
Significance: Systemic reactions are an indication for referral to an allergist for venom desensitization. Venom desensitization can be potentially lifesaving. Ask the parent if they know the type of bee involved with the reaction. (Honey bees are the only bees that leave their stinger at the sting site.)

Question: Does anyone in your family have hayfever (allergic rhinitis), asthma, or eczema?
Significance: Familial history of atopy increases the likelihood of atopy in other family members.

Questions to ask regarding the environment:

Question: Do you have a basement?
Significance: Damp basements are a source of mold spores.

Question: Are there any damp areas in your home?
Significance: Damp areas serve to propagate mold growth in the home.

Question: Do you have forced air or radiator heat?
Significance: Forced air heat tends to blow allergen laden dust around the home.

Question: How do you cool your home?
Significance: Opening outside windows lets the pollens from outside into the house.

Question: Do you have a humidifier?
Significance: Molds can grow in the water, and increased ambient humidity will raise the dust mite population in the home.

Question: Are there any smokers in the home?
Significance: Cigarette smoke is an airway irritant and can exacerbate respiratory difficulties.

Question: Are there any pets in the home, at school, or in daycare?
Significance: Animal dander is a common aeroallergen. Pets should be excluded from the bedroom (a pet that sleeps on the patient's bed is a common problem).

Question: Are there many stuffed animals or books in the bedroom?
Significance: Dust mites love these dust collectors, and they should be removed from the bedroom. Environmental control efforts should be focused on the bedroom. Patients can have significant allergen exposure during sleep.

Question: Does the bedroom have carpeting?
Significance: Hardwood or tile floors are best to keep the dust mite population under control.

Question: How often do you wash the bedding, what type of pillow do you have, and is the mattress encased in plastic?
Significance: To keep the dust mite population under control the bedding should be washed in hot water at least once every two weeks (hot water kills dust mites), the pillow should be fiber filled, and the mattress should be encased in plastic.

Question: Where does the patient spend most of his time?
Significance: Allergenic exposure where most of the patient's time is spent is most important.

Question: Does the patient attend daycare?
Significance: Daycare is a major source of upper respiratory tract infections, which can mimic allergies and exacerbate reactive airway disease.

 ## Physical Examination

A complete physical examination is essential to rule out systemic disease that can mimic allergies (i.e., clubbing, anatomic obstruction, heart murmur, etc.)

Finding: Ocular allergic signs
Significance:

• Allergic shiners are due to passive congestion in the nose, which impedes the venous return to the vessels under the eyes.
• Cobblestoning of the conjunctiva is associated with allergic conjunctivitis.
• Dennie sign (Morgan line), infraorbital folds associated with suborbital edema secondary to atopy.
• Clear stringy discharge is the characteristic eye discharge seen in allergic conjunctivitis.

Finding: Nasal allergic signs
Significance:

• Pale edematous nasal mucosa is characteristic of allergic rhinitis.
• Nasal crease across the bridge of nose is secondary to repeated upward rubbing of the nose.
• Clear nasal discharge with or without occlusion is characteristic of allergic rhinitis.

Finding: Ears allergic signs
Significance: Fluid in the middle ear, or retracted tympanic membranes may be associated with eustachian tube dysfunction seen with allergic inflammation.

Finding: Throat allergic signs
Significance: Cobblestoning of posterior pharynx secondary to submucosal lymphoid hyperplasia can be seen in allergic patients.

Finding: Lungs allergic signs
Significance: Wheezes, rhonchi, decreased air entry, and chronic obstruction can be secondary to allergic responses.

Finding: Skin allergic signs
Significance: Eczema, hives, angioedema, and dermatographism are all characteristic of allergic skin.

 ## Laboratory Aids

Test: Immediate hypersensitivity
Significance:

• Skin prick tests to suspected allergens based on history. These are the study of choice because of their low cost, high sensitivity, rapid results, and documented excellent correlation with clinical sensitivity especially to pollens and animal dander.
• Intradermal skin tests are reserved for patients who have a negative prick test and a suspicious history. This study is more sensitive than prick tests, but less specific and they pose a greater risk of systemic reactions.
• RAST tests (Radioallergosorbent tests) measures free serum IgE to a specific antigen to which a particular patient may be sensitized. These tests are primarily reserved for patients at risk for a severe systemic reaction from skin testing (i.e., Latex allergic patients), or in patients in whom skin testing is not feasible (i.e., patients with extensive skin disease). These tests are less sensitive than skin prick and intradermal tests.
• Serum IgE levels have a low sensitivity and, generally, are of little help.
• Presence of blood eosinophilia. Eosinophils in the blood or respiratory secretions may be indicative of an allergic diathesis.

Test: Baseline laboratory
Significance: Baseline pulmonary function studies should be obtained on asthmatic children.

 ## Emergency Care

ANAPHYLAXIS

• Subcutaneous Epinephrine 1:1000
• Diphenhydramine
• Ranitidine
• Methylprednisolone
• Volume expander to correct hypotension

ACUTE ASTHMA

• Oxygen
• Inhaled B-agonist
• Subcutaneous Epinephrine 1:1000
• Steroids

 ## Common Questions and Answers

Q: Do children outgrow allergies?
A: No. Actually, once a patient is sensitized they are sensitized for life. In addition, the older the patient becomes the greater the chance to develop other sensitivities.

Q: Can allergic children acquire more allergies?
A: Allergic children have the biologic potential to become sensitized to many environmental allergens. The goal should be to limit exposure to these antigens to prevent sensitization.

Q: If a parent is allergic to a specific allergen can the child inherit this allergy?
A: Children inherit the tendency to be allergic, but they do not inherit specific allergies.

Q: What treatments are available?
A: Specific environmental control (as determined by skin testing), antihistamines, topical steroids, and immunotherapy.

Issues for Referral

• Patient failing medical management of upper respiratory or ocular allergies with routine antihistamine/decongestant medications. The allergist can help identify triggers contributing to the allergic symptomatology.
• Poorly controlled asthma not responding to intermittent inhaled B-agonists or an asthmatic who is symptomatic between exacerbations, or one that has an atypical pattern of exacerbations.
• Asthmatics with frequent hospitalizations or steroid-dependent asthmatics should also be referred.
• Patients who miss school frequently due to allergic or asthmatic symptoms.
• Patients with limited activities due to allergies or asthma.
• Strong seasonal history to respiratory complaints
• Systemic reaction to bee sting
• Difficult to manage eczema (atopic dermatitis)
• Recurrent croup
• Food allergy
• History of anaphylaxis
• Egg allergic patient who require Influenza vaccine
• Drug allergy
• Latex allergy

BIBLIOGRAPHY

Fireman P. Diagnosis of allergic disorders. *Pediatr Rev* 1995;16(5):178–183.

Hopkin JM. Asthma and allergy-disorders of civilization? *QJM* 1998;91(3):169–170.

Middleton E, Reed CE, Adkinson NF, Yuninger JW, Busse WW. *Allergic principles and practice,* 4th ed. Philadelphia: Mosby, 1993.

Sites DP, Terr AI, Parslow TG. *Basic and clinical immunology,* 8th ed. Englewood Cliffs, NJ: Prentice Hall, 1994.

Author: Christopher A. Smith

Alopecia (Hair Loss)

 Database

DEFINITION

Alopecia is the loss of hair and can be categorized into four distinct patterns of scalp hair loss: congenital and circumscribed; congenital and diffuse; acquired and circumscribed, 95% of all cases; and acquired and diffuse. In only 1% of all cases is the hair loss diffuse (see Table of Etiologies by Pattern of Hair Loss).

 Differential Diagnosis

CONGENITAL/ANATOMIC

- Sebaceous nevus
- Epidermal nevus
- Hair follicle hamartomas
- Aplasia cutis congenita
- Conradi disease
- Incontinentia pigmenti
- Triangular alopecia of the frontal scalp
- Goltz syndrome (poikiloderma with focal dermal hypoplasia, syndactyly, localized areas of scalp and pubic alopecia, dystrophic nails, dental abnormalities)
- Hair shaft defects such as trichorrhexis nodosa (broomstick fractures), pili torti (twisted hair), monilethrix (beaded hair), trichorrhexis invaginata (bamboo hair)
- Ectodermal dysplasias

INFECTIOUS

- Tinea capitis, including untreated kerion
- Varicella

TOXIC, ENVIRONMENTAL, DRUGS

- Chemotherapeutic agents (anagen effluvium)
- Thallium poisoning
- Heparin
- Coumadin
- Antimetabolites
- Hypervitaminosis A
- Radiation injury (anagen effluvium)
- Chemical or thermal burns

TRAUMA

- Traction alopecia
- Trichotillomania
- Friction
- Scarring from pyoderma

GENETIC/METABOLIC

- Congenital or acquired hypothyroidism
- Hypopituitarism
- Hypoparathyroidism
- Diabetes mellitus
- Progeria
- Marasmus
- Zinc deficiency (acrodermatitis)

ALLERGIC/INFLAMMATORY

- Alopecia areata: thought to be due to dysregulation of the immune system, with all patients having hair antigen autoantibodies
- Lichen planus
- Systemic lupus erythematosis (SLE)
- Darier disease (keratosis follicularis—greasy, crusted papules on scalp, face, neck, trunk, and extremities)
- Porokeratosis of Mibelli (hyperkeratotic plaques with raised border and central atrophy)

MISCELLANEOUS

- Telogen effluvium

Approach to the Patient

GENERAL GOALS

Identify the pattern of hair loss. Utilizing the four categories described previously will help to limit the differential diagnosis.

Phase 1: Examine the skin, scalp, and local lymph nodes for evidence of infection. Does the patient have tinea capitis?

Phase 2: If the history and physical examination are not consistent with tinea capitis, consider trauma related to hair styling practices.

Phase 3: Consider alopecia areata with consistent exam findings.

Hints For Screening Problem

- Recognize that most cases of acquired, circumscribed alopecia are due to three major causes: tinea capitis, alopecia areata, or trauma.
- Always culture acquired circumscribed alopecia for dermatophytes, regardless of clinical presentation, because tinea capitis is by far the most common etiology.

 Data Gathering

HISTORY

Question: Is the hair loss congenital or acquired? Circumscribed or diffuse?
Significance: Most cases of acquired circumscribed alopecia will be tinea capitis, alopecia areata, or traumatic alopecia.

Question: Does the child have any chronic medical conditions?
Significance: Increased incidence of alopecia areata in patients with Down syndrome, thyroiditis, and vitiligo. SLE and endocrinopathies.

Question: Is the child taking any medications?
Significance: Anticoagulants, antimetabolites, and high-dose vitamin A may result in alopecia.

Table of Etiologies by Pattern of Hair Loss

Congenital, circumscribed alopecia
   Birthmarks
   Conradi disease
   Incontinentia pigmenti
   Sutural alopecia in Hallermann-Streiff syndrome
   Triangular alopecia of the frontal scalp
   Goltz syndrome

Congenital, diffuse alopecia
   Hair shaft defects
   Ectodermal dysplasias
   Congenital hypothyroidism
   Progeria

Acquired, circumscribed alopecia (nonscarring forms)
   Tinea capitis
   Alopecia areata
   Trauma

Acquired, circumscribed alopecia (scarring forms)
   Postinfectious: untreated kerion; pyoderma; varicella
   Postinflammatory: lichen planus; systemic lupus erythematosis; Darier disease; porokeratosis of Mibelli
   Postinjury: physical trauma; chemical or thermal burns; radiation injury

Acquired, diffuse alopecia
   Endocrinopathies
   Androgenetic alopecia (male pattern) in adolescents
   Toxins and drugs
   Marasmus
   Zinc deficiency (acrodermatitis)
   Telogen effluvium
   Anagen effluvium (due to chemotherapy or radiation to the head)

Question: Has the child been exposed to anyone with ringworm or any animals such as dogs, cats, or cattle?
Significance: Tinea capitis may be spread from person-to-person and animal-to-person, depending on the type of fungus involved. More than 90% of cases in North America are caused by *Trichophyton tonsurans,* affecting largely prepubertal children. Other infectious agents are *Microsporum canis,* which also affects cats and dogs, and *Trichophyton errucosum,* which affects cattle and humans. With infections caused by *M. canis,* there is no human-to-human transmission, as humans are terminal hosts.

Question: Does the child twist or pull at her hair?
Significance: Trichotillomania is a condition where the person pulls out her own hair. It is more common in girls, with a mean age of onset of 12 years. It is fairly common, with 1 in every 100 children engaging in this activity at some time or another. It may be associated with obsessive-compulsive disorder, an underlying psychiatric disturbance, or a response to a recent traumatic event.

Question: Is there a familial history of alopecia areata?
Significance: There is a familial history of alopecia areata in 10% to 20% of cases.

Question: Has there been a stressful event in the past several months?
Significance: Telogen effluvium is when hairs rapidly convert from growing, or anagen state, to the resting, or telogen, state. It is often precipitated by acute stressful events such as major accidents, fevers, fractures, psychiatric events, crash diets, or major surgery; after 2 to 4 months, the hairs in the telogen state are shed over a period of 3 to 4 months. Trichotillomania sometimes occurs in response to a stressful event.

Question: Does the child have an unusual diet?
Significance: Hypervitaminosis A and zinc deficiency can result in alopecia.

Question: What are the hair care practices of the child (frequency of shampooing, brushing, curling, braiding, or ponytails)?
Significance: Traction alopecia may occur with tight braids or corn rows, tightly pulled pony tails, excessive brushing, tight hair curlers, or frequent shampooing.

 ## Physical Examination

Finding: Is there a circumscribed bald spot that has been present since birth?
Significance: Consider aplasia cutis congenita, sebaceous nevus, or epidermal nevus in the differential diagnosis.

Finding: Are there abnormalities of nails, hair, and teeth?
Significance: Ectodermal dysplasia: hidrotic ectodermal dysplasia consists of hyperkeratosis of the palms and soles, dystrophic nails, and diffuse scalp and body alopecia (more prominent after puberty). Hypohidrotic ectodermal dysplasia includes abnormal dentition and defective or absent sweating.

Finding: In the area of alopecia, are small dark hairs visible, giving the appearance of "black dot" alopecia?
Significance: In tinea capitis, hairs break off at the follicular orifice. This occurs during the non-inflammatory stage of infection.

Finding: Are there scaly, bald patches in scalp?
Significance: These may be seen in tinea capitis, and with atopic dermatitis or seborrhea. The bald patches are traumatic alopecia due to rubbing/scratching.

Finding: Are pustules seen in the scalp?
Significance: These may be seen with pyogenic infections, chronic follicular trauma (e.g., traction), and tinea capitis (inflammatory stage).

Finding: Are pits visible in the nails?
Significance: Nail pits may precede the hair loss seen with alopecia areata.

Finding: Are hairs easily plucked and have tapered proximal shafts ("exclamation point" hairs)?
Significance: This phenomenon may be seen in alopecia areata.

Finding: Are there patches of non-scarring alopecia with irregular, ill-defined borders?
Significance: These are suggestive of trichotillomania or other forms of trauma.

Finding: Are there broken hairs of variable lengths?
Significance: This occurs in trichotillomania.

Finding: Are there perifollicular petechiae or excoriations?
Significance: These may occur in trichotillomania.

 ## Laboratory Aids

Test: Fungal culture
Significance: This is the gold standard for detecting dermatophytes.

Test: Microscopic examination of hair scrapings dissolved in KOH.
Significance: This is an alternative test for dermatophytes infections. This test requires considerable skill and experience.

Test: Microscopic examination of lost hairs.
Significance: In telogen effluvium, the root is non-pigmented and bulb shaped.

Test: Wood light examination
Significance: This is useful only with *Microsporum canis* and *M. audouinii* infections, with the hairs fluorescing bright yellow-green, and *Trichophyton schoenleinii,* fluorescing pale green. *Trichophyton tonsurans* does *not* cause fluorescence.

Test: Thyroid function tests
Significance: Should be performed when there is diffuse alopecia to rule out hypothyroidism.

 ## Common Questions and Answers

Q: Will the child's hair regrow after tinea capitis?
A: Yes. Hair regrowth may begin in 2 weeks, but full regrowth takes 3 to 6 months. Uncommonly, kerions may result in scarring and permanent hair loss.

Q: Will the child with alopecia areata regrow hair?
A: Yes. In 95% of initial cases, hair will regrow completely within 1 year from the onset of symptoms.

Q: What routine blood work-up should be done in evaluating alopecia?
A: None. With diffuse alopecia, history and physical examination should guide the ordering of additional laboratory studies.

Q: What is the first-line therapy for tinea capitis infections?
A: Griseofulvin (20 mg/kg/day) for a minimum of 8 weeks. Addition of selenium sulfide 2.5% shampoo twice weekly may hasten eradication of dermatophyte and decrease spread to others. Topical antifungals have poor penetration into the hair shaft and are, therefore, ineffective in treating tinea capitis.

Q: Is therapy of kerions different than non-inflammatory tinea capitis?
A: No. Studies have shown that the addition of prednisone and/or antibiotics when treating kerions does not hasten resolution.

Issues for Referral

- All but acquired circumscribed alopecia
- Recurrent alopecia areata

Clinical Pearls

- Plucking hairs for culture may cause a false-negative result because hairs long enough to be grasped are uninfected; always use scalp scrapings obtained with a soft sterile brush or curet.
- Up to 5% of children living in crowded cities carry *Trichophyton tonsurans.*
- In performing Wood light examinations, false-negatives may occur if the room is not dark enough, and false-positives may occur if one confuses the bluish or purple fluorescence of hair scale, lint, or petrolatum ointments with the greenish fluorescence of infected hairs.

BIBLIOGRAPHY

Levy ML. Disorders of the hair and scalp in children. *Pediatr Clin North Am* 1991;38(4):905–919.

Suarez S, Fallon Friedlander S. Antifungal therapy in children: an update. *Pediatr Ann* 1998;27(3):177–184.

Vasiloudes P, Morelli JG, Weston WL. Bald spots: remember the "big three." *Contemp Pediatr* 1997;14(10):76–91.

Author: Bruce Oriel

Back Pain

 ## Database

DEFINITION

• Back pain refers to any condition in which a patient has complaints of discomfort of the thoracic, lumbar, or sacral spinal area.
• Back pain can result from a variety of causes, involving the bony or muscular structures of the back, intervertebral discs, spinal cord, or peripheral nerves.
• Inheritance patterns in some of the congenital (scoliosis, Scheuermann disease) and inflammatory/rheumatologic causes of back pain have been described.
• There is a 30% lifetime incidence of back pain in teenage children. Eight percent of adolescents report recurrent or chronic back pain. Discitis is seen almost exclusively in children under 5 years of age.

COMPLICATIONS

Depending on the underlying etiology, complications of missed diagnosis or improper management can include paralysis or other permanent neuromuscular injury, neoplastic/paraneoplastic syndromes, and infectious syndromes.

PROGNOSIS

Prognosis is dependent on the underlying cause of back pain. The vast majority, if properly diagnosed and treated, do well, without significant sequelae.

 ## Differential Diagnosis

CONGENITAL

• Tethered cord

INFLAMMATORY

• Ankylosing spondylitis
• Enteropathic arthritis

INFECTIOUS

• Tuberculosis
• Discitis

TRAUMA

• "Musculotendinous" strain
• Spondylolysis (stress fracture of posterior vertebral elements)
• Spondylolisthesis (anterior displacement or "slip" of the vertebral body, associated with bilateral spondylolysis)
• Herniated disc
• Spinal epidural hematoma (traumatic or due to bleeding diathesis)

NEOPLASTIC

Bony

• Osteoid osteoma, osteoblastoma
• Eosinophilic granuloma
• Leukemia, lymphoma
• Osteosarcoma
• Ewing sarcoma
• Neurogenic
• Glioma
• Neuroblastoma
• Rhabdomyosarcoma

DEVELOPMENTAL

• Scheuermann disease (excessive kyphosis/"hunchback" due to abnormal bone growth causing "wedging" of the vertebral bodies)
• Painful scoliosis

REFERRED

• Pyelonephritis
• Pancreatitis

PSYCHOGENIC

 ## Data Gathering

Warning signs of potentially serious causes of back pain in children include:

• Young age (less than 4 years old)
• Chronic interference with activity (e.g., school, sports, play)
• Duration of pain longer than 4 weeks
• Associated fever, weight loss, or other systemic symptoms
• Postural shift of trunk
• Any neurologic abnormality
• Limitation of spinal motion (e.g., bending forward, straight leg raise)
• Painful or left thoracic scoliosis

HISTORY

Question: Onset, duration, and frequency of pain?
Significance: Fleeting or short duration of pain is rarely serious.

Question: Interference with activity?
Significance: Often a marker of disease severity.

Question: Physical activity and trauma history?
Significance: Spondylolysis and spondylolisthesis are more commonly seen in children who repeatedly twist, bend, or hyperextend their spine (e.g., participate in gymnastics, diving, tennis, contact sports, weightlifting, etc.)

Question: Radiation of pain?
Significance: Pain that shoots down the legs is suggestive of neurologic involvement.

Question: Growth history?
Significance: Adolescents during growth spurts are more prone to musculotendinous strain.

Question: Previous history of scoliosis?
Significance: Idiopathic scoliosis is rarely painful or functionally limiting.

SPECIAL QUESTIONS

Pain that awakes the child from sleep, and/or relief with NSAIDs. Osteoid osteoma and osteoblastoma often presents with night-time back pain and/or recurrent back pain relieved by NSAIDs.

Physical Examination

Finding: Inspect for any occult abnormalities
Significance: Sacral dimples, hair tufts, vascular anomalies, café au lait spots, or discrepancies in limb length.

Finding: With their feet together and knees and hips straight, observe the child from the back and side, both standing and bending over.
Significance: This evaluates the patient for scoliosis, kyphosis, and range of motion. Lumbar lordosis should "reverse" when the child bends over; if it does not, significant pathology should be suspected.

Finding: Palpate for any point or focal tenderness.
Significance: Fractures often manifest with point tenderness.

Finding: Assess lower extremity strength.
Significance: In young children, this may be evaluated by observing gait, heel- and toe-walking, and rising from a squat. A complete neurologic examination of the lower body, including examination of sensation and rectal tone, should be performed to rule out any neurologic involvement.

Finding: With the patient supine, examine the abdomen, deep tendon reflexes, and have the patient perform a straight leg raise.
Significance: Limitation in leg raise, abnormality of reflexes or clonus, or radiating pain is suggestive of neurologic abnormality. Muscle tone should also be assessed, as increased tone may cause limitation in leg raise.

SPECIFIC TESTS

• Standing hyperextension (bending backward) often reproduces the lower lumbar pain of spondylolysis. Hamstring tightness is also commonly seen.
• A bony "ledge"/step-off on palpation of the lumbar spine, or an anterior bony mass on rectal examination, are sometimes appreciated with spondylolisthesis.
• Asymmetry of lower extremity muscle circumference may be a sign of nerve impingement due to a herniated disc.

 ## Laboratory Aids

Test: Plain radiographs (AP and lateral, and if warranted, oblique and flexion/extension views) of the spine are indicated if any worrisome signs or symptoms are present.
Significance: Spondylolysis has the appearance of a "collar" (lucent line) on the "Scottie dog's" neck.

Test: Bone or SPECT scan
Significance: More sensitive for occult or subtle lesions, and should be obtained if a serious etiology is clinically suspected.

Test: MRI
Significance: The preferred examination for suspected neurologic or disc injury.

Test: Blood tests (e.g., sed rate, HLA-B27, ANA, rheumatoid factor, blood culture)
Significance: Indicated only if infectious or rheumatologic etiologies are considered.

Test: Bacterial cultures (needle aspiration or open biopsy)
Significance: Positive in only 25% to 50% of discitis patients. Routine biopsy is, therefore, not recommended in cases of suspected discitis. Staphylococcal species are the most frequently recovered organism.

 ## Therapy

• If none of the warning signs are present, conservative management with rest, ice or heat (whichever is appropriate), acetaminophen or ibuprofen, physical therapy, and close follow-up is reasonable. A back brace may also be helpful.
• Conservative medical treatment is indicated for spondylolysis and spondylolisthesis of less than 50% slip. Surgical treatment is warranted for slip greater than 50% or persistent back pain.
• Anti-staphylococcal medications are indicated in cases of discitis. The choice between oral or intravenous medications depend on the severity of the patient's symptoms.

 ## Follow-Up

• Patients managed conservatively should be re-evaluated within 2 weeks.
• All patients should be instructed to follow-up immediately for any worsening symptoms.

PREVENTION

• When the child has recuperated, back muscle strengthening and hamstring stretching exercises may be helpful.
• When participating in sports, appropriate protective equipment should be used and proper technique should be emphasized.
• In gymnasts, training more than 15 hours per week has been associated with increased risk of injury.

PITFALLS

• Missed diagnosis of a serious cause of back pain.
• Plain films are often normal, even in cases with serious causes.

 ## Common Questions and Answers

Q: When can the child resume activity?
A: Children can resume activity or sports when they are pain free.

Q: Which children should have activity restrictions?
A: "High risk" children (e.g., those with spinal or bony abnormalities, or familial histories of spondylolysis) should avoid hyperextension and contact sports.

BIBLIOGRAPHY

Dyment PG. Low back pain in adolescents. *Pediatr Ann* 1991;20(4):170–178.

Gerbino PG, Micheli LJ. Back injuries in the young athlete. *Clin Sports Med* 1995;14(3):571–590.

Payne WK, Ogilvie JW. Back pain in children and adolescents. *Pediatr Clin North Am* 1996;43(4):989–917.

Sponseller PD. Back pain in children. *Curr Opin Pediatr* 1994;6(1):99–103.

Author: Thomas H. Chun

Bruising

 ## Database

DEFINITION

Bruises are the result of extravasation of blood into the skin. Conventional usage often groups petechiae and bruises (or ecchymoses) together as purpura and defines them as follows:

• Petechiae: flat, red or reddish purple, 1 to 3 mm, non-blanching
• Ecchymoses: larger than petechiae, due to local extravasation, non-pulsatile, sometimes palpable, color depends on age of lesion

 ## Differential Diagnosis

CONGENITAL/ANATOMIC

• Coagulation factor abnormality: Hemophilia, von Willebrand disease
• Platelet defect: Bernard-Soulier syndrome, Glanzmann thrombosthenia, and storage pool defects
• Congenital alloimmune or isoimmune thrombocytopenia
• Neonatal extramedullary hematopoiesis
• Hereditary hemorrhagic telangiectasia

INFECTIOUS

• Meningococcemia
• Viral infections (coxsackieviruses, echoviruses)
• Rocky Mountain spotted fever (RMSF)
• Syphilis
• Pertussis—secondary to severe cough
• Septic or fat emboli
• DIC—acquired factor deficiency

TOXIC, ENVIRONMENTAL, DRUGS

• Warfarin—acquired factor deficiency
• Corticosteroids—striae caused by increased capillary fragility
• Aspirin and ibuprofen—cause a qualitative platelet abnormality
• Sulfonamides
• Bismuth
• Chloramphenicol

TRAUMA

• Normal activity
• Child abuse
• Valsalva, crying, forceful coughing
• Cupping or coin rubbing
• Tight garments

TUMOR (QUANTITATIVE PLATELET ABNORMALITY)

• Bone marrow replacement—leukemia, myelofibrosis

GENETIC/METABOLIC

• Uremia
• Vitamin C deficiency
• Vitamin K deficiency—due to antibiotics, biliary atresia, malabsorption (acquired factor deficiency)

ALLERGIC/INFLAMMATORY/VASCULITIC

• Henoch-Schönlein purpura (HSP)
• Bone marrow failure—aplastic anemia (including Fanconi, PNH)
• Increased destruction—idiopathic thrombocytopenic purpura, Evan syndrome, lupus
• Nephrotic syndrome
• Collagen vascular disease
• Ehlers-Danlos syndrome
• Snake bite (copperhead)

MISCELLANEOUS (DISORDERS THAT SIMULATE BRUISES)

• Ataxia telangiectasia
• Cherry angiomata
• Kaposi sarcoma

Approach to the Patient

GENERAL GOAL

To determine if the etiology of the bruising is due to thrombocytopenia, a coagulation disorder, or an extrinsic factor (such as trauma, infection, etc.).

Phase 1: Determine if the history of bruising and/or petechiae is acute or chronic in onset and if there is known trauma versus spontaneous lesions (see tables Most Common Causes of Bruising and How to Estimate the Age of Bruises).

• The acute onset of diffuse subcutaneous bleeding with bruises of different ages may indicate severe thrombocytopenia. Generally, children will not bruise or develop petechiae spontaneously until the platelet count is under 20,000/mm². ITP, leukemia, aplastic anemia, etc., can cause this bleeding. A hematologist should be consulted, because of the risk of potentially life-threatening bleeding.
• Chronic history of recurrent bleeding, such as mucosal, deep muscle or joint bleeds, may indicate an inherited coagulation defect such as von Willebrand disease or hemophilia. The familial history may be positive, although von Willebrand disease often goes undiagnosed into adulthood if there has been no challenge such as surgery.

Phase 2: Perform screening tests for bleeding disorders to categorize the abnormality.

• Platelet count to assess level of thrombocytopenia
• PT/PTT: Prolongation of either one or both of these may aid in the diagnosis of von Willebrand disease, coagulation factor deficiencies, liver disease, and vitamin K deficiency.
• Bleeding time: Prolongation may indicate the presence of a platelet aggregation disorder or von Willebrand disease.

 ## Data Gathering

HISTORY

Question: At what age was the bruising first noticed?
Significance: Significant bruising in the neonatal period may indicate neonatal thrombocytopenia, congenital infections, and sepsis with DIC. Hemophilia more typically presents with bleeding in the neonatal period, such as with circumcision. Other inherited disorders of coagulation, such as von Willebrand disease, may not be diagnosed until a child is older, as these tend to be mild in nature and may be uncovered with preoperative testing or post-operative bleeding complications. ITP may occur at any age.

Question: What is the pattern or distribution of the bruises?
Significance: The pattern of bruising, especially in a younger child, may indicate normal toddler activity, child abuse, or religious practices such as coining (common among Southeast Asians) in which warm or hot coins are rubbed on the skin to help in the healing process.

Question: What medications is the child taking?
Significance: Use of aspirin, ibuprofen, cough syrups with guaifenesin, and some antihistamines cause platelet dysfunction by inhibiting cyclooxygenase and, therefore, interfering with the release of platelet granules. Use of these drugs may also unmask an otherwise mild inherited bleeding disorder.

Question: Are there any signs or symptoms of systemic illness or infection?
Significance: Infections such as meningococcemia or viruses and collagen vascular diseases may present with ecchymosis or petechiae.

Most Common Causes of Bruising

1. Trauma (either accidental or intentional)
2. Infectious (viral etiology more common than bacterial)
3. Thrombocytopenia
4. Henoch-Schönlein purpura
5. Inherited coagulation defects (hemophilia, von Willebrand disease)

Question: Is there any familial history of a bleeding diathesis, easy bruisability, or heavy menstrual bleeding?
Significance: A positive familial history of inherited disorders of coagulation factors or platelet aggregation may aid in directing the work-up. A negative familial history does not rule out any of these disorders, however.

 ## Physical Examination

Question: Does the child appear well or systemically ill?
Significance: A well appearance is often found in those with ITP, though there is often a history of an antecedent viral illness. An ill appearance should raise concerns about malignancy, infection (especially meningococcemia), or other acquired coagulation factor deficiencies such as those seen with liver failure.

Question: What is the distribution of the bruises?
Significance: Bruising in unusual locations such as the back, genitalia, or thorax should raise suspicions of child abuse, especially if the lesions are in different stages of healing (see table How to Estimate the Age of Bruises) or suggest the pattern of a hand, belt, etc. Purpura confined mostly to the legs are typical of HSP. Most toddlers will have multiple ecchymoses in the pretibial regions that occur with normal activity. Petechiae entirely above the nipple line is consistent with valsalva maneuver, severe cough, and viral infections.

Question: Is the bleeding confined to the skin surface or are deeper tissues such as muscles and joints involved?
Significance: Hemophilia generally causes deeper bleeding, although bruising is common in the infant and younger child.

Question: Are the mucous membranes involved?
Significance: Severe thrombocytopenia, streptococcal pharyngitis, varicella, measles, and other viral infections can cause this finding. Von Willebrand disease can also present with gingival bleeding.

How to Estimate the Age of Bruises

1. New	Purple, dark red
2. 1–4 days	Dark blue to brown
3. 5–7 days	Greenish to yellow
4. >7 days	Yellow

Question: Is there hepatosplenomegaly or lymphadenopathy?
Significance: Involvement of the reticuloendothelial system can be found with malignancies such as leukemia or with viral or bacterial infections.

Question: Are there other congenital abnormalities?
Significance: Syndromes such as Fanconi anemia and thrombocytopenia absent radii (TAR) may present with upper extremity limb malformations and bruising.

 ## Laboratory Aids

Test: CBC
Significance: Platelet count is the most important, however, abnormalities of WBC or Hgb may aid in the diagnosis bone marrow infiltration or failure.

Test: PT
Significance: Elevation may indicate warfarin ingestion or factor VII deficiency.

Test: aPTT
Significance: Prolongation is seen with hemophilia and may be seen in von Willebrand disease.

Test: Both PT and PTT
Significance: Both are prolonged in DIC, liver failure, and vitamin K deficiency.

Test: Bleeding time
Significance: Lengthened in platelet aggregation disorders and with drug effects.

Test: Fibrinogen
Significance: Decreased in liver failure, DIC

Test: Urinalysis
Significance: Hematuria and/or proteinuria may indicate HSP, nephrotic syndrome, or other vasculitis.

 ## Emergency Care

Factors that make this an emergency include:

• Severe thrombocytopenia below 10–20,000/mm³ carries a higher risk of spontaneous internal bleeding including intracranial bleeding.
• Bleeding or bruising accompanied by evidence of leukemia or other malignancy.
• Evidence of sepsis (DIC) or meningococcemia.

 ## Common Questions and Answers

Q: Is hemophilia always diagnosed in the newborn period?
A: No. A familial history may provide clues, but a significant number of patients represent a spontaneous mutation. Additionally, not all boys with hemophilia will bleed with circumcision and the diagnosis may not be made until the infants become more active.

Q: What is a common cause of bruising among girls?
A: Girls may first come to attention at menarche and be diagnosed at that time with von Willebrand disease. Rarely, girls whose fathers have hemophilia may be unfavorably "lyonized" and, therefore, have decreased factor levels consistent with mild hemophilia.

Issues for Referral

• ITP should be referred to a hematologist especially if the child is older, because there is a higher risk of chronic ITP or an underlying disorder such as lupus.
• Prolonged PT/PTT/BT often require referral to work-up an inherited or acquired coagulation defect.
• Any concern about a malignancy, liver failure or child abuse.

Clinical Pearls

• The amount of bruising may or may not correlate with the amount of internal bleeding that has occurred. Hemophiliacs can significantly drop their hemoglobin during a thigh or psoas bleed without having much in the way of ecchymosis.
• A child presenting with ITP may have bruises and petechiae from head to toe without changing the hemoglobin much at all.

BIBLIOGRAPHY

Manno CS. Difficult pediatric diagnoses: bleeding and bruising. *Pediatr Clin North Am* 1991;38(3):637–655.

Author: Julie W. Stern and Lisa Michaels

Chest Pain

 Database

DEFINITION

Chest pain is a common pain syndrome in childhood (see table Most Common Causes of Pediatric Chest Pain). It is less common than abdominal pain and headache.

 Differential Diagnosis

MUSCULOSKELETAL DISORDERS

- Chest wall strain
- Costochondritis
- Direct chest trauma
- Slipping rib syndrome

CARDIAC PATHOLOGY

- Arrhythmia (supraventricular tachycardia, premature ventricular contractions)
- Coronary-artery anomalies
- Coronary-artery aneurysms (Kawasaki syndrome)
- Infections (myocarditis, pericarditis)
- Myocardial infarction/ischemia
- Structural abnormalities

—Aortic stenosis
—Hypertrophic cardiomyopathy
—Pulmonic stenosis
—Mitral valve prolapse
—Severe coarctation of the aorta

GASTROINTESTINAL DISORDERS

- Caustic ingestions
- Esophageal foreign bodies
- Esophagitis (sometimes tetracycline, "pill," induced)

PSYCHOGENIC CAUSES

- Anxiety
- Hyperventilation

RESPIRATORY DISORDERS

- Asthma
- Cough (prolonged)
- Pleural effusion
- Pneumonia

Most Common Causes of Pediatric Chest Pain

Idiopathic
Musculoskeletal
   Chest wall strain
   Costochrondritis
Direct Trauma
Respiratory Conditions
   Asthma, cough, pneumonia
Gastrointestinal problems
   Esophagitis, esophageal foreign body
Cardiac pathology

- Pneumothorax—spontaneous, trauma-related, drug-related (cocaine)
- Pneumomediastinum
- Pulmonary embolism

MISCELLANEOUS

- Breast mass
- Cigarette smoke
- Pleurodynia
- Precordial catch syndrome
- Shingles
- Sickle cell crises
- Thoracic tumor

Approach to the Patient

GENERAL GOAL

Identify the rare child with a serious etiology for chest pain (see tables Important Physical Findings on General Examination of Child with Chest Pain and Important Physical Findings on Chest Examination of Child with Chest Pain).

Phase 1: Is the patient in acute distress? If so, begin emergency management and proceed rapidly to find the cause of pain.

Phase 2: For the majority of stable children with chest pain, determine whether laboratory tests are needed to help identify the etiology.

Phase 3: Treat specific conditions as appropriate. Begin analgesics, reassure the family and arrange for follow-up care.

HINTS FOR SCREENING PROBLEM

Take a thorough history and perform a careful physical exam. Examine the chest last—do not focus only on this area. Use laboratory tests sparingly, only to confirm clinical suspicions.

Important Physical Findings on General Examination of Child with Chest Pain

Severe distress
Chronically ill appearance
Skin rash or bruising
Abdominal pathology
Arthritis present
Anxiety apparent

From: Selbst SM. Evaluation of chest pain in children. *Pediatr. Rev.* 1986;8:56–62.

 Data Gathering

HISTORY

Question: How severe, how often is the pain?
Significance: Constant, frequent severe pain is more likely to be distressing, interruptive of daily activity. Serious etiology is not well correlated with frequency, severity of pain.

Question: What is the type of pain? Its location?
Significance: Burning pain is associated with esophagitis. Sharp, stabbing pain relieved by sitting up or leaning forward is typical of pericarditis. Young children do not describe or localize chest pain well.

Question: When was the onset of pain?
Significance: Acute pain (<48 hours) is more likely to have an organic etiology. Chronic pain (>6 months) is more likely to be psychogenic, idiopathic.

Question: Is the pain induced by exercise?
Significance: Exercise-induced chest pain may be related to serious cardiac disease or asthma.

Question: Recent trauma or muscle overuse?
Significance: Musculoskeletal (chest wall) pain

Question: Eaten spicy foods? Taken tetracycline or other pills?
Significance: Esophagitis

Question: Recent use of cocaine?
Significance: Hypertension, tachycardia, myocardial ischemia, or pneumothorax.

Question: Use of oral contraceptives or recent leg trauma?
Significance: Pulmonary embolism

Question: Recent significant stress (e.g., move, death of loved one, serious illness)?
Significance: Psychogenic pain

Question: Associated complaints?
Significance: Fever may imply pneumonia, myocarditis, pericarditis. Syncope, palpitations may imply cardiac arrhythmias or severe anemia. Joint pain, rash may relate chest pain to collagen vascular disease. Pain that resolves with parental attention may indicate an emotional etiology.

Question: Positive familial history?
Significance: Hypertrophic cardiomyopathy is often familial. Those with a familial history positive for heart disease and chest pain may be concerned about the symptom in a child. Chest pain in such children often has a non-organic etiology.

Important Physical Findings on Chest Examination of Child with Chest Pain

Inspection: trauma, asymmetry, abnormal breathing pattern
Auscultation: tachycardia, dysrhythmia, murmur, rub, rales, wheezing
Palpation: tenderness, subcutaneous emphysema

From: Selbst SM. Evaluation of chest pain in children. *Pediatr Rev* 1986;8:56–62.

Question: Past medical history?
Significance: Previous Kawasaki syndrome, long-standing insulin-dependent diabetes mellitus, and sickle cell disease may have serious cardiac or pulmonary complications leading to chest pain. Marfan syndrome has increased risk for aortic dissection, pneumothorax. Asthma has increased risk for pneumonia, pneumothorax. Collagen vascular disease has increased risk for pleural effusion, pericarditis. Most underlying structural cardiac lesions rarely produce chest pain.

 ## Physical Examination

Finding: Child is in significant distress.
Significance: Requires emergency care; stabilization, consider pneumothorax, arrhythmia.

Finding: Child appears chronically ill.
Significance: Chest pain may be found in serious illness such as malignancy (Hodgkin lymphoma).

Finding: Skin bruising present
Significance: Chest pain may be related to unrecognized trauma.

Finding: Abdominal pathology
Significance: Pain may be referred to the chest

Finding: Arthritis present
Significance: Collagen vascular disease may manifest as pleural effusion, chest pain.

Finding: Unusually anxious child
Significance: Underlying stress may lead to pain.

Finding: Breast enlargement, asymmetry, tenderness
Significance: Physiologic breast changes in young teens may be painful. Consider pregnancy in teenage girls.

Finding: Rubs, decreased breath sounds, wheezing
Significance: May suggest pneumonia, asthma with overuse of chest wall muscles.

Finding: Subcutaneous emphysema palpable on chest or neck
Significance: Pneumothorax, pneumomediastinum

Finding: Heart murmur, rub, arrhythmia
Significance: Congenital heart disease, cardiac infection such as myocarditis, pericarditis, supraventricular tachycardia, ventricular tachycardia.

Finding: Tenderness of chest wall, costochondral junctions
Significance: Musculoskeletal pain

 ## Laboratory Aids

Test: Electrocardiogram
Significance: Obtain if history suggests cardiac pathology, for instance:

- Acute onset of pain
- Pain on exertion
- Pain associated with syncope, dizziness, palpitations
- History of congenital heart disease
- Serious associated medical problems (Kawasaki syndrome, diabetes mellitus)
- Use of cocaine

Obtain also if physical exam is abnormal. For instance:

- Respiratory distress
- Cardiac abnormality
- Fever
- Significant trauma

Test: Chest radiograph
Significance: Same as for electrocardiogram. Also, obtain if history suggests cardiac or pulmonary pathology, tumor, Marfan syndrome, or foreign body (coin ingestion).

Test: Holter monitor
Significance: Arrange for this study if cardiac arrhythmia suspected. Electrocardiogram may fail to detect intermittent arrhythmia.

Test: Exercise stress test, pulmonary function tests
Significance: Obtain if pain induced by exertion.

Test: Drug screen
Significance: Obtain if cocaine use suspected.

 ## Emergency Care

Factors that make this an emergency include:

- Pneumothorax: may present with severe sudden chest pain, respiratory distress, cyanosis, hypotension.
- Cardiac arrhythmia: ventricular tachycardia or supraventricular tachycardia in an older child may progress to heart failure or a lethal rhythm.
- Cocaine intoxication: may present with pneumothorax, cardiac arrhythmia, hypertension.
- Direct chest trauma: may lead to cardiac contusion, and arrhythmia.
- Caustic ingestions or esophageal foreign bodies require prompt attention.

 ## Common Questions and Answers

Q: How common is chest pain in children?
A: Chest pain is a common pain syndrome reported in 6 of 1,000 children who present to an urban emergency department. The complaint is less common than abdominal pain or headache. Although children of all ages may complain of chest pain, the mean age is about 12 years.

Q: Is follow-up important?
A: Yes. Serious pathology is unlikely to be found if not diagnosed initially. However, watch for signs of exercise-induced asthma or for emotional problems that were not obvious initially. Ensure that the child returns to normal activity when appropriate.

Q: What is the prognosis for most children with chest pain?
A: Most children with chest pain have an excellent prognosis. About 40% of children with chest pain will have continued symptoms for 6 to 24 months.

Issues for Referral

- Acute distress
- Significant trauma
- History of heart disease or related serious medical problem
- Pain with exercise, syncope, palpitations, dizziness
- Serious emotional disturbance
- Esophageal foreign body, caustic ingestion
- Pneumothorax, pleural effusion

Clinical Pearls

- If the child is febrile, consider pneumonia, or viral myocarditis.
- Treat specific etiology when found.
- Over-the-counter analgesics (acetaminophen, ibuprofen) suffice for most pain.
- Antacids may be diagnostic and therapeutic for esophagitis pain.
- Rest, heat, relaxation techniques may be useful.
- Avoid expensive, invasive laboratory studies with chronic pain and normal physical examination, benign history.

BIBLIOGRAPHY

Knapp JF, Dowd MD, Tarantino C, Borders J. Case 02-1994: a tall, thin 15 year old male with chest pain. *Pediatr Emerg Care* 1994;10:117–120.

Selbst SM. Chest pain in children, consultation with the specialist. *Pediatr Rev* 1997;18:169–173.

Selbst SM, Ruddy RM, Clark BJ, et al. Pediatric chest pain: a prospective study. *Pediatrics* 1988;82:319–323.

Wiens L, Sabath R, Ewing L, et al. Chest pain in otherwise healthy children and adolescents is frequently caused by exercise-induced asthma. *Pediatrics* 1992;90:350–353.

Author: Steven M. Selbst

Coma

Database

DEFINITION

Coma is defined as an unresponsive state with eyes closed, usually lasting less than 24 hours. This condition signals a medical emergency, and immediate attention/intervention is required for abnormalities in breathing, circulation, glucose, or electrolytes.

- *Lethargy* indicates a patient who is incoherent but arousable and has a tendency to sleep.
- *Stupor* is used when the patient is responsive only to pain.
- *Vegetative state* suggests a chronic state in which sleep–wake cycles persist but there is no evidence of cognition.
- *Locked-in* must be distinguished from coma; that is, cognitive functions are intact, though the patient may appear unconscious.

CAUSES OF COMA

- Trauma: epidural, subdural, intracerebral hematoma, diffuse cerebral swelling
- Poisoning
- Hypoxia/ischemia
- Infection—meningitis, encephalitis, toxic shock
- Subdural empyema
- Hemorrhagic shock
- Metabolic disorders

—Hypoglycemia (salicylate or ethanol intoxication, hyperinsulinemia)
—Diabetic ketoacidosis (DKA): rare catastrophic neurologic deterioration seen on initiation of insulin and/or fluid therapy
—Reye syndrome
—Electrolyte abnormalities (Na, K, Ca, Mg)
—Hepatic/uremic encephalopathy
—Inborn errors of metabolism
—Hormonal abnormalities (thyroid, adrenal, pituitary)
—Hypothermia/hyperthermia

- Tumor
- Seizure
- Vascular: hemorrhage [from arteriovenous malformation (AVM), aneurysm, coagulopathy, infarction, cerebral venous thrombosis, hypertensive encephalopathy]
- Hydrocephalus: ventriculoperitoneal (VP) shunt obstruction
- Mass/bleed obstructing ventricular outflow

PATHOPHYSIOLOGY

Coma implies abnormal brain function, which may be localized to the reticular activating system (RAS) in the brainstem or bilateral cerebral dysfunction. Abnormalities of the protective reflexes of the upper airway or abnormalities of the respiratory pattern may signal impending respiratory failure.

COMPLICATIONS OF ACUTE COMA

- Respiratory failure
- Deep venous thrombosis
- Pneumonia
- Aspiration

Differential Diagnosis

DISORDERS MIMICKING COMA

- Psychogenic coma: patient may resist passive eye opening, regard self in mirror, and avoid passive arm fall over face
- Locked-in state: complete paralysis with normal cerebral function may occur in severe neuromuscular disorders (acute polyneuropathy) or in ventral pontine lesions (hemorrhage, demyelination)

Data Gathering

HISTORY

- Head trauma
- Ingestion
- Drugs/toxins in home
- Fever
- Nausea
- Headache
- Preceding viral illness
- Seizures
- Diabetes
- Preexisting neurologic disease
- Previous episodes of coma

Physical Examination

- Vital signs
- Abnormal respiratory pattern
- Bradycardia
- Hypertension
- HEENT—look for signs of head trauma: raccoon eyes (Battle signs, ecchymosis at mastoid equals basilar skull fracture)
- Retinal hemorrhages
- Bulging fontanelle
- Neck: nuchal rigidity, Kernig and Brudzinski signs associated with meningitis
- Neurologic: verbal or motor response to voice, touch, pain; eye opening/fixation; spontaneous movements/posturing; pupil symmetry/reactivity, abnormal oculocephalic response (doll eyes); worsening signs in any of the above may indicate increased intracranial pressure (ICP)
- Reflexes specific to rostral brainstem function include pupillary light reflex, corneal reflex, jaw jerk
- Reflexes specific to caudal brainstem function include oculocephalic reflex (horizontal eye deviation with passive head rotation), gag, spontaneous respirations

Laboratory Aids

Initial blood studies obtained with placement of an IV line include:

- Glucose
- Electrolytes
- BUN/creatinine
- Calcium
- Arterial blood gas
- CBC
- Toxicology screen
- Ammonia
- Liver transaminases
- Radiology—non-contrast head CT scan first to look for hemorrhage, may be followed by contrasted images for infection/mass lesions
- Cervical spine series (CT or lateral and AP x-ray studies)—indicated if evidence of trauma by history or on examination
- Cervical spine must be stabilized until injury is ruled out
- Lumbar puncture, to rule out infection, bleed; defer until after CT if focal exam or signs of increased ICP
- Question of "traumatic tap" can be settled by spinning out red cells promptly and examining fluid for xanthochromia
- EEG—helpful to rule out non-convulsive status epilepticus

Emergency Care

- First priority is stabilization of respiratory and hemodynamic status.
- Endotracheal intubation is usually required to ensure airway protection and adequate oxygenation.
- Large-bore IV lines should be placed and isotonic fluids administered as needed to replace intravascular volume and maintain adequate blood pressure.
- If finger-stick glucose determination is low, give 2 to 4 mL of 25% dextrose (D25) per kilogram intravenously (D10 if young infant).
- If ingestion is suspected, administer naloxone (0.01 mg/kg IV).

- When there is evidence of increased ICP:
—Hyperventilate to decrease blood CO_2 to 25 to 30 Torr and give mannitol (0.5–1 g/kg IV).
—Dexamethasone, 1 to 2 mg/kg IV, can also be administered.
—All fluids given should be isotonic and the volume limited to that needed to maintain adequate perfusion.
—Head should be elevated 30 degrees above horizontal to maximize cerebral venous drainage.
—Hospitalization is usually in the intensive care unit for close monitoring for changes in respiratory status or signs of increased ICP.
—Drug indications depend on underlying etiology.
—IV antibiotics should be given if infection is suspected.

Follow-Up

PROGNOSIS

Prognosis depends on underlying etiology. Complete recovery is frequently seen after toxic-metabolic coma. In contrast, patients with coma resulting from severe head trauma often have significant neurologic sequelae and may require physical, occupational, and cognitive therapies.

PITFALLS

- Quadriparesis due to neuromuscular weakness may resemble coma; responsiveness is determined by patient questioning, using whatever movements may be preserved (often, eye movements).
- In psychogenic coma, defensive movements may be elicited (resistance to passive eye opening, arm falls away from face); presentation of a mirror may induce involuntary visual fixation.

Common Questions and Answers

Q: What is the role of EEG in the diagnosis of coma?
A: EEG is useful in diagnosis of psychogenic coma (should be normal) and in coma from brainstem lesions, in non-convulsive status epilepticus (shows electrographic seizures), and in possible herpes encephalitis (temporal or frontal sharp activity).

Q: Should anticonvulsants be given to comatose victims of trauma?
A: While there is no clear evidence that anticonvulsants improve outcome or reduce incidence of post-traumatic seizures, they are often given when post-traumatic intracranial hypertension and/or edema is suspected because seizures are known to raise ICP.

Issues for Referral

Neurosurgical intervention may be required in cases of head trauma, hemorrhage, mass lesion, or hydrocephalus. Neurology consultation is usually indicated.

Clinical Pearls

Trauma and near-drowning are leading causes among children, and boys are more often victims of trauma/near-drowning than girls.

BIBLIOGRAPHY

Ashwal S, Bale JF, Coulter DL, et al. The persistent vegetative state in children: report of the Child Neurology Society Ethics committee. *Ann Neurol* 1992;32:570.

Chiappa KH, Hill RA. Evaluation and prognostication in coma. *Electroencephalogr Clin Neurophysiol* 1998;106(2):149–155.

Feske SK. Coma and confusional states: emergency diagnosis and management. *Neurol Clin* 1998;16(2):237–256.

Johnston B, Seshia SS. Prediction of outcome in non-traumatic coma in childhood. *Acta Neurol Scand* 1984;69:417.

Author: Amy R. Brooks-Kayal

Cough

Database

DEFINITION

Cough is a symptom of a variety of underlying conditions, which results from a complex reflex phenomenon initiated by cough receptors and mediated in the brainstem's cough center. These receptors are located throughout the large- to medium-sized airways (and not the lower airways), pharynx, paranasal sinuses, external auditory canal, and stomach, and are triggered by thermal, chemical, mechanical, or inflammatory stimuli. The resultant high velocity expiration, which removes airway secretions, is generally reflexive, but may sometimes be voluntarily initiated or suppressed.

Differential Diagnosis

Infection and reactive airway disease are the most common causes of cough in all age groups and should always be considered.

CAUSES OF ACUTE COUGH

- Infection
- Reactive airway disease (RAD)
- Sinusitis
- Irritative
- Allergic
- Foreign body

CAUSES OF CHRONIC COUGH

- Infection
- Asthma or asthmatic bronchitis
- Sinusitis
- Irritative/Post-infectious
- Allergic
- Foreign body (FB)
- Gastroesophageal reflux (GER)

—Aspiration

- Habitual or psychogenic
- Anatomic abnormalities

—Tracheoesophageal fistula
—Tracheobroncheomalacia
—Laryngeal cleft
—Polyps
—Adductor vocal cord paralysis
—Pulmonary sequestration
—Bronchogenic cyst
—Cystic hygroma
—Vascular ring
—Tumor

- Cystic fibrosis (CF)
- Ciliary dyskinesia syndromes

- Immunodeficiency states

—Human Immunodeficiency Virus (HIV)
—Immunoglobulin deficiencies (IgA, IgG)
—Phagocytic defects
—Complement deficiency

- Pulmonary hemosiderosis
- Angiotensin-converting enzyme inhibitors
- External auditory canal irritation

Approach to the Patient

GENERAL GOAL

The presenting symptom of cough is a familiar one to most physicians and accounts for nearly 7% of chief complaints to pediatricians. Cough is an easily identifiable symptom that frequently provokes parental concern and can be troublesome to the physician. The possible etiologies of cough are diverse, and may range from a minor illness to a life-threatening condition. Therefore, a stepwise approach is required in an effort to prevent a costly and lengthy investigation. In particular, a thorough history and physical examination are of paramount importance in the evaluation.

Phase 1: Complete history and physical examination to determine time course and severity of cough and to ascertain whether it represents a significant problem of respiratory function or a serious underlying disease.

Phase 2: Initiate focused work-up and treatment plan depending on differential diagnosis (see previous section).

Phase 3: Refer to pediatric pulmonologist if cough persists or if concerned about significant pathology (see following section).

Data Gathering

HISTORY

Question: Is the cough acute or chronic?
Significance: Generally considered to be chronic if present longer than 3 weeks. Although there is significant overlap, differential diagnosis varies depending on the time course.

Question: How is this problem different in children as compared with adults?
Significance: Differential diagnosis varies considerably based on the patient's age.

Question: Is there a recent history of upper respiratory infection (URI)?
Significance: Consider serial URIs (children have average of 6 to 8 per year with each lasting up to 2 weeks), post-infectious/irritative or sinusitis (which complicates up to 5% of URIs).

Question: What are the associated symptoms?
Significance:

- Fever, nasal discharge suggest infection.
- Fever with chills or night sweats suggests tuberculosis.
- Sputum production indicates bronchiectasis or other lower airway pathology.
- With headache or facial edema, consider sinusitis.
- With respiratory distress, suspect RAD.

Question: What is the quality of the cough?
Significance:

- Productive cough suggests lower airway infection, CF/bronchiectasis.
- Dry cough suggests RAD, fungal infection.
- Barking cough is usually associated with croup.
- Honking or brassy cough is typical in habitual or psychogenic cough.

Question: What is the pattern of the cough?
Significance:

- Night-time cough suggests RAD.
- With night-time/early morning cough, consider sinusitis.
- Seasonal cough suggests allergy.

Question: Are there any known triggers of cough (e.g., cold air, dust, smoke, URI)?
Significance: Consider irritant, allergic, or reactive airway disease.

Question: Is there any personal or familial history of atopy?
Significance: Consider RAD.

Question: Is there a history of recurrent infections?
Significance: Consider immunodeficiency, CF.

Question: Is there any relation of cough to feedings?
Significance: Consider aspiration, tracheoesophageal fistula.

Question: Is there a history of a choking episode?
Significance: Consider retained foreign body, although there may not be a history of a choking

episode in this case and cough may be episodic as FB moves along respiratory tract.

Question: Is there failure to thrive?
Significance: Rule out CF, immunodeficiency.

 ## Physical Examination

Finding: Patient's general appearance
Significance:

• Evidence of failure to thrive—consider CF, immunodeficiency.
• Cyanosis or pallor—rule out hypoxemia.
• Signs of respiratory distress such as tachypnea, accessory muscle use—most likely RAD or infection.

Finding: Barrel chest
Significance: Suggests air-trapping due to chronic disease.

Finding: Clubbing
Significance: May be seen with bronchiectasis.

Finding: Nasal polyps
Significance: May be associated with allergic conditions or CF.

Finding: Tracheal deviation
Significance: Suggests mediastinal mass or FB aspiration.

Finding: Signs of atopic disease
Significance: Eczema, allergic shiners, transverse nasal crease, rhinitis, mucosal cobblestoning, injected conjunctivae suggest allergy, RAD.

Finding: Periorbital edema, sinus tenderness, purulent posterior pharyngeal drainage, halitosis
Significance: Sinusitis

Finding: Wheezing
Significance: Polyphonic inspiratory or expiratory wheezes suggest RAD, while monophonic or fixed wheezes should make one consider FB or mass/congenital lesion.

 ## Laboratory Aids

Laboratory investigation should reflect a rational, stepwise approach based on likely etiologies after a thorough history and physical examination.

Test: Chest radiograph
Significance:

• Infiltrates may suggest pneumonia, bronchiolitis, pneumonitis, TB, CF, bronchiectasis, FB.
• Volume loss may be seen with FB aspiration; sometimes need to obtain lateral decubitus views in young children who cannot cooperate with inspiratory/expiratory views.
• Hyperinflation suggests RAD or CF.
• Mediastinal nodes may indicate infection (especially TB, fungus) or malignancy.

Test: Mantoux test—purified protein derivative (PPD)
Significance: Rule out tuberculosis

Test: Complete blood count
Significance: Eosinophilia suggests atopic disease or, rarely, parasitic infection; anemia should prompt one to consider chronic disease or, rarely, pulmonary hemosiderosis.

Test: Sputum sample must contain alveolar macrophages
Significance:

• Eosinophils suggest asthmatic process or hypersensitivity reaction of lung.
• Polymorphonuclear cells suggest infection.
• Predominance of macrophages suggests postinfectious hyperresponsive cough receptors.
• Hemosiderin staining suggests pulmonary hemosiderosis.
• Lipid-laden macrophages suggest recurrent aspiration.
• Routine or special cultures based on likely pathogens.

Test: Serum IgE
Significance: Significant elevation indicates allergy or, rarely, parasites.

Test: Sweat chloride test
Significance: Need to be sure that laboratory has experience with this test.

Test: Wright peak flow rate
Significance:

• Easy to perform in the office with the proper flowmeter.
• Helpful to get pre-bronchodilator and post-bronchodilator rates if RAD suspected.
• Standardized tables available with values based on height and race.

Test: Immune work-up
Significance: HIV; immunoglobulins

Test: Barium swallow or pH probe
Significance: Reflux

Test: Bronchoscopy
Significance: To remove FB or obtain tissue samples.

Emergency Care

• Cough should be considered an emergency if there are associated signs or symptoms of respiratory distress.
• Routine emergency airway assessment (i.e., ABCs) should be undertaken on presentation and appropriate supportive measures started in cases in which there is concern.
• Refer for additional treatment as outlined previously.

 ## Common Questions and Answers

Q: Is whooping cough still a problem despite routine childhood immunization?
A: Yes. Pertussis often goes unrecognized as a cause of acute and chronic cough, particularly in infants who have not completed their immunization series and in adolescents (and adults) in whom immunity from vaccination will have waned.

Q: Is it possible for a child to have asthma if they have never wheezed?
A: Yes, there is cough-variant reactive airway disease.

Issues for Referral

Factors that may alert you to make a referral include:

• The cough is unresponsive to treatment.
• The cause is likely to be an anatomic malformation or FB aspiration.
• There appears to be involvement of other organ systems (e.g., failure to thrive, GER, congestive heart failure, immunodeficiency, unusual infection).
• There is hemoptysis.

Clinical Pearls

• The goal is to treat the underlying cause of the cough, not the symptom.
• Educate parents about the beneficial function of cough to remove irritants and about the potential harm of suppressing a productive cough or cough secondary to RAD.
• Specific pharmacologic interventions:

—RAD: bronchodilators ±inhaled antiinflammatory agents (e.g., cromolyn sodium), oral or inhaled steroids, removal of irritants
—Infection: appropriate antibiotics
—Cough suppressants have not been shown to be efficacious in children under 5 years, and have been associated with significant toxicity in this age group.

BIBLIOGRAPHY

Committee on Drugs. Use of codeine and DM-containing cough remedies in children. *Pediatrics* 1997;99(6):918–920.

Kamei RK. Chronic cough in children. *Pediatr Clin North Am* 1991;38(3):593–605.

Katcher ML. Cold, cough and allergy medications: uses and abuses. *Pediatr Rev* 1996;17(1):12–17.

Kemper KJ. Chronic asthma: an update. *Pediatr Rev* 1996;17(4):111–117.

Taylor JA, Novack AH, Almquist JR, Rogers JE. Efficacy of cough suppressants in children. *J Peds* 1993;122(5):799–802.

Author: Margaret McNamara

Crossed Eyes

 ## Database

DEFINITION

• "Crossed eyes" is often a chief complaint indicating inward deviation of the eyes, or esotropia. Because abnormal eye movements of any type may be interpreted as "crossed eyes," this chapter will cover any misalignment of the visual axes, or strabismus (see table Common Presentations of Strabismus).

• Strabismus is reported to occur in approximately 4% of children less than 6 years of age. It may be constant or intermittent; present in all fields of gaze or restricted to only a few; and present with near fixation, far fixation, or both.

 ## Differential Diagnosis

CONGENITAL/ANATOMIC

• Transient sixth nerve palsy: may be seen in neonates, manifesting clinically as a lack of lateral gaze; it typically resolves within the first 6 weeks of life. Many believe this to be secondary to increased intracranial pressure during delivery.

• Pseudoesotropia: not a true strabismus; an optical illusion of asymmetric nasal sclera created by prominent inner eyelid skinfolds and a wide, flat nasal bridge.

• Möbius syndrome: a congenital condition presenting as an esotropia and an expressionless face, caused by unilateral or bilateral sixth and seventh nerve palsies. Associated chest and limb abnormalities may be seen.

• Duane retraction syndrome: congenital esotropia, presents with restriction of lateral gaze.

• Fourth nerve palsy: more commonly congenital than acquired. The affected eye is in upward deviation, secondary to a weakness in the superior oblique muscle. Amblyopia is uncommon because the child usually develops a head tilt in order to maintain ocular alignment.

INFECTIOUS

Acquired sixth nerve palsies: manifesting as lack of lateral gaze, may be transient after a viral illness or can result from increased intracranial pressure from a variety of etiologies, including hydrocephalus, tumor, hemorrhage, and edema.

TUMOR

Intracranial tumors: may manifest as cranial nerve palsies.

GENETIC

Brown superior oblique tendon sheath syndrome: an inability to elevate the eye (most notably seen with an attempt at medial gaze). Children will typically develop a head tilt to maintain binocular vision.

Approach to the Patient

GENERAL GOALS

• Determine if the patient has a history of abnormal eye movements consistent with strabismus or if the patient currently has an abnormal examination.

• Strabismus must be addressed in a timely manner because if left uncorrected, amblyopia (a reduction in visual acuity) may result.

Phase 1: A detailed history must be obtained from the parent or caregiver.

• Abnormal eye movements may be intermittent and difficult to elicit in the office setting. A complete examination must be performed, with special attention to the ophthalmologic and neurologic exams, in order not to miss strabismus.

Phase 2: Consider the age, duration, and findings on physical examination to arrive at a differential diagnosis.

• Provide the appropriate referral to a pediatric and/or neuro-ophthalmologist.

Common Presentations of Strabismus

Esodeviations (esophorias or esotropias, indicating inward or convergent deviation of the eyes):
  due to anatomic, refractive, genetic, and accommodative etiologies are the most common type of pediatric ocular deviation. They are reported to account for more than 50% of ocular misalignments in the pediatric population.
Infantile esotropia (occurring within the first 6 months of life):
  commonly seen with a familial history of esotropia. The angle of deviation is usually large. There is often alternation of fixation from one eye to the other, with good visual development in both eyes. Amblyopia can develop if this alternation is not present. Therapy consists of ocular patching and early surgical intervention.
Accommodative esotropia (due to accommodative attempts to correct for hyperopia):
  occurs between the ages of 6 months and 7 years (most commonly around the age of 2.5 years). Therapy involves the use of corrective lenses.
Exodeviations (divergent misalignment):
  present in 25% of strabismus cases, and usually begin between the ages of 6 months and 6 years. There is often a delay in diagnosis, which may be attributed to the fact that 80% of exotropia cases are intermittent.
Extraocular muscle palsies:
  can present with strabismus of varying degrees. A third nerve palsy may exist, which is more commonly congenital than acquired. A congenital third nerve palsy may be secondary to birth trauma or may be a developmental anomaly. An acquired third nerve palsy may be secondary to an inflammatory or infectious lesion, head trauma, post-viral syndromes, migraines, or an intracranial mass or aneurysm. The third nerve palsy manifests clinically as an exotropia, resulting from an unopposed, lateral rectus muscle and the superior oblique muscle. The eye movement is limited nasally in elevation and depression. Amblyopia is commonly associated with third nerve palsies and requires aggressive treatment to correct visual acuity; the nerve palsy must be corrected surgically.
Duane retraction syndrome:
  the most common cause of permanent limitation of lateral eye movement in the pediatric population. Females are more commonly affected than males. The left eye is more commonly affected than the right. Twenty percent of cases are bilateral. Esotropia, limited abduction of the globe are noted as adduction is attempted. This is secondary to of the lateral rectus muscle from the oculomotor nerve and absence of the sixth nerve.

Data Gathering

HISTORY

Question: When was the onset of symptoms?
Significance: A large percentage of newborns will manifest a transient esotropia or exotropia. Esodeviations or exodeviations persisting after the age of 6 months, or constant deviations, are considered abnormal and warrant additional evaluation.

Question: Is there a history of head tilting?
Significance: Head tilting may represent a vertical eye muscle problem. A full ophthalmologic examination is needed.

Question: Does the deviation occur at a particular time of day?
Significance: Eye fatigue or sleepiness may bring out symptoms of eye crossing.

Question: Does the patient have any other symptoms or change in mental status?
Significance: Vomiting, specifically early morning vomiting, may be a sign of increased intracranial pressure, and warrants immediate evaluation.

Question: Does the child seem to keep their head turned to one side?
Significance: Children with Duane syndrome will frequently keep their head turned to one side in order to keep their eyes aligned and to avoid the side of the eye with limited abduction.

Question: Has the child been noted to close or cover one eye?
Significance: This may be a clue to the presence of diplopia, and may be seen in some types of strabismus.

 ## Physical Examination

Finding: Transient esodeviation
Significance: May be observed in a normal infant less than 2 months of age; not indicative of pathology.

Finding: Esodeviation persisting after 2 months, or constant esodeviation
Significance: Should be evaluated by an ophthalmologist.

Finding: Any suspected defect in ocular motility noted after the age of 3 months
Significance: Warrants additional evaluation.

Finding: The finding of leukokoria (a white pupillary reflex)
Significance: Leukokoria is the most common initial sign of retinoblastoma. Immediate referral is warranted.

Finding: Opacity of the usually clear crystalline lens
Significance: This physical finding suggests the presence of a cataract.

Finding: The presence of a broad epicanthal fold, which may obscure the medial aspect of the sclera. A flat nasal bridge might be noted.
Significance: This finding may create the impression of strabismus. This condition, called pseudostrabismus, does not require referral.

 ## Laboratory Aids

Test: Corneal (Hirschberg method) light reflex is performed by holding a light source 33 cm in front of the patient and noting where the light reflex is on the cornea. The light reflex should be in the same spot in both eyes.
Significance: An esotropic eye will have a temporally displaced light reflex, whereas an exotropic eye will have a nasally displaced reflex. In the case of pseudoesotropia, the light reflection will be symmetrically placed.

Test: Cover-uncover test. Each eye must be tested individually. One eye is covered, and fixation movements are observed in the other eye. The cover is then removed and after a few seconds placed over the other eye. The uncovered eye is observed for movement.
Significance: Accurate to assess the presence of tropia. If movement is not noted, then no tropia exists; if movement is noted, then the diagnosis of heterotropia is made. Outward movement indicates esotropia, inward movement indicates exotropia, upward movement indicates hypotropia, and downward movement indicates hypertropia.

Test: The alternate cover test. Each eye is tested individually. The cover is placed over one eye and is then quickly moved to occlude the other eye, to disrupt coordinated binocular function.
Significance: Similar to cover-uncover test, this test is used to detect phorias and tropias. If movement is noted in the uncovered eye, a phoria or tropia has been elicited. The results of this test and the cover-uncover test will allow the interpretation of the presence of a tropia, phoria, or both.

Test: A complete fundoscopic evaluation
Significance: Detects presence of cataracts or evidence of infections.

Test: Assessment of visual acuity
Significance: Amblyopia occurs even in cases of small-angle strabismus.

 ## Emergency Care

Acute changes in the neurologic status of a patient presenting with a nerve palsy, manifesting clinically as strabismus, may indicate the presence of increased intracranial pressure and warrants emergency neurologic evaluation.

 ## Common Questions and Answers

Q: Up to what age is transient esodeviation considered to be within normal limits?
A: Transient esodeviation may be observed in normal infants up to 2 months of age. Transient esodeviation persisting after the age of 2 months or constant esodeviation should be evaluated by an ophthalmologist.

Q: Could the physical finding of head tilting represent a problem with the visual axis?
A: Head tilting may represent a vertical eye muscle problem and should be referred for evaluation.

Q: Does pseudoesotropia resolve?
A: Frequently, pseudoesotropia will resolve as the child grows and the nasal bridge becomes more prominent.

Issues for Referral

• Strabismus detected by the primary care physician warrants referral to an ophthalmologist for a complete evaluation and properly paced therapeutic intervention.
• If underlying conditions associated with strabismus are suspected, evaluation by other specialists (e.g., neurologist, geneticist) may be indicated.

BIBLIOGRAPHY

Calhoun JH. Eye examinations in infants and children. *Pediatr Rev* 1997;18(1):28–31.

Campbell LR, Charney E. Factors associated with delay in diagnosis of childhood amblyopia. *Pediatrics* 1991;87(2):178–185.

Helveston EM. 19th Annual Frank Costenbader Lecture—the origins of congenital esotropia. *J Pediatr Ophthalmol Strabismus* 1993;30(4):215–232.

Lavrich JB, Nelson LB. Diagnosis and treatment of strabismus disorders. *Pediatr Clin North Am* 1993;40(4):737–752.

Magramm I. Amblyopia: etiology, detection, and treatment. *Pediatr Rev* 1992;13(1):7–15.

Quinn G. In: Schwartz WM, ed. *Pediatric primary care, a problem-oriented approach,* 3rd ed. St. Louis: Mosby-Yearbook, 1997:718–727.

Author: Kathy Wholey Zsolway

Crying

Database

DEFINITION

Crying is usually a normal physiologic response to distress, discomfort, or unfulfilled needs. Crying is felt to be potentially pathologic if it is interpreted by caretakers as differing in quality and duration and/or persists without consolability beyond a reasonable time (generally 1 to 2 hours).

Differential Diagnosis

CONGENITAL/ANATOMIC

- Intussusception
- Gastroesophageal reflux
- Volvulus
- Gaseous distension (2° to improper feeding or burping)
- Incarcerated hernia
- Peritonitis (acute abdomen)
- Testicular/ovarian torsion
- Constipation
- Anal fissure
- Meatal ulceration
- Glaucoma

INFECTIOUS

- Otitis media/externa
- Urinary tract infection
- Stomatitis
- Meningitis
- Gastroenteritis
- Arthritis
- Osteomyelitis
- Balanitis
- Dermatitis (especially pruritic as in scabies or painful as in staphylococcal scalded skin syndrome)

TOXIC, ENVIRONMENTAL, DRUGS

- Neonatal drug withdrawal
- Prenatal/perinatal cocaine exposure
- Immunization reactions (especially DTP)
- Milk intolerance
- Drug reactions (especially antihistamines, pseudoephedrine, phenylpropanolamine), including maternal medications in breast milk
- Vitamin A toxicity
- Emotional/physical neglect

TRAUMA

- Corneal abrasion
- Foreign body (hypopharynx, eye, ear)
- Skull fracture/subdural hematoma
- Intracranial hemorrhage
- Retinal hemorrhage
- Other fractures (especially extremities)
- Hair tourniquet syndrome (encircling finger, toe, penis, clitoris)
- Open diaper pin
- Bite (human, animal, insect)

GENETIC/METABOLIC

- Sickle cell crisis
- Phenylketonuria
- Hypoglycemia
- Electrolyte abnormalities (especially sodium)
- Hypoglycemia
- Hypocalcemia
- Inborn error of metabolism

ALLERGIC/INFLAMMATORY

- Cow milk allergy
- Celiac disease

FUNCTIONAL

- Parental expectations/responses

MISCELLANEOUS

- Overstimulation
- Persistent night awakening
- Night terrors
- Congestive heart failure
- Caffey disease (infantile cortical hyperostosis)
- Dysrhythmia (especially supraventricular tachycardia)
- Autism
- Teething
- Headache
- Temperament
- Colic
- Discomfort (cold, heat, itching, hunger)

Approach to the Patient

GENERAL GOAL

Decide if the crying represents a normal physiologic response, a protracted multifactorial physiologic/developmental response (colic), or a potentially pathologic problem.

Phase 1: How urgent is the need for evaluation? A classic and difficult triage issue. One must identify the periodicity of the problem, associated symptoms, impression of wellness and parental anxiety/reliability.

Phase 2: When in doubt, particularly if "colic" seems unlikely, see the patient as soon as possible.

Data Gathering

HISTORY

Question: Onset after 1 month of age or persistent in infants older than 4 months?
Significance: Colic less likely as a cause.

Question: First episode?
Significance: Recurrent episodes, particularly with a diurnal pattern, are more likely due to colic.

Question: Fever?
Significance: Potential need for evaluation of meningitis, other infections.

Question: Do attempts at consolation make the crying worse?
Significance: Paradoxically increased crying (especially with lifting, rocking) can be seen in meningitis, peritonitis, long-bone fractures, arthritis.

Question: Stridor?
Significance: Implies possible upper airway obstruction (mechanical, functional).

Question: Expiratory grunting?
Significance: Higher likelihood of significant pathologic cause of crying (especially cardiac, respiratory, and/or infectious disease).

Question: Cold symptoms and/or day care attendance?
Significance: Increased likelihood of otitis media.

Question: Vomiting?
Significance: Higher likelihood of pathologic gastrointestinal cause (e.g., obstruction, G-E reflux with possible esophagitis), particularly in infant <3 months, or CNS disease.

Question: What is the pattern of feeding?
Significance: Over/underfeeding, excessive air swallowing, inadequate burping, improper formula preparation may contribute to excessive crying.

Question: Recent fall or trauma?
Significance: Possible fracture, increased intracranial pressure, abuse.

Physical Examination

Finding: Tympanic membrane with loss of landmarks, poor mobility.
Significance: Otitis media

Finding: Tenderness on palpation of extremities or clavicle.
Significance: Suggests fracture or osteomyelitis.

Finding: Conjunctival redness
Significance: Suggests corneal abrasion (fluorescein testing of eye warranted) or foreign body in eye (eversion of lid recommended)

Finding: Impacted or bloody stool on rectal exam, abdominal mass
Significance: Constipation or intussusception

Finding: Geographic scars, frenulum tears, retinal hemorrhages, suspicious bruises, decreased weight/height ratio
Significance: Neglect/abuse (physical, emotional)

Finding: Bulging fontanel
Significance: Possible increased ICP (meningitis, subdural hematoma, vitamin A toxicity)

Finding: Edema of individual toes or fingers
Significance: Hair tourniquet syndrome

Finding: Tender swelling in inguinal or scrotal area
Significance: Incarcerated hernia, testicular torsion

Finding: Heart rate >200 with minimal variability
Significance: Possible supraventricular tachycardia

Laboratory Aids

Test: Stool for occult blood
Significance: Possible intussusception, anal fissure

Test: Fluorescein testing of eye
Significance: Corneal abrasion (may occur without significant conjunctival redness)

Test: Urinalysis/urine culture
Significance: Urinary tract infection

Test: Urine toxicology screen
Significance: Drug withdrawal (neonatal), ingestions, passive exposures (e.g., cocaine)

Emergency Care

Factors that make this an emergency include:

• Suspicion of meningitis: stiff neck, bulging fontanel, fever (especially infants <2 to 3 months)
• Suspicion of intestinal obstruction: vomiting (especially bilious or projectile), mass on abdominal palpation, and/or bloody stools
• Suspicion of incarcerated hernia or testicular/ovarian torsion
• Evidence of cardiac compromise (CHF, SVT): tachycardia, poor perfusion (capillary refill >3 seconds, poor distal pulses), rales
• Evidence of acute dehydration: weight loss, decreased urine output, orthostatic changes, poor perfusion
• Evidence of child abuse or neglect

Common Questions and Answers

Q: What is the most likely cause of inconsolable crying in the first few months of life?
A: Without question, infantile colic. A practitioner needs to be familiar with the clinical pattern of infantile colic, so that deviations from this most common pediatric syndrome are readily recognized.

Q: Is teething a common cause of excessive crying?
A: Grandmothers everywhere insist that it is (as well as a common cause of fever, diarrhea, rashes, etc.). Objective data do not support a strong association. Be careful in ascribing symptoms and signs to teething. Trust the grandmothers, but verify.

Issues for Referral

Factors that may help alert you to make a referral include: Ill versus well-appearing. Although observation alone is less reliable in infants <3 months, judgement of an infant to be ill-appearing (e.g., pallor, grunting, poor arousability, poor response to social overtures) warrants more urgent and extensive evaluation. Weight loss implies a much higher likelihood of an organic cause of repetitive bouts of crying.

Clinical Pearls

• Quality of cry: Objective acoustic analyses of cries may become a common future modality to distinguish pathologic from physiologic crying. However, subjective interpretation can be helpful.

—High-pitched (shrill, piercing) crying in short bursts: associated with CNS pathology, especially with increased intracranial pressure
—High-pitched crying in longer bursts: seen in SGA infants, neonatal drug withdrawal
—Hoarse crying: seen in hypothyroidism, laryngeal diseases, hypocalcemic tetany
—Weak crying: may be seen in neuromuscular disorders, such as Hoffman-Werdnig syndrome, infant botulism, and/or the very ill infant
—Cat-like cry: as noted on every pediatric board exam for the last 35 years, a mewing cry can be associated with cri du chat syndrome (5p syndrome or absence of short arm of chromosome 5)

• Neonatal drug withdrawal has other characteristic findings in addition to excessive crying.

W Wakefulness

I Irritability

T Tremulousness, temperature variation, tachypnea

H Hyperactivity, high-pitched persistent cry, hyperacusis, hyperreflexia, hypertonia

D Diarrhea, diaphoresis, disorganized suck

R Rub marks, respiratory distress, rhinorrhea

A Apnea, autonomic dysfunction

W Weight loss or failure to gain weight

A Alkalosis (respiratory)

L Lacrimation

BIBLIOGRAPHY

Committee on drugs: neonatal drug withdrawal. *Pediatrics* 1998;101(6)72:1079–1088.

Corwin MJ, Lester BM, Golub HL. The infant cry: what can it tell us? *Curr Probl Pediatr* 1996;26(9):325–334.

Poole SR. The infant with acute, unexplained, excessive crying. *Pediatrics* 1991;88(3):450–455.

Author: Mark F. Ditmar

Diarrhea

Database

DEFINITION

Diarrhea should be considered whenever there is an increase in frequency, volume, or liquidity of an individual's stool as compared to their normal bowel movement pattern. While an adult excretes 100 to 200 g of stool each day, a child typically passes 10 g/kg in 24 hours. Diarrhea can also be characterized by duration. Chronic diarrhea is generally defined as the persistence of loose or more frequent stools for more than 2 weeks.

Differential Diagnosis

ACUTE DIARRHEA

- Dietary causes

—Sorbitol, Fructose
—Intolerance to specific foods (beans, fruit, peppers, etc.)

- Infectious causes

—Bacterial (*Salmonella, Shigella, Campylobacter, Yersinia, Plesiomonas, Aeromonas, Escherichia coli*)
—Viral (rotavirus, Norwalk agent, adenovirus)

- Medication

—Antibiotics
—Laxatives: Magnesium-containing

CHRONIC DIARRHEA

- Allergic/autoimmune

—Milk/soy protein allergy
—Eosinophilic enteritis
—AIDS
—IgA deficiency
—Combined immunodeficiency

- Anatomic abnormalities

—Short intestine
—Malrotation

- Bile salt malabsorption
- Celiac disease
- Congenital causes

—Villous atrophy
—Holovisceral myopathy

- Encopresis
- Endocrine disorders

—Hyperthyroidism
—Diabetes
—Congenital adrenal hyperplasia

- Hirschsprung enterocolitis
- Infectious causes

—Bacterial (see Acute Diarrhea)
—Viral (see Acute Diarrhea)
—Parasites (*Giardia, Entamoeba, Cryptosporidium*)
—*Clostridium difficile*
—Bacterial overgrowth

- Inflammatory bowel disease

—Ulcerative colitis
—Crohn disease

- Intestinal lymphangiectasia: primary and secondary
- Irritable bowel syndrome
- Lactose intolerance (primary, secondary, congenital)
- Medication (see Acute Diarrhea)
- Necrotizing enterocolitis
- Pancreatic dysfunction

—Cystic fibrosis
—Shwachman syndrome
—Chronic pancreatitis

- Post-infectious diarrhea
- Pseudo-obstruction
- Secretory tumors (VIPoma, somatostatinoma, gastrinoma)
- Vasculitis

—Hemolytic uremic syndrome
—Henoch-Schöenlein purpura

Tenesmus, perianal discomfort, and incontinence may also occur. While the definition of chronic diarrhea is controversial, chronic diarrhea is defined as more than 2 weeks of constant symptoms. Diarrhea is caused whenever there is an alteration in the normal intestinal fluid-electrolyte balance. Malabsorption, maldigestion, cellular electrolyte pump dysfunction, and intestinal colonization or invasion by microorganisms can cause diarrhea.

Approach to Patient

GENERAL GOAL

Determine the type of diarrhea (osmotic versus secretory).

Phase 1: Secretory Diarrhea Absorption of intestinal fluid and electrolytes is accomplished through multiple cellular pumps transporting sodium, glucose, and amino acids. Factors that interrupt these pumps (cholera toxin, prostaglandin E, VIP, secretin) can cause a severe active isotonic secretory state manifested by profuse diarrhea, dehydration, and acidosis.

Phase 2: Osmotic Diarrhea In general, the solute composition of intestinal fluid is similar to plasma. Osmotic diarrhea occurs when poorly absorbed or non-absorbable solute is present in the intestinal lumen. This can occur with the ingestion of non-absorbable sugars or cathartics, with carbohydrate malabsorption secondary to mucosal damage, with maldigestion secondary to pancreatic or hepatic dysfunction, with rapid transit of intestinal fluid, or with a rare congenital transport defect.

Data Gathering

HISTORY

Question: Has the diarrhea lasted less than 2 weeks?
Significance: A distinction should be made between acute and chronic diarrhea. The cause of acute diarrhea is almost always related to an infection, a medication, or the addition of a new food.

Question: Travel history?
Significance: Questions should be asked regarding travel to areas where drinking water is contaminated (e.g., Mexico—*Entamoeba*) or the ingestion of infected meat (*E. coli*) or fresh water (well water) infected with *Giardia*.

Question: Is the child an adolescent who is concerned about their weight?
Significance: Laxative abuse causing an osmotic diarrhea is common among adolescents who have an eating disorder.

Question: Does the patient have other systemic symptoms?
Significance: Systemic symptoms such as fever, gastrointestinal bleeding, rash, or vomiting should be ascertained. Specific infections and inflammatory bowel disease have associated systemic symptoms.

Question: Hematochezia?
Significance: The occurrence of acute, bloody stools and fever generally indicates a bacterial infection or amebiasis; however, these same symptoms coupled with thrombocytopenia, anemia, and azotemia; or a purpuric rash can indicate hemolytic uremic syndrome or Henoch-Schöenlein purpura (HSP), respectively. Chronic bloody diarrhea, abdominal pain and weight loss are characteristic of inflammatory bowel disease.

Question: What is the age of the child?
Significance: The age of the child is important because a number of diseases present between birth and 3 months of life including congenital villus/transport abnormalities, cystic fibrosis, or milk/soy allergy. In a previously well infant who had a recent viral illness with subsequent protracted diarrhea, the diagnosis of postviral enteritis should be suspected. This disorder is characterized by severe mucosal injury resulting in disaccharidase deficiency and prolonged malabsorption. Chronic non-specific diarrhea should be considered in otherwise normal preschool-aged children who have 2 to 10 watery stools/day without other symptoms and/or etiology. Lactose intolerance commonly occurs in many older children and adults, with over a 95% occurrence rate in some ethnic groups.

Question: Chronic diarrhea with weight loss?
Significance: Inflammatory or immunologic disorders such as ulcerative colitis, Crohn disease, and celiac disease must be considered in older children with chronic diarrhea.

Physical Examination

Finding: What are the child's growth parameters?
Significance: An important part of the physical examination is height, weight, head circumference, and height/weight measurements. Previous measurements are necessary to make an accurate evaluation. Findings of a chronically malnourished child with years of unsuspected weight loss or poor growth velocity would indicate a divergent differential diagnosis from that of a healthy-appearing child with normal growth.

Finding: Does the child have arthritis?
Significance: Arthritis and diarrhea can occur in diseases such as inflammatory bowel disease, celiac disease, HSP, and in specific bacterial infections.

Finding: Is there nailbed clubbing?
Significance: Cystic fibrosis

Finding: Is there a right lower quadrant mass?
Significance: A right lower quadrant mass could suggest an abscess (Crohn disease, appendiceal abscess)

 ## Laboratory Aids

Test: Stool culture
Significance: Stool examination not only for blood/mucous/inflammatory cells but also for microorganisms is important in determining the etiology of the diarrhea. Stool cultures for parasites (*Giardia, Entamoeba*), bacterial pathogens (*Salmonella, Campylobacter, Shigella, Yersinia, Aeromonas, Plesiomonas*) and *Clostridium difficile* toxin should be obtained in all children with unexplained diarrhea.

Test: Stool gram stain
Significance: Useful in determining the presence of polymorphonuclear leukocytes suggesting a colitis.

Test: Stool pH
Significance: Useful in identifying carbohydrate malabsorption; normal stool pH is 5 to 6.

Test: Hemoccult
Significance: Documents blood

Test: 72-hour quantitative fecal fat evaluation
Significance: A sensitive test for steatorrhea. Patients need to be placed on a high-fat diet (3 g/kg) for 3 days. During this time, all stools are collected and frozen, and on completion, the amount of ingested fat is compared to excreted fat. When malabsorption is present, disorders of pancreatic function (cystic fibrosis, Shwachman syndrome) or severe intestinal disease should be suspected.

Test: Lactose breath test
Significance: A non-invasive test that measures hydrogen levels in expired air and is based on the principle that hydrogen gas is produced by colonic bacterial fermentation of malabsorbed carbohydrates. When abnormal in older healthy-appearing children, primary lactose deficiency is suggested. However, in young children, secondary lactase deficiency should be considered and small-bowel disease should be suspected.

Test: D-xylose test
Significance: Based on the principle that D-xylose absorption occurs independently of bile salts, pancreatic secretions, and intestinal disaccharidases. A specific dose of D-xylose (14.5 mg/m², maximum 25 g) is given orally after an 8 hour fast and the serum level of D-xylose is determined after 1 hour. Typically, disorders that alter or disrupt the intestinal mucosa produce abnormal results.

Test: Endoscopy and colonoscopy
Significance: These procedures have become extremely useful tests. These diagnostic tests not only allow direct visualization of the intestinal mucosa but also provide access for intestinal culture, disaccharidase and pancreatic enzyme evaluation, and intestinal biopsy.

Emergency Care

Diarrhea can always lead to dehydration. Any child suspected of clinical dehydration should be closely observed. If oral rehydration is ineffective intravenous therapy is indicated. In addition, rarely acute right lower abdominal pain with diarrhea may indicate appendicitis. Culture negative gastrointestinal bleeding associated with severe abdominal pain and diarrhea should always be treated urgently.

Issues for Referral

Because the occurrence of diarrhea in children is quite common, the decision to pursue an evaluation rests with the primary care physician. Children who present with growth failure, non-infectious heme-positive diarrhea, or unexplained chronic diarrhea should be considered for referral to a pediatric gastroenterologist.

BIBLIOGRAPHY

Ammon HV. Diarrhea. In: Haubrick WS, Schaffner F, Berk JE, eds. *Gastroenterology*, 5th ed. Philadelphia: WB Saunders, 1995:87–101.

Arnold L. Acute diarrhea. In: Schwartz MW, Curry TA, Sargent AJ, Blum NJ, Fein JA, eds. *Principles and practice of clinical pediatrics*. Chicago: Year Book, 1997:227–231.

Baldassano RN, Liacouras CA. Chronic diarrhea: a practical approach for the pediatrician. *Pediatr Clin North Am* 1991;38:667–685.

Rhoads JM, Powell DW. Diarrhea. In: Walker WA, Durie PR, Hamilton JR, Walker-Smith JA, Watkins JB, eds. *Pediatric gastrointestinal disease*. Philadelphia: BC Decker, 1990:62–78.

Vanderhoof JA. Diarrhea. In: Wyllie R, Hyams JS, eds. *Pediatric gastrointestinal disease*. Philadelphia: WB Saunders, 1993:187–197.

Author: Chris A. Liacouras

Dyspnea

Database

DEFINITION

Shortness of breath, a subjective feeling of having difficulty breathing.

Differential Diagnosis

CONGENITAL/ANATOMICAL

- Subglotic stenosis
- Vocal cord paralysis
- Macroglossia
- Pierre Robin syndrome
- Laryngeal atresia
- Pulmonary sequestration
- Pulmonary hypoplasia

INFECTIOUS

- Lower airway

—Bronchiolitis
—Pertussis
—Pneumonia
—Tuberculosis

- Upper airway

—Croup
—Epiglottitis
—Tracheitis
—Peritonsilar abscess

TOXIC, ENVIRONMENTAL, DRUGS

- Aspiration

—Fluid
—Foreign body

- Carbon monoxide poisoning
- Methemoglobinemia
- Smoke inhalation

TUMORS/CYSTS

- Head/Neck

—Dermoid cysts
—Brancial cleft cysts
—Lingual thyroid
—Hemangioma
—Teratoma
—Papilloma
—Brain stem tumor

- Thoracic

—Teratoma
—Cystic hygroma
—Bronchogenic cyst
—Pericardial cyst
—Neurogenic tumor
—Lymphoma
—Leukemia

- Abdominal mass

—Hepatic mass
—Hepatoblastoma
—Neuroblastoma

ALLERGY

- Anaphylaxis

PULMONARY

- Asthma
- Atelectasis
- Pneumothorax
- Pleural effusion
- Hemorrhage
- Embolism

CARDIAC

- Pulmonary edema

RENAL

- Renal failure causing fluid overload
- Metabolic acidosis

HEMATOLOGY

- Anemia
- Sickle cell crisis
- Acute chest syndrome

MUSCLE WEAKNESS

- Duchenne muscular dystropy
- Spinal muscle atrophy

MISCELLANEOUS

- High altitude
- Exercise
- Psychogenic hyperventilation
- Anxiety
- Panic disorders

Approach to the Patient

GENERAL GOALS

To identify the organ system responsible for the dyspnea and to determine whether the process is acute or chronic.

Phase 1: Determine if the cause is respiratory or cardiac in nature. Is the patient clinically stable and can the patient protect their airway? It is important to identify those who will need intensive/emergency care and those who can be worked up in the office.

Phase 2: Inquire about the duration of symptoms the circumstances around the onset of the dyspnea. History and physical examination should focus on respiratory and cardiology. If these two have been ruled out, other etiologies must be evaluated.

Phase 3: Inquire about other medical problems of the patient.

Data Gathering

HISTORY

Question: Onset of dyspnea? What was the patient doing at the time of onset (if acute)?
Significance: In a small child, acute onset may be related to aspiration of a foreign body or liquid. If the patient was unsupervised, foreign body is a high probability. If the dyspnea occurred over days, other respiratory, cardiac, or renal should be suspected.

Question: Any fever, cough, chest pain, runny nose?
Significance: This would suggest an infectious etiology. The chest pain could be related to a pneumothorax, which can occur spontaneously in some individuals.

Question: Anyone at home sick or have respiratory problems and/or illness?
Significance: Leading toward infection. However, in some cases of congenital heart disease a respiratory virus such as RSV can make an otherwise stable patient into a critically ill child.

Question: Is there history of wheezing or asthma?
Significance: Children who have a history of wheezing are likely to reexacerbate their lung disease.

Question: Has the child ever been hospitalized or had respiratory problem in the past?
Significance: Children that have been hospitalized for respiratory problems are likely to have subsequent difficulty with other respiratory problems.

Question: Any history of cardiac problems or ever been diagnosed with a murmur?
Significance: In the absence of an infectious type or wheezing type of history, a murmur can help the examiner focus on the cardiac examination.

Physical Examination

LUNG

Finding: Crackles or rhonchi auscultate
Significance: Lower lung disease such as pneumonia or bronchiolits. Fluid overload can cause bilateral crackles.

Finding: Wheezing auscultated
Significance: Wheezing is usually heard on expiration. Suggest an obstructive lung disease such as asthma or reactive airways disease or anaphylaxis.

Finding: Distant or absent breath sounds
Significance: Foreign body aspiration blocking air movement. Pneumothorax should also be suspected.

Finding: Barking cough
Significance: Croup, which is usually caused by parainfluenza virus. It also could be foreign body.

Finding: Symptoms worse in supine position
Significance: Could be secondary to pulmonary edema or compression by a mediastinal mass.

Finding: Egophony auscultate
Significance: Pleural effusion should be suspected.

HEART

Finding: Loud murmur or gallop auscultated
Significance: Cardiac disease in which pulmonary edema can be etiology of the dyspnea.

Finding: Cyanosis
Significance: Poor oxygen perfusion

Finding: Low blood pressure and poor skin perfusion
Significance: The patient can be in shock. Quick identification of the type of shock is needed to correct the underlying problem.

Finding: Clubbing of the digits
Significance: Suggests chronic disease such as cystic fibrosis or cardiac disease

Finding: Drooling, with mouth open in an ill appearing child
Significance: Suggests epiglotitis and need for careful evaluation (see Epiglotitis)

Finding: Abdominal mass palpated
Significance: Could be causing compression of lungs

Finding: Acites or edema
Significance: Fluid overload either from renal or cardiac etiology

 ## Laboratory Aids

Test: Chest radiograph
Significance: Look for appearance of the lung fields for the different types of pneumonia. Evaluate the heart size and the pulmonary vascularity for fluid overload. Hyperinflation suggest an obstructive pulmonary disease such as asthma. A hyperinflated (usually right lobe) darkened lobe is suspicious of a foreign body present. Seeing a shift in the heart and seeing a lung edge is common in pneumothorax or effusion. Fluid in the costophrenic angle suggests an effusion.

Test: Pulse oximetry
Significance: A quick assessment of oxygen perfusion

Test: Arterial blood gas
Significance: A more detailed assessment of oxygenation and acidosis. A blood gas will also delineate metabolic versus respiratory acidosis and also can show if compensation has occurred.

Test: Complete blood count with differential
Significance: First, an elevated white blood count with a left shift differential can be a sign of infection. If the patient has pallor, the hemoglobin can be evaluated to see if the patient is anemic. A CBC also can be helpful in patients in which leukemia or other oncologic diseases are suspected.

Test: Mantoux (PPD)
Significance: A history of family members with tuberculosis or immigrants from a country where TB is prevalent, a PPD should be placed with anergy panel.

 ## Common Questions and Answers

Q: Is dyspnea, in most cases, pulmonary in nature?
A: Yes, it is in most cases. However, if infectious, foreign body, and asthma etiologies are ruled out, a non-respiratory cause must be investigated

Issues for Referral

• Any patient that has unstable vital signs, inability to oxygenate, and needs critical care services.
• Any patient with a suspected foreign body aspiration will need a bronchcosopy surgical consult.
• If asthma is suspected, use criteria as noted in asthma (see Asthma).
• Any patient with epiglotitis will need an otolaryngologist to evaluate the patient under general anesthesia (see Epiglotitis).
• Anaphylaxis is a medical emergency and mandates immediate action. Epinephrine, benadryl, and possibly steroids are the drugs of choice for treatment.
• Any patient that has a pneumothorax. May need surgical aspiration or chest tube placement (see Pneumothorax).
• Any patient where an oncologic process suspected. Referral to a tertiary care center with a critical care unit and with a pediatric oncologist (see Leukemia).

Clinical Pearls

• A child who presents dyspnea, anxiety, or panic disorder should only be considered once the more serious etiologies have been ruled out.
• If hyperventilation is suspected, a brown paper bag can be useful to break the cycle of hypocarbia.

BIBLIOGRAPHY

Denny FW. Acute respiratory infections in children: etiology and epidemiology. *Pediatr Rev* 1987;9(5):135–146.

Dibs SD, Baker MD. Anaphylaxis in children: a 5-year experience. *Pediatrics* 1997;99(1):E7.

Holroyd HJ. Foreign body aspiration: potential cause of coughing and wheezing. *Pediatr Rev* 1988;10(2):59–63.

McIntosh K. Respiratory syncytial virus infections in infants and children: diagnosis and treatment. *Pediatr Rev* 1987;9(6):191–196.

Schidlow DV, Callahan CW. Pneumonia. *Pediatr Rev* 1996;17(9):300–309.

Segel GB. Anemia. *Pediatr Rev* 1988;10(3):77–88.

Author: Charles I. Schwartz

Dysuria

 Database

DEFINITION

Painful urination

 Differential Diagnosis

CONGENITAL/ANATOMIC

- Meatal stenosis
- Urethral stricture
- Posterior urethral diverticula
- Urethral stones
- Urethral valves
- Ureterocele
- Ectopic ureter
- Vesico-vaginal fistula

INFECTIOUS

- Viral infection
- Gonorrhea
- Herpes simplex
- Tuberculosis
- Cystitis
- Urethritis
- Pinworms
- Prostatitis

TOXIC, ENVIRONMENTAL, DRUGS

- Bubble bath urethritis
- Cytoxin

TRAUMA

- Diaper dermatitis
- Foreign body
- Bicycle injury
- Masturbation
- Sexual abuse

TUMOR

- Sarcoma botroides

GENETIC/METABOLIC

- Cysteinuria

ALLERGIC INFLAMMATORY

- Food allergy
- Stevens-Johnson syndrome
- Contact dermatitis such as poison ivy

FUNCTIONAL

- Attention mechanism

MISCELLANEOUS

- Appendicitis

Approach to the Patient

GENERAL GOALS

Determine the cause and begin treatment.

Phase 1: Rule out common causes such as trauma, infection, chemical irritant, constipation, and masturbation. Consider attention getting behavior.

Phase 2: Continue investigation—look for congential problems that cause infection, strictures. Metabolic disease and allergies.

Phase 3: Begin treatment.

HINTS FOR SCREENING PROBLEMS

Ask about medications and food allergens. Ask about special situations such as sand in bathing suit to cause irritation.

 Data Gathering

HISTORY

Question: Do the symptoms occur at any special time of day?
Significant: May indicate an attention mechanism if occurs before school, etc.

Question: What kinds of medicine do you take?
Significant: Some medications such as cytoxin will cause irritation of the urethra.

Question: Have there been any new foods or known food allergens?
Significant: Milk and citrus fruits can cause dysuria in certain patients. Best determined if symptoms regress on elimination of possible offending food.

Question: Do you use bubble bath?
Significant: Bubble bath is fun but causes the urethra to lose its protecive lipids.

Question: Any signs of bleeding?
Significant: Can indicate trauma, infection, or congenital anomalies. Some feel that calcium exretion can cause dysuria as well as hematuria.

Question: Fever
Significant: Common sign of urinary tract infection.

Question: Frequency
Significant: Both frequency and dysuria are common findings in urinary tract infections.

Question: Past history of urological operations
Significant: Anti-reflux may have a side effect of dysuria

Question: What have you taken for the discomfort?
Significant: Common usage of cranberry juice is used for many urinary problems. The additional volume is usually helpful but the effect of cranberry juice is neglible in the volumes usually consumed.

Question: Quality and strength of the urinary stream
Significant: Patients with posterior urethral valves have small frequent voidings with low pressure because of the obstruction in the posterior urethra.

Physical Examination

Finding: Any signs of redness or ecchymoses?
Significance: May indicate trauma from masturbation or abuse

Finding: Any bleeding?
Significance: Seen in trauma, tumors, and infection

Finding: Any change in behavior?
Significance: This symptom may be an attention seeking device.

Finding: Abnormal swelling?
Significance: May occur in trauma or rare tumors.

Finding: Abnormal urethra?
Significance: Prolapsed urethra or diverticula

Finding: Grape-like stuctures in vagina?
Significance: Sarcoma boitriodes

Finding: Abdominal pain?
Significance: Intra-abdominal abscess or low lying inflamed appendix can cause dysuria

 Laboratory Aids

Test: Urinalysis
Significance: Most urinary tract infections will have white cells in the urine.

Test: Urine culture
Significance: Check for infection.

Test: Ultrasound
Significance: Not routinely requested unless a congenital anomaly is suspected.

Test: Metabolic screens
Significance: If sediment shows crystals; if familial history of metabolic disease.

 Common Questions and Answers

Q: How does bubble bath cause dysuria?
A: The bubble bath removes lipids that protect the urethra causing the tissue to swell and become inflamed.

Q: Can allergies cause dysuria?
A: It is difficult to directly prove allergies as a cause of dysuria. However, in some cases, elimination of certain foods such as spices, citrus fruits, or known skin allergens have improved symptoms.

Q: How do children get infected with gonococcus?
A: This is a red flag of sexual abuse, which must be investigated.

Q: Which viruses cause dysuria?
A: Adenovirus has been identified

Issues for Referral

- Evidence of congenital anomaly
- Increasing severity of symptoms
- Failure to respond to symptomatic or specific treatment

Clinical Pearls

- Sometimes difficult to differentiate dysuria from frequency, which may cause an uncomfortable feeling or pressure that is described by the child as "pain"
- Discharge with dysuria suggests gonococcal or chylamidia infection
- Low lying inflamed appendix may cause bladder irritation and dysuria
- Urethral prolapse may present as hematuria or frequency

BIBLIOGRAPHY

Anonymous. 1998 guidelines for treatment of sexually transmitted diseases. Centers for Disease Control and Prevention. *MMWR Morb Mortal Wkly Rep* 1998;47(RR-1):1–111.

Lee HJ, Pyo JW, Choi EH, et al. Isolation of adenovirus type from the urine of children with acute hemorrhagic cystitis. *Pediatr Infect Dis J* 1996;15(7):633–634.

Rushton HG. Urinary tract infections in children. Epidemiology, evaluation, and management. *Pediatr Clin North Am* 1997;44(5):1133–1169.

Author: M. William Schwartz

Earache

Database

DEFINITION

Earache (otalgia) is a common complaint in the pediatric population (see table Common Causes of Earache). Primary otalgia refers to pain originating from the ear structures. Secondary otalgia arises from referred pain from other areas of the head and neck. Secondary pain is referred through cranial and cervical nerves that share distributions with the ear.

Differential Diagnosis

PRIMARY OTALGIA

Infectious

• Otitis media—most common cause of pediatric otalgia, acute onset
• Otitis externa—more common in summer months; pain increases with traction on pinna
• Serous otitis media—child may complain of pain, fullness, hearing loss, or "hearing things"
• Varicella—chickenpox may involve the auricle and ear canal, as may herpes zoster
• Herpes simplex—appears as grouped vesicles
• Cellulitis
• Furunculosis—localized abscess
• Mastoiditis—complication of otitis media; ear protrudes anteriorly

Trauma

• Foreign body—child may have an intense inflammatory reaction
• Lacerations, abrasions—usually from putting objects in ear or cleaning
• Blunt trauma—may be associated with tympanic membrane perforation, inner ear injury, or basilar skull fractures
• Barotrauma—arising from abrupt changes in middle ear pressure (airplanes, scuba diving)

Tumor

• Rare in pediatric patients, but may involve any of the ear structures including skin, bone, vascular, and neural components

Common Causes of Earache

Otitis media
Otitis externa
Foreign body/trauma
Eustachian tube dysfunction
Teething
Dental infections and trauma
Pharyngitis/Tonsillitis
Sinusitis/Rhinitis

Allergic/Inflammatory

• Dermatologic conditions such as eczema and psoriasis
• Allergy to topical antibiotic and cerumenolytic agents

Functional

• Eustachian tube dysfunction

Miscellaneous

• Impacted cerumen

SECONDARY OTALGIA

Infectious

• Dental infections including abscess and gingivitis
• Stomatitis—herpes simplex and coxsackieviruses are common causes
• Tonsillitis
• Peritonsillar abscess
• Post-tonsillectomy/post-adenoidectomy—pain worsens with swallowing
• Retropharyngeal abscess—drooling, stridor, child usually appears ill
• Mumps
• Sinusitis
• Cervical adenitis
• Laryngitis

Trauma

• Dental trauma
• Penetrating injuries to the oropharynx
• Lacerations
• Burns—caustic, thermal, or electrical
• Injuries to the neck and C-spine including fractures and muscle tension

Tumor

• Oropharyngeal/laryngeal tumors—may be cystic, benign, or malignant
• Rarely intracranial tumors will present with ear pain

Allergic/Inflammatory

• Allergic rhinitis
• Cervical spine arthritis

Miscellaneous

• Foreign body may be lodged in piriform sinus or esophagus
• Esophagitis—usually secondary to severe gastroesophageal reflex (GER)
• Bell palsy—may present as a complication of otitis media
• Temporomandibular joint (TMJ) disease

Approach to the Patient

GENERAL GOALS

Because ear pain arises from a large number of sites, history taking and physical examination should be directed toward assessing symptoms from the entire region, not just the ear (face, oropharynx, larynx, and neck). Preverbal children and children with language delay may present with non-specific symptoms (fever, fussiness, tugging at ears, lethargy, vomiting) that should alert one to consider the possibility of ear pain as the source of the problem.

Phase 1: Each encounter should begin with a careful history and physical examination. The following sections suggest questions that may be helpful, as well as potentially significant physical exam findings. If the examination of the ear does not reveal the cause of pain, thoroughly examine the entire head and neck region.

Phase 2: An abnormal audiogram or tympanogram may help to determine if ear pathology is present in the face of a normal physical exam. Lateral neck films may be helpful in evaluation of a suspected retropharyngeal process. Other laboratory and radiologic evaluations must be guided by your suspicions based on your history and physical.

Phase 3: Referral to an otorhinolaryngologist is indicated in cases of ear pain with no identifiable cause.

Data Gathering

HISTORY

Question: Duration of symptoms?
Significance: Acute onset more likely suggests recent trauma or infection.

Question: Location?
Significance: If referred pain, will likely have symptoms at primary site as well.

Question: Fever?
Significance: Suggestive of infectious etiology.

Question: Trauma?
Significance: Ask about recent ear cleaning, falls, accidents, etc.

Question: History of recurrent otitis media?
Significance: Consider serous otitis media, cholesteatoma.

Question: Tinnitus?
Significance: May represent otitis media with effusion, inner ear abnormalities, vascular lesions or tumors.

Question: Ear drainage?
Significance: Look for primary source such as otitis media with perforation, cholesteatoma, otitis externa, and trauma.

Question: Vertigo?
Significance: Again a primary source from the external, middle, or inner ear is the likely cause, although CNS pathology must be a consideration.

Question: Hearing loss?
Significance: Suggestive of primary problem; however, can be associated with intracranial lesion and multiple other syndromes and diseases.

Question: Hoarseness?
Significance: Suggestive of oropharyngeal or laryngeal pathology including infections, foreign body, and GER.

Question: Drooling?
Significance: Suggestive of oropharyngeal or laryngeal pathology particularly infections, foreign bodies, and caustic ingestion.

Question: Stridor?
Significance: Suggestive of oropharyngeal or laryngeal pathology, which causes airway narrowing. Consider infections, foreign body, mass.

Question: Choking/coughing?
Significance: Consider foreign body, mass, or GER.

 Physical Examination

Finding: Intense pain elicited by traction on pinna.
Significance: Suggestive of otitis externa

Finding: Areas of trauma
Significance: There may be an isolated abrasion or laceration; however, inspect carefully for hemotympanum and associated injuries and evidence of basilar skull fracture.

Finding: Foreign bodies
Significance: May be isolated, or associated with otitis externa

Finding: Bulging, red, immobile tympanic membrane
Significance: Consistent with otitis media

Finding: Retracted, immobile tympanic membrane
Significance: Suggests otitis media with effusion

Finding: Evidence of a mass lesion
Significance: A mass lesion behind the tympanic membrane may represent a cholesteatoma, although other benign and malignant lesions must be considered.

Finding: Neck oropharynx, TMJ, lymph nodes, salivary glands, and neck
Significance: If no findings suggest a primary source, inspect each area carefully for signs of secondary pathology.

Finding: Dental caries
Significance: Multiple dental caries should raise the suspicion of a possible dental abscess.

Finding: Tonsillar asymmetry or uvular deviation from midline
Significance: May represent peritonsillar cellulitis/abscess or mass.

Finding: Trismus, drooling
Significance: May represent a mass/abscess

Finding: Assess facial-nerve function and other cranial nerves
Significance: Bell palsy may be a complication of otitis media. Other cranial nerve dysfunction suggests possible intracranial lesion.

 Laboratory Aids

The history and physical examination are usually enough to make a diagnosis.

Test: Audiometry
Significance: Assess for hearing loss suggestive of primary otalgia

Test: Tympanometry
Significance: Useful in assessment of otitis media with effusion, eustachian-tube dysfunction, and tympanostomy tube obstruction

Test: Lateral neck x-ray studies
Significance: Helpful for symptoms suggestive of retropharyngeal mass/abscess.

Test: Imaging of head
Significance: Rarely needed unless intracranial lesion suspected

Test: Blood screens
Significance: Not routinely useful

 Emergency Care

Disorders with potential to cause airway compromise (mass lesions, foreign bodies, abscess, etc.):

- Establish "ABCs" as indicated
- Consult otorhinolaryngologist (ORL)
- Hospitalize

Trauma resulting in hearing loss, significant bleeding, or fractures:

- Establish "ABCs" as indicated
- Promptly consult ORL
- Do not attempt to remove debris from ear if suspected basilar skull fracture (can introduce bacteria)
- Hospitalize as indicated

Infectious etiologies that cause toxic-appearing or "septic" child:

- Establish "ABCs" as indicated
- Administer intravenous antibiotics as indicated
- Hospitalize

Issues for Referral

Factors that may alert you to make a referral to an ORL include:

- Ear pain without an identifiable source
- Pain with unexplained hearing loss, vertigo, tinnitus
- Pain with unexplained or persistent otorrhea
- Suspected neoplasm
- Otitis media with complications (Otitis Media)
- Foreign bodies that cannot be removed easily from the ear

BIBLIOGRAPHY

LeLiever W. Nonotalgic otalgia (question and answer). *JAMA* 1990;264(17):2302.

Potsic W, Handler S, Wetmore R, Pasquariello P. *Primary care pediatric otolaryngology.* Andover, MA: J. Michael Ryan Publishing, Inc., 1995.

Tunnessen W. *Signs and symptoms in pediatrics.* Philadelphia: J.B. Lippincott Company, 1988:157–163.

Yellon R. The spectrum of reflux-associated otolaryngologic problems in infants and children. *Am J Med* 1997;103(3S):125S–129S.

Author: Lisa M. Biggs

Edema

 Database

DEFINITION

Presence of abnormal amount of fluid in the extracellular spaces of the body. Edema is usually secondary to low albumin, obstruction of venous or lymphatic channels or trauma.

CAUSES

- Excessive losses

—Renal loss of protein
—Gastrointestinal

- Inadequate production

—Liver disease
—Malnutrition

- Local trauma
- Increased hydrostatic pressure

—Congestive heart failure
—Pericardial effusion
—Venous obstruction
—Lymphatic obstruction

 Differential Diagnosis

LOCALIZED

- Trauma—pressure or sun damage
- Infection
- Allergy
- Lymphatic obstruction (less common)
- Bee stings or insect bites

GENERALIZED

Congenital

- Lymphatic obstruction of legs or thoracic duct

Infection

- Hepatitis and liver failure
- Pericarditits

Toxic, Environmental, Drugs

- Sodium poisoning
- Toxic effect on liver and/or heart (chemotherapy)
- Cirrhosis

Tumor

- Obstruction of venous return from enlarged abdominal lymph nodes

Genetic/Metabolic

- Sickle cell renal failure

Allergic Inflammatory

- Protein losing enteropathy

Miscellaneous

- Nephrotic syndrome
- Renal failure
- Congestive heart failure
- Pericarditis
- Gastrointestinal protein loss
- Post-pericardiotomy or congenital heart surgery
- Endocrine—sodium retention, hypothyroidism
- Hepatobiliary diseases

Approach to the Patient

GENERAL GOALS

Determine the cause of swelling. Is it localized, are there any losses of protein or is there underproduction of protein? Determine the serum protein/albumin, which would make you consider increased losses or decreased production.

Phase 1: Is the swelling localized as seen in trauma, lymphatic, or venous obstruction?

Phase 2: Are there urinary or gastrointestinal losses? This will be associated with decreased serum albumin. Most likely the source of the loss is renal disease and less frequently gastrointestinal losses.

Phase 3: Search for other causes of edema such as insect bites, pericardial effusion, metabolic disease.

Data Gathering

HISTORY

Question: Is the edema localized or generalized?
Significance: See Differential Diagnosis section.

Question: Is the patient asymptomatic or in some distress specifically due to the edema?
Significance: Determines treatment urgency

Question: Is there evidence of cardiac, renal, or gastrointestinal disease?
Significance: These are the major causes of edema.

Question: Has waist size become larger? Are shoes difficult to put on?
Significance: Evidence of edema in body.

Question: What is the salt intake in diet?
Significance: In some patients, excess salt contributes to edema.

Question: Is there shortness of breath?
Significance: There may be ascites, which compresses the diaphragm or causes pleural effusions.

Question: Is there chronic diarrhea?
Significance: Seen in protein losing enteropathy or lymphatic obstruction.

Question: Have any urinalyses been performed in the past?
Significance: May help date the onset of the problem.

Question: History of allergies?
Significance: Allergies will commonly cause swelling around the eyes or face.

 ## Physical Examination

Finding: Dependent edema
Significance: Lumbosacral area pretibial pressure to detect edema scrotum/labia

Finding: Percussion of chest
Significance: Pleural effusion

Finding: Shifting dullness
Significance: Early signs of ascites

Finding: Soft ear cartilage
Significance: Common finding in nephrotic syndrome

Finding: Pitting edema
Significance: Pitting edema is seen in cases of protein loss and obstruction of venous/lymphatic flow while non-pitting edema is seen in salt poisoning.

 ## Laboratory Aids

DISCRIMINATING LABORATORY TESTS

Test: Dipstick urinalysis
Significance: If there is generalized edema with heavy proteinuria and hypoalbuminemia, the presumptive diagnosis is always nephrotic syndrome until proven otherwise.

Test: Serum albumin
Significance: If there is generalized edema with no proteinuria but hypoalbuminemia, consider cardiac, gastrointestinal, or hepatobiliary disease and direct additional studies to evaluate these three organ systems specifically. If there is either localized edema or generalized edema but a normal urinalysis and a normal serum albumin, consider other unusual causes for edema such as mechanical or lymphatic obstruction, certain endocrine disorders, or the effects of drugs or toxins.

Test: Stool albumin
Significance: Seen in protein losing enteropathy.

Issues for Referral

Referral to a specialist for edema is indicated for the following reasons:

• Nephrotic edema with impaired glomerular function—pediatric nephrologist
• Protein-losing enteropathy or hepatobiliary disease—pediatric gastroenterologist
• Congestive heart failure secondary to occult cardiac disease—pediatric cardiologist
• Endocrine-mediated edema—pediatric endocrinologist
• Lymphatic or other mechanical obstructions—vascular surgeon or pediatric surgeon, if readily available

 ## Emergency Care

Any child or adolescent with an edema-forming state that compromises either cardiorespiratory function or the vascular integrity of a peripheral organ or limb should be referred immediately to an appropriate specialist for emergency care.

Clinical Pearls

• If edema is massive, the patient may awaken with swollen eyelids. Place blocks under the head of the bed to keep head elevated.
• If there is scrotal edema, jockey shorts will help support scrotum and protect the skin from breaking down.

 ## Common Questions and Answers

Q: At what level of serum albumin, will edema occur?
A: Edema is generally associated with serum albumin below 2.5 Gm/dL.

Q: Why does pericardial effusion cause edema?
A: The pericardial effusion is associated with decreased lymphatic flow and increased venous pressure.

Q: Is there a certain group of allergens that will cause edema?
A: No special allergens are associated with edema. The usual causes include such foods as peanuts and drugs such as penicilin.

BIBLIOGRAPHY

Dudin A, Othman A. Acute periorbital swelling: evaluation of management protocol. *Pediatr Emerg Care* 1996;12(1):16–20.

Jacobs ML, Rychik J, Byrum CJ, Norwood WI Jr. Protein-losing enteropathy after Fontan operation: resolution after baffle fenestration. *Ann Thorac Surg* 1996;61(1):206–208.

Kelsch RC, Sedman AB. Nephrone syndrome. *Pediatr Rev* 1993;14:30–38.

Molina JF, Brown RF, Gedalia A, Espinoza LR. Protein losing enteropathy as the initial manifestation of childhood systemic lupus erythematosus. *J Rheumatol* 1996;23(7):1269–1271.

Rosen FS. Urticaria, angioedema, anaphylaxis. *Pediatr Rev* 1992;13:387–390.

Author: Michael E. Norman

Failure to Thrive

Database

DEFINITION

• Failure to thrive (FTT) is a term used to describe infants and children who fail to meet standards for appropriate growth. FTT is more a sign or symptom of an underlying problem than a final diagnosis or disease state.
• The different criteria for malnutrition are: mild, weight for age 75% to 90% of median; moderate, weight for age 60% to 74% of median; and severe, weight for age less than 60% of median.

Differential Diagnosis

CONGENITAL/ANATOMICAL

• Congenital syndromes
• Chromosomal abnormalities
• Congenital heart disease
• Hirschsprung disease
• Pyloric stenosis
• Malrotation
• Vascular slings

INFECTIOUS

• Hepatitis
• Tuberculosis
• Human immunodeficiency virus (HIV)
• Parasitic infection
• Urinary tract infection
• Chronic sinusitis

TOXIC, ENVIRONMENTAL, DRUGS

• Inadequate caloric intake due to emotional deprivation
• Maternal depression
• Poor feeding techniques
• Poor child–caretaker interactions
• Improper formula preparation
• Household chaos
• Lack of proper environment for mealtimes
• Parental drug/alcohol abuse
• Child abuse/neglect
• Lead/mercury poisoning
• Hypervitaminosis
• Fetal exposure to alcohol/anticonvulsants

GENETIC/METABOLIC

• Malabsorption (lactase deficiency, celiac disease)
• Cystic fibrosis
• Renal tubular acidosis
• Diabetes mellitus
• Thyroid disease
• Pituitary disease
• Adrenal disease
• Parathyroid disease
• Galactosemia
• Aminoacidurias
• Organic acidurias
• Storage diseases
• Hypercalcemia

ALLERGIC/INFLAMMATORY

• Food allergies
• Inflammatory bowel disease
• Chronic lung disease, including aspiration

FUNCTIONAL

• Gastroesophageal reflux (GER)
• Chronic constipation

NEUROLOGIC

• Cerebral palsy
• Oral-motor dysfunction
• Structural abnormalities
• Degenerative diseases
• Diencephalic syndrome

RENAL

• Chronic renal insufficiency

HEMATOLOGIC

• Sickle cell disease
• Thalassemia
• Iron-deficiency anemia

ORTHOPEDIC

• Rickets
• Osteogenesis imperfecta
• Chondrodystrophies

MISCELLANEOUS

• Upper airway obstruction, including adenoidal hypertrophy
• Acquired heart disease
• Dental abnormalities (caries, infection)

Approach to the Patient

GENERAL GOALS

Determine whether the patient has growth failure by measuring the child's weight, height, and head circumference accurately, plotting them on standard growth curves, and comparing them to previous growth points.

Phase 1:

• Is the malnutrition acute or chronic, symmetric or asymmetric? With acute malnutrition, weight is the first parameter to be affected, leading to wasting. After weeks to months of malnutrition, stunted linear growth occurs. Finally, with long-standing and/or severe malnutrition, head circumference is affected. Symmetric FTT suggests long-standing malnutrition, chromosomal abnormalities, congenital infection, or teratogenic exposures as etiologies.

• When growth failure is recognized, the prenatal, developmental, and nutritional history must be complete. Search for indicators of diminished intake, excessive losses, and medical diseases. The physical examination should be thorough. The laboratory evaluation is guided by the results of the history and physical examination. Although some laboratory tests can be useful in the evaluation of FTT, random screening in search of a medical diagnosis is usually unrevealing, and is not recommended.

Phase 2: If the history and physical examination suggest a medical disease as a cause of the growth failure, appropriate diagnostic evaluation should be done. In the majority of cases, the cause of growth failure is environmental or psychosocial. Medical diseases are identified in fewer than 50% of children hospitalized for growth failure and even less frequently in children evaluated in the outpatient setting.

Phase 3: If organic disease is not a consideration, begin education and psychosocial interventions to improve nutrition.

HINTS FOR SCREENING PROBLEM

Always plot growth on the same standardized growth chart so that the child's percentiles are known and can be compared to percentiles at previous ages.

Data Gathering

HISTORY

Question: When did the FTT begin?
Significance: Consideration of the age at which growth failure begins can be helpful in determining the cause of the failure. See the table entitled "Causes of Failure to Thrive" in Section VIII of this book.

Question: Does the child have a medical problem that explains the FTT?
Significance: Ask about symptoms that would lead you to believe the child has a medical illness, including vomiting, chronic diarrhea, abdominal distention, exercise intolerance, developmental problems, etc.

Question: What is the child's typical daily diet?
Significance: Because FTT is more commonly an environmental problem, the child's feeding history may yield clues to the problem. Have the parent describe in detail what the child eats and drinks each day, the daytime schedule, how formula is prepared. Determine who is responsible for meal preparation, when and where the child eats, and what problems the parent identifies related to mealtime.

Question: Are there indications of parental stress, drug abuse, or other family factors that may be contributing to the child's growth failure?
Significance: Children do not live in isolation, and growth failure may be a manifestation of family dysfunction.

Physical Examination

A complete physical examination is mandatory.

Finding: Changing growth patterns on a plotted growth chart.
Significance: In practice, FTT is identified when a child's weight falls below the fifth percentile for age, when the weight falls more than two major percentile groups, or when the weight for height is below 80% of the median.

Finding: Look for wasted, thin extremities, with loose skin hanging from the buttocks; temporal wasting; thin, sparse hair or alopecia.
Significance: Signs of malnutrition.

Finding: Otitis media, respiratory infections
Significance: Children with FTT have more infections than age-matched controls.

Finding: Cheilosis, or cracking and irritation at the corners of the mouth.
Significance: Riboflavin and other vitamin B complex deficiencies.

Finding: Edema
Significance: Protein deficiency

Finding: Oropharyngeal abnormalities (dental caries, tonsillar hypertrophy, submucosal clefts, etc.).
Significance: These factors may interfere with eating.

Finding: Neurologic abnormalities
Significance: Cerebral palsy and other neurologic abnormalities may result in oral-motor dysfunction, swallowing incoordination, and difficulty eating.

Finding: Bruises, burns, patterned cutaneous injuries
Significance: These injuries suggest possible child abuse.

Laboratory Aids

The laboratory evaluation of the child with growth failure should be guided by the history and physical examination findings. Avoid extensive random evaluations.

Test: A complete blood count (CBC)
Significance: Used to identify iron-deficiency anemia

Test: Lead level
Significance: Used to identify lead poisoning

Test: Urinalysis and urine culture
Significance: Screens for urinary tract infection and renal tubular acidosis.

Test: PPD
Significance: Screens for tuberculosis.

Tests: Serum electrolytes, protein, albumin, pre-albumin, calcium, phosophrus, magnesium
Significance: Serum metabolic screening can assess for underlying metabolic problems, renal insufficiency, and are indicated to help prevent the refeeding syndrome. The refeeding syndrome includes potentially dangerous disorders in serum phosphorus, calcium, potassium and other minerals and electrolytes at the time of reintroduction of nutrition, in severely malnourished children.

Emergency Care

SEVERE MALNUTRITION

- Children meeting criteria for severe malnutrition are at risk for refeeding syndrome, and should be hospitalized.
- Early hospitalization of the severely malnourished child focuses on slowly reinstituting nutrition while avoiding potentially life-threatening changes in electrolytes. In the most severe cases, life support and hyperalimentation are needed. Hospitalization provides a controlled environment in which to assess the causes of growth failure, and determine the child's caloric needs for catch-up growth.
- Therapy aimed at improving and sustaining the child's nutrition, however, needs to continue well after the child is discharged from the hospital and requires frequent weight checks, careful monitoring, and support of the family.

CHILDREN WITH EVIDENCE OF ABUSE

- Child welfare should be notified immediately of any child not thought to be safe at home because of evidence of abuse or severe neglect.

Common Questions and Answers

Q: How can you differentiate between FTT and alternative diagnoses related to growth?
A: Recognize that 3% to 5% of the population will naturally fall below the 3rd to 5th percentile using growth charts. These children usually are proportional (normal weight for height). Growth velocity and height for weight determinations can be helpful in identifying children with malnutrition.

Q: How quickly will a child respond to nutritional therapy?
A: Initiation of catch-up growth depends on the severity of the malnutrition. Initially, weight gains of 2 to 3 times the normal growth rate for age may be observed. Weight gain will precede improvements in height. Months of refeeding are required to restore the patient's weight for height, stature, and head circumference.

Issues for Referral

- Suggestion of medical disease: Children should be referred to the appropriate medical or surgical specialist.
- Indications of child abuse or neglect: State laws in every state require that physicians report suspected child abuse and neglect to child welfare agencies for investigation.
- Multidisciplinary team referral: For children with moderate FTT, those who do not improve after therapy has been initiated, or families with psychosocial problems, nutritionists, nurses, social workers, feeding specialists, and psychologists can participate in providing continual assessment and care to the child and family.

Clinical Pearls

- Remember that medical and psychosocial causes of malnutrition often coexist and should be considered.
- Don't forget to ask about how much juice the infant or toddler drinks. This is a common cause of FTT.
- In cases of moderate-severe neglect, it may be necessary to increase the caloric density of the child's foods, as many malnourished children can not increase the volume of food ingested to meet the requirement for catch-up growth. A diet with approximately 30% to 35% more energy and nearly twice the amount of protein is needed for catch-up growth.
- Remember to provide a multivitamin.
- Continued, close follow-up of the malnourished child is essential in order to prevent recurrent growth failure and to monitor the child's development, which can be adversely affected in moderate and severe growth failure.

BIBLIOGRAPHY

Bithoney WG, Dubowitz H, Egan H. Failure to thrive/growth deficiency. *Pediatr Rev* 1992;13:453–460.

Gahagan S, Holmes R. A stepwise approach to evaluation of undernutrition and failure to thrive. *Pediatr Clin North Am* 1998;45(1):169–187.

Maggioni A, Lifshitz F. Nutritional management of failure to thrive. *Pediatr Clin North Am* 1995;42;791–810.

Zenel JA Jr. Failure to thrive: a general pediatrician's perspective. *Pediatr Rev* 1997;18(11):371–378.

Author: Cindy W. Christian

Fever of Unknown Etiology

Database

DEFINITION

Fever of unknown origin (FUO) is defined as a febrile illness (38.5°C on multiple occasions) that has been present for more than 10 days, with no apparent source despite careful history taking, physical examination, and preliminary laboratory studies.

Differential Diagnosis

CAUSES

FUO is more often an unusual presentation of a common disease than a common presentation of an unusual disease. An underlying cause is never established in approximately 10% to 20% of cases. Possible etiologies include:

- Bacterial infections

—Sinusitis
—Urinary tract infection (UTI)
—Tuberculosis (TB)
—Liver or pelvic abscess
—Osteomyelitis
—Endocarditis
—Salmonellosis
—Cat-scratch disease

- Viral infections

—Cytomegalovirus
—Epstein-Barr virus (EBV)
—Viral hepatitis

- Other infections

—Rocky Mountain spotted fever (RMSF)
—Toxoplasmosis

- Collagen vascular disease

—Juvenile rheumatoid arthritis (JRA)
—Systemic lupus erythematosus
—Rheumatic fever
—Serum sickness

- Malignancy

—Leukemia/lymphoma
—Neuroblastoma
—Hodgkin disease

- Other

—Factitious fever
—Drug fever
—Inflammatory bowel disease (IBD)
—Kawasaki syndrome

Uncommon causes of FUO include:

- Bacterial infections

—Endocarditis
—Brucellosis
—Tularemia
—Leptospirosis
—Rat-bite fever

- Other infections

—Disseminated histoplasmosis
—Coccidioidomycosis
—Blastomycosis
—Malaria
—Babesiosis

- Collagen vascular disease

—Sarcoidosis
—Hypersensitivity vasculitis
—Polyarteritis nodosa

- Malignancy

—Atrial myxoma
—Brain tumors

- Other

—Diabetes insipidus
—Thyroiditis
—Familial Mediterranean fever
—Cyclic neutropenia

Approach to the Patient

GENERAL GOALS

Find the cause of the fever and begin treatment of the underlying illness.

Phase 1: Attempt to diagnose more common causes of fever. Also observe the pattern of fever.

Phase 2: Begin invasive studies to seek rarer forms of fever such as lymphoma, burcellosis, babeosis, subacute bacterial endocarditis (SBE).

Phase 3: Reexamine patient and repeat tests to reconsider etiologies such as JRA, sarcoidosis, factitious fever.

Data Gathering

HISTORY

Question: Exposure to animals?
Significance: Cat-scratch disease, brucellosis, tularemia, leptospirosis

Question: Travel history?
Significance: Malaria, fungal infection, coccidiomycosis, blastomycosis

Question: Ingestion of raw meat, fish, unpasteurized milk, or contaminated water?
Significance: Trichinosis, TB, hepatitis, giardiasis

Question: Pica?
Significance: Fungal infection

Question: Change in behavior or activity?
Significance: Brain tumor, TB, EBV, Rocky Mountain spotted fever

Question: Pattern of fever?
Significance: May correlate with underlying etiology, but unlikely.

Question: Height of fever?
Significance: Heat intolerance, typhoid

Question: Medications (including over-the-counter medications and eye drops)?
Significance: Drug fever, atropine-induced fever

Question: Well water ingestion?
Significance: *Giardia* infection

Question: Evidence of behavior problems?
Significance: Factitious fever

Physical Examination

Finding: Impaired weight gain or linear growth
Significance: Collagen disease, malignancy, IBD

Finding: Toxic appearance
Significance: Kawasaki syndrome

Finding: Rash, sparse hair
Significance: Systemic lupus erythematosus

Finding: Conjunctivitis
Significance: Kawasaki syndrome

Finding: Fundoscopic lesions
Significance: Brain tumor, TB, systemic lupus erythematosus

Finding: Sinus tenderness
Significance: Sinusitis

Finding: Nasal discharge
Significance: Sinusitis

Finding: Pharyngitis
Significance: Kawasaki syndrome, EBV

Finding: Tachypnea
Significance: SBE

Finding: Rales
Significance: Histoplasmosis, sarcoidosis, coccidiomycosis

Finding: Cardiac murmur
Significance: SBE

Finding: Hepatosplenomegaly
Significance: Hepatitis, EBV

Finding: Rectal abnormalities
Significance: Pelvic abscess, IBD

Finding: Arthritis
Significance: JRA, IBD

Finding: Bony tenderness
Significance: JRA, leukemia, osteomyelitis

 ## Laboratory Aids

The laboratory evaluation for a child with FUO should be directed toward the most likely diagnostic possibilities. All patients should have:

Test: CBC with differential and careful examination of WBC morphology
Significance: Kawasaki, cyclic neutropenia

Test: Blood cultures
Significance: Endocarditis, salmonellosis

Test: Urinalysis and urine culture
Significance: UTI, Kawasaki

Test: ESR and/or C-reactive protein
Significance: Collagen disease

Test: PPD skin test
Significance: TB

Additional studies to be considered include:

Test: Chest and/or sinus x-ray studies
Significance: TB, sinusitis, histoplasmosis

Test: Stool bacterial culture and examination for ova and parasites
Significance: Salmonella

Test: Bone marrow examination and culture
Significance: Salmonella, histoplasmosis

Test: Slit lamp examination
Significance: Kawasaki

Test: Chest and/or abdominal CT scan
Significance: TB, liver abscess

Test: Gallium scan
Significance: Osteomyelitis

- Cardiac catherization
- Lumbar puncture
- Hepatitis serologies

 ## Common Questions and Answers

Q: How do you explain factitious fever?
A: The patient may twirl the thermometer under their tongue. If left unattended, the child may place the thermometer under hot water or shake it to elevate temperature reading.

Q: When should antibiotics be used?
A: Empiric use of antibiotics should be avoided because of the risk of delaying the discovery of the appropriate underlying diagnosis. A trial of antipyretics may be considered if collagen vascular disease is likely.

BIBLIOGRAPHY

Hoberman A, Wald ER. Urinary tract infections in young febrile children. *Pediatr Infect Dis J* 1997;16(1):11–17.

Lorin MI, Feigin RD. Fever without localizing signs and fever of unknown origin. In: Feigin RD, Cherry JD, eds. *Textbook of pediatric infectious diseases*, 3rd ed. Philadelphia: WB Saunders 1992:1012–1022.

McCarthy PL. The pediatric clinical evaluation and pneumonia. *Curr Opin Pediatr* 1996;8(5):427–429.

McCarthy PL, Klig JE, Shapiro ED, Baron MA. Fever without apparent source on clinical examination, lower respiratory infections in children, other infectious diseases, and acute gastroenteritis and diarrhea of infancy and early childhood. *Curr Opin Pediatr* 1996;8(1):75–93.

McClung HJ. Prolonged fever of unknown origin in children. *Am J Dis Child* 1972;124:544–550.

Miller LC, Sisson BA, Tucker LB, Schaller JG. Prolonged fevers of unknown origin in children: patterns of presentation and outcome. *J Pediatr* 1996;129(3):419–423.

Pizzo PA, Lovejoy FH, Smith DH. Prolonged fever in children: review of 100 cases. *Pediatrics* 1975;55:468–473.

Author: Susan E. Coffin

Hematuria

Database

DEFINITION

Hematuria is defined as an abnormal number of red blood cells in the urine. This means >3 red blood cells per high-power field using a standard urinalysis technique on a centrifuged sample, which correlates with a peroxidase dipstick reaction of 1+ or greater (see table Central Aids in Distinguishing the Origin of Gross Hematuria).

Differential Diagnosis

CAUSES

• Hematuria may originate at any site along the urinary tract.
• Factitious causes, urine appears bloody, but there is no hematuria.

ENDOGENOUS PIGMENTS

• Myoglobin
• Hemoglobin
• Bile pigments
• Urate crystals ("pink diaper" syndrome)

EXOGENOUS PIGMENTS

• Food and beverage dyes
• Drugs that cause urinary discoloration

—Phenazopyridine (Pyridium)
—Deferoxamine
—Rifampin
—Sulfa

GLOMERULAR CAUSES

Common

• Strenuous exercise
• Acute post-infectious glomerulonephrites
• IGA nephropathy
• Thin basement membrane disease (benign familial hematuria)

Uncommon

• Membranoproliferative glomerulophritis
• Nephritis of systemic disease (Henoch-Schönlein or systemic lupus)
• Alport syndrome, hereditary nephritis

NON-GLOMERULAR RENAL CAUSES

Common

• Hypercalciuria/nephrolithiasis
• Renal trauma (contusion)
• Hemoglobinopathies [sickle cell (SC) disease, SC trait, SC disease]
• Ureteropelvic junction obstruction

Uncommon

• Drug-induced interstitial nephritis (penicillins, cephalosporins, NSAIDs, phenytoin)
• Cystic disease
• Neoplasm
• Coagulopathy
• Vascular thrombosis

NON-RENAL CAUSES

Common

• Cystitis (bacterial, viral, occasionally chemical)
• Meatal stenosis in males
• "Terminal hematuria" syndrome (trigonitis)
• Perineal trauma or irritation

Uncommon

• Bladder tumor
• Polyp
• Foreign body in bladder or urethra

External causes of "hematuria"

• Menstrual contamination
• Diaper rash

Approach to the Patient

GENERAL GOALS

Determine the source of the bleeding and select problems that respond to treatment.

Phase 1: Determine if the pigment in urine is from blood or other source.

Phase 2: Determine the source of bleeding, i.e., kidney, bladder, urethra.

Phase 3: Select those who will need treatment versus those who will stop bleeding without treatment.

Data Gathering

HISTORY

Question: Prior episodes of any gross hematuria, or abnormal urinalyses?
Significance: Chronic versus acute process

Question: Medications and diet?
Significance: Food or drug pigment, drug nephrotoxicity. Excessive calcium intake.

Question: Antecedent infection or concurrent infection?
Significance: Antecedent suggests post-infections glomerulonephritis (GN). Concurrent suggests IgA nephropathy, basement membrane disease.

Question: Any precipitating factors (trauma, exercise)?
Significance: Renal contusion, exercise hematuria, or myoglobinuria

Question: Voiding symptoms?
Significance: Suggests lower tract source

Question: Renal colic or other pain?
Significance: Suggests stones

Question: Fever, rash, arthritis?
Significance: Signs or symptoms of systemic illness

Question: Bleeding from any other source?
Significance: Suggests coagulopathy

Question: Hematuria in family members?
Significance: Familial benign hematuria or Alport syndrome

Question: SC disease in family members?
Significance: Sickle nephropathy or hemoglobinuria

Question: Renal stone disease in family members?
Significance: Hypercalciuria or metabolic disease

Question: Cystic kidney disease in family members?
Significance: Autosomal recessive or dominant polycystic kidney disease

Question: Premature deafness in family members?
Significance: Suggestive of Alport syndrome

Question: Anyone in family with kidney failure or identified kidney disease?
Significance: Suggestive of hereditary nephritis, cystic disease or stones

---

Clinical Aids in Distinguishing the Origin of Gross Hematuria

TEST FOR	GLOMERULAR OR RENAL	EXTRARENAL
Urine color	Brown, cloudy	Red
Clots	Usually absent	Frequently present
RBC casts	Frequently present	Never present
Red-cell morphology	Dysmorphic or distorted	Normal RBC shape
Urine stream	Constantly bloody	More bloody at initiation (suggesting distal urethral origin) or termination (suggesting trigonitis)

Physical Examination

Finding: Cardiovascular exam
Significance: Hypertension in glomerulonephritis, renal failure, tachycardia, murmur on gallop in volume overload

Finding: Abdominal exam
Significance: Volume overload ascites, organomegaly, tenderness, or masses

Finding: Genital exam
Significance: External source of bleeding or infection

Finding: Extremities
Significance: Edema or joint swelling

Finding: Skin and mucosal exam
Significance: Petechial, vasculitic rash, ulcerations

 ## Laboratory Aids

Test: Gross and microscopic analyses of fresh urine specimen
Significance: Urinalysis should guide additional evaluation

Test: Screening of the family members for occult hematuria
Significance: Baseline test for child with isolated asymptomatic hematuria

Test: Screening the child for hypercalciuria (random urine calcium:creatinine ratio, 0.2)
Significance: Hypercalcemia causes hematuria

Test: Serum creatinine
Significance: Renal function

Test: Renal ultrasound
Significance: To rule out obvious structural etiology of the hematuria

Test: SC preparation should be considered
Significance:

Test: Evaluation for glomerulonephritis
Significance: Hematuria occurring in combination with proteinuria, edema, hypertension, or signs or symptoms suggestive of a systemic illness

Test: CBC with platelets
Significance: May suggest clotting problem

Test: Serum electrolytes
Significance: Renal function

Test: BUN and creatinine
Significance: Renal function

Test: Streptococcal serology
Significance: Acute GN

Test: Complement studies
Significance: Immune complex disease

Test: Anti-nuclear antibody titer
Significance: Collagen disease (lupus)

Test: Quantitation of proteinuria
Significance: A low C3 complement suggests postinfectious glomerulonephritis or the nephritis of systemic lupus

Test: Urine culture
Significance: Voiding symptoms, fever, and concurrent pyuria

Test: Trauma to the perineum should be avoided and periodic reassessment
Significance: Symptomless "terminal" hematuria, indicating trigonitis

Test: Radiographic evaluation of lower urinary tract
Significance:

ADDITIONAL INVESTIGATIONS

Rarely, additional studies such as cystourethrogram, renal angiography, cystoscopy, or renal biopsy will be required, in conjunction with an appropriate referral. Audiometry may be indicated if hereditary nephritis is suspected. Hematuria without proteinuria is less likely to be renal in origin.

 ## Follow-Up

The well child with asymptomatic isolated hematuria and a negative work-up should be reassessed annually with a complete physical examination and a urinalysis. If hematuria is persistent, periodic assessment of renal function and evaluation for proteinuria should also be performed.

PROGNOSIS

• The majority of children with asymptomatic isolated microscopic hematuria detected on a well-child examination will not be found to have serious underlying pathology and will simply require longitudinal follow-up.
• Children with asymptomatic microscopic or gross hematuria combined with proteinuria have a high likelihood of significant pathology.
• For children with either microscopic or gross hematuria associated with findings suggestive of glomerulonephritis (proteinuria, systemic symptoms), the prognosis will depend on the type of glomerulonephritis identified.

Issues for Referral

• Uncontrollable bleeding—can be seen in SC disease with papillary necrosis or unlocalized source.
• Bleeding after trauma may expose a congenital anomaly such as uretero-pelvic obstruction.
• Bleeding secondary to coagulopathy
• Bleeding and proteinuria

Clinical Pearls

There is usually no treatment for hematuria per se, but in some children with an identified cause of hematuria, specific treatment measures may be indicated for control of the underlying process. In many cases, no specific treatment is indicated, only longitudinal follow-up.

Epidemiology

• Hematuria may be gross or microscopic, symptomless, or associated with a constellation of other complaints and physical findings.
• Asymptomatic microscopic hematuria may be found in 1% to 4% of all healthy school-aged children.
• The complaint of gross hematuria may account for 0.1% to 0.15% of pediatric acute care walk-in visits.
• The majority of children with asymptomatic hematuria will be healthy, and no serious underlying cause will be found.

BIBLIOGRAPHY

Ahn JH, Morey AF, McAninch JW. Workup and management of traumatic hematuria. *Emerg Med Clin North Am* 1998;16(1):145–164.

Feld LG, Meyers KE, Kaplan BS, Stapleton FB. Limited evaluation of microscopic hematuria in pediatrics. *Pediatrics* 1998;102(4):E42.

Feld LG, Waz WR, Perez LM, Joseph DB. Hematuria. An integrated medical and surgical approach. *Pediatr Clin North Am* 1997;44(5):1191–1210.

Grasso SN, Keller MS. Diagnostic imaging in pediatric trauma. *Curr Opin Pediatr* 1998;10(3):299–302.

Mahan JD, Turman MA, Mentser MI. Evaluation of hematuria, proteinuria, and hypertension in adolescents. *Pediatr Clin North Am* 1997;44(6):1573–1589.

Piqueras AI, White RH, Raafat F, Moghal N, Milford DV. Renal biopsy diagnosis in children presenting with haematuria. *Pediatr Nephrol* 1998;12(5):386–391.

Roy S 3rd. Hematuria. *Pediatr Rev* 1998;19(6):209–212; quiz 213.

Ward JF, Kaplan GW, Mevorach R, Stock JA, Cilento BG Jr. Refined microscopic urinalysis for red blood cell morphology in the evaluation of asymptomatic microscopic hematuria in a pediatric population. *J Urol* 1998;160(4):1492–1495.

Author: Roberta S. Gray

Hemolysis

Database

DEFINITION

The premature destruction of red blood cells either intravascularly or extravascularly leading to a shortened red cell survival time.

Differential Diagnosis

See table Common Mechanisms of Hemolysis.

CONGENITAL/ANATOMIC

- ABO and Rh incompatibility between infant and mother
- Cardiac lesions with turbulent flow, left-sided more common than right-sided
- Prosthetic heart valve (especially aortic)
- Kasabach-Merritt syndrome
- Hypersplenism

INFECTIOUS

- Congenital infections with syphilis, rubella, cytomegalovirus (CMV), and toxoplasmosis
- Malaria
- Bartonellosis
- *Clostridium perfringens* (via a toxin)
- *Mycoplasma pneumoniae*
- HIV
- Hemolytic uremic syndrome (HUS)

TOXIC, ENVIRONMENTAL, DRUGS

- Immune-complex "innocent bystander" mechanism

—Quinidine
—Acetaminophen
—Amoxicillin
—Cephalosporins
—Isoniazid
—Rifampin

- Immune-complex drug-adsorption mechanism

—Penicillin
—Cephalosporins
—Erythromycin
—Tetracycline
—Isoniazid

- Drug-induced autoimmune hemolytic anemia

—α-methyldopa

- Toxic drug-induced hemolysis

—Ribovirin (generally mild and not clinically significant)

Common Mechanisms of Hemolysis

ACQUIRED DISORDERS	HEREDITARY DISORDERS
Infectious	Hemoglobinopathies
Drug induced	RBC membrane defects
Immune mediated	RBC enzyme defects
Microangiopathic	

- Snake and spider venoms
- Extensive burns

TRAUMA (MECHANICAL HEMOLYSIS)

- Cardiac hemolysis
- Abnormal microcirculation

—Thrombotic thrombocytopenic purpura (TTP)
—Disseminated intravascular coagulopathy (DIC)
—Malignant hypertension
—Eclampsia
—Hemangiomas
—Renal graft rejection

- "March" hemoglobinuria (due to prolonged physical activity)

TUMOR

- Lymphomas
- Thymoma
- Lymphoproliferative disorders

GENETIC/METABOLIC

- RBC membrane defects

—Hereditary spherocytosis (HS)
—Hereditary elliptocytosis (HE)
—Pyropoikilocytosis
—Paroxysmal nocturnal hemoglobinuria

- Enzyme defects

—Pyruvate kinase deficiency (PK)
—Glucose-6-phosphate dehydrogenase deficiency (G6PD)

- Thalassemias (β-thalassemia major is the most severe)
- Hemoglobinopathies

—Sickle cell anemia (Hgb SS and SC variants)
—Unstable hemoglobins

ALLERGIC/INFLAMMATORY/IMMUNE

- Autoimmune Hemolytic Anemia (AIHA)

—Warm antibody mediated
—Cold antibody mediated
—Hemolytic transfusion reaction

Approach to the Patient

GENERAL GOALS

Establish existence of hemolysis versus other causes of anemia such as blood loss, hypoproduction, etc.

Phase 1: Determine acuity and severity of the hemolysis. If the process has been acute in onset, there will be evidence of unstable vital signs and possibly heart failure. Parents may give a history of a rapid deterioration of the child's physical and/or mental state. Patients with a chronic hemolytic anemia that has progressed slowly over time may have a "critically low" hemoglobin yet be well compensated with fairly normal vital signs (except for tachycardia). A CBC with a corrected reticulocyte count will help determine if there is an appropriate bone marrow response to the level of anemia, and, therefore, whether the process is acute or chronic in onset.

Phase 2: Determine the cause of the hemolysis. Treatment approaches will vary depending on the underlying etiology.

Data Gathering

HISTORY

Question: Is the patient pale, fatigued, or jaundiced? Is there a history of tea colored urine?
Significance: The presence of hemoglobinuria is a sign of intravascular hemolysis, while pallor, fatigue, and jaundice may occur with either intravascular or extravascular hemolysis.

Question: Is there a history of anemia, splenectomy, or early cholrecystectomy in multiple family members?
Significance: While hereditary membrane defects and enzyme deficiencies are autosomal dominant and X-linked disorders, respectively, a negative familial history does not always rule out these diagnoses. In some cases, the diagnosis of HS has not been identified, yet multiple members of a family have had their gallbladders removed at an early age, which may indicate the presence of this defect. Thalassemia (especially β-thal) and sickle cell anemia may present in early childhood with chronic hemolysis with or without a familial history.

Question: Is there a history of travel?
Significance: Malaria is endemic to Africa, India, and parts of Central America.

Question: What drugs is the patient taking? What is the diet history? Specifically ask about exposure to fava beans, mothballs, and antibiotics.
Significance: Drugs can themselves cause hemolysis or can induce hemolysis if there is an underlying disorder such as G-6-PD deficiency.

Question: How old was the child at the first signs and symptoms of hemolysis (pallor or jaundice)?
Significance: Hereditary causes of hemolysis are most often chronic or recurrent, although the diagnosis may be delayed until the child is older if the process is mild. Acute, acquired hemolytic disorders may also recur (such as AIHA, Evan syndrome, lupus, etc.).

Physical Examination

Question: What is the general appearance of the child? Is there any vital sign instability?
Significance: Acute processes such as autoimmune hemolytic anemia (both warm and cold antibody mediated) may present with a child in extremis. Tachycardia is a common finding in nearly all cases of acute hemolysis. Blood pressure instability is a late finding. More chronic processes such as HU, G-6-PD and PK deficiencies, thalassemia or sickle cell disease may be picked up on routine physical or laboratory examination. These children often appear well (except for jaundice) but may become more anemic with an acute illness.

Question: Is there an underlying systemic illness?
Significance: Hemolysis that is a secondary problem (i.e., due to infection, tumors, etc.) may be found incidentally during evaluation of the primary process.

Question: Is there any hepatosplenomegaly or lymphadenopathy?
Significance: Splenomegaly, often impressive, as well as hepatomegaly are common findings in extravascular hemolysis. Hepatomegaly may be more pronounced if the child is in heart failure due to acute, severe anemia. Remember that splenomegaly may be either the cause of, or more frequently, a result of a hemolytic process. If significant lymphadenopathy is present, look for any underlying etiology like lymphoproliferative disorders or other tumors.

Question: What is the skin exam?
Significance: Pallor is nearly a universal finding in acute hemolysis and in exacerbations of chronic hemolysis. Jaundice is more common in intravascular hemolysis. The presence of ecchymoses or petechiae suggest DIC or thrombocytopenia.

Laboratory Aids

Test: CBC with differential and reticulocyte count
Significance: The level of anemia and the reticulocyte count must be interpreted together. Chronic hemolysis due to HS, for example, may have a nearly normal hemoglobin but usually has an increased reticulocyte count. With a rapid fall in Hgb, as in acute autoimmune hemolytic anemia, the reticulocyte count may be low at the start, rise in response to anemia, and fall during recovery. Thrombocytopenia should raise suspicions about TTP or HUS.

Test: Peripheral blood smear
Significance: Fragmented RBCs, schistocytes, and helmet cells are seen in DIC, TTP, HUS, and cardiac valve hemolysis. Other findings on the smear that may be helpful in the diagnosis are spherocytes (HS and warm AIHA), target cells (hemoglobin C and thalassemias), and acanthocytes (anorexia nervosa).

Test: Bilirubin
Significance: Total and unconjugated bilirubins are elevated in most cases.

Test: Urinalysis
Significance: Hemoglobinuria is present in intravascular hemolysis. This is established by a urine dipstick positive for heme with no intact red cells microscopically. Myoglobinuria can also give this picture.

Test: Coombs test
Significance: Direct Coombs test (direct antiglobulin test or DAT) detects antibodies or complement fragments present on the patient's RBCs, while the indirect antiglobulin test detects antibodies in the patient's serum that can bind normal RBCs. The DAT provides direct evidence of immune mediated hemolysis. Warm antibody AIHA is caused by an IgG antibody that coats RBCs, which are subsequently removed by the spleen. Cold antibody AIHA is caused by an IgM antibody that binds RBCs, fixes complement, and can cause both extravascular as well as intravascular hemolysis.

Test: Haptoglobin, hemopexin, and LDH
Significance: In intravascular hemolysis, haptoglobin levels may be undetectable, hemopexin is reduced and LDH is significantly increased. In extravascular hemolysis, haptoglobin is decreased (but detectable) and LDH may be increased, but not to the level seen in intravascular hemolysis.

Test: Bone marrow aspiration
Significance: Rarely indicated, but if performed, erythroid hyperplasia should be present.

Emergency Care

Factors that constitute an emergency include:

• Hemoglobin under 5 g/dL, especially with signs of cardiovascular compromise, requires immediate attention. Attempts to stabilize cardiovascular compromise with volume should be undertaken with care, as hemodilution may occur. Transfusion may be difficult in autoimmune hemolysis because of potential problems with crossmatching.
• Renal failure may accompany severe hemolysis in TTP or HUS.
• Hemolysis in the neonatal period secondary to ABO or Rh incompatibility may require exchange transfusion either for anemia or for hyperbilirubinemia.

Common Questions and Answers

Q: When are blood transfusions indicated in patients with active hemolysis?
A: Patients with severe, acute hemolysis that is causing cardiovascular compromise may require a transfusion if the process cannot be stopped with standard therapy (steroids for warm AIHA, plasmapheresis for TTP, etc.). Transfusions must be given slowly if the hemolytic process has been chronic and the patient's blood volume is expanded.

Q: Can hemolysis always be identified on a peripheral blood smear?
A: No. Schistocytes, fragments, spherocytes, targets, or other morphology may provide clues to specific diagnoses but are not always present. The presence of a hemolytic process is inferred from a fall in hemoglobin, rise in the reticulocyte count and elevation of the bilirubin and LDH levels.

Issues for Referral

• Most patients with severe, acute hemolysis, either primary or due to an underlying chronic hemolytic disorder, will need to be evaluated by a hematologist.
• Suspected RBC membrane and enzyme defects, as well as hemoglobinopathies, should be referred at least for initial evaluation. Ongoing involvement of a hematologist will depend on the ultimate diagnosis.
• A CBC with a reticulocyte count is the most important screening test. Other tests depend on clinical suspicion of the underlying etiology but may include a direct and indirect Coomb test.

Clinical Pearls

• Hereditary RBC membrane defects may be mild and may be diagnosed at an older age. Although these disorders are autosomal dominant, 20% of these patients represent new spontaneous mutations and have no affected family members.
• Blood for diagnostic RBC enzyme studies must be drawn prior to transfusion.

BIBLIOGRAPHY

Berkowitz FE. Hemolysis and infection: categories and mechanisms of their interrelationship. *Rev Infect Dis* 1991;13(6):1151–1162.

Tabbara IA. Hemolytic anemias. Diagnosis and management. *Med Clin North Am* 1992;76(3):649–668.

Author: Julie W. Stern

Hepatomegaly

Database

DEFINITION

Liver enlargement beyond age-adjusted normal values. Can be a common component of many diverse disease processes seen in infants and children.

Differential Diagnosis

CONGENITAL/ANATOMICAL

- Alagille syndrome
- Biliary atresia
- Choledocal cyst
- Congenital hepatic fibrosis
- Obstruction of the common bile duct due to stones, strictures, or tumors

INFECTIONS

- Viral infections

—Hepatitis types A–E
—Cytomegalovirus (CMV)
—Epstein-Barr virus (EBV)
—Coxsackievirus

- Congenital infections

—Toxoplasmosis
—Rubella
—CMV
—Herpes
—Human immunodeficiency virus (HIV)

- Parasitic infections

—Amebiasis
—Flukes
—Schistosomiasis
—Malaria

- Fungal disease

—Candidiasis
—Histoplasmosis

- Sexually transmitted disease

—Gonococcal peri-hepatitis
—Syphilis
—HIV

- Zoonotic diseases

—Brucellosis

- Leptospirosis
- Hepatic abscess
- *Bartonella henselae*
- Pasteurella multocida
- Tuberculosis
- Septicemia

TOXIC, METABOLIC, DRUGS

- Drug-induced hepatitis

—Acetaminophen
—Alcohol
—Corticosteroids
—Erythromycin
—Hypervitaminosis A
—Iron
—Isoniazid
—Nitrofurantoin
—Oral contraceptives
—Phenobarbital
—Valproate

TRAUMA

- Hemorrhage
- Subcapsular hematoma
- Traumatic cyst

TUMOR

- Benign tumors

—Hemangioma
—Hemangioendothelioma
—Mesenchymal hamartoma
—Focal nodular hyperplasia
—Adenoma

- Malignant tumors

—Hepatoblastoma
—Hepatocellular carcinoma

- Metastatic tumors
- Histiocytic disease

GENETIC/METABOLIC

- Alpha₁-antitrypsin deficiency

—Amyloidosis

- Beckwith-Wiedemann syndrome
- Chédiak-Higashi syndrome
- Crigler-Najjar syndrome
- Cystic fibrosis
- Diabetes mellitus
- Galactosemia
- GM₁ gangliosidoses
- Glycogen storage diseases
- Hematochromatosis
- Hereditary fructose intolerance
- Homocystinuria
- Lipodoses
- Mucopolysaccharidoses
- Urea cycle defects
- Wilson disease
- Zellweger syndrome

ALLERGIC/INFLAMMATORY

- Chronic active hepatitis
- Sclerosing cholangitis
- Sarcoidosis
- Systemic inflammatory disease

—Juvenile rheumatoid arthritis
—Systemic lupus erythematosus
—Inflammatory bowel disease

MISCELLANEOUS

- Congestive heart failure
- Extramedullary hematopoesis
- Pulmonary hyperinflation
- Restrictive pericarditis
- Veno-occlusive disease
- Malnutrition
- Reye syndrome
- Total parenteral nutrition

Approach to the Patient

- All patients with hepatomegaly should have a laboratory evaluation including complete blood count with differential, comprehensive metabolic panel (including liver function tests, total protein and albumin, total and direct bilirubin, basic electrolytes and glucose), a prothrombin time and a partial prothrombin time.
- A detailed history and physical will direct the practitioner to any additional laboratory testing or appropriate radiologic evaluation.

Data Gathering

HISTORY

Question: Any prenatal history suggesting possible TORCH infection or HIV infection?
Significance: TORCH infections and HIV may cause hepatomegaly, although the liver involvement with HIV is usually secondary to disseminated opportunistic infections or neoplastic processes, rather than from the primary infection itself.

Question: Any history of blood product transfusions?
Significance: Hepatitis C is the most common cause of transfusion-associated hepatitis and the diagnosis should be considered in any child who had received transfusions prior to 1990.

Question: Any history of sexual activity or intravenous drug use?
Significance: Consider not only hepatitis B and HIV, but also gonococcal peri-hepatitis (Fitz-Hugh–Curtis syndrome), and syphilis.

Question: Any foreign travel?
Significance: Increased risk for parasitic infections or liver abscess.

Question: Any shellfish ingestion?
Significance: Contaminated shellfish has been the source of several large outbreaks of hepatitis A.

Question: What medications is the patient taking?
Significance: Many pharmaceuticals have hepatotoxic side effects. Remember to ask about nonprescription and recreational drug use, as vitamin A, alcohol, and certain mushroom species (*Amanita phalloides*) can be hepatotoxic.

Question: Any other chronic illnesses present?
Significance: Patients with heart disease may have liver enlargement due to congestive heart failure. Patients with cystic fibrosis can have focal biliary cirrhosis. Patients with diabetes mellitus often have hepatomegaly secondary to increased glycogen secretion. Severely anemic patients have hepatomegaly because of extramedullary hematopoesis.

Question: Has the patient received total parenteral nutrition (TPN)?
Significance: Cholestasis, bile duct proliferation, fatty infiltration, and early cirrhosis are all well-described complications of TPN.

Question: Any itching?
Significance: Puritis can be a subtle sign of cholestasis.

 ## Physical Examination

Finding: Where is the liver edge?
Significance: In children younger than 2 years of age, the liver edge can extend from 1 to 3 cm below the right costal margin in the midclavicular line. In older children, the liver edge rarely extends beyond 2 cm. Verify all suspected cases of hepatomegaly by checking the liver span.

Finding: What are signs of chronic liver disease?
Significance: The liver is usually firm and enlarged, though actually may decrease in size eventually with advanced disease. Splenomegaly, caput medusae, spider angiomas, esophageal varices, and hemorrhoids suggest portal hypertension. Ascites may develop due to elevated hydrostatic pressures and decreased oncotic pressures secondary to hypoalbuminemia. Also look for signs of occult bleeding or bruising due to impaired vitamin K production.

Finding: Is splenomegaly present?
Significance: Splenic enlargement in the context of chronic liver disease implies portal hypertension. Splenomegaly in the context of other signs of viral illness like adenopathy, fever, malaise, and pharyngitis suggests acute viral hepatitis. Splenomegaly in the absence of these signs suggests storage disease or hematologic malignancy.

Finding: Are there conditions present that may be mimicking hepatomegaly?
Significance: Pulmonary hyperinflation, subdiaphragmatic abscesses, retroperitoneal mass lesions, or rib cage anomalies may all downwardly displace a normal-sized liver mimicking hepatomegaly.

 ## Laboratory Aids

• Complete blood count with differential (CBC)

Test: Aminotransferase and alanine aminotransferase (AST and ALT).
Significance: Elevations reflect the amount of damage to hepatocytes. Elevations >1000 indicate severe damage.

Test: Prothrombin time and partial prothrombin time (PT and PTT)
Significance: Good indicators of the liver's synthetic function. Elevations can occur with an acute injury or illness. Combined with albumin level, this test can be a sensitive indicator of chronic liver disease as well.

Test: Gamma-glutamyl transferase (GGT) and alkaline phosphatase

Significance: Elevations of GGT out of proportion to elevations in AST and ALT can indicate an obstructive or infiltrative abnormality. If an elevated GGT is associated with elevations in bilirubin, cholesterol, and alkaline phosphatase, an obstructive process is more likely.

Test: Ammonia level
Significance: Rising ammonia levels with a prolongation of the PT and PTT suggests liver failure.

Test: Hepatitis profile
Significance: Should be obtained in all patients with appropriate prodromal illness.

Test: Mono spot
Significance: While this is a non-specific heterophile antibody test for EBV infection, it can be predictive in association with an elevation of the atypical lymphocyte count. There is a high false-negative rate as well in children less than 4 years of age. EBV titer is the only confirmatory test.

Test: Alpha-fetoprotein (AFP) and carcinoembryonic antigen (CEA)
Significance: Tumor markers for hepatoblastoma and hepatocellular carcinoma, respectively.

Test: TORCH titers
Significance: Consider in newborns with hepatomegaly.

Test: Serum immunoglobulins, anti-nuclear antibody (ANA), smooth muscle antibody (SMA), anti-microsomal antibody, etc.
Significance: Additional autoimmune evaluation is indicated for those patients with chronic active hepatitis.

Test: Abdominal ultrasound
Significance: Should be performed on all patients with acholic stools, asymmetric liver enlargement, or abdominal mass.

Test: Serum ceruloplasmin level and urinary excretion of copper
Significance: Decreased ceruloplasmin levels and increased urinary excretion of copper characterize Wilson disease, especially after the administration of oral D-penicillamine. Consider the diagnosis for patients with unexplained liver disease.

 ## Emergency Care/Referral

Indications for immediate hospitalization include:

• Persistent anorexia and vomiting
• Mental status changes
• Worsening jaundice
• Relapse of symptoms after initial improvement
• Known exposure to a liver toxin
• Rising PT
• Rising ammonia level
• Bilirubin >20 mg/dL
• AST >2000
• Development of new ascites
• Hypoglycemia
• Leukocytosis and thrombocytopenia

Common Questions and Answers

Q: Why does cholestasis cause puritis?
A: This probably reflects an abnormal accumulation of bile acids in the skin.

Q: When following patients with chronic liver disease, are there any differences in their nutritional needs?
A: Patients may have impaired fat absorption and, therefore, may have deficiencies of fat soluble vitamins A, D, E, and K, which may become evident as anemia, neuropathy, rickets, pathologic fractures, visual disturbances, or skin changes. Also consider supplementing the diet with medium chain tryglycerides, which are more easily absorbed. There may also be higher than normal requirements of trace minerals as well.

Q: What is the etiology of TPN cholestasis?
A: Certain amino acids present in TPN have been shown to increase the serum levels of bile acids, which may in turn affect peristalsis in the gall bladder. Fasting may also decrease the normal hormonal stimulation of bile secretion.

Clinical Pearls

• Until age 2, girls have a slightly larger liver span than males.
• A Reidel lobe is a normal variant in which the right lobe of the liver appears elongated due to its adhesion to the mesocolon.
• The majority of cases of hepatic failure in children are due to acute viral hepatitis. Toxic exposure accounts for 25% of cases, with the most common drug being acetaminophen.
• Administration of vitamin K in an attempt to correct PT can be a valuable assessment of the liver's synthetic function.
• Fetor hepaticus is a sweetish odor that can be detected on the breath and urine of patients with liver failure.
• Asterixis or liver flap is rare in children.

BIBLIOGRAPHY

Roy C, Silverman A, Alagille D. *Pediatric clinical gastroenterology.* St. Louis: Mosby, 1995.

Walker WA, Mathia RK. Hepatomegaly: an approach to differential diagnosis? *Pediatr Clin North Am* 1975;22:929–942.

Author: John M. Good

Hypogammaglobulinemia

 Database

DEFINITION

Hypogammaglobulinemia is a humoral immuno-deficiency signified by low or absent immuno-globulin levels, as compared with age-matched controls, and defective specific antibody production.

 Differential Diagnosis

- Selective IgA deficiency

—For details, refer to the topics Immune Deficiency, Common Variable Immunodeficiency (CVID), and Immune A Deficiency.

- X-linked agammaglobulinemia (XLA) (Bruton agammaglobulinemia)

—Intrinsic defect in B-cell maturation due to mutations in the gene on the X chromosome encoding a B-cell–associated tyrosine kinase. The protein is involved in cytoplasmic signal transduction.
—All immunoglobulin isotypes are significantly decreased or absent.
—Significant reduction or absence of B cells
—Associated complications include arthritis of the large joints, chronic meningoencephalitis due to echoviruses, chronic diarrhea due to *Giardia lamblia,* neutropenia, autoimmune hemolytic anemia, dermatomyositis, and an increased incidence of lymphoreticular malignancies.
—Patients are also susceptible to viral infections, particularly enteroviruses. Live viral vaccines are contraindicated in these patients because some patients have vaccine-associated poliomyelitis.

- Hyper-IgM syndrome

—Predominantly an X-linked inheritance pattern. Affected females have been described.
—Defect is caused by mutations in the gene encoding the CD40 ligand surface molecule on T cells. This leads to defective T-cell signaling for B-cell immunoglobulin class switching.
—Normal to elevated IgM levels with low to absent IgG, IgA, and IgE
—Associated complications include autoimmune hemolytic anemia/thrombocytopenia/neutropenia, opportunistic infections with *Pneumocystis carinii,* and lymphoproliferative disease.

- Transient hypogammaglobulinemia of infancy

—It is difficult to differentiate this from the normal physiologic nadir of IgG that occurs between 3 and 6 months of age due to the loss of maternally derived immunoglobulin. This nadir is normally short lived.
—Affected infants have abnormally prolonged delay in the onset of their own immunoglobulin production to compensate for this nadir.
—The cause is unknown.
—Self-limited, most infants recover by 18 to 36 months.
—Clinical course is typically benign. Therapy with intravenous immunoglobulin (IVIG) should be considered only in infants with severe recurrent infections.
—This syndrome is frequently seen in infants with a familial history of SCID or other immunodeficiencies.

- Selective IgG subclass deficiency (the four subclasses of IgG, in decreasing order of serum levels: IgG1, IgG2, IgG3, and IgG4)

—Total serum IgG levels can be normal even when one subclass is low or absent.
—Deficiency of IgG3 is most common in adults while deficiency of IgG2 is seen more frequently in children.
—IgG2 deficiency has been associated with an inability to respond to polysaccharide antigens.
—The clinical significance of IgG subclass deficiency has not been fully defined. Many patients have been described as having an increased frequency of upper and lower respiratory tract infections while others are asymptomatic.
—There is no consensus on standard therapy for these patients in regards to replacement IVIG.

- X-linked hypogammaglobulinemia with growth hormone deficiency

—Described in three families
—Immunoglobulin heavy-chain deletion
—Deletions on chromosome 14 in the area of the heavy-chain constant regions
—Most homozygous individuals are asymptomatic. A small subgroup of patients have been noted to have recurrent pyogenic infections

- Kappa-chain deficiency

—Absence of the kappa subtype of light chains in immunoglobulin molecules
—Described in two families
—Associated with variable defects in specific antibody formation

- Immunodeficiency with thymoma

—Seen in adults, typically between 40 and 70 years old
—Associated with significantly decreased to absent IgG, IgA, and IgM

- Secondary causes of hypogammaglobulinemia

—Viruses: Epstein-Barr virus (EBV), cytomegalovirus (CMV), congenital rubella
—The mechanism by which antibody responses and immunoglobulin production are altered in infected patients is not clearly defined.
—Infectious mononucleosis has been associated with defective specific antibody responses to neoantigens and impaired *in vitro* B-cell function in normal individuals. These defects are transient and resolve within 6 to 8 weeks after the onset of the disease. A disastrous response to EBV infection is seen in X-linked lymphoproliferative syndrome. These patients develop fatal infectious mononucleosis, marrow aplasia, B-cell lymphoma, and agammaglobulinemia.
—HIV, CMV, and rubella infections have been associated with abnormal specific antibody responses.

DRUGS

- Immunosuppressive/chemotherapeutic agents, phenytoin
- The associated defects in immune function and antibody production usually resolve after the therapy is discontinued.

OTHER

- Protein-losing enteropathy
- Intestinal lymphangiectasia
- Nephrotic syndrome
- The hypogammaglobulinemia is due to direct loss through the gastrointestinal (GI) tract or kidneys.
- Lymphoreticular malignancies have been associated with various immune defects and decreased immunoglobulin production.

Hypogammaglobulinemia

 Data Gathering

HISTORY

A detailed history for recurrent infection is key to evaluating suspected humoral immunodeficiency.

• Patients with humoral immunodeficiencies usually present with recurrent infections due to encapsulated bacteria, such as *Haemophilus influenzae* type B and *Streptococcus pneumoniae.*
• It is important to rule out hypogammaglobulinemia in patients with recurrent infections because replacement therapy with intravenous IgG is readily available.

Question: At what age did the recurrent infections start?
Significance: Patients with hypogammaglobulinemia usually present after 3 to 6 months of age. Late onset of infections may be more consistent with CVID.

Question: What type of infections have been diagnosed?
Significance: Hypogammaglobulinemia typically results in bacterial infections with encapsulated organisms.

Question: Have there been recurrent severe infections such as meningitis, sepsis, and osteomyelitis?
Significance: Some of the congenital immunodeficiency syndromes are signified by specific infections such as chronic meningoencephalitis with echoviruses, vaccine-associated poliomyelitis, and *Pneumocystis carinii* pneumonia.

Question: Is there a familial history of immunodeficiencies?
Significance: Previously affected males suggests an X-linked inheritance pattern.

Question: Early infant deaths?
Significance: Early infant deaths due to overwhelming infection may indicate a previously undiagnosed congenital immunodeficiency.

Question: Any other associated signs or symptoms?
Significance: Many of the congenital immunodeficiencies have associated arthritis, autoimmune disease, chronic lung disease, and GI manifestations.

 Physical Examination

In general, patients should be examined for signs of acute and chronic infections.

Finding: Growth parameters
Significance: Children with significant, recurrent infections and GI disease related to immunodeficiency may present with failure to thrive.

Finding: Signs of chronic otitis media or conjunctal recurrent disease
Significance: Patients with XLA frequently have signs of chronic conjunctivitis.

Finding: Gingivitis and stomatitis
Significance: May occur with the neutropenia-associated hypogammaglobulinemia syndromes.

Finding: Lymphoid tissue
Significance: Absence of tonsillar tissue and palpable lymph nodes is suggestive of X-linked agammaglobulinemia.

Finding: Lymphadenopathy and tonsillar hypertrophy
Significance: Can be seen in hyper-IgM syndrome and CVID. Persistently enlarged nodes should be investigated.

Finding: Wheezes, rales
Significance: Acute pneumonia or chronic lung disease

Finding: Hepatosplenomegaly or masses
Significance: May be seen in hyper-IgM syndrome and CVID. Abdominal masses should be investigated promptly to rule out malignancy.

Finding: Arthritis, clubbing
Significance: Arthritis can be seen in patients with XLA and CVID. Clubbing can be seen in the presence of chronic lung disease/bronchiectasis.

 Laboratory Aids

Test: Complete blood count with differential
Significance: Autoimmune hemolytic anemia, neutropenia, and thrombocytopenia can be seen in XLA, hyper-IgM, and CVID.

Test: Quantitative immunoglobulin levels
Significance: Each isotype should be measured (IgG, IgA, IgM, IgE). A normal or elevated IgM level in face of low to absent IgG, IgA, is characteristic of hyper-IgM syndrome.

Test: Serial testing of immunoglobulins
Significance: Should be done in infants suspected of transient hypogammaglobulinemia to document subsequent normalization of immunoglobulin levels.

Test: Qualitative antibody levels
Significance: Isohemagglutinins are primarily IgM antibodies to the main blood groups. They should be present in normal patients. However, they will be absent in patients with AB blood type. In addition, their presence is inconstant in children under 1 year of age.

Test: Antibody titers to tetanus, diphtheria, and *Haemophilus influenzae* type B measured post-vaccination.
Significance: Pneumococcal antibody titers post-pneumococcal vaccine has been used by some groups as a measure of response to polysaccharide antigens. However, there is extreme variability from laboratory to laboratory in measurement of titers. In addition, responses to Pneumovax are unreliable in children under 2 years of age.

Test: B-cell enumeration
Significance: Numbers of peripheral B-cell will be decreased to absent in XLA and rare in CVID. They are usually normal in other hypogammaglobulinemia syndromes.

Test: Total lymphocyte count (derived from the CBC with differential)
Significance: Lymphocyte enumeration is done using monoclonal antibodies to cell-specific CD surface markers measured by flow cytometry.

Test: Chest and sinus radiography and CT scans
Significance: May be helpful in evaluating for acute and chronic disease. Bronchiectasis can be a long-term sequela of chronic pulmonary infection.

• Prompt and appropriate antibiotic therapy is an important part of routine treatment.
• There may be a role for prophylactic antibiotics in patients with persistent recurrent infections.
• Replacement therapy with IVIG is the primary therapeutic modality for XLA, hyper-IgM syndrome, and CVID. Usual initiating doses are 200 to 400 mg/kg every 3 to 4 weeks. Nadir IgG levels should be greater than 300 mg/dL.
• Patients receiving IVIG therapy should not receive routine vaccinations; they are passively immunized with the therapy.
• Therapy is usually lifelong in patients with documented humoral immunodeficiency.

 Common Questions and Answers

Q: When should I make a referral?
A: Refer any patient suspected of having a primary humoral immunodeficiency to a specialist in allergy and immunology. These are patients with chronic disease who require prolonged follow-up and good communication between the referring physician and specialist.

BIBLIOGRAPHY

Huston DP, Kavanaugh AF, Rohane PW, Huston MM. Immunoglobulin deficiency syndromes and therapy. *J Allergy Clin Immunol* 1991;87:1–17.

Ochs HD, Wedgwood RJ. Disorders of the B-cell system. In: Stiehm ER, ed. *Immunologic disorders in infants and children*, 3rd ed. 1989:226–256.

Rosen FS, Cooper MD, Wedgwood RJP. The primary immunodeficiencies. *N Engl J Med* 1995;333:431–440.

Schaffer FM, Ballow M. Immunodeficiency: the office work-up. *J Respir Dis* 1995;16:523–541.

Skull S, Kemp A. Treatment of hypogammaglobulinaemia with intravenous immunoglobulin, 1973–1993. *Arch Dis Child* 1996;74(6):527–530.

Author: Alex G. Yip

Immune Deficiency

 Database

DEFINITION

• Immunodeficiencies can be either congenital or acquired.
• Immunodeficiencies often present as an increased susceptibility to infection as well as diarrhea, malabsorption, or failure to thrive; other manifestations can include unusual infections, including unexplained recurrent or chronic thrush.
• Consider immunodeficiencies if a child has two or more bacterial pneumonias per year, five or more episodes of otitis media per year or seven or more episodes in 2 years, recurrent or persistent sinusitis, or frequent, unusual, or unusually severe infections.

 Differential Diagnosis

CONGENITAL OR PRIMARY IMMUNODEFICIENCIES

• Antibody immunodeficiencies (B-cell–associated immunodeficiencies)

—X-linked agammaglobulinemia
—IgG subclass deficiency
—Common variable immunodeficiency
—IgA deficiency
—Transient hypogammaglobulinemia of infancy

• Cellular immunodeficiencies (T-cell–associated immunodeficiencies)

—DiGeorge syndrome—thymic aplasia or hypoplasia
—Chronic mucocutaneous candidiasis

• Combined cellular and antibody (B- and T-cell–associated immunodeficiencies)

—Severe combined immunodeficiency
—Adenosine deaminase (ADA) or nucleoside phosphorylase deficiency
—Ataxia telangiectasia
—Wiskott-Aldrich syndrome

• Natural-killer cell deficiency (abherent cell lysis)
• Phagocytic dysfunction

—Chronic granulomatous disease
—Hyper-IgE syndrome

• Complement deficiencies

BRIEF DESCRIPTIONS OF CONGENITAL OR PRIMARY IMMUNODEFICIENCIES

• X-linked agammaglobulinemia—onset of symptoms after 6 months; infections by bacterial pathogens; respiratory system, skin, bone most commonly infected
• IgG subclass deficiency—infections with bacterial pathogens; IgG2 and IgG4 most common deficiencies in children; usually have normal or increased total IgG levels; may resolve spontaneously between 18 months and 6 years

• Common variable immunodeficiency—may appear in later childhood or adulthood; heterogeneous group of disorders with hypogammaglobulinemia

—B cells fail to mature into plasma cells
—Recurrent and sinopulmonary disease is common

• IgA deficiency—may be asymptomatic; pulmonary and gastrointestinal infections are the most common illnesses; difficult to establish prior to 2 years of age
• Transient hypogammaglobulinemia of infancy—occurs between 3 and 6 months of age; usually transient, although may last up to 8 years; repeated bacterial infections most common presentations
• Immunodeficiency with increased IgM—decreased IgG, IgE, IgA with increased IgM; symptoms begin in first or second year of life; recurrent bacterial infection

—May be seen as associated neutropenia

• DiGeorge syndrome—aplasia of the thymus and hypoparathyroidism, hypothyroidism, congenital heart disease, and abnormal facial features; often present with hypocalcemia.
• Chronic mucocutaneous candidiasis—T-cell-deficient response to candida; 50% with endocrine abnormalities

—NL T-cell response to other antigen

• Severe combined immunodeficiency—illness begins in the first months of life; illnesses include pneumonia, sepsis chronic diarrhea, FTT, thrust *Pneumocystis carini* pneumonia—common initial presentation and cause of pneumonia; at risk for viral and bacterial infection
• ADA deficiency—affects activity of both T- and B-cell function; associated chondro-osseus dysplasia
• Ataxia telangiectasia—progressive cerebellar ataxia; telangiectasis; sinopulmonary infections common; lymphopenia in some cases
• Wiscott-Aldrich syndrome—clinical picture of eczema, thrombocytopenia, and recurrent infections; poor antibody response to polysaccharide antigens and defective T-cell function; small platelets on peripheral blood smear; IgM low; IgG normal or slightly low; IgA and IgE elevated
• Natural-killer cell deficiency—recurrent infections, including severe herpesvirus infections; can be seen in Chédiak-Higashi syndrome, leukocyte adhesion molecule deficiency, and X-linked lymphoproliferative syndrome
• Chronic granulomatous disease—granulomas in skin, lungs, and lymph nodes; impaired bactericidal function of neutrophils; predisposes to infection with catalase-producing organisms; lymphadenopathy with purulent drainage and hepatosplenomegaly are common findings.
• Hyper-IgE syndrome—eczema with bacterial infections of the skin, lungs, middle ears, and sinuses; *Staphylococcus aureus* is a major cause of infection; absolute eosinophilia on peripheral smear is common.

• Complement deficiency—C2 is the most common deficiency; pyogenic infections are the most common problem; deficiency of the terminal components of the cascade C5-C9 are associated with *Neisseria* infections.

SECONDARY IMMUNODEFICIENCIES

• HIV infection
• Malignancy
• Viral suppression
• Nephrotic syndrome

PATHOPHYSIOLOGY

• B-cell dysfunction—leads to antibody deficiency; poor opsonization of bacterial pathogens to allow for phagocytosis.
• T-cell dysfunction—poor response to fungal and viral pathogens
• Complement deficiency—pyogenic infections due to poor opsonization and immune adherence of circulating white blood cells
• Granulocytopenia—poor phagocytosis of bacterial pathogens

GENETICS

• X-linked agammaglobulinemia—X-linked
• IgG subclass deficiency—autosomal recessive?
• Common variable immunodeficiency—autosomal recessive or dominant
• IgA deficiency—autosomal recessive or dominant
• Transient hypogammaglobulinemia of infancy—unknown
• Immunodeficiency with increased IgM—X-linked or autosomal recessive
• DiGeorge syndrome—?
• Chronic mucocutaneous candidiasis—autosomal recessive
• Severe combined immunodeficiency—autosomal recessive or X-linked
• ADA or nucleoside phosphorylase deficiency—autosomal recessive
• Immunodeficiency with ataxia telangiectasia—autosomal recessive
• Wiskott-Aldrich syndrome—X-linked
• Natural-killer cell deficiency—unknown
• Chronic granulomatous disease—X-linked or autosomal recessive
• Hyper-IgE syndrome—autosomal dominant or unknown
• Complement deficiencies—autosomal recessive or dominant

COMPLICATIONS

• Severe invasive bacterial disease
• Recurrent respiratory tract infections
• Failure to thrive
• Unusual infection with unusual organism
• Chronic diarrhea
• Bronchiectasis, chronic or recurrent pneumonia, recurrent bronchitis
• Recurrent or resistant thrush
• Skin lesions—pyoderma or necrotic abscesses

Approach to the Patient

GENERAL GOALS

Screening tests should be directed to evaluate several arms of the immune system including B-cell/antibody function, cell-mediated immunity, neutrophil/phagocytic dysfunction, and complement deficiency.

Data Gathering

HISTORY

Questions

- Familial history
- Number and duration of infections
- Recurrent pneumonias
- Chronic diarrhea
- Association of rashes, diarrhea, failure to thrive
- Neurological problems
- HIV risk factors
- Endocrine disorders B hypothyroidism and hypoparathyroidism seen in DiGeorge syndrome

Physical Examination

Finding: Skin—telangectasia
Significance: Ataxia telangectasia

Finding: Thrush (candidiasis)
Significance: T-cell deficiencies

Finding: Eczema
Significance: Wiskott-Aldrich syndrome, hyper-IgE syndrome

Finding: Pulmonary—chronic lung disease
Significance: IgA deficiency, chronic granulomatous disease, hyper-IgE syndrome, X-linked hypogammaglobulinemia

Finding: Short stature
Significance: Common presentation of immune deficiency

Laboratory Aids

Tests

- Complete blood count with differential
- Quantitative immunoglobulins
- Antibody responses to immunizations (must be certain that the child has been immunized)
- Anergy panel plus PPD—can include trichophyton, *Candida*, tetanus, mumps
- T-cells—total and subsets
- Nitroblue tetrazolium test
- Phagocytic function
- CH50—total hemolytic complement
- Complement levels—C2-C6

- HIV ELISA and Western blot. If positive in children under 15 months of age, HIV infection should be confirmed with HIV PCR and HIV co-culture

THERAPY

In general, therapy should be under the guidance of a pediatric immunologist who is well trained in the treatment of these disorders.

Bone Marrow Transplantation

Tests

- DiGeorge syndrome
- Severe combined immunodeficiency (SCID)
- SCID with ADA deficiency
- Wiskott-Aldrich syndrome
- Chronic granulomatous disease

Thymus Transplantation

Tests

- DiGeorge syndrome
- Gamma globulin replacement therapy
- X-linked agammaglobulinemia
- Immunodeficiency with elevated IgM
- Common variable immunodeficiency
- IgG subclass deficiency
- Prophylactic antibiotics/antifungals
- IgG subclass deficiency
- Chronic mucocutaneous candidiasis
- Ataxia telangiectasia
- Hyper-IgE syndrome
- Complement deficiencies

Common Questions and Answers

Q: Do I have to worry about a previously well child who on routine CBC has neutropenia?
A: It is unlikely that a child who was previously well would have a significant immunodeficiency. The most likely diagnosis is viral suppression of the bone marrow. CBC should be repeated in approximately 2 weeks to confirm a normal neutrophil count.

Q: Does every child who has an episode of varicella-zoster need an immunologic workup?
A: No. One isolated course of non-complicated zoster does not require an immunologic evaluation. However, if more than one dermatome is involved or if the episodes are repeated, an immunologic evaluation is warranted.

Q: Should I be concerned about an immunodeficiency disorder in a 4-year-old child with thrush? How should such a child be evaluated?
A: There is no absolute age at which oral thrush is indicative of an underlying immunodeficiency. Obviously, one should look for predisposing factors such as antibiotic therapy or inhaled steroids as predisposing factors for oral thrush. Many authorities use 2 years as an age beyond which thrush should be evaluated. This evaluation should first include a culture from

the plaque lesions to be certain that the condition is truly oral candidiasis. Immunologic workup should include an HIV ELISA confirmed with a Western blot study when positive, T-cell subsets to include CD4 and CD8, and T-cell mitogen studies. Evaluation of these tests may require the assistance of a pediatric immunologist.

Clinical Pearls

- X-linked agammaglobulinemia—survive to second or third decade
- IgG subclasss deficiency—50% with IgG2 or IgG4 resolve by 18 months to early childhood
- Common variable immunodeficiency—good prognosis; survive to adulthood
- IgA deficiency—the earlier the onset of symptoms: guarded prognosis
- Transient hypogammaglobulinemia of infancy—self-limited with excellent prognosis
- DiGeorge syndrome—good prognosis
- Chronic mucocutaneous candidiasis—severe form: survive to third decade; mild form survive normal life span
- Severe combined immunodeficiency—die by age 1 or 2 years without bone marrow transplantation
- ADA or nucleoside phosphorylase deficiency—die without bone marrow transplantation
- Ataxia telangiectasia—variable
- Wiskott-Aldrich syndrome—variable; may die from massive bleeding at a young age
- Chronic granulomatous disease—survival up to the second decade
- Hyper-IgE syndrome—may survive into adulthood
- Complement deficiencies—usually survive into adulthood

Immunodeficiency should be considered in any child with two or more bacterial pneumonias per year, five or more episodes of otitis media, chronic sinusitis or other pulmonary disease, or unusual or unusually severe infections.

BIBLIOGRAPHY

Hong R. Update on the immunodeficiency diseases. *Am J Dis Child* 1990;144:983–992.

Iseki M, Heiner DC. Immunodeficiency disorders. *Pediatr Rev* 1993;14(6):226–236.

Pacheco SE, Shearer WT. Laboratory aspects of immunology. *Pediatr Clin North Am* 1994;41(4):623–655.

Sorenson RU, Moore C. Immunology in the pediatrician's office. *Pediatr Clin North Am* 1994;41(4):691–714.

Author: Bret J. Rudy

Jaundice

Database

DEFINITION

• Jaundice—a yellow or green/yellow hue to the skin, sclerae, and mucous membranes—becomes recognizable at serum total bilirubin levels of approximately 5 mg/dL (see table Common Causes of Pathologic Jaundice).
• Conjugated hyperbilirubinemia is defined as a direct-reacting fraction of serum bilirubin exceeding 30% to 40% of the total serum bilirubin.
• Unconjugated hyperbilirubinemia, the direct-reacting fraction is <15% of the total serum bilirubin. Patients with direct-reacting bilirubin between 15% to 30% are, therefore, indeterminate.

Differential Diagnosis

UNCONJUGATED HYPERBILIRUBINEMIA

Congenital/Anatomical

• Placental dysfunction
• Upper gastrointestinal (GI) tract obstruction (e.g., pyloric stenosis, duodenal web, stenosis, or atresia)
• Congenital hypothyroidism
• Infants of diabetic mothers

Infectious

• Sepsis

Trauma

• Cephalohematoma; bruising

Genetic/Metabolic

• Inherited red cell enzyme or membrane structural defects (e.g., G6PD deficiency, phosphokinase deficiency, spherocytosis)
• Defect in hepatic bilirubin conjugation (Crigler-Najar syndrome, types I and II)

ALLERGIC/INFLAMMATORY/ IMMUNOLOGIC

• Rh or ABO incompatibility

Functional

• Physiologic jaundice (almost always less than 14 days of age)
• Breast-feeding—associated jaundice

• Swallowed maternal blood; infant bleeding from clotting disorder (increased bilirubin load; see Trauma)
• Familial benign unconjugated hyperbilirubinemia (Lucey-Driscoll syndrome)

CONJUGATED HYPERBILIRUBINEMIA

Congenital/Anatomical

• Biliary atresia
• Biliary hypoplasia
• Congenital or acquired bile duct stenosis
• Choledochal cyst and other anomalies of the choledochopancreaticoductal junction
• Spontaneous perforation of the bile duct
• Bile or mucus plug or "biliary sludge"
• Gallstone
• Cystic dilatation of intrahepatic bile ducts ("Caroli disease")
• Congenital hepatic fibrosis/polycystic kidney and liver disease

Infectious Etiologies

• Bacterial
—Gram-negative sepsis
—Urinary tract infection/pyelonephritis
• Viral
—Cytomegalovirus (CMV)
—Echovirus
—HIV
—Hepatitis B, C
• Toxoplasmosis
• *Pneumocystis carinii*
• Entamoeba histolytica
• Mycobacterium tuberculosis
• M. *avium-intracellulare*
• Syphilis

Toxic/Environmental/Drugs

• Post-necrotizing enterocolitis
• Post-shock or post-asphyxia
• Medications
• Hyperalimentation

Tumor

• Neuroblastoma
• Porta hepatis nodes

Genetic/Metabolic

• Arteriohepatic dysplasia (Alagille syndrome)
• Progressive familial intrahepatic cholestasis (several types including Byler disease, MDR3 deficiency)
• Defects in bile acid metabolism
• Defects in amino acid metabolism
• Defects in lipid metabolism
—Wolman disease (cholesterol ester storage disease)

—Niemann-Pick disease
—Gaucher disease
• Defects in carbohydrate metabolism
—Galactosemia
—Hereditary fructose intolerance
—Glycogenosis type IV
—Zellweger syndrome (cerebrohepatorenal)
• Defects in mitochondrial DNA and respiratory chain enzyme deficiencies
• Alpha$_1$-antitrypsin deficiency
• Cystic fibrosis
• Multiple acyl coenzyme A dehydrogenase deficiency
• Wilson disease (older child only)
• Inherited non-cholestatic conjugated jaundice syndromes (e.g., Dubin-Johnson and Rotor syndromes)
• Familial benign recurrent cholestasis—inborn errors of bile acid synthesis
• Hereditary cholestasis with lymphedema (Aegene syndrome)

Allergic/Inflammatory/Immunologic

• Sclerosing cholangitis

Miscellaneous

• Idiopathic neonatal hepatitis
• Neonatal iron storage disease
• Idiopathic hypopituitarism

Approach to the Patient

GENERAL GOAL

Decide if disorder threatens acute or subacute hepatic failure (conjugated hyperbilirubinemia). Decide if disorder threatens neurologic injury (kernicterus).

Phase 1: Is the jaundice due entirely to unconjugated hyperbilirubinemia?

Phase 2: Is the jaundice due to conjugated hyperbilirubinemia? Obtain values for total, direct, and indirect serum bilirubin; serum aminotransferases (ALT and AST), gammaglutamyltransferase (GGT), prothrombin time (PT), and partial thromboplastin time (PTT).

Phase 3: Rule out those causes of direct hyperbilirubinemia for which delay in diagnosis and treatment may adversely affect outcome, i.e., biliary atresia, tyrosinemia, galactosemia, inborn error of bile acid synthesis, hereditary fructose intolerance, neonatal iron storage disease.

Data Gathering

HISTORY

Question: Does the patient have unexplained itching?
Significance: Suggests cholestatic liver disease (conjugated hyperbilirubinemia).

Common Causes of Pathologic Jaundice

NEWBORN AND EARLY INFANCY PERIOD	OLDER CHILD
Biliary atresia	Autoimmune hepatitis
Idiopathic neonatal hepatitis	Viral hepatitis
Alpha-1-antitrypsin deficiency	Wilson disease
Infection	Biliary obstruction (e.g., gallstone or choledochal cyst)

Question: Does the patient have a change in mental status, handwriting, or school performance?
Significance: Consider Wilson disease (generally children over 4 years of age).

Question: Is there a history of intravenous drug abuse or exposure to blood or blood products, especially prior to 1992?
Significance: The patient may have transfusion associated hepatitis, most likely hepatitis C.

Question: Is there a history of a sibling with prolonged jaundice or hepatic failure in infancy?
Significance: Because many of the causes of neonatal conjugated hyperbilirubinemia are due to recessive disorders, a sibling with prolonged neonatal jaundice, particularly if fatal and left undiagnosed, suggests an inborn error such as tyrosinemia, alpha₁-antitrypsin deficiency, etc., as the cause for the newborn patient's jaundice.

Physical Examination

Finding: Scratch marks
Significance: Possibly attributable to pruritus, suggesting cholestasis.

Finding: Spider angiomata, palmar erythema
Significance: Evidence of chronic liver disease.

Finding: Petechiae, purpura, microcephaly
Significance: Evidence of thrombocytopenia, possibly due to congenital TORCH infection.

Finding: Severe bruising, cephalohematoma
Significance: Increased bilirubin load.

Finding: Pallor
Significance: Indicative of severe anemia, possibly due to ongoing hemolysis as a cause of indirect hyperbilirubinemia.

Finding: Heart murmur
Significance: Alagille syndrome (classically peripheral pulmonic stenosis).

Finding: Hepatosplenomegaly
Significance: Congenital TORCH infection or of significant liver scarring and portal hypertension

Finding: Ascites
Significance: Hypoalbuminemia, generally implying significant chronic liver disease and synthetic dysfunction

Finding: Acholic stool
Significance: Severe cholestasis; in the newborn, suggestive but not pathognomic of biliary atresia; in the older child, may also suggest biliary obstruction due to a gallstone, mass, or other lesion obstructing the flow of bile.

Laboratory Aids

Test: Total bilirubin with fractionation, preferably by HPLC into conjugated, unconjugated, and delta fractions (newborn or young infant).

Significance: If unconjugated hyperbilirubinemia, initiate work-up with:

• Blood type and Rh factor of mother and infant—hemolysis due to blood group or Rh incompatibility
• Hemoglobin, hematocrit, reticulocyte count, peripheral smear for red cell morphology—rule out microsherocytes indicating hemolysis, or evidence of hereditary spherocytosis or elliptocytosis
• Coombs test-assess for autoimmune hemolytic anemia
• PT, PTT, platelet count—assess coagulopathy that may explain lost blood and increased bilirubin load causing unconjugate hyperbilirubinemia
• Sepsis evaluation (blood, urine, and spinal fluid cultures
• T4, T3, TSH—screen for neonatal thyroid disease

Test: Serum aminotransferases (ALT, AST); GGT
Significance: Measures degree of liver inflammation and cholestasis

Test: Serum albumin, PT, PTT, fibrinogen, cholesterol
Significance: Measures degree of liver synthetic function; decrease in albumin, fibrinogen, or very low cholesterol and increases in PT, PTT implies significant liver disease.

Test: Stool color
Significance: Acholic (white) or very pale stools imply possibly obstructive lesion (such as biliary atresia).

• Sepsis evaluation (cultures of blood, urine, and spinal fluid)
• Hepatitis B surface antigen and hepatitis C antibody and RNA by polymerase chain reaction (PCR)

Test: TORCH titers and VDRL
Significance: Congenital infection.

Test: Alpha₁-antitrypsin and Pi (protease inhibitor) type
Significance: Inherited homozygous deficient alleles.

Test: Sweat chloride
Significance: Cystic fibrosis.

Test: Urine and plasma amino acids and urine organic acids
Significance: Screens for inherited amino and organic acidopathies.

Test: Urine dipstick for glucose and Clinitest for reducing substances
Significance: Implying the presence of another sugar such as galactose.

Test: Urine for bile acid analysis
Significance: Assesses for inborn error of bile acid synthesis.

Test: Ultrasonography
Significance: Dilated hepatic ducts implying an obstructive lesion; presence of gallstones or a choledochal cyst.

Test: Hepatobiliary scintigraphy (DISIDA scan)
Significance: The presence of excretion of la-

beled tracer from the liver into the bowel effectively rules out biliary atresia; the absence of excretion does not necessarily rule in an obstructive disorder.

Test: Percutaneous liver biopsy
Significance: Allows with greater than 90% to 95% certainty the assessment of findings that may suggest extrahepatic obstruction, such as biliary atresia which merit surgical exploration and intraoperative cholangiogram.

Common Questions and Answers

Q: Because biliary atresia is an obstructive lesion, are the intrahepatic bile ducts dilated?
A: Never!

Q: What disorders are life-threatening?
A: Biliary atresia, galactosemia, hereditary fructose intolerance, tyrosinemia, sepsis, hypopituitarism, inborn error of bile acid metabolism, neonatal iron storage disease. In the infant with unconjugated hyperbilirubinemia, sepsis and hypothyroidism together with Crigler-Najar syndrome types I and II such as brisk hemolysis that causes a rapid rise of unconjugated bilirubin above 20 mg/dL. In the older child, suspected Wilson disease.

Indications for Referral

• Lack of excretion on hepatobiliary scintigraphy scan.
• Presence of choledochal cyst or dilated biliary ducts seen on ultrasound.
• Abnormal metabolic screen (urine and plasma, amino, or organic acids).
• Evidence of decompensated liver disease, e.g., PT >20 seconds; albumin <3.0, ascites, encephalopathy, bilirubin >20 mg/dL; ALT/AST >300, especially if associated with one or more of the previous criteria.

Clinical Pearls

• Crigler-Najar type II syndrome must be treated promptly with phototherapy and phenobarbital to prevent kernicterus.
• Older children presenting with Wilson disease may present with significant hemolysis and, therefore, with a predominantly unconjugated hyperbilirubinemia but with significant parenchymal liver disease and even liver failure. Do not be fooled!

BIBLIOGRAPHY

Balistreri WF. Neonatal cholestasis. *J Pediatr* 1985;106:171–184.

Lasker MR, Holzman R. Neonatal jaundice: when to treat, when to watch and wait. *Postgrad Med* 1996;99(3):187–193.

Mews C, Sinatra FR. Chronic liver disease in children. *Pediatr Rev* 1993;14(11):436–444.

Author: Eric S. Maller

Learning Problems

 ## Database

DEFINITION

A learning problem exists whenever a child falls behind in school or shows a deterioration from a previous level of performance. Psychosocial factors account for many learning problems, but other learning problems have a direct medical basis. The terms *learning disorder* or *learning disability* refer to conditions in which academic achievement is substantially below that expected for age, schooling, and level of intelligence.

 ## Differential Diagnosis

CONGENITAL/ANATOMICAL

- Premature birth
- CNS malformations (cystic lesions, heterotopias, abnormal gyral morphology, unusual symmetry patterns, hydrocephalus, etc.)

INFECTIOUS

- Subacute sclerosing panencephalitis

TOXIC

- Lead poisoning
- Iron-deficiency
- Drug side effects
- Tumor chemotherapy
- Cranial irradiation
- Anti-epileptic medications
- Bronchodilators

GENETIC/METABOLIC

- Neurodegenerative disorders
- Hypothyroidism
- Unrecognized genetic syndromes

—Velocardiofacial syndrome
—Female carriers of Fragile X syndrome

MISCELLANEOUS

- Hearing impairment
- Vision impairment
- Absence and partial complex seizure disorders
- Narcolepsy
- Chronic malnutrition
- Co-morbidity associated with many chronic illnesses
- Psychosocial difficulties

—family or peer relationship problems

NEUROPSYCHIATRIC DISORDERS

- Specific learning disorders

—Reading disorder
—Mathematics disorder

- Attention deficit hyperactivity disorder
- Oppositional defiant disorder
- Mood disorder

—Depression
—Bipolar disorder

- Borderline mental retardation
- Substance abuse

Approach to the Patient

GENERAL GOAL

Determine whether the learning problems are primary, or whether they result from another medical or psychosocial condition. The pediatrician should coordinate the appropriate medical, psychiatric, and/or psychoeducational evaluation, with consultation as indicated. Early identification of learning problems helps to prevent the cascade of negative consequences triggered by poor academic achievement.

Phase 1: Identify and address medical factors that may affect learning (e.g., sensory impairments, lead intoxication, absence seizures, iatrogenic interventions). Consider subtle genetic syndromes (e.g., Fragile X syndrome in girls) that may cause learning problems without causing other major medical abnormalities.

Phase 2: Screen for psychiatric conditions, and for social and environmental factors that may be associated with learning problems. Psychosocial stresses may exacerbate learning difficulties, or be a primary etiologic factor. If indicated, refer to appropriate consultants.

Phase 3: For patients with learning problems that are suspected to be primary (e.g., reading or math disability, attention deficit disorder), a complete psychoeducational evaluation is indicated. Referral may be made to the school system, or to private professionals. Medical treatment of attention deficit may be undertaken by the primary care physician or by subspecialists.

 ## Data Gathering

HISTORY

Question: How and when does the child fail in daily academic pursuits?
Significance: For specific learning disabilities, problems may occur only in one class. For attention deficit, problems may be minimized with one-on-one teaching.

Question: Deterioration in performance?
Significance: Consider new pathophysiologic processes:

- Psychosocial issues
- Vision/hearing impairment
- Neurodegenerative or seizure process
- Medication side effect

Question: Past medical history? Medications? Review of systems? Psychosocial stresses?
Significance: Identify pre-existing factors that may affect learning.

Question: Early milestones?
Significance: History of language delays is common in children with reading disability.

Question: Family history?
Significance: Attention deficit disorders and learning disorders often carry a heritable component.

HINTS FOR SCREENING

The child may be the only person who can provide important information on their reaction to the learning problems (anxiety, depression, etc.) and on family and school circumstances surrounding these problems. The latter must be addressed with the appropriate confidentiality.

Physical Examination

Finding: Abnormal growth parameters
Significance: May indicate presence of chronic illness or genetic syndrome, or history of neurologic injury.

Finding: Subtle dysmorphology
Significance: Possible teratogenic fetal exposure or unidentified genetic syndrome.

Finding: Abnormal neurological examination
Significance: Any focal signs demand additional evaluation. Soft signs (neuro-maturational signs) are often present in children with learning problems, but are non-specific.

Finding: Abnormal audiology or vision screening
Significance: May be direct cause of learning problem.

Laboratory Aids

Test: Standardized behavior questionnaires
Significance: Diagnosis of attention deficit disorder is critically dependent on input from teachers and parents.

Test: Psychoeducational evaluation
Significance: These data are necessary to establish the presence of a specific learning disability, and to formulate intervention strategies.

Test: Lead level, thyroid functions, EEG
Significance: If history is suggestive, must rule out these etiologies.

Common Questions and Answers

Q: What classroom accommodations can be made for children with learning problems?
A: Depending of the nature of the problem, possible accommodations include preferential seating, extra time for test-taking, use of electronic word processors, provision of written rather than verbal instructions, tutoring, resource room assistance, and alternative classroom placement.

Q: What is the difference between psychoeducational and neuropsychological testing?
A: A typical psychoeducational evaluation includes IQ and academic achievement testing, and behavioral assessment. This testing must be performed individually, by a professional who can establish a good rapport with the student. For most children, this testing is sufficient to identify learning disabilities and to prescribe educational remedies. For children who do not respond to first-line educational interventions, neuropsychological testing may help to define specific cognitive strengths and weaknesses that must be accounted for in working with the student.

Q: How can the family obtain a complete school evaluation?
A: Regulations vary from state to state. Parents can usually start by writing to the principal of their local public school to request a complete evaluation and stating the reasons for their request. (Specific information for each state can be obtained from the National Information Center for Children and Youth with Disabilities (800-695-0285; www.nichcy.org.)

Indications for Referral

• History consistent with seizure disorder or concern about a neurodegenerative disorder.
• Significant symptoms of depression or other psychiatric disorder.
• Dysmorphology on physical examination may indicate referral to genetics.
• Evidence of hearing or visual impairment.
• Unless there is a strong suspicion of a primary medical or psychosocial etiology, consider referral to a clinician experienced in neurodevelopmental disorders. This consultant may assist in comprehensive diagnostic formulation, pharmacologic treatment when indicated, developmental follow-up, and advocacy.
• Federal law requires individualized educational planning for children with the following diagnoses:

—Mental impairment
—Hearing impairments
—Speech or language impairments
—Visual impairments
—Serious emotional disturbance
—Orthopedic impairments
—Autism
—Traumatic brain injury
—Other health impairments
—Specific learning disabilities

• Schools are required by federal law to provide comprehensive evaluations (excepting the medical component), on written request by the parents. Such multi-disciplinary assessments also may be obtained through hospital-based or other private agencies.

Clinical Pearls

• Hyperactivity may be minimal in some children with attention deficit/hyperactivity disorder (ADHD), especially girls. Many children with ADHD show significant difficulties with inattention and distractibility, but little hyperactivity. Good behavior in the doctor's office, and good behavior while playing computer games, do not exclude the diagnosis of ADHD. Even children with severe ADHD may appear attentive in the intimidating and artificial milieu of the doctor's office, and computer games can be motivating and highly reinforcing.
• Comorbidity and symptomatic overlap are common among ADHD, specific learning disabilities, and other psychiatric disorders. Students who have a learning disability, or students who are depressed, may show symptoms of inattention. Academic or attention difficulties may lead to spiraling psychological problems, from damaged self-esteem to conduct disorder to depression.

BIBLIOGRAPHY

Beitchman JH, Young AR. Learning disorders with a special emphasis on reading disorders: a review of the past 10 years. *J Am Acad Child Adolesc Psychiatry* 1997;36(8):1020–1032.

Levy SE. Pediatric evaluation of the child with developmental delay. *Child Adolesc Psychiatr Clin N Am* 1996;5(4):809–826.

Reiff MI. Adolescent school failure: failure to thrive in adolescence. *Pediatr Rev* 1998;19(6):199–207.

Resnick MB, Gomatam SV, Carter RL, et al. Educational disabilities of neonatal intensive care graduates. *Pediatrics* 1998;102(2 Pt 1):308–314.

Shaywitz SE. Dyslexia. *N Engl J Med* 1998;338(5):307–312.

Author: Paul P. Wang

Leukocytosis

 Database

DEFINITION

An increase in white blood cell count above normal for age. The most frequent cause is an increase in the total neutrophil count but leukocytosis may result from an increase in any type of white blood cell, such as lymphocytosis, monocytosis, eosinophilia, basophilia, or atypical monocytosis (see tables Causes of Neutrophilia, Causes of Lymphocytosis, Causes of Eosinophilia, and Causes of Monocytosis).

 Differential Diagnosis

INFECTIOUS

- Bacterial

—*Streptococcus*
—*Staphylococcus aureus*
—*Haemophilus*
—*Neisseria*
—*Brucella*
—*Bartonella* (Cat-scratch disease)
—Pertussis

- Viral

—Infectious mononucleosis
—Cytomegalovirus (CMV)
—Rubella
—Mumps
—Hepatitis

- Fungal

—Aspergillus

- Parasitic

—*Toxocara*
—*Toxoplasma*
—*Trichinella*
—Tapeworms
—*Strongyloides*

- Tuberculosis
- Syphilis

Causes of Neutrophilia

Bacterial infections
Inflammatory states
Acute hemorrhage
Stress
Drugs
   Corticosteroids
   Epinephrine
Metabolic disorders
   Uremia
   Acidosis
Myeloproliferative disorders
   Myelofibrosis
   Polycythemia vera
CML
Sickle cell disease

- Acute infectious lymphocytosis
—Benign viral mediated lymphocytosis (often >25,000/mm³)
- Kawasaki disease

CONGENITAL/ANATOMICAL

- Down syndrome
- Sickle cell disease
- Fanconi anemia
- Thrombocytopenia with absent radii
- Leukocyte adhesion factor deficiency

DRUGS

- Corticosteroids

—Epinephrine
—Lithium

- Granulocyte colony stimulating factor (GCSF)

TRAUMA

- Acute hemorrhage
- Severe burns
- Inflammation

TUMOR

- Leukemia
- Lymphoma
- Myeloproliferative disorders
- Solid tumors

GENETIC/METABOLIC

- Hyperthyroidism
- Acidosis

INFLAMMATORY

- Juvenile rheumatoid arthritis
- Rheumatoid arthritis
- Inflammatory bowel disease

—Ulcerative colitis
—Crohn disease

- Chronic granulomatous disease
- Pulmonary eosinophilic syndromes

—Transient infiltrates associated with a peripheral eosinophilia

ALLERGIC

- Asthma
- Seasonal or drug allergies
- Eczema
- Psoriasis

Causes of Lymphocytosis

Viral infections
Other infections
   Bordetella pertussis
   Tuberculosis
   Syphilis
Acute infectious lymphocytosis
Malignancy
   ALL lymphocytic leukemia
   Lymphoma

HEMATOLOGIC

- Severe hemolysis

ARTIFACTUAL

- Nucleated RBCs
- Clumped platelets on a mechanical differential

Approach to the Patient

Phase 1: Is WBC count dangerously elevated? If the WBC count is greater than 50,000/mm³, consult a pediatric hematologist/oncologist. WBC of 100,000/mm³ can increase blood viscosity causing stroke or infarct.

Phase 2:

- Next, determine which white blood cell line is elevated by reviewing the WBC differential to help direct the workup and therapy.
- The differential diagnosis for a patient with a neutrophilia can be different from a patient in whom lymphocytosis is present. For example, an elevated granulocyte count is more likely with bacterial infections and a lymphocytosis is usually associated with viral infections. Pitfall: Many laboratories provide only machine-generated differentials. If there are any abnormalities a manual differential must be obtained. It may be necessary to review the smear with a hematologist or pathologist especially if there are any significant abnormalities.

Causes of Eosinophilia

Allergic disorders
   Asthma
   Urticaria
   Drug hypersensitivity
Skin disorders
   Eczema
   Psoriasis
   Pemphigus
Parasitic infections
   Aspergillosis
   Toxoplasmosis
   Trichinosis
   Coccidioidomycosis
Hypereosinophilic syndromes
Hereditary eosinophilia
Hematologic disorders
   Fanconi anemia
   Thrombocytopenia with absent radii
   Congenital neutropenias
Inflammatory disorders
   Gastrointestinal
   Sarcoid
   Polyarteritis nodosa

Phase 3: Lastly, the degree of elevation can also be indicative of the diagnosis.

• Most elevations of WBC count are in the 10,000 to 20,000/mm³ range. A WBC count in the 30,000/mm³ range is more consistent with pertussis or pneumococcal bacteremia. Counts higher than that are worrisome for malignant processes or leukemoid reactions.

 ## Data Gathering

HISTORY

Question: Is there any evidence for infection, such as fever, rash, or swelling?
Significance: Infection is the most common etiology for leukocytosis. A thorough history should be taken for apparent or occult infections. Fever can also be a symptom of inflammatory diseases such as JRA or CGD.

Question: What other complaints has the patient had over the preceding weeks to months?
Significance: Infectious etiologies tend to present acutely. If a patient has long-term complaints one should broaden the differential or focus it based on specific complaints. A chronic cough may point to tuberculosis whereas a whooping cough may indicate pertussis.

Question: Does the patient have any other medical problems?
Significance: Patients with sickle cell disease have an elevated WBC count probably secondary to chronic inflammation or marrow expansion. Children with Down syndrome can have a benign leukemoid reaction, especially in the first few months of life, that resolves spontaneously.

Question: Is the patient on any medications?
Significance: Corticosteroids will increase the neutrophil precursors (also called a left-shifted differential). Epinephrine can cause a transitory increase in neutrophil count.

Causes of Monocytosis

Infection
  Tuberculosis
  Malaria
  Brucellosis
  Bacterial endocarditis
Inflammatory disease
  Collagen vascular disease
  Sarcoid
  RA
  Crohn
  Ulcerative colitis
  SLE
Malignancy
  Hodgkin disease
  AML
  Myelodyspastic syndromes

Question: Is there a familial history of any inflammatory diseases?
Significance: For example, collagen vascular disease such as RA, thyroid, Crohn disease.

Question: Has the patient lost weight, been fatigued, had night sweats, or been pale?
Significance: Malignancy such as leukemia must be ruled out.

 ## Physical Examination

Finding: Are there any obvious sources of infection?
Significance: Look for cellulitis, otitis, pharyngitis, or abscesses on examination. A good lung examination on a quiet child is necessary as pneumonia secondary to *Streptococcus* can cause a WBC count as high as 30,000 to 40,000/mm³. A murmur or gallop may be a sign of bacterial endocarditis.

Finding: Lymphadenopathy or hepatosplenomegaly?
Significance: Points toward a possible viral etiology but is also of concern for malignancy.

Finding: Are joints tender or swollen?
Significance: JRA, septic arthritis, SLE

Finding: Mongoloid features?
Significance: Down syndrome.

 ## Laboratory Aids

Test: WBC count including differential and smear.
Significance: If neutrophilia is present think of bacterial infections. One may also see Döhle bodies, toxic granulations, or vacuolization in bacteremia. A recovering or stressed marrow may have an increase in monocytes or eosinophils. Look for leukemic blasts.

Test: Hemoglobin/platelet count
Significance: If either is low, consider a marrow infiltrative process or a hyperstimulated marrow to compensate for a low hemoglobin or platelet count (Fanconi's anemia, thrombocytopenia with absent radii).

Test: Chemistry panel
Significance: Evaluate LFTs for possible viral etiology. Uric acid and LDH are elevated in leukemia and lymphoma.

Test: Cultures
Significance: Blood, urine, stool, throat, etc.

Test: Monospot, Heterophil Ab, EBV titers
Significance: Screen for infectious mononucleosis. Monospot can be falsely negative in younger children.

Test: Leukocyte alkaline phosphatase
Significance: Elevated in infection but not in leukemia. Helps to differentiate CML from a leukemoid reaction.

Test: ANA
Significance: Screen for rheumatologic etiology.

Test: Bone marrow biopsy and aspirate
Significance: Necessary if any other blood cell line is abnormally low or if the WBCs appear dysmorphic. Need to rule out malignancy, myelodysplasia, or other marrow processes. Send cytogenetics when possible.

Test: Chest x-ray
Significance: Pneumonia, tuberculosis.

Issues for Referral

• WBC counts greater than 50,000/mm³
• Any indication of malignancy
• Any indication of a rheumatologic etiology
• Inability to find an etiology with a persistent leukocytosis

 ## Emergency Care

• Antibiotics if a child appears septic.
• Patient should be started on fluids containing bicarbonate and allopurinol if leukemia is suspected, and sent to a pediatric oncology center.

Clinical Pearls

Beware of any differential that has a high percentage of monocytes or atypical lymphocytes whether machine generated or manual. These are the cell types most commonly mistaken for leukemic blasts.

 ## Common Questions and Answers

Q: Infectious mononucleosis (IM) and acute lymphocytic leukemia have many similar signs and symptoms. How can I differentiate them?
A: Both can present with fever, malaise, headache, prominent lymphadenopathy, organomegaly, and suppressed hemoglobin and platelet counts. IM tends to be associated with a sore throat and children with ALL are more likely to complain of bony pain. The easiest way to differentiate the two is a careful exam of the peripheral smear. A heterophil AB or monospot can be sent and, if positive, help with the diagnosis.

Q: What does "left-shifted" mean?
A: There are early granulocyte precursors (metamyelocytes, myelocytes) seen in the peripheral smear with a bandemia and neutrophilia. Often seen with bacteremia or marrow recovery from a suppressing drug/virus.

BIBLIOGRAPHY

Gin-Shaw S, Moore GP. Selected white cell disorders. *Emerg Med Clin North Am* 1993;11(2): 495–516.

Hoffbrand AV, Pettit JE, eds. *Color atlas of clinical hematology*, 2nd ed. Mosby-Wolfe, 1994.

Peterson L, Hrisinko MA. Benign lymphocytosis and reactive neutrophilia. *Clin Lab Med* 1993;13(4):863–877.

Author: Susan R. Rheingold

Lower GI Bleeding

 ## Database

DEFINITION

Lower gastrointestinal (GI) bleeding refers to bleeding from the lower GI tract. It can be hematochezia (passage of bright red or dark blood per rectum) or melena (passage of dark, black or tarry stools).

 ## Differential Diagnosis

- The majority of patients with lower GI bleeding have a fissure or infection.
- Mucosal lesions are more likely to be associated with antecedent occult bleeding.
- In most of patients the bleeding stops spontaneously.

Reasons for Lower GI Bleeding at Different Ages

Neonatal Period

- Anal fissure
- Necrotizing enterocolitis
- Enteric infections
- Allergic colitis
- Lymphonodular hyperplasia (LNH)
- Upper GI source
- Duplication cyst
- Enterocolitis with Hirschsprung disease
- Meckel diverticulum
- Vascular malformations
- Shock with ischemic bowel
- Hemorrhagic disease of the newborn

Infancy

- Anal fissure
- Enteric infections
- Allergic colitis
- Intussusception
- Meckel diverticulum
- Lymphonodular hyperplasia (LNH)
- Upper GI source
- Duplication cyst
- Enterocolitis with Hirschsprung disease
- Vascular malformation
- Shock with ischemic bowel
- Gangrenous bowel

Preschool Aged

- Anal fissure
- Enteric infections
- Polyps
- Parasites
- Meckel diverticulum
- Intussusception
- LNH
- Inflammatory bowel disease (IBD)
- Enterocolitis with Hirschsprung disease
- Hemolytic uremic syndrome
- Shock with ischemic bowel
- Gangrenous bowel
- Vascular malformation
- Child abuse

School Aged

- Anal fissure
- Enteric infections
- IBD
- Intussusception
- Meckel diverticulum
- Polyps
- Henoch Schöenlein purpura (HSP)
- Hemolytic uremic syndrome (HUS)
- Parasites
- Child abuse
- Vascular malformations

Adolescent

- Anal fissure
- Enteric infections
- IBD
- HUS
- Intussusception
- Midgut volvulus
- Vascular malformations
- LNH
- Parasites

Approach to the Patient

GENERAL GOALS

Determine location of bleeding, the cause, and begin stabilization and treatment

Phase 1: Determine if there is blood or other cause of red or black stools. Hematest the stool.

Phase 2: Assess patient to determine etiology; follow history, physical, and laboratory.

Phase 3: Stabilize patient, decide if emergency treatment is needed or if referral is appropriate. (See Emergency Care.)

HINTS FOR SCREENING PROBLEM

- The rate of bleeding will determine the clinical presentation.
- The more rapid the rate, the larger the volume of lower GI bleeding, and greater the drop in hemoglobin and change in pulse and blood pressure.
- Any significant blood loss will lead to pallor, tachycardia, orthostasis, poor capillary refill, CNS changes (restlessness, confusion), and hypotension.
- Hypotension may not be seen even in the face of significant blood loss, because vasoconstriction will occur to maintain blood pressure until decompensation.
- Initial hemoglobin values may be unreliable since a delay in hemodilution may falsely result in near-normal values.
- In newborn, determine if this is swallowed maternal blood.

 ## Data Gathering

HISTORY

Question: Is this really blood?
Significance: Get a history and check if any recently ingested foods resemble blood, e.g., red dye, beets, Jell-O, Kool-Aid.

Question: Color of blood
Significance: If bright red then site of bleeding is probably in left colon, rectosigmoid or anal canal, if darker red then from right colon, if melena or tarry then bleeding is proximal to ileocecal valve.

Question: Check location of blood in relation to the stool
Significance: In colitis the blood will be mixed with the stool, with a fissure it will be in streaks on the outer aspect of the stool.

Question: Determine consistency of the stool
Significance: If diarrhea, more likely to be colitis, if hard then more likely to be a fissure.

Question: Painful stools?
Significance: Suggest anal fissure or local proctitis.

Question: Painless rectal bleeding?
Significance: Associated with polyps and Meckel diverticulum.

Question: Abdominal pain?
Significance: Can be seen with colitis, IBD, or surgical abdomen.

Question: Any underlying known GI disease, previous GI surgery?
Significance: Past history of colitis, Hirschsprung disease, necrotizing enterocolitis.

Question: Any history of jaundice, hepatitis, liver disease, neonatal history?
Significance: Suggestive of portal vein thrombosis (sepsis, shock, exchange transfusion, omphalitis, IV catheters), portal hypertension, and variceal bleeding.

Question: Any familial history of bleeding diathesis?
Significance: von Willebrand disease, hemophilia

- Any medications that can cause bleeding—heparin, warfarin?
- Any associated symptoms?

—Mouth ulcers
—Weight loss
—Joint pains as in IBD
—Petechiae
—Renal insufficiency
—History of ingestion of uncooked meat as in HUS
—Purpuric rash as in HSP
—Severe abdominal pain and vomiting as in a surgical abdomen

Physical Examination

Finding: Skin
Significance:

- Petechiae
- Ecchymosis
- Purpura
- Hemangiomas
- Evidence of chronic liver disease

—Spider angiomata
—Palmar erythema

- Jaundice

Finding: HEENT: freckles on buccal mucosa
Significance: Peutz-Jeghers syndrome

Finding: Mouth ulcers
Significance: Crohn disease

Finding: Abdomen: hepatosplenomegaly, ascites
Significance: Portal hypertension

Finding: Isolated splenomegaly
Significance: Cavernous transformation of the portal vein

Finding: Rectal examination: evidence of any perianal disease
Significance: Source of bleeding

- IBD, bright red blood in the perianal area or on the examining glove
- Polyps bright red blood in stool

Laboratory Aids

Test: CBC
Significance: Iron-deficiency anemia. If there is leukopenia, anemia, and thrombocytopenia think chronic liver disease and portal hypertension. If there is anemia with normal RBC indices, then there is truly an acute cause for bleeding. If RBC indices indicate iron-deficiency anemia, think of varices or a mucosal lesion, i.e., chronic blood loss. If thrombocytopenia, think HUS.

Test: Coagulation profile
Significance: If PT/PTT are abnormal then think of liver disease or disseminated intravascular coagulation (DIC) with sepsis. If DIC screen is negative, think liver disease.

Test: Renal function tests (BUN, creatinine, urine analysis)
Significance: Abnormal in HUS, HSP

Test: Liver function tests
Significance: Abnormal in chronic liver disease

Test: Stool tests
Significance: Stool culture (*Salmonella, Shigella, Campylobacter, Yersinia, Aeromonas, E. coli*), stool for *Clostridium difficile* toxin A and B, three stool samples for ova and parasites (amoeba). Stool smears for white blood cells (not always positive in colitis) and eosinophils (not always positive in allergic colitis).

Test: Abdominal x-ray
Significance: Helpful in surgical abdomen (dilated bowel, air-fluid levels, perforation), constipation (presence of excessive stool), or colitis (edematous bowel, thumb-printing) and toxic megacolon.

Test: Lower and upper endoscopy
Significance: Full colonoscopy to the terminal ileum helpful in diagnosing IBD. Upper endoscopy diagnostic in massive upper GI bleeds presenting with hematochezia.

Test: Barium tests
Significance: Barium enema is diagnostic and therapeutic in intussusception. Contraindicated in moderate and severe colitis. Air contrast barium enema is helpful in diagnosing mucosal lesions (polyps). Upper GI series with small bowel follow through is helpful in evaluating anatomy and Crohn disease and its complications (fistula, sometimes ulcer may be identified). Enteroclysis or small bowel enema provides good mucosal detail.

Test: Meckel scan
Significance: Diagnostic for Meckel diverticulum that secrete acid. There may be false-negatives if the Meckel diverticulum has different tissue expression.

Test: Bleeding scan
Significance: Useful in the patient in whom endoscopy was not diagnostic. Technetium sulfur colloid versus tagged RBC scan. The former detects rapid bleeding but can miss small bleeds, especially if patient is not bleeding during the scan. The latter can detect small bleeds, especially if intermittent.

Test: Angiography
Significance: Useful in detecting vascular causes for GI bleeding. Can also be therapeutic.

Emergency Care

- If patient critical, stabilize the patient with intravenous fluids and blood products.
- Order laboratory tests: CBC, PT/PTT, DIC screen, liver function tests, blood type, and crossmatch.
- Insert an NG tube and lavage with saline if it is unclear whether the patient is having hematochezia due to massive bleeding from the upper GI tract.
- Monitor patient's vital signs and hemoglobin as necessary.
- Make appropriate diagnosis and institute appropriate therapy, i.e., abdominal x-ray, colonoscopy, bleeding scans.

PITFALLS

- Make sure red substance in stool is really blood and not food coloring.
- Initial hemoglobin if normal may be misleading.

Common Questions and Answers

Q: What is the most common cause of lower GI bleeding?
A: Throughout all age groups fissures are the leading cause followed by infections. However, in infancy, the most common cause is a fissure, in toddlers and young children—polyps, and in older children—IBD.

Q: What common foods cause stools to be red? black?
A: Red: Raspberries, cranberries, artificial coloring in cereal. Black: Bismuth, licorice.

Issues for Referral

The following patients should be referred to a specialist:

- Any patient with significant acute lower GI bleeding after initial stabilization
- Patients with less acute bleeding for whom an easily identifiable cause has not been found (e.g., fissures, infection, intussusception, Meckel diverticulum); patients with chronic or recurrent lower GI bleeding.

Clinical Pearls

- Anal fissure: Treat the underlying constipation (mineral oil, lactulose, high-fiber diet). Local therapy consists of sitz baths, local emollient cremes, steroid suppositories.
- Polyp: Colonoscopy and polypectomy
- Intussusception: Barium enema is both diagnostic and permits hydrostatic reduction.
- Parasites.
- Surgery: In cases of massive or persistent bleeding with no identifiable site, exploratory laparotomy may be required.

BIBLIOGRAPHY

Chaibou M, Tucci M, Dugas MA, Farrell CA, Proulx F, Lacroix J. Clinically significant upper gastrointestinal bleeding acquired in a pediatric intensive care unit: a prospective study. *Pediatrics* 1998;102(4 Pt 1):933–938.

Irish MS, Pearl RH, Caty MG, Glick PL. The approach to common abdominal diagnosis in infants and children. *Pediatr Clin North Am* 1998;45(4):729–772.

Silber G. Lower gastrointestinal bleeding. *Pediatr Rev* 1990;12:85–93.

Author: Maria R. Mascarenhas

Mediastinal Mass

Database

DEFINITION

Any mass in the anterior, posterior, or middle mediastinum or in the pulmonary parenchyma

Differential Diagnosis

CONGENITAL/ANATOMICAL

- Thoracic meningocele
- Large normal thymus in neonate
- Bronchogenic cyst
- Pericardial cyst
- Aortic aneurysm

INFECTIOUS

May cause mediastinal adenopathy and/or a pulmonary nodule.

- Tuberculosis
- Histoplasmosis
- Aspergillosis
- Coccidioidomycosis
- Blastomycosis

TOXIC, ENVIRONMENTAL, DRUGS

- Foreign body in the trachea or esophagus

TUMOR

- Benign

—Thymoma
—Teratoma/dermoid cyst
—Lymphangioma/cystic hygroma
—Hemangioma
—Pheochromocytoma
—Ganglioneuroma
—Neurofibroma

- Malignant

—Hodgkin disease
—Non-Hodgkin lymphoma
—Leukemia
—Neuroblastoma
—Rhabdomyosarcoma
—Ganglioneuroblastoma
—Neurofibrosaroma
—Ewing sarcoma

ALLERGIC, INFLAMMATORY

- Sarcoid

COMMON CAUSES OF A MEDIASTINAL MASS

- Benign or malignant tumors
- Foreign bodies
- Infection
- Cysts

Approach to the Patient

GENERAL GOAL

Promptly establish diagnosis and begin treatment as indicated. Leukemia and lymphoma may progress rapidly and become life-threatening.

Phase 1: Identify and treat life-threatening complications promptly.

- Superior vena cava (SVC) syndrome—mass compression of the SVC resulting in decreased blood flow to the heart.
- Tracheal compression
- Spinal cord compression
- Pleural and/or pericardial effusion
- Tumor lysis syndrome—metabolic triad of hyperkalemia, hyperuricemia, and hyperphosphatemia

Phase 2:

- If mass appears solid, attempt to obtain a tissue diagnosis via biopsy or excision of mass
- If mass appears cystic, a surgical consult may be indicated
- If patient exhibits signs of infection (fever, cough, etc.), obtain appropriate cultures, place PPD and anergy panel and begin broad-spectrum antibiotics

HINTS FOR SCREENING

- Be aware that the child may be asymtomatic; the mass may be an incidental finding on chest x-ray.
- A PPD and anergy panel should always be part of the initial evaluation of a mediastinal mass if the etiology is not immediately evident.

COMPLICATIONS

- Superior vena cava (SVC) syndrome: mass compression of the SVC resulting in decreased blood flow to the heart; signs and symptoms include edema and cyanosis of the face, neck, and upper extremities, plethora, distended neck veins, cough, dyspnea, orthopnea, headache, anxiety, and confusion. Symptoms are exacerbated when child is recumbent.
- Tracheal compression: mass compression of the trachea resulting in respiratory compromise; signs and symptoms include stridor, cough, dyspnea, orthopnea.
- Spinal cord compression: symptoms vary depending on the level of the lesion.
- Pleural and pericardial effusions: resulting in respiratory distress or cardiac tamponade.
- Infection: may be the primary mass (tuberculosis) or a complication of the mass (infected cyst, infected nodes).
- Horner syndrome: ptosis, miosis, and anhydrosis resulting from compression of the cervical sympathetic nerve trunk.
- Esophageal narrowing or erosion: may result in feeding difficulty or bleeding.

Data Gathering

HISTORY

Question: Chest pain
Significance: May indicate rapidly enlarging mass

Question: Respiratory distress: stridor cough, dyspnea, orthopnea, wheezing
Significance: May indicate tracheal compression

Question: Headache, syncope, dyspnea, orthopnea, anxiety, facial swelling, eye edema
Significance: SVC syndrome

Question: Fever
Significance: Associated with infection

Question: Weight loss, night sweats
Significance: Associated with malignancies

Question: Fatigue, malaise
Significance: Associated with malignancies or infection

Physical Examination

Finding: Decreased breath sounds, wheezing, stridor
Significance: Mass may be impinging on trachea or bronchi

Finding: Diaphoresis
Significance: Seen in Hodgkin disease

Finding: Edema and cyanosis of face, neck, and upper extremities
Significance: Seen in SVC syndrome

Finding: Venous distention (jugular and superficial chest veins)
Significance: Seen in SVC syndrome

Finding: Conjunctival edema, retinal vessel engorgement
Significance: Seen in SVC syndrome

Finding: Lymphadenopathy and/or hepatosplenomegaly
Significance: Systemic process such as Hodgkin disease

Finding: Generalized bruises, petechiae, mucosal bleeding
Significance: Bone marrow involvement as in leukemia

Finding: Upper extremity and facial petechiae
Significance: Seen in SVC syndrome

PROCEDURE

- Avoid supine position in suspected SVC syndrome.
- In SVC syndrome, when the right arm is elevated the veins may remain full.

Laboratory Aids

Test: CBC with differential
Significance: Anemia, thrombocytopenia, or leukocytosis frequently noted in leukemia or lymphoma syndromes

Test: LDH, uric acid
Significance: Frequently elevated in leukemia or lymphoma syndromes

Test: Arterial blood gas
Significance: Helpful to assess tissue oxygenation if respiratory distress noted

Test: Chest x-ray (lateral film required)
Significance: Establish size and location of mass

Test: Computed tomography (CT) of the chest (if patient can tolerate recumbency)
Significance: Define size, location, and consistency of mass

Test: Magnetic resonance imaging (MRI) of the chest
Significance: Define size, location, and consistency of mass

Test: Diagnostic: lymph node aspiration/biopsy, bone marrow aspiration/biopsy, PPD skin test for tuberculosis
Significance: Establish diagnosis

Test: Diagnostic and therapeutic: pleurocentesis or pericardiocentesis, biopsy or excision of mass
Significance: Establish tissue diagnosis and relieve symptoms

Clinical Pearls

General Therapy

- Chemotherapy and/or radiation therapy for malignant tumors
- Surgical removal to establish diagnosis (pathology may be benign, malignant, or infectious) and relieve symptoms
- Antibiotics for infectious process

Immediate Therapy

If symptoms are progressing rapidly or there is evidence of SVC syndrome, tracheal compression, or spinal cord compression.

- Radiation therapy
- Steroids (may obscure the diagnosis of leukemia/lymphoma)
- Surgery

 ## Follow-Up

- Establish diagnosis and begin treatment promptly when leukemia or lymphoma is suspected because both tumors grow rapidly.
- Monitor for evidence of tumor lysis syndrome (metabolic triad of hyperkalemia, hyperuricemia, and hyperphosphatemia), which may develop early as leukemia or lymphoma is being treated.

PITFALLS

Circulatory collapse or respiratory failure can occur in children with SVC syndrome and/or tracheal compression. Avoid:

- General anesthesia: try to make the diagnosis with local or no anesthesia
- Sedation: may cause irreversible respiratory depression
- Supine position: keep head elevated to increase venous return
- Placing intravenous line in the upper extremities due to poor venous return: try to use lower extremities
- Long delays in establishing diagnosis: leukemia and lymphomas grow quickly and can rapidly impinge on vital structures

 ## Common Questions and Answers

Q: What should be done if the child is asymptomatic and mediastinal mass is an incidental finding on CXR?
A: • Careful history and physical with specific attention to pulmonary, cardiac, and hematologic systems
- Vital signs to include temperature and pulse OX
- CBC, differential, ESR, tumor lysis labs
- PPD, aneray panel
- CT or MRI of chest
- Referral to oncologist, surgeon, or infectious disease specialist, pending above results

Q: When should an oncologist be consulted?
A: With any of the following:

- Rapidly enlarging mass
- Signs and symptoms of tracheal compression, SVC syndrome, or spinal cord compression
- Hepatosplenomegaly, lymphadenopathy, bruises, or petechiae on physical examination
- Anemia, thrombocytopenia, or leukocytosis suggesting bone marrow involvement
- Malignant histology is demonstrated with biopsy
- When help is needed in establishing the diagnosis

BIBLIOGRAPHY

American Thoracic Society. Diagnostic standards and classification of tuberculosis. *Am Rev Respir Dis* 1990;142:725–735.

Bower RJ, Kiesewetter WB. Mediastinal masses in infants and children. *Arch Surg* 1977;112:1003–1009.

Hudson MM, Donaldson SS. Hodgkin's disease. *Pediatr Clin North Am* 1997;44:891–906.

Kelly KM, Lange B. Oncologic emergencies. *Pediatr Clin North Am* 1997;44:809–829.

Maity A, Goldweins JW, Lange BW, D'Angio GJ. Mediastinal masses in children with Hodgkins disease. *Cancer* 1992;69(11):2755–2760.

Schroeder H, Garwicz K, Kristinsson J, Siimer MA, Wesenberg F, Gustafsson G. Outcome after first relapse in children with acute lymphoblastic leukemia: a population-based study of 315 patients from Nordic Society of Pediatric Hematology and Oncology (NOPHO). *Med Pediatr Oncol* 1995;25(5):372–378.

Shad A, Magrath I. Non-Hodgkin's lymphoma. *Pediatr Clin North Am* 1997;44:863–890.

Shamberger RC, Holzman RS, Griscom NJ, et al. Prospective evaluation by computed tomography and pulmonary function tests of children with mediastinal masses. *Surgery* 1995; 118(3):468–473.

Author: Cynthia F. Norris

Pallor

Database

DEFINITION

Pallor is defined as paleness of the skin and may be related either to reduced hemoglobin and/or decreased blood flow to the skin.

Differential Diagnosis

CONGENITAL

- Diamond-Blackfan anemia

—Congenital pure red-cell aplasia (rare)

- Fanconi anemia

—Constellation of varied cytopenias
—Multiple congenital anomalies
—Abnormal bone marrow chromosomal fragility

- Thalassemia syndromes

—Defective globin synthesis

- Erythrocyte membrane defects

—Hereditary spherocytosis
—Elliptocytosis
—Stomatocytosis
—Pyropoikilocytosis
—Infantile pyknocytosis

- Erythrocyte enzyme defects

—Glucose-6-phosphate dehydrogenase (G6PD) deficiency
—Pyruvate kinase deficiency

- Hemoglobinopathies

—Sickle cell syndromes
—Other unstable hemoglobins

INFECTIOUS

- Septic shock
- Infection-related bone marrow suppression

—Parvovirus B19 infection

- Infection-related hemolytic anemias

—Epstein-Barr virus
—Influenza
—Coxsackievirus
—Varicella
—Cytomegalovirus
—*Escherichia coli*
—Pneumococcus
—Streptococcus
—Salmonella typhi
—Mycoplasma

TOXIC/ENVIRONMENTAL/DRUGS

- Iron-deficiency anemia

—Common cause of anemia in children, especially under the age of 3 years and in female adolescents

- Atropine ingestion
- Plumbism

—Anemia usually due to coexisting iron deficiency. Very high lead levels associated with altered heme synthesis

- Vitamin B_{12} and/or folate deficiency

—Results in a megaloblastic anemia

- Medication-induced bone marrow suppression

—Many chemotherapeutic agents for malignancy, antibiotics, especially trimethoprim-sulfamethoxazole

- Drug-related hemolytic anemia

—Antibiotics
—Antiepileptics
—Azathioprine
—Isoniazid
—Non-steroidal anti-inflammatory drugs

TRAUMA

- Acute blood loss

—Chronic blood loss often presents as iron deficiency

TUMOR

- Malignancies include leukemia, a primary bone marrow malignancy as well as any malignancy that metastasizes to the bone marrow, displacing normal marrow cells
- Histiocytosis syndromes

—Disseminated forms, marrow replacement

- Anemia of cancer even without bone marrow invasion

GENETIC/METABOLIC

- Metabolic derangements

—Severe electrolyte disturbance
—pH disturbance
—Inborn errors

- Schwachmann-Diamond syndrome

—Marrow hypoplasia with associated pancreatic insufficiency and associated failure to thrive

- Systemic diseases

—Anemia of chronic disease
—Chronic renal disease
—Uremia

- Hypothyroidism

ALLERGIC/INFLAMMATORY

- Anaphylaxis
- Disseminated intravascular coagulation

OTHER

- Transient erythroblastopenia of childhood

—Acquired pure red blood cell aplasia

- Aplastic anemia

—Bone marrow failure syndrome with at least 2 of the 3 blood cell lines eventually affected

- Sideroblastic anemia

—Defective iron utilization within the developing erythrocytes

- Autoimmune and isoimmune hemolytic anemias
- Microangiopathic hemolytic anemias

—Thrombotic thrombocytopenic purpura (TTP)
—Hemolytic uremic syndrome (HUS)
—Disseminated intravascular coagulation (DIC)

- Mechanical destruction

—Vascular malformation
—Shunts
—Abnormal valves
—Prosthetic valves

Approach to the Patient

Pallor is a common parental complaint. Determine first that the child appears pale, not simply fair-skinned. Decide if there is a medical emergency associated with circulatory failure. If not, the goal is to investigate the etiology and then intervene appropriately.

Phase 1: Quickly assess for signs of shock, indicating circulatory as opposed to hematologic etiology for pallor. If circulatory, initiate emergency procedures as required to support basic vital functions, such as airway, breathing, and circulation.

Phase 2: If patient is stable, perform history, physical examination, and CBC with reticulocyte count to establish time of onset of pallor and associated symptoms, and level of anemia.

Phase 3: Specific diagnostic work-up based on findings in phase 2.

Data Gathering

HISTORY

Question: Rapid onset? (Hours to few days)
Significance: Suggests acute blood loss, autoimmune hemolytic anemia, and/or circulatory compromise.

Question: Weight loss, fever, night sweats, cough, and/or bone pain?
Significance: Suggest an underlying systemic illness, such as leukemia, infection, collagen vascular disease.

Question: Jaundice, dark urine?
Significance: Suggests hemolysis

Question: Age between 6 months and 3 years, or adolescent females?
Significance: Peak age ranges for iron deficiency.

Question: Age less than 6 months?
Significance: May represent a congenital anemia or isoimmunization.

Question: Male?
Signficance: Some red-cell enzyme X-linked defects, such as G6PD and phosphoglycerate kinase deficiencies are sex linked.

Question: African-American?
Significance: Hemoglobins S and C, alpha and beta-thalassemia trait, G6PD deficiency.

Question: Southeast Asian?
Significance: Hemoglobin E and α-thalassemia

Question: Mediterranean descent?
Significance: β-Thalassemia and G6PD deficiency

Question: Premature infant?
Significance: Increased risk of both iron and vitamin E deficiency. Exaggerated hyperbilirubinemia can be the presenting symptom of isoimmune hemolytic or other congenital hemolytic anemia.

Question: Pica?
Significance: Pica is often associated with both plumbism and iron and vitamin deficiency.

Question: Medications?
Significance: Can cause bone marrow suppression and/or hemolysis.

Question: Recent trauma and/or surgery?
Significance: Blood loss can result in iron deficiency.

Question: Recent infection?
Significance: Can be associated with hemolysis or bone marrow suppression.

Question: Familial history?
Significance: Some of the congenital hemolytic anemias are autosomal dominant. Familial history of splenectomy and/or early cholecystectomy can be a clue for a previously undiagnosed hemolytic anemia.

 ## Physical Examination

Finding: Rapid respiratory rate, decreased blood pressure, weak pulses, slow capillary refill
Significance: Vital signs indicate pallor due to acute severe blood loss, shock, or other emergencies.

Finding: Frontal bossing and prominence of the malar and maxillary bones
Significance: Thalassemia, due to extramedullary erythropoiesis

Finding: Glossitis
Significance: Vitamin B_{12} deficiency

Finding: Retinopathy
Significance: Sometimes hemoglobin S or C disease

Finding: Icterus of sclerae and mucous membranes
Significance: May indicate hemolysis

Finding: Systolic flow murmur
Significance: Chronic anemia

Finding: Bruits
Significance: May indicate vascular malformations

Finding: Enlarged spleen
Significance: Hemolytic anemias, malignancy, infection

Finding: Petechiae and bruising
Significance: May indicate an associated thrombocytopenia, coagulopathy, or vasculitis

Finding: Dysmorphic features
Significance: Both Diamond-Blackfan and Fanconi anemias are associated with other congenital defects, including thumb abnormalities, short stature, congenital heart disease.

 ## Laboratory Aids

Test: Hemoglobin or hematocrit
Significance: Establishes the presence of anemia as the etiology for pallor

Test: Mean corpuscular volume (MCV)
Significance: Divides anemias into microcytic, normocytic, and macrocytic

Test: Reticulocyte count
Significance: Distinguishes between decreased production and increased destruction of red cells

Test: Coomb's test and antibody screen
Significance: Identifies immune-mediated red-cell destruction

Test: Peripheral blood smear
Significance: Specific morphologic findings can be diagnostic

Test: Iron studies: iron-binding capacity, serum Fe, ferritin, transferrin
Significance: Diagnosis of iron deficiency anemia or anemia of chronic disease

Test: Hgb electrophoresis, quantitative Hgb A_2 or F
Significance: Diagnosis of hemoglobinopathy

Test: Lead studies: serum lead, free erythrocyte protoporphyrin
Significance: Diagnosis of plumbism

Test: Osmotic fragility
Significance: Diagnosis of red cell membrane defects

Test: Quantitative red-cell enzyme assays
Significance: Diagnosis of inherited RBC enzyme deficiencies

Test: Serum folate, RBC folate, and serum vitamin B_{12} levels
Significance: Diagnosis of deficiency of these vitamins

Test: Bone marrow aspiration and biopsy
Significance: Diagnosis of malignancy or bone marrow failure syndrome

Issues for Referral

- Hemodynamic compromise
- Severe anemia
- Anemias other than dietary iron deficiency or anemia of chronic disease
- All bone marrow failure or infiltrative processes

Tests to prepare for consult

- Complete blood count, reticulocyte count, past blood counts if available

 ## Emergency Care

- If there is circulatory failure without anemia, treatment requires intensive monitoring and access to critical care in an emergency room or ICU. Fluid resuscitation and/or inotropic pressor support as needed.
- Acute blood loss: treat circulatory failure as described. Transfuse with packed red blood cells, platelets, and fresh frozen plasma as needed.
- Severe anemia of unclear etiology with hemodynamic instability: transfuse with packed red blood cells cautiously. In an autoimmune hemolytic process, the child is at significant risk of a hemolytic transfusion reaction. Obtain blood for diagnostic studies before transfusion.
- Malignancies: Emergency care should be directed toward treatment of circulatory failure and possible associated infection, and then to rapid diagnosis and treatment of the malignancy. Consultation with an oncologist should be sought as soon as possible.

Clinical Pearls

- Parents often fail to notice pallor of gradual onset. Grandparents or others who see child less often may be the first to suspect pallor.
- Hematologic pallor: Often well-appearing pale child with anemia. Pallor is clinically apparent when the hemoglobin is less than 9 g/dL.
- Non-hematologic pallor: Generally ill-appearing child. Any condition with peripheral vasoconstriction that alters the distribution of blood flow away from the skin surface.

BIBLIOGRAPHY

Graham EA. The changing face of anemia in infancy. *Pediatr Rev* 1995;15:175–183.

Monzon CM, Beaver D, Dillon TD. Evaluation of erythrocyte disorders with mean corpuscular volume (MCV) and red cell distribution width (RDW). *Clin Pediatr* 1987;26:632–638.

Sills RH. Indications for bone marrow examination. *Pediatr Rev* 1995;16:226–228.

Segal GB. Anemia. *Pediatr Rev* 1988;10:77–98.

Author: Debra L. Friedman

Proteinuria

 ## Database

DEFINITION

Presence of protein in urine. Usually greater than 0.3 g of protein in a 24-hour collection and/or 1 g/L (1+ or greater) on two random urine samples at least 6 hours apart on a mid-stream urine.

 ## Differential Diagnosis

CONGENITAL

- Congenital nephrotic syndrome
- Faconi syndrome
- Congenital syphilis
- Cystinosis

INFECTIONS

- Viral

—Hepatitis B, Epstein-Barr virus, cytomegalovirus, HIV

- Bacterial

—Acute poststreptococcal glomerulonephritis
—Subacute bacterial endocarditis
—Urinary tract infections

- Parasitic

—Malaria
—Schistosomiasis

TOXIC, ENVIRONMENTAL, DRUGS

- Allergens

—Pollens, inhalants

- Venoms

—Bees and snakes

- Immunizations
- Heavy metals
- Heroin
- Medicines

—Captopril
—Penicillamine, non-steroidal anti-inflammatory agents, aminoglycosides

INFLAMMATORY

Renal

Glomerular disease

- Minimal change nephrotic syndrome
- Hereditary nephritis
- Membranoproliferative glomerulonephritis
- Membranous glomerulonephritis
- Messangial proliferative glomerulonephritis
- Focal segmental glomerulosclerosis
- Henoch-Schönlein syndrome
- IGA nephropathy
- Systemic lupus erythematosus nephritis
- Systemic vasculitides
- Shunt nephritis
- Subacute bacterial endocarditis

METABOLIC

- Hypokalemic nephropathy
- Diabetic nephropathy
- Hypothyroidism

TUMOR

- Wilms tumor
- Carcinomas
- Lymphoma
- Leukemia

ISOLATED PROTEINURIA

- Orthostatic proteinuria
- Persistent asymptomatic proteinuria

HEMATOLOGY

- Sickle cell disease
- Renal vein thrombosis
- Hemolytic uremic syndrome (HUS)

MISCELLANEOUS

- Orthostatic proteinuria
- Strenuous exercise
- Fever
- Emotional stress
- Cold exposure
- Congestive heart failure
- Seizure

Tubulointerstitial disease

- Ischemic tubular injury
- Reflux nephropathy
- Interstitial nephritis

Approach to the Patient

GENERAL GOAL

Determine the etiology of the proteinuria and determine what therapy there is to possibly treat the problem.

Phase 1: In most healthy patients proteinuria is a isolated finding that is usually benign, it is important based on the history, physical examination, and laboratory test to determine the severity of the proteinuria in order to determine which can safely be evaluated without referral.

Phase 2: If the finding is severe (e.g., in the nephrotic range proteinuria) it must be decided what should be done for the patient acutely to stabilize, and then whether or not transfer to nephrologist care for additional evaluation.

Phase 3: If the patient is clinically stable, it is up to the primary care physician to do screening tests to help additionally delineate the etiology of the proteinuria. Phone consultation with a pediatric nephrologist may be helpful in this task of initial labs.

Phase 4: Inquire about other medical problems of the patient.

 ## Data Gathering

HISTORY

Question: Is there a pre-existing history of renal disease?
Significance: Obviously, in case of proteinuria a prior history of renal disease will allow the physician to a more aggressive approach to the patient. Even the history of nephritis in the past can be important finding in the evaluation.

Question: Is there a history of abnormal screening urinalyses?
Significance: It is common for primary care physicians to use colormetric urine dip stick at well child check-ups. In the case of proteinuria (1+ or greater), it is important to see if there is a previous history of protein in the urine.

Question: Is there a history of previous or multiple urinary tract infections?
Significance: Urinary tract infection can be associated to other renal/urinary tract problems, such as vesico-ureteral reflux, which leads to damage of the kidneys and thus proteinuria.

Question: Is there history of a preceding illness?
Significance: Occasionally, a disease can precede the onset of nephrosis.

Question: Familial history of renal disease, metabolic disease, or mental retardation?
Significance: Some renal diseases are inherited or associated with genetic diseases, which cause mental retardation.

Question: Recent heavy exercise?
Significance: Strenuous exercise can cause a transient proteinuria trace to 1+ on urine dipstick. Follow-up urinalysis without exercise in previous 24 hours or test for orthostatic proteinuria should be done.

Question: Does the child have an unremarkable previous medical history?
Significance: A majority of children will have no significant past medical history for renal disease. Based on data a small percentage of people will have persistent proteinuria on follow testing.

 ## Physical Examination

Finding: Hypertension
Significance: Hypertension greater than the 95 percentile for gender and age is important to evaluate for renal disease. Proteinuria and hypertension should quickly alert the primary care physician to focus on a renal etiology.

Finding: Edema (usually dependent and pitting)
Significance: In severe proteinuria, edema may be present in the patient. Edema is the result of third spacing of fluid into the interstitial tissues. In general, the appearance of edema can have intravascular hypovolemic dehydration. Potassium sparing diuretics are usually chosen in hypoproteinemic edema. Loop and thiazide diuretics can exacerbate a patient in the intravascular hypovolemic state (*see* Nephrotic syndrome).

Finding: Acites/pleural effusion
Significance: The spacing of fluid usually results of fluid in the peritoneal cavity (ascites). The fluid may move into the pleural cavity from the abdominal cavity. This fluid is at risk for secondary infection.

Finding: Shifting dullness in abdomen
Significance: As the patient is rolled from side to side, percussion of the abdomen will show dullness following the shifting of the ascitic fluid.

Finding: Purpura
Significance: Henoch-Schönlein purpura (HSP) can be a reason for renal disease. Purpura is usually on the buttocks, lower extremities, and dependent areas.

Finding: Suprapubic and costovertebral tenderness
Significance: Urinary tract infections or pyelonephritis can be a cause of isolated proteinuria. White blood cells, nitrites, and blood are also present with infection.

 ## Laboratory Aids

Test: Urine colormetric dip stick
Significance: A quick and reliable method to evaluate proteinuria; 1+ or greater should lead a physician to evaluate a patient for etiology of the finding. This test also allows a family member to follow proteinuria at home and notify the physician or changes in a patient's physiology. If follow-up urines are 100% positive (1+ or greater), the physician should test conduct a 24-hour collection and then consider referral to a nephrologist. See table Relationship Between Urine Protein and Dipstick Results.

Relationship Between Urine Protein and Dipstick Results

GRADE	PROTEIN MEASUREMENTS (MG/DL)
Trace	10–20
1+	30
2+	100
3+	300
4+	1000–2000

Test: 24-Hour collection of urine
Significance: After the collection, an analysis of total protein, creatinine, and electrolytes can be studied. In the evaluation of orthostatic proteinuria, the 24-hour collection can be split into standing and recumbent collections. In this case, the overnight, recumbent sample should be less than 100 mg and the rest of the collection should have protein. However, the standing protein can be 2 to 3 times the level of the recumbent. Normal result is less than 4 mg/m^2 per hour. A pediatric phone consult may necessary to help with the work-up. If the results are greater than 2 g, please see section on nephrotic syndrome. See table 24-Hour Urine Collection Values.

Test: Metabolic serum chemistry including blood urea nitrogen (BUN), creatinine, total protein, albumin, and cholesterol
Significance: Renal failure can be identified with a rise in BUN and creatinine nine as well as hyperkalemia. Hypoproteinemia, hypoalbuminemia and hypercholesteremia are seen in nephrotic syndrome (*see* Nephrotic syndrome).

Test: Urine culture
Significance: In a majority of cases of urinary tract infection, proteinuria can be present. Appropriate antibiotic therapy can treat the infection and in most cases the proteinuria will discontinue. Follow-up urinalysis as well as additional tests should be done if the proteinuria persists.

Test: Additional renal/immunology tests
Significance: Not all the tests are need to evaluate proteinuria, every patient history and physical examination will help determine which tests are needed. They may include an ASO titer, creatinine clearance, urine sediment evaluation by urinalysis, C3, and/or CTXT0 complement level, circulating immune complexes, antinuclear antibody (ANA), hepatitis B surface antigen.

 ## Common Questions and Answers

Q: Is proteinuria serious?
A: In most cases proteinuria is a benign condition usually related to strenuous exercise, orthostatic proteinuria. Most children will need serial physical examinations as well as checking the urine.

24-Hour Urine Collection Values

Normal values: <4 mg/m^2/hr
Abnormal: 4–40/m^2/hr
Nephrotic range: >40 mg/m^2/hour

Q: Are most forms of proteinuria treatable?
A: In the case of orthostatic and transient proteinuria require no treatment. In some cases, autoimmune may be treated with immunosuppressives. Minimal change nephrotic syndrome can be treated (*see* Nephrotic syndrome).

Issues for Referral

• The person who has unstable vital signs or appears to be septic may need referral. Children with ascites are at risk of peritonitis and can develop complications from spreading of the bacteria. Correction of blood pressure should be done after close evaluation fluid intravascular status is understood. Children can have total body fluid overload and have decreased intracellular fluid. In these cases aggressive diuretic therapy can worsen the patient condition.
• Children with signs of kidney failure, electrolyte abnormalities, non-orthostatic persistent proteinuria, hematuria, hypertension, edema, and or purpura/vasculitis.
• The child with positive familial history of severe renal disease and has developed similar symptoms. Renal biopsy may be needed to be performed by a nephrologist.
• Orthostatic, transient, persistent asymptomatic proteinurias are all diseases that should be followed with serial urine dip analysis and blood pressure measurement. Persistent asymptomatic proteinuria should be followed but many will persist without any additional progression.

Clinical Pearls

• In the routine screening of urine colormetric dip sticks first morning urine are preferable. Because orthostatic proteinurias outlook is common, this is the first test that should be done.
• False-positive proteinuria exists and the usual causes can result from alkaline urine (pH >8), overlong emersions in urine, placing in the direct stream of urine, pyuria, false negatives can exist also in case when the urine is too dilute or a different protein is being excreted other albumin.
• The urine dip stick should be read within 1 minute. After that, the color will become darker and give a false-positive test.
• Trace protein is normal.

BIBLIOGRAPHY

Ettenger RB. The evaluation of the child with proteinuria. *Pediatr Ann* 1994;(23)1:486–494.

Norman ME. An office approach to hematuria and proteinuria. *Pediatr Clin North Am* 1987;34(30):545–560.

Author: Charles I. Schwartz

Pruritus

Database

DEFINITION

Itching, an unpleasant cutaneous sensation that provokes the desire to rub or scratch the skin to obtain relief.

Differential Diagnosis

CONGENITAL/ANATOMICAL

• Cholestasis secondary to biliary obstruction

INFECTIONS

• Pinworm (enterobius vermicularis)
• Swimmer itch: due to fresh water mammalian or avian schistosomes
• Herpes viruses: primary Varicella infection or zoster, Herpes simplex
• *Borrelia burgdorferi:* erythema chronicum migrans lesion of Lyme disease
• *Streptococcus pyogenes:* sandpaper rash of scarlet fever
• Tinea
• *Toxocara canis*

TOXIC

• Contact dermatitis

—Allergens
  —Plants (Rhus dermatitis—poison ivy)
  —Cosmetics
  —Dyes
  —Medications
—Irritants
  —Soaps
  —Detergents and other chemicals
  —Excrement
  —Wool
  —Fiberglass

ENVIRONMENTAL

• Papular urticaria: bites of fleas, mosquitoes, etc.
• Pediculosis (lice)
• Mites: scabies (*Sarcoptes scabei*), chiggers (*Enterobicula alfreddugesi*), etc.
• Subcutaneous foreign body
• Phytophotodermatitis occurs when skin is exposed to sunlight after contact with an offending plant

DRUGS

• Systemic use of medications such as aminophylline, aspirin, barbiturates, erythromycin, gold, griseofulvin, iodine contrast dyes, isoniazid, opiates, phenothiazines, vitamin A

ALLERGIC, INFLAMMATORY

• Atopic dermatitis (eczema)
• Psoriasis
• Seborrheic dermatitis

MISCELLANEOUS

• Non-specific urticaria
• Pityriasis rosea
• Asteatotic eczema—"winter itch"
• Xerosis (dry skin)—from excess bathing with or without strong detergents or low humidity, idiopathic

Approach to the Patient

GENERAL GOALS

Determine severity and if the pruritus is isolated or due to an underlying systemic illness primarily by assessing the presence or absence of associated signs and symptoms, especially rash.

Phase 1: Assess the severity of the illness. Pruritus will rarely be an element of a medical emergency except in the cases of anaphylaxis or erythema multiforme-major (i.e., Stevens-Johnson syndrome).

Phase 2: Determine if the itch is isolated or if there are any associated signs or symptoms. Pruritus is most frequently associated with rash. Pruritus with or without rash may be a manifestation of systemic illness. A thorough review of potential precipitating events and the duration of symptoms should be sought. Aside from the obvious need for a thorough examination of the skin, one should pay particular attention to manifestations of underlying diseases and physiologic states. Underlying states may range from hepatic or renal diseases to pregnancy or psychiatric disease. As always, one's differential diagnosis should consider common causes first, then entertain less common and even rare causes.

Phase 3: A thorough history and examination should narrow the differential diagnosis considerably, enabling the clinician to determine the underlying cause of the complaint in the majority of causes. Laboratory tests may be indicated in cases where the diagnosis is unclear.

HINTS FOR SCREENING PROBLEM

One may want to ask if this is a new or recurrent problem. If it is new, one should ask if there is anything new in the child's life that may be associated with the onset of the pruritus (with or without rash). This is often the most revealing question as one may find that the child recently came in contact with a new item, which is known to be a contact irritant (see table below).

Data Gathering

HISTORY

Question: Has anything new or different been introduced to the child, especially anything that comes in contact with their skin?
Significance: See the table on the previous page for a list of potential contact irritants (see table Potential Contact Irritants).

Question: How often is the child bathed and with what?
Significance: Different soaps or detergents contain additives that may be more or less allergenic. Changes in soaps may be important as stated previously. Some soaps cause excessive dryness or possess heavy fragrances. Children who are bathed frequently with anything more than water may develop dry and irritated (pruritic) skin.

Question: Has the child been hiking or camping in a wooded area?
Significance: May be a clue to common skin irritation such as rhus dermatitis or poison ivy.

Question: Are there any underlying illness(es)?
Significance: There is a long list of illnesses that are associated with pruritus (see table Causes of Pruritus in Children).

Question: Is anyone else itching?
Significance: This may identify a common source of a contact irritant. Also, it is common to see more than one family member with scabies or lice.

Question: Accompanied by rash or other signs and symptoms?
Significance: This general question is meant to elicit additional signs and symptoms of any of the systemic diseases listed in the table. For instance, arthritis and athralgias in SLE or JRA, jaundice in the cholestatic disorders.

Question: Has this ever happened before?
Significance: Atopic dermatitis will present as chronic or recurrent pruritic skin lesions.

Physical Examination

Finding: If rash is present, what is the appearance?
Significance:

• Lesions appear in crops with varicella zoster, scabies, insect bites
• Lesions are in groups of 3 or 4 with a central punctum in scabies

Potential Contact Irritants

Shoes	Clothing	Diapers	Cosmetics
Dyes (for hair, etc.)	Detergents	Excrement	Plants (e.g., cacti)
Jewelry (nickel)	Systemic medications	Topical medications	Foods
Wool	Fiberglass	Animals	Capsaicin in hot peppers

- Papular lesions occur with insect bites, chiggers, pediculosis, contact dermatitis, pityriasis rosea, urticaria (wheal), and atopic dermatitis
- Plaque and scale formation occur with psoriasis, xerosis, tinea, atopic dermatitis
- Serpiginous lesions occur with cutaneous larva migrans and myiasis (or maggots)
- Vesicular lesions occur with varicella (generalized), scabies, poison ivy (linear), and atopic dermatitis
- Dry skin (xerosis) occurs with atopic dermatitis
- Christmas tree pattern occurs with pityriasis rosea

Finding: What is the location of the itch and/or rash?
Significance:

- Generalized distribution occurs with varicella
- Anus: consider pinworms
- Back: consider pityriasis rosea
- Axillae and/or diaper area: consider seborrheic dermatitis and scabies
- Dorsal foot: consider shoe dermatitis from rubber or tanning agents
- Exposed surfaces: consider swimmer itch and poison ivy
- Finger, ear lobe, wrist, or necklace distribution: consider irritant contact dermatitis (e.g., nickel)
- Interdigital areas: consider tinea pedis, scabies
- Palms and/or soles: consider biliary cirrhosis
- Plantar foot: consider cutaneous larva migrans
- Scalp: consider pediculosis (nits found cemented to hair shaft) and tinea capitis

Finding: Abnormal affect or mood?
Significance: If after an exhaustive search there appears to be no physiological basis for the itch, one must consider whether the complaint is psychosomatic or due to neurotic excoriation especially in cases of abnormal affect or mood.

 ## Laboratory Aids

Test: Wood light examination, KOH preparation.
Significance: Screen for tinea infections.

Test: Skin scraping in oil under cover slip.
Significance: Verify presence of mites in scabies.

Test: Perianal adhesive tape slide (preferably early morning).
Significance: Verify pinworm.

Test: Serum for hepatic and renal function.
Significance: Screen for underlying disease.

Test: Urine β-HCG
Significance: Investigate presence of cholestasis associated with pregnancy.

Indications for Referral

- Identification of an underlying state, such as pregnancy, or hepatic, renal, or psychiatric disease.
- Some severe cases of atopic dermatitis or psoriasis (may require dermatological referral).
- Identification of pubic pediculosis (may require investigation into abuse).

 ## Emergency Care

- Pruritus due to anaphylaxis will require initial management of airway, breathing, and circulation (ABCs) followed by sympathomimetics (such as epinephrine), antihistamines (such as diphenhydramine), corticosteroids, and possibly fluid resuscitation.
- Pruritus associated with Stevens-Johnson syndrome will require the equivalent of burn management with the need for fluid resuscitation.

Clinical Pearls

- Pruritis that is worse at night points to either scabies or pinworm.
- If the child was recently swimming in fresh water, one should consider swimmer itch, caused by fresh water mammalian or avian schistosomes.

Common Questions and Answers

Q: Is there any symptomatic treatment for pruritus other than antihistamines?
A: There have been a number of anecdotal references to other agents being effective for pruritus including: ursodeoxycholic acid in liver disease, opiate antagonists (such as naloxone and naltrexone), propofol at subhypnotic doses, cholestyramine, rifampin, and serotonin antagonists.

Q: Does the time course of a pruritic rash give any clue in identifying the offending agent?
A: Yes, certain plants will cause an immediate welt on the skin but the urticaria will be short-lived (immediate contact dermatitis). Skin that is traumatized mechanically (e.g., cactus spine) or chemically (e.g., capsaicin in hot peppers) produce more persistent skin reactions. Poison ivy or Rhus dermatitis is a type of allergic contact dermatitis that only occurs in previously sensitized persons. It is due to a cellular immune response and may last several weeks.

BIBLIOGRAPHY

Gilchrist BA. Pruritus: pathogenesis, therapy and significance in systemic disease states. *Arch Intern Med* 1982;142:101.

Greaves MW. Anti-itch treatments: do they work? *Skin Pharmacol* 1997;10:225–229.

Greaves MW, Wall PD. Pathophysiology of itching. *Lancet* 1996;348:938–40.

Hagermark O, Wahlgren CF. Treatment of itch. *Semin Dermatol* 1995;14:320–325.

Author: Mark L. Bagarazzi

Causes of Pruritus in Children

MOST COMMON	LESS COMMON	RARE
Atopic dermatitis (eczema)	Anaphylaxis	Collagen—vascular disorders
Contact dermatitis	Cholestasis	Juvenile rheumatoid arthritis
Allergens: plants ("poison ivy"), cosmetics, dyes, medications	Drug-induced (*e.g.* total parenteral nutrition)	Systemic lupus erythematosus
Irritants: soaps, detergents and other chemicals, excrement, wool, fiberglass	Extrahepatic biliary obstruction	Congenital ectodermal disorders
Cutaneous infections	Biliary cirrhosis	Parvovirus B19 infection
Varicella-zoster virus (chicken pox)	Cutaneous infections	Endocrinological disorders
Tinea infections	Cutaneous larva migrans— "creeping eruption"	Carcinoid syndrome
Pinworm	Hookworm	Diabetes mellitus
Papular urticaria—bites of fleas, mosquitoes, etc.	Cercariasis (Onchocercaria volvulus)	Hyper/hypothyroidism
Pediculosis (lice)	Trichinosis	Hypoparathyroidism
Mites—scabies (*Sarcoptes scabei*), chiggers (*Enterobicula alfreddugesi*), etc.	Myiasis (maggots)	Neurologic syndromes
Seborrheic dermatitis	Neurotic excoriation	Erythropoeitic protoporphyria
Xerosis (dry skin)—due to:	Chronic renal failure—with or without "uremic frost"	Psychosomatic disorders
Excess bathing with or without strong detergents	Hematopoietic neoplasms	Hematopoietic neoplasms
Low humidity	Hodgkin disease	Polycythemia vera
Non-specific urticaria	Lymphoma	Mastocytosis
	Leukemia	Solid organ neoplasms
	Iron deficiency anemia	

Psychiatric or Behavioral Problems

 ## Database

DEFINITION

Behavioral, developmental, or psychosocial problems that require medical or psychiatric treatment, or which cause the child significant impairment.

 ## Differential Diagnosis

ORGANIC CAUSES

- CNS infections or parainfectious syndromes
- Substance abuse, toxic ingestions, medication adverse effects
- Intracranial trauma or other injury
- CNS tumors
- Endocrine disorders

—Thyroid or adrenal dysfunction

- Metabolic disorders

—Abnormal glucose
—Sodium
—Potassium
—Calcium

- Migraines
- Seizure disorders
- Hematologic disorders

—Porphyria
—Severe anemia

- Hypoxia
- Other cardiopulmonary disturbances

Among psychobehavioral disorders, many disorders have similar symptoms. For example:

- Attention deficit/hyperactivity disorder (ADHD) may be difficult to distinguish from mood (depression or bipolar disorder), anxiety (including school phobia), post-traumatic stress, and tic disorders, substance abuse, hearing or vision impairment, and learning disabilities.
- Social withdrawal may be a sign of depression, neglect, PDD, sensory impairment (e.g., deafness), or learning disability.
- Psychotic symptoms are seen not only in psychotic disorders, but also in mood disorders (depression, bipolar disorder), borderline personality disorder, and substance abuse.

Aggressive or violent behavior is not a diagnosis unto itself, but can represent a final common pathway of depression, psychosis, delirium, substance abuse, ADHD (uncommon), physical or sexual abuse, or family dysfunction.

Approach to the Patient

GENERAL GOALS

Phase 1: Rule out organic causes.

Phase 2: As organic causes are being investigated, establish psychiatric/psychological causes as a possible diagnosis.

Phase 3: Work with the family to accept possibility of psychiatric/psychological diagnosis and facilitate referral to mental health services.

HINTS FOR SCREENING PROBLEMS

- There is strong evidence for a heritable/genetic risk of bipolar disorder (manic-depression), schizophrenia, and depression. There is less strong, but growing evidence that other conditions, e.g., anxiety, ADHD, pervasive developmental disorder (PDD), and tic disorders, may be genetically transmissible. Twin studies (monozygotic versus dizygotic) suggest that personality disorders have a significant genetic component.
- Many disorders, e.g., ADHD (between 3:1 to 9:1), depression (1:2), etc., have distinct male:female preponderance.
- Prevalence estimates vary widely, due to differing definitions of "psychopathology." Median rates are 8% for preschoolers, 12% for preadolescents, and 15% for adolescents.
- Suicide is epidemic. Eight percent of high school students attempt suicide, 25% of which require medical attention. Fifty percent of attempters seek medical care in the month preceding their attempt, 25% in the preceding week.
- Conservative estimates of the prevalence of depression in children and adolescents range from 5% to 10%.
- Eating disorders, while relatively uncommon (0.5% to 1% prevalence), have a 5% to 15% mortality rate.

 ## Data Gathering

HISTORY

- A psychobehavioral assessment should include a history of the presenting complaint, a past medical, developmental, and behavioral/psychiatric history, and a complete familial history and review of systems.
- The "SHADSSS" mnemonic is a useful inventory of psychosocial functioning. It is structured such that the least threatening topics are asked first, the most intimate last. All of these areas of psychosocial functioning should be assessed in all patients.

—School (in school? grades? relationships with peers and teachers?)
—Home (living situation? relationship with parents? siblings?)
—Activities (how does the patient spend their free time?)
—Depression
—Substance abuse (including alcohol and tobacco)
—Sexuality (including abuse, STDs, and pregnancy)
—Safety (suicidality, homicidality, plans for revenge or violence)

Children do not exist in a vacuum. All families should receive a family assessment. Families/support systems are crucial for the ultimate success of any treatment plan. At a minimum, a family assessment should include a discussion of:

- Constitution of household, custody/visitation arrangements
- Who supervises the child or provides child care
- Stressors on the family (emotional, financial, interpersonal, violence within the family, involvement with law enforcement or social services, etc.)
- Strategies used by the family in coping with conflicts, problems, stressors, etc.

 ## Physical Examination

A thorough physical examination should be performed on all patients. The goal is to detect any abnormalities suggestive of an organic cause for the patient's symptoms (see Differential Diagnosis).

Laboratory Aids

There is no set of "routine" laboratory tests that should be ordered to rule out an organic etiology of the behavioral or psychiatric symptoms. Tests should be performed on the basis of clinical suspicion.

SPECIFIC RESOURCES

• The use of screening questionnaires (*see* BIBLIOGRAPHY), parent monitoring forms/diaries, and direct observation of parent-child interactions can be used, depending on the practitioners experience, familiarity, and confidence with these modalities, as well as the practice setting. Screening for maternal depression may also be important in detecting psychosocial dysfunction.
• The Pediatric Symptom Checklist (PSC) is a brief, parent completed questionnaire, which has been validated in a number of pediatric settings. A multitude of other screening tools have been developed, which are of varying utility to the pediatric practitioner.
• Conners Rating Scales alone are not sufficient to diagnose ADHD. It is a clinical diagnosis, based on pervasive inattention, hyperactivity, or impulsivity across different settings.
• Published in 1996 by the American Academy of Pediatrics, the *Diagnostic and Statistical Manual for Primary Care* (DSM-PC), child and adolescent version, is the result of collaborative efforts by pediatricians (primary care, and behavioral and developmental specialists), and child psychiatrists, psychologists, and neurologists. It provides a concise, user-friendly guide for diagnosing mental disorders in children and adolescents.

Clinical Pearls

• Children on psychotropic medications should be monitored for adverse effects.
• Stimulants: frequent assessment of growth, heart rate, and blood pressure every 3 to 6 months. Those on pemoline (Cylert) should have LFTs checked every 6 to 12 months.
• Tricyclic antidepressants: baseline ECG (before starting medication), and ECGs 1 month after starting medications and every 6 months thereafter.
• Antipsychotics: reassessment at 2, 4, and 12 weeks after starting medication, and every 3 to 6 months thereafter for adverse effects (dystonia, anti-cholinergic symptoms, movement disorders).

PITFALLS

• Not asking about behavioral or psychiatric problems. Parents are often reluctant to talk about such problems, thinking such problems are stigmatizing.
• Missed psychiatric diagnosis, especially suicidality, homicidality, or plans for revenge or violence.
• Confusing the degree of medical severity of a suicide attempt with the degree of suicide intent, i.e., "(S)he isn't significantly injured, so (s)he isn't seriously suicidal." Children and adolescents often misjudge the lethality of their suicide methods. All attempts must be taken seriously.
• Deciding on a diagnosis and/or treatment without a complete evaluation. Many psychiatric disorders can present in similar fashion (*see* Differential Diagnosis). The success of any treatment plan, as well as avoidance of erroneously "labeling" a child (with an incorrect diagnosis), depends on an accurate diagnosis, based on a thorough bio-psycho-social evaluation.
• Many patients with primary psychiatric disorders will present with vague physical complaints. All patients with such complaints should be screened for psychiatric problems.
• Delay in diagnosis or referral for treatment, e.g., prognosis for learning disabilities and hearing impairment is associated with timely intervention.

Common Questions and Answers

Q: When should a child be referred to a specialist?
A: Whenever there is uncertainty about diagnosis or management, or when the treatment needs of the patient exceed the practitioner's capacity to provide them.

Q: How do you get children and families to talk about their problems?
A: There is no 'trick.' Being a patient, empathetic, non-judgmental listener is the best strategy.

Q: What is constitutes a psychiatric emergency?
A: Any situation where the safety or functioning of the child, family, or another person is endangered.

BIBLIOGRAPHY

Cantwell DP. Attention deficit disorder: a review of the past 10 years. *J Am Acad Child Adolesc Psychiatry* 1996;35(8):978–987.

Clark LR, Ginsburg KR. How to talk to your teenage patients. *Contemp Adolesc Gynecol* 1995;Winter:23–27.

DeGruy FV, Pincus H. The DSM-IV-PC: a manual for diagnosing mental disorders in the primary care setting. *J Am Board Fam Pract* 1996;9(4):274–281.

Dworkin PH. Detection of behavioral, developmental, and psychosocial problems in pediatric primary care practice. *Curr Opin Pediatr* 1993;5(5):531–536.

Finney JW, Weist MD. Behavioral assessment of children and adolescents. *Pediatr Clin North Am* 1992;39(3):369–378.

Kaplan HI, Sadock BJ, Grebb JA, eds. *Synopsis of psychiatry.* Baltimore: Williams & Wilkins, 1994.

Murphy JM, Arnett HL, Bishop SJ, Jellinek MS, Reede JY. Screening for psychosocial dysfunction in pediatric practice. A naturalistic study of the pediatric symptom checklist. *Clin Pediatr (Phila)* 1992;31(11):660–677.

Roberts RE, Attkisson C, Rosenblatt A. Prevalence of psychopathology among children and adolescents. *Am J Psych* 1998;155(6):715–725.

Slap GB, Vorters DF, Khalid N, Margulies SR, Forke CM. Adolescent suicide attempters: do physicians recognize them? *J Adolesc Health* 1992;13(4):286–292.

Spencer T, Wilens T, Biederman J. Psychotropic medications for children and adolescents. *Child Adolesc Psych Clin N Am* 1995;4(1):97–121.

Stancin T, Palermo TM. A review of behavioral screening practices in pediatric settings: do they pass the test? *J Dev Behav Pediatr* 1997;18(3):183–194.

Wolralch ML. Diagnostic and statistical manual for primary care (DSM-PC) child and adolescent version: design, intent, and hopes for the future. *J Dev Behav Pediatr* 1997;18(3):171–182.

Author: Thomas H. Chun

Red Eye

Database

DEFINITION

Erythema of the ocular adnexa, conjunctiva, sclera, cornea, or inflammation of deeper structures.

Differential Diagnosis

OCULAR ADNEXA

Infectious/Inflammatory

- Hordeolum and chalazion
- Dacryocystitis
- Blepharitis
- Phthiriasis (louse)
- Frontal sinus infection or other sinusitis
- Orbital cellulitis
- Periorbital cellulitis
- Dental abscess
- Contact dermatitis
- Seborrhea

Trauma

- Frequent eye rubbing
- Blunt trauma

Tumors

- Neuroblastoma
- Leukemia
- Neurofibroma

Miscellaneous

- Cavernous sinus thrombosis
- Prolonged crying

CONJUNCTIVA

Infection

- Conjunctivitis

Trauma

- Blunt trauma or laceration

Neoplasms

- Orbital tumors (e.g., retinoblastoma)

Toxic/Environmental/Drugs

- Atropine
- Scopolamine
- Smog
- Makeup
- Smoke
- Chemical
- Contact lenses

Allergic/Inflammatory

- Allergic conjunctivitis
- Keratoconjunctivitis sicca and other dry eye disorders
- Nasal inflammation
- Sjögren syndrome and other collagen vascular diseases
- Kawasaki syndrome
- Stevens-Johnson syndrome
- Inflammatory bowel disease
- Juvenile rheumatoid arthritis

Miscellaneous

- Subconjunctival hemorrhage (secondary to severe cough, bacteremia, blood dyscrasia, or vomiting)

CORNEA

Infectious

- Keratitis
- Syphilis

Trauma

- Contact lenses
- Corneal ulcer
- Corneal abrasion
- Chemical irritant

UVEAL TRACT

Infectious

- Iridocyclitis
- Reiter syndrome

PUPIL

Trauma

- Hyphema

Approach to the Patient

GENERAL GOALS

Determine which ocular structure(s) is/are affected. This is critical in reaching an accurate diagnosis given that the differential diagnosis is determined by the site involved.

Phase 1: Determine the acuity and severity of the disease process. For example, cellulitis requires emergency treatment, while most other disorders in the differential diagnosis do not.

Phase 2: Assess whether or not referral is necessary for optimal outcome of non-emergent situations. For example, prolonged symptoms in a contact lens wearer should be referred to an ophthalmologist.

Phase 3: Good follow-up is necessary for all but the most minor eye diseases to ensure that optimal function is maintained.

Data Gathering

HISTORY

Question: Age at onset of illness?
Significance: Ocular inflammation in the first 24 hours of life is most likely the result of chemical irritation. Silver nitrate is the most frequent cause of neonatal chemical conjunctivitis, although other antibiotics used for prophylaxis can also cause conjunctivitis. Inflammation occurring between 2 and 6 days of life is likely due to gonococcal (GC) disease. Between 1 to 3 weeks of age, ocular inflammation usually represents chlamydial conjunctivitis. Older children with conjunctivitis usually have allergic or infectious disease.

Question: History of trauma?
Significance: Patients presenting with a red eye and a history of trauma need to be evaluated for a corneal abrasion.

Question: History of systemic symptoms, including fever or ill appearance?
Significance: Suggests orbital or periorbital cellulitis.

Question: Decrease in the patient's vision?
Significance: Herpes keratitis, orbital cellulitis, scars on the cornea from abrasions or foreign body may affect visual acuity.

Question: Does the patient wear contact lenses?
Significance: Protozoan infections (specifically acanthamoeba), virulent gram-negative infections, and unusual fungal infections are seen almost exclusively in people who wear contact lens.

Question: Is pruritus a prominent symptom?
Significance: May represent allergic conjunctivitis.

Physical Examination

Finding: Edema of the eyelids and conjunctivae (chemosis), local pain, and a copious purulent discharge
Significance: GC conjunctivitis. Swelling and discharge can be so extensive that the orbit may be difficult to view.

Finding: Clusters of vesicles on the face, eyelids, and mucous membranes
Significance: Suggests conjunctivitis due to herpes simplex virus.

Finding: Tearing, purulent discharge, conjunctival hyperemia, and foreign body sensation
Significance: These findings may be seen with bacterial conjunctivitis. The eyelids are often crusted and closed on arising in the morning.

Finding: Subconjunctival hemorrhage
Significance: Haemophilus influenzae and Streptococcus pneumoniae conjunctival infections are often associated with this finding.

Finding: Serous or lightly purulent discharge, profuse tearing
Significance: These findings suggest viral conjunctivitis (non-herpetic).

Finding: Significant erythema and swelling of the lids; diffuse conjunctival hyperemia, rhinitis, and other allergic symptoms may also be present.
Significance: Suggests allergic conjunctivitis.

Finding: A lesion draining on the inside of the eyelid (the conjunctival side)
Significance: This is suggestive of an infected chalazion.

Finding: Diffuse injection of the conjunctiva, watery discharge, pain, decreased visual acuity
Significance: Suggests corneal abrasion. All patients suspected of having a corneal abrasion should have a flourescein examination of the eye.

Finding: Decreased range of motion, of ocular muscles, proptosis, visual changes, or papilledema in association with a tender, erythematous or violaceous eyelid.
Significance: Orbital cellulitis carries a greater risk for damage to the visual axis than periorbital cellulitis. Fever is common.

Laboratory Aids

NEONATAL CONJUNCTIVITIS

• Bacterial culture, including chocolate agar or Thayer-Martin plates, and Gram stain of the purulent material should be obtained. In up to 95% of cases of GC conjunctivitis, gram-negative intracellular diplococci will be identified by Gram stain.
• Chlamydia culture and rapid assay: should be obtained on conjunctival scrapings (not purulent material).
• Conjunctival scrapings for herpes should be obtained if herpes conjunctivitis is part of the differential diagnosis. Culture recovery of the herpes virus is successful in only 70% of patients with herpetic conjunctivitis.

BACTERIAL AND VIRAL CONJUNCTIVITIS

• Culture is necessary only if an unusual or serious pathogen is suspected (e.g., in contact lens wearers). Generally, conjunctivitis in the older child is treated without performing diagnostic tests.

DACRYOCYSTITIS

• Cultures in cases of dacryocysitis, although not routinely indicated, are recommended if the infection does not respond to topical antibiotics.

ORBITAL AND PERIORBITAL CELLULITIS

• Blood culture: should be obtained because an organism may be isolated when there is associated bacteremia.
• Cultures of the purulent discharge: may also aid in identifying the offending organism.

RADIOGRAPHIC STUDIES

• Computed tomography: should be employed whenever orbital cellulitis is considered; is essential when neoplasm is suspected.

Issues for Referral

• Corneal abrasion: if the pain persists for more than 24 hours after the initial.
• GC conjunctivitis: an extremely invasive disease warranting early ophthalmologic input.
• Herpetic conjunctivitis
• Varicella conjunctivitis: the association with corneal destruction and loss of vision makes early referral necessary.
• Foreign body: refer if embedded, or if not easily removed in the office setting.
• Dacryocystitis: if prolonged, or resulting in inflammation/infection (cellulitis) of skin.
• Orbital cellulitis: All cases should be referred.
• Corneal abrasion: lack of improvement in pain over a 24-hour period should result in prompt referral.
• Contact lens wearers: because of the unusual organisms and increased risk for significant morbidity, all patients who wear contact lenses and present with conjunctivitis should be referred to an ophthalmologist within 12 to 24 hours.

Emergency Care

• Neonatal conjunctivitis: While the classic presentation of these infections differ, treatment should be broad until culture, immunologic studies, or clinical presentation have definitively ruled out conditions associated with poor outcomes. This includes frequent (every 1 to 2 hours) irrigation of the eye in GC conjunctivitis, and intravenous antibiotics.
• Herpes conjunctivitis. Treatment should begin immediately and consists of lubrication, patching, and treatment with acyclovir.
• Foreign body: Inability to remove an ocular foreign body should prompt immediate referral to an ophthalmologist. In addition, any open globe injury requires immediate ophthalmologic attention. The eye should be patched using an eye shield WITHOUT pressure.
• Periorbital and orbital cellulitis: Prompt initiation of therapy is important in these two serious diseases. Orbital cellulitis requires hospitalization and intravenous antibiotics. Early periorbital cellulitis can be managed on an outpatient basis if the child is not toxic-appearing and if close (at least daily) follow-up is arranged. Intramuscular ceftriaxone is appropriate for outpatient management. Surgical drainage may be required in cases of orbital cellulitis.
• Presence of a hyphema warrants immediate ophthalmology input.

Clinical Pearls

• Important note: Serious harm can result if steroids are inadvertently prescribed for a patient with herpetic conjunctivitis.

• Bacterial and viral conjunctivitis. Non-herpetic viral conjunctivitis is treated in the same fashion as bacterial conjunctivitis. Treatment involves instillation of antibiotic drops and periodic removal of eye discharge with warm, wet washcloths. Improvement usually occurs within 3–4 days. In the event of treatment failure, a second antibiotic should be chosen, with a significantly different spectrum from the first antibiotic prescribed. Treatment should begin in a timely fashion, but is not urgent or emergent.
• Corneal abrasion: Foreign bodies should be removed by irrigation with sterile saline. All patients suspected of having a corneal abrasion should have a flourescein examination of the eye. When a slit lamp is not available, this is best done with a Wood's lamp. The flourescein will flouresce over any abraded area. After careful evaluation, a sterile, light pressure-dressing should be placed over the eye for approximately 24 hours. Many also recommend topical antibiotic drops. The eye should be examined daily until fully healed. Topical anesthetics should never be given to a patient for repeated home instillation after corneal injury as it delays healing, masks further damage, and can lead to permanent corneal scarring.

Common Questions and Answers

Q: When will congenital dacryostenosis, and the resultant dacryocystitis resolve?
A: Dacryostenosis usually will spontaneously resolve by 1 year of age. If it has not, referral to an ophthalmologist for probing is recommended.

Q: How do I treat lice in the eye lashes (phthiriasis)? Aren't the pediculocides unsafe in the eyes?
A: Lindane, permethrin and other pediculocides should not be used in or near the eyes. To safely kill lice in eye lashes, coat the lashes heavily with petroleum jelly for a 12-hour (or overnight) period.

Q: Do I need to treat or worry about tiny eyelid lacerations?
A: Before choosing a treatment of cleansing and observation only, make sure the laceration does not cross or affect the tear duct which will need to be surgically repaired.

Q: Some children seem to get styes (hordeola) very frequently. What can I do to help?
A: Reduce the bacterial growth in the area by washing the eyelashes daily with baby shampoo.

BIBLIOGRAPHY

Bertolini J, Pelucio M. The red eye. *Emerg Med Clin North Am* 1995;13(3):561–579.

Gigliotti F. Acute conjunctivitis. *Pediatr Rev* 1995;16(6):203–208.

King RA. Common ocular signs and symptoms in childhood. *Pediatr Clin North Am* 1993;40:753–766.

Author: Laura N. Sinai

Short Stature

Database

DEFINITION

Short stature is defined as height below the 3rd percentile, but many pediatricians use the 5th percentile as cut-off. This means 3% or 5% of children are classified as "short." However, most short stature is not associated with pathology.

• Growth failure refers to downward crossing of the height percentile over the normal curves and eventually leads to short stature. With evidence of growth failure, diagnostic evaluation is required, even if short stature is not yet present.

• Failure to thrive refers more to children who fail to meet standards for appropriate growth and are underweight for height. They may or may not be short.

Differential Diagnosis

EXTREMES OF NORMAL GROWTH

• Familial short stature

—Short parent(s)
—Normal height velocity (around the 25th percentile)
—Normal age of onset of puberty
—Normal bone age
—Short stature throughout childhood and adolescence
—Final adult height close to the mid-parental height and around the 3rd or 5th percentile

• Constitutional short stature/delay of growth

—Height percentile below the target range defined by parental heights
—Delayed bone age
—Reduced height velocity (especially in late childhood—below 25th percentile)
—Associated with delay of adolescence
—Positive familial history, boys more often affected
—Final adult height in the normal range and commensurate with target height

• Idiopathic short stature

—Used to categorize patients otherwise normal, but who cannot be diagnosed with a variant of normal growth or any of the causes of short stature
—This is a diagnosis of exclusion and groups patients whose calculated predicted height is more than 2 SD below the mid-parental height, whose height is below the 5th percentile, with delay of skeletal maturation, and without familial history of constitutional delay of growth and adolescence.

PRIMARY SHORT STATURE

• Usually the consequence of an abnormality of the skeletal system. Bone age often not delayed or only delayed mildly.

• Skeletal defect can be primary or secondary (to a metabolic abnormality). In either case this may lead to disproportionate short stature and/or significant dysmorphism. Occasionally, the skeletal abnormalities are subtle and do not lead to disproportionate short stature.

• Skeletal dysplasia

—Osteochondrodysplasia
—Genetic transmission—many cases represent new mutation
—Defects in growth of tubular bones and/or axial skeleton
—Typical radiologic findings on skeletal survey x-ray
—More common forms include: achondroplasia, hypochondroplasia

• Short stature due to congenital error of metabolism

—Diffuse skeletal involvement
—Mostly autosomal recessive inheritance (some X-linked)
—Dysmorphic features
—Typical biochemical abnormalities
—More common type: mucopolysaccharidosis

• Chromosomal abnormalities

—Variations to autosomes or sex chromosomes
—Usually associated with other somatic abnormalities and mental retardation
—Clinical findings may be subtle
—More common forms: Trisomy 21, Trisomy 18, Trisomy 13, and Turner syndrome

• Intrauterine growth retardation (IUGR)

—Often associated with poor postnatal growth
—Cause for IUGR may come from mother, fetus, or placenta
—Primordial dwarfism: due to intrinsic fetal defect leading to both pre- and post-natal growth failure (may be associated with specific genetic anomaly)
—IUGR is seen in: fetal infection, fetal exposure to toxin, placental abnormalities, maternal disease, and fetal hormone abnormalities

SECONDARY SHORT STATURE

• Malnutrition

—Especially under 2 years of age (most common in first 6 months of life)
—Caloric—malnutrition and/or protein—malnutrition
—Vitamin and mineral deficiencies (vitamin D, iron, zinc deficiency)

• Chronic illness

—Many chronic diseases present first with poor growth
—Cardiovascular: VSD, PDA, TOF, TGV, AS, PS, aortic coarctation, AV canal
—Pulmonary: asthma, CF, corticosteroid therapy, BPD
—GI/liver: inflammatory bowel disease, celiac disease, malabsorption, short bowel syndrome, chronic gastroenteritis, CF
—Renal: NS, CGN, RTA, CRF, nephrogenic DI, uropathy, congenital anomalies
—Metabolic: poorly controlled diabetes mellitus, storage disorders
—Chronic infections (HIV) and immune deficiencies
—Hematopoietic: anemia, leukemia, SCD

• Drugs

—Corticosteroids
—Sex steroids
—Methylphenidate, dextramphetamine

• Psychosocial growth retardation
• Endocrine short stature

—Among secondary short stature, endocrine causes are least frequent

Approach to the Patient

GENERAL GOAL

Determine if the patient has short stature and/or growth failure. Determine if height alone is affected, or if growth problem includes weight and head circumference.

Phase 1: Determine if patient's profile fits normal variant of growth.

Phase 2: Determine if patient's profile fits with pathological short stature.

Phase 3: Screening evaluation, referral to pediatric endocrinologist or observation.

Data Gathering

HISTORY

Question: Is the child short for his/her parents?
Significance: Mid-parental height is calculated to estimate the expected target height. To calculate mid-parental height for a boy, add his father's height to his mother's height plus 13 cm, and divide by 2. To calculate mid-parental height for a girl, add her mother's height to her father's height minus 13 cm, and divide by 2. If the child's height percentile is out of keeping with the calculated target height, this is likely significant and a cause for this discrepancy will have to be found.

Question: What is the child's growth (or height) velocity?
Significance: Height velocity for a specific interval can be annualized and plotted on a height velocity curve. This becomes an important criterion in a patient's growth and is different from height at any point in time, which, for a major part, is a representation of the influence of things past.

Question: What is the weight-to-height ratio?
Significance: Usually increased in hypothyroidism, Cushing syndrome, pseudohypoparathyroidism, and growth hormone deficiency. Normal or decreased in emotional deprivation, anorexia, chronic renal failure, renal tubular acidosis, inflammatory bowel disease, malabsorption, malnutrition, lung and heart disease.

Question: Where there any complications during pregnancy, labor, and delivery?
Significance: Clues from the pregnancy can provide information about possible maternal disorders, intrauterine drug exposure, or placental abnormalities (infarction, insufficiency) that lead to IUGR. Birth trauma can be associated with hypopituitarism. An inquiry about the perinatal and neonatal history is also necessary.

Question: Familial history. What are the heights of the parents and grandparents? What are the heights of the siblings? Was puberty on time in both parents? Any history of endocrine disorder or chronic illness affecting a major organ system?
Significance: Calculate mid-parental height. If short stature is running in the family, this could point toward familial or genetic short stature, isolated growth hormone deficiency, or skeletal dysplasia. Delayed pubertal maturation in the parents is important for a diagnosis of constitutional growth delay. Disorders such as diabetes mellitus and insipidus, thyroiditis, hypophosphatemic rickets, arthritis, and inflammatory bowel disease can affect family members in different generations.

Question: What is the social situation of the child?
Significance: Emotional stresses affect growth and development, either directly (abnormal growth hormone production), or indirectly (inadequate nutrition).

Question: What are current eating habits and how was the past eating history? Any evidence of underutilization of calories ingested?
Significance: Estimate approximate total daily caloric intake. Detect deficiencies in certain nutrients, or the existence of abnormal eating habits (malabsorption, vitamin deficiency-rickets, anorexia, inadequate parenting).

Question: Any chronic illness? Any hospitalization, surgery, or trauma to the head?
Significance: Think respectively how chronic disorders could present with growth failure first, without specific symptoms (rheumatoid arthritis, celiac disease), how a previous hospitalization or surgery could be a clue for an underlying pathology (jaundice and hepatitis—chronic liver disease, asthma exacerbations and high-dose corticosteroids, head trauma and pituitary insufficiency).

The history should be completed by obtaining a detailed review of systems, with specific questions inquiring about the occurrence of headache, vomiting, visual disturbance (brain tumor), anorexia, diarrhea, or constipation (bowel disease, hypothyroidism), polyuria and polydypsia (diabetes mellitus, diabetes insipidus, and renal problems), and medication intake, as well as general activity pattern, sleep hygiene, and presence of allergies.

 Physical Examination

Finding: Abnormal upper/lower segment ratio
Significance: Indicative of primary short stature

Finding: Low weight/height ratio
Significance: Points toward malnutrition

Finding: Edema
Significance: Chronic renal failure

Finding: Frontal bossing, flat nasal bridge, and truncal fat deposition
Significance: Growth hormone deficiency

Finding: Abdominal distention and gluteal wasting
Significance: Malabsorption and celiac disease

Finding: Webbed neck, increased carrying angle
Significance: Turner syndrome, Noonan syndrome

Finding: Smooth tongue
Significance: Iron deficiency

Finding: Round face, ear lobe abnormality, and mental retardation
Significance: Pseudohypoparathyroidism

Finding: Temporal thinning of the hair, sparse hair, dry hair
Significance: Hypothyroidism, growth hormone deficiency, hypopituitarism

Finding: Delayed pubertal maturation
Significance: Turner syndrome, constitutional delay, hypopituitarism, hypothyroidism, inflammatory bowel disease, chronic renal disease

Finding: Leg bowing, rachitic rosary, widening of wrists
Significance: Rickets, vitamin D deficiency, malabsorption syndrome

 Laboratory Aids

If no specific cause found, screening tests are indicated.

Test: Complete blood count and differential
Significance: Anemia, infection, inflammation, leukemia

Test: Sedimentation rate
Significance: Infection, inflammation, leukemia

Test: Electrolyte panel, glucose
Significance: Renal disorders, diabetes mellitus, and insipidus

Test: Metabolic panel
Significance: Malnutrition, liver problem, bone disorder, pseudohypoparathyroidism

Test: Urinalysis
Significance: Urinary tract infection, diabetes, renal disorder, metabolic problem

Test: Thyroxine and thyroid-stimulating hormone
Significance: Hypothyroidism, hypopituitarism

Test: X-ray study of the left hand and wrist
Significance: Bone age determination

Test: Karyotype
Significance: Turner syndrome in short girls, chromosomal disorders

Test: IGF-I concentration (growth hormone dependent)
Significance: Shows little fluctuation over 24 hours, but interpretation of values needs to take age-related norms into account. IGF-I is low in GH-deficiency, but can also be low due to hypothyroidism, chronic illness, or poor nutrition. Normal IGF-I concentration makes growth hormone deficiency unlikely.

Additional work-up may be necessary, as determined by history and physical examination (antiendomysial antibodies, sweat chloride test, urine metabolic screening, venous blood gas, lateral skull x-ray, skeletal survey, etc.).

Issues for Referral

- Flat growth curve, grossly delayed bone age, abnormal thyroid test, poorly controlled diabetes, physical findings consistent with growth hormone deficiency, hypothyroidism, rickets—pediatric endocrinologist
- Protein-losing enteropathy, malabsorption, hepatic disorder—gastroenterologist
- Chronic lung disease, abnormal sweat chloride test—pulmonologist
- Congenital heart disease, occult cardiac disease—cardiologist
- Elevated creatinine, low serum bicarbonate, abnormal urinalysis—nephrologist

Growth failure is usually a relatively slow or subacute process and, therefore, does not require emergency work-up. It is of basic importance, however, to pay special attention to correct measurements of height, weight, and head circumference, to evaluate the abnormally growing child adequately.

BIBLIOGRAPHY

Rosenfield RL. Essentials of growth diagnosis. In: Rosenfield RL, ed. *Endocrinology and metabolism clinics of North America.* 1996;25(3):743–758.

Underwood LE, Van Wyk JJ. Normal and aberrant growth. In: Foster DW, Wilson JD, eds. *Williams textbook of endocrinology,* 8th ed. Philadelphia: WB Saunders, 1992;21:1079–1138.

Author: Philippe F. Backeljauw

Sore Throat

Database

DEFINITION

Sore throat or pain with swallowing is a common presenting complaint in the pediatric population. The majority of cases have an infectious etiology, with viral causes being the most common.

Differential Diagnosis

INFECTIOUS

• Pharyngitis/Tonsillitis

—Respiratory viruses: adenovirus/influenza/parainfluenza; Epstein-Barr virus (EBV)
—Bacterial: Group A beta-hemolytic streptococcus (*S. pyogenes*); Diphtheria; *Neisseria gonorrheae*; Chlamydia; Mycoplasma
—Stomatitis: *Herpes simplex virus,* coxsackievirus
—Peritonsillar cellulitis/abscess
—Retropharyngeal abscess
—Epiglottitis/Supraglottitis

ENVIRONMENTAL

• Irritative pharyngitis: exposure to smoke or dry air

TRAUMA

• Foreign body: either retained or causing laceration to posterior pharynx
• Burns: hot liquids/foods
• Voice overuse

TUMOR

• Rare in pediatric population

ALLERGIC/INFLAMMATORY

• Allergens causing chronic postnasal drip which leads to irritant pharyngitis

MISCELLANEOUS

• Psychogenic pain
• Referred pain

Approach to the Patient

GENERAL GOAL

The majority of cases of sore throat have an infectious cause, with most (~80%) of these having a viral etiology. Once the life-threatening and/or non-infectious causes have been excluded, the goal is to determine if the pharyngitis is caused by group A beta-hemolytic streptococci (GABS), which should be treated with antibiotics, or one of the many other infectious etiologies.

Phase 1: Use history and physical exam to separate infectious from non-infectious causes. If etiology seems infectious, consider throat culture for group A streptococci infection.

Data Gathering

HISTORY

Question: Sore throat in association with fever, headache, and/or abdominal pain?
Significance: Common association of symptoms present in group A streptococci pharyngitis

Question: Sore throat in association with fever, URI symptoms (cough, rhinorrhea, conjunctivitis)?
Significance: More suggestive of viral pharyngitis.

Question: Presence of drooling, voice changes?
Significance: Possibility of more severe infectious etiology, including retropharyngeal or peritonsillar abscess, epiglottitis.

Question: Foreign body exposure?
Significance: Retained foreign body (e.g., fishbone) or laceration/irritation from foreign body.

Question: Irritant exposure (e.g., dry air from heating or cooling system)?
Significance: Pharyngeal mucosal drying.

Question: Immunization status and travel history?
Significance: Possibility of Diphtheria in the non- or incompletely immunized patient, especially if recent travel to countries of the former Soviet Union.

Question: Sexual activity (including oral sex and possibility of abuse)?
Significance: Gonococcal pharyngitis.

Physical Examination

Finding: Pharyngeal erythema with or without exudate
Significance: Suggestive of infectious etiology, though does not reliably differentiate viral from bacterial causes

Finding: Tender cervical adenopathy
Significance: Suggestive of infectious etiology; anterior cervical nodes described in classic GABS infection; posterior cervical nodes ±hepatosplenomegaly suggest possibility of EBV

Finding: Stridor/drooling
Significance: Raises concern for etiologies that may cause airway obstruction

Finding: Asymmetric enlargement of tonsillar pillar with deviation of uvula away from enlarged side
Significance: Peritonsillar abscess

Finding: Mild erythema with cobblestoning of posterior pharyngeal mucosa
Significance: Suggests allergic or irritant etiology

Finding: Vesicular or ulcerative lesions in oropharynx
Significance: Suggestive of viral etiologies including herpes simplex (lesions commonly in anterior oropharynx) or coxsackievirus (lesions commonly in posterior oropharynx)

Laboratory Aids

Test: Throat swab for strep antigen test with subsequent culture if antigen test is negative.
Significance: Useful for definitive diagnosis of group A streptococci infection. A negative antigen test should be followed by throat culture to improve sensitivity.

Test: Lateral neck x-ray
Significance: Enlarged epiglottis suggests epiglottitis; widened prevertebral soft tissue space suggestive of retropharyngeal abscess.

Test: Complete blood count and Monospot if indicated
Significance: Atypical lymphocytosis/presence of heterophil antibodies suggestive of EBV infection. EBV titers (if indicated) should be sent in those less than 4 years of age because of low sensitivity (~50%) of Monospot in this age group.

Emergency Care

Factors that make sore throat an emergency include:

• Airway compromise

—Epiglottitis
—Retropharyngeal abscess
—Peritonsillar abscess
—Significant tonsillar hypertrophy
—Diphtheria

The patient may present with toxic appearance, fever, drooling, voice change, and sitting in the sniffing position (to optimize airway). Make NPO, supplemental oxygen; consider airway adjuncts (e.g., NP airway), intravenous access to facilitate airway management (if patient able to tolerate). Consider anesthesia consult for endotracheal intubation in most controlled setting.

Common Questions and Answers

Q: What is the incidence of group A streptococci disease as the cause of pharyngitis?
A: Group A streptococci is the most common bacterial etiology of infectious pharyngitis. The incidence of this disease is approximately 15% to 20% of all cases of infectious pharyngitis.

Q: When must antibiotic therapy begin in group A streptococci pharyngitis in order to prevent rheumatic fever?
A: Antibiotics should be started within 9 days from the onset of symptoms in order to prevent this non-suppurative complication of group A streptococci pharyngitis.

Issues for Referral

• Signs/symptoms of airway compromise—general toxicity, stridor, drooling. Patient may need emergent airway protection/stabilization.
• Fluctuant peritonsillar abscess—drainage may be done by otolaryngologist.
• Presence of foreign body—may need removal by otolaryngologist or x-ray to look for air in retropharyngeal soft tissue

Clinical Pearls

The clinical appearance of a GABS pharyngitis may be indistinguishable from pharyngitis of viral etiologies. The therapy for these illnesses is different: antibiotics for group A streptococci versus symptomatic care for viral pharyngitis. The practitioner should perform diagnostic testing (i.e., rapid strep antigen and/or culture) when GABS pharyngitis is considered. In general, it is not recommended to treat pending the culture results; rather, wait until the GABS pharyngitis is confirmed with a positive antigen or culture before starting antibiotics.

BIBLIOGRAPHY

Bisno AL. Acute pharyngitis: etiology and diagnosis. *Pediatrics* 1996;97(6 Pt 2):949–954.

Fleisher GR. Sore throat. In: Fleisher GR, Ludwig S, eds. *Textbook of pediatric emergency medicine.* Baltimore: Williams & Wilkins, 1993:469–473.

Author: Cynthia R. Jacobstein

Speech Delay

Database

DEFINITION

The failure of progression during infancy and/or early childhood of verbal skills at the expected rate or time.

Differential Diagnosis

See table Most Common Causes of Speech Delay.

CONGENITAL/ANATOMICAL

- Cerebral palsy
- Cleft palate
- Congenital infections (e.g., cytomegalovirus, syphilis, herpes, HIV)
- Lateralized (left-sided) brain lesion
- Mental retardation
- Microcephaly
- Sensorineural impairment (hearing or vision disorder)
- Sturge-Weber syndrome

INFECTIOUS

- Bacterial meningitis
- Human immunodeficiency virus (HIV)
- Recurrent otitis media

TOXIC

- Fetal alcohol syndrome/effects

TRAUMA

- Head injury
- Intracranial hemorrhage
- Stroke

GENETIC/METABOLIC

- Autism
- Pervasive developmental disorder (PDD)
- Developmental language disorder (DLD)
- Fragile X syndrome
- Neuromuscular disease
- Neurodegenerative disorder
- Tuberous sclerosis
- Velocardiofacial syndrome
- Williams syndrome

MISCELLANEOUS

- Environmental deprivation
- Iatrogenic causes: endotracheal tube placement, tracheostomy
- Prematurity

Most Common Causes of Speech Delay

Mental retardation
Hearing loss
Developmental language disorder
Autistic spectrum disorder

Approach to the Patient

GENERAL GOALS

Determine if true delay in acquisition of speech. Determine if treatable etiology.

Phase 1: Determine if delays in attainment of other skills. Assess for impaired hearing.

Phase 2: Evaluate for presence of genetic, neuromuscular, or metabolic disorder.

Phase 3: Refer for treatment or additional evaluation.

HINTS FOR SCREENING PROBLEM

Screening Tools (Appropriate milestones, see the table Patterns of Emerging Speech Development)

- Denver Developmental Screening Test II: agent most commonly used for screening language; less sensitive for identifying delays in expressive language than delays in other areas of development.
- Early Language Milestone Scale (ELM) and Clinical Linguistic and Auditory Milestone Scale (CLAMS): more sensitive measures for children from birth to 36 months of age.
- Other useful screening measures: Peabody Picture Vocabulary Test-III (PPVT-III) and the Receptive-Expressive Emergent Language Screen (REEL). All can be used to assess language in children from 1 to 36 months old.

Data Gathering

HISTORY

Question: At what age did the child demonstrate a social smile? Have first word? Use meaningful words? Demonstrate intelligible speech?
Significance: Knowledge of developmental speech milestones will enable the physician to determine if skills are delayed.

Question: Does the child have normal hearing and vision?
Significance: Children with impaired hearing (and vision to a lesser degree) often suffer from delayed language despite normal oral skills and an otherwise normal neurologic status.

Question: Does the child appear to be developmentally normal in other skills?
Significance: Mental retardation and other developmental disabilities (e.g., cerebral palsy) often present with delayed or aberrant language skills. Some neuromuscular disorders also present with delayed onset of speech with gross motor delay.

Question: Does the child appear medically ill?
Significance: Failure to thrive can signify a multitude of underlying problems (e.g., encephalopathy, chronic neglect), which can cause speech delay.

Question: Does the child exhibit appropriate social relatedness?
Significance: Deviant or delayed speech is a cardinal feature of autism. Children with autism (or pervasive developmental disorder) exhibit a restricted repertoire of activities and interests as well as impairment in social interactions.

Question: Is the child's home environment adequately stimulating?
Significance: Environmental deprivation and neglect are well-documented causes of delayed speech.

Patterns of Emerging Speech Development

AGE	SPEECH
2 months (8 weeks)	coos, social smile, attends to voice
3 months (12 weeks)	some vocal sounds; "aah, ooh"
4 months (16 weeks)	laughs
6 months (28 weeks)	repetitive vowel sounds
9 months (40 weeks)	waves bye-bye, repetitive consonant sounds (e.g., "mama/dada")
12 months (52 weeks)	one or more words besides "mama/dada"
15 months	points, single words
18 months	up to 10 words, jargoning; names pictures, identifies 1 or more body parts
21 months	two-word phrases
24 months	30–50 words, 3-word sentences
30 months	refers to self as "I", knows name
36 months	counts to 3, knows age and sex speech intelligible
48 months	counts four objects, tells story
60 months	counts ten objects correctly, asks meanings of words

Question: Is there evidence of a familial or hereditary condition?
Significance: Hearing impairment, stuttering, and autism are found in higher numbers among first-degree relatives. The effects of fragile X syndrome are also well documented.

Question: Is there any history of seizure activity?
Significance: Seizures may indicate an underlying neurologic impairment (e.g., Landau-Kleffner syndrome) or, if severe and poorly controlled, can themselves directly interfere with achieving milestones.

 ## Physical Examination

Finding: Macrocephaly, microcephaly, hypertelorism, or hair whorls?
Significance: May indicate an underlying brain defect or *in utero* exposure.

Finding: Unusual facies or other dysmorphisms?
Significance: Suggest genetic problem or syndromes, some of which are associated with speech problems and/or mental retardation (e.g., fetal alcohol syndrome, fragile X syndrome, Williams syndrome, velocardiofacial syndrome)

Finding: Abnormal (misshapen), low set, or small ears or eyes?
Significance: May point to a sensorineural impairment and/or a syndrome including mental retardation (e.g., Treacher Collins syndrome, trisomies)

Finding: Scarred tympanic membranes?
Significance: May represent chronic otitis media with resultant prolonged (transient) hearing impairment

Finding: Tracheostomy or suprasternal scar?
Significance: Raises the question of damage to the vocal cords

Finding: Skin abnormalities?
Significance: May represent (e.g., café-au-lait spots, hypopigmented macules, portwine stains) syndrome associated with hearing impairment or mental retardation

Finding: Malnutrition and social withdrawal?
Significance: May point to environmental deprivation or chronic disease

Finding: Abnormal or impaired muscle control?
Significance: May indicate an underlying neurologic process (e.g., facial diplegia in Mobius syndrome, brisk tendon reflexes with clonus in cerebral palsy)

 ## Laboratory Aids

Test: Behavioral audiometry or brainstem auditory evoked response testing
Significance: Children with severe hearing loss will demonstrate speech delay.

Test: Computed tomography (CT) or magnetic resonance imaging (MRI) of the head
Significance: Indicated when speech delay is accompanied by focal neurologic abnormalities, moderate to profound mental retardation, or dysmorphic features.

Test: Karyotype and fragile X screen
Significance: Indicated in the presence of stereotyped or unusual behaviors, dysmorphic features, and developmental delay.

Test: Metabolic screens
Significance: Liver function tests, serum for amino acids, and urine for organic acids are suggested only in the presence of changes in skin or hair, growth failure, lethargy, loss of milestones, organomegaly, or severe developmental delay.

Test: Electroencephalogram (EEG)
Significance: An EEG should be performed if there is a concern or history of seizure activity or regression in or loss of language skills.

Test to Prepare for Consult

• Audiometry
• Office language screen (Denver II, ELM, CLAMS)

 ## Emergency Care

Urgent evaluation is indicated with the presence of seizures, and regression in developmental milestones.

 ## Common Questions and Answers

Q: Do later-born children speak later than first-born children do?
A: No. Parents and siblings often speak for the child in question, but this is a result of, not a cause of the child's delay.

Q: Is the child being "lazy"?
A: Children who are lazy usually demonstrate normal language skills.

Q: Do bilingual children speak later than children in single-language homes do?
A: No. Developmental constants are normal, and by 36 months of age, these children are often fluent in both languages.

Q: Do deaf infants show absence of vocalizations?
A: No. Deaf infants may coo and babble in a normal pattern until 6 months of age.

Special Insight

The initial complaint of parents of preschool-aged children with an autistic disorder is almost always inadequate language. All children with mental retardation exhibit language delay, but not all children with language delay have mental retardation.

Issues for Referral

• Children requiring referral include those without meaningful words by 18 months of age, meaningful phrases by 2 years of age, or those with unintelligible speech at age 3 years.
• Factors that may assist you in making a referral include:

—Speech-language pathologists: evaluate the oral-peripheral mechanism, and provide additional information about communication skills.
—Developmental pediatricians: identify whether there is a discrepancy between communication skills and other developmental skill areas, and evaluate the possible etiologies for the speech problems. This referral is indicated when speech delay is accompanied by other developmental delays.
—Child psychologists or neuropsychologists: evaluate abnormal behaviors and provide information regarding cognitive skills.
—Pediatric neurologists: evaluate seizures, motor abnormalities, and/or neurodegenerative features, and assist in the evaluation and management of unusual behaviors.

BIBLIOGRAPHY

Coplan J. Normal speech and language development: an overview. *Pediatr Rev* 1995;16(3);91–100.

Klein SE. Evaluation for suspected language disorders in preschool children. *Pediatr Clin North Am* 1991;38(6):1455–1467.

McRae KM, Vickar E. Simple developmental speech delay: a follow-up study. *Dev Med Child Neurol* 1991;33:868–874.

Rapin I. Practitioner review: developmental language disorders: a clinical update. *J Child Psychol Psychiatr* 1996;37(6):643–655.

Walker D, Gugenheim S, Downs MP, Northern JL. Early language milestone scale and language screening of young children. *Pediatrics* 1989;83(2);284–288.

Author: H. Lynn Starr

Speech Problems

 Database

DEFINITION

Disorders of word production and language expression. They can be found as isolated difficulties or in conjunction with more complex disorders. See tables Most Common Causes of Speech Problems and Speech Disorders.

 Differential Diagnosis

CONGENITAL/ANATOMICAL

- Cerebral palsy
- Cleft lip/palate
- Hearing impairment
- Intracranial hemorrhage
- Isolated language disorder
- Laryngeal abnormalities
- Midfacial defects
- Mobius syndrome
- Stroke

INFECTIOUS

- Human immunodeficiency virus (HIV)

TOXIC

- Fetal alcohol syndrome/effects

TRAUMA

- Traumatic brain injuries

GENETIC/METABOLIC

- Autism and pervasive developmental disorders
- Mental retardation
- Neuromuscular disease
- Velocardiofacial syndrome
- Williams syndrome

MISCELLANEOUS

- Acquired aphasias (e.g., Landau-Kleffner syndrome)
- Acquired deafness
- Iatrogenic causes: endotracheal tube placement, tracheostomy
- Prematurity
- Severe environmental deprivation

Most Common Causes of Speech Problems

Developmental language disorder
Hearing loss
Mental retardation

Approach to the Patient

GENERAL GOAL

Determine if speech is abnormal, or if the problem is transient, progressive, or static.

Phase 1: Determine if the patient has a hearing impairment or delays in other areas of development.

Phase 2: Determine if problem is an articulation or experience language disorder (see table directly below).

Phase 3: Refer for additional evaluation and treatment if warranted.

 Data Gathering

HISTORY

Question: Does the child have normal hearing and vision?
Significance: Children with sensorineural hearing impairments often have disrupted speech (e.g., articulation disorders) and/or language skills (e.g., semantic-pragmatic disorders).

Question: Is there evidence of developmental delay in other areas of skills?
Significance: Mental retardation and other developmental disabilities (e.g., cerebral palsy) often present with delayed or aberrant skills (dysarthric or dyspraxic speech, lexical-syntactic disorder, and non-verbal and verbal communication impairment).

Question: Does the child have dysmorphic features or other medical conditions?
Significance: Speech problems are manifested in several genetic syndromes such as:

- Williams syndrome
- Fragile X syndrome
- Velocardiofacial syndrome

Question: Does the child exhibit unusual behaviors?
Significance: Children with autism/pervasive developmental disorder may exhibit stereotyped behaviors, with impaired social interactions, as well as deviant speech patterns (delayed language development, non-verbal and verbal communication impairment, semantic-pragmatic disorder).

Question: When was the child noted to have a speech problem?
Significance: Abrupt onset is seen with head trauma, encephalitis, and other acute illnesses.

Question: Has there been any change in the child's speech, especially loss of milestones?
Significance: Progressive loss of speech may be seen in Lindau-Kleffner syndrome and neurodegenerative disorders.

Question: Is there evidence of a familial or hereditary condition?
Significance: Hearing impairment, stuttering, and autism are found in higher numbers among first-degree relatives.

Question: Is there a history of seizure activity?
Significance: Seizures may be indicative of Landau-Kleffner syndrome, a seizure disorder, or of an underlying neurologic impairment.

- Syndromes that include deafness (e.g., Waardenburg: partial albinism, autosomal dominant inheritance) may result in resonance abnormalities, voice disorders, and dysarthric speech.

Speech Disorders

ARTICULATION DISORDERS	
Dysarthria	Articulation impaired by poor oral muscle control
Dyspraxia	Difficulty with the production of speech despite normal oral musculature
Language disorders	An impaired ability to use meaningful words, phrases, or gestures. They include two major types: expressive and receptive language disorders.
Resonance disorders	Difficulty in the volume or tone of speech, often due to abnormalities of the nasal and/or oral airways
Stuttering	Difficulty with the rhythm or fluency of speech, accompanied by signs of distress (e.g., facial grimacing)
Voice disorders	Production of speech impaired by an abnormal larynx
EXPRESSIVE LANGUAGE DISORDERS	
Lexical-syntactic disorders	Difficulties with word-finding and sentence structure
Semantic-pragmatic disorders	Impairment in production and understanding of conversation, including echolalia
Nonverbal and verbal communication impairments	Limited comprehension of language with or without speech
Speech programming deficit	Fluency with interspersed jargon

HINTS FOR THE SCREENING PROBLEM

Children with speech problems may be identified by signs of inadequate language and/or vocabulary, and by evaluation of the conversation skills, comprehension, and syntax in comparison to other children of the same age.

 ## Physical Examination

Finding: Macrocephaly, microcephaly, hypertelorism, or hair whorls?
Significance: May indicate an underlying brain defect, *in utero* exposure to medication (e.g., hydantoin) or infection (e.g., CMV)

Finding: Abnormal (misshapen) or small ears?
Significance: May point to a sensorineural impairment

Finding: Scarred tympanic membranes?
Significance: May represent chronic otitis media and the resultant prolonged (although temporary) hearing impairment

Finding: Cleft lip or palate?
Significance: May cause resonance abnormalities in the production of speech (hypernasal speech)

Finding: Unusual facies or other dysmorphic features?
Significance: Suggest genetic or hereditary syndromes, some of which are associated with speech problems and/or mental retardation (e.g., fetal alcohol syndrome, fragile X syndrome, Williams syndrome, velocardiofacial syndrome)

Finding: Tracheostomy or suprasternal scar?
Significance: May indicate a history of damage to the vocal cords

Finding: Malnutrition and social withdrawal?
Significance: May point to environmental deprivation or chronic disease.

Finding: Abnormal or impaired muscle control?
Significance: May be significant for an underlying neurologic process (e.g., facial diplegia in Mobius syndrome, brisk tendon reflexes with clonus in cerebral palsy)

Finding: Behavioral problems?
Significance: Children with stereotyped behavior, avoidance of eye contact, and poor social skills may have autism or pervasive developmental disorder.

Finding: Shortened frenulum?
Significance: Probably an incidental finding, as this does not result in deviant speech in most instances.

 ## Laboratory Aids

Test: Behavioral audiometry or brainstem auditory evoked response testing
Significance: Hearing loss may impair a child's ability to discriminate between certain speech sounds. This may result in abnormalities of articulation and resonance.

Test: Computed tomography or magnetic resonance imaging of the head
Significance: One of these studies is indicated when speech delay is accompanied by focal neurologic abnormalities (such as hearing loss, abnormal muscle tone, etc.), moderate to profound mental retardation, or dysmorphic features. MRI is the procedure of choice, however, CT scans are superior in imaging cranial bones, and when making the determination of intracranial calcifications.

Test: Karyotype and fragile X screen
Significance: These studies are indicated in the presence of stereotyped or unusual behaviors, dysmorphic features, and developmental delay.

Test: Metabolic screen
Significance: Liver function tests, serum for amino acids, and urine for organic acids are suggested only in the presence of changes in or abnormal skin or hair, growth failure, lethargy, loss of milestones, organomegaly, or severe developmental delay.

Test: Electroencephalogram
Significance: An EEG should be performed if there is a concern or history of seizure activity or regression in or loss of language skills.

Tests to Prepare for Consult

- Audiometry
- Office language screens:

—Denver Developmental Screening Test II: most commonly used for screening language; is most sensitive for detecting severe speech delay.
—The Early Language Milestone Scale (ELM) and the Clinical Linguistic and Auditory Milestone Scale (CLAMS) the preferred measures in screening speech problems.
—The Peabody Picture Vocabulary Test-III is a better measure of receptive than expressive language skills.

Emergency Care

- Acute onset of speech problems (excluding stuttering)
- Presence of seizures
- Loss of developmental milestones

Clinical Pearls

- Dysfluency, or transient loss of normal speech rate and rhythm, is frequently seen in children 2 1/2 to 4 years of age. Dysfluency involves repetition of whole words, without signs of distress, should not be confused with stuttering, which involves repetition of shorter speech segments or difficulty initiating a word, accompanied by signs of distress.
- Males are more likely to exhibit speech problems.

 ## Common Questions and Answers

Q: When should children with stuttering be referred to a speech-language therapist?
A: A child should be referred when dysfluency persists for more than 6 months, has an onset or persistence after 5 years of age, or when stuttering is accompanied by significant distress.

Q: When a child exhibits selective mutism, is a referral to a speech therapist indicated?
A: The first referral should be to a behavioral specialist, preferably a child psychologist.

Issues for Referral

- A speech-language pathologist is needed to evaluate the oral-peripheral mechanism, and to provide additional information about communication skills.
- Referral to an appropriate surgical subspecialist is indicated in the presence of a midline defect (e.g., cleft lip or palate), a syndrome requiring surgical intervention (Treacher Collins syndrome), or recurrent infections.
- Developmental pediatricians are able to identify whether there is a discrepancy between communication skills and other developmental skill areas, evaluate the possible etiologies for the speech problems, and to act as coordinators for needed therapies. This referral is indicated when speech delay is accompanied by other developmental delays.
- Child psychologists or neuropsychologists are able to evaluate abnormal behaviors and to provide information regarding cognitive skills. These specialists are also helpful when behavioral issues are a component of the child's difficulties.
- Pediatric neurologists are able to evaluate seizures, motor abnormalities, and/or neurodegenerative features, and to assist in the evaluation and management of unusual behaviors.
- Referral to a geneticist is indicated when the patient has dysmorphic features, the family has a history of speech/hearing problems, or other findings suggestive of a syndrome.
- School systems may serve as a center for the provision of evaluations and services for children over 3 years of age, and for children with disabilities under the age of 3.

BIBLIOGRAPHY

Coplan J. Normal speech and language development: an overview. *Pediatr Rev* 1995;16(3):91–100.

Klein SE. Evaluation for suspected language disorders in preschool children. *Pediatr Clin North Am* 1991;38(6):1455–1467.

Levy SE, Hyman SL. Pediatric assessment of the child with developmental delay. *Pediatr Clin North Am* 1993;40(3):465–478.

Author: H. Lynn Starr

Splenomegaly

 Database

DEFINITION

A palpable spleen is found in most premature infants and in 30% of term infants. A spleen tip is still palpable in 10% of infants at 1 year of age and in 1% of children 10 years of age. Normal spleens are soft, at the midclavicular line, and often palpable only on deep inspiration. Dullness on percussion beyond the 11th intercostal space suggests splenomegaly. Splenic tenderness is abnormal.

 Differential Diagnosis

INFECTION

- Bacterial
- Bacteremia
- Pneumonia
- Sepsis
- Subacute bacterial endocarditis
- *Salmonella*
- Tuberculosis
- Brucellosis
- Staphylococcal shunt infections
- Tularemia
- Syphilis
- Leptospirosis

VIRAL

- Epstein-Barr virus (mononucleosis)
- Cytomegalovirus
- HIV
- Rubella
- Herpes
- Hepatitis A, B
- Rickettsial/protozoan
- Rocky Mountain spotted fever
- Malaria
- Toxoplasmosis
- Trypanosomiasis
- Babesiosis
- Schistosomiasis
- Visceral larval migrans
- Kala-azar

FUNGAL

- Histoplasmosis
- Coccidioidomycosis

BLOOD DISEASE: HEMOLYTIC DISEASES

- Hereditary spherocytosis
- Sickle cell disease
- Thalassemia major autoimmune hemolytic anemia
- Hemoglobin C disease
- Pyruvate kinase deficiency
- Glucose-6-phosphate dehydrogenase deficiency
- Isoimmunization disorders
- Infantile pyknocytosis
- Iron-deficiency anemia (rare)
- Thrombocytopenic purpura

VASCULAR CONGESTIVE DISORDERS

- Carvernous transformation of the portal vein
- Congential hepatic fibrosis

CIRRHOSIS SECONDARY TO:

- Hepatitis
- Biliary atresia
- Wilson disease
- Cystic fibrosis
- α_1-Antitrypsin deficiency
- Tyrosinemia
- Hereditary fructose intolerance
- Hemosiderosis
- Thrombosis of the hepatic vein
- Budd Chiari syndrome
- Congestive heart failure
- Constrictive pericarditis
- Galactosemia
- Congenital portal vein stenosis or atresia
- Splenic artery aneurysm
- Splenic hematoma
- Splenic hemangioma

METABOLIC DISEASES

- Gangliosidoses
- Mucolipodoses
- Metachromatic leukodystrophy
- Wolman disease
- Gaucher disease
- Niemann-Pick disease
- Amyloidosis
- Hyperlipoproteinemia
- Familial hemophagocytic reticulosis
- Porphyria
- Lysinuric protein intolerance
- Dibasic aminoaciduria
- Cystinosis

NEOPLASTIC DISEASES

- Leukemia
- Lymphoma
- Lymphosarcoma
- Neuroblastoma
- Histiocytosis X

MISCELLANEOUS

- Serum sickness
- Connective-tissue disorders
- Juvenile rheumatoid arthritis
- Systemic lupus erythematosus
- Sarcoidosis
- Beckwith-Wiedeman syndrome
- Infant of a diabetic mother
- Splenic hamartoma
- Cysts: congenital and post-traumatic
- Hyperparathyroidism
- Gingival fibromatosis and digital anomalies

NON-SPLENIC LEFT ABDOMINAL MASSES

- Large kidney
- Retroperitoneal tumor
- Adrenal neoplasm
- Ovarian cyst
- Pancreatic cyst
- Mesenteric cyst

Approach to the Patient

GENERAL GOALS

Determine the etiology of the large spleen.

Phase 1: Establish the presence of enlarged spleen, not a palpable spleen that is pushed down by inflated lungs.

Phase 2: Rule out common causes as a viral infection, bacterial infection, or anemia.

Phase 3: Rule out malignancy or storage disease or other rare causes of large spleen.

Data Gathering

HISTORY

Question: History of acute illness?
Significance: Suggests infection

Question: History of GI bleeding?
Significance: With splenomegaly, suggests increased portal venous pressure.

Question: Familial history of hematologic or immune disease?
Significance: Suggests bleeding disorder or genetic disorder.

Question: Systemic symptoms: fever, jaundice, pallor, bleeding, hematuria, anorexia, abdominal distention?
Significance: Suggests infectious disease

Question: Are there signs of cardiac distress?
Significance: Congenital heart disease or failure.

 ## Physical Examination

Begin the abdominal examination in the lower quadrant as an enlarged spleen may be missed in the upper quadrant exam.

Finding: Auscultate for rub or bruit
Significance: Look for signs of storage disease: retina, facies, etc.

Finding: Complete evaluation of lymph nodes
Significance: Look for ascites

Finding: Pain
Significance: Suggests capsular distention due to infiltration, trauma, or infection

Finding: Prominent abdominal veins or hemorrhoids
Significance: Suggest increased portal venous pressure

 ## Laboratory Aids

Test: Complete blood count with differential and platelets
Significance: Sickle cell, hemolytic anemia, leukemia

Test: Reticulocyte count
Significance: Hemolytic anemia

Test: Liver tests: transaminases: AST, ALT, albumin, bilirubin, PT/PTT, glucose
Significance: Cirrhosis, hepatic obstruction

DISCRIMINATING LABORATORY TESTS

If no hemolytic disease, with signs of infection:

- Blood culture
- Thick smear of blood for malaria
- Viral testing

If no hemolytic disease, no sign of infection, no sign of congestion:

- Ultrasound
- Liver spleen scan
- Biopsy: bone, lymph node, liver

If no hemolytic disease, no sign of infection, but sign of congestion:

- Ultrasound
- Computed tomography
- Magnetic resonance imaging

 ## Emergency Care

- Life-threatening etiologies: sepsis, severe hemolytic anemia, trauma, hypersplenism
- Rapid placement of a large-bore intravenous access route should occur when a life-threatening etiology is suspected.

 ## Common Questions and Answers

Q: How long will the enlarged spleen secondary to a viral infection be present?
A: The enlarged spleen may persist for several months.

SPECIAL INSIGHTS OR CUES

Asthmatic patients may have palpable spleen secondary to overinflation of lungs and depressed diaphragm.

Issues for Referral

- Disproportionate size of spleen
- Increasing size over serial examinations
- Unexplained lymphadenopathy
- Liver dysfunction
- Ascites
- Signs of storage or metabolic disease
- Howell Jolly bodies on peripheral smear, suggesting splenic dysfunction

Author: Andrew E. Mulberg

Teething

Database

DEFINITION

• Teething is the normal developmental process of primary tooth eruption (see table Guidelines for the Time of Tooth Eruption), often characterized by parental reports of fever, fussiness, increased drooling, increased finger sucking, alterations in bowel pattern, and/or decreased appetite.
• Of note, fever >101°F, irritability, or diarrhea should not be attributed to teething and other etiologies should be considered such as otitis media, urinary tract infection, septicemia, meningitis, septic arthritis, or viral infection.

Differential Diagnosis

CONGENITAL/ANATOMICAL

• Natal teeth, neonatal teeth
• Gastroesophageal reflux resulting in esophagitis with decreased appetite

INFECTIOUS

• Primary herpes gingivostomatitis causing pain or drooling
• Human herpes virus 6 causing fever
• Coxsackievirus oral infection causing fever or drooling
• Epiglottitis causing severe drooling with fever
• Viral illness causing fever >101°F, diarrhea, or upper respiratory symptoms

TOXIC

• Toxic ingestion causing drooling

TRAUMA

• "Lancing" of gums (i.e., incising the gum to expose the erupting tooth) causing pain
• Hair tourniquet syndrome causing pain and irritability
• Corneal abrasion causing pain

MISCELLANEOUS

• Drooling, gum rubbing, and finger sucking may be normal developmental behaviors

Approach to the Patient

GENERAL GOAL

Determine if the infant has any other signs or symptoms of another illness that would require additional investigation (e.g., fever >101°F, diarrhea, or irritability); avoid over diagnosing teething, which might delay diagnosis of a more serious illness.

Phase 1: Careful history and physical.

Phase 2: Work-up of specific signs or symptoms suggested by history or physical that are not consistent with teething.

Phase 3: Provide relief of discomfort for the child who is teething.

History

Question: How old is the child?
Significance: The average age for the eruption of the first tooth is approximately 6 months. One percent of infants acquires the first tooth before 4 months and 1% after 12 months. Rule of thumb: age (months) − 6 = average number of teeth (up to 2 years of age). Eruption usually begins with the lower central incisors.

Question: Has the parent noted any swelling or bluish discoloration of the gums?
Significance: Primary tooth eruption is frequently associated with swelling of the gums. A bluish area of gum swelling may represent an eruption cyst secondary to a hematoma. This condition requires parental reassurance only.

Question: Is the infant consolable?
Significance: Infants who are teething may be fussy but should be consolable. An infant who is irritable and not consolable should be evaluated for serious systemic illness such as septicemia, meningitis, septic arthritis, or urinary tract infection.

Question: Have the parents documented any fever?
Significance: Studies have shown that teething may be associated with low grade fever especially over the 3 days prior to tooth eruption. Fevers >101°F cannot be attributed to teething and require work-up for other causes of illness such as upper respiratory infection, otitis media, urinary tract infection, meningitis, septic arthritis, or other viral infection.

Question: What other symptoms is the child experiencing?
Significance: Diarrhea, rashes, seizures, eczema, otitis media, diaper rashes, or upper respiratory symptoms cannot be attributed to teething and should suggest another etiology for the child's symptoms.

Question: How is the child sleeping?
Significance: A teething child should be able to sleep with minimal disturbance. Changes in sleeping habits, such as frequent nighttime awakening, should suggest common problems with sleep associations often seen in young children 6 to 12 months of age.

Question: Are other contacts in the home ill?
Significance: An acute illness should be investigated as the cause of the child's symptoms.

Question: What home remedies or treatments have the parents tried?
Significance: Most over-the-counter preparations marketed for the relief of teething symptoms contain 7.5% to 10% benzocaine as the active ingredient. Excessive use of benzocaine preparations has been associated with methemoglobinemia. Other homeopathic remedies may contain a variety of ingredients including belladonna alkaloids, chamomile, and ground coffee. Depending on the size of the child and the amount of medication or herb ingested, toxicity is possible. Excessive use of topical 2% lidocaine may cause seizures. Other remedies have been associated with salicylate toxicity and lead poisoning. If toxicity is suspected, the local Poison Control center should be consulted.

Question: Have the parents tried applying cold/frozen objects locally onto the gums?
Significance: Though many find that cold objects work well, care must be taken because direct contact with a frozen object may, on occasion, result in local irritation.

Question: What objects have the parents offered the child to chew or bite?
Significance: Choking hazards, such as raw carrots, must be avoided. Teething rings should not be placed around the child's neck as they represent a strangulation hazard.

Guidelines for the Time of Tooth Eruption

TEETH	MAXILLARY ERUPTION	MANDIBULAR ERUPTION
Central incisors	6–8 months	5–7 months
Lateral incisors	8–11 months	7–10 months
Cuspids	16–20 months	16–20 months
First molars	10–16 months	10–16 months
Second molars	20–30 months	20–30 months

Physical Examination

Question: Is there swelling with slight pallor over the gum where the tooth will erupt?
Significance: This is a normal finding.

Question: Is there bluish discoloration overlying the gum where a tooth is expected?
Significance: This represents a hematoma, known as an "eruption cyst," which is a normal finding.

Question: Is the child irritable?
Significance: Irritability on physical examination suggests a more serious illness other than teething. In addition to the infectious etiologies noted, the child should be evaluated for hair tourniquet syndrome and/or corneal abrasion.

Question: Are there oral ulcers?
Significance: Viral enanthems, such as herpes or coxsackie, should be considered.

Question: Is cervical lymphadenopathy present?
Significance: Oral, dental, or pharyngeal infections should be considered.

Question: Are there signs of dehydration, such as dry mucous membranes, absent tears, sunken fontanel, or tenting of the skin?
Significance: Infectious etiologies that result in poor oral intake or diarrhea should be considered.

Question: Is there oral erythema and abrasions with excessive drooling?
Significance: The possibility of caustic ingestion should be explored.

Laboratory Aids

No laboratory tests are indicated in the otherwise healthy child with teething.

Common Questions and Answers

Q: What are some common remedies for relieving the pain caused by teething?
A: Children with teething should find temporary relief from biting or chewing on hard or cold items such as refrigerated plastic teething rings, a cold wet washcloth, or teething biscuits. Gum massage with a clean finger may also provide relief. Over-the-counter products containing benzocaine should be used with caution. Acetaminophen (15 mg/kg by mouth every 4 hours) or ibuprofen (10 mg/kg by mouth every 6 hours) may be used for pain relief but should not be given to mask fever. Remedies that have been used in the past and are no longer recommended include: alcoholic liquors, paregoric, 2% lidocaine solution, lancing the gums, and rubbing the gums with a thimble until the tooth breaks through the gum.

Q: What is the difference between natal teeth and neonatal teeth?
A: Natal teeth are present at birth whereas neonatal teeth erupt during the first month of life. The incidence of natal teeth is 1:2000 to 1:6000 live births and usually involves the lower central incisor. Natal teeth can be associated with various conditions including Pierre Robin sequence, cleft lip or cleft palate. There is often a familial history of natal or neonatal teeth. Ninety-five percent of natal teeth are normal primary incisors that may have formed superficially and erupted early. Only 5% of natal teeth are supernumerary (extra) teeth. Therefore, if a natal tooth is removed, a primary tooth will not erupt in its place in most cases. Because primary teeth act as space holders for the secondary teeth, early loss of a primary tooth may result in significant crowding of the permanent successors.

Q: Does primary tooth eruption in preterm infants occur at the same time as in full-term infants?
A: In healthy preterm infants who had relative uneventful neonatal courses, the first primary tooth erupts at the usual chronological age. In premature infants who required prolonged oral intubation and or who experienced inadequate nutrition due to the severity of neonatal disease may have delayed eruption. The initial eruption sequence remains the same (lower central incisors first).

Issues for Referral

• Children who have delayed eruption of their first primary tooth beyond 12 months require additional investigation for the following: adontia, osteodystrophies, hypothyroidism, hypopituitarism, Down syndrome, rickets, Gardner syndrome. Most of these conditions require referral to a specialist for management.
• Children with premature eruption may have a familial cause, however, referral for evaluation of hyperpituitarism should be considered.
• Referral to a dentist should be considered for children with significant variation in eruption caused by dental infections, additional teeth in the path of eruption, insufficient space in the dental arch, and/or ectopic placement of teeth.
• Natal teeth that are stable and do not interfere with breast-feeding may remain. Loose natal teeth may need to be removed to prevent choking and aspiration. Natal teeth can interfere with breast feeding, causing ulceration, which is another indication for removal.

BIBLIOGRAPHY

Jaber L, Cohen IJ, Mor A. Fever associated with teething. *Arch Dis Child* 1992;67:233–234.

Kates GA, Needleman HL, Holmes LB. Natal and neonatal teeth: a clinical study. *J Am Dent Assoc* 1984;87:67–70.

Mofenson HC, Caraccio TR, Miller H, Greensher J. Lidocaine toxicity from topical mucosal application. *Clin Pediatr* 1983;22:190–192.

Paynter AS, Alexander FW. Salicylate intoxication caused by teething ointment. *Lancet* 1979;2:1132.

Schuman AJ. The truth about teething. *Contemp Pediatr* 1992;9:75–80.

Shusterman S. Pediatric dental update. *Pediatr Rev* 1994;5(15):311–318.

Townes PL, Geertsma MA, White MR. Benzocaine-induced methemoglobinemia. *Am J Dis Child* 1997;131:697–698.

Viscardi RM, Romberg E, Abrams RG. Delayed primary tooth eruption in premature infants: relationship to neonatal factors. *Pediatr Dent* 1994;16:23–28.

Author: Julie A. Boom

Thrombosis

Database

DEFINITION

Pathological arterial or venous intravascular occlusion by thrombus, which interferes with normal blood flow. Arterial events are often embolic.

- Deep venous thrombosis (DVT): involves large systemic veins outside the CNS.
- Dural sinus thrombosis: involves the intracranial venous sinuses often with extension into the cerebral veins.
- Superficial thrombophlebitis.
- Ischemic stroke: arterial occlusion or insufficiency with infarction of brain tissue.
- Hemorrhagic stroke: follows an ischemic event with reperfusion.
- Intracardiac thrombosis: mural, valvular, or hardware associated.
- Neonatal aortic thrombosis: can be spontaneous or catheter associated.
- Renal vein thrombosis: in the neonatal period or in children with nephrotic syndrome.
- Myocardial infarction: Kawasaki disease or with severe familial hypercholesterolemia.
- Budd-Chiari syndrome: thrombosis of the hepatic vein.
- Portal vein thrombosis.

EPIDEMIOLOGY

- The incidence of venous thrombosis in children is approximately 0.7 per 100,000 per year. It is likely that the actual incidence is higher.
- Two-thirds of children with thromboembolic disease have a predisposing underlying condition, the most common being an indwelling catheter.

COMPLICATIONS

- Complications vary depending on the location and severity of the thrombosis.
- For deep venous thrombosis, pulmonary embolism is the most significant acute complication with recurrent thrombosis and post-phlebitic syndrome common chronic complications.
- For arterial thromboembolic disease the ischemic injury to the involved organ determines the acute and long-term complications.

Differential Diagnosis

PRIMARY PROTHROMBOTIC STATES

Inherited

- Factor V Leiden
- Protein C deficiency
- Protein S deficiency
- Anti-thrombin III deficiency
- Plasminogen deficiency
- Dysfibrinogenemia (30% will have thrombotic symptoms)
- Heparin cofactor II deficiency
- Tissue plasminogen activator deficiency

- Plasminogen activator inhibitor type 1 excess
- Homocysteinemia (mild to moderate) from minor defects in enzymes such as methylenetetrahydrofolate reductase (MTHFR)
- Factor XII deficiency
- Activated protein C resistance other than factor V Leiden (Factor V Cambridge, Factor V Hong Kong)

Acquired

- Antiphospholipid antibody syndrome
- Post-infectious protein C or S deficiency
- Severe neonatal acquired protein C or S deficiency
- Lipoprotein(a) excess

RISK FACTORS FOR THROMBOSIS

Neonatal

- Birth trauma
- Prematurity
- Maternal diabetes
- Severe RDS
- Hypernatremic dehydration
- Umbilical catheters
- Sepsis
- Polycythemia
- Perinatal asphyxia

Malignancy/Bone Marrow Disorders

- Leukemia (hyperleukocyrosis, APML)
- Myeloproliferative disorders
- Paroxysmal nocturnal hemoglobinuria

Medications

- L-Asparaginase
- Oral contraceptives

Anatomical

- Indwelling catheters
- Cardiac catheterization
- Congenital heart disease
- Prosthetic heart valves
- Intracardiac baffles
- Tumor compression

Disorders Associated with Thrombosis

- Nephrotic syndrome
- Inflammatory disorders
- Liver disease
- Heart failure/increased venous pressure
- Sickle cell disease
- Behçets disease
- Homocystinuria
- Diabetes mellitus

Miscellaneous Risk Factors

- Infection
- Trauma
- Orthopedic surgery (Hip)
- Strenuous exercise
- Prolonged immobilization or paralysis
- Prolonged sitting

Risk Factors/Conditions Specific for Arterial Disease

- Kawasaki disease
- Takayasu arteritis

- Other vasculitides
- Hyperlipidemia
- Blalock-Taussig shunts
- Organ transplantation

Data Gathering

HISTORY

- Thromboembolic disease is commonly overlooked.
- A familial and/or personal history of thrombosis is an important risk factor for thrombosis.
- Neonatal seizure is a common and often sole presenting sign for dural sinus thrombosis.
- Presenting signs and symptoms of pulmonary embolism can be subtle and include dyspnea and chest pain.

Physical Examination

- Pain, decreased pulses and perfusion, color change.
- Superficial dilated cutaneous veins distal to the site of venous occlusion.
- Unilateral swelling/edema of a limb (may be bilateral if the IVC or SVC is extensively involved.
- Chronic discoloration (darkening) of the skin, ulcerations, pain, intermittent swelling.
- Unexplained hepatosplenomegaly may be the only sign of hepatic or portal vein thrombosis.
- Abdominal pain and ileus may be present with involvement of mesenteric, portal or hepatic vessels.

Approach to the Patient

Phase 1:

- Rapid evaluation of the hemostatic system prior to initiating therapy (CBC, PT/aPTT, fibrinogen).
- Therapy for thromboembolic disease should not be delayed.
- Whenever possible an antithrombin III level, a thrombin time and a screen for the lupus anticoagulant should be drawn before starting heparin. Protein C and S levels should be drawn before starting warfarin and plasminogen levels prior to any thrombolytic therapy.

Phase 2:

- Serial imaging to assess response to treatment.
- Search for an etiology of the thrombosis and evaluate risk factors.
- Test for factor V Leiden and anticardiolipin antibodies if not done with initial blood work.

Phase 3:

- Additional testing if a primary prothrombotic condition is strongly suspected.

Laboratory Aids

General evaluation of the hemostatic system:
- PT/PTT/fibrinogen
- CBC with platelet count
- FSP/d-dimer
- Thrombin time

The following laboratory tests done to investigate for a hypercoagulable state are listed in order of significance:

Phase 1:
- Factor V Leiden mutation analysis by PCR
- Lupus anticoagulant screen
- Dilute Russell Viper Venom time
- Tissue thromboplastin inhibition test
- Anticardiolipin antibodies (IgG, IgM, IgA) by ELISA
- Protein C activity
- Protein S activity and/or free protein S antigen
- Antithrombin III activity
- Lipid profile for arterial disease

Phase 2:
- Prothrombin 20210A allele by PCR
- Plasminogen
- Thrombin time or dysfibrinogenemia screen
- Protein S free antigen should be done if the activity was low
- Plasma homocysteine levels

Phase 3:
- MTHFR-T by PCR
- Factor VIII activity
- Lipoprotein a
- Heparin Cofactor II
- Tissue plasminogen activator (post veno-occlusion)
- Plasminogen activator inhibitor type 1
- Factor XII
- Activated protein C resistance clotting assay

IMAGING
- Ultrasound—least invasive but sensitivity for DVT in upper extremities variable.
- Magnetic resonance imaging with contrast (MRA/MRV)—expensive, time-consuming, and not adequately studied in children against the gold standard.
- Contrast angiography—is the gold standard but invasive and sometimes technically difficult to perform in small children.

PITFALLS
- Normal ranges for coagulation tests are age dependent.
- Diagnosing an inherited deficiency in any of the anticoagulants can be difficult in the neonatal period. Repeat testing at 2 and 6 months of age.
- Consumption can occur during the acute thrombosii, therefore, low levels must be repeated.
- Warfarin will decrease the levels of protein C and protein S.

THERAPY
- Therapy for acute thrombosis and long-term management is individualized.
- Consult a pediatric hematologist or someone with expertise in pediatric anticoagulant therapy.

DRUGS
- Standard Heparin (SH): Standard therapy for acute thrombosis. Given as a bolus followed by an infusion, adjusted to maintain the aPTT at 60 to 85 seconds. The younger the child the more heparin per weight is required to achieve a therapeutic level.
- Low Molecular Weight Heparin (LMWH): More predictable dose response, which is given subcutaneously twice a day. Equivalent in efficacy to SH in the acute management of uncomplicated DVT.
- Urokinase: Thrombolytic agent of choice in pediatric patients. Given as a bolus followed by an infusion for 12 to 24 hours.
- Recombinant tissue plasminogen activator (tPA): a newer thrombolytic agent with theoretical advantages over urokinase.
- Warfarin: an oral anticoagulant given as a loading dose, adjusted to maintenance as the PT prolongs.
- Aspirin

 Follow-Up

- Growth of involved limbs, especially following an arterial event.
- Avoid acquired risk factors for vascular disease.
- Medical risk factors should be controlled: hyperlipidemia, hypertension, etc.

PITFALLS

Central venous catheter related thrombosis may be completely asympyomatic despite extensive damage to the venous system. The long-term consequences of this are not known but recurrent thrombosis years after the line has been removed when the patient is older is a possibility.

 Common Questions and Answers

Q: What is the optimal strategy for preventing thrombosis associated with indwelling catheters?
A: Low-dose warfarin holds some promise in that the rate of thrombosis is decreased with minimal adverse effects. Using urokinase instead of heparin to flush the lines is an option, however, there is no strong evidence to suggest it is better than heparin.

Q: If an inherited prothrombotic condition is identified should family members be tested?
A: If they have other risk factors for thrombo-

sis such as malignancy, major surgery, oral contraceptives, obesity, etc.

Q: When is it appropriate to use LMWH rather than standard heparin?
A: There are several potential advantages to LMWH. The pharmacokinetics are much more predictable and frequent monitoring is not necessary. It is administered subcutaneously, not intravenous. The risk of bleeding may be slightly lower.

Q: When is it appropriate to use thrombolytic therapy?
A: Studies do not clearly demonstrate a role for thrombolytic therapy in DVT. However, if a thrombus extends on heparin therapy, a pulmonary embolus is suspected, or if the disturbance in blood flow causes ischemia, thrombolytic therapy can be used. Intracranial bleeding is a contraindication. For arterial thrombotic events, thrombolytic therapy is often the treatment of choice because of the rapid resolution of the clot and restoration of blood flow.

Q: What precautions should be taken for invasive procedures and for athletics when a patient is on anticoagulant therapy?
A: Lumbar punctures, arterial punctures and surgical procedures should be avoided. If they are necessary then the child should have the anticoagulant partially or fully reversed prior to the procedure. The child should not participate in contact sports such as football, karate, and boxing. For baseball, a helmet should be worn at all times.

Issues for Referral

- Pediatric hematologists should be consulted to assist in evaluating for primary hypercoagulable states and assisting in the management of anticoagulant therapy.
- Interventional radiologists should be consulted for choosing the best imaging study for diagnosis and follow-up.
- Surgical thrombectomy or vascular reconstruction is rarely necessary and carries considerable risk.

Clinical Pearls

Prevention

- Heparin prophylaxis following surgery is not routinely done in pediatrics.
- Awareness of existing risk factors and avoidance of additional acquired risk factors.

BIBLIOGRAPHY

Andrew M, Michelson AD, Bovill E, Leaker M, Massicotte MP. Guidelines for antithrombotic therapy in pediatric patients. *J Pediatr* 1998;132:575–588.

Manco-Johnson MJ. Diagnosis and management of thromboses in the perinatal period. *Semin Perinatol* 1990;14(5):393–402.

Manco-Johnson MJ. Disorders of hemostasis in childhood: risk factors for venous thromboembolism. *Thromb Haemost* 1997;78(1):710–714.

Author: J. Nathan Hagstrom

Upper GI Bleeding

 Database

DEFINITION

Vomiting of blood whether bright red or dark constitutes upper gastrointestinal (GI) bleeding or hematemesis. This usually represents bleeding from the GI tract proximal to the ligament of Treitz. One has to differentiate from hemoptysis (coughing up of blood), nose bleeds, and bleeding from the mouth and pharynx. Sometimes upper GI bleeding can present with malena or the passage of tarry stools.

 Differential Diagnosis

• 95% of the causes of UGI bleeding are due to mucosal abnormalities or esophageal varices.
• Mucosal lesions are more likely to be associated with antecedent occult bleeding.
• In about 80% to 95% of patients the bleeding stops spontaneously.
• Age of the patient is important.

NEONATAL PERIOD

• Swallowed maternal blood
• Hemorrhagic disease of the newborn
• Esophagitis/gastritis
• Stress ulcer
• Foreign body irritation
• Vascular malformation

INFANCY

• Esophagitis/gastritis
• Stress ulcer
• Mallory-Weiss tear
• Pyloric stenosis
• Vascular malformation
• Duplication cysts

PRESCHOOL AGED

• Esophageal varices
• Esophagitis/gastritis/ulcer
• Foreign body/bezoar
• Mallory-Weiss tear
• Vascular malformation

SCHOOL AGED

• Esophageal varices
• Esophagitis/gastritis/ulcer
• Mallory-Weiss tear
• Inflammatory bowel disease

Approach to the Patient

GENERAL GOALS

Determine the cause of the bleeding and begin treatment.

Phase 1: Determine if blood or food coloring, beets, Hematest material.

Phase 2: Assess severity of bleeding. Is there a change in vital signs, hematocrit, blood pressures, capillary filling, pulse?

Phase 3: Determine the site of bleeding and begin treatment. Examine airway for bleeding—epistaxis may contaminate vomitus to appear as upper GI bleeding. Usually will require imaging or endoscopy.

HINTS FOR SCREENING PROBLEM

• Bright red blood signifies active bleeding.
• Darker blood or "coffee grounds" usually means that the blood has had some time to be denatured by gastric acid.
• The rate of bleeding will determine the clinical presentation. The more rapid the rate, the larger the volume of upper GI bleeding, and greater the drop in hemoglobin and change in pulse and blood pressure. Slower bleeding usually presents with anemia and heme positive stools.
• Any significant blood loss will lead to pallor, tachycardia, orthostasis, poor capillary refill, CNS changes (restlessness, confusion), and hypotension. Hypotension may not be seen even in the face of significant blood loss because vasoconstriction will occur to maintain blood pressure until decompensation.
• Initial hemoglobin values may be unreliable because a delay in hemodilution may falsely result in near normal values.
• Absence of blood in the emesis or in nasogastric lavage fluid does not rule out the upper GI tract as the site of bleeding, because a competent pylorus may mask bleeding from a duodenal site. In fact, in some cases of massive UGI bleeding, the patient may not vomit blood but may pass large, black, tarry, or sticky stools, called melena.

 Data Gathering

HISTORY

Question: Amount of blood, i.e., drops versus 1 teaspoon versus 1 tablespoon? Any clots?
Significance: Indicates severity of bleeding.

Question: Vomitus contains blood?
Significance: Indicates bleeding from upper GI tract or swallowed blood.

Question: Any recently ingested foods resemble blood, e.g., red food dye, beets, Jell-o, Kool-Aid, antibiotic syrups, food fibers?
Significance: Vomitus may not have blood.

Question: Can one determine the source of bleeding?
Significance: Hematemesis from the esophagus, stomach, or duodenum versus hemopytsis versus swallowed blood from the nose, mouth, or pharynx.

Question: Was the blood coughed or vomited?
Significance: Indicative of hemoptysis.

Question: Was it from the nose—swallowed and then vomited?
Significance: Not bleeding from the upper GI tract.

Question: Was there prolonged vomiting preceeding the bleeding?
Significance: Prolonged retching prior to hematemesis suggests a Mallory-Weiss tear.

Question: History of recent stress (burns, head trauma, surgery)?
Significance: Suggests an ulcer or gastritis.

Question: History of toxic ingestion?
Significance: May result in an ulcerated esophagus, which can bleed.

Question: Ingestion of certain medications?
Significance: Aspirin, steroids can lead to gastritis and ulcers. Ingestion of drugs (nonsteriodal anti-infammatory drugs) and alcohol can lead to gastritis.

Question: Abdominal pain and vomiting blood?
Significance: Suggests esophagitis, gastritis, and peptic ulcers

Question: Is there breast-feeding?
Significance: Cracked nipples in the mother can lead to the infant swallowing maternal blood and then having hematemesis.

Question: Is there history of gastroesophageal reflux?
Significance: Suggests esophagitis

Question: Is there past history of GI disease?
Significance: Gastroesophageal reflux, peptic ulcer disease, or previous GI surgery may suggest that the current symptoms may be due to recurrence of disease.

Question: Is there history of jaundice, hepatitis, or liver disease?
Significance: Suggests portal hypertension and variceal bleeding

Question: Was there any neonatal history of umbilical vein catherization or infection?
Significance: Portal vein thrombosis (sepsis, shock, exchange transfusion, omphalitis, IV catheters) suggests portal hypertension and bleeding varices due to cavernous transformation of the portal vein.

Question: Familial history of bleeding?
Significance: Familial history of bleeding diathesis, e.g., von Willebrand disease, hemophilia.

Physical Examination

Finding: Are there any skin petechiae, ecchymosis, hemangiomas?
Significance: Evidence of chronic liver disease (spider angiomata, palmar erythema, jaundice). Look for evidence of chronic liver disease and bleeding diathesis.

Finding: HEENT: Nasopharyngeal source of bleeding
Significance: Swallowed blood

Finding: Freckles on buccal mucosa
Significance: Osler-Weber-Rendu syndrome; Peutz-Jeghers syndrome

Finding: Oral thrush
Significance: *Candida* esophagitis

Finding: Oral mucosal lesions
Significance: Corrosive ingestions

Finding: Abdomen

- Hepatosplenomegaly
- Ascites

Significance: Portal hypertension

Finding: Isolated splenomegaly
Significance: Cavernous transformation of the portal vein; portal hypertension

Finding: Rectal examination
Significance: Heme-positive stool may or may not be present. If positive, confirms the presence of UGI bleeding.

Laboratory Aids

Test: Guaiac or Hematest
Significance: If possible check the red substance for blood. In neonates, may need to check for fetal hemoglobin with the Apt test.

Test: CBC
Significance: If there is leukopenia, anemia, and thrombocytopenia think chronic liver disease and portal hypertension. If there is anemia with normal RBC indices, then there is truly an acute cause for bleeding. If RBC indices indicate iron-deficiency anemia, think of varices or a mucosal lesion, i.e., chronic blood loss.

Test: Coagulation profile
Significance: If PT/PTT are abnormal then think of liver disease or disseminated intravascular coagulation (DIC) with sepsis. If DIC screen is negative, think liver disease. Make sure, however, that blood sample was not contaminated with heparin.

Test: Bleeding time
Significance: Abnormal in patients with previous history (or family history) of bleeding disorders.

Test: Liver function tests
Significance: Abnormal in chronic liver disease

Test: Upper endoscopy
Significance: Useful, as diagnosis can be made in 75% to 90% of patients.

Test: Barium tests
Significance: Not as useful as esophagoduodenoscopy (EGD) but can identify a large ulcer. Air-contrast UGI better than regular UGI test.

Test: Bleeding scan
Significance: Useful in the patient with significant bleeding in whom endoscopy was not diagnostic. Can get two types of scans: technetium sulfur colloid or tagged RBC scan. The former detects very rapid bleeding but can miss small bleeds, especially if patient is not bleeding during the scan. The latter can detect small bleeds, especially if intermittent.

Test: Angiography
Significance: Useful in detecting vascular causes for UGI bleeding. Can also be therapeutic, i.e., injection of coils into a vascular malformation to occlude it. Invasiveness and need for specialized training are limitations.

Therapy

Initial management of the emergency depends on diagnosis and clinical condition of the patient.

- Stabilize the patient with intravenous fluids and blood products if neccessary.
- Order laboratory tests: CBC, PT/PTT, DIC screen, liver function tests, blood type, and crossmatch.
- Insert an NG tube and lavage with saline to determine site as well as rate of ongoing bleeding. No need for cold saline.
- Monitor patient's vital signs and hemoglobin as necessary.
- Make appropriate diagnosis and institute appropriate therapy, i.e., EGD, bleeding scans.

DISEASE-SPECIFIC THERAPY

- Peptic ulcer disease

—Proton pump inhibitors
—H_2 blockers
—Sucralfate
—Prokinetic agents

- Esophageal varices

—Vasopressin or somatostatin infusion
—Sclerotherapy or banding
—Sengstaken-Blakemore tube

If bleeding stops quickly, then work-up is less emergent.

Follow-Up

- Monitor hemoglobin in the hospital until stable
- Once patient is discharged, monitor hemoglobin weekly as well as hemoccult cards until stable.
- More specific follow-up depends on the underlying condition.

PREVENTION

- Avoid drugs that are likely to cause bleeding or gastritis especially in a susceptible patient.
- In patients with chronic GI conditions, optimize therapy and monitoring.
- Correct coagulopathy
- Prophylactic sclerotherapy or banding for patients with known variceal bleeds

PITFALLS

- Make sure the vomited material is really blood.
- A negative nasogastric aspirate for blood does not indicate the absence of upper GI bleeding.
- Initial hemoglobin may not be accurate and serial hemoglobins should be obtained.

Common Questions and Answers

Q: When do you refer a patient?
A: Any bleed—immediate referral if bleed is large, the patient is hemodynamically unstable, and bleeding will not stop. Patient with evidence of chronic iron deficiency anemia and heme-positive stools.

Q: What makes upper GI bleeding an emergency?
A: Any persistent bleed with change in vital signs. Significant drop in hemoglobin.

BIBLIOGRAPHY

Ament M. Diagnosis and management of upper gastrointestinal bleeding in the pediatric patient. *Pediatr Rev* 1990;12:107–116.

Sherman PM. Peptic ulcer disease in children—diagnosis, treatment and the implication of *Helicobacter pylori*. *Gastroenterol Clin North Am* 1994;23(4):707–725.

Vinton NE. Gastrointestinal bleeding in infancy and childhood. *Gastroenterol Clin North Am* 1994;23(1):93–122.

Perrault JF, Berry R. Gastrointestinal bleeding. In: Walker WA, Durie PR, Hamilton JR, Walker-Smith JA, Watkins JB, eds. *Pediatric gastrointestinal disease: pathophysiology, diagnosis and management,* 2nd ed. St. Louis: Mosby, 1996:323–342.

Author: Maria R. Mascarenhas

Vomiting

Database

DEFINITION

The expulsion of gastric contents through the mouth in varying degrees. Regurgitation is defined as small, effortless mouthfuls of food or stomach contents. Vomiting is usually associated with large, forceful amounts of stomach contents.

Differential Diagnosis

DISORDERS OF GASTROINTESTINAL TRACT

- Anatomical

—Esophageal: stricture, web, ring, atresia
—Stomach: pyloric stenosis, web, duplication
—Intestine: duodenal atresia, malrotation, duplication
—Colon: Hirschsprung disease, imperforate anus

- Motility

—Achalasia
—Gastroesophageal reflux
—Intestinal pseudo-obstruction

- Foreign Body/Bezoar
- Obstruction

—Intussusception
—Volvulus
—Incarcerated hernia

- Cholecystitis or cholelithiasis
- Eosinophilic enteritis
- Appendicitis
- Necrotizing enterocolitis
- Peritonitis
- Celiac disease
- Peptic ulcer
- Trauma

—Duodenal hematoma
—Pancreatitis (pseudocyst)

NEUROLOGIC

- Intracranial mass lesions

—Tumor
—Cyst
—Subdural hematoma

- Cerebral edema
- Hydrocephalus
- Pseudotumor cerebri
- Migraine (head, abdominal)
- Seizures

RENAL

- Obstructive uropathy

—Ureteropelvic junction obstruction
—Hydronephrosis
—Nephrolithiasis

- Renal insufficiency
- Glomerulonephritis
- Renal tubular acidosis

METABOLIC

- Inborn errors of metabolism

—Galactosemia
—Fructose intolerance
—Hereditary fructose intolerance
—Amino acid or organic acid metabolism
—Urea cycle defects
—Fatty acid oxidation disorders
—Lactic acidosis

INFECTION

- Sepsis
- Meningitis
- Urinary tract infection
- Parasites
- *Giardia*
- Ascaris
- *Helicobacter pylori*
- Otitis media
- Viral/Bacterial

—Gastroenteritis
—Viral hepatitis (A, B, C)
—*Bordatella* pertussis

ENDOCRINE

- Diabetes

—Diabetic ketoacidosis (DKA)
—Gastroparesis

- Adrenal insufficiency

RESPIRATORY

- Pneumonia
- Sinusitis
- Laryngitis

IMMUNOLOGIC

- Milk/soy protein allergy
- *Cryptosporidium* (AIDS)
- Graft-versus-host disease
- Chronic granulomatous disease

OTHER

- Pregnancy
- Rumination
- Bulimia
- Psychogenic
- Cyclic emesis syndrome
- Overfeeding
- Medications

—Drugs
—Vitamin toxicity

- Vascular (superior mesenteric artery syndrome)

Approach to the Patient

Vomiting is a prominent feature of many disorders of infancy and childhood and is often the only presenting symptom of many diseases. Vomiting can occur as a defense mechanism to expel ingested toxins, as an abnormality of the vomiting center related to increased intracranial pressure, as a result of intestinal obstruction or anatomical/mucosal abnormalities, or as the result of a generalized metabolic disease. A full history should include medication and drug use, trauma, and, in adolescents, questions regarding feeding disorders (bulimia) and intercourse (pregnancy).

Data Gathering

HISTORY

Question: Fever?
Significance: Infectious causes of vomiting are common.

Question: Abdominal pain and frequent, forceful or bilious emesis?
Significance: Often associated with anatomic or obstructive intestinal disorder.

Question: Age of patient?
Significance: Pyloric stenosis and inborn errors of metabolism almost always present in infancy with vomiting, dehydration, and biochemical abnormalities.

Question: Mental retardation, pica, and patchy baldness?
Significance: Foreign body or hair ingestion and the development of a gastric bezoar.

Question: Nausea and epigastric pain related to meals?
Significance: Often indicates gastritis, gastric emptying delay, or gallbladder disease.

Question: Alleviated by meals?
Significance: Gastroesophageal reflux and gastric ulcer disease

Question: Alternating vomiting and lethargy?
Significance: Intussusception

Question: Chronic headaches, fatigue, weakness, weight loss, and early morning vomiting?
Significance: Neurologic causes of vomiting secondary to increased intracranial pressure

Question: Right- or left-sided abdominal pain?
Significance: Renal disease, inflammatory bowel disease

Physical Examination

A careful and complete physical examination can often provide excellent clues as to the cause of vomiting in children.

Finding: Visible bowel loops
Significance: Obstruction

Finding: Palpation for a mass effect and tenderness, and auscultation for evidence of absent bowel sounds or borborygmi (rumbling bowel sounds)
Significance: Intestinal obstruction

Finding: Rectal examination
Significance: Testing the stool for occult blood

Finding: Discoloration of skin and sclera
Significance: Jaundice (liver/gallbladder or metabolic disease)

Finding: Orange tint of sclera or skin
Significance: Hypervitaminosis A

Finding: Unusual odor
Significance: Metabolic disease

Finding: Chronic vomiting
Significance: Evidence of neurologic dysfunction, including nystagmus, head tilt, papilledema, abnormal reflexes, and weakness

Finding: Tense anterior fontanelle
Significance: May indicate meningitis, hydrocephalus, or vitamin A toxicity

Finding: Enlarged parotid glands and hypersalivation
Significance: Bulimia and other feeding disorders

Finding: Pelvic examination
Significance: Pregnancy, pelvic inflammatory disease, or ovarian disease

Laboratory Aids

Test: CBC
Significance: Anemia and iron deficiency can occur with intestinal duplication and obstruction, gastritis/esophagitis, and ulcer disease.

Test: Blood chemistry
Significance: Electrolyte abnormalities are found in pyloric stenosis, metabolic abnormalities, while an elevated ALT, total bilirubin, and GGT can indicate liver, gallbladder, or metabolic disease.

Test: Urinalysis
Significance: Pyelonephritis

Test: Amylase
Significance: Pancreatitis

Test: BUN/creatinine
Significance: If elevated—renal disease

Test: Urine culture
Significance: UTI

Test: Plain abdominal x-ray study
Significance: Obstruction

Test: Abdominal ultrasound
Significance: Liver, gallbladder, renal, pancreatic, ovarian, or uterine disease. In infants, abdominal ultrasound is the test of choice for pyloric stenosis. Useful when considering abdominal abscess and appendicitis.

Test: Contrast radiography
Significance: Intestinal anatomic abnormalities (malrotation, intussusception, volvulus)

Test: Computed tomography
Significance: Not generally indicated for evaluation of vomiting, although it is an effective tool when more anatomical abdominal detail is required (abscess, tumor).

Test: Endoscopy
Significance: Esophageal, gastric, and duodenal inflammation (esophagitis, gastritis, ulcer disease, celiac disease, eosinophilic enteritis) as well as for obtaining cultures for unusual infections (duodenal *Giardia*, *Helicobacter pylori*/cytomegalovirus gastritis).

Issues for Referral

- Chronic vomiting (2–3 weeks)
- Weight loss
- Severe abdominal pain or irritability
- Gastrointestinal bleeding
- Evidence of intestinal obstruction
- Serum electrolyte abnormalities
- Abnormal neurologic examination
- Dehydration
- Signs of an acute abdomen
- Lethargy

Emergency Care

Evidence of hematemesis, intestinal obstruction (bilious vomiting), dehydration, neurologic dysfunction, or an acute abdomen should be treated as a medical emergency, and hospitalization should be considered.

BIBLIOGRAPHY

Piccoli DA. Gastroenterology and nutrition. In: Polin RA, Ditmar MF, eds. *Pediatric secrets*. St. Louis: CV Mosby, 1989:93–120.

Silverman A, Roy CC, eds. *Pediatric clinical gastroenterology*, 3rd ed. St. Louis: CV Mosby, 1983.

Sondheimer J. Vomiting and regurgitation. In: Walker WA, Durie PR, Hamilton JR, Walker-Smith JA, Watkins JB, eds. *Pediatric gastrointestinal disease*. St. Louis: Mosby, 1996:19.

Author: Chris A. Liacouras

Weight Loss

 Database

DEFINITION

Weight loss is a documented decrease in weight from a previous measurement. Outside of the newborn period (weight loss in the first 2 weeks is common), acute illnesses resulting in fluid loss, and obese adolescents voluntarily on a designed weight reduction program, weight loss is unusual and worrisome symptom, regardless of the percentage decline.

 Differential Diagnosis

CONGENITAL/ANATOMICAL

- Congenital heart disease
- Pyloric stenosis
- Gastrointestinal malformation (duodenal atresia, annular pancreas, volvulus)
- Short bowel syndrome
- Lymphangiectasia
- Superior mesenteric artery syndrome
- Gastroesophageal reflux
- Immunodeficiency disorders
- Hirschsprung disease

INFECTIOUS

- Urinary tract infection
- Tuberculosis
- Stomatitis
- Osteomyelitis
- Human immunodeficiency virus
- Hepatitis
- Parasitic disease
- Gastroenteritis
- Pericarditis
- Histoplamosis
- Acute severe febrile illness (pyelonephritis, pneumonia, septic arthritis)

TOXIC, ENVIRONMENTAL, DRUGS

- Lead poisoning
- Mercury poisoning
- Vitamin A poisoning
- Chronic methylphenidate, dextroamphetamine, or valproic acid use
- Substance abuse, especially amphetamines and crack cocaine

TRAUMA

- Chronic subdural hematomas

TUMOR

- Diencephalic syndrome
- Leukemia
- Lymphoma
- Pheochromocytoma
- Other neoplasms

GENETIC/METABOLIC

- Diabetes mellitus
- Diabetes insipidus
- Hyperthyroidism
- Cystic fibrosis
- Schwachman syndrome
- Addison disease
- Hypercalcemia
- Congenital adrenal hyperplasia
- Lactose intolerance
- Renal tubular acidosis
- Chronic renal failure
- Hypopituitarism
- Inborn errors of metabolism
- Storage diseases
- Muscular dystrophy
- Lipodystrophy

ALLERGIC/INFLAMMATORY

- Inflammatory bowel disease
- Juvenile rheumatoid arthritis
- Systemic lupus erythematosus
- Sarcoidosis
- Pancreatitis
- Hepatitis
- Celiac disease (gluten enteropathy)

FUNCTIONAL MISCELLANEOUS

- Malnutrition
- Child abuse
- Post-operative
- Dieting
- Depression/affective disorders
- Anorexia nervosa
- Chronic congestive heart failure
- Chronic pulmonary disease
- Chronic renal disease
- Iron deficiency
- Zinc deficiency
- Cerebral palsy
- Post-infectious malabsorption
- Factitious (e.g., scale error)

Approach to the Patient

GENERAL GOAL

Decide as to the acuity, chronicity and severity of weight loss, and the need for hospitalization.

Phase 1: Attempt to narrow the diagnostic possibilities by history and examination, particularly by assessing if the loss might be attributable to diminished intake, diminished absorption, or increased requirements.

 Data History

HISTORY

Question: Is the weight loss real?
Significance: Scale error, different scales, different technique (e.g., clothed versus unclothed)

Question: What is the child's diet?
Significance: A prospective 3-day dietary record can be very useful for demonstrating insufficient caloric intake.

Question: Less than 2 weeks of age?
Significance: Physiological weight loss, underfeeding, inappropriate feeding, inborn errors of metabolism, congenital heart disease, gastroesophageal reflux

Question: Less than 4 months?
Significance: Malnutrition, improper formula preparation, cystic fibrosis, gastroesophageal reflux, pyloric stenosis, congenital heart disease, congenital adrenal hyperplasia, inborn errors of metabolism

Question: 4 months to 8 years?
Significance: Chronic infection, cystic fibrosis, malabsorption, neglect/abuse, renal disease, liver disease, diabetes mellitus

Question: Older than 8 years?
Significance: Eating disorder, chronic infection, neoplasm, renal disease, liver disease, substance abuse, diabetes mellitus, inflammatory bowel disease, collagen vascular disease

Question: Cramping, bloating or abnormally greasy, voluminous stools?
Significance: Possible malabsorption

Question: Vomiting, especially projectile?
Significance: Suggestive of intestinal obstruction, G-E reflux, inborn errors of metabolism

Question: Polyuria, polydipsia and polyphagia?
Significance: Possible diabetes mellitus

Question: Headaches, especially early morning?
Significance: Possible increased intracranial pressure, CNS malignancy

Question: Maternal history of multiple miscarriages, neonatal deaths, or consanguinity?
Significance: Possible inborn error of metabolism

Question: History of severe infections, persistent candidal infections?
Significance: Immunodeficiency, congenital or acquired

Question: Fear of fatness, preoccupation with food, distorted body image, and/or amenorrhea?
Significance: Possible eating disorder

Question: Delayed puberty?
Significance: Suggests chronic severe weight loss, pituitary abnormalities, anorexia nervosa

Question: Foreign travel?
Significance: Possible chronic infection (e.g., tuberculosis, parasitic dissease)

Question: Tiring during feeding or difficulty feeding due to cough and dyspnea?
Significance: Suggests CHF in newborn/infant, hypothyroidism

Question: Increased appetite with weight loss?
Significance: Suggests hyperthyroidism, cystic fibrosis, pheochromocytoma

Question: Altered mental status, seizures, unusual body/fluid odors
Significance: Inborn error of metabolism

Physical Examination

Finding: Clubbing
Significance: Suggests chronic cardiac, pulmonary, or intestinal disease

Finding: Significant abdominal distension
Significance: Suggests celiac disease

Finding: Hypothermia, bradycardia
Significance: Suggests anorexia nervosa, hypothyroidism

Finding: Tachycardia, resting
Significance: Hyperthyroidism, pheochromocytoma, anemia, acute weight loss

Finding: Orthostatic changes
Significance: Significant weight loss, possibly acute

Finding: Hypotension, resting
Significance: Addison disease, anorexia nervosa, significant acute dehydration

Finding: Visual field abnormalities
Significance: Suggests possible CNS malignancy

Finding: Swollen joint
Significance: Juvenile rheumatoid arthritis, inflammatory bowel disease

Finding: Muscle weakness
Significance: Connective tissue disorder, electrolyte abnormality, muscular dystrophy

Finding: Enlarged liver and/or spleen
Significance: Suggests malignancy, chronic infection, storage disease, inborn error of metabolism

Laboratory Aids

Test: Complete blood count
Significance:

• Evidence of

—Anemia—macrocytic associated with folate/B_{12} deficiency, microcytic with iron deficiency or chronic infection
—Polycythemia—suggestive of chronic pulmonary or cardiac disease
—Neutropenia—suggestive of hematologic malignancy, Schwachman syndrome, immunodeficiency
—Lymphopenia—suggestive of immunodeficiency
—Eosinophilia—suggestive of parasitic disease
—Leukocytosis—suggestive of infection
—Thrombocytosis—suggestive of chronic infection, malignancy
—Lymphoblasts—suggestive of leukemia

Test: ESR
Significance: May be elevated in inflammatory bowel disease, chronic infections, rheumatoid diseases

Test: Serum electrolytes
Significance: Abnormalities in dehydration, adrenal insufficiency (low Na, high K), renal disease, anorexia nervosa

Test: BUN, creatinine
Significance: Abnormal in renal disease, dehydration

Test: Stool for occult blood and pH, reducing substances (Clinitest)
Significance: Occult blood suggests inflammatory bowel disease; low pH and positive reducing substances suggest malabsorption

Test: Urinalysis
Significance: Hematuria and/or proteinuria suggest renal disease; glycosuria suggests diabetes mellitus; very low specific gravity suggests diabetes insipidus, chronic renal failure, hypercalcemia; pyuria suggests UTI; pH >6 suggests RTA (type I)

Test: Urine culture
Significance: Evaluation for UTI

Test: Serum protein levels
Significance: Very low levels imply impaired liver function, severe chronic weight loss or protein malabsorption

Test: Tuberculosis skin test
Significance: Possible chronic infection

Test: Liver function tests
Significance: Evaluation for hepatitis, chronic liver disease

Depending on age and clinical findings, other tests to consider include thyroid function tests, sweat test, tests for malabsorption (e.g., lactose breath test, stool fat, stool for trypsin), tests for metabolic disease (e.g., plasma ammonia, lactate, serum/urine amino acids, urine organic acids), imaging studies (e.g., CT, MRI, bone scan), immunologic studies.

Emergency Care

• Significant dehydration: abnormal vital signs with orthostasis, decreased urine output, decreased skin turgor, delayed capillary refill (>3 seconds). Mandates cardiovascular support (intravenous hydration) and a more urgent diagnosis (e.g., inborn error of metabolism, obstructive GI disease, congenital adrenal hyperplasia, diabetic ketoacidosis).
• Abnormal mental status, significant lethargy: May be seen in severe dehydration, hypoadrenalism, hypoxic states, toxic ingestions, renal or respiratory failure, increased intracranial pressure, severe electrolyte abnormalities.
• Increasing vomiting in the setting of known weight loss in infants: High risk for dehydration, hypoglycemia, and electrolyte abnormalities. Need to evaluate for treatable conditions (e.g., obstructive GI disease, inborn errors of metabolism, congenital adrenal hyperplasia, congenital heart disease) in which a delay is life-threatening.
• Severe malnutrition (weight loss >20% of ideal body weight): high risk for metabolic derangements, including dysrhythmias secondary to electrolyte abnormalities. Aggressive evaluation is warranted.

Common Questions and Answers

Q: How common is weight loss in the first 2 weeks of life?
A: Formula-fed babies may lose up to 7% of birth weight and breast-fed newborns up to 10% before regaining their birth weight by 2 weeks of age.

Issues for Referral

Weight loss is a diagnostic exigency—a cause must be found or the loss self-resolved. If a diagnosis is not uncovered in the setting of continued weight loss, referral to a pediatric diagnostic center is indicated.

Clinical Pearls

• Be certain that the weight loss is real. In some studies, up to 25% of weight loss is artifactual as a result of measurement errors (e.g., excessive movement of scale, dressed versus undressed patient).
• Newborns with weight loss, especially at the 2-week visit, may manifest passivity and paradoxical disinterest in breastfeeding, although the reason for their problem is malnourishment due to inadequate intake (often from improper positioning or too infrequent feedings). They may not act "hungry." Observation of the feeding technique (by a practitioner with expertise or a lactation consultant) is vital.

BIBLIOGRAPHY

Kleinman RE, ed. *Pediatric nutrition handbook,* 4th ed. Elk Grove Village, IL: American Academy of Pediatrics, 1998.

Maisels MJ, Gifford K. Breast-feeding, weight loss, and jaundice. *J Pediatr* 1983;102:117–118.

Author: Mark F. Ditmar

Wheezing

Database

DEFINITION

Wheezing is often described as musical in nature, and occurs predominantly during expiration due to airway narrowing in the lower respiratory tract.

Differential Diagnosis

CONGENITAL/ANATOMICAL

- Extrinsic to airway

—Lymphadenopathy
—Tumor/malignancy
—Diaphragmatic hernia

- Intrinsic to airway

—Bronchomalacia
—Endobronchial foreign body
—Endobronchial tuberculosis
—Endobronchial tumors
—Vocal cord dysfunction
—Bronchopulmonary dysplasia
—Congestive heart failure/pulmonary edema
—Pulmonary cysts
—Congenital lobar emphysema
—Pulmonary sequestration

INFLAMMATORY/INFECTIOUS

- Bronchitis
- Bronchiolitis

—Viral bronchiolitis secondary to respiratory syncytial virus (see Bronchiolitis)

- Pneumonia

—Mycoplasma
—Chlamydia
—Aspiration

- Bronchiectasis
- Bronchial papillomas
- Hypersensitivity pneumonitis
- Pulmonary hemosiderosis

GENETIC/METABOLIC

- Cystic fibrosis
- Dyskinetic (immotile) cilia syndrome

—Kartagener syndrome

- Metabolic disturbances

—Hypocalcemia
—Hypokalemia

ALLERGIC

- Asthma (see Asthma)

MISCELLANEOUS

- Psychosomatic illness

—Emotional laryngeal wheezing
—Factitious asthma

Approach to the Patient

GENERAL GOALS

- Characterize the type of abnormal breath sounds heard. Determine the timing of sounds in the respiratory cycle (expiratory and/or inspiratory?) and location (unilateral or bilateral?; are sounds heard best in the region of the neck or chest?). The goal is to distinguish between continuous sounds originating from the upper airway (e.g., stridor) including transmitted upper airway sounds, and lower airway (e.g., wheezing).
- In patients identified with wheezing, determine the likely cause.
- The therapy for wheezing is directed toward a specific cause.

Phase 1: Quickly determine the severity of the patient's illness (e.g., toxicity) including degree of respiratory distress.

Phase 2: Determine the most likely causes of wheezing through careful history and physical examination. The differential diagnoses generated will determine the extent of additional laboratory testing needed. (For additional details, see History.)

Phase 3: There is no one therapy that is effective for all causes of wheezing, therefore, therapy is disease specific. A trial of beta-agonists (e.g., albuterol) may be considered in patients with suspected reactive airway disease or bronchiolitis.

Data Gathering

HISTORY

Question: What is the pattern, if any, of the wheezing over time? New onset versus recurrent? Intermittent versus persistent? Seasonal pattern?
Significance: Episodes of recurrent wheezing with periods of complete resolution suggests reactive airway disease or asthma. Persistent wheezing suggests anatomic (e.g., intrinsic or extrinsic airway compression) or persistent physiological abnormalities (e.g., bronchopulmonary dysplasia, cystic fibrosis, or immotile cilia syndrome).

Question: What was the age of onset of wheezing?
Significance: Onset at birth or during early infancy suggests a congenital/anatomical disease process. Of the infectious etiologies, younger infants and children (especially less than 1–2 years of age) are more susceptible to lower respiratory tract infection with the common viral pathogens (e.g., respiratory syncytial virus bronchiolitis), while mycoplasma pneumoniae is more commonly identified in school-aged children. Foreign body aspiration is more common in children between the ages 1 and 4 years.

Question: Have any triggers of wheezing been identified?
Significance: Upper respiratory infection symptoms (i.e., nasal congestion, cough, fever) can accompany viral bronchiolitis or a virus-triggered reactive airway disease. Common triggers for asthma include allergens (e.g., house dust mites, pollen, animal dander), irritants (e.g., tobacco smoke, pollution), exercise, and changes in humidity or air temperature.

Question: Did an episode of choking precede the onset of wheezing?
Significance: A history of choking mandates consideration of foreign body aspiration.

Physical Examination

Finding: Assess the patient's degree of respiratory distress and toxicity.
Significance: Look for signs of respiratory distress including tachypnea, retractions, nasal flaring, head bobbing, abdominal breathing, cyanosis, the ability to speak in complete sentences, and the adequacy of air entry. Of note, some patients with significant airway obstruction may exhibit relatively little respiratory distress. Also, wheezing may not be audible in patients with severely restricted air movement.

Finding: Determine the timing of abnormal breath sounds in the respiratory cycle, i.e., inspiratory, expiratory, bi-phasic.
Significance: Inspiratory breaths sounds (i.e., stridor) are associated with extrathoracic narrowing of the airway (see Stridor, Croup, Tracheitis, and Epiglottitis).

Finding: Ratio of inspiratory to expiratory phase
Significance: A prolonged expiratory phase indicates obstructive airway disease. In asthma, a prolonged expiration should occur in conjunction with expiratory wheezing.

Finding: Presence of clubbing
Significance: Clubbing indicates chronic cardiopulmonary disease (e.g., congenital or acquired heart disease, cystic fibrosis, bronchopulmonary dysplasia). Clubbing should not be present in children with asthma.

Finding: Presence of allergic shiners, Dennie lines, nasal crease, the "allergic salute" (i.e., rubbing the nose with the palm of the hand), and atopic dermatitis
Significance: The presence of other atopic diseases increases likelihood of coexisting asthma.

Laboratory Aids

Test: Pulse oximetry measurement of oxygen saturation (SaO_2).
Significance: Pulse oximetry can help gauge the degree of respiratory compromise. In asthma, SaO_2 measurements of less than 92% may be seen in severe exacerbations.

Test: Arterial blood gas (ABG)
Significance: ABGs provide a direct measure of oxygenation (paO_2) and ventilation ($paCO_2$). A low $paCO_2$ is expected in a patient with increased work of breathing, therefore, a normal or increasing $paCO_2$ predicts impending respiratory failure. In general, ABG measurements are not necessary in the vast majority of patients seen in the office setting with wheezing.

Test: Pulmonary function testing (PFT)—peak flow meter, spirometry
Significance: PFTs can be used to quantify the degree of airway obstruction. Older children (>6 years old) can cooperate with peak flow measurements, which can be plotted against normal ranges (typically based on height), or personal best (in patients with known asthma).

Test: Microbiologic studies. A variety of cultures, antigen detection, and polymerase chain reaction studies can be performed on nasal washes from infants, for the identification of respiratory viruses (e.g., RSV, adenovirus, parainfluenza virus, influenza), chlamydia, and pertussis. The validity of sputum cultures (especially bacterial cultures) in determining the cause of lower respiratory tract infections in children is limited.
Significance: These tests may allow identification of a specific infectious etiology. However, a delay in getting the results of some of these tests, cost, and a lack of specific therapy for many of the viral agents, may restrict their use and value.

Test: Tuberculosis skin test—Mantoux purified protein derivative (PPD)
Significance: Tuberculosis can produce wheezing through both intrinsic (endobronchial) or extrinsic (lymph node) effects on the airway.

Test: Chest radiography (anteroposterior and lateral)
Significance: Routine chest radiology can demonstrate airway obstruction (e.g., hyperinflation, hyperlucency, flattening of the diaphragms), peribronchial cuffing, infiltrates, atelectasis, bronchiectasis, and radio-opaque foreign bodies. Asymmetry in air-trapping can suggest foreign body aspiration.

Test: Complete blood count including eosinophil count, quantitative immunoglobulins, IgE, complement, HIV testing, allergy skin testing
Significance: Allergy/immunologic evaluation in selected individuals.

 ## Therapy

- A trial of bronchodilator therapy (e.g., albuterol) may be both therapeutic and diagnostic of reversible airway obstruction in patients suspected of having reactive airway disease.
- Antibiotics may be considered in patients with illnesses compatible with *Mycoplasma pneumoniae* or *Chlamydia pneumoniae,* both of which can produce clinical manifestation of wheezing.
- Antiviral agents, such as ribavirin for respiratory syncytial virus, have limited usefulness for the majority of cases.

 ## Emergency Care

Factors that make this an emergency include:

- Respiratory distress—tachypnea, retractions, nasal flaring, head bobbing, abdominal breathing, cyanosis, inability to speak in complete sentences, inadequate air entry.
- Respiratory insufficiency—cyanosis, fatigue, altered mental status (e.g., confusion, agitation), apnea, normal or rising pCO_2 in the face of respiratory distress.
- Management of respiratory emergencies begin with the ABCs—Airway, Breathing, and Circulation. Determine which patients require assisted ventilation (e.g., bag-mask ventilation or endotracheal intubation). Reassess often.

 ## Common Questions and Answers

Q: How common is wheezing in childhood?
A: Wheezing is common in childhood. By 1 year of age, 25% to 30% of infants will have an episode of wheezing. This percentage may increase to 40% by 3 years of age, and nearly one-half by 6 years.

Q: What percent of recurrent wheezing resolves by school age?
A: In one prospective study up to 6 years of age, roughly 40% of children with one or more episodes of wheezing by 3 years of age no longer wheezed by 6 years of age.

Q: Should chest x-rays be routinely obtained in children experiencing their first episodes of wheezing?
A: Admittedly, the decision to obtain a chest x-ray of a patient in this setting is controversial. The reported rate of abnormal x-ray findings (other than those consistent with asthma or reactive airway disease) are in the range of 5% to 6%.

Issues for Referral

Factors that may help alert you to make a referral include:

- Patients requiring surgical intervention. Suspected or confirmed foreign body aspiration requires referral to a surgical service (e.g., pediatric surgery, otolaryngology) for rigid bronchoscopy and removal of the foreign body.
- For patients in whom the diagnosis is not clear after initial evaluation, consider referral to a specialist (e.g., pulmonologist) for additional diagnostic evaluation.
- Patients with specific congenital/anatomic malformations and genetic syndromes.
- Patients with asthma who experience a life-threatening episode, poor control, etc. (*see* Asthma or Expert Panel Report 2, 1997 are recommended to have specialty referral) (e.g., pulmonologist, allergist).
- Patients in whom the identification of specific allergic triggers will help case management may benefit from referral to an allergist for skin testing.

Clinical Pearls

- "All that wheezes is not asthma." While most episodes of wheezing will represent viral infections or asthma, clinicians need to be mindful of alternative diagnoses. This is especially true in patients with first-time, persistent, or atypical episodes of wheezing.
- A high index of suspicion is necessary to make the diagnosis of foreign body aspiration (FBA). While a history of choking is helpful in supporting the diagnosis, the absence of such a history does not rule out the diagnosis.

—Toy safety: Families should be aware of the choking hazards that small toys can be for infants and young children. Parents can screen toys for appropriate size by using a tube from a toilet paper roll. With a diameter of about 1.75 inches, a measurement promoted by the Consumer Product Safety Commission (CPSC), toys which can fit inside are too small for children less than 3 years of age.

BIBLIOGRAPHY

Consumer Product Safety Commission [http://www.cpsc.gov].

Expert Panel Report 2. Guidelines for the diagnosis and management of asthma: National Heart, Lung, and Blood Institute. National Asthma Education Program Expert Panel report. NIH Publication No. 97-4051. April 1997.

Holroyd HJ. Foreign body aspiration: potential cause of coughing and wheezing. *Pediatr Rev* 1988;10(2):59–63.

Marks MB. Differential diagnosis of wheezing in children. *Clin Pediatr* 1974;13(3):225–228.

Martinez FD, Wright AL, Taussig LM, Holberg CJ, Halonen M, Morgan WJ. Asthma and wheeezing in the first six years of life. The Group Health Medical Associates. *N Engl J Med* 1995;332(3):133–138.

Authors: Alan Uba and Gerd Cropp

Specific Diseases

Abdominal Migraine (Epilepsy)

 Database

DEFINITION

Recurrent identical attacks of periumbilical pain, which can include nausea, vomiting, headache, pallor, perspiration, slowing of pulse rate, fever, diarrhea, and/or limb pains. Synonyms include: periodic syndrome, cyclical vomiting, and/or growing pains.

PATHOLOGY

- Controversy exists between migraine versus epileptic pathogenesis. Although non-specific EEG changes are seen more commonly among these children, very few go on to develop signs of epilepsy.
- Children with abdominal migraine are more likely than controls to go on to develop more typical migraine headaches later in life; 10% of children with migraine headaches are found in retrospect to have suffered from unexplained abdominal pain prior to the onset of headache.
- Adult migraine headache sufferers experience abdominal pain more frequently than tension headache sufferers.
- May involve neuronal activity originating in the hypothalamus with involvement of the cortex and autonomic nervous system. Serotonin is implicated, and blockade of serotonin receptors has been shown to act prophylactically in abdominal migraine.
- May involve some, as yet ill-defined, local intestinal vasomotor factors.

EPIDEMIOLOGY

- Mostly occurs in children between the ages of 3 and 10, peaking at about age 9.
- More common in girls.
- May affect as many as 1% to 2% of children at some point in their lives.
- Declining frequency toward adulthood.

GENETICS

Parents of affected children often have history of migraine headaches.

 Differential Diagnosis

INFECTION

- *Giardia*

ENVIRONMENTAL

- Lead intoxication
- Tumors

METABOLIC

- Porphyria
- Lactose intolerance

PSYCHOSOCIAL

- Functional abdominal pain
- Irritable bowel syndrome

SURGICAL

- Appendicitis
- Intussusception
- Biliary colic

INFLAMMATION

- Inflammatory bowel disease
- Peptic ulcer disease
- Mesenteric adenitis

ANATOMICAL

- Meckel diverticulum
- Ureteropelvic junction (UPJ) obstruction

MISCELLANEOUS

- Constipation
- Abdominal epilepsy [but has a shorter duration of pain (minutes), altered consciousness during event, abrupt onset, abnormal discharges in EEG in 80%]

 Data Gathering

HISTORY

- Pain usually lasts less than 6 hours.
- Pain can be located anywhere in abdomen, but more often in upper quadrants.
- No abdominal pain between attacks
- Repetition of identical abdominal crises, anywhere from one per week to several times a year
- Migraine in relatives
- Presence of other migraine-like syndromes such as nausea, vomiting, perspiration, body temperature changes, focal paresthesias, radiation of pain to a limb, malaise
- Absence of impaired consciousness

 Physical Examination

Unremarkable physical findings, with a benign abdomen.

SPECIAL QUESTIONS

Ask about a familial history of migraine headache or unexplained bouts of abdominal pain as children.

Laboratory Aids

Test: CBC, differential, sedimentation rate, urinalysis (to exclude alternative diagnoses)
Significance: R/O infection, i.e., UTI

Test: Stool heme test, and stool for culture
Significance: IBD, GI causes of pain

Test: Lactose breath test
Significance: Lactose intolerance

Test: Lead test, porphyria work-up (depending on situation)
Significance: Poryphyria

Test: EEG
Significance: May help differentiate between abdominal migraine and abdominal epilepsy

Test: Visual evoked response (VER) to red and white flash light
Significance: May be helpful in diagnosing abdominal migraine, as children with clinically diagnosed abdominal migraine display a specific fast-wave activity response compared to normal controls, or children with migraine headaches alone

Test: Obstruction series
Significance: Intermittent or partial bowel obstruction

Test: Upper GI
Significance: To rule out anatomical abnormalities

Test: Ultrasound
Significance: To rule out tumor, chronic appendicitis, etc.

Test: Renal ultrasound
Significance: To rule out UPJ obstruction

Test: Barium enema
Significance: During painful crisis to rule out intussusception

 ## Therapy

DRUGS

• Tricyclic antidepressants, serotonin receptor antagonists or beta blockers, used as in prophylactic treatment of migraine headaches
• Ergotamine, antihistamines, as in abortive medical treatment of migraine headaches

 ## Follow-Up

Most children outgrow abdominal migraines by early adolescence. However, some of them later develop more typical migraine headaches.

PITFALLS

• Abdominal migraine is a diagnosis of exclusion; even if a patient meets most criteria for abdominal migraine, alternative diagnoses should be considered and tested for as appropriate to ensure that a more serious disorder does not exist.
• Patients may go through an unnecessarily extensive work-up to rule out other causes of pain, sometimes including laparotomy.
• Absence of objective abnormalities on laboratory testing does not necessarily indicate neurosis in the patient/family.
• Medications must be given on a daily basis, as they are used in a prophylactic fashion. For the majority of patients, side effects and complications from the use of medications may outweigh the relief of pain, especially in children who are experiencing infrequent episodes.

 ## Common Questions and Answers

Q: Does this mean my child will develop migraine headaches?
A: There is an association between abdominal migraines in childhood and migraine headaches in later life. There is no good way to predict for sure whether your child will experience migraine headaches.

Q: I have two other younger children. What chance do they have of developing abdominal migraines?
A: Although abdominal migraines do tend to run in families, there is no known Mendelian inheritance pattern, as opposed to a disease such as cystic fibrosis, for which a probability can be given.

Q: What can I do to help my child during bouts of pain?
A: The parent should allow the child to do whatever makes him or her comfortable. This may mean rest, positioning, quiet, etc. Acetaminophen and other pain relievers may help to a certain degree. Whether the patient should be excused from school depends on various factors, such as the frequency, severity, and duration of the pain, as well as the age, maturity, and coping skills of the child.

ICD-9-CM 346.2

BIBLIOGRAPHY

Barlow CF. The periodic syndrome-cyclic vomiting and abdominal migraine. *Clin Devel Med* 1984;91:83–84.

Boyle JT. Recurrent abdominal pain: an update. *Pediatr Rev* 1997;18(9):310–320.

Bruyn GW. Migraine equivalents. *Handbook Clin Neurol* 1986;4(48):155–171.

Irish MS, Pearl RH, Caty MG, Glick PL. The approach to common abdominal diagnosis in infants and children. *Pediatr Clin North Am* 1998;45(4):729–772.

Mortimer MJ, Good PA. The VER as a diagnostic marker for childhood abdominal migraine. *Headache* 1990;30:642–645.

Mortimer MJ, Kay J, Janon A. Clinical epidemiology of childhood migraine in an urban general pediatric practice. *Dev Med Child Neurol* 1993;35:243–248.

Symon DY. Abdominal migraine: a childhood syndrome defined. *Cephalalgia* 1986;6:223–228.

Author: Karen Liquornik

Acne

Database

DEFINITION

• Acne is a common disorder of the pilosebaceous glands, characterized by follicular occlusion and inflammation, which affects predominantly adolescents.
• Acne vulgaris is the form of acne most commonly seen in adolescents. It is characterized by various types of lesions, including microcomedones, closed comedos, open comedos, papules, pustules, nodules, and cysts.

Acne can be graded as follows:

• Grade I: noninflammatory acne; comedones
• Grade II: moderate, inflammatory acne with comedones, papules, and occasional pustules
• Grade III: severe localized inflammatory acne
• Grade IV: severe, generalized inflammatory acne with pustules, nodules, and cysts

Other, more rare types of acne include:

• Gram-negative acne
• Cosmetic acne: some moisturizing creams and oil-containing hair care products may produce comedonal acne.
• Occupational acne: certain products can cause obstruction of sebaceous follicles, including mineral oil, petroleum, coal tar, pitch, and halogenated aromatic hydrocarbons.
• Drug-induced acne: seen with use of androgens, steroids, barbiturates, phenytoin, isoniazid, rifampin, bromides, and iodides.
• Acne neonatorum: in infants post-delivery.

PATHOPHYSIOLOGY

Causes

• Androgenic hormones (gonadal and adrenal)
• Bacterial colonization of sebum with anaerobic diphtheroids, *Propionibacterium acnes,* and coagulase-negative staphylococci
• Free fatty acids
• Abnormal keratinization of sebaceous and follicular ducts
• Progesterone may affect acne through a mechanism other than sebum secretion
• Cosmetics, creams, drugs

Lesions Involved in Acne

• Microcomedone: impaction of keratin, lipids, bacteria, and rudimentary hair within the sebaceous follicle. These are small and subclinical, but they are the precursors to all acne lesions.
• Open comedo (blackhead): epithelium-lined sac filled with keratin and lipid with a widely dilated orifice; cylindrical, 1 to 3 mm in length; black from melanin pigment in epidermis.
• Closed comedo (whitehead): flask-shaped, small, skin-colored, slightly elevated papules just beneath the skin's surface. When the follicular wall ruptures, it expels sebum into the surrounding dermis, which initiates the inflammatory process.
• Papules: develop from obstructed follicles that have become inflamed.

• Pustules: these superficial or deep lesions are larger and more inflamed than papules.
• Nodules: formed when deep pustules rupture and form abscesses. These lesions are warm, tender, and painful. Over 8 to 10 weeks, granulation tissue forms, and healing with scar formation occurs. These usually occur at the jawline, earlobes, and neck.
• True cysts: lined by epithelium and usually result as an end product of pustules or nodules. They are not very common.

EPIDEMIOLOGY

• Occurs in 85% of young people from 12 to 24 years of age.

COMPLICATIONS

• Permanent acne scars
• Cellulitis

PROGNOSIS

• Acne improves with age, but 5% to 10% of young adults still complain of significant acne.

Differential Diagnosis

INFECTION

• *Malassezia furfur* (fungus) infection
• Pityrosporum disease

TUMORS

• Adenoma sebaceum from tuberous sclerosis

MISCELLANEOUS

• Flat warts
• Acne rosacea
• Hidradenitis suppurativa

Data Gathering

HISTORY

Question: Onset of acne?
Significance: Normally during Tanner stage II.

Question: Location?
Significance: Gives clues to cosmetic or occupational acne.

Question: Current skin-care regimen?
Significance: Can indicate what level of treatment is necessary.

Question: Use of over-the-counter medications?
Significance: Assesses current therapy.

Question: Use of prescription medications?
Significance: Assesses current therapy.

Question: Evidence of an androgenic disorder (amenorrhea, hirsutism, obesity)?
Significance: Guides therapeutic plan.

Physical Examination

• Examine face, chest, and back. The face is usually affected, but the chest, back, thighs, buttocks, and upper arms can also be affected. Acne spares the hands, forearms, calves, feet, and axilla.
• Determine types of lesions present, number of each type, intensity of inflammation, extent of hyperpigmentation, and scarring.

Laboratory Aids

Adolescent girls with severe acne, with or without evidence of hirsutism, should be evaluated for an androgenic disorder by checking the following: LH, FSH, free and total testosterone, and dehydroepiandosterone sulfate (DHEAS).

Therapy

DRUGS

Topical Agents

• Benzoyl peroxide: bacteriostatic effect on *Propionibacterium acnes;* comedolytic action increases superficial vascular supply, with accelerated healing of lesions. Dose: comes in 1%, 2.5%, 5%, and 10% strengths; aqueous gels are tolerated better than compounds in alcohol or acetone base; start with 5% gel once a day and increase in 2 weeks to twice a day; may use 10% if 5% is not effective. Adverse effects: peeling and irritation; contact dermatitis; potential to bleach clothing.
• Tretinoin (vitamin A derivative): normalizes the epithelial lining of the follicle; increases production of follicular epithelial cells, resulting in expulsion of the compacted debris within the lumen; results in clearing of comedones and microcomedones. Creams are less irritating, followed by gels, then liquid. Start with 0.025% cream or 0.1% microsphere every other day at bedtime 20 minutes after washing with a mild soap. Apply a pea-sized amount only. May increase to higher strength if not effective. After 1 to 2 weeks of therapy, some irritation may occur. If it is severe, discontinue medication for a short time. After 3 to 4 weeks, a pustular eruption can occur, indicating the dislodging of microcomedones; treatment should continue. Adverse side effects: peeling and irritation; hyperpigmentation and hypopigmentation; sun sensitivity.

- Adapalene (Differin; a naphthoic acid with retinoid activity): modulates cell differentiation and formation of keratin within the hair follicle. Dose: available in 0.1% gel. Apply a pea-sized amount nightly after gently washing face with mild soap. Irritation and initial worsening of acne lesions may occur. Adverse side effects: redness, dryness, scaling, pruritis, and burning.
- Other exfoliants: washes and lotions usually contain salicylic acid, resorcinol, sulfur, or phenol; abrasive scrubs contain almond shells, aluminum oxide, or pumice. May cause drying and peeling, and remove oil from the skin, but they fail to prevent new lesions from occurring. Not as effective as benzoyl peroxide and tretinoin.

Topical antibiotics: use for mild to moderate inflammatory acne.

- Erythromycin (2%) and clindamycin (1% phosphate salt) solution, gel, and lotion forms; apply once or twice a day. Use in combination with tretinoin or benzoyl peroxide.
- Azelaic acid 20% (cream) has both antimicrobial and comedolytic properties. Dose: A thin film should be applied twice daily after cleansing with a gentle soap. Adverse side effects: generally well tolerated but may cause a temporary stinging sensation in some patients.

Systemic Therapy

- Antibiotics: decrease population of *Propionibacterium acnes;* reduce amount of free fatty acids. Use: drugs used include tetracycline, minocycline, and erythromycin. Dapsone and clindamycin should be used under the guidance of an experienced dermatologist. Begin with tetracycline or erythromycin at a dose of 500 mg to 1 g daily in two or three divided doses. Minocycline, 50 to 100 mg daily, is also an effective regimen. Doxycycline 50 to 100 mg daily in one or two doses is another option for antibiotic therapy. Decrease dose after 4 weeks if improvement is noted. Some patients may be maintained on 250 mg of tetracycline or erythromycin every 1 to 2 days. May use oral antibiotics in combination with topical therapy. Adverse effects: tetracycline may cause anorexia, nausea, diarrhea, yeast vaginitis; and rare effects include: drug eruption, anemia, neutropenia, phototoxicity. Erythromycin may cause nausea, vomiting, diarrhea, and occasional drug eruptions.
- Isotretinoin (vitamin A derivative): reserved for cases of severe acne because of significant toxicity, and should be used only by doctors familiar with its use. Decreases sebum production to a minimum, normalizes formation of keratin, prevents comedo formation and decreases inflammation. Use: usual daily dose is 0.5 to 1 mg/kg/d divided into two doses; may give up to 2 mg/kg/d; length of therapy is 15 to 20 weeks; improvement continues after stopping the medication. Adverse effects: cheilitis (90%), xerosis (78%), dry mouth (70%), epistaxis (46%), conjunctivitis (40%), desquamation (16%). Isotretinoin is a severe teratogen, and, therefore, requires that female candidates for this therapy have intensive education. They MUST NOT become pregnant during therapy. There is no teratogenic effect on sperm.

SUMMARY OF THERAPY

Grade I Acne

- Topical tretinoin cream at bedtime every other night for 1 week and then every night, or
- Topical adapalene (Differin) gel at bedtime, or
- Topical benzoyl peroxide at bedtime

Grade II Acne

- Topical tretinoin, adapalene, or benzoyl peroxide every night
- Plus topical antibiotics once or twice a day
- If resistant to this therapy add an oral antibiotic

Grade III Acne

- Topical tretinoin or adapalene every night plus benzoyl peroxide every morning
- Topical antibiotics twice a day
- Systemic antibiotics if necessary
- Consider azeleic acid (Azelex) 20% cream, twice a day if pustules or scars are hyperpigmented (use instead of benzoyl peroxide and tretinoin)

Grade IV Acne

- Topical tretinoin or adapalene every night plus benzoyl peroxide every morning
- Topical antibiotics twice a day
- Systemic antibiotics twice a day
- In addition, consider referral to dermatologist for isotretinoin (Accutane).

 Follow-Up

- Superficial papules will resolve in 5 to 10 days with little scarring except for post-inflammatory hyperpigmentation.
- Deep papules usually have more intense inflammation and can take weeks to resolve. There may also be scarring.
- Antibiotics should be tapered and discontinued as soon as possible after significant acne resolution by a trial withdrawal.
- Improvement is seen after 4 to 6 weeks of therapy.

PREVENTION

- Lesions must not be picked at or squeezed. This may result in scarring.
- Avoid cleansers, cosmetics, and moisturizers that are comedogenic.
- Hair products with oil should be avoided. Also avoid wearing hair on the forehead.

PITFALLS

- Frequent, vigorous washing or excessive scrubbing of the face with abrasives is unnecessary, and may lead to dermatitis.
- Astringents and rubbing alcohol make the skin's surface less oily but have minimal beneficial effect on the acne. They may irritate the skin.

 Common Questions and Answers

Q: What types of soaps should those with acne use?
A: It is best to use a gentle cleansing soap, such as Dove, Neutrogena, or Purpose twice a day. Washing with the fingertips is best, rather than using a scrubbing pad or washcloth.

Q: Does the acne have to be moderate to severe to use tretinoin?
A: Actually, tretinoin is one of the best topical medications to use for mild comedonal acne. It should be used every other night for a week and if there is no irritation, it can be increased to every night.

Q: Does diet affect acne?
A: Cola, chocolate, sweets, milk, ice cream, shellfish, nuts, and fatty foods have not been shown to have any effect on severity of acne.

ICD-9-CM 706.1

BIBLIOGRAPHY

Abel EA. Isotretinoin (Accutane) therapy for acne in adolescents. In: *Adolescent medicine: state of the art reviews.* Philadelphia: Hanley & Belfus, 1990;1(2):315–324.

Gibson JR. Azelaic acid 20% cream and the medical management of acne vulgaris. *Dermatol Nurs* 1997;9(5):339–344.

Goos SD, Poche PE. Endocrine aspects of adolescent acne. In: *Adolescent medicine: state of the art reviews.* Philadelphia: Hanley & Belfus, 1990;1(2):289–300.

Hurwitz S. Acne vulgaris: its pathogenesis and management. In: *Adolescent medicine: state of the art reviews.* Philadelphia: Hanley & Belfus, 1990;1(2):301–313.

Kristal L, Silverberg N. Acne: simplifying a complex disorder. *Contemp Pediatr* 1998;(Suppl.):3–10.

Leyden JL. Drug therapy: therapy for acne vulgaris. *N Engl J Med* 1997;336(16):1156–1162.

Strasburger VS. Acne: what every pediatrician should know about treatment. *Pediatr Clin North Am* 1997;44(6):1505–1523.

Author: Liana R. Clark

Acquired Hypothyroidism

 Database

DEFINITION

Hypothyroidism that occurs after the neonatal period.

PATHOPHYSIOLOGY

• There are myriad causes (*see* Differential Diagnosis).
• Decreased synthesis or release of thyroid hormone can result from thyroid gland dysfunction (primary hypothyroidism) or from pituitary/hypothalamic dysfunction leading to under-stimulation of the thyroid gland (secondary and tertiary hypothyroidism).

GENETICS

• A genetic predisposition exists in patients with chronic lymphocytic thyroiditis (CLT), the most common cause of acquired thyroiditis in non-endemic areas; 30% to 40% of patients have a familial history of thyroid disease, and up to 50% of their first-degree relatives have thyroid antibodies.
• Associations of CLT with certain HLA haplotypes are weak and not consistently reproducible.
• Autoimmune thyroid disease may be part of Schmidt syndrome (type II polyglandular autoimmune disease), which also involves Addison disease and type 1 diabetes mellitus. This incompletely penetrant autosomal dominant disorder demonstrates stronger HLA linkage.
• Genetic syndromes associated with higher incidence of autoimmune thyroiditis:

—Down syndrome
—Turner syndrome (especially those with isochromosome Xq)

EPIDEMIOLOGY

• May develop at any age.
• CLT prevalence correlates with iodine intake, such that countries as the United States and Japan with the highest dietary iodine also have the highest CLT prevalence.

COMPLICATIONS

• The most significant complication during childhood is impaired linear growth.
• Myxedema coma may occur.

 Differential Diagnosis

IMMUNOLOGIC

• Chronic lymphocytic thyroiditis (often referred to as Hashimoto thyroiditis)
• Autoimmune polyendocrine syndrome (Schmidt syndrome)

INFECTIOUS

• Post-viral subacute thyroiditis
• Associated with congenital infections

—Rubella
—Toxoplasmosis

ENVIRONMENTAL

• Goitrogen ingestion

—Iodides
—Expectorants
—Thioureas

IATROGENIC

• Following surgical thyroidectomy for thyroid cancer, hyperthyroidism, or extensive neck tumors.
• Following radioiodine ablative therapy for hyperthyroidism or thyroid cancer.
• Following irradiation to the head or neck for cancer treatment.
• Medications: lithium, amiodarone, iodine contrast dyes.

METABOLIC

• Cystinosis
• Histiocytosis X

CONGENITAL

• "Late-onset" congenital-large ectopic gland

GENETIC SYNDROMES

• Down syndrome
• Turner syndrome

SECONDARY OR TERTIARY HYPOTHYROIDISM

• Hypothalamic or pituitary disease

 Data Gathering

HISTORY

Question: Growth pattern?
Significance: Linear growth failure can be the first sign of thyroid dysfunction

Question: Declining school performance?
Significance: Sensitive marker for lethargy and reduced focusing

SYMPTOMS

Question: Any symptoms of hypothyroidism and their duration?
Significance: Early primary hypothyroidism can be asymptomatic. The presence of hypothyroid-related symptoms indicates progression from compensated to uncompensated hypothyroidism.

Question: Notice any thyroid gland enlargement? Its duration? Tenderness?
Significance: Goiter may be the presenting sign of acquired hypothyroidism. Tenderness suggests an infectious process.

Question: Any past medical history factors associated with hypothyroidism? (e.g., genetic syndromes, radiation exposure, medications, history of diabetes)
Significance: Any of these factors should raise the concern for possible acquired hypothyroidism.

Question: Familial history of thyroid disease (hyper or hypo) or other autoimmune endocrinopathies
Significance: Family history of thyroid disease or other autoimmune endocrinopathies increases the risk of developing autoimmune thyroid disease.

Physical Examination

Finding: Bradycardia
Significance: Thyroid hormone has cardiac effects.

Finding: Short stature (or fall-off on growth curve), and increased upper:lower segment ratio
Significance: Euthyroidism is required to maintain normal growth.

Finding: Goiter: note consistency, symmetry, nodularity, signs of inflammation
Significance: Goiter characteristics may give a clue regarding the cause of the hypothyroidism and provide a clinical manner to follow during therapy.

Finding: Myxedema (water retention)
Significance: Myxedema is not limited to the subcutaneous tissue. It may also lead to cardiac failure, pleural effusions, and coma.

Finding: Muscle hypertrophy, yet muscle weakness most obvious in arms, legs, and tongue.
Significance: Hypothyroidism causes disordered muscle function.

Finding: Delayed relaxation phase of deep tendon reflexes
Significance: Due to slowed muscle contraction, not a change in the transmission rate of the nervous impulse.

Finding: Pale, cool, dry, carotenemic skin
Significance: (due to decreased cell turnover)

Finding: Increase in lanugo hair
Significance: Can be seen in children with hypothyroidism and revised with treatment.

SPECIAL QUESTIONS

Sexual development is an important factor because hypothyroidism can be associated with both delayed puberty (due to low thyroid hormone level) as well as precocious puberty and galactorrhea (due to elevated TSH).

 ## Laboratory Aids

TESTS

Test: T4 (low) and TSH (elevated)
Significance: Elevated TSH with normal T4 represents a state of compensated primary hypothyroidism.

Test: Free T4
Significance: The most sensitive marker for secondary/tertiary hypothyroidism (in which case, TSH elevation is lost and total T4 may still be in the low end of the normal range).

Test: Antithyroglobulin and antimicrosomal (antiperoxidase) antibodies
Significance: Markers for CLT.

IMAGING

Test: Head MRI
Significance: Suspected secondary/tertiary hypothyroidism; pituitary or hypothalamic lesion

The following conditions may test false-positive for acquired hypothyroidism:

Test: Thyroid-binding globulin deficiency
Significance: Low total T4, but normal free T4 and TSH

Test: Peripheral resistance to thyroid hormone
Significance: Normal/high total T4

Test: "Euthyroid sick" syndrome
Significance: Low T4 and T3; normal/low TSH; increased shunting to reverse T3

 ## Therapy

L-THYROXINE (SYNTHETIC THYROID HORMONE) REPLACEMENT

• Indicated for the treatment of overt or compensated hypothyroidism.
• 2 to 5 μg/kg/d po, once daily
• Monitor T4 and TSH and titrate dose to maintain normalized TFTs.
• Duration of therapy

—Lifetime
—30% of children with CLT will undergo spontaneous remission, and reassessment of need for treatment can be done after growth is completed.

 ## Follow-Up

CHANGES IN TFTS

• Whenever starting medication or adjusting dose, check T4 and TSH 4 to 6 weeks later, to assess adequacy of the new dose.

WHEN TO EXPECT IMPROVEMENT

• Treated patients often resume growth at a rate greater than normal (catch-up growth).
• Other signs and symptoms resolve at a variable rate.
• Goiters in CLT may not completely regress with treatment (enlargement due to persistent inflammation does not correct, though TSH-mediated hypertrophy will).

SIGNS TO WATCH FOR TO INDICATE PROBLEMS

• Monitor response to treatment by measuring T4 and TSH levels to ensure compliance.

PROGNOSIS

• If patients are compliant, prognosis is excellent.
• In children in whom treatment has been delayed, catch-up growth may not fully normalize height to predicted values.

 ## Common Questions and Answers

Q: What happens if my child forgets a dose?
A: Give the dose as soon as you remember. If it is the next day, give two doses.

Q: How long will my child have to take these pills?
A: Probably for life.

Q: Are there any side effects from the medication?
A: No. The medication contains only the hormone that your child's thyroid gland is not making. The hormone is made synthetically, so there is also no infectious risk.

Q: If my child takes twice the dose, will his or her growth catch up faster?
A: Your child may grow a little faster but will also have adverse effects from having too much thyroid hormone.

Q: Does the medication have to be taken at any particular time of day?
A: No, but consistently choosing the same time of day helps to remember taking it.

ICD-9-CM 244.9

BIBLIOGRAPHY

Betterle C, Volpato M, Greggio AN, Presotto F. Type 2 polyglandular autoimmune disease (Schmidt syndrome). *J Pediatr Endocrinol Metab* 1996;(9 Suppl 1):113–123.

Dayan CM, Daniels GH. Chronic autoimmune thyroiditis. *N Engl J Med* 1996;335:99–107.

LaFranchi S. Thyroiditis and acquired hypothyroidism. *Pediatr Ann* 1992;21(1):29–39.

Rickees SA, Bode HH, Crawford JD. Long-term growth in juvenile acquired hypothyroidism: The failure to achieve normal adult stature. *N Engl J Med* 1988;318:599–602.

Authors: Adda Grimberg and Marta Satin-Smith

Acute Lymphoblastic Leukemia

 Database

DEFINITION

Acute lymphoblastic leukemia (ALL) is a malignant disorder of lymphoblasts occurring as a result of clonal proliferation of a single lymphoblast that has undergone malignant transformation.

CAUSES

- Unknown

Following factors have been associated:

- Exposure to ionizing radiation
- Chemical exposure
- Viral infections

—HTLV I associated with adult T cell leukemia
—HTLV II associated with hairy cell leukemia

- Immunodeficiencies

—Wiskott-Aldrich syndrome
—Ataxia telangiectasia
—Congenital hypogammaglobinemia
—Prolonged immunosuppressive therapy is related to lymphoid malignancies

PATHOLOGY

- Bone marrow aspirate shows >30% leukemic lymphoblasts
- French American British (FAB) Classification: based on morphology
- Immunologic Classification

—B cell lineage

—80% to 85% of childhood cases, mostly early pre-B cell or pre-B cell
—Pre-B and early pre-B cell usually common

- ALL antigen (CALLA) positive
—Immunological markers for B cell lineage are CD19, CD20, CD21, and CD24

—T cell lineage

—15% to 20% of all cases
—10% of these are CALLA positive
—Immunological markers for T cell lineage are CD1, CD2, CD3, CD4, CD5, CD7, and CD8

- Cytochemistry

—ALL blasts usually periodic acid-Schiff (PAS) positive
—Always negative for Sudan black and Myeloperoxidase

- Cytogenetics

—Karyotype of malignant cells is normal in 50% of cases
—Others have several translocations

—t (4;11) associated with infant ALL
—t (1;19), t (9;22) Philadelphia chromosome
—t (11;18) associated with T cell disease
—t (8;14) associated with B cell disease

—Hyperdiploid (> 50 chromosomes) state associated with good prognosis

GENETICS

Increased risk of leukemia with:

- Trisomy 21
- Fanconi anemia
- Bloom syndrome
- Ataxia telangiectasia
- Klinefelter syndrome
- Schwachmann Diamond syndrome
- 20% risk of ALL in monozygotic twin if one twin develops ALL before 5 years of age
- 2- to 4-fold higher risk in siblings than in general population

EPIDEMIOLOGY

- Acute leukemia is most common cancer of childhood
- Incidence of ALL is 4/100,000 children younger than 5 years old
- >75% of acute leukemia in childhood is ALL
- Peak incidence at 4 years of age
- More common in whites and boys
- Higher incidence in industrialized countries

COMPLICATIONS

- Due to disease:

—Failure of remission induction—uncommon
—Central nervous system (CNS) relapse
—Testicular relapse
—Bone marrow relapse
—Infections, sepsis, and hemorrhage

- Due to therapy:

—Cranial radiation (XRT) and intrathecal methotrexate (IT MTX)

—Leukoencephalopathy and deterioration of intellectual functions
—Growth retardation

—Prednisone

—Avascular necrosis of bones
—Cushingoid habitus
—Hypertension

—Vincristine (VCR)

—Syndrome of inappropriate antidiuretic hormone
—Footdrop (reversible)
—Hair loss

—L-asparaginase

—Pancreatitis
—Coagulopathy leading to cerebral infarcts

—Adriamycin

—Cardiac toxicity

—Cyclophosphamide

—Hemorrhagic cystitis
—Sterility

—Methotrexate (MTX)

—Hepatotoxicity

PROGNOSIS

Remission induction in all risk categories with presently available therapy is 95%.

- Long-term survival in standard risk group is about 70% (>5 years after completion of therapy).
- Long-term survival is about 60% to 65% for high-risk group.

 Differential Diagnosis

NON-MALIGNANT CONDITIONS

- Juvenile rheumatoid arthritis
- Infectious mononucleosis
- Idiopathic thrombocytopenic purpura
- Pertussis and parapertussis
- Aplastic anemia

MALIGNANT CONDITIONS

- Neuroblastoma
- Lymphoma
- Rhabdomyosarcoma
- Retinoblastoma
- Acute myeloid leukemia

 Data Gathering

HISTORY

Question: Fever
Significance: Infection

Question: Bleeding (cutaneous and mucosal)
Significance: Low platelet count, coagulopathy

Question: Bone pains; Arthralgia, limp
Significance: Infiltrative disease of marrow

Question: Fatigue and pallor
Significance: Anemia

Question: Lymphnode enlargement
Significance: Infiltration with leukemia

Question: Stridor, orthopnea, shortness of breath
Significance: Mediastinal mass

Question: Oliguria
Significance: Renal failure

- Headache, vomiting, seizures

 Physical Examination

Finding: Pallor
Significance: Anemia

Finding: Lymphadenopathy (generalized)
Significance: Infiltration with leukemia

Finding: Hepatosplenomegaly
Significance: Infiltration with leukemia

Finding: Sternal tenderness
Significance: Bone marrow infiltration

Finding: Petechiae and purpura
Significance: Thrombocytopenia

Finding: Subconjunctival and retinal hemorrhages
Significance: Thrombocytopenia

Finding: Testicular enlargement in boys
Significance: Testicular infiltration

Finding: Papilledema in CNS leukemia
Significance: Meningeal infiltration

Finding: Congestive heart failure
Significance: Severe anemia

Finding: Swelling of the face, orthopnea
Significance: Superior venacaval syndrome in presence of mediastinal mass

 Laboratory Aids

Test: CBC
Significance: Increased white blood count

- >10,000/mm³ in 50% cases
- >50,000/mm³ in 20% cases

Neutropenia (<500/mm³) common
Hb <10 g/dL in 80% cases
Thrombocytopenia (<100,000/mm³) in 75% cases

Test: Bone marrow aspirate
Significance: >25% leukemic lymphoblasts is diagnostic

Test: Immunophenotyping and cytogenetic studies on bone marrow aspirate
Significance: Prognostic

Test: Biochemical abnormalities
Significance: Tumor lysis syndrome

- Hyperuricemia
- Hyperphosphatemia
- Hypocalcemia
- Hyperkalemia
- Increased LDH
- Slight abnormality of liver function tests due to leukemic infiltrate

Test: Chest x-ray
Significance: 5% to 10% cases have mediastinal mass

Test: CSF examination with lymphoblasts
Significance: CNS leukemia (5% at diagnosis)

PROGNOSTIC FACTORS

Patients with any of the following criteria belong to high risk group.

- Age <1 year or >10 years of age
- WBC count >50,000/mm³
- Mediastinal mass or other bulky disease
- T or mature B cell disease
- Translocations—t (9;22), t (4;11), t (1;19)
- Hypodiploidy (<46 chromosomes by karyotype)

 Therapy

Stratified according to risk groups.

- Standard risk or high risk
- Four phases of therapy

—Induction
—Consolidation
—Delayed intensification
—Maintenance

- Induction

—To achieve remission (<5% blasts in bone marrow)
—Usually with 3 or 4 drugs

  —VCR
  —Prednisone
  —L-asparaginase with or without doxorubicin

—Intrathecal methotrexate

- Consolidation and CNS prophylaxis

—To prevent CNS disease
—Intrathecal MTX along with oral 6-mercaptopurine (6MP) and MTX in standard risk
—Intrathecal MTX along with cranial radiation (1800 cGy), oral 6MP and MTX for high risk patients

- Delayed Intensification

—To further decrease leukemic burden
—VCR
—Prednisone
—L-asparaginase
—Doxorubicin
—Cyclophosphamide
—Cytosine arabinoside (ARA-C)
—6 thioguanine (6TG)
—Intrathecal MTX

- Maintenance

—Daily oral 6MP
—Weekly MTX and monthly pulses of VCR and Prednisone
—Intrathecal MTX for 2.5 to 3 years

- CNS leukemia at diagnosis

—Cranial radiation (2400 cGy)
—Triple intrathecal (MTX, ARA-C, Hydrocortisone), in addition to therapy above.

- Bone marrow transplant to be considered for relapsed patients.

SUPPORTIVE CARE

Hydration and alkalization with NaHCO₃ to keep urine pH 6.5–7.0 in first few days of induction.

- Blood and platelet transfusions as required.
- Broad spectrum antibiotics for fever and neutropenia.
- Pneumocystis prophylaxis with Trimethoprim/Sulphamethoxyzole.
- Varicella zoster immune globulin prophylaxis within 72 hours of exposure to varicella.
- No live viral vaccine to anyone in household.
- No vaccination to the affected child while on therapy.

 Follow-Up

CBC every month for first year and then every 3 months for second year, then every 6 months for 5 years. Liver and renal function tests every 3 to 6 months. Cardiac evaluation yearly. Endocrine evaluation in children close to puberty.

 Common Questions and Answers

Q: Can the child on treatment for ALL go to school?
A: Yes.

Q: Will the hair fall out and child be sick for all 3 years on chemotherapy?
A: The hair usually falls out only in first 6 months. Most children feel well during the maintenance chemotherapy.

Q: Does the child need to be isolated from other children?
A: The child should be isolated from any child who has varicella or is obviously sick due to any other infection.

Q: What do we do if we skip one dose of maintenance chemotherapy?
A: Continue to take the medication as recommended. Skipping one dose does not increase risk of relapse. However, missing doses should not become a habit.

ICD-9-CM 204.0

BIBLIOGRAPHY

Pui CH. Clinical and biological relevance of Immunological marker studies in childhood acute lymphoblastic leukemia. *Blood* 1993;82(2):343–362.

Pui CH. Acute lymphoblastic leukemia. *Pediatr Clin North Am* 1997;44(4):831–846.

Pui CH, Christ WM. Biology and treatment of acute lymphoblastic leukemia. *J Pediatr* 1994;124(4):491–503.

Silverman LB, Weinstein HJ. Treatment of childhood leukemia. *Curr Opin Oncol* 1997;9(1):26–33.

Author: Sadhna M. Shankar

Acute Myeloid Leukemia

 ## Database

DEFINITION

Acute myeloid leukemia (AML) is a clonal proliferation of malignant myeloblasts.

CAUSES

- Exact cause unknown.
- Predisposing factors

—Exposure to ionizing radiation.
—Exposure to Benzene.
—Exposure to alkylating agents

  —Cyclophosphamide
  —Nitrogen mustard
  —Chlorambucil
  —Melphalan

—Exposure to epipodophyllotoxins

  —VP16
  —VM26

PATHOLOGY

- Bone marrow aspirate must contain >30% myeloblasts.
- Immunophenotyping

—Blasts positive for myeloid antigens
—CD11, CD13, CD14, CD15, CD33, CD34
—CD41 and CD42 (megakaryocytic)

- Morphology

—Large blasts with low nuclear/cytoplasmic ratio
—Multiple nucleoli and cytoplasmic granules

- Cytochemistry

—Blasts are positive for myeloperoxidase and sudan black and usually negative for periodic acid. Schiff (PAS) and terminal deoxynuleotide transferase (TdT)

GENETICS

Following disorders predispose to AML

—Fanconi anemia
—Down syndrome
—Bloom syndrome
—Kostman syndrome
—Diamond Blackfan anemia
—Neurofibromatosis

EPIDEMIOLOGY

- 15% to 20% of childhood acute leukemia is AML
- Leukemia in first 4 weeks of life is usually AML
- Incidence slightly increased in teens
- Ratio of AML to ALL throughout childhood is 1:4
- Boys and girls equally affected

COMPLICATIONS

- Bleeding
- Disseminated intravascular coagulation (DIC) occurs in some varieties of AML
- Infection

—40% patients are febrile at diagnosis

- Leukostasis

—Intravascular clumping of blasts causing hypoxia, infarction, and hemorrhage.
—Usually with white blood count (WBC) >200,000/mm^3

- Tumor lysis syndrome and renal failure due to hyperuricemia
- Failure to induce remission in 15% to 20% of pediatric cases

PROGNOSIS

- 85% achieve remission with intensive chemotherapy
- About 30% to 40% achieve long-term survival (more than 5 years after diagnosis)

 ## Differential Diagnosis

- Myeloid blast crisis of chronic myeloid leukemia (Philadelphia chromosome positive)
- Acute lymphoblastic leukemia
- Leukemoid reaction
- Exaggerted leukocytosis

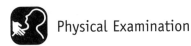 ## Data Gathering

HISTORY

Question: Fever (40% cases)
Significance: Infection

Question: Pallor (25% cases)
Significance: Anemia

Question: Anorexia and weight loss (22% cases)
Significance: Systemic symptoms of malignancy

Question: Fatigue (19% cases)
Significance: Anemia

Question: Bleeding (33% cases)
Significance: Cutaneous and mucosal thrombocytopenia

Question: Bone pain (18% cases)
Significance: Bone marrow infiltration

Question: Headache/vomiting
Significance: Meningeal leukemia, intracranial bleeding

Question: Repeated infections
Significance: Persistant neutropenia due to leukemia

Physical Examination

Finding: Pallor
Significance: Anemia

Finding: Petechiae, purpura, bleeding
Significance: Thrombocytopenia

Finding: Purple skin lesions
Significance: Leukemic infiltrate (leukemia cutis)

Finding: Swollen gingiva
Significance: Leukemic infiltration

Finding: Mass lesions
Significance: Chloromas (leukemic tumors)

Finding: Lymphadenopathy (<25% cases) or Hepatosplenomegaly (50% cases)
Significance: Leukemic infiltration

Finding: Testicular enlargement (rare)
Significance: Testicular infiltration

Acute Myeloid Leukemia

 ## Laboratory Aids

Test: CBC
Significance: Anemia, thrombocytopenia, WBC count usually >10000/mm^3

Test: Peripheral smear
Significance: Myeloblasts may be seen.

Test: Bone Marrow aspirate
Significance: Diagnostic; >30% myeloblasts; confirmed by immunophenotyping and cytochemistry

Test: PT, PTT and fibrin split products (FSP) increased. Fibrinogen may be decreased
Significance: Coagulopathy, disseminated vascular coagulation

Test: Hyperkalemia, hypocalcemia, hyperphosphatemia and hyperuricemia
Significance: Presence of tumor lysis

Test: Cerebrospinal fluid cytology
Significance: >5 WBC/mm^3 suggestive of central nervous system (CNS) disease; 5% to 15% of cases have CNS disease at diagnosis.

PROGNOSTIC FACTORS

Factors associated with low remission induction rate:

- WBC count >100,000/mm^3
- Monosomy 7
- Secondary AML or prior myelodysplastic syndrome

 ## Therapy

INDUCTION

- Most effective drugs for remission induction in AML.
- Anthracyclines

—Doxorubicin
—Daunomycin

- Cytosine Arabinoside (ARA-C) with or without 6-thioguanine (6TG)
- VP16 and Dexamethasone added in some regimen
- High rate of remission induction with Trans retinoic acid in Acute promyelocytic leukemia
- Consolidation therapy usually with ARA-C and L-asparaginase
- Intrathecal ARA-C for CNS prophylaxis
- Maintenance with VP16, ARA-C, 6TG, Daunomycin, Dexamethasone
- Duration of therapy is usually 6–9 months
- Allogeneic bone marrow transplant may be the best treatment for AML in first remission

SUPPORTIVE CARE

- Hydration, alkalization, and Allopurinol during induction
- Blood product support

—Avoid products from family members if possibility of allogeneic bone marrow transplant

- Broad spectrum antibiotics and antifungal therapy for fever and neutropenia
- Prophylactic trimethoprim/sulphamethoxyzole for *Pneumocystis*
- Nystatin/fluconozole for fungal prophylaxis
- Heparin may be needed for treatment of DIC.

 ## Follow-Up

Monthly for first year then every 3 months for the second year and then every 6 months. CBC is done on each visit. Liver and kidney function tests are done every 3 months. Cardiac function should be checked every 6 to 12 months. Endocrine function should be tested in pubertal children.

 ## Common Questions and Answers

Q: Is an indwelling line required for therapy?
A: Always.

Q: Are repeated hospitalizations likely?
A: Repeated hospitalizations are needed for chemotherapy and infectious complications.

Q: Can the child go to school?
A: May be able to go intermittently during therapy.

ICD-9-CM 205.0

BIBLIOGRAPHY

Ebb DH, Weinstein HJ. Diagnosis and treatment of childhood AML. *Pediatr Clin North Am* 1997;44(4):847–862.

Hurwitz CA, Mounce KG, Grier HE. Treatment of patients with AML: review of clinical trials of past decade. *J Pediatr Hematol Oncol* 1995;17(3):185–197.

Kersey JH. Fifty years of studies of biology and therapy of chilhood leukemia. *Blood* 1997;90(11):4243–4251.

Author: Sadhna M. Shankar

Adenovirus Infection

Database

DEFINITION

Adenoviruses are ubiquitous double-stranded DNA viruses. There are 47 human serotypes.

PATHOPHYSIOLOGY

Adenoviruses may cause a lytic or chronic/latent infection. They have also been shown to be capable of inducing oncogenic transformation of cells, although the clinical significance of this observation is unclear at present.

EPIDEMIOLOGY

- Primary infection usually occurs early in life (by age 10 years) and is most often characterized by upper respiratory symptoms.
- Military trainees are especially susceptible to infection, probably due to crowded living conditions.
- Respiratory and enteric infections may occur at any time of year. Epidemics of respiratory disease occur in winter and spring.
- Transmission of respiratory disease occurs via contact with infected secretions. Transmission of enteric adenoviruses is via fecal–oral route.
- Outbreaks of pharyngoconjunctival fever have been associated with inadequately chlorinated swimming pools.

COMPLICATIONS

- Bronchiolitis obliterans (rare), corneal opacities with visual disturbance (usually resolves spontaneously)

PROGNOSIS

Most syndromes are self-limited.

ASSOCIATED ILLNESSES

- Respiratory infection responsible for 10% of all pediatric respiratory illnesses; may cause upper respiratory symptoms, whooping cough syndrome; pneumonitis; lower respiratory tract disease associated with adenovirus types 4 and 7.
- Pharyngoconjunctival fever: low-grade fever associated with conjunctivitis, pharyngitis, rhinitis, and cervical adenitis; 15% of patients may have meningismus; increased incidence in summer months; common-source outbreaks most often associated with type 3.
- Epidemic keratoconjunctivitis: bilateral conjuncitivitis with preauricular adenopathy; may persist for up to 4 weeks; corneal opacities may persist for several months; associated with types 8, 19, and 37.
- Hemorrhagic cystitis may cause microscopic or gross hematuria; if present, gross hematuria persists on average for 3 days; often associated with dysuria and urinary frequency; more common in males than females; associated with types 11 and 21.
- Infantile diarrhea: watery diarrhea associated with fever; symptoms may persist for 1 to 2 weeks; associated with types 40 and 41.
- Central nervous system (CNS) infection epidemics (associated with outbreaks of respiratory disease) and sporadic cases of encephalitis and meningitis have been observed; often associated with pneumonia.
- Miscellaneous adenoviruses have been associated with intussusception (isolated in up to 40% of cases), fatal congenital infection, disseminated disease in immunocompromised patients.

Differential Diagnosis

- Respiratory infection

—Influenza
—Parainfluenza
—Pertussis
—Mycoplasma
—Bacterial pneumonia

- Pharyngoconjunctival fever group A streptococcus

—Epstein-Barr virus
—Parainfluenza
—Enterovirus
—Measles

- Epidemic keratoconjunctivitis herpes simplex

—Chlamydia
—Enterovirus

- Hemorrhagic cystitis glomerulonephritis

—Vasculitis
—Renal tuberculosis

- Infantile diarrhea rotavirus

—Norwalk agent
—Astrovirus
—Salmonella
—Shigella
—Campylobacter

- CNS infection herpes simplex virus

—Enterovirus
—Mycoplasma
—Bacterial meningitis

Data Gathering

HISTORY

Question: Fever
Significance: Nonspecific

Question: Rhinitis
Significance: URI

Question: Laryngitis, sore throat
Significance: URI

Question: Non-productive or croupy cough
Significance: Respiratory infection

Question: Headache, myalgias
Significance: CNS infection

Question: Hematuria (gross or microscopic), dysuria, urinary frequency
Significance: Hemorrhagic cystitis

Question: Watery diarrhea
Significance: Enteric adenovirus

 ## Physical Examination

Finding: Head and neck conjuctivitis, rhinitis, pharyngitis, exudate, meningismus
Significance: Typical findings of adenovirus

Finding: Pulmonary tachypnea, wheezing, rales
Significance: Pneumonia

Finding: Abdomen tenderness, distension
Significance: Gastroenteritis

 ## Laboratory Aids

Test: CBC
Significance: Leukocytosis or leukopenia, often with left shift in the differential count.

Test: Erythrocyte sedimentation rate
Significance: Often elevated

Test: Chest radiograph
Significance: Bilateral patchy interstitial infiltrates (lower lobes).

Test: Serology
Significance: Diagnosis may be made by a documented 4-fold rise in serum antibody.

Test: Viral isolation
Significance: From nasopharyngeal secretions, urine, conjuctivae, or stool.

Test: Viral identification
Significance: Either visualization of virion by electron microscopy or demonstration of viral antigen in infected cells by immunofluorescence; highest yield from nasopharyngeal swab or stool.

 ## Therapy

PREVENTION

Precautions Should be Used for Hospitalized Patients

SYMPTOMS	TYPE OF PRECAUTIONS
Respiratory disease	Contact
Gastrointestinal	Enteric disease
Conjunctivitis	Drainage and secretion

Oral vaccines have been used by the military.

ICD-9-CM 079.0
Diarrhea secondary to adenoviral infection 008.62
Conjunctivitis-pharyngoconjuctival fever 077.2
Conjunctivitis 077.3

BIBLIOGRAPHY

Baum SG. Adenovirus. In: Mandell GL, Douglas RG, Bennett JE, eds. *Principles and practice of infectious diseases,* 4th ed. New York: Churchill Livingstone, 1995:1382–1387.

Claesson BA, Trollfors B, Brolin I, et al. Etiology of community-acquired pneumonia in children based on antibody responses to bacterial and viral antigens. *Pediatr Infect Dis J* 1989;8(12):856–862.

Krajden M, Brown M, Petrasek A, Middleton PJ. Clinical features of adenovirus enteritis: a review of 127 cases. *Pediatr Infect Dis J* 1990;9:636–641.

Wirsing von Konig CH, Rott H, Bogaerts H, Schmitt HJ. A serologic study of organisms possibly associated with pertussis-like coughing. *Pediatr Infect Dis J* 1998;17(7):645–649.

Author: Susan E. Coffin

Alcohol (Ethanol) Intoxication

 Database

DEFINITION

• Alcohol intoxication is the ingestion of toxic quantities of ethanol (ethyl alcohol), which results in common signs, including lack of coordination, slurred speech, ataxia, nausea, vomiting, increased urination, vasodilatation, coma, shock, hypoglycemia, and seizures.
• Ingestion of 1 g/kg yields peak blood level 100 mg/dL (legal limit defining intoxication).
• Blood level of 50 mg/dL can cause intoxication in children.

ETIOLOGY

• Alcoholic beverages contain 20% to 50% alcohol (hard liquor), 10% to 14% (wine), and 3% to 8% (beer); 1% = 1 mg/dL.
• Ethanol is also in liquid cold remedies, mouthwashes, aftershave lotion, liniments, tinctures, some rubbing alcohols, perfumes, colognes, glass cleaners, and paint removers.
• When ingestion is intentional, it often occurs concurrent with multiple drug ingestion and trauma from risk-taking behaviors.

PATHOPHYSIOLOGY

• Ethanol is rapidly absorbed (20% in stomach, 80% in small intestine)
• Blood levels peak 30 to 60 minutes after ingestion
• It is metabolized primarily in the liver utilizing alcohol dehydrogenase
• 2% to 10% of ethanol is excreted unchanged by the kidneys
• Ethanol depresses the central nervous system (CNS) via the reticular activating system by interfering with ion transport at the cell membrane and interacting with γ-aminobutyric acid receptors.
• Hypoglycemia is caused by impaired gluconeogenesis and lactic or keto-acidosis may develop. Seizures are a frequent manifestation of hypoglycemia in children.

EPIDEMIOLOGY

• Intentional intoxication is most common in adolescents
• Accidental intoxication occurs most frequently in toddlers

COMPLICATIONS

• Death: associated with ingestion of >3 g/kg (which corresponds to an approximate serum level of 300 mg/dL)
• CNS depression: apnea, hypoxia, poor judgment, and risk taking
• Vomiting and aspiration
• Vasodilatation and hypotension
• Increased urinary losses and dehydration
• Hypoglycemia and seizures and coma

PROGNOSIS

• Blood levels <300 mg/dL: survival expected if treated
• Blood levels >500: high risk of death despite therapy

 Differential Diagnosis

INFECTION

• Meningitis
• Encephalitis
• Overwhelming infection

ENVIRONMENTAL

• Inhalations and toxic exposures (e.g., carbon monoxide poisoning)
• Other ingestions

TUMOR

• Brain tumor and sudden increase in intracranial pressure secondary to obstruction by mass

TRAUMA

• Head trauma

METABOLIC

• Other causes of hypoglycemia
• Ketoacidosis
• Hyperammonemic states

Data Gathering

HISTORY

Question: Assess the quantity and time of ingestion
Significance: May help in determining expected blood level and the development of additional symptoms.

Question: Other possible ingestions?
Significance: Concurrent ingestions are common and effects can vary as well as treatment.

Question: Did the ingestion occur as an intentional or unintentional act?
Signficance: Assess risk of suicidal ideation

Question: Past medical problems?
Significance: Because alcohol may exacerbate underlying conditions (e.g., diabetes, liver disease, renal failure), it is important to obtain a history on past medical problems.

Question: When did the patient last eat?
Significance: Determines the risk for aspiration.

Physical Examination

Finding: Complete neurologic examination
Significance: Assesses level of consciousness, ability to protect airway

Finding: Signs of trauma
Significance: Head trauma can occur concurrently or mimic symptoms of ethanol intoxication. Falls and motor vehicle accidents are also common secondary problems.

Laboratory Aids

Test: Estimated peak ethanol level
Significance: Calculated as mg ingested/(volume of distribution $\times$ body weight), where volume of distribution is 0.6 L/kg in adults and 0.7 L/kg in children

Test: Drug screen
Significance: Usually includes drugs of abuse, antidepressants, benzodiazepines, and others.

Test: Electrolytes, glucose, renal function (BUN, creatinine), liver enzymes, arterial blood gas
Significance: Dehydration, hypoglycemia, renal impairment, liver toxicity, metabolic and respiratory acidosis can occur.

RADIOGRAPHIC IMAGING

Computed tomography of head: if head trauma suspected

Therapy

- ABCs (airway, breathing, circulation); life support measures including mechanical ventilation may be required.
- Gastric lavage if within 30 to 60 minutes of ingestion (do not induce emesis because of CNS depression).
- Activated charcoal if ingestion of other substances suspected; not useful in alcohol intoxication alone.
- Treat hypoglycemia with IV dextrose. Treat until clinically stable and blood ethanol level is <50 mg/dL.
- Treat dehydration and hypotension with intravenous fluids.
- Monitor for hypothermia.
- Hemodialysis may be required if levels exceed 300 to 350 mg/dL.
- No specific antidote exists

Follow-Up

- If ingestion was intentional, psychiatric evaluation is highly recommended.
- Accidental ingestions require parental education about child safety.

PREVENTION

- Child safety caps on medicine bottles
- Locks on medicine and liquor cabinets
- Avoid purchasing medicines containing alcohol for use by children

PITFALLS

Ingestion of other toxic substances may be missed.

BIBLIOGRAPHY

Ernst AA, Jones K, Nick TG, Sanchez J. Ethanol ingestion and related hypoglycemia in a pediatric and adolescent emergency department population. *Acad Emerg Med* 1996;3(1):46–49.

Leung AK. Ethyl alcohol ingestion in children. *Clin Pediatr* 1986;25(12):617–619.

Raroque SSU, Weibe, RA. Household products and environmental toxins. In: Levin DL, Morriss, FC, eds. *Essentials of pediatric intensive care*, 2nd ed., New York: Quality Medical Publishing and Churchill Livingston. 1997:922–923.

Rodgers GC, Matyunas NJ. *Handbook of common poisonings in children*, 3rd ed. Committee on Injury and Poison Prevention. Evanston, Illinois: American Academy of Pediatrics, 1994:149–152.

Author: Deborah L. Silver

Alpha-1 Antitrypsin Deficiency

 Database

DEFINITION

Alpha-1 antitrypsin deficiency is a disease characterized by the deficiency of the serum protease inhibitor, α-1-antitrypsin, leading to premature development of lung emphysema and chronic liver disease.

CAUSES

• Deficiency of α-1 antitrypsin, a serum protease inhibitor, a glycoprotein of approximately 52 kD, which inhibits the activity of elastase, an enzyme involved in the remodeling of connective tissue.
• In the absence of regulated protease activity, alteration in the structure of end organs, lung, and liver can develop and cause disease.

EPIDEMIOLOGY

• Most common metabolic cause of emphysema in adults and liver disease in children, for which they receive orthotopic liver transplantation.
• Incidence and prevalence change with the population studied, ranging from 1:1639 live births in Sweden to 1:2000 individuals in the United States.

GENETICS

• Autosomal recessive inheritance
• Multiple structural forms of the α-1 antitrypsin protein are encoded on chromosome 14.
• 75 Different alleles with the most common phenotypes are characterized as Pi, protease inhibitors, by gel electrophoresis.
• The most common normal variant is referred to as M.
• Individuals with the most severe deficiency have an α-1 antitrypsin alleleic variant, referred to as Z.

COMPLICATIONS

• Cirrhosis and emphysema are common
• Individuals expressing the homozygous ZZ alleles
• Infants are often diagnosed with neonatal hepatitis and jaundice and may develop one of three patterns of disease in the future: death, continuing evidence of liver damage, possibly necessitating liver transplantation for development of normal liver function.
• In adults with cirrhosis and chronic active hepatitis, the heterozygous alleleic variant, MZ, may be detected.

 Differential Diagnosis

Alpha-1 antitrypsin deficiency in infancy and childhood may have diverse presentations, including jaundice and hepatosplenomegaly or ascites and cirrhosis in the neonatal period to asymptomatic hepatosplenomegaly in adulthood. Differential diagnosis of idiopathic neonatal hepatitis, cholestasis, and cirrhosis should be considered for the varying presentation of α-1 antitrypsin deficiency (see Jaundice and Cirrhosis chapters).

 Data Gathering

HISTORY

Question: Was there jaundice in the newborn?
Significance: Neonatal hepatitis and jaundice may be the first signs of α-1 antitrypsin deficiency

Question: Was there prolonged jaundice?
Significance: Common to see persistent elevation of neonatal bilirubin level, often within the first 4 months of life

Question: What is the significance of resolved cholestasis in infants?
Significance: May then have long asymptomatic periods

Question: What is adult presentation?
Significance: Adulthood present with cirrhosis and ascites

 Physical Examination

Finding: Jaundice and hepatosplenomegaly
Significance: Evidence of chronic liver disease in older children and adults

 Laboratory Aids

Test: The diagnosis of the alleleic variants is made by serum protein electrophoresis, which characterizes the most common of the protein forms.
Significance: The most common variants are the normal alleleic variant, M; deficient variant, Z and S, the latter leading to lung disease and the former leading to both liver and lung disease; and the null and dysfunctional variants.

Test: MM
Significance: Gives a serum α-1 antitrypsin level of 20 to 53 mmol/L, the normal state.

Test: PiZZ
Significance: Gives a low concentration of 2.5 to 7 mmol/L.

Test: Pinull/nul
Significance: Gives zero levels.

Test: PiSZ
Significance: Gives a mildly increased risk.

IMAGING TECHNIQUES

Testing for diagnosis for complications of α-1 antitrypsin deficiency may include ultrasonography with Doppler study to evaluate a candidate for transplantation or the presence of portal hypertension.

Therapy

DRUGS

- No appropriate drug therapy currently exists for the deficient state.
- Ursodeoxycholic acid, a choleretic agent, is used in doses of 20 to 30 mg/kg/day in one or divided doses for management of cholestasis and pruritus.
- Other medications for treatment of complications of chronic liver disease may be necessary.
- Future treatment options will include definitive gene therapy for ZZ and possibly other genotypes.

DURATION

- Lifelong expectant management and treatment of complications

SURGICAL

- Only definitive therapy is orthotopic liver transplantation

 ## Follow-Up

PROGNOSIS

- One-fourth of children will need a future liver transplantation as a result of worsening liver function and evidence of cirrhosis and portal hypertension.
- One-fourth will stabilize and liver function will normalize.
- One-fourth will slowly develop chronic liver disease and cirrhosis.
- One-fourth will have less severe liver function and live into adulthood.

 ## Common Questions and Answers

Q: What is the usual course for my child with this problem?
A: In general, one-fourth of children will need future liver transplantation as a result of worsening liver function and evidence of cirrhosis and portal hypertension; one-fourth will stabilize and liver function will normalize; one-fourth will slowly develop chronic liver disease and cirrhosis; and one-fourth will have less severe liver function and live into adulthood.

Q: Is there a cure for my daughter at present?
A: Yes; at present treatment options range from treating for complications and definitively performing a liver transplantation to remove the affected organ. Since prognosis can change for children, we wait until the liver is no longer functioning before it is replaced.

ICD-9-CM 277.6

BIBLIOGRAPHY

α-1-Antitrypsin deficiency. In: Sherlock S, Dooley J, eds. *Diseases of the liver and biliary system.* London: Blackwell Scientific, 1992:425–427.

Balistreri W. Neonatal cholestasis. *J Pediatr* 1987;106:171.

Balistreri W. Liver disease associated with a α-antitrypsin deficiency. In: Balistreri W, Stocker J, eds. *Pediatric hepatology.* New York: Hemisphere, 1990:159–175.

Marcus N, Teckman JH, Perlmutter DH. α-Antitrypsin deficiency in childhood disease. *J Pediatr Gastroenterol Nutr* 1998;27(1):65–74.

Perlmutter DH. α-Antitrypsin deficiency. In: Walker WA, Durie PR, Hamilton JR, Walker-Smith JA, Watkins J, eds. *Pediatric gastrointestinal disease.* Philadelphia: BC Decker, 1991:976–991.

Author: Andrew E. Mulberg

Altitude Illness

 Database

DEFINITIONS

- Acute mountain sickness (AMS)
—Failure to adapt to the hypoxic demands of altitude

- Mild Mountain Sickness
—Headache in morning and on exertion, anorexia, nausea, dizziness, vomiting, shortness of breath on exertion, insomnia, irritability, periodic breathing, poor performance

- Moderate Mountain Sickness
—Severe headache, lassitude, weakness, anorexia, nausea, ataxia, decreased urine output, diminished judgment and coordination
—Capable of activities with difficulty

- Severe Mountain Sickness
—Insidious or acute onset, usually 2 to 4 days after ascent
—Can progress to life-threatening within hours

- High-Altitude Cerebral Edema (HACE)
—Headache, vomiting, lassitude, irritability, drowsiness, ataxia, slurred speech, cranial nerve paralysis, hypo or hyperreflexia, hemiparesis, hemiplegia, mental status changes (confusion, unreasonableness, depression, disorientation, amnesia, hallucinations, severe nightmares), decreased urine output, seizures, papilledema, coma, death

- High-Altitude Pulmonary Edema (HAPE)
—Initially with dyspnea on exertion, then at rest, decreased exercise capability, dry cough, fatigue, tachypnea, low grade temperature (<38.5°C)
—Develop pink frothy sputum, cyanosis, wheezing, rales, tachycardia, low-grade fever, orthopnea

- Other altitude related issues
—High-altitude syncope, edema (facial and extremity), retinopathy (hemorrhages), pharyngitis and bronchitis, flatus, immune suppression, thrombosis, coagulation abnormalities, platelet changes

PATHOPHYSIOLOGY

- Hypoxia, hypoventilation, hypercapnia, fluid, and electrolyte balance
—Fluid shifts
—Latent period of 12 to 72 hours between altitude exposure and symptoms
—Usual remission period of 3 to 4 days coincides with fluid changes

- Increased sympathetic nervous system activity

PROGNOSIS AND COMPLICATIONS

- Excellent if recognized quickly, ascent stopped, and/or descent and treatment begun
- Can be poor if symptoms not recognized or appreciated and appropriate descent and therapy not initiated

- Symptoms insidious or acute onset, usually 2 to 4 days after ascent
—Can progress to life-threatening within hours

ASSOCIATED ILLNESSES

- Ophthalmologic
—Retinal vessel engorgement
—Retinal hemorrhages
—Usually resolves in 7 to 10 days without symptoms
—100% of people at 6500 m (>21,000 ft)
—Macular hemorrhages
—More severe
—Associated with visual changes
—Ultraviolet keratitis

- Other
—Pharyngitis
—Bronchitis
—Productive cough
—Immunosuppression

 Differential Diagnosis

ENVIRONMENTAL

- Alcohol toxicity
- Hangover
- Drug effects
- Hypothermia
- Carbon monoxide poisoning

METABOLIC

- Dehydration

PSYCHOSOCIAL

- Exhaustion
- Personality traits (irritability)
- Insomnia

 Data Gathering

HISTORY

Question: Previous altitude illness?
Significance: Suggests symptoms in future with ascent to similar altitude.

Question: Location (altitude) where symptoms occurred, how did the patient arrive at that altitude, and what was the rate of ascent?
Significance: Rapid ascent minimizes time for natural acclimatization and increases risk of developing altitude illness.

Question: Exertion level?
Significance: Increased exertion on ascent may increase speed of symptom development.

Question: Medication, drug or alcohol use, predisposing medical illness (asthma, restrictive lung disease)?
Significance: Underlying medical conditions may predispose one to development of altitude illness. Medication use or presumed medical illness may mask signs and symptoms of altitude illness.

Question: Symptom complex (variable)?
Significance: Altitude illness is a variable and progressive disease. Recognition of the early signs and symptoms can alert one to seek care prior to disease intensification.

Question: Morning headache, progressive with ascent?
Significance: Suggests HACE.

Question: Insomnia, difficulty falling asleep, frequent waking?
Significance: Suggests hypoxia and development of altitude illness.

Question: Periodic breathing (hyperpnea to apnea)?
Significance: Suggests moderate to more advanced altitude illness.

Question: Gastrointestinal: anorexia, nausea, vomiting, abdominal cramps, flatus?
Significance: Potentially related to ascent.

Question: Pulmonary: dry cough, shortness of breath, sore throat, dyspnea on exertion and at rest, decreased exercise capability?
Significance: Potential progression to HAPE.

Question: Neurologic: lassitude, weariness, indifference, fatigue, irritability, dizziness, ataxia, weakness?
Significance: Progression to HACE.

Question: Decreased urine output, fluid retention?
Significance: Indicative of fluid shifts, fluid losses, inadequate replacement, and dehydration.

Question: Peripheral edema: eyes, face, hands, ankles, feet (greater incidence in females)?
Significance: Suggests fluid shifts/retention with ascent. Should alert one to potential development of more significant altitude illness.

 Physical Examination

Finding: Normal in early AMS
Significance: Physical examinations are non-descript early in development.

Finding: Abnormalities usually occur after 12 to 24 hours at altitude (range 2 to 96 hours)
Significance: Tachycardia, tachypnea, dry cough, wheezing, rales, pink frothy sputum, cyanosis, low-grade fever, vomiting, ataxia, slurred speech, cranial nerve paralysis, hypo or hyperreflexia, hemiparesis, hemiplegia, mental status changes (confusion, lassitude, unreasonableness, drowsiness, depression, disorientation, amnesia, hallucinations), decreased urine output, retinal hemorrhage, seizures, papilledema and/or coma.

Laboratory Aids

Test: Chest x-ray study (CXR)
Significance: Vasocongestion, patchy or diffuse infiltrates; often worse than physical examination would suggest

Test: ECG
Significance: Rule out myocardial etiology of symptomatology or consequence of ascent.

Test: Toxicologic screen
Significance: Rule out medication effect for presenting symptomatology.

Test: Electrolytes
Significance: Assess hydration status and fluid shifts.

Test: Carbon monoxide level
Significance: Ensure carbon monoxide poisoning not a factor in presentation.

Test: CBC
Significance: Assess oxygen carrying capacity of blood. Look for anemia and platelet abnormalities.

Test: Ventilation and perfusion scan
Significance: Structural pulmonary assessment.

Test: Brain CT
Significance: Assess for structural abnormalities and cerebral edema.

 ## Therapy

GENERAL

- Suspect AMS
- Stop ascent
- Partial or full descent
- Oxygen if available
- Fluids
- Consider acetazolamide to hasten acclimatization
- Avoid alcohol, codeine, sedative-hypnotics
- Avoid respiratory depressants

SPECIFIC

- Mild AMS
—Treatment may not be needed
—Symptomatic headache relief with ibuprofen, acetaminophen, aspirin, prochlorperazine (Compazine)
—Temporal artery massage

- Moderate to severe AMS
—Oxygen (relieves hypoxia, reduces pulmonary hypertension)
—Furosemide (be careful of volume depletion)
—Acetazolamide
—Consider dexamethasone (if allergic to Sulfa or cannot take acetazolamide)
—Vasodilators (nifedipine, morphine)

- HACE
—Descend immediately
—Oxygen
—Furosemide

—Dexamethasone
—Consider intubation and hyperventilation

- HAPE
—Descend immediately
—Oxygen
—Furosemide
—Acetazolamide
—Vasodilators (nifedipine, morphine) may be useful
—Consider antibiotics
—Positive-pressure breathing
  —Pursed-lip breathing, mask, intubation
  —Knee-chest position with abdominal squeeze
  —Symptoms may recur when positive pressure removed

MEDICATIONS

- Acetazolamide (Diamox) (a carbonic anhydrase inhibitor)
—Hastens natural respiratory changes that occur during acclimatization
—Can help prevent AMS
—Effectiveness in treating established AMS not clear
—General guidelines for use
  —Use in conjunction with (not in place of) gradual ascent, with passive transport to 3000 m (9850 ft) and rapid active transport
  —Prophylaxis if previous history of AMS, history of periodic breathing, insomnia
  —Treatment of early AMS
  —May be useful if sulfa allergy is present
  —Dosage: 5 to 10 mg/kg/day divided b.i.d. (maximum 250 mg/dose), 24 hours prior to ascent and 1 to 2 days at altitude
  —Side effects: polyuria, paresthesias, nausea, drowsiness, taste changes

- Dexamethasone (Decadron)
—Helpful for AMS treatment and early cerebral edema
—Dosage: 4 mg b.i.d. to q.i.d.

- Oxygen
—Helpful at low flow at night (for headache, insomnia, cyanosis)
—Increases PaO_2

- Nifedipine
—Dosage: 20 mg sustained release q 8 hours may be useful for treatment and prevention of HAPE, 24 hours prior to ascent and for 2 to 3 days at altitude

- Diet
—Increase fluid consumption with altitude and exertion
—Carbohydrate diet

 ## Follow-Up

- Expect improvement with mild mountain sickness in 1 to 2 days
- Moderate mountain sickness clears with descent and acclimation
- Severe mountain sickness clears with descent and therapy

PROGNOSIS

- Good if recognized and treated appropriately
- Poor if not recognized or treated appropriately

PREVENTION

- Avoid rapid ascent
—Do not go too high too fast
—Do not fly or drive to heights >3000 m (>10,000 ft)

- Gradual acclimatization
—Limit ascents to 300 m (1000 ft) per day above 3000 m (10,000 ft)
—Allow at least 24 hours for each 1000 m (3300 ft) gained
—Exercise is not a substitute for acclimatization

- Be aware and respectful of symptoms (even if minor)
—Assume symptoms secondary to AMS unless proven otherwise
—Go no higher until symptoms resolve
—Descend if worsening

- Climb high, sleep low
- Avoid alcohol, codeine, sedative-hypnotics, respiratory depressants
- Exercise within individual capacity; avoid heavy exercise after passive ascent for at least 24 hours

 ## Common Questions and Answers

Q: Can one develop AMS at moderate altitudes, such as during a ski vacation?
A: Yes, although the altitudes encountered rarely lead to the development of severe symptoms in this population.

Q: Will physical conditioning prior to ascent decrease the risk of developing altitude illness?
A: No, in fact better conditioning may inadvertently increase the risk of developing altitude illness as one may achieve higher altitudes more quickly.

Q: Should everyone in whom a headache develops when at a higher than usual altitude be treated (pretreated) with acetazolamide?
A: No. One must weigh other options and severity of illness prior to decision to treat or prophylax for AMS.

BIBLIOGRAPHY

Hackett PH, Roach RC. Medical therapy of altitude illness. *Ann Emerg Med* 1987;16:980–986.

Johnson TS, Rock PB. Acute mountain sickness. *N Engl J Med* 1988;319:841–845.

Richalet JP. High altitude pulmonary oedema: still a place for controversy? *Thorax* 1995;50:923–929.

Author: George Anthony Woodward

Amblyopia

Database

DEFINITION

From "amblyos" meaning "dullness of vision" (lazy eye)
A neuropathologic process unique to infancy and childhood resulting in decreased vision in one or both eyes; initiated by any condition resulting in abnormal or unequal visual input between birth and about 9 years of age.

PATHOPHYSIOLOGY

• Normal and equal visual input is necessary (trophic) for proper cell growth and synaptogenesis of the postchiasmal visual pathways in the brain (lateral geniculate, visual cortex).
• Visual system cell growth and synaptogenesis ("cortical vision") is initiated at birth and is finished by 9 years of age. If, during this period, one eye (or both) is not capable of normal and equal visual input, synaptogenesis and cell growth is disturbed, resulting in deficient vision.
• The younger the cortical vision system the more sensitive it is to abnormal input.
• Amblyopia will develop after only 1 week of abnormal visual input in an infant less than 1 year old.
• The clinical rule is that a week of abnormal visual input per year of life is amblyogenic. The period of cortical visual development between birth and 17 weeks of life is the "sensitive, or critical period."
• If a congenital or neonatal amblyogenic stimulus is not treated before the end of the sensitive period it is impossible to recover full and normal vision. A congenital or neonatal amblyogenic stimulus is more potent and leads to irreversible neuronal changes if not treated by about 4 months of age.

CLASSIFICATION

There are three major types of amblyopia that reflect a common interruption in visual development.

• Image-degradation amblyopia: there is usually either a structural problem involving the lids and periocular tissues (ptosis, hemangioma, orbital tumor, orbital inflammation), or poor image processing (retinal edema and inflammation, optic nerve dysplasia and atrophy).
• Strabismic amblyopia: infants and children (up to 9 years of age) with strabismus develop a neuro-adaptive mechanism to prevent diplopia. This is called "suppression" and is a facultative scotoma (blind spot) centered on the fovea of the non-fixing eye. This scotoma switches from one eye to the other when the patient changes fixation. When one eye becomes dominant the other is suppressed, leading to amblyopia (50% of patients with strabismus). In patients who regularly switch fixation between eyes amblyopia does not occur (50% of patients with strabismus).

• Ametropic amblyopia: This type of amblyopia results from abnormal cortical visual input due to uncorrected significant refractive errors. Children with significant myopia (nearsightedness), hyperopia (farsightedness), or astigmatism are unable to position themselves or the world so it is in focus on the retina. Amblyopia occurs when the retina transmits only a blurred image to the brain. A potent amblyogenic stimulus occurs when only one eye has a refractive error or there is a significant difference between the eyes (anisometropic amblyopia).

PATHOLOGY

The lateral geniculate body layers serving the amblyopic eye(s) are atrophic. The visual cortex serving the amblyopic eye(s) is atrophic, less organized, and synaptically aberrant.

GENETICS

There is no hereditary predisposition to primary amblyopia, as this is an acquired disease. There is an increased prevalence in family members due to similar amblyogenic conditions strabismus, which can cause strabismus secondarily.

EPIDEMIOLOGY

Amblyopia is present in 2% of the population and is the leading cause of preventable visual loss in children. Strabismic amblyopia is the most common (occurring in 50% of patients with strabismus), followed by ametropic (mostly anisometropia), and image degradation (lenticular and corneal disease are most common).

COMPLICATIONS

Untreated amblyopia results in irreversable visual loss with an increased risk of complete visual disability if the good eye is traumatized or affected by disease.

PROGNOSIS

Final visual acuity is dependent on the combination of amblyogenic factor, age at presentation, and compliance with amblyopia treatment. In general, the earlier the diagnosis and treatment the better the prognosis.

Differential Diagnosis

• Other causes of cortical visual loss
—Structural disease involving the visual cortex
  —Tumors
  —Vascular malformations
  —Demyelination
  —Trauma
• Clinically silent ocular disorders
—Retinal degenerations and dystrophies
—Posterior optic atrophy
—Glaucoma
—Early corneal dystrophy
• Hysterical visual loss or conversion reaction

Data Gathering

HISTORY

Question: How, when, and where was visual loss first noticed?
Significance: Age of onset and duration of vision loss is crucial in reversibility of amblyopia.

Question: How has this changed?
Significance: Worsening acuity may imply an organic component to the amblyopic vision loss.

Question: Other ocular abnormalities noted or treated?
Significance: These may contribute to the etiology of the amblyopic vision loss.

Question: Familial ocular history?
Significance: There are forms of amblyopia with higher prevalence in families.

Question: The presence of any trauma, prenatal, perinatal, or postnatal medical or surgical problems?
Significance: These questions will aid with determining the etiology of the amblyopia.

Question: Current and past medications and known allergies?
Significance: These routine questions may be important in the medical management of the strabismus, e.g., use of certain topical eye drops.

Question: Exposures to toxins or new climates/travel/day care, or recent systemic illness?
Significance: These historical questions also aid in determining organic causes of vision loss in addition to amblyopia, e.g., toxoplasmosis.

Physical Examination

Finding: Accurate monocular and binocular visual acuities are the most sensitive indicators of amblyopia. Snellen (letter), Allen (picture), or HOTV charts are the most accurate testing methods.
Significance: The ultimate diagnosis of amblyopia is determined by an accurate measurement of visual acuity.

Finding: Other important diagnostic signs are the presence of head posture, strabismus, nystagmus, abnormal pupillary responses, photophobia, and absent or asymmetric red fundus reflexes.
Significance: All of these physical signs can help with differentiating organic vision loss from amblyopia.

Finding: A general developmental and neurological examination
Significance: Helps rule out obvious central nervous system pathology.

Laboratory Aids

Test: Hematologic
Significance: There are no hematologic tests or blood chemistries that will help with diagnosis. These are ordered as indicated by the diagnosed amblyogenic stimulus (e.g., uveitisblood analysis).

Test: Radiologic
Significance: No imaging is helpful for diagnosis, but may be used to define associated condition (trauma, developmental or acquired orbital and lid abnormalities).

Test: Electrophysiologic
Significance: Visual evoked responses and electroretinography (*see* Strabismus chapter) are useful to diagnose and characterize any associated organic disease of the afferent visual system (retinal degeneration, optic nerve dysplasia, anoxic encephalopathy). The presence of both amblyopia and organic disease affects the prognosis of visual recovery from amblyopia treatment.

Therapy

• Amblyogenic condition: Once the diagnosis of amblyopia is made, treatment is first directed toward reversing or decreasing the amblyogenic stimulus. Image-degradation amblyopia is treated by medically or surgically clearing the ocular media (lid hemangioma reduction, cataract extraction, ptosis surgery, corneal transplantation). Strabismic amblyopia is treated prior to surgery as part of the general treatment. This usually consists of a combination of spectacles and penalization. Ametropic amblyopia is first treated by giving the patient full correction of the optical error either with spectacles or contact lenses full time. As long as vision improves no additional treatment is needed.

• Penalization: If treating the amblyogenic condition alone does not restore normal vision then penalization is added. Occlusion of the good eye with an adhesive patch on the eye is the most effective method. This is started for all but 1 hour a day (to prevent amblyopia in the good eye). The patient is followed closely, 1 week for every year of age to a maximum of once a month. Patching is then tapered based on the patient's response. Many children will not tolerate a patch, although alternatives (contact lenses, tinted glasses, optical blurring, plaster casts) all prove inadequate. It has been shown that pharmacologic cycloplegia of the good eye (atropine drops daily) is effective at stabilizing vision and improving vision in some cases. Atropine cycloplegia of the good eye results in poor near vision, forcing the patient to use the amblyopic eye for close vision. This is effectively a "near patch." Experimental treatment of amblyopia in older children and adults with a systemic dopamine agonist (L-dopa) resulted in improved visual function, thus opening a new avenue of research for treatment after visual maturation.

Follow-Up

• The effectiveness of treatment should be closely monitored, as the most common reason for a poor response with penalization is noncompliance. Frequent visits provide positive reinforcement, reassurance, and encouragement needed by both the family and the patient.
• Patients are followed at intervals according to their age. A general rule is 1 week for each year of life up to 4 to 4 to 6 weeks for children over 4. Once vision is stabilized, visits and penalization can be tapered to maintain best vision until 8 to 9 years of age.
• Contact with social services for blind and visually handicapped individuals must be made for children even if they are only suspected of being visually impaired. Encourage families to make the contact even when the child may be too young to provide objective data of the extent of handicap.

PREVENTION

• Screening children as soon as possible, testing visual acuity in school and by the primary care physician, is currently the best method of identifying possible amblyopia and improving the treatment prognosis.
• The general compliance rate with penalization is 50%, effectively reducing the prognosis for attainment of normal vision.

PITFALLS

Testing visual acuity in children is often inconsistent. Reliable and repeatable methods must be used to test vison in the office setting.

Common Questions and Answers

Q: What will be the final vision of an amblyopic eye?
A: The greater the structural or visual difference between the two eyes the less the chance of achieving normal vision. Obtaining 20/200 vision from counting fingers vision with treatment gives the patient a functional eye.

Q: Will the eye see normal after successful treatment?
A: An amblyopic eye which is 20/20 after treatment remains subjectively different from the normal eye to the patient for his or her lifetime.

ICD-9-CM 368.0

BIBLIOGRAPHY

Ching FC, Parks NMN, Friendly DS. Practical management of amblyopia. *J Pediatr Ophthalmol Strab* 1986;23:12–17.

Hubel DH. Deprivation and development. In: Hubel DH, ed. *Eye, brain, and vision.* New York: WH Freeman, 1989:191–218.

Vaegan K, Taylor TD. Critical period for deprivation amblyopia in children. *Trans Am Ophthalmol Soc UK* 1979;99:432–455.

Verecken EP, Brabant P. Prognosis for vision in amblyopia after loss of the good eye. *Arch Ophthalmol* 1984;102:220–227.

von Norden GK. Mechanisms of amblyopia. *Adv Ophthalmol* 1977;34:93–110.

Author: Richard W. Hertle

Anaerobic Infections

 Database

DEFINITION

Anaerobes are organisms capable of growing in a reduced oxygen tension, either exclusively (obligate anaerobes) or in addition to growing in air (facultative anaerobes). They are the predominant organisms in normal bacterial flora.

PATHOPHYSIOLOGY

- Usually caused by endogenous organisms
- Occurs when there is a break in a mucocutaneous barrier
- Infections are often polymicrobial and include aerobic organisms
- Increased risk associated with impaired host immunity or presence of devitalized tissue (due to surgery, trauma, vascular insufficiency)
- Numerous virulence factors including exotoxins (e.g., *Clostridia* spp.), antiphagocytic capsule (e.g., *Bacteroides* spp.), endotoxin (gram-negative anaerobes)
- Infections may be characterized by suppuration, abscess formation, or tissue destruction

EPIDEMIOLOGY

- Less frequent in children than in adults
- Responsible for up to 10% of significant bacteremic episodes in infants and children

COMPLICATIONS

- Vary with nature of infection

PROGNOSIS

- Determined by speed with which infection is appropriately treated with surgery and antibiotics
- Up to 40% mortality associated with clinically apparent anaerobic bacteremia
- Soft-tissue infections caused by *Clostridial* spp. may cause up to 20% mortality despite aggressive therapy

ASSOCIATED ILLNESSES

- Central nervous system (CNS) infections

—Brain abscess
—Subdural empyema
—Epidural abscess

- Head and neck infections

—Sinusitis
—Chronic otitis media
—Ludwig angina
—Cervical adenitis
—Peritonsillar abscess
—Dental abscess
—Gingivitis

- Pleuropulmonary infections

—Aspiration of oral and/or gastrointestinal fluids
—Secondary to aspirated foreign bodies
—Actinomycosis

- Peritonitis/peritoneal abscess

—Appendiceal abscess
—Perforated viscus
—Postoperative complication
—Trauma related

- Cholangitis

—Ascending infection may occur following Kasai procedure
—Infection is often polymicrobial

- Bacteremia

—Often associated with underlying GI disease

- Soft-tissue infection

—Paronychia
—Crepitant cellulitis
—Necrotizing fasciitis
—Gas gangrene

- Infected bite wounds

—Anaerobes isolated from 50% of human or animal bites

 Differential Diagnosis

- Likely pathogens not recovered from aerobic cultures
- Failure of empiric antibiotic coverage that is not active against anaerobes

 Data Gathering

HISTORY

Question: Impaired mental status?
Significance: Increased risk of aspiration.

Question: History of thumbsucking?
Significance: Anaerobes frequently isolated from paronychia.

Question: Recent surgery or trauma?
Significance: Poor drainage leads to infection.

Question: Underlying immunodeficiency or chronic illness?
Significance: Impaired phagocytic function.

Question: Discharge with foul odor?
Significance: Characteristic of anerobic infection.

Physical Examination

Finding: Location of infection
Significance: Increased incidence of anaerobic infections associated with oropharyngeal, abdominal, and female genital tract

Finding: Poor dentition
Significance: Increased colonization of oropharyax with anaerobic organisms

Finding: Gas in tissue, crepitus
Significance: Infection with gas-forming organism

Finding: "Dishwater" pus
Significance: Characteristic of anaerobic infections

 ## Laboratory Aids

Test: Gram stain
Significance: Small, pleomorphic gram-negative bacilli (*Bacteroides* spp.); large gram-positive organisms with "box-car" morphology (*Clostridia* spp.)

Test: Anaerobic cultures
Significance: Should be performed on tissue or aspirated fluid obtained in a sterile fashion from the infected site. Avoid sending a swab for culture. Specimens need to be transported promptly to the microbiology laboratory.

Test: Antibacterial susceptibility testing
Significance: Due to usual efficacy of empiric regimens, susceptibility studies should be limited to organisms involved in potentially life-threatening or difficult-to-treat infections.

Test: X-ray studies
Significance: Air-fluid level, cavity formation, gas in tissue

Test: Special imaging studies
Significance: CT and/or MRI scans often important to define anatomical location and extent of disease.

 ## Therapy

EMPIRIC DRUG THERAPY

- CNS infections
—Cefotaxime/metronidazole or oxacillin/chloramphenicol
- Head and neck infections
—Penicillin or clindamycin
- Pleuropulmonary infections
—Penicillin or clindamycin or ampicillin/sulbactam
- Peritonitis/peritoneal abscess
—Ampicillin/sulbactam or cefoxitin
- Cholangitis
—Ampicillin/sulbactam and gentamicin
- Bacteremia
—Isolate-dependent
- Soft-tissue infection
—Site-dependent
- Infected bite wounds
—Amoxicillin/clavulinic acid

ADJUNCTIVE THERAPY

- Surgery
—Effective drainage of abscesses and debridement of devitalized tissue essential
- Hyperbaric oxygen
—Especially for extensive *Clostridial* infections

ICD-9-CM 041.84

BIBLIOGRAPHY

Dunkle LM. Anaerobic infections. In: Feigin RD, Cherry JD, eds. *Textbook of pediatric infectious diseases,* 3rd ed. Philadelphia: WB Saunders, 1992:1044–1052.

Finegold SM. Anaerobic bacteria: general concepts. In: Mandell GL, Douglas RG, Bennett JE, eds. *Principles and practice of infectious diseases,* 4th ed. New York: Churchill Livingstone, 1995:2156–2173.

Goldstein EJ. Selective nonsurgical anaerobic infections: therapeutic choices and the effective armamentarium. *Clin Infect Dis* 1994;18:S273–S279.

Gorbach SL. Antibiotic treatment of anaerobic infections. *Clin Infect Dis* 1994;18:S305–S310.

Nichols RL, Smith JW. Anaerobes from a surgical perspective. *Clin Infect Dis* 1994;18:S280–S286.

Author: Susan E. Coffin

Anaphylaxis

 Database

DEFINITION

Anaphylaxis is an explosive antigen specific IgE-mediated response resulting in the release of potent biologically active mediators from mast cells and other inflammatory cells. However, non-IgE mediated direct mast cell degranualtion can result in the same response. Patients may develop any combination of the following symptoms: cutaneous (urticaria/angioedema), respiratory (bronchospasm/laryngeal edema), cardiovascular (hypotension, arrhythmias, myocardial ischemia), and gastrointestinal (nausea, vomiting, pain, diarrhea).

PATHOPHYSIOLOGY

Inducing agents stimulate mast cells to release inflammatory mediators either via an antigen-specific or antigen non-specific manor. These mediators may then act either locally or systemically. Mediator release results in the table Pathophysiology of Anaphylaxis.

GENETICS

Atopy can be familial and atopics are at more risk for anaphylaxis.

EPIDEMIOLOGY

• Incidence 0.4 cases per million individuals annually
• Increased hospital incidence of 0.6 cases per 1000 patients
• 400 to 800 deaths annually in the United States

COMPLICATIONS

• Pulmonary edema, pulmonary hemorrhage, and pneumothorax
• Laryngeal edema with or without airway obstruction
• Myocardial ischemia and infarction
• Death may result from asphyxiation from upper airway obstruction or profound shock or both.

PROGNOSIS

Excellent provided the trigger can be avoided.

 Differential Diagnosis

GENETIC/METABOLIC

• Hereditary angioedema
• Systemic mastocytosis
• Pheochromocytoma
• Carcinoid

ALLERGIC/IMMUNOLOGICAL

• Idiopathic
• IgE-mediated
• Non-immunologic mast-cell degranulation
• Exercise-related
• Sulfiting agents
• Non-steroidal anti-inflammatory drug reaction
• Serum sickness

MISCELLANEOUS

• Vasovagal collapse

COMMON CAUSES

• IgE mediated

—Antibiotics (penicillin and others)
—Foreign protein agents (bee sting venom, latex antigens, fire ant venom and others)
—Therapeutic agents (allergen extracts, vaccines and others)
—Foods (peanuts, nuts, shellfish, and others)

• Non-IgE mediated (activates histamine release from mast cells without IgE)

—Radiocontrast media
—Opiates
—Dextran
—Vancomycin
—Polymyxin B
—Quaternary ammonium muscle relaxants (i.e., methylscopolamine bromide, homatropine methylbromide, methantheline bromide, and probanthine bromide)

Approach to the Patient

GENERAL GOAL

Rapidly decide whether the symptoms the patient is experiencing are consistent with anaphylaxis (profuse rhinorrhea, urticaria, wheezing, throat tightness, tachycardia, and hypotension).

Phase 1: Initiate therapy for anaphylaxis. This generally includes: Epinephrine 1:1000 administered subcutaneously, H_1 antihistamines, and H_2 antihistamines (refractory cases).

Phase 2: Attempt to identify the agent that induced the anaphylactic reaction.

 Data Gathering

HISTORY

Question: How long does it take for a patient to react to an offending allergen?
Significance: Anaphylactic reactions usually begin within seconds to minutes after contact with offending antigen. This can help the physician identify the responsible antigen.

Question: Can a patient have an anaphylactic reaction on their first exposure to an allergen?
Significance: A patient must have had a previous exposure to the offending allergen for sensitization to occur. Therefore, anaphylactic reactions should not occur on first exposure.

Question: What does the patient sense during an anaphylactic reaction?
Significance: Patients commonly describe an impeding doom. This may be the first sign of an impending anaphylactic reaction.

Question: What organ systems are affected in an anaphylactic reaction?
Significance: The target organs may include: the heart, the lungs, the skin and the gastrointestinal tract. Any or all of these target organs may be affected.

Question: What is the mechanism of fatal anaphylaxis?
Significance: Death may occur from upper airway obstruction and/or shock. When treating a patient with anaphylaxis upper airway obstruction, and hypotension should be taken very seriously.

Question: Has the patient had anaphylaxis in the past?
Significance: The patient likely knows the responsible allergen. Efforts should be directed towards allergen avoidance.

Question: Does the patient have autoinjectable epinephrine?
Significance: Most deaths from anaphylaxis are associated with delayed administration of epinephrine. Most patients with a history of anaphylaxis are candidates for autoinjectable epinephrine.

Pathophysiology of Anaphylaxis

PATHOLOGIC PROCESS	SIGN OR SYMPTOM	PUTATIVE MEDIATOR RESPONSIBLE
Vascular permeability	Urticaria, angioedema, laryngeal edema, abdominal swelling, cramps	Histamine (H_1), leukotrienes, prostaglandins
Vasodilation	Flushing, headache	Histamine (H_1 and H_2), leukotrienes, prostaglandins
Smooth-muscle contraction	Wheezing, gastrointestinal cramps, diarrhea	Histamine (H_1), leukotrienes, prostaglandins
Congestion	Rhinorrhea, bronchorrhea	Histamine (H_2), prostaglandins, leukotrienes

Source: From Atkinson et al., with permission.

Question: Did the patient experience a bee sting, or are they allergic to any foods?
Significance: Bee venom allergy can result in anaphylaxis. It is important to identify the bee (remember honey bees leave their stinger at the sting site). Immunotherapy is indicated and effective for Bee venom allergic patients. Any food can cause anaphylaxis, but peanuts, nuts, and shellfish are notorious.

Question: Does the patient have asthma or heart disease?
Significance: Asthma and cardiovascular disease are risk factors for death during anaphylaxis.

Question: Does the patient take any medications?
Significance: B-blockers make treatment of anaphylaxis more difficult. Alternative medications should be sought in patients with a history of anaphylaxis.

 ## Physical Examination

Finding: Angioedema
Significance: May be noted anywhere during a systemic allergic reaction, but it is much more significant if it involves the lips, tongue, mouth or larynx (can result in airway obstruction).

Finding: Urticaria
Significance: Cutaneous manifestation of a systemic allergic reaction.

Finding: Profuse rhinorrhea
Significance: May signal upper respiratory tract involvement in a systemic allergic reaction.

Finding: Wheezing
Significance: May signal lower respiratory tract involvement in a systemic allergic reaction.

Finding: Tachycardia, and hypotension
Significance: May signal cardiovascular involvement in a systemic allergic reaction. Tachycardia usually represents a compensatory mechanism in order to maintain the patient's blood pressure.

 ## Laboratory Aids

The treatment of anaphylaxis should never be withheld while awaiting laboratory confirmation.

Test: Plasma histamine
Significance: Plasma histamine is elevated during anaphylaxis.

Test: Serum tryptase
Significance: Serum tryptase becomes elevated during anaphylaxis.

Test: Complete blood count
Significance: Hemoconcentration (as judged by an increased hematocrit or hemoglobin) is common as fluid exits the intravascular space during an anaphylactic reaction.

Test: Chest x-ray
Significance: The bronchospasm associated with anaphylaxis may result in air trapping and hyperinflated lung fields on chest x-ray.

Test: ECG
Significance: Anaphylaxis may show rhythm abnormalities, ischemic changes or infarction on an ECG.

Test: Cardiac enzymes
Significance: Myocardial ischemia during anaphylaxis may result in a myocardial infarction, and elevated cardiac enzymes.

Referral

Factors that may help alert you to make a referral include:

• History of idiopathic anaphylaxis. The allergist can help by testing to likely triggers.
• History of anaphylaxis to bees. Anaphylaxis to bees is an indication for venom desensitization.
• History of food anaphylaxis. The allergist can assist with an appropriate avoidance diet and support resources.
• History of latex anaphylaxis. The allergist can assist with strict latex avoidance precautions, and latex testing if the history is unclear.

 ## Therapy

• Subcutaneous epinephrine 1:1000 concentration. Early administration of epinephrine is very important.
• Maintain airway. Laryngeal edema can be managed with racemic epinephrine from a meter dose inhaler or nebulizer.
• A tourniquet may be applied (above the injection or sting site) to decrease venous blood return from the site of antigen entry.
• Supplement with oxygen, place in recumbent position and elevate legs. Patients during anaphylaxis have an increased oxygen consumption.
• Diphenhydramine IV. H1 blockade is very important in the control of an anaphylactic reaction.
• Cimetidine IV or Ranitidine IV. H2 blockade may be helpful in refractory anaphylaxis.
• Maintain blood pressure with volume expanders or pressors. Hypotension is a serious manifestation of anaphylaxis.
• Aminophyline may be added for wheezing.
• Hydrocortisone or another systemic steroid should be started. These are most helpful to prevent a late phase reaction, and they are of little help during an immediate anaphylactic reaction.

 ## Follow-Up

• All patients who have had anaphylaxis should be discharged with epinephrine in an autoinjecting apparatus.
• Patients with a known trigger should be counseled on strict avoidance.
• All patients should follow up with an allergist.
• Patients not admitted to the hospital should be observed for several hours because late reactions can begin as late as 12 hours after the initial anaphylaxis. These patients are at risk for a second episode of anaphylaxis. These patients, therefore, should be bolused with steroids during the acute treatment, and they should be given a short course of oral corticosteroids to finish at home. In addition, these patients must be discharge with autoinjecting epinephrine (this will provide temporary relief so the patient will have time to seek medical assistance). Patients must know to seek immediate medical help if symptoms return.

 ## Common Questions and Answers

Q: When should the autoinjectable epinephrine be used?
A: It is intended for severe allergic reactions as manifested by any of the following: bronchospasm, angioedema of the lips or tongue, or hypotension (dizziness). The patient must seek immediate medical help if the autoinjectable epinephrine is required.

Q: Do patient's outgrow this condition?
A: No. Subsequent reactions tend to have a more rapid onset, and tend to be more severe.

Q: Who should be referred to an allergist?
A: All patients who have experienced anaphylaxis would benefit from consultation with an allergist. Patients with anaphylaxis from bee stings, and certain antibiotics can be desensitized. In addition, the allergist can be helpful in identifying obscure triggers of anaphylaxis.

BIBLIOGRAPHY

Atkinson TP, Kaliner MA. Anaphylaxis. *Med Clin North Am* 1992;76:841–853.

Bochner BS, Lichtenstein LM. Anaphylaxis. *N Engl J Med* 1991;324:1785–1790.

Cahaly RJ, Slater JE. Latex hypersensitivity in children. *Curr Opin Pediatr* 1995;7(6):671–675.

Kaliner MA. Anaphylaxis. In: Lockey RF, Bukantz SC, eds. *Fundamentals of immunology and allergy.* Philadelphia, WB Saunders, 1987:203.

Middleton E, Reed CE, Ellis EF, Adkinson NF, Yunginger JW, Busse WW. *Allergy principles and practice,* 4th ed. Philadelphia: Mosby, 1993.

Stites DP, Terr AI, Parslow TG. *Basic and clinical immunology,* 8th ed. Englwood Cliffs: Prentice Hall, 1994.

Author: Christopher A. Smith

Anemia of Chronic Disease

 Database

DEFINITION

Anemia that accompanies a variety of systemic diseases.

PATHOPHYSIOLOGY

- Associated with infections, collagen vascular diseases, inflammatory diseases, and malignancies.
- Shortened red-cell survival due to extracellular destructive process. Possible enhanced phagocytic activity of macrophages.
- Impaired bone marrow erythropoietic response to the anemia with a blunted increase in red-cell production of only once to twice normal. Decreased marrow response to erythropoietin.
- Impaired erythroid progenitor response.
- Impaired mobilization of reticuloendothelial system iron stores.
- Suppression of erythropoiesis by one or more of the inflammatory cytokines such as IL-1, γ-IFN, and TNF-α.

EPIDEMIOLOGY

May be associated with chronic infectious, collagen vascular disorders and other chronic inflammatory diseases, and with cancer.

COMPLICATIONS

If severe, patients may be transfusion dependent and thus be at risk for complications associated with packed red blood cell transfusions.

 Differential Diagnosis

- Main differential is iron deficiency anemia.
- In both iron deficiency and anemia of chronic diseases

—Decreased plasma iron
—transferrin saturation
—marrow sideroblasts
—elevated free erythrocyte protoporphyrin (FEP)
—low reticulocyte count.

- In anemia of chronic disease

—low iron-binding capacity
—normal or elevated reticuloendothelial iron
—normal serum ferritin
—increased hemosiderin within the macrophages

- In iron deficiency

—high iron-binding capacity
—low reticuloendothelial iron
—low serum ferritin.

 Data Gathering

HISTORY

- Underlying disease process exists. Disease entities often associated with anemia of chronic disease include infections, both acute and chronic; inflammatory disease; collagen vascular diseases; malignancies, and renal failure.
- The anemia develops over the first month of the disease process and then remains fairly stable over time.

 Physical Examination

Various abnormal physical findings may be present depending on the underlying chronic disease process.

Finding: Mild pallor.
Significance: Because the onset of anemia of chronic disease is insidious and the level of anemia tends to stabilize, the degree of pallor is mild.

Finding: No signs of circulatory compromise.
Significance: Increased cardiac output to compensate for anemia.

Laboratory Aids

- Complete blood count with indices: Normocytic, normochromic (can be microcytic, hypochromic) anemia with hematocrit rarely less than 20%
- Reticulocyte count: Usually in the normal range, but low for the level of anemia.
- Iron studies: Low plasma iron, with low total iron-binding capacity, low transferrin saturation by iron, normal or high ferritin, elevated FEP.
- Hemosiderin in bone marrow macrophages is increased if bone marrow aspiration is done and the aspirate is viewed with iron stains. This is generally not indicated.
- Albumin and transferrin: Both low.
- Acute-phase reactants like C-reactive protein may be elevated.

PITFALLS

- If only the serum iron is obtained without the remainder of iron studies, the child may be inappropriately diagnosed with iron deficiency.
- Anemia of chronic disease often coexists with other causes of anemia, including: occult blood loss, dietary iron deficiency and drug-related marrow suppression.

 ## Therapy

DRUGS

- Iron: There is no role for iron therapy unless there is coexisting iron-deficiency anemia.
- Recombinant human erythropoietin: Effective, but indications for use are still not universally accepted. Clearly utilized in chronic renal failure. Should be used for more severe and symptomatic anemia where the underlying disease is likely to be prolonged and difficult to treat. Should be used in patients who are otherwise transfusion-dependent. Often used in childhood cancer to decrease the exposure to blood products.

OTHER THERAPIES

- Treatment should be directed at the underlying disease process.
- Transfusion of packed red blood cells is sometimes indicated intermittently in severe anemia with hemodynamic compromise.

 ## Follow-Up

- Treatment of underlying disease process may promote slow resolution of associated anemia.
- Hematocrit increase about 6-8 weeks after start of recombinant human erythropoietin therapy. Continues to rise over 6 months.

 ## Common Questions and Answers

Q: Does anemia that is associated with a chronic disease require further evaluation?
A: If the anemia fits within the general guidelines of diagnosis as outlined above, there is no need to pursue further investigation, except in specific cases. If there is an associated malignancy where marrow metastasis is possible, a bone marrow aspirate and biopsy should be done. In conditions with malabsorption, nutritional deficiencies and blood loss should be ruled out.

ICD-9-CM 281.9

BIBLIOGRAPHY

Bertero MT, Caligaris-Cappio F. Anemia of chronic disorders in systemic autoimmune diseases. *Haematologica* 1997;82:375–381.

Means RT. Clinical application of recombinant erythropoietin in the anemia of chronic disease. *Hematol Oncol Clin North Am* 1994;8:933–944.

Mean RT. Erythropoietin in the treatment of anemia in chronic infectious, inflammatory, and malignant disease. *Curr Opin Hematol* 1995;2:210–213.

Shine JW. Microcytic anemia. *Am Fam Phys* 1997;55:2455–2462.

Author: Debra L. Friedman

Angioedema

 Database

DEFINITION

Angioedema is an autosomal dominant disorder in which mutations in the C1-INH (C1 esterase inhibitor) gene results in a deficiency (or an inactive form) of plasma C1-INH. This permits unregulated activation of the complement and plasma kinin-forming pathways leading to angioedema.

COMMON CAUSES

Classic Hereditary Form

• Defect in one of the two genes coding for C1-INH on chromosome 11.

Acquired Forms

• In one form, normal amount and functionally normal C1-INH is secreted into the plasma, but it is bound to circulating antibodies which inactivate it (associated with benign and malignant monoclonal B cell lymphoproliferative disorders)
• In the other form, an autoantibody not associated with lymphoproliferative disorders binds to C1-INH, which makes the C1-INH-C1s complex unstable resulting in increased degradation of C1-INH.

PATHOPHYSIOLOGY

• Deficiency of C1-INH leads to unopposed activation of the first complement component, resulting in the formation of bradykinin, which produces angioedema.
• Angioedema may occur in the upper airway, gastrointestinal tract, and extremities.
• Life-threatening upper airway obstruction may develop.

GENETICS

• Autosomal dominant
• Mutations may be in either of two genes for C1-INH located on chromosome 11.
• Acquired forms lack a genetic predisposition (there is no mutation in the C1-INH gene).

COMPLICATIONS

• Life-threatening upper airway obstruction.
• Severe abdominal pain often mistaken for a surgical abdomen.

PROGNOSIS

Good with prophylactic and recombinant C1-INH therapies.

 Differential Diagnosis

TOXIC, ENVIRONMENTAL, DRUGS

Patients on angiotensin-converting enzyme (ACE) inhibitors

ALLERGIC INFLAMMATORY

• IgE-mediated allergic reactions

—Drug allergy
—Food allergy
—Contact allergy

• Transfusion reaction

TUMOR

Associated with neoplasms via unknown mechanism

GENETIC/METABOLIC

• Urticaria pigmentosa/mastocytosis
• Familial cold urticaria
• C3b inactivator deficiency
• Amyloidosis with deafness and urticaria
• Hereditary vibratory angioedema

PHYSICAL

• Physical urticarias

—Cold urticaria
—Cholinergic urticaria
—Pressure urticaria (angioedema)
—Vibratory angioedema
—Solar urticaria
—Aquagenic urticaria

• Exercise-induced anaphylaxis

RHEUMATOLOGIC

Collagen vascular disease

PSYCHOLOGICAL

• Panic attacks
• Globus hystericus
• Vocal cord dysfunction

MISCELLANEOUS

Idiopathic angioedema

 Data Gathering

HISTORY

Question: At what age did the recurrent episodes of subcutaneous and submucosal edema begin?
Significance: Recurrent episodes of angioedema usually begin at puberty.

Question: How are the episodes of angioedema characterized?
Significance: Angioedema episodes are characterized by edema of the upper airway, extremities or bowels (can cause severe abdominal pain).

Question: Are the angioedema episodes associated with hives?
Significance: Episodes of angioedema are not associated with hives.

Question: How long do the episodes of angioedema last?
Significance: The duration of an angioedema episode usually last 1 to 4 days.

Question: What triggers the angioedema episode?
Significance: Episodes of angioedema can be triggered by emotional stress and physical trauma.

Question: Do other familial members have similar episodes of angioedema?
Significance: Angioedema can be inherited in an autosomal dominant fashion. There may be other affected familial members.

Question: Do the episodes of angioedema respond to epinephrine, antihistamines, or corticosteroids?
Significance: Angioedema related to angioedema responds poorly to epinephrine, antihistamines, and corticosteroids.

 Physical Examination

Aside from angioedema, the physical examination is normal.

Laboratory Aids

GENERAL GOAL

Decide if the patient's symptoms are consistent with angioedema (recurrent angioedema after minor trauma, familial history, onset at puberty, lack of hives, poor response to epinephrine).

• Measure C1 esterase inhibitor level.
• If C1 esterase inhibitor level is normal, and an acquired deficiency is suspected, order a functional assay of C1 esterase inhibitor. Samples for complement assays must be placed on ice immediately, otherwise, the results may be falsely low.

Test: Direct measurement of C1-INH (study of choice to identify the hereditary form of C1-INH deficiency).
Significance: This is an antigenic assay. Affected patients will have a minimal quantity of C1-INH detected, and heterzygotes (carriers) will have approximately one-half normal levels detected.

Test: Direct measurement of C4 and C2 during attacks.
Significance: In acquired C1-INH deficiency the direct measurement of C1-INH is normal, but the C2 and C4 levels are decreased during attacks.

Test: CH50
Significance: The CH50 is a general screen of the complement system, and if abnormal can indicate a deficiency of any of the complement components.

REFERRAL

Factors that may help alert you to make a referral include:

• Any patient diagnosed with angioedema. An allergist can help evaluate these patients for possible androgen prophylaxis therapy. In addition, they can assist in the creation of an emergency plan for recombinant C1 esterase infusion.
• Patients with difficult to control angioedema without an identified trigger. An allergist/immunologist can assist with the appropriate evaluation.

THERAPY

Prophylaxis

• Anabolic steroids (Danazol or Stanozolol) cause increased production of C1-INH resulting in near normal C2 and C4 levels (decreased degradation by activated C1), and a significantly decreased episode frequency. This therapy is indicated in patients with frequent or life-threatening episodes.
• Plasmin inhibitors (Epsilon-Aminocaproic acid or Tranexamic acid) do not correct C2 and C4 levels, but are clinically effective.
• Recombinant C1-INH concentrate recently available.

Acute Attacks

• Recombinant C1-INH concentrate
• Intermittent administration of subcutaneous epinephrine (this type of angioedema is usually poorly responsive, but in an emergent situation this may be considered).

MEDICAL MANAGEMENT

Treatment of the underlying condition will often result in resolution of the angioedema.

Follow-Up

• Patients should be seen at least annually.
• Follow-up should include:

—Review of triggers
—Prospective genetic counseling
—Reinforcement of the need for prophylaxis
—Review of attacks during the previous year
—Creation of an emergency plan for the administration of recombinant C1 esterase inhibitor during severe attacks

• Regular follow-up with an endocrinologist is indicated for patient's requiring androgen steroid therapy

Common Questions and Answers

Q: What is a good screening test for angioedema?
A: The CH50 is a good screening test. Patients with angioedema will have a low CH50. Remember that the specimen must be placed on ice immediately. Failure to ice the specimen will result in a falsely low CH50.

Q: What are the side effects of the prophylactic androgen therapy?
A: The side effects include: masculinization, menstrual irregularities, enhanced epiphyseal growth plate closure, water retention, hypertension, cholestatic hepatitis, hepatic carcinoma, decreased spermatogenesis, and gynecomastia.

BIBLIOGRAPHY

Agostoni A, Cicardi M. Hereditary and acquired C1-inhibitor deficiency: biological and clinical characteristics in 235 patients. *Medicine* 1992;71:206–215.

Borum ML, Howard DE. Hereditary angioedema. Complex symptoms can make diagnosis difficult. *Postgrad Med* 1998;103(4):251–256.

Frank MM, Gelfand JA, Atkinson JP. Hereditary angioedema: the clinical syndrome and its management. *Ann Intern Med* 1976;84:580–593.

Middleton E, Reed CE, Ellis EF, Adkinson NF, Yunginger JW, Busse WW. *Allergy principles and practice,* 4th ed. Philadelphia: Mosby, 1993.

Sim TC, Grant JA. Hereditary angioedema: its diagnostic and management perspectives. *Am J Med* 1990;88:656–664.

Stites DP, Terr AI, Parslow TG. *Basic and clinical immunology,* 8th ed. Englewood Cliffs: Prentice Hall, 1994.

Author: Christopher A. Smith

Animal Bites

 Database

DEFINITION

Spider Bites

- Though there are about 20,000 species of predominantly venomous spiders in the United States, most lack fangs capable of penetrating human skin or toxin strong enough to produce more than a mild reaction.
- Two species, however, can cause significant harm.
- The black, red, and brown widow spiders (*Latrodectus mactans* species) and brown recluse spiders (*Loxosceles reclusa* species) can cause severe local and systemic reactions, including death.

Snake Bites

- While there are about 120 snake species in this country, only 15% envenomate poisonous substances capable of causing fatal reactions.
- About 8,000 people annually in the United States sustain a poisonous snake bite, and 12 to 15 fatalities occur.
- Four of the 20 species of poisonous snakes found in North America are responsible for the majority of bites: Crotalinae (pit viper family: rattlesnakes, cottonmouths, copperheads), and Elapidae (coral snake).

PATHOPHYSIOLOGY

Animal Bites

Rarely, depressed skull fracture, major vessel injury, visceral penetration, and chest trauma

Insect Stings

- Small local reactions: painful, pruritic, urticarial lesion at the sting site
- Large local reaction: swelling and erythema, about 5 cm in diameter. May cross joint boundary and decrease function.
- Systemic anaphylactic reaction: some combination of generalized cutaneous manifestations (urticaria, edema, pruritus), gastrointestinal symptoms, upper or lower airway compromise, and hypotension

Spider Bites

- Local reaction: pain, erythema, swelling, and pruritus.
- Ischemia and skin necrosis: A bright red papule appears within a few hours of the bite and can evolve within 48 to 72 hours into a hemorrhagic vesicle surrounded by purple discoloration (necrosis) or blanching (vasospasm). Shortly after, a firm, star-shaped, purple necrotic lesion appears, and within 7 to 14 days black eschar is visible. Ulcer healing can take weeks to months.

- Systemic reaction of black widow bites: muscle cramping, hypertension, tachycardia, and cholinergic effects (diaphoresis, salivation, lacrimation, and bronchorrhea) may be accompanied by abdominal rigidity or chest tightness. Nausea and vomiting are seen. Mortality in young children is as high as 50% and results from cardiovascular collapse.

Snake Bites

- Crotalidae (pit viper) bites

—Intense local pain and burning occur initially, followed by edema and perioral numbness that extends to the scalp and periphery.
—Local ecchymosis and vesicles appear within the first few hours, and by 24 hours hemorrhagic blebs are present.
—Necrosis extending throughout the bitten extremity generally ensues without treatment.
—Nausea, vomiting, weakness, chills, and sweating can also occur.
—Within several hours neuromuscular involvement can develop (diplopia, dysphagia, lethargy, etc.).
—The dramatic and life-threatening effects are hypovolemic shock, hemorrhagic diathesis, and neuromuscular dysfunction.

- Elapidae (coral snake) bites

—Characterized by mild local signs and symptoms (pain, swelling), but significant neurologic effects that include extremity paresthesias, weakness, fasciculations, and bulbar dysfunction that can progress to flaccid paralysis.

PROGNOSIS

Animal Bites

- Fortunately, most injury from animal bites is trivial, but infections are not uncommon, and fatalities do occur rarely.

Insect and Spider Bites

Most bites do not produce serious effects; some bites can cause severe local and systemic reactions, including death. The most severe reactions and the rare fatalities occur with greater frequency in children.

Snake Bites

Because only 15% of all snake bites are from poisonous snakes, and only about two-thirds of those involve true envenomation, the majority of bites cause only local injury.

EPIDEMIOLOGY

- Dogs are responsible for 90% to 95% of cases, while the remainder of cases are divided as follows: cats, 3% to 8%; rodents or rabbits, 1%; and raccoons and other animals, 1%. Ninety percent of the offending animals are well-known to the victim.

- Though fatalities from animal bites are rare, the majority occur in the pediatric population. Considerable morbidity does occur: 10% require suturing, 5% to 50% develop into infections, 30% cause disability, and 50% leave scars.

 Differential Diagnosis

- Brown recluse spider bite: other spider bites, insect bites and stings, poison ivy/oak, Stevens-Johnson syndrome, toxic epidermal necrolysis, erythema nodosum, chronic herpes simplex, purpura fulminans, diabetic ulcer
- Black widow spider bites: acute abdomen, renal colic, opioid withdrawal, and tetanus
- Poisonous snake bites: non-poisonous snakebite (leaves scratches, not punctures), rodent bites, thorn wounds

 Data Gathering

HISTORY

Animal Bites
History-taking should include:

- Type of animal
- Apparent health of the animal
- Any provocation for the attack
- Location of the bite
- Rabies immunization status of the animal
- Tetanus immunization status of the child

Insect and Spider Bites

- A description of the offender is important (particularly spiders).
- The black widow, about the size of a quarter, should be described as glossy black, gray, or brown with a red, orange, or yellow hourglass-shaped marking on the ventral surface of the abdomen.
- The brown recluse spider is small (1 to 1.5 cm), with a characteristic brown violin-shaped mark on the dorsum of the cephalothorax (*see* Associated Diseases and Complications, for details of presenting signs and symptoms).

Snake Bites

- A pit just in front of the eye
- Fangs instead of rows of small teeth
- Elliptical or slitlike pupil
- Single row of subcaudal plates
- Somewhat triangular shape to the head
- Presence of rattles (at times)
- The Elapidae (coral snakes) are red, yellow, and black striped (specifically, red stripes bordered by yellow stripes) snakes. They have round pupils and rows of small teeth.
- Non-poisonous snakes also have round pupils, rows of small teeth, no pit, and a double row of subcaudal plates.

Physical Examination

All snake bite wounds should be inspected for fang punctures. When present, the distance between them should be measured.

Laboratory Aids

ANIMAL BITES

Test: No laboratory tests routinely done.

INSECTS STINGS

Test: No laboratory tests routinely done.

SPIDER BITES

Test: Brown recluse spider bites—platelet count for evidence of hemolysis is needed as well as monitoring of hemoglobin, urine sediment, blood urea nitrogen (BUN), and creatinine.
Significance: Evidence of hemolysis and renal failure.

Test: Black widow spider bites—follow complete blood count (leukocytosis may be seen), hemoglobin, hematocrit, reticulocyte count, tests for hematuria (urinalysis, renal profile), blood glucose, and electrolytes.
Significance: In severe cases, elevated creatine kinase has been reported.

SNAKE BITES

Test: Appropriate laboratory monitoring should include CBC, PT/PTT, fibrinogen, fibrin split products, type and cross-match electrolytes, BUN, creatinine, and urinalysis for hematuria.

Therapy

ANIMAL BITES

Wound Care

- Copious irrigation of the wound should be performed with at least 500 mL lactated Ringer solution or normal saline with a 19-gauge angiocatheter attached to a syringe.
- Devitalized tissue needs debridement.
- Primary closure of wounds by suturing is controversial, but the consensus now appears to be in favor of bite wound closure.
- Because of the propensity for infection, hand wounds are an exception and probably should not be sutured.

Antibiotics

- Are indicated for wounds with obvious infection and wounds at high risk for becoming infected; deep punctures, cat bites, non-superficial hand wounds, and non-superficial facial wounds.

- Treatment with amoxicillin and clavulinic acid (Augmentin) or penicillin plus a penicillinase-resistant penicillin is suggested.
- Rabies prophylaxis (*see* Rabies chapter): recommended for bites by bats, skunks, raccoons, foxes, coyotes, and unknown, unobservable dogs and cats. It is not recommended following bites by observable healthy dogs and cats or most rodents and lagomorphs (hares and rabbits). Human rabies immune globulin (RIG): 20 IU/kg body weight (one-half infiltrated into wound, the remainder intramuscularly); human diploid cell rabies vaccine (HDCV): 1.0 mL intramuscularly on days 0, 3, 7, 14, and 28. (Rabies vaccine adsorbed [RVA] can be used alternatively at the same dosage.)
- Tetanus prophylaxis: Most children are fully immunized. Those who are not may require adsorbed tetanus (and diphtheria) toxoid. Tetanus immune globulin, a human product used for passive immunization, is required only in dirty wounds sustained by children with inadequate or uncertain immunization history.

Insect Stings

- If the stinger remains in the skin, it should be removed by flicking or scraping with a fingernail. Mild reactions can be treated with ice or cold compresses. Moderate reactions may require an antihistamine such as diphenhydramine orally for several days. Mild or severe anaphylactic reactions require epinephrine 1:1000 solution 0.01 mL/kg (maximum, 0.3 mL) subcutaneously followed by diphenhydramine and a corticosteroid PO or IV.

Spider Bites

Black Widow Bites

- To alleviate muscle pain and cramping, an opioid (morphine or meperidine) alone or in combination with a benzodiazepine can be used.
- 10% calcium gluconate may also be given slowly by intravenous with electrocardiographic monitoring.
- Methocarbanol (Robaxin) is a muscle relaxant, and can be given q6h if needed.
- *Lactrodectus* antivenom is available and should be administered as soon as possible. For children less than 40 kg the usual dose is 2.5 mL (one vial). For children weighing more than 40 kg, the following are specific indications for antivenom use: age >16 years, respiratory difficulties, or significant hypertension.

Brown Recluse Spider Bites

- Mild bites: Frequent cleaning with soap and water, ice compresses initially, immobilization and elevation, use of diphenhydramine for pruritus, and an analgesic may also be considered.
- Large necrotic areas may require surgical excision and skin grafting.
- Antivenom is not yet commercially available.
- The use of dapsone is controversial. Current recommendations are to limit its use to adults with proven brown recluse bites. Dapsone should not be used in children because of the risk of methemoglobinemia.

Snake Bites

Pit Viper (Crotalidae) Bites

- Rapid transport to medical facility, removal of jewelry/clothing from affected extremity, immobilization of the area in position of function below level of heart.
- A constriction band is indicated when incision and suction are called for or when anticipated transport will be longer than 30 to 60 minutes.
- Incision and suction are helpful only for pit viper bites when started within 5 to 10 minutes of the bite.
- After constriction band placement, linear incisions (1 × 0.05 cm deep) should be made through the fang marks, and suction with a snake bite kit suction cup applied for 30 to 60 minutes.
- If possible, the snake should be killed and brought in for identification. The head of a dead snake must be handled with care because it can deliver a venomous bite for up to 1 hour after death/decapitation.
- The use of antivenom is the mainstay of treatment.
- There are two types of antivenom, one for North American pit vipers and the other for Eastern coral snakes.
- Three to 20 vials may be required after skin testing for sensitivity to horse serum.
- Intravenous dosing is guided by serial measurements of the circumference of the extremity.
- The following should also be considered:

—Treatment of shock with intravenous fluids
—Analgesic use
—Broad-spectrum antibiotic administration for extensive tissue involvement
—Tetanus prophylaxis

ICD-9-CM
Spider venomous 989.5
Snake 989.5

BIBLIOGRAPHY

Avner JR, Baker MD. Dog bites in urban children. *Pediatrics* 1991;88(1):55–57.

Hall CB, Powell KR. Infections from animal and human bites. *Rep Pediatr Infect Dis* 1992;2:9–12.

Koh WL. When to worry about spider bites. Inaccurate diagnosis can have serious, even fatal, consequences. *Postgrad Med* 1998;103(4):235–6, 243–4, 249–50.

Talan DA, Citron DM, Abrahamian FM, et al. Bacteriologic analysis of infected dog and cat bites. *N Engl J Med* 1999;340:85–92.

Wright SW, Wrenn KD, Murray L, Seger D. Clinical presentation and outcome of brown recluse spider bite. *Ann Emerg Med* 1997;30(1):28–32.

Author: Susan Dibs

Ankylosing Spondylitis

 Database

DEFINITION

Ankylosing spondylitis is an inflammatory arthritis that tends to be asymmetric peripherally and to involve the insertion of tendons, ligaments, as well as the sacroiliac joints and spine.

CAUSES

- Idiopathic

PATHOLOGY

- Inflammatory synovitis of joints and calcification of the anterior and posterior longitudinal ligaments of the spine

EPIDEMIOLOGY

- Typically affects adolescent males
- About 1 per 1000 white boys
- Much less common in blacks

GENETICS

- HLA-B27 associated

COMPLICATIONS

- Acute anterior uveitis
- Aortic insufficiency

 Differential Diagnosis

INFECTION

- Reiter syndrome caused by *Enterobacteriaceae* or *Chlamydia*
- Whipple disease
- Intestinal-bypass—associated arthritis
- Diskitis
- Pott disease

TUMORS

- Osteoid osteoma

TRAUMA

- Traumatic injury causing low back pain/spasm
- Herniated disk

METABOLIC

- Ochronosis

CONGENITAL

- Kyphosis

IMMUNOLOGICAL

- Inflammatory bowel disease—associated arthropathy
- Pauciarticular juvenile rheumatoid arthritis

PSYCHOLOGICAL

- Feigning low back pain/stiffness

MISCELLANEOUS

- Psoriasis-associated arthritis
- SEA (seronegative enthesopathy and arthropathy) syndrome

 Data Gathering

HISTORY

Question: Ankylosing spondylitis
Significance: Signified by back pain of insidious onset that has been present for at least 3 months. There is usually a familial history of a male relative with disease and inactivity stiffness resulting in gelling of peripheral joints and back.

 Physical Examination

Finding: Sacroiliac tenderness
Significance: Indicates site of inflammation

Finding: Pain on direct palpation at insertion of Achilles tendon and plantar fascia at calcaneal insertion
Significance: Indicates site of inflammation

Finding: Schober test of lumbar spine flexibility
Significance: Mark 15-cm span at mid-low back at level of iliac crest while patient is standing. Have patient flex back as far as possible. Remeasure span. Abnormal if less than 5 cm increase in span.

Laboratory Aids

Test: CBC, ESR, HLA-B27, rheumatoid factor (RF), and antinuclear antibody (ANA) tests should be done.
Significance: Note that ESR is occasionally not elevated. RF and ANA are typically negative.

Test: Imaging
Significance: Sacroiliac views should be obtained to demonstrate evidence of pseudowidening and/or sclerosis.

Test: False Positives
Significance: HLA-B27 occurs in 8% of whites and 6% of blacks.

 ## Therapy

DRUGS

- NSAIDs: naproxen, indomethacin, meclofenemate
- Disease-modifying drugs: sulfasalazine, methotrexate

PHYSICAL THERAPY

Physical therapy is an essential component of treatment. Must encourage range-of-motion exercises and avoid prolonged neck flexion.

DURATION OF THERAPY

- May be lifelong

DIET

- Food intake should be good with NSAIDs
- Ensure folate intake with methotrexate

 ## Follow-Up

WHEN TO EXPECT IMPROVEMENT

Over weeks to several months should see some improvement in stiffness, synovitis, and range of motion.

SIGNS TO WATCH FOR TO INDICATE PROBLEMS

- Worsening stiffness
- Acute or chronic eye pain
- Chest pain or shortness of breath

PROGNOSIS

- Poor if disease remains active for 10 years or more

PITFALLS

Overdiagnosis in HLA-B27-positive individuals in whom other causes for joint swelling should be considered.

 ## Common Questions and Answers

Q: Should HLA-B27 be checked routinely in boys with back pain?
A: Detection of HLA-B27 alone should not precipitate an extensive work-up because it is so common in the normal healthy population. However, the risk for developing a spondyloarthropathy is 16 times greater than in the HLA-B27-negative individual.

Q: Can affected individuals play contact sports?
A: This is probably not a good idea because as the spine fuses, the risk for fracture of the spine (especially the C-spine) increases.

ICD-9-CM 720.0

BIBLIOGRAPHY

Cabral DA, Malleson PN, Petty RE. Spondyloarthropathies of childhood. *Pediatr Clin North Am* 1995;42(5):1051–1070.

Case records of the Massachusetts General Hospital. Weekly clinicopatholgical exercises. Case 17-1990. A 16-year-old boy with painful swelling of the left knee joint and calf. *N Engl J Med* 1990;322:1214–1223.

Flato B, Aasland A, Vinje O, Forre O. Outcome and predictive factors in juvenile rheumatoid arthritis and juvenile spondyloarthropathy. *J Rheumatol* 1998;25(2):366–375.

Spondyloarthropathies and psoriatic arthritis in children. *Curr Opin Rheumatol* 1993;5:634–643.

Author: Gregory F. Keenan

Anomalous Coronary Artery

 Database

DEFINITION

In this disorder, the left coronary artery arises from the pulmonary trunk rather than the aorta.

CAUSES

• Abnormal septation of the conotruncus into aorta and pulmonary artery.
• Persistence of the pulmonary buds and involution of the aortic buds that will eventually form the coronary arteries.

PATHOPHYSIOLOGY

• Left ventricle is perfused with desaturated blood.
• Collateral flow tends to steal blood from the myocardial blood vessels into the pulmonary artery, resulting in myocardial ischemia.

EPIDEMIOLOGY

• Rare anomaly
• 87% of patients with this anomaly present in infancy

 Differential Diagnosis

• Cardiomyopathy
• Mitral-valve incompetence
• Left ventricular failure from other causes
• Colic
• Bronchiolitis

CLINICAL FEATURES

• Intractable congestive heart failure
• Paroxysms of poor feeding, pallor, and sweats
• Irritability
• Sometimes asymptomatic
• Occasionally may be symptomatic in infancy and then gradually improve (with adequate coronary collateralization)
• Older children and adults may have dyspnea, syncope, or angina pectoris on effort
• Sudden death

 Physical Examination

• Signs of congestive heart failure
• Loud P2 component of S2
• Gallop rhythm
• Murmur: mitral incompetence or a continuous murmur reminiscent of a coronary arteriovenous fistula
• Diagnosis should be entertained in any infant presenting with cardiomegaly or perplexing cardiorespiratory symptoms.

Laboratory Aids

Test: Chest x-ray study
Significance: Cardiomegaly, pulmonary edema

Test: Nuclear imaging
Significance: Thallium myocardial perfusion imaging shows reduced uptake in ischemic regions.

Test: Electrocardiography
Significance: Anterolateral infarct pattern in an infant (Q in I, aVL, V4–V6), abnormal R wave progression in precordial leads

Test: Echocardiogram
Significance: Attachment of coronary artery to pulmonary artery by two-dimensional Doppler interrogation shows flow passing from coronary artery to great artery rather than vice versa.

- Large right coronary artery
- Function and wall-motion abnormalities of left ventricle
- Echogenic papillary muscles
- Mitral regurgitation
- Cardiac catheterization
- Low cardiac output
- High filling pressures
- Pulmonary hypertension
- Aortic root angiography shows passage of contrast medium from left coronary to pulmonary artery

Test: Pulmonary artery angiogram
Significance: Shows reflux of contrast medium into the left coronary artery.

 Therapy

The first priority is stabilization of the patient.

SURGERY

- Ligation of origin of left coronary artery and reconstitution of flow with saphenous or internal mammary graft.
- Direct reimplantation of the left coronary (with a button of pulmonary artery around the origin) into the aorta.
- Creation of an aortopulmonary window and tunnel that directs blood from aorta to the left coronary ostium (Takeuchi procedure).
- Ligation of the origin of the left coronary artery to prevent steal in very sick infants

PROGNOSIS

- Untreated, 65% to 85% die before the age of 1 year, usually after 2 months of age (when pulmonary vascular resistance falls).
- Few improve spontaneously.
- Late results after surgery are fairly good.
- Mitral-valve incompetence may progress in spite of surgery and its repair may be required later.

ICD-9-CM 746.85

BIBLIOGRAPHY

Emmanouilides GC, Riemenschneider TA, Allen HD, Gutgesell, HP, eds. *Moss and Adams' heart disease in infants, children and adolescents including the fetus and young adult,* 5th ed. Baltimore: Williams & Wilkins, 1995:776–780.

Fyler C. *Nadas' pediatric cardiology.* Philadelphia: Henley & Belfins, St. Louis: Mosby, 1992;51:715–718.

Author: Maully Shah

Anorexia Nervosa

 Database

DEFINITION

Illness characterized by:

- Refusal to eat, with resultant weight loss or failure to gain weight
- Intense fear of gaining weight or becoming fat
- Misperception of body size
- In females, amenorrhea

Restricting Type

- Person does not usually engage in binge eating or purging behaviors.
- Patients are characterized as more obsessive-compulsive, stoical, perfectionistic, introverted, and emotionally inhibited.

Binge Eating/Purging Type

- Person regularly engages in binge eating or purging behavior
- Patients are described as impulsive, depressive, socially dysfunctional, sexually adventurous, and as substance misusers, with high levels of general emotional distress.

Mild

- Mildly distorted body image
- Weight >90% of average weight for height
- No symptoms or signs of excess weight loss
- Healthy weight loss methods
- (>1000 cal/day, moderate exercise, no purging)

Moderate

- Moderate distortion of body image unchanged with weight loss
- Weight 90% of average weight for height with refusal to stop additional weight loss
- Symptoms or signs of weight loss associated with denial of any problem existing
- Unhealthy means to lose weight (consuming <1000 cal/day, excessive exercise or purging)

Severe

- Grossly distorted body image unchanged with weight loss
- Weight 85% of average weight for height associated with refusal to stop weight loss
- Symptoms or signs of extreme malnutrition, often coexisting with denial regarding thinness
- Unhealthy means of losing weight (consuming <1000 cal/day, excessive exercise or purging)

GENETICS

There is some evidence of genetic vulnerability to anorexia nervosa.

EPIDEMIOLOGY

Incidence

- Worldwide: 1 case/100,000 people
- White, pubertal females in Western countries: 1 case/200 people

- Prevalence rate for adolescent girls in the United States is 0.48%
- Female to male ratio: 9–10:1
- Mean onset is 13.75 (range 10–25) years
- Coincides with changes of puberty

COMPLICATIONS

Endocrine

- Hypothyroidism
- Hypogonadotropic hypogonadism
- Hypoestrogenism

Cardiac (Related to Malnutrition and Electrolyte Disturbance)

- Bradycardia
- Nodal rhythm
- First- and second-degree heart block
- Intraventricular conduction disturbances
- Bundle-branch block
- Ventricular ectopic beats

Gastrointestinal

- Delayed gastric emptying
- Decreased intestinal motility

Renal

- Hypochloremic, hypokalemic metabolic alkalosis

Neurological

- Muscle weakness
- Peripheral neuropathy
- Abnormal thermoregulation
- Reduced basal temperature

Cognitive

- Impaired concentration and alertness
- Distractibility
- Apathy
- Sleeping problems

Gynecological

- Amenorrhea

Musculoskeletal

- Osteopenia

Dental

- Enamel erosion
- Salivary gland enlargement

Dermatological

- Lanugo hair
- Pedal or pretibial edema
- Orange skin
- Brittle hair and nails
- Calluses on knuckles (Russell syndrome; due to vomiting)

PROGNOSIS

- Mortality: 5.9%
- 50% have good outcome, 25% have intermediate outcome, and 25% do poorly.

Good Prognosis for Those With:

- High educational achievement
- Early age of onset
- Good emotional adjustment
- Improvement in body image after weight gain
- Good initial ego strength
- Supportive family

Poor Prognosis for Those With:

- Late age of onset
- Continued distortion of body image
- Premorbid obesity
- Vomiting or laxative abuse
- Significant depression, obsessive behavior
- Family dysfunction
- Male gender
- Very low body mass indexes at initiation of therapy

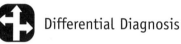 Differential Diagnosis

INFECTION

- Tuberculosis

TUMORS

- Cerebral neoplasm

METABOLIC

- Hyperthyroidism or hypothyroidism
- Addison disease
- Diabetes mellitus

PSYCHOSOCIAL

- Depression
- Malabsorptive states
- Gastroesophageal obstruction

 Data Gathering

HISTORY

Special Questions

Question: Assess self-esteem, reason for dieting, ways of controlling weight, and frequency of weighing.
Significance: Determine degree of eating disorder psychopathology.

Eating-Disorder Specific

Question: Does patient exercise, binge/purge, use laxatives, diuretics, or emetics, or have food rituals or particular eating behaviors?
Significance: Assesses eating disorder stereotypical behavior

General

Question: Does patient have symptoms of weakness, fatigue, cold intolerance, headaches, dizziness, abdominal pain, or constipation?
Significance: Addresses common physical symptoms of anorexia nervosa

Psychiatric

Question: Is there any history of depression, mood disorder, anxiety disorder, suicide attempt, or substance use by the patient?
Significance: Addresses common psychological symptoms of anorexia nervosa.

 ## Physical Examination

Finding: Vital signs to assess for hypotension, bradycardia, hypothermia
Significance: Signs of malnutrition and dehydration

Finding: Weight 15% below ideal
Significance: Consider hospitalization

Finding: Short stature
Significance: Malnutrition, reduced growth, retardation

Finding: Degree of emaciation
Significance: Consider hospitalization

Finding: Dry skin
Significance: Hypothyroidism

Finding: Edema
Significance: Hypoproteinemia

Finding: Yellow skin
Significance: Carotenemia

 ## Laboratory Aids

Laboratory assessment should be done as part of the initial diagnostic evaluation.

Test: Electrolytes, including calcium, magnesium, phosphate
Significance: Demonstrates electrolyte abnormalities from poor intake or laxative and/or diuretic use

Test: BUN and creatinine
Significance: Assess degree of dehydration

Test: Liver function tests
Significance: Patient may have mild elevation of hepatic enzymes

Test: Cholesterol, lipids
Significance: May have hypercholesterolemia

Test: Total protein, albumin
Significance: May be hypoproteinemic

Test: Thyroid function tests, LH and FSH
Significance: Tend to see hypothyroidism and hypogonadotropic hypogonadism

RADIOGRAPHIC AND OTHER STUDIES

Test: Electrocardiogram
Significance: All patients should have a baseline ECG because cardiac abnormalities are the major medical cause of morbidity and mortality.

Test: Chest x-ray (optional)
Significance: Evaluates for TB

 ## Therapy

• A multidisciplinary approach is needed to make the diagnosis of anorexia nervosa. Include a psychotherapist and a nutritionist when evaluating and treating these patients.
• Malnourished adolescents with anorexia nervosa are hypometabolic, and initial energy requirements may be as low as 800–1000 kcal/d.
• Calorie intake should be increased by 200–300 kcal every 2 to 3 days as tolerated.
• Expected rate of weight gain will vary, but a rate of 0.36 lb/d has been shown to be safe in adolescents with anorexia nervosa.

Mild Anorexia Nervosa

• Assess and monitor diet and weight loss plan.
• Refer to nutritionist, if indicated, for education and meal planning.
• Establish weight loss limit at patient's own weight goal.
• Reevaluate in 1 to 2 months.

Moderate Anorexia Nervosa

• Perform medical and nutritional assessment of weight loss, including laboratory studies.
• Establish weight gain goal (target weight, 85% of average; rate of weight gain, 1–2 lb/week).
• Provide specific guidelines for structure of daily activities (e.g., eating schedule, exercise, after-school activities, sports, and recreation).
• Provide medical, nutritional, and mental health counseling that considers the developmental stage and needs of the patient.
• Establish follow-up every 1 to 2 weeks to monitor health and to maintain therapeutic relationship with patient and parents.
• Consult with eating disorder specialists, with referral if necessary.
• Establish criteria for hospitalization.

Severe Anorexia Nervosa

• Perform medical and nutritional assessment of weight loss, including laboratory studies.
• Refer to eating disorder specialists.

Criteria for Hospitalization

• Hypovolemia and hypotension
• Hypothermia (temperature <36°C)
• Electrolyte imbalance, dehydration
• Heart rate <55 beats/min
• Grey-out (a fuzzy light-headed feeling) or syncope
• Weight below 75% ideal body weight (IBW)
• Uncontrollable binging and purging
• Acute food refusal
• Persistent weight loss

MEDICATIONS

• Estrogen and calcium replacement to correct osteopenia
• Stool softeners for constipation; no laxatives
• Antidepressants such as fluoxetine (Prozac) have been helpful in treatment if there is concomitant depression.

 ## Follow-Up

Weight gain should occur gradually over several weeks.

SIGNS TO WATCH FOR TO INDICATE PROBLEMS

• Weight loss or failure to gain weight after institution of dietary program
• Electrolyte abnormalities
• Willful behavior and acting out
• Increased depression or mood disturbance

PITFALLS

• Gonadotropins are usually at a prepubertal level.
• T_3 is low and reverse T_3 is elevated, reflecting increased conversion of T_4 to reverse T_3 and decreased conversion of T_4 to T_3.
• Liver transaminases rise during refeeding.
• Acute decreases in phosphorus during refeeding can indicate refeeding syndrome. Use supplementation if necessary.

 ## Common Questions and Answers

Q: Should the patient with amenorrhea be started on hormonal replacement?
A: Yes, adolescents should begin hormone therapy. Oral contraceptive pills are easiest to use. Often the patient does not wish to take hormones because she is fearful that she will gain weight.

Q: Should the patient be allowed to exercise as an outpatient?
A: Exercise should be restricted until the patient's weight has improved sufficiently to preclude bradycardia or other cardiac arrhythmias. Often exercise can be used as a bargaining tool in the behavioral management of these patients. If the patient maintains a minimum of 91% ideal body weight, he or she may exercise. If the weight decreases, exercise is again restricted.

ICD-9-CM 307.1

BIBLIOGRAPHY

Garner DM. Pathogenesis of anorexia nervosa. *Lancet* 1993;341(8861):1631–1635.

Harper G. Eating disorders in adolescence. *Pediatr Rev* 1994;15(2):72–77.

Sullivan PF. Mortality in anorexia nervosa. *Am J Psychiatry* 1995;152(7):1073–1074.

Author: Liana R. Clark

Aortic Valve Stenosis

 Database

DEFINITION

Aortic valve stenosis occurs as a congenital anatomical deformity of the aortic valve, which causes obstruction of the left ventricular outflow tract.

• Incidence 3% to 6% of all congenital cardiac defects, increases with age. Congenital bicuspid aortic valve not always recognized in childhood, often presents as valve becomes stenotic in older age.
• Male/female ratio of 4:1.
• Associated cardiac anomalies up to 20%. Most commonly, coarctation of the aorta and patent ductus arteriosus, as well as bicuspid aortic valve. Ventricular septal defect and pulmonary stenosis also occur. Aortic valve stenosis associated with other left heart obstructive lesions; the most severe form is hypoplastic left heart syndrome.

CAUSES

• Acquired aortic valve stenosis also occurs, usually secondary to rheumatic heart disease.
• Acquired aortic stenosis (AS) from rheumatic fever not usually seen in early childhood, rare even in the first decade. Often associated with aortic insufficiency. Mitral valve usually involved.

ANATOMY

• Congenital AS most often from decreased commisural separation between cusps of the aortic valve. Fusion results in bicuspid aortic valve with eccentric orifice. Impaired excursion of aortic valve leaflets causes obstruction to left ventricular ejection of cardiac output.
• In infants, aortic valve often unicommisural, associated with severe left ventricular (LV) outflow tract obstruction.

PATHOPHYSIOLOGY

• Hemodynamic significance related to the degree of LV outflow tract obstruction.
• Pressure gradient between LV cavity and aorta directly related to the flow across the aortic valve squared. Elevated LV cavity pressure causes LV hypertrophy (LVH). Pressure load and LVH creates potential subendocardial ischemia. This can be the substrate for ventricular arrhythmias and sudden death.
• Increased risk of subacute bacterial endocarditis, incidence increases with severity of the obstruction.

PROGNOSIS

• Varies with severity of obstruction. Disease in infancy is usually the most severe.
• Frequently progressive over time. Mild AS (<25-mm Hg gradient) often followed medically. A gradient of >50 mm Hg has an increased risk of arrhythmia and sudden death.
• Lifelong requirement for subacute bacterial endocarditis prophylaxis.
• Relief of most LV outflow tract obstruction accomplishable with catheter-based and/or surgical intervention. Treatment may include valve replacement.

 Differential Diagnosis

• Subvalvar AS

—Subaortic membrane
—Abnormal AV valve attachments
—Malalignment of the infundibular septum
—IHSS (hypertrophic obstructive cardiomyopathy)

• Supravalvar AS

—Williams syndrome
—Idiopathic infantile hypercalcemia (± familial form)

• Chest pain syndromes

—Coronary abnormalities causing myocardial ischemia, especially with exercise

 Data Gathering

HISTORY

Question: Mild to moderate AS?
Significance: Usually asymptomatic, normal growth and development.

Question: Fatigue, exertional dyspnea, chest pain, and syncope?
Significance: May develop with severe AS. Less frequently abdominal pain, sweating, and epistaxis. Sudden death, especially with exertion.

Question: Severe cardiac dysfunction?
Significance: In infants, severe cardiac dysfunction associated with non-immune hydrops fetalis. Signs of decreased systemic output including hypotension, tachycardia, cardiomegaly, pulmonary vascular congestion, and respiratory distress. Impaired LV function may be associated with myocardial ischemia and/or infarction.

Question: Critical AS?
Significance: In newborns represents systemic circulation dependent on flow across patent ductus arteriosus. May require urgent catheter or surgical intervention.

Aortic Valve Stenosis

 ## Physical Examination

Finding: Loud harsh systolic murmurs at base of heart radiating to jugular notch and carotid arteries.
Significance: Turbulent flow past aortic valve

Finding: Palpable thrill
Significance: Associated with a gradient >25 mm Hg from LV to aorta.

PLYNEAL FINDINGS

• Opening ejection click
• S2 can be narrowly split and may be single with delayed aortic closure.
• A lift or palpable pre-systolic expansion if left atrial pressure is elevated.
• Diastolic murmur with associated aortic insufficiency.
• In infants with critical AS, a systolic murmur may not be audible because of severe LV dysfunction and poor cardiac output.

 ## Laboratory Aids

Test: Electrocardiography
Significance: Left ventricular hypertrophy (large S wave in V1, large R wave in V6). Signs of myocardial perfusion abnormalities with strain pattern (abnormal QRS-T vector angle).

Test: Chest radiograph
Significance: Possible cardiomegaly with LVH, size correlates poorly with gradient. Left atrial enlargement in severe AS. Signs of congestive heart failure such as pulmonary vascular congestion, pulmonary artery dilation, and right ventricular hypertrophy, especially in infants. Poststenotic dilation of the aortic valve (rare in children). Adults may have calcification of the aortic valve.

Test: Echocardiography
Significance: Defines aortic valve anatomy. Fusion of aortic valve commissures with impaired leaflet excursion. Identifies degree of stenosis and associated regurgitation.

Test: Exercise testing
Significance: Non-invasive modality to test symptoms such as dyspnea, chest pain, dizziness, or palpitations associated with exertion. Cardiovascular response to exercise in terms of heart rate, blood pressure, and electrocardiographic (ST-T) changes measured.

Test: Cardiac catheterization
Significance: Direct measurement of pressure gradient between LV-aorta, and cardiac output. Angiography demonstrates valve anatomy. Potential intervention by transcatheter balloon dilation of the aortic valve. The major risk of aortic valve dilation is the development of aortic insufficiency.

 ## Therapy

• Balloon dilation via cardiac catheterization
• Surgical valvotomy
• Valve replacement

—Prosthetic aortic valve
—Aortic homograft (Does not require systemic anticoagulation, especially desirable in women of childbearing years.)
—Pulmonary autograft in the aortic position (Ross procedure) (Does not require systemic anticoagulation, especially desirable in women of childbearing years.)

• There is an incidence of homograft degeneration. Right ventricular to pulmonary artery conduit may require replacement with patient growth.

 ## Common Questions and Answers

Q: How likely is endocarditis in patients with AS?
A: The presence of aortic valve stenosis represents moderate risk for development of subacute bacterial endocarditis. The Second Natural History Study reported 22 cases in 462 patients with AS, for an incidence of 27.1 per 10,000 person-years. Of these 20/22 occurred in patients with >50 mm Hg gradient across the aortic valve.

Q: Should activity be limited in individuals with aortic stenosis?
A: Recommendations for activity restrictions are based on the degree of AS, extent of symptomatology, and ECG findings. Patients with severe AS should be counseled not to participate in competitive sports.

ICD-9-CM 746.3

BIBLIOGRAPHY

Awadallah SM, Kavey RW, Byrum CJ, Smith FC, Kveselis DA, Blackman MS. The changing pattern of infective endocarditis in childhood. *Am J Cardiol* 1991;68:90–94.

Dajani AS, Taubert KA, Wilson W, et al. Prevention of bacterial endocarditis: recommendations by the American Heart Association. *JAMA* 1997;277:1794–1801.

Egito EST, Moore P, O'Sullivan J, et al. Transvascular balloon dilation for neonatal critical aortic stenosis: early and midterm results. *J Am Coll Cardiol* 1997;29:442–447.

Gerosa G, McKay R, Davies J, Ross DN. Comparison of the aortic homograft and the pulmonary autograft for aortic valve or root replacement in children. *J Thorac Cardiovasc Surg* 1991;102:51–61.

Gersony WM, Hayes CJ, Driscoll DJ, et al. Second natural history of congenital heart defects study (NHS-2): bacterial endocarditis in patients with aortic stenosis, pulmonary stenosis, or ventricular septal defect. *Circulation* 1993;87(Suppl I):I-121–I-126.

Graham TP Jr, Bricker JT, James FW, Strong WB. 26th Bethesda Conference: recommendations for determining eligibility for competition in athletes with cardiovascular abnormalities, Task Force 1: congenital heart disease. *J Am Coll Cardiol* 1994;24:867–873.

Moore P, Egito E, Mowrey H, Perry SB, Lock JE, Keane JF. Midterm results of balloon dilation of congenital aortic stenosis: predictors of success. *J Am Coll Cardiol* 1996;27:1257–1263.

Author: Alexa N. Hogarty

Aplastic Anemia

 Database

DEFINITION

Aplastic anemia is a disorder in which the bone marrow fails to produce red blood cells, white blood cells, and platelets. The disorder exists in both acquired or constitutional forms in childhood.

CAUSES

Acquired

- Unknown/idiopathic (50%–75%)
- Hepatitis (and untypable), EBV, CMV, Parvovirus B19, HIV
- Drugs, e.g., chloramphenicol, oxyphenylbutazone, quinacrine, cimetidine, carbamazepine
- Toxins, e.g., heavy metals, aromatic hydrocarbons (benzenes)
- Radiation
- Autoimmune diseases

Constitutional

- Fanconi anemia
- Dyskeratosis congenita
- Paroxysmal nocturnal hemoglobinuria

PATHOPHYSIOLOGY

- Hematopoietic stem cell has an intrinsic proliferative defect
- Autoimmune reaction against the stem cell
- Abnormal stromal cells of the bone marrow microenvironment
- Genetic predisposition

GENETICS

- Most cases are sporadic
- Several rare disorders are associated with aplastic anemia; of these, Fanconi anemia is a congenital disorder in which most patients are predisposed to develop aplastic anemia within the first decade and is generally associated with multiple congenital anomalies; inheritance is autosomal recessive with variable penetrance and genetic heterogeneity

EPIDEMIOLOGY

- Incidence in United States and Europe is 3.5 to 5.4 cases per million per year
- Two major age peaks: 15 to 25 years and above 60 years
- Males and females affected equally
- Increased incidence in Asia presumably related to environmental factors

COMPLICATIONS

- Infection: especially fungal (*Aspergillus*) or gram negative bacteria
- Hemorrhage: intracranial, especially if refractory to platelet transfusions
- Hemosiderosis secondary to long-term red blood cell transfusions, with subsequent organ dysfunction if untreated

PROGNOSIS

- In patients with severe aplastic anemia, 90% fatal within first year if untreated
- Bone marrow transplant (HLA identical matched sibling) group

—70% overall survival
—80% to 90% survival for the young, uninfected, and minimally transfused group of patients

- Medical immunosuppressive therapy

—75% survival

- Factors associated with poor outcome:

—Bleeding at presentation
—Acute onset with severe pancytopenia
—Pancytopenia greater than 1 month
—Male sex
—MCV not elevated

 Differential Diagnosis

- Acute leukemia
- Myelodysplastic syndrome
- Paroxysmal nocturnal hemoglobinuria
- Folate or B$_{12}$ deficiency
- Acute drug reaction with bone marrow suppression
- Acute infection (viral) with bone marrow suppression, e.g., HIV-1, CMV, Parvovirus B19, Epstein-Barr virus
- Marrow infiltration by malignant tumors, e.g., non-Hogkin lymphoma, neuroblastoma
- Hemophagocytic lymphohistiocytosis (also known as Familial Erythrophagocytic Lymphohistiocytosis)

 Data Gathering

HISTORY

Evidence of Bone Marrow Failure

Question: Lethargy
Significance: Symptom of anemia

Question: Pallor
Significance: Sign of anemia

Question: Bruising
Significance: Due to thrombocytopenia

Question: Bloody stools
Significance: Thrombocytopenia, mucosal ulceration

Question: Nosebleeds
Significance: Thrombocytopenia

Question: Gum bleed
Significance: Thrombocytopenia

Question: Fevers
Significance: Infection associated with neutropenia

Evidence of Cause

- Drug or toxin exposure (although usually not identified)
- History of hepatitis or jaundice

 Physical Examination

Finding: Skin bruising, petechiae, pallor, jaundice
Significance: Thrombocytopenia

Finding: Fundal exam
Significance: Detects retinal hemorrhages

Finding: Sinus tenderness
Significance: Infection

Finding: Gum bleeds, thrush, petechiae, oral ulcerations
Significance: Neutropenia, candida colonization

Finding: Adenopathy
Significance: Suggests leukemia, cancer

Finding: Liver/spleen enlarged
Significance: Suggests leukemia, cancer

Finding: Perianal ulcerations infection
Significance: Infection and/or neutropenia

Finding: Skeletal anomalies (as seen in Fanconi anemia)
Significance: Seen in Fanconi anemia

Laboratory Aids

TO CONFIRM THE DIAGNOSIS

Test: CBC with differential and reticulocyte count
Significance:

- Severe (2 of the following):

—Granulocyte count <500 cells per fL
—Platelet count <20,000 per fL
—Reticulocyte count (corrected for hematocrit) <1%

- Mild or moderate (hypoplastic anemia)

—Mild or moderate cytopenia

Test: Bone marrow aspirate and biopsy
Significance:

- Severe aplastic anemia:

—Hypocellular

- Mild or moderate aplastic anemia: normal or increased cellularity may be seen

Test: MRI of lumbar/thoracic spine (investigational)
Significance: T_1-weighted images reveal marrow cellularity based on fat content

TO EXCLUDE OTHER CAUSES

Test: Bone marrow aspirate and chromosomes for karyotype
Significance: Myelodysplastic syndrome/acute leukemia

Test: Peripheral blood lymphocytes to assess chromosomal breakage
Significance: Fanconi anemia

Test: Ham test
Significance: Paroxysmal nocturnal hemoglobinuria

Test: Folate and B_{12} levels
Significance: Macrocytic anemia with neutropenia

Test: Chemistry panel with liver function tests, hepatitis serology
Significance: Hepatitis associated with aplastic anemia

 ## Therapy

- Bone marrow transplantation

—Therapy of choice for severe aplastic anemia
—For patients with HLA identical sibling (15%–20% of U.S. population)

- Immunosuppressive therapy

—Anti-thymocyte globulin and cyclosporine

- Androgens

—Used for the treatment of aplastic anemia associated with Fanconi anemia

- Supportive therapy

—Growth factors (G-CSF, GM-CSF, erythropoietin, IL-3, IL-11, stem cell factor, thrombopoietin)
—Transfusion support: no first degree relatives (could interfere with bone marrow transplantation), CMV negative, irradiated, leukodepleted, try to have a limited donor pool and minimize the number of transfusions
—Infectious disease support: pan culture and institute broad spectrum antibiotics if febrile and neutropenic, antifungal oral prophylaxis, handwashing, cooked food, nail care, avoid construction sites (often a source of fungus)

Follow-Up

Time to Recovery

Most responders to medical therapy will recover within 70 to 100 days, although some may be dependent on cyclosporine.

Signs of Recovery

The signs of recovery include increased mean corpuscular volume (MCV), reticulocyte count, neutrophil and monocyte count, then increased platelet count or reduced need for transfusions. Partial recovery is possible.

PITFALLS

Relapse

- Rate 10%; most are still salvageable
- Salvage therapy: unrelated donor bone marrow transplant (prognosis 30%–40%)

Other

- 5%–10% risk of myelodysplastic syndrome or paroxysmal nocturnal hemoglobinuria

 ## Common Questions and Answers

Q: Can family members donate blood for a child with aplastic anemia?
A: This is not recommended as transfusion with blood products from parents or siblings increases the risk of nonengraftment of bone marrow in the setting of bone marrow transplantation.

Q: What activities should a child with aplastic anemia avoid?
A: Patients with low red blood cell counts should avoid excessive exercise or going to high altitudes. Patients with low white blood cell counts are more susceptible to infection with bacteria but not with viruses. Patients should avoid dental work as this may introduce bacteria into the blood stream through the mouth. Patients with low platelet counts should avoid contact sports, including football, hockey, skiing, roller blading, etc.

Q: How does one learn more about experimental therapies for the treatment of aplastic anemia?
A: Inquiries to the National Institute of Health in Bethesda, Maryland, or to the Hematology division of the nearest medical school or NIH designated cancer center should result in information about the availability of experimental therapies.

ICD-9-CM 284.9

BIBLIOGRAPHY

Guinan EC. Clinical aspects of aplastic anemia. *Hematol Oncol Clin North Am* 1997;11(6):1025–1044.

Young NS, Alter BP. *Aplastic anemia, acquired and inherited,* 1st ed. Philadelphia: WB Saunders, 1994.

Young NS, Maciejewski J. The pathophysiology of acquired aplastic anemia. *N Engl J Med* 1997;336(19):1365–1372.

Author: Kara M. Kelly

Apnea

Database

DEFINITION

Breathing disorder characterized by cessation of airflow lasting more than 20 seconds

Central Apnea

• Lack of airflow secondary to cessation of breathing
• Absence of drive to breath from the central nervous system

Obstructive Apnea

• Lack of airflow secondary to airway obstruction
• Paradoxical chest-wall motion frequently seen
• Respiratory drive present

Mixed Apnea

• Central and obstructive events occurring together

PATHOPHYSIOLOGY AND CAUSES

Central Apnea

• *Physiological*

—Prematurity or immature respiratory control center

• *Infection*

—Meningitis
—Viral meningoencephalitis
—Respiratory syncytial virus (RSV)
—Pertussis

• *Gastrointestinal*

—Reflux
—Aspiration

• *Neurological*

—Asphyxia
—Laryngeal chemoreflex
—Seizure
—CNS malformations
—Cerebral or intraventricular hemorrhage
—Masses and congenital central hypoventilation

• *Pharmacological*

—Accidental drug ingestion
—Ethanol
—Sedatives
—Narcotics
—Toxins

• *Metabolical*

—Hypoglycemia
—Hypoxia
—Hypocarbia
—Overheating

• *Anemia*

—*Genetic/Familial Disorders*
  —Werdnig-Hoffmann
  —Familial dysautonomia

—*Behavioral*
  —Breath-holding spells
  —Excitement
  —Agitation
—*Epidemiology*
  —Over 50% of premature infants will develop apnea.
  —Premature infants usually outgrow their apnea when they reach term age.
  —Some infants may exhibit apnea of over 20 seconds in duration without apparent adverse effects.
  —Pathological apnea in full-term infants not caused by gastroesophageal reflux (GER) is rare.
—*Complications*
  —Apparent life-threatening events (ALTE) refer to apneic events that to the child's caretaker appear life-threatening [incorrectly referred to as "near-miss" SIDS (sudden infant death syndrome) or "aborted SIDS" events]

PROGNOSIS

• In general, good. Most infants outgrow apnea of prematurity/immaturity at term or within 1 to 2 months of age.
• Obstructive apnea is often cured with surgery (tonsil and adenoidectomy; uvulopharyngopalatoplasty)
• Resolution of apena otherwise dependent on its cause (i.e., GER, infection, etc.) and available treatment.
• Less than 10% of infants who die of SIDS had an ALTE prior to their death (SIDS by definition gives no warning).

Differential Diagnosis

• Periodic breathing: respiratory pattern in which three or more central apneas lasting 3 seconds in duration occur in a regularly repeating pattern within a 20-second period.
• Primary snoring: snoring without associated apnea, hypoxemia, or hypoventilation.
• Central hypoventilation syndrome: decrease in central ventilatory drive leading to abnormal increase in carbon dioxide tension
• Obesity hypoventilation syndrome (Pickwickian syndrome): etiology is multifactorial; morbidly obese subjects who exhibit restrictive pulmonary disease, decreased central respiratory drive, with airway obstruction.
• Breath-holding spells

Data Gathering

HISTORY

Many times, the patient will have been in excellent health prior to the apneic event; the history is most useful in describing the event.

Questions for Assessment of the Apneic Event

• Was the baby moving his or her chest with or without evidence of airflow?
• Was the motion paradoxical?
• Was the patient awake or asleep when the event occurred?
• Was there a color change (pale, cyanotic, red)?
• Was there a change in the patient's muscle tone (floppy versus stiff)?
• Was the episode related to feeding or preceded by coughing, choking, gagging, vomiting, or crying?
• Was there a change in the patient's mental status during or after the event?
• Was there any urinary or stool incontinence during the event?

Questions for Assessment of Health Prior to the Apneic Event

• Evidence of infection (i.e., fever, rhinorrhea, nasal congestion, cough, diarrhea)?
• Gestational age (full-term or premature)
• Prior history of seizures or GER?
• Presence of snoring (snoring is never normal in a child)?
• Does the patient have headaches or daytime somnolence?
• Has there been a change in the patient's school performance?

Physical Examination

Most often normal in newborns and infants

GENERAL EXAMINATION

• Craniofacial abnormalities

—Micrognathia
—Macroglossia
—Choanal atresia/stenosis

• Evidence of nasal obstruction

—Congestion
—Rhinorrhea
—Foreign body

• Enlarged tonsils and adenoid tissue in toddlers/older children

CARDIOVASCULAR EXAMINATION

• Heart rate
• Murmur
• Cyanosis

PULMONARY EXAMINATION

• Respiratory rate
• Chest mounts
• Quality of breath sounds

SPECIAL QUESTION

Finding: Was the child truly apneic?
Significance: Frequently, the parents see the child "not looking well" and assume the child is not breathing, rather than checking for respiratory effort.

Laboratory Aids

BLOOD TESTS

Test: CBC with differential
Significance:

- Anemia
- Polycythemia
- Infection

Test: Electrolytes
Significance: Bicarbonate, glucose

Test: Arterial blood gas
Significance: May be helpful in estimating significance of the event

Test: Polysomnography
Significance: Should be performed in any child with suspected obstructive or central sleep apnea

VARIABLES TO BE MONITORED

- O_2 saturation
- End-tidal CO_2 tension
- Respiratory movements (abdomen, chest)
- Airflow
- pH probe (if GER suspected)
- Record for minimum of 6 hours

IMAGING

Test: Chest radiography
Significance: Usually normal. Look for evidence of infection or aspiration.

Test: Lateral neck radiography
Significance:

- Helpful in obstructive apnea
- Assess tonsillar and adenoid size
- Assess patency of nasopharyngeal airway

Test: CT or MRI of head
Significance: Indicated if CNS pathology suspected as cause of central apnea

REQUIREMENTS FOR TESTING

- NPO for 4 hours prior to pH probe study
- Make sure child does not take a nap prior to overnight study

 ## Therapy

DRUGS

Stimulants (Useful for Apnea of Prematurity)

- Caffeine

—Loading dose: 10 mg/kg
—Maintenance dose: 2.5 mg/kg/day
—Therapeutic level: 5 to 20 mg/L

- Theophylline

—Loading dose: 4 to 5 mg/kg
—Maintenance dose: 3 to 5 mg/kg/d divided t.i.d.
—Therapeutic level: 6 to 10 mg/L

- Supplemental O_2 is helpful for both obstructive and central apnea, especially if oxygen desaturation is occurring.

ANTI-REFLUX THERAPY

- Thickened feeds (1–3 teaspoons of rice cereal/oz of formula)
- Positioning (prone position for sleeping)
- Reglan (dose: 0.1 mg/kg/d given q.i.d.)
- Cisapride (dose: 0.3 mg/kg/d given q.i.d.)

MECHANICAL VENTILATION

- Continuous positive airway pressure (CPAP) to stint open the airways in obese patients with obstructive apnea.
- Bilevel positive airway pressure (BiPAP) as mode of non-invasive ventilation is occasionally needed.

CENTRAL HYPOVENTILATION SYNDROME

May require tracheostomy and mechanical ventilation

SURGERY

If enlarged tonsillar and/or adenoid tissue is cause of obstructive apnea, tonsillectomy and/or adenoidectomy may be curative.

HOME APNEA MONITORS

- Use is controversial.
- Monitoring technology now allows for the storing of information on a microchip, which can be downloaded for the physician to review.
- Indications

—Any infant perceived to be at high risk for SIDS: severe ALTE (Note: no study has demonstrated efficiency of home monitoring therapy in preventing SIDS.)
—One or more siblings who died of SIDS
—Symptomatic premature infants
—Central hypoventilation syndrome
—Infants and young children who have tracheostomies

WHEN TO DISCONTINUE MONITORING (HIGHLY CONTROVERSIAL)

Duration of Therapy

- Dependent on underlying cause of apnea
- Possible conflicts with other treatments
- GER may be exacerbated in patients requiring therapy with theophylline

 ## Follow-Up

WHEN TO EXPECT IMPROVEMENT

- Dependent on underlying cause of apnea
- Premature infants usually outgrow apnea of prematurity by term to 4 weeks postgestational age.
- In obstructive apnea due to enlarged tonsils/adenoids, symptoms improve soon after surgery.

PROGNOSIS

- In premature infants: excellent
- In children with enlarged tonsils/adenoids: excellent
- In obese patients: variable, due to difficulty in obtaining and maintaining weight loss

PITFALLS

- Many false alarms with home monitors (stick-on electrodes have fewer false-positive alarms than electrodes attached to wraparound belts).
- Two-channel pneumography (heart rate and respirations) used to assess apnea in young infants can miss oxygen desaturation and obstructive apnea.

 ## Common Questions and Answers

Q: When can monitoring be discontinued?
A: This is dependent on the underlying reason for monitoring. When the infant is no longer thought to be at increased risk of cardiorespiratory arrest or sudden death or when the infant has tolerated at least one respiratory infection without significant events, monitoring may be discontinued. Unfortunately, medicolegal issues also affect the decision to discontinue monitoring.

Q: Does monitoring prevent SIDS?
A: Monitoring can prevent death from other causes, but it has not been shown to decrease the incidence of SIDS.

ICD-9-CM 770.8
Newborn 786.09 CS

BIBLIOGRAPHY

Freed GE, Steinschneider A, Glassman M, et al. Sudden infant death syndrome prevention and an understanding of selected clinical issues. *Pediatr Clin North Am* 1994;41:967–990.

Keens TG, Davidson Ward SL. Apnea spells, sudden death, and the role of the apnea monitor. *Pediatr Clin North Am* 1993;40:897–911.

National Institute of Health Consensus Development Conference on Infantile Apnea and Home Monitoring. *Pediatrics* 1986;79:292–299.

Author: Hakon Hakonarson

Appendicitis

 Database

DEFINITION

Acute inflammation of the appendix.

CAUSES

• Obstruction of appendiceal lumen by fecalith, calculi, or hyperplastic lymphoid tissue
• Torsion of appendix, leading to ischemic necrosis

PATHOLOGY

• Acute obstruction raises intraluminal pressure, leading to ischemia.
• Bacteria invade the appendiceal wall at sites of ulceration producing inflammation.
• Necrosis of the wall results in perforation with fecal contamination of the peritoneum.

EPIDEMIOLOGY

• Usually occurs in children over 2 years
• Peak incidence in teens and young adults

GENETICS

• Familial tendency toward appendicitis

COMPLICATIONS

• Perforation occurs in up to three-fourths of patients under age 4 and in two-thirds of patients between the ages of 5 and 8.

 Differential Diagnosis

INFECTION

• Gastroenteritis (e.g., *Yersinia, Campylobacter*)
• Constipation
• Right lower lobe pneumonia
• Mesenteric adenitis
• Typhlitis
• Urinary tract infection
• Pelvic inflammatory disease, tubo-ovarian abscess, or ectopic pregnancy

INFLAMAMATORY

• Inflammatory bowel disease exacerbation
• Anaphylactic purpura
• Hemolytic uremic anemia

GENETIC/METABOLICAL

• Diabetes
• Sickle and Sickle C disease
• Renal stone
• Hypernatremia

MISCELLANEOUS

• Functional abdominal pain
• Fecalith
• Tortion of testes
• Tortion of ovary
• Ovarian cyst
• Endometriosis

 Data Gathering

HISTORY

Question: Is there vomiting?
Significance: Many surgeons feel that vomiting is the cardinal symptom associated with appendicitis.

Question: Is there fever?
Significance: Low-grade fever is common in appendicitis; higher fever can be an abscess or other infectious disease.

Question: Does the pain move?
Significance: Typically, there is poorly localized, crampy midabdominal pain that migrates to right lower quadrant (RLQ).

Question: Ask about other classic features?

• Nausea, anorexia
• Patient prefers to lie still
• Rarely secretory diarrhea
• Change in bowel habits, especially diarrhea

Significance: Appendicitis may be presenting with unusual features.

Physical Examination

Finding: Focal peritoneal signs
Significance: Peritoneal irritation

Finding: Pain at McBurney point
Significance: Peritoneal irritation

Finding: Hypoactive bowel sounds
Significance: Decreased motility secondary to inflammation

Finding: Focal tenderness on rectal examination
Significance: Appendicitus or abscess

Finding: Following perforation, abdomen becomes rigid and tender with absent bowel sounds; patients often febrile, tachypneic, and tachycardic
Significance: Peritonitis

SPECIAL QUESTIONS

Finding: Was car ride painful, e.g., going over bumps?
Significance: Another way to elicit peritoneal irritation

PHYSICAL EXAMINATION TRICKS

- Palpation with stethoscope
- Jiggling bed should produce RLQ pain
- Pain may be elicited by asking patient to cough or to hop on right foot.

 ## Laboratory Aids

TESTS

Test: CBC
Significance: Elevated WBC count with left shift

IMAGING

Test: Abdominal x-ray
Significance:

- often normal
- 8% to 10% show calcified fecalith
- Cecal-wall thickening
- Air-fluid levels
- Indistinct psoas margins

Test: Barium enema
Significance: May show evidence of RLQ mass or partial or complete non-filling of appendix.

Test: Ultrasound
Significance: Edema, inflammation, and/or abscess formation

 ## Therapy

- IV fluids to correct hypovolemia, electrolyte abnormalities
- Emergency appendectomy
- Broad-spectrum antibiotics should be used if perforation is suspected.
- Nasogastric tube and pain medications may provide comfort preoperatively.
- Abscess may require external drainage.

 ## Follow-Up

- Recovery rapid
- Prognosis excellent without perforation, very good with perforation (mortality, 1%)

PITFALLS

- Position of appendix may vary, i.e., location of pain may vary.
- Retroiliac appendix—poorly localized pain
- Retrocecal appendix—RUQ pain
- Appendix in gutter—flank pain
- Pelvic appendix—pain on rectal examination, or diarrhea caused by direct irritation of sigmoid colon
- Appendicitis progresses rapidly in children; perforation often occurs due to delayed diagnosis
- Pain may resolve briefly following perforation

 ## Common Questions and Answers

Q: Why is perforation more commonly observed in children with appendicitis?
A: There is a more rapid progression of symptoms that may not follow the classic pattern of RLQ pain. Young children may not be capable of describing their pain. The mesentery in children is thin walled and less effective at walling off an infection.

Q: Is appendicitis genetically inherited?
A: Appendicitis does show a tendency to occur in families.

ICD-9-CM 540.9

BIBLIOGRAPHY

Brender JD, Marcuse EK, Koepsell T, Hatch EI. Childhood appendicitis: factors associated with perforation. *Pediatrics* 1985;76:301–306.

Ravitch MM. Appendicitis. *Pediatrics* 1982;70:414–419.

Schnaufer L, Mahboubi S. Abdominal emergencies. In: Ludwig S, Fleisler G, eds. *Pediatric emergency medicine*, 3rd ed. Philadelphia: Williams & Wilkins 1993:1309–1313.

Shandling B, Fallis J. Acute appendicitis. In: Behrman RE, ed. *Nelson textbook of pediatrics*, 4th ed. Philadelphia: WB Saunders, 1992:987–990.

Author: Andrew E. Mulberg

Arthritis—Juvenile Rheumatoid

 Database

DEFINITION

- Juvenile rheumatoid arthritis (JRA) is chronic synovial inflammation of unknown etiology in at least one joint, for at least 6 weeks. Age of onset must be less than 16 years old. It can be subdivided into three major types.
- Pauciarticular JRA is JRA affecting less than 5 joints.

—Type I usually affects young girls who are antinuclear antibody (ANA)-positive and usually begins in girls less than 6 years old.
—Type II (spondyloarthropathies) generally affects boys, many of whom are HLA-B27-positive, in late childhood or adolescence.

- Polyarticular JRA affects 5 or more joints and can occur at any age.
- Systemic-onset JRA is characterized by high, spiking quotidian or diquotidian fevers and an evanescent pink/salmon-colored macular rash. These children may also have lymphadenopathy, hepatosplenomegaly, pericarditis, or pleuritis. The arthritis may not appear until weeks to months after the onset of the systemic symptoms. Systemic-onset JRA can occur at any age.

CAUSES

The etiology of JRA is unknown, but genetic predisposition, autoimmunity, infection, and trauma may all play a role.

PATHOLOGY

- Chronic synovial inflammation

EPIDEMIOLOGY

- JRA affects approximately 70,000 children in the United States.
- Affects girls twice as often as it affects boys, but pauciarticular type II usually affects boys (male:female ratio, 10:1).
- Approximately 50% of children with JRA have the pauciarticular type.
- 40% have the polyarticular type.
- 10% have systemic-onset JRA.

GENETICS

Some studies have indicated that various HLA markers may be associated with different subtypes of JRA. For example, HLA-DR4 seems to be associated with rheumatoid factor-positive (RF1) polyarticular JRA, HLA-DR1 is associated with pauciarticular disease without uveitis, and HLA-DR5 is associated with pauciarticular JRA with uveitis.

COMPLICATIONS

- Joint degeneration with loss of articular cartilage
- Soft-tissue contractures
- Leg-length discrepancies
- Micrognathia
- Cervical spine dislocations
- Rheumatoid nodules
- Growth retardation

Pauciarticular JRA, especially with a positive ANA, is also associated with a chronic uveitis, which can lead to loss of vision if not detected early with routine slit-lamp eye examinations. Pericarditis and pleuritis, as well as severe anemia, may develop in patients with systemic-onset JRA.

 Differential Diagnosis

- Monoarticular JRA

—Septic joint
—Trauma
—Hemarthrosis
—Villonodular synovitis

- Monoarticular or pauciarticular JRA

—Lyme disease
—Acute rheumatic fever
—Malignancies
—Sarcoidosis
—Inflammatory bowel disease

- Polyarticular JRA

—Viral or post-viral illness (especially parvovirus)
—Lyme disease
—Lupus

- Systemic-onset JRA

—Infection
—Oncological process (leukemia)
—Inflammatory bowel disease
—Lupus

 Data Gathering

HISTORY

- Morning stiffness that improves after a hot shower/bath or with stretching and mild exercise is common in JRA.
- The joints often become sore/painful again in the late afternoon or evening.
- Patients with JRA generally do not complain of severe pain, but rather they avoid using certain joints that are particularly affected. If a child has severe pain in a joint, especially pain that seems out of proportion to the physical findings, diagnoses other than JRA should be entertained.
- In systemic JRA the fever curve is important to document. Between fever spikes the child is completely afebrile. The rash is evanescent and the patients often have a history of fatigue, malaise, and weight loss.

 Physical Examination

- Arthritis must be present in at least one joint. There may be restricted range of motion in the affected joints and soft-tissue contractures as well.

—Enthesitis and sacroiliac tenderness are often seen in spondyloarthropathies.

- In systemic JRA the rash, if present, is almost pathognomonic for this disease.
- Lymphadenopathy and hepatosplenomegaly may be seen.
- A careful cardiac and pulmonary examination must be done to look for pericarditis and pleuritis.

Laboratory Aids

- No laboratory finding is diagnostic for JRA.
- Many patients with JRA, especially the polyarticular and systemic types, have elevated sedimentation rates and anemia.
- Patients with systemic JRA often have a leukocytosis, predominantly neutrophils, and thrombocytosis as well.
- ANA is a useful test in classifying patients with JRA.

—Positive in 80% of pauciarticular type I
—40% to 60% polyarticular
—10% normal population

- RF will be positive in 15% to 20% of patients with polyarticular arthritis. RF1 patients tend to behave like adult patients with rheumatoid arthritis with more aggressive and persistent arthritis and a worse prognosis.

IMAGING

- Radiography is often normal early in JRA.
- Later, if arthritis persists, loss of articular cartilage, joint fusion, and bone demineralization may be seen, as well as bone cysts and erosions.

Therapy

DRUGS

- Non-steroidal anti-inflammatory drugs (NSAIDs)

—First-line therapy for JRA
—If there is no response to the initial NSAID after 4 to 6 weeks of an adequate dose, a different one should be tried. Patients will often respond differently to the various nonsteroidal drugs.

- If NSAIDs are ineffective in controlling the disease, a second-line agent should be added, such as hydroxychloroquine, sulfasalazine, or methotrexate.
- Methotrexate: If the arthritis is severe, methotrexate is often started. Laboratory values must be monitored closely in these patients, looking for bone marrow suppression or elevation of transaminase levels.
- Glucocorticoids: In systemic JRA with high fevers, glucocorticoids are often necessary, either as oral (daily or every other day) doses or as intravenous pulses, every 2 to 8 weeks. Steroids are also used for patients with polyarticular JRA whose arthritis is unresponsive to other medications. Because of the many side effects of systemic steroids, patients should be weaned off steroids as soon as possible.

PHYSICAL AND OCCUPATIONAL THERAPY

Physical and occupational therapy are important in the management of JRA. The goal is to maintain range of motion, muscle strength, and function.

DIET

Patients with systemic or polyarticular JRA, especially those on steroids, should maintain adequate calcium intake to minimize osteoporosis. Patients on methotrexate should take folate supplements daily, except on the days that the methotrexate is given.

WHEN TO EXPECT IMPROVEMENT

- Responses to treatments for JRA vary tremendously.

—Some patients may respond to NSAIDs within a week or two.
—Others take 4 to 6 weeks to improve, or they may not respond at all.
—Steroids usually start to relieve symptoms within a few days.
—Hydroxychloroquine, can take 8 to 12 weeks until the maximum benefit is seen.

- The waxing and waning nature of JRA itself adds to the variability of patient responses to treatments.

PROGNOSIS

- Varies considerably
- Children with pauciarticular JRA usually do very well and often go into remission within a year or two of starting treatment. They may have flareups, however, even up to 10 years after being symptom-free and off all medications.
- Patients with polyarticular JRA who are RF1 often develop a severe arthritis that may persist into adulthood.
- RF2 polyarticular patients generally do better.
- 50% of patients with systemic-onset JRA will develop chronic polyarticular disease.

PITFALLS

Overdiagnosis: arthritis must be present for at least 6 weeks before a patient can be diagnosed with JRA. Many viral illnesses can give joint pain and swelling that mimics JRA, but resolves within 4 to 6 weeks.

Common Questions and Answers

Q: Will the patient outgrow JRA?
A: In some studies, up to 50% of patients with JRA still had active disease 10 years after diagnosis. Only 15%, however, had any loss of function.

Q: Will siblings of patients with JRA develop the disease?
A: Rarely, but it can occur.

ICD-9-CM 714.30

BIBLIOGRAPHY

Aaron S, Fraser PA, Jackson JM, et al. Sex ratio and sibship size in juvenile rheumatoid arthritis kindreds. *Arthritis Rheum* 1985;28:753.

Singsen BH. Epidemiology of rheumatic diseases of childhood. *Rheum Dis Clin North Am* 1990;16:581–599.

Towner SR, Michet CJ JR, O'Fallon WM, et al. The epidemiology of juvenile rheumatoid arthritis in Rochester, Minnesota. *Arthritis Rheum* 1983;26:1208.

Wallace CA, Levinson JE. Juvenile rheumatoid arthritis: outcome and treatment for the 1990s. *Pediatr Rheum* 1991;17:891–905.

Author: Elizabeth Candell Chalom

Ascaris Lumbricoides

 Database

DEFINITION

Ascaris lumbricoides is a large roundworm, 15 to 40 cm in length, which infects humans via eggs found in soil. Animals are not affected. Approximately one-fourth of the world's population is infested with this worm.

PATHOPHYSIOLOGY

• The lifecycle begins when eggs are ingested from soil contaminated with human feces.
• Subsequently, the larvae are liberated in the small intestine.
• The rhabdoid larvae invade the venous system and travel to the portal circulation, inferior vena cava, and finally, pulmonary capillaries.
• They penetrate the alveoli, and are subsequently expelled by coughing across the epiglottis and swallowed. During the migration of the parasite through the pulmonary vessels, an eosinophilic response is evoked.
• The larvae become adult worms in the small intestine.
• The cycle takes 2 months.
• In the intestinal stage, mechanical obstruction from the mass of worms in the gut may be observed in children.

EPIDEMIOLOGY

• One female worm produces 200,000 eggs per day.
• Fertilized eggs must incubate in the soil for 2 to 3 weeks.
• The eggs are viable for up to 6 years in temperate climates; they survive freezing but not direct sunlight.
• All ages may be affected; however, children are more frequent hosts due to oral behavior.
• Ascariasis is more common where sanitation is poor and population dense.

COMPLICATIONS

• Bronchopneumonia may be seen during the migrational stage, producing fever, cough, dyspnea, wheeze, eosinophilia, and pulmonary infiltrates.
• Heavy infestations may cause abdominal pain, malabsorption, and growth failure.
• Children may experience obstruction (ileocecal), malabsorption, or intussusception.
• Perforation of a viscus, or migration into the appendix, biliary, or pancreatic ducts may rarely occur.

PROGNOSIS

• Once intestinal infection is detected and treated, the prognosis is excellent. If obstructive or respiratory complications have occurred, the prognosis is less favorable.
• The case fatality rate in the United States is 3%.

 Differential Diagnosis

• Ascariasis should be considered in the differential diagnosis when a patient presents with pneumonia and peripheral eosinophilia.
• The diagnosis of Ascaris infection should be considered whenever intestinal obstruction is seen in an endemic area.
• This infection may be associated with other parasites acquired from contaminated soil.

 Data Gathering

HISTORY

Question: Do patients infected with ascaris always have symptoms?
Significance: The majority of patients with moderate infections are asymptomatic.

Question: Do patients actually see worms in their stool?
Significance: History or passage of large worms in the stool or vomitus is suggestive.

Question: What are pulmonary symptoms?
Significance: During the pulmonary stage, cough, dyspnea, fever, and pulmonary infiltrates in the presence of eosinophilia suggest the diagnosis.

Question: Are there symptoms of obstruction?
Significance: Rarely, the infection presents as intestinal obstruction, with an incidence of approximately 2 children per 1000 infected.

Laboratory Aids

Test: Microscopic examination of stool specimens
Significance:

• Will demonstrate the characteristic eggs.
• During the pulmonary phase, eosinophils and larvae may be seen.
• No serological tests are necessary, and are poorly specific to the diagnosis.

 ## Therapy

• A single dose of pyrantel pamoate (11 mg/kg; maximum, 1 g) is effective.
• Mebendazole (100 mg twice daily for 3 days) is effective, but not recommended for children under age 2.
• Piperazine citrate (75 mg/kg/d for 2 days; maximum, 3.5 g) is suggested in cases of obstruction due to large worm bezoars to aid passage. It should not be administered with pyrantel pamoate.

PREVENTION

Infection Control

• With appropriate disposal of human excrement and handwashing, this infection could be eliminated.
• In communities with high *Ascaris* carriage, biannual administration of pyrantel pamoate or mebendazole is effective.

 ## Follow-Up

Treatment as specified above is highly effective. Reinfection is problematic in endemic areas.

ICD-9-CM 127.0

Reference

Katz M. Nemahelminthes. In: Feigin RD, Cherry JD, eds. *Textbook of pediatric infectious diseases*. Philadelphia: WB Saunders, 1987:2087–2099.

Oski FA, ed. *Principles and practice of pediatrics*. Philadelphia: JB Lippincott, 1990:1288–1289.

Peter G, ed. *1997 red book: report of the committee on infectious disease, American Academy of Pediatrics*. Elk Grove Village, IL: American Academy of Pediatrics, 1997:142–143.

Plorde J. Intestinal nematodes. In: Braunwald E, et al., eds. *Harrison's principles of internal medicine*. New York: McGraw-Hill, 1987:817–818.

Author: Janet H. Friday

Ascites

Database

DEFINITION

Ascites is defined as effusion and accumulation of fluid in the abdominal cavity. Peritoneal fluid formation is a dynamic process of production and absorption. See table Analysis of Ascitic Fluid.

PATHOPHYSIOLOGY

The development of ascitic fluid may be sudden or insidious associated with nonhepatic etiologies or an acute reduction in hepatocellular function in a marginally compensated liver (cirrhosis secondary to severe metabolic disturbances, i.e., tyrosinemia). Accumulation of fluid occurs with:

- Inflammatory conditions, i.e., mesenteric adenitis, tuberculosis, pancreatitis secondary to inflammation of visceral and/or parietal peritoneum
- Obstruction of portal vein flow and/or lymphatic flow by mass, tumor, or obstruction; tumors of abdominal viscera, retroperitoneum, thorax, or mediastinum (often characterized by chylous ascites)
- Primary (congenital) abnormalities of the lymphatics (Milroy disease); congenital neonatal ascites secondary to GI tract trauma (ureteral rupture); hematologic (hydrops secondary to hemolysis from blood-type incompatibility); gastrointestinal or heart disease; and lysosomal storage diseases including sialidosis (neuraminidase deficiency), Salla disease, GM1 gangliosidosis, Gaucher disease, and Niemann-Pick type C
- Decreased plasma oncotic pressure secondary to hypoalbuminemia (increased losses: renal, gastrointestinal tract; decreased production: hepatic failure)
- Rupture of intraabdominal viscus or peritoneal/mesenteric cyst

COMPLICATIONS

- Spontaneous bacterial peritonitis is an infection of the peritoneal fluid of patients with ascites and may present with signs of peritoneal inflammation or more subtle findings. A high index of suspicion is necessary in order to make the diagnosis. Abdominal paracentesis is indicated, especially to establish the fluid's white blood cell count and to obtain cultures. The blood culture bottle should be injected with peritoneal fluid at the bedside in order to increase the culture's yield. Mortality is high.

—Treatment includes antibiotics, and paracentesis should be performed 48 hours after the introduction of treatment.
—An indication for therapeutic response will be a decrease in the neutrophil count in the ascitic fluid by 50% from that detected on presentation. It is appropriate to treat according to sensitivities when cultures are available. The length of therapy depends on clinical response but should be a minimum of 10 days.

- Respiratory distress from decreased lung volume and diaphragmatic limitation

PROGNOSIS

Depends on the etiology. If from nephrotic syndrome, will regress as proteinuria clears. If from liver failure, will depend on recovery of liver function.

Differential Diagnosis

- Enlarged liver or spleen
- Mesenteric cyst: does not have shifting dullness when position is changed
- Intestinal obstruction

Data Gathering

HISTORY

- The etiology for acute decompensation in hepatocellular function, i.e., massive bleeding, sepsis, superimposed infections, should be investigated.
- Use of umbilical catheters in newborn period
- Respiratory distress
- Exposure to hepatotoxins

Physical Examination

- Vital signs
- Abdominal cavity circumference
- Weight
- Auscultation of the pericardium
- Neurologic examination to evaluate for encephalopathy
- Skin changes suggestive of chronic liver disease
- Special attention should be directed toward identification of a distended abdomen, fullness in the flanks, inverted umbilicus, and development of hernias, scrotal edema, rectal prolapse, and a prominent anterior wall.
- Techniques to detect free intraabdominal fluid include presence of a fluid wave, shifting dullness, and puddle sign (percuss abdomen with patient flexed at hip to detect dullness that may accurately detect fluid over 1 L).
- Other physical examination signs include splenomegaly and prominent abdominal veins (portal hypertension), cor pulmonale (congestive heart failure), pericardial friction rub (pericarditis), diffuse abdominal pain (peritonitis or visceral perforation), abdominal pain radiating to the back (pancreatitis), and lymphedema (lymphatic obstruction/trauma to the thoracic duct).

Analysis of Ascitic Fluid

	COLOR	TRIGLYCERIDES	TOTAL FAT	WHITE-BLOOD-CELL COUNT
Cirrhotic	Straw	<250 mg/dL		WBC/mL (more than 75 leukocytes [PMNs] suggests inflammation)
Chylous	Yellow-white Creamy	400 mg/dL	Two times that of plasma	
Traumatic	Blood, bile, air, or intestinal contents			

Laboratory Aids

TESTS

Laboratory Tests

- Complete white blood cell count
- Electrolytes
- Liver-function tests: transaminases, PT/PTT
- Amylase and lipase (to exclude pancreatitis)
- Creatinine and blood urea nitrogen
- Blood cultures
- Urine for specific gravity
- Viral serologies, including hepatitis B virus, coxsackievirus, enteroviruses

Imaging

- Abdominal radiography
- Ultrasound of the abdomen to differentiate between free and loculated fluid collection and the presence of intraabdominal masses
- Abdominal computed axial tomography

Abdominal Paracentesis

Abdominal paracentesis is a safe procedure in the evaluation of etiologies of ascites. The two complications are perforation of the bowel and hemorrhage. With sterile conditions, a narrow-bore angiocatheter, usually 23-gauge, is inserted through the linea alba 2 cm below the umbilicus, using the Z-technique. Paracentesis is done for routine studies, including white blood cell count, culture, LDH, total protein, albumin, glucose, Gram stain, amylase, cholesterol with triglycerides, and cytology. These tests will require approximately 10 to 20 mL of fluid. Interpretation of these data are reflected in the table below.

- When glucose in the ascitic fluid is below 30 mg/dL, tuberculous peritonitis must be excluded.
- When ascitic amylase is greater than the normal serum amylase, pancreatitis is suggested.

 ## Therapy

The management of the ascites should be directed toward the underlying etiology. In a patient with cirrhosis, accumulation of ascites should be avoided by preventing complications such as esophageal hemorrhage, spontaneous bacterial peritonitis, hepatorenal syndrome, inferior vena cava obstruction, and renal and cardiac circulatory disturbances.

- Sodium intake should be restricted to 1 to 2 mEq/kg/d (low-salt diet).
- Water should be restricted to 75% of maintenance requirements.
- Diuretics may be used to promote negative sodium and water balance. When diuretics are used, urine output and serum electrolytes should be monitored to prevent prerenal azotemia and decrease effective blood flow to the kidneys.
- Therapeutic abdominal paracentesis should be used only in resistant cases, because ascitic fluid tends to reaccumulate. Paracentesis of volumes greater than 1 L should be accompanied by the IV infusion of salt-poor albumin during the procedure.
- LeVeen shunt (peritoneal venous shunting) is rarely used as a therapeutic option because of the high frequency of infection, obstruction, and other complications.
- Portosystemic shunting may be valuable in cases where portal hypertension is felt to be the underlying etiology of ascitic accumulation.

 ## Follow-Up

Weight and effects of diuretics should be assessed closely with attention to preservation of renal function. Urine and serum electrolytes should be monitored. Abdominal girth should be measured frequently. In cases of infection or peritonitis, a repeat paracentesis should be performed approximately 48 hours after the initiation of antibiotics for culture and white blood cell count.

PITFALLS

- With congenital ascites, evaluate for lysosomal storage diseases.
- When performing paracentesis, make certain that the fluid is ascitic and not intraluminal.
- Ultrasonography may be helpful to determine the location of this fluid.
- With new onset of ascites, make certain to evaluate for abdominal neoplasia.
- With marginally compensated liver disease, attempt to identify the source of the patient's acute decompensation.

 ## Common Questions and Answers

Q: What is the common thought regarding neonatal ascites?
A: Exclude lysosomal storage and/or other metabolic diseases.

Q: What is the best test to discriminate the type of ascites?
A: Analysis of the peritoneal fluid collected by abdominal paracentesis is required for this purpose. Differentiation of a serous effusion versus exudate is thus achieved.

ICD-9-CM 789.5

BIBLIOGRAPHY

Clark, JH, Fitzgerald JF, Kleinman MB. Spontaneous bacterial peritonitis. *J Pediatr* 1984;104(4):495–500.

Fitzgerald JF. Ascites. In: Wyllie R, Hyams J, eds. *Pediatric gastrointestinal diseases*. Philadelphia: WB Saunders, 1993:151–160.

Gillan JE, Lowden JA, Gaskin K, et al. Congenital ascites as a presenting sign of lysosomal storage disease. *J Pediatr* 1984;104:225–231.

Hoefs JC, Runyon BA. Spontaneous bacterial peritonitis. *Disease-A-Month* 1985;31(9):1–48.

Machin GA. Diseases causing fetal and neonatal ascites. *Pediatr Pathol* 1985;4(3–4):195–211.

Wasserman D. Ascites. In: Altshuler S, Liacouras C, eds. *Clinical pediatric gastroenterology*. Philadelphia: Churchill Livingstone, 1997:323–325.

Author: Dror Wasserman

Aspergillosis

 ## Database

DEFINITION

Aspergillosis is infection caused by *Aspergillus* species. The two most common etiologic agents are *Aspergillus fumigatus* and *Aspergillus flavus*.

PATHOPHYSIOLOGY

- Macrophage phagocytic response is the first and main line of defense against infection with *Aspergillus*.
- Relative lack of importance of cell-mediated immunity in host defense for this infection (therefore, not a common infection in patients with acquired immunodeficiency syndrome)
- The lung is the most common site of both noninvasive and invasive *Aspergillus* infection.

ASSOCIATED ILLNESSES

- *Allergic bronchopulmonary aspergillosis* is characterized by periodic episodes of wheezing, low-grade fever, eosinophilia on peripheral smear, transient infiltrates on chest x-ray film, and a cough productive of brown mucus plugs. It occurs when patients with chronic respiratory disease trap *Aspergillus* spores in mucus, which leads to an immune response and a worsening of respiratory symptoms.
- *Paranasal sinusitis* and *otomycosis* in healthy hosts in warm, wet climates
- *Aspergillomas* are noninvasive pulmonary fungus balls that grow in bronchogenic cysts or other lung cavities. They are the most frequent form of pulmonary aspergillosis.
- *Invasive aspergillosis* occurs in the immunocompromised host, most commonly in patients treated with long-term broad-spectrum antibiotics, cytoxic chemotherapy, or immunosuppressive therapy, or in patients with an underlying disease that causes neutrophil or macrophage dysfunction (i.e., acute leukemia or chronic granulomatous disease). In the immunocompromised host, invasion of blood vessels by *Aspergillus* leads to infarction, necrosis, and hematogenous dissemination.

EPIDEMIOLOGY

- *Aspergillus* species are ubiquitous and worldwide, growing in soil, grain, dung, bird droppings, and decaying plant matter.
- Spores are resistant to desiccation, lightweight, and easily dispersed in air currents.
- Main route of transmission is via inhalation of airborne spores; person-to-person spread does not occur.
- Other than those with otomycosis or allergic bronchopulmonary disease, most patients infected with *Aspergillus* are immunocompromised in some way (see above).
- Nosocomial outbreaks have occurred when ventilation or heating systems become contaminated, or when large numbers of spores become airborne during building construction or renovation.
- The incubation period in the human host has not been defined.

COMPLICATIONS

- Disseminated infection: defined as infection of two or more organs, and can involve any of the previously discussed sites, as well as the CNS, heart, bones, or skin. Invasiveness depends on the immune state of the host, as well as the period of time and number of spores in the exposure.
- Patients with underlying diseases that predispose them to pulmonary cavitations, blebs, or cysts (such as asthma, chronic bronchitis, TB, sarcoid, histoplasmosis, and bronchiectasis) may develop an aspergilloma (fungus ball) after seeding their pulmonary secretions with *Aspergillus*. When the mass is large enough to be demonstrated on chest x-ray study, serum levels of IgG antibody to *Aspergillus* will be characteristically high. Patients may present with hemoptysis, exacerbation of their underlying disease, or rarely, invasion or dissemination.

Prognosis

- Good in noninvasive disease, such as simple otomycosis or paranasal sinusitis
- Immunosuppressed or severely neutropenic patients can have rapid extension or dissemination of disease; prognosis is often very poor. Early recognition and aggressive treatment and debridement are necessary.

 ## Differential Diagnosis

- Other overwhelming systemic infections, both bacterial and fungal
- Allergic pneumonitis (other causes)
- Neoplasm

 ## Data Gathering

HISTORY

Question: Is there a history of the chronic otitis externa?
Significance: Associated with otomycosis

Question: Is there history of sinusitis that does not clear?
Significance: Indolent or noninvasive paranasal sinusitis presents with signs and symptoms of chronic sinusitis that is unresponsive to antibiotic therapy.

Question: Does an asthmatic patient cough up large, dark mucus plugs?
Significance: Allergic bronchopulmonary aspergillosis should be considered in the asthmatic patient with a history of expectorating dark mucus plugs, or a history of fleeting pulmonary infiltrates on chest x-ray (due to bronchial plugging).

 ## Physical Examination

- Otomycosis is characterized by a mass of black spores (*A. niger*) that start close to the eardrum and eventually fill the external canal, pain on tragal movement, and occasionally a purulent discharge. It is only rarely an invasive disease.
- Invasive sinus aspergillosis may present with severe pain, proptosis, monocular blindness, and bony destruction on x-ray films, with evidence of direct extension to the anterior fossa or orbit, or with widespread dissemination.

Laboratory Aids

- Isolation of *Aspergillus* species by culture is required for definitive diagnosis.
- *Aspergillus* can be recovered from samples of blood, CSF, sputum, urine, BAL sample, or tissue biopsy. Types of specimens collected are guided by history and physical examination.
- Microscopic examination of specially stained tissue samples, or of 10% potassium hydroxide wet preparation samples, that are positive for branching, septate hyphae are suggestive of *Aspergillus* or other fungal invaders.
- Elevated serum IgE eosinophilia, serum antibody for *Aspergillus,* and an immediate-type skin test response to *Aspergillus* antigen are often present in patients with allergic aspergillosis and are helpful in establishing the diagnosis.
- Recent developments in early diagnosis include the use of: high-resolution chest CT, new rapid stain techniques and monoclonal antibodies for BAL samples, and serum ELISA for *Aspergillus galactomannan*.
- *Aspergillus* can be a contaminant of laboratory stains or other preparative agents, but a positive culture or a microscopic examination positive for hyphae in an immunocompromised patient should be considered of likely clinical significance.

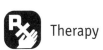 Therapy

- Allergic bronchopulmonary aspergillosis is frequently managed with oral or inhaled corticosteroids.
- If paranasal sinusitis is noninvasive, surgical drainage or debridement usually results in clearance of the infection.
- Otomycosis (most commonly secondary to *A. niger*) is often found in association with a bacterial external otitis. Debridement of the external canal and treatment of underlying bacterial external otitis usually produces a good therapeutic response.
- Invasive or systemic disease is treated with amphotericin B, with recommended doses ranging from 0.5 to 1.5 mg/kg/d (after initial test dose and subsequent incremental increases in therapeutic doses until total daily dose is reached; see hospital pharmacy protocol).
- The addition of flucytosine or rifampin to amphotericin B therapy is sometimes recommended.
- Itraconazole has been used as an alternative in patients unable to tolerate amphotericin B, but adequate therapeutic trials in invasive aspergillosis have not been performed.
- Surgical excision, in addition to amphotericin B, is sometimes required for localized debridement in invasive disease.

 Follow-Up

The course of illness is variable, depending on host immune function and location and invasiveness of disease.

PITFALLS

- Any immunocompromised patient with persistent fevers or signs of invasive infection not improving on treatment with broad-spectrum antibiotics must be evaluated for fungal infection and the empiric use of antifungal medications considered.
- The rare finding of diffuse nodular pneumonia in children may be indicative of an underlying diagnosis of chronic granulomatous disease and aspergillosis.

PREVENTION

INFECTION CONTROL

- Hospitalized, immunosuppressed patients are at risk for invasive aspergillosis.
- Environmental measures to control airborne spread of conidiospores in hospitals during construction are indicated.
- Laminar-flow rooms with appropriate filters will significantly decrease contact with airborne conidiospores.

 Common Questions and Answers

Q: What are rare complications of aspergillosis?
A: Endocarditis, osteomyelitis, and cutaneous disease.

Q: Does person-to-person spread occur?
A: No. The principle route of transmission is inhalation of airborne spores.

ICD-9-CM 117.3

BIBLIOGRAPHY

American Academy of Pediatrics. Aspergillosis. In: Peter G, ed. *1997 red book: report of the Committee on Infectious Diseases,* 24th ed. Elk Grove Village, IL: American Academy of Pediatrics, 1997:144–145.

Bennett JE. Aspergillus species. In: Mandell GL, et al., eds. *Principles and practice of infectious diseases,* 3rd ed. New York: Churchill Livingstone, 1990:1958–1961.

Blum MD, Wiederman BL. Aspergillus. In: Feigen RD, Cherry JD, eds. *Textbook of pediatric infectious diseases,* 3rd ed. Philadelphia: WB Saunders, 1992:1891–1896.

Author: Molly (Martha) W. Stevens

Asplenia/Hyposplenia

 Database

DEFINITION

Hyposplenia and asplenia are defined by the functional capacity of the spleen to filter blood and perform immunogenic functions.

PATHOPHYSIOLOGY

• Hyposplenia/asplenia occurs in association with a number of illnesses and after splenectomy.

• Most patients with hyposplenism process antigens without difficulty.

• If the spleen is minimally functional, an inability to handle infections results from defective antibody synthesis and removal of opsonized organisms.

• Encapsulated microorganisms, such as *Pneumococcus, Meningococcus,* and *Haemophilus,* are usually handled by this mechanism.

• Under the age of 4 years, significant morbidity and mortality can result for the patient with impaired splenic function.

However, the asplenia syndrome should be viewed separately. Asplenia syndrome is characterized by complex congenital heart disease, asplenia, and abdominal heterotaxy. Common associated anomalies include atrioventricular canal defects, conotruncal anomalies, anomalous systemic pulmonary venous connections, and visceroatrial situs inversus. Its morbidity is distinctly unfavorable.

GENETICS

• Most causes of hyposplenia or asplenia are not inherited.

• A disturbance in embryogenesis in the fifth week of gestation results in bilateral right-sidedness with abnormal pulmonary lobation in 80% of patients and abdominal heterotaxy in 72%. An autosomal recessive inheritance pattern is suggested based on family studies and mouse models of heterotaxy. A review of 519 autopsy cases calculated survival to be 2.6 months, with death typically resulting from cardiorespiratory failure or infection.

 Differential Diagnosis

Diminished splenic function is found in/with:

• Normal infants
• Congenital asplenia
• Asplenia syndrome
• Old age
• Sequestration crises (sickle cell hemoglobinopathies, essential thrombocytosis, malaria, thrombosis of the splenic vessels)
• Autoimmune disorders (glomerulonephritis, systemic lupus erythematosus, rheumatoid arthritis, graft-versus-host disease, and sarcoidosis)
• Gastrointestinal disorders (celiac disease [30%–50% are hyposplenic], Crohn disease, ulcerative colitis, dermatitis herpetiformis)
• Space-occupying lesions (tumors, amyloid, cysts)
• Splenic irradiation
• Postsplenectomy

 Data Gathering

HISTORY

• Has there been an underlying disease such as sickle cell disease or Crohn disease?
• Is there a history of recurrent fevers?

 Physical Examination

• Physical examination may reveal that the spleen may be normal, large, or atretic and cannot be used as an index of splenic function.

• The size of the spleen is most closely linked to the underlying etiology.

• Complete splenic replacement by cysts, neoplasm, or amyloid are examples of hyposplenic splenomegaly.

• Sequestration crises such as that associated with sickle cell disease and malaria clog the spleen with cellular debris, resulting in an increased spleen size and decreased function.

Laboratory Aids

- In the apparently healthy child with no identified risk factors who presents with an overwhelming infection with an encapsulated organism, the hematologic smear should be examined.
- Reduction or absence of splenic function can be determined by specific hematologic changes.
- Nonspecific changes include a modest increase in WBC and platelet count. Target cells, Howell-Jolly bodies (nuclear fragments that normally are removed in the spleen), and pitted erythrocytes can be visualized on peripheral blood smear.
- Pits or pox on the red-cell surface are the most sensitive indicator of hyposplenism.

—These are submembranous vacuoles that can be seen only in wet preparations of red cells using direct interference–contrast microscopy.

- ^{51}Cr-labeled, heat-damaged red blood cells can be used to measure the capacity of the spleen to clear particulate matter from the bloodstream.
- The size of the spleen can be determined by either ultrasound or computed tomography (CT) scan.

 Therapy

- Immunization with a polyvalent pneumococcal vaccine should be carried out in all patients with hyposplenism.
- Those who will be undergoing splenectomy should receive the vaccine prior to the operation.
- No revaccination is needed according to the present recommendations.
- Children should also receive *Haemophilus influenzae* vaccine.

PITFALLS

Under the age of 4 years, splenectomy is contraindicated because of the risk of developing bacterial infection.

 Common Questions and Answers

Q: What should I do if my child has a fever?
A: In hyposplenic patients, especially those under the age of 4 years, all fevers should be taken seriously. If the child is not on prophylactic penicillin, he/she should be treated for all symptomatic infections.

Q: Are there any special times I need to worry about infections?
A: In these patients, dental work, especially tooth extraction, should always be preceded by a course of prophylactic antibiotics.

ICD-9-CM 459.0

BIBLIOGRAPHY

Phoon CK, Neill CA. Asplenia syndrome: insight into embryology through an analysis of cardiac and extracardiac anomalies. *Am J Cardiol* 1994;73:581–587.

Phoon CK, Neill CA. Asplenia syndrome—risk factors for early unfavorable outcome. *Am J Cardiol* 1994;73:1235–1237.

Author: Barbara Haber

Asthma

 Database

DEFINITION

- Characterized by three components:

—Reversible airway obstruction
—Airway inflammation
—Airway hyperresponsiveness to a variety of stimuli

PATHOPHYSIOLOGY AND CAUSES

- Immune and inflammatory responses in the airways triggered by inhalation of an array of environmental allergens and/or infectious antigens
- Hereditary factors play a role.
- Atopy plays a role.

—Ability to make excess IgE in response to antigen is associated with increased airway reactivity.
—Asthma is more common in children who have allergic rhinitis and eczema.

- Viral (especially respiratory syncytial virus [RSV]) infections during infancy are associated with the development of asthma.
- Exposure to cigarette smoke and other fumes or chemicals is associated with asthma.
- IgE response is involved in initiating inflammation and bronchospasm.
- Airway is invaded by inflammatory cells (mast cells, basophils, eosinophils, macrophages, neutrophils, B and T lymphocytes).
- Inflammatory cells respond to and produce various mediators (cytokines, leukotrienes, lymphokines), augmenting the inflammatory response.
- Airway epithelium is disrupted and basal membrane is thickened.
- Airway smooth muscle ultimately becomes hyperresponsive, and bronchospasm ensues.
- Airway smooth muscle hypertrophy and hyperplasia are characteristic of chronic asthma.

GENETICS

- Little is known about why some subjects develop asthma and others do not.
- Epidemiologic studies have shown clear evidence for a genetic component in asthma.
- Children of asthmatics have higher incidence of asthma:

—6% to 7% risk if neither parent has asthma
—20% risk if one parent has asthma
—60% risk if both parents have asthma

- Current evidence supports the environment having a greater influence than genetics.
- Atopic asthma tends to run in families.
- Several genes are known to be associated with the development of atopy.

EPIDEMIOLOGY

- Most common chronic illness in children
- Recent increases in asthma prevalence, morbidity, and mortality
- Death rate of asthma among children rose over 30% between 1980 and 1987.
- Wheezing in children is extremely common in the industrialized world (cumulative prevalence, 30%–60%).
- Most episodes occur during viral infections.
- Most children outgrow their wheeze by age 6 years.
- 5% to 7% of all children (30%–40% of those who wheeze) continue to wheeze and asthma develops.
- Asthma is more common in boys than in girls up to 10 years, but incidence is equal thereafter.

COMPLICATIONS

- Morbidity

—Frequent hospitalizations and absence from school
—Chronic symptoms affect activity level and function.
—Psychologic impact of having a chronic illness
—Chronic recurrent atelectasis may lead to the development of localized bronchiectasis.

- Mortality

—Increase in asthma mortality of unknown cause in all age groups in recent years
—Increase in number of life-threatening episodes

PROGNOSIS

- With proper therapy and good compliance: excellent

 Differential Diagnosis

INFECTIONS

- Pneumonia
- Bronchiolitis (RSV)
- *Chlamydia* infection
- Laryngotracheobronchitis

MECHANICAL

- Obstructive mass
- Vascular ring
- Foreign body
- Vocal cord dysfunction

MISCELLANEOUS

- Cystic fibrosis
- Bronchopulmonary dysplasia
- Pulmonary edema
- Gastroesophageal reflux (GER)
- Recurrent aspiration
- Bronchiolitis obliterans

 Data Gathering

HISTORY

Inquire about these symptoms:

- Coughing
- Wheezing
- Shortness of breath
- Chest tightness

Pattern of Symptoms

- Perennial versus seasonal
- Continuous versus acute
- Duration and frequency of episodes
- Diurnal variation/nocturnal symptoms

Do any of the following set off the breathing difficulty?

- Infections (upper respiratory, sinusitis)
- Allergies to:

—Dust mites
—Animal dander
—Pollen
—Mold

- Cold air or weather changes
- Exercise (exercise asthma)
- Environmental stimulants

—Cigarette smoke
—Strong odors
—Pollutants

- Emotional factors

—Laughing
—Crying
—Fear

- Drug intake

—Aspirin
—NSAIDs
—β-blockers
—ACE inhibitors

- Food additives
- Endocrine factors

—Menses
—Pregnancy
—Thyroid dysfunction

- Family history of asthma or atopy

Impact of Asthma

- Number of hospitalizations/ICU admissions
- Number of ER visits/doctor's office visits
- Asthma attack frequency
- Number of missed school days
- Limitation on activity
- Number of courses of systemic steroids needed

Environmental History

- Type of home
- Location of home (urban, suburban, rural)
- Heating system/air conditioning
- Fireplace
- Carpeting
- Stuffed animals
- Pets
- Exposure to cigarette smoke

 ## Physical Examination

- Pulmonary examination may be normal when asymptomatic.
- Assess work of breathing

—Level of distress
—Intercostal/supraclavicular muscle retractions

- Chest shape (i.e., normal vs. barrel-shaped)
- Lung auscultation

—Wheezing
—End-expiratory involuntary cough
—Prolonged expiratory phase
—Rhonchi or rales

- HEENT examination: Signs of allergies or sinusitis

—Watery or itchy eyes
—Allergic shiners
—Dennie lines
—Nasal congestion
—Boggy nasal turbinates
—Nasal polyps
—Postnasal drip

- General examination: Vital signs

—Blood pressure (pulsus paradoxus)
—Respiratory rate (tachypnea)

- Skin: Evidence of eczema

Physical Examination Trick

Forced exhalation maneuver to observe for rhonchi or wheezes or for precipitating coughing

 ## Laboratory Aids

TESTS

- Pulmonary function tests

—Essential for the diagnosis and ongoing care of children with asthma
—Measure the degree of airway obstruction and the response to bronchodilators
—Values obtained can measure absolute degree of airway obstruction.
—Serial values can follow progress of disease and response to treatment.
—Children 4 years old can usually perform airway conductance test.
—Children 6 years old can usually perform spirometry and lung volume tests.

- Provocational testing

—Exercise challenge: determines effect of exercise on triggering bronchospasm
—Methacholine challenge: confirms diagnosis of asthma (positive test); useful in cases where history is equivocal and pulmonary function test is normal; measures the degree of airway hyperreactivity

- Pressure-volume curves determine lung compliance; useful in selected cases.
- Allergy evaluation

—Blood tests (eosinophilic count, IgE level)
—Skin testing (best test for assessing allergen sensitivity)
—RAST testing (not as accurate as skin testing)
—Sputum/nasal examination for presence of eosinophilia

- Other studies

—GER evaluation
  —pH probe
  —Milk scan
  —Barium swallow

—Bronchoscopy to rule out:
  —Anatomic malformations
  —Foreign bodies
  —Mucus plugging
  —Vocal cord function

—Assess for aspiration (lipid-laden macrophages)

Imaging

- Chest radiograph should be obtained at least once for all children to rule out congenital lung malformations or obvious vascular malformations. Findings can be normal. Common findings are peribronchial thickening, subsegmental atelectasis, and hyperinflation.
- Sinus radiography is useful if symptoms suggest sinusitis.
- Chest CT should be performed in selected cases: right middle lobe syndrome, bronchiectasis, and anatomical abnormality.

Home Testing

- Peak flow meter

—Measures peak flow rate (PEFR)
—Correlates well with FEV_1 of spirometry
—Useful in treating patients with difficult-to-control or labile asthma
—Dips in PEFR precede onset of clinical asthmatic symptoms.
—PEFR should be performed at least once a day.
—PEFR values are divided into three zones:
  —Green: 80% of baseline
  —Yellow: 50% to 80% of baseline
  —Red: 50% of baseline

—Specific PEFR guidelines should be individualized for each patient.

Asthma

 Therapy

DRUGS

Bronchodilators

- Relaxes airway smooth muscle
- Three classes described below

β_2-Agonists

- Main indication is for relief of acute broncho-spasm.
- Used PRN in asthmatics who have infrequent symptoms
- Used intermittently or routinely in conjunction with antiinflammatory agents in patients with frequent exacerbations or chronic airway obstruction
- Used prior to exercise in exercise-induced bronchospasm
- Regular use or overuse associated with:

—Worsened control of asthma
—Increased airway hyperresponsiveness
—Increased mortality (highly controversial)

- Routes

—Inhaled (most effective): nebulizer
—Metered-dose inhaler (MDI): spinhaler
—Oral (least effective; most side effects)

- Preparations: Short-acting (effect lasts 4–6 hours):

—Albuterol (Ventolin, Proventil)
—Terbutaline (Brethaire, Brethine)
—Metoproterenol (Alupent)

- Preparation: Long-acting (lasts up to 12 hours)

—Salmeterol (Serevent)

Theophylline

- Has lost some of its popularity in recent years due to more effective and safer β_2-agonists and the current focus on antiinflammatory therapy
- Indications

—Chronic, poorly controlled asthma
—Nocturnal asthma (if no GER)
—Adjunctive therapy with β_2 drugs and steroids in hospitalized patients in selected cases

- Route: oral or IV
- Serum levels must be routinely monitored

—Therapeutic levels: 5 to 15 mg/mL
—Side effects are seen with increased levels.
—Many factors affect theophylline levels.
  —Increased levels seen with:
    —Erythromycin
    —Ciprofloxacin
  —Cimetidine
    —Viral illnesses
    —Fever
  —Decreased levels seen with:
    —Phenobarbital
    —Phenytoin
    —Rifampin

Anticholinergic Agents

There is little information to support the adjunctive use of anticholinergic drugs in children.

- Preparations

—Nebulized atropine
—Ipratropium bromide MDI (Atrovent)

Antiinflammatory Agents

- First line of therapy for moderate-to-severe asthma
- Three classes described below

Mast-Cell Stabilizers

- Preparations

—Short-acting: cromolyn sodium (Intal)
—Long-acting: nedocromil sodium (Tilade)

- Decrease bronchial hyperresponsiveness
- Effective in both allergic and nonallergic asthma
- Used prior to exercise in exercise-induced bronchospasm
- No significant side effects
- Routes

—Inhaled: nebulizer
—MDI
—Spinhaler

Corticosteroids

- Preparations

—Inhaled (dosage individualized to each patient)
  —Beclomethasone (42 mg/puff) (Beclovent, Vanceril)
  —Triamcinolone (100 mg/puff) (Azmacort)
  —Flunisolide (250 mg/puff) (Aerobid)
  —Fluticazone (44; 110; 220 μg/puff) (Flovent)
  —Budesonide (200 μg/puff) (Pulmicort)
—Oral
  —Prednisone 2 mg/kg/d 3 to 5 days; should be tapered if 5 days of therapy required
—Intravenous
  —Solumedrol 1 mg/kg IV q6h until condition improves

- Potent antiinflammatory drugs
- Inhaled corticosteroids reduce airway inflammation and hyperresponsiveness more than does cromolyn.
- Inhibit production and release of cytokines and arachidonic acid—associated metabolites
- Enhance β-adrenoceptor responsiveness
- Routes

—Inhaled: used for management of chronic asthma
—MDI
—Oral or intravenous (used for management of acute asthma attacks)

Leukotriene Modifiers

- First asthma-specific drugs on the market that are effective in preventing asthma
- Block the synthesis and/or action of leukotrienes; experience from clinical use is growing
- 5-Lipoxyenase inhibitors; zileuton. Other inhibitors are in clinical trials.
- Leukotriene (LT-1) receptor antagonists; zafirlukast and montelukast. Other antagonists are in clinical trials.

MISCELLANEOUS DRUGS

Steroid-Sparing Agents

Troleandomycin (Tao)

- Macrolide antibiotic
- Decreases clearance of corticosteroids, thus prolonging the effects of corticosteroids on the lung
- Lower corticosteroid dosing required

Methotrexate

- Potent immunosuppressive drug
- May have potential role as adjunct to steroid therapy
- Needs further investigation in children

Cyclosporine

- Has been shown to have steroid-sparing effect in adult population with asthma
- Side effects are significant and may limit use.

IV IgG

- High-dose therapy under investigation

MgSO$_4$

- Used as a bronchodilator in severe asthma attacks
- Few, if any, benefits in most patients with asthma

HELIUM

- May improve airflow in severe asthma
- Can improve ventilation and potentially oxygenation
- Confirmatory studies are not available.

EDUCATION/ENVIRONMENTAL CONTROL

- First step in managing asthma is to educate the patient and his or her family about avoiding known triggers.
- Avoid airborne irritants (tobacco smoke, wood stoves, noxious fumes).
- Minimize dust-mite exposure

—Remove carpets (if possible) or use 3% tannic acid solution or benzyl benzoate for cleaning.
—Use plastic (vinyl) coverings on mattresses and box springs.
—Wash pillows, blankets, and sheets in hot water.

- Avoid molds by decreasing relative humidity to 50%.
- Remove pets (if necessary).

IMMUNOTHERAPY

- Efficacy in asthma is controversial.
- Use only in selected cases if medical management and environmental control measures are ineffective.

Duration of Therapy

- Depends on severity of the patient's asthma
- Bronchodilators

—Should be PRN (if able)
—In URI-triggered flares: 7 to 14 days
—Monitor PEFR

- Antiinflammatory agents

—Use every day.
—May be weaned in many patients as asthma comes under long-standing control

DIET

- Avoid foods or food additives (if truly allergic).
- Food-induced asthma is uncommon.

POSSIBLE CONFLICTS WITH OTHER TREATMENTS

- Theophylline kinetics are altered by many drugs.
- Use of theophylline can worsen GER.

 Follow-Up

WHEN TO EXPECT IMPROVEMENT

- In acute asthma attacks, with appropriate therapy, improvement is usually seen within 24 to 48 hours.
- In chronic asthma, control of symptoms can usually be obtained within 1 month.

SIGNS THAT MAY INDICATE PROBLEMS

- Decrease in PEFR
- Increasing use of inhaled bronchodilators
- Subject not improving on enhanced home therapy

PITFALLS

- Not recognizing that asthma can manifest as chronic cough
- "Recurrent pneumonias" many times are actually virus-triggered asthma attacks with coughing and subsegmental atelectasis on chest radiography.
- Pulmonary function testing is effort-dependent.
- Suboptimal effort may result in artificially decreased pulmonary function values, overestimating the amount of bronchospasm present.

 Common Questions and Answers

Q: Will my child outgrow his or her asthma?
A: Family history and allergies affect the ultimate outcome. Wheezing during the first 3 years of life is extremely common, with 40% to 50% of all children wheezing at some time. Many of these children do not develop asthma and "outgrow" their illness by school age. Some patients develop asthma again as young adults.

Q: Can my child become dependent on asthma medications?
A: Children do not become "dependent" on these medications as they would with narcotic agents. Daily asthma medications are required to maintain airway patency and to control airway inflammation.

Q: Will my child be on medications for the rest of his or her life?
A: This depends on the severity of the asthma. The types, doses, and frequency of asthma medications will change over a patient's lifetime.

Q: Do inhaled steroids affect patient growth?
A: There is no convincing evidence of long-term growth suppression or bone demineralization in school-aged children receiving up to 400 mg/d of inhaled steroids. Further studies are in progress.

ICD-9-CM 493.01

BIBLIOGRAPHY

Bloomberg GR, Strunk RC. Crisis in asthma care. *Pediatr Clin North Am* 1992;39:1225–1241.

Hakonarson H, Grunstein MM. Management of childhood asthma. In: Barnes P, Grunstein MM, Leff A, Woolcock A, eds. *Asthma,* vol. 2. New York: Raven Press, 1997:1847–1868.

Hill M, Szefler SJ. Asthma pathogenesis and the implications for therapy in children. *Pediatr Clin North Am* 1992;39:1205–1224.

Koenig P. A step-wise approach to the changing drug therapy of asthma. *Pediatr Ann* 1992;21:565–571.

Morgan WJ, Martinez FD. Risk factors for developing wheezing and asthma in children. *Pediatr Clin North Am* 1992;39:1185–1203.

National Asthma Education and Prevention Program. *Expert Panel Report 2: Guidelines for the diagnosis and management of asthma.* Washington, DC: US Government Printing Office, February 1997 (NIH-NHLBI publication).

Reid MJ. Complicating features of asthma. *Pediatr Clin North Am* 1992;39:1327–1341.

Richards W. Asthma, allergies, and school. *Pediatr Ann* 1992;21:575–585.

Shapiro GG. Childhood asthma: update. *Pediatr Rev* 1992;13:403–412.

Workshop on Early Childhood Asthma. What are the questions? *Am J Respir Crit Care Med* 1995;151:S1–S42.

Author: Hakon Hakonarson

Ataxia

 ## Database

DEFINITION

Ataxia is defined as any problem with orientation of movement. Though cerebellar dysfunction is the most common cause of ataxia in children, other sites of pathology should also be considered: peripheral nerve, dorsal-root ganglion, brainstem, and inner ear (labyrinth).

- Appendicular ataxia affects limb movement.
- *Truncal ataxia, gait ataxia, dysarthria,* and *nystagmus* often occur together in cerebellar ataxia.

CLINICAL PRESENTATION

- Acute cerebellar ataxia following a benign viral infection is common in children.
- *Chronic ataxia* usually signals serious underlying pathology (tumor, hereditary or metabolic disorder).

PATHOPHYSIOLOGY

The cerebellum "fine tunes" all coordinated movement and is sensitive to any structural (e.g., tumor, stroke) or metabolic (e.g., intoxication) injury. Ataxia is involved in any disturbance of pathways to (e.g., vestibular nerve, proprioceptive sensory nerves, dorsal-root ganglion cells) or from (e.g., superior cerebellar peduncles, brainstem) the cerebellum. It may impair coordination.

GENETICS

Hereditary causes of chronic ataxia include Friedreich ataxia, ataxia telangiectasia, mitochondrial disease, and aminoacidopathies.

ASSOCIATED CONDITIONS

- *Acute ataxia,* in association with opsoclonus-myoclonus syndrome, may be symptomatic of underlying neuroblastoma/ganglioneuroma.
- Friedreich ataxia is associated with cardiomyopathy, diabetes, and peripheral neuropathy.
- Mitochondrial disorders: short stature, retinopathy, heart block, myopathy

 ## Differential Diagnosis

Chorea, tremor, or athetosis may be mistakenly diagnosed as ataxia.

ACUTE ATAXIA

- Intoxication: depressed mental status; toxicologic screen; medications at home
- Posttraumatic: history/physical findings
- Postinfectious: acute cerebellar ataxia (dysarthria, mild hypotonia)
- Paraneoplastic: more indolent/subacute onset; ataxia may precede opsoclonus/myoclonus; neuroblastoma/ganglioneuroma
- Migraine: resolves in hours; headache may precede ataxia
- Labyrinthitis: fast phase of nystagmus is unidirectional
- Acute disseminated encephalomyelitis (ADEM) white matter changes on MRI, variable on CT
- Acute polyneuropathy: GBS (arreflexia, signs of sensory ataxia)
- Stroke: focal deficits; abnormal imaging studies
- Postictal: rapidly resolving ataxia with negative studies, slowing on EEG; history of convulsion
- Familial periodic ataxia: family history
- Acute ataxia: can be a rare presentation of meningitis/encephalitis
- Psychogenic: "astasia abasia" (variable effort; no pathologic nystagmus, characteristic gait)

CHRONIC ATAXIA

- Brain tumor (especially under 10 years): associated cranial neuropathies, papilledema, headache, pyramidal tract signs
- Friedreich ataxia: onset 5 to 15 years; family history, associated cardiomyopathy, polyneuropathy, diabetes
- Leukodystrophy: adrenoleukodystrophy, metachromatic leukodystrophy, Pelizaeus-Merzbacher disease (abnormal MRI signal in white matter)
- Other metabolic diseases: Niemann-Pick, maple syrup urine disease (MSUD), Hartnup disease (amino acid screen)
- Abetalipoproteinemia: onset in second decade; hypocholesterolemia/decreased LDL
- Hereditary neuropathy: decreased reflexes, weakness usually more prominent, family history, molecular diagnosis
- Hereditary ataxia: autosomal dominant, molecular diagnosis
- Long-term phenytoin: primarily adults
- Metabolic: variable onset; may be episodic, with other systemic symptoms; Hartnup disease, MSUD, organic acidemias, Niemann-Pick C (visceromegaly?, foam cells in marrow)
- Intermittent or chronic ataxia may be a feature of mitochondrial disease, usually in association with other systemic signs/symptoms: retinopathy, sensorineural hearing loss, diabetes, growth delay, seizures, myopathy.
- Rare: ataxic cerebral palsy, brain dysgenesis, Joubert syndrome, multiple sclerosis, Gerstmann-Straussler (familial; prion disease)

 ## Data Gathering

HISTORY

You must establish acute versus chronic onset of ataxia to narrow the differential diagnosis.

- In acute ataxia, history should be directed to possible intoxication, head trauma, or migraine.
- History of episodic change in consciousness or convulsions points to seizure disorder (postictal ataxia).
- Recent varicella or other infection suggests postviral cerebellar ataxia, labyrinthitis, or Guillain-Barré syndrome (GBS) (see chapter on Guillain-Barré syndrome).
- Congenital heart disease or other known circulatory disorder raises the possibility of cerebellar stroke.
- In chronic ataxia, history of extreme irritability or progressive macrocrania (from well-care records) in an infant or toddler suggests brain tumor.
- History of recurrent vomiting (metabolic disorders), psychiatric disturbance (conversion disorders), or other family members with neurologic disease (hereditary neuropathies, ataxia telangiectasia) may all lead to the diagnosis.

Physical Examination

The neuroanatomic localization of the ataxia must be determined.

• *Cerebellar ataxia* often interferes with speech; consciousness is normal despite "drunken" movements and gait. Signs include:

—Intention tremor: oscillations seen (e.g., on finger-nose testing) when agonists and antagonists cocontract to orient limb movement
—Disdiadohokinesia: impairment of rapid, alternating movements
—Titubation, truncal ataxia, and pathologic nystagmus: point to cerebellar or vestibular disease
—Cranial nerve findings, especially third, sixth, or lower cranial nerves: point to possible brain tumor; hyperreflexia or upgoing toes may be present.
—Asymmetric ataxia or weakness: may signify tumor, stroke, or demyelinating disease

• Sensory ataxia also spares consciousness; other signs include:

—Romberg fall: ataxia worsened by eye closure; indicates sensory dysfunction, either proprioceptive (peripheral nerves, dorsal-root ganglia), or vestibular (inner ear, vestibular nerve).
—Arreflexia: not seen in central causes of ataxia; key sign in distinguishing sensory ataxia (as in GBS) from cerebellar ataxia

• Toxic/metabolic causes: intoxications, postictal ataxia, and sleep drunkenness usually alter consciousness.

 ## Laboratory Aids

• Toxicologic screen is usually a good initial screen in acute ataxia.
• Radiologic studies are necessary when intoxication has been ruled out (rule out tumor, stroke, demyelination); MRI is superior to CT for imaging the cerebellum, though contrast CT is adequate to rule out posterior fossa tumor.
• Spinal tap may reveal a few cells/mild increase in protein in benign acute cerebellar ataxia of childhood or in acute demyelinating encephalomyelitis.
• EEG if postictal ataxia is a possibility.
• Full work-up for neuroblastoma in ataxia opsoclonus/myoclonus includes body CT, serum ferritin, urine homovanillic/vanillylmandelic acid (HVA/VMA).
• Low cholesterol in chronic ataxia suggests abetalipoproteinemia.
• Genetic test for Friedreich (chronic) ataxia may soon become available.
• Laboratory testing for mitochondrial ataxia, which may produce intermittent *or* chronic ataxia, usually with other systemic abnormalities (see above) includes urine organic acids, plasma lactate/pyruvate, genetic testing on blood, muscle biopsy.

 ## Therapy

• As indicated for any underlying condition; precautions and limitation of activity to decrease the chance of injury/aspiration
• Steroids (2 mg/kg IV prednisolone) often used for ADEM, though there is no proven benefit.
• Immunomodulatory therapies have been tried (plasmapheresis, IVIG) for paraneoplastic ataxia-opsoclonus/myoclonus, since the movement disorder may persist long after therapy for the tumor.
• Acetazolamide may be helpful for familial periodic ataxia.

 ## Follow-Up

• Acute postinfectious cerebellar ataxia usually resolves over days to weeks; if imaging studies show demyelination, recovery may take longer and the chance of recurrence may be higher.
• If initial studies in opsoclonus/myoclonus do not reveal a neoplasm, follow-up studies should be repeated.

PITFALLS

• Children with acute recurrent ataxia should be evaluated for metabolic disease, even if examination is normal between attacks. Possibilities include ornithine transcarbamoylase deficiency, mitochondrial disorders.
• Inadvertent intoxication with anticonvulsants in the household may not be detected on routine toxin screen. Ask about carbamazepine, phenytoin.
• Symptoms of progressive herniation of the cerebellar tonsils in a child or adolescent with Arnold-Chiari type 1 malformation may mimic migraine. A head scan should be done on a child with ataxia and a headache.

 ## Common Questions and Answers

Q: What intoxications are most likely to cause ataxia?
A: Benzodiazepines, the major anticonvulsants (except valproate), ethanol, tricyclics, antihistamines, others.

Q: How long can postinfectious cerebellar ataxia last?
A: Rarely, it may last for months, but should be improving during that time.

Q: What is the role of physical therapy for cerebellar ataxia?
A: Physical therapy for ataxia is of limited value.

ICD-9-CM 334.3

BIBLIOGRAPHY

Connolly AM, Dodson WE, Prensky AL, Rust RS. Course and outcome of acute cerebellar ataxia. *Ann Neurol* 1994;35(6):673–679.

DeAngelis C. Ataxia. *Pediatr Rev* 1995;16(3):114–115

Salih AM, Ahlsten G, Stalberg E, et al. Friedreich ataxia in 13 children: presentation and evolution with neurophysiologic, electrocardiographic, and echocardiographic features. *J Child Neurol* 1990;5:321–326.

Steinlin M, Zangger B, Boltshauser E. Nonprogressive congenital ataxia with or without cerebellar hypoplasia: a review of 34 subjects. *Dev Med Child Neurol* 1998 40:148–154.

Author: Peter M. Bingham

Atelectasis

 Database

DEFINITION

- State of collapsed and airless alveoli
- May be subsegmental, segmental, or lobar, or may involve the whole lung
- A radiographic sign of disease and not a diagnosis in itself

CAUSES (TYPES/MECHANISMS)

- Resorption atelectasis (also called obstructive atelectasis); obstructed communication between alveoli and trachea

—Large airway obstruction
  —Intrinsic: e.g., foreign-body aspiration, mucus plug, inflammatory (TB, sarcoid), tumor
  —Extrinsic: e.g., hilar adenopathy, mediastinal masses, cardiomegaly, congenital malformations

—Small airway obstruction
  —Altered mucociliary clearance: e.g., pain, CNS depression, smoke inhalation
  —Chronic obstructive airway disease: e.g., asthma, cystic fibrosis
  —Acute infection: e.g., acute bronchiolitis, pneumonia

- Adhesive atelectasis: stems from surfactant deficiency

—Diffuse surfactant deficiency: e.g., hyaline membrane disease, ARDS, smoke inhalation
—Localized surfactant deficiency: e.g., acute radiation pneumonitis, pulmonary embolism, pneumonia

- Passive atelectasis: e.g., loss of lung volume due to shifts in intrapleural pressure

—Simple pneumothorax

- Diaphragmatic abnormalities: e.g., paralysis, congenital eventration

—Hypoventilation: e.g., post-anesthesia; inherent neuromuscular weakness (e.g., muscular dystrophy)

- Compressive atelectasis: mechanical compression of the pulmonary parenchyma or pleural space

—Intrathoracic: e.g., tension pneumothorax, pleural effusion, lobar emphysema, intrathoracic tumors, diaphragmatic hernias
—Abdominal distension: e.g., large intraabdominal tumors, hepatosplenomegaly, massive ascites, morbid obesity

- Cicatrization atelectasis: stems from decreased lung compliance secondary to fibrosis

—Generalized pulmonary fibrosis: e.g., sarcoidosis, collagen vascular diseases, idiopathic pulmonary fibrosis
—Localized pulmonary fibrosis: e.g., bronchiectasis, chronic tuberculosis and fungal diseases

- Gravity-dependent atelectasis: result of gravity-dependent alterations in alveolar volume (e.g., bedridden patients with poor mucociliary clearance; pulmonary edema)

PATHOPHYSIOLOGY

- Reduced lung compliance
- Loss of alveoli (if extensive) may lead to hypoxia.
- Intrapulmonary shunting develops from hypoxia-induced pulmonary arterial vasoconstriction.
- If atelectasis is extensive, pulmonary hypertension may develop.
- Atelectatic areas are prone to bacterial overgrowth.

GENETICS

Depends on the underlying disease causing atelectasis

EPIDEMIOLOGY

- Depends on the underlying disease causing atelectasis; resorption atelectasis most common

COMPLICATIONS

- Recurrent infections
- Bronchiectasis
- Hemoptysis
- Abscess formation
- Fibrosis of the pulmonary parenchyma

PROGNOSIS

- Depends on underlying disease process
- In general, excellent

 Differential Diagnosis

- Pneumonia

—Viral pneumonia versus subsegmental atelectasis
—Bacterial pneumonia versus segmental or lobar atelectasis

- Thymus (atelectasis in upper lobe)
- Congenital malformations (i.e., sequestration, bronchogenic cyst)
- Pleural effusion

 Data Gathering

HISTORY

Special Questions

Question: Is there history of asthma, chronic lung disease, exposure to smoke or toxic fumes?
Significance: These are some of the conditions that may cause atelectasis.

Question: Is there fever or difficulty breathing?
Significance: These may be asymptomatic.

Question: Is there a cough?
Significance: Cough can be present, but not in all cases.

Question: Is there any dyspnea or chest pain?
Significance: Acute pneumothorax may cause atelectasis.

 Physical Examination

- May be normal
- Tachypnea
- Rales or rhonchi
- The most specific sign is localized loss of breath sounds.
- Dullness to percussion if large area involved
- Tracheal deviation and shift of heart sounds toward atelectatic side
- Localized wheezes in cases of partial obstruction
- Cyanosis in those with extensive atelectasis, causing impairment of oxygenation

Special Question

- Is the atelectasis acute, recurrent, or chronic?

Laboratory Aids

TESTS

Depending on Underlying Disease

- Bronchoscopy can be useful for evaluation of possible:

—Foreign body aspiration
—H-type tracheoesophageal fistula (TEF)
—Bronchial stenosis

Infection

- Cultures (sputum, blood)
- Nasal washing (especially for viruses)
- Skin testing (PPD if tuberculosis suspected)
- Asthma
- Spirometry
- Cystic fibrosis
- Sweat test

Immunodeficiency

- CBC with differential
- Immunoglobulins (IgG, IgA, IgM)

Lung Malformations

- CT scan of chest

Imaging

Chest Radiography

- Most important diagnostic tool
- Radiographic signs of atelectasis

—Direct signs, i.e., crowded pulmonary vessels, crowded air bronchograms, displacement of interlobar fissures
—Indirect signs, i.e., pulmonary opacification, elevation of diaphragm, displacement of trachea, hilum; approximation of ribs; compensatory hyperexpansion of surrounding lung

CT of Chest

- Confluence of bronchi and blood vessels that converge toward the atelectatic side
- Provides information in regard to precise location and extent of obstructing process

PITFALLS

- If the proximal bronchi are occluded or filled with secretions, air bronchograms may not be seen, and displacement of the interlobar fissures may be the only direct sign of atelectasis.
- The indirect signs of atelectasis are not constant, and one or more signs might be absent. Lung opacification may not be apparent until a considerable amount of volume loss has occurred. When atelectasis is bilateral, the trachea and the mediastinum usually remain in the midline. Close approximation of the ribs may also occur from poor positioning—this sign by itself may be an unreliable indicator of atelectasis.

 Therapy

- Treat underlying disease: e.g., removal of aspirated foreign body
- Chest physical therapy with bronchodilators—usually for at least 1 month
- If no improvement with conservative therapy, bronchoscopy with lavage to remove possible mucus plug
- Surgery to remove affected region if chronic, unresponsive to therapy, or significant morbidity seen
- Prevention: directed toward underlying cause, when applicable; e.g., in atelectasis secondary to altered mucociliary clearance or chronic airway obstruction such as in cystic fibrosis or asthma, chest physical therapy should be given.

 Follow-Up

WHEN TO EXPECT IMPROVEMENT

- 1 to 3 months

 Common Questions and Answers

Q: When is the optimal time for bronchoscopy?
A: There are no established criteria. Bronchoscopy should be done early in the course of disease if there is high suspicion of a foreign body or significant respiratory distress, or if atelectasis is extensive and conservative treatment is ineffective. Most isolated atelectatic areas will improve during a 3-month period with appropriate therapy; thus, bronchoscopy should be postponed, if possible, for at least this period.

BIBLIOGRAPHY

Karlson KH. *Pediatric respiratory disease: diagnosis and treatment*. Philadelphia: WB Saunders, 1993:436–440.

Oermann CM, Moore RH. Foolers: things that look like pneumonia in children. *Semin Respir Infect* 1996;11:204–213.

Redding GJ. Atelectasis in childhood. *Pediatr Clin North Am* 1984;31:891–905.

Woodring JH, Reed JC. Types and mechanisms of pulmonary atelectasis. *J Thorac Imaging* 1996;11:92–108.

Authors: Elizabeth C. Uong and Richard Mark Kravitz

Atopic Dermatitis

 ## Database

DEFINITION

Atopic dermatitis or eczema is a chronic, pruritic, papulosquamous eruption seen in individuals with associated personal or family history of atopy—asthma, allergies, hay fever, or rhinitis. There are often intermittent acute flares of atopic dermatitis. It most commonly begins in infancy or early childhood.

CAUSES

• Etiology of atopic dermatitis is multifactorial, with genetic, environmental, physiologic, and immunologic factors.
• Decreased resistance to sensitization and increased viral and dermatophyte infections seen in these patients suggest decreased cell-mediated immunity.
• Patients often have elevated IgE levels and decreased chemotaxis of neutrophils.
• Up to 70% of patients have a family history, but the mode of inheritance is not well defined.

PATHOLOGY

• Histologic findings are dependent on the stage of atopic dermatitis—acute or chronic.
• The acute form is characterized by epidermal psoriasiform hyperplasia with intercellular edema and spongiosis that can lead to vesicle formation.
• Lymphocytes can be seen infiltrating the epidermis.
• The chronic form shows acanthosis, hyperkeratosis, and lymphocytes in the epidermis.

GENETICS

• There is a genetic trait seen in atopic dermatitis, with 30% to 70% of family members having atopy—allergies, asthma, eczema, or hay fever.
• The exact mode of inheritance is not well defined and appears to be multifactorial.

EPIDEMIOLOGY

• Atopic dermatitis is a common disease, occurring in up to 7% of children.
• Approximately 60% of patients with atopic dermatitis will develop it in the first year of life, and 30% between the ages of 1 and 5 years.
• A family history of atopy—allergies, asthma, eczema, or hay fever—is present in 30% to 70% of patients.
• Atopic dermatitis is usually worse in the winter.

COMPLICATIONS

• Decreased cell-mediated immunity and decreased chemotaxis can result in increased infection—viral, dermatophyte, and bacterial. Patients with atopic dermatitis have a high density of *Staphylococcus aureus* on their skin, and given the fissures and open excoriations, there is a risk of superinfection of these lesions.
• The decreased integrity of the skin can result in widely spread cutaneous infections such as herpes simplex infection, known as Kaposi varicelliform eruption or eczema herpeticum. Similar problems can also be seen with coxsackievirus or molluscum contagiosum and used to occur with vaccinia.
• Cataracts can be found in patients with atopic dermatitis, and a severe, rare complication of the disease is the development of Sézary syndrome or mycosis fungoides.

 ## Differential Diagnosis

Diagnostic criteria have been established for atopic dermatitis. The differential diagnosis of atopic dermatitis includes:

• Severe seborrheic dermatitis
• Contact dermatitis
• Allergic or irritant, psoriasis
• Wiskott-Aldrich syndrome
• Histiocytosis X
• Acrodermatitis enteropathica
• Scabies
• Xerosis
• Hyper-IgE syndrome
• Metabolic deficiencies

—Carboxylase
—Prolidase deficiencies

 ## Data Gathering

HISTORY

• Age of onset
• Location
• Prior treatment
• Bathing habits
• Family history of atopy—allergies
• Asthma
• Eczema
• Hay fever

 ## Physical Examination

• Acute flares reveal weeping and crusted erythema.
• Chronic disease is characterized by hyperpigmentation or hypopigmentation, lichenification, and scaling.
• The distribution of the disease is dependent on age.

—During infancy to approximately 2 years of age, the disease is widespread and includes cheeks, forehead, scalp, and extensor surfaces.
—In children from approximately 3 to 11 years, the disease involves the more characteristic flexural sites with lichenification.
—The hands and face can also be involved.
—From adolescence to adulthood, the flexures, neck, hands, and feet are frequently involved, with the face and neck flaring occasionally.

• When the disease is severe, it can present as exfoliative erythroderma with diffuse scaling and erythema.
• Other associated findings include geographic tongue, Dennie-Morgan folds (infraorbital folds), pityriasis alba, (dry white patches), hyperlinear palms, facial pallor, infraorbital darkening, follicular accentuation, keratosis pilaris (dry, rough hair follicles on extensor surfaces of upper arms and thighs).

Special Questions

Excessive dryness exacerbates this disease; therefore, inquiry about bathing habits, frequency, and emollients is helpful.

 ## Laboratory Aids

• No tests are diagnostic of atopic dermatitis.
• Biopsy can be helpful to rule out other papulosquamous disease, such as psoriasis.
• IgE levels are often elevated. Cultures can help identify superinfection during acute flares and viral cultures, and Tzanck smear can identify complications of eczema herpeticum.
• Patch testing can help differentiate atopic dermatitis from contact dermatitis.

Therapy

- There is no cure for atopic dermatitis.
- Patients must understand that this is a chronic disease with intermittent flares and that control is the aim of treatment.
- Good skin care is critical to maintenance and includes use of mild soaps, frequent use of emollients, and avoidance of excessive bathing.
- Avoidance of irritants from the environment, such as wool sweaters or blankets, is recommended. Protective clothing at night to avoid scratching while sleeping is also helpful, as is trimming the nails. Antihistamines such as hydroxyzine or diphenhydramine help to decrease itching.
- Topical steroids control inflammation and mid- to high-potency steroids can be used during acute flares, with tapering of steroids to milder potency when control is achieved. Once cleared, topical steroids can be held and substituted with emollients. Long-term use of steroids can lead to atrophy, telangiectasias, tachyphylaxis, and occasionally, stunting of growth. Oral antibiotics are indicated when there is superinfection of lesions.
- Antivirals are needed for cases of eczema herpeticum. During acute flares with oozing and crusting and when there is superinfection with bacteria or herpes simplex virus, compresses can be helpful.
- Systemic steroids are generally not used because of the chronicity of atopic dermatitis, and are reserved for when control of the eruption is very difficult, and then use should be of short duration.
- Phototherapy with ultraviolet B can be used in patients with extensive disease resistant to other therapy.

 Follow-Up

It should be emphasized to patients that atopic dermatitis is a chronic disease and that good skin care is necessary to control disease activity. Up to 40% to 50% of children will outgrow their atopic dermatitis after the age of 5 years.

 Common Questions and Answers

Q: Will the child outgrow this?
A: Up to 40% to 50% of children will outgrow their atopic dermatitis after the age of 5 years. In some patients, however, the disease will persist to variable extents throughout adulthood.

Q: When atopic dermatitis is controlled, is any treatment necessary?
A: Excessive dryness can exacerbate or flare disease; therefore, less use of soaps and frequent use of emollients is recommended.

Q: Do food hypersensitivities play a role in atopic dermatitis?
A: This is a debated issue. In general, the majority of patients are probably not adversely affected by foods. However, some individuals, particularly those unresponsive to routine therapy, may benefit from screening for food hypersensitivity and a trial of avoidance to any foods that test positive. The most common foods associated with exacerbation when an association can be made are eggs, milk, wheat, soy, peanuts, and fish.

ICD-9-CM 691.8

BIBLIOGRAPHY

Boguniewicz M. Advances in the understanding and treatment of atopic dermatitis. *Curr Opin Pediatr* 1997;9(6):577–581.

Bondi EE, Jegasothy BV, Lazarus GS. *Dermatology diagnosis and therapy*. Norwalk, CT: Appleton & Lange, 1991.

Burks AW, James JM, Hiegel A, Wilson G, Wheeler JG, Jones SM, Zuerlein N. Atopic dermatitis and food hypersensitivity reactions. *J Pediatr* 1998;132(1):132–136.

Fitzpatrick TB, Eisen AZ, Wolfe K, et al. *Dermatology in general medicine,* 4th ed. New York: McGraw-Hill, 1993:1543–1564.

Hill DJ, Hosking CS. Emerging disease profiles in infants and young children with food allergy. *Pediatr Allergy Immunol* 1997;8(10 Suppl):21–26.

Lever WF, Schaumberg-Lever G. *Histopathology of the skin,* 7th ed. Philadelphia: Lippincott, 1990.

Oakes RC, Cox AD, Burgdorf WH. Atopic dermatitis: a review of diagnosis, pathogenesis, and management. *Clin Pediatr* 1983;22(7):467–475.

Author: Christen Mowad

Atrial Septal Defect

 Database

DEFINITION

An opening in the atrial septum, other than a patent foramen ovale (PFO).

- Three major types of atrial septal defects (ASDs):

—Ostium secundum
—Ostium primum
—Ostium venosus defect.

- A PFO usually does not cause a significant intracardiac shunt.
- Ostium secundum defects make up 50% to 70% of all ASDs; usually there is a shunt from the left atrium to the right atrium.
- Ostium primum defects occur in about 30% of all ASDs. They are usually associated with a cleft left AV valve.
- Sinus venosus defects (located at the SVC-RA junction) occur in about 10% of all ASDs. The right pulmonary vein may drain anomalously.

ASSOCIATED LESIONS

An ASD may be associated with partial or total anomalous pulmonary venous drainage, mitral valve anomalies including prolapse, transposition of the great arteries or tricuspid atresia.

PATHOPHYSIOLOGY

A left-to-right shunt occurs through the ASD, resulting in right atrial and right ventricular (RV) volume overload. There is usually increased pulmonary blood flow. The left-to-right shunt generally increases with time as pulmonary resistance drops and RV compliance normalizes. Moderate and large defects are associated with a Qp/Qs ratio of more than 2:1. The direction of atrial shunting is determined by the relative compliance of the RV and LV.

GENETICS

Although usually spontaneous, ASDs may occur as part of a syndrome (Holt-Oram [autosomal dominant]).

EPIDEMIOLOGY

ASDs usually occur sporadically in 5% to 10% of all congenital heart diseases. The ratio between female and male is 2:1.

PROGNOSIS

- The prognosis of small ASDs seems excellent without specific therapy.
- Spontaneous closure of some small secundum ASDs can occur in up to 87% of infants in the first year of life. Isolated secundum ASDs of moderate and large size do not typically cause symptoms in most infants and children.
- Pulmonary hypertension is rare in childhood.
- Atrial flutter and fibrillation present in up to 13% of unoperated patients over 40 years of age.
- Bacterial endocarditis is rare in children with isolated ASD.
- Paradoxical emboli may occur, and should be considered in patients with cerebral or systemic emboli.

 Differential Diagnosis

- Ventricular septal defect
- Patent ductus arteriosus
- AV canal defect

 Data Gathering

HISTORY

- Most infants are asymptomatic.
- Older children with moderate left-to-right shunts are often asymptomatic, but may have mild fatigue or dyspnea.
- Children with large left-to-right shunts may complain of fatigue and dyspnea, which may become noticeable when the child gets older.
- Growth failure is uncommon. Older patients with large atrial shunts may develop atrial arrhythmias.

 Physical Examination

- Inspection and palpation of the precordium are usually normal.
- Older children with a large shunt may have a hyperdynamic precordium.
- Auscultation reveals three important features:

—Wide and "fixed" splitting of S2
—A soft systolic murmur at the upper left sternal border
—A diastolic rumble at the lower sternal border, indicating a Qp/Qs ratio of at least 2:1.

Laboratory Aids

ECG

Usually normal sinus rhythm with right axis deviation. There is often an rSr' indicating RV volume overload. First-degree AV block may be present. A monophasic R wave in lead V1 may suggest pulmonary hypertension.

CXR

Cardiomegaly, increased pulmonary vascular markings, and a dilated pulmonary trunk in patients with significant left-to-right shunts.

ECHO

A two-dimensional echo study is diagnostic; it reveals the location, size, and associated defect, if any. It may demonstrate dilated right-heart structures. Color Doppler generally permits visualization of the direction of shunt flow.

Cardiac Catheterization

Generally unnecessary; it is indicated when pulmonary vascular disease is suspected (determination of pulmonary vascular resistance) or for associated cardiac defects.

 ## Therapy

Infants with congestive heart failure should be treated with digoxin and diuretics. Elective surgical repair is indicated for ASDs associated with large left-to-right shunts, cardiomegaly, or symptoms. Other indications may include: prevention of paradoxical emboli and cerebrovascular accidents or refractory supraventricular arrhythmias. High PVR (i.e., >8 Wu/M^2) increases the morbidity and may worsen the prognosis. Sinus venosus and ostium primum defects require elective surgery regardless of the defect size. The timing of the repair is usually deferred until 3 to 4 years of age. The mortality of surgical repair for an uncomplicated ASD approaches 0%. For some secundum ASDs, device closure of the defect can be done in the cardiac catheterization laboratory.

 ## Follow-Up

- Children with typical auscultation and ECG findings should undergo an echocardiographic evaluation to determine the location and size of the ASD.
- Children with ASDs should have regular follow-up to assess for signs of congestive heart failure or RV volume overload. Restriction on activity is unnecessary. SBE prophylaxis is not indicated in isolated secundum ASDs.
- SBE prophylaxis is indicated for the first 6 months (assuming no residual defect) after closure of a secundum defect.
- Complications related to surgery include sinus node dysfunction. Venous obstruction (facial or pulmonary edema) may occur after a sinus venous ASD repair. Postpericardiotomy syndrome, which manifests with nausea, vomiting, abdominal pain or fever, may occur even weeks after the initial repair. Although a friction rub may not be present, CXR may demonstrate cardiomegaly, and ECHO may reveal a pericardial effusion. Residual ASD after surgery is rare and usually without significant hemodynamic consequence.

 ## Common Questions and Answers

Q: When should a moderate secundum ASD be closed?
A: This can generally be performed in children prior to their starting grade school.

Q: What is the significance of a patient having gastrointestinal complaints (nausea and vomiting) 1 to 2 weeks after surgical closure of an ASD?
A: This may represent a pericardial effusion (post-pericardotomy syndrome).

ICD-9-CM 745.61

BIBLIOGRAPHY

Chang AC, Hanley FL, Wernovsky G, Wessel DL. *Pediatric cardiac intensive care.* Baltimore: Williams & Wilkins, 1998:207–211.

Garson A, Bricker J, McNamara D. *The science and practice of pediatric cardiology.* Philadelphia: Lea & Febiger, 1990:1023–1036.

Radzik D, Davignon A, van Doesburg N, et al. Predictive factors for spontaneous closure of atrial septal defect diagnosed in the first 3 months of life. *J Am Coll Cardiol* 1993; 22:851–853.

Author: Song-Gui Yang

Attention-Deficit Hyperactivity Disorder

 Database

DEFINITION

Attention-deficit hyperactivity disorder (ADHD) is a syndrome characterized by persistent and developmentally inappropriate levels of inattention and/or hyperactivity and impulsivity. The following disorders have been associated with an increased prevalence of ADHD:

- Toxin exposures (lead toxicity, fetal alcohol syndrome)
- Brain injury (traumatic, infectious)
- Tourette syndrome
- Genetic and metabolic disorders
- Recurrent otitis media
- Iron deficiency
- Malnutrition

PATHOPHYSIOLOGY

Research suggests that some cases may be related to decreases in the activity of certain brain regions, particularly the frontal lobes.

- The catecholamine neurotransmitters, dopamine and norepinephrine, are likely to be important, as the medications that are most effective for ADHD alter the levels of these neurotransmitters.
- Family and school environments can have a major influence on ADHD symptoms

GENETICS

- Risk of ADHD in first-degree relatives is approximately 25%.
- Concordance in monozygotic twins: 59% to 81%; concordance in dizygotic twins: 33%

EPIDEMIOLOGY

- Affects 3% to 5% of school-aged children
- Male:female ratio: 4:1
- Affects 1% to 2% of adults (less well studied)

COMPLICATIONS

- School failure (33% kept back a grade before reaching high school)
- Poor peer relationships
- Sleep problems (over 50%)
- Poor fine motor skills
- Increased risk of accidental injury
- Additional psychiatric diagnosis (over 50%)
- Learning disabilities (30%)

PROGNOSIS

Many individuals with ADHD are quite successful. As a group, however, individuals with ADHD tend to complete fewer years of school and have lower occupational ranks. Children with ADHD and aggressive or antisocial behaviors are at relatively high risk for continuing to demonstrate these behaviors as adults. Thus, these children will usually need to be referred for intensive treatment, including pharmacotherapy, counseling, academic interventions, and family therapy.

 Differential Diagnosis

- Medical
—Seizures (absence)
—Hypothyroidism
—Hyperthyroidism
—Hearing impairment
—Visual impairment
—Medication side effects
—Neurodegenerative disorders (early in course)
- Developmental
—Mental retardation
—Pervasive developmental disorders (autism)
- Educational
—Learning disabilities
- Psychiatric
—Depression
—Mania
—Anxiety disorders
—Oppositional defiant disorder
—Conduct disorder
—Obsessive-compulsive disorder
- Family
—Disorganized/chaotic family environment

 Data Gathering

HISTORY

Ask for a detailed description of behaviors (frequency, duration, intensity).

- When was the onset of symptoms? Symptoms of ADHD usually present prior to age 7.
- Obtain developmental, medical, family, and social history, focusing on diseases in differential diagnoses.
- Does the child finish work, chores?
- Does the child squirm or fidget?
- Does the child lose or forget things needed for homework or other tasks?
- Does the child interrupt games, questions, or conversations?
- Does the child have difficulty waiting his/her turn?
- How does the child attend to activities at home versus school? Discrepancy, especially if worse at home, suggests that other diagnoses should be considered.
- Do problem behaviors vary across activities such as tasks versus play activities? Many children with ADHD can pay attention during play activities, but not while performing tasks.

 Physical Examination

- May have "soft" neurologic signs such as overflow movements, choreiform movements, finger gnosis. These are more common in children with ADHD than in controls, but are not specific.
- The remainder of physical and neurological examination is usually normal.
- To rule out other diagnoses: examine skin for neurocutaneous syndromes, do a thorough mental status and developmental examination, and conduct hearing and vision tests.

 Laboratory Aids

TESTS

Rating Scales

- There are many rating scales to assess ADHD (see Barkley, 1998).
- Parent and teacher ratings are routine components of the assessment.
- Significant discrepancy between parent and teacher ratings is a red flag.

Other Tests

- Computerized continuous performance tasks are sometimes used, but scores on these tests are not sensitive in detecting ADHD.

 Therapy

Behavioral counseling and educational interventions are important components of treatment (see Mercugliano et al., 1998, for an in-depth discussion).

DRUGS

Methylphenidate (Ritalin)

- Efficacy
—Eighty percent of children with ADHD improve significantly; individual response is highly variable. Teacher rating scales are helpful in documenting positive response to the medication.

- Pharmacokinetics

—Onset, 20 to 30 minutes; duration, 3 to 4 hours. Slow-release form with longer duration is available.

- Dose

—0.3 to 0.6 mg/kg per dose; higher doses may be needed in some patients.

- Side effects

—Common:

- —Appetite suppression
- —Insomnia
- —Stomachaches
- —Headaches
- —Note: Somatic complaints are common in children with ADHD and should be inquired about before medication is started.

—Less Common:

- —Rebound (increased activity or moodiness as medication wears off)
- —Dizziness
- —Growth suppression (at high doses)
- —Dysphoria
- —Tics (5%–10%)
- —Tourette syndrome (1%; medication may unmask underlying disorder)
- —Excessive dose may result in tired or withdrawn appearance

- Interactions

—May inhibit metabolism of anticonvulsants, coumadin, tricyclic antidepressants
—Should not be used with MAO inhibitors
—Other sympathomimetic medications (e.g., ephedrine, pseudoephedrine) may increase side effects.
—Antihistamines may decrease efficacy.

Dextroamphetamine (Dexedrine, Adderall)

- Effects and side effects are similar to those of methylphenidate; usual dose range, 0.15 to 3 mg/kg per dose.
- Adderall and Dexedrine spansule capsules are long acting (start at 2.5–5.0 mg/d; unusual for total daily dose to exceed 30 mg).

Pemoline (Cylert)

- Onset, 1 to 2 hours
- Plasma half-life, 5 to 6 hours.
- Usual dose, 1 to 3 mg/kg/d. Liver function tests need to be monitored. Liver failure resulting in death or liver transplantation has occurred.

OTHER MEDICATIONS

Alpha-Adrenergic Agonists

- Clonidine (Catapress), Guanfacine (Tenex)
- Indications

—Nonresponders to stimulants
—Hyperactivity or aggression is the major problem.
—ADHD with tics or Tourette syndrome

- Side effects

—Sedation (very common)
—Rebound hypertension if medications are stopped suddenly
—Decreased blood pressure (dizziness)
—Depression

Tricyclic Antidepressants

- Imipramine (Tofranil), Nortriptyline (Pamelor), Desipramine (Norpramin)
- Indications

—Nonresponders to stimulants
—ADHD with tics or Tourette syndrome
—ADHD with anxiety or mood disorders

- Side effects

—Anticholinergic effects
—Cardiac arrhythmias (must monitor ECGs)
—Fatigue

- Warn families that overdoses can be fatal.

Atypical Antidepressants

- Bupropion (Wellbutrin)
- Indications

—Nonresponders to stimulants
—ADHD with anxiety or mood disorders

- Side effects

—Irritability
—Insomnia
—There is limited experience in children, but in adults, drug-induced seizures can occur, especially at high doses.

 Follow-Up

- Assess school performance.
- Check for associated behavior problems.
- Assess family and peer relationships.
- Check for medication side effects.
- Assess continuing need for medication yearly.

PITFALLS

- Lack of information on symptoms from both school and home
- Missing associated learning problems and/or psychiatric disorders
- Individual response to stimulant medication is idiosyncratic; higher doses do not always result in improvement in symptoms.

 Common Questions and Answers

Q: At what age can you begin to make the diagnosis of ADHD?
A: No lower limit has been identified. There is a wide range of normal activity levels and attention spans in preschool-aged children. Be cautious about making the diagnosis in children under the age of 4 years.

Q: Should stimulant medication be prescribed on weekends and over the summer?
A: Family and peer relationships of some children with ADHD benefit from use during these times; periods off medication may minimize the long-term effects on weight and growth. Children engaged in school-like or school-related tasks during the summer or on weekends may need to be on medication for these activities.

Q: Can methylphenidate be used to treat ADHD in children with tics or Tourette Syndrome?
A: Methylphenidate will cause an exacerbation of tics in some children with chronic tic disorder or Tourette syndrome. However, many children will not experience any significant change in tic frequency on methylphenidate. When methylphenidate is used for the treatment of ADHD in children with tics, the effects of the medication on the ADHD symptoms and the tics must be monitored. Tic rating scales are available to help with this monitoring.

Q: Can methylphenidate be used to treat ADHD in children with seizures?
A: Although the *Physicians' Desk Reference* states that methylphenidate lowers the seizure threshold, the medication can be used in children with well-controlled seizure disorders.

ICD-9-CM 314.01

BIBLIOGRAPHY

American Psychiatric Association. *Diagnostic and statistical manual of mental disorders,* 4th ed. Washington, DC: American Psychiatric Association, 1994.

Barkley RA. *Attention deficit hyperactivity disorder: a handbook for diagnosis and treatment,* 2nd ed. New York: Guilford, 1998.

Culbert TP, Banez GA, Reiff MI. Children who have attentional disorders: interventions. *Pediatr Rev* 1994:15:5–15.

Mercugliano M, Power TJ, Blum NJ. *The clinician's practical guide to attention-deficit/hyperactivity disorder.* Baltimore: Brookes, 1998.

Author: Nathan J. Blum

Atypical Mycobacterial Infections

 Database

DEFINITION

Atypical mycobacterial (ATM) infection refers to disease caused by *Mycobacterium* other than *tuberculosis, bovis,* and *leprae,* and usually involves *Mycobacterium avium-intracellularae* or *M. scrofulaceum.* These diseases are also referred to as nontuberculous mycobacterial infections, environmental mycobacterial infections, and mycobacteria other than tuberculosis (MOTT) infections.

CAUSES

• The most common associated illness is unilateral chronic cervical adenopathy/adenitis in preschool-aged children.
• In adults, ATM infection may cause a chronic single pulmonary nodule or more extensive chronic lung disease.
• In children and adults infected with HIV, disseminated disease is common, yet it is not common in other acquired or congenital immunodeficiencies that affect T-cell function.
• Rarely, it may cause otitis/mastoiditis in immunocompetent children.
• Chronic skin, bone, or soft-tissue infections may develop after trauma/surgery, usually with *M. chelonei* or *M. fortuitum* as the etiologic agents.

PATHOPHYSIOLOGY

• Organisms are ubiquitous in the environment: soil, fresh water, ocean water, home and hospital water, dust, and food (eggs, dairy products, meat).
• It is spread by aerosol inhalation or ingestion of contaminated food, dust, or water.
• Person-to-person spread has never been documented and is not a concern.

EPIDEMIOLOGY

• 80% to 90% of cases of adenitis caused by ATM infection occur in preschool-aged children (ages 1–5 years).
• Early in the HIV epidemic, the incidence rate of disseminated disease in HIV-infected adults was approximately 40%; in HIV-infected children, 10% to 20%. This rate has decreased markedly in recent years through the routine use of prophylaxis and because of the improved immunologic function in HIV-infected individuals on newer antiretroviral agents.

COMPLICATIONS

• Chronic draining of infected cervical nodes
• Rarely, pulmonary disease or dissemination
• Chronic skin/bone infections
• Disseminated disease

PROGNOSIS

• For localized adenopathy: excellent
• For disseminated disease, generally treatable in the rare immunocompetent individual
• In patients with AIDS, treatable in terms of symptom relief, but requires lifelong therapy

 Differential Diagnosis

• For unilateral adenopathy/adenitis:
—Viral/bacterial adenitis-affected nodes are tender, warm, and erythematous; usually associated with upper respiratory symptoms and/or fever.
—Cat-scratch disease (contact with cat, usually kitten). Frequently, child will have scratch/puncture mark on arm. There are rarely any systemic signs/symptoms.

• Neoplastic disease

 Data Gathering

HISTORY

• Region of residence
• Recent travel
• Length of time of adenopathy, associated systemic symptoms
• Contact with cats (for differential of cat-scratch disease or toxoplasmosis)
• Systemic symptoms, such as fever and weight loss, make neoplastic disease more likely.
• Chronic cough would suggest *M. tuberculosis.*
• Recent upper respiratory symptoms/fever suggest viral or bacterial cause.

Atypical Mycobacterial Infections

 ## Physical Examination

- Most common: Single or regional cervical adenopathy, 90% of the time, is unilateral, firm, not fixed, and not especially tender nor warm; occasionally, there is spontaneous drainage.
- Generalized adenopathy makes ATM disease unlikely.
- Systemic signs of infection are absent.
- Hepatosplenomegaly indicates other diagnosis, especially neoplastic disease or HIV-related illness.
- Normal nutritional status

 ## Laboratory Aids

- Specific PPD tests are not readily available at this time. Many children with ATM adenitis will have 5- to 10-mm reactions to standard PPD.
- Definitive diagnosis is made by isolation and identification of organism. The most frequently identified strains are: *M. avium-intracellularae, M. kansasii, M. chelonei, M. fortuitum,* and *M. scrofulaceum.*
- Normal chest radiograph
- In disseminated disease, cultures are positive from blood and bone marrow aspirates.

 ## Therapy

- Complete surgical excision for isolated adenopathy secondary to ATM; chemotherapy unnecessary in most cases.
- For disseminated or pulmonary disease, three- or four-drug treatment regimens based on sensitivity. Combinations generally include several of the following antibiotics: rifampin, isoniazid, rifabutin, clarithromycin or azithromycin, ethambutol, ciprofloxin, and amikacin.

PREVENTION

For HIV-infected children with severe immunodeficiency, prophylaxis with daily clarithromycin or rifabutin, or once-weekly azithromycin, decreases the risk of development of disseminated disease.

 ## Follow-Up

Routine follow-up should be done for 1 year after excision to monitor for possible local/contralateral recurrence.

PITFALLS

Use of incision and drainage/aspiration for treatment of adenitis, which can lead to chronically draining node. Aspiration may be needed to make the original diagnosis, but total excision results in almost 100% cure rates.

 ## Common Questions and Answers

Q: Should all cases of cervical adenitis be tested for ATM?
A: The typical case of cervical adenitis, presenting with the usual prodrome, responds rapidly to appropriate oral or parenteral antibiotics, which would not be the case if ATM were the culprit. Certainly, a PPD test should be done on all children with cervical adenitis. If the node is aspirated, in addition to routine bacterial cultures, fluid should be sent for mycobacterial culture.

Q: Should patients with disease secondary to ATM undergo a chest x-ray study?
A: Yes. Though uncommon, ATM-related pulmonary disease can be seen in children.

Q: If the node is excised, should oral therapy be instituted?
A: Most studies suggest that oral therapy is unnecessary following total excision.

ICD-9-CM 031.9

BIBLIOGRAPHY

Saitz EW. Cervical lymphadenitis caused by atypical mycobacteria. *Pediatr Clin North Am* 1981;28:823–839.

Smith MHD, Starke JR, Marquis JR. Tuberculosis and opportunistic mycobacterial infections. In: Feigin R, Cherry J, eds. *Pediatric infectious diseases,* 3rd ed. Philadelphia: WB Saunders, 1992:1354–1356.

Schaad UB, Votteler TP, McCracken GH, Nelson JD. Management of atypical mycobacterial lymphadenitis in childhood: a review based on 380 cases. *J Pediatr* 1979;95:356–360.

Taha AM, Davidson PT, Bailey WC. Surgical treatment of atypical mycobacterial lymphadenitis in children. *Pediatr Infect Dis J* 1985;4:664–667.

Author: Richard M. Rutstein

Autistic Spectrum Disorders

 Database

DEFINITION

Autism is a chronic, nonprogressive developmental disability with a classic triad of impairment in social interaction, communication, and behavior. DSM-IV categorizes autistic disorder under the more general rubric of pervasive developmental disorders, which have in common impairments in social and communicative interaction with restricted interests or repetitive behavior. IQ ranges from retarded to above average. Most, but not all, children with autism have some degree of mental retardation and may develop epilepsy.

EPIDEMIOLOGY

The estimated prevalence of autism ranges from 4 to 5 cases per 10,000 to 15 cases per 10,000.

ETIOLOGY

No single underlying cause for autism has been identified. Disorders found to be either in association with or causative for autism include:

- Prenatal: toxemia, rubella, cytomegalovirus, toxoplasmosis
- Perinatal: anoxia, trauma, hyperbilirubinemia
- Chromosomal: fragile X syndrome, trisomy 21, XYY syndrome, tuberous sclerosis
- Metabolic: phenylketonuria, hyperthyroidism, lead ingestion, histidinemia, lipidosis
- Congenital: microcephaly, hydrocephalus, Dandy-Walker syndrome
- Acquired: infantile spasms, meningitis, encephalitis

Of the hereditary diseases associated with autism, fragile X is the most commonly reported. The frequency of fragile X syndrome among autistic males is 7.7% and among autistic females is estimated at 12.3%.

CLINICAL PRESENTING SIGNS AND SYMPTOMS

- Speech and language delay
- Limited eye contact
- Severe sleep problems
- Feeding difficulties
- Signs of deafness
- Temper tantrums
- Stereotypies (i.e., rocking, hand flapping)
- Fascination with parts of toys (i.e., rotating wheels)
- Attachment to unusual objects
- Hyperactivity or hypoactivity
- Distress with changes in routine
- Little pretend or imitative play

 Differential Diagnosis

Major differential diagnoses of autistic behaviors include:

- Mental retardation
- Rett syndrome occurs only in females initially. Normal development followed by deceleration in head growth ("progressive microcephaly"), marked regression in development. Autistic features may develop with loss of purposeful hand movements, followed by repetitive hand-wringing or other repetitive behavior.
- Evidence of schizophrenia (hallucinations, delusions) excludes autism. Mental retardation is characterized by IQ,70 with delayed early milestones and delayed adaptive skills, with communication and social skills that are appropriate for mental age. Schizophrenia is characterized by periods of remission, without mental retardation; development may be normal.
- Diagnosis of attention-deficit hyperactivity disorder (ADHD) and autism are mutually exclusive diagnoses according to DSM-IV, though autistic syndromes may encompass symptoms of ADHD.

 Data Gathering

HISTORY

A complete prenatal, neonatal, and childhood history helps to detect risk factors.

- Failure to thrive due to peculiar eating habits may be noted.
- Diagnosis is frequently based on a history of impaired verbal/nonverbal communication, social isolation, poor eye contact, stereotyped behavior, resistance to change, and tactile defensiveness.
- A history of incoordination, paroxysmal disturbance suggesting epilepsy (staring spells, convulsions), and fragmented sleep are frequently present.

 Physical Examination

- Secondary growth disturbance (due to reflux, aversive feeding behavior) should be sought in growth curves.
- Evidence of self-injurious behavior (excoriations, bruising, hair loss)
- Physical findings may suggest alternate (metabolic) disorders or the underlying basis of autism:

—Long, thin face and prominent ears are characteristic of fragile X, and macroorchidism may not be present until after puberty.
—Pigmented lesions may suggest neurocutaneous syndromes, especially hypopigmented macules or fibromas indicating tuberous sclerosis.
—Microcephaly suggests TORCH infection (toxoplasmosis, rubella, cytomegalovirus, herpes infection), Angelman syndrome, or Rett syndrome.
—Macrocephaly suggests neurocutaneous disorder, storage disease, or hydrocephalus, or it may have no clear underlying cause.
—Neurologic examination: Spasticity, visual loss, or ataxia suggests leukodystrophy. Neurologic examination is necessary for assessment of stereotypic behavior, involuntary movements, abnormalities in motor coordination, and mirror or other overflow movements.
—Ophthalmologic and audiologic evaluations are necessary to rule out visual and hearing deficits.

Laboratory Aids

Neurodiagnostic tests may not be useful unless specific neurologic disorders are suspected. While some studies suggest minor structural abnormalities of the brain in autism (e.g., small cerebellum, open operculum), such findings are of limited diagnostic or practical value.

TESTS

- EEG

—*Significance:* 20% to 40% of autistic patients develop seizures.

- Chromosomes/fragile X

—*Significance:* appropriate for all autistic patients; helpful for genetic counseling

- Inborn error screen

—*Significance*: to detect PKU, other amino acid disorders.

- Head MRI/CT

—*Significance:* focal neurologic deficit to evaluate structural CNS abnormalities of cortex, cerebellum, brainstem, microcephaly/macrocephaly

- TORCH (toxoplasmosis, rubella, cytomegalovirus, herpesvirus) titers

—*Significance:* microcephaly

- Complete blood count

—*Significance:* growth delay, hyperactivity, pica

- Blood lead level

—*Significance:* lead intoxication

- Thyroid function tests

—*Significance:* for hypothyroidism

- Audiogram/BAER

—*Significance:* speech and language delay, signs of hearing loss

 ## Therapy

MEDICAL MANAGEMENT

Though pharmacological therapy is frequently unsuccessful, target symptoms for a trial of medical therapy include:

- Self-injurious behavior: fenfluramine, naltrexone
- Sleep disturbances: benzodiazepines, melatonin
- Seizures: barbiturates (may worsen hyperactivity), carbamazepine, phenytoin, valproate, others
- Motor hyperactivity: clonidine, tricyclic antidepressants, methylphenidate (may worsen symptoms)
- Violent rages: lithium, tricyclic antidepressants, L-dopa. Autistic children generally get worse on stimulants, with increased stereotypies and worsening behavior. Neuroleptics (dopamine blockers) such as haloperidol and fluphenazine and resperidone decrease behavioral symptoms and can increase learning; morbidity includes movement disorders (tardive dyskinesias), risk of neuroleptic malignant syndrome. Clonidine is often the mainstay of treatment.

EDUCATIONAL/PSYCHOSOCIAL/MEDICAL MANAGEMENT

- A complete psychoeducational assessment and treatment plan for intellectual, developmental, adaptive, functional, communication, and social skills is warranted.
- Psychotherapy has not been effective.
- Behavioral therapies may improve patient/family outcomes.

PITFALLS

- Social deficits—not speech, language, or IQ—are the hallmarks of the disease.
- Symptoms of autism—especially social isolation—may worsen on stimulants.
- Subclinical seizure types, including absence spells, may be detected only on EEG.

 ## Follow-Up

Development of language in the preschool years is the best prognostic indicator. If there is no language by age 5 to 6 years, language development is unlikely and the probable outcome is poor. Prognosis is closely linked to cognitive ability and acquisition of social and communication skills; autistic children require lifelong treatment and support.

 ## Common Questions and Answers

Q: What are the chances of having a second child with autism?
A: Several studies do show an increased risk of autism in families with a single case, even without any other features of a heritable cause of autism.

Q: What is the value of brain imaging in autism?
A: MRI may help diagnose a heritable syndrome with genetic counseling implications (e.g., leukodystrophy, tuberous sclerosis).

ICD-9-CM 299.0

BIBLIOGRAPHY

Edwards DR, Bristol MM. Autism: early identification and management in family practice. *Am Fam Pract* 1991;44(5):1755–1764.

Freeman BJ, Ritvo ER. The syndrome of autism: establishing the diagnosis and principles of management. *Pediatr Ann* 1984;13:284–290.

Minshew NJ, Payton JB. New perspectives in autism: Part II. The differential diagnosis and neurobiology of autism. *Curr Probl Pediatr* 1988;18:613–694.

Olsson I, Steffenburg S, Gilberg C. Epilepsy in autism and autisticlike conditions: a population based study. Arch Neurol 1988;45:666–668.

Piven J. The biological basis of autism. *Curr Opin Neurobiol* 1997;7(5):708–712.

Wing L. The autistic spectrum. *Lancet* 1997;350(9093):1761–1766.

Author: Patricia T. Molloy

Autoimmune Hemolytic Anemia

 Database

DEFINITION

Autoimmune hemolytic anemia (AIHA) is characterized by shortened red-cell survival that is caused by autoantibodies directed against red blood cells, with or without the participation of complement on the red-cell membrane.

CAUSES

- Idiopathic
- Passive transfer of maternal antibodies
- Secondary to an underlying disorder

—Infection: viral (e.g., *Mycoplasma,* Epstein-Barr virus [EBV], cytomegalovirus [CMV], hepatitis, HIV) or bacterial (e.g., *Streptococcus,* typhoid fever, *Escherichia coli* septicemia)
—Drugs: antimalarials, antipyretics, sulfonamides, penicillin, rifampin
—Hematologic disorders: leukemia, lymphoma
—Immunopathic/autoimmune disorders: lupus, Wiskott-Aldrich syndrome, ulcerative colitis, rheumatoid arthritis, scleroderma
—Tumors: ovarian, carcinomas, thymomas, dermoid cysts

PATHOPHYSIOLOGY

- Warm autoantibodies

—Maximal activity of in vitro red-cell binding at 37°C
—IgG-class antibody usually with relative specificity for Rh erythrocyte antigens
—IgG-coated RBCs cleared predominantly in the spleen by macrophages
—Complement not required for clearance, although complement fixation may contribute to clearance

- Cold autoantibodies (cold agglutinins)

—Maximal activity of in vitro red-cell binding at temperatures between 0°C and 30°C
—Almost always caused by IgM antibody with specificity for antigens of the i/T system on RBCs
—Anti-i antibodies characteristic of *Mycoplasma pneumoniae*-associated hemolysis
—Anti-i antibodies usually found in infectious mononucleosis
—IgM-coated RBCs are cleared primarily in the liver by hepatic macrophage C3b receptors.
—Hemolysis is complement-dependent.

- Paroxysmal cold hemoglobinuria (PCH)

—IgG autoantibody binds RBC at cooler areas of the body (i.e., extremities), causing irreversible binding of complement components (C3 and C4). When coated RBCs enter warmer areas of the body, IgG falls off and complement causes hemolysis (Donath-Landsteiner biphasic hemolysin).
—Unusual IgG antibody with anti-P specificity
—Most frequently found in children with viral infections (30%)

EPIDEMIOLOGY

- Occurs at an incidence of about 1:50,000 to 80,000 persons per year
- Less common in children and adolescents than in adults
- No apparent racial or sexual preponderance (in childhood)
- Peak incidence in childhood is in first 4 years of life with warm AIHA.
- Mortality in pediatric series ranged from 9% to 19%.

COMPLICATIONS

- Heart failure may be seen in severe anemia; requires aggressive supportive care.
- Morbidity is usually secondary to treatment (see Therapy section).

PROGNOSIS

Dependent on age, underlying disorder (if any), and response to therapy. See also in Data Gathering section, Natural History.

 Differential Diagnosis

- Defects intrinsic to RBC

—Membrane defects
—Enzyme defects
—Hemoglobin defects
—Congenital dyserythropoietic anemias
—Paroxysmal nocturnal hemoglobinuria

- Defects extrinsic to RBC

—Immune-mediated
  —Isoimmune: hemolytic disease of the newborn, blood-group incompatibility
  —Autoimmune: see in Database section, Causes
—Drug-dependent red-cell antibodies
—Nonimmune mediated
  —Idiopathic
  —Secondary to an underlying disorder (i.e., hemolytic uremic syndrome [HUS], thrombotic thrombocytopenic purpura [TTP])
  —Mechanical: march hemoglobinuria, heart valves

 Data Gathering

NATURAL HISTORY

- Acute disease

—Onset with rapid fall in hemoglobin level over hours to days
—Usual course: complete resolution of disease within 3 to 6 months
—Resolution more likely in children who present between 2 and 12 years of age

- Chronic disease

—Slower onset of anemia over weeks to months, with some having persistence of hemolysis or intermittent relapses
—More likely to be associated with underlying disorder
—More common in adults and children <2 years or >12 years of age

HISTORY

- Pallor
- Jaundice
- Dark urine
- Fever
- Weakness
- Dizziness
- Syncope
- Exercise intolerance

 Physical Examination

- Pallor
- Jaundice
- Splenomegaly
- Hepatomegaly
- Tachycardia, systolic flow murmur
- Orthostasis in acute onset

 Laboratory Aids

- CBC: Hb level decreased (occasionally, thrombocytopenia seen in Evan syndrome); MCV may be normal
- Reticulocyte count increased
- Peripheral smear: spherocytes, polychromasia, macrocytes, rouleaux formation
- Direct antiglobulin test (Coombs): positive

—Single most important test
—Warm AIHA will have IgG ± C3 positive
—Cold AIHA and PCH will have C3 positive

- Haptoglobin level decreased
- Indirect hyperbilirubinemia
- Elevated LDH
- Urinalysis: hemoglobinuria, increased urobilinogen
- Bone marrow aspiration—erythroid hyperplasia (to rule out leukemia or lymphoma associated with AIHA)
- Cold agglutinin titer: positive (usually 1:64)
- Donath-Landsteiner test should be performed in cases of suspected PCH.

PITFALLS

A negative Coombs test can occur when small numbers of IgG or C3 molecules are present on the red-cell membrane (i.e., in cases of less severe hemolysis). Radiolabeled Coombs test or enzyme immunoassays are more sensitive diagnostic tests in these circumstances. Reticulocytopenia may occur in most severe cases where the antibody coats and removes reticulocytes.

Therapy

PATIENT MONITORING

- Hemoglobin level q4h to q12h (depending on severity)
- Reticulocyte count: daily
- Spleen size: daily
- Hemoglobinuria: daily
- Coombs test: weekly

BLOOD TRANSFUSION

- Indication

—Blood transfusion is indicated in cases of physiologic compromise from the anemia (usually only in severe acute onset) or with continued blood loss.

- Complications

—The blood bank may be unable to find compatible blood. In IgG-mediated disease, autoantibody is usually panreactive; therefore, you must use the least incompatible unit of blood. In cold agglutinin disease, you must prewarm all infusions to decrease IgM binding and must monitor for acute hemolysis during transfusion.

- Dose

—Use only a volume of blood sufficient to relieve compromise from anemia.

CORTICOSTEROIDS

- Indication

—In IgG-mediated disease, steroids have been shown to interfere with macrophage Fc and C3b receptors responsible for RBC destruction. They also have been shown to elute IgG Ab from the RBC surface (improving survival).
—In chronic warm AIHA, pulsed high-dose dexamethasone has been shown to be effective in some cases.

- Complications

—There are both short- and long-term side effects of steroids. Corticosteroids are generally not effective in cold agglutinin disease.

- Dose

—Start prednisone PO/methylprednisolone IV at 2 mg/kg/d in divided doses. Tapering of steroids should begin once a therapeutic response is achieved (may take several weeks to months). Alternative treatments should be considered for patients unresponsive to steroids or who require high doses for maintenance of hemoglobin level.

- Goal

—The goal is initially to return to normal hemoglobin level with nontoxic levels of steroid, or no steroids. However, in some patients, the goal may be achieving decreased hemolysis and a clinically asymptomatic state with minimal steroid side effects.

INTRAVENOUS IMMUNE GLOBULIN (IVIG)

- Indication

—IVIG may be useful in selected cases of immune hemolytic anemia unresponsive to steroids. The mechanism of action is not entirely clear.

- Complications

—The effect is usually temporary; retreatment may be required q3 to q4 weeks. There may be a risk of hepatitis C. IVIG is expensive.

- Dose

—Up to 1 g/kg/d for 5 days has been required to achieve a beneficial effect.

PLASMAPHERESIS/EXCHANGE TRANSFUSION

- Indication

—This treatment will slow the rate of hemolysis in severe disease.

- Complications

—It is only of short-term benefit and is expensive.

- Dose

—The frequency and duration depend on response.

SPLENECTOMY

- Indication

—Patients unresponsive to medical management, who require moderate to high maintenance doses of steroids or who develop steroid intolerance may be candidates for splenectomy. It is not effective in cold agglutinin disease.

- The response rate is about 50% to 70%, with the majority only partial remissions.
- Complications

—There is a high morbidity rate for the surgical procedure and during the postoperative period.
—There is an increased risk of sepsis.

IMMUNOSUPPRESSIVE AGENTS (ANTIMETABOLITES, ALKYLATING AGENTS)

- Indication

—When there is a clinically unacceptable degree of hemolysis that is refractory to steroids and splenectomy, immunosuppressive agents are indicated. Some have been effective in cold agglutinin disease.

- Complications

—There are varying side effects dependent on the agent used. Therefore, clinical indications must be strong and exposure to drug should be limited.

- Dose

—Adjusted to maintain WBC>2000, ANC>1000, and platelet count at 50,000 to 100,000 cells/mm³

PROGNOSIS

Dependent on age, underlying disorder (if any), and response to therapy. See also in Data Gathering section, Natural History.

 Common Questions and Answers

Q: Will the anemia go away?
A: Children with cold autoantibodies tend to have short-lived illness, whereas children with warm antibodies often have a chronic clinical course characterized by periods of remissions and relapses.

Q: Is this contagious?
A: No. Another child may acquire the same viral illness, however the body's response to produce an autoantibody is dependent on the individual patient.

ICD-9-CM 283.0

BIBLIOGRAPHY

Domen RE. An overview of immune hemolytic anemias. *Cleve Clin J Med* 1998;65(2):89–99.

Engelfriet CP, Overbeeke MAM, Kr. von dem Borne AEG. Autoimmune hemolytic anemia. *Semin Hematol* 1992;29(1):3–12.

Lanzkowsky P. Hemolytic anemia. In: Lanzkowsky P, ed. *Manual of pediatric hematology and oncology.* New York: Churchill Livingstone, 1989:83–122.

Mathew P, Chen G, Wang W. Evans syndrome; results of a national survey. *J Pediatr Hematol Oncol* 1997;19(5):433–437.

Meyer O, Stahl D, Beckhove P, Huhn D, Salama A. Pulsed high-dose dexamethasone in chronic autoimmune hemolytic anemia of warm type. *Br J Haematol* 1997;98(4):860–862.

Ware RE, Rosse WF. Autoimmune hemolytic anemia. In: Nathan DG, Oski FA, eds. *Hematology of infancy and childhood,* 5th ed., Philadelphia: WB Saunders, 1998:499–522.

Author: Deborah L. Kramer

Avascular (Aseptic) Necrosis of the Femoral Head (Hip)

 Database

DEFINITION

Avascular (aseptic) necrosis (AVN) results from the interruption of the blood supply of bone (either traumatic or nontraumatic occlusion). The femoral head is the most common site of AVN.

CAUSES

- Traumatic

—After fracture
—After hip dislocation
—After slipped capitol femoral epiphysis
—After casting, bracing, surgery

- Nontraumatic

—Idiopathic (older, after physeal closure); similar to adult AVN
—Idiopathic (younger, before physeal closure); see Perthes
—Caisson disease
—With sickle cell disease
—After septic arthritis
—With steroids or chemotherapy

PATHOPHYSIOLOGY

- Death and necrosis of bone with gradual return of blood supply
- Necrotic bone gradually resorbed and replaced by new bone

EPIDEMIOLOGY

- Variable, depending on cause

GENETICS

- Variable, depending on cause

COMPLICATIONS

- Decreased range of motion
- Osteoarthritis
- Physeal arrest with growth disturbance

PROGNOSIS

- Variable, depending on cause

 Differential Diagnosis

- Trauma

—Osteochondral fracture
—Impaction fracture
—Epiphyseal/physeal fracture

- Infection

—Osteomyelitis
—Septic arthritis

- Neoplastic process

—Epiphyseal tumors (chondroblastoma, Trevoir disease, et al.)

- Rheumatologic processes

 Data Gathering

HISTORY

- Onset (gradual or after traumatic event)
- Association with:

—Trauma
—Medications (steroids or chemotherapy)
—Casting, splinting, surgery (iatrogenic)
—Pain, limping?
—Stiffness (decreased range of motion)

 Physical Examination

- Gait

—Limping
—Antalgic
—Trendelenburg gait

- Range of motion

—Flexion and extension
—Abduction and adduction
—Internal and external rotation

- Hip joint irritability (short arc rotation)
- Sign of other disease process (e.g., sickle cell disease)
- Physical examination trick

—Loss of internal rotation is usually the first and most affected loss of motion seen.

Avascular (Aseptic) Necrosis of the Femoral Head (Hip)

 Laboratory Aids

TESTS

Laboratory examinations should be normal in most forms of AVN of the femoral head.

Imaging

- Usual

—Sclerosis
—Subchondral fracture
—Collapse
—Reossification
—Repair

- Variable

—Cysts
—Physeal growth arrest (young)
—Early osteoarthritis
—Subluxation

 Therapy

DRUGS

- NSAIDs may be effective in decreasing associated inflammation.
- If associated with steroid use, discontinuation or elimination if possible

TREATMENT PRINCIPLES

- Maintain range of motion (physical therapy, traction, continuous passive motion).
- Contain the femoral head in the acetabulum (see Perthes principles).
- Surgery
- Redirectional osteotomy
- Femoral or acetabular (see containment operations of Perthes)
- Core decompression to introduce new blood supply

DURATION OF THERAPY

- Variable, depending on cause

DIET

- Thought not to alter disease process; recommend general balanced diet

 Follow-Up

WHEN TO EXPECT IMPROVEMENT

- Variable, depending on cause

SIGNS TO WATCH FOR

- Subluxation
- Early osteoarthritis
- Growth arrest

PROGNOSIS

- Overall, good if mild involvement (usual) and patient is young
- See Prevention below

PREVENTION

- Traumatic

—After fracture: early anatomic reduction and stable internal fixation is key.
—After hip dislocation: early reduction is key.
—After slipped capitol femoral epiphysis: associated with unstable grade 3 slips.
—After casting, bracing, surgery: prevention is key.

- Nontraumatic

—Idiopathic (older, after physeal closure); similar to adult AVN
—Idiopathic (younger, before physeal closure): see Perthes disease
—Caisson disease: rare now
—With sickle cell disease: good medical management key
—After septic arthritis: early surgical drainage of hip key to prevention
—With steroids or chemotherapy: do not use unless no other alternatives.

Common Questions and Answers

Q: What type of medication is associated with AVN of the hip?
A: Steroids

Q: For AVN in children, is younger or older age associated with a better prognosis?
A: Younger age

ICD-9-CM
Legg Perthe 732.1
Avascular necrosis 733.40

BIBLIOGRAPHY

Lahdes-Vasama T, Lamminen A, Merikanto J, Marttinen E. The value of MRI in early Perthes' disease: an MRI study with a 2-year follow-up. *Pediatr Radiol* 1997;27(6):517–522.

Author: John P. Dormans

Babesiosis

 Database

DEFINITION

Human babesiosis is a tick-borne malaria-like illness characterized by fever, malaise, and hemolytic anemia. Most infected individuals are asymptomatic.

CAUSES

- Human babesiosis is caused by the intra-erythrocytic parasite of the *Babesia* genus.
- In the northeast United States, *Babesia microti* is transmitted by *Ixodes dammini*, the same tick responsible for Lyme disease.
- A babesiosis-like syndrome caused by the WA1 protozoan is found in the western part of the United States.
- Rarely, the disease has been acquired through transfusion of contaminated blood products or vertical transmission from mother to fetus.

PATHOPHYSIOLOGY

- A bite from an infected tick transmits the protozoa.
- The incubation period is usually 1 to 4 weeks but can be as long as 9 weeks.
- Infection of the erythrocyte causes membrane damage and lysis, which promotes adherence to the endothelium and microvascular stasis.
- The spleen plays an important role in decreasing the protozoal load by filtering abnormally shaped infected red blood cells (RBCs) and antibody production.

EPIDEMIOLOGY

- The first case in the United States was reported from California in 1966.
- The most severely affected are those who are at the extremes of age, functionally or anatomically asplenic, or otherwise immunocompromised.
- Transmission usually occurs in the summer and early fall.
- Most cases have been reported from the northeast United States and the West Coast. Endemic areas include Rhode Island, Massachusetts, and New York. There also have been cases from Maryland, Virginia, Georgia, Wisconsin, and Minnesota.

COMPLICATIONS

- Rarely fatal in the United States.
- Pancytopenia and overwhelming secondary bacterial sepsis may occur.
- Other unusual complications in adults include:

—Pulmonary edema and adult respiratory distress syndrome, often happening after treatment has begun.
—Renal failure
—Hemophagocytic syndrome
—Seizures

- Those coinfected with Lyme disease are more susceptible to more severe disease and complications.

ASSOCIATED ILLNESSES

It is estimated that 23% of patients have concurrent Lyme disease.

 Differential Diagnosis

- Infection
- Nonspecific viral syndrome
- Malaria

 Data Gathering

- Few patients recall a tick bite.
- Patients live in or have had recent travel to an endemic region.
- Initial symptoms are vague and may include progressive fatigue, malaise, and anorexia, accompanied by intermittent fevers as high as 40°C.
- Chills, myalgias, and arthralgias may follow these symptoms.
- Less common complaints include headache, cough, sore throat, abdominal pain, and emotional lability.

 Physical Examination

- Often, fever is the only finding.
- Some may have a mildly enlarged liver and/or splenomegaly.
- Jaundice or hematuria may also be seen.
- Petechaie and ecchymosis are rare.

 Laboratory Aids

SPECIFIC TESTS

- Giemsa- or Wright-stained thick and thin blood smears can be used to microscopically identify the organism.
- Indirect immunofluorescent assay (IFA) is antigen-specific for *B. microti* and can be used when blood smears are negative. In general, a titer ≥1:64 indicates exposure, and titers ≥1:256 suggest acute infection. In endemic areas, the IFA test has a sensitivity of 91% and a specificity of 99%.
- Polymerase chain reaction (PCR) is highly specific.
- Isolation of the parasite can be done by intraperitoneal injection of a patient's blood into a golden hamster, but this takes weeks to perform.

OTHER TESTS

Most of the abnormal routine tests are the result of hemolysis.

- Urinalysis: proteinuria, hemoglobinuria
- Complete blood count: normocytic/normochromic anemia, thrombcytopenia, and atypical lymphocytosis
- Possible positive Coombs test
- Elevated erythrocyte sedimentation rate
- Liver function tests: elevated bilirubin, lactate dehydrogenase, and liver transaminases

In asymptomatic patients, these tests are often normal.

FALSE NEGATIVES

- The blood smears may not demonstrate the protozoan at low levels of parasitemia.
- Serologic false positives for *B. micoti* include cross-reactivity with other *Babesia* species or malarial organisms.
- Theoretical serologic false positives for WA1: rheumatoid factor, antinuclear antibody and antibody to *Toxoplasma gondii*.

Therapy

- Those with mild clinical disease usually recover without treatment.
- Asplenic, immunodeficient, or symptomatic patients should be treated with clindamycin and quinine.

—The dose of clindamycin is 20 to 40 mg/kg/day divided into three doses for 7 days.
—Quinine is dosed 10 to 25 mg/kg/day divided into three doses for 7 days.

- For life-threatening infections, exchange transfusion has been successful. Progressive respiratory distress may require mechanical ventilation.

 ## Follow-Up

WHEN TO EXPECT IMPROVEMENT

- Those who are only mildly affected usually have resolution of their symptoms over a few weeks.
- For the severely affected and immunodeficient patients, the convalescent period may be as long as 18 months.

SIGNS TO WATCH FOR

- Respiratory distress, especially after treatment has begun
- Pancytopenia and lymphadenopathy: may indicate the development of hemophagocytic syndrome

PITFALLS

- Children who are from endemic areas and have an acute febrile illness may be misdiagnosed with a nonspecific viral illness.
- One should be suspicious for a coinfection with Lyme disease in those who are not responding to standard therapy.
- Delayed recognition of this uncommon disease may be life threatening in the immunocompromised patient.

PREVENTION

- Prevention begins with avoidance of tick bites.
- For most individuals, simple measures include wearing long-sleeved shirts and long pants, with pants tucked into the socks in tick-infested areas.
- Light clothing will make ticks easier to see.
- Spraying the bottoms of one's pants with a tick repellent may also be helpful.
- Children and dogs should be inspected for ticks after being outside.
- High-risk individuals may want to avoid endemic areas from May to September.
- In endemic regions, transfusion-related cases can be decreased by PCR screening of blood or rejecting donors who have had a recent tick bite or fever.
- Currently, no prophylaxis treatment after a tick bite is recommended.

 ## Common Questions and Answers

Q: How long does a tick have to be attached for infection to occur?
A: In general, successful transmission requires at least 24 hours of attachment.

Q: How should a tick be removed?
A: The tick should be grasped with forceps as close to its head as possible and pulled straight up. If possible, it should be saved for identification.

Q: Does infection confer lifetime immunity?
A: Reinfection is possible.

ICD-9-CM 088.82

BIBLIOGRAPHY

American Academy of Pediatrics. *Babesiosis. Red book: report of the Committee of Infectious Diseases.* Washington, DC: American Academy of Pediatrics, 1997:146–147.

Boustani MR, Gelfand JA. Babesiosis. *Clin Infect Dis* 1996;22:611–615.

Krause PJ, Telford SR, Pollack RJ, Ryan R, Brassard P, Zemel L, Spielman A. Babesiosis: an underdiagnosed disease in children. *Pediatrics* 1992;89:1045–1048.

Krause PJ, Telford S, Spielman A, et al. Comparison of PCR with blood smear and inoculation of small animals for diagnosis of Babesia mictoi parasitemia. *J Clin Microbiol* 1996;34:2791–2794.

Krause PJ, Telford SR, Spielman A, Sikand V, et al. Concurrent Lyme disease and babesiosis. Evidence for increased severity and duration of illness. *JAMA* 1996;275:1657–1660.

Krause PJ, Ryan R, Telford S, Persing D, Spielman A. Efficacy of immunoglobulin M serodiagnostic test for rapid diagnosis of acute babesiosis. *J Clin Microbiol* 1996;34:2014–2016.

Author: Frances M. Nadel

Balanitis

 Database

DEFINITION

- Inflammation of glans penis and foreskin
- Posthitis: inflammation of the mucous membrane surface of prepuce
- Balanoposthitis: inflammation of the penile skin

CAUSES

- Infectious agents: anaerobic fusospirochetal organisms, skin flora; *Staphylococcus, Streptococcus*
- Sexually transmitted organisms: *Chlamydia, Mycoplasma, Trichomonas*
- Yeasts: *Candida*
- Miscellaneous: amoeba
- Chronic irritation: wet diapers, poor hygiene, smegma, soap
- Traumatic etiologies: zipper injuries

 Differential Diagnosis

- Infectious
- Traumatic
- Irritative

 Data Gathering

HISTORY

- May have malodorous purulent discharge
- Ulcers with erosion of mucosa
- Trauma (i.e., hair around coronal sulcus) or use of chemical irritants
- Sexual intercourse
- Chlamydial: may be associated with proctitis or nongonococcal urethritis
- Candidal: history of diabetes mellitus in host; 10% are recurrent
- Trichomonal: often have urethritis

 Physical Examination

- Erythema of glans and prepuce
- Discharge with edema of glans
- Gangrenous balanoposthitis: anaerobic infection of glans penis, causing erosion and ulceration
- Candidal: glazed appearance with satellite pustules
- Syphilitic-multilocular pustules

COMPLICATIONS

- Preputial fissures and fibrosis if recurrent (i.e., candidal)
- Rupture of prepuce associated with amoebal infection

Laboratory Aids

- Darkfield examination to rule out *Treponema pallidum*
- Gram stain
- Cultures for specific organisms

 Therapy

SYMPTOMATIC

- Frequent sitz baths
- Hydrogen peroxide soaks: help reverse the anaerobic process
- If superficial, topical antibiotic ointment may be adequate.
- If cellulitis is present with fever, systemic antibiotics are indicated, including coverage for *Staphylococcus* and *Streptococcus*.
- Spirochetal: penicillin
- Candidal: anticandidal agents; partner should be treated
- Trichomonal: metronidazole; partner should be treated
- Mycoplasmal or chlamydial: tetracycline; partner should be treated
- Amoebal: emetine

 Follow-Up

- Penile hygiene is reviewed.
- The condition often is not recurrent; therefore circumcision after one episode is not absolutely necessary.

SURGICAL THERAPY

- Circumcision is recommended if there are recurrent episodes, and is performed after edema subsides from acute episode.
- In the acute phase, a dorsal slit may be required because of edema causing phimosis (i.e., amoebal).

 Common Questions and Answers

Q: Can swimming in swimming pools cause this?
A: No.

ICD-9-CM 607.1

BIBLIOGRAPHY

Brown MR, Cartwright PC, Snow BW. Common office problems in pediatric urology and gynecology. *Pediatr Clin North Am* 1997;44(5):1100.

Vohra S, Badlani G. Balanitis and balanoposthitis. *Urol Clin North Am* 1992;19:143.

Author: Christina Lin Master

Barotitis

Database

DEFINITION

Barotrauma of the middle or inner ear, most often caused by scuba diving or flying.

PATHOPHYSIOLOGY

• The eustachian tube is responsible for equalizing pressure of middle ear to external ear or environment. Differences in the atmospheric pressure between the inner ear, middle ear, and the environment result in injury to the middle and/or inner ear. When ambient pressure decreases (e.g., airplane ascent) the tympanic membrane bulges outward and the eustachian tube vents the excess middle ear pressure. (With a functioning eustachian tube, barotitis does not develop; the pressure is easily equalized.) When ambient pressure increases (e.g., scuba diving, airplane descent) the tympanic membrane bulges inward and the eustachian tube resists inward flow of air to the middle ear. (Even with a normally functioning eustachian tube, pressure equalization is difficult.)
• Middle ear barotitis results in vascular engorgement, bleeding, and exudate formation.
• Inner ear barotrauma can cause labyrinthine window rupture.
• At a pressure differential of 60 mm Hg (greater ambient to middle ear pressure), subjective discomfort is reported. At a pressure differential of 90 mm Hg, the eustachian tube becomes "locked," because the palatal musculature is not strong enough to open the tube and air will not be able to enter the middle ear to equalize the pressure. The tympanic membrane can rupture at pressure differentials over 100 to 500 mm Hg.
• Barotitis is sometimes classified using Teed's classification of disease severity; see Physical Examination section.

EPIDEMIOLOGY

• Significant disease is uncommon in commercial (pressurized) aircraft, although mild negative pressure of the middle ear is common after flying.
• Significant symptoms or injury can occur in scuba divers, and those who fly military aircraft and experience rapid altitude changes during tactical maneuvers.

COMPLICATIONS

• Vertigo
• Hearing loss
• Tympanic membrane rupture
• Oval or round window rupture
• Hemorrhage

PROGNOSIS

• Complete spontaneous resolution in mild cases
• Rarely, tympanotomy or tympanostomy is required to relieve pressure and pain, as well as prevent complications.
• Variable outcome for auditory and vestibular symptoms and injuries to inner ear

Differential Diagnosis

INFECTION

Otitis media with effusion can cause decreased hearing, sensation of fullness, tympanic membrane hyperemia, and pain.

TRAUMA

• Blunt trauma to the tympanic membrane (e.g., cotton swabs) can cause rupture and bleeding.
• Exposure to extremely loud noise can result in pain and hearing loss.

Data Gathering

HISTORY

• Questions regarding exposure to pressure change (diving or flying) or trauma (ear clapping, "heavy metal" concert) are critical to making the proper diagnosis.
• Ear pain, sensation of pressure, and decreased hearing are the most common symptoms.
• Symptoms of inner ear damage may include vestibular and/or auditory complaints.

Physical Examination

Teed's Classification:

Grade 0: Normal

Grade 1: Retraction, redness in Schrapnell membrane and along manubrium

Grade 2: Retraction, with redness of entire ear drum

Grade 3: Grade 2 plus hemotympanum or clear exudate

Grade 4: Perforation of tympanic membrane

• Nystagmus
• Hearing loss

Laboratory Aids

TESTS

Hearing Tests

• Should be performed on all patients who have signs of barotrauma, and on patients with normal physical examinations but who are symptomatic.

Radiographic Studies

• MRI: may be indicated in patients with vestibular symptoms or hearing loss to rule out inner ear damage.

 ## Therapy

• When diving or descending in an airplane, performing a Valsalva maneuver (blowing the nose while pinching the nostrils closed) will force air into the middle ear via the eustachian tube, thereby equalizing the pressure between the middle ear and the environment.
• Swallowing, yawning, and chewing can aid release of pressure through the eustachian tube when ascending in an airplane or when returning to the surface when scuba diving.
• A Politzer bag is an instrument used for clearing pressure disequilibrium that has not improved with Valsalva maneuvers and a trial of decongestants. (See Brown, 1994, for a description of the device and its use.)
• Otovent is another instrument that can be used for treatment or prevention. Usage can be taught to children as young as 2 to 6 years of age.
• Severe disease may require tympanotomy or tympanostomy to relieve pressure.
• For the patient with excruciating pain or unrelenting eustachian tube dysfunction, myringotomy is effective. It is best performed by an otorhinolaryngologist.

DRUGS

• Nasal decongestant sprays may be helpful by constricting mucosal arterioles and enhancing eustachian tube function. Topical decongestants are used 1 hour prior to plane travel/diving and one-half hour prior to plane descent.
• Oral decongestants may be helpful through the same physiologic pathway as topical agents. They should be initiated 1 to 2 days prior to the expected pressure change.
• Antihistamines may also be helpful by reducing mucosal edema and enhancing the eustachian tube orifice. They can be used on the day of the expected pressure change.

 ## Follow-Up

• Pressure differential without damage to the middle or inner ear usually resolves within a few days of returning to normal atmospheric pressure.
• Barotitis that resulted in injury to the middle or inner ear has a variable rate of improvement; some damage is permanent (e.g., organ of Corti), while other injury is reversible (e.g., tympanic membrane).

PREVENTION

• Travel in commercial aircraft will generally not result in severe barotitis.
• Most items in the Therapy section can be used as prevention: antihistamines, decongestants, avoidance of dehydration, frequent Valsalva maneuver, Otovent use, and so on.
• Ascend and descend carefully when scuba diving.
• Avoid dehydration and the resulting thickened secretions that may interfere with eustachian tube function.

 ## Common Questions and Answers

Q: Is the Valsalva maneuver also effective on plane ascent?
A: Yes, creating even greater pressure in the middle ear by performing the Valsalva maneuver can overcome a resistant eustachian tube and result in sudden venting of increased middle ear pressure.

Q: Can children with otitis media travel in airplanes?
A: Yes, Weiss and Frost (1987) have shown that commercial air travel did not result in worsening of symptoms, and, in fact, the presence of otitis media with effusion seemed protective against barotitis.

Q: How can I help my baby not have ear pain when traveling in an airplane?
A: Have the child nurse, take a bottle, or eat during ascent and descent. This will result in pharyngeal movements that will repeatedly open the eustachian tube and equalize middle ear pressure to environmental pressure. Also, if the child is currently experiencing an upper respiratory infection, use of decongestants prior to flight may be helpful.

ICD-9-CM 993.0

BIBLIOGRAPHY

Brown TP. Middle ear symptoms while flying: ways to prevent a severe outcome. *Postgrad Med* 1994;96:135–142.

Nakashima T, Itoh M, Sato M, Watanabe Y, Yanagita N. Auditory and vestibular disorders due to barotrauma. *Ann Otol Rhinol Laryngol* 1988;97:146–152.

Stangerup SE, Tjernstrom O, Harcourt J, Klokker M, Stokholm J. Barotitis in children after aviation: prevalence and treatment with Otovent. *J Laryngol Otol* 1996;110:625–628.

Weiss MH, Frost O. May children with otitis media with effusion safely fly? *Clin Pediatr* 1987;26:567–568.

Author: Laura N. Sinai

Bell Palsy

 Database

DEFINITION

An acute, unilateral palsy of the upper and lower musculature of the face due to involvement of the facial nerve.

- Many cases are likely secondary to a virally induced neuritis. Causative agents include herpes simplex virus (HSV), varicella-zoster virus (VZV), Epstein-Barr virus (EBV), and coxsackie, influenza, and mumps viruses.
- Other cases may occur as a result of trauma or Lyme disease.
- Ramsay Hunt syndrome: characterized by unilateral facial paralysis and severe otalgia, associated with the appearance of a periauricular/auricular vesicular eruption (12% of all facial paralysis).

PATHOPHYSIOLOGY

- Facial nerve (Cranial Nerve VII) has motor, sensory, and autonomic components.
- In viral infections, viral reactivation followed by replication within the ganglion cells leads to inflammation of Schwann cells. Ultimately, an autoimmune response leads to demyelinization and hypofunction of the involved nerve.
- Blunt trauma to the temporal bone/mastoid area can also directly injure the facial nerve.

EPIDEMIOLOGY

- Incidence is 2.7 per 100,000 in children less than 10 years of age; and 10.1 per 100,000 in children 10 to 20 years of age.
- In children 10 to 20 years of age, girls are affected twice as much as boys.
- Less than 1% of cases are bilateral.
- The recurrence rate is 10%.

COMPLICATIONS

- Corneal abrasions
- Keratitis
- Facial contractures
- Synkinesis
- Facial tics
- Gustatory tearing (crocodile tears)
- Recurrent facial palsy (should cause one to reconsider the diagnosis)

PROGNOSIS

- More than 60% of children will recover completely.
- Improvement in symptoms usually begins within 2 to 4 weeks, and reaches its maximum within 6 to 12 months.
- Facial paralysis associated with Ramsay Hunt syndrome has a worse prognosis. In patients with complete paralysis, only 10% will recover normal facial function. Among those with incomplete paralysis, only 66% will recover completely. The simultaneous onset of paralysis and the vesicular eruption is a negative prognostic sign.

 Differential Diagnosis

CONGENITAL

- Möbius syndrome
- Congenital unilateral lower-lip paralysis (CULLP)
- Hemifacial microsomia
- Aural atresia/microtia
- Chiari malformation

ENVIRONMENTAL

- Teratogenesis (drugs, infectious agents)

INFECTIOUS

- Acute otitis media
- Chronic otitis media
- Lyme disease
- Epstein-Barr virus
- *Mycoplasma pneumoniae* infection
- Mastoiditis: bacterial, tuberculosis
- Osteomyelitis of the skull

TRAUMA

- Birth trauma, including damage due to forceps assistance
- Temporal bone fractures
- Penetrating head/neck wounds
- Iatrogenic injury during otologic surgery

NEOPLASTIC

- Astrocytoma
- Medulloblastoma
- Pontine glioma
- Parotid gland tumors

METABOLIC

- Hyperparathyroidism
- Hypothyroidism
- Osteopetrosis
- Idiopathic infantile hypercalcemia

IMMUNOLOGIC/INFLAMMATORY

- Guillain-Barré syndrome
- Sarcoidosis
- Multiple sclerosis
- Myasthenia gravis

MISCELLANEOUS

- Melkersson-Rosenthal syndrome: recurrent swelling of the lips/face, intermittent facial nerve paralysis, and fissured tongue (lingua plicata)

 Data Gathering

HISTORY

- Birth history: mode of delivery, associated trauma?
- Ask about preceding viral illness.
- Early symptoms may include facial numbness, watery eyes or decreased tearing, facial pain, impairment of taste, and hyperacusis.
- Difficulty hearing
- History of trauma
- Acute versus chronic onset (Bell palsy is usually acute)
- Tick exposures

 Physical Examination

- Differentiate central from peripheral facial nerve palsy. The forehead muscles are innervated by both cerebral hemispheres via nerve fibers traveling in each peripheral facial nerve. Therefore, central lesions will cause paralysis of only the lower face. Peripheral lesions will involve both the upper and the lower face.
- Involvement of other cranial nerves
- Complete neurologic examination
- Rash (periauricular vesicles seen in Ramsay Hunt syndrome)
- Evaluate for acute/chronic otitis media

Laboratory Aids

• Lyme titers, especially if living in an endemic area
• Lumbar puncture: usually not indicated with an isolated CN VII palsy. However, should be performed if neurologic examination is abnormal (aside from CN VII) or if meningitis/encephalitis is suspected.

RADIOGRAPHIC AND OTHER STUDIES

• Head magnetic resonance imaging (MRI): only indicated if neurologic examination is abnormal aside from CN VII palsy.
• Electrodiagnostic testing (nerve excitability, facial nerve latency, and electroneuronography) can determine the rate/severity of neural degeneration distal to the site of injury. It is most often used after a traumatic facial nerve injury to determine the timing of surgical exploration. It must be done more than 72 hours from the development of paralysis.
• Modified tear test: used to determine the ability for tear production, between the affected and unaffected eye. Involves a 1-minute filter paper measurement of tear production after ammonia fume exposure. It is indicated if spontaneous tear production is not witnessed.
• Stapedial reflex: only useful if the tympanic membrane is normal. Impedance is measured after an intense sound stimulation. An intact stapedial reflex indicates paralysis is incomplete, predicting a better prognosis.

Therapy

• Prednisone (2 mg/kg/day): the mainstay of therapy. Studies have shown better prognosis when steroids are used in both idiopathic Bell palsy and HSV-related facial nerve palsy. Prognosis is better with earlier onset of therapy. Most would treat with a 10-day course, with a tapering dose over the last few days. Reevaluate the patient after 5 to 6 days to ensure that the symptoms are not progressing.
• Acyclovir (p.o.): should be started in patients with Ramsay Hunt syndrome, usually as a 10-day course. Some studies advocate its use in all cases of idiopathic Bell palsy, in conjunction with p.o. prednisone.
• Antibiotics: to treat otitis media, Lyme disease, if applicable
• Eye care: the eye must be protected during the day with "artificial tears," (e.g., Tears Naturale) and with an ointment (e.g., Lacri-Lube) at night.
• Facial nerve decompression: not often recommended, because Bell palsy is not an entrapment syndrome.
• Electrotherapy: electrical stimulation of the paralyzed muscles is not recommended. It may actually slow the growth of neurofibrils.

Follow-Up

• Patients should be reevaluated on days 5 to 6. If progression of the paralysis has occurred, the diagnosis of Bell palsy should be reconsidered.
• Stapedial reflex: returns less than 3 weeks after onset of the paralysis; indicates that facial nerve function is returning.
• Maximal nerve excitability stimulation test: can be used to help indicate prognosis. It is only useful during the first few weeks; thereafter, degeneration occurs, making the test inaccurate.

PITFALLS

• Waiting to start therapy (prednisone/acyclovir). If therapy is delayed, a patient with severe disease may develop irreversible nerve damage.
• Failing to consider a different diagnosis with either prolonged or recurrent facial paralysis.

PREVENTION

Currently, there are no preventative strategies for Bell palsy.

Common Questions and Answers

Q: Should acyclovir be started only in those patients with vesicular eruptions?
A: Certainly, acyclovir should be given to all children with facial palsy and a periauricular vesicular eruption. In addition, severe pain may be an indication of zoster, and acyclovir should be given. Studies have also indicated that empiric treatment with prednisone and acyclovir in idiopathic facial palsy did result in a better return of facial function.

Q: What should be considered with recurrent facial palsy?
A: Recurrent, unilateral facial palsy requires the physician to search for an alternate diagnosis. Neoplasms, vascular malformations, sarcoidosis, diabetes, and infectious mononucleosis should all be considered. One should also consider Melkersson-Rosenthal syndrome with recurrent paralysis.

ICD-9-CM 351.0

BIBLIOGRAPHY

Adour K. Medical management of idiopathic (Bell's) palsy. *Otolaryngol Clin North Am* 1991;24(3):663–673.

Bauer C, Coker N. Update on facial nerve disorders. *Otolaryngol Clin North Am* 1996;29(3):445–454.

Orobello P. Congenital and acquired facial nerve paralysis in children. Otolaryngol Clin North Am 1991;24(3):647–651.

Smith S. *Pediatric neurologic diseases,* 2nd ed. St. Louis: Mosby, 1994.

Author: Debra Boyer

Bezoars

 Database

DEFINITION

Bezoars are concretions of swallowed foreign material formed in the gastrointestinal tract.

- The peak age of onset reported in the literature is 10 to 19 years.
- Ninety percent of patients reportedly are women.

CAUSES

The classification of bezoars is dependent on the most prominent substance from which they are formed. This includes:

- Trichobezoars: patient's own hair
- Phytobezoars: indigestible fruit and vegetable matter
- Lactobezoars: milk
- Foreign bodies
- Fungal
- Less common materials include vitamins, antacids, psyllium, sucralfate, cimetidine, and nifedipine.

 Data Gathering

TRICHOBEZOARS

- Associated with trichotillomania and trichophagia
- Bezoars may become large and form a cast of the stomach.
- The bezoar may extend through the pylorus into the small bowel. This "tail" may obstruct the papilla of Vater, leading to jaundice and pancreatitis.

PHYTOBEZOARS

- Most common form among adults
- Associated with gastric dysmotility and poor gastric emptying (either primary or following gastric surgery) and hypochlorhydria
- Composed primarily of cellulose, hemicellulose, lignins, and tannins

LACTOBEZOARS (MILK)

Most often reported in premature, low-birth-weight infants (although there are reports in full-term infants and exclusively breast-fed infants)

- Factors contributing to lactobezoar formation include:

—Formulas with a high casein content
—Early and rapid feeding advancement in small infants
—High-caloric-density formulas
—Formulas with high calcium/phosphate content
—Continuous tube feedings
—Altered gastric motility in low-birth-weight infants

 Physical Examination

HISTORY

Symptoms and signs of bezoar formation include:

- Pain
- Nausea
- Vomiting
- Diarrhea
- Gastric ulceration
- Upper gastrointestinal bleeding and perforation

TRICHOBEZOARS

- Unusual patterns of balding
- Palpable left upper quadrant mass in the abdomen is often detected.

PHYTOBEZOARS

Abdominal mass is palpable in less than half of patients.

Laboratory Aids

- Iron-deficiency anemia, steatorrhea, or protein-losing enteropathy
- Plain abdominal radiography of the abdomen
- Upper gastrointestinal studies may outline the mass.
- Endoscopy may provide both the diagnosis of the specific type of bezoar and a method of treatment through fragmentation with biopsy forceps or snares.

Therapy

TRICHOBEZOARS

Surgical: they are normally too large, and hair is not dissolvable.

PHYTOBEZOARS

- Diet alteration
- Medications such as prokinetic agents to stimulate gastric motility
- Enzyme therapy to help dissolve the material
- Acetylcysteine treatment via nasogastric tube has been documented in one case report.
- Papain has shown to be approximately 87% effective. (Papain tablets are not currently available in the United States, so monosodium glutamate [MSG] dissolved in clear liquids has been used.) Complications of this therapy include the development of gastric ulceration and hypernatremia secondary to the high sodium content of MSG.
- Endoscopic fragmentation or extraction
- Surgical extraction

LACTOBEZOARS

- Withholding feedings for approximately 48 hours while the patient is sustained on IV fluids

Common Questions and Answers

Q: What are some commonly used medications that can lead to bezoar formation?
A: Vitamins, antacids, psyllium, sucralfate, cimetidine, and nifedipine.

Q: What may place an infant at risk for formation of a bezoar?
A: The literature suggests that formulas with a high casein contact may be linked with lactobezoar formation. Other possible contributing factors include early and rapid feeding advancement in small infants, high-density formulas, formulas with high calcium/phosphate content, continuous tube feedings, and altered gastric motility in low-birth-weight infants.

ICD-9-CM 938

BIBLIOGRAPHY

Walker-Renard P. Update on the medicinal management of phytobezoars. *Am J Gastroenterol* 1993;88(10):1663–1666.

Wyllie R, Hyams J. *Pediatric gastrointestinal disease: pathophysiology, diagnosis, management.* Philadelphia: WB Saunders, 1993.

Author: Donna Zeiter

Biliary Atresia

 Database

DEFINITION

Biliary atresia is a progressive obliteration of the lumen of the extrahepatic (EHBA) and intrahepatic biliary duct systems of the liver.

PATHOPHYSIOLOGY

The etiology is unclear. Each of the following etiologies has been suggested but has never been substantiated:

- Infection (reovirus 3, cytomegalovirus [CMV])
- Vascular insufficiency
- Autoimmune obliteration of the bile ducts
- Pancreatic reflux leading to destruction of the biliary duct system

Pathology

Gross Anatomy

EHBA can affect all or any part of the extraheptic biliary tree. When the affected portion is limited to the distal common bile duct, cystic duct, or gall bladder, the form is considered correctable because biliary drainage may be established. This situation occurs in less than 10% of patients. Coexisting anomalies are found in 10% to 20% of patients. Reported associated findings include:

- Absence of the inferior vena cava with azygous continuation
- Preduodenal portal vein and symmetric liver
- Malrotation
- Situs inversus
- Bronchial anomalies
- Multiple spleens

Histology

Because this is a progressive disease, the pathologic findings vary with stage. Extrahepatic biliary obstruction begins near the time of birth and progresses. Early in the course of the disease (approximately the first year), the liver biopsy shows cholestasis, interlobular bile duct proliferation, and a mononuclear infiltrate invading the periductal tissue. Later biopsies show degeneration and loss of bile ducts. If the biopsy is performed prior to 4 weeks of age, the pathology may be confused with other causes of neonatal cholestasis, such as giant-cell hepatitis.

GENETICS

- No clear genetic inheritance can be demonstrated, as indicated by discordance for both monozygotic and dizygotic twins.
- However, HLA-B12, HLA-A9-B5, and HLA-A28-B35 are found with a higher frequency in affected individuals.

EPIDEMIOLOGY

EHBA accounts for 25% to 30% of the cases of neonatal cholestasis and occurs with a frequency of 1 per 8,000 to 15,000 live births. It is the most common cause of neonatal jaundice for which surgery is indicated.

 Differential Diagnosis

The differential diagnosis includes all causes of neonatal cholestasis (NC).

EXTRAHEPATIC CAUSES OF NEONATAL CHOLESTASIS

- Biliary atresia
- Choledochal cyst
- Sclerosing cholangitis
- Bile duct stenosis
- Anomalies of the choledochopancreatico-ductal junction
- Spontaneous perforation of the common bile duct
- Obstructing neoplasia or stone
- Inspissated bile or mucus plug

INTRAHEPATIC DISORDERS OF NEONATAL CHOLESTASIS

Infection

- Sepsis
- Urinary tract infection (UTI)
- TORCH
- Coxsackie B virus, echovirus

Metabolic Abnormalities

- Tyrosinemia
- Galactosemia
- Hereditary fructose intolerance
- Inborn errors of bile acid metabolism
- Zellweger syndrome
- Benign familial recurrent cholestasis
- α_1-Antitrypsin deficiency
- Neonatal iron-storage disease
- Cystic fibrosis
- Hypopituitarism
- Bile duct paucity (Alagille syndrome and non-syndromic paucity)
- Trisomy 17, 18, 21 and Turner syndrome

Drugs/Toxins

- Medications
- Total parenteral nutrition (TPN)

Systemic Disease

- Post-shock
- Post-asphyxia
- Congestive heart failure

Inherited Jaundice Syndromes

- Dubin-Johnson syndrome
- Rotor syndrome
- Idiopathic neonatal giant-cell hepatitis

 Data Gathering

HISTORY

Typically, the patient is an otherwise healthy infant who develops jaundice within the first 90 days of life, and laboratory data demonstrate a conjugated hyperbilirubinemia.

 Physical Examination

- Jaundice is best visualized by examination of the hard palate, buccal mucosa, or sclera and may not be present until the bilirubin exceeds 5 to 7 dL in the newborn period and 2 dL in the older child.
- Acholic stools, hepatomegaly, and abnormal liver consistency are variable findings and do not need to be present to establish the diagnosis of biliary atresia.

Laboratory Aids

- Conjugated hyperbilirubin is defined as a conjugated fraction greater than 2.0 dL or a conjugated/total greater than 15%.
- Any child with a conjugated hyperbilirubinemia should undergo the following examinations:

—Fractionated bilirubin
—AST, ALT, PT/PTT, total protein, albumin, CBC
—Bacterial cultures (blood, urine, stool)
—Viral studies (hepatitis B, hepatitis C, Epstein-Barr virus [EBV], TORCH, HIV, adenovirus, enterovirus)
—α_1-Antitrypsin with Pi typing
—Urine and serum amino acids
—Urine organic acids
—Urine for reducing substance while the child is taking lactose-containing formula; if positive, assay of galactose-1-phosphate uridyl-transferase
—X-ray studies to exclude evidence of congenital infections and Alagille syndrome (i.e., calcifications of brain and butterfly vertebrae)
—Eye examination for congenital infections
—Sweat test
—HIV serology
—Thyroid-function tests
—Abdominal ultrasound
—Hepatobiliary scintigraphy
—Liver biopsy
—Operative cholangiogram, if nonexcreting scintigraphy

Therapy

- General approach

—Once the diagnosis of EHBA is established, a surgical drainage procedure is performed.
—Subsequent management is directed at providing nutrition and monitoring for common problems.
—Although surgical intervention is helpful, liver disease progresses and the majority of patients will ultimately require liver transplantation.

- Surgical drainage

—Correctable biliary atresia occurs in up to 10% of patients and is defined as obstruction limited to the distal common bile duct, cystic duct, and/or gallbladder. These patients may undergo a more limited operation linking the patent distal portion of the tree to the intestine, bypassing the obstruction.
—Noncorrectable biliary atresia occurs most frequently and is manifested as an absent extrahepatic biliary tree. The standard surgical procedure is the hepatoportoenterostomy (Kasai procedure).

- Nutrition

—Malabsorption due to decreased concentration of bile acids within the duodenal lumen is common and leads to fat-soluble vitamin deficiency and malnutrition. Patients receive routine supplementation with vitamins A, D, E, and K. The diet should be enriched with medium-chain triglycerides to ensure adequate fat ingestion. Nasogastric tube feedings should be implemented.

- Pruritus is common and develops when there is increased serum bile acid concentration. Many approaches to treatment with only limited success have included ursodeoxycholic acid, antihistamines, cholestyramine, improved nutrition (e.g., nasogastric supplements), rifampin, phenobarbital, naloxone, and biliary diversion.
- Hyperlipidemia/xanthomas: Hyperlipidemia develops as a complication of chronic liver disease and can be treated with choleretic agents such as ursodeoxycholic acid as well as with improved nutrition.
- Ascites

—Spironolactone, chlorothiazide, and furosemide are commonly used diuretics. Acute changes in fluid balance or a rapid diuresis can be achieved by the use of furosemide in conjunction with albumin replacement

- Liver transplantation: indications for transplantation include life-threatening hemorrhage from portal hypertension, failure to thrive, intractable pruritus, and liver failure.

 Follow-Up

Common long-term problems:

- Poor growth
- Fat-soluble vitamin deficiency
- Cholangitis
- Portal hypertension
- Pruritus
- Progression of liver damage despite a surgical drainage procedure

The clinician should:

- Keep notes in a flow chart.
- Monitor growth parameters and fat-soluble vitamins.
- Monitor liver span, liver texture, and spleen size to follow progress of disease.
- Follow liver-function tests and CBC.
- Watch closely for cholangitis: the most important findings suggestive of cholangitis are fever and elevated transaminases and GGT levels.

PITFALLS

Because age at the time of surgical intervention is the most important determinant of outcome, a delay in diagnosis can be tragic. Surgery is successful in 86% of infants prior to 8 weeks, 36% of infants between 8 and 12 weeks, and only 20% for those over 12 weeks.

 Common Questions and Answers

Q: When should a patient with neonatal jaundice have a fractionated bilirubin test?
A: If hyperbilirubinemia has not resolved by 6 weeks, fractionation should be performed to allow ample time for evaluation of neonatal cholestasis and the possible need for surgical intervention.

Q: Can the physician prioritize the diagnostic evaluation?
A: In general, the answer is no. Because the diagnosis must be made as early as possible and because many tests are performed only in special laboratories, the full workup should be complete within a few days to 2 weeks, depending on the age of the child.

Q: Will a Kasai operation hurt the chances of successful liver transplantation?
A: No. A review of children who underwent transplantation at Boston Children's Hospital reported an 89% 10-year survival for patients who had the Kasai procedure.

ICD-9-CM 751.61

BIBLIOGRAPHY

Gitnick G, LaBrecque DR, Moody FG. *Diseases of the liver and biliary tract*. Philadelphia: Mosby–Year Book, 1992.

Haber BA, Lake A. Neonatal cholestasis. *Clin Perinatol* 1990;17:483–506.

Mowat AP. *Liver disorders in childhood*. Boston: Butterworth–Heinemann, 1987.

Suchy F. *Liver disease in children*. Philadelphia: Mosby–Year Book, 1994.

Loomes K, Mulberg AE. The infant with cholestasis: diagnosis and management. In: Brandt LJ, Daum F, eds. Clinical practice of gastroenterology. Philadelphia: Churchill Livingstone, 1999.

Author: Barbara Haber

Biliary Dyskinesia

 Database

DEFINITION

Clinical diagnosis is based on pain that seems to emanate from the biliary tract, but no gallstones or anatomic abnormalities of the extrahepatic biliary tree are found. Biliary dyskinesia is also referred to as sphincter of Oddi dysfunction, post-cholecystectomy syndrome, and biliary dyssynergia.

CAUSES

It is poorly understood, but thought to result from abnormal responses of the sphincter of Oddi to the usual stimuli or meals or cholecystokinin (CCK).

PATHOPHYSIOLOGY

It is postulated that relative obstruction to flow through the sphincter of Oddi results in bile duct or pancreatic duct distension, which gives rise to pain with or without pancreatitis.

CHARACTERISTIC FEATURES

Five patterns of biliary dysfunction have been identified:

- Spasm: high basal sphincter pressure
- Tachyoddia: high frequency of phasic contractions (>10 per second)
- Bradyoddia: low frequency of phasic contractions (<1 per second)
- Nutcracker: phasic contractions that are prolonged (>10 seconds) and of a high amplitude (>300 mm Hg; normal is <30 mm Hg)
- Retrograde propagation of contractions

GENETICS

Unknown; however, a recessive gene of variable penetrance has been suggested in some family clusters.

EPIDEMIOLOGY

- Biliary dyskinesia is being recognized with increasing frequency in late childhood and the teenage years.
- Females are disproportionately more affected than are males.

PROGNOSIS

It is not a life-threatening disorder; however, affected patients may be severely debilitated.

DIFFERENTIAL DIAGNOSIS

Includes causes of right upper quadrant pain:

- Acute cholangitis, cholecystitis, or cholelithiasis
- Hepatitis
- Peptic ulcer disease, *Helicobacter pylori,* gastritis from NSAIDs
- Reflux esophagitis
- Renal disease, UTI
- Pneumonia
- Pancreatitis
- Irritable bowel syndrome
- Lactose intolerance
- GI anatomical abnormalities (i.e., intestinal malrotation)

 Data Gathering

HISTORY

To be classified as biliary in origin, the pain must last longer than 15 minutes and be located in the right upper quadrant or mid-abdomen.

- The major symptom is pain, which is usually epigastric, radiating to the right upper quadrant and into the back.
- Pain is often related to a fatty type meal but may also occur spontaneously.
- Nausea and vomiting may accompany the pain.
- There may be an increased sensitivity to opiate-type medication (e.g., codeine and morphine). Even small doses of codeine, such as occurs in cough mixtures, may initiate a severe episode of pain.
- In some patients, the symptoms may be accompanied by a rise in serum amylase, and a diagnosis of recurrent pancreatitis is made.
- Pain is not relived by antacids, ranitidine, or dietary manipulations.
- There may be a history of cholecystectomy for a similar pain.

Physical Examination

- Not febrile
- Mild tenderness in the right upper quadrant and epigastrium
- Remainder of physical examination usually normal

Laboratory Aids

- Transiently abnormal liver transaminases (alkaline phosphatase)
- Abnormal amylase in association with pain episode is also an objective finding.
- The common bile duct may be dilated on ultrasonography, but, usually, no abnormal findings are seen.
- The gold standard for definitive diagnosis is abnormal findings on sphincter of Oddi manometry, generally done during endoscopic retrograde cholangiopancreatography (ERCP).
- Quantitative hepatic scintigraphy is sensitive for distal common duct obstruction, but it is only applicable in postcholecystectomy patients with normal liver function.

Therapy

Medical therapy is empirical, and most patients end up requiring cholecystectomy and or sphincterotomy.

- Avoid narcotic analgesics because of their potential to exacerbate the symptoms as well as their addictive potential. Nonnarcotic analgesics (e.g., acetaminophen, aspirin, ibuprofen) may be used to relieve pain.
- Smooth muscle relaxants (e.g., trinitroglycerin and calcium channel blockers) may be effective in "spasm" or "nutcracker" sphincter.
- Laparoscopic cholecystectomy is the treatment of choice for biliary dyskinesia.
- Endoscopic sphincterotomy relieves symptoms in patients with abnormal manometric findings.

Follow-Up

- Best response to therapy is seen in patients with sphincter of Oddi spasm or stenosis.
- Persistence of pain and disability despite endoscopic or surgical therapy may require referral to specialized pain management center.

Common Questions and Answers

Q: What should raise suspicion of the possibility of biliary pain?
A: Usually, female patient with fatty meal–related epigastric or RUQ pain that is nonresponsive to antacids. Liver enzymes and ultrasound may be normal.

Q: Can symptoms develop or recur after cholecystectomy?
A: Yes. Some patients get long-lasting relief after cholecystectomy, but others have recurrence of symptoms and are best treated with endoscopic sphincterotomy.

Q: What pain relievers should be avoided in biliary dyskinesia?
A: Narcotics, including codeine (Tylenol 1, 2, and 3), because these may stimulate spasm of the sphincter of Oddi and worsen symptoms. Some over-the-counter cough suppressants that contain codeine will cause similar symptoms

Q: What is an indication for referral?
A: Patients who are dependent on or fail to get relief with NSAIDs.

ICD-9-CM 575.8

BIBLIOGRAPHY

Everson GT. Disorders of the biliary system. In: Gitnick G, Hollander D, Samloff IM, Schoenfield LJ, Vierling JM, eds. *Principals and practice of gastroenterology and hepatology*, 2nd ed. Norwalk, CT: Appleton & Lange, 1994:545–555.

Rescorla JF. Cholelithiasis, cholecystitis, and common bile duct stones. *Curr Opin Pediatr* 1997;9:276–282.

Rizk TA, Deshmukh N. Familial acalculous gallbladder disease. *South Med J* 1993;86(2):183–186.

Toouli J. What is sphincter of Oddi dysfunction? *Gut* 1989;30:753–761.

Toouli J, Baker RA. Innervation of the sphincter of Oddi: physiology and considerations of pharmacological intervention in biliary dyskinesia. *Pharmacol Ther* 1991;49:269–281.

Author: Timothy A.S. Sentongo

Blastomycosis

 Database

DEFINITION

Blastomycosis is infection caused by the dimorphic soil fungus *Blastomyces dermatitidis*.

PATHOPHYSIOLOGY

• Blastomycosis is a chronic disease characterized by granulomatous and suppurative lesions.
• It may cause asymptomatic infection or be associated with acute, chronic, or rapidly progressive systemic disease.
• It causes a large number of different presenting symptoms and different radiographic appearances.

EPIDEMIOLOGY

• Infection occurs after inhalation of conidia (spores of mycelial form).
• No person-to-person transmission
• Human infection is not uncommon. It is endemic in the United States in the southeast and central states and in the towns bordering the Great Lakes, with the highest incidence in the United States in Arkansas, Kentucky, Louisiana, Mississippi, North Carolina, Tennessee, and Wisconsin. Other reported areas of infection include parts of Canada (Ontario, Manitoba), Africa, India, and South America.
• Natural infection occurs only in two mammalian species: humans and dogs.
• It may be associated with immune compromise, but is not common in patients with HIV.
• Uncommon in the pediatric age group (<4% of cases in the most extensive patient review)
• Incubation period estimated at 30 to 45 days

COMPLICATIONS

• Dissemination is the main complication of the infection.
• Systemic infection may be well advanced before symptoms are noted, making eradication more difficult. Long-term therapy and follow-up may be necessary.

PROGNOSIS

• Self-limited pulmonary infection is often undiagnosed and resolves without dissemination (almost 50% of those infected may be asymptomatic).
• Early treatment with amphotericin B in progressive, severe, or disseminated disease is effective, with excellent rates of cure.
• The prognosis for chronic cutaneous disease is better than that for systemic disease.
• The number of deaths from blastomycosis is decreasing with the use of antifungal agents. Prevalence of blastomycosis remains high, however, in endemic areas.

ASSOCIATED ILLNESSES

• *Pulmonary blastomycosis:* most common form of infection by *Blastomyces* in children; can be acute, subacute, or chronic. Illness severity can vary greatly, from asymptomatic to presentations of URI, bronchitis, pleuritis, pneumonia, or severe respiratory distress.
• *Cutaneous blastomycosis:* skin manifestations are variable and include nodules, verrucous lesions, subcutaneous abscesses, or ulcerations. Cutaneous disease occurs following pulmonary inoculation in most cases, but can be inoculated primarily to skin.
• *Disseminated blastomycosis:* usually begins as pulmonary infection, with subsequent spread to involve skin (most commonly), bone, GU tract, and CNS.

 Differential Diagnosis

• Tuberculosis
• Neoplasm
• Sarcoidosis
• Other bacterial, viral, and fungal infections causing URI, bronchitis, pleuritis, and pneumonia

 Data Gathering

HISTORY

• Symptoms of common respiratory infections (nonproductive cough, pleuritic chest pain, poor appetite) that last more than 2 weeks. There may also be a history of fever, chills, weight loss, fatigue, night sweats, or, rarely, hemoptysis.
• History of residence or travel to an endemic area

Physical Examination

- Initial pulmonary infection may present as a mild respiratory infection. Respiratory signs and symptoms often have resolved by the time cutaneous manifestations are apparent.
- Skin involvement appears as nodules, nodules with ulceration, and, finally, granulomatous lesions with advancing borders.
- Sites in disseminated disease include lung, skin, bone, GU tract, CNS, and, infrequently, liver and spleen, lymph nodes, thyroid, heart, adrenals, omentum, GI tract, muscles, and pancreas.
- CXR indicated by physical examination or history may show localized consolidation in acute disease, and cavitations or pulmonary nodules with a more chronic course.

 ## Laboratory Aids

- Direct visualization of the yeast form may be performed on samples of sputum, urine, CSF, BAL sample, or tissue biopsy after 10% potassium hydroxide preparation.
- Culture of the organism from samples can be performed and a DNA probe used to identify *B. dermatitidis*.
- Serologic testing may be helpful in disseminated disease.
- Immunodiffusion testing is reliable for indication of infection, but a negative test does not rule out infection with *Blastomyces*.
- Severe pulmonary infection may develop with cavitation, pneumonia, or pulmonary nodules apparent on chest x-ray films.

 ## Therapy

- Mild or moderate disease is treated with oral itraconazole or ketoconazole, with or without an initial short course of amphotericin B.
- Severe or CNS or other severe infection should be treated with intravenous amphotericin B.
- Length of therapy is site-dependent: at least 6 months for pulmonary disease and at least 12 months for bone disease.

PREVENTION

- INFECTION CONTROL
- No special precautions for hospitalized patients are indicated.
- Outbreaks have occurred, with clustering of cases occurring at the same place and time.
- A natural reservoir is undetermined.

ICD-9-CM 116.0

BIBLIOGRAPHY

American Academy of Pediatrics. Blastomycosis. In: Peter G, ed. *1997 redbook: report of the Committee on Infectious Diseases,* 24th ed. Elk Grove Village, IL: American Academy of Pediatrics, 1997:154–155.

Chapman SW. Blastomyces dermatitis. In: Mandell GL, et al., eds. *Principles and practice of infectious diseases,* 3rd ed. New York: Churchill Livingstone, 1990:1999–2007.

Maxson S, Jacobs RF. Community-acquired fungal pneumonia in children. *Semin Respir Infect* 1996;11(3):196–203.

Mitchell TG. Blastomycosis. In: Feigin RD, Cherry JD, eds. *Textbook of pediatric infectious diseases,* 3rd ed. Philadelphia: WB Saunders, 1992:1898–1904.

Varkey B. Blastomycosis in children. *Semin Respir Infect* 1997;12(3):235–242.

Author: Molly (Martha) W. Stevens

Blepharitis

 Database

DEFINITION

Inflammation or infection of the eyelid margins, characterized by erythema, crusting, and scaling at the lid margins, with irritation, burning, and itching of the eye. There are two main types of blepharitis:

• *Simple squamous blepharitis* is often called seborrheic blepharitis. It tends to occur in the older child who has other signs and symptoms of seborrhea. It has a predilection for areas with increased sebaceous gland activity.
• *Ulcerative blepharitis* is often called staphylococcal blepharitis. It is usually due to a secondary infection with *Staphylococcus aureus* or *S. epidermidis*. Purulent inflammation of the glands of the lid margin results in ulcerations.

PATHOPHYSIOLOGY

• Thirty meibomian glands are located in each tarsal plate. Pilosebacious glands of Zeis and apocrine glands of Moll are located anterior to the meibomian glands within the distal eyelid margin.
• Bacteria and meibomian gland secretions play an integral role in the development of blepharitis.
• Occlusion of the glands of the eye will cause an accumulation of secretions.

EPIDEMIOLOGY

• Blepharitis is the most common cause of chronic conjunctivitis in children.
• Children who rub their eyes frequently are at risk for developing blepharitis.
• It is associated with contact lens use, as well as use of cosmetics.

COMPLICATIONS

• Chalazion: the most common complication, which results from the spread of infection to the meibomian gland and obstruction of the orifices
• Hordeolum (or stye): obstruction of the glands of Zeis
• Partial loss of eyelashes (madarosis) from recurrent rubbing and pulling on the lashes
• Secondary blepharoconjunctivitis
• Thickening of the lid margins (tylosis ciliaris)

PROGNOSIS

• Frequently recurrent or chronic

 Differential Diagnosis

• Atopic dermatitis (accounts for 90% of eyelid dermatitis)
• Contact dermatitis
• Trauma may primarily appear as an inflamed eyelid or may exacerbate an already inflamed eyelid.
• Psoriasis may rarely affect the eyelids.
• Chalazion
• Stye
• Rosacea: chronic hyperemic disease that often involves the eyelids. Look for persistent erythema, telangiectasias, and episodes of papulopustule formation.
• Systemic lupus erythematosus may cause dermatitis of the eyelid.
• Drugs
• Photosensitive dermatitis
• Infections, such as cellulitis or impetigo
• Acute conjunctivitis (bacterial or viral)
• Lice can cause an inflammatory reaction of the eyelid, with marked pruritus.

 Data Gathering

HISTORY

• Chronology and development of the inflammation; often recurrent
• Change in size or appearance
• Chemicals or medications used on or near the eyes
• Scratching or rubbing of the eyes
• Handwashing practices
• Eyelid hygiene
• Allergic or atopic history in the patient or the family
• Crusting pattern; symptoms often worse in the morning
• Contact lens use
• Makeup use

 Physical Examination

• Evaluate eyelid margins for thickening, crusting, erythema, and ulcerations; commonly bilateral.
• Usually, an associated papillary conjunctivitis is present.
• Loss of eyelashes
• Edema around the lid develops because of redundancy of eyelid skin and loose connection to underlying tissue; however, it remains localized because the surrounding skin is tightly adherent.
• Grouped vesicle on the eyelid suggests herpes simplex virus.
• Evidence of nits or adult lice suggests pubic lice.
• Evaluate for seborrhea in the scalp.
• Examine the skin for signs of atopic dermatitis.
• Hypertrophy and desquamation of the epidermis near the lid margin, with erythema and scaling near the lid border, are seen with seborrheic blepharitis.

PITFALLS

• Ulcerative blepharitis can be a manifestation of herpes simplex infection (grouped vesicles).
• Pubic lice can reside in the eyelashes and cause blepharitis. Itching is the predominant complaint.

Laboratory Aids

- Giemsa stain of conjunctival scrapings: helps confirm the diagnosis. Neutrophils are present in blepharitis.
- Bacterial and viral culture of the lid margins

 ## Therapy

- A combination of antimicrobials and eyelid hygiene (e.g., soap, dilute baby shampoo, or lid scrub) provides the best results.
- Most patients prefer a commercial preparation of lid scrub for the convenience and ease of use.
- Warm compresses for 15 minutes, twice a day (use caution to avoid causing a first-degree burn)
- Tarsal massage
- Removal of the scales and crust with a moist cotton swab
- Topical anti-staphylococcal antibiotic, two to three times a day (ophthalmic ointment is more soothing than solution, but ointment will cause blurring of vision)
- Oral medications may be required in severe cases.
- Continue treatment for several weeks, until blepharitis is completely resolved.
- Treat underlying seborrhea of the scalp and eyebrows with selenium sulfide shampoo.
- Use hypoallergenic makeup.

 ## Follow-Up

- As needed to assure compliance with prescribed regimen
- Improvement may be seen in as short a time as a few days.
- Any child with recurrent chalazions or a chronic stye should be evaluated for blepharitis.

PREVENTION

- Avoidance of eye rubbing
- Maintenance of good eye hygiene
- Isolation of hospitalized patient: standard universal precautions
- Control measures: frequent handwashing in children who rub their eyes

 ## Common Questions and Answers

Q: How did my child get blepharitis?
A: The pathophysiology of blepharitis is unclear at present. There may be an interaction of host mechanisms, such as composition of tears, with colonizing bacteria.

Q: Will it go away?
A: Blepharitis is usually a chronic condition. With good eyelid hygiene, it can be controlled. The eyelid hygiene will need to be continued for life.

Q: Is it contagious?
A: No. Children and other family members will not get blepharitis from the patient. However, it is recommended that they wash their hands frequently to prevent spread of bacteria.

Q: What is the difference between a chalazion and a stye?
A: Both chalazions and styes are accumulations of secretions from the glands of the eyelid. A chalazion is found on the inner surface of the eyelid and is due to blocked meibomian glands. Chalazions often appear as a subcutaneous nodule within the eyelid. If the chalazion gets large enough, it can distort vision by producing astigmatism from pressure exerted on the globe. Surgical removal of a chalazion is recommended if it distorts vision or is considered a cosmetic blemish. It may resolve spontaneously. A stye is an accumulation of secretions from the gland of Zeis and is found on the outer surface of the eyelid. The treatment for both lesions is application of warm compresses twice daily.

ICD-9-CM 373.00

BIBLIOGRAPHY

Carter SR. Eyelid disorders: diagnosis and management. *Am Fam Physician* 1998;57:2695–2702.

Key JE. A comparative study of eyelid cleaning regimens in chronic blepharitis. *CLAO J* 1996;22(3):209–212.

Nelson LB, Calhoun JH, Harley RD. *Pediatric ophthalmology,* 3rd ed. Philadelphia: WB Saunders, 1991:352.

Parkinson RW. Eyelid dermatitis: a common, often confounding rash. *Postgrad Med* 1996;100:231–240.

Weiss AH. The swollen and droopy eyelid; signs of systemic disease. *Pediatr Clin North Am* 1993;40(4):789–804.

Weiss AH. Chronic conjunctivitis in infants and children. *Pediatr Ann* 1993;22(6):366–374.

Author: Philip R. Spandorfer

Bone Marrow Transplantation

 Database

DEFINITION

Treatment with marrow-ablative chemoradiotherapy followed by an infusion of marrow from:

- The patient (autologous)
- An identical twin (syngeneic)
- A histocompatible donor (allogeneic)

INDICATIONS

- Accepted indications if a human leukocyte antigen (HLA) identical sibling is available:

—Acute lymphoblastic leukemia (ALL) in second complete remission (CR) and in certain patients in first CR (Philadelphia chromosome positive ALL)
—Acute myelogenous leukemia in first CR
—Chédiak-Higashi and other severe neutrophil defects
—Chronic myelogenous leukemia (CML)
—Diamond-Blackfan anemia (resistant to medical therapy)
—Fanconi anemia
—Juvenile myelomonocytic leukemia (formerly called JCML)
—Myelodysplasia
—Myelofibrosis
—Osteopetrosis
—Severe aplastic anemia
—Severe combined immunodeficiency and other congenital immunodeficiencies
—Thalassemia major (treatment of choice in Italy)
—Wiskott-Aldrich syndrome

Autologous transplantation is an accepted treatment for lymphoma in second CR and for unfavorable neuroblastoma in CR or very good partial response.

- Under investigation:

—Autologous bone marrow transplantation (BMT) is also under investigation for treatment of relapse in Wilms tumor, germ-cell tumors, and selected brain tumors and sarcomas.
—Sickle cell disease: A national trial is studying BMT in patients who have developed significant sequelae, such as stroke. European investigators have successfully performed BMT on asymptomatic patients, but the risk:benefit ratio is unknown.

—Mucopolysaccharidoses, lipidoses, and mucolipidoses

- BMT can lead to restoration of enzymatic activity in white cells and removal of accumulated substrate in affected tissues. In some diseases, such as adrenoleukodystrophy (childhood onset), it has been successful. In others, such Krabbe disease (infantile form), it has been a failure. Of concern is that improvement in organ function has not always led to improvement in intellectual function.

DONOR SELECTION (IN ORDER OF PREFERENCE)

- Identical twin: The increased risk of relapse of leukemia is offset by decreased treatment-related mortality.
- HLA identical sibling
- Other family members

—Rarely (i.e., in 5% of families), a nonsibling relative who is phenotypically mismatched for one antigen—will be found. Such transplantations have comparable results to HLA-identical sibling BMT.

- Haploidentical transplantations have been performed but require depletion of T cells from the graft to avoid fatal graft-versus-host disease (GVHD). They are associated with a lower survival than conventional BMT.
- Unrelated donors

—The National Marrow Donor Program (NMDP) presently has over 2 million volunteers registered and maintains a cooperative search agreement with European registries. Over 60% of preliminary searches yield at least one potential donor, although this percentage is lower for minority patients.

- Autologous

—Gene-marking studies have shown that infused marrow containing tumor can contribute to relapse. Better methods of purging marrow are needed.

PREPARATIVE REGIMENS

- The purpose of the preparative regimen is twofold:

—To eradicate malignancy and/or ablate the patient's bone marrow
—To suppress the patient's immune system so that it will accept a foreign bone marrow

- Agents used primarily for immunosuppression:

—Cyclophosphamide
—Antithymocyte globulin (ATG)

- Agents used primarily for antineoplastic effects or bone marrow ablation:

—Busulfan
—Cytarabine (ARA-C)
—Etoposide (VP-16)
—Carmustine (BCNU)
—Carboplatin
—Melphalan

- Agents used for both purposes:

—Total-body irradiation (TBI)
—Thiotepa

Note: Few randomized trials have compared one regimen to another. Choice depends on the disease being treated, the type of donor available, and previous treatment received.

STEM-CELL COLLECTION METHODS

- Conventional marrow harvesting from the iliac crests under general anesthesia
- Peripheral blood stem-cell (PBSC) collections via apheresis

—Hematopoietic stem cells normally circulate in the peripheral blood in small numbers but can be mobilized by chemotherapy and/or growth factors. Previously used for autografts, successful allogeneic transplantations have now been performed with PBSCs.

- Umbilical cord blood

—A rich source of hematopoietic stem cells; even 45 mL of cord blood is sufficient to reconstitute the hematopoietic system of a child.

TOXICITIES

• Chemoradiotherapy

—Universal: nausea/vomiting/diarrhea, alopecia, pancytopenia
—Possible and agent-specific:
  —TBI: skin erythema, parotitis
  —Cyclophosphamide: hemorrhagic cystitis, SIADH, cardiomyopathy
  —ATG: allergy, serum sickness
  —Busulfan: seizures, pulmonary fibrosis, bronzing of the skin
  —ARA-C: fever, neurologic symptoms, acute respiratory distress syndrome (ARDS)
  —VP-16: allergic reactions
  —BCNU: pulmonary fibrosis

• Graft failure

—Can occur early (failure to engraft) or even after successful engraftment
—Rare in HLA-identical sibling transplantations
—Risk increases with unrelated donors (6%) or T-cell depletion (approximately 14% but depends on the degree of T-cell depletion)
—Usually fatal

• Graft-versus-host disease (see chapter on GVHD)
• Infection: the major cause of nonrelapse mortality

—In the first month posttransplantation, bacterial and fungal infections predominate.
—In the second and third months, viral infections predominate, which include cytomegalovirus (CMV), adenovirus, herpesvirus, and polyomaviruses.
—After 3 months: herpes zoster and bacterial infections in patients with chronic GVHD

Note: After T-depleted transplantations, the risk of fatal Epstein-Barr virus infection is significant.

• Hepatic veno-occlusive disease

—Clinical criteria met when two of the following are present:
  —Hepatomegaly and/or right upper quadrant pain
  —Hyperbilirubinemia (>2.0 mg/dL)
  —Greater than 5% weight gain and/or ascites
  —Incidence of approximately 25% (range, 1%–54%) and mortality of 30% (range, 3%–67%) have been reported.

—Therapy is largely supportive. Some striking reports of improvement after treatment with recombinant tissue plasminogen activator and, more recently, defibrotide have been published.

• Interstitial pneumonitis

—Typically appears 40 to 80 days post-BMT as rapid-onset tachypnea associated with bilateral interstitial infiltrates
—Common etiologies include:
  —CMV
  —*Pneumocystis carinii*
  —Idiopathic: when no bacterial, viral, fungal, or protozoan cause is identified. Radiation to the lungs probably plays a role in the development of "idiopathic" pneumonitis.

LATE COMPLICATIONS

• Endocrine

—Hypothyroidism: seen in approximately 20% of patients after TBI; rare after chemotherapy alone
—Growth hormone deficiency: seen in over half of patients receiving TBI
—Primary gonadal failure and absence of development of secondary sexual characteristics are common, especially if the recipient was prepubertal at the time of transplantation or received TBI.

• Infertility: Sterility is expected after TBI; fertility may be preserved after cyclophosphamide alone.
• Opthalmologic: Cataracts are seen in 40% of patients after TBI and in 20% after chemotherapy alone. A higher incidence is seen in those who also receive steroids.
• Dental: Poor calcification of teeth and root blunting have been seen. The defects are more severe in children younger than age 7 at transplantation.
• Renal

—Radiation nephritis
—Hemolytic uremic syndrome and thrombocytopenic purpura occur, especially during treatment with cyclosporine

• Secondary malignancies: Fifteen-year cumulative incidence rates are 6% and 20% after regimens with and without TBI, respectively.
• Intellectual function: Few prospective studies published

 Common Questions and Answers

Q: When should I immunize a patient after transplantation?
A: At 1 year post-BMT, patients free of chronic GVHD should begin a primary immunization schedule with DPT/Salk/HiB/hepatitis B. MMR is usually given at 2 years post-BMT.

Q: If my patient relapses after BMT, can a second BMT be done?
A: Previously, there were few therapeutic options for patients who relapsed less than 1 year post-BMT. Remissions after an infusion of buffy coat (containing T cells) from the patient's donor can been achieved. Although the majority of successful infusions have been in patients with CML, success has also been seen in acute leukemia. Chronic GVHD will often result.

BIBLIOGRAPHY

Armitage JO. Bone marrow transplantation. *N Engl J Med* 1994;330:827–838.

Kernan KA, Bartsch G, Ash RC, et al. Analysis of 462 transplantations from unrelated donors facilitated by the National Marrow Donor Program. *N Engl J Med* 1993;328:593–602.

Sanders JE. Bone marrow transplantation in pediatric oncology. In: Pizzo PA, Poplack DG, eds. *Principles and practice of pediatric oncology,* 3rd ed. Philadelphia: Lippincott Williams & Wilkins, 1997:357–373.

Vannatta K, Zeller M, Noll RB, Koontz K. Social functioning of children surviving bone marrow transplantation. *J Pediatr Psychol* 1998;23(3):169–178.

Author: Ann Marie Leahey

Botulism

 ## Database

DEFINITION

An illness produced by neurotoxins elaborated by *Clostridium botulinum*, which causes an acute, descending, flaccid paralysis. The neurotoxin may be ingested or absorbed from infected wounds, or ingested spores germinate, producing toxin. There are three types of illness.

• In infant botulism, ingested spores germinate and colonize the infant's colon and elaborate toxin.
• In adults, the patient ingests preformed toxin while eating improperly prepared or stored foodstuffs.
• In wound botulism, spores germinate in an infected wound and toxin is absorbed.

CAUSES

C. botulinum, the etiologic agent, is a gram-positive, spore-forming, obligate anaerobic bacteria that is found in soil throughout the world.

PATHOPHYSIOLOGY

• Botulinum toxin is one of the most lethal of naturally occurring compounds.
• Neurotoxin is taken up by nerve endings and irreversibly blocks acetylcholine release in peripheral cholinergic synapses.
• Cranial nerves are usually affected first and most severely, leading to difficulty swallowing and loss of airway protective reflexes. Respiratory failure develops.
• Botulinum toxin does not cross the blood-brain barrier; therefore, the sensorium remains clear.
• Recovery occurs with the regeneration of terminal motor neurons and the formation of new motor end plates.
• Infants are particularly prone to colonic colonization with *C. botulinum* due to differences in the intestinal flora in infants. When foods other than breast milk are introduced in breast-fed infants, changes in flora may be especially important.

EPIDEMIOLOGY

• *Infant botulism* occurs in the first year of life, with more than 95% of cases reported in the first 6 months.
• Infants are usually white, breast-fed, and from middle-class families. Infants who have less than one bowel movement per day may be at increased risk. Cases are seen more frequently in rural and suburban areas.
• Most cases have been reported in California, Utah, and Pennsylvania.
• There often is a history of a recent change in feeding practice (addition of formula or solids or changing from breast to bottle feeding).

• Honey seems to be a particularly contaminated food and has been implicated in California.
• Breast-fed infants get ill at an older age than do bottle-fed infants; all cases of sudden infant death syndrome (SIDS) associated with infant botulism have been in bottle-fed infants.
• *Food-borne* cases are usually associated with the use of home-processed foods—especially vegetables, fruits, and condiments.
• *Wound botulism* is very rare.

COMPLICATIONS

• The most serious and fatal complication is respiratory failure due to paralysis of the respiratory muscles.
• Bulbar dysfunction in infant botulism may lead to dehydration before presentation.
• The loss of airway protective reflexes can lead to aspiration and pneumonia.
• Constipation and urinary retention may precede the onset of paralysis and may complicate later management as well.
• The earliest symptoms in adults and older children may be visual changes, including blurred vision, loss of accommodation, and diplopia.
• SIADH and urinary tract infections have been reported in infants with infant botulism.

PROGNOSIS

• *Food-borne* botulism carries a mortality rate of 20% to 25%. This rate is lower in patients less than 20 years old (about 10%).
• Patients with a shorter incubation period usually have more severe involvement and a worse prognosis, probably related to an increased amount of toxin ingested.
• If recognized early and treated aggressively, botulism carries a good prognosis, and complete recovery can be expected. Fatigability may persist for up to 1 year.
• *Infant botulism* has an estimated mortality rate of less than 5% in hospitalized patients. Complete recovery can be expected when disease is recognized early and treated appropriately.

 ## Differential Diagnosis

INFECTIONS

• In noninfants, bacterial sepsis, meningitis, poliomyelitis, tick paralysis, and diphtheric polyneuritis.
• Absence of fever and a clear sensorium make sepsis and meningitis less likely. The descending and symmetrical nature of the paralysis and a history of ingestion of home-processed foods are clues to the diagnosis of botulism, as are the early and more severe involvement of the cranial nerves.

NEUROLOGIC

• Myasthenia gravis usually spares the pupillary response, while it is fatigable in botulism, if not absent.
• Guillain-Barré syndrome usually presents with an ascending paralysis, and patients often complain of muscle cramps and paresthesias. Elevated CSF protein levels are not usually seen in botulism. EMG is very helpful in distinguishing between these disorders.
• In Werdnig-Hoffman disease (type I spinal muscle atrophy), facial muscles are spared.

TOXINS

Drug ingestions may lead to weakness and lethargy. Usually, the patient's level of consciousness is also affected, and a history of ingestion may be obtained.

Data Gathering

HISTORY

• The first symptom of *infant botulism* is usually constipation. There is a progressive course of lethargy, weakness, and poor feeding.

—In breast-fed children, the mother often notes breast engorgement.
—Occasionally, the progression may be quite rapid, and the abrupt onset of lethargy and weakness may suggest the diagnosis of bacterial sepsis or meningitis.

• *Food-borne* cases result in complaints of emesis in about 50% of patients.

—There may initially be complaints of diarrhea followed by constipation.
—The incubation period from ingestion to the onset of symptoms is usually 18 to 36 hours (range, a few hours to several days).
—Patients complain of weakness and dry mouth.
—Visual complaints include blurry vision, loss of accommodation, and diplopia.
—Patients may complain of dysphagia or dysarthria.
—Patients may have urinary retention.
—Fever is absent.
—Within 3 days, there is the onset of the characteristic descending, symmetrical paralysis. The cranial nerves are usually affected first.
—Mentation is clear, except for understandable anxiety and agitation.

• *Wound botulism* has an incubation period of 4 to 14 days.

—Fever may or may not be present.
—Patients often report constipation but rarely nausea or vomiting.
—They may complain of unilateral sensory changes and of purulent discharge from the wound.
—The duration of symptoms prior to hospitalization ranges between 1 and 20 days.

Physical Examination

- Older children and adults often appear alert and are afebrile.
- Ptosis, extraocular palsies, and fixed and dilated pupils are often the first signs of descending paralysis. Loss of airway protective reflexes and respiratory muscle weakness lead to respiratory failure.
- The triad of bulbar palsies, a lucid sensorium, and the absence of fever should prompt one to consider strongly the diagnosis of botulism.
- Infant botulism presents in a similar way. Patients are usually afebrile. They are usually weak, with decreased spontaneous activity at presentation. They have an expressionless (masklike) face, ptosis, a weak cry, poor head control, and generalized weakness and hypotonia.
- Pupils are often midposition initially and may be at least weakly reactive. The pupillary response is fatigable. The pupils become fixed and dilated for a period in many cases. Except for the symmetric, descending paralysis, the remainder of the physical examination is normal.
- Signs of autonomic instability include unexpected fluctuations in skin color, blood pressure, and heart rate.

SPECIAL QUESTIONS

- Home-prepared foods?
- The history of constipation followed by progressive weakness and decreased activity in an afebrile infant should prompt consideration of botulism.

PHYSICAL EXAMINATION TRICK

In infants, early in the course of the disease, pupillary and corneal reflexes may fatigue easily.

Laboratory Aids

TESTS

- Tests for the presence of toxin or the organism can be conducted on patient samples (serum, gastric aspirates, feces, or wound exudate) or suspected foodstuffs.
- Anaerobic cultures of a wound or the GI tract may yield the organism.
- Electromyography (EMG) shows a characteristic pattern of brief duration, sharp amplitude, overly abundant motor unit action potentials (BSAPs).
- EEG, MRI, and CT are nonspecific and usually normal in the absence of any complications.

Requirements for Testing

- Most tests for toxin and cultures are conducted by state health departments.
- The most common test performed is an assay for botulinum toxin in stool.
- Specimens must be shipped in sealed, breakproof, and leakproof containers. Even small amounts of toxin, if inhaled or ingested, can lead to disease.
- Suspect foods should be shipped refrigerated and in their original containers if possible.

Therapy

- All patients with suspected botulism should be admitted to the hospital and have continuous monitoring of their heart rate, respiratory rate, and oxygenation, as well as frequent assessment of their respiratory effort and airway protective reflexes.
- The mainstay of therapy is meticulous supportive care. Particular attention is paid to respiratory and nutritional needs.
- Endotracheal intubation may be necessary both for patients with frank respiratory failure and when airway protective reflexes are lost.
- Wounds should be explored and debrided, and anaerobic cultures should be obtained.
- Cases of suspected toxin ingestion should be treated early with induced emesis and/or gastric lavage in an attempt to decrease toxin exposure.
- All cases should be reported to the state health department and the CDC.

DRUGS

- Antibiotics are not helpful in *infant botulism*.
- Equine antitoxin is not recommended for *infant botulism*. A human-derived antitoxin is being evaluated and may be obtained under a Treatment Investigational New Drug protocol from the California Department of Health Services at 510-540-2646 (24 hours a day).
- Antibiotics are indicated only for documented complications such as pneumonia.
- Cathartics are not beneficial, and enemas may cause colonic distention and increased toxin absorption.
- Cases of botulism resulting from *ingested toxin* or *wound infection* should be treated with trivalent (ABE) botulinum antitoxin, available from the CDC. Antitoxin should not be administered to asymptomatic individuals who have only eaten suspect foods.
- Wound botulism should be treated with IV penicillin G 250,000 units/kg/d.

DURATION

- In wound botulism, antibiotics should be continued for 10 to 14 days.
- Supportive care should be continued until the patient is able to be weaned from respiratory support and begin PO feedings.

Follow-Up

The nadir of the paresis in infants is usually 1 to 2 weeks after presentation. Infants remain at their nadir for 1 to 3 weeks. Infants are ready for discharge when gag, suck, and swallow reflexes are adequate to protect against aspiration. In food-borne and wound botulism, recovery may be prolonged, with symptoms of fatigability persisting for up to 1 year.

PREVENTION

- Honey should not be fed to infants.
- Botulinum toxin is heat-labile; 5 minutes of boiling will destroy the toxin.
- Home-canned foods should be boiled for at least 10 minutes before serving.
- Spores are more resistant to heat. Home canners must use temperatures well above boiling to destroy spores effectively (120°C for 30 minutes). Pressure cookers are needed to achieve these conditions.

Common Questions and Answers

Q: Can infant botulism recur?
A: True recurrence in infant botulism has not been documented.

Q: Should antitoxin be given to persons who have ingested food that they think might be contaminated with botulinum toxin?
A: Since the antitoxin carries a significant risk of serum sickness, it should be given only to persons with neurologic symptoms.

Q: Where is antitoxin obtained?
A: Antitoxin may be obtained from the Centers for Disease Control and Prevention, Atlanta, Georgia; 404-639-3753 (days), 404-639-2888 (nights).

ICD-9-CM 005.1

BIBLIOGRAPHY

Glatman-Freedman A. Infant botulism. *Pediatr Rev* 1996;17:185–186.

Passaro DJ, Werner SB, Mcgee J, et al. Wound botulism associated with black tar heroin among injecting drug users. *JAMA* 1998;279:859–863.

Schreiner MS, Field E, Ruddy R. Infant botulism: a review of 12 years' experience at the Children's Hospital of Philadelphia. *Pediatrics* 1991;87:159–165.

Shapiro RL, Hatheway C, Swerdlow DL. Botulism in the United States: a clinical and epidemiologic review. *Ann Intern Med* 1998;129:221–228.

Author: James M. Callahan

Brain Abscess

 Database

DEFINITION

A brain abscess is a suppurative infection involving the brain parenchyma; it may be a single or multiple lesion.

CAUSES

• Bacteria are the most common causes of brain abscesses.
• *Streptococcus sp.* and *Staphylococcus sp.* are the two most common cultured microorganisms.
• Neonates typically develop abscesses after a gram-negative meningitis (*Proteus* and *Citrobacter*)
• A single organism is found in about 70% of patients.
• Anaerobic organisms are being found with increasing incidence with improved laboratory and culture techniques.
• Fungi and protozoa are common with immunocompromised patients.

PATHOPHYSIOLOGY

• Microorganisms enter the brain parenchyma by contiguous or hematogenous (metastasis) pathways.
• Cyanotic congenital heart disease patients tend to have abscesses in the middle meningeal artery distribution: frontal, parietal, and temporal lobes.
• Frontal abscesses are commonly seen with frontal sinusitis.
• Temporal, parietal, or cerebellar abscesses tend to occur with mastoiditis or otitis media infections.
• Brain abscesses can occur anywhere in the brain parenchyma, regardless of a predisposing risk factor.

PREDISPOSING RISK FACTORS

• Cyanotic congenital heart disease (CCHD)
• Otolaryngologic infections such as sinusitis, mastoiditis, chronic otitis media, or cholesteatomas
• Meningitis (especially with neonates)
• Penetrating head trauma
• Surgical manipulation of the brain (ventriculoperitoneal shunts)
• Esophageal manipulation (sclerotherapy or dilation)
• Cystic fibrosis
• Dental infections
• Lung infections
• Any site of infection (osteomyelitis, orbital, cellulitis, etc.)
• Immunocompromised patients
• Unknown etiology is found in about 30% of patients.

EPIDEMIOLOGY

• Incidence is about 2 to 3 per 10,000 general hospital admissions.
• A majority of children are male (2:1 male-to-female predominance).
• Average age of presentation is about 7 years of age.
• About 2% to 4% of children with CCHD will develop a brain abscess. (Tetralogy of Fallot is the most common CCHD.)

COMPLICATIONS

These arise from the location, size, and number of intracranial abscesses and can vary from SIADH and seizures, to focal neurological deficits.

PROGNOSIS

• A *high* index of suspicion is required to diagnose a brain abscess. A delay in diagnosis or performing a lumbar puncture (LP) for suspected meningitis increases mortality and morbidity.
• With the advent of computed tomography (CT) and magnetic resonance imaging (MRI) scans, the mortality rate has dropped from 30% to 14% or less.
• Multiple abscesses, coma on presentation, less than 2 years of age, performance of an LP, and rupture of abscess into the ventricle carry a higher mortality rate.
• About 30% to 40% of patients will have some morbidity. This ranges from seizures, hemiparesis, focal neurological deficits, and hydrocephalus, to cognitive/behavior problems.

 Differential Diagnosis

• Infectious: meningitis, encephalitis, subdural empyema, epidural abscess
• Vascular: venous sinus thrombosis, migraine, cerebral infarct, cerebral hemorrhage
• Miscellaneous: primary or secondary tumor, pseudotumor cerebri

 Data Gathering

HISTORY

• It should be noted that the location of the brain abscess or abscesses will often influence the history of presentation and physical examination.
• The classic triad of fever, headache, and focal neurologic findings occurs in less than 30% of cases.
• Headache is the most common complaint.
• The average duration of symptoms prior to diagnosis is about 4 weeks.
• Vomiting and mental status changes can often be the presenting chief complaints.
• Neonates often have a history of meningitis before developing a brain abscess.
• Questions should focus on acute or chronic otolaryngologic infections such as sinusitis, chronic otitis media, and mastoiditis, as well as a history of cholesteatomas.
• Cyanotic congenital heart disease (CCHD) should be determined, as well as a partially repaired CCHD

Physical Examination

• Neonates may present with a full fontanel, increasing head circumference, seizures, or vomiting.
• Older children may have signs of increasing intracranial pressure, such as papilledema, focal neurologic deficit, and hemiparesis.
• Meningeal signs are found in 30% of patients.
• Ataxia is seen in cerebellar lesions.

PITFALLS

• About 40% of children will not have fevers.
• In older children, consider the possibility of a frontal abscess extending from a bacterial sinusitis, especially with complaints of severe headache and symptoms of prolonged sinusitis.

Laboratory Aids

TESTS

Laboratory Tests

• CBC may be mildly elevated, and less than 10% will show a left shift.
• Sedimentation rates (ESR) are poor indicators of brain abscesses.
• Electrolytes may show a low sodium, indicating SIADH.
• A lumbar puncture (LP) is contraindicated if any mass lesion is suspected, but if CSF is obtained, it may show a mild-to-moderate pleocytosis (20% of patients may have normal values); the opening pressure is always elevated; glucose may be decreased in 30% of patients; the protein is elevated in 70% of cases; and only 10% of cultures are positive, unless the abscess ruptures into the ventricles.

Imaging

A CT or MRI scan are the studies of choice in diagnosing brain abscesses.

 Therapy

• Broad-spectrum antibiotics should be started at the time of diagnosis until identification of the microorganism is determined. At that time, the antibiotics can be tailored to the offending microorganism.
• Most brain abscesses are surgically removed. A few may require CT-guided aspiration.
• When multiple abscesses are found on CT scan, one lesion should be aspirated to determine the identification of the microorganism.
• Some patients are managed successfully with antibiotics alone.
• Antifungals should be considered with immunocompromised patients.
• The use of steroids is controversial.
• If a patient is manifesting signs and symptoms of increased intracranial pressure (Cushing triad: bradycardia, hypertension, and abnormal respirations), or if the patient is comatose and is unable to protect his/her airway, the patient should be intubated, hyperventilated, and given mannitol.
• Those patients with unknown predisposing factors should be evaluated by cardiology, dental, and otolaryngology.

 Follow-Up

• Neonates and older patients may be discharged with home physical therapy and home nursing for intravenous antibiotics.
• Patients will need intravenous antibiotics for a total of 3 to 4 weeks; some may require longer courses of antibiotics.
• Some children will need follow-up CT scans.
• Follow-up with neurosurgical, rehabilitation, and neurology clinics is usually required.
• Some children may need in-patient rehabilitation services.

PREVENTION

Wearing helmets may prevent penetrating head trauma while bike riding, roller blading, and so on.

 Common Questions and Answers

Q: Do all brain abscesses require surgery?
A: No. Some will regress with antibiotics and follow-up with MRI.

Q: What is the best way to diagnose an abscess.
A: Performing a CT or MRI. LP is contraindicated with mass lesions.

ICD-9-CD 324.0

BIBLIOGRAPHY

Carmel PW. Purulent focal infections. In: Rudolph AM, ed. *Rudolph's pediatrics,* 19th ed. Stamford, CT: Appleton & Lange, 1991:1845–1849.

Jadavji T, Humphreys RP, Prober CG. Brain abscesses in infants and children. *Pediatr Infect Dis J* 1985;4:394–398.

Kaplan K. Brain abscess. In: Symposium on infections of the central nervous system. *Med Clin North Am* 1985;69:345–360.

Patrick CC, Kaplan SL. Current concept in the pathogenesis and management of brain abscesses in children. In: New concepts in pediatric infectious disease. *Pediatr Clin North Am* 1988;35:625–636.

Renier D, Flandin C, Hirsch E, et al. Brain abscesses in neonates. *J Neurosurg* 1988;69:877–882.

Rennels MB, Woodward CL, Robinson WL, et al. Medical cure of apparent brain abscesses. *Pediatrics* 1983;72:220–224.

Saez-Llorens XJ, Umana MA, Odio CM, et al. Brain abscess in infants and children. *Pediatr Infect Dis J* 1989;8:449–458.

Yogev R. Focal suppurative infections of the central nervous system. In: Long SS, Pickering LK, Prober CG, eds. *Principles and practice of pediatric infectious diseases,* 1st ed. New York: Churchill Livingstone, 1997:349–358.

Author: Jeffrey P. Louie

Brain Injury—Traumatic

 Database

DEFINITION

Traumatic brain injury is damage to the brain sustained as a result of accidental or nonaccidental trauma. Manifestations may include loss of consciousness, seizures, posturing, syncope, hemiparesis. *Concussion* implies loss of consciousness at the time of impact. *Head injury* frequently is associated with trauma to the face, neck, or other parts of the body without permanent brain injury.

PATHOPHYSIOLOGY

- Rapid acceleration/deceleration injuries, causing contusions, skull fractures, diffuse axonal injury (DAI), subdural hematoma, and cervical spine injuries; penetration injuries, causing brain lacerations; intracerebral hemorrhage; brain fungus
- Secondary phenomena (e.g., as a result of circulatory failure in the setting of body trauma or as a result of air/fat emboli after body/extremity trauma)

Age-Specific Pathophysiology

Infants

- A large head causes vulnerability to injury.
- A deformable, expansile skull usually protects from herniation due to cerebral edema or hematoma.
- The most commonly seen injuries are shear injuries and subdural hematoma (SDH) secondary to venous sinus tears in nonaccidental trauma.
- Diffuse axonal injury secondary to shaken impact syndrome can lead to cerebral swelling with secondary infarction and/or decreased central respiratory control, leading to apnea, hypoxia, and cerebral edema.
- Birth trauma commonly results in subgaleal hematoma, cephalhematoma, and caput succedaneum.
- More severe birth trauma can result in SDH due to tearing of the dura of falx.

Children/Adolescents

- Usually due to motor vehicle accidents
- Projectile injuries in adolescent population
- Can result from nonaccidental trauma (usually correlated with other stigmata of assault)

EPIDEMIOLOGY

- Incidence of general trauma is approximately 86 per 1,000, of which, 50% is head trauma.
- In children, 2 years of age, falls are the most common cause of trauma.

ASSOCIATED CONDITIONS

- Intoxications (of child, caretaker, others in the environment)
- Physical abuse/neglect
- Epilepsy

 Differential Diagnosis

- Neurologic presentation is similar to that of other hypoxic—ischemic brain injuries (e.g., near-drowning), other causes of stupor/coma (see chapter), seizure activity (postictal encephalopathy).
- Distinction between simple concussion, DAI, and hypoxic—ischemic injury may be difficult at initial presentation but will clear as clinical picture/neuroimaging evolves.

Data Gathering

HISTORY

- Eyewitness accounts are invaluable.
- A history of previous concussions or seizures, and details of who was caring for the child and when are all useful.
- Try to determine if the patient fell and injured the head or collapsed from a neurologic problem and fell with no additional injury.
- *Laboratory testing* depends on the problem list, but may include:

—MRI: to evaluate posttraumatic hydrocephalus, or to evaluate extent and nature of injury for prognosis
—EEG: to evaluate suspected seizures
—Audiometry: especially with speech delay after head trauma
—CSF tracer study: for suspected CSF leak

- Other complications

—Infants can sustain growing fractures due to prolapse of meninges into the skull fracture, leading to formation of a leptomeningeal cyst.
—The pediatrician should refer any patient with a known skull fracture who manifests a new swelling in area of old fracture to neurosurgery for three-dimensional CT imaging of the head.
—Approximately 2% of persons with severe head injury will develop seizures.
—Studies in adults showed no prophylactic benefit to phenytoin beyond 1 week postinjury.
—Mild head injury (Glasgow coma score [GCS] of 13–15) was found to have no long-term effects on cognition in a large British study (n = 513,000).
—Patients who have sustained moderate-to-severe head injury (GCS,13) often have academic difficulties, memory abnormalities, disinhibition, and other complications as described above.
—Moderate-to-severe injury (with associated hemiplegia) can, in rare instances, cause symptomatic dystonia.
—Static encephalopathy after head injury can be manifested as any combination of learning disabilities, seizure disorder, speech disorder, memory disturbance, and visual/hearing loss.

 Physical Examination

- Stabilization of neck to avoid exacerbation of potential spine injury is an immediate concern once airway, breathing, and circulation are ensured.
- Elevation of the head to 30 degrees may help to alleviate intracranial hypertension.
- Vital sign changes indicative of Cushing reflex (bradycardia, hypertension, irregular respirations) suggest intracranial pressure/impending brain herniation; these signs warrant prompt intubation and IV access.
- A C-spine collar should be worn until x-ray studies are done and found to be negative.
- HEENT examination for ecchymoses, retinal hemorrhages, bullet holes, penetrating bone fragments, herniating brain, hemotympanum, CSF leak (nasal or otic)
- Neurologic examination should document responsiveness (to voice, touch, pain), resting posture (flaccid, extensor, flexor), spontaneous movements (convulsions, writhing/agitated movements, purposeful), and oculomotor findings (see below).
- When carefully documented over time, these observations provide far more useful information to other caretakers than do coma scores.
- Papilledema may take 6 hours or more to develop if there is intracranial hypertension.
- Pupils: Marked asymmetry suggests brain herniation causing third-nerve palsy (see Follow-Up section, Pitfalls). Reactivity of pupils is best examined through an otoscope.
- Eye movements: Dysconjugate gaze is common in the unconscious patient and may not indicate a focal structural problem or elevated ICP. Absence of contraversive, lateral movement of eyes with passive head-turning (doll's-eyes maneuver—if cervical spine has been cleared) suggests midbrain damage due to hemorrhage or axonal shear.
- Heart: Narrow pulse pressure or hypotension may be due to shock or pericardial tamponade. Bradycardia or irregular respirations may be due to intracranial hypertension.
- Careful examination for trauma or other clues: ecchymoses, open fractures, hematuria

Laboratory Aids

- Plain films and CT scans are the imaging studies of choice on initial evaluation of a patient with suspected traumatic brain injury. They usually are readily accessible and provide key information for emergent patient management.
- C-spine plain film to evaluate bones from base of skull to C7 in whiplash injury or suspected shaken impact injuries
- Skull film (and long-bone films) if degree of injury is not consistent with history or history of fall from unclear height
- CT scan to evaluate for head and/or spine injury, including SDH as well as basilar, depressed, or facial bone fractures
- CT scan showing normal brain/ventricular spaces: observation only; may want to consider EEG and lumbar puncture
- In all patients with suspected traumatic brain injury, one should obtain:

—CBC (infants can have a large amount of intracranial blood loss)
—PT/PTT (to evaluate a possible bleeding disorder as a possible preoperative laboratory test)
—Electrolytes (to look for evidence of impending SIADH, which can be seen in patients with cerebral edema as well as meningitis)

 ## Therapy

- Once laboratory values are obtained, appropriate corrective measures should be undertaken as needed (e.g., packed RBC or platelet transfusion, fluid restriction).
- Anticonvulsants may be used in those with persistent coma and elevated intracranial pressure (ICP), and in those with intracranial hemorrhage, since seizures cause ICP spikes. Otherwise, anticonvulsant therapy is reserved for children with documented seizure(s).
- Radiologic findings may prompt specific interventions, including:

—*CT scan showing focal hematoma* or skull films showing hairline fracture over the middle meningeal artery: neurosurgery consultation, close monitoring overnight with frequent neurologic checks, seizure precautions
—*CT scan showing structural injury,* including cerebral edema, hemorrhage, hypodense white matter: Transport to ICU for medical management of elevated ICP; measures may include fluid restriction, heart monitoring, SIADH monitoring with frequent electrolyte checks and strict fluid balance, mannitol, and hyperventilation as needed for progression of neurologic symptoms; neurosurgery consult for evaluation of hematoma and consideration of placement of ICP monitor.
—*Normal neuroimaging* in coma due to trauma may still be present in the setting of major CNS injury and attendant complications; alternate diagnoses (meningitis, epilepsy) and other laboratory investigation (spinal tap, EEG) should be considered if the traumatic basis of stupor/coma remains in doubt.
—Immobilize C-spine as necessary.

 ## Follow-Up

Monitoring for sequelae cognitive difficulties, hyperactivity, seizures, hydrocephalus, movement disorders, paralysis, visual/hearing disturbance, headache; psychologists, neurologists, neurosurgeon, ophthalmologists, audiologists, and physical therapists may be helpful.

PITFALLS

- Pupil asymmetry in an awake patient may be due to pharmacologic treatment (i.e., mydriatic agents for examination).
- Bacterial meningitis in a child who has had TBI may signal a CSF leak.
- Basilar skull fracture may be missed on routine CT scan—review bone windows or skull films.
- Witnesses and or primary caregivers may have personal reasons to conceal part or all of the circumstances regarding the child's injury.

 ## Common Questions and Answers

Q: What are the specific signs of increased intracranial pressure?
A: Cushing's reflex in association with deterioration in mental status. A change in pupils or ocular motility, or onset of posturing may also indicate increased ICP.

Q: When is mannitol used?
A: In patients with increased ICP in the absence of intracranial hemorrhage, mannitol may exacerbate elevated ICP if extravascular blood is present.

ICD-9-CM 854.0

BIBLIOGRAPHY

Bijur PE, Haslum M, Golding J. Cognitive and behavioral sequelae of mild head injury in children. *Pediatrics* 1990;86:337–344.

Duhaime A-C, Gennarelli TA, Thibault LE, et al. The shaken baby syndrome. *J Neurosurg* 1987;66:409–415.

Lee MS, Rinne JO, Ceballos-Baumann A, et al. Dystonia after head trauma. *Neurology* 1994;44:1374–1378.

Zimmerman RA, Bilaniuk LT. Pediatric head trauma. *Neuroimag Clin North Am* 1994;4:349–366.

Author: D. Elizabeth McNeil

Brain Tumor

 Database

DEFINITION

A brain tumor is a primary neoplasm arising in the central nervous system (CNS).

PATHOPHYSIOLOGY

• No specific causative agents are known, but there is an increased risk associated with radiation, chemical exposure, other malignancies, familial diseases.

The majority of tumors are classified based on their histology. The most common:

• Glioma

—Arise from astrocytes (supportive tissue)
—50% of childhood CNS tumors
—Range from benign or low grade, often in the cerebellum or optic pathway, to malignant or grade III to IV, in the cerebrum or brainstem.
—Locally recurrent and invasive when malignant

• Primitive neuroectodermal tumor (PNET)

—Malignant embryonal tumor arising from poorly differentiated neuroepithelial cells
—Comprise about 30% of childhood CNS tumors
—Occur more frequently in the midline of the cerebellum (referred to as medulloblastoma)
—Predisposition for leptomeningeal dissemination

• Ependymoma

—Arise from ependymal cells that line the ventricular system
—Comprise about 5% to 10% of childhood CNS tumors
—Most commonly occur in the fourth ventricle; adults have a higher incidence in the spinal cord
—Locally recurrent and invasive; prone to spinal metastases late in the course of the disease

• Rhabdoid or atypical teratoid tumor

—Rare embryonal tumor arising from unknown cell type
—Comprise less than 3% of childhood CNS tumors
—Occur most often in infants less than 2 years of age
—Propensity to arise in the posterior fossa with aggressive clinical pattern; reported in association with malignant rhabdoid tumors of the kidney

• Tumors of the choroid plexus and pineal gland
• Neuronal tumors

—Ganglioglioma
—Neuroblastoma

• Meningioma and hemangioblastoma, rare in children

GENETICS

• Not a heritable condition
• Primary CNS tumors are associated with several familial syndromes:

—Neurofibromatosis with optic pathway tumors and meningiomas
—Tuberous sclerosis with gliomas and rarely ependymomas
—Li-Fraumeni syndrome with astrocytomas

EPIDEMIOLOGY

• Most common solid neoplasm of childhood (second to leukemia in overall incidence)
• Incidence rising (about 1,700 new cases/yr)
• Peak age between 3 to 9 years old
• Slight male predominance

—Majority arise infratentorially (within cerebellum or brainstem) in children older than 1 year of age

COMPLICATIONS

• Increased intracranial pressure (ICP)

—Obstruction of cerebrospinal fluid (CSF) flow
—Requires immediate neurosurgical evaluation

• Diencephalic syndrome

—May be seen in infants with tumors involving the hypothalamus
—Results in failure to thrive and emaciation in a euphoric child with increased appetite

• Cognitive and neuroendocrine deficits

—Dependent on location of tumor, age, and therapy used

• Additional therapy-related complications:

—Chemotherapy
  —Risks associated with bone marrow suppression (infection, bleeding, anemia)
  —Hearing loss
  —Risk of secondary leukemia

—Radiation
  —Risk of second malignancies (meningioma, osteosarcoma, glioma, other sarcomas)
  —Neuropyschological damage is age and dose-related

PROGNOSIS

Dependent on histology of tumor, location, and extent of initial resection.

• Glioma

—Low grade: 90% survival
—High grade: 25% survival
—Brainstem: 10% survival

• PNET or medulloblastoma

—80% survival at 3 years if localized
—Less than 50% survival if disseminated (improving with autologous "bone marrow transplantation")

• Ependymoma

—60% to 70% survival at 5 years with total resection
—Less than 30% survival with subtotal resection.

• Infants overall have a worse prognosis, possibly due to the limitations of therapy versus the aggressiveness of the tumor.

 Differential Diagnosis

INFECTION

• Cerebral abscess

TUMORS

• Metastatic tumor to brain uncommon in childhood solid tumors

TRAUMA

• Hemorrhage unlikely to be confused with tumor

CONGENITAL

• Arteriovenous malformation
• Hamartoma

PSYCHOSOCIAL

• Some patients with nausea, vomiting, or behavior changes are first diagnosed with psychiatric disorders (anorexia nervosa) prior to discovery of a brain tumor.

 Data Gathering

HISTORY

Question: Headache frequency, intensity and vomiting?
Significance: Associated with increased intracranial pressure (ICP).

Question: New onset of neurological symptoms, difficulty chewing or swallowing.
Significance: Brainstem tumor.

Question: Diplopia
Significance: Cranial nerves or nodei affected.

Question: Visual field cuts ("bumps into things")
Significance: Optic tract lesion

Question: Weakness
Significance: Pyramidal tract lesion

Question: Ataxia
Significance: Cerebellar lesion

Question: Changes in behavior or school performance, new onset seizures.
Significance: Supratentorial lesion

Physical Examination

Finding: Head circumference/macrocephaly or bulging fontanelle and/or papilledema
Significance: Increased ICP

Finding: Focal deficit on neurological examination
Significance: Localizes mass lesion

Finding: Cranial nerves, palsies, parreflexia
Significance: Brainstem tumor

Finding: Coordinations; gait disturbances; head tilt
Significance: Cerebellar mass

Finding: Eye movements; nystagmus
Significance: Optic tract tumor

Finding: Changes in mental status
Significance: Supratentorial lesion

Finding: Signs of neurocutaneous disease (e.g., café au lait spots, Lisch nodules)
Significance: Syndrome like fibromatosis

 ## Laboratory Aids

IMAGING

Test: MRI with and without gadolinium enhancement
Significance: Gold standard image for identification, localization, and characterization of tumor

Test: CT
Significance: Can be used as a screen, but if negative with a high index of suspicion, follow with MRI

FALSE POSITIVES

Abscess, dysplastic brain, hamartoma

STAGING OF TUMOR

Test: Post-op head MRI within 48 to 72 hours
Significance: To determine residual disease

Test: Spine MRI; CSF cytology
Significance: Neuraxial staging for tumors with high risk of leptomeningeal dissemination

Test: Alpha-fetoprotein (AFP), B-HCG
Significance: Serum and CSF markers for germ cell tumors

 ## Therapy

SURGERY

• Both for histology and to attempt maximal tumor debulking, should be performed by experienced pediatric neurosurgeon
• Contraindicated in pontine (brainstem) glioma
• Ventriculoperitoneal (VP) shunt when needed for obstructive hydrocephalus (risk of peritoneal seeding minimal)

DRUGS

• Dexamethasone to control increased intracranial pressure (0.5 mg/kg divided q6h)
• Chemotherapy

—Drugs are most often used in combination

• New protocols currently under development

—CCNU, vincristine, procarbazine for high-grade glioma
—Cisplatin, CCNU, vincristine for medulloblastoma or PNET
—Carboplatin, vincristine, ± etoposide for low-grade glioma

RADIATION THERAPY (XRT)

• XRT to the tumor bed is used for most patients with brain tumors.
• Medulloblastoma/PNET patients need craniospinal XRT. The one exception is in infants and young children (<3 years of age) in whom cognitive deficits from XRT can be devastating.

Duration of Therapy

• Radiation therapy: 6 weeks
• Chemotherapy: 1 to 2 years

Possible Conflicts with Other Treatments

Chemotherapy can alter anticonvulsant levels.

• XRT (limited to structures in XRT field)

—Hair loss
—Otitis externa

 ## Follow-Up

• Neurological deficits can take months to improve or stabilize with permanent deficit.
• Any relapse or worsening of symptoms must be evaluated for tumor recurrence.
• MRI imaging every 3 months the first year, every 6 months for the next 4 years, and annually thereafter. Benefit of routine surveillance imaging is controversial.

PITFALLS

• New onset of psychoses should prompt imaging to rule out tumor.
• Not referring the patient to a pediatric brain tumor/oncology center at diagnosis (preoperatively). This requires an experienced (pediatric) neurosurgeon.

 ## Common Questions and Answers

Q: Are my other children at risk for getting a brain tumor?
A: No.

Q: Did something I do cause this?
A: No. In addition, the claims made about high-power lines and cellular phones causing brain tumors or cancer are unproven.

Q: Is this inherited?
A: No, except tumors associated with neurofibromatosis.

ICD-9-CM 191.9

BIBLIOGRAPHY

Cohen ME, Duffner PK. *Brain tumors in children,* 2nd ed. New York: Raven Press, 1994.

Gilles FH. Classifications of childhood brain tumors. *Cancer* 1985;56:1850–1857.

Gurney JG, Severson RK, Davis S, Robison LL. Incidence of cancer in children in the United States. *Cancer* 1995;75:2186–2195.

Heideman RL, Packer RJ, Albright LA. Tumors of the central nervous system. In: Pizzo PA, Poplack DG, eds. *Principles and practice of pediatric oncology,* 3rd ed. Philadelphia: JB Lippincott, 1997,633–697.

Packer RJ. Childhood tumors. *Curr Opin Pediatr* 1997;9(6):551–557.

Reddy AT. Packer RJ. Pediatric central nervous system tumors. *Curr Opin Oncol* 1998;10(3): 186–193.

Author: Deborah L. Kramer (Michael Needle, first edition)

Branchial Cleft Fistula

 Database

DEFINITION
- Remnant of the embryonic branchial system
- Part of a spectrum that includes:

—Branchial cyst (remnant of the cervical sinus)
—Branchial fistula (connection between the branchial cleft and pouch)
—Branchial sinus (sinus tract from the cervical sinus to the:
  —Neck (external branchial sinus)
  —Pharynx (internal branchial sinus)

PATHOPHYSIOLOGY
- Develops if the closing membrane between a branchial cleft and pouch is perforated
- Allows for the development of a tract between the neck and pharynx
- By 4 weeks' gestation, the embryo develops a system of branchial arches, clefts, and pouches that develop into the structures of the head and neck.
- Second branchial arch grows caudally over the second, third, and fourth branchial clefts, forming the cervical sinus.
- Cervical sinus usually involutes from within; if it persists, a branchial cyst is formed.
- If the closing membrane is perforated, a branchial cleft fistula forms.
- Fistula is lined by squamous and nonciliated columnar epithelium.
- Yellow mucoid secretions may arise from a fistula or sinus.
- Branchial fistulas always follow the same route:

—External opening at the lower third of the neck along the anterior border of the sterno-cleidomastoid muscle.
—Penetrates the platysma muscle.
—Runs along the carotid sheath and then passes between the internal and external carotid arteries.
—Crosses over the hypoglossal and glossopharyngeal cranial nerves.
—Passes below the stylohyoid ligament.
—Enters the pharynx at the posterior tonsillar fossa.

- Branchial cysts or sinuses are always found along this route.

GENETICS
- Familial history of branchial defects occasionally noted

EPIDEMIOLOGY
- 95% of defects arise from the second branchial system.
- Defects from the third or fourth branchial system are much less common.
- Branchial cysts are more common than sinuses or fistulas (complete fistulas are uncommon).
- Branchial defects usually present in childhood:

—Fistulas present earlier than sinuses (in most cases, <5 years old).
—Sinuses present earlier than cysts

- 67% of fistulas unilateral; 33% bilateral
- 60% of fistulas right-sided; 40% left-sided
- Sexual predominance:

—Slight female predominance for sinuses and fistulas
—Equal predominance for cysts

COMPLICATIONS
- Cysts, sinus tracts, and fistulas can become recurrently infected (especially with abscess formation).
- Surgery is more difficult if there has been previous infections or previous surgery.
- Damage to hypoglossal and glossopharyngeal nerves or carotid artery can occur during surgical repair.
- Recurrence of the lesion seen if not fully removed.

PROGNOSIS
- If lesion completely excised: excellent

 Differential Diagnosis

INFECTIONS
- Reactive lymphadenopathy (secondary from pharyngitis, tonsillitis, or otitis media)
- Neck abscess
- Tuberculosis

TUMORS
- Lymphoma
- Rhabdomyosarcoma

MISCELLANEOUS
- Thyroglossal duct cyst (laterally displaced)
- Lymphangioma
- Hemangioma

 Data Gathering

HISTORY
- Tender if infected
- Recurrent neck infections?
- Intermittent discharge from neck?
- Usually present since birth?
- Rule out possibility of malignancy.
- Fevers
- Night sweats
- Weight loss
- Other sites of adenopathy or masses

 Physical Examination

- Mass usually mobile
- Lesion usually non-tender (unless actively infected)
- Assess for sites of drainage:

—At the anterior border of the sternocleidomastoid muscle
—In the posterior pharynx at the tonsillar fossa

- Assess for signs of malignancy:

—Other sites of adenopathy (especially axillary or inguinal nodes)
—Hepatomegaly
—Splenomegaly

Laboratory Aids

Test: CBC with differential
Significance: Increased WBC with left shift seen with infection.

IMAGING

Test: Chest radiography
Significance: Assess for hilar adenopathy, suggesting a systemic process (such as tuberculosis or malignancy).

Test: Lateral neck radiography
Significance: Assess for airway compromise (not usually seen).

Test: Fistulogram
Significance: Inject contrast into the fistula to delineate its course.

Test: CT scan of neck
Significance:

• Helpful for evaluation of neck masses (especially abscesses)
• Characteristic appearance of branchial cyst:

—Posterior or posterolateral displacement of the sternocleidomastoid muscle.
—Medial or posteromedial displacement of the carotid artery and jugular vein
—Anterior displacement of the submandibular gland

Test: Ultrasound
Significance: Also helpful for neck masses

 ## Therapy

DRUGS

Antibiotics are indicated if the defect is infected.

SURGERY

• Excision of the entire lesion
• Surgery should be delayed if infection present

 ## Follow-Up

• Post-operative follow-up as outpatient for wound inspection
• Observation for recurrence or reinfection

PITFALLS

• Lesion may recur if not completely excised.
• High incidence of reinfection if not properly treated.

 ## Common Questions and Answers

Q: Can the cyst, fistula, or sinus recur?
A: Only a 3% recurrence rate is seen if the lesion is completely excised. A higher rate of recurrence is seen in cases of incomplete excision or with previous surgeries.

Q: Should the lesion be removed as soon as it is discovered?
A: The lesion should not be removed if there is an active infection present; treat the infection first. Should be scheduled as elective surgery.

ICD-9-CM 744.41

BIBLIOGRAPHY

Chandler JR, Mitchell B. Branchial cleft cysts, sinuses, and fistulas. *Otolaryngol Clin North Am* 1981;14:175–186.

Ford GR, Balakrishnan A, Evans JNG, Bailey CM. Branchial cleft and pouch anomalies. *J Laryngol Otol* 1992;106:137–143.

Harnsberger HR, Mancuso AA, Muraki AS, et al. Branchial cleft anomalies and their mimics: computed tomographic evaluation. *Radiology* 1984;152:739–748.

Karmody CS. Developmental anomalies of the neck. In: Bluestone CD, Stool S, Kenna M. *Pediatric otolaryngology*, 3rd ed. Philadelphia: WB Saunders, 1996:1497–1511.

Langman's Medical Embryology, 6th ed. Baltimore: Williams & Wilkins, 1990:298–327.

Lusk RP. Neck masses. In: Bluestone CD, Stool S, Kenna M. *Pediatric otolaryngology*, 3rd ed. Philadelphia: WB Saunders, 1996:1488–1496.

Thaler ER, Tom LWC, Handler SD. Second branchial cleft anomalies presenting as pharyngeal masses. *Otolaryngol Head Neck Surg* 1993;109:941–944.

Todd NW. Common congenital anomalies of the neck. *Surg Clin North Am* 1993;73:599–610.

Author: Richard Mark Kravitz

Breast Abscess

 ## Database

DEFINITION

Breast abscess is breast inflammation with pus localized in the breast bud or breast tissue.

ETIOLOGY

- Infection is most often due to *Staphylococcus aureus* in newborn infants and in adolescents.
- In newborns, *Escherichia coli, Pseudomonas aeruginosa,* and Group B Streptococcus, should also be considered.
- In adolescents, tuberculosis, *Neisseria gonorrhea,* and syphilis must also be considered. Trauma (sexual manipulation, nipple rings), mammary duct ectasia, epidermal cysts, mastitis and acne are predisposing factors.

PATHOPHYSIOLOGY

- Potentially pathogenic bacteria may colonize the skin and move retrograde into the ducts and deeper tissues.
- In newborns, breast hypertrophy secondary to maternal hormones appears to increase the risk of breast abscess formation. Abscesses are usually unilateral.

EPIDEMIOLOGY

- Most often neonates, 1 to 5 weeks old
- Neonatal male to female ratio is 1:2
- Occur in 2% of all postpartum women

COMPLICATIONS

- Bacteremia and sepsis, especially in newborns
- Cellulitis
- Necrotizing fasciitis
- Destruction of mammary gland with scar formation

PROGNOSIS

- Excellent, with appropriate treatment

 ## Differential Diagnosis

INFECTION

- Cellulitis
- Mastitis

TRAUMA

- Fat necrosis with painless, firm, circumscribed, mobile mass
- Contusion with firm tender poorly defined mass
- Hematoma as a sharply defined mass with ecchymosis

MISCELLANEOUS

- Mondor disease is a superficial phlebitis in the skin, often due to trauma (e.g., a biopsy), which resolves spontaneously.
- Carcinoma

 ## Data Gathering

HISTORY

Question: Manipulation of breast, trauma, a sudden onset of swelling, warmth, tenderness, and erythema are often reported.
Significance: Signs of infection

Question: Fever, irritability, nipple discharge?
Significance: Signs of infection

 ## Physical Examination

- Breast tissue may have fluctuance, warmth, swelling, erythema and tenderness
- Fever
- Purulent nipple discharge
- Regional adenopathy

 ## Laboratory Aids

- Nipple discharge from aspirates or incisional specimens, and send for bacterial culture.
- In neonates, send blood for bacterial culture to rule out bacteremia; consider full sepsis work-up. Consider culturing the throat and nose for evidence of colonization by *S. aureus.*

RADIOGRAPHIC STUDIES

- Ultrasound as needed

Therapy

DRUGS

- Neonates: IV Oxacillin or other β-lactamase resistant penicillin, with or without an aminoglycoside
- Adolescents: IV β-lactamase resistant penicillin (oxacillin, methicillin)

OTHER TREATMENTS

- Incision and drainage if fluctuance present
- Warm compresses
- For adolescents, who are breast-feeding infants, continued expression of milk is necessary to avoid engorgement and areas of milk stasis

DURATION

- Neonates: 10 to 14 days of oral antibiotics, given at home
- Adolescents: more than 14 days total of antibiotics

 ## Follow-Up

- Expect improvement within 48 hours of initiation of intravenous antibiotics
- Need to follow all patients closely given the risk of recurrence

PREVENTION

Avoid manipulation of breast tissue.

PITFALLS

- Superficial phlebitis can be confused with a breast abscess
- Fever is not always present on presentation

 ## Common Questions and Answers

Q: Is fluctuance always found on examination?
A: No, yet breast swelling and/or warmth/ erythema is nearly universally present.

Q: Is fever necessary for the diagnosis?
A: No, not always present at time of presentation.

Q: May a mother continue to breastfeed if she has a breast abscess?
A: The *1997 Red Book* recommendations are to discontinue breast feeding from the affected breast, but the unaffected breast may be used for breast feeding. After treatment is complete, the affected breast can be utilized in breast feeding again.

ICD-9-CM 611.03

BIBLIOGRAPHY

American Academy of Pediatrics. Peter G, ed. *1997 red book: report of the Committee on Infectious Diseases,* 24th ed. Elk Grove Village, IL: American Academy of Pediatrics; 1997:74.

Bailey LA, Waecker NJ Jr. Pseudomonas aeruginosa mastitis in a neonate. *Pediatric Infect Dis J* 1993;12(1):104.

Bodemer C, Panhans A, Chretien-Marquet B, Cloup M, Pellerin D, de Prost Y. Staphylococcal necrotizing fasciitis in the mammary region in childhood: a report of five cases. *J Pediatrics* 1997;131(3):466–469.

Bodsworth NJ, Price R, Nelson MJ. A case of gonococcal mastitis in a male. *Genitourin Med* 1993;69:222–223.

Greydanus DE, Parks DS, Farrell EG. Breast disorders in children and adolescents. *Pediatr Clin North Am* 1989;36(3):601–638.

Walsh M, McIntosh K. Neonatal mastitis. *Clin Pediatr* 1986;25:395–399.

Author: Andrea McGeary

Breast Feeding

 Database

DEFINITION

Human lactation produces breast milk, a species-specific nutrient for infants, term and preterm. Depending on the gestational age of the infant, milk varies in composition regarding fat, protein, carbohydrate, and minerals. Unique components of breast milk:

- Antibodies
- Interferon
- Growth factors that confer maturational factors to gut
- Live cells including polymorphonuclear neutrophils, lymphocytes, and macrophages

See table Comparison of Nutrients.

Studies have shown the following to be benefits of breast feeding in the first 6 to 12 months of life:

- Reduced incidence of diarrheal illnesses
- Reduced incidence of otitis media

Many studies support the plausibility that prolonged and exclusive breast feeding would protect against atopic disease.

PATHOPHYSIOLOGY

- In pregnancy: maternal prolactin is elevated leads to increase in secretory cells plus prolactin receptors in breast; and significantly elevated progesterone levels inhibit prolactin action (production of breast milk). After birth, placenta delivery leads to prolactin surge while progesterone and estrogen levels decrease. Prolactin leads to stimulates secretory cells leads to milk production.
- With each nursing session there is a prolactin burst. Prolactin remains elevated for the duration of breastfeeding the infant.

EPIDEMIOLOGY

- 60% of mothers initiate breastfeeding at birth, by 6 months only 18% are still nursing
- Factors associated with higher prevalence and longer duration breastfeeding include higher level of maternal education and greater maternal age.
- Factors negatively associated with breastfeeding include:

—Single motherhood whether widowed, divorced, or never married
—African-American ethnicity
—Maternal employment outside of home.

COMPLICATIONS

- Engorgement: breasts are firm, hard, hot, painful. They may be so firm that the infant cannot latch on.
- Sore and/or cracked nipples: nipples erythematous, with or without fissures, sometimes scabs may form; pain may be mild to pronounced.
- Candidiasis of maternal nipples: nipples may be erythematous, have deep burning or soreness.
- Inadequate milk supply.
- Poor weight gain in the infant may result from inadequate supply or poor feeding technique.

PROGNOSIS

- Breastfed infants in first 3 months have similar increase in weight, length, and head circumference, compared to formula-fed infants but proportionately slower weight gain for the next 9 months, resulting in a leaner infant with height and head circumference being maintained.

 Data Gathering

HISTORY

Consider the following decision factors that contribute to feeding practices:

- Maternal preference, knowledge base
- Paternal preference, knowledge base
- Cultural/societal supports including mother's mother
- Parity: feeding method of mother's previous infants

For the mother uncertain about how much milk infant is getting:

Question: How long does the infant nurse on each side?
Significance: Infants should nurse for 10 to 15 minutes on each side.

Question: Do her breasts feel softer after each feeding?
Significance: Breasts should feel softer if milk has been removed adequately by the infant.

Question: Does the infant seem satisfied?
Significance: To ensure that a baby has received enough, they should seem satisfied after a feeding.

Question: How many wet diapers a day is the infant making?
Significance: Infants receiving adequate hydration should void 6 to 8 times per day.

Question: Mother complaining of sore or cracked nipples?
Significance: Determine frequency of feeds, varied positions when feeding, and the nature of any home therapy attempted. Also, ask about concomitant infant oral thrush or infant diaper rash consistent with Candida dermatitis.

Question: Mother concerned about the quantity of milk being provided to the baby?
Significance: Confirm she is supplementing breast milk, offering breast at least q2h initially, drinking enough fluids herself, eating a balanced diet, and getting adequate rest.

 Physical Examination

Finding: Ensure that the neonate has not lost more than 10% of his/her birth weight in the first couple of weeks, and that she/he has regained his/her birth weight by the end of the second week.
Significance: Minimal criteria for adequate breast milk supply.

Finding: Assess for jaundice.
Significance: Infants who breast feed are at risk for breast feeding jaundice.

- Observe the infant's feeding, positioning, adequacy of latch-on, and suck.

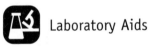 Laboratory Aids

Test: Electrolytes
Significance: Infant appears dehydrated

Test: Bilirubin
Significance: Infant jaundice is present

Comparison of Nutrients

	PROTEIN	FAT	CHO	Ca	Fe
per 100 mL	Total (whey/casein)		(Lactose)		
colostrum	2.3 g (total)	2.9 g	5.3 g	39 mg	70 μg
term	1.1 g (20%/80%)	3.8 g	7.0 g	35 mg	100 μg
preterm	1.81 g	4.0 g	6.95 g	22 mg	100 μg
cow milk	3.3 g (80%/20%)	3.3 g	4.8 g	130 mg	70 μg

(Adapted from Lawrence RA, with permission.)

Therapy

• Engorgement (due to production of milk, and increased circulation of blood and lymph in breasts)

—Feed infant often, avoid supplements (e.g., formula, sugar water), express milk if infant must skip feeding
—When time to wean, do so gradually.
—Use warm, moist compresses just before nursing, gently massage breasts during feeding. After nursing, reduce swelling with ice packs.

• Sore and/or cracked nipples

—Prevent by changing nursing positions often (various nursing styles should be demonstrated by lactation consultant before mother and baby are discharged from hospital)
—Ensure that the baby has much of the areola in his/her mouth when nursing, allow nipples to air dry completely between feedings, and always break suction seal before removing infant from breast.
—If pain occurs with nursing, change positioning (e.g., cradle position to football position). The infant's suck in one position may irritate a region of the nipple, which is uninvolved when the suck is from a different angle.
—Clean nipples with clear water, dry completely, and apply expressed breast milk to nipple. Pure lanolin cream may be helpful.
—If mother has fever, malaise, and/or discharge from affected area, she may have mastitis and should seek care from her health care provider.

• Nipple candidiasis or "thrush nipples"—after each feed massage nystatin cream into nipple(s); concurrently treat infant with nystatin suspension for 10 days.

• Inadequate milk supply, poor feeding, and weight gain: mother should drink 32 to 40 oz. fluids daily, preferably water; eat balanced diet (2500 kcal/day). Offer breast q1–2h to increase milk supply; wake infant at least once between 12 A.M. and 6 A.M. to nurse; sleep when baby sleeps to maximize mother's rest necessary for milk production.

• For the sleepy infant: change diaper, undress to diaper only, increase mother-baby skin-to-skin contact. Rule out infant illness.

 Follow-Up

• Aggressive follow-up by primary care provider is ideal. In addition, if mother does not have adequate sources for a lactation consultant from nursery, local directories are available. Women Infants and Children (WIC) programs in many regions have developed strong lactation support staff.
• Monitor weight on a weekly basis, if necessary, until milk supply is well established and infant is nursing successfully.
• Women who return to work may continue exclusively breastfeeding their infants. Support of her employer including a time and place to express milk is paramount for successful breastfeeding. For milk expression, an electric double pump is ideal for time considerations and for maintaining milk supply.
• Weaning: nutritional and developmental studies suggest exclusive breastfeeding for up to 6 months. Weaning should be done gradually both for mother's physical comfort and her infant's psychological acceptance.

PREVENTION

Contraindications to breast feeding include:

• Galactosemia
• Maternal neoplasm, life-threatening or debilitating illness
• Maternal medications: recreational drugs, chemotherapeutic drugs, bromocriptine, ergotamine, lithium, phenindone
• Maternal infection: HIV—absolute contraindication in developed world

PITFALLS

• Inadequate support of nursing mother who may give up and have a sense of failure
• Dispensing of formula samples on hospital discharge to breastfeeding mothers promotes acceptance of formula feeding as cultural norm

 Common Questions and Answers

Q: How frequently should I feed the baby? What does "on-demand" mean?
A: At first, newborn infants should be offered the breast at least every 1.5 to 2 hours as the milk supply is established. In the first 2 weeks, newborns should nurse 8 to 12 times/day and should be awakened to nurse if the baby sleeps more than 4 hours.

Q: How much is too much? Can I overfeed the baby?
A: An infant will usually stop eating if full but may continue to suck with less vigor for comfort. This less vigorous sucking is called "grazing." The mother will soon notice the difference and should cease nursing and choose to cuddle and rock the infant at that time.

Allowing "grazing" at the nipple can lead to obesity or even nursing caries; by the end of the first month the infant should take most of the feed in 10 to 15 minutes.

Q: Does my baby need vitamins?
A: If the mother continues her prenatal vitamins and eats a well-balanced diet, vitamin supplementation for the infant may not be necessary. Vitamin D is not in sufficient amounts in breast milk; however, its precursor is in the infant's skin and is converted to the active metabolite if the infant is exposed to sunlight at least 15 minutes/day. For a dark-skinned infant in winter, it is recommended to give liquid vitamin drops with 5 to 7.5 μg vitamin D daily. Vitamin drops are safe for all babies when used at the recommended dosage. Fluoride is recommended for the breastfed infant greater than 6 months of age if the baby is not receiving any fluoridated water. The recommended dosage in this setting is 0.25 mg fluoride daily.

Q: Is it not just easier to bottle feed?
A: Breastfeeding is convenient, always available, sterile, at the proper temperature, and mother may modestly nurse in most settings. It is also inexpensive. Compare the nominal increase of maternal nutrition costs to more than $1,000/year of infancy spent on proprietary formula.

BIBLIOGRAPHY

Banta-Wright SA. Minimizing infant exposure to and risks from medications while breastfeeding. *J Perinat Neonat Nurs* 1997;11(2):71–84.

Campbell C. Breastfeeding and health in the western world. *Br J Gen Pract* 1996;46:613–617.

Dewey KG. Cross-cultural patterns of growth and nutritional status of breast-fed infants. *Am J Clin Nutr* 1998;67:10–17.

Dillon AE, Wagner CL, Wiest D, Newman RB. Drug therapy in the nursing mother. *Clin Obstet Gynecol* 1997;24(3):675–696.

Golding J, Rogers I, Emmett P. Association between breast feeding, child development and behaviour. *Early Hum Dev* 1997;49(Suppl):S175–S184.

Jacobsen SW, Jacosen JL. Breast feeding and intelligence. *Lancet* 1992;339:926.

Krishna RV, Plichta SB. The role of social support in breastfeeding promotion: a literature review. *J Hum Lact* 1998;14:41–45.

Lawrence RA. *Breastfeeding: a guide for the medical profession.* St. Louis: Mosby-Year Book, 1999:Appendix A.

Vandenplas Y. Myths and facts about breastfeeding: does it prevent later atopic disease? *Acta Pediatr* 1997;86:1283–1287.

Xanthou M. Human milk cells. *Acta Pediatr* 1997;86:1288–1290.

Author: Stephanie D. James

Breast Feeding Jaundice and Breast Milk Jaundice

 Database

DEFINITION

There is significant overlap between breast feeding jaundice (BFJ) and breast milk jaundice (BMJ).

- BFJ: unconjugated hyperbilirubinemia with peak bilirubin level exceeding normal physiological range (6–10 mg/dL) in the third to fifth day of life in otherwise healthy infants who are exclusively breastfed.
- BMJ: prolonged unconjugated hyperbilirubinemia beginning after 1 week continuing up to the sixth week of life in otherwise healthy infants who are exclusively breastfed.

PATHOPHYSIOLOGY

- BFJ: reduced caloric intake, starvation, and relative dehydration
- BMJ: icterogenic breast milk from mothers whose infants have the BMJ syndrome is abnormal in at least three ways:

—Competitive inhibition of hepatic glucuronyl transferase by an unusual metabolite of progesterone, pregnane-3-alpha, 20 beta-diol.
—Inhibition of glucuronyl transferase activity by increased concentration of non-esterified (free) fatty acids especially unsaturated long chain and all medium chain, due to increased or abnormal lipase activity.
—Increased enterohepatic circulation of bilirubin due to either increased concentration of beta glucuronidase (deconjugates bilirubin glucuronides) activity in breastmilk or some unknown factor.

EPIDEMIOLOGY

- BFJ

—More common in certain racial groups, such as Native American, Asian (Chinese, Japanese, Korean, etc.)
—Incidence: approximately 12% to 13%

- BMJ

—Preterm and term infants equally affected
—Male to female, 1:1
—True incidence (in U.S.) unknown, approximately 0.5% to 2.4% of live births
—No known risk factors
—Highest serum bilirubin concentration reported: 50 mg/dL, does not exceed 20 mg/dL in most infants

GENETICS

- BFJ: N/A
- BMJ: familial predisposition noted, genetics unknown.

COMPLICATIONS

Rare occurrences of overt bilirubin encephalopathy (kernicterus) due to BMJ syndrome in otherwise healthy full-term infants when serum bilirubin levels were 40 mg/dL or higher.

PROGNOSIS

Excellent in almost all healthy full-term neonates for long-term neurodevelopment and auditory function. However, there is a risk of kernicterus if serum bilirubin exceeds 40 mg/dL, a rare event.

 Differential Diagnosis

INFECTION

- Sepsis
- Urinary tract infection

TOXINS

- Vitamin K_3
- Sulfonamides
- Oxytocin
- Nitrofurantoin

METABOLICAL

- Hypothyroidism
- Galactosemia (early)
- Inherited hepatic glucuronyl transferase deficiencies (types I and II)

HEMATOLOGIC

- Blood group incompatibility
- Rh incompatibility, and minor group antigen incompatibility
- Enzyme defects

—G6PD
—Pyrtivate kinase

- Red blood cell membrane defects
- Hereditary spherocytosis
- Hemoglobinopathies

—Alpha thalassemia
—Beta thalassemia

MISCELLANEOUS

- Extravasation of blood
- Swallowed maternal blood
- Cephalohematoma
- Polycythemia
- Transient familial neonatal hyperbilirubinemia (Lucey-Driscoll syndrome)
- Intestinal obstruction

—Meconium plugs
—Meconium ileus
—Hirschsprung disease

- Intestinal atresia

—Pyloric stenosis

 Data Gathering

HISTORY

Pregnancy

- Length of gestation?
- Maternal illness (diabetes, hypertension)?
- Medication (oxytocin), drug use?

Labor

- Instrumentation used?
- Apgar scores?
- Cephalohematoma?
- Swallowed maternal blood?

Sepsis

- Maternal urinary tract infection?
- Rupture of membranes over 18 hours?
- Chonoammonitis?
- Group B streptococcal status?
- Maternal temperature?

Perinatal Hospital Course

- Passage of meconium?
- Timing of appearance of jaundice?
- Phototherapy?

Current State of Being

- Feeding?
- Activity?
- Hydration?
- Stools?
- Weight gain?

Familial History of Hemolytic Disorders

- Jaundice in siblings?

 Physical Examination

Conduct a careful, complete examination. See table Relation of Physical Findings and Bilirubin Level

Finding: Overall good health in infant
Significance: Differentiates BMJ from most other causes of prolonged jaundice.

 Laboratory Aids

Test: Total bilirubin with direct and indirect components
Significance: In hemolysis, indirect bilirubin is high.

Test: Complete blood count (with smear)
Significance: Helps determine degree of hemolysis.

Test: Reticulocyte count.
Significance: Keep in inind that this test is elevated in the neonatal period.

Test: Blood type
Significance: Direct and indirect Coombs test (in presence of "set up" but a negative direct Coombs, diagnosis of ABO incompatibility can be made from antibody titers in mother or detection of antibody on RBC by elution technique).

Test: Check G6PD activity
Significance: G6PD deficiency may present in the neonatal period as jaundice.

Breast Feeding Jaundice and Breast Milk Jaundice

 ## Therapy

More frequent nursing, up to 12 times a day, effective in reducing serum bilirubin levels.

SUPPORTIVE CARE

• Close monitoring of serum bilirubin concentration.
• Maintain serum bilirubin concentration below 25 mg/dL.
• Maintain hydration, urine output greater than 2 cc/kg/h and specific gravity less than 1.010. (An alternative therapy is to offer formula after breast feeding until the milk production is optimal. *See* Academy of Pediatrics Committee Report on breast feeding.)
• If bilirubin greater than 20 mg/dL: replace breast feeding with formula for 48 hours, or supplement breast feeding with small frequent formula feeds (best achieved with "nursing supplementor," a thin flexible tube attached to the breast immediately adjacent to the nipple and connected to a reservoir of formula).
• If serum bilirubin level rises to 20 mg/dL begin phototherapy. Always administer phototherapy at an irradiance dose between 10 to 12 μw/cm^2/nm. (*See* AAP Practice Parameter, 1994, which provides treatment guidelines.)
• If mother prefers not to interrupt nursing, start phototherapy at 18 to 20 mg/dL.
• If serum bilirubin level exceeds 30 mg/dL or does not show a fall after 4 to 6 hours of phototherapy when greater than 25 mg/dL.

DURATION OF THERAPY

• Phototherapy is continued until bilirubin has decreased to safe range, which is dependent on age, gestation, and weight.
• Bilirubin should be followed (at least once) within 12 to 24 hours after phototherapy has been discontinued to check for rebound.

POSSIBLE CONFLICTS WITH OTHER TREATMENTS

• In presence of existing dehydration, administration of high dose phototherapy may increase the infant's temperature and worsen the hydration status; intravenous fluids are indicated.
• Phototherapy should be given concurrently with exchange transfusion when bilirubin level exceeds 30 mg/dL.

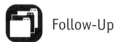 ## Follow-Up

WHEN TO EXPECT IMPROVEMENT

• When breast feeding is temporarily discontinued in infants with BMJ, serum bilirubin concentration declines within 24 hours and usually reaches one-half of the original level within 2 to 3 days
• When nursing resumes, serum bilirubin concentration rises by 1 to 3 mg/dL in next 48 hours and remains steady before beginning a gradual decline.
• Wallaby blankets often result in slower decline in bilirubin level than other forms of phototherapy.

PROGNOSIS

• Neurodevelopmental sequelae and auditory dysfunction (kernicterus) extremely rare in healthy full-term neonates.
• Risk of kernicterus is significant if serum bilirubin exceeds 40 mg/dL.
• Prolonged unconjugated hyperbilirubinemia in subsequent siblings likely.

PITFALLS

• None of the laboratory tests accurately identify infants at risk of kernicterus because maximal serum bilirubin is only weakly associated with the true risk factors—free brain tissue bilirubin and duration of hyperbilirubinemia.
• There has been a resurgence of kernicterus recently in healthy non-hemolytic jaundiced newborns discharged home early (before 48 hours of life), and jaundice remains a major cause of readmission to the hospital in the first 2 weeks of life (4.2 per 1000 discharges).
• Although not statistically significant, a recent study pointed to a less than adequate fluid and caloric intake as a cause in jaundiced newborns. The general guideline that is being applied for discharge is to repeat a serum bilirubin level in 24 hours after discharge in all newborns with bilirubin level ≥8 mg/dL and ≥13 mg/dL on day 1 and day 2, respectively; and to ensure follow-up of all newborns, especially those exclusively breastfed, within 2 to 3 days of discharge.

 ## Common Questions and Answers

Q: Does direct sunlight help babies with BMJ?
A: Yes. However, there is a risk of sunburn from UV radiation if exposure is not monitored or if the baby is exposed to strong sunlight.

Q: Does estimation of "free" or unbound bilirubin help in predicting infants at risk for kernicterus?
A: Many tests have been developed in an attempt to predict bilirubin encephalopathy. These tests include free bilirubin, bilirubin binding capacity, bilirubin/albumin ratio (indicates availability of bilirubin anion to bind to cell membranes), blood carboxyhemoglobin or exhaled CO (indicate bilirubin load), and many neurophysiological tests such as brain stem auditory evoked potentials, cry analysis, Brazelton behavioral assessment scale and others. None of these were consistently found to correlate with kernicterus and many are unavailable in clinical settings.

Q: Is transcutaneous bilirubinometry accurate enough to replace laboratory estimations of bilirubin?
A: Transcutaneous bilirubinometry can be accurate, provided it is well standardized for the population under consideration and can replace serum bilirubin measurement as a screening test and for monitoring the effect of the therapy. However, values provided by the bilirubinometer can vary considerably depending on the technique, skin color and exposure to phototherapy.

ICD-9-CM 774.39

BIBLIOGRAPHY

American Academy of Pediatrics. Practice parameter: management of hyperbilirubinemia in the healthy term newborn. *Pediatrics* 1994;94:558–562.

Gartner LM, Auerbach KG. Breast milk and breast feeding jaundice. *Adv Pediatr* 1987;34:249–274.

Maisels MJ, Kring E. Length of stay, jaundice and hospital readmission. *Pediatrics* 1998;101:995–998.

Maisels MJ, Newman TB. Kernicterus occurs in full term, healthy, newborns without apparent hemolysis. *Pediatr Res* 1994;35:239A.

Martinez JC, Maisels J, Otheguy L, Garcia H, Savorani M, Mogni B. Hyperbilirubinemia in the breast-fed newborn: a controlled trial of four interventions. *Pediatrics* 1993;91:470–473.

Newman TB, Klebanoff MA. Neonatal hyperbilirubinemia and long term outcome: another look at the Collaborative Perinatal Project. *Pediatrics* 1993;92:651–657.

Author: Sameer Wagle

Relation of Physical Findings and Bilirubin Level

DISTRIBUTION	AVERAGE SERUM BILIRUBIN LEVEL
Limited to head and neck	6
Upper trunk	9
Lower trunk and thighs	12
Arms and legs below knee	15
Hands and feet	≥15

This is not valid once infant has begun phototherapy.

Breath-Holding Spells

 Database

DEFINITION

- Simple breath-holding spells (BHS) are an involuntary (reflexive) event in which the child becomes apneic and often bradycardic at end expiration
- BHS are classified as severe when they are prolonged and associated with loss of consciousness, seizure activity
- Often divided into cyanotic spells or pallid spells, based on child's appearance during episodes

ETIOLOGY

- Usually brought on by anger, frustration, fear, or minor injury
- Cyanotic spells thought to be related to an autonomic dysregulation leading to prolonged expiratory apnea
- Pallid spells thought to be related to an overactive vagal response resulting in bradycardia or asystole
- Anemia has been reported to worsen the severity and frequency of BHS

EPIDEMIOLOGY

- Lifetime prevalence of up to 25% during childhood
- Severe BHS occur in less than 1% of the population
- Onset is typically between 6 months and 2 years of age
- Rare after age 6 years
- Cyanotic spells more common than pallid spells

COMPLICATIONS

- No clear evidence of long-term sequelae
- Reports of neurodevelopmental abnormalities, and rarely, death in children with severe BHS do exist, but the association of these outcomes with the BHS is very controversial.

 Differential Diagnosis

- Seizures: the presence of a precipitating event and the occurrence of cyanosis or pallor prior to the tonic-clonic movements usually allows BHS to be distinguished from seizures by history
- Familial dysautonomia
- Long QT syndrome
- Brain stem lesions: tumor, Arnold-Chiari malformation

 Data Gathering

HISTORY

Focus on preceding circumstances and parents' reaction to the event(s)

Question: Was there an injury, anger, frustration?
Significance: Helps identify situations likely to preceed the spells.

 Physical Examination

Finding: Results of the general physical examination are normal. To rule out other disorders, brain stem and spinal cord function should be evaluated on neurological examination.
Significance: Familial dysautonomia is a rare disorder that causes symptoms from infancy. Symptoms include failure to thrive, chronic aspiration, insensitivity to pain, and crying without tears.

 Laboratory Aids

Test: CBC
Significance: Check for anemia and iron deficiency

Test: EEG
Significance: Helpful in distinguishing BHS from seizure disorder when history unclear

Test: ECG
Significance: Indicated to rule out long QT syndrome when there is syncope and history is atypical for BHS.

Therapy

- Reassure parents that these spells will not harm the child.
- Parental education for severe BHS. Normal breathing resumes after loss of consciousness.
- Place child on the floor to prevent falling
- Clear the mouth of food/foreign bodies during episode to prevent aspiration.
- Activate the emergency medical system if the loss of consciousness is longer than 1 minute.

DRUGS

- Iron: treatment with ferrous sulfate (5 mg/kg/day) for 16 weeks resulted in a cessation of BHS in over 50% of cases. Not all responders were iron deficient on laboratory evaluation. Mechanism of action were unknown.
- Atropine: used in severe pallid BHS to prevent bradycardia and loss of consciousness.

 Follow-Up

- Based on the amount of support the parents need in learning to manage these spells
- Referral to a mental health professional if parents unable to discipline child for fear of inducing BHS

PITFALLS

- Child may learn to trigger spells, if they result in the child getting what he or she wants.
- Attempts to give mouth-to-mouth resuscitation to children with BHS is unnecessary and has been reported to have led to aspiration.

 Common Questions and Answers

Q: Are children with BHS more stubborn or disobedient than other children?
A: No. Recent studies found no difference in the behavioral profiles of children with BHS and controls.

Q: Will BHS occur in other children in the family?
A: There does seem to be a tendency toward having BHS that can be inherited. Twenty percent to 30% of first-degree relatives of probands with severe BHS will have a current or past history of severe BHS.

ICD-9-CM 786.9

BIBLIOGRAPHY

Daoud AS, Batieha A, Al-Sheyyab M, Abuekteish F, Hijazi S. Effectiveness of iron therapy on breath-holding spells. *J Pediatr* 1997;130:547–550.

DiMario FJ. Breath-holding spells in childhood. *Am J Dis Child* 1992;146:125–131.

DiMario FJ, Burleson JA. Behavior profile of children with severe breath-holding spells. *J Pediatr* 1993;122:488–491.

McWilliam RC, Stephenson JBP. Atropine treatment of reflex anoxic seizures. *Arch Dis Child* 1974;59:473–475.

Schmitt BD. *Instructions for pediatric patients.* Philadelphia: WB Saunders, 1992.

Author: Nathan J. Blum

Bronchiolitis

 Database

DEFINITION

Acute lower respiratory illness that causes obstruction of the small conducting airways of the lung.

PATHOPHYSIOLOGY AND CAUSES

- Respiratory synsytical virus (RSV) is the most common cause of this illness.
- RSV is transmitted by:

—Direct contact with nasal secretions from an infected individual.
—Aerosol spread (less common).

- RSV induces damage to the bronchial epithelium, resulting in inflammation of the smaller airways.
- Leukocytes (predominantly lymphocytes) infiltrate the peribronchial epithelial tissue, causing airway edema.
- Inflammation causes necrosis of the respiratory epithelium with replacement by nonciliated epithelial cells, which diminish the proximal movement of secretions to the larger airways and results in airway obstruction.
- IgE-mediated hypersensitivity may play a role.
- Other agents associated with bronchiolitis include:

—Parainfluenza viruses? Influenza A
—Adenovirus
—Rhinovirus
—Mycoplasma pneumoniae

EPIDEMIOLOGY

- Seen in all geographic areas
- Peaks during the winter and early spring
- Most children infected in the first 3 years of life; 80% within the first 12 months
- More common in infants with:

—Lower socioeconomic status
—Crowded living conditions
—Delayed immunizations
—Exposure to cigarette smoke
—Bottle-feeding versus breast-feeding

- More serious the younger the child (6 months)
- Rarely fatal in otherwise healthy infants
- Approximately one-half of infants with bronchiolitis develop subsequent wheezing.

GENETICS

- Genetic background is unclear.

Complications

- Most serious/common complications:

—Pneumonia
—Respiratory failure
—Apnea

- Highest risk of complications seen with:

—Congenital heart disease
—Bronchopulmonary dysplasia (BPD)
—Chronic lung disease
—Cystic fibrosis
—Prematurity
—Immunodeficiency

PROGNOSIS

- For most infants: excellent, self-resolving disease
- Death occurs rarely in infants and babies with no underlying disease (usually as a result of unrecognized apnea, respiratory failure, or superinfection)
- Morbidity and mortality is considerable in patients with an underlying chronic disease.
- 40% to 50% of infants will have recurrent episodes of wheezing until 2 to 3 years of age:

—Some will develop asthma.
—Others have abnormal lung function later in childhood.

 Differential Diagnosis

- Pneumonia (viral or bacterial)
- Asthma
- Gastroesophageal reflux (GER)
- Foreign body
- Noxious agents (chemicals, fumes, toxins)

 Data Gathering

HISTORY

Question: Rhinorrhea with thick nasal secretions?
Significance: Characteristic of disease

Question: Coughing?
Significance:

- Initially hoarse cough for 3 to 5 days
- Progresses to deep, wet cough of increased frequency

Question: Poor feeding?
Significance: Possible dehydration

Question: Low-grade fever?
Significance: Characteristic of disease

Question: Restlessness or lethargy?
Significance: May indicate low oxygen saturation

Question: Apnea (seen in younger patients)?
Significance: Impending failure

Question: Color change/cyanosis?
Significance: Impending failure

Question: Development of respiratory distress?
Significance: Impending failure

 Physical Examination

PULMONARY EXAMINATION

- Cough
- Tachypnea
- Accessory muscle retractions
- Hyperresonance to percussion
- High-pitched wheezing
- Prolonged expiratory phase
- Fine inspiratory crackles

HEENT EXAMINATION

- Nasal flaring
- Nasal congestion with thick, purulent secretions

OTHER FINDINGS

- Low-grade fever
- Tachycardia
- Possible cyanosis of nail beds and oral mucosa
- Liver and spleen typically pushed down by hyperinflated lungs

 Laboratory Aids

BLOOD TESTS

Test: CBC with differential
Significance: Rarely helpful

Test: Pulse oximetry
Significance: To assess oxygenation

Test: Arterial blood gas
Significance: Useful for assessing:

- Oxygenation
- Evidence of respiratory failure acidosis with CO_2 retention

RAPID VIRAL IDENTIFICATION

- Immunofluorescence or ELISA

VIRAL CULTURE

Test: Culture of nasopharynx
Significance: Should be done for all patients with negative rapid respiratory studies.

IMAGING

- Chest radiography
- Hyperinflation
- Flattened diaphragms
- Patchy or more extensive atelectasis
- Possible collapse of a segment or a lobe
- Diffuse interstitial infiltrates commonly seen

Therapy

GENERAL MANAGEMENT

• Most cases are mild and can be treated at home.
• Only 1% to 5% of previously healthy children require hospitalization.
• Hospitalization should be considered for infants and young children who:

—Were born prematurely.
—Appear ill or toxic.
—Are <3 months of age
—Have decreased oxygen saturation
—Have an underlying disease such as:
   —Bronchopulmonary dysplasia
   —Congenital heart disease
   —Chronic lung disease (i.e., cystic fibrosis)
   —Immunodeficiency

DRUGS

Supplemental Oxygen

• Given to any patient with hypoxia

Bronchodilators

• All infants with bronchiolitis with significant wheezing should receive a trial of at least one aerosolized β-adrenergic treatment to see if there is any relief of symptoms.
• Infants with history of prior wheezing or a familial history of asthma are more likely to respond to a bronchodilator.
• Theophylline not usually useful as a bronchodilator but should be considered if apnea is present (keep level 5–10 mg/mL).

Corticosteroids

• Use in children with bronchiolitis has not been evaluated adequately.
• Does not appear to be helpful

Antibiotics

• Superimposed bacterial infection is rare.
• Not usually indicated

Antiviral Agents (Ribavirin)

• Ribavirin is a synthetic nucleoside with activity against several viruses, including RSV.
• Use is controversial (beneficial effect most evident in the more severely ill patients).
• Benefits

—Improves oxygenation
—Shortens duration of illness
—Shortens period of viral shedding

• Indications

—Patients at increased risk for severe or complicated RSV infection
—Patients requiring mechanical ventilation
—Premature patients
—Patients <6 weeks of age
—Bronchopulmonary dysplasia
—Chronic lung disease
—Congenital heart disease
—Heart failure
—Pulmonary hypertension
—Patients with immunodeficiency
—Patients receiving chemotherapy
—Patients who have recently undergone transplantation
—Multiple congenital anomalies
—Neurological disorders
—Metabolical disorders

• Dosing

—Delivered via small-particle aerosol generator.
—Dosage: 6 g in 300 mL sterile H_2O given over 12 to 20 hours for 3 to 7 days
—Precautions: pregnant women should avoid exposure due to possible teratogenic effects.

RSV Hyperimmunoglobulin (RSV-IVIG)

• Recommended for premature infants and infants with chronic pulmonary disease (e.g., BPD)
• Human monoclonal antibodies for intramuscular injection are currently under investigation with promising results to date
• This therapy has not yet been approved by the FDA

Duration

• Continue bronchodilators until oxygenation normalizes and/or bronchospasm resolves.
• Ribavirin (if indicated) should be started as early in the illness as possible and continued for 5 days.

 Follow-Up

WHEN TO EXPECT IMPROVEMENT

• Most infants improve within 3 to 5 days.
• Those who need mechanical ventilation may have difficulties with extubation due to excessive secretions and atelectasis.

SIGNS TO WATCH FOR

• Impending respiratory failure (increased work of breathing, retractions, hypoxemia, CO_2 retention, lethargy).
• Sudden deterioration suggesting atelectasis due to mucous plugging.
• Fatigue may occur in infants who have prolonged and extensive disease.
• Fatigue will manifest with increased pCO_2 and worsening hypoxemia.

PITFALLS

• Hypoxia is common, so always follow oxygen saturation.
• Be aware of apnea.
• Respiratory failure may have a sudden presentation
• In cases of clinical bronchiolitis, causes of false-negative ELISA tests:

—Poor quality of sample
—Sample contamination
—Insufficient sample
—Non-RSV bronchiolitis

 Common Questions and Answers

Q: How did my child get bronchiolitis?
A: RSV bronchiolitis is a common, seasonal, lower respiratory tract infection that is easily transmissible.

Q: Can my child become reinfected?
A: Children can become reinfected with RSV bronchiolitis, and infection can occur more than once during the same respiratory season.

Q: Do patients with bronchiolitis need to be isolated?
A: Hospitalized patients who are RSV-positive need to be isolated with other RSV-positive patients and from uninfected patients. Patients who are receiving ribavirin should be kept in isolation.

Q: Will my child develop asthma?
A: Significant numbers of infected children will develop recurrent wheezing. Some will end up with asthma.

ICD-9-CM 466.19

BIBLIOGRAPHY

American Academy of Pediatrics. *1994 red book: report of the Committee on Infectious Diseases.* Elk Grove Village, IL: American Academy of Pediatrics, 1994:396–398, 570–575.

Holberg CJ, Wright AL, Martinez FD, et al. Risk factors for respiratory syncytial virus-associated lower respiratory illness in the first year of life. *Am J Epidemiol* 1991;133:1135–1151.

Shaw KN, Bell LM, Sherman NH. Outpatient assessment of infants with bronchiolitis. *Am J Dis Child* 1991;145:151–155.

Welliver JR, Welliver RC. Bronchiolitis. *Pediatr Rev* 1993;14:134–139.

Author: Hakon Hakonarson

Bronchopulmonary Dysplasia

 ## Database

DEFINITION

Subsequent improvements in the care of premature neonates have decreased incidence of severe bronchopulmonary dysplasia (BPD), as described by Northway, and many authors have proposed refinement in the original definition, making the precise definition of BPD somewhat controversial.

PATHOPHYSIOLOGY

• Barotrauma is the result of positive-pressure applied to a surfactant-deficient lung, causing unequal pressures and thus unequal aeration of the tracheo-bronchial tree.
• Terminal bronchioles and alveolar ducts are prone to damage and rupture when subjected to higher than normal pressures.
• Ruptured bronchioles can lead to pulmonary interstitial emphysema (PIE), which increases the risk of BPD six-fold.
• Free radical damage is increased in premature lung, from hyperoxia and impaired antioxidant activity.

GENETICS

• Premature infants with a strong familial history of asthma and eczema are more likely to develop BPD.
• There is an association with HLA-A2.

EPIDEMIOLOGY

• Risk is inversely proportional to birth weight.
• Rare in infants weighing more than 1500 grams; common in infants weighing less than 1000 grams.
• Most common form of chronic lung disease in infancy.

COMPLICATIONS

• Prolonged intubation may cause subglottic stenosis and tracheomalacia.
• Pulmonary hypertension may occur as a result of vasculature damage and subsequent intimal proliferation, which may, in turn, produce right ventricular hypertrophy and, if severe enough, cor pulmonale.
• Pulmonary edema often occurs secondary to increased pulmonary capillary permeability and increased pulmonary pressures.
• Reactive airways, bronchospasm, and altered pulmonary mechanics due to a poorly compliant lung may result in abnormal pulmonary function testing and increased work of breathing.
• Malnutrition and growth failure may occur as a result of increased work of breathing and a subsequently high caloric expenditure.
• Impaired lung defenses result in an increased susceptibility to infection, especially respiratory syncitial virus (RSV).

PROGNOSIS

• Majority of survivors demonstrate slow, steady improvement.
• High death rate (17%–47%) for patients with severe disease requiring prolonged mechanical ventilation.
• Despite multiple and varied treatment modalities, none have shown significant impact on the long-term outcome of chronic BPD.
• BPD survivors often have long-term pulmonary sequelae including hyperinflation, reactive airways, and exercise intolerance.
• Even older children and young adults who were felt to be asymptomatic have been shown to have abnormal responsiveness to exercise.
• Newer technologies, in particular the use of high-frequency ventilation and the widespread use of exogenous surfactant, have definitely improved survival rates for premature infants; however, concomitant reduction in the incidence and severity of BPD has been difficult to demonstrate.

 ## Differential Diagnosis

• Asthma
• Bronchiolitis obliterans
• Congenital heart disease
• Cystic adenomatoid malformation
• Cystic fibrosis
• Ideopathic pulmonary fibrosis
• Infections
• Meconium aspiration syndrome
• Recurrent aspiration

 ## Data Gathering

HISTORY

• Maternal use of antenatal steroids?
• Gestational age, birth weight, APGAR score?
• Initial resuscitative efforts, need for intubation, use of surfactant, duration in intubation, type of ventilation, duration of supplemental oxygen therapy, and other factors? These may have influenced the type and degree of lung injury.
• Familial history of asthma, atopy, or other children with BPD?
• Social support structure?
• Any potentially exacerbating factors such as exposure to smoking?

 ## Physical Examination

• Review of systems to include careful assessment of work of breathing both at rest and during activity
• Feeding and sleeping history, and a review of growth charts.
• Vitals to include respiratory rate and pulse oxymetry both at rest and with activity.
• Signs of pulmonary hypertension, including peripheral edema, hepatomegaly, and venous distention.

 ## Laboratory Aids

Test: Changes on chest radiography
Significance: Include hyperinflation, emphysema, cyst formation, pulmonary edema, fibrosis, and cardiovascular changes. The severity of these changes may help predict the severity of the disease.

Test: Chest computed tomography scan
Significance: May help provide more detailed information.

Test: Electrocardiogram
Significance: Often followed serially to assess for right ventricular hypertrophy (RVH).

Test: Echocardiogram
Significance: Often a useful adjunct to follow those patients with RVH.

Test: Cardiac catheterization
Significance: Reserved for those patients with evidence of pulmonary hypertension and cardiac dysfunction.

Test: Pulmonary function testing
Significance: Often used to follow patients and evaluate responsiveness to interventions.

Test: Blood gases
Significance: Useful both in the acute and chronic management of BPD to follow the degree of hypoxia and hypercapnia.

Test: Bronchoscopy, barium swallow, PH probe, and sleep studies
Significance: May reveal other underlying conditions possibly contributing to pulmonary dysfunction.

 ## Therapy

DIURETICS

• Diuretics are used for treating pulmonary edema, often improving lung mechanics and gas-exchange.
• Furosemide may have other non-diuretic benefits, including effects on prostaglandin synthesis, direct vasodilitation, and improved surfactant production.

- There are many side effects from long-term furosemide therapy including azotemia, ototoxicity, electrolyte abnormalities, excessive urinary calcium loss, osteopenia, and nephrocalcinosis.
- Thiazide diuretics, usually used in conjunction with a potassium-sparing diuretic such as spironolactone, are generally considered to be not as effective as furosemide.
- Routine monitoring of electrolytes recommended for patients on long-term diuretic therapy.
- Electrolyte supplementation often required with long-term diuretic usage.

BRONCHODILATORS

- Inhaled beta-agonists are effective treatment for reversible bronchospasm, though the safety and efficacy of long-term usage of these agents has yet to be established.
- Albuterol is often the drug of choice, though longer acting agents often used as well.
- Muscarinic antagonists, such as ipratropium, may be useful adjuncts, especially in patients who are not significantly responsive to albuterol. Felt to work on large- and medium-sized airways.
- Cromolyn, though not a bronchodilator, is often used for its anti-inflammatory effects and has a low side-effect profile.
- Methylxanthines, such as caffeine and theophylline, are often used in the treatment of apnea because of their effects on respiratory drive, also have a mild diuretic effect and help improve diaphragmatic contractility, making them a potentially useful adjunct in BPD as well.

PULMONARY VASODILATORS

Supplemental oxygen is an effective vasodilator and remains a mainstay of treatment for infants with either chronic or intermittent hypoxia.

STEROIDS

- Steroid usage in BPD is controversial.
- Increased risk for sepsis has probably been overstated.
- Often used successfully in short regimens to wean ventilatory support and hasten extubation.
- No long-term benefits of steroid therapy have been demonstrated, including reduced hospitalization, improved survival, or reduced incidence of BPD.
- Inhaled steroids may provide the desired anti-inflammatory effects, without systemic side effects, though their usage is unstudied and not routinely indicated.

NUTRITION

- Infants with BPD may have increased caloric needs as much as 150 kcal/kg/d.
- Premature and critically ill infants may be deficient in antioxidants such as vitamin A, vitamin E, and superoxide dismutase (SOD).

- Supplementation of vitamin A, vitamin E, and SOD at therapeutic and supratherapeutic levels have not yet shown to affect outcomes in BPD, though anti-oxidant supplementation remains an area of ongoing research.

 Follow-Up

- A multidisciplinary approach is recommended for all patients with moderate and severe BPD.
- Team may include primary care physician, pediatric pulmonologist, pediatric cardiologist, nutritionist, speech, respiratory, occupational, and physical therapists.
- Monitor growth and nutritional status.
- Monitor neurodevelopmental status, including NICU "high-risk" follow-up.

PREVENTION

- Antenatal steroids for all mothers with irreversible pre-term labor, less than 35 weeks gestation.
- Surfactant administration clearly improves mortality, though a reduction in the incidence or severity of BPD has been difficult to demonstrate.
- A change in ventilatory strategy toward "permissive hypercapnia," which favors the acceptance of lower pH and higher PCO_2 in exchange for lower peak inspiratory pressures and less barotrauma, has been widely adopted.
- High frequency ventilation, with either oscillatory or jet technology, may prevent barotrauma, though has yet to be shown to affect the incidence or severity of BPD.
- Avoidance of pulmonary edema, including the prophylactic and early treatment of patent ductus arteriosis may be of benefit.
- Early nutritional support, including the supplementation of anti-oxidant vitamins and minerals at therapeutic and supratherapeutic levels, may be of benefit.

PITFALLS

- Ensure adequate calcium and phosphorus intake in patients at risk for hyperparathyroidism and rickets.
- Patients less than 2 years old are candidates for RSV immune globulin prophylaxis, if not contraindicated.
- Patients older than 6 months are candidates for influenza vaccine, if not contraindicated.
- Chest physiotherapy may cause pathological fractures in patients with osteopenia.

 Common Questions and Answers

Q: Will antibiotics help my child?
A: While some evidence suggests that infection with ureaplasm may be important in the pathogenesis of BPD, it remains to be seen whether or not treatment of this particular organism affects outcome. Excessive usage of antibiotics increases occurrence of antibiotic resistance.

Q: Which babies should get RSV immune globulin (Respigam or Synagis)?
A: Immunoprophylaxis has been recommended by the AAP Committee on Infectious Diseases for infants with BPD who are less than 2 years old at the onset of RSV season or for other premature infants, regardless of BPD status, who are either former 28 week gestation or less infants, and are now younger than 1 year, or former 32 week gestation or less infants, and are younger than 6 months at the onset of RSV season.

Q: Will anti-RSV immunoprophylaxis prevent my baby from getting RSV?
A: It won't prevent RSV, but it will help your child's own immune system attack the virus.

Q: What is the difference between Respigam and Synagis?
A: Respigam is a human-derived RSV specific hyperimmune globulin, which is administered intravenously over a several hour period. Synagis (generic name is palivizumab) is an RSV-specific monoclonal antibody produced by recombinant technology and is 50 to 100 times more potent than Respigam and, therefore, able to be given as an intramuscular injection.

Q: Will my child have asthma when he grows up?
A: Asthma occurs in over 50% of older children who survived BPD.

Q: What types of additional therapies can help my child?
A: Chest physiotherapy may be of benefit in infants with both early and late BPD, helping to mobilize secretions and to prevent atelectasis. Speech and occupational therapy may be of benefit as infant who have had prolonged intubation or other interventions that may interfered with oral functioning may have some degree of oral-motor dysfunction and oral aversion. Other infants simply with increased work of breathing may have discoordinated suck and swallow, making oral feedings difficult. Physical therapy may be of benefit to help infants with gross and fine motor delays, poor tone, and abnormal posture. Parents can learn many of the therapies in order to incorporate therapeutic exercises and positioning into their daily routines.

ICD-9-CM 770.7

BIBLIOGRAPHY

Bader D, Ramos AD, Lew CD, Platzker AC. Childhood sequelae of infant lung disease: exercise and pulmonary function abnormalities after bronchopulmonary dysplasia. *J Pediatr* 1987;10:693–699.

Hageman JR, ed. *The pediatric clinics of North America: neonatolgy update.* Philadelphia: WB Saunders Co., 1998.

Northway WH Jr, Rosan RC, Porter DY. Pulmonary disease following respirator therapy of hyaline-membrane disease. *N Engl J Med* 1967;276:357–368.

Author: John M. Good

Brucellosis

 Database

DEFINITION

Brucellosis is caused by infection with the bacteria of the genus *Brucella*. The organism was first isolated from the spleen of patient who died of Malta fever in 1887, by Sir David Bruce of the British Royal Army Medical Corps.

- Four species of brucella cause human disease: *B. abortus* (cattle), *B. melitensis* (goats and sheep), *B. suis* (hogs), and *B. canis* (dogs).
- Organisms are small fastidious gram-negative coccobacilli.

PATHOPHYSIOLOGY

- While humans are not a usual host, infection with *Brucella* species may occur following contact with infected domesticated or wild animals.
- Subsequently, the bacterium replicates inside the phagocytic cells of the host.
- Routes of infection include abraded skin, oral membranes, respiratory tract, or conjunctiva inoculation.
- Virulence factors in the bacteria and host factors (nutritional, immunological) may predict severity of infection.
- Incubation period is usually 3 to 4 weeks.

EPIDEMIOLOGY

- Approximately 200 cases are reported in the United States yearly; less than 10% in children.
- Brucellosis may be acquired from non-pasteurized dairy products, particularly in Mexico, the Mediterranean, the Far East, and South America.
- Veterinarians are occasionally inoculated with live vaccine (via needle or airborne routes) during occupational accidents, producing mild disease.

COMPLICATIONS

- Localized disease may result in osteomyelitis (usually vertebral), arthritis, splenic abscess, epididymoorchitis, meningoencephalitis, pleural effusion, pneumonia, and bacterial endocarditis.
- Chronic brucellosis may occur more than 1 year after the onset of disease. A subset of these patients have no objective evidence of infection.
- An erythematous macular, papular, or pustular rash may be seen on the hands and arms of veterinarians following the removal of placentas from infected animals.

PROGNOSIS

- Even prior to the advent of treatment with antibiotics, most patients recovered from a *Brucella* infection within 3 months.
- If the duration of illness with appropriate treatment exceeds 2 months, other diagnoses should be considered.

 Differential Diagnosis

- Diagnosis should be considered when evaluating persons with evidence of localized or systemic infection and risk of contact through domestic animals (especially cattle and swine).
- More common diseases with similar presentations include:

—Influenza
—Infectious mononucleosis
—Tuberculosis
—Leptospirosis
—Toxoplasmosis
—Rheumatic fever
—Systemic lupus erythematosus
—Viral hepatitis
—Disseminated gonococcal disease

 Data Gathering

HISTORY

- Infection with brucellosis is often asymptomatic.
- Onset may be insidious, although certain species produce a severe form.
- Low-grade fever?
- Fatigue?
- Headache?
- Malaise?
- Weakness?
- Sweats?
- Chills?
- Arthralgias?
- Myalgias?
- Abdominal pain?

 Physical Examination

Physical findings infrequent, but include

- Splenomegaly
- Lymphadenopathy
- Hepatomegaly.

 Laboratory Aids

Test: Culture of the *Brucella* species
Significance: Can be isolated from the blood, lymph nodes, spleen, liver, or bone marrow.

Test: Blood culture
Significance: More likely to be positive early in infection, and usually requires 1 to 3 weeks of growth time.

Test: Culturing *Brucella* specimens
Significance: Can be hazardous to laboratory personnel, and should be labeled "Caution: Possible Brucellosis."

Test: Serologic evidence
Significance: Infection can be demonstrated with the serum agglutination test (SAT), prepared from *B. abortus* antigens. An early light peak, followed by rising lag titers is usual. A single titer of 1:160 is significant, although not diagnostic.

Therapy

- Course of the illness can be shortened and incidence of complications reduced by treatment with one of the tetracyclines.
- Usual dosage is administered for 4 to 6 weeks.
- Tetracyclines should be avoided in pregnant women and children less than 8 years old.
- Trimethoprim-sulfamethoxazole can be used in children safely in its usual dosage.
- Streptomycin has traditionally been added to a tetracycline, but may not be necessary.
- Abscesses should be surgically drained.
- Splenectomy may be required in patients with splenomegaly and multiple relapses.

 Follow-Up

Titers may be followed to ensure appropriate response to therapy.

PREVENTION

Isolation of the Hospitalized Patient

- Contact precautions are necessary for the patient with draining wounds.

Control Measures

- Domesticated animals can attain immunity to *Brucella* through vaccination with a live attenuated vaccine.
- Pasteurization of milk and milk products prevents infection.
- Meat workers, veterinarians, and cattle workers should reduce risk by appropriate bandaging of wounds, and by wearing gloves and goggles.

PITFALLS

Initial treatment may be accompanied by a Jarisch-Herxheimer reaction.

 Common Questions and Answers

Q: What are the other names for brucellosis?
A: Malta fever, Mediterranean fever, and Undulant fever

Q: What is the cause of relapses?
A: Usually caused by discontinuing antibiotics prematurely.

ICD-9-CM 023.9

BIBLIOGRAPHY

Kaye D, Petersdorf R. Brucellosis. In: Braunwald E, et al., eds. *Harrison's principles of internal medicine.* New York: McGraw-Hill, 1987:610–613.

Mikolich DJ, Boyce JM. Brucella species. In: Mandell GL, Douglas GR, Bennet JE, eds. *Principles and practice of infectious diseases.* New York: Churchill Livingstone, 1990:1635–1642.

Oski FA, ed. *Principles and practice of pediatrics.* Philadelphia: JB Lippincott, 1990:1308.

Peter G, ed. *1997 red book: report of the Committee on Infectious Disease.* Elk Grove Village, IL: American Academy of Pediatrics, 1997:157–159.

Young EJ, Yow MD. Brucellosis. In: Feigin RD, Cherry JD, eds. *Textbook of pediatric infectious diseases,* 2nd ed. Philadelphia: WB Saunders, 1987:1107–1111.

Author: Janet H. Friday

Bulimia

 Database

DEFINITION

Bulimia nervosa is an eating disorder characterized by binge eating, combined with behavior intended to produce weight loss. To counteract the effects of the binge eating, the patient self-induces vomiting, abuses laxatives, exercises excessively, diets rigorously, and fasts for prolonged periods. Binges are characterized by:

• Rapid consumption of large amounts of food in discrete periods of time, usually less than 2 hours.
• Fear of being unable to stop eating.
• Food of high caloric value, often swallowed without chewing.
• Associated feelings of guilt, anxiety, and depression.
• Frenzied quality, often occurring alone and secretively.

Criteria for diagnosis of bulimia: minimum average of two binge-eating episodes per week for at least 3 months

PATHOPHYSIOLOGY

• Some authors posit that bulimic behavior services unmet needs, such as providing intense stimulation to relieve tension.
• Personality traits of low self-esteem, self-regulatory difficulties, frustration intolerance, and impaired ability to recognize and directly express feelings have been described in patients with bulimia nervosa.

GENETICS

No inheritance patterns have been found.

EPIDEMIOLOGY

• Onset in late adolescence to early adulthood (range: 13–58 years of age)
• Females account for 90% to 95% of cases
• Affects 1% to 3% of young females in Western countries
• Ten times more common than anorexia nervosa

COMPLICATIONS

Pulmonary

• Aspiration pneumonia
• Pneumomediastinum

Gastrointestinal

• Pancreatitis
• Parotid-gland enlargement
• Gastric and esophageal irritation
• Mallory-Weiss syndrome
• Paralytic ileus (due to laxative abuse)
• Cathartic colon

Metabolic

• Hypokalemia (due to laxative abuse)
• Electrolyte imbalances, including hypomagnesemia
• Fluid imbalances
• Hyperamylasemia

Dental

• Enamel erosion
• Caries and periodontal disease

PROGNOSIS

• Very low mortality: 0.3%
• No studies of long-term prognosis in adolescents
• Adult studies:

—Normal weight at follow-up (24 and 72 months)
—29% to 87% reported binge eating at follow-up (2–35 months)
—28% to 77% reported at least one vomiting episode at follow-up (12–50 months)
—3% to 13% reported laxative abuse at follow-up (12–50 months)

 Differential Diagnosis

PSYCHOSOCIAL

• Psychogenic vomiting

MISCELLANEOUS

• Gastrointestinal obstruction
• Hiatal hernia

 Data Gathering

HISTORY

Eating-Disorder Specific

• Eating habits
• Rituals, behaviors
• Body image
• Actual and desired weights, minimum and maximum weights
• Use of laxatives, diuretics, diet pills, emetics
• Presence of binge or purge behavior
• Menstrual history
• Use of exercise

General

• Weakness or fatigue
• Headaches
• Abdominal pain, fullness, or nausea
• Constipation

Psychiatric

• Mood disorder
• Substance abuse
• Anxiety
• Personality disorders
• Suicidal tendencies

Family

• Medical and psychiatric histories

Physical Examination

Finding: Vital signs
Significance: Check for hypotension

Finding: Edema of hands and feet
Significance: Evidence of low albumin

Finding: Calluses on knuckles or hands
Significance: Russell sign

Finding: Muscle cramps or weakness
Significance: Hypokalemia

SPECIAL QUESTIONS

- How much do you want to weigh?
- How do you control your weight?
- How do you feel about yourself?
- How often do you vomit, use diuretics or laxatives?

 Laboratory Aids

Perform a laboratory evaluation as part of the diagnostic work-up.

Test: CBC
Significance: Iron deficiency anemia

Test: Electrolytes, including calcium, magnesium, and phosphate: abnormalities may occur as a result of prolonged vomiting or use of laxatives
Significance: Iron deficiency anemia

Test: BUN and creatinine
Significance: Fluid imbalance and dehydration common

Test: Glucose
Significance: Patient may be hypoglycemic

Test: Cholesterol, lipids
Significance: Evidence of malnutrition

Test: Amylase
Significance: Pancreatitis

Test: Total protein, albumin
Significance: Evidence of malnutrition

Test: Liver function tests
Significance: Evidence of malnutrition

Test: Urine toxicology screen, optional
Significance: May be positive, as this disorder often is associated with substance abuse

Test: ECG with rhythm strip
Significance: May reveal cardiomyopathy caused by use of ipecac for emesis

RADIOGRAPHIC STUDIES

- Upper GI series with small-bowel follow-through, optional

 Therapy

- Outpatient therapy
- Behavioral treatment with initial goal of breaking or decreasing the binge-purge cycle
- Individual psychotherapy
- Family treatment
- Group therapy
- Emphasize bingeing, not purging, as primary target symptom

DRUGS

- Antidepressants

—Decrease the binge-purge behavior
—Improve attitudes about eating
—Lessen preoccupation with food and weight
—Fluoxetine (Prozac), sertraline (Zoloft), and fluvoxamine (Luvox) have been used with good results in patients with bulimia nervosa.

- Stool softeners may be used for constipation, but avoid laxatives.

- Hospitalize in cases of:

—Hypovolemia
—Severe electrolyte disturbances
—Intractable vomiting
—Acute psychiatric emergencies (e.g., suicidal ideation, acute psychosis)
—Medical complication of malnutrition (e.g., aspiration pneumonia, cardiac failure, pancreatitis, Mallory-Weiss syndrome, etc.)
—Comorbid diagnoses that interfere with the treatment of the eating disorder (e.g., severe depression, obsessive-compulsive disorder, severe family dysfunction)

 Follow-Up

- Reduction in binge and purge episodes may take months or years.
- Behavioral and thought disorders associated with bulimia nervosa may be of long duration.

SIGNS TO WATCH FOR

- Weight loss or major weight fluctuations
- Electrolyte abnormalities
- Muscle cramps
- Fatigue
- Depression or mood disturbance
- Willful behavior or acting out

PREVENTION

- Emphasize healthy self-esteem and body image during visits with preadolescents and adolescents.

PITFALLS

- During treatment, patients and their families may cause "splitting" of the hospital staff. To avoid this, always be supportive and maintain consistency in stating goals.

 Common Questions and Answers

Q: How do I determine if a patient has anorexia with vomiting, or bulimia?
A: The key feature of bulimia nervosa is the binge episode, which distinguishes it from anorexia nervosa. If there are not at least two binge eating episodes per week for at least 3 months, the diagnosis is not bulimia.

Q: What laboratory abnormalities should I look for in my patients with bulimia?
A: Electrolyte abnormalities, particularly hypokalemia. Patients may develop a hypochloremic metabolic alkalosis. If electrolytes are significantly abnormal, the patient should be hospitalized until they have normalized.

ICD-9-CM 133.6

BIBLIOGRAPHY

Fisher M. Medical complications of anorexia nervosa and bulimia nervosa. *Adolesc Med: State Art Rev* 1992;3(3):487–501.

Fisher M, Golden NH, Katzman DK, et al. Eating disorders in adolescents: a background paper. *J Adolesc Health* 1995;16:420–437.

Haller E. Eating disorders: a review and update. *West J Med* 1992;157:658–662.

Harper G. Eating disorders in adolescence. *Pediatr Rev* 1994;15(2):72–77.

Hersog DB, Keller MB, Lavori PW. Outcome in anorexia nervosa and bulimia nervosa: a review of the literature. *J Nerv Ment Dis* 1988;176(3):131–143.

Schebendach J, Nussbaum MP. Nutrition management in adolescent with eating disorders. *Adolesc Med: State Art Rev* 1992;3(3):541–557.

Walsh BT, Wilson GT, Loeb KL, et al. Medication and psychotherapy in the treatment of bulimia nervosa. *Am J Psychiatry* 1997;154(4):523–531.

Author: Liana R. Clark

C1 Esterase Inhibitor Deficiency

 Database

DEFINITION

• C1 esterase inhibitor deficiency is a hereditary and acquired form of recurrent angioedema. The attacks are usually without urticaria.

• C1 esterase inhibitor deficiency has now been classified into a number of types including:

—Hereditary angioedema (HAE) type I (transmitted as an autosomal dominant)
—HAE type II (transmitted as an autosomal dominant)
—Acquired angioedema (AAE) type I
—AAE type II

• HAE type I accounts for approximately 85% of the C1 esterase deficiencies and is a genetic alteration that leads to impairment of mRNA transcription or translation and, therefore, decreased enzyme synthesis.

• HAE type II is a genetic alteration that leads to production of an inactive protein.

• In acquired deficiency of C1 esterase inhibitor, there appears to be a normal ability to synthesize the enzyme; however, the enzyme is metabolized at an increased rate. This syndrome may be seen in patients with autoimmune diseases or malignancy and usually occurs after the fourth decade of life.

• AAE type I is a very rare syndrome usually associated with lymphoproliferative (usually B cell), carcinomas, autoimmune diseases, and paraproteinemias. Because of the other disease processes, complement-activating factors and idiotype-antiidiotype complexes act to increase consumption of C1 esterase inhibitor.

• AAE type II develops when an auto antibody is produced against the C1 esterase inhibitor protein. When these antibodies adhere to the C1 esterase molecule and conformational change occurs leading to decreased function or enhanced metabolism.

• AAE forms may be differentiated from HAE by genetic studies and serologically by significantly decreased C1q, C1r, C1s levels and decreased functional activity of the enzyme in AAE.

PATHOPHYSIOLOGY

• C1 esterase inhibitor is a single chain polypeptide with a molecular weight of 108 kd. The gene has been identified on chromosome 11 (11q12-q13.1)

• This protein inhibits the classic complement pathway by inhibiting activation of C2 and C4. In the fibrinolytic system, C1 esterase inhibitor inhibits formation of plasmin, the activation of C1r and C1s, and the formation of bradykinin from kininogen.

• With a deficiency of this enzyme, the classic complement system becomes activated along with fibrinolysis and kinin formation, which is felt to participate in the production of angioedema.

• Kinin is known to cause similar histologic lesions to histamine but without pruritis.

• The complement activation leads to production of C2b, a product which also has kinin-like activity, and bradykinin, a vasoactive peptide which may also participate in the formation of angioedema.

GENETICS

HAE type I and II are transmitted as an autosomal dominant.

 Data Gathering

HISTORY

Question: What is presentation?
Significance: Patients with HAE usually present in the second decade of life with angioedema involving the subcutaeous tissues (mostly involving the extremities).

Question: What gastrointestinal effects are present?
Significance: Angioedema involving the gastrointestinal tract may lead to severe pain, vomiting, and diarrhea.

Question: Are there respiratory complications?
Significance: Two out of three patients will have orofacial or laryngeal swelling.

Question: Can there be hives?
Significance: The edema usually occurs without evidence of inflammation; however, episodes of urticaria have also been documented.

• The variability of clinical manifestations, even among individuals with the same genetic mutation, is striking, implicating non-genetic factors or other genes as possible mediators of clinical presentation.
• Emesis?
• Diarrhea?
• Hypotension from extravasation of plasma into the skin?
• Hemoconcentration?
• Azotemia?
• Central nervous system complaints including headache, hemiparasis, and seizures, may be triggered by trauma or stress.
• AAE presents in the same way but usually in the fourth decade of life, not associated with a familial history.

Laboratory Aids

- C1 esterase inhibitor concentration
- C1 esterase inhibitor activity
- C4 concentration
- C1q concentration (usually lower in patients with AAE)

 Therapy

- For these entities, therapy is divided into management of the acute attack, maintenance therapy for HAE, and more specific interventions for those with AAE.
- During an acute episode, management focuses on adequate respiratory and fluid resuscitation, and the treatment of pain.
- In HAE, acute attacks are treated with replacement of the C1 esterase inhibitor with IV concentrates. Fresh frozen plasma may also be used.
- For prophylaxis, androgens (such as danazol and stanozolol) are used in postpubertal patients with HAE of both types.
- These androgens stimulate the synthesis of C1-INH, and, while the level of activity is not normalized, it is increased sufficiently to be clinically efficacious.
- In prepubertal children, androgens are used only in those with severe attacks or purified C1-INH if available.
- For those patients who do not tolerate androgens, tranexamic acid and epsilon-aminocaproic acid (antifibrinolytic inhibitors or plasmin activity) may be used although they carry the risk of significant side effects.
- AAE type I requires an intensive search for malignancy, although this form of AAE occasionally appears before the development of clinical signs of the malignancy.
- Androgens are also effective in preventing attacks in individuals with this syndrome.
- AAE type II requires immunosuppression to decrease formation of the autoantibody.
- Androgen treatment has not led to good clinical response.

ICD-9-CM
Hereditary angioedema 277.6
Angioedema 955.1

BIBLIOGRAPHY

Heymann WR. Acquired angioedema. *J Am Acad Dermatol* 1997;36:611–615.

Huston DP, Bressler RB. Urticaria and angioedema. *Med Clin North Am* 1992;76(4):805–840.

Oski FA, DeAngelis CD, Feign RD, Warshaw JB. *Principles and practice of pediatrics*. Philadelphia: JB Lippincott Co., 1990.

Winnewisser J, Rossi M, Spath P, Burgi H. Type I hereditary angio-oedema. Variability of clinical presentation and course within two large kindreds. *J Intern Med* 1997;241:39–46.

Zuraw BL. Urticaria, angioedema, and autoimmunity. *Clin Lab Med* 1997;17(3):559–569.

Author: Donna Zeiter

Campylobacter Infections

 Database

DEFINITION

• *Campylobacter* species involved in human infections include *C. jejuni* (which causes enteritis), *C. fetus* (implicated in systemic illness), and *C. pylori* (a causative agent in antral gastritis).
• *Campylobacter* is a motile, curved, microaerophilic, non–lactose-fermenting, gram-negative rod that requires oxygen and carbon dioxide for optimal growth.

PATHOPHYSIOLOGY

• *C. jejuni* adheres to epithelial cells and mucus, secretes cytotoxins (which play a role in the development of watery diarrhea), and induces an inflammatory ileocolitis.
• *C. pylori* specifically adheres to the antral gastric mucosa, inducing an active chronic gastritis; cytotoxin produced by the organism may account for vacuolization in cultured intestinal mucosa cells. This mucosal invasion with subsequent inflammation impairs the protection of gastric mucosa against the acid milieu.
• Enteritis, the most well-known disease of *C. jejuni,* has been isolated as often as or more often than *Salmonella* or *Shigella*, with an incidence of 4% to 12% of diarrheal illness.
• Antral gastritis from *C. pylori* is often an underdiagnosed entity, since diagnosis is made by endoscopic biopsy, revealing the characteristic type B gastritis with subsequent culture isolation of *C. pylori*.
• Bacteremia, although uncommon, can occur, especially in the neonate and immunocompromised host; *C. fetus* is the species most likely to be isolated.

EPIDEMIOLOGY

• *Campylobacter* infections equal and perhaps exceed the number of cases of inflammatory enteritis due to other causes, with the highest attack rates observed in young children.
• 30% to 100% of chickens, turkeys, and water fowl are infected asymptomatically in addition to swine, cattle, sheep, horses, rodents, and household pets (especially young). Contaminated water and milk sources also act as reservoirs for infections.
• Transmission of disease is by the fecal-oral route from contaminated food and water or by direct contact with fecal material from animals or persons infected with the organism.
• Person-to-person transmission of *C. jejuni* has been reported when the index cases were young children who were incontinent of feces; vertical transmission from mother to neonate has also been reported.
• Asymptomatic hospital personnel or food handlers have not been implicated as sources.
• The peak rate of isolation occurs in the warmer months of the year (late summer, early fall).

COMPLICATIONS

• Post-infectious immunological complications include reactive arthritis, Guillain-Barré syndrome, Reiter syndrome, and erythema nodosum.
• *C. jejuni* is the most frequently identified cause of Guillain-Barré syndrome with serotype 0:19.
• HLA-B27 antigen is associated with reactive arthritis.
• Seizures may develop in young children with enteritis and high fevers.
• A typhoid-like syndrome and meningitis have also been reported in patients with *Campylobacter* infection.

PROGNOSIS

• For patients with enteritis, the prognosis is very good, regardless of whether antibiotic treatment is given.
• For patients with gastritis, if the infection with *C. pylori* is not eradicated, a chronic phase can persist for months.

 Differential Diagnosis

Campylobacter infection should be considered in all patients with a diarrheal illness, especially those with a history of bloody or mucous stools, as well as in patients with chronic abdominal pain or acute, recurrent gastritis.

 Data Gathering

HISTORY

Question: Exposure to unpasteurized milk products?
Significance: Source of campylobacter infection.

Question: Well water used?
Significance: Contaminated water serves as a reservoir.

Question: Inadequately cooked poultry
Significance: Chickens are asymptomatic carriers.

Question: Fever, abdominal pain, bloody diarrhea?
Significance: Illness is characterized by fever, abdominal pain, and bloody diarrhea. Symptoms can last for 24 hours and be indistinguishable from a viral gastroenteritis, or can be relapsing, thus mimicking inflammatory bowel disease.

Question: Inflammatory ileocolitis?
Significance: The most common manifestation in children.

Question: Duration of symptoms?
Significance: Incubation period is 1 to 7 days and is usually self-limited by 5 to 7 days.

Physical Examination

Finding: Chronic abdominal pain
Significance: An index of suspicion for *C. pylori* infection should exist in any patient with chronic abdominal pain, especially when there is concern about gastritis. At least 90% of patients with duodenal ulcer disease reveal documented *C. pylori* infection, and approximately 70% of patients with gastric ulcer are infected.

Finding: Colicky, epigastric pain, bloating, nausea, vomiting, and halitosis.
Significance: Signs and symptoms of *C. pylori* infection. If the infection is not eradicated, a chronic phase results, which can persist indefinitely.

 ## Laboratory Aids

Test: Examination of fecal specimen for darting motility of *C. jejuni* by darkfield or phase-contrast microscopy
Significance: If examined within 2 hours of passage, it can permit presumptive diagnosis.

Test: Stool culture
Significance: Can be used, but selective media (Skirrow, Butzler, or campy-BAP) must be used to isolate *Campylobacter* species.

Test: Serology using tube agglutination, bactericidal assays, and indirect immunofluorescence can be helpful.
Significance: ELISA tests specific for IgG antibodies to *C. pylori* have a sensitivity and specificity of 90%.

Test: Culture of gastric mucosal biopsy
Significance: The gold standard for isolating *C. pylori*.

 ## Therapy

• If treated early in the course of disease (less than 4 days) erythromycin for 5 to 7 days appears to be effective in eradicating the organism from the stool within 2 to 3 days.
• Ciprofloxacin, tetracycline, aminoglycosides, clindamycin, chloramphenicol, and cefotaxime are alternative antimicrobials if resistant or bacteremic strains are present.

 ## Follow-Up

• Once treated, symptoms should improve in 2 to 3 days.
• In the untreated patient, the median excretion of organism is up to 2 to 3 weeks, and it was 3 months before all patients in one study were free of the organism. Asymptomatic carriage is uncommon.
• The expected course of treatment of *C. pylori* infection is variable since *in vitro* sensitivities are not reliable predictors of the response to treatment.

PREVENTION

• The importance of handwashing after contact with animals or animal products, proper cooling and storage of foods, pasteurization of milk, and chlorination of water supplies will decrease the overall risk for infection.
• In the hospital setting, enteric precautions are recommended for infected infants and children who are incontinent of stool and should be maintained until the patient receives at least 48 hours of antibiotic treatment.

PITFALLS

Not all bacterial colitis presents with blood or mucus appearing diarrhea. Therefore, suspicion should exist if the diarrhea is prolonged or environmental exposures pose a risk for developing infection.

 ## Common Questions and Answers

Q: Is treatment necessary if the child is asymptomatic by the time the *Campylobacter* is isolated as the pathogen causing the enteritis?
A: No treatment is needed in this situation. Therapy for symptomatic patients, although it may be of benefit, has not been proven efficacious.

Q: Are there any risks of *Campylobacter* infection to the pregnant patient?
A: Women infected symptomatically or asymptomatically may experience recurrent abortions or pre-term deliveries. Life-threatening infections to the fetus or newborn are also possible.

Q: Can you develop immunity to *Campylobacter* infections?
A: Immunity to *C. jejuni* is acquired after one or more infections. For children living in endemic areas, effective natural immunity is due to significant repeated early exposure with a progressive decrease in the illness—infection ratio as age increases.

ICD-9 CM 559.008.43

BIBLIOGRAPHY

Allos BM. *Campylobacter jejuni* infection as a cause of Guillain-Barré syndrome. *Inf Dis Clin North Am* 1998;12:173–184.

Blaser MJ, Reller LB. *Campylobacter* enteritis. *N Engl J Med* 1981;305:1444–1452.

Drumm B, Sherman P, Cutz E, Karmali M. Association of *Campylobacter pylori* on the gastric mucosa with antral gastritis in children. *N Engl J Med* 1987;316:1557–1561.

Hughes RAC, Rees JH. Clinical and epidemiologic features of Guillain-Barré syndrome. *J Inf Dis* 1997;176(Suppl. 2):S92–S98.

Peter G, Halsey NA, Marcuse EK, Pickering LK. *Campylobacter* infections. In: *1994 red book: report of the Committee on Infectious Diseases*, 23rd ed. Elk Grove Village, IL: American Academy of Pediatrics, 1994:146–147.

Ruiz-Palacios G, Pickering LK. *Campylobacter* infections. In: Feigin RD, Cherry JD, eds. *Pediatric infectious diseases*, 3rd ed. Philadelphia: WB Saunders, 1992:1073–1081.

Tauxe RV, Hargrett-Bean N, Patton CM, Wachsmuth IK. *Campylobacter* isolates in the United States, 1982-1986. *MMWR* 1987;37:10–25.

Thorson SM, Lohr JA, Dudley S, Guerrant RL. Value of methylene blue examination, dark-field microscopy, and carbol-fuchsin gram stain in the detection of campylobacter enteritis. *J Pediatr* 1985;106:941–943.

Author: Philip V. Scribano

Candidiasis

 ## Database

DEFINITION

There are more than 80 species of the *Candida* genus, but only a few cause clinical human infection. *Candida albicans* is by far the most common. Other non-albicans species that cause disease include *C. tropicalis, C. pseudotropicalis, C. paratropicalis, C. guilliermondii, C. parasilosis,* and *C. stellatoidea*. *Candida* is a ubiquitous organism of low virulence, rarely causing severe disease in the immunocompetent host.

PATHOPHYSIOLOGY

• Rarely causes severe disease in the immunocompetent host. It becomes a pathogen when changes or host defense (locally or systematically) allow for overgrowth and invasion of the organism.
• Not part of the normal flora of skin
• Frequently found as normal flora in mouth, gastrointestinal (GI) tract, respiratory tract, and vaginal tract.

ASSOCIATED DISEASES

Candida may cause disease at any site. Infection is most commonly discussed topographically.

Thrush (Acute Pseudomembranous Candidiasis)

Very common candidal infection in pediatrics; occurs in up to 30% to 40% of healthy newborns. It may be asymptomatic, or cause pain, anorexia, or poor nursing. Outside the newborn/infant period it is associated with changes in normal host resistance from several causes, including the use of antibiotics or immunosuppressive drugs, conditions of endocrine or immune dysfunction, diabetes, and neoplasm.

Diaper Dermatitis

Most common in the first several months of life due to predisposing factors found with diaper use.

Other Oropharyngeal Candidiases

• Include *acute atrophic candidiases* (glossitis) and *angular cheilosis* (perleche).
• Candidal glossitis occurs secondarily to broad-spectrum oral antibiotic therapy and commonly includes the complaint of glossodynia. Perleche results from chronic licking of the corners of the mouth, severe overbite, or occasionally from orthodontic braces.

Intertrigenous Candidiasis

Intertrigenous candidiasis is characterized by a confluent, intensely erythematous, weeping rash with a scaling edge found at skin folds: axillae, groin, gluteal folds, infra- or intramammary region, interdigital, umbilical, nuccal, and glans penis. Predisposing factors in healthy patients include chronic moisture, recent antibiotic use, and obesity.

Candidal Vaginitis

Candidal vaginitis is characterized by local pruritus and a thick/cheesy or watery white discharge. It is often accompanied by labial edema, mucosal erythema, dysuria, and a vulvar burning sensation. It is common in immunocompetent individuals, especially after antibiotic use, while on anovulatory meds, and in pregnancy.

Disseminated or Systemic Candidiasis

Disseminated or systemic candidiasis occurs in the immunocompromised host: patients with malignancies; immune system disorders; insulin-dependent diabetes mellitus (IDDM) and other endocrine disorders; on prolonged broad-spectrum antibiotics, steroids, or cancer chemotherapy; on chronic hyperalimentation with chronic indwelling catheters; and after x-irradiation therapy, organ transplantation, or complex invasive surgery. Most frequent sites include the GI tract, lungs, kidneys, liver, spleen, and brain. Fungal sepsis may occur. Peritoneal, urinary tract, and cardiac candidal infections are most frequently related to instrumentation or catheterization in the immunocompromised host.

EPIDEMIOLOGY

• Colonization in healthy children of the oral mucosa, GI tract, respiratory tract, and vaginal mucosa are fairly common. Rates of colonization have been shown to increase substantially in hospitalized or chronically ill patients.
• Transmission appears to require direct contact with susceptible mucous membranes or cutaneous sites.
• Systemic or disseminated dz is usually hematologically spread from oral or GI lesions, or skin puncture sites.

COMPLICATIONS

Allergic Reactions to Candida

• The most common of the allergic response syndrome to *Candida* are the candidids (id rashes), characterized by a papulovesicular or scaling plaque-like eruption that can include flexor or extensor surfaces of the upper extremities, extensor surfaces of thighs, and occasionally the hands, face, or trunk.
• Other clinical allergic syndromes include mucous colitis, generalized pruritus (with or without characteristic rash), chronic asthma exacerbations, and possibly a cause of erythema annulare.

 ## Differential Diagnosis

• Other diaper rashes: atopic, seborrheic, bacterial, or occlusional.
• Mouth lesions: aphthous stomatitis, acute necrotizing gingivitis (trench mouth or Vincent angina), herpes gingivostomatitis or other viral causes of stomatitis (i.e., coxsackievirus)
• Intertrigenous infections: serborrheic and atopic dermatidites
• Vaginitis: gonorrhea, trichomonas, chlamydia, gardnarella, shigella, streptococcus, chemical or mechanical irritants
• Systemic disease: bacterial infection or sepsis

 ## Data Gathering

HISTORY

Question: Is the thrush recurrent?
Significance: Reinoculation can occur from bottle or mother's nipples, pacifiers, or toys (*see* Therapy).

Question: Were antibiotics used?
Significance: Oral thrush and monilial diaper dermatitis are forms of candidiasis in infants, but can occur in older children after treatment with systemic antibiotics.

Question: Was the vaginal discharge accompanied by itching?
Significance: Candidal vulvovaginitis, the first clinical manifestation is usually labial pruritus, progressing to a local burning sensation, swelling of the labia, external dysuria, and a white watery or cheesy (curd-like) vaginal discharge.

 ## Physical Examination

Finding: Oral lesions
Significance: Can be of the buccal or lingual mucosa, gingiva, or tongue and have a characteristic white, friable, cheesy pseudomembrane that when scraped away reveals reddened, denuded, and sometimes ulcerated mucosa.

Finding: Rash
Significance: The rash of monilial diaper dermatitis is initially scattered, erythematous papules that progress and coalesce into a deeply erythematous, weeping, confluent rash, classically with a scalloped vesiculopapular or scaling border and papular, erythematous satellite lesions.

Laboratory Aids

Test: Direct light microscopic observation
Significance: The diagnosis of mucosal, cutaneous, and vaginal candidiasis depends on clinical observation but can be confirmed by direct light microscopic observation of material scraped gently from the lesions and Gram stained or mounted with 10% or 20% potassium hydroxide (to lyse cellular debris) for the long, branching hyphae of *C. albicans*.

Test: Cultures
Significance: Mucosal or cutaneous scrapings, blood, urine, CSF, bone marrow, tissue biopsy, abscess aspirate, and bronchial lavage fluid can be cultured for *C. albicans* to confirm infection.

Test: CT scan
Significance: Is used to help identify deep organ lesions (liver, spleen, brain, kidney).

Therapy

Treatment of candidiasis is dependent on the location of tissue invasion and on host immunocompetence or risk of dissemination.

ORAL CANDIDIASIS

• Removal of the white pseudomembranous material with a plain tongue blade or with a cotton-tipped applicator dipped in nystatin suspension after feeds will often clear lesions after several days.
• More extensive, recurrent, or persistent oral lesions can be treated with nystatin suspension, 1 to 2 mL (of 100,000 units/mL) solution in each cheek, after meals, four to six times a day until 2 days after the lesions have cleared. Miconazole oral gel has been shown to be more effective, but is not available in the United States.
• Bottle nipples and pacifiers should be boiled for 5 minutes, at the beginning and end of a course of treatment, to avoid reinoculation.
• Recurrent thrush in a breast-fed infant may be indicative of colonization of the mother's nipples with *C. albicans*; this can be eliminated by topical treatment of the nipples with nystatin cream four times a day for 5 to 7 days.
• In older patients, nystatin suspension is used as a swish swallow of 500,000 units every 4 to 6 hours for at least 7 days, or in oral tablet form, 500,00 to 1,000,000 units three times a day. Clotrimazole lozenges are also effective for older patients; 10 mg dissolved in mouth every 4 to 6 hours for 1 week.
• Gentian violet is no longer recommended for the treatment of oral candidiasis.
• For severe or persistant infection (immunocompromised host): fluconizole or ketoconazole are effective.

CUTANEOUS OR INTERTRIGENOUS CANDIDIASIS AND MONILIAL DIAPER DERMATITIS

Both are treated successfully by allowing the area to be dry as much as possible and the use of nystatin cream (100,000 units/g) applied four times daily until the rash has cleared. A similar regimen of clotrimazole 1%, miconazole 2%, ketoconazole 2%, econazole 1%, or ciclopirox 1% is also effective.

CANDIDAL VULVOVAGINITIS

Intravaginal and vulvar applications of vaginal creams or suppositories of clotrimazole (qd for 7 to 14 days or b.i.d. for 3 days), miconazole (qhs for 7 days), butoconazole (qhs for 3 days), or terconazole will clear the majority of symptomatic vaginal infections of *C. albicans*.

SYSTEMIC OR DISSEMINATED CANDIDIASIS

• Usually treated in an inpatient setting due to severity of illness, underlying disease process, and/or need for the intravenous route of drug administration.
• Treatment should also address removal of iatrogenic or predisposing factors if possible (e.g., removal of contaminated indwelling line or catheter).
• Antifungal agents commonly used:

—Amphotericin B: 0.25 to 1.0 mg/kg/d, or 1.5 mg/kg every other day; given over 4 to 6 hours intravenously (after initial test dose; see hospital formulary) for 4 to 6 weeks for systemic infections.
—Flucytosine: 150 mg/kg/d in four divided doses, given orally. Used to supplement amphotericin B in severe infections, alone for treatment of oropharyngeal or esophageal candidiasis (check susceptibility testing)
—Ketoconazole: used for immunocompromised children with thrush or esophagitis at 3.3 to 6.6 mg/kg/d, given orally, until lesions clear (maximum of 400 mg/d).

• The toxicity of amphotericin (rigors, anemia, thrombocytopenia, and nephrotoxicity) requires close monitoring and may limit its use.

PREVENTION

• INFECTION CONTROL
• Sterilization of bottle nipples and toys to prevent reinoculation of oral candidiasis as previously mentioned
• Avoidance of long courses of broad-spectrum antibiotics
• Careful attention to the maintenance of sterility of intravenous catheters and their skin entrance sites

Follow-Up

No follow-up necessary if clinical resolution is noted by parents or patients for all but systemic or disseminated candidiasis.

PITFALLS

• Need to maintain a high index of suspicion for systemic or disseminated disease in the immunocompromised host.
• Consider in any patient with predisposing factors who has persistent fevers despite antibiotic therapy, a diffuse maculopapular rash, or unexpected eye complaints.

Common Questions and Answers

Q: When should an older child with thrush be worked up for possible immunodeficiency?
A: The cause for thrush in an older child (out of the infant period) should be carefully sought. Most often the cause is a recent course of antibiotic therapy.

Q: Is Nystatin effective therapy for vaginal candida?
A: No. Clortrimazole and other azole drugs are more effective.

ICD-9-CM 112.9

BIBLIOGRAPHY

American Academy of Pediatrics. Candidiasis. In: Peter G, ed. *1997 red book: report of the Committee on Infectious Diseases,* 24th ed. Elk Grove Village, IL: American Academy of Pediatrics; 1997:162–164.

Feign RD, Cherry JD, eds. *Textbook of pediatric infectious diseases,* 3rd ed. Philadelphia: WB Saunders, 1992:805–808, 1907–1913.

Hoppe JE. Treatment of oropharyngeal candidiasis and candidal diaper dermatitiis in neonates and infants: review and reappraisal. *Pediatr Infect Dis J* 1997;16(9):885–894.

Hurwitz S. *Clinical pediatric dermatology.* Philadelphia: WB Saunders, 1981. Chapters 2, 3, 13.

Author: Molly (Martha) W. Stevens

Cardiomyopathy

 Database

DEFINITION

Cardiomyopathy is defined as a disease of the myocardium, which can be either a primary process or secondary to an associated disorder.

- Dilated cardiomyopathy (DCM): Impairment of biventricular systolic function with predominant involvement of the left ventricle eliciting congestive heart failure.
- Hypertrophic cardiomyopathy (HCM): Characterized with an asymmetric hypertrophy of the left ventricle with 20% to 25% of the patients exhibiting left ventricular outflow tract obstruction.
- Restrictive cardiomyopathy (RCM): Cardiac muscle disease that impairs ventricular filling (normal or decreased diastolic volume of the ventricles), yet systolic function generally remains normal.

PATHOPHYSIOLOGY

- DCM: There are many associated diseases that cause DCM, which are grouped as inborn errors of fatty-acid oxidation, disorders of mitochondrial oxidative phosphorylation, X-linked muscular dystrophies, toxin-induced cardiomyopathy (i.e., anthracycline), post-infectious (viral myocarditis associated with coxsackievirus B or echovirus), nutritional deficiencies, primary and secondary carnitine deficiency, and chronic tachyarrhythmias. Similarly, idiopathic DCM is manifested by abnormally dilated ventricular chambers with frequently noted mural thrombi and atrioventricular valve leaflet scarring with secondary annulus dilatation, and hypertrophy and degeneration of myocytes.
- HCM: This disease is manifested by ventricular hypertrophy, which is often asymmetrical and involves the interventricular septum most commonly but may also affect the free walls. Dynamic obstruction of the left ventricular outflow tract can occur and anatomically relates to the presence of mitral valve systolic anterior motion causing subaortic obstruction.
- RCM: Causes of RCM include amyloidosis, infiltrative and storage diseases (Gaucher disease, Hurler syndrome, Fabry disease), carcinoid syndrome, and radiation-induced fibrosis. Idiopathic RCM can also be familial. The disease is manifested by increased stiffness of the myocardium; therefore, small increases in volume will cause a disproportionately greater increase in ventricular pressure.

GENETICS

- DCM: A portion of cases of idiopathic DCM may have a genetic cause with approximately 20% of patients with the disease having a first-degree relative with abnormalities of myocardial function.

- HCM: A familial hypertrophic cardiomyopathy is known and is an autosomal dominant disease with variable penetrance. Other studies have noted areas of chromosome 1, 14, and 15 to be involved, and can document 60% of patients who have a first-degree relative with morphological evidence of HCM.
- RCM: Idiopathic cases may have a familial occurrence and may be associated with a skeletal myopathy. Also, an autosomal dominant form of the disease with variable penetrance has been associated with Noonan syndrome.

EPIDEMIOLOGY

- DCM: Idiopathic DCM has a prevalence of 36/100,000. Overall survival of 50% to 60% at 2 years.
- HCM: Prevalence of 1/500 with a heterogeneous natural history of the disease.
- RCM: Least common of the cardiomyopathic disorders.

COMPLICATIONS

- In some studies, the overall actuarial survival of those with DCM is 63% to 90% at 1 year with a 5-year survival of 20% to 80%.
- Arrhythmias may be seen and are most often ventricular in origin.
- Thrombus formation can be seen in DCM due to the stasis of blood in a hypocontractile state and, therefore, systemic or pulmonary emboli are possible.

PROGNOSIS

- A general rule for idiopathic DCM is that one-third exhibit improved cardiac function, one-third have stable cardiac dysfunction, and one-third progress to significant cardiac dysfunction.
- Overall rate of sudden death is 2% to 4% in HCM with deaths occurring most commonly in children and young adults.
- The reported median survival in RCM is 1.4 years in children.

 Differential Diagnosis

- DCM: Children and young adults often present with symptoms that mimic other disease states. For example, abdominal distention, right upper quadrant pain, nausea, and anorexia that indicates right heart failure could be mistaken for hepatic or gallbladder disease. Dyspnea on exertion may mimic exercise-induced asthma. The cardiomegaly on chest radiograph may be mistaken for a large pericardial effusion.
- HCM: This disease must be differentiated from the left ventricular hypertrophy that is seen in an athlete.
- RCM: Must be distinguished from constrictive pericarditis (a history of tuberculosis, trauma, or cardiac surgery may suggest constrictive pericarditis).

 Data Gathering

HISTORY

Question: Respiratory distress?
Significance: A manifestation of congestive heart failure.

Question: Irritability?
Significance: A manifestation of congestive heart failure on a pericardiol effusion.

Question: Diaphoresis?
Significance: A manifestation of congestive heart failure.

Question: Gastrointestinal complaints (nausea, emesis)?
Significance: Right-sided congestive heart failure; pericardial effusion or decreased systomic output.

Question: Tachypnea with feeding, pallor, and poor weight gain?
Significance: A manifestation of congestive heart failure.

Question: Chest pain?
Significance: Carditis, pericardial effusion, or arrhythemia.

Question: Syncope?
Significance: Low cardiac output or arrhythemia.

Question: Palpitations?
Significance: Arrhythemia.

Question: Orthopnea, paroxysmal nocturnal dyspnea?
Significance: A manifestation of congestive heart failure.

Question: Peripheral edema?
Significance: Right-sided heart failure.

Question: Reduced exercise capacity?
Significance: Congestive heart failure or low cardiac output.

Question: Neurological changes (delayed development)?
Significance: Systemic emboli in DCM.

Question: Recent febrile illness?
Significance: In DCM, 50% of cases have a history of fever within 3 months of the diagnosis.

 Physical Examination

CARDIAC

Finding: DCM: tachycardia, cardiomegaly, hepatomegaly, S3 or S4 gallop
Significance: Evidence of heart failure and decreased cardiac output.

Finding: HCM: Can be normal.
Significance: The presence of outflow tract obstruction produces a systolic ejection murmur of variable intensity related to the degree of obstruction, the murmur increases in intensity with Valsalva and decreases in magnitude with squatting. A parasternal or carotid thrill may be present

Finding: RCM: Jugular venous pulse either fails to fall versus rises in inspiration (Kussmaul sign), S3 or S4
Significance: Advanced cases may exhibit weak peripheral pulses as evidence of low cardiac output.

RESPIRATORY

Finding: Tachypnea, rales, or cardiac wheezing
Significance: Signs of congestive heart failure

ABDOMINAL

Finding: Hepatomegaly, ascites, tenderness to palpation
Significance: Right-sided congestive heart failure.

EXTREMITIES

Finding: Peripheral edema in advanced cases
Significance: Congestive heart failure.

 ## Laboratory Aids

NON-SPECIFIC TESTS

Test: Chest radiograph
Significance: Cardiomegaly, pulmonary edema, Kerley B lines, and pleural effusions

Test: Electrocardiogram
Significance: Non-specific ST-T wave changes, hypertrophy or enlargement of chambers (although generalized low voltages may be seen), ventricular and supraventricular tachyarrhythmias, atrioventricular block, localized Q waves

SPECIFIC TESTS

Laboratory tests aimed at a specific etiology or an associated disease state should be accomplished in certain cases. For example, carnitine levels may prove helpful as well as polymerase chain reaction assay testing (evidence for an enteroviral infection) on endomyocardial biopsies performed on selected cases of DCM. Storage and metabolic disease states should be investigated if there is clinical suspicion.

Test: Echocardiography
Significance: Allows for measurement of systolic function, ventricular dimensions, outflow tract obstruction, and diastolic filling properties.

Test: Cardiac catheterization
Significance: DCM: Low cardiac output with possible alterations in pulmonary vascular resistance, performance of endomyocardial biopsies, aortography to assure usual coronary anatomy (rule out anomalous coronary origin) HCM: Determination of the presence or absence of left ventricular outflow tract obstruction, hypertrophy, "spike and dome" arterial pulse tracing, Brockenbrough phenomenon (a beat following a premature ventricular contraction exhibits an arterial pulse pressure less than that of the control beat) RCM: Atrial pressures are elevated and equal, the ventricular pressure exhibits a rapid and deep early decline at the onset of diastole followed by a rapid rise to a plateau in early diastole (so-called "square-root sign")

 ## Therapy

• DCM: Vasodilators (enalapril, hydralazine), anticoagulation to avoid embolic complications, antiarrhythmics as needed, inotropic agents (Digoxin), beta-adrenergic blockers (Metoprolol, Carvedilol), and at the time of diagnosis, a trial of prednisone and/or intravenous gamma globulin.
• HCM: Beta-adrenergic blockers, Verapamil, Nifedipine, Diltiazem, antiarrhythmics as needed. If medical therapy is not effective, other options may include myotomy-myectomy or atrioventricular sequential pacing to relieve outflow tract obstruction.
• RCM: Diuretics can be used with caution to treat venous congestion, antiarrhythmics as needed, anticoagulation to avoid embolic complications, regulated physical activity, and supportive care.
• Patients can be successfully transplanted.

 ## Follow-Up

All of these patients require careful follow-up by a cardiologist in addition to their primary care physician to note any adverse alterations in their cardiac status including arrhythmia control and surveillance. Patients should be referred for a transplant evaluation if deemed necessary by their clinical status.

PREVENTION

There is no specific prevention, however, a physician should evaluate individuals with a familial history of cardiomyopathy even if they are asymptomatic.

PITFALLS

In cases of HCM, the cardiac examination can be completely normal, therefore, those patients that raise suspicion for the disease either by family or clinical history should be carefully evaluated.

 ## Common Questions and Answers

Q: Should family members be evaluated once a cardiomyopathy is diagnosed in a first degree relative?
A: Yes. In some types of cardiomyopathy, there is a strong genetic component and family members should be evaluated. Certainly the diagnosis of certain subtypes of cardiomyopathy (i.e., post-infectious DCM, toxin-induced DCM) do not require evaluation of relatives.

Q: Does the cardiomyopathy of infants of diabetic mothers carry the same clinical course and outcome as that of patients with HCM?
A: No. The pathophysiology initially is similar in that asymmetric hypertrophy of the ventricular septum is often seen in the cardiomyopathy in infants of diabetic mothers and can be obstructive to left ventricular outflow. However, the clinical course of the cardiomyopathy in infants born to diabetic mothers is usually benign and resolves within the first 6 months of life.

Q: What are the differentiating features of HCM and the benign physiological hypertrophy of an athlete's heart?
A: Several criteria are used to make this distinction. For example, a familial history of HCM leads one to be suspicious of this entity. Studies have suggested specific left ventricular dimensions by echocardiography to differentiate benign hypertrophy and HCM (i.e., a wall thickness of ≥15 mm or left ventricle cavity dimensions of <45 mm are more consistent with HCM). Also, echocardiographic evidence of abnormal mitral valve inflow is suggestive of HCM.

ICD-9-CM 425.4

BIBLIOGRAPHY

Akagi T, Benson LN, Lightfoot NE, Chin K, Wilson G, Freedom RM. Natural history of dilated cardiomyopathy in children. *Am Heart J* 1991;121:1502–1506.

Chan DP, Allen HD. Dilated congestive cardiomyopathy. In: Emmanouilides GC, ed. *Moss and Adams heart disease in infants, children, and adolescents including the fetus and young adult,* 5th ed. Baltimore: Williams & Wilkins, 1995:1365–1381.

Dec GW, Fuster V. Medical progress: Idiopathic dilated cardiomyopathy. *N Engl J Med* 1994; 331(23):1564–1575.

Kelly DP, Strauss AW. Mechanisms of disease: Inherited cardiomyopathies. *N Engl J Med* 1994;330(13):913–919.

Kushwaha SS, Fallon JT, Fuster V. Medical progress: Restrictive cardiomyopathy. *N Engl J Med* 1997;336(4):267–276.

Lewis AB, Chabot M. Outcome of infants and children with dilated cardiomyopathy. *Am J Cardiol* 1991;68:365–369.

Maron BJ. Hypertrophic cardiomyopathy. In: Emmanouilides GC, ed. *Moss and Adams heart disease in infants, children, and adolescents including the fetus and young adult,* 5th ed. Baltimore: Williams & Wilkins, 1995:1337–1365.

Pelliccia A, Maron BJ, Spataro A, Proshan MA, Spirito P. The upper limit of physiologic cardiac hypertrophy in highly trained elite athletes. *N Engl J Med* 1991;324:295–301.

Spirito P, Seidman CE, McKenna WJ, Maron BJ. Medical progress: The management of hypertrophic cardiomyopathy. *N Engl J Med* 1997;336(11):775–785.

Author: Timothy M. Hoffman

Cataracts

Database

DEFINITION

A cataract is any opacification of the clear, crystalline lens of the eye. Some are small and non-progressive and do not cause visual symptoms, but those that are clinically significant and decrease visual acuity in children represent a major challenge.

CAUSES

• Of the congenital variety, about one-third are inherited, one-third are associated with systemic genetic, metabolic, or maternal infectious disorders, and about one-third are idiopathic.
• A small number occur associated with other primary ocular abnormalities.
• Developmental cataracts can result from some metabolic disorders, toxic agents (steroids, radiation), and localized trauma.

PATHOPHYSIOLOGY

• Represent a derangement of the normal developmental growth of the crystalline fibers of the central lens nucleus or peripheral cortex
• Frequently classified according to their morphology or etiology.
• Age at which they began or occurred is often determined by the location of the opacity within the lens.
• Any central opacity of 3 mm or more produces substantial visual disability.

GENETICS

It is estimated that 8% to 23% of cases are familial, and primary inherited congenital cataracts usually follow an autosomal dominant mode of inheritance, but there are also autosomal and, rarely, X-linked recessive varieties.

EPIDEMIOLOGY

Cataracts occur in about 0.4% of children, and it has been variously estimated that between 10% and 40% of all blindness in children is because of cataracts.

COMPLICATIONS

• Lack of removal of a visually significant cataract at the appropriate early time can lead to irreversible deprivation amblyopia so that no amount of surgery, optical correction, and amblyopia therapy is of any help.
• Surgical removal of a cataract, while technically not usually difficult with today's microsurgical instruments, leaves the eye without a lens (aphakic) and unable to focus without some type of optical correction (spectacles, contact or intraocular lenses). Unless rapid restoration of optical correction occurs, irreversible deprivation amblyopia may still occur after the cataract is removed. This is especially true when cataracts are unilateral.

• The aphakic pediatric eye is more prone to elevated intraocular pressures (glaucoma) and early retinal detachments, either of which can cause permanent visual loss, than a normal eye with its own lens.

PROGNOSIS

• Prior to 1980, the majority of children treated for monocular cataracts had their best corrected vision only in the 20/200 to 20/800 range (legal blindness—best corrected visual acuity of 20/200 or worse); and bilateral cataracts usually obtained only best corrected visual acuities in the 20/80 to 20/200 range.
• Early surgery, better surgical techniques, and rapid optical correction now affords frequent corrected visual acuities in the 20/40 or better range for bilateral cataracts, and in the 20/40 to 20/200 range for monocular cataracts.
• In all cases, the onset or presence of nystagmus before the cataract is removed is an ominous sign for poor outcome.
• In general, successful treatment of the cataract in a child can be extremely difficult and must be accomplished very early in life if the cataract is congenital.
• Useful vision in children with unilateral cataracts in the newborn period can be restored/obtained only if the surgery is completed within the first 8 to 12 weeks of life.
• After 8 to 12 weeks, because of irreversible deprivation amblyopia, visual restoration becomes progressively more difficult to impossible.
• With congenital bilateral cataracts, the prognosis for visual rehabilitation is slightly better providing surgical removal and optical correction is also accomplished early, preferably by 3 months of age.
• Later onset has better prognosis because the visual system is more mature.

Differential Diagnosis

The differential diagnosis of cataracts in children is more concerned with the underlying cause of the leukokoria itself rather than the presence of some other entity, as the cataract is readily defined by the ophthalmologist. Retinoblastoma, retinopathy of prematurity, juvenile retinoschisis, persistent hyperplastic primary vitreous, severe uveitis, and retinal detachment can all cause primary leukokoria or result in a cataract. In addition, the cataract may be an expression of some more severe underlying, previously undiagnosed systemic disease that must be defined to benefit the child's overall health.

ASSOCIATED DISEASES

Systemic disorders include the TORCH syndromes, especially congenital rubella.

• Fetal alcohol syndrome
• Chromosomal disorders such as Down syndrome, trisomy 13-15, Turner syndrome
• Many craniofacial and mandibulofacial syndromes
• Dermatological syndromes such as congenital ichthyosis, hereditary ectodermal dysplasia, infantile poikiloderma
• Skeletal syndromes such as Marfan and Conradi syndromes
• Renal disorders such as Lowe or Alport syndrome
• Neurofibromatosis
• Myotonic dystrophy
• Metabolic and endocrine disorders such as galactosemia, hypoglycemia, diabetes mellitus
• Fabry disease and hypoparathyroidism
• Local ocular disorders with cataracts include aniridia, many of the anterior chamber dysgenesis syndromes, trauma, and those associated with ocular inflammatory processes (chronic iritis, uveitis) such as juvenile rheumatoid arthritis.

Data Gathering

HISTORY

Question: Decreased visual responses
Significance: Cataracts may decrease vision

Question: Sun sensitivity (squinting in bright light)
Significance: Cataracts may increase light sensitivity

Question: Strabismus
Significance: Strabismus may indicate loss of vision in one eye

Question: White pupil
Significance: White pupil cataracts appear as white object in pupil

Question: Unequal or abnormal pupillary reflections in photographs
Significance: Cataract will block red reflex

Question: Nystagmus
Significance: Nystagmus is an ominous sign for degree of vision loss

Question: Careful family and prenatal history
Significance: 8% to 23% of cataracts are genetic

Question: Positive familial history or known history of disorder associated with cataracts
Significance: See associated disease section

Physical Examination

Finding: Decreased vision
Significance: Cataracts may decrease visual acuity

Finding: Strabismus
Significance: May indicate loss of vision in one eye

Finding: White pupil (leukokoria) on flashlight examination
Significance: Cataracts appear as white pupil

Finding: Unequal or poor red fundus reflections by direct ophthalmoscopy
Significance: Cataract will interfere with seeing red reflex

Finding: Visual acuity assessment
Significance: Determine if cataracts caused visual loss

Finding: Presence/absence of nystagmus
Significance: Nystagmus is poor prognostic sign

Finding: Bilaterality of disease
Significance: Most bilateral cataracts are idiopathic, hereditary, or secondary to systemic disease

Finding: Size of globe
Significance: Micropthalmia suggests congenital cataracts

Finding: Thorough physical examination for systemic syndrome
Significance: Many diseases are associated with cataracts. See associated disease sections

Laboratory Aids

Complete ophthalmic examination.

- Bicromicroscopy
- Ultrasonography to visualize media behind opacity
- Electrophysiological analysis of visual system
- Selective work-up
- TORCH titers, including syphilis
- Urine for reducing substance (galactosemia), protein, and pH (Lowe syndrome)
- Blood glucose, calcium, phosphate
- Quantitative amino acids, RBC enzyme levels (galactokinase, gal-1-uridyltransferase)
- Genetic consultation; chromosome analysis

Therapy

- With monocular, small cataracts, sometimes simple dilatation of the pupil of the cataractous eye and occlusion of the normal eye help overcome mild amblyopia and preserve acceptable vision without surgical removal of the cataract. Glasses may or may not be of additional help.
- With visually significant cataracts, surgical removal is the only way to begin therapy. However, without optical correction of the operated, aphakic eye, visual rehabilitation is impossible.
- Prior to age 2, optical correction of aphakia is most frequently accomplished with contact lenses or spectacles when the cataracts are bilateral. In unilateral cases, successful visual rehabilitation always requires extensive occlusion therapy to the normal eye for years. In this instance, optical correction of the unilateral aphakia is best obtained with a contact lens. Even when visual rehabilitation of the monocular aphakia is successful, normal binocular vision with three-dimensional and perfect depth perception is rarely possible.
- Refractive corneal surgery for optical correction of the aphakic is only rarely indicated in children and is not very successful.
- In children older than 2 years, especially those with unilateral cataracts, intraocular lenses (IOLs) have proved successful in appropriate cases, and are now used more frequently. They do afford faster visual rehabilitation and excellent chances of normal binocular vision.

PREVENTION

There is currently no known way to prevent cataracts.

Follow-Up

- Without treatment, progressive visual loss is the natural course of a visually significant cataract. When the opacity is present at birth or very early in life, the visual loss quickly becomes irreversible.
- Once surgical removal and optical correction is started, the child, parents, and physician enter into an intensive and long rehabilitation period, lasting until visual maturity and stability is reached (usually, around 9 years old). Following this, yearly eye examinations are the minimum requirement.
- Parental and educational support services may be needed for those with residual visual handicap.
- Special local, state, and federal services for the visually handicapped and/or blind may be required, as not all children who have successful surgical results will have good vision.

PITFALLS

- Lack of early diagnosis and treatment
- Lack of understanding of irreversible deprivation amblyopia

Common Questions and Answers

Q: Is surgical removal the same as visual cure?
A: No. This is the beginning of treatment that includes optical correction and amblyopia therapy.

Q: Once the cataract is removed, is intensive, extensive follow-up needed?
A: Yes. The visual prognosis is directly related to post-surgical treatment compliance.

Q: Is the cataract easier to treat when the child is older?
A: No. Irreversible deprivation amblyopia develops when the child is older, which precludes the chance for normal vision.

ICD-9-CM 366.9

BIBLIOGRAPHY

Childhood cataracts and other lens disorders. In: Del Monte MA, eds. *Pediatric ophthalmology and strabismus: basic and clinical science course,* section 6. San Francisco: American Academy of Ophthalmology, 1994–95:93–95.

Gimbel HV, Basti S, Ferensowicz M, DeBroff BM. Results of bilateral cataract extraction with posterior chamber intraocular lens implantation in children. *Ophthalmology* 1997;104:1737–1743.

Hertle RW, Quinn GE, Schaffer DB, Markowitz GD, Granet DB, Napolitano JA. Visual rehabilitation after cataract extraction in children using intraocular lenses. From the Proceedings of the Joint ISA & AAPO&S Meeting, Vancouver, Canada, June 19–23, 1994. In: Lennerstrand G, ed. *Update on strabismus and pediatric ophthalmology.* Boca Raton: CRC Press, Inc., 1995: 511–515.

Hiles DA, Hered RW. Disorders of the lens. In: Isenberg SJ, ed. *The eye in infancy.* Chicago: Year Book, 1989:284–319.

Nelson LB, Ullman S. Congenital and developmental cataracts. In: Tasman W, Jaeger EA, eds. *Duane's clinical ophthalmology.* Philadelphia: JB Lippincott, 1994:1–10.

von Noorden GK, Crawford MLJ. The effects of total unilateral occlusion versus lid suture on the visual system of infant monkeys. *Invest Ophthalmol Vis Sci* 1981;21:142–146.

Wiesel TN, Hubel DH. The period of susceptibility to the physiological effects of unilateral eye closure in kittens. *J Physiol* 1970;206:419–436.

Author: David B. Schaffer

Cat-Scratch Disease

 Database

DEFINITION

Cat-scratch disease (CSD) is a subacute, regional lymphadenitis syndrome that occurs following cutaneous inoculation. The majority of patients have had an identifiable contact with a cat, most notably in the form of a scratch or bite.

CAUSES

The etiologic agent for CSD is now referred to as *Bartonella henselae* (previously, *Rochalimaea henselae*), a pleomorphic gram-negative rod. Skin inoculation with the organism through cat contact is the typical mechanism of infection.

PATHOPHYSIOLOGY

Following infection, both the primary inoculation site and the affected lymph nodes show a characteristic central avascular necrotic area surrounded by lymphocytes with some giant cells and histiocytes. Involved nodes develop generalized enlargement, cortex thickening, and germinal-center hypertrophy. Progression leads to pus-filled sinuses within the affected nodes.

EPIDEMIOLOGY

- Occurs in patients of all ages, with 80% of cases being in those less than 21 years old
- Approximately 24,000 cases each year and likely represents the most common cause of chronic benign adenopathy
- More common when scratched by a cat less than 12 months of age

COMPLICATIONS

- Unilateral subacute or chronic tender nodes of the axillary, epitrochlear, and preauricular area support a diagnosis of CSD, especially in the face of a consistent cat contact.
- Regional lymphadenitis
- Parinaud oculoglandular syndrome. This occurs when the site of primary inoculation is the conjunctiva or eyelid. A mild to moderate conjunctivitis develops along with preauricular lymph nodes.
- Encephalopathy/encephalitis: may occur suddenly 2 to 6 weeks after the initial symptoms of CSD, and seizures may be the heralding symptom. Patients may become delirious and then comatose for several days before recovering. Spinal fluid is typically normal or shows minimal WBC and protein elevation. Recovery is generally complete.
- Erythema nodosum: likely represents a delayed hypersensitivity reaction to the infection. Most often involves the subcutaneous fat of the legs and, at times, dorsum of arms, hands, and feet.
- Osteolytic bone lesions occur as a rare complication.
- Other rare complications include thrombotic thrombocytopenic purpura, erythema marginatum, mesenteric lymphadenitis, pneumonia, arthralgias, subacute iriditis, urethritis, lymphedema, thyroiditis, and anicteric hepatitis.

PROGNOSIS

Most patients with CSD have a benign course. Patients with significant complications such as encephalopathy, thrombocytopenic purpura, or bone lesions usually have a more prolonged course, but also have a good long-term prognosis.

 Differential Diagnosis

Most known causes of lymphadenopathy (*see* Neck masses). Location of the abnormal lymph nodes may supply a strong clue.

 Data Gathering

HISTORY

Question: Cat contact?
Significance: The majority of patients have an antecedent cat contact.

Question: A skin rash?
Significance: May describe the appearance of a papule on the skin at the site of inoculation 3 to 5 days after the initial injury.

Question: Changes in rash?
Significance: This papule generally progresses through a vesicular and crusty stage.

Question: When did large lymph nodes appear?
Significance: Within 1 to 2 weeks, lymphadenopathy in the region of drainage may be noted.

Question: Other symptoms?
Significance: Mild associated symptoms of generalized achiness, malaise, anorexia may also be present. Fever is present in less than 10%.

Physical Examination

- One or more red papules at the inoculation site may be detectable.
- The true sign of CSD (present in 10% of cases) is chronic or subacute lymphadenitis involving the first or second set of nodes draining the inoculation site.
- The groups affected, in decreasing order of frequency, are the axillary, cervical, submandibular, periauricular, epitrochlear, femoral, and inguinal lymph nodes.
- Usually tender with overlying erythema, warmth, and induration.
- Less than one-half become suppurative or form a sinus tract to the skin.

 ## Laboratory Aids

Test: Direct fluorescence antibody testing
Significance: For detection of antibodies to *B. henselae,* conducted on serum samples at the Centers for Disease Control and Prevention. This test should be used to confirm a CSD diagnosis.

Test: Enzyme immunoassay
Significance: For detection of IgG antibodies to *B. henselae,* also commercially available (Specialty Laboratories, Santa Monica, CA).

Test: Blood cultures
Significance: Using lysed or centrifuged blood may at times yield *B. henselae* growth from infected individuals in whom bacteremia is suspected.

Isolation of organism from skin lesions and nodal aspirates may be possible.

 ## Therapy

Antibiotic therapy for CSD is somewhat controversial. Some authors still suggest the use of an oral antibiotic such as trimethoprim-sulfamethoxazole (TMP-SMX), 6 to 8 mg/kg of TMP b.i.d. to t.i.d. for 7 days. Or Azithromycin 500 mg initially then 250 mg for a total of 5 days in patients more than 45.5 kg and 10 mg/kg on the first day and 5 mg/kg for the subsequent 4 days in children for uncomplicated CSD, or many experts suggest conservative, symptomatic treatment only. Percutaneous drainage of tender, fluctuant adenitis can provide relief of pain. For immunocompromised patients and those with severe disease (including encephalitis) gentamicin sulfate, 5 mg/kg/d divided q8h intramuscularly or intravenously, is recommended. The duration of treatment should be based on response.

PREVENTION

Measures to prevent CSD should be directed toward minimizing contact between infected cats and people. Keeping kittens and older cats indoors and avoiding rough play may decrease the likelihood of infection. Avoidance of stray animals and good local care of any sustained bite or scratch is essential.

 ## Follow-Up

Most patients will have a benign course and can expect resolution of systemic symptoms in less than 2 weeks. Slow resolution of enlarged or painful lymph nodes will occur over weeks to months. As mentioned, percutaneous drainage of tender, fluctuant lymph nodes may be required to relieve pain. As stated previously, the course for patients with severe complications, including encephalitis, will be more prolonged, but without lasting sequelae.

 ## Common Questions and Answers

Q: Can a sibling develop CSD from an infected patient?
A: No. Person-to-person transmission is not reported.

Q: Should the parents of a child with cat-scratch disease get rid of the cat?
A: In general, this is not recommended. These animals are not ill. The capacity to transmit disease appears to be transient, and recurrent disease is rare.

ICD-9-CM 078.3

BIBLIOGRAPHY

Adal KA, Cockerell CJ, Petri WA. Cat-scratch disease, bacillary angiomatosis, and other infections due to Rochalimaea. *N Engl J Med* 1994;330:1509–1515.

Bass JW, Freitas, BC, Freitas AD, et al. Prospective randomized double blend placebo-controlled evaluation of azithromycin for treatment of cat-scratch disease. *Pediatr Infect Dis J* 1998;17:447–452.

Boyer KM, Cherry JD. Cat-scratch disease. In: Feigin RD, Cherry JD, eds. *Textbook of pediatric infectious diseases,* 3rd ed. Philadelphia: WB Saunders, 1992:1084–1088.

Carithers HA. Cat-scratch disease: an overview based on a study of 1,200 patients. *Am J Dis Child* 1985;139:1124–1133.

Carithers HA. Cat-scratch disease: acute encephalopathy and other neurologic manifestations. *Am J Dis Child* 1991;145:48–101.

Case records of the Massachusetts General Hospital. Weekly clinicopathological exercises. Case 1-1998. An 11-year-old boy with a seizure [clinical conference] [published erratum appears in *N Engl J Med* 1998;338(7):483] *N Engl J Med* 1998;338(2):112–119.

Kelly CS, Kelly RE Jr. Lymphadenopathy in children. *Pediatric Clinics of North Am* 1998;45(4):875–888.

Margileth AM. Antibiotic therapy for cat-scratch disease: clinical study of therapeutic outcome in 268 patients and a review of the literature. *Pediatr Infect Dis J* 1992;11:474–478.

Stone JE. Encephalitis associated with cat-scratch disease—Broward and Palm Beach Counties, Florida, 1994. *JAMA* 1995;273:614.

Author: Susan Dibs

Cavernous Sinus Syndrome

 Database

DEFINITION

The cavernous sinus syndrome (CSS) includes a variety of disease processes that localize to the cavernous sinus—a venous plexus that drains the face, mouth, tonsils, pharynx, nasal cavity, paranasal sinuses, orbit, middle ear, and parts of the cerebral cortex. Small lesions in this region may produce dramatic neurological signs.

PATHOPHYSIOLOGY

The cavernous sinus is located lateral to the pituitary gland and sella turcica, superior to the sphenoid sinus, and inferior to the optic chiasm. Within the cavernous sinus are the carotid artery, the pericarotid sympathetic fibers, and the abducens nerve (VI); within its lateral wall are the oculomotor nerve (III), the trochlear nerve (IV), and the ophthalmic and maxillary divisions of the trigeminal nerve (V1, V2). CSS is typically caused by septic or aseptic sinus thrombosis, neoplasm or trauma. Acute obstruction by mass or thrombosis may progress rapidly if not diagnosed and treated quickly.

COMPLICATIONS

Complications are dependent on the etiology of CSS. Septic CSS thrombosis and fungal infections may rapidly evolve to life-threatening sepsis and meningitis. Mucormycosis, usually seen in patients with diabetic ketoacidosis, is especially devastating. Aseptic CSS thrombosis may evolve to more extensive intracranial venous sinus thrombosis. Local spread of neoplasms will continue if not treated appropriately.

PROGNOSIS

Prognosis depends on the underlying etiology. Bacterial infections usually respond if diagnosed and treated promptly.

 Differential Diagnosis

- Other disorders that may resemble CSS include orbital cellulitis, sphenoid sinusitis, thyroid eye disease, cavernous carotid aneurysm, orbital apex tumor, orbital pseudotumor, ocular migraine, and ocular trauma.
- CSS may be due to septic or aseptic venous thrombosis, neoplasms, carotid-cavernous fistulas, or idiopathic inflammation.
- First priority is to rule out septic cavernous sinus thrombosis, a life-threatening complication of infections of the face, sinuses, middle ear, teeth, and orbit.
- Infectious agents include *Staphylococcus aureus, Streptococcus pneumoniae,* gram-negative rods, and anaerobes.
- *Mucormycosis* and *Aspergillus* may be found in immunocompromised patients.
- Aseptic venous thrombosis has been associated with sickle cell anemia, trauma, dehydration, vasculitis, pregnancy, oral contraceptive use, congenital heart disease, inflammatory bowel disease, and hypercoagulable states.
- Neoplasms involving the cavernous sinus include pituitary adenomas, meningiomas, craniopharyngiomas, lymphomas, neuromas, chordomas, chondrosarcomas, and nasopharyngeal carcinomas. Neoplasms may present with diplopia, visual-effect deficits, headache, or isolated cranial nerve deficits. The lateral extension of pituitary neoplasms into the cavernous sinus usually affects the third cranial nerve, with the fourth and sixth nerves less commonly involved. Rupture of a cystic craniopharyngioma may appear as acute CSS.
- Carotid-cavernous fistulas, which often have a more chornic course, are direct high-flow shunts between the internal carotid artery and the cavernous sinus. Almost always sequelae of trauma, they may present with a history of ocular motility deficits, arterialization of conjunctival vessels, and a bruit usually heard best over the orbit.
- Non-specific and idiopathic inflammation of the cavernous sinus, also called idiopathic cavernous sinusitis or Tolosa-Hunt syndrome, has been reported in patients as young as 3½ years. This is a diagnosis of exclusion.

 Data Gathering

HISTORY

Question: History of a recent local infection?
Significance: Facial furuncle or cellulitis, sinusitis, dental infection, otitis, or orbital cellulitis may predispose to CSS.

Question: Are local or systemic symptoms present?
Significance: Fever, headache, eye pain, diplopia, and facial parasthesias may be present.

 Physical Examination

Finding: Conjunctival injection with lid swelling and proptosis.
Significance: Signs of cavernous sinus venous congestion

Finding: Ptosis, anisocoria, ophthalmoparesis, and facial sensory changes
Significance: Signs of cranial nerve involvement

Finding: Horner syndrome.
Significance: Sympathetic nerve fibers traveling with V1 may be affected

Finding: Begin unilaterally
Significance: May rapidly spread bilaterally.

Finding: Optic nerve and visual acuity are spared early in CSS.
Significance: Can be affected as it progresses.

Finding: Funduscopic findings include venous dilatation and hemorrhages.
Significance: Papilledema is rare in acute cavernous sinus disease.

Finding: Resistance to retropulsion
Significance: May be very painful to elicit, but is a helpful sign.

Finding: Ocular bruit
Significance: May be heard in any acute CSS, but especially in carotid-cavernous fistula.

Finding: Signs of meningitis and systemic toxicity
Significance: These rapidly evolve if infections are untreated.

Laboratory Aids

Test: CBC, ESR, PT/PTT, blood culture
Significance: Basic studies in any child with suspected acute CSS. A lumbar puncture should be performed if there is no contraindication and infection is suspected.

Test: MRI or CT
Significance: Any child with proptosis, cranial-nerve findings, or an ocular bruit should have an urgent MRI or CT. MRI, with and without gadolinium, with special attention to the cavernous sinus and parasellar region, is the imaging study of choice. Magnetic resonance venography (MRV) may be helpful.

Test: Angiography
Significance: Suspected carotid-cavernous fistulas require angiography.

Test: Nasopharyngeal biopsy and culture
Significance: Helpful if *Mucormycosis* or *Aspergillus* is suspected.

Test: Blood cultures
Significance: Positive in 70% of cases of septic venous sinus thrombosis.

 ## Therapy

• For septic cavernous sinus thrombosis, broad-spectrum antibiotics, including anaerobe coverage, are begun immediately. Duration of therapy is usually 2 to 4 weeks beyond the resolution of symptoms.
• Amphotericin B is given if *Mucormycosis* or *Aspergillus* is suspected.
• Surgical drainage of the primary infection (i.e., sinusitis) may be indicated (avoiding surgical manipulation of the cavernous sinus itself).
• Anticoagulation is controversial, but one study in adults found heparin reduced morbidity from septic cavernous sinus thrombosis.
• Post-traumatic carotid-cavernous fistulas rarely close spontaneously and have been treated with endoarterial balloon embolization.
• Consultation with a neuro-oncologist and a neurosurgeon are important for suspected neoplasms or surgical lesions.
• Idiopathic cavernous sinusitus, a diagnosis of exclusion, responds to corticosteroids. Treatment should not be started until neoplasm and infection have been ruled out.

 ## Follow-Up

• Septic cavernous sinus thrombosis may relapse, or embolic abscesses may develop, 2 to 6 weeks after therapy has been stopped. Mortality remains 13% to 30%, and less than 40% of patients recover fully from cranial-nerve deficits.
• Patients with carotid-cavernous fistulas frequently have persistent cranial-nerve deficits even after embolization.
• Idiopathic cavernous sinusitis responds to steroids, but relapses can be problematic. Clinical follow-up and serial MRI scans are indicated to rule out a low-grade neoplasm or fungal infection.

PREVENTION

• Local bacterial infections—sinusitis, facial cellulitis, dental abscesses, otitis, pre-septal cellulitis and orbital cellulitis—should be treated promptly.
• Patients with suspected hypercoagulable states should be evaluated fully; dehydration must be avoided in such patients and anticoagulation may be necessary.

PITFALLS

• Ophthalmoplegic migraine must be distinguished from CSS by neuroimaging studies and history. Proptosis does not occur in migraine. This is a diagnosis of exclusion, especially on first presentation.
• Acute infection and hemorrhage of the pituitary gland—pituitary apoplexy—may present with acute bilateral ophthalmoplegia and signs of acute pituitary insufficiency. This most commonly occurs with pituitary neoplasms, but may also occur in pregnant women at the time of delivery. Chronic granulomatous disorders and tuberculosis may underlie CSS.

 ## Common Questions and Answers

Q: Will my child's eye movements return to normal?
A: In most cases, oculomotor nerves regain function as other signs improve, though they may take the longest to recover.

Q: Can more pain medicine be given?
A: There is often an attempt to balance side effects of sedation and hypoventilation against the need for pain control, especially when intracranial pressure is a concern.

BIBLIOGRAPHY

Berge J, Louail C, Caille JM. Cavernous sinus thrombosis diagnostic approach. *J Neuroradiol* 1994;21:101–117.

Doyle KJ, Jackler RK. Otogenic cavernous sinus thrombosis. *Otolaryngol Head Neck Surg* 1991;104:873–877.

Galetta SL. Cavernous sinus syndromes. In: Margo CE, ed. Diagnostic problems in clinical ophthalmology. Philadelphia: WB Saunders, 1994:609–615.

Karlin RJ, Robinson WA. Septic cavernous sinus thrombosis. *Ann Emerg Med* 1984;13:449–455.

Keane JR. Cavernous sinus syndrome—Analysis of 151 cases. *Arch Neurol* 1996;53:967–971.

Odabasi AO, Akgul A. Cavernous sinus thrombosis: A rare complication of sinusitis. *Intl J Pediatr Otorhinolaryngol* 1997;39:77–83.

Author: Dennis J. Dlugos

Cavernous Transformation and Portal Vein Obstruction

 Database

DEFINITION

Cavernous transformation is defined as the collection of collaterals that develop around an obstructed vessel. In pediatrics, the obstruction is most typically of the portal vein. In portal vein obstruction the main portal vein or splenic vein is obstructed somewhere along its course, between the hilum of the spleen and the porta hepatis.

PATHOPHYSIOLOGY

Patients present with asymptomatic splenomegaly or upper gastrointestinal hemorrhage, resulting from portal hypertension. Less commonly, the patient presents with ascites or failure to thrive. And 50% of portal vein obstructions are idiopathic. Identified etiologies include:

- Congenital lesions
—Web
—Vascular anomaly
- Clot that develops as a result of hypercoagulable states
—Malignancy
—Protein C deficiency
—Protein S deficiency
—Anti-thrombin III deficiency
- Clot from other etiologies
—Omphalitis
—Umbilical-vein catheterization
- Portal pyelophlebitis
- Intra-abdominal sepsis
—Surgery near the porta hepatis
—Sepsis
—Cholangitis
—Dehydration
—Trauma

GENETICS

A genetic basis of this problem has not been identified. Congenital abnormalities of the heart, major blood vessels, biliary tree, and renal system are found in 40% of cases.

EPIDEMIOLOGY

Even if the lesion developed in infancy, patients present at any age. Patients in the 70th decade have been reported, but most patients present between birth and 15 years of age. Bleeding is more typical of patients presenting before 7 years of age; splenomegaly in the absence of symptoms is more typical for patients between ages 5 and 15.

COMPLICATIONS

Most of the complications are secondary to portal hypertension, such as variceal hemorrhage and splenomegaly with hypersplenism. In some cases, steatorrhea and protein-losing enteropathy occur secondary to venous congestion of the intestinal mucosa. Ascites may also develop around the time of the onset of portal hypertension. Often, it develops in the period immediately following an upper gastrointestinal (GI) hemorrhage due to acute hepatic decompensation and decreasing albumin. Both the albumin and the ascites resolve in several weeks.

 Differential Diagnosis

The differential diagnosis must exclude other causes of splenomegaly and portal hypertension. Once portal vein obstruction has been identified, a search for the underlying etiology must be pursued.

 Data Gathering

Clinical examination reveals no jaundice or other evidence of chronic liver disease. Splenomegaly is the only intra-abdominal abnormality that can be identified. Ascites is rarely present.

HISTORY

Question: Other causes of splenomegaly?
Significance: Exposure to infectious mononucleosis, metabolic storage disease, and malignancy.

 Physical Examination

Finding: Splenomegaly and possible hemorrhoids
Significance: The spleen is measured from the left anterior axillary line at the costal margin diagonally toward the umbilicus.

Cavernous Transformation and Portal Vein Obstruction

 Laboratory Aids

Test: CBC
Significance: Leukopenia and thrombocytopenia will be present if there is hypersplenism

Test: AST/ALT/GGT
Significance: Should be normal

Test: PT/PTT
Significance: May be abnormal if malabsorption is present

Test: Protein C, protein S, anti-thrombin III
Significance: Associated with hypercoagulable states

Test: Ultrasound with Doppler
Significance: To examine portal vein flow and to identify collateral veins if there is cavernous transformation of the portal vein. The liver may be slightly small, but may be normal in texture.

Test: Liver biopsy
Significance: Exclude other etiologies.

Test: Upper endoscopy
Significance: To define extent of varices

Test: Bone marrow examination
Significance: To determine if there is an underlying myeloproliferative disease

 Therapy

Therapy is designed to manage variceal hemorrhage and to identify an underlying etiology to determine if the patient is at risk for additional venous thrombosis or malignancy. The therapy for GI hemorrhage is:

- Prophylactic sclerotherapy
- β-blocker therapy
- Shunt in order to decompress varices

 Follow-Up

Follow-up by the pediatrician should focus on growth parameters and early detection of malabsorption. The gastroenterologist will manage GI hemorrhage and supplemental nutrition, if needed.

PITFALLS

The patient should be advised about activity restrictions due to splenomegaly and should be told to avoid medicines that interfere with platelet function.

 Common Questions and Answers

Q: What is the long-term prognosis?
A: Good. Upper GI hemorrhage becomes less problematic as the child becomes older. Shunting is rarely recommended. Most patients undergo prophylactic sclerotherapy. As liver function is normal, it is rare for encephalopathy to develop.

Q: Should I restrict my child's activities?
A: Contact sports should be limited or a spleen guard used. NSAIDs, including aspirin, should be avoided because of the risk of hemorrhage.

ICD-9-CM 747.49

BIBLIOGRAPHY

Gitnick G, LaBrecque DR, Moody FG. *Diseases of the liver and biliary tract*. Philadelphia: Mosby-Year Book, 1992.

Mowat AP. *Liver disorders in childhood*. Boston: Butterworths, 1987.

Suchy F. *Liver disease in children*. Philadelphia: CV Mosby, 1994.

Author: Barbara Haber

Celiac Disease

 Database

DEFINITION

This is defined as a lifetime sensitivity to gluten, a protein fraction that is present in wheat, barley, rye and possibly in oats.

CLINICAL PRESENTATION

• Typical presentation is in the toddler under the age of 2 years who presents with failure to thrive, malabsorption, wasting of muscles, bloated abdomen, fractious and unhappy behavior. The stools are explosive, foul and vomiting is common. About 80% of all children with celiac disease present with this picture.
• Atypical forms are:

—Late presentation in school children with recurrent abdominal pain
—Recurrent aphthous stomatitis
—Cryptogenic hepatitis
—Dental defects

• Disease also causes:

—Iron deficiency anemia resistant to iron therapy
—Gastrointestinal bleeding
—Short stature
—Joint problems
—Dermatitis herpetiformis without obvious symptoms of malabsorption

• With increasingly sensitive methods for detection more cases of celiac disease have been found where the disease is clinically silent when the enteropathy is found incidentally in a healthy child. With detailed studies of these patients, there is a higher prevalence of these patients with vague symptoms such as behavioral problems, anemia, fatigue, and osteopenia.
• In latent celiac disease, patients have mild symptoms of celiac disease but on endoscopy there is no evidence of enteropathy, but once challenged with 20 g of gluten there is obvious enteropathy. These probably represent patients with a milder form of the disease.
• Finally, some toddlers present with classic celiac disease on endoscopy and gluten challenge but after a few years they tolerate a gluten-containing diet with no endoscopic evidence of enteropathy. This is probably a form of transient protein intolerance, such as with milk protein intolerance.

PATHOPHYSIOLOGY

Small bowel biopsy is done by direct endoscopy with forceps or with the Crosby capsule. The Crosby capsule takes better aligned biopsies to demonstrate the entire crypt-villus architecture but using a dissecting microscope, it is quite easy to align the biopsy for the pathologist. The aligning is crucial since the diagnosis is made based on visualizing flattening of the villus, which can be easily mimicked by a poorly aligned biopsy from a healthy patient. Features that characterize celiac disease are:

• Total villus atrophy
• Crypt hyperplasia
• Increased crypt cell mitosis
• Infiltration of Lamina propria with excess lymphocytes (CD4 T cells mainly)

EPIDEMIOLOGY

• Prevalence of 90 per 100,000
• Women more affected than men
• Uncommon in the United States but more common in Europe
• Including asymptomatic patients may affect as many as 1 in 300 people based on blood donor studies.

GENETICS

• There is 5% to 15% of first-degree concordance in first degree relatives with celiac disease and 75% concordance in twins demonstrating the genetic causality.
• In addition 90% of patients have the HLA DQ2 molecule coded by the alleles DQA1*0501 and DQB1*0201 and 5% carry the HLA DR4, DQ8 haplotype.

OTHER ASSOCIATED DISEASES

• Ankylosing spondylitis, scleroderma systemic lupus erythematosus (SLE), Sjögren syndrome
• Chromosomal anomalies such as Down and Turner syndrome
• Addison disease, autoimmune thyroiditis, Graves disease, parathyroid adenoma, diabetes mellitus
• Alopecia, atopic eczema, dermatitis herpetiformis, psoriasis
• Mouth diseases such as cancer, lichen planus, and recurrent stomatitis
• Inflammatory bowel disease and oropharyngeal cancers
• Chronic active hepatitis, primary biliary cirrhosis, primary sclerosing cholangitis
• Neurological and behavioral disorders
• IgA deficiency
• Asthma, alveolitis, sarcoidosis

 Differential Diagnosis

• Milk protein intolerance
• Toddler's diarrhea
• Giardiasis
• Gastritis
• Gastroenteritis
• Eosinophilic gastroenteritis
• Autoimmune enteropathy
• Immunodeficiency
• Cystic fibrosis
• Inflammatory bowel disease
• Celiac disease has been associated with other diseases including:

—Diabetes mellitus
—Thyrotoxicosis
—Hypothyroidism
—IgA deficiency
—Sarcoidosis
—Vasculitits
—Dermatitis herpetiformis
—Pernicious anemia

Data Gathering

HISTORY

Question: Diet?
Significance: Determine the relationship between intake of gluten and symptoms. Find out the amount of wheat, rye and barley.

Question: Growth pattern?
Significance: Most patients have short stature.

Question: Description of stools?
Significance: Stools tend to be explosive and foul smelling.

Question: Description of behavior
Significance: Patients tend to be irritable.

 ## Physical Examination

Finding: Growth pattern
Significance: Often have short stature

Finding: Classic presentation is large abdomen with wasted buttocks
Significance: Many patients do not have that appearance.

 ## Laboratory Aids

Test: Antibody testing
Significance: Because 2% of patients with celiac disease are IgA deficient, it is best to check both IgG and IgA antigliadin antibodies concurrently.

Test: Antigliadin antibody (AGA) IgA and IgG
Significance: 90% with active celiac disease are positive

Test: Anti-reticulin antibody (AR) IgA
Significance: More specific but less sensitive than antigliadin Ab

Test: Anti-endomysial antibody (AEA) IgA
Significance: More specific than AGA but in treated patients titers fall more than AGA.

BIOPSY

• Before a biopsy is done it is usual to check all the celiac antibodies as a screening test. With diagnosed patients AGA and AEA titers are useful monitoring tools for compliance and recovery.
• Should be performed on a regular diet.
• Reveals flattened villi with plasma cell infiltrate.

CBC

• Microcytic anemia is common

DIAGNOSIS

• Because AEA are so specific for celiac disease, some people have advocated treatment based on positive AEA antibodies alone. The current standard for diagnosis is the typical small bowel biopsy findings on a gluten-containing diet with symptoms resolving on a gluten-free diet with reversal of enteropathy on subsequent endoscopy.
• Additional monitoring is done with symptoms and antibody testing.
• Finally, to diagnose transient gluten intolerance, a gluten challenge is carried out after an interval. There is no consensus as to when this should be performed.

TREATMENT

Gluten-free diet with normalization of symptoms and enteropathy, which can take up to 6 months.

PROGNOSIS

On patients with strict diet there is very little risk of malignant lymphoma and other malignancies. Therefore, in patients with proven celiac disease it is advisable to remain on gluten-free diet for life.

 ## Common Questions and Answers

Q: Why do you do a gluten challenge when celiac disease is a lifelong disease?
A: This is to exclude the diagnosis of transient gluten intolerance, which is more like a milk protein intolerance and disappears when the gut heals. In such patients, a gluten challenge is normal.

Q: Are oats included in the gluten containing cereal?
A: Strictly speaking wheat, rye, barley, and oats are more closely related in their development from the primitive grains such as rice, corn, sorghum, and millets, which do not activate celiac disease. Gluten-free means a diet devoid of all wheat, rye, barley, and oats but some adult studies have shown that ingestion of even up to 50 g of oats did not cause clear-cut histological or clinical deterioration in celiac patients. It appears that of the four grains, oats is the least "toxic" to celiac patients.

Q: Can patients with celiac disease drink beer?
A: Not if the beer is derived from barley, rye, wheat or oats.

ICD-9-CM 579.0

BIBLIOGRAPHY

Catassi C, Fabiani E. The spectrum of coeliac disease in children. In: Walker-Smith JA, ed. *Paediatric gastroenterology, Bailliere's clinical gastroenterology international practice and research.* Bailliere Tindall, 1997:485–507.

Kagnoff MF. Genetic basis of celiac disease: role of HLA genes. In: Marsh M, ed. *Coeliac disease.* Boston: Blackwell Scientific Publications, 1992:215–238.

Revised criteria for diagnosis of coeliac disease. Report of Working Group of European Society of Paediatric Gastroenterology and Nutrition. *Arch Dis Child* 1990;65(8):909–911.

Authors: John Tung and Donna Zeiter

Cellulitis

 Database

DEFINITION

- Inflammation/infection of the skin/subcutaneous tissues
- Often classified by body area involved

—Periorbital
—Orbital
—Buccal
—Peritonsillar
—Extremity
—Breast

CAUSES

- *Staphylococcus aureus*
- Streptococcal (group A β-hemolytic and *S. pneumoniae*)
- *Haemophilus influenzae* type b (rare since advent of childhood immunization)
- *Pseudomonas aeruginosa,* other gram-negative bacilli, anaerobic bacteria (immunocompromised children)

PATHOPHYSIOLOGY

- Most commonly secondary to local trauma

—Abrasions
—Lacerations
—Bites
—Excoriated dermatitis
—Other breach in the integument

- May develop secondary to local invasion or infection (e.g., sinusitis leading to orbital cellulitis)
- Hematogenous dissemination (classically *H. influenzae* type b)

EPIDEMIOLOGY

- Cellulitis secondary to local trauma of the integument is by far the most common cause of cellulitis in children.
- Incidence of hematogenous disease is dramatically declining as *H. influenzae* type b disease disappears.

ASSOCIATED ILLNESSES

- Periorbital

—Usually secondary to local trauma
  —Impetigo
  —Varicella
  —Eczema

—Much less common, hematogenous
—Rarely associated with infectious conjunctivitis

- Orbital

—Most commonly associated with severe sinusitis
—Less common, dental abscess

- Buccal

—Same pathophysiology and epidemiology as periorbital cellulitis (not including conjunctivitis)

- Peritonsillar

—Commonly secondary to severe group A β-hemolytic streptococcal pharyngitis
—Often progresses or associated with a peritonsillar abscess

- Extremity

—Almost always secondary to local trauma

- Breast

—Usually with mastitis

COMPLICATIONS

- Local as well as distant spread of infection is possible.
- Suppuration and abscess formation may occur (e.g., peritonsillar abscess).
- Extremity cellulitis may extend into the deep tissues to produce an arthritis or osteomyelitis, or it may extend proximally as a lymphangitis.
- Orbital cellulitis may be complicated by visual loss and/or cavernous sinus thrombosis.
- Prior to widespread immunization against *Haemophilus influezae* type b, the bacteremia associated with facial cellulitis was not uncommonly associated with pneumonia, meningitis, pericarditis, epiglottitis, as well as arthritis and osteomyelitis.

PROGNOSIS

- The prognosis for complete recovery is good as long as appropriate antimicrobials are administered in a timely fashion.

 Differential Diagnosis

- Allergic angioedema is the most common entity; it can usually be excluded by its lack of tenderness and the absence of fever.
- Contact dermatitis, similarly, is distinguished by its painlessness, pruritus, and the Koebner phenomenon (appearance of isomorphic lesions in the lines of scratching).
- A traumatic contusion may be mistaken for cellulitis, but the history should be confirmatory.
- Severe conjunctivitis may mimic periorbital cellulitis; conjunctival injection, chemosis, and discharge usually implicate a conjunctivitis.
- "Popsicle panniculitis," a cold-induced fat injury to the cheeks of infants, may be almost indistinguishable from buccal cellulitis; a history of cold weather exposure, or ice or popsicle sucking should be sought.
- A primary eye malignancy (retinoblastoma), locally invasive tumor (rhabdomyosarcoma), or metastatic disease (neuroblastoma, leukemia, lymphoma), may simulate periorbital or orbital cellulitis.

 Data Gathering

HISTORY

Question: An expanding, red, painful area of swelling, with or without fever
Significance: The common presentation

Question: Mild constitutional symptoms
Significance: May occur with local disease; serious systemic symptoms, with bacteremic disease.

Question: History of local trauma to the integument
Significance: This is the clue to the portal of bacterial entry

Physical Examination

Finding: Erythema, edema, tenderness, and warmth
Significance: Usual presentations

Finding: A red, lymphangitic streak
Significance: May extend proximally from the extremity

Finding: Regional adenopathy
Significance: Is not uncommon

 ## Laboratory Aids

Test: CBC
Significance: May be normal or show leukocytosis in more severe cases.

Test: Blood cultures
Significance: Though the incidence of invasive *H. influenzae* type b disease is rapidly declining, blood cultures still should be obtained in facial and other serious cases of cellulitis; in children with *H. influenzae* type b cellulitis, 80% to 90% of blood cultures are positive.

Test: Needle aspiration and culture
Significance: "Leading edge" cultures, etc., are generally not indicated.

Test: Lumbar puncture
Significance: Indicated only in ill-appearing children and young infants (rule out sepsis)

Test: X-ray studies
Significance: Sometimes helpful to rule out complications such as arthritis or osteomyelitis

Test: Head CT scan
Significance: Important in orbital cellulitis to delineate extent of disease, and also in some cases when distinction from periorbital cellulitis is clinically difficult

Test: Bone marrow aspirate and biopsy (as well as CT scan)
Significance: To rule out malignancies

 ## Therapy

• Most cases of uncomplicated cellulitis can be treated with oral antibiotics active against *Staphylococcus* and *Streptococcus* (e.g., amoxicillin-clavulanate, cephalexin, erythromycin).
• Ill-appearing children or extensive cellulitic lesions require intravenous antibiotics.
• Initial intravenous therapy should be directed against *S. aureus* and *Streptococcus* (e.g., oxacillin, nafcillin, or cefazolin).
• When hematogenous dissemination is a strong possibility, an agent active against *H. influenzae* type b also should be added (e.g., ceftriaxone, cefotaxime, cefuroxime, or chloramphenicol).
• Neonates (<7 weeks of age) should have gram-positive and gram-negative coverage (e.g., oxacillin or nafcillin and gentamicin or oxacillin or nafcillin and cefotaxime) to cover the enterics as well.
• The duration of antibiotics (intravenous and oral) should generally be 7 to 10 days.
• Abscesses should be surgically drained.

 ## Follow-Up

• Rapid, steady improvement should be expected.
• If daily improvement is not noted, inappropriate antimicrobial therapy, a deeper infection or abscess, or some other complication should be suspected.

PREVENTION

• Good wound care can prevent most cases of cellulitis.
• Parents should be instructed to cleanse all wounds thoroughly with soap and water, then cover with a clean, dry cloth.
• Topical antibiotic ointment is optional.

PITFALLS

• Avoid trying to make distinction between staphylococcal and streptococcal by clinical presentation—it is always safest to cover cellulitis patients with an agent active against both (i.e., penicillin and amoxicillin are not good empiric choices).
• The "violaceous hue" touted as an indicator of *H. influenzae* type b cellulitis is neither sensitive nor specific.

 ## Common Questions and Answers

Q: Is ophthalmology consultation necessary in all cases of periorbital cellulitis?
A: Ophthalmology consultation is not necessary in simple, uncomplicated cases of periorbital cellulitis that clearly have no associated proptosis, limitation in extraocular eye movement, or visual impairment that would suggest a more serious orbital cellulitis; if, however, the diagnosis is in question, consultation is indicated.

Q: Is cefuroxime adequate coverage in cases of facial cellulitis?
A: If meningitis is suspected, cefuroxime should not be used, as its CSF penetration is suboptimal.

ICD-9-CM 682.9

BIBLIOGRAPHY

Barone SR, Aiuto LT. Periorbital and orbital cellulitis in the Haemophilus influenzae vaccine era. *J Pediatr Ophthalmol Strabismus* 1997;34(5):293–296.

Bisno AL. Cutaneous infections: microbiologic and epidemiologic considerations. *Am J Med* 1984;76(52):172–179.

Brown GC, ed. Current concepts in ophthalmology. *Pa Med* 1995;Supplement.

Ciarallo LR, Rowe PC. Lumbar puncture in children with periorbital and orbital cellulitis. *J Pediatr* 1993;122(3):355–359.

Fleisher GR, Ludwig S, eds. *Textbook of pediatric emergency medicine,* 3rd ed. Baltimore: Williams & Wilkins, 1993.

Lessner A, Stern GA. Preseptal and orbital cellulitis. *Infect Dis Clin North Am* 1992;6(4):933–952.

Meislin HW. Pathogen identification of abscesses and cellulitis. *Ann Emerg Med* 1986;15(3):329–332.

Pownall KR. Periorbital and orbital cellulitis. *Pediatr Rev* 1995;16(5):163–167.

Schwartz GR. Wright SW. Changing bacteriology of periorbital cellulitis. *Ann Emerg Med* 1996;28(6):617–620.

Author: Nicholas Tsarouhas

Cerebral Palsy

Database

DEFINITION AND CLASSIFICATION

- Cerebral palsy (CP) encompasses non-progressive motor impairment syndromes that result from damage to or dysfunction of the developing brain.
- Subtypes are defined by type of neurological impairment and anatomic distribution:

—Spastic CP (pyramidal CP) (40%): increased deep tendon reflexes, sustained clonus, hypertonia, and the clasp-knife response; spastic diplegia—lower extremity involvement; spastic hemiplegia—one side of the body involved; and spastic quadriplegia—total-body involvement.
—Dyskinetic CP (30%): fluctuating tone, rigidity (coactivated antagonists). Total-body involvement by definition. Persistent primitive reflex patterns [e.g., asymmetric tonic neck reflex (ATNR), labyrinthine] often seen. Subtypes—athetoid CP: slow writhing movements (or chorea: rapid, random, jerky movements), and dystonic CP: posturing of the head, trunk, and extremities.
—Ataxic CP (10%): characterized by cerebellar signs (ataxia, dysmetria, past-pointing, tremor, nystagmus) and abnormalities of voluntary movement
—Mixed CP (10%): two or more types codominant, most often spastic and dyskinetic

- Other CP (10%): criteria for CP met but specific subtype cannot be defined
- Extrapyramidal CP: sometimes applied to non-spastic types of CP as a group

EPIDEMIOLOGY

- Prevalence approximately 2 per 1000
- Approximately 50% of cases are associated with prematurity.
- Increased incidence with multiple gestation (10% were twins in one study)
- Increased concordance among monozygotic versus dizygotic twins in some studies (not in others)
- Intrauterine growth retardation (IUGR) more common in CP than controls, especially for full-term infants in whom CP develops.
- Male:female ratio, 1.3:1
- Inconsistent correlation to maternal age, socioeconomic status, and parity
- Epidemiological studies suggest that prenatal factors are more strongly associated with subsequent CP than perinatal or postnatal factors; however, individual risk factors are poorly predictive of subsequent CP in the individual child.
- Diagnosis of perinatal asphyxia requires evidence of multiorgan system hypoxic-ischemic insult and severe encephalopathy (e.g., neonatal seizures, severe hypotonia), and accounts for only about 9% of cases of CP.

ETIOLOGY

- In majority of cases, etiology not apparent
- Epidemiological studies indicate two types of vulnerability to CP: prematurity-related and IUGR-related.

—Prematurity-related: unique vulnerability of the periventricular white matter between 28 and 32 weeks of gestation results in periventricular leukomalacia
—IUGR-related: in full-term infants, fetal abnormalities associated with CNS dysgenesis, non-CNS malformation, teratogens, growth retardation, evidence of hypoxic-ischemic encephalopathy more often seen

ASSOCIATED IMPAIRMENTS

- Sensory

—Sensorineural and conductive hearing loss
—Impairments of visual acuity
—Oculomotor dysfunction
 —Strabismus
—Somatosensory impairments

- Cognitive

—Mental retardation (MR) in about 50%, especially in spastic quadriparesis
—High incidence of learning disabilities
 —Attention deficit/hyperactivity disorder
 —Sleep and behavioral disturbances

- Neurological

—Seizures
—Hydrocephalus

- Musculoskeletal

—Contractures
—Hip subluxation/dislocation
—Scoliosis

- Cardiorespiratory

—Upper airway obstruction
—Aspiration pneumonitis
—Restrictive lung disease
 —Secondary to thoracic deformity
—Reactive airway disease

- Gastrointestinal tract/nutrition

—Failure to thrive
—Gastroesophageal reflux
—Constipation
—Oral motor dysfunction/dysphagia

- Gastrourinary tract

—Neurogenic bladder

- Skin

—Decubitus ulcers

- Dental

—Caries
—Gingival hyperplasia
—Abnormalities of enamel (congenital)

Differential Diagnosis

- Motor impairment syndromes related to spinal cord, lower motor neuron, peripheral nerve, or primary muscular disease

- Connective-tissue disorders (primary and secondary) resulting in musculoskeletal abnormalities (e.g., arthrogryposis multiplex, skeletal dysplasias)
- Inborn errors of metabolism and CP: protean manifestations, dyskinesia, ataxia, postnatal growth failure, neurologic deterioration (especially associated with recurrent vomiting) are clues, but presentation can be insidious.

Data Gathering

HISTORY

Question: Prenatal history
Significance: Exposure to toxins/drugs, infections or fever, HIV/STD risk, vaginal bleeding, abnormal fetal movement, pre-eclampsia (especially proteinuria), breech position, poor maternal weight gain, premature labor, fetal distress, IUGR, prenatal testing, placental disorders

Question: Perinatal history
Significance: Premature delivery, neonatal resuscitation, low Apgar scores (7 at 5 and 10 minutes), birth trauma, evidence of neonatal encephalopathy (seizures, severe hypotonia), complicated neonatal course (intraventricular hemorrhage, prolonged respiratory support, meningitis, sepsis, hyper-bilirubinemia)

Question: Post-natal history
Significance: Hospitalization for severe infection or trauma, periodic or persistent deterioration in function (suggests neurodegenerative/metabolic disease)

Question: Development
Significance: Severe delay in motor milestones (e.g., not rolling at 7 months, not sitting at 8 months, not walking at 15 months) associated with persistent primitive reflexes (e.g., prominent tonic neck and labyrinthine responses at 1 year of age) and delayed or absent development of protective reactions (e.g., lateral prop at 7 months, parachute at 13 months). Associated delays in language, play, social, and adaptive behavior.

Physical Examination

GENERAL

Finding: Respiratory pattern
Significance: Obstruction, aspiration risk, evidence of dysmorphism/pigmentary skin changes and growth abnormalities contribute to assessment of etiology.

Finding: Head circumference
Significance: To evaluate for microcephaly/macrocephaly/hydrocephaly

Finding: Strabismus/cataracts/iris or retinal abnormalities
Significance: Either cranial nerve damage, muscle imbalance, metabolic disease, or congenital infection.

MUSCULOSKELETAL

Finding: Range of motion
Significance: Decreased with contractures

Finding: Leg-length discrepancy
Significance: Hip dislocation

Finding: Spinal curvature
Significance: Neuromuscular imbalance

NEUROLOGICAL

Finding: In addition to formal examination, documentation of best level of visual motor/manipulative skills (i.e., able to run, transfer, hold a cup, etc.)
Significance: Helpful in following the course of the motor impairment.

Finding: Cranial nerves
Significance: Especially strabismus, speech and swallowing, vision and hearing

Finding: Tone
Significance: Spasticity versus rigidity versus hypotonia

Finding: Strength
Significance: Often decreased

Finding: Clasp-knife response
Significance: Hyperactive deep tendon reflexes, and clonus in spasticity; Babinski reflex (extensor response to plantar stimulation)

Finding: Persistent primitive reflexes
Significance: CNS damage

Finding: Protective reactions
Significance: Head and trunk righting, prop reactions, parachute; cerebellar signs

Finding: Postural stability
Significance: Neuromuscular imbalance

Finding: Gait abnormalities, subtle seizures
Significance: Motor or CNS damage

 Laboratory Aids

Test: Hearing and vision
Significance: All in first year with regular follow-up examinations (identification of sensory deficits and clues to etiology)

Test: Brain imaging
Significance: Should be performed when hydrocephalus is suspected; frequently useful in determining etiology

Test: Genetic and metabolic studies
Significance: Indicated when the history and physical examination suggest a progressive or hereditary disorder.

Test: X-ray studies
Significance: Should be done routinely in spastic diparesis for hip dislocation; usefulness of scoliosis films depends on physical findings.

Test: Audiological evaluation
Significance: Required for those with language delay or those who manifest hearing impairment.

Test: Radionucleotide studies or pH probe
Significance: "Milk scan"; evaluate gastroesophageal reflux (GER), gastric emptying, aspiration

Test: Blood tests—chemistries, liver-function studies, cell counts
Significance: Evaluate nutritional/metabolic status, anticonvulsant levels

Test: Urodynamic studies
Significance: Spastic bladder, indicated in those with recurrent urinary tract infections or voiding dysfunction.

Test: Sleep study
Significance: May disclose treatable obstructive sleep apnea in those with excessive somnolence or abnormal sleep-wake cycles.

Test: Pulmonary-function studies
Significance: Helpful in documenting progressive restrictive pulmonary dysfunction (e.g., in severe scoliosis).

Test: EEG
Significance: Seizure disorder is suspected

 Therapy

- Family-centered care is directed toward optimizing function/minimizing handicap (habilitation).
- Interdisciplinary clinics: to provide multiple services (medical, surgical, therapy, etc.) coordinated with primary care physician.
- Education services: recent emphasis on inclusion/mainstreaming; for many children, special education services are still required and appropriate.
- Physical, occupational, speech/language therapy, other allied health professionals: therapy provided in home, school, and hospital settings, directed primarily at improved functioning in the areas of mobility, self-care, and communication; orthodontists for braces.
- Social services: provided in a variety of contexts to aid in the coordination of care

 Follow-Up

- Requirements for follow-up vary greatly with the degree of disability and the scope of impairments. An interdisciplinary clinic setting may be more appropriate for a child with severe CP.
- Early referral to a pediatric orthopedist is indicated, especially for monitoring of early hip subluxation, which is best managed before progression to frank dislocation.
- Early referral for developmental assessment to establish need for early intervention, to optimize development, and to promote family coping

PITFALLS

- Overdiagnosis of CP in infants with spastic hypertonia (especially those born prematurely): normalization of tone/function may take up to 2 years.
- Slowly progressive neurogenerative disease may masquerade as CP.
- Cervical cord lesions may masquerade as quadriparetic spastic CP. Swallowing reflexes may be preserved, cognitive development is normal.
- Determination of ideal body weight may be complex in CP; growth standards according to CP type are under development.

 Common Questions and Answers

Q: Is severe clumsiness a form of CP?
A: Mild spastic diplegia or hemiplegia may present this way, but spasticity and contractures distinguish these from developmental coordination disorders.

Q: Do children with CP also have mental retardation?
A: Not necessarily; although 50% have mental retardation, it is not a part of the definition of CP.

Q: What about surgery for CP?
A: Spasticity in the lower extremities may be addressed directly with selective dorsal rhizotomy (interruption of afferent limb of stretch reflex arch). Otherwise, surgical therapy in CP is directed at associated conditions; many children with CP undergo orthopedic procedures for hip dislocation, release of contractures, and scoliosis. Surgery for correction of strabismus or placement of a gastrostomy tube is commonly performed.

BIBLIOGRAPHY

Badawi N, Watson L, Petterson B, et al. What constitutes cerebral palsy? *Dev Med Child Neurol* 1998;40(8):520–527.

Freeman JM, Nelson KB. Intrapartum asphyxia and cerebral palsy. *Pediatrics* 1988;82:240–249.

Golden CG. Apgar scores as predictors of chronic neurologic disability, by Karin B. Nelson, MD, and Jonas H. Ellenberg, PhD, *Pediatrics,* 1981;68:36–44. *Pediatrics* 1998;102(1 Pt 2):262–264.

Kuban KC, Leviton A. Cerebral palsy. *N Engl J Med* 1994;330:188–195.

Nelson KB, Ellenberg JH. Antecedents of cerebral palsy: multivariate analysis of risk. *N Engl J Med* 1986;315:81–86.

Author: Louis Pelligrino

Cervicitis

Database

DEFINITION

Cervicitis is infection of the endocervix resulting in inflammation leading to mucopurulent cervical discharge, edema, erythema, and friability of the cervix and endocervical canal.

CAUSES

In the majority of young women, no pathogen is isolated. Common identifiable causes include:

- *Chlamydia trachomatis*
- *Neisseria gonorrhoeae*
- *Herpesvirus hominis*
- *Trichomonas vaginalis*
- *Candida albicans*

ASSOCIATED DISEASES

The presence of other sexually transmitted diseases must be considered including *T. vaginalis*, syphilis, hepatitis B, HIV, and bacterial vaginosis.

EPIDEMIOLOGY

The true incidence of mucopurulent cervicitis is unknown; however, it is quite common. As many patients are asymptomatic and the interpretation and presence of the clinical signs is quite variable, many cases go undiagnosed.

COMPLICATIONS

The patient with endocervical infection is at risk for reinfection and symptomatic or asymptomatic upper genital tract disease with all its sequelae, including infertility, ectopic pregnancy, and chronic pelvic pain. In addition, these patients are at risk for reinfection, other sexually transmitted diseases, and pregnancy.

PROGNOSIS

If treated appropriately, these patients are cured and have no sequelae from the infection.

Differential Diagnosis

- The differential diagnosis includes potential causes of inflammation of the vulva, the urethra and/or bladder, the vagina, and the endocervical canal. In patients presenting with abnormal menstrual bleeding, these infectious causes are common.
- However, there are numerous other causes including pregnancy. (*See* Dysfunctional Uterine Bleeding.)

Data Gathering

HISTORY

Symptoms

Question: Abnormal vaginal bleeding and/or discharge
Significance: Result of infection

Question: Dysuria
Significance: Urethritis

Question: Vulvar itching
Significance: Irritation from infection

Question: Dyspareunia
Significance: Pain from mobility of tender cervix

Medical History

Question: Previous sexually transmitted disease (STD)
Significance: Common association

Question: Gravity
Significance: May lead to infertility

Question: Parity
Significance: May lead to infertility

Question: Last menstrual period
Significance: May lead to ectopic pregnancy

Question: Birth control method
Significance: Condoms are protective

Question: Exposure to infected partner
Significance: Important to treat both partners

Physical Examination

Abdomen

Finding: No tenderness
Significance: Infection is limited to cervix

Pelvic

Finding: Mucopurulent discharge from the cervical os or yellow exudative discharge present on a cotton-tipped swab from the endocervical canal
Significance: Classic finding for cervicitis

Finding: No cervical motion or adenexal tenderness or masses
Significance: Infection has not spread beyond cervix

- Friability of the exocervix

Laboratory Aids

Test: Cervical Gram stain from cervical discharge (uncontaminated by vaginal secretions) with >.10 polymorphonuclear leukocytes per high-power field and/or gram-negative intracellular diplococci
Significance: Typical findings

Test: Cervical gonococcal culture or LCR
Significance: Gonococcus is a common infection cause

Test: Cervical chlamydia culture or fluorescence antibody test or LCR
Significance: Chlamydia is a common infection cause

Test: HSV culture
Significance: Herpes is a common infection cause

Test: Wet preparation or culture for *T. vaginalis*
Significance: Test for trichomonas

Test: Potassium hydroxide preparation for budding hyphae
Significance: Test for candida

Etiology of Infection of Tumors

VULVITIS	VAGINITIS	CERVICITIS	URETHRITIS	CYSTITIS
Herpes simplex	Gardnerella	*C. Trachomatis*	*C. Trachomatis*	Coliform
Human papillomavirus (HPV)	*C. albicans*	*N. gonorrhoeae*	*N. gonorrhoeae*	*Staphylococcus*
Sapprophyticus	*C. Albicans*	*T. Vaginalis*		
Foreign body	HSV	HSV		

Therapy

• Patients should receive therapy for *N. gonorrhoeae* and *C. trachomatis*. Treat other pathogens if clinically indicated or if documented by laboratory studies.

• Gonorrhea

—Cefixime, 400 mg PO
—Ceftriaxone, 125 mg IM
—Ciprofloxacin, 500 mg PO
—Doxycycline, 100 mg PO b.i.d. for 7 days

• *C. trachomatis*

—Azithromycin, 1 g PO
—Doxycycline, 100 mg PO b.i.d. for 7 days
—Erythromycin base, 500 mg PO q.i.d. for 7 days

• *T. vaginalis*

—Metronidazole, 2 g PO
—Metronidazole, 500 mg PO b.i.d. for 7 days

• *H. hominis*

—Acyclovir, 200 mg PO five times daily for 7 to 10 days, or until resolution

• *C. albicans*

—Clotrimazole 1% cream, 5 g intravaginally for 3 days
—Clotrimazole 100 mg vaginal tablet, for 7 days

 Follow-Up

The recommended treatment regimens have an excellent cure rate. The patient should have resolution of symptoms 3 to 5 days after starting therapy. Routine follow-up cultures are not necessary unless the patient remains symptomatic. Reculturing may be considered 2 to 3 months following therapy to identify reinfection.

PITFALLS

Failure to recognize the importance of evaluating the internal pelvic organs by physical examination with the presenting symptoms of dysuria, vaginal discharge, or abnormal menstrual bleeding in the postpubertal female.

 Common Questions and Answers

Q: How much cervical motion tenderness is present in patients with cervicitis?
A: None. Patients with cervicitis have inflammation and infection of the cervix only. They do not have any evidence of peritoneal inflammation on physical examination. Therefore, patients with tenderness should be treated with the protocols set forth by the CDC for pelvic inflammatory disease. This does not include the use of a single dose of azithromycin.

BIBLIOGRAPHY

Holmes KK. Lower genital tract infections in women: cystitis, urethritis, vulvovaginitis, and cervicitis. In: Holmes KK, Mardh P, Sparling PF, et al., eds. *Sexually transmitted diseases,* 2nd ed. New York: McGraw-Hill, 1990:527–545.

Neinstein LS. *Adolescent health care: a practical guide,* 2nd ed. Baltimore: Urban and Schwarzenberg, 1991.

US Department of Health and Human Services. 1998 Guidelines for treatment of sexually transmitted diseases. *MMWR* 1998 Jan 23:47(RR-1).

Author: Jane Lavelle

Chanchroid

 Database

DEFINITION/CAUSES

Infection with the gram-negative rod *Haemophilus ducreyi* resulting in painful genital ulcers.

PATHOPHYSIOLOGY

Trauma and abrasion allow the organism to penetrate the epidermis, leading to infection, ulcer formation, and lymphadenitis with a pyogenic inflammatory response.

ASSOCIATED DISEASES

- Associated with HIV transmission and infection
- Coinfection with syphilis and human herpesvirus can occur.

EPIDEMIOLOGY

Initially considered a rare disease in developed countries, but over the past decade there has been a dramatic rise in the number of cases in the United States. It is transmitted via sexual contact with an individual with an ulcer. It is seen more commonly in males.

COMPLICATIONS

- Draining bubo

 Differential Diagnosis

- Common causes of genital ulcers include infection with *Treponema pallidum* or herpes simplex.
- Uncommon etiologies include:

—Trauma
—Fixed drug eruptions
—Lymphogranuloma venereum
—Inflammatory bowel disease
—Behçet syndrome

 Data Gathering

HISTORY

- Males usually present with symptoms referable to an ulcer.
- Females present with nonspecific symptoms such as dysuria, dyspareunia, vaginal discharge or rectal pain, or bleeding.

 Physical Examination

Classic findings include:

- Presence of an extremely painful ulcer with an irregular border and a gray, necrotic center.
- Males: prepuce and coronal sulcus
- Females: entrance to the vagina
- Inguinal lymphadenopathy
- Present in 50%, may spontaneously drain (bubo)
- Extragenital sites
- Very rare

 Laboratory Aids

Test: Gram stain from the base of the ulcer
Significance: May show short gram-negative bacilli in parallel "school of fish" arrangement. This is non-specific.

Test: Culture diagnosis
Significance: This is the gold standard, but it is difficult to perform, not widely available and insensitive.

- Specimens are taken from the base of the ulcer using a cotton or calcium alginate swab.
- Diagnosis is made on clinical suspicion.
- Herpes culture and RPR should be sent.
- Coinfections occur in up to 10% of patients.

Therapy

- Azithromycin, 1 g PO
- Ceftriaxone, 250 mg IM
- Ciprofloxacin, 500 mg b.i.d. for 3 days (patients >18 years)
- Erythromycin base, 500 mg q.i.d. for 7 days

PREVENTION

- Condom use, consider HIV testing.
- Partners should be treated whether or not symptoms are present.

 Follow-Up

- Patients are symptomatically improved within 48 to 72 hours.
- Ulcers themselves heal between 1 and 4 weeks.
- Lymphadenopathy may take longer to regress and may progress to fluctuation in spite of adequate therapy.
- Patients should be followed weekly until symptoms resolve.
- In patients who do not follow the typical course, consider other causes of genital ulcers, non-compliance, presence of a coexisting STD, especially HIV infection, and rarely, presence of a resistant organism.
- Recent sexual partners, within the preceding 10 days, should be treated.

 Common Questions and Answers

Q: How do the ulcers of chancroid differ from those caused by herpes simplex and *T. pallidum*?
A: The ulcers caused by chancroid have irregular margins and deep undermined edges. They are very painful and occur singularly or in small numbers. Herpes simplex lesions occur as grouped vesicles that when ruptured leave behind painful shallow ulcers. The ulcers of syphilis are painless and solitary and have smooth margins surrounding a clean indurated base.

BIBLIOGRAPHY

Piot P, Plummer FA. Genital ulcer adenopathy syndrome. In: Holmes KK, Mardh P, Sparling PF et al., eds. *Sexually transmitted diseases,* 2nd ed. New York: McGraw-Hill, 1990.

US Department of Health and Human Services. 1998 Guidelines for treatment of sexually transmitted diseases. *MMWR* 1998 Jan 23:47(RR-1).

Author: Jane Lavelle

Chickenpox (Varicella, Herpes Zoster)

Database

DEFINITION

Varicella-zoster virus (VZV) is a herpesvirus. Only one strain is recognized. Humans are the only source of infection.

PATHOPHYSIOLOGY

• The virus can be demonstrated in the vesicular lesions by immunofluorescence, viral culture, and polymerase chain reaction (PCR) in specimens obtained from these lesions.
• Humoral immunity is sometimes insufficient to provide protection. Severe varicella is due more to impairment of the cell-mediated immune response than to a defect in humoral immunity.
• Healthy children in whom a cell-mediated immune response develops after the varicella exanthem have mild primary VZV infection, whereas in immunodeficient children in whom VZV-specific lymphocytes fail to proliferate progressive disseminated varicella develops.
• Adults have impaired cell-mediated responses and are, consequently, 35 times more likely to die of varicella than healthy children who contract chickenpox.
• Elderly adults and patients on immunosuppressive therapy have lower VZV-specific lymphocyte proliferation and are more likely to reactivate VZV, resulting in herpes zoster. A decrease in cell-mediated immunity is a necessary but not a sufficient setting for the development of zoster. Reactivation of the virus in the ganglia may occur sporadically without regard to immune function, but may be more likely to be symptomatic if cell-mediated immunity is depressed.

ASSOCIATED DISEASES/COMPLICATIONS OF VARICELLA INFECTION

• Secondary bacterial infection—especially virulent Group A streptococcal infections and *Staphlococcal* (drug resistance, an increasing problem)
• *Varicella pneumonitis* (more common in adults and infants)
• Gastrointestinal complications associated with viscous involvement, such as pancreatitis, appendicitis and hepatitis, idiopathic thrombocytopenia (ITP), and bleeding diathesis
• Nephritis
• Transverse myelitis
• Encephalitis, 60 cases per year
• Disseminated intravascular coagulation (Hemorrhagic VZV)
• Individuals with AIDS may have chronic VZV
• Arthritis, which can become superinfected usually with *Staphlococcus aureus*
• Congenital varicella syndrome that occurs in the first or second trimester of pregnancy, characterized by limb atrophy and scarring of the extremity. Central nervous system and eye manifestations also occur.
• Death—1 to 2 deaths per week in the United States, Varicella is the most common vaccine preventable cause of death.
• These complications are associated with significant morbidity and may occur irrespective of the use of acyclovir.

EPIDEMIOLOGY

• Person-to-person transmission occurs by direct contact with varicella or zoster and respiratory secretions.
• Varicella is most common during late winter and early spring.
• The introduction of an index case of varicella into a home results in transmission of the virus to suceptible persons and secondary cases of disease in 98% of susceptible persons.
• Secondary cases in this situation usually have more severe disease.
• Most reported cases occur between the ages of 5 and 9 years, although in areas of the United States, where many 1 to 4 year olds are in child care, this age group predominates with an increase in complications.
• Immunity from natural disease is usually lifelong, but symptomatic reinfections do occur; more common are asymptomatic reinfections, with a four-fold boost in antibody level.
• Immunocompromised individuals with either primary varicella or zoster are at risk for severe disease.
• Disease is also more severe in infants more than 3 months of age, adolescents, adults, those on oral and/or intravenous steroids or long-term aspirin therapy, or those with pulmonary disorders including asthma.
• Congenital varicella syndrome risk is about 2%, and is greatest in the first trimester. Incubation 10 to 21 days after contact; cases most contagious 2 days before the rash appears and until 5 days after lesions stop cropping (longer in immunocompromised patients)

Differential Diagnosis

• The appeerence of a typical rash that occurs in successive crops of macules, papules, and vesicles is distinctive.
• With limited or mild rash, the differential diagnosis includes other causes of vesiculation:
• Coxsackievirus infection with hand, foot, and mouth disease
• Rickettsial pox
• *Mycoplasma*
• *Pseudomonas* (in immunocompromised individuals)
• Eczema herpeticum
• Herpes zoster with dissemination
• Toxic epidermal necrosis, and various noninfectious vesicular conditions of the skin

Data Gathering

HISTORY

Question: Time of year
Significance: More common in winter and spring

Question: Typical rash that has multiple stages identified
Significance: Classic finding

Question: History of not previously having had varicella usually make the diagnosis.
Significance: Varicella infection provides immunity

Laboratory Aids

• Immunofluorescence of the vesicular fluid
• Culture of the vesicular fluid
• PCR of any tissue of vesicular fluid (reference labs include Dr. Philip LaRussa, NY.)
• The complement-fixation test is not reliable in determining immunity, and has been abandoned.

Test: Acute and convalescent sera for antibody testing by a number of assays, including enzyme immunoassay (EIA), immunofluorescence assay (IFA), latex agglutination (LA), and fluorescent antibody to membrane antigen (FAMA).
Significance: These tests can also be used to determine immunity.

Chickenpox (Varicella, Herpes Zoster)

 Therapy

- Acyclovir, vidarabine, famvir, foscarnet, and a number of antiviral agents-pending licensure have been shown in clinical trials to be effective against VZV.
- Acyclovir is the drug of choice in children
- Who benefits? Any child who is ill enough to warrant hospitalization and whose rash demonstrates new vesicle formation should be treated with acyclovir (IV dose is 1500 mg/m² divided into three doses q8h).
- Consider oral acyclovir (80 mg/kg divided in four doses q6h) for children over 12 years of age, those with chronic cutaneous or pulmonary disorders, persons on short or intermittent corticosteroids or aerosolized cortico-steroids, newborn infants, and selected immunocompromised persons at risk for severe varicella.
- Children with varicella should not receive salicylates because of the association with Reye syndrome. Acetaminophen may be used to control the fever. NSAIDs may increase complications from bacterial superinfection.

ISOLATION OF HOSPITALIZED PATIENTS

- Strict isolation for the duration of vesicular eruption (usually 5 days, longer in immunocompromised patients)
- Patients should be in negative-pressure rooms if possible.
- Exposed susceptible persons should be in strict isolation for 8 to 21 days after the onset of the rash in the index patient.
- Those who received varicella zoster immune globulin (VZIG) should be kept in isolation for 28 days after exposure.
- Immunocompromised patients who have zoster (localized or generalized) and normal patients with disseminated zoster should remain in strict isolation for the duration of the illness. For normal patients with localized zoster drainage and secretion, precautions are recommended until all lesions are crusted.

PREVENTION

- This is now a vaccine preventable disease and is incorporated in the harmonized immunization schedule recommended by the AAP and ACIP since 1995, and is covered by the vaccine for children's program
- Extensive clinical trials conducted in Japan, Belgium, and the United States evaluating the safety, immunogenicity, and transmissibility of vaccine virus, including comparative studies of various vaccine preparations, dose titration, efficacy (of which there is only one placebo-controlled study), consistency, and persistency of the immune response resulted in licensure of the varicella vaccine in March 1995.

- The vaccine is recommended for routine immunization of all healthy suceptible children, adolescents, and adults.
- One dose (0.5 mL subcutaneously) is required for children 12 months to 13 years of age.
- Individuals over 13 years of age require 2 doses, 1 to 2 months apart.
- The vaccine is safe <4% rash rate from immunization. Post-licensure surveillance has documented one incidence of transmission in 9.5 million doses.
- The vaccine is 93% efficacious against natural disease in clinical trials, and field experience using the secondary family attack rate methodology has shown 84% efficacy.
- Duration of immunity from individuals followed in the clinical trials has shown that both humoral and cell-mediated immune responses persist for at least 10 years (USA data) and 20 years (Japanese data).
- The vaccine is not currently recommended for immunocompromised individuals, but there are studies in process.
- Vaccine is available by protocol for acute lymphatic leukemia in remission (Tel: 215-283-0897).
- For those individuals who cannot recieve VZV vaccine because of an immunocompromised state, varicella-susceptible pregnant women (until the VZV vaccine registry has data to make alternate recommendations), and newborns, VZIG would continue to be recommended.

 Follow-Up

For normal healthy individuals follow-up is not necessary.

PROGNOSIS

- 50 to 100 previously healthy children die each year (1–2 each week) from varicella. This rate is about 35 times higher in the immunocompromised and adult populations.
- For most children, this childhood exanthem is a benign disease that lasts 6 to 8 days.
- With the advent of universal immunization, complications of varicella will become historical, as those associated with measles as we reach for the goal of measles eradication.

 Common Questions and Answers

Q: What do you do for a patient on corticosteroids who has not had VZV and is exposed to VZV?
A: These patients are immunosuppressed (if the dose of steroids is >.2 mg/kg/d) and would require VZIG or treatment with acyclovir within 72 hours of developing VZV, if VZIG had not been administered.

Q: What about asthmatics on inhaled steroids? Can they be immunized safely and are they at risk of more severe varicella if not immunized?
A: Asthmatics on inhaled steroids can be immunized as the dose of inhaled steroids is not immunosuppressive. Recent data does show asthmatic children who are unimmunized do get more severe varicella.

Q: Is there any patient who should not receive VZV vaccine?
A: Yes. Immunosuppressed individuals (still under study protocols), pregnant patients, and infants <1 year.

Q: Will a booster dose of VZV vaccine be necessary?
A: Surveillance procedures must be put into place to track the baseline incidence of varicella prior to licensure of the varicella vaccine and follow the patterns of disease post-licensure. Current data do not support the need for a "booster" dose because seroconversion following one dose in children and 2 doses in those individuals over 13 occurs in 98% of vaccinees. However, trials with two dose series demonstrates higher titers and lower breakthrough rates. In the near future a combination mmrv vaccine maybe available, making this question mute.

ICD-9-CM 052.9

BIBLIOGRAPHY

Arvin AM. Cell-mediated immunity to varicella-zoster virus. *J Infect Dis* 1992;166(Suppl. 1): S35–S41.

Fleisher G, Henry W, McSorley M, et al. Life threatening complications of varicella. *Am J Dis Child* 1982;135:896–899.

Lieu TA, Cochi SL, Black SB, et al. Cost-effectiveness of a routine varicella vaccination program for US children. *JAMA* 1994;271:375–381.

Watson B, Gupta R, Randall T, Starr SE. Persistence of cell-mediated and humoral immune responses in healthy children immunized with the live attenuated varicella vaccine. *J Infect Dis* 1994;169:197–199.

Watson B, Haupt R. Roadblocks to varicella vaccine. *Contemp Pediatr* 1997;14:167–181.

Author: Barbara Watson

Child Physical Abuse

Database

DEFINITION

Injuries or illnesses that occur to children as a result of family dysfunction. In practice, it is considered nonaccidental injury of children at the hands of their caretakers. Physical abuse is legally defined by state laws.

- Multifactorial etiology:

—Include societal, familial, and individual factors
—Associated with poverty, family stress, family isolation

- Associated problems:

—Domestic violence
—Sexual abuse
—Neglect
—Emotional abuse
—Juvenile delinquency
—Poverty
—Parental substance abuse, including alcohol

EPIDEMIOLOGY

- Approximately 250,000 substantiated cases identified in the US each year
- Almost 2,000 deaths/year, by conservative estimates
- Parents who were abused as children are at much greater risk for abusing their own children. It is estimated that 30% of abused children become abusive parents.

COMPLICATIONS

- Death
- Mental retardation
- Cerebral palsy
- Seizures
- Learning disabilities
- Emotional problems

PROGNOSIS

Varies greatly depending on injuries sustained, family problems, available support systems.

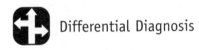

Differential Diagnosis

Varies depending on injury sustained.

INFECTION

- Sepsis
- Meningitis
- Congenital syphilis
- Osteomyelitis
- Impetigo
- Staphylococcal scalded-skin syndrome
- Purpura fulminans

ENVIRONMENTAL

- Phytophotodermatitis
- Coining: rubbing oiled coin over the child's body as part of a medicinal ritual. Seen in some Asian cultures.
- Cupping: a cup with a small amount of alcohol is ignited and inverted over the skin. As the heated air cools, a vacuum is produced. It is believed that this suction from the cup will draw out illness. This is a folk remedy used by Mexican-American, Southeast Asian, and other cultures.
- Moxibustion: Chinese folk remedy in which cones or balls of the moxa herb are burned on the skin.

TRAUMA

- Accidental injury

METABOLIC

- Copper deficiency
- Rickets
- Scurvy
- Vitamin K deficiency

CONGENITAL

- Osteogenesis imperfecta
- Ehlers-Danlos syndrome
- Familial dysautonomia, with congenital indifference to pain
- Mongolian spots
- Minor skeletal anomalies

IMMUNOLOGICAL

- Henoch-Schönlein purpura
- Immune thrombocytopenic purpura

MISCELLANEOUS

- Apparent life threatening event (ALTE)
- Epidermolysis bullosa
- Erythema multiforme

HEMATOLOGICAL

- Leukemia
- Hemophilia
- von Willebrand disease
- Disseminated intravascular coagulation (DIC)

Data Gathering

HISTORY

The following should raise the question of child abuse:

Question: History provided does not correlate with findings
Significance: Makes one suspect the truthfulness of the historian

Question: Denial of trauma to child
Significance: Typical response of child abuse

- Child's development not compatible with mechanism described
- History of events changes with time
- Unexpected delay in seeking care
- A detailed history of injury is essential for comparing the mechanism provided by the historian to the injuries sustained
- If no history of trauma is provided, ask when the child was last well, and who the caretakers were around that time. This may be helpful in identifying when the child was injured, and by whom.
- Search for indications of family stress, isolation, substance abuse, and violence, including domestic violence.

Physical Examination

Always perform a complete examination in a well lit room. Assess child for:

- Growth failure
- Bruises
- Burns
- Retinal hemorrhages
- Oral injuries
- Palpable rib fractures
- Abdominal injuries
- Genital injuries
- Are the findings explained by any medical condition?

Laboratory Aids

For children with bruising and/or bleeding:

Test: CBC, including a platelet count
Significance: Evaluate for anemia and thrombocytopenia

Test: PT/PTT
Significance: Evaluate for hemophilia and other bleeding disorders

Test: Bleeding time
Significance: Screen for Von Willebrand disease

Test: For those with abdominal trauma:
Significance: Noninvasive evaluation of intra-abdominal injury

Test: Liver function tests
Significance: Evaluate for possible liver injury

Test: Amylase, lipase
Significance: Evaluate for pancreas injury

Test: Urinalysis
Significance: Screen for genitourinary injury or myoglobinuria

Test: Creatine kinase (if muscle injury)
Significance: Evaluate for muscle injury; possible myoglobinuria

Test: Lumbar puncture
Significance: Evaluate for meningitis; identify bloody CSF

Test: Toxicology screens
Significance: Child may have been poisoned

RADIOGRAPHIC STUDIES

• Skeletal survey: useful for all children <2 years old, for some children 2 to 5 years old. Not generally used for children older than 5 years. Bony injuries highly suggestive of abuse include rib, metaphyseal, scapular, sternal, and spinous process fractures.
• Clavicle, long bone shaft, and linear skull fractures are common fractures and are sometimes related to abuse, but have low specificity for abuse.
• Radionuclide bone scan: serves as an adjunct to skeletal survey
• Computed tomography (CT) and magnetic resonance imaging (MRI): for suspected head, thoracic, or abdominal trauma. Subdural hemorrhage is a hallmark of inflicted head injury. Subdural hemorrhages associated with abuse can be located anywhere around the brain, but are often found in the posterior interhemispheric fissure.

Therapy

• Report all suspected abuse to local child welfare agency.
• Report abuse to law enforcement when injuries warrant police investigation.
• Consult social worker.
• Children with head injury should be examined by an ophthalmologist.
• Subdural hemorrhages do not usually require surgical evacuation.

DRUGS

• Dependent on injury sustained
• Pain medication

Follow-Up

• Cases will be investigated by child welfare agents and/or the police.
• Need for foster care placement and/or ongoing supervision decided by investigators.
• Changes in family functioning often require intensive, long-term intervention.
• Improvement of individual injuries varies according to the injury; family functioning may improve with intervention for some families, but may never improve for others.
• Non-compliance with medical follow-up or additional injuries to child may indicate ongoing abuse, parental substance abuse, etc.

PREVENTION

• Much of what is considered prevention is actually early intervention in high-risk families.
• Primary prevention would include universal parenting education and home visitation for all families. Currently, families thought to be at risk for abuse are identified and offered services.

PITFALLS

• Failing to consider abuse in the differential diagnosis of all pediatric trauma.
• Failing to consider abuse in the differential diagnosis of all infants and toddlers with mental status changes (especially ALTEs), even in the absence of bruising.
• Failing to consider alternative medical diagnoses in children who are thought to be abused.
• Acute (<10 days) rib fractures are easily missed on plain films.

Common Questions and Answers

Q: What are the signs of Shaking Impact Syndrome (also known as "Shaken Baby Syndrome")?
A: Shaking impact syndrome is a clinical diagnosis based on history, physical examination findings and radiologic data. The hallmark of shaking impact syndrome is subdural hemorrhage, which is often a marker for diffuse, acceleration-deceleration brain injury. The majority of victims have retinal hemorrhages, which tend to be bilateral and are sometimes severe. Some, but not all children have old and/or new skeletal or skin injuries, although these are not needed to make the diagnosis. The symptoms of head trauma in young children are nonspecific, and include mental status changes, ALTEs, vomiting, lethargy, irritability, seizures, etc. Abusive head injury in infants is often missed by physicians who fail to consider the diagnosis in babies with the above mentioned symptoms, leading to further injury or death of abused infants.

Q: Are retinal hemorrhages pathognomonic for physical abuse?
A: No, retinal hemorrhages may be seen in a variety of diseases and in some normal newborns. They occur in approximately 30% of newborns delivered vaginally. In these children they usually resolve in a few days, but may rarely last for 5–6 weeks. Outside of the newborn period, severe inflicted injury is the leading cause of retinal hemorrhages in children. Retinal hemorrhages may also result from increased intracranial pressure, severe hypertension, carbon monoxide poisoning, meningitis, vasculitis, endocarditis, and coagulopathy, but severe, bilateral hemorrhages are almost always due to abuse.

Q: What is the differential diagnosis for subdural hemorrhages?
A: It includes birth injury, accidental trauma, coagulopathy, hemorrhagic disease of the newborn, and vascular malformations. Trauma remains the leading cause of subdural hemorrhages in children.

Q: When is a child abuse report filed?
A: Whenever there is a suspicion, based on the history, physical examination, laboratory data, and/or psychosocial assessment, that a child's injuries or illnesses were a result of abuse or neglect. Certainty regarding the diagnosis is not needed.

Q: Can I be held liable for reports that are made that are not substantiated?
A: No. Health care workers who report suspected abuse "in good faith" are protected from civil and criminal litigation arising from allegations of false reports.

ICD-9-CM 995.81

BIBLIOGRAPHY

Duhaime AC, Christian CW, Rorke LB, Zimmerman RA. Nonaccidental head injury in infants—the "Shaken-Baby Syndrome." *N Engl J Med* 1998;338:1822–1829.

Giardino AP, Christian CW, Giardino ER. *A practical guide to the evaluation of child physical abuse and neglect*. Thousand Oaks: Sage, 1997.

Helfer ME, Kempe RS. *The battered child*, 5th ed. Chicago: University of Chicago Press, 1997.

Kleinman PK. *Diagnostic imaging of child abuse*. St. Louis: Mosby Yearbook, 1998.

Ludwig S, Kornberg A, eds. *Child abuse and neglect: a medical reference*. New York: Churchill Livingstone, 1991.

Reece R, ed. *Child abuse medical diagnosis and management*. Philadelphia: Lea & Febiger, 1994.

Reece R. Child abuse. *Pediatr Clin North Am* 1990;37:797–1011.

Author: Cindy W. Christian

Chlamydial Pneumonia

 Database

DEFINITION

Obligatory intracellular bacteria with a unique developmental cycle capable of producing pulmonary infections

- The genus *Chlamydia* has three species known to affect humans:

—*C. trachomatis* (CT)
—*C. psittaci*
—*C. pneumoniae* (CP).

- They usually produce the clinical manifestations of the so-called atypical or interstitial pneumonia.
- CT is one of the most frequent causes of afebrile pneumonia in early infancy. It is a complication of the maternal genital tract infection by this organism. Some patients develop inclusion conjunctivitis.
- *C. psittaci* is mainly pathogenic for birds and occasionally affects humans. CP can cause acute bronchitis, pneumonia, pharyngitis, and otitis media.
- Together with *Mycoplasma pneumoniae*, they probably account for most of the community-acquired pneumonias (CAP) in school-age children and adolescents.

EPIDEMIOLOGY

Chlamydia trachomatis

There are at least 15 serologic types (serovars).

- This is the most common sexually transmitted infection in the United States.
- CT pneumonia usually develops in infected infants under 2 months of age (2 weeks to 5 months).
- Half of the neonates born to infected mothers via vaginal delivery will acquire CT.

—Conjunctivitis may develop in 25% to 50%.
—Pneumonia may develop in 5% to 20%.

- Chronic conjunctival infection by some serovars can lead to blindness, which is rare in the United States.
- Incubation period: at least 1 week

Chlamydia psittaci (Psittacosis/Ornithosis)

- Healthy and sick birds can disperse the bacteria by their excrement or secretions.
- Infection occurs presumably through the airborne route.
- This is an occupational disease for workers in close contact with live birds or at poultry meat-processing plants. Pet owners can be also at risk. Though usually rare in children, it should be considered in any child with the environmental exposure who develops an atypical pneumonia.

Chlamydia pneumoniae

- Various strains are recognized; the original one is known as TWAR.
- It is presumed to be transmitted from person to person through aerosolized respiratory secretions.
- Age-detection of serum CP-specific antibodies in healthy children peak around 5 to 14 years of age, and they are present in most adults.
- In US studies of CAP in children, *C. pneumoniae* was found in 13% to 28% of cases.
- The majority of infections are thought to be asymptomatic. A carriage state has been detected, and may be more frequent in patients with immunodeficiencies.
- Coinfection with other respiratory pathogens like viruses or mycoplasma was reported. In middle ear fluid, copathogenicity was frequent with the common agents that cause middle ear infection.
- CP-specific IgE was demonstrated and may mediate the mechanism leading to bronchospasm.
- CP was isolated from cystic fibrosis patients during pulmonary exacerbations.
- Incubation period: about 21 days.

COMPLICATIONS

- Chlamydial pneumonia can have a protracted course for weeks or months if left untreated.
- Episodes of reactive airways disease may develop after pneumonia in infants.

PROGNOSIS

- In general, good
- Infection with CT has been associated with an increased risk of developing airways hyperreactivity.

 Differential Diagnosis

CHLAMYDIA TRACHOMATIS

- Viral respiratory pathogens:

—Respiratory syncytial virus (RSV)
—Adenovirus
—Influenza A and B
—Parainfluenza

- Other agents that can cause pneumonitis:

—Cytomegalovirus
—*Pneumocystis carinii*
—*Ureaplasma urealyticum*
—Pertussis

CHLAMYDIA PNEUMONIAE

- *Mycoplasma pneumoniae*
- Influenza A and B
- Parainfluenza
- Adenovirus
- RSV
- Can resemble typical bacterial pneumonia
- Less frequently: *C. psittaci*, *Coxiella burnetii*, or *Legionella pneumophila*

 Data Gathering

HISTORY

Chlamydia trachomatis

- Insidious onset
- Afebrile illness
- Rhinorrhea
- Repetitive cough

—Staccato type in more than 50% of infants
—Sometimes pertussis-like coughing spells

- Conjunctivitis
- Mild-to-moderate respiratory distress

Chlamydia pneumoniae

- Often insidious onset
- Sore throat
- Fever
- Hoarseness
- Prolonged cough; can be productive
- Also described, a biphasic course where cough follows the gradual decline of the initial symptomatology

 Physical Examination

CHLAMYDIA TRACHOMATIS

- Afebrile
- Half of the patients will have conjunctivitis with discharge (can be seen up to several weeks after birth)
- Rhinitis with mucoid discharge or nasal stuffiness, sometimes causing significant obstructive breathing
- Hypoxia frequently present
- Tachypnea is usually moderate (50–60 breaths/min)
- Frequent cough during examination
- Scattered rales on chest auscultation
- Wheezing is an uncommon finding.

CHLAMYDIA PNEUMONIAE

- Most patients are mildly to moderately ill.
- Cervical lymphadenopathy
- Postnasal discharge
- Pharyngitis without exudate
- Wheezing frequently without rales on chest auscultation

Laboratory Aids

TESTS

Chlamydia trachomatis

- Definitive diagnosis is by identification of the organism in cell culture (inclusion bodies). A specimen can be obtained from the nasopharynx or conjunctiva.
- Polymerase chain reaction (PCR)is a nucleic acid amplification method that has proven equal or more sensitive than culture. A specimen can be obtained from the infant's conjunctiva.
- DNA probe, direct fluorescent antibody (DFA), and enzyme immunoassay (EIA) are the most common direct antigen-detection tests. Useful in conjunctival specimens. These nonculture methods can have false-positive results.
- Serum antibody detection can be performed by microimmunofluorescence (MIF).

—Chlamydia-specific IgM titer of 1:32 or greater is diagnostic for CT pneumonia.

- Eosinophilia of 300 to 400/mm^3 and elevation of IgM (>110 mg/dL) and IgG (>500 mg/dL) are indirect laboratory evidence that suggest CT pneumonia.

Chlamydia pneumoniae

- Definitive diagnosis is by isolation of the organism in cell culture (inclusion bodies) or the proven, more sensitive, nested PCR (unfortunately not yet commercially available).

- Can use sputum or nasopharyngeal specimens. CP has been recovered from bronchioalveolar lavage fluid.
- Serologic diagnosis by MIF, probably the best standarized test. Evidence of acute infection:

—Fourfold elevation of paired convalescent antibody titers
—Specific IgM titer of 1:16 or greater
—Specific IgG titer of 1:512 or greater

- WBC count is usually normal.

Imaging

- Chest radiography

—C. trachomatis usually has bilateral diffuse infiltrates with hyperinflation.
—C. pneumoniae presents with focal to bilateral infiltrates; pleural effusions have been reported.

 Therapy

DRUGS

Chlamydia trachomatis

- Erythromycin, 50 mg/kg/d divided q.i.d for 14 days (therapy is effective in 80% of cases).
- If the patient does not tolerate erythromycin, oral sulfonamides may be used after the immediate neonatal period.

Chlamydia pneumoniae

- Erythromycin, 50 mg/kg/d divided q.i.d for 14 days. For adolescent patients, erythromycin 500 mg q.i.d for 14 days or 250 mg q.i.d for 21 days.
- An alternative for children over 9 years of age is doxycycline 100 mg b.i.d for 14 days.
- Clarithromycin 15 mg/kg/d divided b.i.d for 10 days was proven as effective as erythromycin.
- Azithromycin 10 mg/kg on day 1 (maximum, 500 mg) followed by 5 mg/kg days 2 to 5 (maximum, 250 mg) has been shown as efficacious as erythromycin in pediatric studies.

 Follow-Up

- Recovery is usually slow.
- Cough and malaise may persist for several weeks.

PREVENTION

Adequate surveillance and treatment of CT colonizing the genital tract of pregnant women is the best way of preventing the infant's disease.

PITFALLS

Chlamydia trachomatis

- Infection can occur in infants delivered by cesarean section, even without rupture of amniotic membranes.
- Ocular prophylaxis at birth does not reliably prevent Chlamydial conjunctivitis, even if erythromycin ointment is used. Topical treatment alone is not recommended because it does not eradicate the nasopharyngeal colonization.
- Antibiotic treatment failure rate is about 20%. A second course of therapy is sometimes needed.

Chlamydia pneumoniae

- Lack of commercially reliable test for diagnosis. MIF is proven diagnostic in only less than 50% of infected children. Early antimicrobial therapy may interfere with the development of detectable antibodies.
- Sometimes is difficult to differentiate between infection and carriage state, or recent and past infection.
- Patients have been shown to remain culture-positive after treatment, despite clinical improvement.
- Isolation: standard precautions
- Control measures: In infants infected with CT, the mother and her sexual partner should be treated. None for CP pneumonia.

 Common Questions and Answers

CHLAMYDIA TRACHOMATIS

Q: If the mother has an untreated genital infection, should we treat the asymptomatic newborn?
A: Yes. The child should receive oral erythromycin for 14 days.

Q: Do we need to pursue the diagnosis of other sexually transmitted diseases?
A: Yes. Gonorrhea, syphilis, hepatitis B, and HIV infection need to be ruled out. If conjunctivitis, an ocular swab to exclude Neisseria gonorrhoeae infection must be included.

Q: When do we need to suspect CT pneumonia?
A: In any infant less than 4 months of age that presents with cough, tachypnea, and rales on examination, when the chest x-ray shows bilateral infiltrates with hyperinflation.

ICD-9-CM 483.1

BIBLIOGRAPHY

American Academy of Pediatrics. 1997 red book: report of the Committee on Infectious Diseases. Elk Grove Village, IL: American Academy of Pediatrics, 1997:168–174.

Hammerschlag MR. Atypical pneumonias in children. Adv Pediatr Infect Dis 1995;10:1–39.

Darville T. Chlamydia. Pediatr Rev 1998;19(3).

Schidlow DV, Callahan CW. Pneumonia. Pediatr Rev 1996;17(9).

Author: Roberto V. Nachajon

Cholelithiasis

 Database

DEFINITION

Cholelithiasis, defined as cholesterol and/or pigment stones in the gallbladder, is primarily a disease of adulthood. Since the introduction of ultrasonography in the late 1970s, incidental or silent gallstones are detected more often in children.

CAUSES

- Hemolytic disease (17%–29% of children with sickle cell disease)
- Total parenteral nutrition
- Prematurity
- Necrotizing enterocolitis
- Cystic fibrosis
- Obesity
- Pregnancy
- Oral contraceptives
- Down syndrome

PATHOLOGY

- Bile is composed of five major components: water, bilirubin, cholesterol, pigments, and phospholipids and calcium salts. Stones are of two types: pigment and cholesterol stones. The formation of cholesterol stones is associated with sludge and cholesterol supersaturation. Other important factors include:

—Gallbladder stasis
—Excess lecithin
—Increased biliary mucus secretion
—Rapidity of nucleation time

- Total parenteral alimentation is associated with decrease in bile flow, stasis, sludge, and stone formation.
- The formation of gallstones secondary to ileal disease and resection has been reported in children and adults because of a decreased bile acid pool and cholesterol supersaturation of the bile.

EPIDEMIOLOGY

- Cholelithiasis is relatively uncommon in childhood; however, gallstones have even been detected in utero.
- Pigment stones are more prevalent in prepubertal children, whereas cholesterol stones are predominant in adolescence and adulthood.
- The incidence of gallstones remains negligible in males throughout childhood and adolescence to adulthood.
- In females, the incidence is 0.27% during ages 6 to 19 years and increases to 2.7% between the ages of 18 and 29; gallstones predominate in females.
- Canadian Eskimos and native Africans have the lowest risk of cholelithiasis.
- Native Americans, Swedes, and Czechs have the highest risk.

SYMPTOMS

- Silent gallstones present in infancy and pre-school-age children.
- The classic symptoms of right-upper-quadrant pain and vomiting exist in older children and adolescents.
- Younger children present with nonspecific symptoms, including obstructive jaundice.
- Fever is unusual in all age groups and often indicates the development of complications such as cholecystitis, choledocholithiasis, cholangitis, or gallbladder perforation, all of which are rare in children.
- Pancreatitis exists in 8% of patients with gallstones and is the most common complication. Pancreatitis is more common in obese adolescents who have undergone rapid weight reduction, as reported in the adult population.

 Data Gathering

HISTORY

- Most gallstones are incidental findings on abdominal ultrasound and are clinically silent.
- Biliary colic, pancreatitis, obstructive jaundice, cholangitis, or other complications should be excluded.
- Intolerance to fatty food rarely exists in children.

The history should always include questions concerning:

- Previous episodes of right-upper-quadrant abdominal pain
- Any risk factors for hemolysis
- History of necrotizing enterocolitis
- Total parenteral nutrition
- Diuretic use
- Short gut syndrome
- History of resection of the terminal ileum.

Physical Examination

- The physical examination may be completely normal or may uncover the acute abdomen of pancreatitis.
- In adolescents, the Murphy sign (tenderness on palpation of the RUQ of the abdomen associated with inspiration) may be elicited.

Laboratory Aids

TESTS

- Blood testing is usually unrewarding.
- Occasionally, a leukocytosis, elevation in liver enzymes, or elevated amylase/lipase may be detected.
- Abdominal radiography may show the presence of a gallstone; 50% of these are radiopaque.
- Ultrasound is the diagnostic procedure of choice—noninvasive, sensitive, and specific.
- Endoscopic retrograde cholangiopancreatography (ERCP) is especially good for evaluation of choledocholithiasis and removal of common bile duct stones.

Therapy

- In children with asymptomatic gallstones, observation is the best therapy.
- In infants, there is a chance for spontaneous stone dissolution, especially in cholelithiasis linked to total parenteral nutrition (TPN). In children who are dependent on TPN, such as patients with short-bowel syndrome, pseudo-obstruction, and inflammatory bowel disease, gallstones should be removed.
- Cholecystectomy remains the procedure of choice in children with symptoms or in the presence of silent gallstones.
- Laparoscopic cholecystectomy may decrease the length of the hospital stay and the extent of the required abdominal incision.
- Medical treatment for cholesterol gallstones in children may include chenodeoxycholic acid and ursodeoxycholic acid. This treatment is not recommended in the pediatric age group because of low success rate.
- Prevention of gallstone formation is linked to recognition of possible underlying risk factors and attempts to limit these risk factors (small enteral feeds in addition to TPN, early pancreatic enzyme supplements in patients with cystic fibrosis, using alternative forms of contraception in high-risk populations, and weight control in obese infants and children with known hemolytic disease).
- Pigment stone formation increases with age. Cholecystectomy, even for the asymptomatic patient, is warranted. In patients with sickle cell disease, the gallbladder should be removed once stones are identified. This will decrease the risk of cholecystitis and other complications, and will also help to differentiate between biliary colic and sickle cell abdominal pain crisis.
- Patients with a history of cholecystitis are at increased risk for further episodes (69% will have biliary colic within 2 years, and 6% will require cholecystectomy).

Follow-Up

- Asymptomatic patients: Follow up every year; monitor for onset of symptoms.
- Symptomatic patients: Consider cholecystectomy.

Common Questions and Answers

Q: Does my child with cystic fibrosis have a greater problem with gallstones?
A: Yes, children with CF may have more frequent development of gallstones than will normal children. Reports of gallstones while on ursodeoxycholic acid therapy have also been noted.

Q: Why does my child with sickle cell disease have gallstones?
A: Because the process involves breakdown of hemoglobin, which is then derived into bilirubin, this process may accelerate the formation of gallstones.

Q: If my child has repeated attacks of abdominal pain and there are gallstones in the gallbladder, should he have surgery? What kind?
A: Yes; in older adolescents, laparascopic cholecystomy is being recommended. For younger children or infants, open cholecystectomy is the preferred choice of treatment. There is no role for Actigall in their therapy.

ICD-9-CM 574.20

BIBLIOGRAPHY

Gilger MA. Cholelithiasis and cholecystitis. In: Wyllie R, Hyams J, eds. *Pediatric gastrointestinal diseases*. Philadelphia: WB Saunders, 1993:931–944.

Haller JO. Sonography of the biliary tract in infants and children. Am J Roentgenol 1991;157(5):1051–1058.

Heubi JE, Lewis LG. Diseases of the gallbladder in infancy, childhood, and adolescence. In: Suchy F, ed. *Liver diseases in children*. Chicago: Mosby–Year Book, 1994:609–621.

Irish MS, Pearl RH, Caty MG, Glick PL. The approach to common abdominal diagnosis in infants and children. *Pediatr Clin North Am* 1998;45(4):729–772.

Kasirajan K, Obermeyer RJ, Kehris J, Lopez J, Lopez R. Microinvasive laparoscopic cholecystectomy in pediatric patients. *J Laparoendosc Adv Surg Techniques Part A* 1998;8(3):131–135.

Rescorla FJ. Cholelithiasis, cholecystitis, and common bile duct stones. *Curr Opin Pediatr* 1997;9(3):276–282.

Rescorla FJ, Grosfeld JL. Cholecystitis and cholelithiasis in children. *Semin Pediatr Surg* 1992;1(2):98–106.

Author: Dror Wasserman

Chronic Active Hepatitis

 Database

DEFINITION

Chronic active hepatitis is defined as a continuing inflammation of the liver that in time may become cirrhotic. It covers any cause of inflammation not due to acute self-limiting infection or past drug exposure. There are persistent abnormal liver function tests characterized by raised transaminases, histological evidence of hepatitis, which leads to irreversible changes over time (usually at least 6 months, although irreversible damage can occur over a shorter period).

CAUSES

- Autoimmune liver disease
- Chronic viral hepatitis
- Bile acid synthetic defects
- Progressive familial intrahepatic cholestasis syndromes (PFIC)
- Wilson disease
- Tyrosinemia
- Persistent biliary disease: post Kasai, choledochal cyst
- Sclerosing cholangitis
- Immunodeficiency
- Glycogen storage disease
- Cystic fibrosis
- Iron storage disorders/chronic transfusion
- Mitochondrial respiratory chain defects
- Peroxisomal defects

PATHOPHYSIOLOGY

Pathology has been traditionally classified as chronic persistent hepatitis, chronic aggressive hepatitis, and chronic lobular hepatitis. The hepatocytes are damaged, with inflammatory cellular infiltration accompanied by liver regeneration.

Chronic Persistent Hepatitis

Minimal portal tract fibrosis, slightly widened portal tracts. The limiting plate is intact and inflammation does not extend beyond this. There is no bridging fibrosis between portal tracts.

Chronic Aggressive Hepatitis

Perilobular hepatitis, with inflammatory cells extending from portal tracts into parenchyma with fibrosis. Piecemeal necrosis refers to dying hepatocytes surrounded by lymphocytes and fibroblasts. In advanced disease, fibrosis bridges the portal tracts (bridging fibrosis). Cirrhosis occurs when there is loss of architecture due to fibrosis.

Chronic Lobular Hepatitis

Liver architecture is preserved with scattered changes of acute hepatitis with hepatocyte necrosis in the lobules (perivenular regions). These changes are most often associated with hepatitis B and NANB hepatitis.

EPIDEMIOLOGY

- More common in females

 Differential Diagnosis

INDICATED FURTHER INVESTIGATIONS

- Congenital hepatic fibrosis, Niemann-Pick type C, or other storage disorders
- Lysosomal storage disease, glycogen storage disease
- Congenital or acquired venous or arterial malformations
- Wilson disease
- Cystic fibrosis
- Byler disease (PFIC-1)
- Alagille syndrome

 Data Gathering

HISTORY

- Symptoms of chronic illness, poor growth, intermittent jaundice, abdominal pain, bleeding, malabsorption, fever, amenorrhea, poor school achievement, and itching
- Variceal bleeding can be a presenting syndrome in patients with portal hypertension.
- A history of jaundice in infancy, family history of liver disease or autoimmune liver disease, blood transfusions, intravenous drug abuse, or multiple sexual partners can suggest an etiology of hepatitis.
- Chronicity is often defined by the persistence of hepatitis for at least 6 months.

 Physical Examination

Stigmata of chronic liver disease are:

- Spider nevi
- Cutaneous shunts
- Palmar erythema
- Cyanosis (hepatopulmonary syndrome)
- Jaundice
- Itching
- Enlarged liver or small, shrunken liver
- Splenomegaly
- Ascites
- Rickets

 Laboratory Aids

TESTS

Laboratory Tests

- Albumin, creatinine, GGT, AST, ALT, bilirubin, PT, FBC, blood group, Coombs test
- Serum ceruloplasmin, serum copper, 24-hour urine copper (penicillamine challenge), liver copper
- Cholesterol, triglycerides
- Immunoglobulins
- Complement levels (C3, C4)
- Tissue autoantibodies
- Virology: Hep A, Hep B, Hep C, Hep D
- α_1-Antitrypsin phenotype
- Urinary succinylacetone
- Urinary bile acids
- Sweat test
- AFP

Imaging

- CXR
- Ultrasound scan of abdomen, focusing on liver, spleen, and kidney
- Echocardiogram
- Liver biopsy

INDICATED FURTHER INVESTIGATIONS

- PTC or ERCP (or MRCP): congenital hepatic fibrosis, sclerosing cholangitis
- Colonoscopy: sclerosing cholangitis associated with inflammatory bowel disease
- Bone marrow aspirate: exclude Niemann-Pick type C or other storage disorders
- Enzyme from white cells or cultured fibroblasts (skin biopsy): to exclude lysosomal storage disease, glycogen storage disease
- Angiography: congenital or acquired venous or arterial malformations, assessment of portosystemic shunt
- Cardiac cathetherization: to assess pulmonary hypertension and cardiac status
- Microaggregate albumin scan: to assess hepatopulmonary syndrome and hepatic encephalopathy
- Muscle biopsy: respiratory chain enzymes in mitochondrial disorders
- Genotyping: where the technology is available (e.g., Wilson disease, cystic fibrosis, Byler disease (PFIC-1), Alagille syndrome)
- Active hepatitis is diagnosed
- Patients present with fatigue, nausea, malaise, anorexia, weight loss, pruritis, arthralgia, rash, and fever, but 10% have no symptoms. Findings include jaundice, hepatomegaly, cutaneous stigmata, splenomegaly, edema, ascites, cirrhosis, GI hemorrhage, dark urine, and pale stools. Active hepatitis is commonly associated with HLA B8, DR3 haplotype; younger patients have the DR3 haplotype, while older patients have the DR4 haplotype. Patients with the DR3 haplotypes have more severe disease and frequent relapses.

• Liver biopsy can be postponed until coagulopathy improves. Patients may deteriorate rapidly if not treated aggressively, and in some cases develop fulminant liver failure. Corticosteroids are started, and the dose slowly weaned over 4 to 6 weeks to maintain normal transaminases. This can take about 6 months. Remission is induced in 70% of patients within 24 months of therapy, but relapses occur in 50% in 6 months and in 70% in 36 months. Azathioprine is used when corticosteroid doses cannot be weaned. Liver function tests, immunoglobulin levels, and autoantibody titers are monitored closely. In one report, discontinuation of treatment occurred in 20% of Type 1 active hepatitis but not in Type 2. Repeat biopsies have shown histological relapse rates to be very high—87% to 100%. Forty percent of treated patients develop cirrhosis after 10 years. Malignancies developed in 5%, with the mean time of onset 9.7 years after diagnosis. In rare instances, in which the autoimmune process cannot be controlled by steroids and azathioprine, cyclosporine or tacrolimus may be tried. ERCP is done routinely in some centers on all patients with active hepatitis, and when changes of sclerosing cholangitis are detected, patients are started on ursodeoxycholic acid. The success of liver transplantation is the same as for other causes, but the disease occasionally recurs.

Therapy

The management of patients is that of any chronic liver disease and treatment specific to a diagnosis.

GENERAL MANAGEMENT

• Maintaining growth and development is of paramount importance to optimize the physical and mental well-being of the patient. Fat-soluble vitamins given orally are poorly absorbed and levels must be monitored. Anthropometric parameters must be recorded, including skinfold thickness. The use of medium-chain triglycerides for fat malabsorption and branch-chain amino acids in hepatic encephalopathy are useful nutritional maneuvers.
• Proactive involvement of the clinical psychologist and play therapist can help alleviate some of the problems, such as depression and fear. Chronic debilitating pruritis is an indication for liver transplantation after failure of medical therapy, which may include antihistamines, cholestyramine, naltrexone, rifampicin, and ursodeoxycholic acid.
• Monitoring portal hypertension by assessment of portal flow on ultrasound and splenic size may provide some indication of disease progression. Airplane cabin pressures are maintained at levels lower than atmospheric, and this can predispose to variceal bleeding.

• The physician must be vigilant in monitoring for spontaneous bacterial peritonitis in patients with ascites; it carries a mortality rate between 55% and 78% and a recurrence rate of 69% after 1 year.

SPECIFIC MANAGEMENT

• Chronic viral hepatitis B and C: Hepatitis B that causes chronic active hepatitis is currently treated with alpha-interferon for at least 6 months. The success rate based on adult studies is 33% and 37% for the loss of HBeAg and HBV DNA, respectively. In patients with cirrhosis, the use of interferon is risky, because it can cause liver disease decompensation, and should be given only in centers that are familiar with and have access to liver transplantation. There may be a role for Lamivudine, an oral nucleoside analogue that inhibits viral DNA replication; it has been shown to markedly reduce HBV DNA levels in 98% of patients during therapy, but there is a high recurrence rate after the drug is discontinued. Treatment of hepatitis C with interferon in children is not established. In adults, it is licensed for use, with good response in the region of 41% improvement in ALT; 70% of patients show improved histology, but with a 50% to 70% relapse rate.
• The treatment for end-stage liver failure is liver transplantation.

DRUGS

• Azathioprine: 1 to 2 mg/kg/d (od)
• Cholestyramine: 240 mg/kg/d in three divided doses; avoid giving with other medications because it can bind and reduce absorption. Give other medications 1 hour before or 4 hours after cholestyramine.
• Cyclosporine: 1 to 2 mg/kg/d orally (bd)
• Interferon alpha (dose from published pediatric trials):

—Chronic HBV: 5 to 10 μ/m^2 given three times a week for 6 to 12 months
—Chronic HCV: 3 μ/m^2 given three times a week for 6 to 12 months

• Interferon is not licensed for use in children. Very common side effects are hematologic, infectious, autoimmune, neuropsychiatric, and systemic with myelosuppression. If platelets fall below 50,000/m^3 and neutrophils below 1,500/m^3, then interferon dose is lowered or temporarily discontinued.
• Lamivudine (trial basis): 25 to 100 mg/d in adult for 1 year
• Naltrexone: 25 to 50 mg/d in adults (tablets, 50 mg)
• Tacrolimus: 0.15 mg/kg/d orally (bd)
• Ursodeoxycholic acid: 10 to 20 mg/kg/d (bd)

Common Questions and Answers

Q: Can patients with autoimmune liver disease be transplanted? Will the disease not recur?
A: Patients who end up with end-stage liver failure should be transplanted. It is not common to see the recurrence of the original autoimmune liver disease after transplant, but it occurs.

Q: What are the risks of providing very young patients with a liver transplant?
A: There is a theoretical advantage in transplanting the very young, in that less rejection occurs and immunosuppression requirements are less. Using split liver techniques, outcomes of OLT in infants has improved.

Q: Why should we be aggressive with vitamin supplementation?
A: There is significant malabsorption of vitamins A, D, E, and K. Vitamin D and E deficiencies are the most significant with rickets and neuropathy.

Q: Oral supplements of vitamins are sometimes very difficult to administer in the very young. How can I overcome this problem?
A: It is common practice in some centers to give Vitamins D and E as an intramuscular injection on a monthly basis, with levels done in between.

Q: Why do jaundiced children scratch?
A: It is the accumulation of bile salts that causes pruritis.

Q: Are the stigmata of chronic liver disease also seen in children?
A: It is very common to find spider nevi, liver palms, splenomegaly, cutaneous shunts, and clubbing.

ICD-9-CD 571.40

BIBLIOGRAPHY

Hyams KC. Risks of chronicity following acute hepatitis B virus infection: a review. *Clin Infect Dis* 1995;20(4):992–1000.

Johnson PJ, McFarland IG, et al. Meeting report: International Autoimmune Hepatitis Group. *Hepatology* 1993;18:998–1005.

Lai, CL, Chien RN, Leung NW, et al. One year trial of lamivudine for chronic hepatitis B. *N Engl J Med* 1998;339(2):61–68.

Ruiz-Moreno M, Rua MJ, Castillo I, et al. Treatment of children with chronic hepatitis C with recombinant interferon α: a pilot study. *Hepatology* 1992;16:882–885.

Trivedi P, Mowat AP. Chronic hepatitis. In: Suchy FJ, ed. *Liver disease in children*, 1st ed. St. Louis: Mosby, 1994:510–523.

Vergani GM, Vergani D. Immune mechanisms in pediatric liver disease. In: Suchy FJ, ed. *Liver disease in children*, 1st ed. St. Louis: Mosby, 1994:173–180.

Author: John Tung

Chronic Granulomatous Disease

 Database

DEFINITION

Chronic granulomatous disease is a rare inherited defect involving phagocytes. The defective phagocytes (neutrophils and monocytes) have a decreased or absent ability to generate reactive oxygen intermediates, leaving the host susceptible to recurrent bacterial and fungal infections.

PATHOPHYSIOLOGY

The associated defects involve the NADPH oxidase complex of the neutrophil. Neutrophils in chronic granulomatous disease have an impaired ability to combat infection via an impaired respiratory burst. The NADPH oxidase complex is composed of four subunits, any of which may be defective in chronic granulomatous disease. Sixty percent of patients with chronic granulomatous disease have a defect in the gp91-*phox* subunit, which is inherited in an X-linked manner. Thirty-three percent of patients have a defect in the p47-*phox* subunit, which is inherited in an autosomal recessive manner. Defects occur less frequently in the p22-*phox* and p67-*phox* subunits.

GENETICS

- Gene mutations may occur spontaneously and are inherited as an X-linked variant, or autosomal recessive variant.
- Mutations may occur in any one of the four subunits of the neutrophil NADPH oxidase complex:

—gp91-*phox:* X chromosome
—p22-*phox:* chromosome 16
—p47-*phox:* chromosome 7
—p67-*phox:* chromosome 1

EPIDEMIOLOGY

- Prevalence: approximately 1 in 500,000 individuals

COMPLICATIONS

These patients have an increased susceptibility to bacterial and fungal infections that usually are not pathogenic in normal hosts

- Recurrent skin infections
- Sepsis
- Chronic lung disease (secondary to recurrent infections)
- Chronic liver disease (secondary to recurrent infections)
- Chronic osteomyelitis of large and small bones
- Malabsorption
- Systemic and discoid lupus erythematosus: increased incidence in female carriers

The diagnosis of chronic granulomatous disease should be considered in patients with:

- Recurrent lymphadenitis
- Staphylococcal hepatic abscess
- *Aspergillus* or *Nocardia* pneumonia
- *Serratia marcescens* osteomyelitis
- Infections with *Pseudomonas cepacia*
- *Salmonella* sepsis
- Perirectal abscesses
- Brain abscesses

PROGNOSIS

Survival beyond the fourth decade is common. Bone marrow transplantation is curative.

 Differential Diagnosis

INFECTIOUS

Infections are related to the immune deficiency.

GENETIC/METABOLIC

- Leukocyte glucose-6-phosphate dehydrogenase deficiency
- Myeloperoxidase deficiency
- Humoral immune deficiencies
- Complement deficiencies

COMMON CAUSES

- Chronic granulomatous disease is not acquired; it is inherited as an X-linked variant or as an autosomal variant.

 Data Gathering

HISTORY

Question: At what age did the patient present?
Significance: Patients with chronic granulomatous disease usually present before 2 years of age with marked lymphadenopathy, hepatosplenomegaly, draining lymph nodes, and pneumonias.

Question: What is the infecting organism?
Significance: Patients with chronic granulomatous disease tend to develop infections with unusual organisms, such as: *S. aureus, S epidermidis, S. marcescens, Pseudomonas, Escherichia coli, Candida, Aspergillus, Nocardia,* and *Salmonella.*

Question: Are there other affected family members?
Significance: Chronic granulomatous disease is inherited in an X-linked and autosomal recessive pattern. Therefore, there may be other affected family members.

Question: Does the mother have lupus?
Significance: There is a higher incidence of lupus in females who are carriers for chronic granulomatous disease.

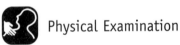 Physical Examination

Finding: Skin abscess or boils
Significance: Patients with chronic granulomatous disease develop frequent skin infections.

Finding: Mucous membrane and perirectal infections
Significance: Patients with chronic granulomatous disease commonly develop infections at mucous membrane and epidermal junctions, especially in the perirectal area.

Finding: Lymphadenopathy
Significance: Patients with chronic granulomatous disease commonly develop lymphadenopathy and draining lymph nodes.

Finding: Hepatosplenomegaly
Significance: Hepatosplenomegaly is a common finding in patients with chronic granulomatous disease.

Finding: Abnormal lung examination
Significance: Pulmonary disease is common in patients with chronic granulomatous disease.

Laboratory Aids

APPROACH TO THE PATIENT

- General goal: Decide whether the patient's type of infections (osteomyelitis, perirectal abscess, etc.) and infecting organisms are consistent with the diagnosis of chronic granulomatous disease.
- Order a nitroblue tetrazolium (NBT) test.
- If abnormal, initiate sulfamethoxazole/ trimethoprim prophylaxis.

Test: The NBT
Significance: The NBT is the most widely available test for chronic granulomatous disease. Neutrophils from normal individuals can reduce the dye, resulting in a color change. Neutrophils from patients with chronic granulomatous disease cannot reduce the dye, and it remains colorless. Neutrophils and monocytes from patients with chronic granulomatous disease have an impaired hexose monophosphate shunt. Therefore, they have a decreased conversion of NADP to NADPH, and a decreased oxidative burst, which results in an inability to reduce the NBT in this study.

Test: The 2,7 Dichlorofluorescin (DCF)
Significance: DCF can directly measure the production of hydrogen peroxide utilizing a fluorescent label and flow cytometry. Patients with chronic granulomatous disease have decreased hydrogen peroxide production.

Test: Immunoblotting
Significance: Immunoblotting can be used to quantify the amount of each NADPH subunit present.

ISSUES FOR REFERRAL

Factors that may help alert you to make a referral include:

- A new diagnosis of chronic granulomatous disease: An immunologist can assist with antibiotic prophylaxis and with parameters for when to seek medical attention, and they can help identify which genetic variant is responsible for the patient's disease.
- Pregnant carrier for chronic granulomatous disease: An immunologist can help with prenatal diagnosis. Furthermore, some centers may consider in utero bone marrow transplantation for an affected fetus.
- Fever or suspected infection: Patients with chronic granulomatous disease tend to develop infections in unusual sites with unusual organisms. An immunologist can help with the evaluation and appropriate antibiotic coverage.

 ## Therapy

- *Antibiotic prophylaxis:* Trimethoprim-sulfamethoxazole is the antibiotic of choice, because both components are concentrated in the neutrophil, and for its bacterial spectrum.
- *Recombinant gamma interferon:* This is reserved for patients with severe disease. This therapy may decrease the incidence of infection.
- *Bone marrow transplant:* Chronic granulomatous disease has been cured in patients with matched transplants.
- *Acute infections:*

—*Broad-spectrum intravenous antibiotics:* There should be a low threshold to start this therapy. Severe infections should be treated with broad-spectrum intravenous antibiotics until an organism is identified. Good initial antibiotics include intravenous penicillins, aminoglycosides, and antipseudomonal antibiotics.
—*Amphotericin B:* This should not be withheld if a fungal infection is suspected, or if the patient's clinical status is deteriorating despite broad-spectrum antibiotics.
—*Leukocyte transfusions:* These are reserved for severe infections, and efficacy is controversial.

 ## Follow-Up

Chronic granulomatous disease is a lifelong disease. These patients tend to develop chronic lung disease; therefore, pulmonary function studies should be followed at least annually. Liver disease is also common; therefore, liver function studies should also be followed at least annually. Female carriers should be observed for signs of lupus erythematosis.

 ## Common Questions and Answers

Q: How do you interpret an NBT test reported as 50% of normal?
A: This is generally consistent with a carrier state. The carrier is not at increased risk for infection. However, carrier females have an increased risk of developing lupus.

Q: What do the infecting organisms have in common?
A: Patients with chronic granulomatous disease are most susceptible to catalase-positive organisms.

Q: Are all chronic granulomatous disease patients with fever admitted automatically?
A: No. It is true that these patients are more prone to invasive and systemic infections, but these patients are not admitted with every febrile episode (especially if there is evidence of a minor bacterial or viral infection). However, subtle signs of an invasive infection must be taken very seriously, and these patients are certainly admitted.

Q: Can a prenatal diagnosis be made?
A: Yes. However, currently this can only be done in a limited number of research laboratories, and the testing is not commercially available. Testing involves chorionic villus sampling, and it can only be done on families in which the specific mutation has been mapped.

ICD-9-CM 288.1

BIBLIOGRAPHY

Candotti F, Blaese RM. Gene therapy of primary immunodeficiencies. *Springer Semin Immunopathol* 1998;19(4):493–508.

Curnutte JT. Chronic granulomatous disease: the solving of a clinical riddle at the molecular level. *Clin Immunol Immunopathol* 1993;67 (3 pt 2):S2–S15.

Heyworth PG, Curnutte JT, Noack D, Cross AR. Hematologic important mutations: X-linked chronic granulomatous disease—an update. *Blood Cells Mol Dis* 1997;23(3):443–450.

Kamani N, Douglas SD. Natural history of chronic granulomatous disease. *Diagn Clin Immunol* 1988;5:314–317.

Middleton E, Reed CE, Ellis EF, Adkinson NF, Yunginger JW, Busse WW. *Allergy principles and practice,* 4th ed. Philadelphia: Mosby, 1993.

Sites DP, Terr AI, Parslow TG. *Basic and clinical immunology,* 8th ed. Englewood Cliffs, NJ: Prentice Hall, 1994.

Author: Christopher A. Smith

Cirrhosis

 Database

DEFINITION

Cirrhosis is a process characterized by increased fibrous tissue and nodule formation following necrosis of the hepatocyte within the liver.

CAUSES

The number of etiologic agents is numerous and detailed below:

- Infectious

—Hepatitis B, C, and D
—Syphilis (neonates)

- Alcohol
- Metabolic

—Wilson disease (copper overload)
—α_1-Antitrypsin deficiency
—Type IV glycogenesis
—Galactosemia
—Tyrosinemia

- Hepatic venous outflow obstruction

—Budd-Chiari syndrome
—Congestive heart failure

- Immunologic

—Chronic active hepatitis

- Toxins and medications

—Methotrexate
—Amiodorone

- Indian childhood cirrhosis
- Prolonged cholestatic syndromes

—Sclerosing cholangitis

GENETICS

In several disorders, including sclerosing cholangitis and hemochromatosis, there have been identified HLA markers. However, no specific markers correlate with cirrhosis.

EPIDEMIOLOGY

Based on the varying etiologies, no specific epidemiologic pattern can be identified.

COMPLICATIONS

The final common pathways of hepatic dysfunction secondary to cirrhosis are related to hepatocyte and vascular insufficiency. These include encephalopathy, ascites, liver failure, and portal hypertension leading to hemorrhage.

PROGNOSIS

The prognosis for cirrhosis leading to decompensation depends on the etiologic agent. Poor prognostic features include elevated PT, ascites, gastrointestinal hemorrhage, encephalopathy, poor nutrition, hypoalbuminemia, and neurologic changes.

 Data Gathering

HISTORY

Based on the varying etiologic agents, one should elicit pertinent historical features characteristic of each specific problem as detailed:

- Exposure to hepatitis
- Exposure to hepatotoxins
- Family history of metabolic disease
- Neurologic problems (Wilson disease)

Physical Examination

Estimation of liver size may be helpful in suggesting cirrhosis. Helpful diagnostic clues include:

- Hepatomegaly or small liver
- Spider angiomata
- Dupuytren contracture
- Testicular atrophy
- Palmar erythema
- Splenomegaly
- Venous outflow obstruction suggested by collaterals on the anterior abdominal wall
- Clubbing
- Hypertrophic osteoarthropathy

Laboratory Aids

TESTS

Imaging

There are various options available to the clinician for diagnosing cirrhosis of the liver.

- Direct visualization through laparoscopy will facilitate liver biopsy.
- Radioisotope scanning reveals decreasing uptake, increased flow to spleen and bone marrow, and irregular texture.
- Ultrasound reveals increased echogenicity.
- A CAT scan is most sensitive for detecting altered liver texture and size as well as vascular appearance.

 ## Therapy

DRUGS

Diuretics and decreased sodium content of foods will enhance the resolution of ascites, a complication of cirrhosis.

DURATION

Medical therapy is performed until the clinical status requires advancement of therapy, including hepatic transplantation or stabilization of clinical status.

SURGICAL

For management of portal hypertension, the diversion of portal blood flow to the systemic system can be established but is associated with complications and increased morbidity and mortality. Varying shunt procedures include mesocaval, portocaval, and distal splenorenal shunts. In the setting of decompensated cirrhosis, hepatic transplantation may be necessary.

 ## Common Questions and Answers

Q: Will my child with cystic fibrosis develop cirrhosis?
A: The medical literature cite a 5% to 20% incidence of cirrhosis in children with cystic fibrosis. Many factors seem to relate to the development of cirrhosis in these children, but the genetic type of cystic fibrosis does not seem to be a cause only.

Q: Will every child with cirrhosis need a liver transplant?
A: Most children who develop cirrhosis from causes such as biliary atresia or metabolic disease will ultimately require a liver transplant.

ICD-9-CD 571.0

BIBLIOGRAPHY

Ernst O, Gottrand F, Calvo M, Michaud L, Sergent G, Mizrahi D, L'Hermine C. Congenital hepatic fibrosis: findings at MR cholangiopancreatography. *Am J Roentgenol* 1998;170(2): 409–12.

Perisic VN. Long-term studies on congenital hepatic fibrosis in children. *Acta Paediatr* 1995;84(6):695–696.

Sherlock S, Dooley J. Hepatic cirrhosis. In: Sherlock S, Dooley J, eds. *Diseases of the liver and biliary system,* 9th ed. London: Blackwell Science, 1993:357–369.

Author: Andrew E. Mulberg

Cleft Lip and Palate

 Database

DEFINITION

A cleft lip (CL) is a deformity of the upper lip that may include a discontinuity of vermilion, skin, muscle, and mucosa, as well as the underlying gingiva and bone. It can be unilateral or bilateral. A complete cleft extends into the nose, while an incomplete cleft has at least some bridge of intact tissue separating the oral and nasal cavities. A cleft palate (CP) usually represents a visible separation between the two halves of the roof of the mouth, involving mucosa, muscle, and often the bones of the hard palate. A submucous CP has intact mucosa, but the underlying muscle and bone are at least partially divided.

ETIOLOGY

• Cleft lip may result from failure of the medial nasal and maxillary processes to join in utero, or possibly from lack of adequate mesenchymal reinforcement, leading to subsequent breakdown and separation. Cleft palate results from failure of the palatal shelves to fuse.
• Lower-than-expected incidence of CL and CP has been noted with prenatal dietary supplementation with folic acid and vitamin B_6. Folic acid supplementation has also been clearly associated with a decreased incidence of neural tube defects.

PATHOPHYSIOLOGY

Muscle fibers are atrophic and disorganized in the region of the cleft, and mitochondrial abnormalities are noted at the cleft margins by histochemical and electromyographic studies.

GENETICS

• One-third of patients with cleft lip and/or palate have a positive family history; positive family history is noted twice as often in CL with or without CP as in CP alone.
• Two-thirds of cases have no clear genetic basis and are presumed to be environmental. Clefting may be present as a feature of a number of recognized patterns of malformations attributable to alcohol, anticonvulsants (phenytoin), and isotretinoin. Isolated clefting has not been associated with prenatal exposure to a single substance.

Clefting inheritance is multifactorial or multigenic. Syndromes are more common with isolated CP than with CL with or without CP.

• The most common is Stickler syndrome (17.5% of syndromic clefts), characterized by autosomal dominance, CP, epicanthal folds, flat facies, severe myopia, retinal detachment, and glaucoma, caused by a mutation of the gene for type 2 collagen (chromosome 12q).

• Other syndromes linked to specific chromosomal abnormalities include velocardiofacial (22q11), Van der Woude (autosomal dominant, CP and/or CL, lower lip pits, 1q32), and Smith-Lemli-Opitz (defect in cholesterol synthesis, 7q34).

EPIDEMIOLOGY

• Incidence of CL with or without CP is 1 in 700 births.
• Racial heterogeneity noted in CL and CP (Asians, 2.1 in 1,000 births; whites, 1 in 1,000; blacks, 0.41 in 1,000)
• Isolated CP is in 1 in 2,000 births across races.
• Bilateral CL is associated with CP in 86% of cases, and unilateral CL is associated with CP in 68% of cases.
• CL1CP is more common on the left side, particularly in boys.
• Incidence of CL with or without CP increases with parental (especially paternal) age greater than 30 years. Some association with low socioeconomic class may be nutrition-related.

COMPLICATIONS

• Airway obstruction and feeding disorders, particularly with Pierre-Robin sequence (micrognathia, glossoptosis, airway obstruction, with or without CP)
• Chronic otitis media
• Speech problems
• Associated defects
• About one-third of patients with CP have associated anomalies, with isolated having the highest. CNS, cardiac, and urinary tract malformations and club foot are commonly associated with clefting.

 Data Gathering

HISTORY

Prenatal exposure to alcohol, cigarettes, phenytoin, isotretinoin; family history of CL or CP, or speech problems in first-degree relative

 Physical Examination

• Incomplete or complete cleft of lip, alveolus, hard and soft palate, or uvula. Soft palate and uvula clefts are always midline, while lip, alveolar, and hard palatal clefts can be unilateral or bilateral.
• A bifid uvula may indicate a submucous cleft.
• A small mandible and retropositioned tongue may indicate a risk for airway obstruction.
• Look for associated anomalies of the face, heart, and extremities that may indicate a clefting syndrome.

 Physical Examination

TRICKS

Examine the palate from the top of the patient, with the head in your lap, using a tongue depressor and flashlight. Palpate the posterior hard palate for a possible notch in the bone. Palpate the gums and maxilla for a possible notch in the floor of the nose.

 Laboratory Aids

The following tests should be performed if indicated by history and physical examination:

• Complete ophthalmologic examination to check for myopia, glaucoma, retinal detachment
• Pulse oximetry to check for desaturation while feeding or while supine
• Polysomnography to distinguish central from obstructive apnea
• Increased serum 7-dehydrocholesterol and decreased serum cholesterol to rule out Smith-Lemli-Opitz syndrome
• Karyotype to rule out specific genetic abnormalities
• Echocardiography, renal ultrasound, IV pyelography if indicated

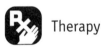 Therapy

NEONATAL

Airway management, prone positioning if tongue is causing airway obstruction. Cleft patients may have significant feeding problems because of inability to generate negative intraoral pressure necessary to feed efficiently. Preemie nipples with enlarged or cross-cut openings, or soft plastic squeezable bottles, can facilitate milk flow. Poor weight gain may necessitate NG tube feedings.

SURGICAL

• Significant airway obstruction and desaturation in the neonatal period refractory to prone positioning may indicate the need for a tongue-lip adhesion, release of the floor of the mouth musculature, or tracheostomy.
• Wide clefts of the lip may benefit from preliminary lip adhesion at 23 months of age. Timing of definitive lip repair varies from 2 to 6 months of age.
• Palate repair is generally done prior to 1 year of age to decrease speech and language difficulties.
• Otitis media is more common with CP, and bilateral myringotomy tubes can be inserted at the time of cleft repair.

• Correction of secondary deformities may include lip scar revision, cleft nasal deformity correction (infancy to adulthood), alveolar bone grafts (usually when permanent canines are erupting), pharyngoplasty for soft palate—pharyngeal incompetence, closure of palatal fistulas, and orthognathic surgery for severe jaw deformities.

ORTHODONTICS

May include obturators to facilitate feeding and speech, palatal expansion prior to bone grafting, conventional orthodontics (appliances, prosthetic teeth, bridgework), and preorthognathic surgery manipulation of the dentition

 Follow-Up

MULTIDISCIPLINARY TEAM

- Pediatrician
- Plastic surgeon
- Speech pathologist
- Orthodontist
- Pediatric dentist
- Psychologist
- Social worker
- Nurse practitioner
- Anthropologist (facial growth specialist)
- Geneticist
- Support groups

POTENTIAL PROBLEMS

• Hypernasal quality with vowel sounds and nasal air emission during consonant production may indicate velopharyngeal incompetence or palatal fistula. Thirty percent of patients may require additional palatal or pharyngeal surgery following initial palate repair.
• Multiple ear infections may require prolonged use of myringotomy tubes to prevent hearing impairment.
• Delays in speech and language development may require detailed evaluation, early intervention programs, and speech therapy.
• Poor dentition, occlusal problems (crossbite), gingivitis, and crowding have been noted. Behavior disorders and psychosocial adjustment disorders may require attention.

PROGNOSIS

Good, for normal growth and development with long-term follow-up by a multidisciplinary team and with good parental support

PITFALLS

• Failure to diagnose life-threatening airway problems in the neonate can be fatal.
• Failure to diagnose associated anomalies may lead to missed syndromes and inaccurate genetic counseling.
• A submucous cleft palate can be easily missed until hypernasal speech is noted later in life.

 Common Questions and Answers

FOR NONSYNDROMIC CL WITH OR WITHOUT CP

Q: What is our risk of having a second child with a cleft, if neither of us has a cleft?
A: Two percent.

Q: What is my child's risk of later having a child with a cleft?
A: Four percent.

Q: What is our risk of having a third child with a cleft, if we have two affected children, but neither of us is affected?
A: Nine percent.

Q: What is our risk of having a second child with a cleft, if one of us also has a cleft?
A: Seventeen percent.

FOR NONSYNDROMIC ISOLATED CP

Q: What is our risk of having a second child with a cleft, if neither of us has a cleft?
A: Two percent.

Q: What is my child's risk of later having a child with a cleft?
A: Six percent.

Q: What is our risk of having a third child with a cleft, if we have two affected children, but neither of us is affected?
A: One percent.

Q: What is our risk of having a second child with a cleft, if one of us also has a cleft?
A: Fifteen percent.

Q: Will my child look normal?
A: All cleft lip repairs will leave some type of permanent scar, with potential asymmetry that may benefit from later additional lip scar revision. The goal is to create a lip that does not attract undue attention. The nose is often the most difficult to correct, because of asymmetry in cartilage and skin contour.

Q: Will my child speak normally?
A: Most children will achieve velopharyngeal competence and normal speech, but may require additional speech therapy to achieve this goal.

*ICD-9-CM 749.10
749.20*

BIBLIOGRAPHY

Byrd HS. Cleft lip I: primary deformities. *Select Read Plast Surg* 1994;7(21):1–34.

Hardesty RA, ed. Advances in the management of cleft lip and palate. *Clin Plast Surg* 1993; 20(4):597–821.

Hobar PC. Cleft lip II: secondary deformities. *Select Read Plast Surg* 1994;7(22):1–28.

Hodges PL, Pownell PH. Cleft surgery and velopharyngeal function. *Select Read Plast Surg* 1994;7(23):1–36.

Kaufman FL. Managing the cleft lip and palate patient. *Pediatr Clin North Am* 1991;38(5): 1127–1147.

Witt PD, Marsh JL. Advances in assessing outcome of surgical repair of cleft lip and cleft palate. *Plastic Reconstr Surg* 1997;100(7): 1907–1917.

Authors: Christine A. Carman-Dillon and David W. Low

Clubfoot

 ## Database

DEFINITION

Clubfoot is a congenital or neuromuscular deformity in which the hindfoot is fixed in equinus and varus and the forefoot is fixed in varus.

CAUSES

• Most cases are idiopathic (multifactorial inheritance pattern with significant environmental influence).
• Infrequently, neuromuscular imbalance may underlie the deformity (cerebral palsy, myelomeningocele, lipomas of the cord, caudal or sacral agenesis, polio, arthrogryposis, fetal alcohol syndrome).

PATHOPHYSIOLOGY

• Many anatomic abnormalities have been postulated as causing clubfoot: anomalous or deficient muscles, myoblasts, mast cells, abnormal primary bone formation, joint and muscle contractures, vascular anomalies (absent dorsalis pedis artery), nerve anomalies, and abnormalities of the fibrous connective tissue.
• Interruption of the development of the embryonic foot has also been suggested.

EPIDEMIOLOGY

• Prevalence is 1 to 1.4 per 1,000 live births.
• The risk of deformity increases by 20 to 30 times where there is an affected first-degree relative. Male:female ratio is 2:1.

 ## Differential Diagnosis

• Distinguish other deformities of the foot:

—Metatarsus adductus or varus (heel is in neutral position)
—Calcaneovalgus (foot is in valgus)
—Vertical talus (foot is in valgus, heel in equinovalgus)

• Many children with clubfoot will also have tibial tortion.

 ## Data Gathering

HISTORY

• Family history of clubfoot (3%)
• Onset of deformity (congenital or developmental)

 ## Physical Examination

Careful examination is called for, especially

• The neuromuscular system for neuromuscular etiologies such as lumbosacral sinuses, dimples, and lipomas
• The hips for hip dysplasia
• The neck for torticollis

PHYSICAL EXAMINATION TRICKS

Push the foot into a corrected position. Is the deformity fully correctable? Overcorrectable?

 ## Laboratory Aids

• X-ray studies (after 3 months of age)
• Tarsal bones are poorly ossified in the newborn. Diagnosis is clinical.
• At 3 to 6 months of age, anteroposterior (AP) and lateral x-ray films in dorsiflexion (maximal correction) may help in defining residual deformity. The beam should be focused on the hindfoot for both the AP and lateral x-rays, as the measured angles will be hindfoot angles.
• Decreased talocalcaneal angle on the AP and lateral views (25 degrees or less) confirm persistent deformity.
• Medial displacement of the cuboid on the calcaneus and persistent plantar flexion of the forefoot on the hindfoot (talar to first metatarsal angle) indicate more complex deformities.

Therapy

- Initial treatment is serial (weekly) manipulation and casting.
- Taping may be useful for treatment of the infant requiring ICU care; access to the feet should be maintained for blood tests.
- Failure to correct the deformity completely by manipulation within 3 to 9 months should lead to surgical treatment.

Follow-Up

- Realignment of the deformity is the goal and should be achieved at surgery or by casting.
- Most surgeons cast the feet for 3 months postoperatively.
- Some brace the feet for 6 months.
- Remember, the cause of the deformity is not corrected. Only the alignment of the bones and lengthening of the soft tissues are corrected.
- Depending on the severity of the deformity, calf narrowing and weakness, and ankle and subtalar stiffness, a difference between the feet of one to two shoe sizes and even a leg-length discrepancy will be present in all corrected clubfeet.
- There will also be decreased ankle and subtalar motion as compared to the normal.
- Adolescent children with clubfeet often will get leg cramps and will tire easily while doing normally strenuous activities in sports.
- All true recurrences should lead to further evaluation for neuromuscular or syndrome causes that might have been missed in the infant.

Common Questions and Answers

Q: How can a rigid clubfoot be distinguished from a positional clubfoot?
A: During initial evaluation of the child, it is important to assess the amount of flexibility in a clubfoot. This can be most easily done by flexing the hip to 90 degrees, flexing the knee to 90 degrees, and then gently trying to turn the forefoot into a straight position lined up with the thigh. If the foot easily spins around into a normal position, it can be assumed that this is a flexible or positional clubfoot. If deformity persists, this is a rigid deformity. If possible, the examining physician should palpate the heel to see if the os calsis comes out of its equinus position filling the heel pad. In some children, particularly with a rocker bottom sole, the heel pad looks as if it is in the correct position, but the os calsis remains in equinus with the posterior aspect of the os calsis proximal to the heel pad.

Q: What percentage of clubfeet are successfully treated by casting?
A: To some extent, the amount of success depends on how much correction is desired. Occasionally, cast correction will provide a partial correction. Some feet, after casting, can be held in the corrected position, only to spin back to the clubfoot deformity when released. Positional clubfeet are likely to improve with casting in perhaps 80% of cases. Rigid clubfeet are much less likely to be corrected by casting. The success rate in the rigid feet is likely to be about 10% to 20%.

Q: What will be the permanent disability of a congenital clubfoot deformity?
A: While casting and surgical correction of a congenital clubfoot can realign the bones, the surgery does little to correct the underlying neuromuscular problems. As a result, all children with rigid clubfeet are likely to have a leg-length inequality (usually less than 1.5 in.), a smaller foot (usually one to two sizes), calf narrowing that cannot be significantly improved with exercise, and joint stiffness (ankle, subtalar, and midfoot). Even children with optimal realignment of the deformity will notice their inability to perform gymnastic activities or running activities requiring normal range of motion of the ankle and foot. Many will complain of the inability to keep up with their peer group during adolescent and young-adult sports activities.

Q: How soon should an infant with congenital clubfoot be referred to an orthopedic surgeon?
A: If casting is to be even partially successful, cast treatment should begin within the first week or two of life. Clearly, medical and life-threatening conditions will take precedence over the treatment of the clubfoot. Access to the feet for IV or blood studies will interfere with a casting regimen. Casting should begin as soon as is practical. It may even be possible to begin taping of the foot as an alternative to casting, which will still allow IV access to the feet. Referral to an orthopedic surgeon should therefore follow as soon as is practical.

ICD-9-CM 754.70

BIBLIOGRAPHY

Hamel J, Becker W. Sonographic assessment of clubfoot deformity in young children. *J Pediatr Orthop B* 1996;5(4):279–286.

Johnston CE II, Hobatho MC, Baker KJ, Baunin C. Three-dimensional analysis of clubfoot deformity by computed tomography. *J Pediatr Orthop B* 1995;4(1):39–48.

Napiontek M. Clinical and radiographic appearance of congenital talipes equinovarus after successful nonoperative treatment. *J Pediatr Orthop* 1996;16(1):67–72.

Yamamoto H, Muneta T, Morita S. Nonsurgical treatment of congenital clubfoot with manipulation, cast, and modified Denis Browne splint. *J Pediatr Orthop* 1998;18(4):538–542.

Author: Richard S. Davidson

Coarctation of Aorta

 Database

DEFINITION

Discrete stenosis of the upper thoracic aorta, usually just opposite the site of insertion of the ductus arteriosus (juxtaductal). A defect in the vessel media giving rise to a prominent posterior infolding ("the posterior shelf"). The lesion is most often discrete, but may be long-segment or torturous in nature. It is usually juxtaductal but may occur in other sites (ascending or abdominal aorta).

PATHOPHYSIOLOGY

• Decreased systemic blood flow to lower extremities after ductal closure
• Increased resistance to left ventricular outflow causes systolic hypertension and LV hypertrophy.
• If the coarctation of the aorta (CoA) is severe, left ventricular dysfunction and congestive heart failure result, with low cardiac output and increased left ventricular end-diastolic pressure.
• Decreased myocardial perfusion may be present in cases of very low output.

GENETICS

• Multifactorial; occurs in 35% of patients with Turner syndrome (XO)
• Has been described in cases of monozygotic twins

EPIDEMIOLOGY

Approximately 6% to 8% of patients with congenital heart disease have CoA. Male:female ratio is 1.2 to 2.0:1.

COMPLICATIONS

• Systemic hypertension
• Shock
• Congestive heart failure
• Cerebrovascular accident

PROGNOSIS

Untreated CoA has a poor natural history, with the onset of congestive heart failure. Claudication is common in older children with previously undiscovered CoA. Clinical conditions that may affect long-term prognosis after repair of CoA include:

• Residual or recurrent coarctation
• Hypertension (rest and exercise)
• Aortic aneurysm
• Associated intracardiac lesions

Generally, the prognosis following successful repair in infancy or childhood is excellent.

ASSOCIATED LESIONS

• Patent ductus arteriosus (PDA)
• Ventricular septal defect
• Valvar or subvalvar aortic stenosis
• Bicuspid aortic valve occurs in 85% of patients with CoA.
• Mitral stenosis: often associated with structural mitral valve abnormalities (i.e., supravalvar mitral ring, thickening of mitral leaflet, single papillary muscle with parachute deformity, or short dysplastic chordae tendinae)
• Shone syndrome: multiple left-sided obstructive lesions, including mitral stenosis, subaortic membrane, aortic valve stenosis, and coarctation
• Berry aneurysm of the circle of Willis
• Renal artery stenosis associated with abdominal coarctation

 Differential Diagnosis

• Other left-heart obstructive lesions
• Hypoplastic left-heart syndrome
• Critical aortic stenosis

 Data Gathering

HISTORY

There are two typical patterns of the clinical presentation of CoA:

• An infant with congestive heart failure or shock—"A small, pale, irritable child in respiratory distress." It is caused by closure of PDA and is more common in infants with complex CoA (20%–30%).

—Poor feeding
—Dyspnea
—Diaphoresis
—Poor weight gain
—Oliguria

• An otherwise asymptomatic child with systolic hypertension and/or a heart murmur (70%–80%).

—Lower extremity claudication
—Headaches

 Physical Examination

• Tachypnea and tachycardia
• Discrepant arterial pulses and systolic blood pressure in the upper and lower extremities
• Weak "thready" pulses
• Grades 2 to 3/6 systolic ejection murmur
• Gallop rhythm in an infant with congestive heart failure
• Ejection click from bicuspid aortic valve

—The most important finding: decreased or absent lower extremity pulses. (Always put your fingers on femoral pulses.) Are pulses present? Is there a delay between the brachial and femoral pulses?
—Heart murmur: best heard at the upper LSB, at the base and radiating to the left interscapular area posteriorly
—An infant with critical CoA with PDA: "differential cyanosis" The lower part of the body appears cyanotic because the descending aortic flow is provided by the right ventricle through PDA (check postductal saturation).

 Laboratory Aids

• ECG: Right ventricular hypertrophy is usually present in symptomatic infants. ECG is often normal in children. Left ventricular hypertrophy is apparent with more severe coarctation or coarctation of longer standing.
• Chest x-ray: in the infant, moderate-to-severe cardiomegaly with increased pulmonary vascular markings (PVM). In an asymptomatic child, the heart size is often normal with normal PVM. Rib notching may be seen in older children secondary to erosion of the ribs by dilated intercostal collateral vessels.
• Echocardiography: localization and degree of CoA and associated findings; PDA, isthmus hypoplasia. Assessment of associated left-sided obstruction (severity of which may be underestimated in patients with congestive heart failure, low cardiac output, or the presence of a PDA): mitral valve abnormality, left ventricular outflow obstruction, and aortic stenosis (bicuspid aortic valve)
• MRI: clearly defines the location and severity of CoA. May be useful for serial follow-up postoperatively (especially aortic aneurysms)
• Cardiac catheterization and angiography: usually not indicated unless there are further questions to be answered and/or a planned intervention.

Therapy

MEDICAL

For the sick neonate who presents with severe congestive heart failure or shock (ductal-dependent left-sided obstructive lesion):

- Prostaglandin infusion: 0.05 μg/kg/min
- Inotropes: digoxin
- Diuretics for pulmonary venous hypertension or pulmonary edema: furosemide
- Correction of metabolic disturbances caused by systemic hypoperfusion
- Surgical intervention should follow as soon as possible.

For the asymptomatic child, elective repair and medical management of hypertension are appropriate.

SURGICAL

Infancy

- Surgical repair of CoA and associated intracardiac anomalies
- The surgical mortality rate for infants with CoA and a large VSD ranges from 5% to 15% and is higher for children with more complex intracardiac anomalies.

Childhood

- Elective CoA repair between ages 3 and 5 years in asymptomatic children without severe upper extremity hypertension. Later repair is associated with increased risk of sustained hypertension and atherosclerosis.

Types of Surgical Repair

- End-to-end anastomosis
- Subclavian flap aortoplasty
- Prosthetic patch aortoplasty
- Bypass graft

Nonsurgical Option

- Percutaneous balloon angioplasty of native CoA is still controversial because of concern about recurrent stenosis and aneurysm formation.

POSTOPERATIVE COMPLICATIONS

- Bleeding
- Postcoarctectomy syndrome/mesenteric arteritis
- Paradoxical hypertension
- Spinal cord ischemia (0.4%)
- Residual coarctation
- Chylothorax
- Stridor
- Diaphragm paralysis
- Subclavian steal
- Aortic aneurysm or dissection

 Follow-Up

- Reexamine every 6 to 12 months.
- Residual or recurrent CoA (25%–60%); occurs most commonly after repair in infancy: Percutaneous balloon angioplasty can be performed as early as 2 months postoperatively.
- Residual systemic hypertension; most commonly in patients whose CoA repair is delayed beyond late childhood
- Aneurysm formation
- Cerebrovascular accidents
- Monitor four-extremity blood pressure for recoarctation or residual hypertension.
- Antibiotic prophylaxis to prevent endocarditis or endarteritis
- May have hypertension with exercise, even if normotensive at rest
- Exercise-induced hypertension without anatomic stenosis may respond to beta-blocker therapy.

PITFALLS

- The most reliable clinical findings to diagnose CoA are the presence of pressure differences in upper and lower extremities and decreased or absent femoral pulses. Palpable pulses do not exclude coarctation. What one palpates is pulse pressure, not absolute systolic pressure.
- Four-extremity blood pressure measurement is very important in assessing infants and children with possible congenital heart disease. Proper cuff size must be used.

 Common Questions and Answers

Q: When is the most appropriate time to perform surgical repair of simple CoA?
A: Currently, it is recommended that elective CoA repair be performed between 3 and 5 years of age in asymptomatic children without severe upper extremity hypertension, based on the risk of recoarctation (higher incidence under 3 years, especially under 1 year, of age) and residual hypertension and subsequent atherosclerotic cardiovascular disease.

Q: What is the incidence of residual hypertension after surgical repair of CoA?
A: The incidence of late residual hypertension may be reduced to approximately 6% if CoA repair is performed under 5 years of age, as opposed to 30% to 50% in patients whose CoA is repaired at an older age.

ICD-9-CM 747.10

BIBLIOGRAPHY

Beekman RH. Coarctation of aorta. In: Moss, Adams. *Heart disease in infants, children, and adolescents,* 5th ed., 1111–1113.

Chang AC, Hanley FL, Wernovsky G, Wessel DL. *Pediatric cardiac intensive care.* Baltimore: Williams & Wilkins, 1998:247–254.

Fyler DC. *Nadas' pediatric cardiology.* Philadelphia: Hanley and Belfur, Inc., 1992:535–556.

Liberthson RR. Coarctation of the aorta: review of 234 patients and clarification of management problems. *Am J Cardiol* 1979;43:835–840.

Morriss MJH, McNamara DG. Coarctation of the aorta and interrupted aortic arch. In: Gasson A, Jr., Bricker JT, Fisher DJ, Neish SR, eds. *The science and practice of pediatric cardiology.* Philadelphia: Lea & Febiger, 1990:1353–1381.

Author: Jennifer C. Shores

Coccidioidomycosis

 Database

DEFINITION

Coccidioidomycosis is infection by the dimorphic fungus *Coccidioides immitis*.

PATHOPHYSIOLOGY

- Inhalation of arthrospores from disturbed, arid soil is major route of infection.
- Sixty percent of acute infections are subclinical (asymptomatic).
- Most patients have infection limited to a localized area of lung and hilar nodes after mounting an intense inflammatory response with granuloma formation.
- Dissemination occurs in a minority of patients (<1% cases) via lymphatic or hematologic spread, causing widespread granulomatous lesions.
- The course of illness is highly variable and dependent on host immune response and amount of exposure. HIV-infected patients and other patients with immunosuppression due to T-lymphocyte dysfunction (lymphoma, organ transplantation) are particularly susceptible to severe forms of pulmonary and extrapulmonary coccidioidomycosis.

EPIDEMIOLOGY

- *Coccidioides immitis* is found in abundance in soil in the southwestern United States (west Texas, New Mexico, Arizona, California), northern Mexico, and parts of South and Central America. Estimations (by skin testing) of infection in up to one-third of the population in endemic areas.
- There is no person-to-person spread.
- The average incubation period is 10 to 16 days, with a range of approximately 6 to 30 days.
- Primary infection is most commonly seen in the summer and fall months.
- Susceptibility is unaffected by age, race, or sex, but dissemination rates after infection vary considerably (see Complications section below).

COMPLICATIONS

- Localized complications of primary pulmonary infection are infrequent and include pleural effusions and pericarditis.
- Factors increasing the susceptibility of a patient for disseminated coccidioidomycosis include immunosuppression; infancy; Filipino, African-American, or Hispanic populations; and patients in whom infection is characterized by mediastinal adenopathy or fever greater than 1 month in duration.
- Hydrocephalus is common after spread of infection to the CNS.

PROGNOSIS

- Primary infection of the lungs is usually self-limited, with a course of illness lasting 1 to 3 weeks; complications (see above) may prolong the course.
- Dissemination is infrequent (see above for risk factors). Morbidity and mortality have improved with use of amphotericin B, but immunocompromised patients with poor T-cell function still have a poor prognosis after the development of disseminated infection.
- Dissemination of disease to the CNS can cause a rapidly fatal meningitis if not recognized and treated.

ASSOCIATED DISEASES

- *Primary pulmonary coccidioidomycosis* is usually a nonapparent, asymptomatic infection.
- *Symptomatic pulmonary infection* is characterized by cough, fever, and chest pain and may be accompanied by rash or arthralgias. Chronic pulmonary lesions are rare in children.
- Skin is a second, infrequent, primary site of infection, which occurs via direct inoculation (trauma).
- Progressive systemic disease can spread from the lungs to involve lymph nodes, bones, joints, abdominal organs, skin, and CNS.
- Limited dissemination (spread to one or more sites) is common in children.
- Disseminated coccidioidomycosis in children resembles progressive tuberculosis, with spread weeks to months after primary infection. Children receiving chemotherapy and those with HIV may reactivate previous infection.
- Disseminated disease is less common in children than in adults. It is characterized by persistent fevers, toxicity, and development of granulomatous lesions outside the chest. Common extrapulmonary sites of infection include bone (fingers, toes, ribs, vertebrae), skin, and CSF.

 Differential Diagnosis

Tuberculosis (lung or CSF)

- Mycoplasma
- Other pulmonary fungal diseases, such as histoplasmosis
- Influenza
- Other viral or bacterial infections that present as bronchopneumonia

 Data Gathering

HISTORY

- History of travel or residence in endemic areas
- Initial symptoms: fever, dry or productive cough, and pleuritic chest pain, which may be accompanied by myalgia, arthralgia, chills, night sweats, headache, and anorexia
- Hemoptysis is rare in children, but is reported in up to 15% of symptomatic adults.

Coccidioidomycosis

 Physical Examination

- The severity of symptomatic illness is widely variable in acute infection: from mild flulike illness lasting a few days, to severe lower tract respiratory disease with lobar pneumonia, pleural effusions, and, rarely, pericarditis.
- Symptomatic children often have an erythematous maculopapular rash, usually limited to the lower trunk and thighs, but occasionally it is more diffuse and resembles measles.
- Erythema nodosum may occur later in the course of the infection, especially in children in the San Joaquin Valley.
- Young children may have a clinical finding of stridor after infection of subglottic tissues.

 Laboratory Aids

- Hematologic findings include elevated ESR, leukocytosis, and, often, eosinophilia.
- Coccidioidin or spherulin skin test positivity (delayed type hypersensitivity), along with characteristic signs and symptoms of coccidiodomycosis, is strongly suggestive of the infection.
- Skin tests can be positive 10 to 21 days after infection, but are frequently negative in progressive or disseminated disease.
- Culture of organism is possible in qualified laboratories.
- Visualization of large spherules is possible in stained specimens of sputum, tracheal aspirates, CSF, urine, or tissue biopsy.
- IgM agglutination tests are rapid and sensitive but not specific. Tube precipitin and immunodiffusion can also evaluate IgM response.
- IgG is detected by immunodiffusion or complement fixation from serum or CSF: High and persistent complement fixation titers are seen in severe disease; decreasing titers suggest resolution of infection.
- No characteristic CXR findings. Most common: well-circumscribed nodules, pulmonary infiltrates, pleural effusions, hilar adenopathy, and cavitations

 Therapy

- Uncomplicated or minor disease is self-limited and should not be treated with antifungal therapy (>95% of cases).
- Surgical debridement is used for localized and persistent lesions in bone and lung.
- Amphotericin B is recommended for severe progressive disease, for disease in immunocompromised patients (e.g., those with neoplasm or AIDS), and for patients with disseminated or CNS infection.
- Intrathecal amphotericin B is useful in CNS infections.
- High-dose ketoconazole with intraventricular or intrathecal miconazole has been used alternatively for CNS coccidioidomycosis.

PREVENTION

Infection Control

- No special isolation or precautions for the hospitalized patient
- Contaminated dressings from skin lesions should be handled and discarded with care.
- Preventive efforts are aimed at dust control and trials to eliminate organisms from soil.
- Avoidance of field activities or travel in highly endemic areas is recommended for children with a negative skin test.

PITFALLS

- Skin test in disseminated disease may be negative.
- Diagnosis in nonendemic areas can easily be missed due to low clinical suspicion or missed travel history. Clinicians in endemic areas should maintain a high level of clinical suspicion.

ICD-9-CM 114.9

BIBLIOGRAPHY

American Academy of Pediatrics. Coccidioidomycosis. In: Peter G, ed. *1997 red book: report of the Committee on Infectious Diseases,* 24th ed. Elk Grove Village, IL: American Academy of Pediatrics, 1997:181–183.

Libke RD, Granoff DM. Coccidioidomycosis. In: Feigin RD, Cherry JD, eds. *Textbook of pediatric infectious diseases,* 3rd ed. Philadelphia: WB Saunders, 1992:1916–1925.

Stevens DA. Coccidioidomycosis. *N Engl J Med* 1995;332(16):1077–1082.

Stevens DA. Coccidioides immitis. In: Mandell GL, et al., eds. *Principles and practice of infectious diseases,* 3rd ed. New York: Churchill Livingstone, 1990:2008–2016.

Author: Molly (Martha) W. Stevens

Colic

Database

DEFINITION

A poorly defined and incompletely understood state of prolonged or excessive crying in young infants who are otherwise well

- No standard definition of this phenomenon
- Best definition available: more than 3 hours a day of irritability, fussing, or crying on more than 3 days in any 1 week during the first 3 to 4 months of life in an infant who is otherwise healthy and well fed. Some add the criterion of a duration of 3 weeks or more.
- Crying is not qualitatively different, but quantitatively, it is considerably more than the average.

PATHOPHYSIOLOGY

- No single cause is always found.
- Typically, the problem lies in the interaction between factors in the infant and the environment.

—In infant: There is a normal physiologic or temperamental predisposition to be more sensitive, irritable, intense, or harder to soothe than average for the age.
—Parents generally have not yet learned how to read correctly and respond appropriately to the infant's needs. They may be manipulating the infant in ways that increase rather than decrease the amount of crying.

- Colic generally occurs in the absence of any abnormality in the infant or the parents, but rather when the parents have not yet learned to interact harmoniously with the infant.
- There is no evidence that the bowel is at fault; flatus is more likely to be the result of the crying than the cause.
- Psychosocial risk factors, such as poor support for the mother and various stressors, are probably more common than in noncolicky infants, but they are not necessary.

—When such external factors present, they seem to exert their effects by reducing the parent's ability to respond appropriately to the infant.

- In the case of a physical problem in the infant, such as milk allergy, the prolonged crying is, by definition, not colic.

GENETICS

No genetic influence has been discovered, but it has not been investigated. Temperamental traits are known to be largely inherited, however.

EPIDEMIOLOGY

- Colic typically begins shortly after a baby comes home from a newborn nursery.
- It can last until 3 to 4 months of age if not successfully managed.
- If excessive crying lasts after 4 months, other diagnoses should be considered.

COMPLICATIONS

- Excessive crying does not turn into any other condition, but the factors that caused it may contribute to sleep problems and other behavioral concerns in the infant after the colic has gone.
- Parents are usually exasperated by it.
- The most serious outcome is that, due to parental exasperation, the infant may be physically abused.
- The infant is likely to be overfed.

PROGNOSIS

The long-term outcome of these infants has not been studied adequately. Predictions are hazardous.

Differential Diagnosis

- Normal crying. Average, normal infants cry about 2 hours a day at 2 weeks of age, just under 3 hours at 6 weeks, and then decrease to about 1 hour by 12 weeks. Normal crying, like colic, tends to occur predominantly in the evening.
- Prolonged or excessive crying from physical causes:

—Faulty feeding techniques: overfeeding or underfeeding and inadequate burping or sucking
—Physical problems in the infant: acute disorders such as otitis media, intestinal cramping with diarrhea, corneal abrasion, and incarcerated hernia; or chronic ones such as gastroesophageal reflux
—Cow's-milk allergy, lactose intolerance, or transmission of irritating substances such as caffeine via breast milk

Data Gathering

HISTORY

- Define symptoms: intensity, duration, and frequency of crying. Some parents complain more than others about the crying.
- Ask parents to describe a typical day.

—Description of a typical day or keeping a crying diary is helpful.
—This will give insights into the daily routine, feeding, rest, and interpretive skills of parents.

- Ask parents to describe and demonstrate their soothing techniques.
- Information on the baby's temperament can be obtained by asking the parents to describe the baby's typical reaction patterns.
- Medical history should include concerns about the pregnancy and the newborn period, anxieties related to parents' own experiences as children or with previous children, and the quality of family supports and other stressors.

Physical Examination

- No findings are expected if the child has colic. However, examination should always be performed in order to reassure both parents and physician.
- Attempts at management over the telephone without a physical examination are likely to be unsuccessful.

Laboratory Aids

No tests are indicated unless specifically suggested by history and physical examination.

Therapy

- The most effective form of treatment is counseling, which should consist of these main points:

—*The infant is not sick.* Crying may be persistent, but there is no evidence of a physical problem. There is no proof the infant is having pain, just distress. Avoid iatrogenic problems caused by suggesting that something is wrong with the infant. The infant is probably just overaroused and tired.

—*Education about infant crying.* Parents need to know how much normal infants cry and how they vary in sensitivity, irritability, and soothability. The way parents react to their infants can affect the amount of crying. Parents often do not understand that a common reason for infant crying is fatigue and a need to be left alone.

—*The excessive crying can be reduced.* Parents have to learn to tune in more sensitively to infants' needs and to be more effectively responsive to them.

- Basic strategy: Soothe more, as by a pacifier, repetitive sound, or a hot water bottle, and stimulate less by decreasing the picking up, holding, and feeding the infant when it is not appropriate.

—A quiet environment, correction of any faulty feeding techniques, and a minimum of unnecessary handling without changing the composition of the feedings. Pertinent psychosocial issues should be dealt with.

- Expression of optimism by the pediatrician about the immediate outcome is justified and in itself improves chances of success. Simply saying that the colic will be gone by 3 to 4 months of age is not comforting and may be quite the opposite.
- Extra carrying does not help.
- Drugs, such as phenobarbital or diphenhydramine, are seldom necessary. Some observers have reported beneficial effects, when used for a week or two in conjunction with counseling, but these results have not as yet been subjected to double-blind studies. Simethicone has not been shown to be helpful.
- Formula changes are frequently attempted by physicians hoping for a simple solution, but they rarely are effective. Sometimes they seem to be helpful for a few days, only to cease being so a day or two later.
- Almost any procedure done with conviction is likely to be followed by a temporary reduction in crying because of the placebo effect.

 Follow-Up

- It is important to keep in close touch with parents of an excessively fussy baby. Telephone contact every 2 to 3 days is essential until improvement. Reexamination is rarely needed.
- Standard pediatric textbooks state that colic usually goes away by itself by 3 to 4 months of age and that little can be done to change that pattern. However, several studies report that colic can be sharply reduced within 2 to 3 days if management such as that described above is used. Some infants take longer, but virtually all respond to suitable management.

PREVENTION

No study has yet demonstrated any certain way of preventing this prolonged or excessive crying. Two methods that are likely to be helpful are education of all parents about infant crying and soothing, and dealing with parental anxieties whenever they occur.

PITFALLS

Numerous pitfalls await the unprepared physician:

- Overdiagnosing the condition of the infant or caretaking inadequacies of parents
- Overtreatment of the infant with changes of feedings, medications, and various inappropriate procedures such as enemas and rectal manipulations. Despite the widely held, popular view that cow's-milk allergy is a principal reason for excessive crying, no study of acceptable double-blind design has demonstrated its occurrence in infants who are free of respiratory, gastrointestinal, or cutaneous manifestations of allergy.

 Common Questions and Answers

Q: What is wrong with my baby? What can we do to relieve the pain? Why is he/she so gassy? How do you know that it is not due to an allergy? Shouldn't we strengthen the formula? You mean it's all my fault? Will this ever stop? What will he/she be like later?
A: All the answers are to be found above.

ICD-9-CM 789.0

BIBLIOGRAPHY

Carey WB. "Colic": prolonged or excessive crying in young infants. In: Levine MD, Carey WB, Crocker AC, eds. *Developmental–behavioral pediatrics,* 3rd ed. Philadelphia: WB Saunders, 1999.

Carey WB. The effectiveness of parent counseling in managing colic. *Pediatrics* 1994;94: 333–334.

Lester BM, Barr RG, eds. Colic and excessive crying. 105th Ross Conference on Pediatric Research, 1997, Columbus, OH: Ross Products Division, Abbott Laboratories.

Wessel MA, Cobb JC, Jackson EB, et al. Paroxysmal fussing in infants, sometimes called "colic." *Pediatrics* 1954;14:421–434.

Author: William B. Carey

Common Variable Immunodeficiency

 ## Database

DEFINITION

Common variable immunodeficiency (CVID) is a heterogeneous immunodeficiency syndrome characterized by hypogammaglobulinemia, recurrent infections, and a wide spectrum of immunologic abnormalities, including autoimmune disease. Other terminology for this disease includes:

- Acquired hypogammaglobulinemia
- Adult-onset hypogammaglobulinemia
- Dysgammaglobulinemia
- Common variable hypogammaglobulinemia

ETIOLOGY

- The primary immunologic defect(s) leading to this syndrome is (are) unknown.
- Most patients have impaired immunoglobulin and specific antibody production despite normal B-lymphocyte numbers.
- Functional defects of both B and T lymphocytes occur.

GENETICS

- Usually, no clear inheritance patterns
- Some families have a pattern consistent with autosomal recessive inheritance.
- Increased prevalence of two rare MHC Class III haplotypes in a large number of CVID kindreds
- Family members of patients with CVID have an increased incidence of other immunologic defects, including IgA deficiency and autoimmune disease.

EPIDEMIOLOGY

- Incidence is estimated to be 1 in 100,000 in the general population.
- Can present at any age, but usually seen in the second to third decade of life. CVID has been described in patients as young as 6 months.
- Diagnosis is usually made several years after the onset of recurrent infections.
- A subgroup of children has been described in which the onset of disease was most often before 5 years of age. This group was characterized by a relapsing and remitting course in which autoimmune disease predominated.

COMPLICATIONS

- Autoimmune disease in 20% of CVID patients. Most common are autoimmune hemolytic anemia and thrombocytopenia.
- GI complications include chronic diarrhea and malabsorption.
- Lymphoproliferative disease: Overall risk is 8% to 10%. The most common are lymphomas and leukemia.
- Chronic sinusitis and lung disease with abnormal PFTs
- Progressive decline in T-lymphocyte function

 ## Differential Diagnosis

- Other primary antibody-deficiency disorders: X-linked agammaglobulinemia and transient hypogammaglobulinemia of infancy
- Severe malabsorption with protein-losing enteropathy
- HIV infection
- Chronic lung disease: cystic fibrosis, immotile cilia syndrome, and α_1-antitrypsin deficiency
- Primary autoimmune diseases: immune thrombocytopenic purpura (ITP), autoimmune hemolytic anemia (AIHA), systemic lupus erythematosus (SLE), and thyroiditis

 ## Data Gathering

HISTORY

- Recurrent sinopulmonary infections, especially sinusitis and pneumonias, with encapsulated bacteria
- Autoimmune diseases such as AIHA, ITP, thyroid disease, and chronic active hepatitis
- Persistent diarrhea of infectious (e.g., *Giardia lamblia*) or noninfectious etiologies
- Severe or unusual viral infections with herpes simplex, cytomegalovirus (CMV), and varicella, such as pneumonitis, hepatitis, or encephalitis. Chronic meningoencephalitis can be seen with enteroviral infection.

 ## Physical Examination

- Evaluation should focus on the presence of infection.
- Thirty percent of patients will have lymphadenopathy and/or splenomegaly.

 ## Laboratory Aids

TESTS

- IgG, IgA, IgM, and IgE below age-appropriate norms
- CBC with differential: Examine smear for evidence of hemolysis in AIHA.
- Autoimmune antibody screen: ANA, autoantibody panel
- Stool culture for bacteria and ova/parasites to evaluate chronic diarrhea
- Isohemagglutinins as well as functional antibody titers to bacterial antigens such as tetanus, diphtheria, and pneumococcus are usually low to absent.
- Spirometry may be helpful in following chronic lung disease.
- Mitogen/antigen stimulation studies will help assess lymphocyte function.
- T- and B-lymphocyte enumeration by flow cytometry
- Absent B lymphocytes suggests X-linked agammaglobulinemia (XLA) rather than CVID.
- Appropriate cultures based on site of infection

IMAGING

Chest and sinus x-ray studies/CT scans may be warranted for evaluation of chronic disease.

DIAGNOSTIC PROCEDURES

- GI endoscopy with biopsies for cases of idiopathic persistent diarrhea
- Lymph node biopsy in suspected malignancy

Therapy

- Appropriate antibiotics for acute infections. Prophylactic antibiotics may be helpful in chronic/recurrent infections.
- Monthly IV immunoglobulin (IVIG) replacement: Nadir IgG levels should be greater than 300 mg/dL.
- Cautious use of corticosteroids may be necessary in the treatment of GI and autoimmune manifestations.

 ## Follow-Up

- Close and frequent follow-up is warranted for patients with severe, recurrent symptoms. It may be as frequent as monthly, depending on symptoms.
- Signs and symptoms suggesting malignancy (e.g., persistent adenopathy in absence of infection, significant weight loss, or abdominal mass) should be evaluated expeditiously.

 ## Common Questions and Answers

Q: What is the life expectancy of patients with the diagnosis of CVID?
A: Since the clinical presentations and symptoms are variable, it is difficult to predict the life expectancy in individual patients. The availability of IVIG, in addition to antibiotic therapy, has greatly improved the outlook for these patients. However, despite adequate therapy, a large percentage of patients with CVID have a progressive decline in immune function. Major morbidity and mortality usually result from the associated complications of malignancy, chronic lung disease, and severe autoimmune disease.

Q: Do children differ in their presentation compared with adults?
A: In a subgroup of children with CVID, autoimmune disease may be the major clinical problem rather than infections.

Q: Should patients with CVID receive live viral vaccines?
A: In general, patients receiving IVIG therapy do not require any vaccinations. Live viral vaccines should be avoided in these patients, especially if they have deteriorating immune function.

Q: Can CVID be diagnosed prenatally?
A: Since there are no clear genetic inheritance patterns, prenatal diagnosis is unavailable.

ICD-9-CM 279.06

BIBLIOGRAPHY

de Asis ML, Iqbal S, Sicklick M. Analysis of a family containing three members with common variable immunodeficiency. *Ann Allergy Asthma Immunol* 1996;76(6):527–529.

Conley ME, Park CL, Douglas SD. Childhood common variable immunodeficiency with autoimmune disease. *J Pediatr* 1986;916:915–922.

Eisenstein EM, Sneller MC. Common variable immunodeficiency: diagnosis and management. *Ann Allergy* 1994;73:285–294.

Hausser C, et al. Common variable hypogammaglobulinemia in children. *Am J Dis Child* 1983;137:833–837.

Sneller MC, et al. New insights in common variable immunodeficiency. *Ann Intern Med* 1993;118:720–730.

Winkelstein JA, et al., eds. *Patient and family handbook for the primary immune deficiency diseases*, 2nd ed. Immune Deficiency Foundation, 1993.

Yocum MW, Kelso JM. Common variable immunodeficiency: the disorder and treatment. *Mayo Clin Proc* 1991;66:83–96.

Author: Alex G. Yip

Complement Deficiency

 Database

DEFINITION

Complement consists of plasma and cell membrane proteins that function as cofactors in defense against pathogenic microbes and in the generation of many immunopathogenic disorders. Biologic actions include:

- Cytolysis: destruction of cells by disrupting cell membrane
- Opsonization of organisms, which facilitates phagocytosis
- Inflammation by generation of peptides, which can up-regulate chemotaxis and can cause vasodilatation
- Clearance of immune complexes

PATHOPHYSIOLOGY

- Two pathways, the classic and the alternate, that converge on same terminal pathway—the membrane attack complex
- Primary or congenital deficiencies of complement
- Secondary deficiencies of complement
- Usually secondary to a consumptive or decreased productive state:

—Newborn state
—Malnutrition, anorexia nervosa
—Liver cirrhosis
—Reye syndrome
—Nephrotic syndrome

See the table Complement Deficiency and Related Clinical Problems.

GENETICS

- Deficiencies of either pathway are usually autosomal recessive traits.
- Properdin deficiency is X-linked.
- Heterozygotes are usually phenotypically normal.

EPIDEMIOLOGY

Prevalence of known primary immunodeficiency is 1 per 100,000. Complement accounts for approximately 2% of all primary immunodeficiencies.

SYMPTOMS/COMPLICATIONS

Deficiencies can lead to:

- Recurrent infection
- Immune complex disease
- Autoimmunity

 Differential Diagnosis

Humoral deficits such as immunoglobulin deficiency or dysfunction, consumptive process such as sepsis

 Data Gathering

HISTORY

Indications for Evaluating Complement System

- SLE, juvenile rheumatoid arthritis (JRA), or other immune complex disease
- Recurrent pyogenic infections
- Second episode of bacteremia at any age
- Second episode of meningococcal meningitis or gonococcal arthritis
- Recurrent angioedema
- Pneumococcal bacteremia after infancy

 Physical Examination

- Failure to thrive
- Scars from various infections
- Joint destruction

Complement Deficiency and Related Clinical Problems

DEFICIENCY	CLINICAL MANIFESTATIONS
C2	Systemic lupus erythematosus (SLE), vasculitis, glomerulonephritis
C4	SLE, glomerulonephritis
C3	Glomerulonephritis, pyogenic infection, immune complex disease
C1(qrs)	SLE, pyogenic infections, hereditary angioedema
Properdin	Neisserial infections
Factor D	Neisserial infections
C5, C6, C7, C8	Disseminated neisserial infections

Laboratory Aids

- CH50: to assess integrity of classical pathway. It is the quantity of serum required to lyse 50% of an aliquot of antibody-sensitized sheep RBC. Handling of the specimen is paramount because complement components are thermolabile, and a common cause of an abnormal value is improper handling. Procedure may require use of dry ice.
- APH50: to assess integrity of alternate pathway
- C3, C4, and other individual components

 ## Therapy

- Fresh-frozen plasma for acute severe infections
- Aggressive work-up and management of infections
- Prophylactic antibiotics may be useful for recurrent infections.
- Immunization for pneumococci, *Haemophilus influenzae,* and *Neisseria meningitidis* for patient and household members
- Close monitoring for onset of autoimmune disease
- Study other family members for genetic counseling.

PITFALLS

- Special care is required for the proper handling of blood test to prevent falsely low values.
- Sometimes the complement cascade can be activated and consume the complement factor, leading to the improper diagnosis of a complement deficiency.

 ## Common Questions and Answers

Q: How common are complement deficiencies?
A: Very uncommon. They account for 2% of all immunodeficiencies.

Q: When should I evaluate for a complement deficiency?
A: Any child with recurrent sinopulmonary infections or more than one episode of a Neisserial infection.

ICD-9-CM 279.3

BIBLIOGRAPHY

Berger M, Frank MM. The serum complement system. In: Stiehm ER, ed. *Immunologic disorders in infants and children,* 3rd ed. Philadelphia: WB Saunders, 1989:97–115.

Colten HR. Complement deficiencies. *Annu Rev Immunol* 1992;10:809–834.

Ernst T, Spath PJ, Aebi C, Schaad UB, Bianchetti MG. Screening for complement deficiency in bacterial meningitis. *Acta Paediatr* 1997;86(9):1009–1010.

Frank MM. Complement deficiencies. In: Stites DP, Terr AI, eds. *Basic and clinical immunology.* Norwalk, CT: Appleton & Lange, 1991:36–366.

Frank MM. Detection of complement in relation to disease. *J Allergy Clin Immunol* 1992;89:641–648.

Author: Michelle M. Klinek

Condyloma (Condyloma Acuminata)

 Database

DEFINITION

Members of the Papovaviridae family, the human paillomaviruses, cause warts. Exophytic venereal warts or condylomata acuminata are caused by human papillomavirus (HPV) types 6 and 11. Virus types 16, 18, 31, 33, and 35 cause subclinical infection in the anogenital region and have been associated with genital carcinomas.

PATHOPHYSIOLOGY

- Transmission is primarily through sexual contact.
- It can also be acquired during the birth process.
- The incubation period ranges from 3 months to several years.
- The virus is trophic for epithelial cells and infects the basal layer of actively dividing cells.
- Infection results in koilocytosis, nuclear atypia, and so forth. These changes may progress to severe dysplasia and CIS (carcinoma in situ).

EPIDEMIOLOGY

- HPV infection is not a reportable disease.
- It is the most common viral STD.
- A minimum of 10% to 20% of sexually active women are infected with HPV.
- Genital warts and HPV infection are diseases of young adults 16 to 25 years of age.

PROGNOSIS

Therapy will not eradicate the virus; thus, HPV causes recurrent disease.

ASSOCIATED DISEASES

- Laryngeal papillomas
- Other sexually transmitted diseases

 Differential Diagnosis

- Condyloma lata
- Molluscum contagiosum
- Pink pearly papules or hypertrophic papillae of the penis
- Lipomas
- Fibromas
- Adenomas

 Data Gathering

HISTORY

- Most patients have no symptoms.
- Presence of warts
- Vaginal or urethral discharge, bleeding, local pain.
- Dysuria
- Pruritis

 Physical Examination

- Warts appear as soft, sessile tumors with surfaces ranging from smooth to rough with many finger-like projections.
- HPV may also cause flat keratotic plaques that project only slightly with a hyperpigmented surface and are difficult to identify without the addition of acetic acid.
- Subclinical infection is common, causing many foci of epithelial hyperplasia invisible to the examiner.
- In males, infection is found on the penis, urethra, scrotum, perianal, and rectal area.
- In females, infection involves the vulva, vagina, cervix, perianal area, and rectum.
- Diagnosis is made by visual inspection of the anogenital region and/or Pap smear.

 Laboratory Aids

- Application of 3% to 5% acetic acid for 5 minutes causes lesions to appear white and thus more readily apparent.
- Tissue specimens may show koilocytosis typical for HPV infection.
- Colposcopy aids the diagnosis of cervical lesions.
- No cultures are available currently.

 Therapy

- To date, no therapy exists that eradicates the virus.
- All available therapies have equal efficacy in eradicating warts, ranging from 22% to 94%, with the significant rate of relapse of 25% within 3 months (see table).

—Consider size, location, number of warts, previous treatment, and patient preference.
—Also consider patient preference, expense, and side effects.
—Patients with extensive lesions should be referred to physicians who routinely treat these lesions.

SURGICAL EXCISION

- External: see table below
- Meatal: cryotherapy or podophyllin
- Anal: cryotherapy or TCA
- Vaginal: TCA
- Cervical: Refer to an expert.

PREVENTION

- Condom use may diminish transmission.
- Examine partners; treat those infected.

Specific Therapies

MEDICATION	PROCEDURE	SIDE EFFECT
Podofilox 0.5%	Apply with cotton swab b.i.d. for 3 days. After 4 days, repeat as necessary for four cycles total; should not exceed 0.5 mL/d.	Local
Imiquimod 5% cream	Patients apply at bedtime 3 times per week for up to 16 weeks. Wash off after 6–10 hours.	Local
Podophyllin 10%–25%	Applied by practitioner and then washed off 1–4 hours later. Dose is limited, 0.5 mL per treatment, to avoid systemic toxicity.	Local
Trichloroacetic acid (TCA) 80%–90%	Applied to warts directly, then talc is applied to remove unreacted acid. Washed off after 4 hours.	Local
	Need special equipment	Mode
Laser surgical excision	Requires special equipment and training; often requires general anesthesia; controlled tissue destruction	Local

Condyloma (Condyloma Acuminata)

Follow-Up

- Follow up for expected course of disease.
- Scheduled follow-up is not necessary.
- Latent infection and recurrent disease are common.

Common Questions and Answers

Q: What treatment is indicated during pregnancy?
A: Most experts recommend surgical removal if necessary. Podophyllin is absolutely contraindicated.

Q: Should partners of patients with genital warts be referred for examination?
A: Recurrence is due to reactivation of the virus; reinfection plays no role. Therefore, partner examination is not necessary. However, they may benefit from treatment and counseling. The majority of them have subclinical infection. It is important that female partners have routine PAP smears.

Q: Are genital warts in children always indicative of sexual abuse?
A: No. The HPV virus has an incubation period of many months. Thus, warts transmitted to infants at the time of birth may not become clinically apparent for 1 to 2 years. Whether the incubation period can be longer than this remains unknown. Thus, maternal history and, potentially, examination are both important factors. Children older than 2 years with anogenital warts should be carefully evaluated by experienced clinicians for child abuse. It is possible that caregivers may transmit the virus to children through close but nonsexual contact; thus, this history is also important in older children.

ICD-9-CM 078.0

BIBLIOGRAPHY

Emans SJ, Goldstein DP. Human papillomavirus (HPV) and human immunodeficiency virus (HIV). In: Emans SJ, Goldstein DP, eds. *Pediatric and adolescent gynecology,* 3rd ed. Boston: Little, Brown, 1990:385–410.

Nienstein LS. *Adolescent health care, a practical guide.* Baltimore: Urban & Schwarzenberg, 1991.

Oriel D. Genital human papillomavirus infection. In: Holmes KK, Mardh P, Sparling PF, et al., eds. *Sexually transmitted diseases,* 2nd ed. New York: McGraw-Hill, 1990:433–441.

1998 guidelines for treatment of sexually transmitted diseases. *MMWR* 1998;47(RR-1).

Author: Jane Lavelle

Congenital Hepatic Fibrosis

 Database

DEFINITION

Congenital hepatic fibrosis (CHF) is an inherited, noncirrhotic liver disease associated with cystic disease of the kidneys. Prominent clinical features include portal hypertension and an increased risk of ascending cholangitis. Liver biopsy shows the classic lesion of ductal plate malformation. Patients are typically divided into two groups: those presenting in infancy with severe renal disease (autosomal recessive polycystic kidney disease, or ARPKD) and those presenting later in childhood with symptoms of liver disease predominating. Mortality is high in the group presenting early, but if these patients survive, they later demonstrate hepatic lesions identical to those seen in CHF. The patients presenting in later childhood typically have more mild renal disease. The relationship of ARPKD to CHF is controversial, but many believe that these two developmental disorders of the liver and kidneys represent a single disease entity.

PATHOPHYSIOLOGY

• Ductal plate malformation is a characteristic histologic lesion of the liver, implying a disturbance of the normal formation of the bile ducts. Hallmarks on pathology include persistence of the ductal plate, or increased numbers of large and abnormally shaped duct elements, and increased amounts of noninflammatory fibrosis in the portal tracts. Hepatocytes and lobular architecture appear normal.
• Genetic etiology is currently unknown, but the gene locus has been identified. The developmental abnormalities involve the liver and kidneys, as well as, less commonly, the vasculature and the heart.
• Portal hypertension is thought to result from the fibrosis in the portal tracts, as well as, in some patients, from portal vein abnormalities.

GENETICS

• Inheritance is autosomal recessive in most families.
• The gene causing ARPKD/CHF has not yet been identified, but the locus has been mapped to chromosome 6p21-p12.

EPIDEMIOLOGY

The incidence of ARPKD is 1 per 4,000 to 1 per 8,000 live births.

COMPLICATIONS

• Portal hypertension with hypersplenism and variceal bleeding
• Cholangitis
• Renal and/or hepatic failure
• Associated vascular anomalies in the liver and brain
• Increased risk of hepatocellular or cholangiocarcinoma
• May be associated with congenital heart disease
• Systemic hypertension due to renal involvement

 Differential Diagnosis

• Varies with presentation. Usually differential diagnosis is that of cirrhosis.
• Liver histology is highly characteristic.

 Data Gathering

HISTORY

• CHF most commonly presents with hematemesis or melena, generally between the ages of 5 and 13 years.
• Patients may present with fever and jaundice (cholangitis) or, rarely, with signs of liver failure.
• The majority have hepatosplenomegaly or GI bleeding within the first decade.

Physical Examination

- Firm, enlarged liver with a prominent left lobe
- Splenomegaly
- Kidneys may be palpable.

Laboratory Aids

TESTS

Blood Tests

- Thrombocytopenia and leukopenia associated with hypersplenism
- Liver enzymes and bilirubin are typically normal, although transaminases may be mildly elevated in some patients.
- Usually hepatic synthetic functions (albumin, PT) are normal.
- May see elevated BUN and creatinine with renal involvement

Imaging

- Ultrasound with Doppler: increased echogenicity, splenomegaly, and evidence of portal hypertension
- Angiography: may show duplication of intrahepatic branches of the portal vein
- Renal ultrasound and IVP: minor abnormalities in up to 70% of patients

Liver Biopsy

- Characteristic histology of ductal plate malformation
- Send specimen for bacterial culture.

Therapy

- Suspected cholangitis should be managed with liver biopsy, culture, and appropriate antibiotics. Some patients with chronic cholangitis may require antibiotic prophylaxis.
- Choleretic agents, including ursodeoxycholic acid, are used in bile stasis and refractory cholangitis.
- Prophylactic sclerotherapy provides relief from variceal hemorrhage in many cases.
- Portosystemic shunting may be required.
- Liver transplant may be indicated for chronic cholangitis, recurrent bleeding, or progressive hepatic disease.

Follow-Up

- Watch for recurrent upper gastrointestinal tract bleeding.
- Morbidity occurs mainly from portal hypertension and cholangitis.
- Mortality often results from ascending cholangitis associated with sepsis and hepatic failure.
- Those presenting in infancy may develop chronic renal failure.
- The prognosis is good when the disease presents in older children.

Common Questions and Answers

Q: Will other children of mine be affected?
A: Maybe. The inheritance pattern is autosomal recessive, with the possibility of an affected sibling being 1:4.

Q: Is my child at increased risk if he contracts viral hepatitis?
A: Yes, the underlying liver disease places these patients at increased risk. They should be immunized against hepatitis A and B.

Q: If my child has a fever, does she need to be seen by her doctor?
A: Yes. Patients with CHF who have fever without an obvious source should be evaluated for possible cholangitis, at least by obtaining a blood culture and liver enzymes.

ICD-9-CM 571.5

BIBLIOGRAPHY

Desmet VJ. Congenital diseases of the intrahepatic bile ducts: variations on the theme "ductal plate malformation." *Hepatology* 1992; 16(4):1069–1083.

Mucher G, Becker J, Knapp M, et al. Fine mapping of the autosomal recessive polycystic kidney disease locus (PKHD1) and the genes MUT, RDS, CSNK2b, and GSTA1 at 6p21.1-p12. *Genomics* 1998;48(1):40–45.

Perisic VN. Long-term studies on congenital hepatic fibrosis in children. *Acta Paediatr* 1995; 84:695–696.

Piccoli DA, Witzleben CL. Cystic disease of the liver. In: Suchy FJ, ed. *Liver disease in children*. St. Louis: Mosby, 1994:638–652.

Authors: Kathleen M. Loomes and Andrew E. Mulberg

Congenital Hypothyroidism

 ## Database

DEFINITION

• Primary thyroid failure that is present at birth

PATHOPHYSIOLOGY

• Thyroid gland malformation

—Agenesis: absent thyroid gland
—Dysgenesis: ectopic (e.g., sublingual) or incorrectly formed (e.g., hemigland) thyroid

• Dyshormonogenesis

—Fifteen known defects of thyroxine synthesis, including those in iodide transport and iodide organification

• Transient hypothyroidism

—Maternal ingestion of antithyroid drugs
—Transplacental transfer of maternal antithyroid antibodies (can be transient or permanent damage)
—Exposure to high levels of iodine (povidine) in neonatal period

GENETICS

• Dysgenesis sporadic, with a familial occurrence in 1%
• Dyshormonogenesis is inherited in an autosomal recessive pattern. Most commonly:

—Chromosome 2p: Mutations in the thyroid peroxidase gene result in partial or complete loss of iodide organification function.
—Chromosome 19p: Mutations in the sodium-iodide symporter gene result in an inability to maintain the normal thyroid-to-plasma iodine concentration difference.

EPIDEMIOLOGY

• Worldwide, the incidence of congenital hypothyroidism is 1 in 3,000 to 4,000 births; in North America, it is 1 in 3,700.
• Male:female ratio is 1:2 to 3.
• Eighty percent dysgenesis or agenesis; 20% dyshormonogenesis
• Racial differences in athyreotic hypothyroidism: 1 in 5,526 whites yet 1 in 32,377 blacks.

COMPLICATIONS

• If untreated:

—Severe mental retardation (cretinism)
—Poor motor development
—Poor growth

• Children with hypothyroidism as part of hypopituitarism do not seem to be as significantly affected by their low thyroid hormone levels as do those with primary hypothyroidism.

PROGNOSIS

Excellent, if treatment is started within the first 4 weeks of life. Level of T_4 at birth is an important indicator of long-term sequelae.

 ## Differential Diagnosis

• Developmental

—Transient hypothyroxinemia in the first weeks of life in premature babies

• Metabolic

—Sick euthyroid syndrome in severely ill neonates

• Secondary or tertiary hypothyroidism

—Panhypopituitarism

• Genetic

—Thyroid-binding globulin (TBG) deficiency (X-linked recessive)

• Environmental

—Iodine exposure (e.g., delivery by cesarean section, surgery in the neonatal period)
—Maternal ingestion of antithyroid drugs

• Immunologic

—Transfer of maternal antithyroid and TSH–receptor blocking antibodies

 ## Data Gathering

Most children are diagnosed by the neonatal screening program.

• Five percent to 10% false-negative rate
• Neonatal screening protocols differ state to state (i.e., whether screen T_4 levels, TSH levels, or both).
• Beware in severely ill neonates who are transferred from one unit or hospital to another that sending off the state screen is not overlooked! If missed by the state screening procedure, the findings below are seen within the first 2 months of life.

HISTORY

• Symptoms that may relate to hypothyroidism:

—Prolonged jaundice
—Poor feeding
—Constipation
—Sedate or placid child
—Poor linear growth

• Family history of thyroid disorders:

—Autoimmune thyroid disease
—Vague histories of "mild hypothyroidism" not requiring treatment are often found in families with TBG deficiency.

• Maternal medications
• Birth history
• Results of the newborn screen

 ## Physical Examination

• Signs that may relate to hypothyroidism:

—Hypothermia
—Large fontanelles (especially posterior) with wide cranial sutures
—Coarse facial features, including macroglossia
—Hoarse cry
—Hypotonia
—Delayed deep tendon reflex release
—Distended abdomen
—Umbilical hernia

• Examine for possible goiter; helpful tricks:

—Inspect the base of the tongue for an ectopic gland.
—While supporting the posterior neck and occiput, allow the infant's head to hang back over a parent's arm or examination table. This will extend the neck and allow better visualization of the anterior region.

 ## Laboratory Aids

TESTS

Neonatal Screening Program (Filter Card)

• Although methods vary from state to state, most screen for T_4 and then run TSH levels on the lowest tenth percentile of that day's T_4 values.
• Abnormal results on state screen should prompt *immediate* examination and confirmatory tests.

Confirmatory Tests

• Serum T_4 and TSH are preferable to a repeated filter screen, which may result in delayed diagnosis and treatment.
• If abnormalities in binding are suspected, also check TBG level and free T_4 level or T_3 resin uptake.
• Free T_4 level is the most sensitive indicator of secondary or tertiary hypothyroidism (hypopituitarism).

Imaging

• ^{123}I or technetium thyroid scan will define gland anatomy (agenesis, dysgenesis, or ectopic gland).
• ^{123}I scan with perchlorate washout may also help to identify dyshormonogenesis (especially organification defects).
• ^{123}I scan must be obtained prior to the initiation of thyroxine replacement therapy. If this significantly delays the commencement of treatment, defer scanning until brain growth is complete (2 years of age), when a period off medication can be more safely pursued.

False-Positives

- Blood specimens obtained before 48 hours of life may have "elevated" TSH as a result of the normal postnatal surge.
- TBG deficiency: total T_4 is low, but TSH is normal. Especially consider in males (X-linked).

 Therapy

DRUGS

- L-thyroxine

—10 to 15 μg/kg/d once a day. Titrate dose to keep T_4 in the upper range of normal.
—TSH levels may not come into the normal range for several weeks, even with good T_4 values.

Duration

- Lifelong
- If medication is started without imaging studies and diagnosis is not clear-cut, can stop L-thyroxine following completion of brain growth (2–3 years of age). Reevaluate need for continued supplementation after a 6-week trial off.

DIET

- No restrictions
- Soy formulas may interfere with absorption.

 Follow-Up

WHEN TO EXPECT IMPROVEMENT

- Most children are asymptomatic at diagnosis.
- Parents may note an increase in activity, improvement in feeding, and increase in urination and bowel movements soon after starting treatment.

SIGNS TO WATCH FOR

Poor growth and low T_4 and elevated TSH values suggest poor compliance or undertreatment.

PITFALLS

- X-linked TBG deficiency: low total T_4, normal TSH, and normal free T_4. Diagnose with low TBG level or low T_3 resin uptake. No treatment is necessary!
- Panhypopituitarism: low T_4 and low or low-normal TSH (i.e., loss of the negative feedback loop). Screen with free T_4. Treat with L-thyroxine as would primary hypothyroidism, and investigate for other pituitary hormone deficiencies.

 Common Questions and Answers

Q: Will my child be retarded?
A: It depends on when the diagnosis was made and how quickly treatment was started. Some long-term studies have suggested an increase in learning disabilities when compared with siblings, even in patients treated within the first 4 weeks of life.

Q: What if I forget a dose?
A: Give it as soon as you remember. If it is the next day, give two doses.

Q: How do I give this medicine to my baby?
A: L-thyroxine is only available in tablet form. Crush the tablet between two spoons and dissolve the powder in a small amount of formula or breast milk, which you offer to the baby at the *start* of a feeding to ensure complete ingestion.

Q: Are there side effects from the medication?
A: None. The tablet contains only the hormone that your child's thyroid is not making. It is synthetically produced, so there are no infectious risks.

Q: Should the transient hypothyroxinemia of prematurity be treated with L-thyroxine?
A: Severe hypothyroxinemia in preterm infants has been associated with increased problems in neurologic and mental development later in childhood, but causality has not been established. A randomized, placebo-controlled, double-blind trial of thyroxine supplementation in 200 infants born before 30 weeks' gestation, revealed no improvement in mental, motor, or neurologic outcome at 2 years of age, though higher developmental testing was seen for those born before 27 weeks' gestation.

ICD-9-CM 243

BIBLIOGRAPHY

AAP Section on Endocrinology and Committee on Genetics, and American Thyroid Association Committee on Public Health. Newborn screening for congenital hypothyroidism: recommended guidelines. *Pediatrics* 1993;91(6): 1203–1210.

Brown AL, Fernhoff PM, Milner J, McEwen C, Elsas LS. Racial differences in the incidence of congenital hypothyroidism. *J Pediatr* 1981; 99:934–936.

Fisher DA, Dussault JH, Foley TP, et al. Screening for congenital hypothyroidism: results of screening one million North American infants. *J Pediatr* 1979;94:700–705.

Heyerdahl S, Kase BF, Lie SO. Intellectual development in children with congenital hypothyroidism in relation to recommended thyroxine treatment. *J Pediatr* 1991;118:850–857.

Klett M. Epidemiology of congenital hypothyroidism. *Exp Clin Endocrinol Diabetes* 1997;105[Suppl 4]:19–23.

Kooistra L, Laane C, Vulsma T, et al. Motor and cognitive development in children with congenital hypothyroidism: a long-term evaluation of the effects of neonatal treatment. *J Pediatr* 1994;124:903–909.

Macchia PE, Felice MD, Lauro RD. Molecular genetics of congenital hypothyroidism. *Curr Opin Genet Dev* 1999;9:289–294.

Polk DH. Diagnosis and management of altered fetal thyroid status. *Clin Perinatol* 1994;21: 647–662.

Reuss ML, Paneth N, Pinto-Martin JA, Lorenz JM, Susser M. The relation of transient hypothyroxinemia in preterm infants to neurologic development at two years of age. *N Engl J Med* 1996;334:821–827, 857–858 [editorial].

Van Vliet G. Neonatal hypothyroidism: treatment and outcome. *Thyroid* 1999;9:79–84.

Van Wassenaer AG, Kok JH, deVijlder JJM, et al. Effects of thyroxine supplementation on neurologic development in infants born at less than 30 weeks' gestation. *N Engl J Med* 1997;336:21–26.

Willi SM, Moshang T. Diagnostic dilemmas: results of screening tests for congenital hypothyroidism. *Pediatr Clin North Am* 1991;38(3): 555–566.

Authors: Adda Grimberg and Marta Satin-Smith

Congestive Heart Failure

 Database

DEFINITION

Congestive heart failure (CHF) is the pathophysiologic state in which the heart is unable to pump sufficient blood to meet the metabolic demands of the body.

ETIOLOGY

• Excessive workload (volume and/or pressure) secondary to congenital heart disease (CHD) or acquired heart disease in the presence of normal myocardial function
• Normal workload in the presence of myocardial dysfunction

CAUSES

In Utero

• Arrythmias: supraventricular or ventricular tachycardia, complete heart block (CHB)
• Volume overload: atrioventricular (AV) valve regurgitation or arteriovenous malformations (AVM)
• Primary myocardial disease: cardiomyopathy, myocarditis
• Anemia: Rh disease, fetomaternal and twin-twin transfusion
• Premature closure of foramen ovale or ductus arteriosus

In Neonates

• Myocardial dysfunction: asphyxia, sepsis, myocarditis, hypoglycemia
• Pressure overload: left-sided obstructive lesions (e.g., aortic stenosis, coarctation of the aorta, hypoplastic left-heart syndrome)
• Volume overload: patent ductus arteriosus, truncus arteriosus, aortopulmonary window, total anomalous pulmonary venous return, AVM
• Arrythmias: supraventricular or ventricular arrythmias, CHB

In Infants

• Volume overload: left-to-right shunt physiology (e.g., patent ductus arteriosus, truncus arteriosus, aortopulmonary window, ventricular septal defect, common AV canal defect, total anomalous pulmonary venous return)
• Myocardial dysfunction: endocardial fibroelastosis, glycogen storage disease, myocarditis, Kawasaki syndrome, anomalous left coronary artery from pulmonary artery
• Secondary causes: renal disease, hypertension, hypothyroidism, sepsis
• Arrhythmias: supraventicular

—Ventricular tachycardia, complete heart block

• Pressure overload: coarctation of the aorta, residual aortic stenosis, subaortic membrane

In Childhood and Adolescence

• Unrepaired CHD with volume and/or pressure overload
• Repaired CHD with residual defects that result in volume and/or pressure overload
• Acquired heart disease: pericarditis, myocarditis, endocarditis, acute rheumatic fever
• Secondary causes: hypertension, thyrotoxicosis, chemotherapy (doxorubicin, radiation), sickle cell anemia, cor pulmonale, neuromuscular disease (e.g., Duchenne muscular dystrophy)

 Differential Diagnosis

• Respiratory disease
• Hypoalbuminemia
• Anemia
• Hypothyroidism
• Poisoning: parathione, salicylates
• Arrythmias
• Viral myocarditis
• Syndromes: Marfan, Hurler, Noonan
• Sepsis

 Data Gathering

HISTORY

Infants and Neonates

• Prolonged feedings associated with tachypnea, retractions, and excessive perspiration
• Emesis, inadequate caloric intake, and failure to thrive
• Irritability with feeding and frequent respiratory infections

Childhood and Adolescence

• Exercise intolerance with exertional dyspnea
• Chronic cough, wheezing, orthopnea, fatigue, weakness, anorexia, nausea, and edema
• Weight loss secondary to anorexia and nausea
• Weight gain secondary to fluid retention

 Physical Examination

Infants and Neonates

• Tachycardia
• Gallop
• Tachypnea
• Wheezing
• Crackles
• Retractions
• Nasal flaring
• Grunting
• Hepatomegaly
• Splenomegaly
• Edema (periorbital)
• Cool and/or mottled extremities
• Poor capillary refill
• Weak pulses

Childhood and Adolescence

• Tachycardia
• Gallop
• Tachypnea
• Cool and pale extremities, with cyanosis and poor capillary refill
• Jugular venous distension
• Wheezing ("cardiac asthma")
• Hepatomegaly
• Splenomegaly
• Edema (periorbital or peripheral)
• Pulsus alternans
• Pulsus paradoxus

Laboratory Aids

TESTS

Chest X-Ray

Cardiomegaly, increased pulmonary vascular markings, hyperinflation, pleural effusion

Electrocardiography

- Abnormal P-waves and nonspecific ST-T wave changes
- May help in the diagnosis of a cardiac anomaly (e.g., anomalous left coronary, pericarditis, arrhythmia)

Echocardiography

- Rule out CHD
- Assessment of cardiac function

Cardiac Catheterization

- Delineation of cardiac hemodynamics and anatomy (used only in selected cases)
- Cardiac biopsy may be helpful in the diagnosis of myocarditis or cardiomyopathy
- Electrophysiologic study to delineate arrhythmia

Other Laboratory Findings

- Abnormalities in the pH, PaO_2, and $PaCO_2$ may be seen.
- Hyponatremia, hypokalemia, and/or hypochloremia (2^0 to chronic diuretic therapy)
- Anemia, leukocytosis, or leukopenia (e.g., viral myocarditis)
- Elevation of ESR (e.g., rheumatic fever or Kawasaki syndrome)
- Proteinuria, high urine specific gravity, microscopic hematuria

 Therapy

TREATMENT OF UNDERLYING CAUSE

- Surgical palliation or correction of structural abnormality
- Radiofrequency ablation of arrythmia
- Interventional cardiac catheterization (e.g., balloon dilation of aortic or pulmonary stenosis, coil embolization of patent ductus arteriosus, device closure of atrial septal defect)
- Medical treatment of endocarditis, myocarditis, anemia, or hypertension

MANAGEMENT

- General measures: restriction of physical activity, oxygen, tube feedings, increase in caloric content of feedings, limit of salt intake
- Pharmaceutical management

—Inotropic agents (digoxin, dopamine, dobutamine)
—Diuretics (loop diuretics: e.g., furosemide)
—Afterload reducing agents (angiotensin converting enzyme inhibitors: e.g., captopril and enalapril)

 Follow-Up

Depends on the etiology and degree of CHF

PREVENTION

- Intravenous immunoglobulin (IVIG) for myocarditis
- Limited use of cardiac anthracycline drugs
- SBE prophylaxis to prevent infective endocarditis
- Controlling arrhythmias with pharmacotherapy, or
- Treatment of tachyarrythmias with radiofrequency ablation and bradyarrythmias (CHB) with pacing

PITFALLS

- In patients with CHF, on the basis of left-to-right shunting, spontaneous clinical improvement of CHF may indicate the development of pulmonary vascular disease.
- Patients with a VSD can develop a right ventricular muscle bundle even if the VSD spontaneously closes. Some patients may also develop a subaortic membrane or prolapse of a coronary cusp with subsequent aortic insufficiency.
- In ductal dependent lesions, an increase in PaO_2 with metabolic acidosis may be 2^0 to increased pulmonary blood flow with decreased systemic blood flow.

 Common Questions and Answers

Q: My child has a large ventricular septal defect and is on digoxin and Lasix. Should I take salt out of his diet?
A: No. Excessive salt restriction is not necessary. A no-added-salt diet is sufficient.

Q: What is the importance of tachycardia and bradycardia in heart failure?
A: Tachycardia limits diastolic filling time and may result in a decreased output. However, bradycardia may be poorly tolerated in patients with heart failure and a relatively fixed stroke volume who are dependent on heart rate to maintain an appropriate output.

BIBLIOGRAPHY

Emmanoulides GC, Riemenscheider TA, Allen HD, Gutgesell HP, eds. In: *Moss and Adams. Heart disease in infants, children, and adolescents, including the fetus and the young adult,* 5th ed. Baltimore: Williams & Wilkins, 1995.

Fyler DC, ed. *Nadas' pediatric cardiology.* Philadelphia: Hanley & Belfus, 1992.

Author: Hae-Rhi Lee

Conjunctivitis

 Database

DEFINITION

Conjunctivitis is an inflammatory (usually infectious) process involving the mucous membrane of the eye (conjunctiva). It is manifested by redness and swelling of the conjunctiva, with associated discharge.

PATHOPHYSIOLOGY

Bacterial, viral, allergic, or toxic activation of the inflammatory response, which causes dilation and exudation from conjunctival blood vessels

PATHOLOGY

• Dilated conjunctival capillaries with leukocytic infiltration and edema of conjunctiva and substantial propria
• In children with competent lymphocyte function (>3 months of age), visible conjunctival lymphoid follicles may develop.

GENETICS

No clear genetic profile

EPIDEMIOLOGY

• Viral conjunctivitis is extremely common, and highly contagious. Adenovirus is the common cause.
• Contagious conjunctivitis may also be caused by bacteria (staphylococci, streptococci, and *Haemophilus*). Serious complications are rare.
• Ophthalmia neonatorum (neonatal conjunctivitis) remains a significant cause of blindness worldwide.
• *Chlamydia*, herpes simplex, and chemicals such as silver nitrate are other causes.

COMPLICATIONS

• Extremely rare for common bacterial, viral, or allergic conjunctivitis
• Blindness may result from untreated neonatal conjunctivitis.

 Differential Diagnosis

FOR NEONATAL CONJUNCTIVITIS

• Chemical conjunctivitis

—Noninfectious, mild, self-limited
—Result of silver nitrate administration (Credé prophylaxis)

• Birth trauma

—Unilateral, often with associated eyelid contusion
—History of forceps use or difficult delivery

• Congenital glaucoma

—Mild conjunctival redness, minimal discharge
—Look for enlarged eye, cloudy cornea, tearing, and photophobia

• Nasolacrimal duct obstruction

—Unilateral or bilateral discharge
—May be clear to mucopurulent with reflux from nasolacrimal sac
—Usually, conjunctiva is white and uninflamed

FOR ALL CONJUNCTIVITIS

• Preseptal cellulitis

—Early eyelid edema/erythema
—Looks like conjunctivitis, especially in young children, who are difficult to examine
—Motility deficit, proptosis, decreased vision, afferent pupillary defect—orbital cellulitis

• Keratitis

—Keratitis signifies corneal infection and may have associated conjunctivitis.
—Primary herpes keratitis is associated with vesicular eyelid rash and pain.
—Consult an ophthalmologist for specific treatment. Bacterial keratitis may be caused by staphylococci, streptococci, and *Pseudomonas;* Lyme spirochete; or vitamin A deficiency.

• Iritis

—Usually unilateral, with or without a history of trauma
—Photophobia, decreased vision, and constant pain (except associated with juvenile rheumatoid arthritis)
—A contagious history is rare.
—Consult an ophthalmologist for full examination, including pupillary dilation.

 Data Gathering

HISTORY

• Type I ophthalmia neonatorum (<40–60 days of age)

—Acute perinatal conjunctivitis with purulent discharge

• Type 2 ophthalmia neonatorum

—"Pink eye"
—Red, watery eyes with acute onset, with or without upper respiratory tract infection
—Often, history of similar infection in siblings or contacts
—Usually viral, occasionally bacterial, commonly self-limited

 Physical Examination

• Discharge ranges from clear, watery (often viral) to mucopurulent (often bacterial).
• Conjunctiva are inflamed and edematous.
• May have eyelid swelling or submandibular and preauricular lymphadenopathy
• Cornea clear
• Vision, pupils, and motility are normal.
• Refer to an ophthalmologist if vesicular rash is present on eyelids and corneal changes are present (possible herpes simplex).

 Laboratory Aids

TESTS

• Gram stain of discharge (always in ophthalmia neonatorum):

—Gonococcus (GC): gram-negative intracellular diplococcus
—Polymorphonuclear leukocytes without bacteria likely chemical (neonatal) or viral conjunctivitis
—Intracytoplasmic, paranuclear inclusion bodies on Gram stain: *Chlamydia*

• Culture

—Thayer-Martin test for GC
—Viral cultures for herpesvirus and adenovirus are not clinically useful.
—*Chlamydia* culture techniques are not widely available.

• Immunofluorescence staining

—May be useful in identifying *Chlamydia* infection

Therapy

- *GC:* Aqueous penicillin G, 100,000/kg/d IV q.i.d for 7 days *or* ceftriaxone, 28 to 50 mg/kg/d IV q8 to 12h *and* ocular irrigation followed by topical 0.5% erythromycin or 1.0% tetracycline ophthalmic ointments q.i.d for 14 days.
- *Chlamydia:* Oral erythromycin syrup, 12.5 mg/kg/d in four doses for 14 days. Topical 0.5% erythromycin *or* 1.0% tetracycline ophthalmic ointment q.i.d both eyes for 14 days. Recurrence or intolerance is treated with trimethoprim-sulfamethoxazole, 0.5 mL/kg/d in two divided doses for 14 days and topical ointments as above.
- *Herpes simplex:* Topical trifluorothymidine (viroptic solution), nine times a day for at least 14 days with or without systemic acyclovir (IV solution)
- *Chemical*

—Close observation only
—Self-limited

- *Viral or epidemic keratoconjunctivitis*

—Cool compresses
—May use empiric antibiotic treatment if bacterial infection is suspected, including erythromycin 0.5%, tetracycline 1% ointment, or polymyxin B solution four times a day.
—No specific antiadenovirus treatment is available.

 Follow-Up

- Daily follow-up is necessary for GC, *Chlamydia,* and herpes simplex virus.
- For epidemic viral conjunctivitis, frequency is dictated by severity (daily to weekly).

NATURAL HISTORY

- GC conjunctivitis is benign if recognized early, and devastating if misdiagnosed or delayed.
- *Chlamydia* chronic infection leads to scarring and corneal opacity; *chlamydial* pneumonia develops in 20% of these patients.
- Viral: usually benign course, but may rarely lead to conjunctival scarring
- HSV may lead to significant visual loss from recurrence and corneal scarring, even with proper therapy.

PITFALLS

- Failure to diagnose GC conjunctivitis may lead to corneal perforation (ocular disaster).
- Recommending no follow-up routinely

—Follow atypical conjunctivitis closely until a more serious disease can be excluded.
—A nonresponsive or worsening condition needs ophthalmic consultation.

- Treating any red eye with steroids

—Activates or accelerates unrecognized HSV infection
—Chronic administration may raise intraocular pressure or cause cataracts.

- Chronic use of empiric broad-spectrum antibiotics for self-limited conjunctivitis promotes bacterial resistance.
- It is critical to rule out GC infection because of the destructive nature of eye disease *and* associated systemic infection.

 Common Questions and Answers

Q: Is conjunctivitis contagious?
A: All infectious conjunctivitis is contagious, but to varying degrees. Viral or epidemic keratoconjunctivitis (EKC) is the most contagious. Careful handling of secretions, tissues, towels, bed linens, and strict hand washing usually prevent spread. Wipe surfaces with isopropyl alcohol or dilute bleach to prevent recontamination. GC, *Chlamydia,* and HSV can be transmitted through infected discharge or secretions, but this is less common. The most common source is the infected birth canal.

Q: Should the patient with "pink eye" (non-GC, non-*Chlamydia,* non-HSV conjunctivitis) be treated with empiric antibiotics?
A: Empiric treatment with topical antibiotics does little harm except for sulfa-containing compounds. Antibiotic toxicity, including Stevens-Johnson reactions, can occur from sulfa antibiotics, and use of antibiotics long term promotes selection of resistant strains of bacteria.

ICD-9-CM 372.30

BIBLIOGRAPHY

Bell TA, Grayston JT, Krohn MA, Krommal RA, Eye Prophylaxis Study Group. Randomized trial of silver nitrate, erythromycin and no prophylaxis for the presence of conjunctivitis among newborns not at risk for gonococcal ophthalmitis. *Pediatrics* 1993;92:755–760.

Brown ZA, Vontrer LA, Bonchetti J, et al. Effects on infants of a first episode of genital herpes during pregnancy. *N Engl J Med* 1977;317:1246–1251.

Crede CSF. Reports from the obstetrical clinic in Leipzig: prevention of eye inflammation in the newborn. *Am J Dis Child* 1971;121:3–4.

Isenberg SJ, Apt L, Yoshimori R, et al. The source of the conjunctival flora at birth and implications for ophthalmia neonatorum prophylaxis. *Am J Ophthalmol* 1988;106:458–462.

Chen JY. Prophylaxis of ophthalmia neonatorum: comparison of silver nitrate, tetracycline, erythromycin and no prophylaxis. *Pediatr Infect Dis J* 1992;11(12):1026–1030.

Author: Martin C. Wilson

Constipation

Database

DEFINITION

Constipation is the passage of infrequent bowel movements, which may be hard or painful. It also may refer to a decrease in frequency of bowel movements compared with the patient's usual bowel pattern. Constipation can result in pain, rectal bleeding, and encopresis or soiling.

CAUSES

• Most patients will have idiopathic or functional constipation with no identifiable cause.

—There is usually an acute event followed by chronicity.

• Hard stools cause anal pain or a fissure, leading to intentional or subconscious withholding.

—This results in rectal dilatation, decreased sensation, shortening of the anal canal, decreased tone of the external anal sphincter, and leaking.

• Precipitating events include the following:

—Transition from breast milk to cow's milk in infants

—Power struggle in toddlers

—Refusal to use toilets outside the home

—Streptococcal infection of the anus and perianal area

—Transient viral illness (diarrhea followed by constipation)

—Zealous toilet training

• Constipation also can be caused by anatomic anomalies in the lower gastrointestinal (GI) tract, decreased propulsion, impaired rectal sensation (primary or secondary), or a functional outlet obstruction (muscular spastic levator ani or impaired relaxation of the puborectalis).

• Neurologic causes (abnormalities of the myenteric plexus, intestinal pseudoobstruction, congenital aganglionosis, intestinal neuronal dysplasia, muscular diseases (familial and nonfamilial visceral myopathies), and lesions of the spinal cord result in loss of rectal tone and sensation and reduced anal closure, affecting the sacral reflex center (e.g., myelomeningocele, spina bifida occulta, tethered cord).

• Anatomic disorders of anus and rectum (stricture, stenosis, mass, ectopic anus, imperforate anus)

• Endocrine abnormalities (hypothyroidism), drugs, electrolyte abnormalities

PATHOPHYSIOLOGY

• Retention of stool allows water to move out of stool, increasing size and firmness.

• Decreased motility will lead to retention of stool. See Causes.

GENETICS

Often a family history of motility disturbances or constipation can be found. A genetic basis for Hirschsprung disease and certain forms of intestinal pseudoobstruction has been found.

COMPLICATIONS

• Anal fissures: Infrequent hard stools can cause a tear of the anal mucosa, causing pain and withholding.

• Encopresis: Chronic constipation leads to progressive rectal dilatation and decreased rectal sensation. Fecal impaction results with secondary soiling or encopresis.

• Intestinal obstruction manifests as vomiting, abdominal pain, and constipation, with abdominal x-ray (AXR) films showing intestinal obstruction and presence of large amounts of stool.

• Sigmoid volvulus: A chronically constipated child may present with symptoms of acute abdomen, fever, tender abdomen, and palpable mass. AXR shows obstruction in the colon. Barium enema may be both diagnostic as well as therapeutic by achieving reduction.

• Hirschsprung enterocolitis can occur in an infant with a history suspicious for Hirschsprung disease, who is now toxic, febrile with abdominal distention, and has bloody diarrhea. AXR can show a dilated colon.

PROGNOSIS

For functional constipation, the success rate is variable (45%—90%), depending on the treatment and follow-up. Presence of abdominal pain at the time of presentation, close follow-up, and use of mineral oil were good prognostic factors. Presence of soiling, use of Senokot, and lack of follow-up were associated with failure and recurrences.

Differential Diagnosis

• Hirschsprung disease: congenital aganglionic megacolon (i.e., the absence of ganglion cells)

• Neuromuscular causes: tethered spinal cord

• Anal abnormalities: anteriorly displaced anus, ectopic anus, imperforate anus

• Endocrine abnormalities: hypothyroidism and hyperparathyroidism

• Electrolyte imbalance: hypokalemia, hyponatremia, hypomagnesemia, hypercalcemia

• Lead ingestion: can present with anemia, constipation, and abdominal pain

• Infant botulism: constipation, aphonia, and weakness in a previously well infant

• Chronic intestinal pseudoobstruction syndrome: can present with abdominal distention, diarrhea, and constipation; usually a diagnosis of exclusion

• Abdominopelvic mass: can cause constipation by pressure (i.e., distended bladder or pelvic tumor)

• Surgical conditions: Malrotation, congenital intestinal bands, intestinal stenoses, acquired colonic strictures resulting from inflammatory bowel disease (IBD), necrotizing enterocolitis (NEC), pyloric stenosis

• Drugs: calcium supplements, barium, opiates; always get a careful drug history to avoid missing drug-related constipation.

Data Gathering

HISTORY

Question: What is the timing of the passage of meconium?
Significance: If it is delayed for more than 24 to 48 hours, consider Hirschsprung disease.

Question: Is the child able to pass a bowel movement unaided by a suppository or enema?
Significance: If rectal stimulation is required for passage of a bowel movement, think of Hirschsprung disease or habituation to rectal stimulation.

Question: What are the size, frequency, and consistency of bowel movements?
Significance: One to three normal (in size and consistency) painless bowel movements may be passed every 1 to 3 days. The size of bowel movements reflects the caliber of the colon.

Question: Does the child experience frequent urination, bed wetting, or urinary tract infections?
Significance: These are seen frequently with chronic constipation.

Question: Is there soiling?
Significance: Soiling occurs if the stool is impacted or with nerve damage involving the anus.

Question: Is there presence of rectal sensation?
Significance: Patients with long-standing constipation or withholding who develop a dilated rectum will often lose the sensation of rectal distention.

Question: Is there a history of painful bowel movements or rectal fissure?
Significance: This could be the cause of withholding secondary to fear of painful bowel movements.
Some children are too busy playing to take the time to have a bowel movement. Some children do not want to use the toilet in school because of hygiene issues.

Question: Is the child experiencing any stressful events (i.e., new sibling, death in family)?
Significance: Stress can precipitate stool withholding, leading to constipation.

Question: Does the child have an unsteady or clumsy gait?
Significance: This may suggest neuromuscular problems.

Question: Did the child experience difficult toilet training?
Significance: Some children with encopresis have a history of difficult toilet training.

Question: What is the diet history for fluid, milk, caffeine, and fiber intake?
Significance: Excessive amounts of milk (calcium) and caffeine may be constipating in some individuals. Diets low in fiber and fluid can cause constipation.

Physical Examination

- **General:** Look for evidence of systemic illness.
- **Abdomen:** Abdominal distension (indicative of the presence of stool or gas), presence of stool masses (size, location), distended bladder and bowel sounds (may be decreased in intestinal pseudoobstruction).
- **Rectal examination:** Perianal soiling, size and position of anus (may suggest imperforate or ectopic anus), presence of skin tags and fissures and perianal or anal erythema (streptococcal proctitis), or evidence of child abuse. On digital examination, assess anal tone (in functional constipation, anal tone is decreased; Hirschsprung disease may cause the anal canal to appear very long and tight), amount and consistency of stool, size of rectum (dilated rectum suggestive of chronic constipation; tight and empty anus suggestive of Hirschsprung disease), and presence of blood. Absence of anal wink suggests neurologic abnormalities.
- **Neurologic examination:** Check reflexes in the lower extremities.
- **Back:** Check for sacral dimple, tuft of hair (suggestive of underlying sacral abnormality), flat buttocks, and patulous anus.

PITFALLS

- "Grunting baby syndrome": Infants with this syndrome cry, scream, and draw up their legs during a bowel movement. They respond to rectal distention by contracting their pelvic floor. This is not constipation.
- Always rule out an organic cause for constipation.
- Compliance and good follow-up are key to successful management of functional constipation.

Laboratory Aids

TESTS

- **Abdominal x-ray study:** Look for presence and location of stool and evidence of bowel obstruction.
- **Unprepped barium enema:** useful in Hirschsprung disease; will show a narrow transition zone (affected bowel) with proximal dilated colon or small bowel, depending on extent of the disease. In very young infants, a transition zone may not be seen.
- **Anorectal manometry:** may be useful in Hirschsprung disease (failure of relaxation of the internal anal sphincter) and in patients with encopresis who do not respond to conventional therapy
- **Suction rectal biopsy:** useful in identifying patients with Hirschsprung disease. Absence of ganglion cells is suspicious; always needs to be confirmed by a full-thickness surgical rectal biopsy

Therapy

TREATMENT OF FUNCTIONAL CONSTIPATION

- **Clean-out:** If patient is impacted, then a series of three to five enemas may be required, depending on the amount of retained stool. In general, children over 2 to 3 years of age require adult-size phosphate enemas. Younger children should get pediatric-size enemas. Oral or nasogastric polyethylene glycol solution (Go-Lytely) given over 6 to 8 hours may be used for clean-out. The solution is given until the effluent is clear.
- **Stool softeners:** Infants up to 1 year of age may be given dark Karo syrup or Maltsupex (1 tsp/8 oz of formula) several times a day. Children over 1 year of age may get mineral oil, lactulose, or milk of magnesia several times a day to soften stools and make their passage easier.
- **Stimulant laxatives:** Sennokot may be used as a stimulant for short periods of time. Long-term use has been associated with colonic nerve damage in adults.
- **Diet:** A high-fiber diet is recommended (toddler: 10–12 g/d; school-aged: 12–16 g/d; adolescent: 16–20 g/d). In some patients, caffeine and excessive milk-product intake may be constipating. Milk intake should be limited to 16 ounces a day.
- **Toilet sitting:** regular toilet sitting twice a day for 10 minutes, preferably after meals, to help retrain the bowel
- **Calendar:** It is important to keep a record of stools, accidents, toilet sitting, and medication intake. It is hard for parents to remember details, which may be important in identifying causes of failure.
- **Fluid intake:** High fluid intake is important.
- **Biofeedback** is helpful in patients who fail conventional therapy and have the following abnormalities on anorectal manometry: decreased sensory threshold to rectal distension, paradoxical contraction of the external anal sphincter and puborectalis muscle during simulated defecation.

TREATMENT OF COMPLICATIONS

- **Encopresis (soiling or "diarrhea"):** Abdominal x-ray (AXR) film shows large amounts of stool in the colon, including a dilated rectum. Disimpaction or clean-out, followed by treatment of constipation, is recommended (see above).
- **Intestinal obstruction:** vomiting, abdominal pain, and constipation. AXR film shows intestinal obstruction. Make NPO, give IV fluids, and rule out an acute abdomen. Then give enemas and clear out stool from below. Never give oral laxatives or a polyethylene glycol solution in a case of obstruction.

- **Sigmoid volvulus:** chronically constipated child with symptoms of acute abdomen, fever, tender abdomen, and palpable mass. AXR shows obstruction in the colon. Barium enema may reveal a volvulus and may reduce the volvulus.
- **Hirschsprung enterocolitis:** in an infant who presents with a history suspicious for Hirschsprung disease, who is now toxic, febrile with abdominal distention, and has bloody diarrhea. AXR shows dilated colon with or without a transition zone: NPO, IV fluids, antibiotics. Rectal tube and enemas are controversial. Obtain a surgical consult.

Follow-Up

- Schedule regular visits to make sure therapy is maintained.
- Have parents call as soon as problems develop.
- Once patient is doing well, decrease the frequency of visits.

PREVENTION

- **Dietary measures:** high-fiber diet, plenty of fluids, avoidance of excessive caffeine intake

Common Questions and Answers

Q: When is constipation an emergency?
A: When intestinal obstruction, sigmoid volvulus, or Hirschsprung enterocolitis occur.

ICD-9-CM 564.0

BIBLIOGRAPHY

Abi-Hanna A, Lake AM. Constipation and encopresis in childhood. *Pediatr Rev* 1998;19(1): 23–30; quiz 31.

Loening-Baucke V. Chronic constipation in children. *Gastroenterology* 1993;105:1557–1564.

Seth R, Heyman MB. Management of constipation and encopresis in infants and children. *Gastroenterol Clin North Am* 1994;23(4): 621–636.

Staiano GS. The long term follow up of children with chronic idiopathic constipation. *Arch Dis Child* 1992;67:340.

Author: Maria R. Mascarenhas

Contact Dermatitis

 Database

DEFINITION

Contact dermatitis is an eczematous eruption that may result from two different processes: direct irritation to the skin or a delayed hypersensitivity reaction to a contact allergen.

PATHOPHYSIOLOGY

- Direct irritation to the skin commonly results from harsh soaps, acids, certain foods, saliva, urine, and feces.
- Common allergens resulting in delayed hypersensitivity reactions include:

—Vinyl
—Cosmetics
—Preservatives
—Fragrances
—Dyes
—Metals (particularly nickel)
—Topical medications
—Plasticizers in rubber products
—Poison ivy

- Results in nonspecific findings of intracellular edema and inflammation, indistinguishable from other forms of eczema

GENETICS

Susceptibility to certain contact allergens for delayed hypersensitivity is in part genetically determined.

EPIDEMIOLOGY

Contact dermatitis can occur at any age, although young infant skin is more easily irritated by a primary irritant, but seems to be less likely to develop a delayed hypersensitivity response.

COMPLICATIONS

Generally, there are no long-term complications, although secondary bacterial infections may occur.

PROGNOSIS

Complete resolution can be expected after elimination of further exposure to the allergen.

 Differential Diagnosis

- Infection

—Impetigo (bacterial infections of the skin, usually caused by *Staphylococcus* or *Streptococcus*, with characteristic yellow, crusty lesion)
—Scabies: Skin lesions from itching and topical therapies may resemble atopic dermatitis.

- Tumors

—Letterer-Siwe (or Langerhans cell histiocytosis) is an uncommon disease that may present with a rash that begins with a scaly erythematous eruption on the scalp, behind the ears, or in the intertriginous regions, and is differentiated by the presence of small reddish-brown papules or vesicles, purpuric lesions, hepatosplenomegaly, and adenopathy.

- Metabolic

—Acrodermatitis enteropathica (deficiency of zinc, in addition to vesiculobullous lesions of the hands and feet, and surrounding mouth and diaper areas). These patients have failure to thrive, diarrhea, alopecia, and frequent bacterial and candidal infections.

- Immunologic

—Atopic dermatitis usually affects infants at a later onset, is very pruritic, and is often accompanied by a family history of atopy.
—Seborrheic dermatitis: erythematous, scaly, or crusting lesions that are characteristically yellow or salmon-colored and greasy; it tends to involve the scalp, face, and postauricular and intertriginous areas.
—Nummular eczema, named for its characteristic "coin-like" lesions that develop on areas of dry skin, usually begins as tiny papules and vesicles.
—Psoriasis (known for its silvery adherent scale and underlying reddish hue; these lesions have well-delineated margins and usually affect the scalp, extensor surfaces, and genital regions. Guttate (teardrop-shaped) psoriasis is often seen after bacterial and viral infections (especially streptococcal).

 Data Gathering

HISTORY

- The diagnosis is made by determining contact of an offending allergen with the areas of skin involved.
- Obtaining the history of offending allergens is often difficult.
- Depending on the distribution of skin involved, particular allergens may be specifically asked about.
- Having the patient keep a diary may provide clues to other allergens as inciting agents.

 Physical Examination

- Diagnosis is determined by the recognition of the erythematous, edematous, and papular-vesicular eczematous lesions and the distribution of the rash.
- Contact dermatitis commonly shows sharp delimitation or bizarre asymmetric distributions.
- Determining the distribution of the rash may give clues to the etiology. Areas where clothes contact the skin, such as wrist or waist, may suggest detergent or flame-retardant allergies; eruptions on the face and hands suggest a soap dermatitis.

 Laboratory Aids

TESTS

The patch test is the controlled exposure of an antigen to the skin. It should be used only to confirm a suspected allergen. After removal of the patch (generally 48 hours) the skin is examined 20 to 60 minutes later for erythema, papules, vesicles, or bullae.

PITFALLS

- The patch test may be falsely positive if done during times when the skin is acutely inflamed or if it is performed too closely to the previously existing dermatitis.
- The patch test should not be done while the patient is on antihistamines.

Therapy

- Mainstay therapy is eliminating future exposure to the irritant or allergen.
- Application of cool compresses and topical antipruritic lotions such as calamine can be helpful.
- Topical corticosteroids will help with the pruritus but will not accelerate resolution of the rash.
- The therapy should be continued for as long as the rash is present. Systemic antihistamines are generally not helpful for treating contact dermatitis.
- In severe cases, systemic corticosteroids may be used for a short course, with a tapering course to avoid a rebound of the dermatitis.

 ## Follow-Up

- Follow-up depends on the severity of the dermatitis and elimination of continued exposure to the allergen.
- Generally, improvement is seen in 5 to 7 days.

PREVENTION

Prevention is the only approach to reduce the incidence of contact dermatitis. Use of lotions with potential topical sensitizers, such as benzocaine and antihistamines, should be avoided. Desensitization, using systemic administration of the allergen, is not effective.

 ## Common Questions and Answers

Q: Can the fluid from blisters caused by poison ivy spread the rash to other parts of the body?
A: The contents of the vesicles and bullae from rhus dermatitis are not contagious. After exposure to poison ivy is eliminated, new lesions appear because of the variable sensitivity of various areas of the body to the allergen.

ICD-9-CM 692.9

BIBLIOGRAPHY

Beltrani VS, Beltrani VP. Contact dermatitis. *Ann Allergy Asthma Immunol* 1997;78:160–173.

Friedlander SF. Contact dermatitis. *Pediatr Rev* 1998;19:166–171.

Hurwitz S. *Clinical pediatric dermatology,* 2nd ed. Philadelphia: WB Saunders, 1993.

Author: Robert Kamei

Contraception

Database

DEFINITION

Contraception is the prevention of conception or pregnation. The "ideal" contraceptive is 100% effective (prevents pregnancy over a 1-year period in all of 100 patients with typical use), has no side effects, can be easily reversed, and can be easily used by teen-agers.

CLASSES OF CONTRACEPTIVES AND THEIR HEALTH BENEFITS

• *Abstinence* (only "ideal" contraceptive)

—Very effective method of preventing transmission of HIV, viral hepatitis, syphilis, *Neisseria gonorrhea, Chlamydia trachomatis*

• *Barriers methods* to sperm entry (male and female condoms, diaphragm)

—Male condoms are 88% effective with typical use. The female condom and diaphragm with spermicide are 75% and 85% effective, respectively.
—Male and female condom use prevents spread of sexually transmitted diseases (STDs) such as HIV, viral hepatitis, syphilis, *N. gonorrhea*, and *C. trachomatis*.

• *Spermicidal agents* (foam, film, vaginal inserts)

—Nonoxynal-9 is the active agent most widely used.
—Seventy-nine percent effective in preventing pregnancy with typical use.
—Reduce transmission of *C. trachomatis* and *N. gonorrhea*.
—Spermicides used with condoms will increase efficacy to 93% with typical use.

• *Hormonal agents* (oral contraceptives [OCPs], Depo-Provera, Norplant, and emergency contraception)

—Three categories of OCP's include fixed dose combination pills, combination phasic preparations, and the progestin only mini-pill.

—Fixed-dose combination pills containing a steady dose of estrogen and progestin
—Combination phasic preparations containing varying doses of estrogen and progestin. They vary to simulate the normal physiologic cycle.

—The mini-pill contains only a small dose of progestin. This is an appropriate method for patients at increased risk for estrogen-dependent complications (e.g., sickle cell patients, patients with a history of thromboembolic phenomena).
—The progestin-only mini-pill, Depo-Provera, and Norplant contain only progesterone.
—Estrogen/progestin combined OCPs are 94% to 97% effective in preventing pregnancy with typical use (99.9% effective with perfect use).

—Estrogen/progestin combined OCPs have been shown to reduce the incidence of endometrial and ovarian cancers after as little as 3 months of use, protect against salpingitis (PID) and subsequent ectopic pregnancies, and decrease incidence of benign breast disease and dysmenorrhea, and are effectively used to treat problems such as dysfunctional uterine bleeding and polycystic ovary syndrome.
—Depo-Provera and Norplant contain only progesterone.

—Depo-Provera and Norplant are 99.7% and 99.9% effective, respectively, in preventing pregnancy.
—Emergency contraception, also called post-coital contraception, is a safe back-up method of contraception.

—Failure rates of emergency contraception are 2% per single use and 24% if repeated each month.

—Failure rates of emergency contraception are 2% per single use and 24% annually if repeated each month. Emergency contraception should be used only as a backup method.

• *Intrauterine devices* (not currently recommended for teen-agers)

PATHOPHYSIOLOGY

• The spermicides nonoxynol-9 and octoxynol-9 act by destroying sperm-cell membranes.
• Most spermicide preparations contain an inert base (foam, cream, or jelly) to support the spermicidal agent and provide a barrier to sperm entry.
• Hormonal therapy suppresses ovulation by directly decreasing release of GnRH from the hypothalamus, and FSH and LH from the pituitary.
• Progesterone causes thickening of the cervical mucus, a thin endometrium, and decreased tubal motility.

COMPLICATIONS

Barrier Methods

• Latex allergy: Patients may use polyurethane rather than latex condoms.
• Breakage or permeability: Oil-based lubricants used with latex condoms will increase the risks of these complications.
• Irritation, urinary tract infections (if the wrong size is used), and toxic shock syndrome (if left in place longer than 24 hours) may be seen with diaphragm use.

Spermicides

• Local irritation or allergic reaction

Hormonal Contraceptives

• Mortality from gynecologic and related causes of 15- to 19-year-olds was 7.0 (per 100,000 women) if no fertility control measures were used, 0.3 in nonsmoking OCP users, and 2.2 in smoking OCP users.
• Menstrual irregularities

• Spotting
• Nausea, breast changes, fluid retention, leukorrhea, headache, and hepatocellular adenoma are estrogen dose-dependent side effects.
• Thromboembolic events (MI, PE, and CVA) related to estrogen
• Increased appetite, depression, fatigue, decreased libido, and headache are progesterone-related side effects.
• Nausea and/or vomiting occurs in most patients using emergency contraception or "doubling up" on OCPs.

PROGNOSIS

• Compliance is poor in teen-agers.
• Within 3 months of OCP use, only 44% to 45% of patients remain compliant. After 1 year, only 33% are compliant.

Data Gathering

HISTORY

General considerations in method selection include the following:

• What is the teen's sexual history?
• Is sexual activity spontaneous or planned?
• Does the patient feel that she/he can be compliant with a daily pill or barrier methods?
• Does the patient require absolute confidentiality?
• Is the patient comfortable touching genitals?
• Does the patient have open communication with the partner?
• Does the patient want pregnancy? Does the partner?

Absolute contraindications to *estrogen-containing* OCPs include the following:

• History of cholestatic jaundice or hepatic tumor
• History of estrogen-dependent neoplasm
• History of MI, CVA, PE, or DVT
• Angina pectoris
• Undiagnosed vaginal bleeding
• Pregnancy

Relative contraindications to *estrogen-containing* OCPs include the following:

• Migraine or other vascular headache
• Cardiac, gallbladder, or renal disease
• Untreated hypertension
• Mental depression
• Insulin-dependent diabetes
• Elevated cholesterol or triglycerides
• Seizure disorder
• Sickle cell or other hemoglobinopathies
• Use of medication or drug with interactive effect

Physical Examination

• Obtain baseline weight and blood pressure.
• Document normal anatomy.

Laboratory Aids

- Pregnancy test prior to initiating hormonal contraceptives
- Lipid profile if there is a family history of sudden death or cardiovascular disease

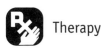 ## Therapy

BARRIER METHODS

Trained personnel can teach the proper technique for application of male and female condoms.

SPERMICIDES

- These must be inserted near the time of intercourse; some formulations require 10 to 15 minutes for activation, and most have an unpleasant taste.
- Trained office personnel can teach the proper technique for insertion.

ORAL CONTRACEPTIVES

- OCP monthly packages contain 3 weeks of hormone, followed by 1 week of placebo.
- Menstruation begins after 2 or 3 days of placebo.
- OCPs are taken as a daily pill, preferably at the same time every day (at night with food, to minimize nausea).
- OCPs are usually started on the first Sunday after the menstrual period begins.
- OCPs may not offer protection during the first cycle; therefore, a backup barrier method should be used.
- Fertility returns, on average, 2 to 3 months after discontinuation. One percent to 2% of patients will experience a delay in fertility for up to 1 year.

OTHER HORMONAL AGENTS

- Depo-Provera, an injectable form of medroxyprogesterone acetate, is given intramuscularly in the deltoid or gluteus maximus.

—Each shot has a 3-month duration, with subsequent shots occurring every 12 weeks.
—The shot should be given within 5 days after the start of the last menstrual period.
—Depo-Provera offers contraceptive protection immediately.
—Fertility (and ovulatory cycles) should return within 6 months of the last injection.

- Norplant is an implant of levonorgestrel.

—It employs six matchstick-sized implants placed subcutaneously.
—Contraceptive protection extends for 5 years or until removal.

EMERGENCY CONTRACEPTION

- Emergency contraception, or post-coital contraception, does not include synthetic chemicals, such as RU486.

- The Yuzpe regimen is safe and well studied. It consists of two fixed dose combination pills (usually Ovral), containing at least 50 μg of estrogen each, taken within 72 hours of unprotected intercourse. This is followed by two additional pills in 12 hours.
- This high dose of estrogen (200 μg total) will almost always cause nausea and vomiting, therefore, pretreatment with an antiemetic is recommended.
- The FDA has approved the marketing of emergency contraception (Preven). It consists of four pills that contain concentrations of estrogen/progestin similar to those of the Yuzpe regimen.

DRUG INTERACTIONS

- Drugs that activate the cytochrome P-450 enzyme will diminish the efficacy of hormonal contraceptives. This is of greatest concern with low-dose preparations and can be remedied by using higher doses.
- Drugs that diminish hormonal contraceptive effects include phenobarbital, carbemazepine, primidone, rifampin, griseofulvin, and tetracyclines (including doxycycline). Hormonal contraceptives can increase levels of phenytoins, benzodiazepines, antidepressants, corticosteroids, β-blockers, theophylline, and alcohol. Hormonal contraceptives can decrease the efficacy of acetaminophen, oral anticoagulants, guanethidine, hypoglycemics, and methyldopa.
- Practitioners should refer to the *Physician's Desk Reference* for any question of drug interactions.

 ## Follow-Up

- Patients using hormonal contraceptives should be seen within 6 weeks to 3 months of initiation to evaluate compliance and side effects.
- Patients should contact a health-care professional immediately if they experience severe headaches; a change in vision; shortness of breath; chest, arm, or leg pain; tingling or numbness; dizziness; or nausea.
- Blood pressure should be monitored at every visit.

PREVENTION

- Only male and female condoms protect against STDs.
- Encourage the consistent use of latex condoms.
- Patients using OCPs must be strongly encouraged to cease tobacco use. Methods of treating nicotine dependence should be employed if indicated.

PITFALLS

- Contraceptive use may lead to patients discontinuing use of condoms. Providers should emphasize at every visit that only condoms protect against STDs.

- Practitioners who are reluctant to use of contraceptives in adolescents should balance the risks of pregnancy with that of contraceptive method. Risks are usually much greater with pregnancy.

 ## Common Questions and Answers

Q: My patient asks for confidentiality regarding contraception. Should I give it to her?
A: Yes, teenagers have the right to confidentiality regarding contraception and treatment of STDs. It may be in the patient's best interest to have a caring adult involved.

Q: If there are so many potential side effects to hormonal methods, shouldn't I just recommend barrier methods?
A: Choice of contraceptive method should occur on a case-by-case basis. Hormonal contraceptives are a more effective means of contraception than are barrier methods. Side effects are much lower than those associated with pregnancy.

Q: What should I tell my patient if she misses a dose of her oral contraceptive?
A: If she has missed one pill, she should take it as soon as she remembers; then take the next pill at the regular time. If she has missed two doses, she should take two when she remembers, and then two the next day. She should use a backup method during the cycle in which she had to "double up." If she has missed three or more pills, she will probably menstruate. After discarding the last pack, she should start a new pack on the first Sunday after the start of her next period. She is not protected during the remainder of this cycle.

ICD-9-CM
Family planning advice V025.09
Oral prescription V025.01
Other agents V025.02

BIBLIOGRAPHY

Glasier A. Emergency postcoital contraception. *N Engl J Med* 1997;337(15):1058–64.

Nelson A, Neinstein LS. Oral contraceptives. In: Neinstein LS, ed. *Adolescent health care: a practical guide,* 3rd ed. Baltimore: Williams & Wilkins, 1996:695.

Polaneczky M. Adolescent contraception. *Opin Obstet Gynecol* 1998;10(3):213–219.

Strasburger VC, Brown RT. Adolescent sexuality and health related problems. In: *Adolescent medicine: a practical guide.* Philadelphia: Lippincott-Raven, 1998:151.

Trussell J, Rodriguez G, Ellertson C. New estimates of the effectiveness of the Yuzpe regimen of emergency contraception. *Contraception* 1998;57(6):363–369.

Author: Jonathan R. Pletcher

Cor Pulmonale

 Database

DEFINITION

Cor pulmonale is right ventricular (RV) failure secondary to an altered cardiopulmonary process, resulting in excessive pulmonary artery pressure and resistance (PVR). Cor pulmonale is not the result of a primary congenital heart defect.

CAUSES

- Parenchymal lung disease (most common)
- Chronic obstructive pulmonary disease

—Cystic fibrosis
—Asthma

- Restrictive lung disease

—Infectious pulmonary toxins
—Pulmonary fibrosis
—Bronchopulmonary dysplasia (combined)

- Upper airway diseases
- Tonsillar/adenoidal hypertrophy
- Syndromes (Down, Treacher-Collins)
- Neuromuscular disorders
- Duchenne muscular dystrophy
- Pulmonary vascular abnormalities
- Collagen vascular diseases
- Pulmonary venoocclusive diseases
- Pulmonary thromboembolism
- Chest wall deformities
- Primary pulmonary hypertension (PPHN)

PATHOPHYSIOLOGY

Chronic hypoxia is the principal factor, resulting in a cascade of endothelial dysfunction with pulmonary vasoconstriction, followed by the development of pulmonary hypertension. A variety of vasoactive mediators may be responsible for the effect on vasomotor tone. Alveolar hypoventilation, hypoxemia, hypercarbia, and acidemia all result in increased RV afterload and decreased RV systolic function.

EPIDEMIOLOGY

Cor pulmonale may be found at any age, but is typically due to a long-standing pulmonary process. PPHN is most often diagnosed in the second or third decade of life. There is a female predominance, and it is often diagnosed during pregnancy.

COMPLICATIONS

Aside from the underlying lung process, the chronic hypoxia results in anemia, polycythemia-decreased systemic oxygen delivery, and RV failure secondary to the inability of the RV to handle the excessive afterload.

PROGNOSIS

Patients with reversible lung disease usually have a better prognosis. Patients with cor pulmonale are at risk for sudden death because of the inability to augment cardiac output with exercise secondary to a relatively fixed PVR. Numerous medical therapies and lung transplantation may improve long-term survival.

 Differential Diagnosis

Congenital heart disease with pulmonary hypertension and right-to-left shunting (Eisenmenger syndrome) should be ruled out.

 Data Gathering

HISTORY

- Fatigue, dizziness, and/or syncope
- Deterioration of exercise tolerance from that of baseline
- Chest pain (secondary to RV ischemia)
- Palpitations
- Hemoptysis

 Physical Examination

- Tachycardia
- Parasternal RV impulse
- Cyanosis may be evident.
- Hepatomegaly, jugular venous distention, peripheral edema
- A loud, narrowly split or single second heart sound (P2), gallop, holosystolic murmur right of the sternum (tricuspid regurgitation), and diastolic murmur at the left upper sternal border (pulmonary insufficiency)

 Laboratory Aids

NONSPECIFIC TESTS

- ECG: may show right atrial enlargement, RV hypertrophy, and T-wave inversion
- Decreased PaO_2, increased $PaCO_2$, and a compensatory metabolic alkalosis
- Polycythemia may be consistent with chronic hypoxemia.
- Chest x-ray: cardiomegaly from RV dilation and main pulmonary artery enlargement
- Echocardiography: RV dilation, hypertrophy, pulmonic insufficiency, and if tricuspid regurgitation is present, an RV pressure can be estimated.
- Cardiac catheterization, while invasive, remains the gold standard.

Therapy

- The primary goal is reduction of the abnormally elevated pulmonary artery pressure and the RV workload.
- If at all possible, address the primary etiology (i.e., tonsillectomy/adenoidectomy in a patient with obstructive upper airway disease).
- Oxygen (nocturnal oxygen)
- Diuretics (if pulmonary congestion)
- Bronchodilators (theophylline)
- Digoxin (may improve RV contractility)
- Anticoagulants
- Pulmonary vasodilators

—Nitric oxide
—Prostacyclin
—Calcium channel blockers

- Atrial septostomy (in select cases, may improve cardiac output at the expense of hypoxemia)
- Lung or heart-lung transplantation

 ## Follow-Up

PROGNOSIS

Long-term survival is variable because of the age of onset for pulmonary changes and the underlying conditions (e.g., Down syndrome) that may adversely affect survival. Death often occurs in the second or third decade of life.

PITFALLS

In newborns, the RV muscle mass is comparable to the LV. RV failure from pulmonary hypertension is rare in newborns. RV failure in newborns is usually a consequence of hypoxemia, ischemia, and metabolic acidosis (e.g., persistent fetal circulation).

 ## Common Questions and Answers

Q: Is cardiac catheterization indicated in all patients with cor pulmonale?
A: Yes. While a great deal of information can be learned from echocardiography, direct pulmonary artery pressure/resistance measurements require an invasive procedure. In addition, assessment of the reactivity of the pulmonary vascular bed to various agents (oxygen, prostacyclin, and calcium channel blockers) is best performed in the catheterization laboratory.

Q: Is nocturnal oxygen therapy beneficial?
A: Nocturnal oxygen has been speculated to delay the progression of cor pulmonale in some select patients with obstructive sleep hypoxemia.

ICD-9-CM 416.9
Chronic 415.0

BIBLIOGRAPHY

Brouillette RT, Fernback SK, Hunt CE. Obstructive sleep apnea in infants and children. *J Pediatr* 1982;100:31.

Perkin RM, Anas NG. Pulmonary hypertension in pediatric patients. *J Pediatr* 1984;105:511.

Wessel DL, Adatia I, Thompson JE, Hickey PR. Delivery and monitoring of inhaled nitric oxide in patients with pulmonary hypertension. *Crit Care Med* 1994;22(6):930–938.

Author: Mitchell I. Cohen

Costochondritis

 Database

DEFINITION

Costochondritis is chest pain that emanates from a costal cartilage and is reproducible on compression of that cartilage.

PATHOPHYSIOLOGY

- Inflammation of unknown etiology (histologic examination is usually normal)
- Infection

—Complication of median sternotomy
—Can present months to years after surgery (the costal cartilage is avascular, making it vulnerable to infection if it has been exposed, injured, or denuded of perichondrium)
—Occurs by spread from adjacent osteomyelitis or may arise de novo during surgery

- —Bacterial
    —*Staphylococcus aureus* (especially after thoracic surgery)
    —*Salmonella* (in sickle cell disease)
    —*Escherichia coli*
    —*Pseudomonas* species
    —*Klebsiella* species

- —Fungal
    —*Aspergillus flavus*
    —*Candida albicans*

- —Posttrauma

EPIDEMIOLOGY

- Costochondritis accounts for 10% to 22% of all pediatric chest pain.
- Peak age for chest pain in children is 12 to 14 years old.
- Incidence of sternal wound infections following median sternotomy is 0.1% to 1.6%.

PROGNOSIS

- Inflammatory costochondritis: excellent
- Infectious costochondritis: prognosis relates to:

—Underlying clinical condition of the patient (i.e., immunocompromised, postradiation therapy for cancer, postcardiac surgery)
—Extent of surgery required to reconstruct the area damaged by the infection

 Differential Diagnosis

ETIOLOGIES

- Cardiovascular

—Myocardial infarction
—Pericardial effusion
—Dissecting aneurysm

- Pulmonary

—Pneumonia
—Pulmonary embolism
—Pneumothorax

- Mechanical

—Muscle strain
—Stress fractures
—Trauma

- Rheumatologic

—Rheumatoid arthritis
—Ankylosing spondylitis

- Oncologic

—Rhabdomyosarcomas

- Leukemia

—Ewing sarcoma

- Miscellaneous

—Tietze syndrome
—Psychogenic chest pain
—Breast tissue pain (both sexes)

 Data Gathering

HISTORY

Inflammatory Costochondritis

- Pain usually preceded by exercise or an upper respiratory tract infection
- Description of pain:

—Usually sharp
—Affects the anterior chest wall
—Localized or radiates to the back or abdomen
—Usually unilateral (left side greater than right side)

- The fourth to sixth costochondral junction is the usual site of pain.
- Motion of the arm and shoulder on the affected side elicits the pain.
- Girls are affected more often than are boys.

Tietze Syndrome

- Onset is usually abrupt, but can be gradual.
- Believed to be caused by a minor trauma, though etiology is unknown
- Description of pain:

—Radiates to arms or shoulder
—May last up to several weeks
—Swelling at the sternochondral junction may persist for several months to years.

- Usually affects the second or third costochondral joint
- Pain is aggravated by sneezing, coughing, deep inspiration, or twisting motions of the chest.
- No differences in frequency between sexes

Infectious Costochondritis

- Slow, insidious course
- Usually unimpressive clinical symptomatology

Physical Examination

- Usually normal
- Inspect for evidence of trauma, scars, bruising, and swelling.
- Palpation and percussion of the costochondral and costosternal junctions should reproduce and localize the pain.
- In Tietze syndrome, spindle-shaped swelling is visible at the sternochondral junction.

Laboratory Aids

TESTS

- WBC not helpful (even when infection present)

Imaging

- Radiologic studies (chest radiography, CT) not helpful
- Gallium scan:

—May be useful in some cases of infectious origin
—Not highly specific
—May show increased radionuclide uptake
—No evidence of osteomyelitis of the sternum in most cases

- Technetium bone scan:

—Not highly specific

Therapy

INFLAMMATORY COSTOCHONDRITIS

- Antiinflammatory and analgesic agents
- Reassurance
- If pain disturbs normal activities and sports, infiltration with local anesthetic may prove useful.

INFECTIOUS COSTOCHONDRITIS

- Prolonged course of IV antibiotics
- Prompt surgical resection of all involved cartilage
- Reconstructive surgery with muscular flaps should be done.

Follow-Up

WHEN TO EXPECT IMPROVEMENT

- Inflammatory costochondritis

—Long-lasting condition
—Follow-up once a year is recommended.

- Infectious costochondritis

—Long-term follow-up after surgery is mandatory.

PITFALLS

- Inflammatory costochondritis

—Important cause of school absence
—Adolescents tend to limit physical activity unnecessarily for long periods.
—Restriction of activities is usually not required.
—Most adolescents still worry about cardiac problems, even after the diagnosis has been made.

- Infectious costochondritis

—Long-term IV antibiotics alone do not resolve the problem; surgical resection and repair also are required.
—There is a tendency for the infection to spread to adjacent costal cartilages and across the sternum to the contralateral chest wall.
—In general, avoid costochondral junctions when performing surgical procedures in the chest (i.e., chest-tube placement).

Common Questions and Answers

Q: Am I having or will I have a heart attack?
A: Chest pain does not imply a heart problem. This pain arises from the chest wall; there is no risk of a myocardial infarction.

Q: Is costochondritis related to arthritis?
A: There is no relation to any form of arthritis.

ICD-9-CM 733.6

BIBLIOGRAPHY

Brown RT. Costochondritis in adolescents. *J Adolesc Health Care* 1981;1:198–201.

Brown RT, Jamil K. Costochondritis in adolescents: a follow-up study. *Clin Pediatr* 1993;32: 499–500.

Caruana V, Swayne LC. Gallium detection of salmonella costochondritis. *J Nucl Med* 1988;29: 2004–2007.

Chicarilli ZN, Ariyan S, Stahl RS. Costochondritis: pathogenesis, diagnosis and management considerations. *Plast Reconstr Surg* 1986;77:50–59.

Culliford AT, Cunningham JN, Jeff RH. Sternal and costochondral infections following open heart surgery: a review of 2,594 cases. *J Thorac Cardiovasc Surg* 1976;72:714–726.

Fraz M. *Pediatric respiratory disease: diagnosis and treatment.* Philadelphia: WB Saunders, 1993:162–172.

Mendelson G, Mendelson H, Horowitz SF, et al. Can ^{99m}technetium methylene diphosphate bone scans objectively document costochondritis? *Chest* 1997;111:1600–1602.

Miller JH. Accumulation of gallium-67 in costochondritis. *Clin Nucl Med* 1980;5:362–363.

Selbst SM, Ruddy RM, Clark BJ, et al. Pediatric chest pain: a prospective study. *Pediatrics* 1988;82:319–323.

Author: Richard Mark Kravitz

Crohn Disease

 Database

DEFINITION

Crohn disease is a chronic inflammatory disease that affects the entire gastrointestinal tract, but most commonly the terminal ileum and proximal colon.

CAUSES

- Unknown

PATHOPHYSIOLOGY

- The intestinal wall is edematous, with wall thickening and strictures.
- Mesentery can be thickened, with enlarged lymph nodes.
- Normal bowel can exist in continuity with affected bowel (skip areas).
- Matting together of inflamed bowel and organs
- Abscesses/fistulas
- Inflammatory cells infiltrate all layers of the intestine.
- Epithelioid granulomas are found in 40% of biopsies of patients and are pathognomonic.

GENETICS

- First-degree relatives have a 5% to 25% higher risk than normal population.
- Family members of patients with Crohn disease have increased risk for both Crohn disease and ulcerative colitis.
- Offspring have an 8.9% and siblings an 8.6% of developing IBD.
- Concordance in monozygotic twins is 50%.

EPIDEMIOLOGY

- The incidence rate in children is 10 per 100,000 in North American 10- to 19-year-olds.
- Forty percent of patients first present in childhood or adolescence.
- Males and females are equally affected in adulthood, but in childhood, there is a 2:1 male:female ratio.

COMPLICATIONS

- Toxic megacolon is a rare but serious complication.
- Obstruction (8%–40%) due to strictures, phlegmon, adhesions, giant polyposis, gallstones, lymphoma
- Abscess due to fistula and perforation
- Enteroenteric, enterovesical, enterovaginal, and enterocutaneous fistulas occur.
- Perianal disease affects 25% to 50% of patients.
- Malabsorption occurs in small bowel disease. The nutrient affected depends on the site of disease (e.g., B12 deficiency: terminal ileum; iron deficiency: duodenum).
- Incidence of adenocarcinoma is reported to be 4 to 20 times that of the general population.

- Massive hemorrhage is rare (1%). Rectal bleeding is common.
- Growth failure is frequent; final height is reduced and puberty is delayed in Crohn disease affecting prepubertal children.

 Differential Diagnosis

- Ulcerative colitis
- Appendicitis
- Infection: *Mycobacteria, Salmonella, Shigella, Campylobacter, Aeromonas, Yersinia, Clostridium difficile, Escherichia coli, Giardia, Cryptosporidium*
- Hemolytic-uremic syndrome
- Henoch-Schönlein purpura
- Irritable bowel syndrome
- Peptic ulcer disease
- Constipation
- Autoimmune enteropathy, immunodeficiency
- Primary lactase deficiency
- Psychosocial disturbance

 Data Gathering

HISTORY

- Frequency of signs and symptoms

—Weight loss, 85%
—Diarrhea, 80%
—Abdominal pain, 75%
—Rectal bleeding, 50%
—Growth failure, 35%
—Nausea and vomiting, 25%
—Rectal disease, 25%
—Extraintestinal signs, 25%
—Perianal disease, 15%

- Symptoms depend on the site of disease activity.
- The sites most often affected in decreasing frequency are terminal ileum, right colon, isolated colon, proximal small bowel, and gastroduodenum.

SPECIAL CONCERNS

- Recurrent abdominal pain
- Diarrhea
- Weight loss
- Recent travel (enteric infections)
- Antibiotic use (*C. difficile*)
- Rectal bleeding
- Family history of IBD
- Appendectomy
- Growth failure: Careful charting of recent growth parameters, especially growth velocities from school or medical records, is essential.

—Patients with small bowel disease have emesis, nausea, pain, and diarrhea. Diarrhea is secondary to malabsorption and bacterial overgrowth. Growth retardation is more frequent in these patients.

—Patients with distal disease have symptoms of diarrhea, rectal bleeding, and urgency.

- Extraintestinal disease: arthritis, erythema nodosum, pyoderma gangrenosum, mouth ulcers, uveitis, hypercoagulable states, vasculitis, renal stones, amyloidosis, sclerosing cholangitis
- Extraintestinal symptoms:

—Aphthous ulcers
—Arthritis
—Erythema nodosum
—Pyoderma gangrenosum

 Physical Examination

- Decreasing height and weight percentiles over the past few years
- Abdominal examination: hyperactive bowel sounds, RLQ mass and tenderness
- Rectal examination: perirectal disease (tag, fissure, hemorrhoids, abscesses)

 Laboratory Aids

TESTS

Laboratory Tests

- Blood count: microcytosis, macrocytosis suggesting nutrient deficiency: iron, B12, folate, zinc levels
- ESR (disease activity)
- Electrolytes (hydration, renal function)
- Transaminases
- Alkaline phosphatase
- γ-Glutamyl transpeptidase (hepatobiliary disease)
- pANCA Crohn disease (19% positive) and UC (80% positive)
- ASCA (anti-*Saccharomyces cerevisiae* antibody) Crohn disease (70% positive)
- Stool for occult blood and presence of white cells
- Stool cultures, *C. difficile* toxin A and B

Imaging

- Consider plain abdominal radiograph in acute presentation.
- Barium upper GI and small bowel follow-through; this shows extent of disease in small bowel that is not accessible to endoscopy.
- Barium enema has been replaced by colonoscopy in acute colitis; useful in evaluation of complications such as strictures and fistulas.
- CT scan and ultrasound are useful tools for evaluating complications and disease severity.
- Endoscopy with multiple biopsy enables visualization and tissue diagnosis and is the test of choice for initial evaluation of colonic Crohn disease. Upper endoscopy with biopsy is indicated in patients with symptoms of gastroduodenal disease.

Therapy

DRUGS

• Prednisone can control intestinal inflammation. Dosage is 1 to 2 mg/kg/d oral prednisone (maximum, 60 mg). Initially, patient is treated for 4 to 6 weeks and tapered 5 mg weekly to the lowest amount tolerated.
• Sulfasalazine, a biologically active congener of sulfapyridine and 5-aminosalicylate, the latter being antiinflammatory. It may be useful in prophylaxis in adult disease. Dose is 50 to 75 mg/kg/d t.i.d (maximum, 4 g/d). Folate (1 mg/d) supplementation is also used.
• There are many ASA preparations used according to their sites of efficacy to correspond to diseased bowel:

—Asacol (terminal ileum, colon) 30 to 50 mg/kg/d (maximum 4.8 g/d for active disease and 3.2 g/d to maintain remission)
—Pentasa (duodenum, jejunum, ileum, colon), 50 to 60 mg/kg/d (maximum, 4 g/d for active disease and 3 g/d to maintain remission)
—Dipentum (colon)
—Rowasa, 4-g enemas and 500-mg suppositories

• Azathioprine, 2.0 to 2.5 mg/kg/d, and its metabolite 6-mercaptopurine, starting with 1.0 to 1.5 mg/kg/d to maintain white cell count greater than 4×10^9/L and platelets greater than 100×10^9/L, can maintain remission and is steroid-sparing. It is also useful for treating fistulas.
• Cyclosporine: unclear utility in Crohn disease in children; nutritional management is as follows:

—Bowel rest with parenteral nutrition
—Elemental diet reported to be effective in inducing remission in active disease
—To correct growth failure, an increase in caloric intake is recommended and can be given as overnight nasogastric feeds if oral supplements are not tolerated. An elemental formula is recommended.

• Antibiotics

—Metronidazole and Ciprofloxacin are useful for intestinal and perianal disease.

• Topical hydrocortisone is useful in localized left-sided disease and is available in liquid and foam enemas. Absorption is dependent of degree of inflammation and length of exposure, but up to 75% may be absorbed. Poorly absorbed topical steroids, such as budesonide, are not yet available.
• cA$_2$ (anti-TNF): recently FDA-approved medication. Initial use will be for patients unresponsive to the above medical therapies (5 mg/kg IV infusion). Potentially will be given every 2 to 3 months if necessary.

SURGERY

Crohn disease is a chronic recurrent disease with recurrence at sites of anastomosis and ostomies. With obstruction, abscess, fistulas, growth retardation, and bleeding failing to respond to medical therapy, surgery is considered.

Follow-Up

• The morbidity of this disease is very high. The majority of patients experience recurring disease.
• In adults, 55% of patients will have mild-to-severe disease at any one time, with the remainder in remission.
• Patients with colonic disease seem to suffer more from extraintestinal disease and are more refractory to treatment.
• Exacerbation of disease in children often follows intercurrent viral illness, such as EBV and adenovirus.
• The cause of poor growth is multifactorial, including anorexia, malabsorption, increased energy expenditure, and prolonged corticosteroid use.
• Most patients have good general health in between disease and go on to lead productive lives.
• Death is a rare complication (2.4% in a large series).
• After 5 and 20 years of disease, the probability of survival was 98% and 89% of expected survival, respectively.
• In terms of risk of neoplasia, incidence of adenocarcinoma of the rectum and colon is reported to be 4 to 20 times that of the general population.
• There are no good population base studies looking at the incidence of lymphoma in IBD. One study of 2,000 patients found that 1 in 300 Crohn disease patients develops lymphoma.

Common Questions and Answers

Q: Will my child have this disease forever?
A: There are many different clinical presentations of Crohn disease. Some people will have only the initial attack and then are symptom-free, but usually an individual will have episodes of recurrences and remissions. Presently, research is being done to identify the genetic factors in Crohn disease; once the genes can be identified, a cure will be possible.

Q: What is the cause of Crohn disease?
A: Both genetic and environmental factors are important in the development of Crohn disease. Possible environmental factors include aseptic environment in the first few years of life, lack of breast feeding, frequent use of antibiotics or aspirin, and diet.

Q: Where can I learn more about Crohn disease?
A: The Crohn and Colitis Foundation of America (CCFA) is a nonprofit organization dedicated to the care of people with Crohn disease and ulcerative colitis.

Q: What new therapies will be used in the near future?
A: Biologic agents, which is a type of therapy that uses our recently improved knowledge of the immune system, either down-regulate inflammatory mediators or up-regulate immunomodulatory mediators. It is hoped that this new class of therapies will greatly improve our care of people with IBD.

ICD-9-CM 558.9

BIBLIOGRAPHY

Greenfield SM, Punchard NA, Teare JP, Thompson RPH. Review article: the mode of action of aminosalicylates in inflammatory bowel disease. *Aliment Pharmacol Ther* 1993;7:369–383.

Grybovski JD. Crohn disease in children 10 years old or younger: comparison with ulcerative colitis. *J Pediatr Gastroenterol Nutr* 1994;18(2):174–182.

Hildebrand H, Karlberg J, Kristiansson B. Longitudinal growth in children with IBD. *J Pediatr Gastroenterol Nutr* 1994;18(2):165–173.

Hofley PM, Piccoli DA. Inflammatory bowel disease in children. *Med Clin North Am* 1994;78(6): 1281–1302.

Hyams JS. Crohn disease. In: *Pediatric gastrointestinal disease: pathophysiology, diagnosis, management.* Philadelphia: WB Saunders, 1993:742–764.

Hyams JS. Extraintestinal manifestations of IBD in childhood (review). *J Pediatr Gastroenterol Nutr* 1994;19(1):7–21.

Seidman E, Laleiko N, Ament M, et al. Nutritional issues in pediatric inflammatory bowel disease. *J Pediatr Gastroenterol Nutr* 1991;12: 424.

Telander RL, Schmeling DJ. Current surgical management of Crohn disease in childhood (review). *Semin Pediatr Surg* 1994;3(1):19–27.

Author: Robert N. Baldassano

Croup (Laryngotracheobronchitis)

 Database

DEFINITION

- Croup (laryngotracheobronchitis) is an acute viral infection classically characterized by a triad of symptoms: a barking cough, inspiratory stridor, and hoarseness that result from variable degrees of subglottic stenosis.
- *Spasmodic croup* is characterized by the acute onset of inspiratory stridor, usually occurring at night for several hours and recurring over the next several nights. The child is often not ill or has mild upper respiratory symptoms. It may be a variant of viral laryngotracheobronchitis.

ETIOLOGY

- Human parainfluenza virus type 1, most commonly identified
- Human parainfluenza virus types 2 and 3
- Respiratory syncytial virus (RSV)
- Adenovirus
- Influenza viruses A and B
- Enteroviruses
- *Mycoplasma pneumoniae* (rare)

PATHOPHYSIOLOGY

- The virus enters the body via respiratory droplets on the epithelium of the nasopharyngeal airway.
- The host defense mechanism is to cause an immune response, resulting in increased mucus production, which leads to airway narrowing.
- Edema and erythema of the mucosa of the subglottic region and vocal cords further narrow the airway.
- Airway narrowing may be severe in the subglottic region because the cricoid cartilage limits the lumenal diameter in this area.
- The process of endothelial damage, swelling, and mucus production may extend to the small airways, with resulting atelectasis.

EPIDEMIOLOGY

- Most commonly occurs in the first 3 years of life (6–36 months)
- Peak incidence: second year of life (4.7/100)
- The male:female ratio is 3:2.
- Most prevalent in the late fall and winter
- Fewer children are requiring hospitalization

COMPLICATIONS

- Poor oral intake/dehydration
- Hypoxia
- Upper airway obstruction
- Respiratory failure (rare)

PROGNOSIS

- The vast majority of patients does not require hospitalization.
- Almost all patients go on to complete recovery.

 Differential Diagnosis

- Congenital
—Tracheoesophageal fistula
—Foregut duplication
—Laryngomalacia
—Tracheomalacia
—Vocal cord paralysis
—Arnold-Chiari malformation
—Vascular ring
—Laryngeal web

- Infection
—Epiglottis (although less common since universal HiB vaccine)
—Bacterial tracheitis
—Retropharyngeal abscess
—Adenotonsillitis
—Diphtheria
—Pneumonia

- Toxins
—Foreign-body aspiration
—Caustic material ingestion (very alkaline products)
—Smoke inhalation

- Trauma
—Subglottic edema/stenosis post intubation
—Laryngeal fracture

- Tumor
—Papillomatosis
—Hemangioma
—Cystic hygroma
—Lymphoma
—Rhabdomyosarcoma
—Thymoma
—Teratoma

- Genetic/metabolic
—Hypocalcemia

- Allergic/inflammatory
—Asthma
—Angioneurotic edema (anaphylaxis)
—Spasmodic croup
—Microaspiration secondary to gastroesophageal reflux

 Data Gathering

HISTORY

Question: How long have the symptoms been present? Is the process acute or chronic?
Significance: Croup is an acute illness.

Question: Any fever?
Significance: Croup is often associated with fever. If no fever, do not forget foreign-body or caustic ingestions.

Question: When did the stridor begin or occur?
Significance: If the child awakens at night, this supports the diagnosis of croup. If the child is playing at the onset of stridor, consider foreign-body aspiration.

Question: How have the symptoms progressed?
Significance: Ask about URI prodrome, sore throat, change in quality of voice, dysphagia/drooling (consider epiglottitis), dysphonia, particular position of comfort.

Question: Is there a history of previous airway problems or recurrent stridor?
Significance: Recurrence or a prolonged history should lead one to consider subglottic stenosis or gastroesophageal reflux.

 Physical Examination

- In general, the child with croup is often anxious and ill-appearing. Allow them to sit in a comfortable position and in their caregiver's (parent's) lap, this will hopefully reduce the agitation provoked by examination.
- It is important initially to assess level of consciousness, irritability, color, and respiratory distress.
- Vital signs: Check for pulsus paradoxicus (large inspiratory drop in systolic blood pressure because of fall in pleural pressure secondary to airway obstruction).
- What is the preferred position? Sitting in a tripod position with the neck extended to "sniff" is concerning for epiglottis.
- Assess work of breathing, including respiratory rate, nasal flaring, retractions, abdominal breathing, and head bobbing.
- Assess air entry into the chest.
- Listen for audible stridor at rest.
- Listen for the presence of wheezing.
- Observe for drooling.
- Assess the quality of the voice.
- Neck masses or bruising suggest bacterial infection or trauma.
- The Croup Score (as developed by Westley, et al. and modified by Super, et al.) is utilized by many clinicians to describe the severity of symptoms (see table Severity Score of Croup Patients).

 Laboratory Aids

TESTS

Laboratory Tests

- In general, laboratory tests are not required to make this diagnosis.
- Blood testing, such as arterial blood gas or complete blood count with differential, is not helpful in diagnosing croup. In fact, the pain and fear of the testing will likely heighten the child's anxiety and worsen respiratory distress.

Croup (Laryngotracheobronchitis)

Severity Score of Croup Patients

INDICATOR OF SEVERITY OF ILLNESS	SCORE
Inspiratory stridor	
None	0
At rest, with stethoscope	1
At rest, without stethoscope	2
Retractions	
None	0
Mild	1
Moderate	2
Severe	3
Air entry	
Normal	0
Decreased	1
Severely decreased	2
Cyanosis	
None	0
With agitation	4
At rest	5
Level of consciousness	
Normal	0
Altered mental status	5
Mild	0–3
Moderate to severe	>3

Radiographic Studies

Anteroposterior and lateral view x-rays of the neck: The anteroposterior view classically demonstrates the "steeple" sign in patients with croup. The lateral view is useful in ruling out epiglottis, retropharyngeal cellulitis/abscess (fullness or free air in the retropharyngeal space), and a radiopaque foreign body

Other Procedures

Pulse oximetry: helpful for children in respiratory distress to determine if hypoxia is present

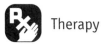 Therapy

- Most do well with conservative management at home or, much less commonly, after a short stay in the emergency department.
- In the child with impending respiratory failure, prompt intubation and direct visualization of the airway *in the operating room* is imperative. Do not wait for x-rays to confirm a diagnosis.
- Humidity: humidified air delivered by tent or face mask in the hospital, or by cool mist vaporizer or a steam-filled bathroom at home. In the cold of winter, walking outside into the crisp, cold air is often very effective.
- Racemic epinephrine: A nebulized, racemic epinephrine treatment offers immediate reduction in swelling of the laryngeal airway in children who present in extreme respiratory distress or in whom humidified air does not improve stridor (croup score >3) after 20 to 30 minutes. Dose: 0.5 mL of 2.25% solution in 2.5 mL normal saline delivered via nebulizer.

- Steroids: Utilized in the emergency room and inpatient settings, steroids have resulted in decreased length of hospital stay and decreased number of admissions due to croup. Dexamethasone (half-life 36–54 hours) given intramuscularly (IM) in the setting of moderate-to-severe croup (croup score >3): 0.6 mg/kg as a single dose is the recommended dose.

 Follow-Up

- In most cases, the illness is self-limited, lasting 3 to 5 days.
- A "rebound phenomenon" with worsening of stridor and respiratory distress after initial relief with the racemic epinephrine treatment may be seen up to 2 hours posttreatment in some patients. Several studies have shown that children can be safely discharged home 3 to 4 hours after racemic epinephrine treatment.

PITFALLS

Recurrent croup may have an underlying anatomic problem associated. In younger children (infants), congenital anomalies and gastroesophageal reflux are more likely contributors.

 Common Questions and Answers

Q: Should all children with croup receive steroids in an attempt to prevent hospitalization?
A: The literature certainly is convincing for the use of IM dexamethasone in combination with mist and racemic epinephrine for children with moderate-to-severe croup scores. There is no evidence to date, however, supporting the use of steroids in the mild cases as a preventative measure. Steroids have not been shown to shorten the course of the illness; however, the severity is diminished.

Q: Do children who receive racemic epinephrine for croup require hospitalization?
A: No. Several studies now have shown that after a 3- to 4-hour period of observation and dexamethasone, children can be safely discharged home. Any rebound effects should occur within the first 2 hours.

Q: Do steroids need to be given IM?
A: The bioavailability of steroids is excellent, whether IM or orally administered. The half-life of dexamethasone is much longer (36–54 hours) than that of prednisone (12–36 hours). With croup, many patients have poor oral intake exacerbated by respiratory distress. Gastric irritation with enteral dosing is not uncommon, making compliance poor. Most of the large studies evaluating croup and steroid dosing have looked at the IM dosing of dexamethasone. Oral steroid dosing for croup has not been established.

Q: What's new in the treatment of croup?
A: Budesonide, a glucocorticoid available in a nebulized form, has recently been used successfully in the treatment of croup. The ease of administration and rapid onset of action make it an exciting prospect for management. This medication is, however, not available in the United States.

ICD-9-CM 464.4

BIBLIOGRAPHY

Connors K, Gavula D, Terndrup T. The use of corticosteroids in croup: A survey. *Pediatr Emerg Care* 1994;10(4):197–199.

Geelhoed GC. Sixteen years of croup in a western Australian teaching hospital: effects of routine steroid treatment. *Ann Emerg Med* 1996; 28(6):621–626.

Kairys SW, Olmstead EM, O'Connor GT. Steroid treatment of laryngotracheitis: a meta-analysis of the evidence from randomized trials. *Pediatrics* 1989;83(5):683–693.

Klassen TP, Feldman ME, Watters LK, et al: Nebulized budesonide for children with mild-to-moderate croup. *N Engl J Med* 1994;331(5): 285–289.

Kunkel NC, Baker MD. Use of racemic epinephrine, dexamethasone, and mist in the outpatient management of croup. *Pediatr Emerg Care* 1996;12(3):156–159.

Ledwith CA, Shea LM, Mauro RD. Safety and efficacy of nebulized racemic epinephrine in conjunction with oral dexamethasone and mist in the outpatient treatment of croup. *Ann Emerg Med* 1995;25(3):331–337.

Macdonald WBG, Geelhoed GC. Management of childhood croup. *Thorax* 1997;52:757–759.

Marx A, Torok TJ, Holman RC, Clarke MJ, Anderson LJ. Pediatric hospitalizations for croup (laryngotracheobronchitis): biennial increases associated with human parainfluenza virus 1 epidemics. *J Infect Dis* 1997;176:1423–1427.

Steele DW, Santucci KA, Wright RO, Natarajan R, McQuillen KK, Jay GD. Pulsus paradoxus: an objective measure of severity in croup. *Am J Respir Crit Care Med* 1998;157:331–334.

Super DM, Cartelli NA, Brooks LJ, Lembo RM, Kumar ML. A prospective randomized double-blind study to evaluate the effect of dexamethasone in acute laryngotracheitis. *J Pediatr* 1989;115:323–329.

Waki EY, Madgy DN, Belenky WM, Gower VC. The incidence of gastroesophageal reflux in recurrent croup. *Int J Pediatr Otorhinolaryngol* 1995;32:223–232.

Westley CR, Cotton EK, Brooks JG: Nebulized racemic epinephrine by IPPB for the treatment of croup. *Am J Dis Child* 1978;132:484–487.

Author: Shannon Connor Phillips

Cryptococcal Infections

Database

DEFINITION

Cryptococcal infections can involve several organ systems, including the lungs, bones, visceral organs, and skin, with the most commonly involved organ system being the central nervous system with meningeal involvement.

CAUSES

- *Cryptococcus neoformans,* a yeastlike fungus

PATHOPHYSIOLOGY

- Cellular immunity is the key defense against infection with *Cryptococcus.*
- Pulmonary involvement may be either focal or widespread.
- Meningeal involvement with *Cryptococcus* results from hematogenous spread through the lungs. It can get direct spread from the meninges into the parenchyma of the brain.
- Local reactions can lead to granulomatous formations, which can be seen in both the meninges and the lung.

EPIDEMIOLOGY

- Some association exists with exposure to pigeon droppings, although many individuals who are diagnosed with *Cryptococcus* do not remember a direct exposure.
- Increased risk of cryptococcal infection exists in individuals with a compromised cellular immune system, although it is seen less commonly in young children infected with HIV as compared with adolescents and adults with HIV. There is no person-to-person spread of the infection, with most infections thought to be acquired through aerolization from either contaminated pigeon droppings or contaminated soil.

COMPLICATIONS

- Meningeal involvement is one of the most common clinical manifestations of the disease. Meningitis can present with any of the following: fever, headache, malaise, and, at times, photophobia and meningismus. Patients may demonstrate changes in personality and may have papilledema, retinal exudates, decreased hearing, or a facial nerve palsy.
- Cutaneous involvement presents as acneiform lesions that ulcerate and may result from hematogenous spread of the organism or from direct extension from an infected bone. Pulmonary involvement may be asymptomatic and determined at autopsy in up to 50% of cases. It may manifest as cough with a small amount of sputum production, with small amounts of hemoptysis.
- Bone involvement presents with pain and swelling, with a radiographic picture very similar to that for osteogenic sarcoma and requiring biopsy to confirm the diagnosis.

PROGNOSIS

- Prognosis is good with treatment with amphotericin B. However, there is some risk for residual neurologic deficits in up to 40% of patients.
- Left untreated, however, cryptococcal meningitis is fatal. Individuals with impaired cellular immunity, especially those infected with HIV, are at great risk for relapse after initial treatment, with up to 65% experiencing recurrence of infection. Thus, long-term maintenance therapy with fluconazole is recommended.

ASSOCIATED DISEASES

- Cryptococcal infection is the most common cause of fungal meningitis in the United States and is a particular problem in immunocompromised hosts, especially those with HIV. Cryptococcal meningitis can manifest as headache, nausea and vomiting, fever, and general malaise, with only 30% presenting as meningismus. It is uncommon to see focal neurologic disease, although individuals can present with changes in personality, confusion, disorientation, ataxia, or lethargy.
- Pulmonary *Cryptococcus* may be asymptomatic but can be manifest with a cough that is productive of small amounts of mucus. Pleural effusions can be found associated with pleuritic-type chest pain.
- Cutaneous involvement can mimic acne-type eruptions, which can ulcerate. *Cryptococcus* of the bone manifests as pain and swelling, with diagnosis made by biopsy.

Differential Diagnosis

- Cryptococcal meningitis should be in the differential diagnosis of any aseptic meningitis, especially in individuals with chronic or recurrent episodes.
- It should be included in any individual with an underlying immunodeficiency who presents with headache, lethargy, fever, or changes in personality.
- Viral encephalitis
- Tuberculous meningitis
- Neoplasia
- *Cryptococcus* should be considered in the differential diagnosis of chronic cough with or without hemoptysis or in individuals with an isolated pulmonary nodule.

Data Gathering

HISTORY

- Cryptococcal meningitis may present as either an indolent infection or as an acute illness.
- In patients infected with HIV, up to 90% will complain of headache and fever.
- Although not common, focal neurologic symptoms can result from cryptococcal meningitis, including decreased hearing, facial nerve palsy, and diplopia.
- Pulmonary disease may be asymptomatic in up to 50% of people infected, or it may present as cough and hemoptysis.

Physical Examination

More global changes can be seen, such as disorientation, confusion, lethargy and fatigue, and hallucinations. Hydrocephalus may occur at any point in the disease. Osseous *Cryptococcus* is present in 10% of cases.

 ## Laboratory Aids

TESTS

- CSF should be obtained to confirm the diagnosis; it should be sent for cell count and differential; protein; glucose; cultures for bacterial, fungal, and viral pathogens; India ink stain; and cryptococcal antigen.
- India ink stain of the CSF reveals budding yeast in at least 50% of the cases.
- CSF evaluations in HIV-infected individuals may be relatively unremarkable; however, in most others, CSF abnormalities exist with a mild mononuclear pleocytosis, mildly elevated protein, and depressed glucose.
- Blood and CSF samples should be sent for fungal culture.

 ## Therapy

Combination therapy, especially for CNS disease, is recommended as follows:

- Amphotericin, 0.3 to 1 mg/kg/d plus 5-fluorocytosine (5-FC), 37.5 mg/kg q6h. This regimen should be continued for a minimum of 6 weeks.
- In patients with HIV, maintenance therapy is recommended with fluconazole at 400 mg/d.
- Treatment of pulmonary *Cryptococcus* is recommended in the immunocompromised host. Treatment of bone or isolated visceral infection is also recommended with 6 to 8 weeks of amphotericin B.

 ## Follow-Up

Follow-up is important for normal hosts due to the risk of relapse. Thus, patients should be seen at 3-month intervals for 12 to 18 months following treatment, with cultures obtained for fungal isolation. Patients with immunodeficiencies should be followed every 2 to 3 months, even while on suppressive therapy, to monitor for clinical signs or symptoms of relapse.

 ## Common Questions and Answers

Q: What are the sources of *Cryptococcus* in nature?
A: Pigeon droppings and soil.

Q: Can "normal" (immunocompetent) people get this infection? How long should it be treated?
A: Yes. Treat for 6 weeks.

Q: Should all patients with *Cryptococcus* be worked up for immunodeficiency?
A: Yes.

ICD-9-CD 117.5

BIBLIOGRAPHY

Aberg JA, Powderly WG. Cryptococcal disease: implications of recent clinical trials on treatment and management. *AIDS Clin Rev* 1997–1998;229–248.

Chuck SL, Sande MA. Infections with *Cryptococcus neoformans* in the acquired immunodeficiency syndrome. *N Engl J Med* 1989;321:794–799.

Dismukes WE. Cryptococcal meningitis in patients with AIDS. *J Infect Dis* 1988;157:624–628.

Saag MS, Powderly WG, Cloud GA, et al. Comparison of amphotericin B with fluconazole in the treatment of acute AIDS-associated cryptococcal meningitis. *N Engl J Med* 1992;326:83–89.

Wittner M. Cryptococcal disease. In: Feigen RD, Cherry JD, eds. *Textbook of pediatric infectious diseases,* vol. 2. Philadelphia: WB Saunders, 1992:1934–1939.

Author: Bret J. Rudy

Cryptorchidism

 Database

DEFINITION

- Undescended testes

CAUSES

- Hypogonadotropic hypogonadism

—Boys with cryptorchidism lack the normal post-natal gonadotropin surge at 60 to 90 days. As a result, there is no proliferation of Leydig cells, no testosterone surge, and no maturation of germ cells.
—Higher incidence of central nervous system (CNS) abnormalities in boys with bilateral cryptorchidism than those with unilateral cryptorchidism or normal testes, possibly related to a pituitary abnormality causing hypogonadotropism

- Gubernaculum also influences testicular descent, possibly due to innervation by the genitofemoral nerve, which promotes descent

—Only 17% of cryptorchid testes have normal gubernacular attachment

- Different possible locations of a cryptorchid testis:

—Intra-abdominal—at least 1 cm above internal inguinal ring
—High annular—just at internal ring
—Canalicular
—Within superficial inguinal pouch of Denis Browne—the most common location
—High scrotal
—25% are descended testes missed by palpation
—20% absent
—Ectopic testes have taken an aberrant course of descent—prepenile, superficial ectopic, transverse scrotal, femoral or perineal location

PATHOLOGY

- Cryptorchid testes have normal histology at birth.
- By 1 year of life there is atrophy with lack of development.
- By 2 years of life there are greatly reduced numbers of germ cells due to increased temperatures and the damage appears to be irreversible.
- Undescended testes are smaller than descended; damage is irreversible.
- More histological changes are noted the higher the testis is located.
- Some germ cell loss is also noted in the contralateral descended testis; up to 40% of contralateral descended testes may have decreased germ cells if the undescended testicle is not corrected.

EPIDEMIOLOGY

- Incidence greater in premature infants and low birthwieght infants—3.4% in full-term; 17% in premature infants weighing 2 to 2.5 kg; 100% in infants, 900 g.

—Normal descent occurs in the seventh month of gestation.

- 0.7% incidence in children. 1 year old and adults

—Post-natal increases of luteinizing hormone (LH) and follicle-stimulating hormone (FSH) may result in late descent that occurs in about 50% of cryptorchid testes in first 12 months.
—Spontaneous descent does not appear to occur beyond 1 year.
—Most descend by 3 months of age; for premature babies, within 3 months of their due date; the post-natal surge of gonadotropin and testosterone play an important role in the descent of testes in the first 3 months of life.
—70% descend by 1 year

- 66% of boys with cryptorchidism may have retractile testes
- 30% are bilateral

GENETICS

- Incidence of 1% to 4% in siblings of boys with cryptorchidism
- 6% of fathers of boys with cryptorchidism had cryptorchidism
- Increased incidence in disorders of gonadotropin deficiency (i.e., Kallmann, Prader-Willi, Lawrence-Moon-Biedl syndromes)
- Also increased incidence in Klinefelter and Noonan syndromes, and neural-tube disorders

 Differential Diagnosis

- Retractile testes—normally descended testes that may be noted on initial physical examination because the cremasteric reflex is weak.

—Subsequently, may be difficult to palpate because of exaggerated cremasteric reflex at about 3 months of age; may be bilateral
—Testes are positioned outside of scrotum, but can be brought down into and remain in the scrotum with out tension
—Human chorionic gonadotropin (hCG) stimulation test often results in descent
—Normal-sized testes with normally developed scrotum
—Histologically normal
—Testes usually remain in the scrotum by early puberty

- If testes are not palpable, absent testes must be considered:

—20% of undescended testes are not palpable—50% are inguinal, 25% intra-abdominal, 15% below the external inguinal ring, 10% absent
—45% of non-palpable testes are due to absent gonad
—Anorchia occurs in 5% of bilateral cryptorchidism
—Usually occurs due to vascular accident prenatally or soon after birth—analogous to testicular torsion
—Spermatic vessels and vas deferens end blindly in inguinal canal or scrotum.
—48% to 59% of unilateral non-palpable testis are due to testicular absence associated with significant contralateral hypertrophy of testis

Physical Examination

Finding: Non-palpable testes
Significance: Repeated annual examination is necessary, however, because descended testes may spontaneously come to occupy an extra-scrotal position where it is prone to the same degenerative changes seen in cryptorchidism

Finding: Associated hypospadias with unilateral or bilateral cryptorchidism
Significance: Increases the risk of an intersex disorder such as mixed gonadal dysgenesis or male pseudohermaphroditism

Finding: Bilateral non-palpable gonads
Significance: Should trigger evaluation for anorchia, female androgenital syndrome, or hypothalamic-pituitary insufficiency

PHYSICAL EXAMINATION TRICKS

• To detect retractile testes, use a warm room, and seated, cross-legged, or squatting position.
• Begin palpation in the area of internal inguinal ring, and walk fingers down the canal toward the scrotum.
• Lubricating jelly may help decrease friction.

 ## Laboratory Aids

Usually none needed.

TESTS

Test: hCG Stimulation
Significance: Normal response of testicular tissue is a fourfold increase in serum testosterone. No response in anorchia.

Test: Basal gonadotropin levels
Significance: These are 3 standard deviations above the mean in anorchia in boys<9 years old.

Test: Anorchia
Significance: This is also associated with elevated LH and FSH levels.

Test: Venography
Significance: Is successful in locating testes in 75% of cases of non-palpable testes, but is limited by size of gonadal vessels to older children.

Test: Laparoscopy
Significance: This is 95% accurate in locating non-palpable testes.

IMAGING

• Ultrasound and CT scanning have been useful in older boys, although MRI seems to be more accurate.

 ## Therapy

CONSERVATIVE THERAPY

• Hormonal therapy involves use of hCG and/or gonadotropin-releasing hormone (GnRH) to bring down testes by stimulating testosterone but without inducing pubertal changes.

—GnRH has few side effects and does not cause virilization, but is not approved for use in the United States.
—GnRH alone results in descent in 28% in studies in Europe
—hCG successful in 10%, but relatively ineffective for intra-abdominal testes
—Bilateral cryptorchidism is more responsive to hCG therapy than unilateral
—10% to 20% ascend after hCG therapy, requiring a repeat course or surgery
—Combination of GnRH followed by hCG is successful in 80%
—Combined use produces better results than monotherapy; best results in low-lying testes
—50% relapse rate at 7 years
—Hormonal therapy may improve future fertility
—Recommended doses are biweekly injection of 250 IU hCG for infants, and 500 IU up to age 6 years and 1000 IU for older children for a total course of 5 weeks.
—Therapy must be initiated by 10 months of age so that treatment failures can be referred for orchiopexy.
—Side effects of hCG include epiphyseal plate fusion, accelerated development of secondary sex characteristics and retarded growth with large doses.

SURGICAL THERAPY

• Goal is to locate testis and to relocate the testis to the scrotum if possible:

—Options include traditional orchiopexy or microvascular autotransplantation.
—Surgery recommended between 6 and 18 months because of progressive damage that occurs to testes with time.
—Complications—injury to the vas deferens may affect fertility.

• Laparoscopy can be both diagnostic and therapeutic—if spermatic cord and vessels end blindly, no additional exploration necessary.
• If testes are intra-abdominal, orchiectomy is recommended because of future cancer risk.

PROGNOSIS

• Infertility if bilateral and untreated

—If bilateral and treated—50% are fertile
—If unilateral and treated—75% are fertile
—Earlier orchiopexy may improve fertility, but there are conflicting data

• Risk of cancer is 22× greater than the general population in third or fourth decade in undescended testes, especially if untreated or corrected after or during puberty:

—Risk is increased sixfold if testis is intra-abdominal versus other cryptorchid locations
—60% of tumors of undescended testes are seminomas
—Cancer is rare before puberty
—25% of tumors occur in contralateral normally descended testis
—No evidence that orchiopexy alters malignancy potential, but orchiopexy renders testis accessible for regular self-examination
—Earlier age at orchiopexy reduces the excess risk of malignancy

• Carcinoma *in situ* found in 2% to 3% of all men with a history of cryptorchidism:

—Treat with orchiectomy or radiation
—Ultrasonography may be used to screen for irregularities indicative of carcinoma *in situ*
—Invasive cancer develops in 50% in 5 years.

ICD-9-CM 752.51

BIBLIOGRAPHY

Gill B, Kogan S. Crytporchidism. Current concepts. *Pediatr Clin North Am* 1997;44(5):1211–1227.

Kelalis P, King L, Belman A, eds. *Clinical pediatric urology*. Philadelphia: WB Saunders, 1992.

Palmer J. The undescended testicle. *Endocrinol Metab Clin North Am* 1991;20:231–240.

Rozanski T, Bloom D. The undescended testis: theory and management. *Urol Clin North Am* 1995;22:107–118.

Author: Christina Lin Master

Cryptosporidiosis

 Database

DEFINITION

In an immunocompetent patient disease is manifested as a self-limiting gastroenteritis. However, immunocompromised patients can develop protracted severe gastroenteritis, which can lead to severe wasting and ultimately death.

CAUSES

Most commonly, gastrointestinal illness is caused by ingestion of the oocysts of *Cryptosporidium parvum*; a coccidian protozoa that is frequently found in the feces of animals as well as some insects.

PATHOLOGY/PATHOPHYSIOLOGY

• Transmission occurs when oocysts contaminating food or water are ingested or, more commonly, through fecal-oral transmission from person to person.
• The infectious dose for humans is low, estimated at less than 10 oocysts. The incubation period is approximately 5 to 21 days and oocyst shedding may occur for weeks to months.
• Invasion of intestinal epithelial cells of the upper gastrointestinal tract leads to a secretory diarrhea. The exact mechanism by which this occurs is still unclear.

EPIDEMIOLOGY

• Typically children under 5 years of age are most often affected. Severe disease is usually seen in the immunocompromised; such as patients with impaired cell mediated immunity (in particular those who are HIV positive or taking immunosuppressive medications), those with immunoglobulin deficiencies as well as gamma interferon deficiencies.
• A significant seasonality has been reported, with peaks occurring in North America during the late summer and early fall.
• Outbreaks have been associated with swimming pools, lakes, water recreation parks, drinking water supplies, day camps, unpasteurized apple cider, exposure to farm animals, and day care attendance.
• Other risk factors include exposure to dogs, cats, deers, cockroaches, and traveling abroad.

COMPLICATIONS

• In immunocompromised patients, infection can lead to severe protracted diarrhea with malnutrition and wasting. Biliary tract disease and systemic dissemination such as pulmonary disease can also be seen in the immunocompromised.

PROGNOSIS

• For immunocompetent hosts, gastrointestinal disease is self-limited usually lasting 10 to 14 days. Supportive therapy is usually all that is necessary.
• For immunocompromised patients, diarrhea can be severe, debilitating, and often life-threatening. Aggressive supportive therapy is usually required along with a trial of antimicrobial therapy. Unfortunately, there are no agents that are uniformally effective against *Cryptosporidium parvum*.

 Differential Diagnosis

INFECTIOUS

• Viral gastroenteritis including but not limited to:

—Rotavirus
—Adenovirus
—Astrovirus
—Norwalk
—Cytomegalovirus (CMV)

• Bacterial gastroenteritis including but not limited to:

—*Salmonella*
—*Shigella*
—*Yersinia*
—*Campylobacter*
—*Aeromoas*
—*Pleisomonas*
—Enterotoxigenic *E. coli*
—*Vibrio cholerae*

• Parasitic gastroenteritis including but not limited to:

—*Giardia*
—*Entamoeba*
—*Cyclospora*
—*Isospora*
—*Microsporidia*
—*Dientamoeba fragilis*
—*Blastocystis hominis*
—*Clostridium difficile enterocolitis*

NON-INFECTIOUS

• Allergic
• Autoimmune
• Anatomical
• Endocrine
• Iatrogenic/Medications
• Inflammatory bowel disease
• Malabsorption
• Neoplastic

 Data Gathering

HISTORY

• Onset: Acute onset of watery non-bloody diarrhea, crampy abdominal pain, low-grade fever, and occasionally nausea and vomiting.
• Exposure: Exposure to ill contacts, public swimming pools, lakes or wave parks, animals, day care attendance, travel history, dietary history such as consumption of unpasteurized beverages and drinking water supply.
• Evidence of immunosuppression: Immunosuppression secondary to disease or medication as well as exposure to immunosuppressed individuals in the household or, if patient is old enough, through occupation.

 Laboratory Aids

Test: Modified acid fast stain
Significance: Diagnosis is made by observing the 4 to 5 μm cysts in preserved stool specimens. Immunofluorescent antibody or rapid (3 minute) direct antigen detection tests are also available. Stool specimens should be performed three times on alternate days to exlude the diagnosis.

Test: Must specifically request that the microbiology lab test for this organism.
Significance: A recent national survey of clinical laboratories revealed only 5% routinely tested for *C. parvum*.

Test: Sputum specimen
Significance: For respiratory infections, diagnosis is made by finding the oocysts in sputum specimens.

Test: H and E staining of small intestinal biopsies
Significance: May show the organism protruding from the microvillus border of enterocytes.

Therapy

• Fluid and electrolyte replacement. For protracted cases, patients will eventually require hyperalimentation.
• The antibiotic paromomycin, an aminoglycoside, can improve symptoms and decrease parasite excretion in the feces of some immunocompromised patients and this has become the treatment of choice for immunosuppressed patients. The dosage is 25 to 30 mg/kg/day three times a day for 7 days. Spiromycin is not effective.
• Some patients have been shown to have improvement in their clinical symptoms with the gastrointestinal hormone octreotide. The dosage is 300 to 500 mcg three times a day.
• *Cryptosporidium* is on the CDC recommended reporting list of infectious diseases; however, not all states in the United States mandate reporting *Cryptosporidium*.

Follow-Up

• Since the oocysts can be shed in the stool for a long time after clinical resolution, it is not necessary to check follow-up convalescent stools. However, it is important to realize that asymptomatic patients can still transmit the infection to household and day care contacts.
• Requiring patients whose diarrhea has resolved to have a negative stool test for *Cryptosporidium* before reentry to day care has not been evaluated as an outbreak control measure. Repeated testing is expensive.

PREVENTION

• Isolation of hospitalized patient

—Contact precautions (i.e., gown and gloves for all patient contact) are recommended for the length of the hospital stay. If possible, a single bedroom would be optimal so that a bathroom does not need to be shared.

• Community prevention

—Public water supplies should be adequately filtered in order to ensure oocyst removal.
—Communities that do not use filtration systems are at increased risk for outbreaks, the most recent of which was the Milwaukee epidemic, where an estimated 400,000 people were affected.
—Homeowners with well water should consider installing drinking water filtration systems.
—Sources of drinking water should be protected from possible fecal contamination.
—Garden hoses should not be used to provide drinking water.
—All juices should be pasteurized. *Cryptosporidium* has been shown to survive in unpasteurized apple cider for up to 4 weeks.

—Symptomatic patients should not be allowed to swim in public pools.
—Good handwashing after contact with animals.

• Control measures

—Hand washing especially after changing diapers.
—Separation of diapering and food handling areas.
—Disinfection of diapering areas after each use, frequent (at least twice daily) disinfection of toys, table tops, and high chairs during outbreaks is recommended.
—Oocysts can survive for long periods and are resistant to many disinfectants such as: pine oil, cresylic acid, ethanol, n-propanol, isopropanol, lysol, phenol, iodophores, aldehydes, benzylkonium chloride, and quaternary ammonia compounds. Exposure of oocysts to 5.25% sodium hypochoride (full strength bleach) will destroy infectivity after 10 minutes. However, normally used concentrations of bleach have been shown to be poor disinfectants for *Cryptosporidium*. And 3% hydrogen peroxide is felt to be more effective and is recommended for outbreak control; 5% ammonia is also effective, however, it has a strong odor and if mixed accidentally with chlorine containing solutions (such as bleach) can produce hazardous chlorine gas.
—Temporarily excluding or, if possible, cohorting symptomatic children. Since fecal shedding can be quite prolonged, it is generally recommended that once symptoms have resolved children should be allowed to return to their regular settings.

• During an outbreak, screening should be considered for children and caregivers who are in a household or in close contact with immunocompromised persons.
• Swimming pools found to be contaminated with *Cryptosporidium* require closing and hyperchlorination. The level of chlorination required to kill cryptosporidium oocysts is approximately 640 times greater than that required to kill *Giardia* cysts. Maintaining this level of chlorination is not feasible and, therefore, swimming in public pools places an immunocompromised patient at increased risk.

PITFALLS

• Not considering the diagnosis in patients with acute diarrhea.
• Not sending the appropriate number of stool specimens to exclude the diagnosis.
• Assuming the microbiology lab will routinely test for *C. parvum*.
• Forgetting to test for other parasites if *C. parvum* is found in the stool.

Common Questions and Answers

Q: For whom should Cryptosporidiosis as a differential diagnosis be considered?
A: For anyone with acute onset of watery diarrhea with any of the mentioned risk factors.

Q: When is it safe for a child with *Cryptosporidium* to return to day care?
A: When the diarrhea has resolved.

ICD-9-CM 559.007.4

BIBLIOGRAPHY

Cordel RL, Addiss DG. Cryptosporidiosis in child care settings: a review of the literature and recommendations for prevention and control. *Pediatr Infect Dis* 1994;13:310–317.

Cryptosporidium. *1997 Redbook: report of the Committee on Infectious Diseases,* 24th ed. Academy of Pediatrics. 1997:185–186.

LaVia W. Parasitic gastroenteritis. *Pediatr Ann* 1994;(23):556–560.

Outbreak of cryptosporidiosis at a day camp. *MMWR* 1996;45(21):442–444.

Outbreaks of *Eschericheria coli* 0157:H7 infection and cryptosporidiosis associated with drinking unpasteurized apple cider. *MMWR* 1997;46(1):4–8.

Author: Jane M. Gould

Cushing Syndrome (Adrenal Excess)

 Database

DEFINITION

An excess in the secretion of cortisol by the adrenal cortex. This may be associated with excess production of other adrenal hormones, such as androgens and mineralocorticoids.

PATHOPHYSIOLOGY

- Cushing disease—pituitary ACTH oversecretion, usually due to pituitary adenoma, with resultant bilateral adrenal hyperplasia.

—Adrenal tumors
—Adrenal adenomas—secrete mainly cortisol
—Adrenal cortical carcinomas—usually large, rapidly growing tumors, which produce a variety of hormones including cortisol and androgens.

EPIDEMIOLOGY

- Incidence

—0.1 to 0.5 new pediatric cases per million population/year
—Ten times more common in adults

- Gender

—Cushing disease—female predominance
—Adrenocortical carcinoma—female predominance

- Age

—Cushing disease—accounts for 80% of Cushing syndrome in adults and children greater than 7 years of age.
—Adrenal tumor—adrenocortical carcinomas account for more than 50% of Cushing syndrome in children less than age 7.

- These tumors are less common in adults and children older than 7 years of age.

COMPLICATIONS

- Cushing syndrome:

—Growth arrest
—Obesity
—Pubertal arrest
—Glucose intolerance
—Osteoporosis
—Adrenal carcinomas—metastatic spread

PROGNOSIS

- The prognosis for cure is good with Cushing disease and adrenal adenoma.
- The prognosis for adrenal carcinoma is poor because of the frequency of micrometastases and high recurrence rate.

 Differential Diagnosis

- Cushing disease
—Pituitary ACTH oversecretion
- Adrenal tumors
—Adrenal adenomas
—Adrenal cortical carcinomas
- Exogenous glucocorticoid treatment

 Data Gathering

HISTORY

- Weight gain, gradual onset
- Weakness and fatigue

Question: What emotional/mental changes are seen?
Significance: Cortisol exceess can cause emotional changes.

 Physical Examination

Finding: Growth arrest
Significance: Most consistent finding

Finding: Obesity
Significance: Cervicodorsal fat (localized: moon facies, truncal obesity)

Finding: Thin skin with striae, facial plethora
Significance: Sign of cortisol excess

Finding: Hirsutism, acne
Significance: Sex hormone effect

Finding: Pubertal arrest/menstrual disorders
Significance: Common finding

Finding: Hypertension
Significance: Mineralocorticoid effect

Finding: Bruising
Significance: Capillary friability

Finding: Hyperpigmentation
Significance: ACTH effect

Finding: Virilization/feminization
Significance: Sex hormone effect

 Laboratory Aids

DIAGNOSTIC TESTS

Test: Urinary 24-h free cortisol greater than 90 gg/24 h (preferred test). Correct for creatinine and surface area. Two or three separate collections are preferable.
Significance: Establishes the diagnosis of hypercortisolism.

Test: Urinary 24-h 17-hydroxysteroids greater than 6 mg/g creatinine
Significance: Establishes the diagnosis of hypercortisolism

Test: Overnight dexamethasone suppression test (15 gg/kg)
Significance: Screening only; 8:00 A.M. plasma cortisol $\geq$5 μg/L, suspect hypercortisolism

Test: Loss of diurnal variation of plasma cortisol in older children.
Significance: Normally, the 11:00 P.M. cortisol is less than 50% of 8:00 A.M. value. The majority of patients with Cushing syndrome have mean elevated plasma cortisol, without diurnal variation.

DIFFERENTIATE CAUSES

Test: ACTH levels
Significance: Cushing disease: increased ACTH with hypercortisolism. Adrenal tumor: low ACTH and hypercortisolism.

Test: Androgen levels
Significance: Often high in adrenocortical carcinoma. These patients are often virilized. Androgen levels are low in benign cortisol secreting adenomas.

Test: Dexamethasone suppression tests. Low dose (30 gg/kg/day) divided q6h PO ×2 days, followed by high dose (120 ltg/kg/day) divided q6h PO ×2 days. A 24-h urine collection for cortisol and 17-hydroxysteroids throughout.
Significance: Non-Cushing states usually suppress urinary-free cortisol and 17 hydroxysteroids to 50% to 90% of baseline values after low dose.

- Majority of pituitary tumors suppressible after high dose
- Adrenal source: Hypercortisolism will not suppress.

TUMOR LOCATION

Test: Pituitary MRI with gadoliniurn
Significance: May demonstrate a pituitary adenoma

Test: Abdominal CT/MRI
Significance: Will demonstrate adrenal carcinoma, adrenal adenomas, or bilateral hyperplasia/nodules resulting from Cushing disease.

Test: Cavernous sinus sampling for ACTH
Significance: Will help to lateralize pituitary microadenomas

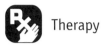 Therapy

CUSHING DISEASE

• Transphenoidal pituitary surgery

—70% to 80% success, may be less in some series
—Perioperative glucocorticoid replacement required

• Pituitary radiation—6 to 18 months for effect

—Remission in 45% to 85% of individuals
—Remission rate improved if combined with o,p'DDD

• Bilateral adrenalectomy

—High rate of surgical complications
—May result in Nelson syndrome--pituitary adenoma growth and hyperpigmentation, long-term glucocorticoid and mineralocorticoid replacement.

• Drug therapy

—Ketoconazole—inhibits multiple adrenal enzymes
—o,p'DDD—adrenolytic agent
—Metyrapone—11-hydroxylase inhibitor
—Aminoglutethimide—20,22 desmolase inhibitor
—Trilostane—3 B-hydroxysteroid dehydrogenase inhibitor
—RU 486—Glucocorticoid receptor antagonist
—Drug combinations may lower individual doses and lessen side effects

• Adrenal tumors

—Aggressive surgical resection
—Chemotherapy for carcinoma: Cytoxan, Adriamycin, 5FU, MTX

• Drug therapy to control hypercortisolism

—o,p'DDD at high doses—may improve recurrence risk in patients with complete tumor resection. In those with residual or recurrent disease, it may improve hypercortisolism, but not survival

• Glucocorticoid and possibly mineralocorticoid replacement.

 Follow-Up

• Chronic glucocorticoid replacement 10 to 12 mg/m^2/day divided as b.i.d. to t.i.d. until recovery of hypothalamic/pituitary function (6–12 months). Triple for stress; fever illness, vomiting. Injectable hydrocortisone for emergency use taper corticosteroid treatment gradually.
• Reassess 24-h urinary cortisol/ketosteroid secretion during the first week after treatment and at 6 weeks.
• In the week after effective pituitary surgery, cortisol should be undetectable and ACTH less than 5 pg/mL, 24 hours after last hydrocortisone dose. Stimulation and suppression tests are performed 6 weeks post-surgery (holding hydrocortisone dose).
• Frequent follow-up to monitor for recurrence. Monitor for cortisol withdrawal symptoms, hypopituitarism. Consider medical treatment for persistent hypercortisolism.

PITFALLS

• False-positive tests for hypercortisolism

—Stress—lack of suppression
—Depression
—Anorexia
—Primary glucocorticoid resistance

• False-negative tests

—Incomplete urine collection
—Periodic hormonogenesis
—Slow metabolism of dexamethasone

• Aberrant renal metabolism
• Repeat if suspicion is strong

 Common Questions and Answers

Q: What clinical features help distinguish patients with pituitary Cushing disease from patients with adrenal tumors?
A: Cushing syndrome and hyperpigmentation suggests an ACTH effect. Cushing syndrome and virilization suggests adrenal carcinoma.

Q: What physical characteristics most clearly differentiate children with exogenous obesity from those with Cushing Syndrome?
A: Exogenous obesity is associated with robust linear growth while Cushing Syndrome is associated with growth failure.

ICD-9-CM 255

BIBLIOGRAPHY

Cacciari E, Cicognani A, Pirazzoli P, et al. Adrenocortical tumours in children: our experience with nine cases. *Acta Endocrinol Suppl (Copenh)* 1986;279:264–274.

Gomez MT, Malozowski S, Winterer J, Vamvakopoulos C, Chrousos GP. Urinary free cortisol values in normal children and adolescents. *J Pediatr* 1991;118(2):256–258.

Magiakou MA, Mastorakos G, Oldfield EH, et al. Cushing's syndrome in children and adolescents: presentation, diagnosis, and therapy. *N Engl J Med* 1994;331:629–636.

Orth DN. Cushing's syndrome. *N Engl J Med* 1995;332(12):791–803.

Author: Lorraine Katz

Cutaneous Larva Migrans

 Database

DEFINITION

Infestation of the epidermis by the infectious larvae of certain nematodes. Humans are accidental hosts, with the primary hosts being dogs and cats.

CAUSES

• Most common organism is the dog or cat hookworm, *Ancylostoma braziliense*.
• Other species include *A. canium, Uncinaria stenocephala*, and *Bunostomum phlebotomum*.

PATHOPHYSIOLOGY

• Humans are accidental hosts.
• Filariform larvae penetrate the epidermis either through hair follicles or fissures or through intact skin with the use of proteases.
• Diagnosis is usually clinical. Organisms rarely recovered from biopsy and antibody titers unreliable because symptoms are due to hypersensitivity to the organism or its excreta, and immunity usually does not develop.

ASSOCIATED DISEASES

• Most common manifestation is an intensely pruritic, linear, serpiginous skin lesion known as a "creeping eruption."
• Most common complication is secondary bacterial infection of the involved skin.
• Rare cases of a peripheral eosinophilia with pulmonary infiltrates (Loffler syndrome) occur when dermal penetration by the larvae occurs and the bloodstream is invaded.

EPIDEMIOLOGY

• Contracted from contaminated soil.
• Worldwide distribution, but most frequent in warmer climates, including the Caribbean, Africa, South America, Southeast Asia, and Southeastern United States.
• Occupational exposures occur from crawling under buildings, such as plumbers and pipefitters.
• Route of spread:
—Primary host (dog or cat) passes eggs to ground through feces.
—Warm, sandy soil acts as an incubator.
—Eggs mature into rhabditiform larvae (noninfectious), which molt in 5 days to filariform larvae (infectious).
—Incubation period from infection to symptoms usually 7 to 10 days, although can range up to several months.

COMPLICATIONS

• Most common complication is secondary bacterial infection of the skin. Self-limited disease—if untreated, larvae die within 2 to 8 weeks but may persist for up to 1 year.
• Rarely, the larvae can invade the dermis and, subsequently, the bloodstream, leading to a peripheral eosinophilia and pulmonary infiltrates (Loffler syndrome).

PROGNOSIS

• This is a self-limited disease and without treatment will resolve when the larvae die.
• There is a 98% response rate to topical thiabendazole and a 99% response rate reported with oral thiabendazole.

 Differential Diagnosis

• Cutaneous larva migrans should be considered in anyone with an intensely pruritic, raised, serpiginous, linear cutaneous eruption.
• Hookworm infections (*Strongyloides stercoralis, Uncinaria stenocephala, Bunostomum phlebotomum, Gnathostoma spinigerum*)
• Free living nematodes (*Pelodera strongyloides*), and insect larvae.
• Other cutaneous eruptions which may mimic cutaneous larva migrans include erythema chronicum migrans of Lyme disease, jelly fish stings, and photosensitivity.

 Data Gathering

HISTORY

Question: What is the incubation period?
Significance: Usual time from infection to symptoms is 7 to 10 days but may last for up to several months.

Question: Is there rash?
Significance: It is intensely pruritic, raised, serpiginous, and linear. Often located on the feet and extremities, buttocks, and genitalia.

Question: Is there pruritis?
Significance: Symptoms typically begin with some tingling in the affected area with the development of the typical rash with intense pruritus.

Question: How fast does rash spread?
Significance: Rash typically lengthens by 2 to 3 cm daily.

Laboratory Aids

Test: Biopsy
Significance: Rarely yields organisms

Test: Serologic testing
Significance: Not helpful

Diagnosis based on clinical presentation

 ## Therapy

• First-line treatment is topical thiabendazole, supplied as a 10% suspension of 500 mg/5 mL applied four times per day for 10 days.
• Alternatively, oral thiabendazole in a dose of 25 to 50 mg/kg/day q12h for 2 days
• Albendazole, not approved for use in the United States, is available in other countries and is administered as 400 mg/day for 3 days in adults.

 ## Follow-Up

• Symptoms persist for 8 weeks but up to 1 year in untreated patients.
• Those with extensive involvement should be seen after treatment to be certain of improvement in symptoms.

 ## Common Questions and Answers

Q: Can children spread the infection to each other?
A: The usual spread of infection is from direct contact with the larvae. Spread from one individual to another usually does not occur.

ICD-9-CM 126.9

BIBLIOGRAPHY

Davies HD, Sakuls P, Keystone JS. Creeping eruption: a review of clinical presentation and management of 60 cases presenting to a tropical disease unit. *Arch Dermatol* 1993;129(5): 588–591.

Jones SK. Cutaneous larva migrans—'recurrens' [Letter]. *Br J Dermatol* 1994;130(4):546.

Jones WB. Cutaneous larva migrans. *South Med J* 1993;86(11):1311–1313.

Uppal A, Liebers D, Tobin EH. Tracking the itch. When to suspect migrating larvae. *Postgrad Med* 1997;101(5):281–282, 288.

Van den Enden E, Stevens A, Van Gompel A. Treatment of cutaneous larva migrans. *N Engl J Med* 1998;339(17):1246–1247.

Author: Bret J. Rudy

Cystic Fibrosis

 Database

DEFINITION

Autosomal recessive disease, characterized by chronic obstructive lung disease, pancreatic exocrine deficiency, and elevated sweat chloride concentrations.

PATHOPHYSIOLOGY

- Cystic fibrosis transmembrane regulator (CFTR)
—Functions as a cyclic AMP-activated chloride channel.
—Allows for the transport of chloride out of the cell water molecules passively following chloride ion out of the cell, keeping secretions well hydrated.
—An abnormality in CFTR blocks chloride transport. Inadequate hydration of the cell surface results, causing thick secretions and organ damage.
- In the respiratory system
—Lungs usually normal early in illness
—Hypertrophy of mucus-secreting glands
—Mucus plugging
—Bronchiectasis
—Cyst formation (especially in upper lobes)
—Bacterial colonization
- In the gastrointestinal tract
—Atrophy of the pancreas
—Focal biliary cirrhosis of the liver
—Hypoplasia of the gallbladder

GENETICS

- CFTR gene
—Located on the long arm of chromosome 7
—Most common deletion is 3 base pairs, resulting in absence of phenylalanine at codon 508.
—This F508 mutation is seen in over 70% of the cystic fibrosis population in North America.
—Currently, over 300 mutations reported

EPIDEMIOLOGY

- Most common lethal inherited disease in the white population
- Incidence of abnormalities in the CFTR gene
—1:25 individuals of the white race
- Incidence of cystic fibrosis:
—1:2500 in white population
—1:17,000 in black population
—1:10,000 in the population of hispanic origin
—Less common in African blacks and Asians

COMPLICATIONS

- Respiratory complications
—Recurrent bronchitis and pneumonia
—Chronic sinusitis
—Pneumothorax
—Hemoptysis
- Gastrointestinal complications
—Pancreatic insufficiency:
  —Patients usually have steatorrhea.
  —Decreased levels of vitamins A, D, E, and K
  —Poor growth

—Clinically significant hepatobiliary disease
—Found in 3% of the affected population, cirrhosis of the liver is the most commonly seen complication in patients with advanced liver disease, findings may include:
  —Esophageal varices
  —Splenomegaly
—Cholestasis
—Hypersplenism
  —Reproductive complications:
   —Sterility in 98% of the males due to absence or atresia of the vas deferens
   —Infertility rate for females is 70% to 80% due to thick, tenacious mucus occluding the cervical os.
  —Endocrine complications:
   —Diabetes mellitus seen in up to 12% of patients as they approach the young adult years

PROGNOSIS

- Variable
- Mean lifespan is approximately 29 years
- Course of the disease varies patient to patient

 Differential Diagnosis

PULMONARY

- Recurrent pneumonia or bronchitis
- Severe asthma
- Aspiration pneumonia

GASTROINTESTINAL

- Gastroesophageal reflux
- Celiac sprue
- Protein-losing enteropathy

OTHER

- Failure to thrive due to:
—Social problems
—Poor caloric intake
—Feeding problems

 Data Gathering

HISTORY

Question: Have there been respiratory symptoms?
Significance: The most common presenting respiratory symptoms:

- Chronic cough
- Recurrent pneumonia
- Nasal polyps
- Chronic pansinusitis

Question: Have there been gastrointestinal symptoms?
Significance: Most common presenting gastrointestinal symptoms:

- Meconium ileus (15% to 20% of patients present with this symptom).

- Pancreatic insufficiency occurs in 85% of patients
- In infants, fat malabsorption may lead to failure to thrive.
- In older patients, pancreatitis.
- Rectal prolapse
—Occurs in 2% of the patients
—Must consider CF until proven otherwise
—Commonly seen between 1 and 5 years
- Meconium ileus equivalent:
—Distal obstruction of the large intestine
—Seen in older children

Question: Dietary history?
Significance: Soy bean formula may lead to edema.

Question: Evidence of acute onset of weakness?
Significance: In summer, increased sweating may lead to hyponatremia or hypochloremic metabolic alkalosis.

 Physical Examination

Finding: Respiratory findings
Significance:

- Cough, frequently productive of mucopurulent sputum
- Rhonchi
- Rales
- Hyperersonance to percussion
- Barrel-chest deformity of thorax in severe cases
- Nasal polyposis
- Cyanosis (in later stages)

Finding: Other common findings:

- Digital clubbing
- Hepatosplenomegaly in patients with cirrhosis
- Growth retardation
- Hypertrophic osteoarthropathy
- Teenage patients may have:
—Delayed puberty
—Amenorrhea
—Irregular menstrual periods

 Laboratory Aids

Test: Sweat test
Significance: "Gold standard" for the diagnosis of cystic fibrosis; sweat chloride greater than 60 mEq/L is considered abnormal.

- False-positives seen in:
—Severe malnutrition
—Ectodermal dysplasia
—Adrenal insufficiency
—Nephrogenic diabetes insipidus
—Hypothyroidism
—Hypoparathyroidism
—Mucopolysaccharidoses
- False-negatives seen in:
—Patients with edema and hypoproteinemia

Test: Genetic testing
Significance:

- Uses polymerase chain reaction technology
- Can detect over 90% of the abnormal geno-types and lack of a positive genotype reduces, but does not eliminate, the possibility of cystic fibrosis.
- Collection methods include blood samples or cheek bruisings

Test: Sputum cultures
Significance: Frequently recovered organisms include:

- *Escherichia coli*
- Haemophilus influenzae
- Staphylococcus aureus
- Pseudomonas aeruginosa (non-mucoid and mucoid)
- *Pseudomonas cepacia*
- Aspergillus species

Test: Pulmonary function tests
Significance: Usually reveals obstructive lung disease, although some patients may have a restrictive pattern.

Test: Pancreatic function tests
Significance: Degree of pancreatic disease

Test: 72-hour fecal fat measurement
Significance: Fat malabsorption

Test: Measurement of serum para-aminobenzoic acid (PABA) levels
Significance: Usually reveal evidence of pancreatic insufficiency. One 72 hour fecal fat measurement is the gold standard. Other tests include para-amniobenzoic acid (PABA) level, stool trypsin, serum immune trypsin (IRT)

Test: Stool trypsin levels
Significance: trypsin deficiency

IMAGING

- Chest radiography
- Often non-specific
- Typical features include:
  - Hyperinflation
  - Peribronchial thickening
  - Atelectasis
  - Cystic lesions filled with mucus
  - Bronchiectasis (in advanced cases)

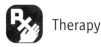 Therapy

DRUGS

- Antibiotic therapy (based on sputum culture results)
- Oral antibiotics
  - Cephalexin
  - Cefaclor
  - Trimethoprim-sulfamethoxazole
  - Chloramphenicol
  - Ciprofloxacin
  - Inhaled tobramycin in selected patients

- Intravenous antibiotics
  - To cover *Staphylococcus aureus*—oxacillin, nafcillin, or vancomycin
  - To cover *Pseudomonas aeruginosa* and *B. cepacia*—semisynthetic penicillin or cephalosporin; ticarcillin, piperacillin, or ceftazidime plus aminoglycoside (for synergistic action); gentamicin, tobramycin, or amikacin
  - Severe cases with resistant strains may benefit from imipenem or meropenern
  - Synergistic antibiotic studies should be performed in patients with multi-resistant strains

CLEARANCE OF PULMONARY SECRETIONS

- Aerosolized bronchodilator therapy (to open airways)
- Mucolytic agents to help break up viscous pulmonary secretions; benefit is controversial. Agents currently available include:
- N-acetylcysteine
- rhDNase (Pulmozyme, Genentech, San Francisco, CA)
- Chest physiotherapy with postural drainage. This can be given either manually, or with mucus-clearing devices such as a percussor vest or a Flutter valve.

LIVER DISEASE

- Patients with cholestasis may benefit from therapy with ursodieoxycholic acid (Acrisall, Novartis, Summit, NJ)
- Phenobarbital has also been tried, but it interferes with vitamin D metabolism
- Pancreatic enzyme replacement therapy:
- Used in patients who are pancreatic-insufficient
- Dosage adjusted for the frequency and character of the stools and for growth pattern
- Generic substitutes are not bioequivalent to name brands
- The maximum recommended dose is 2,000 units of lipase/kg/meal
- Vitamin supplements:
- Multivitamins
- Fat-soluble vitamin replacement (usually E and K)

DIET

- High-calorie diet with nutritional supplements

DURATION

- Usually lifelong nutritional support required
- Duration of antibiotic therapy is controversial; more chronic use is required as pulmonary function deteriorates.

 Follow-Up

CARE PLAN

- Specialized care should be at a cystic fibrosis center.
- Frequency of visits depends on severity of illness: usually every 2 to 4 months.

PROGNOSIS

- Long-term prognosis is poor
- Current mean life span is 29 years
- Due to new antibiotics, maintenance of good pulmonary toilet with chest physiotherapy and bronchodilators, and enzyme replacement therapy. The mean age of survival has been increasing for the past three decades.

PREVENTION

- Isolation of hospitalized patient
- Need to isolate from immunocompromised patients, otherwise standard universal precautions. If the affected patient has an antibiotic-resistant organism, then contact precautions.
- Control measures: none

PITFALLS

- Most common pitfall is failure to diagnose.
- Not uncommon to delay in making the diagnosis in patients with mild symptoms who do not have evidence of malabsorption.

 Common Questions and Answers

Q: Should relatives be tested?
A: All siblings should have a sweat test. It is assumed that the parents are healthy carriers if asymptomatic.

Q: How well will a child do?
A: The course of the illness is variable. It is impossible to predict the course of the disease in a specific person.

Q: How should borderline sweat tests be interpreted?
A: Borderline sweat tests should always be repeated. If still borderline, genetic testing should be performed. All results should be correlated with other findings such as physical examination, sputum cultures, pulmonary function, radiographic findings, and nutritional evaluation.

ICD-9-CM 277.0

BIBLIOGRAPHY

Colin AA, Wohl MEB. Cystic fibrosis. *Pediatr Rev* 1994;115:192–200.

Cystic Fibrosis Genetic Analysis Consortium. World-wide survey of the F508 mutation. *Am J Hum Genet* 1990;47:354–359.

Fick RB, Stillwell PC. Controversies in the management of pulmonary disease due to cystic fibrosis. *Chest* 1989;95:1319–1327.

Mouton JW, Kerrebijn KF. Antibacterial therapy in cystic fibrosis. *Med Clin North Am* 1990;74: 837–850.

Author: Hector L. Flores-Arroyo

Cytomegalovirus Infection

 Database

DEFINITION

Cytomegalovirus (CMV) is a ubiquitous double-stranded DNA virus that is a member of the herpesvirus family. Establishes latency in peripheral mononuclear cells.

PATHOPHYSIOLOGY

Infection leads to intranuclear inclusions with massive enlargement of cells. Almost any organ may become infected with CMV in severe disseminated infection.

EPIDEMIOLOGY

• Seroprevalence varies with socioeconomic status; 50% of middle and 80% of lower socioeconomic status adults are seropositive.
• Increased rates of primary infection seen in early childhood, adolescence, and child-bearing years.
• Transmission may occur via contact with infected respiratory secretions, urine, or breast milk, sexual contact, solid organ transplantation, or infusion of infective blood products.

COMPLICATIONS/PROGNOSIS

Varies with nature of infection (see subsquent text).

ASSOCIATED DISEASES

Congenital Infection

• Occurs in 1% of newborns.
• 10% of infected infants are symptomatic at birth, with severe cytomegalic inclusion disease characterized by growth retardation, hepatosplenomegaly, thrombocytopenia, and central nervous system (CNS) involvement.
• 10% to 20% of infants who are asymptomatically infected at birth will develop long-term sequelae.
• Most common cause of congenital deafness.

Mononucleosis Syndrome

• CMV can cause a mononucleosis-like syndrome similar to that caused by Epstein-Barr virus (EBV) infection.
• Pharyngitis and splenomegaly may be less severe than that associated with EBV-induced mononucleosis.

Interstitial Pneumonitis

• Primarily seen in immunosuppressed children and adults.
• Usually begins with fever and non-productive cough, but may progress to dyspnea and severe hypoxia over 1 to 2 weeks.
• Mild, self-limited pneumonitis may occur in immunocompetent patients.

Retinitis

• Seen in approximately 30% of infants with symptomatic congenital infection.
• May complicate CMV disease in patients with severe immunodeficiency.

Hepatitis

• Occurs in healthy individuals with primary infections and immunosuppressed patients with either primary or reactivated disease.
• Characterized by mildly elevated liver function studies, mild hepatomegaly, and fever.
• Jaundice and severe hepatitis uncommon.

Gastrointestinal Disease

• Severely immunosuppressed patients may experience esophagitis, gastritis, colitis, or pancreatitis.

CNS Disease

• Commonly seen in infants with symptomatic congenital infection.
• Characterized by microcephaly, periventricular calcifications, seizures, developmental delay, and sensorineural hearing loss.
• Encephalitis or meningoencephalitis may occur postnatally in either healthy or immunocompromised patients.

 Differential Diagnosis

Congenital Infection

• Congenital rubella syndrome
• Toxoplasmosis
• Syphilis
• Neonatal herpes simplex virus
• HIV
• Enteroviral infection

Mononucleosis Syndrome

• EBV infection
• Toxoplasmosis
• Hepatitis A or B infection

Interstitial Pneumonitis

• Respiratory syncytial virus
• Adenovirus
• Measles
• Varicella
• *Pneumocystis carinii*
• Chlamydia
• Mycoplasma
• Fungal
• Drug/toxin-induced

Retinitis

• Ocular toxoplasmosis
• Candidal retinitis
• Syphilis
• Herpes simplex virus

Hepatitis

• EBV infection
• Hepatitis A, B, or C infection
• Enterovirus
• Adenovirus
• Herpes simplex virus
• Drug/toxin-induced

Gastrointestinal Disease

• Herpes simplex virus
• Adenovirus
• *Salmonella*
• *Shigella*
• *Campylobacter*
• *Yersinia*
• *C. difficile*
• *Giardia*
• *Cryptosporidium*

CNS Disease

• Congenital disease (see Congenital infection)
• Meningoencephalitis in immunocompetent host: herpes simplex virus, EBV, varicella-zoster virus, enterovirus, arbovirus
• Meningoencephalitis in immunocompromised host: in addition to organisms listed previously, differential diagnosis should include HIV encephalitis, fungal meningitis (due to *Cryptococcus, Candida, Aspergillus, Histoplasma*), toxoplasmosis.

 Data Gathering

HISTORY

Question: Day care attendance?
Significance: Increased risk of infection

Question: Recent blood transfusion?
Significance: Transfusion-associated CMV

Question: Use of immunosuppressive medications
Significance: Increased use of serious infection

Question: Prolonged fever?
Significance: Mononucleosis-like syndrome

Question: Blurred vision?
Significance: CMV retinitis

Question: Cough, dyspnea, wheezing?
Significance: CMV pneumonitis

Question: Vomiting, abdominal pain, diarrhea (watery or bloody)?
Significance: CMV colitis

Physical Examination

- Strabismus

Finding: Microcephaly
Significance: Congenital infection

Finding: White, perivascular retinal infiltrates and hemorrhage
Significance: Retinitis

Finding: Deafness (may require audiogram, brainstem evoked auditory responses, etc.)
Significance: Congenital infection

Finding: Photophobia, headache, nuchal rigidity
Significance: Meningitis

Finding: Tachypnea, rales
Significance: Pneumonitis

Finding: Hepatomegaly and/or splenomegaly
Significance: Mononucleosis-like syndrome

Finding: Rash
Significance: Petechiae, purpura, "blueberry muffin" lesions, rubelliform rash

Finding: Adenopathy
Significance: Mononucleosis-like syndrome

Laboratory Aids

Test: Viral culture
Significance: Virus may be isolated from nasopharyngeal/oropharyngeal secretions, urine, stool, white blood cells. Isolation of virus may take up to 4 weeks.

Test: Shell-vial assay
Significance: Enhanced viral culture through the use of centrifugation. Allows detection of virus 24 to 72 hours after inoculation.

Test: Direct immunofluorescence
Significance: Detection of CMV-infected cells in specimens from biopsy or bronchoalveolar lavage.

Test: Quantitative antigenemia assay
Significance: Detection of circulating CMV-infected mononuclear cells by indirect immunofluorescence. In an immunocompromised patient, may monitor response to therapy or identify viral reactivation.

Test: DNA hybridization
Significance: Detection of viral nucleic acid in tissue or other specimens

Test: Histological examination
Significance: Presence of typical enlarged cells with intranuclear inclusions ("owl's eye" nuclear inclusion)

Test: Serology
Significance: ELISA or indirect fluorescent antibody assay to detect the presence of CMV IgM or IgG. CMV IgM usually persists for 6 weeks following primary infection although may persist up to 6 months.

PITFALLS

- Due to frequency of asymptomatic shedding, mere isolation of virus does not necessarily establish an etiological association.
- Severely immunocompromised patients who are actively infected with CMV may be seronegative.
- Four-fold rise in CMV IgG not diagnostic of primary infection. Increased antibody titers may occur with reactivation.
- False-positive detection of CMV IgM may occur due to production of cross-reactive antibodies.
- Congenital CMV infection should be established by viral isolation from urine or nasopharyngeal secretions within the first 2 weeks of life.

Therapy

DRUGS

- Ganciclovir will suppress replication but not eradicate virus (virostatic agent).

—Indications: CMV chorioretinitis in immunocompromised patients; tissue diagnosis (hepatitis, enteritis, pneumonitis) of CMV infection or isolation of CMV from buffy coat of immunocompromised patient; not indicated for symptomatic neonate with congenital CMV disease (clinical trials in progress at present)
—Side effects: neutropenia ($\approx$50%), thrombocytopenia ($\approx$5%)

- Foscarnet—virostatic agent

—Indications: CMV chorioretinitis, pneumonitis, hepatitis, enteritis (biopsy-proven) in an immunocompromised patient who has failed to improve on ganciclovir therapy or has experienced significant bone marrow toxicity related to ganciclovir use
—Side effects: renal impairment (25%), headache (25%), seizures (10%)

PREVENTION

- Drainage and secretion, and pregnant women precautions should be instituted for hospitalized patients known to be shedding CMV.
- Seriously ill CMV seronegative neonates should receive blood products from CMV-negative donors.
- CMV-seronegative solid organ or bone marrow transplantation recipients should receive organs (and all blood products) from CMV-negative donors whenever possible.
- Controversy exists over role of hyperimmune γ-globulin to prevent disseminated CMV disease in CMV-negative recipient of CMV-positive transplantation.

Common Questions and Answers

Q: Should children with congenital CMV infection be excluded from daycare settings?
A: No. Due to the high frequency of shedding of CMV in the urine and saliva of asymptomatic children, especially under 2 years of age, exclusion from out-of-home care is not justified for any child known to be infected with CMV. Careful attention to hygienic practices, especially handwashing, is important.

ICD-9-CM 078.5

BIBLIOGRAPHY

Boppana SR, Pass RF, Britt WJ, Stagno S, Alford CA. Symptomatic congenital cytomegalovirus infection. *Pediatr Infect Dis J* 1992;11: 93–99.

Brown HL, Abernathy MP. Cytomegalovirus infection. *Semin Perinatol* 1998;22(4):260–266.

Cullen A, Brown S, Cafferkey M, O'Brien N, Griffin E. Current use of the TORCH screen in the diagnosis of congenital infection. *J Infect* 1998;36(2):185–188.

Demmler GJ. Acquired cytomegalovirus infections. In: Feigin RD, Cherry JD, eds. *Textbook of pediatric infectious diseases,* 3rd ed. Philadelphia: WB Saunders, 1992:1532–1547.

Demmler GJ. Congenital cytomegalovirus infection. *Semin Pediatr Neurol* 1994;1(1):36–42.

Fowler KB, Stagno S, Pass RF, Britt WJ, Boll TJ, Alford CA. The outcome of congenital cytomegalovirus infection in relation to maternal antibody status. *N Engl J Med* 1992;326(10): 663–667.

Author: Susan E. Coffin

Dehydration

Database

DEFINITION

- Dehydration is a negative balance of body fluid, usually expressed as a percentage of body weight. Mild, moderate, and severe dehydration correspond to deficits of <5%, 5% to 10%, and >10%, respectively.
- Dehydration is classified into three types based on the serum sodium concentration: isotonic (Na <130–150 mmol/L), hypotonic (Na <130 mmol/L), and hypertonic (Na >150 mmol/L).

PATHOPHYSIOLOGY

Dehydration is caused by either excessive fluid losses or inadequate intake. Some conditions leading to dehydration include:

- Gastrointestinal losses—vomiting, diarrhea (most common cause of dehydration in pediatric patients);
- Renal losses—diabetes mellitus, diabetes insipidus, diuretic agents;
- Insensible losses—sweating, fever, tachypnea, increased ambient temperature, large burns;
- Poor oral intake—stomatitis, pharyngitis, anorexia, oral trauma, altered mental status.

Note that infants and debilitated patients are at particular risk due to lack of ability to satisfy their thirst freely.

EPIDEMIOLOGY

Approximately 10% of children in the United States with acute gastroenteritis develop at least mild dehydration. Although it accounts for 10% of all non-surgical hospital admissions for children under 5 years of age, up to 90% of cases can be managed on an outpatient basis.

COMPLICATIONS

- Severe dehydration may lead to hypovolemic shock and acute renal failure.
- Hyponatremia is associated with hypotonia, hypothermia, and seizures.
- Overly rapid correction of hypernatremia can produce cerebral edema.

PROGNOSIS

Excellent with appropriate rehydration therapy.

Data Gathering

HISTORY

Question: Frequency and duration of emesis and/or diarrhea?
Significance: This will give a rough estimate of risk of dehydration.

Question: Amount and type of liquids taken?
Significance: If there were large quantities of water, be alert for hyptonic dehydration. If excessive electrolyte solution used for hydration, may have hypertonic dehydration.

Question: Frequency and quantity of urination (may be difficult to estimate in infants with diarrhea)?
Significance: Decreased urination indicates possibility of dehydration.

Question: Fever?
Significance: Fever increases insensible water loss.

Question: Exertion or heat exposure?
Significance: Increases insensible water loss.

Physical Examination

Acute change in weight is the best indicator of the fluid deficit. If the child's recent pre-illness weight is not available for comparison, a reasonable estimate of the degree of dehydration may be made from physical findings.

Finding: General appearance
Significance: Lethargy, irritability, thirst

Finding: Vital signs
Significance: Tachycardia; orthostatic increase in heart rate or hypotension; hyperpnea

Finding: Skin
Significance: Prolonged capillary refill at fingertip (<2 seconds is normal in warm environment); mottling; poor turgor

Finding: Eyes
Significance: Decreased or absent tears; sunken eyes

Finding: Mucous membranes
Significance: Dry or parched

Finding: Anterior fontanelle
Significance: Sunken

DIAGNOSTIC PITFALLS

- Physical signs generally appear when the deficit is at least 2% to 3%.
- No single finding is pathognomonic of dehydration. A reasonable guideline is that the presence of three or more findings indicates at least mild dehydration. The number and severity of physical signs increase with the degree of dehydration.
- Urine output decreases early in the course of dehydration, and a history of decreased urination is a non-specific finding.
- Capillary refill time is a specific indicator, but may be falsely prolonged by cool ambient temperature (<20°C or <68°F). It is not affected by fever.
- Children with a deficit greater than 15% will show signs of cardiovascular instability such as severe tachycardia and hypotension.
- Physical findings are more significant for a given degree of dehydration in children with hyponatremia, leading to overestimation of the deficit. Conversely, the clinical picture is somewhat moderated in hypernatremia.

Laboratory Aids

Diagnosis of dehydration is best made on clinical grounds. The following laboratory tests are sometimes helpful adjuncts.

Test: Serum sodium
Significance: Classifies type of dehydration. Hyponatremia and hypernatremia are uncommon (<5% of cases). Measure sodium levels in cases of clinically severe disease, or if risk factors are present (e.g., young infant, history of excessive free water intake).

Test: Rapid glucose test or serum glucose
Significance: To detect hypoglycemia due to prolonged fasting

Test: Urine specific gravity
Significance: This is elevated early in dehydration, but may not become elevated at all in young infants or children with sickle cell disease.

Test: Serum bicarbonate
Significance: This is frequently low with diarrheal illness, even in the absence of dehydration. Useful to detect significant acidosis when dehydration is clinically severe.

Test: Blood urea nitrogen (BUN)
Significance: Rises only late in dehydration in children.

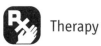 ## Therapy

ORAL REHYDRATION THERAPY (ORT)

Most children can be successfully managed with ORT.

• Use rehydration solution containing 2% to 2.5% glucose and 75 to 90 mmol/L Na (e.g., WHO solution), or 45 to 50 mmol/L Na (e.g., Pedialyte [Ross Laboratories, Columbus OH], Infalyte, [Mead Johnson, Evansville, IN]).
• Replace entire deficit in 4 to 6 hours—for mild dehydration, 50 mL/kg; for moderate to severe dehydration, 80 to 100 mL/kg. Include ongoing losses, approximately 5 mL/kg for each diarrheal stool.
• Begin with slow administration, with strict limits when vomiting is present—5 mL every 1 to 2 minutes. For infants, use a syringe or spoon rather than a bottle. After 1 hour, if the oral liquids have been tolerated, increase the volume and rate.
• Have the child's caregiver participate in giving the fluids, and provide education regarding fluid replacement and signs of dehydration.
• Monitor weight, intake and output, and clinical signs. Failure of ORT includes intractable vomiting, clinical deterioration, or lack of improvement after 4 hours.

INTRAVENOUS FLUID THERAPY

Intravenous fluids are required when ORT fails or is contraindicated, such as in severe dehydration or shock, poor gag or suck, depressed mental status, preterm infant, severe hypernatremia (Na >160 mmol/L), suspected surgical abdomen.

• Administer intravenous bolus of normal saline or Ringer lactate, 20 mL/kg, over 10 to 30 minutes. Repeat as needed to restore cardiovascular stability. Avoid dextrose-containing solutions for boluses except to correct documented hypoglycemia.
• Calculate maintenance fluid requirements: 100 mL/kg for the first 10 kg, plus 50 mL/kg for the next 10 kg, plus 20 mL/kg over 20 kg.
• Calculate fluid deficit based on clinical estimate or known weight loss. For isotonic or hypotonic dehydration, give one-third to one-half normal saline with 5% dextrose, at a rate to provide maintenance and replace deficit over 24 hours. For hypertonic dehydration, replace deficit over 48 hours, using one-fifth to one-fourth normal saline with 5% dextrose.
• Monitor weight, intake and output, and clinical signs. With hypernatremia, measure serum sodium every 4 to 6 hours; do not exceed rate of fall of 1 mmol/L/h.

 ## Follow-Up

After rehydration, children with ongoing losses, as in gastroenteritis, should receive a maintenance solution in addition to regular feedings to maintain a positive fluid balance. Recommend 5 to 10 mL/kg for each diarrheal stool. Avoid clear liquids with excessive glucose, such as fruit juices, punches, and soft drinks, as these can promote osmotic fluid losses in the stool. In infants less than 6 months old, do not give large amounts of plain water, which can lead to hyponatremia.

PREVENTION

Many cases of frank dehydration may be prevented by early institution of adequate oral maintenance fluid therapy in children with gastroenteritis, with particular attention to replacement of ongoing stool losses and slow administration of fluids to children with vomiting. Use of appropriate solutions is essential to prevent electrolyte disturbance and worsening of diarrhea.

 ## Common Questions and Answers

Q: How can an oral rehydration solution be prepared at home?
A: An acceptable rehydration solution (2.2% glucose, 70 mmol Na/L) can be prepared with the following: ½ teaspoon of table salt, ½ teaspoon of baking soda, and 1 cup of orange juice, added to 3 cups of water. For maintenance solution, decrease the table salt to ¼ teaspoon.

Q: Can commercially available maintenance solutions be used for rehydration as well as maintenance?
A: Data suggest that reduced-osmolarity maintenance solutions, with a sodium concentration of 45 to 50 mmol/L, are equally effective for rehydration as solutions with a higher sodium content.

Q: How can oral rehydration solution be made more palatable?
A: Rehydration solutions may be more palatable if iced, or flavored with apple or orange juice (1 part juice to 4 parts rehydration solution) or unsweetened Kool-Aid powder (2.5 mL powder per 240 mL of solution).

ICD-9-CM 276.5

BIBLIOGRAPHY

American Academy of Pediatrics Provisional Committee on Quality Improvement, Subcommittee on Acute Gastroenteritis. Practice parameter: the management of acute gastroenteritis in young children. *Pediatrics* 1996;97:424–436.

Feld LG, Kaskel FJ, Schoeneman MJ. The approach to fluid and electrolyte therapy in pediatrics. *Adv Pediatr* 1988;35:497–536.

Gorelick MH, Shaw KN, Murphy KO. Validity and reliability of clinical signs in the diagnosis of dehydration in children. *Pediatrics* 1997; 99(5):e6. (URL:http://www.pediatrics.org/cgi/content/full/99/5/e6)

Grisanti KA, Jaffe DM. Dehydration syndromes: oral rehydration and fluid replacement. *Emerg Med Clin North Am* 1991;9:565–588.

International Study Group on Reduced-Osmolarity ORS Solutions. Multicentre evaluation of reduced-osmolarity oral rehydration salts solution. *Lancet* 1995;345:282–285.

Kallen RJ. The management of diarrheal dehydration in infants using parenteral fluids. *Pediatr Clin North Am* 1990;37:265–286.

MacKenzie A, Barnes G, Shann F. Clinical signs of dehydration in children. *Lancet* 1989;2: 605–706.

Author: Marc H. Gorelick

Dermatomyositis/Polymyositis

 Database

DEFINITION

The dermatomyositis/polymyositis complex includes a number of conditions in which muscle becomes damaged by a non-suppurative lymphocytic inflammatory process. Juvenile dermatomyositis (JDM) is the most common seen in the pediatric population.

DIAGNOSTIC CRITERIA FOR JDM

Diagnosis requires the presence of the pathognomonic rash plus three additional criteria.

- Progressive symmetric weakness of proximal muscles
- Dermatitis-heliotrope rash over eyelids, Gottron papules over extensor surfaces of joints
- Elevated serum level of muscle enzymes
- Electromyograph (EMG) findings of myopathy and denervation
- Biopsy demonstration of inflammatory myositis

PATHOPHYSIOLOGY

- Unknown
- Several potential mechanisms include the following:

—Abnormal cell-mediated immunity
—Immune-complex formation
—Immunodeficiency
—Infection
  —Toxoplasma gondii
  —Coxsackievirus B
  —Others

EPIDEMIOLOGY

- Incidence: 1:200,000
- The average age of onset is 7 years
- Overall male-female ratio is 1.0:1.7; however, equal in children under 10 years of age

COMPLICATIONS

- Myositis
- Rash
- Arthritis
- Calcinosis
- Raynaud syndrome
- Dysphagia and dysphonia
- Restrictive lung disease and aspiration pneumonia
- Myocarditis (rare)
- Gastrointestinal tract vasculitis
- Osteoporosis

PROGNOSIS

- Normal-good, 65% to 80%
- Minimal atrophy and joint contractures, 24%
- Calcinosis, 20% to 40%
- Wheelchair dependent, 5%
- Death, 7% to 10%

 Differential Diagnosis

POST-INFECTIOUS

- Influenza A and B, coxsackievirus B, schistosomiasis, trypanosomiasis, toxoplasmosis
- Bacterial/pyomyositis-focal

MYOSITIS WITH OTHER CONNECTIVE TISSUE DISEASES

- Overlap with JRA
- Systemic lupus erythematosus

CHILDHOOD NEUROMUSCULAR DISEASES

If no rash consider

- Muscular dystrophy
- Congenital myopathies
- Metabolic disorders

—Glycogen storage disease
—Carnitine deficiency
—Myoadenylate deaminase

- Neurogenic atrophies

—Spinal muscular atrophy and anterior horn
—Peripheral nerve dysfunction

- Neuromuscular transmission disorders
- Inclusion body myositis

 Data Gathering

HISTORY

Question: Fever?
Significance: Evidence for systemic illness

Question: Anorexia and weight loss?
Significance: Gastrointestinal involvement

Question: Fatigue
Significance: Sign of muscle weakness

Question: Weakness
Significance: Difficulty rising from floor, climbing stairs, swallowing, regurgitation through nose

Question: Dysphonia
Significance: Sign of muscle weakness

Question: Rash
Significance: Clue to diagnosis

 Physical Examination

Finding: Muscle weakness
Significance: Proximal and symmetric tenderness strength

- 0—no contractility
- 1—contracts, no joint movement
- 2—Full range of motion (FROM) without gravity
- 3—FROM against gravity
- 4—complete ROM with some resistance
- 5—normal

Finding: Rash
Significance: 75% have pathognomonic rash, which usually appears several weeks after muscle weakness.

Finding: Facial rash
Significance: Violaceous, heliotropic changes over eyelids

Finding: Extremities
Significance: Gottron papules over extensor surfaces

Finding: Nail-fold telangiectasia
Significance: Simultaneous dilated loops, dropout, and arborized capillary loops

PHYSICAL EXAMINATION TRICKS

- Gower sign: Inability to rise from floor without using hands
- Use ophthalmoscope to examine nail-fold for telangiectasia
- Objective measure of strength: duration of straight leg raise (n = 20 seconds)

Laboratory Aids

Test: Auto-antibodies
Significance:

- Normal-RF, Jo-1, complement and dsDNA
- ANA: 10% to 50%
- PM-1 60% adult polymyositis; however, rare children

Test: Muscle enzymes
Significance:

- Elevated in 95% cases
- Creatine kinase
- AST
- Aldolase
- LDH

PATHOLOGY

- Skeletal muscle

—Group atrophy or perifascicular myopathy
—Variation in fiber size due to concomitant degeneration and regeneration
—Inflammatory exudate in perivascular distribution
—Necrotizing vasculitis of arterioles, capillaries, and venules; probably due to immune complex deposition

- Skin

—Epidermal atrophy
—Vascular dilatation
—Lymphocyte infiltration of the dermis

ELECTROMYOGRAPHY

- Myopathic motor units
- Denervation potentials
- High-frequency repetitive discharges
- Do not biopsy same muscle as used for EMG

MRI

- Inflamed muscles are identified by signal enhancement
- Useful to direct biopsy

BARIUM SWALLOW

- To identify palatal or proximal esophageal weakness

PULMONARY FUNCTION TESTS/PEAK FLOW

- To evaluate pulmonary musculature

 ## Therapy

PHYSICAL THERAPY/OCCUPATIONAL THERAPY

- Initially to maintain ROM
- Strengthening only after acute inflammation resolves

DRUGS

- 2 mg/kg of steroids per day for 1 month, taper over 2 years
- Intravenous gammaglobulin, controversial, efficacious for rash
- Plaquenil, particularly useful for the rash
- Methotrexate, PO or IV, avoid IM, which may alter serum levels of muscle enzymes
- Cyclosporine

SUPPORTIVE CARE

- Monitor for swallowing difficulty
- Respiratory compromise/occasionally requires mechanical ventilation
- Treatment of calcinosis may include Colchicine

 ## Follow-Up

- Function
- Muscle strength
- Joint ROM
- Development of calcinosis
- Muscle enzyme levels

PITFALLS

- Steroid-induced myopathy
- Insidious onset
- Proximal and distal muscles, often large muscle groups such as hip flexors
- Normal serum muscle enzymes
- Minimal myopathic changes on EMG
- Type II fiber atrophy on muscle biopsy

 ## Common Questions and Answers

Q: Is it mandatory to perform a muscle biopsy to confirm the diagnosis?
A: No.

Q: How long should you treat with prednisone?
A: The usual practice is 2 years minimum.

Q: Is there an associated risk of malignancy as for adults with this disorder?
A: No.

ICD-9-CM 710.3

BIBLIOGRAPHY

Cassidy JT, Petty RE. Juvenile dermatomyositis. In: *Textbook of pediatric rheumatology,* 3rd ed. New York: Churchill Livingstone, 1995:223–364.

Spiro AJ. Childhood dermatomyositis and polymyositis. *Pediatr Rev* 1984;6(6):163–172.

Author: Emily von Scheven

Developmental Disabilities

 Database

DEFINITION

Developmental delay is a descriptive term, not a specific diagnosis, comprising many disorders and encompassing a broad category of etiologies. The term describes any situation where a child is not meeting age appropriate milestones as expected in one or more streams of development. These streams of development include gross motor, fine motor, receptive and expressive language, adaptive and social. The key feature is that the rate of progress has been slow over time in the area(s) of delay.

PATHOPHYSIOLOGY

This is highly variable depending on etiology, which can include genetic, familial, metabolical, infectious, endocrinological, traumatic, anatomic brain malformations, environmental toxins and degenerative disorders as causes. These disorders often result in some neurological or neuromuscular injury causing the delay. In many cases etiology is never determined. Prevalence of this group of disorders may vary depending on how inclusive the definition. The milder delays are quite common and can be found in any pediatric practice. Some disorders in this grouping are more prevalent in boys. The long-term outcome depends on the severity and type of delay with the more severe children usually having lifelong disability.

ASSOCIATED FINDINGS

There are numerous associated findings including, seizures, sensory impairments, feeding disorders, psychiatric disorders (especially depression), and behavioral disorders. Having a child with significant developmental delays also can add stress to the family in terms of time, finances, and emotions.

 Differential Diagnosis

The differential can be extensive and may become more evident with additional work-up. Broad diagnoses include:

- Mental retardation
- Developmental language disorder
- Autism
- Learning disability
- Cerebral palsy
- Attention deficit hyperactivity disorder
- Significant visual or hearing impairment
- Degenerative disorders

Specific etiologies are too numerous to list completely but a partial list of the more common causes would include:

- Genetic/familial

—Fragile X syndrome
—Trisomy 21 (Down syndrome)
—Other chromosomal abnormalities

—Tuberous sclerosis
—Neurofibromatosis
—PKU
—Muscular dystrophy

- Nervous System Anomalies

—Hydrocephalus
—Lissencephaly
—Spina bifida
—Seizures

- Infections

—Prenatal cytomegalovirus
—Rubella
—Toxoplasmosis
—HIV
—Postnatal bacterial meningitis
—Neonatal herpes simplex

- Endocrinological

—Congenital hypothyroidism

- Environmental

—Heavy metal poisoning such as lead

- *In utero* drug or alcohol exposure
- Trauma/injury

—Closed head trauma
—Asphyxia
—Stroke
—Perinatal cerebral hemorrhages

HINTS FOR SCREENING PROBLEMS

- Children with behavioral problems may also be masking developmental delays.
- Children with delays in one stream of development may also have delays in other areas of development. For example, language delay may be an indication of general cognitive delays.
- Hearing impairment may present as a delay in development.

 Data Gathering

HISTORY

Pregnancy History

Question: Maternal age and parity?
Significance: Chromosomal defect associated with older age groups.

Question: Maternal complications?
Significance: May contribute to malformations on prematurity.

Question: Infections and exposures?
Significance: Congenital infection torches.

Question: Medications/drugs used?
Significance: Defects related to seizure medications.

Question: Tobacco or alcohol used, along with quantities?
Significance: Increased prematurity and malformations.

Question: Fetal activity?
Significance: Decreased fetal activity associated with neuromuscular disease.

Birth History

Question: Gestational age?
Significance: Prematurity associated with developmental delay.

Question: Birth weight?
Significance: Increased developmental delay in low birth weight.

Question: Route of delivery?
Significance: CNS injury incurred in breech and difficult deliveries.

Question: Maternal or fetal complications/distress?
Significance: Herpes association with CNS damage.

Question: Apgar scores?
Significance: 5 minute Apgar <5 is correlated with developmental delays.

General Health

- Significant illnesses, hospitalizations, or surgeries?
- Accidents or injuries?
- Hearing and vision status?
- Medications used?
- Known exposures to toxins?
- Any new or unusual symptoms?

Developmental History

- Current developmental achievement in each stream of development?
- SAge when developmental milestones were achieved?
- Any loss of skills?
- Where parents think their child is functioning developmentally?

Educational History

- Type of schooling and services received, if any?
- Any previous educational/developmental testing?

Behavioral History

- Any perseverative or stereotypical behaviors?
- Interaction skills?
- Attention and activity level?

Familial History

- Anyone with developmental delays, neurological disorders, syndromes, consanguinity?

Physical Examination

A complete physical examination including growth perimeters is needed looking for etiology.

- Observation of interactions and behavior
- Head circumference
- Skin examination looking for neurocutaneous lesions
- Major or minor dysmorphic features
- Neurological examination

Look for cranial nerve deficits, neuromuscular status, reflexes, balance and coordination and any soft signs.

Laboratory Aids

There is no specific laboratory test battery for general developmental delays. The testing needs to be tailored to the individual situation based on the history and physical examination. A high index of suspicion should be maintained for any associated findings and delays in the other streams of development. Listed below are some of the more common studies ordered for developmental delay work up.

Test: Developmental testing
Finding: Although considerable information will already be available on history and observation, a more formal developmental screening or testing should be done.

Test: Possible office tests would be the Denver Developmental Screening Test, the CAT/CLAMS or the ELM.
Significance: The latter test is basically for language screening.

Test: Hearing
Significance: Should be checked in any child with speech and language and/or cognitive delays.

Test: Genetic testing
Significance: Warranted for any dysmorphic features or a familial history of delays or genetic disorder. A karyotype and Fragile X DNA should be considered particularly for significant cognitive delays.

Test: Metabolic tests
Significance: Quantitative plasma amino acids, quantitative urine organic acids, lactate, pyruvate or ammonia should be considered if there is any loss of skills or indication of a metabolic disorder.

Test: Hypothyroidism
Significance: Most infants have screening for hypothyroidism shortly after birth. This should be rechecked if symptoms indicate.

Test: EEG
Significance: Consider if there is any concern about seizures.

Test: Head MRI
Significance: Consider for head abnormalities, significant neurological findings, loss of skills or for work up of a specific disorder such as trauma or leukodystrophy.

Referral to other medical specialists may also be indicated. These specialists may include developmental pediatrics, neurology, genetics, orthopedics, or ophthalmology.

Therapy

Therapy should include appropriately treating any medical conditions and associated findings. For example, anticonvulsants for seizures or hearing aids when appropriate for hearing impairment. In addition, traditional therapy has included Early Intervention or Special Education services specifically addressing the areas of delay. Therapy could include physical therapists, occupational therapists, speech/language therapists, special educators, psychologists, and audiologists depending on the needs of the child.

REFERRAL

Referral to a specialist or a multidisciplinary team for more detailed testing would be indicated when delay is suspected.

Follow-Up

General pediatric care for well child visits and to monitor any underlying medical conditions is indicated. In addition, these children need ongoing monitoring of their therapy and educational programs to assure that it is still meeting their individual needs, as these needs change over time. The families will also need ongoing counseling and support in dealing with a child having special needs.

Common Questions and Answers

Q: When do you test a child for delays?
A: A child can have developmental assessments at any age, including infancy. Making a specific diagnosis, for example, level of mental retardation, may need to wait until the child is older.

Q: When can a child start receiving services?
A: Children who qualify can receive therapy services starting at birth and in some cases extending up to age 21 years.

Q: The parents are raising a concern about delays, but the general impression in the office is that he or she is doing okay. What should be done next?
A: Parents or grandparents may be the first to express concerns, especially in a child with milder delays. A more detailed developmental history and more formal developmental screening or testing would be indicated as an initial step.

ICD-9-CM 315.9

BIBLIOGRAPHY

Gilbride KE. Developmental testing. *Pediatr Rev* 1995;16:338–345.

Johnson CP, Blasco PA. Infant growth and development. *Pediatr Rev* 1997;18:224–242.

Levy SE, Hyman SL. Pediatric Assessment of the child with developmental delay. *Pediatr Clin North Am* 1993;40:465–477.

Liptak GS. The pediatrician's role in caring for the developmentally disabled child. *Pediatr Rev* 1996;17:203–210.

Author: Rita Panoscha

Developmental Dysplasia of the Hip

 Database

DEFINITION

A range of congenital hip disorders: from mild acetabular dysplasia to dislocation of the femoral head from the acetabulum.

CAUSES

- Perinatal factors

—Breech presentation
—Ligamentous laxity
—Collagen vascular disorders

- Neonatal factors

—Hip positioned in extended, adducted fashion

PATHOLOGY

Due either to mechanical forces or to underlying laxity. Femoral head not positioned correctly within acetabulum, resulting in a shallow acetabulum, unable to contain the femoral head.

EPIDEMIOLOGY

Incidence of hip dysplasia is 0.5% to 2% of live births; however, true dislocation occurs in 0.1% to 0.2% of live births.

GENETICS

Most patients are first-born females, with familial history of affected first-degree relative.

COMPLICATIONS

- If left untreated, congenital hip dysplasia results in limp, pain, and accelerated degenerative disease of the hip.
- Rarely, there is avascular necrosis of the femoral head.

 Differential Diagnosis

- Infection
- Environmental

—Culture-associated neonatal swaddling

- Congenital

—Arthrogryposis
—Lumbosacral agenesis
—Spina bifida
—Neonatal Marfan syndrome
—Fetal hydantoin syndrome
—Larsen syndrome

 Data Gathering

HISTORY

Question: Breech delivery?
Significance: Higher incidence of developmental dysplasia of the hip in breech delivery.

Question: Familial history of hip dysplasia?
Significance: 10% to 20% of patients have familial history.

 Physical Examination

GLUTEAL AND THIGH SKIN-FOLD ASYMMETRY

Finding: Ortolani test
Significance: Have infant supine, stabilize pelvis, abduct and externally rotate hip with examiner's middle finger over greater trochanter. Palpable click is positive sign produced by reduction of dislocated hip.

Finding: Barlow test
Significance: Passive dislocation of hip on adduction and internal rotation. Palpable click is positive sign as hip dislocates.

PHYSICAL EXAMINATION TRICKS

Examination may be normal initially, in spite of the presence of hip dysplasia. Consequently, hip evaluation should be performed as part of neonatal physical examination through 4 months of age.

Laboratory Aids

IMAGING

Test: X-ray studies
Significance: Not useful prior to 3 months, and may be normal because of difficulty determining hip/acetabulum relation in unossified femoral head.

Test: Ultrasound both static and dynamic imaging
Significance: Can determine hip joint spacial relationships. Ultrasound is useful in monitoring progress of therapy.

FALSE POSITIVES

Hip clicks will be present in 10% of infants; only a small percentage will have hip dysplasia.

PITFALLS

Overdiagnosis is a problem because avascular necrosis of femur can occur (rarely) as a result of therapeutic interventions.

REQUIREMENTS FOR TESTING

Ultrasonographer must be experienced in hip imaging.

 ## Therapy

- Triple diaper: Not effective in moderate or severe dysplasia
- Pavlik harness: Effective if used prior to 6 months of age
- Complications include avascular necrosis of proximal femur, femoral nerve palsy, and medial knee instability.
- Closed or open reduction: If diagnosis/therapy delayed beyond 6 months.
- Duration: If harness is used prior to 4 months of age, the average therapy takes 3 to 4 weeks.

 ## Follow-Up

WHEN TO EXPECT IMPROVEMENT

In children treated early (age < 4 months), duration of splinting is 3 to 4 weeks, with subsequent weaning from splint.

SIGNS TO WATCH FOR

- Ultrasound or x-ray evidence of ongoing subluxation/dislocation

PROGNOSIS

If diagnosed early, prognosis is uniformly excellent.

PITFALLS

- Overdiagnosis early
- However, any infant with a hip click deserves an evaluation by an orthopedist.
- Missed early diagnosis can result in more complicated management and less favorable outcome.

 ## Common Questions and Answers

Q: If my patient has a hip click at birth demonstrating an unstable hip joint, what is the likelihood the infant will have hip dysplasia?
A: About 10% (1.5 children per 1000 live births).

Q: How effective is the Pavlik harness used within the first 4 months of life?
A: In patients with reducible hip dysplasia, results are excellent.

ICD-9-CM 755.63

BIBLIOGRAPHY

Bennet GC. Screening for congenital dislocation of the hip. *J Bone Joint Surg Br* 1992;74:643–644.

Cotillo JA, Molano C, Albinana J. Correlative study between arthrograms and surgical findings in congenital dislocation of the hip. *J Pediatr Orthop B* 1998;7(1):62–65.

Darmonov AV, Zagora S. Clinical screening for congenital dislocation of the hip. J Bone Joint Surg Am 1996;78(3):383–388.

Donaldson JS, Feinstein KA. Imaging of developmental dysplasia of the hip. *Pediatr Clin North Am* 1997;44(3):591–614.

Poul J, Bajerova J, Sommernitz M, et al. Early diagnosis of congenital dislocation of the hip. *J Bone Joint Surg Br* 1992;74:695–700.

Author: Gregory F. Keenan

Diabetes Insipidus

 Database

DEFINITION

Polyuria and polydipsia caused by inability to produce or respond to anti-diuretic hormone (ADH) also called arginine vasopressin.

CAUSES

Insufficient ADH Secretion

- Traumatic or post-surgical
- Related to tumor invasion of posterior pituitary:

—Extension from anterior pituitary/suprasella: optic glioma, rarely adenomas
—Hypothalamic: germinoma, craniopharyngioma, meningioma
—Lymphoma
—Granulomas: histiocytosis X, sarcoidosis
—Metastatic carcinoma

- Post-severe ischemic or hypoxic injury to the brain
- Familial (autosomal dominant)
- Congenital malformation of central nervous system
- Infection

—Viral encephalitis
—Meningitis
—Tuberculosis

- Increased metabolic clearance of ADH (gestational diabetes insipidus)
- Drug- or toxin-related: snake venom, tetrodotoxin
- Autoimmune disorders
- Psychogenic: excessive water drinking
- Idiopathic: must observe for many years to exclude slow-growing tumors

Unresponsive to ADH

- Familial or "nephrogenic" (X-linked dominant and autosomal recessive forms)
- Tumor-related
- Urinary tract obstruction, especially in utero
- Renal medullary cystic disease
- Electrolyte disturbances: hypokalemia, hypercalcemia (hypercalciuria)
- Drugs: usually reversible

—Diuretics
—Diphenylhydantoin
—Reserpine
—Cisplatin
—Rifampin
—Lithium: may become permanent
—Demeclocycline
—Ethanol
—Chlorpromazine
—Volatile anesthetics
—Foscarnet
—Amphotericin B

- Loss of the medullary concentrating gradient due to successive free water intake relative to solute intake

PATHOPHYSIOLOGY

- ADH stimulates the formation of cyclic adenosine monophosphate (cAMP) in the renal collecting ducts, thereby increasing water permeability and increasing reabsorption of free water.
- Lack of ADH effect results in urinary loss of free water.
- Patients with an intact thirst mechanism drink copiously (polydipsia) to compensate for free water loss.
- If the thirst mechanism is not present or if access to free water is limited (e.g., infants or vomiting), severe dehydration can occur.

GENETICS

- Rare cases of autosomal dominant transmission of ADH deficiency
- Nephrogenic diabetes insipidus (DI) is usually familial (either autosomal recessive or X-linked dominant)

EPIDEMIOLOGY (AGE-RELATED)

Because most cases are secondary to another disease, the incidence depends on the primary causes.

COMPLICATIONS

- Without treatment and without access to water:

—Hypernatremia
—Dehydration
—Coma

- When overdosed with water:

—Hyponatremia
—Seizures
—Cerebral edema

PROGNOSIS

- Generally good but depends on the primary cause

 Differential Diagnosis

- Psychogenic polydipsia
- Abnormal thirst mechanism (dipsogenic DI)
- Hypernatremic dehydration
- Diabetes mellitus
- Polyuric renal failure (e.g., renal tubulopathy)
- Hypercalcemia
- Adrenal insufficiency
- Cerebral salt wasting

 Data Gathering

HISTORY

Question: Is the child growing normally?
Significance: Abnormal growth can be a sign of DI.

Question: Does the patient wake up during the night to drink or void? If so, what does the patient prefer to drink?
Significance: True DI is associated with polyuria throughout the day and night. Enuresis may be the first sign in a child who previously acquired bladder control. Patients, including infants, prefer water over other liquids such as juice, soda, or milk

Question: How many hours can the patient go without drinking?
Significance: Patients with complete DI do not voluntarily stop drinking for more than 1 to 2 hours, unless the thirst mechanism is also abnormal.

Question: Volume of urine output in a day (not just frequency of urination)?
Significance: The daily volume of urine can be as high as 4 to 10 liters. Younger or dehydrated children with DI tend to make less urine daily than older or hydrated children with DI.

Question: Familial history of DI?
Significance: Nephrogenic DI will typically affect maternal uncles during infancy.

Question: Has the child had frequent episodes of dehydration requiring medical attention?
Significance: Families may disregard the polydyisia as normal behavior. Repeated episodes of severe dehydration can damage the brain.

 Physical Examination

Finding: Signs of dehydration
Significance: DI is typically associated with dry, pale skin and mucus membranes.

Finding: Complete neurological examination
Significance: Check for impaired visual fields which can be the first sign of brain tumor.

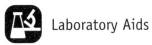

Laboratory Aids

SPECIFIC TESTS

Test: Morning urinary osmolality with simultaneous serum sodium and serum osmolality.
Significance: If urine osmolality is at least two times higher than serum osmolality, patient does not have complete DI.

Test: Water-deprivation test
Significance: Though definitive, it requires admission to the hospital for controlled testing under the close supervision of a pediatric endocrinologist. Patient fails test if either:

• Urinary osmolality cannot concentrate more than twice serum osmolality at the same time that serum osmolality exceeds 305 mOsm/kg
• Serum osmolality exceeds 305 mOsm/kg at any time
• Patient loses more than 5% of body weight and becomes symptomatic from hypovolemia

Once patient fails the water deprivation test, a dose of aqueous vasopressin should be given followed by close monitoring of urinary osmolality to document responsiveness to ADH.

NON-SPECIFIC TEST

Test: Urinary specific gravity
Significance: Insufficient by itself and non-diagnostic during a water deprivation test.

IMAGING

Test: MRI of the head
Significance: To confirm the "bright spot" normally seen in the posterior pituitary and to search for tumors.

HOME TESTING

Test: 24-hour urine collection
Significance: To obtain accurate urinary volume while patient has free access to water.

Do not restrict water intake unless the patient is in the hospital under close surveillance!

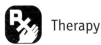

Therapy

DRUGS

• DDAVP: intranasal spray or oral tablets
• Aqueous vasopressin: subcutaneous
• Duration of action of DDAVP is variable from patient to patient. Titration and frequency of dosing should be made by the family under the supervision of an endocrinologist.
• Control of DI in infants is more difficult because these patients may increase fluid intake due to hunger or increase caloric intake due to thirst, thereby causing an imbalance between free water intake and output. Some infants can be treated with diluted formula—the volume

and frequency of feedings will be increased, but intake of free water will better match urine output. Strict record keeping of intake/output and accurate daily weighing are usually necessary for infants or patients without an intact thirst mechanism.
• Nephrogenic DI has been treated with diuretics since these patients are resistant to DDAVP.

SIDE EFFECTS OF DDAVP

• Facial flushing
• Increase in blood pressure
• Headache
• Nasal congestion
• Hyponatremia: caused by water overdose (intoxication), not by overdose of drug. Taking a higher dose of DDAVP will generally extend the period of anti-diuresis but will not cause hyponatremia. Drinking too much water in the setting of anti-diuresis causes hyponatremia. Water intoxication most often occurs in anti-diuresed patients who also are on intravenous fluids, lack an intact thirst mechanism, or have psychogenic polydipsia.

DURATION

Lifelong generally. Some tumors regress with radiation allowing recovery of ADH secretion.

DIET

• Patients with an intact thirst mechanism should drink only when thirsty.
• Patients without an intact thirst mechanism should drink only a carefully calculated fluid volume.

POSSIBLE CONFLICTS WITH OTHER TREATMENTS

Nasal congestion or gastrointestinal illness can affect the absorption of DDAVP administered.

Follow-Up

Depends on the patient and underlying disease causing DI

WHEN TO EXPECT IMPROVEMENT

• Effects of DDAVP are immediate.
• Most cases of DI are lifelong. One exception is DI that occurs during the 7 to 10 days immediately after neurosurgery, since this post-surgical DI may resolve spontaneously within 1 to 2 weeks after surgery.

SIGNS TO WATCH FOR

• Lethargy
• Somnolence
• Irritability
• Hyperpyrexia
• Any sign of dehydration
• Seizures

PITFALLS

• Management of patients without an intact thirst mechanism and of newborns is difficult.
• Patients with psychogenic polydipsia may fail a water deprivation test because prolonged excessive water intake can wash out the renal medullary gradient required for concentrating the urine.
• Surreptitious water intake during water deprivation test.
• Idiopathic, acquired DI can be due to slowly growing brain tumors not visible on the initial MRI.

Common Questions and Answers

Q: In a patient with intact thirst mechanism and partial DI is the use of DDAVP necessary?
A: No, as long as the patient has constant access to free water.

Q: How does therapy of DI affect daily life? Is it easily integrated into normal activity and eating patterns?
A: DDAVP is used in a patient with intact thirst mechanism to facilitate the daily routine as well as to allow patients to sleep without the need to void frequently during the night.

Q: Is there a longer acting preparation or an implantable pump for dosing?
A: The longest-acting form of ADH is an injected medication and can have effects for 3 days, increasing the risks of hyponatremia. Home use of the nasal spray or tablets is, therefore, easier and safer than the use of injections.

ICD-9-CM 253.5

BIBLIOGRAPHY

Mootha SL, Barkovich AJ, Grumbach MM, et al. Idiopathic hypothalamic diabetes insipidus, pituitary stalk thickening, and the occult intracranial germinoma in children and adolescents. *J Clin Endocrinol Metab* 1997;82(5):1362–1367.

Kirchlechner V, Koller DY, Seidl R, Waldhuser F. Treatment of nephrogenic diabetes insipidus with hydrochlorothiazide and amiloride. *Arch Dis Child* 1999;80(6):548–552.

Leger J, Velasquez A, Garel C, Hassan M, Czernichow P. Thickened pituitary stalk on magnetic resonance imaging in children with central diabetes insipidus. *J Clin Endocrinol Metab* 1999;84(6):1954–1960.

Robertson GL. Diabetes insipidus. *Endocrinol Metab Clin N Am* 1995;24(3):549–572.

Siegel AJ, Baldessarini RJ, Klepser MB, McDonald JC. Primary and drug-induced disorders of water homeostasis in psychiatric patients: Principles of diagnosis and management. *Harv Res Psychiatry* 1998;6(4):190–200.

Authors: Robert J. Ferry, Jr. and Paulo F. Collett-Solberg

Diabetic Ketoacidosis

 Database

DEFINITION

• State of severe metabolic derangement that occurs in patients with insulin-dependent diabetes mellitus secondary to insulin deficiency and stress hormone excess.
• Hyperglycemia (blood glucose >200 mg/dL)
• Ketonemia (>3 mmol in serum or ketonuria)
• Acidosis (pH <7.3 or HCO_3 >15 mEq/L)

CAUSE/PATHOLOGY

• Insulin deficiency and excess of the counter-regulatory hormones glucagon, cortisol, and epinephrine lead to unregulated catabolism.
• Glycogenolysis and gluconeogenesis lead to hyperglycemia.
• Lipolysis and ketone production lead to metabolic acidosis.
• Hyperosmolar state leads to osmotic diuresis, dehydration, and electrolyte loss.

EPIDEMIOLOGY

• 30% of new diabetic children present in diabetic ketoacidosis (DKA); higher percentage in children under 5 years.
• Overall mortality ~3% to 5% per episode
• 65% of all hospital admissions in diabetic children under 19 years old
• Most common cause of death (>50%) in diabetic children

COMPLICATIONS

• Cardiovascular collapse

—Caused by osmotic diuresis and dehydration
—Treated with prompt initiation of fluid resuscitation

• Overwhelming acidosis

—From ketoacid accumulation
—Treated with bicarbonate and insulin infusion

• Hypoglycemia from insufficient dextrose supplementation, treated by increasing dextrose
• Hypokalemia

—Caused by loss of potassium in the urine and correction of acidosis with insulin
—Treated by intravenous potassium supplementation

• Cerebral edema

—Most serious complication of DKA and most frequent cause of death
—Rapid changes in serum osmolarity lead to influx of water into brain tissue
—Occurs 6 to 18 hours after initiation of therapy, as patient is improving
—Heralded as headache, change in mental status, or abnormal neurological signs
—May progress rapidly to brain herniation and death
—Treatment is supportive, aimed at reducing intracranial pressure with mannitol, and hyperventilation

PROGNOSIS

• Overall, 5% mortality with each episode of DKA

 Differential Diagnosis

• Gastroenteritis
• Severe intraabdominal process (e.g., ulcer, pancreatitis, appendicitis)
• Urinary tract infection
• Pneumonia
• Stress hyperglycemia
• Hypercalcemia
• Salicylate ingestion
• Inborn error of metabolism
• Non-ketotic hyperosmolar coma

 Data Gathering

HISTORY

Question: Polyuria, polydipsia, and polyphagia with weight loss
Significance: Symptom of hyperosmolar state.

Question: Nausea, vomiting, abdominal pain
Significance: Related to acidosis and electrolyte disturbance.

Question: Changes in breathing patterns (Kussmaul respirations)
Significance: Related to acidosis and respiratory correction.

Question: Precipitating event, such as an intercurrent illness or psychosocial stress
Significance: Increased need for insulin in these states.

• Lethargy, obtundation

 Physical Examination

Finding: Vital signs—tachycardia, hypotension
Significance: Seen in dehydration

Finding: Dry mucous membranes, sunken eyes, poor skin turgor, poor distal perfusion, weak pulses
Significance: Dehydration

Finding: Fruity odor to breath indicates ketosis
Significance: Ketosis

Finding: Deep, sighing, hyperpneic (Kussmaul) respirations
Significance: Respiratory regulation of acid base disturbance

Finding: Abdominal tenderness
Significance: Related to electrolyte disturbance and increased lipids

Finding: Altered mental status
Significance: Acidosis and hyperglycemia

 Laboratory Aids

Test: Glucose more than 200 mg/dL
Significance: Indicates insulin deficiency

Test: Urinalysis—glycosuria and ketonuria
Significance: Glucose level exceeds renal threshold

Test: Sodium—serum levels low
From electrolyte losses and artifact of hyperlipidemia; actual Na level = measured Na + 1.6 ×
Significance: [glucose − 200)/100]

Test: Potassium—serum levels may be elevated, normal, or low; total body is potassium-depleted.
Significance: Potassium deletion from hyperaldosterone. Serum level is dependent on state of hydration.

Test: Bicarbonate less than 15 mEq/L
Significance: Acidosis

Test: Phosphate—low, secondary to osmotic diuresis
Significance: Acidosis

Test: ABG—low pH (<7.3), low pCO_2, and low HCO_3
Significance: Acidosis

Test: CBC—elevated WBC count even in the absence of infection
Significance: Strep reaction

Therapy

- Resuscitation

—Assess adequacy of airway and breathing.
—Restore circulation if necessary with normal saline bolus of 10 to 20 mL/kg.
—Cannot gauge hydration status initially by urine output because of osmotic diuresis.
—Avoid aggressive fluid resuscitation—too-rapid correction of hyperosmolarity increases risk of cerebral edema.

- Monitoring

—ICU admission for infants, toddlers, initial pH <7.1, hemodynamic, or neurological instability
—ECG monitoring for hypokalemia or hyperkalemia
—Serial neurological examinations q1h, with special attention to headache, declining mental status, any neurological symptoms
—Serial blood sugars hourly
—pH and electrolytes q1–2h until stable

- Fluids

—Assume 10% dehydration, 15% in infants
—Aim to replace losses plus maintenance fluids evenly over 48 hours
—Replacement fluids should always be normal saline, not ½ normal saline
—Ongoing renal losses greater than 3 mL/kg/h may be replaced if significant

- Electrolytes

—Assume Na and K losses of approximately 5 to 10 mEq/kg
—Hyponatremia will correct as fluids and insulin are given
—Continued drop in Na is associated with increased risk of cerebral edema
—Replace potassium as an equal mixture with chloride and phosphate:

K+ > 5.5, 20 mEq/L in replacement fluids

K+ = 4.0–5.5, 40 mEq/L

K+ < 4.0, 60 mEq/L

—Potassium replacement should never exceed 0.5 mEq/kg/h

- Acidosis

—Usually corrects once adequate insulin and fluids are given
—Consider bicarbonate if arterial pH <7.1 or there is inadequate respiratory compensation rule of thumb: (i.e., if $pCO_2 > (1.5 \times [HCO_3]) + 8$)
—Give as slow infusion over 1 to 2 hours at dose of 1 to 2 mEq/kg

- Insulin

—Prompt initiation critical in terminating ongoing ketone and acid production
—Initial dose is 0.1 U/kg/h as continuous intravenous infusion
—Do not give subcutaneously in DKA, as skin perfusion may be suboptimal
—Aim to lower serum glucose by 50 to 100 mg/dL/h

- Glucose

—Add 5% dextrose to intravenous stock when blood glucose <300 mg/dL
—Change to 10% dextrose when blood glucose <200 mg/dL

- Duration

—Stop infusion when pH > 7.3, HCO₃ > 15, glucose < 300, and patient is tolerating oral fluids
—Convert to subcutaneous therapy by adding up total insulin given over 24 hours and dividing into two to four injections or return to usual home regimen of with frequent monitoring and extra insulin as needed

 ## Follow-Up

- New diabetics should be followed closely after hospital discharge to assess adequacy of insulin regimen.
- Children with recurrent DKA shoud be evaluated for treatment failure (familial dysfunction, knowledge gaps).

PREVENTION

- Timely referral for children with symptoms of polyuria, polydipsia, and weight loss
- Surveillance with frequent blood sugar and urine ketone monitoring, supplemental insulin dosing, phone contact with pediatrician or endocrinologist should avert almost all episodes of DKA in children known to have diabetes.

 ## Common Questions and Answers

Q: What are the usual triggers for DKA?
A: Intercurrent illnesses, such as gastroenteritis, urinary tract infections, pneumonia; psychosocial stressors; failure to take insulin on schedule.

Q: Does an episode of DKA mean that the insulin regimen is inadequate?
A: DKA always implies insulin deficiency; insulin regimen may be adequate when child is well, but additional stresses of illness or psychosocial factors often require supplemental insulin.

ICD-9-CM 250.1

BIBLIOGRAPHY

Green SM, Rothrock SG, Ho JD, et al. Failure of adjunctive bicarbonate to improve outcome in severe pediatric diabetic ketoacidosis. *Ann Emerg Med* 1998;31(1):41–48.

Kaufman FR. Diabetes in children and adolescents. Areas of controversy. *Med Clin North Am* 1998;82(4):721–738.

Kecskes S. Diabetic ketoacidosis. *Pediatr Clin North Am* 1993;40(2):355–363.

Krane E. Diabetic ketoacidosis: biochemistry, physiology, treatment, and prevention. *Pediatr Clin North Am* 1987;34(4):935–960.

Author: Stuart A. Weinzimer

Diabetes Mellitus

 Database

DEFINITION

Diabetes mellitus (DM) is a disorder of absolute or relative insulin deficiency that results in disruptions in normal energy storage and metabolism. This causes impaired glucose tolerance, hyperglycemia, ketosis, and acidosis, which can ultimately lead to dehydration, shock, and death.

CAUSES

- Type I DM: In genetically susceptible individuals, an environmental trigger (believed viral) causes an autoimmune-mediated destruction of pancreatic β-cells, leading to absolute insulin deficiency.
- Type 2 DM: Insulin resistance at tissue level leads to relative insulin deficiency.

PATHOLOGY (TYPE I DM)

- Induction of expression of DR antigens on β-cell surface following viral infection.
- Recruitment of cytotoxic lymphocytes.
- Production of anti-insulin and anti-islet-cell antibodies.
- Progressive loss of β-cell mass and insulin supply, resulting in insulin deficiency.

EPIDEMIOLOGY

- Most common endocrine/metabolic disorder of childhood
- 1 to 2 in 1000 school-aged children, but increases with age such that:

—1 in 1500 children by age 5 are affected
—1 in 350 by age 16

- Type I DM: More common in Northern Europeans, less common in Asians, African-Americans
- Type 2 DM: More common in African-Americans, often with strong family history
- Boys and girls equally affected
- Incidence: 16 new cases per 100,000 children per year
- Incidence of Type 2 DM increasing, may be as high as 10% of new cases

GENETICS

- Susceptibility associated with HLA region of chromosome 6 (Type I DM)
- Five-fold greater risk with MHC antigen types DR3 and DR4 (Type I DM)
- Genetic defect in Type 2 DM unknown, but some have defects in insulin secretion (maturity-onset diabetes of the young)

COMPLICATIONS

- Diabetic ketoacidosis (DKA): profound metabolic derangement characterized by hyperglycemia, ketosis, and acidosis, leading to osmotic diuresis, dehydration, shock, and death
- Hypoglycemia: complication of insulin therapy
- Long-term effects:

—Nephropathy—microalbuminuria, proteinuria, chronic renal failure
—Retinopathy—microvascular proliferation, visual loss
—Neuropathy—progressive diminution of nerve conduction velocity
—Vasculopathy—accelerated atherosclerosis, large-vessel disease
—Embryopathy--infants of diabetic mothers at increased risk of birth defects
—Growth failure (Mauriac syndrome) and delayed sexual maturation
—Rate of development of chronic complications related to degree of metabolic control

 Differential Diagnosis

- Urinary tract infection (polyuria)
- Renal glycosuria
- Hypercalcemia (polyuria, weight loss)
- Chronic illness (weight loss, malaise)
- Stress-related hyperglycemia
- Drug-induced hyperglycemia (steroids)
- Pneumonia (in DKA)
- Sepsis (in DKA)
- Acute abdominal event (in DKA)

 Data Gathering

HISTORY

Question: Polyuria, nocturia, enuresis?
Significance: Related to hyperglycemia.

Question: Polydipsia?
Significance: Increased thirst follows polyuria and dehydration.

Question: Polyphagia
Significance: Increased appetite related to loss of calories from glucosuria.

Question: Weight loss, poor growth
Significance: Dehydration, loss of calories

Question: Malaise, weakness
Significance: Electrolyte disturbance and acidosis.

Question: Changes in behavior, school performance
Significance: Mental status changes related to acidosis.

 Physical Examination

- Usually normal in Type I DM
- Obesity and acanthosis nigricans (hypertrophic skin pigmentation of the neck) in Type 2 DM
- In DKA, signs of dehydration and acidosis (Kussmaul respirations)

 Laboratory Aids

- Blood glucose more than 200 mg/dL (2-hour post-prandial is most sensitive).
- Glycosuria, ketonuria (latter is variable in Type 2 DM)
- Hemoglobin A_{1c} (gives approximation of average blood glucose level over previous 2 to 3 months)

Test: Measurement of insulin and C-peptide levels
Significance: Islet cell antibodies may differentiate Type I versus Type 2 DM.

Therapy

INSULIN

- Usually given in combination of short-acting and long-acting preparations b.i.d. to t.i.d.
- Total daily dose (TDD) usually about 1 U/kg/day, less during "honeymoon period"
- Often given as: two-thirds of TDD in morning (one-third of that as short-acting and two-thirds long-acting), and one-third of TDD in evening (with one-half of that as short-acting and one-half as long-acting, split between dinner and bedtime)
- Oral anti-diabetic agents may be effective in Type 2 DM

DIET

- Consistency of amount and timing of meals is important:

—20% of daily calories from breakfast and lunch
—30% from dinner
—10% from snacks evenly spaced between meals and before bedtime

- Balance of source of calories is important:

—55% from carbohydrates (of which 70% complex)
—30% from fats
—15% from protein

- American Diabetes Association system of "exchanges" of different food groups
- Carbohydrate "counting"

EXERCISE

- Regular exercise helps to reduce insulin requirements and reduce blood glucose.

HOME MONITORING

- Checking blood glucose q.i.d. (before meals and bedtime snack), more often if necessary.
- Checking urine for ketones whenever blood glucose more than 240 mf/dL or during intercurrent illnesses.

 ## Follow-Up

- Regular appointments with diabetologist or nurse specialist every 3 months to assess growth and development and trouble-shoot management problems
- Meetings with nutritionist periodically to reassess meal plan
- Meetings with psychologist as needed to address psychosocial and family stressors
- Monitoring of glycosylated hemoglobin every 3 months to assess long-term control and compliance
- Yearly urine collections to evaluate microalbuminuria
- Yearly ophthalmologic examinations to evaluate retinopathy
- Yearly blood tests to evaluate for hyperlipidemia

 ## Common Questions and Answers

Q: What is the "honeymoon period"?
A: The period of "remission" following initial stabilization of metabolism with exogenous insulin. It is marked by the presence of residual endogenous insulin secretion; insulin doses usually drop to 0.5 U/kg/day or less. The honeymoon phase usually lasts weeks to months, but may persist 1 to 2 years.

Q: What is the risk of diabetes in a sibling or child of a person with Type I DM?
A: It is 2% to 5% in first-degree relatives (siblings, offspring); 25% to 35% in identical twins, higher in certain genetic haplotypes.

Q: What are the goals of glucose control?
A: Preprandial blood glucose 80 to 120 mg/dL; postprandial blood glucose less than 180 mg/dL; avoidance of episodes of hypoglycemia; maintenance of a reasonably non-restrictive lifestyle and psychological adjustment.

Q: Does having diabetes necessarily mean that one will develop the long-term complications?
A: The Diabetes Control and Complications Trial showed that intensive management and tight control (average blood sugar < 140 mg/dL) reduces the risk of complications (retinopathy, nephropathy, and neuropathy) by 50% to 75%.

ICD-9-CM 250.0

BIBLIOGRAPHY

American Diabetes Association. Standards of medical care for patients with diabetes mellitus. *Diabetes Care* 1994;17(6):616–623.

Diabetes Control and Complications Trial Research Group. The effect of intensive treatment of diabetes on the development and progression of long-term complications in insulin-dependent diabetes mellitus. *N Engl J Med* 1993;329:977–986.

Kaufman FR. Diabetes in children and adolescents. Areas of controversy. *Med Clin North Am* 1998;82(4):721–738.

Liss DS, Waller DA, Kennard BD, McIntire D, Capra P, Stephens J. Psychiatric illness and family support in children and adolescents with diabetic ketoacidosis: a controlled study. *J Am Acad Child Adolesc Psychiatry* 1998;37(5):536–544.

Malone J. Understanding diabetes in children. *Adv Pediatr* 1994;41:33–52.

Sperling M. Outpatient management of diabetes mellitus. *Pediatr Clin North Am* 1987;34(4):919–933.

Author: Stuart A. Weinzimer

Diaper Rash

 Database

DEFINITION

Commonly known as diaper rash, it is a collection of dermatoses defined by its etiology and distribution.

PATHOPHYSIOLOGY

Diaper rashes are the result of several different processes, alone and in combination:

- Friction: Rubbing of wet diapers against exposed skin areas such as the inner surface of the thighs, genitals, buttocks, abdomen, results in an erythematous, shiny rash that spares the intertriginous areas.
- Irritation: Confined to the exposed areas under the diaper, sparing the intertriginous areas, secondary to irritants such as feces/urine, cleaning materials.
- Allergic: Contact allergies are unusual in this age group and may be the result of detergents, topical medicines.
- Atopic: Usually later onset in infants, is pruritic and is often accompanied by a familial history of atopy.
- Seborrhea: Typical yellow-salmon-colored greasy rash especially affecting the intertriginous areas, and may be seen in other areas such as the scalp, face, neck, and flexural areas.
- Candidal: Especially common during or immediately after antibiotic administration, this rash is beefy red, with a raised sharp margin, and characteristic pinpoint erythematous, satellite lesions.

GENETICS

Dependent on the individual causes of diaper dermatitis, such as predisposition for allergic-based rashes.

EPIDEMIOLOGY

This dermatitis is by definition exclusive to individuals wearing diapers, and generally resolves when diapers are no longer worn.

COMPLICATIONS

Generally none, although secondary bacterial or fungal infections may lead to ulceration.

PROGNOSIS

Diaper rash resolves once the child is potty trained and out of diapers.

 Differential Diagnosis

Although any rash under a diaper can be considered a diaper rash, the following are other diseases that may present on the skin of the anogenital region but are not common causes of diaper dermatitis.

- Infection

—Congenital syphilis: Less commonly seen now because of maternal screening, this infection may manifest with a macular, papular, or bullous lesion in the diaper area. The palms and soles may also reveal lesions.
—HIV infection: May first present with erosive and ulcerated lesions, especially in the gluteal cleft. May be associated with other infections such as cytomegalovirus or herpes, may be pruritic. Other findings such as anemia, hepatosplenomegaly are often present.

- Tumors

—Letterer-Siwe (Langerhans cell histiocytosis) may present as a diaper rash with small reddish-brown papules or vesicles.

- Metabolic

—Acrodermatitis enteropathica: Deficiency of zinc. In addition to vesiculobullous lesions of the hands and feet and surrounding mouth and diaper areas, these patients have failure to thrive, diarrhea, alopecia, and frequent bacterial and candidal infections.

- Immunological Finding

—Psoriasis: Although unusual, may affect the diaper area with dark red, well-marginated plaques with silvery scales. Other areas of the body are usually similarly affected.

- Other

—Granuloma gluteal infantum, the etiology is not well understood, probably an inflammatory response to a variety of irritants. Results in discrete red painless nodules up to 4 cm in size.

 Data Gathering

HISTORY

Question: Any skin disorders at other sites
Significance: Skin disorders such as atopic dermatitis or seborrhea located elsewhere on the body suggest involvement in the diaper area as well.

Question: Use of medications (especially oral antibiotics, or topical medications)?
Significance: Medications can directly effect the diaper area, or leave it more susceptible to rashes. Oral antibiotics change the normal bowel and skin flora, and may cause diarrhea which can irritate the skin. Topical medications such as steroid ointments may change the appearance of the rash, or may cause changes in the skin (such as thinning).

Question: Use of detergents or soaps on skin or clothes?
Significance: These substances are often not recognized by parents as containing irritants (such as perfumes) which can damage the skin, leaving it susceptible to diaper rash

Question: Any current medical problems (such as diarrhea) which might irritate the skin?
Significance: Many medical problems manifest themselves in the skin, and may affect the diaper rash.

Question: Review skin care techniques: what is put on the skin and how is it used?
Significance: Parents often think a diaper rash represents poor hygiene, and as a result increase the cleaning of the area around the rash. Depending on how it is done and what is used, this cleaning may instead result in further irritation and damage to the skin.

Physical Examination

Finding: Location of the rash should be carefully noted.
Significance: Is it predominately in the exposed surfaces (contact, friction) or in the intertriginous areas (seborrhea, candidal)?

Finding: The margins of the rash should be inspected for satellite lesions.
Significance: Candida classically has satellite lesions.

Finding: Appearance of lesions
Significance: The lesion is dry or moist appearing (candidal); if it has a shiny parchment paper-like appearance (friction or atopic dermatitis)

Finding: A thorough examination of other areas of skin (e.g., looking for atopic or seborrheic dermatitis).
Significance: May give clues to the underlying skin of the diaper area and determine etiological factors of the rash.

Laboratory Aids

Almost always a clinical diagnosis. Candidal infections may be verified by skin scraping and viewed with potassium hydroxide under a microscope.

Therapy

Proper skin care is the primary treatment modality. When soiled, the skin should be gently washed with a mild soap and patted dry or air-dried. The diaper should be kept off and the rash exposed to air as much as possible. Any moderate to severe rash will invariably be secondarily infected with Candida and should be treated with topical nystatin, miconazole, or clotrimazole. If the skin is very inflamed and especially if there is evidence of contact, atopic, or seborrheic dermatitis, a small amount of topical corticosteroid cream (such as 1% hydrocortisone) can be used for a few days.
Although gentle skin care techniques should be permanently adopted, the use of topical antifungal medication and ointments should be continued until the rash completely resolves. Steroid medications should be stopped after a few days, when the intense acute inflammation has improved.

Follow-Up

With proper treatment, the rash should be noticeably better within 4 to 7 days. Failure of resolution of rash indicates that another dermatologic process may be complicating the diaper rash.

PREVENTION

Proper skin care with gentle cleaning and mild soap should be used. Superabsorbent diapers may be suggested, along with frequent diaper changes. Barrier creams such as zinc oxide may help protect the skin from external irritants after resolution of the rash.

PITFALLS

General pitfall to avoid is the use of laboratory aids to help diagnose this disorder, because it is almost always a clinical diagnosis. Topical steroid used alone may worsen a candidal infection.

- Often the caretaker believes the rash is a result of inadequate cleansing of the skin and, subsequently, attempts to wash the skin more. This additionally irritates and exacerbates the rash. Topicals that strongly adhere to the skin do not need to be scrubbed completely clean before putting on another treatment.
- Steroids marketed by drug companies in combination with antifungal creams are often more potent than necessary. In addition, the action of topical steroids is potentiated when used under "occlusion" (the diaper). When topical steroids are used, they are best given as a separate prescription that can be stopped at an earlier time than the antifungal medication.
- Talcum powder can worsen the irritation, and may be aspirated by both baby and caretaker. Its use should be discouraged.
- If a candidal diaper infection is resistant to treatment, and thrush (monilia infection of the mouth) is present, oral nystatin may be used q.i.d.

Common Questions and Answers

Q: Should I switch from cloth to disposable diapers (or vice versa)?
A: This is controversial, although there are some studies that indicate that the superabsorbent disposable diapers may be better for controlling diaper rashes. Cloth diapers used with plastic overpants probably irritate the skin more because they trap moisture against the skin.

Q: Is the diaper rash due to not keeping the skin clean enough?
A: Although the combination of stool and urine may release enzymes that help break down skin integrity, probably more harmful to skin is vigorous and frequent scrubbing with relatively abrasive materials on the macerated, easily damaged skin typically found in the diaper area. This rough cleaning allows introduction of bacteria and yeast into the skin and results in a diaper rash. Parent should be advised to use soft cleaning materials (such as cotton balls) to gently clean stool from the diaper area. It is not usually necessary to clean the skin of urine every time, rather patting the infant dry with a soft cloth and then replacing the diaper is all that is generally required.

ICD-9-CM 691

BIBLIOGRAPHY

Hurwitz S. *Clinical pediatric dermatology,* 2nd ed. Philadelphia: WB Saunders, 1993.

Singalavanija S, Frieden I. Diaper dermatitis. *Pediatr Rev* 1995;16:142–147.

Wong LD, Brantly D, Clutter LB, et al. Diapering choices: a critical review of the issues. *Pediatr Nurs* 1992;18:41–54.

Author: Robert Kamei

Diaphragmatic Hernia (Congenital)

 Database

DEFINITION

• Herniation of abdominal contents into the thoracic cavity through an opening in the diaphragm
• Two types of congenital diaphragmatic hernias

—Bochdalek hernia (posterolateral location)
—Morgagni hernia (retrosternal location)

CAUSES

• Diaphragm forms between 7 to 10 weeks of gestation
• Diaphragm is composed of two parts:

—Pleuroperitoneal folds attach to the chest wall, develop a muscular lining and become the lateral and dorsal portions of the diaphragm
—Septum transversum, which becomes the central tendon of the diaphragm

• Anything that interferes with the formation of the diaphragm allows an abdominal hernia to develop
• Bochdalek hernia develops when:

—Midgut returns to the abdominal cavity prematurely or diaphragmatic development is delayed
—Bowel is trapped in the thoracic cavity, preventing the pleuroperitoneal folds from connecting with the thoracic wall
  —This allows a communication to exist between the thoracic and abdominal cavities

• Morgagni hernia develops when:

—A defect develops in the septum transversum

PATHOPHYSIOLOGY

• Bochdalek hernia

—Usually occurs on the left side (left-sided pleuroperitoneal folds close later than the right)
—Bowel in the thoracic cavity
—Bilateral lung hypoplasia (ipsilateral lung hypoplasia worse than contralateral side)

• Morgagni hernia

—Usually occurs on the right side (left-sided defects are covered by the heart)
—Hernia can contain: liver, bowel, and omentum
—Less lung hypoplasia seen than with Bochdalek hernias

EPIDEMIOLOGY

• Bochdalek hernia

—Accounts for 90% of cases of congenital diaphragmatic hernias
—Incidence: in 1/2200 to 1/5000 live births
—80% to 90% of cases on the left side (bilateral cases are rare)
—Slightly more common in males
  —40% of cases associated with some type of congenital malformation
  —5% to 16% of cases with chromosomal abnormality
  —18% associated with a congenital heart disease

• Morgagni hernia

—Accounts for 2% of all diaphragmatic hernias more common in females

GENETICS

• Estimated 2% recurrence rate in first degree relatives

COMPLICATIONS

• Bochdalek hernia

—Pulmonary hypertension
—Persistent fetal circulation with right to left
—Shunting
—Pulmonary insufficiency
—Death

• Morgagni hernia

—10% incidence of strangulation of the bowel if not repaired

 Differential Diagnosis

PULMONARY

• Pulmonary cysts
• Cystic adenomatoid malformation
• Pneumatocele
• Congenital lobar emphysema
• Pulmonary sequestration
• Eventration of the diaphragm
• Hiatal hernia
• Laryngotracheal obstruction
• Atelectasis
• Pneumothorax
• Anterior mediastinal mass
• Pneumonia
• Pleural effusion

CARDIAC

• Dextrocardia
• Congenital heart disease

 Data Gathering

HISTORY

Question: Bochdalek hernia?
Significance: Presents at birth; patient frequently presents in severe cardiopulmonary distress.

Question: Morgagni hernia?
Significance: Usually asymptomatic. If symptomatic, usually presents later in life. May have complaints of: vague abdominal discomfort, vomiting, failure to thrive, chest pain, dyspnea, cough, and recurrent respiratory infections.

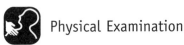 Physical Examination

Finding: Bochdalek hernia
Significance:

• Severe respiratory distress
• Cyanotic
• Tachypnea
• Decreased breath sounds on the affected side
• Hyperresonance to percussion on the affected side
• Asymmetry of the chest wall (enlarged on the affected side)
• Increased anterior-posterior diameter of the chest
• Occasional bowel sounds heard in the chest
• Tachycardia
• Cardiac point of maximal impulse shifted away from the affected side
• Scaphoid abdomen (abdominal contents in thoracic cavity)

Finding: Morgagni hernia
Significance: Examination may be normal

Laboratory Aids

TESTS

Test: Arterial blood gas
Significance:

- pO_2 shows evidence of severe hypoxia
- pCO_2 elevated
- pH reveals significant acidosis (both respiratory and metabolic)

IMAGING

Test: Chest radiograph
Significance:

- Bochdalek hernia

—Mediastinal structures shifted away from the affected side
—Heart shifted away from the affected side
—Decreased lung volumes (ipsilateral lung more than contralateral lung)
—Atelectasis of the contralateral lung
—Unable to visualize the diaphragm on the ipsilateral side
—Loops of bowel in the thoracic cavity
—In left-sided hernias, a nasogastric tube inserted into the stomach will be seen in the thoracic cavity
—Abdominal bowel is usually gasless

- Morgagni hernia

—A mass is seen in the anterior mediastinum: may be solid or gas-filled

Test: Fetal ultrasound
Significance: Abdominal viscera in the thoracic cavity; polyhydramnios

 Therapy

- Bochdalek hernia

—Resuscitation of the patient
—Stabilization of the patient:
  —Oxygenation
  —Correction of acidosis
  —Normalization of blood pressure
  —Decompression of the intrathoracic bowel (placement of a nasogastric tube to low suction allows the bowel to decompress, thus letting the ipsilateral hypoplastic lung expand)
—Surgical repair of the defect:
  —Decreased morbidity and mortality if the patient can be stabilized prior to surgical repair

—Post-operative management
—ECMO (extracorporeal membrane oxygenation)
  —May prove useful in the peri-operative management:
  —Pre-operative: for patient stabilization
  —Post-operative: to allow the lungs to fully expand after the compressing intrathoracic bowel has been removed

—If the diagnosis of a Bochdalek hernia is made early enough in gestation (i.e., 24–28 weeks gestation), fetal surgery to repair the defect may be considered

- Morgagni hernia

—Surgical repair is indicated, even if the patient is asymptomatic, due to the high rate of strangulation of the intrathoracic bowel (10%)

 Follow-Up

WHEN TO EXPECT IMPROVEMENT

Dependent on the extent of pulmonary hypoplasia and pulmonary hypertension.

SIGNS TO WATCH FOR

- The development of pulmonary hypertension in the post-operative period
- Rapid development of hypoxia is associated with the development of a pneumothorax

PROGNOSIS

- Bochdalek hernias:

—Dependent on the degree of pulmonary hyperplasia and pulmonary hypertension:
  —If not surgically repaired: 100% mortality
  —If patient survives the peri-operative period: 33% to 65% survival

—Poor prognostic factors:
  —Polyhydramnios *in utero*
  —Fetal stomach in the thoracic cavity
  —Early presentation (i.e., presenting in the first 6 hours versus after 24 hours)
  —Persistent elevated pCO_2 and decreased pO_2

- Morgagni hernias: excellent

PITFALLS

Bochdalek hernias

—Not being able to stabilize the patient (suggestive of severe pulmonary hypoplasia and/or pulmonary hypertension)
—Delay in getting the patient to an appropriate medical center
—Not recognizing other congenital malformations or chromosomal abnormalities that may affect the patient's ultimate outcome or which would represent a contraindication for surgical repair (i.e., Trisomy 18)

Morgagni hernias

—Not considering the diagnosis when abnormalities seen on chest radiograph

 Common Questions and Answers

Q: What is the long-term pulmonary function in survivors of Bochdalek hernias?
A: Dependent on the degree of pulmonary hypoplasia; pulmonary function testing shows evidence of both obstructive and/or restrictive lung disease. Decreased perfusion on the affected side.

Q: What long-term problems can be seen in survivors of Bochdalek hernias?
A: Dependent on the degree of pulmonary hypoplasia; recurrent respiratory infections of the hypoplastic lungs.

ICD-9-CM 553.3

BIBLIOGRAPHY

Adzick NS, Vacanti JP, Lillehei CW, et al. Fetal diaphragmatic hernia: ultrasound diagnosis and clinical outcome in 38 Cases. *J Pediatr Surg* 1989;24:654–658.

Cunniff C, Jones KL, Jones MC. Patterns of malformation in children with congenital diaphragmatic defects. *J Pediatr* 1990;116:258–261.

Harrison MR, Adzick NS, Longaker MT, et al. Successful repair in utero of a fetal diaphragmatic hernia after removal of herniated viscera from the left thorax. *N Engl J Med* 1990;322:1582–1584.

Harrison MR, Langer JC, Adzick NS, et al. Correction of congenital diaphragmatic hernia in utero, V. Initial clinical experience. *J Pediatr Surg* 1990;25:47–57.

Hudak BB. *Respiratory disease in children: diagnosis and management.* Baltimore: Williams & Wilkins, 1993:501–532.

Lierl M. *Pediatric respiratory disease: diagnosis and treatment.* Philadelphia: WB Saunders Co., 1993:457–498.

Molenaar JC, Bos AP, Hazebroek FWJ, Tibboel D. Congenital diaphragmatic hernia, what defect? *J Pediatr Surg* 1991;26:248–254.

Puri P. Congenital diaphragmatic hernia. *Curr Probl Surg* 1994;31:787–846.

Salzberg AM, Krummel TM. *Kendig's disorders of the respiratory tract in children.* Philadelphia: WB Saunders Co., 1990:227–267.

Schumacher RE, Farrell PM. Congenital diaphragmatic hernia: a major remaining challenge in neonatal respiratory care. *Perinat Neonat* 1985;9:29–41.

Authors: Mayra Bustillo and Richard Mark Kravitz

Diarrhea Acute

 Database

DEFINITION

• Short in duration; usually lasts less than 2 weeks
• In infants, stool volume in excess of 10 g/kg/d is considered diarrhea.
• In children older than 3 years of age, the stool volume is equivalent to adult levels and greater than 200 g/d of stool volume is considered diarrhea.

CAUSES

• Most common cause for acute diarrhea is a viral infection:

—Rotavirus
—Norwalk
—Enteric adenovirus
—Calicivirus

• Bacterial infections:

—Salmonella
—Escherichia coli
—Shigella
—Campylobacter
—Clostridium
—Yersinia
—Cholera

• Parasitic infections also common
• Variety of less common causes:

—Antibiotic-associated diarrhea
—Toxin exposure (food poisoning)
—Overfeeding in newborns
—Hirschsprung colitis
—Hyperthyroidism

PATHOPHYSIOLOGY

• In acute diarrhea, impairment of the normal absorptive and secretory balance of the different regions of the gut resulting in diarrhea.
• Viral pathogens generally produce injury to the proximal small bowel and bacterial pathogens usually cause colonic injury.
• Bacterial pathogens cause injury through:

—Invasion of the mucosa, causing cell death as they replicate (invasive)
—Cytotoxicity (direct cell death)
—Toxigenicity (producing toxins that alter water balance)
—Adherence to the mucosal surface, causing disruption of normal cell function

EPIDEMIOLOGY

• Diarrhea remains one of the most significant global medical problems.
• In developed countries such as the United States, the overall problem is less severe than in other developing countries because improved sanitation systems reduce transmission.
• There are approximately 20 to 40 million episodes of diarrhea in the United States in children less than 5 years of age annually. An estimated 200,000 need hospitalization, and 200 to 400 die each year.
• Worldwide, an estimated 4 million children die from diarrheal disease annually.
• Most transmission is via the fecal-oral route.
• Other organisms are transmitted via direct person-to-person contact (day care centers). Some are transmitted via infected food or water.
• Most common viral pathogens occur in the winter months and the common bacterial pathogens in the summer.

COMPLICATIONS

• The most common complication is dehydration. If severe enough, this may be associated with electrolyte abnormalities and acidosis.
• Some bacterial pathogens may also lead to bacteremia and may even cause seizures by either an infectious or a toxin-mediated process.
• Certain pathogens, namely *Escherichia coli* 0157 subtype H7 can cause the hemolytic uremic syndrome.
• In cases in which the small-bowel mucosa has been significantly injured, a protein-losing enteropathy can occur.
• Meningitis and osteomyelitis are less frequent complications.

Differential Diagnosis

• The major cause of acute diarrhea is viral gastroenteritis.

—Rotavirus is most common between the ages of 6 and 24 months. It is the most common cause of diarrheal illness in the pediatric population.

• There is an increase in incidence during the winter months, and symptoms last between 2 and 8 days.
• Most children have developed antibodies to the virus by the age of 2; this explains the decrease in incidence seen in older patients.

—Norwalk virus seems to affect older children and adults and has no seasonal variation. Duration of symptoms is between 1 and 2 days.
—Enteric adenovirus is predominantly seen in children less than 2 years of age and occurs mainly in the summer months. Symptoms may last up to 14 days.

—Calicivirus accounts for about 3% of diarrheal disease that requires hospitalization. It mainly affects children between 3 months and 6 years. Symptoms last between 2 and 8 days.
—Cytomegalovirus has been associated with diarrhea and colitis, but is pathogenic predominantly in the immunocompromised host.

Bacterial pathogens include:

—Salmonella is the most common cause of bacterial diarrhea in children in the United States. Its highest incidence is in infancy.
—Shigella accounts for approximately 20% of diarrhea due to a bacterial pathogen. It occurs mainly between the ages of 6 months and 10 years. It is the most common cause of bacterial outbreaks in the day care center setting. A large number of complications can be seen with *Shigella* infections, such as seizures, bacteremia, meningitis, and osteomyelitis.
—Campylobacter is a common pathogen, but at times is underdiagnosed because it requires specific media and conditions to grow. It appears to have two peaks of infection: children under 1 year of age and young adults.
—Yersinia is a fairly common organism worldwide and causes symptoms most frequently in young children.
—Cholera isa major pathogen in developing nations.
—Escherichia coli is a species with a diverse group of organisms in which some are non-pathogenic and part of the normal intestinal flora. The four pathogenic types that cause diarrhea include:

—Enteropathogenic *E. coli*
—Enterotoxigenic *E. coli*
—Enteroinvasive *E. coli*
—Enterohemorrhagic *E. coli*

—Clostridium difficile has been noted primarily but not exclusively in patients in whom there has been an alteration in their normal intestinal flora by the use of antibiotics.
—Aeromonas and *Plesiomonas* are less common bacterial pathogens. The latter has been diagnosed in immunocompromised hosts.
—Giardiasis is the most common protozoal cause of acute diarrhea.

• Several other causes of acute diarrhea must be considered along with the infectious causes. These less common etiologies are listed.

—Antibiotics may cause diarrhea by altering the intestinal flora. In many cases of antibiotic use, diarrhea can still occur without the presence of *C. difficile*.
—Overfeeding, especially in small newborns, may lead to diarrhea.
—Hirschprung disease/colitis can lead to acute bloody, mucous diarrhea when the mucosa of the colon becomes inflamed. These patients tend to appear ill.
—Toxic ingestions such as with over-the-counter laxatives may be considered in the appropriate clinical setting.
—Hyperthyroidism can also cause diarrhea.

Data Gathering

HISTORY

Question: Exposure history?
Significance: Needs to be obtained, focusing on possible exposures to other affected individuals, especially children in day care centers.

Question: Diet history?
Significance: Focusing on water source, poultry intake, milk intake, and fish sources needs to be performed.

Question: Antibiotic use?
Significance: Presence of C. difficile

Question: Travel history?
Significance: Important for endemic causes and seasonal variations.

Question: Stool pattern and symptoms?
Significance: May be beneficial in helping to focus on a specific etiology.

Physical Examination

There are few findings that may assist in determining the causative agent of the diarrhea.

• Signs consistent with dehydration

Finding: Stools with occult or gross blood
Significance: Shigella, Salmonella, E. coli, Campylobacter

Finding: Abdominal tenderness
Significance: E. coli

Finding: Extraintestinal findings such as seizures, mental status changes
Significance: Shigella

Finding: Bone and joint pain
Significance: R/O osteomyelitis, salmonella

Finding: Rashes
Significance: Typhoid

Laboratory Aids

Test: Stool evaluation
Significance: Stool should be evaluated for:

• Occult blood and WBC
• Ova and parasites
• Rotavirus (Rotazyme test)
• *C. difficile* (toxin A and B)
• *Shigella*
• *E. coli*

Test: X-ray study
Significance: In more severe cases or in the appropriate clinical setting abdominal x-ray studies may be helpful.

Test: Endoscopy and/or colonoscopy
Significance: In the most complex and difficult cases more invasive procedures may be helpful in making the diagnosis.

Test: Blood tests
Significance: CBC, blood culture, and electrolytes may be helpful in management but are not diagnostic.

Therapy

• Most cases of acute, infectious diarrhea seen in pediatric offices in developed countries are mild and self-limited and can be managed on an outpatient basis with close follow-up.
• The goal of therapy is to treat the underlying cause of the diarrhea if identifiable and treatable and to provide adequate hydration in order to maintain euvolemia, electrolyte balance, and acid-base balance.
• The hydration status in dehydrated patients can be altered by oral or intravenous replacement therapy based on the clinical situation. Support with total parenteral nutrition (TPN) or elemental tube feeds may be necessary in patients with severe episodes of diarrhea.
• Antimicrobial agents do not greatly affect the overall course of gastroenteritis in most cases. Specific antibiotic therapies do exist for certain organisms and do help lessen the severity of the episode as well as decrease the fecal shedding and, therefore, the spread of the organism. In certain clinical settings, such as infection with *Salmonella*, antibiotics are not indicated.
• The best possible therapy for acute, infectious diarrhea is prevention. The best way to prevent transmission is to interrupt the fecal-oral pathway. For the most part, this requires an increased awareness of sanitation and hygiene as well as the proper handling and cooking of meat, fish, and poultry products.

REHYDRATION

During rehydration, the estimated fluid deficit based on clinical assessment is replaced. This is done with appropriate rehydration fluids.

• In cases in which the dehydration is below 5%, oral replacement therapy is used. In cases in which the dehydration is severe (<10%), intravenous fluids should be used. Between 5% to 10% dehydration, each individual clinical situation should be considered and at times a combination of oral and intravenous therapy have the best outcome.
• Other limitations to oral rehydration would include intractable vomiting, high stool output, and carbohydrate malabsorption.
• Reassessment of a patient with dehydration should be very vigilant and continuous, and adjustments should be made every 2 to 4 hours as needed.
• In addition to replacement of the deficit, ongoing losses should initially be replaced on a 1:1 basis.

MAINTENANCE THERAPY

In this phase, maintenance fluids and energy nutrient requirements are met.

• At this point, advancement in diet should begin and should proceed as tolerated. Special care should be taken with patients who may initially be lactose-intolerant. Soon after resolution of diarrhea an appropriate lactose-free formula may be used in the initial refeeding phase.
• Ongoing fluid losses should continue to be replaced until the diarrhea has resolved.

Follow-Up

• The majority of episodes of acute diarrhea are mild and self-limited and with close supervision and education of hydration status, patients can do well.
• In more severe cases, close monitoring and reassessment of hydration status is required.
• Once symptoms have improved and the diarrhea resolved, there is no routine follow-up needed.

PITFALLS

• Reassess therapy frequently and adjust therapy based on clinical setting.
• Use appropriate electrolyte solutions during rehydration and maintenance therapy.

ICD-9-CM 558.9

BIBLIOGRAPHY

Bhatnagar S, Singh KD, Sazawal S, Saxena SK, Bhan MK. Efficacy of milk versus yogurt offered as part of a mixed diet in acute noncholera diarrhea among malnourished children. *J Pediatr* 1998;132(6):999–1003.

Blacklow NR, Greenberg HB. Viral gastroenteritis. *N Engl J Med* 1991;325:252–264.

Guerrant RL, Lohr JA, Williams EK. Acute infectious diarrhea: I. Epidemiology, etiology and pathogenesis. *Pediatr Infect Dis* 1986;5(3):353–359.

Meyers A, Sampson A, Saladino R, Dixit S, Adams W, Mondolfi A. Safety and effectiveness of homemade and reconstituted packet cereal-based oral rehydration solutions: a randomized clinical trial. *Pediatrics* 1997;100(5):E3.

Rautanen T, Isolauri E, Salo E, Vesikari T. Management of acute diarrhoea with low osmolarity oral rehydration solutions and Lactobacillus strain GG. *Arch Dis Child* 1998;79(2):157–160.

Authors: Edisio Semeao and Andrew E. Mulberg

DiGeorge Syndrome

 Database

DEFINITION

DiGeorge syndrome is characterized by thymic aphasia or hypoplasia resulting in a spectrum of immunodeficiency, absent or hypoplastic parathyroid glands, and cardiac malformations.

- Complete DiGeorge syndrome involves all these abnormalities.
- Partial DiGeorge syndrome occurs when the immune system is intact.

PATHOPHYSIOLOGY

DiGeorge is believed to be a developmental defect of the third and fourth pharyngeal arches.

GENETICS

- Heterogeneous
- Some reported cases of autosomal dominant, autosomal recessive, and X-linked modes of inheritance
- Most common associated chromosomal abnormalities are microdeletions of 22q11.

COMPLICATIONS

In the newborn period, hypocalcemic tetany, manifestation of cardiac abnormality, and recurrent infections. Later on, developmental delay and arthralgias.

PROGNOSIS

Prolonged survival is seen in many patients after the spontaneous improvement of T cell immunity. These patients are considered to have partial DiGeorge syndrome. However, other patients may have more severe T cell dysfunction. Complications may include an increase in auto-immune phenomena and neurological sequelae.

 Data Gathering

HISTORY

- Neonatal hypocalcemia secondary to hypo-parathyroidism
- Recurrent infections: diarrhea, candidiasis
- Heart murmurs
- In particular, interrupted aortic arch, septal defects, patent ductus arteriosus, and truncus arteriosus.
- Failure to thrive

 Physical Examination

Finding: Facial dysmorphism
Significance: Small recessed chin; low, rotated ears; "fish-shaped mouth"; micro-gnathia; short philtrum, anteverted nares, and hypertelorism.

- Cleft lip and palate
- Heart murmur
- Hydronephrosis
- Colobomas
- Central nervous system malformations
- Major immunological features present at birth:

—Lymphopenia
—T cell dysfunction
—Antibody levels and function are variable

Laboratory Aids

Test: Chest x-ray study
Significance: To evaluate for cardiac malformation and also for the presence of a thymic shadow

Test: CBC
Significance: Immediately after birth, a lymphocyte count, 1200/mm^3 is suspicious.

Test: Serum levels of calcium and para-thormone
Significance: Check for hypocalcemia part of syndrome.

Test: Lymphocyte markers
Significance: To determine absolute numbers of T and B cells and their subsets

Test: Mitogen studies
Significance: To study the functional abilities of T and B cells, often depressed response to phytohemagglutinin, concanavalin A, and pokeweed mitogen.

Test: Quantitative immunoglobulins (IgG, IgA, IgM, and IgE)
Significance: Often the humoral system will be abnormal if there is extensive T cell dysfunction.

Test: FISH (fluorescence *in situ* hybridization) for 22q11 deletion
Significance: Most common chromosomal defect.

 ## Therapy

Depending on the defects or deficiencies the child manifests, some of the following issues may need to be addressed:

- Cardiology for the cardiac malformations
- Otolaryngology and feeding specialist for cleft palate
- Endocrinology for follow-up of hypoparathyroidism
- Immunology to monitor T cell disorder and recurrent infections

SPECIAL CONSIDERATION WITH INFECTIONS

Children with the complete DiGeorge syndrome are at increased risk of morbidity and mortality from viral infections either from vaccines such as oral polio or natural infections such as varicella. It is advisable to:

- Avoid live viral vaccines
- Consider varicella immune globulin in a patient either with unknown humoral immunity status or definitive humoral abnormalities. Intravenous acyclovir may be necessary if varicella develops and patient has a low T cell count or abnormal mitogens.

SPECIAL CONSIDERATION WITH BLOOD TRANSFUSIONS

Because these patients are at risk for graft-versus-host disease, it is best to use cytomegalovirus-negative, irradiated blood.

 ## Common Questions and Answers

Q: Is there a definitive test to distinguish between partial and complete DiGeorge syndrome?
A: Over time, patients with partial DiGeorge syndrome will reconstitute their T cells and acquire improved function based on mitogen and antigen studies.

ICD-9-CM 279.11

BIBLIOGRAPHY

Amman AJ. T cell immunodeficiency disorders. In: Stites DP, Terr AI, eds. *Basic and clinical immunology.* Norwalk, CT: Appleton & Lange, 1991:335–338.

Conley ME, Beckwith JB, Mancer JF, Tenckhoff L. The spectrum of the DiGeorge syndrome. *J Pediatr* 1979;94:883–890.

Driscoll DA, Budarf ML, Emanuel BS. A genetic etiology for DiGeorge syndrome: consistent deletions and microdeletions of 22q11. *Am J Hum Genet* 1992;50:924–933.

Radford DJ. The DiGeorge syndrome and the heart. *Curr Opin Pediatr* 1991;3:828–831.

Author: Michelle M. Klinek

Diphtheria

 Database

DEFINITION

Diphtheria is an acute infectious disease caused by Corynebacterium diphtheriae and affects primarily the membranes of the upper respiratory tract with the formation of a gray-white pseudomembrane.

CAUSES

The causative organism, *Corynebacterium diphtheriae*, is a gram-positive pleomorphic bacillus.

PATHOPHYSIOLOGY

The initial entry site for *C. diphtheriae* is via airborne respiratory droplets, typically the nose or mouth, but occasionally the ocular surface, genital mucous membranes, or pre-existing skin lesions. Following 2 to 4 days of incubation at one of these sites, the bacteria elaborates toxin. Locally, the toxin induces formation of a necrotic coagulation of the mucous membranes (pseudomembrane) with underlying tissue edema. Respiratory compromise may ensue. Elaborated exotoxin may also have profound effects on the heart, nerves, and kidneys in the form of myocarditis, demyelination, and tubular necrosis, respectively.

EPIDEMIOLOGY

• The single known reservoir for *C. diphtheriae* is humans; disease is acquired by contact with either a carrier or a diseased person.
• Though the disease is distributed throughout the world, it is endemic, primarily in developing regions of Africa, Asia, and South America. In the Western world, the incidence of diphtheria has changed dramatically in the past 50 to 75 years, as a result of the widespread use of diphtheria toxoid after World War II. The incidence has declined steadily and is now a rare occurrence.
• Recent outbreaks have occurred, most notably in the new independent states of the former Soviet Union, and supply additional evidence that disease occurs among the socioeconomically disadvantaged living in crowded conditions.
• The majority of cases occur during the cooler autumn and winter months in individuals less than 15 years of age who are unimmunized.

ASSOCIATED ILLNESSES

• Respiratory tract diphtheria:
—Nasal diphtheria starts with mild rhinorrhea that gradually becomes serosanguineous, then mucopurulent, and often malodorous. This form occurs most often in infants.
—Tonsillar and pharyngeal diphtheria begins with anorexia, malaise, low-grade fever, and pharyngitis. A membrane appears within 1 to 2 days. Cervical lymphadenitis and edema of the cervical soft tissues may be severe. Disease course varies with extent of toxin elaboration and membrane production. Respiratory and cardiovascular collapse may occur.
—Laryngeal diphtheria most often represents extension of a pharyngeal infection and clinically presents as typical croup. Acute airway obstruction may occur, and in severe cases, the membrane may invade the entire tracheobronchial tree.
—Cutaneous diphtheria occurs in warmer tropical regions. It is characterized by chronic non-healing ulcers with gray membrane and may serve as a reservoir in endemic and epidemic areas of respiratory diphtheria.

• Other sites: rarely vulvovaginal, conjunctival, or aural forms occur.

COMPLICATIONS

• Cardiac toxicity: myocarditis may develop secondary to elaborated toxin anytime between the first and sixth week of illness. Though cardiac failure can occur, the majority of cases are transient.
• Neurological toxicity again occurs secondary to toxin elaboration and mainly reflects bilateral motor involvement.
• Paralysis of the soft palate is most common, but ocular paralysis, diaphragm paralysis, peripheral neuropathy of the extremities, and loss of deep tendon reflexes also occur.
• The frequency of all complications, including those listed above, increases with increasing time between symptom onset and antitoxin administration and also with extent of membrane formation.

PROGNOSIS

• Most strongly dependent on the immunization status of the host. Those without prior adequate immunization have significantly higher morbidity and mortality.
• Delay to onset of treatment also increases mortality. When appropriate treatment has been administered on day 1 of illness, mortality may be as low as 1%. When treatment has been delayed until day 4, the mortality rate is up to 20-fold higher.
• Organism virulence: toxigenic strains are associated with more severe disease and a poorer prognosis.
• Location of membrane: laryngeal diphtheria has a higher mortality owing to airway obstruction.
• A megakaryocytic thrombocytopenia and WBC .25,000 are associated with poor outcome.

 Differential Diagnosis

• Nasal diphtheria can present much like the common cold, nasal foreign body, sinusitis, adenoiditis, or snuffles (congenital syphilis).
• Tonsillar or pharyngeal diphtheria may be confused with streptococcal pharyngitis, infectious mononucleosis, primary herpetic tonsillitis, thrush, Vincent angina, post-tonsillectomy faucial membranes, or the oropharyngeal involvement caused by toxoplasmosis, cytomegalovirus, tularemia, and salmonellosis.
• Laryngeal diphtheria: differential diagnosis includes croup, acute epiglottitis, aspirated foreign body, peripharyngeal and retropharyngeal abscess, laryngeal papillomas, or other masses.

 Data Gathering

HISTORY

Question: Exposure?
Significance: Exposure to an individual with diphtheria is not necessarily elicited because contact with an asymptomatic carrier may be the only source of infection.

Question:
Significance: The incubation period is 1 to 6 days. Respiratory diphtheria, depending on the site of infection, may begin with nasal discharge alone or with pharyngitis accompanied by mild systemic symptoms. Progression of symptoms thereafter occurs as outlined under "Associated Illnesses."

 Physical Examination

Finding: Nasal discharge, nasal or pharyngeal membrane, heart rate out of proportion to body temperature, respiratory distress, stridor, cough, hoarseness, palatal paralysis, neck swelling, and cervical lymphadenitis. Attempts to remove any membrane present will result in bleeding.
Significance: Classic findings.

Finding: Conjunctival diphtheria
Significance: Gives palpebral conjunctival involvement with a red, edematous, membranous appearance.

Finding: Aural diphtheria
Significance: Presents as otitis externa with a purulent, malodorous discharge.

Finding: Cutaneous diphtheria
Significance: See Associated Illnesses.

SPECIAL QUESTIONS

Previous diphtheria immunization history, diphtheria exposure.

Diphtheria

 Laboratory Aids

Test: Diagnosis should be on clinical grounds.
Significance: Delay in treatment increases morbidity and mortality.

Test: Culture of material from the membrane or beneath the membrane should be attempted.
Significance: If a strain of *C. diphtheriae* is isolated, additional testing for presence or absence of toxin production should be conducted by a laboratory prepared to conduct an animal neutralization test or, alternatively, neutralization (with antitoxin) in tissue culture.

Test: Examination of a methylene blue-stained lesion
Significance: Metachromatic granules can be helpful, if performed by an experienced technician.

Test: Fluorescent antibody testing and counter-immunoelectrophoresis
Significance: Previously performed in state laboratories, are no longer widely available.

 Therapy

DIPHTHERIA ANTITOXIN (DAT)

DAT antiserum, produced in horses, must be administered as soon as possible as follows. (Note: For patients with known horse serum sensitivity, a test dose should be administered first, and if positive, the patient should be desensitized.)

- Pharyngeal or laryngeal disease of <48 hours; duration, 20,000 to 40,000 units IV
- Nasopharyngeal lesions, 40,000 to 60,000 units IV
- Extensive disease of 3 or more days duration or diffuse neck swelling, 80,000 to 100,000 units IV

ANTIBIOTIC THERAPY

- Antibiotic therapy should be used in addition to DAT, not in place of it, as follows:
- Respiratory diphtheria

—Penicillin G
  —Aqueous crystalline, 100,000 to 150,000 U/kg/d in four divided doses ×14 days
  —Procaine, 25,000 to 50,000 U/kg/d in two divided doses ×14 days
  or
  —Erythromycin, 40 to 50 mg/kg/× (maximum 2 gm/d) PO or parenterally ×14 days

- Cutaneous diphtheria: requires local care of the lesion with soap and water and administration of antimicrobials for 10 days.

PREVENTION

Active immunization with diphtheria toxoid is the cornerstone of population-based diphtheria prevention. The current recommendations from the Immunization Practices Advisory Committee of the Centers for Disease Control are:

- 2 months to 7 years: five doses of diphtheria vaccine, the first three given as DTP vaccine 0.5 mL IM at 2-month intervals beginning at 2 months of age. The fourth dose should be either DTaP or DTP at 15 to 18 months of age, and a fifth dose of DTaP or DTP at 4 to 6 years of age.
- 7 years: primary immunization of those >7 years should be conducted with adult-type diphtheria and tetanus toxoids, adsorbed (Td) with two doses given IM at least 4 weeks apart and a booster dose 1 year later.
- Booster doses of Td should be given at 10-year intervals to all immunized individuals. Isolation of patients with diphtheria is required until culture from the site of infection is negative on three consecutive specimens.

 Follow-Up

- In mild cases of diphtheria, after membrane sloughs off in 7 to 10 days, recovery is usually uneventful.
- In more severe cases, recovery may be slower and serious complications can occur.

 Common Questions and Answers

Q: Are there currently places in the world where diphtheria is a problem?
A: Yes. A diphtheria epidemic began in 1990 in Russia, spread in 1991 to the Ukraine, and during 1993 and 1994 spread to the remaining New Independent States of the former Soviet Union. During 1994, provisional totals of 47,802 cases (39,907 in Russia) and 1746 deaths due to diphtheria were reported throughout the New Independent States.

Q: What is the incidence of diphtheria in the United States?
A: From 1980 to 1993, only 40 cases of diphtheria were reported in the United States, an average of three per year (all respiratory disease).

Q: What precautions should be taken by travelers to areas of the world with diphtheria outbreaks?
A: The Advisory Committee on Immunization Practices (ACIP) of the Centers for Disease Control and Prevention recommends that travelers to such areas should be up-to-date for diphtheria immunization. Infants traveling to areas where diphtheria is endemic or epidemic should receive three doses of DTP or DT before travel.

ICD-9-CM 032.9

BIBLIOGRAPHY

Bisgard KM, Hardy IR, Popovic T, et al. Respiratory diphtheria in the United States, 1980 through 1995. *Am J Public Health* 1998;88(5):787–791.

Enhanced surveillance of non-toxigenic Corynebacterium diphtheriae infections. *CDR Weekly* 1996 Jan 26:6(4):29, 32.

Feigin RD, Stechenberg BW, Strandgaard BH. Diphtheria. In: Feigin RD, Cherry JD, eds. *Textbook of pediatric infectious diseases,* 3rd ed. Philadelphia: WB Saunders, 1992:1110–1115.

MacGregor RR. Corynebacterium diphtheriae. In: Mandell GL, Douglas RG Jr, Bennett JE, eds. *Principles and practice of infectious diseases,* 3rd ed. New York: Churchill Livingstone, 1990:1574–1581.

Toxigenic Corynebacterium diphtheriae—Northern Plains Indian Community, August–October 1996. *MMWR* 1997;46(22):506–510.

Author: Susan Dibs

Diskitis

 Database

DEFINITION

• Benign, self-limited inflammatory process of an intervertebral disk

CAUSES

• Idiopathic or initiated by low-grade infection

PATHOLOGY

• Probably of infectious etiology by an indolent organism
• Usually none identified, occasionally *Staphylococcus aureus, Moraxella,* or the enterobacteraceae are cultured.

EPIDEMIOLOGY

• Over one-half of cases occur in children less than 4 years old.
• Peak incidence is between 1 and 3 years of age.

GENETICS

• No specific predispositions identified

COMPLICATIONS

• Occasionally, scoliosis, kyphosis
• Rarely, facet joint degenerative disease

 Differential Diagnosis

INFECTION

• Vertebral osteomyelitis (*Staphylococcus, Salmonella,* etc.)
• Potts disease (tuberculous spondylitis)

ENVIRONMENTALTrauma

—Fracture
—Disk herniation
• Tumors
—Osteoid osteoma
• Metabolic
—Avascular necrosis of vertebral body
Congenital
—Spondylolisthesis
• Immunological
—Ankylosing spondylitis

MISCELLANEOUS

• Scheuermann disease (osteochondritis of the vertebral bodies)

 Data Gathering

HISTORY

• Uncomfortable child?
• Refuses to walk?
• History of fever?
• Back or abdominal pain?
• Symptoms are of short duration prior to presentation?

 Physical Examination

• Usually rigid posture, and pain elicited on movement
• Focal tenderness to palpation
• Most common locations: L4-5 and L3-4

Laboratory Aids

TESTS

- PPD
- WBC
- ESR
- Blood cultures

IMAGING

Test: Plain x-ray studies
Significance: Usually normal, though may demonstrate disk narrowing as illness progresses.

Test: Bone scan
Significance: Demonstrates increased uptake at affected area.

Test: MRI
Significance: Useful in atypical situations to confirm location of pathology (demonstrates disk edema).

 ## Therapy

DRUGS

- Usually quite responsive to NSAIDs
- Rarely, antibiotics are indicated.

DURATION

- Follow CBC and ESR.
- Continue treatment until child is asymptomatic.

PHYSICAL AND OCCUPATIONAL THERAPY

- Patient should be immobilized during acute period.
- Casting may be required.

DIET

- No special changes

 ## Follow-Up

WHEN TO EXPECT IMPROVEMENT

Most patients are asymptomatic in 6 to 8 weeks.

SIGNS TO WATCH FOR

- Recurrence of symptoms due to reactivation of the disease
- Progressive loss of disk height
- Destruction of adjacent vertebral bodies

PROGNOSIS

- Usually excellent
- Scoliosis can occur
- Rarely, facet joint symptoms occur years later.

PITFALLS

- Difficulty separating early vertebral body osteomyelitis from diskitis

 ## Common Questions and Answers

Q: When is a biopsy and tissue culture indicated?
A: If there is bony destruction of adjacent vertebral bodies or if clinical course is prolonged.

Q: When are antibiotics indicated?
A: Obviously in situations with positive cultures, or if course is atypical or prolonged.

ICD-9-CM 722.90

BIBLIOGRAPHY

Bradford DS, Hensinger RM, eds. *The pediatric spine.* New York: Thieme, 1985.

Cassidy JT, Petty RE. *Textbook of pediatric rheumatology.* Philadelphia: WB Saunders, 1995.

Mandell GA. Imaging in the diagnosis of musculoskeletal infections in children. *Curr Probl Pediatr* 1996;26(7):218–237.

Payne WK 3rd, Ogilvie JW. Back pain in children and adolescents. *Pediatr Clin North Am* 1996;43(4):899–917.

Ventura N, Gonzalez E, Terricabras L, Salvador A, Cabrera M. Intervertebral discitis in children: a review of 12 cases. *Int Orthop* 1996;20(1):32–34.

Author: Gregory F. Keenan

Disseminated Intravascular Coagulation

 Database

DEFINITION

Disseminated intravascular coagulation (DIC) is a profound hemorrhagic disorder associated with concurrent activation of procoagulant, anticoagulant, and fibrinolytic mechanisms.

PATHOPHYSIOLOGY/PATHOLOGY

Dysregulation of procoagulant, anticoagulant, and fibrinolytic pathways due to various initiating events.

- Microvascular hemorrhages and thrombosis.
- Procoagulant factors released in the blood may initiate DIC in acute promyelocytic leukemia.
- Endotoxins released during infections cause activation of coagulation factor XII, endothelial injury, platelet aggregation, and inhibition of fibrinolysis.
- Following disease processes can cause DIC:

—Infections
  —Meningococcemia
  —Gram negative and positive sepsis
  —Malaria
  —Viral and fungal sepsis

—Tissue injury
  —Massive brain injury
  —Shock or asphyxia
  —Hypothermia or hyperthermia

—Malignancies
  —Acute promyelocytic leukemia
  —Metastatic carcinomas

—Obstetric causes
  —Intrauterine fetal death
  —Amniotic fluid embolism

—Gastrointestinal
  —Fulminant hepatitis
  —Reyes syndrome

—Neonatal
  —Necrotizing enterocolitis
  —Congenital viral infections
  —Group B strep infection
  —Erythroblastosis fetalis

—Miscellaneous
  —Acute hemolytic transfusion reaction
  —Kasabach Merritt syndrome
  —Snake bite

EPIDEMIOLOGY

- Exact incidence not known.
- Most commonly secondary to infections.
- Snake bite may be most common cause world wide.

COMPLICATIONS

- Hemorrhage

—Pulmonary
—Intracranial

- Renal failure

- Multiorgan system failure

PROGNOSIS

Poor unless underlying disease is treated.

 Differential Diagnosis

- Coagulopathy of liver disease
- Pathological fibrinolysis
- Thrombotic thrombocytopenic purpura

 Data Gathering

HISTORY

- Presence of one of the underlying conditions listed in causes.
- Abrupt onset of bleeding?
- Pulmonary or intracranial hemorrhage?
- Oliguria
- Prolonged bleeding from venipuncture sites.
- Major organ dysfunction
- Pulmonary, renal, hepatic.

Physical Examination

- Signs of underlying disease.
- Generally a very sick child.
- Ecchymosis and petechiae.
- Bleeding from previously intact venipuncture sites.
- Skin infarctions (purpura fulminans) secondary to thrombosis of dermal vessels.
- Pulmonary hemorrhage, gastrointestinal bleeding, bleeding from surgical wounds, hematuria.
- Intraperitoneal and pleural hemorrhages.

 Laboratory Aids

All these tests should be checked every 8 to 12 hours as they change rapidly.

Test: CBC
Significance: Decreased platelet count, often earliest abnormality.

Test: Peripheral smear
Significance: Schistocytes, microspherocytes (50% of cases).

Test: PT, PTT, and Thrombin time
Significance: Prolonged

Test: Fibrinogen
Significance: Decreased

Test: Fibrin degradation products
Significance: Increased

Test: Factor VIII and V
Significance: Decreased, Factor VIII is normal in coagulopathy of liver disease.

 Therapy

- Treat the underlying disorder.
- Cryoprecipitate, platelets and fresh frozen plasma to control bleeding.
- Fresh frozen plasma also replaces anticoagulants—protein C and S.
- Heparin used for management of purpura fulminans due to meningococcemia.
- Routine use of heparin for DIC is debatable.

SUPPORTIVE CARE

Manage other organ system failure.

ICD-9-CM 286.6

BIBLIOGRAPHY

Levi M, van der Poll T, van Deventer SJ. Pathogenesis of disseminated intravascular coagulation in sepsis. *JAMA* 1993;270(8):975–979.

Wheeler A, Rubenstein EB. Current management of disseminated intravascular coagulation. *Oncology* 1993;8(9):69–79.

Wintrobe's clinical hematology, 10th ed., Vol. II. Baltimore: Lippincott Williams & Wilkins, 1998, 1480–1493.

Author: Sadhna M. Shankar

Down (Trisomy 21) Syndrome

 Database

DEFINITION

- Syndrome consisting of multiple abnormalities, including hypotonia, flat facies, upslanting palpebral fissures, and small ears
- First described by John Langdon Down in 1866
- Trisomy for chromosome 21

Multiple abnormalities found in Down syndrome:

- Congenital heart disease (50%; most not symptomatic as newborn), in decreasing frequency: atrioventricular (AV) canal (60%), ventriculoseptal defect (VSD), patent ductus arteriosus (PDA), atrioseptal defect (ASD), aberrant subclavian artery, tetralogy of Fallot
- Hearing loss (75%): sensorineural and conductive.
- Strabismus (33%)
- Nystagmus (15%)
- Fine lens opacities (by slit-lamp examination 59%), cataracts (1 to 15%)
- Refractive errors (50%)
- Stenotic nasolacrimal duct
- Delayed tooth eruption
- Tracheoesophageal fistula
- Gastrointestinal atresia (12%)
- Meckel diverticulum
- Hirschsprung disease (less than 1%)
- Imperforate anus
- Renal malformations
- Hypospadias (5%)
- Cryptorchidism (25% to 50%)
- Thyroid disease (15%): congenital hypothyroidism, hyperthyroidism
- Transient myeloproliferative disorder, neonatal (leukemoid reaction)
- Neonatal polycythemia
- Leukemia (less than 1%; 10 to 30 times greater risk than general population)
- Retinoblastoma and testicular germ-cell tumors (slightly greater risk than general population)
- Infertility, especially in males
- Obesity
- Alopecia areata (10% to 15%)
- Seizures (5% to 10%), usually myoclonic
- Alzheimer disease (nearly all over age 40 years)
- Mild to moderate mental retardation (IQ range 40–70)

PATHOPHYSIOLOGY

Specific to the associated findings.

EPIDEMIOLOGY

- Incidence: 1/600 to 1/800 live births
- Male:female ratio is 1.3:1
- For specific maternal ages, incidence is 1 in 1,500 live births for maternal ages 15 to 29 years, 1 in 800 for ages 30 to 34, 1 in 270 for ages 35 to 39, and 1 in 100 for ages 40 to 44
- Best recognized and most frequent chromosomal syndrome of humans
- One of the three most common autosomal trisomies (also trisomy 18 and 13) in humans
- Most common autosomal chromosomal abnormality causing mental retardation
- More than 50% of trisomy 21 fetuses are spontaneously aborted in early pregnancy

GENETICS

- 95% to 97% of cases are due to chromosomal non-disjunction (failure to segregate during meiosis) in the maternal DNA
- Less than 5% of cases are due to paternal non-disjunction
- 1% with trisomy 21/normal mosaicism (non-disjunction occurs after conception; two cell lines are present); generally less severely affected
- Remainder due to translocations between chromosome 21 and 14 [t(14q21q)]; rarely between 21 and 13 or 15; 50% of translocations are sporadic de novo events; 50% result from balanced translocations in one parent.

COMPLICATIONS

- Serous otitis media (50% to 70%)
- Conjunctivitis (frequent)
- Sinusitis
- Tonsillar and adenoidal hypertrophy
- Obstructive airway disease with associated sleep apnea, cor pulmonale
- Obstructive bowel disease (12%, newborn period)
- Constipation (due to low tone and decreased gross motor mobility)
- Subluxation of the hips (secondary to ligamentous laxity)
- Atlantoaxial instability (10% to 20%; secondary to ligamentous laxity)

PROGNOSIS

- Dependent on the associated findings
- Life expectancy is mildly decreased, with many living into the sixth decade
- Alzheimer disease affects approximately 15% after the fourth decade
- Recurrence is approximately 1% if parents are not translocation carriers
- As adults, the majority of patients with Down syndrome can work in supported positions

 Data Gathering

HISTORY

Check for previous history of infant with Down syndrome in the family.

 Physical Examination

The phenotype is variable from person to person.

Finding: General
Significance: Short stature; hypotonia (80% to 100%), with an open mouth and a protruding tongue; midface hypoplasia.

Finding: Head
Significance: Brachycephaly with a flattened occiput, microcephaly, false fontanel (95%).

Finding: Eyes
Significance: Upslanting palpebral fissures (98%), inner epicanthal folds, Brushfield spots (speckling of the iris), fine lens opacities on slit-lamp examination, cataracts, refractive error, strabismus, nystagmus.

Finding: Ears
Significance: Small, prominent; low-set; over-folding of upper helix; small canals with difficulty visualizing tympanic membranes.

Finding: Nose
Significance: Small (85%); flat nasal bridge.

Finding: Tongue
Significance: Relative macroglossia, but not true macroglossia (tongue mass is normal); fissuring.

Finding: Mouth
Significance: High-arched palate, abnormal palate.

Finding: Teeth
Significance: Missing (50%), small, hypoplastic; irregular placement.

Finding: Neck
Significance: In infancy, excess skin at the nape; short appearance; occasionally webbed.

Finding: Lungs
Significance: Check for signs of infection or congestive heart failure.

Finding: Heart
Significance: Assess for murmur, arrhythmia, cyanosis.

Finding: Abdomen
Significance: In neonate, distention may be present if obstruction or atresia is present; diastasis recti.

Finding: Genital
Significance: In adolescents, straight pubic hair; in males, small penis, cryptorchidism.

Finding: Extremities
Significance: Hands, broad with short metacarpals and phalanges; fifth finger with hypoplasia of the midphalanx (60%) and clinodactyly (50%); simian crease (single transverse palmar crease) in approximately 50%; wide gap between the first and second toes (96%); syndactyly of second and third toes; hyperflexibility of joints. A newborn with a simian crease has a 1 in 60 chance of having Down syndrome.

Finding: Skin
Significance: Cutis marmorata (43%); in older children, hyperkeratotic dry skin (75%); fine, soft, sparse hair.

Down (Trisomy 21) Syndrome

Laboratory Aids

Test: Prenatal karyotyping via amniocentesis or chorionic villus sampling
Significance: Is typically offered to women >35 years of age given the increased incidence of Down syndrome in the fetus

Test: Chromosomal karyotype on cultured lymphocytes from peripheral blood
Significance: May be performed postnatally if there is a clinical suspicion of Down syndrome

Test: Tissue sample other than blood (usually skin)
Significance: To check for mosaicism

Test: CBC
Significance: In the newborn period to check for polycythemia and transient myeloproliferative disorder; Down syndrome patients may have an increased mean corpuscular volume (MCV) on CBC, making the diagnosis iron-deficiency anemia difficult

Test: Thyroid-function tests
Significance: To rule out hypo- or hyperthyroidism

RADIOGRAPHIC STUDIES

Test: Fetal ultrasound
Significance: May show polyhydramnios if bowel obstruction is present

Test: Echocardiography and chest x-ray study.
Significance: Done in the first month of life to rule out cardiac disease.

Test: Lateral cervical spine x-ray studies in flexion/neutral/extension
Significance: To rule out atlantoaxial instability (defined as greater than 5-mm space between atlas and odontoid process of the axis).

OTHER STUDIES

Test: Electrocardiogram (ECG)
Significance: Done within the first month of life to rule out cardiac disease.

Test: Auditory brainstem response within the first 6 months of life
Significance:

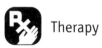

Therapy

Not applicable except for treatments specific to complications/associated illnesses

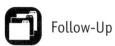

Follow-Up

GROWTH AND DEVELOPMENT

Specific growth charts for Down syndrome are available; average age for acquiring developmental milestones differs from normal population; late closure of fontanels; consider early intervention program for hypotonia and developmental delay.

GENETICS

Genetic counseling recommended.

CARDIAC

Early evaluation in newborn period, with follow-up until the presence or absence of disease is evident; subacute bacterial endocarditis prophylaxis for patients with certain types of cardiac disease.

OPHTHALMOLOGICAL

Early evaluation for cataracts and glaucoma, with routine visit at 6 to 12 months, and then every 1 to 2 years.

EAR, NOSE, AND THROAT (ENT)/ AUDIOLOGICAL

Annual audiological evaluation in the first 3 years of life, then every other year; ENT referral to visualize tympanic membranes with microscopic otoscope if small narrow external canals.

ORTHOPEDIC

Screen for atlantoaxial instability with x-ray studies in preschool years, then every decade. Prior to participation in sports (e.g., Special Olympics), must evaluate for atlantoaxial instability.

ENDOCRINE

Thyroid-function tests in newborn period, followed by yearly thyroid-stimulating-hormone levels.

OTHER

Multiple organizations (e.g., Down Syndrome International) are available to families of children with Down syndrome.

PITFALLS

- Caution with endotracheal intubation if absence or presence of atlantoaxial instability is not known to avoid spinal cord injury, which may be seen in rare cases.
- Hearing loss may be misinterpreted as a behavioral problem.
- Care with atropine and pilocarpine use for ophthalmological evaluation because of cholinergic hypersensitivity that may be seen.

Common Questions and Answers

Q: Why was Down syndrome referred to as mongolism in the past?
A: There was a mistaken notion about a racial cause for this syndrome due to the facial appearance, which was thought to be similar to that of those from Mongoloid origin.

Q: Do all children with Down syndrome have mental retardation?
A: No. Though all persons with non-mosaic Down syndrome have some degree of cognitive disability, some have IQs greater than 70 and are not considered to have mental retardation.

Q: Do children with this syndrome have an increased susceptibility to infection?
A: The literature on this subject is unclear and has been subject to debate. Midface hypoplasia may contribute to an increased incidence of ear, sinus, and nasolacrimal duct infections. There may be an increased risk of lower respiratory tract infection for children with unrepaired heart disease.

Q: Can a normal cardiac examination rule out the presence of a cardiac anomaly?
A: No, all patients with Down syndrome should have a cardiac evaluation within the first month of life. Timely surgery may be necessary to prevent serious complications.

Q: Are patients with atlantoaxial instability symptomatic?
A: No, most are asymptomatic, but symptoms of cord compression may be seen in 1% to 2% of patients.

Q: I have seen growth charts for Down syndrome patients that allow for plotting of lengths, heights, and weights. Are there special growth charts available for plotting head circumference?
A: Yes. If appropriate growth charts are not used for plotting head circumference, head growth may appear abnormal. Head circumference growth charts are available through the Internet: http://www.growthcharts.com.

BIBLIOGRAPHY

American Academy of Pediatrics. Health supervision for children with Down syndrome. *Pediatrics* 1994;93:855–859.

Cooley WC, Graham JM. Down syndrome: an update and review for the primary pediatrician. *Clin Pediatr* 1991;30:233–253.

Cronk C, Crocker AC, Pueschel SM, et al. Growth charts for children with Down syndrome: 1 month to 18 years of age. *Pediatrics* 1988;81:102–110.

Hayes A, Batshaw ML. Down syndrome. *Pediatr Clin North Am* 1993;40:523–535.

Jones KL. Down syndrome. In: Smith DW ed. *Smith's recognizable patterns of malformation,* 4th ed. Philadelphia: WB Saunders, 1988:10–15.

Satge D, Sommelet D, Geneix A, Nishi M, Malet P, Vekemans M. A tumor profile in Down syndrome. *Am J Med Genet* 1998;78(3):207–216.

Author: Esther K. Chung

Dysfunctional Uterine Bleeding/Menorrhagia

 Database

DEFINITION

• Endometrial bleeding beyond the range of normal menses: duration of 2 to 8 days, occuring every 21 to 40 days, with blood loss of 20 to 80 mL/cycle.
• Dysfunctional uterine bleeding (DUB) can vary in presentation, from heavy, long menses followed by long periods of amenorrhea, to short, heavy menses occurring every 1 to 2 weeks.
• Most commonly associated with anovulatory cycles resulting from immature hypothalamic-pituitary-ovarian axis.

PATHOPHYSIOLOGY

• In most cases of DUB presenting within 2 years of menarche, anovulation results in absence of corpus luteum.
• Without the secretory effect of progesterone from the corpeus luteum, endometrial proliferation continues due to unopposed estrogen.
• The thickened endometrium eventually outgrows support from basal endometrium, resulting in sloughing of highest endometrial levels.
• As subsequent levels of endometrium are shed, bleeding increases. Profuse bleeding can result when the basal endometrium is exposed.

GENETICS

• Familial history of anovulatory cycles is common.
• Patients with disorders such as blood dyscrasias and polycystic ovary syndrome (PCOS) usually have a positive familial history.

EPIDEMIOLOGY

• Most commonly occurs within 2 years of menarche when more than 50% of cycles are anovulatory.
• Later age at menarche results in greater length of anovulation.
• Most females do not develop DUB during their anovulatory cycles.
• DUB can develop in 20% to 30% of patients with PCOS (Stein-Levinthal).

COMPLICATIONS

• Mild to severe anemia resulting from blood loss

 Differential Diagnosis

The differential diagnosis can be divided into three categories based on cycle length and timing of bleeding.

CATEGORY I

• Normal cyclic intervals with increased bleeding during each cycle

Infection

• Endometritis due to *Neisseria gonorrhea* or *Chlamydia trachomatis*
• Pelvic inflammatory disease (PID)

Primary Gynecological

• Intrauterine abnormalities, such as polyps, submucousal myomas, or fibroids
• Endometriosis
• Complication of pregnancy, such as ectopic pregnancy, spontaneous abortion, or placenta previa

Hematological

• Inborn coagulopathies, such as von Willebrand disease
• Clotting disorders resulting from systemic disease, such as immune thrombocytopenic purpura, systemic lupus erythematosus, chronic renal failure, hepatic disease, or leukemia
• Medicine or poisons affecting coagulation (e.g., aspirin, Coumadin)

CATEGORY II

• Normal cyclic intervals with bleeding between cycles

Infection

• PID

Primary Gynecological

• Endometriosis
• Complications of pregnancy

Tumors

• Endometrial adenocarcinoma [Exceedingly rare tumor associated with *in utero* exposure to diethylstilbesterol (DES), discontinued in 1974]
• Benign uterine tumors

Trauma

• Vaginal laceration
• Intrauterine device (IUD)
• Foreign body

CATEGORY III

Abnormal cycle intervals or no apparent cycle.

Primary Gynecological

• Premature ovarian failure
• Complications of pregnancy

Tumors

• Craniopharyngioma
• Pituitary adenoma

Endocrine

• Anovulatory cycle
• PCOS (Stein Leventhal)
• Thyroid disease
• Pituitary disease, such as prolactinoma
• Adrenal disorders

Psychosocial

• Anorexia nervosa
• Excessive exercise

 Data Gathering

HISTORY

Question: Initial history and evaluation?
Significance: Focus on assessing amount and site of bleeding and hemodynamic stability.

Question: Complete menstrual history?
Significance: The pattern of DUB in relation to menstrual cycle can help narrow the diagnostic work-up (*see* Differential Diagnosis).

Question: Cramping?
Significance: The presence of cramping suggests ovulation and the presence of progesterone.

Question: Time lapse between menarche?
Significance: Increased time lapse since menarche lessens the likelihood of anovulatory cycles.

Question: Quality of bleeding?
Significance: The presence of clots suggests non-endometrial bleeding, while brown, or prune-colored, blood suggests endometrial blood.

Question: Bruising history?
Significance: Easy bruisability, epistaxis, or bleeding gums suggests a clotting disorder.

Question: A complete familial history should be obtained.
Significance: A family history of thyroid disease, bleeding disorder, PCOS, or DUB can help to guide the laboratory work-up.

Question: A thorough review of systems is an integral part of the work-up.
Significance: Seemingly unrelated symptoms may reveal cryptic chronic or systemic disease processes.

Question: The sexual history should also assess the likelihood of sexual abuse.
Significance: Not only can sexual abuse result in bleeding from trauma, but can also be a source of sexually transmitted diseases and pregnancy.

Physical Examination

Finding: Vital signs, including orthostatic blood pressures
Significance: Severe blood loss.

Finding: Pelvic Examination
Significance: A pelvic examination is essential in determining the source of bleeding. It should include a speculum examination looking for signs of trauma, foreign body, or adenosis. The bimanual examination should be performed to assess for ovarian mass, uterine fibroids, signs of PID, or signs of pregnancy.

Finding: Hirsutism and acne
Significance: May indicate a hyperandrogenic state.

• Assessing for signs of thyroid, liver, or hematologic disease.

Laboratory Aids

TESTS

Test: Urine or serum β-HCG should be obtained, regardless of sexual history.
Significance: Urine β-HCG testing can reliably detect pregnancy as early as 2 weeks postconception; however, may be positive for up to 2 weeks following an abortion.

Test: Wet prep and cervical testing for *C. trachomatis* and *N. gonorrhea*
Significance: STD.

Test: Pap test
Significance: A Papanicolaou smear should be performed to rule-out cervical neoplasia as a source of bleeding.

Test: Examination of cervical mucus
Significance: An experienced provider can evaluate cervical mucus in the absence of active bleeding for signs of estrogen or progesterone dominance.

Test: Consider prolactin level and thyroid function tests
Significance: Hyperprolactinemia can have several causes, including pituitary microadenoma, and result in amenorrhea or DUB.

Test: PT, PTT, platelet count, and bleeding time.
Significance: Severe bleeding and anemia, or with a familial history of bleeding.

Test: Endometrial biopsy
Significance: Rarely warranted for adolescents.

RADIOGRAPHIC IMAGING

Test: Pelvic ultrasound
Significance: Indicated when ectopic pregnancy is suspected. And should be considered when a pelvic mass is felt, uterine anomaly is being considered, or bimanual examination cannot be completed.

Test: MRI
Significance: Indicated for patients with a suspected pelvic mass when ultrasonography does not clearly define the anatomy.

Therapy

• If attributed to anovulatory cycles, or a complete work-up fails to yield a diagnosis, treatment is guided by the severity of DUB and the presence of active bleeding.
• For mild DUB (inconvenient, unpredictable bleeding with a normal hemoglobin): Reassurance until ovulatory cycles resumes. Encourage maintenance of a menstrual calendar with follow-up in 3 to 6 months.
• Iron supplementation
• If inconvenience and anxiety are unresponsive to reassurance, use of an oral contraceptive should be considered to regulate menstrual cycle. Combination OCPs can be used in sexually active patients, or medroxyprogesterone acetate (Provera, Upjohn, Kalamazoo, MI), 10 mg daily for 5 to 7 days every 35 to 40 days for patients who are not sexually active.
• For moderate DUB (irregular, prolonged, heavy bleeding with a hemoglobin >10 g/dL); hormonal therapy, as described previously.
• Menstrual calendar with follow-up every 1 to 2 months
• For severe DUB (heavy, prolonged bleeding with a hemoglobin <10 g/dL), treatment depends on the presence of active bleeding.
• If not actively bleeding, hemodynamically stable patients can be started on OCPs, iron supplementation, and have follow-up in 1 to 2 months.
• In the presence of active bleeding:

—Hospitalization of patient to monitor patient during treatment.
—Blood transfusion as necessary.
—Hormonal therapy should be started immediately, and can be either IV or PO.
—Conjugated estrogen can be given intravenously, 20 to 25 mg every 6 hours for a maximum of 6 doses. Norgestrel/ethinyl estradiol, 1 tablet every 6 hours, should be given concurrently, then tapered as bleeding resolves Norgestrel/ethinyl estradiol can be given, as described, in the absence of IV estrogen. Tapering can begin when bleeding stops, and can be easily remembered as 1 pill q.i.d. for 4 days, 1 pill t.i.d. for 3 days, then 1 pill b.i.d. for 2 weeks.
  —After taper, OCPs should be continued for 6 to 12 months.
  —If hormonal therapy fails, dilation and curettage may be necessary.
  —Patients should be monitored monthly after an episode of severe DUB.

POSSIBLE SIDE EFFECTS

• Estrogen, given in high doses, will cause nausea and/or vomiting. Patients receiving high-dose estrogen should be prophylaxed against this with an appropriate anti-emetic.

Follow-Up

WHEN TO EXPECT IMPROVEMENT

• Bleeding usually tapers after the first few doses of hormones.
• After 6 to 12 months have passed, and the patient does not wish to remain on OCPs, a trial off of medication might reveal normal ovulatory cycles.
• DUB persists for 2 years in 60% of patients, 4 years in 50%, and up to 10 years in 30%.

PITFALLS

• Neglecting to perform testing for pregnancy in an adolescent who denies sexual activity.
• All home pregnancy tests should be repeated.
• If there is a prolonged course of DUB, consider PCOS.

Common Questions and Answers

Q: If most girls have anovulatory cycles, why do only some present with DUB?
A: Most girls do have an irregular menstrual cycle during the first 2 years after menarche. However, in a majority of those girls, the negative-feedback system of estrogen will lead to endometrial shedding and a cyclic pattern.

Q: If DUB from anovulatory cycles is caused by lack of progesterone, why does the initial treatment of severe DUB with active bleeding involve large doses of estrogen?
A: In severe DUB, the exposed endometrial base is bleeding profusely. For progesterone to exhibit its secretory effects, the endometrium in that area must be restored by estrogen. Therefore, the estrogen effectively acts as a bandage.

Q: When hormonal therapy fails, and the basal endometrium continues to bleed, how does a dilatation and curettage act as the final treatment?
A: The curettage removes any remaining bleeding vessels and stimulates local prostaglandins to create a uterine contracture that tamponades bleeding.

ICD-9-CM 626.8

BIBLIOGRAPHY

Muram D. Vaginal bleeding in childhood and adolescence in menstrual cycle disorders. *Obstet Gynecol North Am* 1990;33:389–408.

Polaneczky MM, Slap GB. Menstrual disorders in the adolescent: dysmenorrhea and dysfunctional uterine bleeding. *Pediatr Rev* 1992;13:83–87.

Authors: Kenneth R. Ginsburg and Jonathan R. Pletcher

Dysmenorrhea

 Database

DEFINITION

- Pain associated with menstrual flow characterized by spasmodic lower abdominal cramping with radiation to the back and anterior aspect of thighs
- Primary dysmenorrhea: pain with menstrual flow without evidence of organic pelvic disease
- Secondary dysmenorrhea: pain with menses secondary to an organic disease such as endometriosis, ovarian cysts, adhesions, genital tract abnormalities or pelvic inflammatory disease

Grading of Severity

- Grade I: mild dysmenorrhea that does not interfere with participation in everyday activity
- Grade II: moderate dysmenorrhea, with minimal systemic symptoms; interferes with participation in some activities
- Grade III: severe discomfort, often associated with systemic symptoms; individual is unable to participate in normal activities for several days

Causes

- Thought to be due to uterine contractions combined with prostaglandin excess

Associated/Predisposing Illnesses

- Endometriosis
- Ovarian cysts
- Pelvic adhesions
- Pelvic inflammatory disease
- Reproductive tract malformations

PATHOPHYSIOLOGY

- During menses the uterus undergoes infrequent labor-like contractions of 100 to 120 mm Hg, which can lead to dysmenorrhea. Higher basal uterine pressures and higher levels of uterine contractions and/or dysrhythmic contractions are found in patients who suffer from dysmenorrhea.
- Prostaglandins E_2 and F_2, synthesized in endometrial tissue, are believed to be responsible for dysmenorrhea. The former causes vasodilation and bleeding; and the latter, myometrial contractions, vasoconstriction, and ischemia. Higher levels of prostaglandins are found in the endometrium of patients with dysmenorrhea. Prostaglandin synthesis is enhanced by progesterone and the presence of a secretory endometrium.
- Primary dysmenorrhea usually does not begin until 2 to 4 years after the onset of menses, when the adolescent begins to ovulate regularly and produce progesterone.

EPIDEMIOLOGY

- 43% to 90% of all women have some degree of dysmenorrhea. 10% of these women are incapacitated for 1 to 3 days a month.
- 38% of adolescents at Sexual Maturity Rating SMR-3, and 66% of those at SMR-5 experience dysmenorrhea.
- Risk factors for developing dysmenorrhea

—Early age at menarche
—Long menstrual periods
—Smoking
—Alcohol use
—Weight >90th percentile

COMPLICATIONS

- Pain
- Interference with everyday activities
- Systemic symptoms (50%), including:

—Nausea and vomiting (90%)
—Fatigue (85%)
—Nervousness (67%)
—Dizziness (60%)
—Diarrhea (60%)
—Backache (60%)
—Headache (50%)

PROGNOSIS

Dysmenorrhea often lessens in the mid to late 20s.

 Differential Diagnosis

INFECTION

- Endometritis
- Pelvic inflammatory disease

TUMORS

- Uterine polyps
- Fibroids

CONGENITAL

- Reproductive tract abnormalities

PSYCHOSOCIAL

- Functional abdominal pain

MISCELLANEOUS

- Endometriosis
- Intrauterine device (IUD)

 Data Gathering

HISTORY

Menstrual History

- Age at menarche?
- Regularity of cycle?
- Amount of bleeding?
- Duration of bleeding?
- Day of cycle when pain begins and ends?
- Presence of large blood clots?

Sexual History

- Age at first coitus?
- Number of partners?
- Contraceptive method?
- Frequency of use of barrier methods?
- Pregnancy history?
- Sexually transmitted disease/pelvic inflammatory disease history?
- Dyspareunia?

Gastrointestinal and Genitourinary History

- Dysuria or other urinary tract signs?
- Constipation, diarrhea, or other GI-tract signs?
- Gastrointestinal or genitourinary surgery?

SPECIAL QUESTIONS

- How bad are the cramps?
- Do the cramps interfere with going to school or other activities?
- Are there other symptoms that accompany the cramps?

 Physical Examination

- Evidence of endometriosis, endometritis, polyps, fibroids, or uterine or cervical abnormalities.
- If not sexually active, pelvic examination is indicated only if symptoms are not responsive to standard medical therapy.

 Laboratory Aids

If endometritis or pelvic inflammatory disease is suspected:

- CBC
- ESR
- Endocervical cultures

Therapy

Include education and reassurance.

DRUGS

• Grade I–II dysmenorrhea: aspirin, acetaminophen, or over-the-counter prostaglandin inhibitors (ibuprofen, naproxen sodium). If the patient wishes contraception, oral contraceptive pills will provide both contraception and relief from primary dysmenorrhea.
• Grade II–III dysmenorrhea: prescription prostaglandin inhibitors with or without oral contraceptive pills:

—Tolmetin (Tolectin, McNeil, Fort Washington, PA), 400 mg t.i.d.
—Sulindac (Clinoril, Merck, West Point, PA), 200 mg t.i.d.
—Ibuprofen (Motrin, Hoffman Roche, Nutley, NJ), 400 to 600 mg t.i.d. to q.i.d.
—Naproxen sodium (Anaprox), 550 mg to start then 275 mg t.i.d. to q.i.d.

• Fenamates

—Mefenamic acid (Ponstel), 500 mg to start then 250 mg q.i.d.
—Meclofenamate (Meclomen), 100 mg to start, then 50 to 100 mg q.i.d.

• Try one class of prostaglandin inhibitors for three cycles before switching to another class.
• Patients should start medication 1 to 2 days before menses begins.
• Other treatments:

—Omega-3 fish oil
—Calcium antagonists
—Glyceryl trinitrate
—Transcutaneous electrical nerve stimulation (TENS)
—Acupuncture
—Herbal remedies

 Follow-Up

• Should see improvement within 3 to 4 menstrual cycles. If there is no response to medical management, referral to gynecologist for laparoscopic evaluation should be strongly considered.
• Monitor patients taking prostaglandin inhibitors for gastrointestinal distress.

PREVENTION

• Regular exercise has been shown to decrease the severity of dysmenorrhea symptoms.
• Avoid high-salt diet and caffeine.

PITFALLS

• Avoid missing diagnosis of PID.
• Consider endometriosis in adolescent patients. Recently, adolescents have been presenting more frequently with atypical endometriosis.

 Common Questions and Answers

Q: When should I consider oral contraceptive pills for a patient with dysmenorrhea?
A: If the patient has Grade II or higher dysmenorrhea that is not responding to medication, or if she has many systemic symptoms. Oral contraceptives should also be suggested to sexually active adolescents with any grade of dysmenorrhea. The advantages are lessening of dysmenorrhea, less menstrual flow, and less iron-deficiency anemia.

Q: How do I distinguish primary from secondary dysmenorrhea?
A: Primary amenorrhea usually begins gradually 2 to 4 years after the onset of menses. In contrast, an adolescent with isolated atypical, painful, menstrual periods should be evaluated for complications of pregnancy and/or genital tract infections. The older adolescent with a long history of increasingly painful menstrual periods should be evaluated for endometriosis. Congenital malformations of the genital tract are very rare and usually cause severe pain with the first menstrual period, unlike primary dysmenorrhea and endometriosis. Most malformations that cause dysmenorrhea include some blood flow outlet obstruction, and pelvic masses are often detected by examination or ultrasound.

Q: What are the characteristics of endometriosis in adolescents?
A: Adolescents with endometriosis often display dysmenorrhea of increasing severity. Other symptoms include abnormal vaginal bleeding, dyspareunia, and intestinal and bladder dysfunction. They may have no findings on pelvic examination, but some display posterior cul de sac tenderness and a smaller percentage display posterior cul de sac nodularity. The diagnosis is best made by laparoscopic evaluation.

ICD-9-CM 625.3

BIBLIOGRAPHY

Campbell MA, McGrath PJ. Use of medication by adolescents for the management of menstrual discomfort. *Arch Pediatr Adolesc Med* 1997; 151(9):905–913.

Coupey SM, Ahlstrom P. Common menstrual disorders. *Pediatr Clin North Am* 1989;36(3): 551–558.

Emans SJ, Laufer MR, Goldstein DP. *Pediatric and adolescent gynecology*, 4th ed. Philadelphia: Lippincott-Raven, 1998:371–375.

Gidwani GP. Longitudinal study of risk factors for occurrence, duration and severity of menstrual cramps in a cohort of college women. *Clin Pediatr* 1998;37(1):51.

Harel Z, Biro FM, Kottenhahn RK, Rosenthal SL. Supplementation with omega-3 polyunsaturated fatty acids in the management of dysmenorrhea in adolescents. *Am J Obstet Gynecol* 1996; 174(4):1335–1338.

Hurd SJ, Adamson GD. Pelvic pain: endometriosis as a differential diagnosis. *Adolesc Pediatr Gynecol* 1992;5:3–7.

Kennedy S. Primary dysmenorrhea. *Lancet* 1997;349(9059):1116.

Neinstein LS. *Adolescent health care: a practical guide.* Baltimore: Urban & Schwarzenberg, 1991:653–657.

Author: Liana R. Clark

Ehrlichiosis

 Database

DEFINITION

A zoonotic infection caused by two microorganisms of the genus *Ehrlichia*. The two human ehrlichiosis are monocytic ehrlichiosis (HME) caused by *Ehrlichia chaffeensis* and human granulocytic ehrlichiosis (HGE) caused by an organism of the genus Erhlichia but of an unknown species. The genus *Ehrlichia* is found within the family Rickettsiacceae.

CAUSES

HME and HGE are both carried by tick vectors. HME is thought to be transmitted by *Amblyomma americanum*, the Lone star tick. The vector for HGE is believed to be either *Ixodes scapularis*, the deer tick, or *Dermacentor variabilis*, the brown dog tick.

PATHOPHYSIOLOGY

- Obligate intracellular, pleomorphic, coccobacilli bacteria
- Transmission to a human by a tick vector
- Incubation period ranges from 1 to 21 days
- HME infects mononuclear phagocytes, while HGE infects granulocytes
- The ehrlichiae reside within a phagosome, where the bacteria divide by binary fission
- The infected cell is destroyed by the ehrlichiae releasing more ehrlichiae into the phagocyte system

EPIDEMIOLOGY OF EHRLICHIOSIS

- Most patients contract illness during April through September, the months of greatest tick and human outdoor activity
- HME and HGE are geographically separate

EPIDEMIOLOGY OF HME

- Males are more often infected (57%)
- Average age is 6.7 (range 7 months to 13.7 years)
- Most children reside in rural areas
- HME has been found in 30 states throughout the southeastern and south-central United States
- HME is found in similar states where Rocky Mountain spotted fever (RFSF) occurs
- The states with the most cases are Missouri, Tennessee, Oklahoma, Texas, Arkansas, Virginia, and Georgia
- Data from Oklahoma found ehrlichiosis was as common as RMSF, with an incidence of 3.3 per 100,000
- Data from Georgia revealed ehrlichiosis was more common than RMSF, with an incidence of 5.3 per 100,000
- HME has also been identified in Pennsylvania, Massachusetts, and Washington state

EPIDEMIOLOGY OF HGE

- Prevalence and incidence are not known, only 12 cases have been reported since 1995
- The majority of HGE infections have occurred in states where Lyme disease is very prevalent: Wisconsin, Minnesota, and Connecticut
- Infections are also thought to have occurred in California, New York, Maryland, Rhode Island, and Florida

COMPLICATIONS

Neurological Sequelae

- Headache, described as severe
- Mental status changes
- Seizures
- Coma
- Focal neurological findings
- Cognitive learning deficits

Hematological

- Disseminated intravascular coagulopathy (DIC)
- Thrombocytopenia
- Leukopenia
- Lymphopenia
- Anemia

Gastrointestinal

- Gastrointestinal hemorrhage
- Elevated liver enzymes
- Hepatosplenomegaly

Respiratory

- Pulmonary hemorrhage
- Interstitial pneumonia
- Pleural effusions
- Noncardiogenic pulmonary edema

Infectious

- Fungal superinfection
- Nosocomial infections
- Opportunistic infections

Renal

- Renal failure
- Proteinuria
- Hematuria

Cardiac

- Cardiomegaly
- Cardiac murmurs

Metabolic

- Hyponatremia

PROGNOSIS

- The majority of patients are hospitalized (>60%)
- Case fatality for HME is 2% to 5%, HGE is 7% to 10%
- One report of a pediatric fatality
- Elevated BUN and creatinine have been associated with a more severe course
- Children appear to have an excellent outcome
- Blood, renal, and liver abnormalities resolve in 1 to 2 weeks after initiating antibiotics
- Cognitive and behavioral problems have been reported
- Neuropathy has also been described

 Differential Diagnosis

TICK BORNE INFECTION

- RMSF
- Tularemia
- Relapsing fever
- Lyme disease
- Colorado tick fever
- Babeiosis

INFECTION

- Toxic shock syndrome
- Kawasaki disease
- Meningococcemia
- Pyelonephritis
- Gastroenteritis
- Hepatitis
- Leptospirosis
- Epstein-Barr virus
- Influenza
- Cytomegalovirus
- Enterovirus
- Strep throat

MISCELLANEOUS

- Leukemia
- Idiopathic thrombocytopenia purpura (ITP)
- Hemolytic uremic syndrome (HUS)

 Data Gathering

HISTORY

Question: Tick-bite history
Significance: Exposure to wooded areas with ticks is very helpful

Question: Classic presentation is described as fevers, headache, myalgias, followed by the development of a progressive leukopenia, thrombocytopenia, and anemia.
Significance:

Question: Fever?
Significance: Fevers are found in all children with Ehrlichiosis.

Question: Rash?
Significance: Rash occurs in about 66% of patients and is pleomorphic. It has been described as macular, macularpapular, petechial, erythematous, vesicular, scarletiform or in a combination. The distribution is usually located on the trunk and on the extremities.

Question: Myalgia?
Significance: Myalgia is found in the majority of children.

Question: Headache?
Significance: Often described as severe.

Question: Gastrointestinal?
Significance: Abdominal pain, vomiting, anorexia, diarrhea is often elicited.

Question: Arthralgia?
Significance:

Question: Cough and sore throat?
Significance: Is often described.

Physical Examination

- Mental status changes/irritability
- Nuchal rigidity
- Cardiac murmur (II/VI systolic ejection murmur at the LLSB)
- Hepatosplenomegaly
- Poor perfusion with hypotension (shock) has been described in a few children as a presenting symptom.
- Conjunctival or throat injection
- Rash as described

Laboratory Aids

Test: CBC with differential (with smear)
Significance: Thrombocytopenia, <150,000/mm^3 (77% to 92% incidence); Lymphopenia, <1500/mm^3 (75%); Leukopenia, <4000/mm^3 (58% to 68%); Anemia, Hct <30% (38% to 42%)

Test: Electrolytes with BUN and Creatinine
Significance: Hyponatremia (33% to 65%)

Test: Liver function tests
Significance: Elevated ALT, >55U/L (90%)

Test: Coagulation labs, type and cross as indicated
Significance: Detect DIC, thrombocytopenia, and anemia

Test: Cerebral spinal fluid (CSF)
Significance: Leukocytosis, with an average cell count of 100/mm^3; lymphocytic predominance; elevated protein and borderline low glucose; microbiology cultures are negative.

- Bone marrows are usually hypercellular, but normocellularity and hypocellularity have also been found.

SERUM STUDIES

- Titers for *E. chaffeenis* have been developed to diagnose HME, while titers for *E. equi* are being used to diagnose HGE
- Titers are available through state health departments at the Centers for Disease Control and Prevention or a reference laboratory
- Acute and convalescent titers of ehrlichiae (a fourfold rise or fall is considered positive), obtained 2 to 4 weeks apart
- An acute titer of ≥1:64 is considered diagnostic
- Polymerase chain reaction (PCR) has been developed in research laboratories
- The detection of morulae (inclusion) bodies in peripheral blood monocytes or granulocytes can aid in the diagnosis

Therapy

- Supportive care and medical management
- Volume and blood pressure medications as needed
- Intubation for respiratory failure
- Dialysis for renal failure
- Platelets for thrombocytopenia
- Packed red blood cells for anemia
- Fresh frozen plasma, cryoprecipitate, and vitamin K for DIC
- Anti-fungal or antibiotics for secondary infections

DRUGS

- Doxycycline is the drug of choice: 3 mg/kg/d in two divided doses (oral or intravenous) regardless of the age of the child
- Chloramphenicol is effective for HME, but little data of the effectiveness with HGE
- Treatment for a minimum of 5 to 7 days and should continue for 3 days after defervescence
- Doxycycline is a tetracycline and is associated with permanent dental staining and enamel hypoplasia, although with the short courses of treatment dental staining is unlikely. Other side effects of doxycycline are photosensitivity, hepatotoxicity, nausea, and pseudotumor cerebri

PREVENTION

- Avoidance of tick-infested areas
- Clothes should cover arms and legs
- Tick repellents, but use with caution in young children
- A thorough body search should always be done after returning from a tick-infested area.
- If a tick is found, the area should be cleaned with a disinfectant. To remove the tick, grasp the tick at the point of origin with forceps, staying as close to the skin as possible. Applying steady, even pressure, the tick is pulled off the skin. Once the tick is removed, the skin should be cleaned with a disinfectant
- Instruct parents to seek medical attention if symptoms develop
- No vaccine available

PITFALLS

- Simultaneous infections have been documented of *Ehrlichia* and Lyme disease, therefore, in patients diagnosed with Ehrlichiosis, Lyme titers should be sent to determine if there is a dual infection
- Failing to consider the diagnosis of Ehrlichiosis or a delay in treatment pending confirmatory serum titers

Common Questions and Answers

Q: What is the most common chief complaint in children with Ehrlichiosis?
A: Intense unremitting headache. In patients with headache and flu-like illness in the spring to early fall, consider the diagnosis. Laboratory abnormalities of leukopenia, thrombocytopenia, and hepatitis should lead to presumptive therapy until the diagnosis is clear.

ICD-9-CM 066.8

BIBLIOGRAPHY

Barton LB, Rathore MH, Dawson JE. Infection with Ehrlichia in childhood. *J Pediatr* 1992;120:998–1001.

Dumler JS, Bakken JS. Ehrlichial diseases of humans: emerging tick-borne infections. *Clin Infect Dis* 1995;20:1102–1110.

Fichtenbaum CJ, Peterson LR, Weil GJ. Ehrlichiosis presenting as a life-threatening illness with features of the toxic shock syndrome. *Am J Med* 1993;95:351–357.

Harkess JR, Ewing SA, Brumit T, et al. Ehrlichiosis in children. *Pediatrics* 1991;87:199–203.

Jacobs RF, Schultze GE. Ehrlichiosis in children. *J Pediatr* 1997;131:184–192.

Olson JC, Dalton MJ. Ehrlichia Species (Ehrlichiosis). In: Long SS, Pickering LK, Prober CG, eds. *Principles and practice of pediatric infectious diseases*, 1st ed. New York: Churchill Livingstone, 1997:1014–1016.

Schutze GE, Jacobs RF. Human monocytic ehrlichiosis in children. *Pediatrics* 1997;100:e10.

Author: Jeffrey P. Louie

Encephalitis

 Database

DEFINITION

Encephalitis is inflammation of the brain parenchyma due to infection. Meningoencephalitis is inflammation of the brain and the meninges.

PATHOPHYSIOLOGY

- Direct or delayed (postinfectious) reaction by the immune system to a virus, bacteria, fungus, or parasite
- Organisms enter the CNS via the systemic circulation, direct inoculation (trauma), or neural pathways (rabies, herpes simplex virus [HSV]).
- Infiltration of inflammatory cells into the CNS
- Inclusion bodies (intranuclear; HSV, subacute sclerosing panencephalitis [SSPE], viral, intracytoplasmic; rabies), CSF, and serology changes

EPIDEMIOLOGY

- Depends on age, geographic location, and season
- The most common causes of encephalitis are viruses:

  —Summer (enteroviruses)
    —Summer and fall (Western and Eastern equine encephalitis, St. Louis encephalitis, La Crosse encephalitis)
  —Winter (varicella)

- Nonviral causes (tuberculosis, Lyme disease, toxoplasmosis, cat-scratch disease, rickettsial disease, tick-borne infections) are associated with specific environmental or geographic exposure.
- The most common cause of sporadic encephalitis is HSV (rabies and HIV also occur in all seasons).

COMPLICATIONS

Seizure disorders, focal or generalized, quadriparesis/hemiparesis, ataxia, learning disabilities, and aphasias can result from encephalitis.

PROGNOSIS

Outcome can range from complete recovery to coma, persistent vegetative state, and death.

 Differential Diagnosis

Several toxic, metabolic, vascular, or epileptic syndromes may resemble encephalitis:

- Ingestions
- Reye syndrome
- Acute hemorrhagic leukoencephalitis (postinfectious, etiology unknown, associated *Mycoplasma* infection, destruction of white and gray matter)
- Intracranial hemorrhage
- Pituitary infarction
- Acute obstructive hydrocephalus or ventriculoperitoneal shunt obstruction
- Sinus thrombosis
- Subdural empyema
- Stroke or septic embolization (endocarditis)
- Brain abscess or subdural empyema
- Malignant hyperthermia
- Status epilepticus
- Other considerations include bacterial meningitis (*Neisseria meningitidis, Haemophilus influenzae* type b, group B streptococcus in the neonate, *Escherichia coli* in the neonate) parasites, acute disseminated encephalomyelitis (ADEM), and vasculitis.
- Diagnosis of specific causes of true encephalitis depends on geographic location, age, and clinical and associated laboratory findings.
- Microbes to consider:

  —Herpes viruses (in the child and adult, herpes has preference for the medial temporal lobe)
  —Lyme disease; possible coinfection with ehrlichiosis, babesiosis
  —Varicella (postinfectious encephalitis)
  —Cat-scratch and rickettsial diseases
  —Tuberculosis
  —Fungal (cryptosporidiosis)
  —Parasitic (amebae, *Toxoplasma*, cysticercosis)
  —Toxoplasma

- Meningitis:

  —Meningitis may cause secondary parenchymal inflammation of the brain
  —Mental status changes are usually more prominent in primary encephalitis as compared with meningitis

 Data Gathering

HISTORY

- Ask about a viral prodrome with symptoms such as upper respiratory infection, cough, coryza, malaise, anorexia, decreased enteral intake, diarrhea, nausea, and vomiting.
- Encephalitis is often heralded by headaches, photophobia, a stiff neck, increased sleeping, a change in mental status, irritability, confusion, hallucinations, and seizures.
- Prodromal symptoms can range from hours to weeks.
- Inquire about recent travel history, pets, and tick bites.

 Physical Examination

- Changing vital signs may suggest impending herniation due to brain swelling (hypertension, bradycardia, apnea).
- Neck: The patient may have meningismus and positive Kernig and Brudzinski signs.
- Diffuse adenopathy
- Chest: signs of pneumonia, rales, rhonchi
- Abdomen: hepatosplenomegaly
- Skin: may show various types of rashes, from petechial in meningococcemia to an erythematous nonspecific viral rash
- Neurologic examination: rapid or slow changes in mental status ranging from mild confusion to hallucinations to stupor and coma
- Aphasia (suggestive of herpes) is distinguished from psychomotor slowing by prominence of grammatic errors and dysarthria and normal alertness.
- There may be pupillary abnormalities with nystagmus: Funduscopic examination may reveal papilledema as a sign of increased intracranial pressure (ICP). Cranial neuropathies, increased muscle tone, pathologic deep tendon reflexes, Babinski sign, clonus, ataxia, and so forth, may be encountered.

PITFALLS

A CSF sample without any RBCs does not rule out herpes simplex.

- Never assume that a CSF pleocytosis is secondary to seizures. Institute antiviral and antibacterial therapy promptly; it can always be discontinued once an organism is identified or cultures are negative.
- Children with immunodeficiency are at higher risk for fungal meningoencephalitis, which may be missed unless appropriate studies are sent.
- Amebic infection of the brain should be considered in children with exposure to fresh water sources.
- Cysticercosis is common in tropical and underdeveloped areas. Ring-enhancing lesions may point to this diagnosis.

Laboratory Aids

TESTS

A decision about laboratory testing depends partly on the severity of symptoms.

Radiologic

• CT or MRI of the brain with and without contrast medium should be performed urgently to rule out surgically remediable conditions (empyema, abscess).
• Typical changes in encephalitis include parenchymal, meningeal, and focal or diffuse enhancement of the brain. (HSV has a preference for the medial temporal lobe, with hemorrhagic and cystic changes.)
• Hydrocephalus, obstructive or communicating, may occur as a result of the encephalitis.

Spinal Tap

A CSF spinal tap should be deferred if imaging shows subfalcine herniation (left-to-right shift of lateral ventricles), cerebral edema, obstructive hydrocephalus (lateral ventricles large, fourth ventricle relatively small), or central herniation (asymmetry or effacement of fourth ventricle/basilar cystern).

Lumbar Puncture

Once radiologic evidence for increased intracranial pressure has been ruled out, a lumbar puncture should be performed

• Opening pressure is frequently elevated.
• Pleocytosis is lymphocytic if viral, and usually neutrophilic if bacterial.
• Protein will be increased, glucose will be decreased, and RBCs may be present (particularly in HSV).
• CSF should be sent for bacterial and viral culture. Order a fungal culture if suspected.
• If HSV is suspected, PCR should be obtained, as the virus is difficult to grow in vitro.
• Gram stain and acid-fast bacillus, cryptococcal antigen, and yeast tests also should be ordered.

Other Routine Tests

• Blood electrolytes, BUN, glucose, calcium, magnesium, phosphorus, blood count with differential, blood and urine culture, and toxicology screen
• An EEG may be helpful, particularly if HSV is suspected; it may show periodic lateralizing epileptiform discharges (PLEDs), which are suggestive, but not diagnostic, of herpes.

 ## Therapy

• General: Patients with encephalitis frequently require ICU care with cardiorespiratory support. Mini-dose subcutaneous heparin is standard for prophylaxis of intravascular thrombosis in acutely ill adults, but is untested in the pediatric age group. Early involvement of physical and occupational therapy is important.
• Treatment of intracranial hypertension includes mannitol and hyperventilation, usually with assistance from intensivists or neurology/neurosurgery consultants; these measures should be reserved for situations in which vital or neurologic signs indicate impending herniation.
• Antiinfective agents: Initial treatment should be with antibacterial and antiviral agents (acyclovir: monitor renal function) until the cause becomes clear or cultures are negative.
• Fluids: Avoidance of fluid overload, which may exacerbate cerebral edema, requires strict attention to fluid/osmotic balance. Normal saline is preferred; electrolytes are closely monitored, anticipating possible SIADH or diabetes insipidus.
• Anticonvulsants are reserved for clinical or electrographic evidence of seizure/epileptic activity; usual choices include phenytoin, phenobarbital, and carbamazepine. Treatment of PLEDs without associated convulsions is controversial. Potential side effects and sedation from anticonvulsants should be considered in this decision.
• Consultation with an infectious disease specialist, neurologist, or neurosurgeon may be helpful.

 ## Follow-Up

The outcome from encephalitis varies greatly and depends on age and degree of CNS involvement/destruction. Physical and occupational therapy should be consulted early in the course of the hospitalization. Patients who appear to have recovered completely physically may still have cognitive deficits. Neuropsychologic testing is helpful to identify the deficits and to create long-term treatment plans, which will maximize the patient's recovery.

PREVENTION

• Completion of routine immunizations (varicella, H-flue type b, etc.) and routine hygiene (hand washing) are the best preventive measures.
• Other measures should be taken according to the infection (e.g., skin testing contacts in cases of tuberculosis).
• Isolation of hospitalized patient: depends on organism suspected. Airborne, droplet, and contact precautions are frequently used together during the first 24 hours, pending a more specific diagnosis from cultures. The infectious disease department will determine type and duration of isolation and whether family members need to be treated.

 ## Common Questions and Answers

Q: My child has been diagnosed with encephalitis; will he be mentally retarded?
A: The complications following encephalitis vary greatly from severe mental retardation and cerebral palsy to full recovery. There is a correlation between degree of brain destruction and outcome. However, children frequently recover better than adults with a similar degree of illness.

ICD-9-CM 323.9

BIBLIOGRAPHY

Bertram M, Schwartz S, Hacke W. Acute and critical care in neurology. *Eur Neurol* 1997;38(3): 155–166.

Calisher CH. Medically important arboviruses of the United States and Canada. *Clin Microbiol Rev* 1994;7(1):89–116.

Whitley RJ, Lakeman F. Herpes simplex virus infections of the central nervous system: therapeutic and diagnostic considerations. *Clin Infect Dis* 1995;20(2):414–420.

Author: A.G. Christina Bergqvist

Encopresis

 Database

DEFINITION

Encopresis is overflow incontinence resulting from chronic constipation.

PATHOPHYSIOLOGY

Chronic constipation with fecal impaction results in overflow incontinence and reduced sensation secondary to rectal distention. The pattern of holding fecal matter, leading to chronic constipation and overflow incontinence, may result from a variety of etiologies, such as a painful experience from a fissure or refusal to use school bathrooms. However, the history often does not reveal a triggering event.

GENETICS

Monozygotic twins have a fourfold higher incidence than do dizygotic twins.

EPIDEMIOLOGY

The ratio of boys to girls is approximately 6:1. There is no association with family size, ordinal position in the family, age of parents, or socioeconomic status.

COMPLICATIONS

- Social problems
- Urinary tract infections, especially in girls
- Abdominal discomfort
- Decreased appetite

 Differential Diagnosis

The physician must determine if stool leakage is due to functional constipation or an underlying anatomic, metabolic, or endocrinologic abnormality.

- Anatomic

—Anterior displaced anus
—Fistula secondary to inflammatory bowel disease
—Stricture (after necrotizing enterocolitis or inflammatory bowel disease)
—Abdominal pelvic mass (sacral teratoma, meningomyelocele)

- Neurologic

—Hirschsprung disease
—Meningomyelocele
—Spinal cord tumor
—Hypotonia (cerebral palsy, amyotonia congenita, familial visceral myopathy)
—Amyloidosis

- Metabolic

—Hypothyroidism
—Panhypopituitarism
—Diabetes mellitus
—Constipating drugs

 Data Gathering

HISTORY

- Timing in the neonatal period of meconium passage, as well as past surgeries, medical history, and medications, are relevant.
- The review of systems should be unremarkable, except for possible mild abdominal discomfort and a small amount of blood on the outside of the stool or separate from the bowel movement if a fissure has developed.

 Physical Examination

- Demonstrates a dilated rectum but a normally positioned anus
- Should include deep tendon reflexes, anal wink, rectal examination, and documentation of normal growth

Laboratory Aids

No laboratory tests are needed if both the history and physical examination are consistent with functional constipation and associated encopresis. If the patient's history or physical is atypical and Hirschsprung disease is suspected, an unprepped barium enema and rectal suction biopsy may be warranted.

 Therapy

Management combines pharmacology, behavioral modification, and dietary alterations.

• Pharmacology

—Remove fecal impaction via enemas, cathartic regimens, including laxatives.
—Stool softener

• Behavior modification

—Decrease family stress.
—Have the child sit on toilet for 5 to 10 minutes one to two times per day (tailored to the age of the child).
—Delay toilet training if the child is in diapers (to reduce stress).
—Motivate
—Biofeedback (reserved for very difficult cases)

• Diet

—High-fiber diet
—Adequate fluid

 Follow-Up

The first follow-up is at 2 weeks to ensure compliance and success with the initial management. If the fecal impaction has been successfully removed, a reward system is started. The patient is followed at monthly intervals to ensure motivation and to be supportive. Treatment with stool softeners is needed until behavior and diet have improved and until rectal dilatation has resolved. Medication is often needed for 6 months or longer.

PITFALLS

• Parents may misconstrue stool-withholding behavior as an attempt to defecate.
• Parents think that their child's soiling is deliberate. They do not understand that the child can neither feel the passage of stool nor prevent it. The usual urge to defecate, which comes from stretching of the ampulla and internal anal sphincter, is not felt because the rectal ampulla is massively distended.
• Patients or their parents often stop stool softeners as soon as a normal stool pattern starts. If therapy has been ended prematurely, the patient's constipation and encopresis returns immediately, because rectal tone is still poor and no other behavior or dietary modifications have been made.

 Common Questions and Answers

Q: Is the medicine addictive?
A: Stool softeners rather than cathartics are chosen for long-term therapy because the colon does not become dependent.

Q: Will my child become sick if this problem is not resolved?
A: Most children with chronic constipation and encopresis grow well and do not develop other health problems. The major problems are social and should be taken seriously. Social development is crucial for the school-aged child.

ICD-9-CM 787.6

BIBLIOGRAPHY

Wyllie R, Hyams JS. *Pediatric gastrointestinal disease*. Philadelphia: WB Saunders, 1993.

Author: Barbara Haber

Endocarditis

Database

DEFINITION

Endocarditis is microbial infection of the endocardium of the heart.

PATHOGENESIS

- Endocarditis primarily is seen in patients with a preexisting congenital or acquired heart disease who develop bacteremia with organisms that are likely to cause infection.
- Intravenous drug abusers and patients with intravenous lines may develop endocarditis in the absence of a cardiovascular abnormality.
- Local turbulence secondary to the cardiovascular abnormality is thought to result in damage to the endocardial surface.

—Followed by the development of a network of fibrin and platelets in which bacteria then can become entrapped, causing the nidus of infection.

- Bacteremia can be a complication of a focal infection (e.g., pneumonia, cellulitis, or urinary tract infection) or can be associated with various dental and surgical procedures. Bacteremia, however, can occur spontaneously and has been documented with activities such as chewing hard candy and brushing teeth.

MICROORGANISMS

- Gram-positive cocci account for 90% of culture-positive endocarditis.

—Alpha-hemolytic streptococci (*Streptococcus viridans*) are responsible for most cases of endocarditis in all age groups.
—Staphylococci (*S. aureus* and coagulase-negative staphylococci) are the second largest group.
—Other organisms that can cause endocarditis are beta-hemolytic streptococci, pneumococci, enterococci, *Pseudomonas* species, the HACEK bacteria, *Neisseria* species, and *Candida* species.

- Approximately 5% of endocarditis cases are reported as culture-negative.

EPIDEMIOLOGY

- Endocarditis is relatively uncommon. Studies have reported incidences between 1 in 1,280 and 1 in 4,500 of all pediatric hospital admissions.
- The overall incidence of endocarditis seems to have decreased in the current era of antibiotics, but some have actually suggested an increase in incidence with the higher survival of patients with congenital heart disease and the wide and often prolonged use of central intravascular lines.

COMPLICATIONS

Despite improvements in diagnosis and treatment of endocarditis, it continues to be a disease with significant morbidity and mortality (approximately 10%).

- Cardiac

—Damage to the valve leaflets may result in valvar regurgitation, heart failure, or conduction abnormalities.

- Embolic

—Embolic events can occur to multiple organ systems (central nervous system, kidneys, spleen, skin, lungs).

PROGNOSIS

If diagnosed in timely fashion and appropriate therapy is instituted, prognosis is relatively good for bacterial endocarditis. Fungal endocarditis is associated with a higher morbidity and mortality.

Differential Diagnosis

- Other infections (e.g., acute rheumatic fever)
- Malignancy
- Connective tissue disorders

Data Gathering

HISTORY

Fever, general malaise, fatigue, weight loss, myalgias, arthralgias, night sweats, headache, and anorexia. Occasionally, a focal infection or a preceding dental or surgical procedure can be identified.

Physical Examination

- General

—Fever (usually low grade with alpha-hemolytic streptococci and high grade with *S. aureus*) and pallor

- Embolic or immunologic phenomena

—Splinter hemorrhages, retinal hemorrhages, Osler nodes, Janeway lesions, splenomegaly, clubbing, arthralgia, and arthritis

- Cardiac

—New or changing murmurs and symptoms of congestive heart failure

- Neurologic

—Neurologic symptoms can be seen on the basis of central nervous system emboli and hemorrhage, and can sometimes mimic the picture of an abscess, aseptic meningitis, or cerebral infarct.

Laboratory Aids

TESTS

Blood Cultures

- Blood cultures are the gold standard for diagnosing endocarditis.
- Blood cultures are positive in 85% to 90% of the reported cases of endocarditis and remain the most important tool in making the diagnosis of endocarditis.
- At least three sets of blood cultures should be obtained over a 24-hour period. Each set should be obtained from separate venipuncture sites via strict sterile technique.
- As large a volume as clinically reasonable should be collected.
- The bacteremia of endocarditis is continuous; therefore, it is not necessary to obtain the blood cultures during a fever spike.

Nonspecific Laboratory Data

Elevated ESR, rheumatoid factor, anemia, hematuria, leukocytosis, and decreased complement

Echocardiography

- Transthoracic echocardiography is a valuable noninvasive technique in the identification of vegetations.
- The sensitivity and specificity of transthoracic echocardiography, however, is not 100%; therefore, a negative echocardiogram does not rule out endocarditis.
- Transesophageal echocardiography (useful in older or obese patients) may visualize smaller vegetations as well as areas that are inadequately seen with standard transthoracic imaging.
- In patients with a nonconclusive transthoracic study but a high index of suspicion for endocarditis, transesophageal echocardiography is recommended.

PITFALLS

- The absence of vegetation(s) by echocardiography does not rule out endocarditis.
- In patients with a prosthetic valve, echocardiography is not always helpful, as there is frequently artifact from the prosthetic valve. Abnormal movements of the valve leaflets may suggest a vegetation.
- The ESR may remain elevated for some time, even after cessation of bacteremia.

Therapy

- General

—Rest; antipyretics; transfusion, if needed; optimal nutrition; fluid and electrolyte balance; dental hygiene

- Antibiotics

—Prolonged therapy (4–8 weeks) with intravenous antibiotics is needed. The choice of antibiotic(s) and the duration of antibiotic treatment depend on the infecting organism and its sensitivity pattern. For fungal SBE, intravenous amphotericin B is given for a minimum of 6 to 8 weeks.

- Surgery: potential indications for surgical therapy

—Severe congestive heart failure
—Worsening heart failure
—Endocarditis that is uncontrollable with antibiotics
—More than one serious systemic embolus
—Local suppurative complications (e.g., abscess with conduction abnormalities)
—Development of a mycotic aneurysm
—Fungal endocarditis may require replacement of the infected valve and excision of infected tissue.

Follow-Up

Repeat blood cultures should be obtained after a few days of antibiotic or antifungal therapy to ensure the eradication of bacteria. After completion of a full course of antibiotics, blood cultures should be again obtained in the first 2 months after discontinuation of therapy.

Prevention

- Dental hygiene
- Minimal use of central lines
- Correction of the cardiovascular anomaly by surgery or interventional catheterization techniques
- SBE prophylaxis

SBE PROPHYLAXIS

For Dental, Oral, Respiratory Tract, or Esophageal Procedures

- Amoxicillin (50 mg/kg orally 1 hour before procedure; maximum, 2.0 g). If unable to take oral medications, ampicillin (same dose) may be given 30 minutes before the procedure.
- Clindamycin (20 mg/kg orally 1 hour before procedure; maximum, 600 mg) may be used if the patient is allergic to penicillin.

For Genitourinary/Gastrointestinal (Excluding Esophageal) Procedures

- High-risk patients: Ampicillin (50 mg/kg; maximum, 2.0 gm IM/IV) plus gentamicin 1.5 mg/kg (maximum, 120 mg) within 30 minutes of starting procedure; 6 hours later, 25 mg/kg/IV ampicillin (maximum, 1 g) or amoxicillin 25mg/kg/PO (maximim, 1g). Vancomycin plus gentamicin may be used for patients allergic to amoxicillin/ampicillin.
- Moderate-risk patients: Amoxicillin (50 mg/kg/PO; maximum, 2.0 g) 1 hour prior to the procedure, or ampicillin 50 mg/kg IM/IV (maximum, 2.0 g) within 30 minutes of starting the procedure. Vancomycin may be used for patients allergic to amoxicillin/ampicillin.

Cardiac Conditions That Require SBE Prophylaxis

- High-risk group: prosthetic valves, previous SBE, cyanotic heart disease, surgically constructed shunts or conduits
- Moderate-risk group: most other congenital heart disease, acquired valvar disease (e.g., rheumatic valvar disease), hypertrophic cardiomyopathy, mitral valve prolapse with regurgitation or thickened leaflets

Cardiac Lesions That Do Not Require SBE Prophylaxis

- Isolated secundum atrial septal defect
- Surgically repaired patent ductus arteriosus
- Ventricular septal defect and atrial septal defect beyond 6 months (without residual)
- Previous coronary artery bypass surgery
- Mitral valve prolapse without regurgitation
- Previous Kawasaki syndrome without vulvar dysfunction
- Rheumatic fever without valvar dysfunction
- Pacemakers and defibrillators

Procedures That Require SBE Prophylaxis

- Tonsillectomy, adenoidectomy, surgery of respiratory mucosa, rigid bronchoscopy
- Sclerotherapy for esophageal varices, esophageal dilation, biliary tract and intestinal surgery, endoscopic retrograde cholangiography
- Prostatic surgery, cytoscopy, urethral dilation
- Dental extractions, periodontal procedures, dental implant, endodontic procedures, dental cleaning, intraligamentary injections, initial placements of orthodontic bands, subgingival placement of antibiotic fibers/strips

Procedures That Do Not Require SBE Prophylaxis

These may be recommended in high-risk patients.

- Endotracheal intubation, flexible bronchoscopy, ear tubes, transesophageal echocardiography, GI endoscopy
- Vaginal hysterectomy, vaginal delivery, cesarean section, urethral catheterization, uterine dilation and curettage, abortion, sterilization, intrauterine devices
- Cardiac catheterization
- Circumcision
- Shedding of primary teeth

Common Questions and Answers

Q: I forgot to give my child antibiotics prior to the procedure. Should I give him a dose afterwards?
A: In regard to preventing endocarditis, no data exist on the benefit of administering antibiotics after a procedure.

Q: My child has an innocent heart murmur. Does he need SBE prophylaxis?
A: SBE prophylaxis is not indicated.

BIBLIOGRAPHY

Dajani AS, Taubert KA, Wilson W, et al., Prevention of bacterial endocarditis; recommendations by the American Heart Association. *JAMA* 1997;277:1794–1801.

Emmanoulides GC, Riemenscheider TA, Allen HD, Gutgesell HP, eds. *Moss and Adams, heart disease in infants, children, and adolescents, including the fetus and the young adult,* 5th ed. Baltimore: Williams & Wilkins, 1995.

Author: Hae-Rhi Lee

Enuresis

 ## Database

DEFINITION

Enuresis is involuntary urination after the age of expected bladder control, and is generally reserved for children 5 to 6 years of age or older.

- In the majority, incontinence occurs only at night (nocturnal enuresis or "bedwetting"); a smaller group also is incontinent during the day (diurnal enuresis).
- *Primary enuresis:* Continence is never achieved.
- *Secondary enuresis:* Incontinence recurs after a dry period of at least 6 months.

PATHOPHYSIOLOGY

- For primary nocturnal enuresis (PNE), several theories, with different mechanisms probably playing greater or lesser roles in specific individuals

—A maturational delay of neurodevelopmental processes, with bladder emptying at lower volume secondary to smaller functional bladder capacity
—Other studies suggest that decreased secretion of ADH at night causes some patients to produce urine at the same rate night and day, compared with dry peers, who have decreased rates of urine production at night, due to an increase in ADH secretion.
—Abnormalities of sleep have not been proven to play a role.

- Daytime wetting may be related to detrusor muscle instability, reflux of urine into the vagina with back-seepage after voiding, giggle incontinence, and poor toileting habits.
- Underlying medical or surgical causes are much less common in primary than secondary enuresis.

GENETICS

- Seventy percent of children with enuresis have a parent who was enuretic.
- If both parents were enuretic, 77% of children are enuretic.
- If one parent was enuretic, 43% to 47% of children are enuretic.
- If neither parent was enuretic, only 15% of children are enuretic.
- Incidence in monozygotic twins is twice the incidence in dizygotes

EPIDEMIOLOGY

- Twenty percent of children have primary nocturnal enuresis at age 5 years, 10% at age 7 years, and 5% at age 10 years; primary nocturnal enuresis persists in approximately 1% of adults.
- Daytime wetting occurs in only 1% of 7- to 12-year-olds.
- Nocturnal enuresis is two to three times more common in males; daytime wetting is more common in females.

COMPLICATIONS

Embarrassment, poor self-esteem, and reluctance to participate in overnight activities with peers

PROGNOSIS

- Prognosis is very good, even without treatment.
- The spontaneous cure rate is 15% per year.

 ## Differential Diagnosis

Several underlying diseases or conditions can present with enuresis:

- Urinary tract infection
- Diabetes mellitus
- Diabetes insipidus
- Sickle cell disease
- Structural genitourinary tract defects, including ectopic ureter, ureteral duplication, neurogenic bladder
- Spinal cord pathology
- Constipation
- Excessive caffeine, methylxanthines or other medications
- Any condition causing polyuria can present as enuresis.

 ## Data Gathering

HISTORY

- Onset (primary versus secondary)
- When it occurs—nighttime, daytime, or both—and how often
- Toileting habits, frequency of voiding and stooling
- Pattern of urination: dribbling, dysuria, hesitancy, urgency (suggest structural defects, dysfunctional voiding, UTI)
- Associated signs and symptoms: stool incontinence, polydipsia, polyuria
- History of other medical problems, including UTIs
- Behavioral/developmental history: age milestones obtained, toilet training methods, behavioral problems
- Medications (especially caffeine or medications with diuretic effects)
- Typical fluid intake (looking for excessive intake in evening)
- Recent environmental stressors (if secondary enuresis)
- Effect of enuresis on child: Does child sleep over with friends or at camp? Is child teased at school?
- Parents' attitude toward the problem
- Family history of enuresis? If positive, is the child aware?
- Family history of other diagnoses in differential
- Treatments (or punishments) attempted

 ## Physical Examination

- Vital signs and growth parameters
- Abdominal examination to rule out masses, renal enlargement, palpable bladder, constipation
- Genitalia: irritation, adhesions, rash, or other signs of constant dampness; balanitis; stenosis; foreign bodies; trauma
- Observe voiding for character of stream, dribbling
- Rectal: perianal sensation, anal sphincter tone, impaction
- Palpate spine for bony defects and cutaneous signs of underlying spinal defects.
- Neurologic: deep tendon reflexes, gait, strength and tone of lower extremities

 ## Laboratory Aids

TESTS

- Urine for specific gravity, urinalysis (especially glucose), microscopic examination and culture to exclude UTI, diabetes mellitus, and diabetes insipidus. In the majority of cases, this is the only investigation needed
- If there is a history of UTIs, voiding abnormalities, or voiding symptoms, a voiding cystourethrogram and renal ultrasound should be performed to rule out anatomic defects. The plain scout film can also show constipation or vertebral bony anomalies.
- If findings are suggestive of neurologic dysfunction, urodynamic studies should be performed.

Therapy

- Treat any underlying condition.
- Education, reassurance, and support
- Avoid punishment.
- Encourage positive reinforcement: praise, star charts, and so on.
- Avoid aggressive therapy in those less than 7 years old.
- Fluid restriction in the evenings is unproven but logically appealing.
- Retention training/bladder stretching exercises are controversial
- Alarm systems: most effective and most cost effective of all interventions; require several weeks to months to achieve complete dryness
- Desmopressin (DDAVP): remains controversial but is used in PNE when other therapies fail, if use can be monitored appropriately

—Response is generally quick, but enuresis recurs in most subjects after the medication is stopped.
—Concerns remain regarding potential for hyponatremia and volume overload.
—Not recommended in children less than 9 years of age
—Expensive

- Imipramine: useful but potentially lethal if used inappropriately

—Prescribe only nonlethal quantities to prevent accidental ingestions.

- Oxybutynin: may be useful in the small population of patients with documented detrusor instability
- Night waking exercises and other behavior modification techniques may also be useful in some patients.

 Follow-Up

- Timely and regular phone follow-up to answer questions, assess progress, and offer encouragement
- See the patient in the office in 1 month if medications are begun.

PITFALLS

- Remember the natural course of the symptoms, and balance the use of potentially dangerous medications (if used inappropriately) against the social/emotional impact on the individual.
- Do not overdo laboratory studies: Balance risks and costs with the likelihood of yield. Extensive work-up of isolated PNE seldom yields an organic etiology; work-up should generally be limited to examination of the urine.

 Common Questions and Answers

Q: Isn't DDAVP dangerous? What about hyponatremia and volume overload?
A: While the most common side effects noted with DDAVP have been headaches, abdominal pain, and nasal stuffiness, concern remains regarding the potential for hyponatremia and water intoxication. While studies show a safe side-effect profile, there have been scattered reports of serious side effects. Use of DDAVP needs to be monitored carefully, especially since the significance of variations in ADH levels is unclear in the pathophysiology of PNE.

Q: Won't enuresis recur when DDAVP is stopped?
A: While a significant number of children respond to some degree at the initiation of treatment, results of long-term response to prolonged medication use have varied from study to study. In most instances, long-term cure rates have been only slightly better than spontaneous cure rates.

ICD-9-CM 788.30

BIBLIOGRAPHY

Bloom DA. The American experience with desmopressin. *Clin Pediatr* 1993;Special Issue:28-31.

Friman PC. A preventive context for enuresis. *Pediatr Clin North Am* 1986;33:871–886.

Ilyas M, Jerkins GR. Management of nocturnal childhood enuresis in managed care: a new challenge. *Pediatr Ann* 1996;25:258–264.

Moffatt ME, Harlos S, Kirshen AJ, Burd L. Desmopressin acetate and nocturnal enuresis: how much do we know? *Pediatrics* 1993;92:420–425.

Norgaard JP, Djurhuus JC. The pathophysiology of enuresis in children and young adults. *Clin Pediatr* 1993;Special Issue:5–9.

Novello AC, Novello JR. Enuresis. *Pediatr Clin North Am* 1987;34:719–731.

Rappaport L. The treatment of nocturnal enuresis—where are we now? *Pediatrics* 1993;92:465–466.

Robson WLM. Diurnal enuresis. *Pediatr Rev* 1997;18:407–412.

Rushton HG. Evaluation of the enuretic child. *Clin Pediatr* 1993;Special Issue:14–18.

Schmitt BD. Nocturnal enuresis. *Pediatr Rev* 1997;18:183–190.

Shortliffe LMD. Primary nocturnal enuresis: introduction. *Clin Pediatr* 1993;Special Issue:3–4.

Wan J, Greenfield S. Enuresis and common voiding abnormalities. *Pediatr Clin North Am* 1997;44:1117–1131.

Author: Suzette Surratt Caudle

Eosinophilic Pneumonia

 Database

DEFINITION

Infiltrates on chest radiograph with either:

- Peripheral eosinophilia (pulmonary infiltrate with eosinophilia—PIE syndrome)
- Increased eosinophils (>5%) in bronchoalveolar lavage (BAL) fluid
- Eosinophilic infiltrate in lung biopsy

PATHOPHYSIOLOGY

Simple Pulmonary Eosinophilia (Loffler Syndrome)

- Characterized by:

—Migratory pulmonary infiltrates
—Eosinophilia
—Minimal pulmonary symptomology

- Usually caused by:

—Drug reaction (i.e., ampicillin, sulfasalazine, crack cocaine, cromolyn)
—Parasitic infection (i.e., *Ascaris*, *Toxocara*, *Strongyloides*, *Ancylostoma*)
—No etiology found (33% of cases)

Chronic Eosinophilic Pneumonia

- Characterized by:

—Cough
—Systemic symptoms
—Long duration
—Eosinophilia (blood/BAL/tissue)

- Unknown etiology

Allergic Bronchopulmonary Aspergillosis (ABPA)

- Characterized by:

—History of asthma or cystic fibrosis
—Worsening control of asthma or cystic fibrosis
—Colonization of bronchi by *Aspergillus*
—Eosinophilia with elevated IgE level
—Bronchiectatic changes frequently seen

- Usually caused by *Aspergillus fumigatus*

Acute Eosinophilic Pneumonia

- Characterized by:

—Acute febrile illness
—Rapid progression
—Respiratory failure
—Peripheral eosinophilia usually absent early in course; BAL, however, is positive for eosinophilia

- Unknown etiology (possibly due to an acute hypersensitivity reaction after exposure to an unknown inhalant)

Asthma with Vasculitis (Churg-Strauss Syndrome)

- Characterized by:

—History of allergic disease and asthma
—Significant eosinophilia
—Multiple-organ vasculitis (necrotizing giant-cell vasculitis of small arteries and veins)

- Unknown etiology

PATHOLOGY

- Infiltration of alveolar and interstitial spaces with eosinophils
- Specific findings dependent on the underlying etiology:

—Infection: The organism might be found.
—APBA: Bronchiectatic changes are usually seen.
—Churg-Strauss syndrome: necrotizing giant-cell vasculitis of small arteries and veins

EPIDEMIOLOGY

- Incidence of ABPA:

—One percent to 2% of patients with chronic asthma
—Five percent to 15% of patients with cystic fibrosis

- Drug reactions are some of the most commonly reported causes of PIE.
- Most of the other forms of eosinophilic lung disease are more common in the adult population.

COMPLICATIONS

- Pulmonary fibrosis, if left untreated
- Death can occur in severe cases.

PROGNOSIS

- Loffler syndrome: excellent
- Infectious process: good, if infection is under control
- Drug reaction: excellent
- Acute eosinophilic pneumonia: good, if promptly treated
- Chronic eosinophilic pneumonia: excellent, if properly treated; tapering of steroid dose must be done carefully.
- ABPA is a chronic disease that can lead to pulmonary fibrosis and severe bronchiectasis.
- Churg-Strauss syndrome:

—Mean survival of steroid-treated patients is 9 years.
—Without steroid therapy, 50% die within 3 months of onset of vasculitis.

 Differential Diagnosis

- Pulmonary

—Asthma (especially with allergies)
—Cystic fibrosis
—Adult respiratory distress syndrome (ARDS)
—Hypersensitivity pneumonitis

- Infectious

—Pneumonia (viral, bacterial, fungal)
—Tuberculosis
—*Pneumocystis carinii* pneumonia (PCP)

- Connective-tissue disease

—Sarcoidosis
—Wegener granulomatosis

- Malignancies

—Lymphoma
—Leukemia

 Data Gathering

HISTORY

- Depends on the specific form of eosinophilic pneumonia
- Minimal respiratory symptoms with short duration suggest Loffler syndrome.
- Travel history may suggest parasitic infection.
- Close contact with a dog or cat can suggest *Ancylostoma* or *Toxocara* infection.
- Prolonged cough, fever, dyspnea, and weight loss suggest chronic eosinophilic pneumonia.
- Acute presentation with respiratory compromise suggests acute eosinophilic pneumonia.
- HIV risk factors suggest PCP infection.
- Systemic symptoms suggest vasculitis, malignancy, or chronic eosinophilic pneumonia.
- Inquire if patient is currently, or has been recently, taking any medications
- Asthma history suggests ABPA or Churg-Strauss syndrome

 Physical Examination

- Lung examination can be normal (Loffler syndrome).
- Cough
- Prolonged expiratory phase
- Wheezing
- Rales
- In some cases, respiratory distress is observed.
- If the underlying cause is a systemic disease, findings may include:

—Fever
—Weight loss
—Multiple-organ involvement

Laboratory Aids

TESTS

- Blood tests

—CBC with differential: to assess for eosinophilia
—IgE levels: total IgE, IgE specific for *Aspergillus*
—Serology studies: for *Strongyloides, Toxocara*

- Multiple stool samples for ova and parasites
- Skin testing for *Aspergillus*
- Pulmonary function testing

—Obstructive lung diseases: asthma, ABPA, bronchiolitis obliterans, Churg-Strauss syndrome
—Restrictive lung diseases: acute eosinophilic pneumonia, chronic eosinophilic pneumonia, drug reaction

- Bronchoalveolar lavage (BAL)

—Cytology: Greater than 20% eosinophils in BAL fluid is diagnostic for eosinophilic pneumonia.
—Culture: viral, bacterial, fungal, parasitic
—Pathologic stains: parasites, PCP, and fungus

- Lung biopsy for suspected cases of:

—Vasculitis
—Malignancy
—Interstitial lung disease

IMAGING

Chest Radiography

- Migratory pulmonary infiltrates
- Hyperinflation
- Bronchiectasis can be seen in ABPA.
- Peripherally located lesions are characteristic for chronic eosinophilic pneumonia.

Chest CT

- Parenchymal or interstitial infiltrates:

—Diffuse in acute eosinophilic pneumonia
—Peripheral in chronic eosinophilic pneumonia

- Mediastinal lymphadenopathy (50% of cases of chronic eosinophilic pneumonia)
- Bronchiectasis (in ABPA)

PITFALLS

- Cases of eosinophilic pneumonia can present without blood eosinophilia, so a normal differential on white blood cell count does not exclude PIE.
- Some parasites (i.e., *Ancylostoma* and *Toxocara*) cannot be diagnosed by stool examination.
- Other parasites (i.e., *Ascaris*) may cause pulmonary eosinophilia weeks before the first ova can be detected in stool samples.

 ## Therapy

DRUGS

- Therapy should be directed to the underlying disease.
- If a drug reaction is suspected, the drug should be discontinued.
- Loffler syndrome rarely requires treatment.
- Antiparasitic agents are used if parasitic infection is present.
- Corticosteroids are indicated for:

—ABPA
—Acute eosinophilic pneumonia
—Chronic eosinophilic pneumonia
—Churg-Strauss syndrome
—Drug reactions (if discontinuation of the offending drug did not help)

DURATION

- Dependent on the underlying disease and the clinical response
- Duration of steroid therapy is usually short:

—Two weeks to 3 months, followed by a tapering period
—If tapering is done slowly, remissions are uncommon.
—In acute eosinophilic pneumonia, patients never experience a relapse.

- Treatment may be prolonged or even permanent in some cases (i.e., ABPA, chronic eosinophilic pneumonia, and Churg-Strauss syndrome).

 ## Follow-Up

WHEN TO EXPECT IMPROVEMENT

- Loffler syndrome: spontaneous resolution within 1 month
- Acute and chronic eosinophilic pneumonia often show dramatic response to steroids within 24 to 48 hours.
- Churg-Strauss syndrome: Response to steroid therapy is seen within several weeks.

SIGNS TO WATCH FOR

- Reappearance of symptoms or worsening of infiltrates while tapering the steroid dose

 ## Common Questions and Answers

Q: How long will the patient need to be on steroids?
A: It depends on the underlying etiology.

ICD-9-CM 518.3

BIBLIOGRAPHY

Allen JN, Davis WB. State of the art: eosinophilic lung diseases. *Am J Respir Crit Care Med* 1994;150:1423–1438.

Amin RS, Wilmott RW. *Kendig's disorders of the respiratory tract in children.* Philadelphia: WB Saunders, 1998:731–753.

Greenberger PA. Immunologic aspects of lung diseases and cystic fibrosis. *JAMA* 1997;278:1924–1930.

Hayakawa H, Sato A, Toyoshima M, et al. A clinical study of idiopathic eosinophilic pneumonia. *Chest* 1994;105:1462–1466.

Naughton M, Fahy J, FitzGerald MX. Chronic eosinophilic pneumonia: a long-term follow-up of 12 patients. *Chest* 103:162–165.

O'Sullivan BP, Nimkin K, Gang DL. A fifteen-year-old boy with eosinophilia and pulmonary infiltrates. *J Pediatr* 1993;123:660-666.

Pope-Harman AL, Davis WB, Allen E, et al. Acute eosinophilic pneumonia: A summary of 15 cases and review of the literature. *Medicine* 1996;75:334–342.

Shannon JJ, Lynch JP. Eosinophilic pulmonary syndromes. *Clin Pulm Med* 1995;2:19–38.

Authors: Richard Mark Kravitz

Epiglottitis

 Database

DEFINITION

Epiglottitis is an acute, life-threatening bacterial infection consisting of cellulitis and edema of the epiglottis, aryepiglottic folds, arytenoids and hypopharynx, resulting in narrowing of the glottic opening.

PATHOPHYSIOLOGY

- Etiologic agents include: *Haemophilus influenzae* type B (accounted for >90% of cases in pre-vaccine era), *Staphylococcus aureus*, *Streptococcus pneumoniae*, *Streptococcus pyogenes* (group A β-hemolytic streptococcus), and group C β-hemolytic streptococcus (rare). *Candida albicans* may be an etiologic agent in immunocompromised patients. *Pasteurella multocida* has been implicated in a handful of cases after exposure to nasopharyngeal secretions from a cat.
- The inhaled anesthetic, sevoflurane, has been implicated in a few cases of epiglottitis.
- Erythema and edema of the uvula, aryepiglottic folds, arytenoids, epiglottis, and vocal cords include an exudate rich in neutrophils and fibrin, which usually proceed to organization and fibrous scarring.

EPIDEMIOLOGY

- Disease due to *H. influenzae* type B occurs most often between the ages of 2 and 7 years (overall range: infancy to adulthood).
- Epiglottis and other invasive disease (including epiglottitis) secondary to *H. influenzae* have been reduced by 98% since the introduction of the conjugate vaccines in 1989 (approved at 15 months) and 1990 (approved at 2, 4, and 6 months)
- Year-round occurrence
- Affects boys and girls equally
- All geographic areas
- Rare in populations in which the peak incidence of meningitis is shifted towards infancy (i.e., Alaskan Eskimos, Native Americans)
- Occasional secondary cases in households or daycare centers
- May be more frequent in children with sickle cell anemia, asplenia, immunoglobulin defects, or leukemia
- Disease due to *S. pyogenes* occurs most often in early school-age children during the winter and early spring.

COMPLICATIONS

- Without prompt medical intervention, complete airway obstruction leading to respiratory arrest, hypoxia, and death
- Necrotizing cervical fasciitis (rarely)
- Therapeutic complications include: aspiration, endotracheal tube dislodgment and extubation, tracheal erosion or irritation, pneumomediastinum, pneumothorax, and pulmonary edema.
- Complications of *H. influenzae* type B bacteremia include: septic shock, pneumonia, cervical lymphadenopathy, and, rarely, arthritis and pericarditis.

PROGNOSIS

- Mortality is estimated at 8% in hospital series.
- Virtually all cases in which arrest occurred prior to transfer to tertiary center resulted in fatality.
- Mortality should approach zero with appropriate airway management.

 Differential Diagnosis

- Viral laryngotracheobronchitis (croup) with secondary bacterial tracheitis
- Severe parainfluenza or influenza infection
- Peritonsillar or retropharyngeal abscess
- Uvulitis
- Retropharyngeal abscess
- Peritonsillar abscess
- Foreign-body aspiration in a child with an upper respiratory infection
- Upper respiratory infection, including croup, in a child with a congenital or acquired airway problem (e.g., premature infant with subglottic stenosis, laryngeal web, vascular ring, tracheal stenosis)
- Diphtheria: rare in United States
- Laryngeal infections, including laryngeal tuberculosis

 Data Gathering

HISTORY

- Abrupt onset of high fever (39°C–40°C), sore throat, and dysphagia
- Very limited or no prodrome of mild upper respiratory illness
- Rapid onset of toxicity and respiratory distress
- Cough and hoarseness are late symptoms, if they occur at all.
- Time from onset of symptoms to presentation with progressive respiratory distress is generally less than 12 hours.
- Has the child been immunized against *H. influenzae* type B?
- How does the child prefer to hold itself? (i.e., sitting upright, leaning forward with chin hyperextended)

 Physical Examination

- Extremely anxious appearance
- Child prefers to remain sitting up.
- Child often leaning forward with chin hyperextended to maintain airway
- Slow and labored respiratory effort
- Drooling is seen as a manifestation of dysphagia.
- Inspiratory stridor, retractions, and late cyanosis
- Diagnosis can be suspected on history and observation of child's appearance alone.
- Do *not* attempt to examine the throat if epiglottitis is a serious consideration.

 Laboratory Aids

TESTS

- CBC: increased white blood cell count with left shift
- Cultures of blood (positive in up to 90%) and epiglottis (only performed in the operating room): may be positive for the causative organism.

IMAGING

- Lateral neck radiograph: showing characteristic "thumb sign" of edematous epiglottis, with narrowing of the posterior airway and ballooning of the hypopharynx

Therapy

- Airway management: maintain child upright, *never supine*. Personnel experienced in airway management should accompany the child at all times, including during transport and in radiology.
- Rapid assembly of a team, which should include an anesthesiologist, an otolaryngologist, and a pediatrician, if possible.
- Allow the child to assume his or her most comfortable position (usually in the mother's arms).
- Oxygen by mask or blown by face
- Transport to operating room as soon as possible for anesthesia and intubation, followed by positive pressure ventilation as necessary.
- Institute intravenous catheterization and blood collection and culturing of epiglottis only after the airway is secured.
- Perform emergent cricothyrotomy if obstruction occurs prior to controlled airway management.
- Use fluid resuscitation in cases of septic shock.

DRUGS

- Empiric antibiotic coverage to include gram-positive cocci and β-lactamase-producing *H. influenzae* type B. Duration of therapy: 7 to 10 days for all but staphylococcal disease (14–21 days). Switch may be made to oral medication after extubation and resumption of feeding.
- Cefuroxime: 150 mg/kg/d divided every 8 hours
- Ampicillin/sulbactam: 200 mg/kg/d divided every 6 hours
- Chloramphenicol: 75 to 100 mg/kg/d divided every 6 hours
- Ampicillin: 100 to 200 mg/kg/d divided every 6 hours for non-β-lactamase-producing *H. influenzae* type B (approximately 80% of isolates)
- Penicillin: 100,000 to 200,000 U/kg/d divided every 4 to 6 hours for streptococcal disease
- Oxacillin: 100 to 200 mg/kg/d for staphylococcal disease

Follow-Up

- Extubation is usually possible within 24 to 48 hours. Criteria include: decreased epiglottis erythema and edema upon direct inspection, and development of an air leak around the endotracheal tube.
- Defervescence is usually prompt after initiation of appropriate antimicrobial therapy.

PREVENTION

- Rifampin: 20 mg/kg/d in single dose for 4 days to eradicate colonization
- Universal immunization with *H. influenzae* type B capsular polysaccharide conjugate vaccines at 2, 4, and 6 months, with booster at 12 to 18 months

ISOLATION OF HOSPITALIZED PATIENT

Droplet precautions should be continued for at least 24 hours from the initiation of effective therapy.

CONTROL MEASURES

- Prophylaxis for index case and susceptible children in household, child care setting, and intimate contacts

PITFALLS

- A radiograph is indicated only when the diagnosis is in doubt, and should not delay airway management.
- Blood collection should be avoided until the airway has been secured, so as not to upset the child unnecessarily.
- Failure to ensure appropriate airway management prior to any other interventions, including laryngeal examination, radiographs, and laboratory studies

Common Questions and Answers

Q: What is the incidence of epiglottitis since the introduction of conjugate vaccines against *H. influenzae* type B?
A: Because *H. influenzae* type B caused 90% of epiglottitis, and the incidence of all invasive disease due to *H. influenzae* type B has decreased by 98% in children under 5 years of age, one can estimate that the incidence of epiglottitis has been reduced by almost 90%.

Q: Have there been reports of epiglottitis caused by *H. influenzae* type B after complete vaccination?
A: Yes, eight cases due to *H. influenzae* type B were reported in the United States during the 2-year period of 1994 to 1995.

Q: How many of the cases of invasive disease due to *H. influenzae* type B occur in children with inadequate vaccination?
A: During 1994 and 1995, 47% of children under 4 years of age were too young (aged 5 months or younger) to have completed a primary series with an Hib-containing vaccine. Among children old enough to be fully vaccinated, 63% of those developing disease were undervaccinated, and the remainder (37%) had completed a primary series in which vaccine failed.

Q: Should a fully vaccinated child who develops invasive disease due to *H. influenzae* type B be tested for an underlying immunodeficiency?
A: Probably. In one study, about one-third of children diagnosed with invasive disease due to *H. influenzae* type B were found to have a previously undiagnosed immunoglobulin deficiency.

Q: Can epiglottitis recur?
A: Yes, but rarely.

Q: Are corticosteroids of any value in the management of epiglottitis?
A: There appears to be no benefit.

ICD-9-CM 464.30

BIBLIOGRAPHY

American Academy of Pediatrics. *Haemophilus influenzae* infections. In: Peter G, ed. *1997 red book: report of the Committee on Infectious Diseases*, 24th ed. Elk Grove, IL: American Academy of Pediatrics, 1997:220–230.

Blackstock D, Adderly RJ, Steward DJ. Epiglottitis in young infants. *Anesthesiology* 1987;67:97–100.

Gonzalez-Valdepena H, Wald ER, Rose E, et al. Epiglottitis and *Haemophilus influenzae* immunization: the Pittsburgh experience—a 5-year review. *Pediatrics* 1995;96:424–427.

Grodin M. *Epiglottitis. J Emerg Med* 1983;1:13–19.

Hickerson SL, Kirby RS, Wheeler JG, Schutze GE. Epiglottitis: a 9-year case review. *South Med J* 1996;89:487–490.

Wenger JK. Supraglottitis and group A streptococcus. *Pediatr Infect Dis J* 1997;16:1005–1007.

Author: Mark L. Bagarazzi

Epstein-Barr Virus (Infectious Mononucleosis)

 Database

DEFINITION

Epstein-Barr virus (EBV) is a double-stranded DNA virus, and was implicated as the causative agent for infectious mononucleosis by 1968.

PATHOPHYSIOLOGY

- EBV replicates initially in the oropharyngeal epithelium.
- Selective infection of B-lymphocytes occurs.
- The clinical syndrome of infectious mononucleosis results from proliferation of cells in the tonsils, lymph nodes, and spleen.
- Nonspecific humoral immune responses include the formation of heterophil antibodies and autoantibodies.
- Specific antibodies to EBV antigens are produced.
- Despite humoral responses, cellular immunity is responsible for controlling EBV infection.
- Latent, lifelong infection of B-lymphocytes occurs.
- Latent virus can be reactivated during periods of immunosuppression.

EPIDEMIOLOGY

- Worldwide distribution
- Humans are the only known reservoir.
- EBV spreads between individuals in saliva, and occasionally via blood transfusions.
- The incubation period is 30 to 50 days.
- Antibodies to EBV are almost universally present in adult populations.
- Populations with a high population density or low socioeconomic status usually become primarily affected within the first 3 years of life.
- In developed countries, acquisition of EBV is biphasic:

—The initial peak in incidence occurs before the age of 5 years.
—The second peak occurs during adolescence, coinciding with an increased frequency of intimate oral contacts.

COMPLICATIONS

- Dehydration

—Severe pharyngitis often limits fluid intake.
—Is the most common problem requiring hospitalization

- Streptococcal pharyngitis

—Between 5% and 25% of patients with acute EBV infection may have concomitant group A streptococcal pharyngitis.

- Antibiotic-induced rash

—Morbilliform in appearance
—Most common after administration of ampicillin or amoxicillin
—Rare association with penicillin
—Usually benign, resolves with discontinuation of the aminopenicillin

- Splenic rupture

—Incidence of approximately 1 in 1,000 patients
—More common in males
—Half of the cases of splenic rupture are spontaneous; half follow blunt trauma.

- Airway obstruction

—May result from massive lymphoid hyperplasia and mucosal edema

PROGNOSIS

- Most patients with primary EBV infection will recover uneventfully in 1 to 4 weeks.
- Long-lasting immunity generally ensues.
- Prognosis of patients with unusual manifestations of EBV infection depends on the severity of the illness and the organ system involved.
- Patients with inherited or acquired immunodeficiency are at higher risk of complications and neoplasms.

ASSOCIATED ILLNESSES

- Subclinical infection

—The majority of EBV infections in children, and even in adolescents, are clinically inapparent.
—Mild, nonspecific symptoms may include coryza, diarrhea, and/or fever.
—Immunologic seroconversion does occur.

- Infectious mononucleosis ("glandular fever")

—Most commonly observed with late primary acquisition of EBV
—The classically defined illness is characterized by:
    —Fatigue
    —Malaise
    —Fever
    —Tonsillopharyngitis (often exudative)
    —Lymphadenopathy
    —Splenomegaly
—Usually associated with increased numbers of atypical lymphocytes in the peripheral blood

- Rare illnesses of the nervous system have been reported:

—Guillain-Barré syndrome
—Bell palsy
—Aseptic meningitis
—Meningoencephalitis
—Peripheral and/or optic neuritis

- Hematologic disorders have been reported in rare association with EBV:

—Aplastic anemia
—Hemolytic anemia
—Hemolytic-uremic syndrome

- Other illnesses associated with EBV in case reports:

—Hepatitis
—Pancreatitis
—Myocarditis
—Mesenteric adenitis
—Orchitis
—Genital ulcerative disease

- Congenital infection

—Primary EBV infection during pregnancy is uncommon.
—Although rare, TORCH-like congenital defects may conceivably be linked to EBV.

- Lymphoproliferative disorders

—EBV is suspected of occasionally playing a role in the etiology of the lymphoproliferative disorders:
    —Burkitt lymphoma
    —Nasopharyngeal carcinoma
    —Lymphoma and non-Hodgkin lymphoma (in immunocompromised children)
    —Virus-associated hemophagocytic syndrome
    —Lymphomatoid granulomatosis

- Chronic fatigue syndrome

—EBV, as well as many other infectious and environmental agents, have been proposed to contribute to this vague clinical syndrome.

 Differential Diagnosis

- Infectious mononucleosis is an illness with characteristic clinical features caused by EBV. Other causes of the infectious mononucleosis syndrome include:

—Adenovirus
—Cytomegalovirus
—*Toxoplasma gondii*
—Human herpes virus-6
—Human immunodeficiency virus
—Rubella

 Data Gathering

HISTORY

- A prodrome may occur:

—Commonly lasts 2 to 5 days
—Malaise, fatigue, 6 ± fever

- The following features are common:

—Fatigue
—Malaise
—Anorexia
—Fever
—Sore throat
—"Swollen glands"

- Young children are more likely to have a rash or abdominal pain.

Physical Examination

- Tonsillopharyngitis

—May be exudative and mimic streptococcal pharyngitis
—Often accompanied by palatal petechiae

- Lymphadenopathy

—Most prominent in cervical chains
—May be diffuse
—Usually nontender

- Hepatosplenomegaly

—Splenomegaly occurs in over half of cases.
　—Even if not palpable, splenomegaly may be demonstrated on ultrasound.
　—Most prominent in second to fourth week of illness
—Hepatomegaly is less common.

Laboratory Aids

TESTS

- CBC with differential

—Leukocyte count up to 20,000/mm³
—Lymphocytosis
—Atypical lymphocytes often comprise more than 10% of total leukocyte count.
—Thrombocytopenia may occur.

- Liver enzymes

—Mild hepatitis often is found.
—Jaundice is rare.

- "Monospot" (mononucleosis rapid slide agglutination test for heterophil antibodies)

—Detects heterophil antibodies (nonspecific IgM antibodies to unrelated antigens)
—Often negative in children under 6 years of age
—Detects 90% of cases in adolescents and adults

- EBV serology

—Usually reserved for heterophil-negative patients where strong clinical suspicion persists
—Antibodies detected by indirect immunofluorescence or ELISA techniques
—Acute or past infection can usually be detected and differentiated.

- Other technology

—Tissue culture of EBV is difficult and therefore not clinically useful.
—Polymerase chain reaction may detect EBV genetic material.

False Positives

- CBC

—Atypical lymphocyte counts greater than 10% of the total leukocyte count also occur with cytomegalovirus and toxoplasmosis infections.

- Monospot

—False-positive tests are infrequent.
—Heterophil antibodies are also produced in serum sickness and neoplastic processes.
—Heterophil antibodies may persist for months after acute infection and be indicative of past illness.

PITFALLS

- Heterophil antibodies may not appear early in the illness.
- Up to 10% of patients with acute EBV infection may have no heterophil response 3 weeks into the illness.
- The heterophil response is less common in infants and children.

Therapy

- Supportive care and symptomatic treatment will be sufficient for most cases of primary EBV infection.
- Acetaminophen or ibuprofen will reduce fever and provide analgesia.
- Oral, and sometimes IV, rehydration is often indicated.
- Corticosteroids (prednisone, 1 mg/kg/d divided into two doses) may reduce swelling of lymphoid tissues (see section, Common Questions and Answers)

—Indicated for patients with impending airway obstruction
—May be considered for patients with severe tonsillopharyngitis requiring IV hydration
—May be considered for patients with rare, life-threatening manifestations of EBV infection, such as hepatitis, aplastic anemia, and CNS dysfunction

- Acyclovir has not been shown to provide clinical benefit.

PREVENTION

- No vaccine is clinically available.
- Hospitalized patients need not be isolated when rigorous handwashing is employed.
- Restriction of intimate contact with immunosuppressed individuals may be advisable.
- Patients with recent EBV infection, either proven or suspected, should not donate blood.

Follow-Up

- Immunocompetent individuals usually recover uneventfully in 1 to 4 weeks.
- Recovery is often biphasic, with a worsening of symptoms after a period of improvement.
- Splenomegaly may persist for weeks after primary infection (see section, Common Questions and Answers).
- Fatigue may persist months after recovery.

Common Questions and Answers

Q: Should all patients with infectious mononucleosis be given corticosteroids?
A: Even though children may feel tired, weak, and ill, symptomatic EBV infection is most often self-limited with only symptomatic care. Long-term effects from the use of steroids to treat EBV are not known. EBV has been linked to certain lymphoproliferative disorders, and theoretical risks to modulating the host immune response with corticosteroids have been proposed.

Q: How long after infectious mononucleosis may a patient return to athletic activity?
A: Over half of patients with "mono" will have a boggy, enlarged spleen. This enlarged spleen is prone to rupture even if it is not palpable. All athletic activity should be restricted until no evidence exists for a clinically enlarged or tender spleen. If this criterion is met, and the patient feels subjectively better, light (noncontact) activities may be resumed. Return to contact sports is not advised until at least 4 to 6 weeks after resolution of all signs and symptoms of illness. Some experts recommend ultrasound study of the spleen before a return to heavy contact sports such as rugby, football, lacrosse, and hockey.

ICD-9-CM 075

BIBLIOGRAPHY

Chetham MM, Roberts KB. Infectious mononucleosis in adolescents. *Pediatr Ann* 1991;20:206–213.

Durbin WA, Sullivan JL. Epstein-Barr virus infection. *Pediatr Rev* 1994;15:63–68.

Hickey SM, Strasburger VC. What every pediatrician should know about infectious mononucleosis in adolescents. *Pediatr Clin North Am* 1997;44:1541–1556.

Peter J, Ray CG. Infectious mononucleosis. *Pediatr Rev* 1998;19:276–279.

Sumaya CV. Epstein-Barr virus infections in children. *Curr Probl Pediatr* 1987;Dec:682–722.

Author: Kevin C. Osterhoudt

Erythema Multiforme

 Database

DEFINITION

Erythema multiforme (EM) is an acute self-limited cutaneous eruption with many different multiform lesions. It is characterized classically as a target or iris lesion, but can appear as erythematous macules, papules, vesicles, and bullae with mucosal involvement. There are many triggers of EM, which is thought to encompass a spectrum of disease from relatively mild disease (EM minor) to severe forms with more than one mucosal surface involved (EM major or Stevens-Johnson syndrome). Some authors include toxic epidermal necrolysis (TEN) as the most severe form of EM, characterized by widespread erythema, bullae, and sloughing of large sheets of skin, with significant morbidity and mortality.

CAUSES

• The major causes of EM, which is thought to be an immune-mediated reaction, include drugs such as sulfa, penicillin, and phenytoin, and infections such as herpes simplex virus and *Mycoplasma*.
• There are a host of other etiologic factors, including exposure to various chemicals and tumors. The eruption usually occurs 1 to 2 weeks after the initial exposure.
• Often, the causative factor is not identified.
• Recurrent EM is generally secondary to herpes simplex virus.

GENETICS

Although simultaneous cases in family members have been reported, the disease is not genetic.

PATHOLOGY

The pathologic findings vary according to the lesion examined. Biopsy reveals necrosis of keratinocytes to varying degrees, depending on the clinical lesion biopsied. There is moderate-to-severe papillary dermal edema with mild-to-moderate perivascular dermal infiltrate composed predominantly of mononuclear cells and also some eosinophils (particularly if drug-related). Subepidermal blistering may be seen. Extravasated blood cells are found, but there is no evidence of vasculitis. Hydropic degeneration of the basement membrane also can be seen, as can epidermal spongiosis.

EPIDEMIOLOGY

• Erythema multiforme is seen in approximately 1% of all dermatology patients and has an equal incidence in men and women. (Some studies suggest a slightly higher incidence of EM minor in women.)
• The disease occurs predominantly in young adults and is believed by some to occur more frequently in spring and summer, with the more severe form of EM major occurring in the winter.

COMPLICATIONS

• Erythema multiforme minor is generally self-limited, with rare complications.
• In EM major, mucosal involvement can lead to stricture formation of the urethra, trachea, and esophagus, as well as conjunctivitis, corneal erosions, and, rarely, blindness.
• Pneumonitis, nephritis, hepatitis, and infection are other reported complications.
• In TEN, mortality and morbidity are high, with death occurring from sepsis.

 Differential Diagnosis

Classic presentation with targetoid lesions and mucosal involvement is generally not a diagnostic challenge; however, given the many forms of presentation, the diagnosis of EM can be difficult. The differential diagnosis can be extensive, depending on the presentation, and includes:

• Viral exanthem
• Bullous impetigo
• Staphylococcal scalded-skin syndrome
• Bullous pemphigoid
• Urticaria
• Urticarial vasculitis
• Systemic lupus erythematosus
• Serum sickness
• Pemphigus vulgaris
• Secondary syphilis
• Chicken pox
• Rocky mountain spotted fever

 Data Gathering

HISTORY

The cutaneous findings are sometimes preceded by a prodrome with fever and malaise. A careful drug and exposure history, as well as any signs or symptoms of infection or herpetic lesions, may reveal the etiologic cause. Inquire in detail about the patient's drug history, over-the-counter preparations, and signs or symptoms of infection or herpetic lesions.

Physical Examination

- Erythema multiforme classically appears as target lesions characterized by a dark, dusky center surrounded by a pale zone and then a zone of erythema. The lesions are typically acrally distributed.
- The lesions occur in many forms and can appear as red macules, papules, urticarial lesions, or vesicles and bullae.
- Mucosal involvement with superficial denudation can occur in the eyes, nasopharyngeal mucosal, or anogenital region.

 ## Laboratory Aids

TESTS

- There are no diagnostic laboratory tests; however, biopsy is often helpful, and other tests may help identify a cause.
- A WBC count with differential, looking for eosinophilia, may help identify a drug as causative.
- Cultures and chest x-ray study to evaluate for herpes or pneumonia
- Cold agglutinins associated with *Mycoplasma*
- Antistreptolysin-O titers and leukocytosis may identify a particular infectious cause.
- ESR may be elevated, but is nonspecific.
- A chest x-ray study may help identify an infectious cause of EM.

 ## Therapy

MILD FORMS

- Mild forms of EM resolve spontaneously without scarring and require only supportive therapy, including antihistamine or topical steroid for pruritus associated with the lesions.
- Oral lesions are often painful, and oral preparations to swish and spit, made of viscous lidocaine or diphenhydramine, may provide relief.
- Treatment of the underlying process is helpful (e.g., acyclovir for herpes simplex virus-associated cases).

ERYTHEMA MULTIFORME MAJOR

- May be life-threatening and can require hospitalization
- Supportive care, ophthalmology consultation, monitoring of fluid and electrolyte balance, and vigilant watch for infection are necessary.
- Antibiotics, analgesics, and local care including compresses with acetic acid soaks or saline will help decrease the incidence of infection.
- The use of systemic steroids is controversial, but when helpful, they are given early in the course of disease for approximately 2 weeks when there is no contraindication, such as infection.

TOXIC EPIDERMAL NECROLYSIS

- High associated mortality is often secondary to infection.
- Care is ideally at a burn center, with careful attention to infection and to fluids and electrolytes.
- Antibiotics, local compresses with acetic acid, or saline can help prevent superinfection.
- The use of systemic steroids is controversial, and is most effective when started early. The benefits and risks, including infection, must be weighed.

 ## Follow-Up

- Mild forms of EM are acute and self-limited, with lesions resolving in 2 to 4 weeks, with postinflammatory hyperpigmentation or hypopigmentation.
- Sequelae due to mucosal scarring can occur.
- Severe forms of EM major or TEN have associated morbidity and mortality.
- When recurrent, EM is often associated with herpes simplex virus.

ICD-9-CM 695.1

BIBLIOGRAPHY

Bondi EE, Jegasothy BV, Lazarus GS. *Dermatology diagnosis and therapy*. Norwalk, CT: Appleton & Lange, 1991.

Duvic M. Erythema multiforme. *Dermatol Clin* 1983;1(2):493–496.

Huff JC, Weston WL, Tonnessen MG. Erythema multiforme: a critical review of characteristics, diagnostic criteria and causes. J *Am Acad Dermatol* 1983;8(6):763–775.

Lever WF, Schaumberg-Lever G. *Histopathology of the skin*, 7th ed. Philadelphia: Lippincott, 1990.

Weston WL, Badgett JT. Urticaria. *Pediatr Rev* 1998;19(7):240–244.

Author: Christen Mowad

Erythema Nodosum

 ## Database

DEFINITION

Erythema nodosum is a delayed, cell-mediated hypersensitivity syndrome characterized by red, tender, nodular lesions that are usually on the pretibial surface of the legs and occasionally on other areas of the skin where subcutaneous fat is present.

CAUSES

• Thought to be a result of a host hypersensitivity immune response to circulating immune complexes secondary to infectious and/or inflammatory stimuli, resulting in chronic injury to the blood vessels of the reticular dermis and subcutaneous fat
• There are many associated triggering/underlying diseases:

—In children
    —Streptococcal infection and tubercular infection are the most common causes.

—In older patients
    —Streptococcus and sarcoidosis are most common.
    —Drugs (oral contraceptives, sulfonamides, iodides/bromides, phenytoin)
    —Infection (streptococcal infection, tuberculosis, psittacosis, histoplasmosis, yersiniosis, lymphogranuloma venereum, cat-scratch disease, coccidioidomycosis, upper respiratory infection)

• Systemic (sarcoidois, inflammatory bowel disease, Hodgkin disease, Behçet disease)
• Pregnancy

PATHOLOGY

• Septal panniculitis: lymphocytic perivascular infiltrate in the dermis; lymphocytes and neutrophils in the fibrous septa in the subcutaneous fat
• In older lesions, histiocytes, giant cells, and occasionally plasma cells are seen.
• No fat-cell destruction or vasculitis is present.

EPIDEMIOLOGY

• Girls are affected more often than boys.
• Most cases seen in the third decade, but not uncommon after age 10
• Greatest seasonal incidence in spring and fall

 ## Differential Diagnosis

• Infection
—Erysipelas/cellulitis
—Superficial or deep thrombophlebitis
—Erythema induratum
—Deep fungal infection
—Angiitis

• Environmental (poisons)
• Tumors
• Trauma
• Bruise
• Metabolic

—Panniculitis secondary to pancreatic disease
—Congenital

• Immunologic

—Major insect bite reaction
—Psychosocial

• Miscellaneous
• Weber-Christian (thighs and trunk) lesions may suppurate and heal with atrophy/localized depression.

PROGNOSIS

• Most individual lesions will completely resolve in 10 to 14 days.
• In general, erythema nodosum resolves in 3 to 6 weeks with or without treatment, unless the underlying cause is a chronic infection or systemic disorder.
• Aching of legs and swelling of ankles may persist for weeks; rarely, symptoms may persist for up to 2 years.
• In children, the recurrence rate is 4% to 10% and is often associated with repeated streptococcal infection.

 ## Data Gathering

HISTORY

• In over 50% of patients, a history of arthralgia is noted 2 to 8 weeks prior.
• Prodromal symptoms of fatigue/malaise or upper respiratory infection precedes by 1 to 3 weeks.
• Patients often present with pain and tenderness of extremities, sometimes to the point of difficulty in ambulation.

 ## Physical Examination

• Red nodules on anterior lower legs, 2 to 6 cm in diameter
• Overlying skin is normal except for erythema.
• Initially, lesions are bright to deep red with palpable warmth.
• Later, lesions develop a brownish red or violaceous, bruiselike appearance.
• Smaller lesions are slope-shouldered nodules.
• Larger lesions are flat-topped plaques.

SPECIAL QUESTIONS

• Medication history (oral contraceptives, sulfonamides, iodides/bromides)
• Last menses (erythema nodosum is seen in pregnancy)
• History of diarrhea (inflammatory bowel disease or infectious diarrhea)
• TB exposure

PHYSICAL EXAMINATION TRICKS

• Erythema nodosum never ulcerates or suppurates.
• Usually, there are no more than six lesions at a time.
• As a rule, both legs are affected.

Laboratory Aids

TESTS

- Throat culture
- Antistreptolysin-0 titer
- PPD
- CBC
- ESR
- Stool culture, if history of diarrhea
- Serologic testing, if yersiniosis, histoplasmosis, or coccidioidomycosis suspected
- Chest x-ray study, if diagnosis is in doubt
- Excisional biopsy specimen for histopathology, bacterial and fungal cultures is helpful

False Positives

Bilateral hilar adenopathy may also be seen with coccidioidomycosis, histoplasmosis, TB, streptococcal infection, or lymphomamatosis.

 ## Therapy

- Identification and treatment of underlying cause
- Bed rest and leg elevation

DRUGS

- Salicylates or other NSAIDs, such as naproxen or indomethacin
- Potassium iodide, 300 mg PO tid for 3 to 4 weeks, especially for cases diagnosed early in course
- Corticosteroids are effective, but rarely necessary.
- Duration: 2 to 4 weeks

 ## Follow-Up

WHEN TO EXPECT IMPROVEMENT

- Within 2 to 3 days
- Return visit in 1 week

SIGNS TO WATCH FOR

If lesions recur after cessation of treatment, underlying infection may worsen as well.

 ## Common Questions and Answers

Q: Will the lesions leave a scar?
A: Erythema nodosum virtually always heals without scarring.

ICD-9-CM 695.2

BIBLIOGRAPHY

Hurwitz S. *Clinical pediatric dermatology: a textbook of skin disorders of childhood and adolescence,* 2nd ed. Philadelphia: WB Saunders, 1993.

Author: Carmen M. Parrott

Ewing Sarcoma

 Database

DEFINITION

Ewing sarcoma is the second most common malignant bone tumor in children and adolescents. It represents a family of tumors, including Ewing sarcoma of bone, extraosseus Ewing sarcoma (arises in soft tissue adjacent to bone), and peripheral neuroectodermal tumor (PNET) of bone or soft tissue. The cause of Ewing sarcoma is unknown.

PATHOLOGY

• One of the "small round blue" cell tumors of childhood
• In approximately 90% of cases, the characteristic translocations t(11;22) and the minority t(21;22) can be detected
• Often a large soft-tissue component is present.
• Necrosis and hemorrhage are common.
• The PNET variant has more neural differentiation.

GENETICS

• Majority of cases occur sporadically
• Not associated with familial cancer syndromes

EPIDEMIOLOGY

• Second most common malignant bone tumor of children and young adults
• Approximately 110 new cases are diagnosed in the United States each year.
• Sixty-four percent occur in the second decade of life.
• More common in males than in females
• Ninety-six percent of cases in Caucasian population; extremely rare in Asians and blacks
• Associations (rare): skeletal anomalies (endochondroma, aneurysmal bone cyst), genitourinary anomalies (hypospadius, duplicated renal collecting system), Down syndrome, hereditary retinoblastoma

COMPLICATIONS

• Pathologic fracture
• Cord compression secondary to vertebral involvement
• Metastatic spread is seen in 20% at diagnosis. Sites include lung, bone, and bone marrow; liver and lymph nodes are less often involved.

PROGNOSIS

• Overall, 50% to 70% of patients can be cured.
• Favorable prognostic features

—Localized disease
—Primary site: distal bones, rib
—Tumor size less than 100 mL or 8 to 10 cm
—Age less than 10 years
—Histologic response to chemotherapy: no viable tumor at time of surgical resection

• Unfavorable prognostic features

—Metastatic disease at diagnosis, especially involving bone or bone marrow (<30% disease-free survival)
—Primary site: pelvis
—Elevated LDH
—Presence of neural differentiation

 Differential Diagnosis

• Malignant

—Osteosarcoma
—Neuroblastoma
—Non-Hodgkin lymphoma
—Rhabdomyosarcoma

• Nonmalignant

—Osteomyelitis
—Trauma/fracture
—Langerhans cell histiocytosis (eosinophilic granuloma)
—Benign bone tumor (giant-cell tumor) or cyst

 Data Gathering

HISTORY

• Presenting symptoms and their frequency of occurrence:

—Local pain (85%)
—Local swelling (60%)
—Fever (30%)
—Paraplegia, back pain (2%)

• Systemic symptoms (fever, weight loss) are more common in patients with metastatic disease
• Delay between first symptom and diagnosis is quite common; the duration of symptoms ranges from 4 weeks to 4 years, with an average of 9 months.

 Physical Examination

• Can develop in any bone of the body, with equal involvement of flat and long bones (unlike osteosarcoma, which arises more commonly in long bones)
• Distribution of primary sites include the following:

—Extremities (53%): usually begins in the midshaft; lower extremities affected more than upper extremities
—Central axis (47%): pelvis (45%), chest wall (34%), spine or paravertebral (12%), head or neck (9%)

 Laboratory Aids

TESTS

Laboratory Tests

• CBC
• Electrolytes, liver and renal function tests, serum calcium, phosphorus in anticipation of starting chemotherapy

Imaging and Other Tests

To evaluate primary site and confirm diagnosis

• X-ray (bony destruction with "onion skinning" appearance most often seen)
• CT scan or, preferably, MRI scan
• ^{99m}Tc-diphosphonate bone scan
• Serum LDH
• Biopsy: In addition to routine morphologic and immunohistochemical stain assessments, analysis of tumor chromosomes by traditional cytogenetics, fluorescent in situ hybridization, or reverse transcriptase PCR is helpful in making the diagnosis and may provide information regarding prognosis. Because of the importance of these studies, consultation with a pediatric oncologist *before* the biopsy is strongly encouraged.

To evaluate for evidence of distant metastases (present in 20% of patients at diagnosis)

• Chest radiograph and CT scan
• ^{99m}Tc-diphosphonate bone scan
• Bilateral aspiration and biopsy of iliac bone marrow

Therapy

- Therapy is a multimodal approach based on location and extent of disease: surgery; chemotherapy (common agents used include vincristine, doxorubicin, cyclophosphamide, etoposide, and ifosfamide); and radiation therapy.
- All patients with localized disease at diagnosis also have tumor cells outside the primary site that cannot be detected by standard measures; chemotherapy is therefore essential for cure.
- Duration of therapy depends on location and extent of disease.
- The surgical trend is toward less radical surgery, with limb preservation.
- Most children are treated according to large cooperative group protocols at pediatric oncology centers.
- Treatment is characterized by significant side effects, including increased susceptibility to infection, severe mucositis, and poor nutritional status.
- Most patients require placement of an indwelling central venous catheter for the duration of their therapy.

Follow-Up

WHEN TO EXPECT IMPROVEMENT

All patients with Ewing sarcoma require approximately 30 to 48 weeks of chemotherapy to prevent recurrence in the original site of tumor or distant spread. However, some improvement in signs and symptoms is usually seen within the first several weeks of therapy.

ACUTE EFFECTS OF THERAPY

Therapy for Ewing sarcoma is intensive. Patients can expect many of the following side effects:

- Frequent admissions to the hospital for chemotherapy or complications of the therapy
- Complications from bone marrow suppressive effects of chemotherapy or radiotherapy:

—Anemia: Blood transfusions are usually necessary; erythropoietin (a stimulator of erythropoiesis) is given to many patients to reduce the number of transfusions required.
—Thrombocytopenia: Platelet transfusions are often necessary to reduce the risk of serious bleeding.
—Neutropenia: Increased risk of bacterial and fungal infections; G-CSF (granulocyte colony stimulating factor) is usually administered daily following chemotherapy to shorten the duration of neutropenia.

- Complications from the gastrointestinal side effects of chemotherapy or radiotherapy:

—Nausea and vomiting; relieved with ondansetron and other antiemetic agents

—Malnutrition secondary to reduced appetite and mucosal ulcerations; nutritional supplements (oral, nasogastric or parenteral) may be necessary.

- Complications from radiotherapy

—Skin erythema or breakdown
—Pathologic fracture or poor function

LATE EFFECTS OF THERAPY

Therapy for Ewing sarcoma is intensive, and is associated with significant long-term adverse effects. Regular follow-up with a pediatric oncologist is strongly recommended. These late effects of therapy include the following:

- Cardiomyopathy

—Anthracyclines (doxorubicin) weaken cardiac muscle, leading to reduced left ventricular function many years after therapy.
—Approximately 5% of patients receiving cumulative doses of doxorubicin greater than 500 mg/m² will develop congestive heart failure.
—Radiation to the heart can lower the cumulative dose threshold to 300 mg/m².
—Any patient who has received an anthracycline should be cautioned against initiating strenuous physical activity without adequate preparation.
—Pregnant women who have received anthracyclines in the past should inform their obstetrician so that appropriate cardiac assessment can be completed prior to vaginal delivery.

- Kidney and bladder damage

—Urinalysis should be performed to detect hemorrhagic cystitis or tubular damage with spilling of sugar, protein, and phosphate into the urine.
—Blood pressure should be monitored in patients who received irradiation to the kidneys; vascular damage and hypertension may develop many years after therapy.

- Infertility and delayed puberty

—Reduced or absent gonadal function is related to high doses of alkylating agents (cyclophosphamide, ifosfamide): Males are at high risk of azoospermia; females may be fertile, but are at risk for premature menopause.
—Low-dose estrogen therapy with oral contraceptive medications may be necessary for amenorrheic women.

- Second malignant neoplasms

—Sarcomas may occur within the radiation field.
—Myelodysplastic syndromes and acute myeloid leukemia may occur secondary to radiation or chemotherapy (cyclophosphamide, etoposide).

- Growth abnormalities/functional defects at the primary site

—Radiation doses greater than 20 Gy will cause growth retardation in prepubertal children.
—Scoliosis can occur if the vertebrae are involved in the radiation field.

Common Questions and Answers

Q: At what time point is a child with Ewing sarcoma considered cured?
A: Typically, cure is measured as 5-year survival without evidence of disease. However, late relapses or second tumors do occur in children with Ewing sarcoma.

Q: Should a Ewing sarcoma be completely resected at the time of diagnosis?
A: Most times, this is not recommended, as Ewing sarcoma is very sensitive to chemotherapy, facilitating an improved delayed surgical resection.

Q: Should children with Ewing sarcoma take vitamins?
A: There is little information on the necessity and safety of vitamin supplementation during chemotherapy for Ewing sarcoma and other childhood malignancies. In general, supplementation at standard RDA dosing is safe, but high doses are not recommended.

ICD-9-CM 170.4

BIBLIOGRAPHY

Grier HE. The Ewing family of tumors: Ewing sarcoma and primitive neuroectodermal tumors. *Pediatr Clin North Am* 1997;44(4):991–1004.

Womer RB. Problems and controversies in the management of childhood sarcomas. *Br Med Bull* 1996;52(4):826–843.

Author: Kara M. Kelly

Exstrophy of the Bladder

 Database

DEFINITION

Exstrophy is a complex of developmental anomalies of the cloacal membrane, affecting the genitourinary, musculoskeletal, and gastrointestinal systems. It is part of the epispadias-exstrophy complex that includes epispadias, bladder exstrophy, and cloacal exstrophy. In bladder exstrophy, there are defects in the abdominal musculature, exposing the bladder, with genital defects and possible rectal abnormalities. In cloacal exstrophy, the hindgut and bladder are exposed through the abdominal wall defect. Cloacal exstrophy is often associated with cardiac, gastrointestinal, renal, limb, and neurologic defects such as myelomeningocele and hydrocephalus. In epispadias, the urethral meatus is located on the dorsal aspect of the shaft of penis.

CAUSES

• Mesodermal tissue fails to reinforce the cloacal membrane caudally, which is necessary for the development of the lower abdominal wall musculature and pelvis, affecting the division of the cloaca into the bladder and the rectum by the urorectal septum.
• The cloacal membrane is thus predisposed to rupture; the timing of the rupture determines which variant of the epispadias-exstrophy complex develops.

GENETICS

• There is a 1 in 100 chance of recurrence in a family with an index case.
• There is a 1 in 70 chance of exstrophy in children of parents with exstrophy; this is a 500-fold greater incidence than in the general population.

EPIDEMIOLOGY

• Bladder exstrophy has an incidence of 1 in 30,000 live births.
• Male:female ratio is 2:1.
• Sixty percent of those born with this complex have classic bladder exstrophy.
• Thirty percent have a variant of epispadias (1 in 40,000–118,000 live births)
• Ten percent have cloacal exstrophy (1 in 400,000 live births)

—Other minor variants (i.e., superior vesical fissure): musculoskeletal defects like exstrophy but with opening of persistent cloacal membrane only at the uppermost portion
—Pseudoexstrophy: musculoskeletal defects but no major defect in the genitourinary tract

• Tends to occur in infants of younger mothers
• At higher parity there is an increased incidence of exstrophy, but not epispadias.

PROGNOSIS

• If left untreated, total urinary incontinence; in severe cases, death
• Increased incidence of bladder adenocarcinoma
• Sexual disability
• Broad-based gait due to widely spaced ischial rami
• In females, the main complications include cervical and uterine prolapse in pregnancy.
• Cesarean section is recommended in those who underwent functional bladder closure to preserve reconstructed urinary sphincter.
• After staged reconstruction

—Urinary continence, 43% to 82%
—Preserved renal function, 97%
—Satisfactory erection in males, 83%

 Physical Examination

BLADDER EXSTROPHY

• Widened symphysis pubis, widened distance between the hips, outwardly rotated lower limbs, resulting in a waddling gait

—Triangle-shaped defect in abdominal wall exposing bladder mucosa (may appear glistening or polypoid); with increased exposure, there is increased thickening of the epithelium.
—Divergent rectus muscles: At the top of the triangle is the umbilicus, which is downwardly displaced.
—A small umbilical hernia usually present.
—Indirect inguinal hernia due to persistent patent processus vaginalis and large diameter of internal and external inguinal rings

• Anorectal anomalies

—Short perineum, anteriorly displaced anus, at risk for rectal prolapse
—Defects in levator ani and puborectalis cause anal incontinence and rectal prolapse, especially if untreated; usually transient and easily reduced; usually resolves with surgical closure of bladder

• Male genital anomalies

—Short penis due to widely separated crura; open dorsally, exposing the urethra
—Dorsal chordee, short urethral groove
—The penis may be very small.
—Vas deferens and ejaculatory ducts are normal, with normal fertility possible.
—Most have retractile testes, shallow scrotum

• Female genital anomalies

—Usually less complex than male defects
—Short urethra and vagina
—Narrow and anteriorly displaced vaginal opening
—Bifid clitoris, widely separated labia, and mons pubis
—Normal uterus, fallopian tubes, and ovaries with normal fertility
—Occasional occurrence of uterine duplication

• Urinary anomalies

—Bladder mucosa is initially normal at birth, but ectopic bowel mucosa may be present.
—Mucosal changes may occur due to persistent infection.
—Bladder may be small and fibrosed.
—Usually normal upper urinary tract
—Horseshoe, pelvic, hypoplastic, solitary, or dysplastic kidney occasionally occurs.
—The distal portion of the ureter enters the bladder with little angulation, causing reflux in almost 100% of children with bladder exstrophy.

CLOACAL EXSTROPHY

- Exstrophic cecum and terminal ileal segment separating bladder into exstrophic halves
- Omphaloceles are seen and may include bowel, liver, or spleen.
- In boys, the penis is small and widely separated into two, making reconstruction often impossible, so female gender assignment is often recommended.
- In girls, there is a separated clitoris, bifid uterus, duplicate vagina, or exstrophic vagina.
- All have imperforate anus because the hindgut remains open.

EPISPADIAS

- In male epispadias, the urethral meatus may be penopubic, penile, or glanular.

—In penile or glanular, the bladder neck is competent, so continence is usually achieved.
—In penopubic epispadias, the bladder neck is often incompetent, so incontinence is common.
—Dorsal penile curvature is present in most.
—Epispadias may be concealed by foreskin or labia.

- In female epispadias, the urethra is large and patulous, with a bifid clitoris.

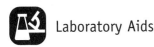

Laboratory Aids

TESTS

Imaging

- Prenatal sonography at 20 weeks gestation is very useful. Findings of absence of fluid in the bladder on repeat examinations, or presence of an echogenic mass on the lower abdominal wall, or a low-set umbilicus are consistent with the presence of bladder exstrophy.
- Radionuclide scans and ultrasound studies are needed to evaluate renal function and drainage of the collecting system.

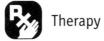

Therapy

CONSERVATIVE

- Ligate umbilical cord with suture, not a plastic clamp, in order to minimize trauma to bladder mucosa.
- Cover the bladder mucosa with plastic wrap at birth to minimize insensible fluid losses.
- Avoid petroleum jelly gauze and saline, which adhere to the mucosa.
- Ensure drainage of the urinary tract with a Foley catheter.

THREE STAGES OF SURGICAL REPAIR

- **Stage 1:** Attain initial closure within 72 hours of life, before there are permanent changes in the bladder wall.

—Bony structures are more pliable in newborns due to the maternal hormone, relaxin, and pelvic osteotomy may be avoided
—Reapproximate the ischial rami; reconstruct the bladder and urethra; close the abdominal wall.
—Provide prophylaxis with antibiotics postoperatively for at least 6 months because of vesicoureteral reflux.
—Evaluate the urinary tract with a radionuclide scan; if normal, follow up vesicoureteral reflux with ultrasound at 3 and 6 months, then at 12-month intervals for the next 2 years.
—May not be able to achieve functional closure if bladder is very small, but bladder size may be augmented with a colon graft
—The most common postoperative complication is bladder prolapse.
—Converts bladder exstrophy into complete epispadias with incontinence

- **Stage 2:** Penile and urethral reconstruction

—Repair epispadias at 1 to 2 years by releasing dorsal chordee, lengthening urethral groove and penis.
—The most common postoperative complication is the development of a fistula, which can be surgically repaired.
—Leaves child with total incontinence

- **Stage 3:** bladder neck reconstruction with bilateral ureteral reimplantation, usually at about 3 years of age

—The goal is to improve continence and prevent vesicoureteral reflux, and thereby preserve renal function by preventing upper tract infection.

Antibiotic prophylaxis is indicated, with regular follow-up evaluation of the upper tract and renal function.

- Staged reconstruction may not be possible if the bladder is extremely small, if there are upper tract changes (i.e., hydronephrosis), or if there are complex congenital anomalies that preclude extensive surgery.
- If the penis is very dystrophic, sex reassignment should be considered.
- If staged correction is not possible, urinary diversion is indicated.
- Ureterosigmoidostomy: Reimplantation of normal-sized ureters into the colon. Complications include pyelonephritis, hyperchloremic acidosis, rectal incontinence, ureteral obstruction, and late development of colonic tumors (22% in one study). Advantages are that no abdominal stoma is required, and continence and preservation of renal function may be adequately achieved.
- Ileocecal ureterosigmoidostomy has the advantages of ureterosigmoidostomy but without an apparent increased risk of cancer.
- Trigonosigmoidostomy does not have the complications of electrolyte imbalances or increased cancer risk but still maintains renal function and urinary continence.
- Ureterointestinal anastomosis with a colonic conduit: External stoma and appliance are required. Once rectal continence is achieved and reflux is shown to be absent, at 4 to 6 years, the conduit may be undiverted. Complications include postoperative colonic or ureteral obstruction (19% and 6%, respectively, in one study). No incidences of stomal complications, pyelonephritis, or persistent reflux are noted.
- Major postoperative complications include ureteral obstruction and bladder-outlet obstruction.

—In females, vaginal dilatation or episiotomy may be required for vaginal stenosis.
—Complications of staged repair include urinary tract infection in association with vesicoureteral reflux, which places upper tract and long-term renal function at risk

ICD-9-CM 753.5

BIBLIOGRAPHY

Kelalis P, King L, Belman A, eds. *Clinical pediatric urology.* Philadelphia: WB Saunders, 1992.

Zaontz MR, Packer MG. Abnormalities of the external genitalia. *Pediatr Clin North Am* 1997; 44(5):1267.

Author: Christina Lin Master

Floppy Infant Syndrome

Database

DEFINITION

"Floppy infant" connotes neuromuscular weakness, though central nervous system or nonneurologic problems must also be considered. This syndrome typically presents with decreased movement, abnormal posture due to weakness, or CNS dysfunction.

PATHOPHYSIOLOGY

There are two major categories of hypotonia:

• Hypotonia without significant weakness (nonparalytic)
• Hypotonia with significant weakness (paralytic)

GENETICS

• Numerous genetic, metabolic, and dysmorphic syndromes with varying patterns of inheritance may underlie hypotonia in infancy.
• The most common causes include the "central" causes, involving the cerebellum, brainstem, basal ganglia, and hemispheres.
• Less common causes are those afflicting peripheral nerves.
• Often, central hypotonia that is not due to CNS injury is benign in nature.

COMPLICATIONS

• Respiratory difficulties
• Recurrent pneumonia
• Poor nutritional status resulting from sucking and swallowing difficulties

ASSOCIATED ILLNESSES

• Metabolic disorders
• Hip dislocation
• Gastroesophageal reflux
• Motor delay

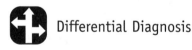

Differential Diagnosis

COLLAGEN DISEASES AND SYSTEMIC ILLNESSES

• Ehlers-Danlos syndrome
• Marfan syndrome
• Osteogenesis imperfecta
• Congenital laxity of ligaments

SYSTEMIC DISORDERS

• Sepsis
• Malnutrition
• Cyanotic heart disease
• Renal acidosis
• Hypercalcemia
• Rickets
• Hypothyroidism
• Cystic fibrosis
• Malnutrition
• Sepsis

• Intestinal obstruction (volvulus, intussusception)
• Disorders of connective tissue and other systemic illnesses may produce hypotonia without weakness.
• Hypotonia may be the sole presenting sign in infectious, metabolic, or gastrointestinal illness.
• "Benign congenital hypotonia" denotes a common clinical picture of nonparalytic hypotonia in older infants whose physical examination reveals only hypotonia. These infants have, at most, only mild motor delay and no other neurologic or pertinent physical abnormalities. By definition, the creatine kinase level is normal. Laboratory and diagnostic studies are normal, and prognosis is good.

FLOPPY INFANT SYNDROME (<6 MONTHS OF AGE) BY SYSTEM

Disorders Involving Cerebral Cortex, Cerebellum, Brainstem

• Nonspecific mental retardation
• Hypotonic cerebral palsy
• Intracranial hemorrhage
• Malformations
• Infections
• Toxic
• Metabolic encephalopathies
• Hypoxic-ischemic encephalopathies
• Genetic/chromosomal anomalies such as Down and Prader-Willi syndromes
• Aminoacidurias
• Mucopolysaccharidoses
• Organic acidurias
• Sphingolipidoses

Disorders Involving Spinal Cord

• Myelodysplasias (meningomyeloceles, diplomyelia, diastematomyelia)
• Traumatic transection (often seen with breech deliveries)

Paralytic Hypotonia

• Floppy infants whose physical examination reveals significant motor weakness and decreased or absent deep tendon reflexes
• Differential diagnosis in this category involves mainly disorders of anterior horn cell, peripheral nerve, neuromuscular junction, and muscle.

Disorder of Anterior Horn Cell

• Hereditary spinal muscular atrophy (Werdnig-Hoffman)
• Poliomyelitis (polio or other enteroviridae)

Disorders of Peripheral Nerve

• Dejerine-Sottas disease
• Guillain-Barré syndrome
• Rare causes include giant neuroaxonal dystrophy, congenital hypomyelinating neuropathy, familial dysautonomia (Riley-Day syndrome), metachromatic and Krabbe leukodystrophy, and neonatal Guillain-Barré syndrome.

Disorders of Neuromuscular Junction

• Transient and congenital myasthenia gravis
• Botulism
• Toxic blockade secondary to aminoglycoside antibiotics (especially in infants with renal failure), nondepolarizing neuromuscular blockers (prolonged postoperative hypotonia)
• Hypermagnesemia secondary to treatment of preeclampsia in the mother

Disorders of Muscle

• Congenital structural myopathies such as:

—Central core
—Nemaline rod
—Myotubular
—Mitochondrial
—Glycogenosis
—Lipid storage disease
—Congenital myotonic dystrophy
—Congenital muscular dystrophy
—Metabolic myopathies

PITFALLS

• Hypermagnesemia is a common cause of apnea in the intensive care nursery.
• Fasciculations are overdiagnosed and should be included in the clinical picture only when they are noticed at rest.
• Airway protection is of primary concern in all hypotonic infants.

Data Gathering

HISTORY

Important factors to obtain in the history include:

• Fetal movements
• Delivery
• Gestational maturity
• Apgar scores
• History of the perinatal period
• Infections, recent illnesses, and medications
• Family history
• Motor milestone achievement

Physical Examination

The physical examination usually indicates whether floppy infant syndrome is due to a neurologic dysfunction, and, if so, whether it is centrally or peripherally based. It should include the following:

• Evaluation of mental status
• Infants with hypotonia secondary to a neuromuscular process often appear very bright and alert despite their weakness.
• Those with CNS dysfunction will likely have cognitive involvement.

• In nonparalytic hypotonia, the infant may initially appear weak and floppy, but spontaneous movements of the limbs occur readily against gravity. Posture and tone should be noted in the supine position, in ventral suspension, and with traction. Look for the presence of a "scarf" sign.

• Reflexes may be difficult to obtain in the newborn; the presence of brisk tendon reflexes in a hypotonic child almost always signifies that hypotonia is due to cerebral dysfunction. Further development may reveal spastic cerebral palsy.

• Tongue fasciculations are best seen at the lateral margins of the tongue as spontaneous rippling movements; the infant is still (not crying). They are most commonly associated with denervation as seen in spinal muscular atrophy.

• Facial weakness (decreased expression) is often seen with congenital myotonic dystrophy, myotubular myopathy, congenital muscular dystrophy, congenital facial diplegia, trauma, or Moebius syndrome.

• Ptosis/opthalmoplegia suggests myotubular myopathy, mitochondrial myopathy, congenital muscular dystrophy, myasthenia gravis, or congenital fibrosis syndrome.

• Arthrogryposis and contractures are seen in congenital muscular dystrophy, myotonic dystrophy, and neuropathies.

• Hip dislocation should be considered in any hypotonic child. To screen for this, Ortolani maneuver and hip x-ray studies should be done.

• Weakness and respiratory problems are seen in many conditions, such as spinal muscular atrophy, myotonic dystrophy, myotubular myopathy, nemaline myopathy, and congenital muscular dystrophy.

• Swallowing/sucking difficulties can be seen in myotubular myopathy, myotonic dystrophy, nemaline myopathy, and neonatal myasthenia.

• Weakness and loss of tone in the lower extremities with active use of the upper extremities suggests spinal cord injury.

 ## Laboratory Aids

TESTS

• Specifics of the presentation will guide laboratory studies. Initial work-up may include a urinalysis, electrolytes, creatine kinase (CK), thyroid studies, and amino and organic acid screen.

• EMG/nerve conduction velocity (NCV) is very useful to localize neuromuscular involvement. If both the CK and EMG/NCV are abnormal, a muscle biopsy should be done to better define the underlying pathology. If the CK and EMG/NCV are normal and the clinical examination points toward CNS involvement, an MRI should be considered.

• A tensilon test may be done if repetitive stimulation on the EMG suggests myasthenia. Acetylcholine receptor antibodies may also be obtained in the work-up of myasthenia.

• Stool samples should be evaluated for *Clostridium* when botulism is suspected.

• A lumbar puncture may be carried out to rule out systemic illnesses, as well as look for increased protein, which may be seen in peripheral nerve disease.

• An MRI or CT with contrast of the spine should be done in a child with a suspected spinal cord injury.

• Elevated lactate and pyruvate levels may be helpful in looking for mitochondrial disease.

 ## Therapy

• Acute respiratory distress or hypoventilation in a weak, hypotonic infant must be anticipated and may require oxygen support as well as aggressive pulmonary toilet, antibiotic therapy, and perhaps even ventilator assistance.

• Sucking and swallowing difficulties may necessitate nutritional support via NG tube feedings and supplementation.

• Underlying toxic or metabolic causes should be addressed and treated appropriately.

• Spinal cord injury may also cause respiratory embarrassment. Steroid therapy should be considered within the first 8 hours of the injury.

• For transient myasthenia gravis, medical therapy is often not needed. However, anticholinesterase medications and plasmapheresis may be necessary for infants with significant respiratory or feeding difficulties.

• Immunotherapy may also be appropriate for infants with Guillain-Barré syndrome or polymyositis. Immunosuppressive agents used in the acute phase include IV immunoglobulin and plasmapheresis.

• Botulism antitoxin trivalent is used in some centers to treat infantile botulism.

• For many of the congenital myopathies and other neuromuscular disorders, treatment is primarily supportive, and active physical therapy is needed to minimize contractures and maximize strength and mobility. Spinal deformities such as scoliosis should be evaluated on a regular basis, as surgical intervention may be necessary.

• Orthopedic consultation to evaluate hips, and contractures may be helpful.

 ## Follow-Up

• In infants whose hypotonia is secondary to CNS involvement, developmental milestones and early intervention will need to be closely monitored in order to evaluate the degree of motor and cognitive impairment.

• Spinal cord injury can have a devastating effect on a child; this will depend on the location and severity of the injury as well as on treatment.

• Generally, in infants with spinal muscular atrophy Type I (Werdnig-Hoffman), the earlier the onset, the poorer the prognosis. Approximately 60% die by the age of 2 years, and 80% by the age of 4. Outcome for many of the con-

genital myopathies and dystrophies depends not only on the specific disease, but also on the age of onset and associated respiratory and feeding difficulties.

• Transient neonatal myasthenia with any of the symptoms listed earlier usually resolves by 8 weeks of age. However, infants with congenital myasthenia gravis usually require long-term therapy, depending on the underlying pathology. Symptoms may persist into childhood and adulthood.

• Infants with botulism may recover completely in weeks to months if adequate medical and supportive therapy is administered.

PITFALLS

• Hypermagnesemia is a common cause of hypotonia in neonates whose mothers were treated for eclampsia. Intensive care monitoring is required because of the risk of apnea.

• Infants with acute/subacute onset of paralytic hypotonia (e.g., botulism, Guillain-Barré syndrome) may lose airway protective reflexes before neurogenic hypoventilation. Pooling of secretions/decreased gag may prompt intubation.

• Intussusception may present with hypotonia. Rectal examination may reveal the diagnosis.

 ## Common Questions and Answers

Q: By what age should one expect resolution of benign congenital hypotonia?
A: Hypotonia should not be evident by the time the infant is walking; a delay in walking beyond 15 months casts doubt on the diagnosis.

Q: When and how should spinal muscular atrophy (SMA) be ruled out?
A: SMA is a consideration in any infant with insidious onset of significant weakness with arreflexia. Electrophysiologic and (muscle) pathology findings are usually definitive.

ICD-9-CM 781.9

BIBLIOGRAPHY

Brooke M. *A clinician's view of neuromuscular diseases,* 2nd ed. Baltimore: Williams & Wilkins, 1986.

Dubowitz V. *Muscle disorders in childhood.* Chicago: Year Book, 1989.

Parush S, Yehezkehel I, Tenenbaum A, Tekuzener E, Bar-Efrat-Hirsch I, Jessel A, Ornoy A. Developmental correlates of school-age children with a history of benign congenital hypotonia. *Dev Med Child Neurol* 1998;40(7):448–452.

Stiefel L. Hypotonia in infants. *Pediatr Rev* 1996;17(3):104–105.

Weiner H, Bresnan M, Levitt L. *Pediatric neurology for the house officer,* 2nd ed. Baltimore: Williams & Wilkins, 1982.

Author: Meena Scavena Baldi

Food Allergy

 Database

DEFINITION

"Food allergy" is often implicated in many gastrointestinal symptoms of children. This belief may lead to extreme elimination diets, placing children at significant nutritional risk. Food hypersensitivity is defined as a reproducible response to food in which an immunologic mechanism is incriminated. Food intolerance is defined as symptoms that are modulated by nonimmunologic mechanisms (i.e., lactose intolerance).

PATHOPHYSIOLOGY

• The pathophysiology of food allergy is poorly understood and may involve both the classic Type I immediate hypersensitivity reaction (linked to IgE) or Type IV delayed-type hypersensitivity reaction (non-IgE-mediated).
• The gastrointestinal mucosal immune system is complex, involving antigen presentation via M cells, macrophages, and dendritic cells to lymphocytes in Peyer's patches, which further subspecialize into B cells, which secrete IgA and IgM, and T cells, which secrete cytokines such as IL-5, which act as eosinophil chemoattractants. Both eosinophils and mucosal mast cells also may play roles in allergic responses to food.

EPIDEMIOLOGY

• The prevalence of true food hypersensitivity has been estimated between 1% and 3%.
• Approximately half of patients with atopic dermatitis had at least one food allergen exacerbating their disease.

 Differential Diagnosis

Any pathologic process leading to colitis in infancy should be considered in the differential diagnosis of allergic colitis, including:

• Infectious colitis
• Hirschsprung enterocolitis
• Inflammatory bowel disease
• Behçet syndrome

In patients with eosinophilic gastroenteropathy, the differential includes:

• Inflammatory bowel disease
• Drug allergy
• Hypereosinophilic syndrome
• Celiac disease
• Autoimmune enteropathy

 Data Gathering

• A careful history is important for identifying suspected food allergens; however, it is important to remember that less than half of the reported food reactions will be confirmed on double-blinded placebo-controlled challenges.
• Key pieces of information include type of symptoms, frequency of symptoms, timing of symptoms from ingestion, and quantity of food leading to response.
• In the acute reaction, urticaria, angioedema, exacerbation of atopic dermatitis, and certainly hypotension will lead to supportive evidence for true food allergic response.
• Anaphylaxis is one of the more dramatic presentations of food allergy. It may be systemic or limited to the oropharynx. Systemic anaphylaxis presents with vomiting, pallor, urticaria, listlessness, and respiratory and cardiovascular compromise. Oral allergy syndrome is localized to the oropharynx and consists of urticaria and angioedema. The symptoms of oral anaphylaxis tend to resolve rapidly.
• IgE-ediated reactions:

—Type I reactions are more common in infants, with 50% of these reactions occurring in the first year, 20% in the second, and 10% after 2 years.
—Egg, milk, peanuts, soy, nuts, wheat, and fish account for 90% of food reactions in children.
—Forty percent of these patients developed tolerance to the offending food with in 1 to 2 years.

• Non-IgE-mediated reactions:

—Eosinophilic colitis most commonly secondary to cow's milk/soy protein allergy. Infants present with diarrhea associated with blood and mucus in the stool in an otherwise healthy patient. The syndrome has been described in exclusively breast-fed infants who are exposed to antigens transmitted through the breast milk.
—Eosinophilic gastroenteropathy may also occur in patients with cow's milk/soy allergy. These infants often present with protracted vomiting, diarrhea, failure to thrive, iron deficiency anemia, and hypoalbuminemia. The disease process may involve the mucosa, muscularis, or serosa of the bowel.
—Eosinophilic esophagitis presents with gastroesophageal reflux, dysphagia, and poor growth. Intense eosinophilic infiltration of the mucosa is seen on biopsy. Often, pH probe studies are negative or equivocal. The family history may be remarkable for atopy. Both IgE- and non-IgE-related mechanisms for the development of this entity are under investigation.
—Respiratory symptoms as the only manifestation of food allergy are rare. Often, respiratory symptoms accompany other systemic or gastrointestinal symptoms. No studies at this time have proven a link between food allergy and chronic cough or wheezing.

Laboratory Aids

• In patients with suspected IgE-mediated food hypersensitivity, skin prick testing may be helpful in defining the offending allergen. A panel of common allergens is often used, including milk, soy, egg, peanuts, fish, and wheat.

• Testing with the natural foods may be necessary if there is a high index of suspicion and the commercially prepared extracts do not elicit a response.

• Age is an important factor in interpreting skin-prick tests:

—For patients less than 1 year of age, a response is highly significant because the presence of IgE in this age group is unusual; a negative skin test will not rule out allergy in this group.

—For those patients over 1 year, skin testing is 90% to 100% sensitive; therefore, a negative test makes IgE-mediated reactions highly unlikely. In non-IgE-mediated food hypersensitivity, skin-prick tests will be negative. Radioallergosorbent (RAST) testing does not appear to add to the diagnostic yield when performed with skin testing.

—Open, single, or double-blinded food challenges are helpful if there is no improvement on elimination of the suspected food allergen from the diet.

—Double-blinded food challenges may be best way to define a reproducible reaction.

—Further laboratory aids under investigation include lymphocyte proliferation assays and patch skin testing.

Therapy

• For anaphylaxis:

—Full monitoring of vital signs
—Diphenhydramine for milder symptoms
—Epinephrine, if significant respiratory or cardiovascular symptoms persist. All patients at risk for anaphylaxis to foods should have epinephrine for home use and a Medi-Alert bracelet.

• For nonanaphylactic reactions:

—Elimination of the suspected food allergen from the diet. This must be done carefully to maintain adequate nutrition for the child. If the symptoms resolve with elimination, the next step is to reintroduce the allergen to determine if the symptoms are reproducible. If the patient responds to dietary restriction, the elimination diet may be continued for 1 to 3 months. The patient may then be rechallenged at that time to determine if tolerance to the offending agent has been established. If the symptoms persist, the pediatrician should consider referral to a specialist for further evaluation and management. Education of the family and caregivers is vital to this therapy. It may be very difficult to identify those foods that may contain the offending allergen. Referral to a dietitian or nutritionist may aid in this education.

Follow-Up

A prolonged elimination diet is usually not necessary. Tolerance to allergens usually develops over time. In one study, 28% were tolerant at 2 years, 56% by 4 years, and 78% by 6 years. IgE-mediated disease tends to persist longer. Even children with a history of severe allergic reactions will most likely eventually outgrow them.

Common Questions and Answers

Q: Do you recommend elimination diets?
A: No, because doing so often can result in malnutrition without identifying the exact allergen in any specific circumstance. Double-blinded food challenges are the best way to identify the offending agent.

Q: What are the common allergens?
A: Most initial blood tests will screen for allergy to milk, egg, soy, chocolate, fish, nuts, and egg white.

ICD-9-CM 693.1

BIBLIOGRAPHY

Bischoff SC, Herrmann A, Manns MP. Prevalence of adverse reactions to food in patients with gastrointestinal disease. *Allergy* 1996;51:811–818.

Bischoff SC. Mucosal allergy: role of mast cells and eosinophil granulocytes in the gut. *Baillieres Clin Gastroenterol* 1996;10(3):443–459.

Bishop JM, Hill DJ, Hosking CS. Natural history of cow's milk allergy: clinical outcome. *J Pediatr* 1990;116:862–867.

Bock A, Sampson H. Food allergy in infancy. *Pediatr Clin North Am* 1994; 41(5):1047–1067.

Burks AW, Sampson HA. Diagnostic approaches to the patient with suspected food allergies. *J Pediatr* 1992;121:S64–S71.

Justinich C. Food allergy and allergic enteropathy. In: Hyams JS, Wyllie R, eds. *Pediatric gastrointestinal disease: pathophysiology, diagnosis, and management.* (in press).

Odze RD, Wershil BK, Leichter AM, et al. Allergic colitis in infants. *J Pediatr* 1995;126(2):163–170.

Sampson HA, McCaskill CC. Food hypersensitivity and atopic dermatitis: evaluation of 113 patients. *J Pediatr* 1985;107:669–675.

Young E, Stoneham MD, Petruchevitch A, et al. A population study of food intolerance. *Lancet* 1994;343:1127–1130.

Author: Donna Zeiter

Food Poisoning

 Database

DEFINITION

Rapid onset of diarrhea, vomiting, and fever 12 to 72 hours after the ingestion of contaminated food

CAUSES

• See the table Epidemiologic Aspects of Food Poisoning in Section VIII of this book.
• Variety of bacteria: most common are *Campylobacter*, *Salmonella* (non-typhoid), and *Shigella*.

PATHOLOGY

• Ingestion of preformed toxin
• Elaboration of toxin from bacteria into the gastrointestinal tract
• Direct invasion of mucosa by bacteria

EPIDEMIOLOGY

At least 300 outbreaks of food-borne disease are reported each year.

 Differential Diagnosis

INFECTION

• Parental infections:

—Upper respiratory tract
—Urinary tract infections
—Otitis media

• *Escherichia coli*
• *Vibrio*
• *Clostridium difficile*
• *Yersinia enterocolitica*
• *Aeromonas hydrophilia*
• *Giardia lamblia*
• *Entamoeba histolytica*
• Rotavirus
• *Campylobacter jejuni*, most common
• *Listerosis*
• *Vibriosis*
• *Yersinia*

FOOD INTOLERANCE/FOOD ALLERGIES

• Cow's milk protein allergy
• Carbohydrate intolerance (most common is lactose)

MISCELLANEOUS

• Use of antibiotics
• Malnutrition

—Altered mucosal structure
—Defective disaccharidase activity
—Abnormal motility
—Changed intestinal bacterial flora

DIETARY MANIPULATIONS

• Hyperosmolar formulas
• Food additives (dyes, processing materials, coloring)
• Caffeine
• Overfeeding
• Low fat intakes (especially during recovery phase)
• Excessive fluids

 Data Gathering

HISTORY

• Outbreak of illness following ingestion of a meal
• Others in family with similar symptoms
• Time of onset of vomiting after ingestion—relates to type of bacterial toxins (see the table Clinical Aspects of Food Poisoning in Section VIII of this book)
• *E. coli*, *Campylobacter*, and *Salmonella* are more frequent in summer months

 Physical Examination

• See table Clinical Aspects of Food Poisoning in Section VIII of this book.
• Botulism

—Severity related to host susceptibility and to amount of toxin ingested
—Disease may be so mild that consultation is not obtained; in other cases, it is fatal within a few hours.
—Generalized hypotonia
—Absent deep tendon reflexes
—Dilated, reactive pupils
—Poor suck
—Decreased to absent gag reflex
—Ptosis

 Laboratory Aids

TESTS

• Isolation of the organism from stools and the suspected food
• Demonstrating the toxin in the suspected food
• Identifying 10^5 organisms per gram of suspected food
• Finding 10^6 organisms or spores per gram of patient's stool or vomitus
• Lesions on the hands of food handlers may be the source of contamination and should be cultured.

Botulism

• Toxin in stools is diagnostic.
• Stool culture for *Clostridium botulinum*
• Electromyography with repetitive stimulation
• Lumbar puncture to exclude other diagnoses

Enterohemorrhagic E. coli *O157:H7*

• Latex agglutination test

Food Poisoning

 Therapy

- No specific treatment
- Intramuscular antiemetics
- If clinically dehydrated, rehydration can be accomplished in 4 to 6 hours, using an oral solution containing 75 to 90 mEq Na/L.
- IV fluids for patients unable to be rehydrated via the oral route (because of ileus, circulatory failure, CNS complications), or with stool losses greater than 10 mL/kg/hr
- Most foods (except for lactose) should be tolerated in the pediatric patient recovering from food poisoning.
- The "BRATT" diet (bananas, rice, applesauce, toast, tea) is inappropriate for the management of acute diarrheal episodes, due to low calorie, protein, and fat contents.
- A balanced, varied diet, providing easily digestible, complex carbohydrates, will promote increased stool consistency.

DRUGS

Antibiotics

Salmonella

- Not used in patients with uncomplicated gastroenteritis
- Does not shorten the duration of the disease
- Can prolong the duration of excretion of *Salmonella* organisms
- Antimicrobial therapy is warranted for *Salmonella* gastroenteritis occurring in patients with an increased risk of invasive disease and other complications:

—Infants under 3 months of age
—Patients with malignancies
—Hemoglobinopathies
—AIDS
—Recipients of immunosuppressive therapy
—Persons with chronic gastrointestinal tract disease
—Patients with severe colitis

- Ampicillin, amoxicillin, trimethoprim-sulfamethoxazole, cefotaxime, or ceftriaxone is recommended for susceptible strains in patients for whom therapy is recommended.

Botulism

- Supportive care
- Monitor cardiac and respiratory function.
- Endotracheal intubation and assisted ventilation
- Avoid aminoglycosides.

 Follow-Up

PROGNOSIS

- Most gastroenteritis secondary to food poisoning is mild and self-limited.
- Recovery is complete in 2 to 5 days in most individuals.
- In the very young, the prognosis is more guarded, because these patients can become dehydrated quickly.
- Once the patient has survived the paralytic phase of botulism, the outlook for complete recovery is excellent.

PREVENTION

- Parenteral vaccines are not recommended for use in children.
- Botulism in infants, 1 year:

—Wash objects placed in infants' mouths (pacifiers, toys, etc.).
—Wash or peel skin of fruits and vegetables.
—Avoid honey.

 Common Questions and Answers

Q: What are the most common causes of food poisoning?
A: Bacteria (*Salmonella, Staphylococcus*).

Q: How are the signs and symptoms of food poisoning different from a viral gastroenteritis?
A: The signs and symptoms of food poisoning and gastroenteritis are similar in that the patient displays diarrhea, vomiting, and fever. Usually, food poisoning occurs after ingestion of a meal, at which time several people can be affected.

Q: Which foods are most likely to be contaminated?
A: Dairy products that are not refrigerated properly and meat that is not cooked at high enough temperatures.

ICD-9-CM 005.9

BIBLIOGRAPHY

Salmonella infections, staphylococcal infections. In: Peter G, ed. *1994 Red book: report of the Committee on Infectious Diseases,* 23rd ed. Elk Grove Village, IL: American Academy of Pediatrics, 1994:412, 423.

Todd EC. Epidemiology of food-borne diseases: a worldwide review. World Health Stat Q 50(1–2):30–50.

Wolfle J. Kowalewski S. Epidemiology of ingestions in a regional poison control center over twenty years. *Vet Hum Toxicol* 1995;37(4):367–368.

Authors: Timothy A.S. Sentongo and Andrew E. Mulberg

Frostbite

Database

DEFINITION

Frostbite is localized injury of the epidermis and underlying tissue resulting from exposure to extreme cold or contact with extremely cold objects. Distal extremities and unprotected areas (fingers, toes, ears, nose, and chin) are most commonly affected. Frostbite is classified according to severity:

• Superficial, first-degree: partial skin freezing
• Superficial, second-degree: full-thickness skin freezing
• Deep, third-degree: full-thickness skin and subcutaneous tissue freezing
• Deep, fourth-degree: full-thickness skin, subcutaneous tissue, muscle, tendon and bone freezing

PATHOPHYSIOLOGY

• Tissue damage and cell death result from the initial freeze injury and the inflammatory response that occurs with rewarming.
• Direct cellular damage can occur from frostbite. As the temperature of freezing tissue approaches minus 2°C, extracellular ice crystals form and cause increased osmotic pressure in the interstitium. This leads to cellular dehydration. As freezing continues, these shrinking, hyperosmolar cells die due to abnormal intracellular electrolyte concentrations. With rapid freezing, intracellular ice crystal formation occurs, resulting in immediate cell death.
• Indirect cellular damage results from progressive microvascular insult. Initial tissue response to extreme cold exposure is vasoconstriction. Blood flow to the extremities is reduced as freezing continues. Ice crystals form in the plasma, blood viscosity increases, and cessation of circulation occurs in the distal extremities, resulting in hypoxia and tissue damage.
• Oxygen free radicals and inflammatory mediators, especially prostaglandin F2 and thromboxane A2, contribute to tissue injury following rewarming and reperfusion of the damaged tissue.

EPIDEMIOLOGY

• Frostbite is most common in adults aged 30 to 49 years.
• The feet and hands account for 90% of frostbite injuries.
• The following are persons at-risk:

—Mentally ill patients
—Patients with impaired circulation
—Winter sport enthusiasts and fans
—Homeless persons
—Malnourished people
—Outdoor laborers
—Military personnel exposed to cold, wet climates
—Elderly and very young patients

• Risk factors include:

—Alcohol
—Arthritis
—Atherosclerosis
—Constricting clothing
—Diabetes
—Hypothermia
—Immobilization
—Previous cold injury
—Smoking
—Vasoconstrictive drugs

COMPLICATIONS

• Arthritis
• Changes in skin color
• Chronic pain
• Digital deformities
• Gangrene
• Growth plate abnormalities (only in children)
• Hyperesthesias
• Tetanus
• Tissue loss
• Wound infection
• Squamous cell carcinoma (rare)

PROGNOSIS

• Dependent on degree of cold injury
• Favorable indicators: sensation in affected area, healthy-appearing skin color, blisters filled with clear fluid
• Unfavorable indicators: cyanosis, blood-filled blisters, unhealthy-appearing skin

Differential Diagnosis

• Frostnip: mild form of cold injury with pallor and painful, tingling sensation. Warming of the cold tissue results in no tissue damage.
• Hypothermia
• Thermal injury: easily excluded based on history, but can result from warming techniques

Data Gathering

HISTORY

Special Questions

• Was there prolonged exposure to cold environment? In frostbite, there is typically a history of prolonged cold exposure.
• Was there contact with a cold object, especially metal? Metal will drain heat from skin through conduction and increase the risk of frostbite.
• What was the timing and duration of exposure?
• Was there any treatment prior to presentation?

Symptoms depend on severity:

• Superficial, first-degree: transient tingling, stinging and burning followed by throbbing and aching with possible hyperhidrosis
• Superficial, second-degree: numbness with vasomotor disturbances in more severe cases
• Deep, third-degree: no sensation initially, followed by shooting pains, burning, throbbing, and aching
• Deep, fourth-degree: absent sensation and muscle function, pain, and joint discomfort

Physical Examination

• Superficial, first-degree: waxy appearance, erythema, and edema of involved area without blister formation
• Superficial, second-degree: erythema, significant edema, blisters with clear fluid within 6 to 24 hours. Desquamation may occur with eschar formation 7 to 14 days after initial injury.
• Deep, third-degree: hemorrhagic blisters, necrosis of the skin and subcutaneous tissues, skin discoloration in 5 to 10 days.
• Deep, fourth-degree: initially, little edema with cyanosis or mottling; eventually, complete necrosis, then becomes black, dry, and mummifies; occasionally results in self-amputation.

Laboratory Aids

TESTS

Laboratory tests usually are not necessary but may be indicated when infection is suspected.

Radiographic Studies

• No diagnostic studies done immediately after rewarming can accurately predict the amount of nonviable tissue.
• Radionucliotide angiography with ^{99}mTc-pertechnetate or bone scanning with ^{99}mTc-methylene diphosphonate 1 to 2 weeks after initial injury is advocated by some to assess tissue viability in cases of third- and fourth-degree frostbite.

Therapy

IMMEDIATE

• Do not rub the area; this may cause mechanical injury.
• Do not expose the area to direct heat; this may cause burn injury.
• Remove wet clothing and constricting jewelry.

MEDICAL CARE

- Check core temperature to rule out hypothermia, which would need to be addressed first.
- Rapid rewarming in warm water (40°C–42°C) for 15 to 45 minutes. *Do not* rewarm slowly. Rewarming is complete when skin is soft and sensation returns. Usually this is all that is needed for superficial, first-degree frostbite.
- Apply dry, sterile dressings to affected areas and between frostbitten toes and fingers.
- Drain clear-fluid blisters (thromboxane-containing) to avoid ongoing tissue injury.
- Leave hemorrhagic blisters intact in order to avoid infection.
- Elevate affected parts to minimize edema.
- Daily hydrotherapy with hexachlorophene or povidone-iodine added to the water
- Topical application of aloe vera to debrided blisters and intact hemorrhagic blisters to minimize further thromboxane synthesis
- Tetanus prophylaxis: dT or DT, depending on age, and tetanus immunoglobulin if patient never fully immunized
- NSAIDs are recommended by some to prevent prostaglandin-induced platelet aggregation and vasoconstriction.
- Analgesics, as indicated
- Antibiotics: given prophalactically by some, while others recommend waiting for signs of infection
- High-protein, high-calorie diet to promote healing
- Prohibit nicotine because of vasoconstrictive properties.
- Physical therapy after edema resolves

SURGICAL CARE

- Conservative surgical intervention is recommended because it usually takes 6 to 8 weeks for injured tissue to declare viability.
- Escharotomy is performed on digits with impaired circulation or movement.
- Fasciotomy is performed if significant edema causes a compartment syndrome.
- Early amputation and debridement with closure of the wound site are necessary for uncontrolled infection.
- Debridement of mummified tissue is performed after 1 to 3 months.

FUTURE TREATMENT

Experimental work is being done to identify agents that interrupt vasoconstriction, cell injury, and vascular stasis and those that inhibit prostaglandins and free radicals.

 Follow-Up

WHEN TO EXPECT IMPROVEMENT

- Superficial, first-degree frostbite heals in a few weeks.
- More severe frostbite needs to be followed closely for signs of infection.
- Physical therapy and rehabilitation are needed with severe frostbite.

PREVENTION

- Avoid prolonged cold exposure whenever possible.
- Dress appropriately for cold weather. Dress in layers: Undergarments should be made of material that absorbs perspiration and prevents heat loss, and outer garments should be windproof and water repellent/proof. Cover head, ears, and neck. Mittens help conserve heat better than gloves. Footwear should be water repellent and insulated.

PITFALLS

- Refreezing after thawing leads to increased injury.
- Rubbing tissue that is frostbitten increases injury through mechanical injury.

 Common Questions and Answers

Q: How can I protect my child from getting frostbite?
A: Limit the amount of time the child spends outdoors during extremely cold days—especially wet, cold, and windy days. Dress your child appropriately with layers of clothing. Outer garments should be waterproof. Make sure he or she is wearing a hat, scarf, and mittens. Have the child come inside frequently to warm up and for you to check for signs of cold injury.

Q: If my child has had frostbite in the past, can she get it again?
A: Yes, children who have had a previous frostbite injury are at increased risk for repeat injury, especially in the location of previous damage. Appropriate clothing and limitation of cold exposure should be strictly enforced.

Q: Are there any long-term effects of frostbite?
A: Severe, deep frostbite can lead to stunted growth of the affected area, especially the digits, resulting in deformities. Arthritis, chronic pain, skin discoloration, and cold sensitivity can also occur.

Q: How can I tell if my child has frostbite or just cold fingers?
A: Cold fingers are red and may be painful but do not become numb or white. Frostbitten fingers are painful, white, and waxy prior to rewarming and turn red with rewarming. The sequential development of digital blanching, occasional cyanosis, and erythema of the fingers or toes following cold exposure and subsequent rewarming is known as Raynaud's phenomenon. All types of cold injury should be treated by immersing the fingers in warm water for 15 to 45 minutes. If blisters form or there is no sensation in the fingers, medical care is needed.

Q: If I suspect frostbite in my child and we are stuck outdoors without access to warm water, are there any options for treatment?
A: Of course you would want to get indoors as soon as possible. If that is not possible, you can start to thaw your child's body part by using your body as a warmer, by placing the exposed body part under your armpit and keeping it there until further care can be initiated.

Q: When should I call the doctor?
A: The doctor should be called if, after rewarming, the skin is not soft and/or sensation does not return to normal. Call the doctor immediately if the skin is discolored and cold, blisters develop during rewarming, or there are signs of infection, such as the appearance of red streaks leading from the affected area, pus accumulation, or fever.

Q: What is chilblain?
A: Chilblain is a severe form of cold injury that commonly occurs on the face, anterior tibial surfaces, and dorsum of hands. It is a form of chronic vasculitis of the dermis that is provoked by repeated exposure to cold temperatures above freezing.

Q: Is frostnip the same thing as frostbite?
A: No, frostnip is the mildest form of cold injury that commonly occurs on exposed parts of the body, such as the fingers, nose, and ears. The symptoms of frostnip are numbness and pallor of the involved body parts. Warming of these areas is the only treatment that is needed, and there is no associated tissue damage.

ICD-9-CM 991.3

BIBLIOGRAPHY

Bracker MD. Environmental and thermal injury. *Clin Sports Med* 1992;2:419–436.

Britt LD, Dascombe WH, Rodriguez A. New horizons in management of hypothermia and frostbite injury. *Surg Clin North Am* 1991;71: 345–370.

Brown FE, Spiegel PK, Boyle WE. Digital deformity: an effect of frostbite in children. *Pediatrics* 1983;71:955–959.

Carrera GF, Kozin F, McCarthy DJ. Arthritis after frostbite injury in children. *Arthritis Rheum* 1979;22:1082–1087.

Holmer I. Work in the cold: review of methods for assessment of cold exposure. *Int Arch Occup Environ Health* 1993;65:147–155.

Reamy BV. Frostbite: review and current concepts. *J Am Board Fam Pract* 1998;11:34–40.

Author: Denise Salerno

Fungal Skin Infections
(Dermatophyte Infections, Candidiasis, and Tinea Versicolor)

 Database

DEFINITION

• Superficial mycoses (fungal infection) involving the skin, hair, or nails

ETIOLOGY

• Dermatophyte infections

—Tinea capitis: greater than 90% *Trichophyton tonsurans* in North America; *Microsorum canis* a predominant organism in other geographic regions
—Nonhairy sites: *M. canis, T. tonsurans, T. rubrum, M. audouinii*

• Candidiasis: usually *Candida albicans*
• Tinea versicolor: *Malassezia furfur* (also called *Pityrosporum ovale*)

PATHOPHYSIOLOGY

• Fungal elements penetrate skin, hair shaft, or nail.
• Predisposing factors may include moisture, macerated skin, and immune compromise.
• Fungistatic fatty acids in sebum after puberty may offer protection against tinea capitis.
• Host immune response is usually able to contain infection.
• Inflammatory response is variable; highly inflammatory forms may lead to pustular lesions and kerion (a large inflammatory mass) formation.

GENETICS

• Frequency and severity of infection are possibly determined by unclear genetic factors.
• Increased glycogen granules in the normal skin of patients with tinea versicolor suggests an underlying disorder or genetic predisposition.

EPIDEMIOLOGY

• Dermatophyte infections

—Etiology varies by geographic region.
—Tinea capitis is most common in prepubertal children.
—Tinea corporis is usually seen in younger children; tinea cruris, tinea pedis, and onychomycosis are uncommon in preadolescent children.
—Fomites and pets may be a source of infection.

• Candidiasis: vast majority of infants colonized with *C. albicans*.
• Tinea versicolor: usually seen in adolescents and young adults

COMPLICATIONS

• Dermatophyte infections

—Secondary bacterial infection (which may obscure the diagnosis of dermatophyte infection)
—Kerion may lead to scarring alopecia.

• Candidiasis

—Scarring in severe disease
—Fungemia in immunocompromised host

 Differential Diagnosis

• Dermatophyte infections

—Dermatologic conditions

—Tinea capitis: seborrheic dermatitis, psoriasis, alopecia areata, trichotillomania, folliculitis, impetigo
—Tinea corporis: herald patch of pityriasis rosea, nummular eczema, psoriasis, contact dermatitis, tinea versicolor, granuloma annulare

—Systemic diseases: cutaneous T-cell lymphoma, histiocytosis, primary skin cancer, sarcoid

• Candidiasis

—Dermatologic conditions: contact dermatitis, seborrheic dermatitis, atopic dermatitis, bacterial infection
—Systemic diseases: acrodermatitis enteropathica, histiocytosis

• Tinea versicolor

—Dermatologic conditions: pityriasis alba, postinflammatory hypopigmentation, vitiligo, seborrheic dermatitis, pityriasis rosea

PROGNOSIS

• Relapses and recurrences are not uncommon.
• Areas with a significant inflammatory component may lead to scarring and permanent alopecia.

 Data Gathering

HISTORY

• Onset is usually gradual, except for candidal diaper rash, which is often abrupt
• Usually pruritic

 Physical Examination

• Dermatophyte infections

—Tinea corporis
  —Skin lesions usually annular, hence the term *ringworm*
  —May be flesh-colored, erythematous, or violet to brown
  —Highly inflammatory forms may be frankly pustular.

—Tinea capitis may have various presentations:
  —Round to oval patches of alopecia with erythema
  —Seborrheic dermatitis-like pattern with minimal or no alopecia
  —Follicular pustules with crusting, resembling bacterial folliculitis
  —Boggy, tender plaque with follicular pustules (kerion)
  —Diffusely, dry scalp

—Onychomycosis
  —White, yellow, or silvery discoloration of lateral border or distal portion of nail
  —Nail eventually becomes discolored, thickened, and deformed.
  —Affects toes more often than fingers

• Candidiasis

—Diffuse erythema (often "beefy" red)
—Raised edge with a sharp margin
—Pustulovesicular, satellite lesions
—Prefers dark, warm, moist environments; favors skin folds/creases (axillae, groin, below the breasts, and in infants, the diaper area)

• Tinea versicolor

—Scaling, oval macular patches
—Hypopigmented or hyperpigmented, depending on sunlight exposure and complexion
—Distributed on upper trunk, neck, and proximal arms (high amount of sebum and free fatty acids which the organism requires); occasionally occurs on the face

 Laboratory Aids

TESTS

Diagnosis is usually made by characteristic lesions; if in doubt, may do Wood's lamp examination, potassium hydroxide (KOH) preparation, or fungal culture.

Wood's Lamp Examination (Short-Wave Ultraviolet Light)

- Examine in a completely darkened room.
- Dermatophytes: Hair infections caused by *Microsporum* species will give a green fluorescence; not helpful for skin or nail infections.
- Tinea versicolor: yellow, coppery-orange, or bronze fluorescence.

KOH Preparation

- Clean the site with alcohol.
- Scrape the lesion along the scaling edge with a blade; obtain material from hair follicles and crusts.
- Place material on glass slide with one drop of 10% KOH.
- Warm the slide gently or let it sit for 30 minutes.
- Place a cover slip on the slide.
- Examine the slide under the microscope at low power under low light.

Results

- Dermatophytes: arthrospores around or within hair shaft; long branching hyphae for skin infections
- Candidiasis: budding yeast, pseudohyphae
- Tinea versicolor: hyphae and spores ("spaghetti and meatballs")

Fungal Culture

- Obtain a specimen with scalpel blade or sterile toothbrush as described above.
- Results are available in several weeks.
- Some laboratories offer susceptibilities in addition to identification of fungus.
- It may be difficult to distinguish normal skin colonization from infection.

 Therapy

DRUGS

Dermatophyte Infections

- Tinea capitis

—First-line: Griseofulvin 15 to 20 mg/kg once daily, taken with high-fat food (e.g., milk or ice cream) for 6 to 12 weeks; concomitant therapy of 2.5% selenium sulfide shampoo twice weekly will suppress viable spores and decrease spread.
—Second-line: oral itraconazole 3 to 5 mg/kg once daily for 4 to 6 weeks.
—Kerion: Treat as tinea capitis; may require oral steroids if significant inflammation present

- Tinea corporis

—Drug of choice: topical imidazole applied twice daily for 2 to 4 weeks.
—Oral therapy may be used for persistent or extensive involvement.

- Onychomycosis

—Griseofulvin orally for 6 to 18 months (6 months for fingernails and 12–18 months for toenails)
—Itraconazole in weekly pulses for 3 to 4 months is effective; 200 mg twice daily for 7 days, then off for 3 weeks.

Candidiasis

- Topical nystatin three to four times daily for 7 to 10 days

Tinea Versicolor

- Selenium sulfide 2.5% applied to the affected skin for 10 minutes. Wash off thoroughly. Monthly applications may help prevent recurrences.
- Topical imidazoles are effective but more expensive.
- Oral ketoconazole 200 to 400 mg/d for 5 to 10 days, or itraconazole 200 mg/d for 5 to 7 days may be used if extensive, recurrent, or persistent.

POSSIBLE CONFLICTS WITH OTHER TREATMENTS

Many antifungals have drug interactions. Consult a reference (e.g., *Physician's Desk Reference*) when prescribing them to a patient already on medication.

 Follow-Up

WHEN TO EXPECT IMPROVEMENT

- Dermatophyte: Inflammation should improve within several days, but may take several weeks to completely resolve; nail infections may take 6 to 12 months to show improvement.
- Candidal skin lesions improve within 24 to 48 hours and resolve by 1 week.
- Tinea versicolor may take weeks to improve; repigmentation may take months and requires exposure to sunlight.

SIGNS TO WATCH FOR

- Watch for signs of secondary bacterial infection.
- Highly inflammatory lesions may require systemic steroids.

PREVENTION

- Children should be discouraged from sharing clothing (especially hats).
- Hair utensils and hats should be washed in hot, soapy water at the onset of therapy.
- Pets should be watched and treated early for any suspicious lesions.
- Isolation of the hospitalized patient is not necessary.

PITFALLS

- Tinea capitis requires systemic therapy.
- Application of topical steroids will decrease inflammation and may mask infection ("tinea incognito"). Use only mild steroids, if necessary.
- Repeated infection may indicate a source that needs to be diagnosed and treated (e.g., family member or pet).

 Common Questions and Answers

Q: When is oral therapy indicated for the treatment of dermatophyte infections?
A: Topical therapy is usually effective for infections of the skin; however, it penetrates hair and nails poorly. Tinea capitis and onychomycosis require oral therapy. Disease that is persistent and not responding to topical antifungals, or extensive disease, which makes topical application impractical, are also indications for systemic therapy.

Q: What is the role of topical and systemic steroids in the treatment of dermatophyte infections?
A: Topical corticosteroids may be helpful with antifungal therapy to reduce inflammation. Only mildly potent steroids should be used. Combination products containing a potent corticosteroid and an antifungal should be avoided, especially in the diaper area, where absorption may be increased.

Q: What can be done to prevent recurrent tinea versicolor in an adolescent?
A: *M. furfur* is a ubiquitous organism and is present on the skin of postpubertal individuals. Humid environments, excessive sweating, and unclear genetic factors result in infection. Recurrences are common and can be prevented by monthly application of selenium sulfide 2.5%.

ICD-9-CM

Dermatophyte 110.9
Candidiasis 112.9
Tinea Versicolor 111.0

BIBLIOGRAPHY

Friedman A. Superficial bacterial and fungal infections of the skin. *Adv Pediatr Infect Dis* 1990;5:205–219.

Goldgeier M. Fungal infections of the skin, hair and nails. *Pediatr Ann* 1993;22:253–259.

Rosenthal J. Pediatric fungal infections from head to toe: what's new? *Curr Opin Pediatr* 1994;6:435–441.

Smith M. Tinea capitis. *Pediatr Ann* 1996;25:101–105.

Suarez S. New antifungal therapy for children. *Adv Dermatol* 1997;12:195–209.

Authors: William R. Graessle and Jill A. Foster

Gastritis

 Database

DEFINITION

Gastritis is inflammation of the mucosa of the stomach. It is the most common cause of upper gastrointestinal tract hemorrhage in older children.

CAUSES

- *Helicobacter pylori* (children more likely to have more severe gastritis)
- Stress (e.g., in CNS disease, ICU patients)
- Idiopathic
- Caustic ingestions (e.g., lye, strong acids, pine oil)
- Drug-induced (e.g., NSAIDs, steroids, valproate)
- Ethanol
- Protein sensitivity (e.g., cow's milk protein allergy)
- Eosinophilic gastroenteritis
- Crohn disease
- Infection (e.g., tuberculosis, *H. pylori*, cytomegalovirus, parasites)

EPIDEMIOLOGY

- One of the most frequent GI diagnoses

COMPLICATIONS

- Bleeding (from mild to hemorrhagic)
- When gastritis caused by acid/alkali ingestions, outlet obstruction may result from prepyloric strictures.

 Differential Diagnosis

- Peptic ulcer disease
- Gastroesophageal reflux with esophagitis
- Pancreatitis
- Inflammatory bowel disease
- Lactose intolerance

 Data Gathering

HISTORY

- Epigastric pain
- Vomiting postprandially
- Irritability
- Poor feeding and weight loss
- Less often: chest pain, hematemesis, or melena

 Physical Examination

- Epigastric tenderness

 Laboratory Aids

TESTS

- Heme-test all stools.
- Anemia with other signs of chronic blood loss on CBC (e.g., microcytosis, low reticulocyte count)
- *H. pylori* antibody
- Culture of homogenized gastric biopsy for *H. pylori*
- Silver or hematoxylin and eosin stain of gastric biopsy for *H. pylori*

PROCEDURES

- Upper endoscopy with biopsies: sensitivity greatest
- When endoscopy not available, upper GI radiography

Gastritis

 Therapy

DRUGS

• Antacids or H₂ blockers to maintain gastric pH greater than 4

—Ranitidine, 2 to 3 mg/kg tid in children
—Cimetidine, 10 mg/kg qid
—Famotidine, 0.5 to 2.0 mg/kg/d divided twice
—Omeprazole, lansoprazole for resistant cases

• Discontinue NSAIDs.
• Eliminate alcohol and tobacco.

DIET

• Dietary changes not helpful
• Stress gastritis with hemorrhage
• Vigilant supportive care with close monitoring of hemodynamics, fluids, and electrolytes
• H. pylori

—H₂ blocker therapy for 8 weeks
—If symptoms persist, amoxicillin, bismuth, and metronidazole for 10 days
—Drug regimens change frequently.

 Follow-Up

• Monitor for hemoccult-positive stools.
• Follow complete blood counts.
• May elect to repeat endoscopy in severe cases

PITFALLS

• Antacids are not palatable to children and can lead to diarrhea or constipation.
• Ranitidine is less effective and can increase toxicity when given to patients receiving other medicines metabolized by the cytochrome P-450 system (e.g., theophylline)
• Significant relapse rates for H. pylori

 Common Questions and Answers

Q: Will a bland diet help to resolve gastritis?
A: Dietary changes have not been shown to affect the natural course of gastritis.

Q: What is Helicobacter pylori?
A: H. pylori is a bacterium frequently found in the gastric mucosa of patients with gastritis and peptic ulcer disease. Relapse rates for gastritis secondary to this cause are high and can be diagnosed by a combination of upper endoscopy and urea breath tests.

ICD-9-CM 558.9

BIBLIOGRAPHY

Berquist WE. New, improved Helicobacter pylori eradication therapy in children. J Pediatr Gastroenterol Nutr 1998;26(3):360–361.

Cox K, Ament ME. Upper gastrointestinal bleeding in children and adolescents. Pediatrics 1979;63:408–413.

Czinn SJ. Helicobacter pylori gastroduodenal disease in infants and children. In: Wyllie R, Hyams JS, eds. Pediatric gastrointestinal disease. Philadelphia: WB Saunders, 1993:429, 434.

Eule AR. Gastritis. In: Wyllie R, Hyams JS, eds. Pediatric gastrointestinal disease. Philadelphia: WB Saunders, 1993:435–446.

Hassall E, Dimmidk JE. Unique features of Helicobacter pylori disease in children. Dig Dis Sci 1991;36:417–423.

Author: Andrew E. Mulberg

Gastroesophageal Reflux

 ## Database

DEFINITION

Gastroesophageal reflux (GER) is defined as effortless regurgitation of gastric contents; it is extremely common in infants. GER occurs physiologically at all ages, and most episodes are brief and asymptomatic. It is important to identify the rare child with pathologic reflux, to perform the appropriate diagnostic studies, and to start effective therapy.

• GER is divided into a pathologic and a physiologic process. Physiologic reflux (the normal GER of infancy) is the more common form. Most infants will eventually outgrow the symptoms. Pathologic reflux is defined by quantity of reflux according to the age and the frequency of the reflux episodes. Complicated GER is pathologic reflux associated with irritability, pain, esophagitis, esophageal bleeding, failure to thrive, reactive airway disease, near-miss SIDS, or aspiration pneumonias.

• GER may be asymptomatic and still carry the risk of complications. GER is the most common cause of vomiting in infancy but may also indicate other disorders.

 ## Differential Diagnosis

Other causes of vomiting in infancy include:

• Infection

—Gastroenteritis
—Urinary tract infection
—Sepsis

• Neurologic

—Meningitis/encephalitis
—Intracranial injury
—Brain tumor
—Hydrocephalus
—Subdural hematoma

• Metabolic

—Uremia
—Aminoacidopathies
—Adrenal hyperplasia
—Phenylketonuria
—Galactosemia

• Food intolerance

—Milk/soy protein allergy
—Celiac disease

• Anatomic malformation

—Gastric-outlet obstruction
—Pyloric stenosis
—Volvulus/malrotation
—Esophageal atresia
—Meconium ileus
—Enteral duplications
—Intussusception
—Trichobezoar

DRUGS THAT AFFECT LOWER ESOPHAGEAL SPHINCTER PRESSURE

• Nitrates
• Nicotine
• Narcotics
• Theophylline
• Anticholinergic
• Estrogen
• Somatostatin
• Prostaglandins

 ## Data Gathering

HISTORY

• Should identify episodes of near-miss SIDS, aspiration pneumonia, chronic cough, laryngitis, stridor, and reactive airways disease
• Should exclude bowel obstruction (bile in the emesis, polyhydramnios during pregnancy)
• If the vomiting begins after the first few weeks of life, it is important to rule out infection, metabolic disease, allergy, and neurologic disease.

Special Questions

• Presence of polyhydramnios
• Bile in emesis
• Family history of metabolic disease
• Family history of allergies
• Perinatal asphyxia (and other neurologic disorders)
• History of prematurity, skin rash (atopic dermatitis), and reactive airways disease

 ## Physical Examination

• May be normal
• Growth failure
• Blood in the stool
• Reactive airways disease and other manifestations of pulmonary complications
• Anemia

Laboratory Aids

TESTS

Diagnosis of GER is made clinically. Testing is needed to identify potential causes or complications. Evaluation should include:

- Stool hemoccult
- Growth parameters

Radiographic Studies

- Barium swallow, tracheoesophageal fistulogram
- Chest radiography
- Nuclear medicine studies
- Milk scan
- Gastric emptying study
- Salivagram

pH Probe

- Simple (single-channel)
- Double-channel
- pH/Thermistor (apnea) study

Endoscopy

- Esophagogastroduodenoscopy (EGD)
- Laryngoscopy
- Bronchoscopy

Manometric Studies

- Esophageal manometry
- Antroduodenal manometry

Therapy

Several modes of therapy are available, depending on the severity, duration of reflux, and complications. The treatment should be individualized and should consider cost efficacy. Traditional treatment includes:

- Small frequent feeds
- Thickening of the feeds (approximately 1 teaspoon of cereal per ounce of formula)
- Positioning: head elevation
- Consider use of a hypoallergenic formula for patients with associated food allergy.

PROKINETIC THERAPY

- Cisapride (Propulsid), 0.2 to 0.25 mg/kg/dose qid. Alert: cardiac toxicity, drug interaction
- Metaclopramide (Reglan), 0.1 mg/kg/dose qid
- Antacids

—Require multiple dosing, carry risk of diarrhea, and may also lead to malabsorption of other medications

- H$_2$ Blockers

—Cimetidine (Tagamet), 10 to 12.5 mg/kg/dose qid
—Ranitidine (Zantac), 2 to 3 mg/kg/dose bid to tid
—Famotidine (Pepcid), 0.3 to 0.5 mg/kg/dose bid

- Proton pump inhibitors

—Omeprazole (Prilosec)
—Lansoprazole (Prevacid)

- Binding Agents

—Sucralfate (Carafate): maximally effective at pH 4 and on mucosal lesions

- Medication interactions

—Cisapride has adverse drug interactions with erythromycin; clarithromycin and ketoconazole may lead to ventricular fibrillation.
—Reglan may cause oculogyric crisis.
—Antacids may lead to diarrhea and constipation.
—H$_2$ blockers may cause headache, rash, diarrhea.

SURGERY AND REFLUX

- The goal of surgery is to increase lower esophageal sphincter tone by wrapping a portion of the cardia around the lower esophagus. This is done to prevent reflux mechanically. Usually, this is associated with a gastric-emptying procedure (i.e., pyloroplasty) and gastric tube placement.
- The indications for surgery can be divided into patients with poor response to medications (i.e., failure to thrive, refractory and severe esophagitis, recurrent aspiration pneumonia, inability to wean from medications) and patients with no need for failure of medical trial (i.e., esophageal stricture, large and symptomatic diaphragmatic hernia, high-grade intestinal metaplastic changes, as in Barrett esophagus). Complications of fundoplication include retching, bowel obstruction, dumping syndrome, difficulty in feeding, paraesophageal hernia, sliding of the wrap, and recurrent GER.

Common Questions and Answers

Q: How long will my baby suffer with GERD?
A: Most physiologic GERD resolves by 9 to 12 months of age. If GER persists after 1 year, it is highly likely that it is associated with a complication.

Q: Should I fear the use of Propulsid?
A: No; it is a safe drug, and with the proper precaution of an ECG prior to its use, the drug is highly effective and safe.

Q: How effective is the Nissen fundoplication in the resolution of GER?
A: The Nissen fundoplication has greater morbidity associated with it in the cohort of children with severe physical and mental disabilities. If performed by a surgeon with vast experience, the procedure is a last effort subsequent to GERD refractive to medical therapy.

ICD-9-CM 530.81

BIBLIOGRAPHY

Jolley S, Halpem L, Tunnell W, et al. The risk of sudden infant death from gastroesophageal reflux. *J Pediatr Surg* 1991;26:691–696.

Orenstein SR. Gastroesophageal reflux. In: Wyllie R, Hyams J, eds. *Pediatric gastrointestinal diseases*. Philadelphia: WB Saunders, 1993:337–369.

Orenstein SR. Gastroesophageal reflux. *Curr Probl Pediatr* 1991;May/June:193–241.

Author: Dror Wasserman

German Measles (Third Disease Rubella)

 Database

DEFINITION

Rubella is derived from Latin, meaning "little red," and was initially considered a variant of measles. Infection is characterized by mild symptoms (often subclinical), with an erythematous rash progressing from head to toes. Prevention of congenital rubella syndrome (see below) is the main objective of vaccination programs.

CAUSE

Rubella virus is classified in the togavirus family as from the genus *Rubivirus*.

- It is an RNA virus with a single antigenic type.
- It was first isolated in 1962 by Parkman and Weller.

PATHOPHYSIOLOGY

- Respiratory transmission
- Replication in the nasopharynx and regional lymph nodes
- Viremia 5 to 7 days after exposure with spread of the virus throughout the body
- In congenital rubella syndrome (CRS), transplanted infection of the fetus occurs during viremia.

EPIDEMIOLOGY

- Spread person to person via airborne transmission; a worldwide infection
- In temperate regions, incidence peaks in the late winter and early spring.
- Infection is most contagious when rash is erupting. However, the virus may be shed, beginning 7 days before the rash to 14 days after.
- Infants with CRS may shed virus for up to 1 year.
- In the prevaccine era, the incidence of infection in the United States was approximately 58 per 100,000 population.
- Currently, fewer than 1,000 cases per year are reported. In 1993, 192 cases were reported.
- Infection occurs equally in the following age groups: under 5 years, 5 to 19 years, and 20 to 39 years.
- CRS was reported rarely during the 1980s, with fewer than five cases annually. From 1990 to 1991, approximately 30 cases were reported annually.
- The rubella vaccine was licensed in 1969.

COMPLICATIONS

Complications tend to occur in adults, and are uncommon, but include:

- Arthritis or arthralgia

—Occurs in 70% of adult women, lasting up to 1 month
—Usually affects small joints

- Encephalitis

—1 in 5,000 cases
—May be associated with mortality

- Bleeding

—1 in 3,000 cases
—Occurs in children more than in adults

- Thrombocytopenia is commonly noted.

—Rarely see orchitis and neuritis

- Congenital rubella syndrome (CRS)

—In 1964, there were 20,000 newborns with CRS.
—Rubella infection in early gestation can lead to fetal death, premature delivery, and congenital defects.
—The severity of defects is worse the earlier in gestation the infection occurs.
—Eighty-five percent of infants are affected if infection occurs in the first trimester.
—Defects are rare if infection occurs after the twentieth week.
—Common defects of CRS include:

  —Deafness: the most common defect
  —Ophthalmologic defects: cataracts, glaucoma, microphthalmia
  —Cardiac defects: patent ductus, arteriosus, ventricular septal defect, pulmonic stenosis, coarctation of the aorta
  —Neurologic defects: mental retardation, microcephales
  —Some manifestations of CRS (diabetes mellitus, progressive encephalopathy) may be delayed for years.

PROGNOSIS

- Quite good. As many as 50% of infections are asymptomatic.
- Rubella infection in a pregnant woman can be devastating for the infant (see above).

ASSOCIATED DISEASES

- Congenital rubella syndrome (see Complications section)

 Differential Diagnosis

Infections that are sometimes confused with rubella include:

- Modified measles
- Scarlet fever
- Roseola
- Erythema infectiosum (fifth disease, parvovirus B19 infection)
- Enteroviral infections
- Infectious mononucleosis
- Drug eruptions

 Data Gathering

HISTORY

- In children, the prodrome is not often recognized.
- In adults, a 1- to 5-day prodrome of low-grade fever, malaise, and cervical adenopathy may precede the rash.
- Inquire about immunizations and exposures.

Physical Examination

- The rash begins on the face, then progresses to the trunk and extremities. The rash does not usually coalesce, and lasts for 3 days.
- Adenopathies, especially postauricular, posterior cervical, and suboccipital, are commonly noted, along with conjunctivitis.
- Arthralgia/arthritis may be seen in adolescents and adults.

 Laboratory Aids

- Viral isolation from throat or urine
- A fourfold or greater rise in specific rubella antibodies, IgG, or a single IgM antibody is diagnostic.

 Therapy

- Supportive care

PREVENTION

- The rubella vaccine was licensed in 1969. The current strain of the vaccine (RA 27/3, developed at the Wistar Institute in Philadelphia) was licensed in 1979 and has replaced all other strains.
- Immunity occurs in 95% of vaccines and is thought to be lifelong.
- The vaccine virus is not communicable, except in breast-feedings. Persons who are immunodeficient (except HIV infection) should not receive the vaccine.

PITFALLS

- Not ensuring full vaccination for preschool-aged children
- If suspicious of rubella, it should be reported to the local public health authorities.

 Common Questions and Answers

Q: While pregnancy is a contraindication to rubella vaccination, if a pregnant woman is inadvertently vaccinated, will there be harm to the fetus?
A: Data collected since 1979, by the Centers for Disease Control and Prevention, show no evidence of CRS in 321 susceptible women who were vaccinated while pregnant.

ICD-CM 056.9

BIBLIOGRAPHY

American Academy of Pediatrics. Rubella. In: Peter G, ed. *1994 Red book: report of the Committee on Infectious Diseases,* 23rd ed. Elk Grove Village, IL: American Academy of Pediatrics, 1994:406–412.

Atkinson W, Furphy L, et al., eds. *Epidemiology and prevention of vaccine-preventable diseases,* 2nd ed. Bethesda, MD: Centers for Disease Control and Prevention, 1995.

Plotkin SA. Rubella vaccine. In: Plotkin SA, Mortimer EA, eds. *Vaccines.* Philadelphia: WB Saunders, 1988:235–262.

Author: Louis M. Bell

Giardiasis

 Database

DEFINITION

Giardiasis is the symptomatic infection of the duodenum and jejunum with the flagellated protozoon *Giardia lamblia*.

PATHOPHYSIOLOGY

- *Giardia lamblia* is not a normal inhabitant of the upper small intestine and a frequent cause of diarrhea throughout the world. The life cycle has a multiplying intraduodenal trophozoite and an excreted cyst stage.
- Infection occurs after cyst ingestion from fecally contaminated water or by direct fecal-oral transmission in poor sanitary conditions.

GENETICS

- No confirmed predisposition
- Blood group A, certain human leukocyte antigen alleles are risk factors.

EPIDEMIOLOGY

Direct person-to-person transmission accounts for the very high prevalence rates over the past decade. High prevalence rates have recently been reported in patients with cystic fibrosis as well as Crohn disease.

COMPLICATIONS

- Malabsorption syndrome
- Steatorrhea
- Lactose deficiency
- Deficiencies of iron, folic acid, and vitamins A, B12, and E
- Protein-losing enteropathy
- Urticaria
- Arthralgia

PATHOLOGY AND PATHOGENESIS

- Mucosal lesions vary from normal to subtotal villus atrophy with crypt hyperplasia and proliferation of intraepithelial and lamina propria lymphocytes. Trophozoite may be seen on biopsies as an S-like curled shape on longitudinal sections. Certain factors that could possibly be related to pathogenesis are:

—Small bowel bacterial overgrowth
—Deconjugation of intraluminal bile salts
—Breast milk that has anti-*Giardia* properties related to free fatty acids cleaved from milk triglyceride by a bile salt-stimulated lipase present in human milk

PROGNOSIS

- Remains good for symptomatic patients
- Combination therapy with two medications has been successful when repeated courses of a single drug have failed.

 Differential Diagnosis

- Celiac disease
- Cystic fibrosis
- Lactose intolerance

 Data Gathering

HISTORY

- Exposure to well water
- Living in endemic area
- Asymptomatic infection can occur.
- Common manifestations are watery, foul-smelling diarrhea without blood, abdominal cramps, and bloating.
- A chronic course is associated with weight loss, abdominal distention, anorexia, and flatulence.
- Malabsorption syndrome may include steatorrhea; secondary lactase deficiency; deficiencies of iron, folic acid, vitamins A, B12, and E; and protein-losing enteropathy.

 Physical Examination

- Abdominal distention
- Urticaria
- Arthralgia

 Laboratory Aids

- Stool microscopy for detection of cysts and/or trophozoite
- A commercial ELISA test for detection of *Giardia lamblia* antigen in stools is available.
- In the case of strong suspicion of giardiasis, but there are three negative stool samples, a small intestinal sample may be obtained from the duodenum. The string test is the most useful. Consideration of empiric antiparasitic therapy may be recommended in endemic areas.
- If immunodeficiency is suspected, check immune function, especially IgA.

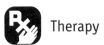

Therapy

PREVENTION

- Metronidazole is the most effective and best tolerated. Dose: 15 mg/kg/d divided tid for 7 days
- Furazolidone has lower efficacy but is better tolerated and is available in liquid suspension.
- For recurrent infection, combination therapy of metronidazole and quinacrine is used.
- Asymptomatic giardiasis, in the absence of risk factors, should not be treated.

INFECTION CONTROL

- Maintenance of good sanitary conditions
- Family members and close contacts should be examined and treated if necessary.
- Examine the water source in endemic areas.

Follow-Up

- The incubation period is usually 1 to 2 weeks.
- Reinfection is common if the source is not eradicated.
- If symptoms persist, with negative diagnostic studies, consider an alternative etiology or another enteropathogen.

Common Questions and Answers

Q: Where is a likely place that the infection occurs?
A: Well water is a common place.

Q: What do I do if I suspect giardia, but the stool sample is negative?
A: Three samples are needed. If you are in an endemic area, you may chose to treat empirically.

ICD-9-CM 007.1

BIBLIOGRAPHY

Fraser D. Epidemiology of *Giardia lamblia* and *Cryptosporidium* infections in childhood. *Isr J Med Sci* 1994;30(5–6):356–361.

Hill DR. Giardiasis issues in diagnosis and management. *Infect Dis Clin North Am* 1993;7(3): 503–525.

Reeder MM. Radiological diagnosis of giardiasis. *Semin Roentgenol* 1997;32(4):291–300.

Thielman NM, Guerrant RL. Persistent diarrhea in the returned traveler. *Infect Dis Clin North Am* 1998;12(2):489–501.

Author: Helen Anita John-Kelly

Gingivitis

Database

DEFINITION

Gingivitis is a reversible or chronic inflammation of the gum tissue margin surrounding the teeth. Symptoms may include bleeding, swelling, ulceration, and pain; though, gingivitis is usually mild and asymptomatic.

ETIOLOGY

- Poor dental hygiene
- Caries
- Bacterial plaque, calcified and uncalcified
- Mouth breathing
- Orthodontic appliances
- Malocclusion
- Crowded teeth
- Poor nutrition: vitamin deficiencies (e.g., vitamin C deficiency), diet low in coarse detergent-like foods (e.g., raw carrots, celery, apples)
- Infections: herpes simplex virus (HSV) type I, *Candida albicans*, HIV, bacterial pathogens
- Drugs: phenytoin, cyclosporin, nifedipine
- Trauma

PREDISPOSING CONDITIONS

- Diabetes mellitus
- Chronic renal failure
- Immunologic deficiency (HIV, Chediak-Higashi, cyclic neutropenia)
- Histiocytosis X
- Scleroderma
- Secondary hyperparathyroidism
- Neurologic problems: cerebral palsy, mental retardation, seizures. Routine dental care is often difficult due to poor cooperation and is often complicated by gingival hyperplasia caused by phenytoin.

PATHOPHYSIOLOGY

- Bacteria and food deposits adherent to the teeth (plaque) may accumulate, eroding the area where the gum and teeth meet.
- Incomplete dental care over time may result in this margin becoming inflamed.
- Inflammation may be more severe in children with altered immune function.
- If allowed to progress, the connective tissue attachment of the teeth and the root surface may become involved, resulting in irreversible periodontal disease.
- Microscopic changes include edema, exudate, ulceration, and proliferation of the epithelium surrounding the tooth.

EPIDEMIOLOGY

- Affects more than 90% of children between the ages of 7 and 13 years
- Thirteen percent to 40% of children 6 to 36 months of age have eruption gingivitis, which commonly resolves after teeth erupt.
- Boys have more severe and prevalent gingivitis until the early teens.
- Peak incidence is in adolescence, possibly due to hormonal influences and inconsistent dental hygiene.

COMPLICATIONS

- Osteomyelitis
- Tooth decay
- Sepsis, particularly in patients who are immunocompromised

PROGNOSIS

- Good oral hygiene may reverse mild-to-moderate gingivitis within several months.
- Periodontal disease is not reversible; therefore, prevention is essential.

Differential Diagnosis

- Infection
—Abscess
- Trauma
—Food impaction
—Orthodontic appliances
—Self-inflicted minor injury
- Hematologic
—Gingival bleeding due to hemophilia (Factor VIII or IX deficiency)
—Thrombocytopenia
- Immunologic
—Neutrophil disorders
—Leukemia
—HIV
—Graft versus host (infiltrative gingivitis)
- Miscellaneous
—Gingival hyperplasia due to medications, including phenytoin and nifedipine

Data Gathering

HISTORY

Question: Is there any bleeding along the gum line with routine brushing and flossing?
Significance: This is very common with gingivitis.

Question: Is there any gingival pain, spontaneous bleeding, or loose teeth?
Significance: This may be seen with gingival disease, but one must consider other diagnoses.

Review the frequency of dental care visits and home dental hygiene regimen.

Question: Are any dental appliances worn by the patient?
Significance: Orthodontic equipment makes gingiva more difficult to clean, and reactive tissue growth is more common.

Question: Are any regular medications taken?
Significance: As mentioned, phenytoin may result in gingival hyperplasia, and chemotherapeutic agents may result in gingivitis.

Question: Has the patient undergone pubertal changes?
Significance: This seems to worsen gingival inflammation.

- Review significant medical history, asking about bleeding disorders and immunodeficiency.
- Assess the diet of the child to determine if there might be nutritional deficiencies.

Physical Examination

- Examine the face and neck for signs of swelling, erythema, and warmth, which may all be signs of more extensive bacterial infection.
- Evaluate the gingival tissue for erythema, swelling, ulceration, fluctuance, or drainage.
- Evaluate the teeth for caries, fractures, looseness, malocclusion, pain, and plaque.
- Assess the patient's oral hygiene technique in the office. This is the single largest contributor to gingivitis.

Laboratory Aids

TESTS

• Complete blood count with differential: if there is a concern of excess bleeding, which may be due to thrombocytopenia or pancytopenia
• Blood culture: if there is a concern of sepsis complicating the picture
• Direct fluorescent antibody testing for HSV 1: if herpes is suspected (stomatitis is usually present); swab the base of a stoma/vesicle and smear on a slide.
• Biopsy is rarely necessary.

Radiographic Studies

Panoramic or individual tooth radiographic imaging is important to assess the bones for evidence of periodontal extension of the gingivitis.

Therapy

MILD GINGIVITIS

• Mechanical plaque removal
• Careful daily dental hygiene, including meticulous brushing and flossing

MODERATE-TO-SEVERE GINGIVITIS

• Care as outlined for mild gingivitis
• Should be evaluated by a pedodontist (if available) or by a general dentist
• Mouth rinses for plaque inhibition (e.g., chlorhexidine 0.12%)
• Irrigation devices
• Sonic toothbrushes
• Gingivectomies in cases of overgrowth to permit better cleaning
• Antibiotics to cover mouth flora organisms in the more severe cases when bacterial superinfection is suspected

Follow-Up

• Routine dental care with professional cleaning and plaque removal is recommended for all children and adults.
• Appliances to keep gingival growth contained may be used in certain cases.

PREVENTION

• Consistent daily oral hygiene. For infants: gum massage, washcloth to remove plaque; in young children: assistance with brushing with a small amount of fluoridated toothpaste; in school-aged children: supervise brushing and assist if necessary.
• Fluorides: Supplements are appropriate if the water supply is not fluoridated.
• Sealants: adherent plastic coating applied to the pits and fissures of the permanent teeth to provide a mechanical barrier
• Begin regular dental checkups every 6 months at 3 years of age. Children with gingival overgrowth, HIV, or ongoing chemotherapy need visits to the dentist every 3 months to assure good hygiene. Routine daily care may be inconsistent and often impossible in children with motor and cognitive limitations; these children also need more frequent visits to the dentist.
• Mouthguards for competitive sports
• Counseling about dangers of smoking

PITFALLS

Success in preventing and treating gingivitis requires consistent daily care, which may be very difficult in children and adolescents.

Common Questions and Answers

Q: Are there differences among toothpastes and prevention of gingivitis?
A: Yes. A recent study demonstrated that stabilized stannous fluoride toothpaste is effective in preventing gingivitis. When essential oil mouthwashes (e.g. Listerine) are added, there is additional reduction in the amount of gingivitis noted.

Q: What dietary changes may improve gingival health?
A: Avoiding frequent carbohydrate intake may reduce gingivitis. Carbonated beverages, sugared chewing gum, and candy often adhere to teeth. When daily dental care is inconsistent, plaque formation is increased and gingivitis is much more likely.

ICD-9-CM 523.1

BIBLIOGRAPHY

Beiswanger BB, McClanahan SF, Bartizek RD, et al. The comparative efficacy of stabilized stannous fluoride dentifrice, peroxide/baking soda dentifrice and essential oil mouthrinse for the prevention of gingivitis. *J Clin Dentistry* 1997;8(2 Spec No):46–53.

Bimstein E. Periodontal health and disease in children and adolescents. *Pediatr Clin North Am* 1991;38(5):1183–1207.

Eaton KA, Rimini FM, Zak E, et al. The effects of a 0.12% chlorhexidine-digluconate-containing mouthrinse versus a placebo on plaque and gingival inflammation over a 3-month period. A multicentre study carried out in general dental practices. *J Clin Periodontal* 1997;24(3):189–197.

Griffen AL, Goepferd SJ. Preventive oral health care for the infant, child, and adolescent. *Pediatr Clin North Am* 1991;38(5):1209–1226.

Ivanovic M, Lekic P. Transient effect of a short-term educational programme without prophylaxis on control of plaque and gingival inflammation in school children. *J Clin Periodontal* 1996;23(8):750–757.

McDonald RE, Avery DR, Weddell JA. Gingivitis and periodontal disease. In: *Dentistry for the child and adolescent,* 6th ed. St. Louis: Mosby-Year Book, 1994:455–502.

Ramberg P, Axelsson P, Lindhe J. Plaque formation at healthy and inflamed gingival sites in young individuals. J Clin Periodontol 1995; 22(1):85–88.

Author: Shannon Connor Phillips

Glaucoma—Congenital

 Database

DEFINITION

Congenital glaucoma is the improper development of the drainage system for aqueous humor, leading to elevated intraocular pressure with enlargement of the eye and damage to the optic nerve.

CAUSES

• Aqueous humor, a clear fluid produced by the ciliary body at the posterior base of the iris, passes through the pupil and exits through the trabecular meshwork and Schlemm's canal, located at the junction of the cornea and the iris anteriorly.
• Blockage of outflow of the aqueous humor for any reason causes the pressure to build in the eye, resulting in enlargement of the eye in younger children and destruction of fibers of the optic nerve in children with abnormally high intraocular pressures.

PATHOPHYSIOLOGY

• Primary congenital glaucoma caused by structural abnormalities of trabecular meshwork, iris, or cornea
• Glaucoma associated with systemic abnormalities such as aniridia, rubella, Sturge-Weber
• Glaucoma acquired secondary to ocular abnormality such as cataract

EPIDEMIOLOGY/GENETICS

• 1:10,000 births
• 1:2 female to male ratio
• Seventy percent bilaterally affected
• Primary congenital glaucoma accounts for approximately one-half of all cases of glaucoma in children.

COMPLICATIONS

If glaucoma is controlled:

• Unrecognized and untreated amblyopia (the most serious threat to child's vision)
• High degrees of myopia
• Anisometropia (difference in refractive error between fellow eyes)
• Buphthalmos and corneal scarring

PROGNOSIS

Guarded; even if pressure is well controlled, the child must be carefully followed for amblyopia, abnormal refractive errors, and recurrence of glaucoma.

ASSOCIATED DISEASES

Aniridia, Sturge-Weber, neurofibromatosis, Marfan syndrome, Pierre Robin syndrome, homocystinuria, Lowe syndrome, rubella, chromosomal abnormalities, persistent hyperplastic primary vitreous

 Differential Diagnosis

• Excessive tearing, most commonly due to nasolacrimal duct obstruction
• Megalocornea

—May be associated with high myopia
—Often familial

• Corneal haze
• Birth trauma, forceps
• Congenital corneal dystrophies, developmental anomalies, intrauterine inflammation (rubella, syphilis), mucopolysaccharidoses, cystinosis

 Data Gathering

HISTORY

Question: Is there tearing, light sensitivity, or lid squeezing?
Significance: Epiphora (tearing), photophobia (light sensitivity), and blepharospasm (lid squeezing) may be present due to corneal edema from increased intraocular pressure.

 Physical Examination

• General signs of many systemic syndromes associated with glaucoma (neurofibromatosis, Sturge-Weber)
• Corneal enlargement (11 mm suspicious below age 1 year)
• Corneal haze from edema and/or scarring, often seen with acute ruptures in Descemet's membrane
• Myopia, often extreme degrees
• Optic nerve cupping develops rapidly in infants but may be reversible with control of glaucoma.

INTRAOCULAR PRESSURE MEASUREMENT

• Prefer awake child; use bottle or breast to quiet along with low lighting.
• If examination under anesthesia is needed, check intraocular pressure as soon as possible after induction, because pressure drops with anesthetic agents.

CORNEAL INSPECTION

• Diameter measure with calipers

—Normal newborn, 10.0 to 10.5 mm
—Over 11.5 mm suspicious
—Watch for asymmetry.

• Clarity

—Haze may be due to edema or breaks in Descemet's membrane (called Haab's striae).

• Refractive error

—High myopia common
—Useful as an office measure of change over time

• Optic disc assessment

—Cupping of nerve head is an early sign.
—May reverse with good intraocular pressure control

 Laboratory Aids

TESTS

• Gonioscopy: evaluation of anterior chamber angle (between iris and cornea)

—In trabeculodysgenesis, the insertion of the iris into the corneoscleral angle is often flat or concave.
—Iris defects may suggest the type of abnormality causing glaucoma.
—Abnormal iris vessels may influence the surgical plan.

• Ultrasound: axial length using A-scan

—Eye usually abnormally long for age
—Longitudinal data very useful in determining continued presence of glaucoma

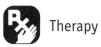 Therapy

IMMEDIATE

• Medical treatment for glaucoma in children is usually a temporizing measure prior to surgical intervention.

• In other types of glaucoma, medical treatment involves the use of the same medications as those used in adults, such as beta-blockers, adrenergic agents, and carbonic anhydrase inhibitors. In general, miotics are not used because they may cause a paradoxical rise in intraocular pressure.

SURGICAL PROCEDURES

• Goniotomy/trabeculotomy: Both of these procedures open portions of Schlemm's canal (goniotomy approaches Schlemm's canal from inside the eye and trabeculotomy from the outside) into the anterior chamber, allowing easier outflow of aqueous humor to the subconjunctival space.

• Trabeculectomy: This is similar to trabeculotomy but includes excision of a small portion of Schlemm's canal and the trabecular meshwork.

• Seton procedures: Various devices are inserted from the subconjunctival space into the anterior chamber, allowing free flow of aqueous humor from the eye.

• Cyclodestructive procedures: Procedures involving destruction of the ciliary body (which produces aqueous humor) decrease aqueous production.

• Iridectomy: If the mechanism of glaucoma is limited outflow of aqueous humor from posterior to iris through the pupil, then removal of a portion of the iris may eliminate obstruction.

 Follow-Up

EARLY POSTOPERATIVE

• Postoperative steroids and cycloplegic drops are essential to prevent adhesions due to inflammation and to decrease pain.

• Corneal edema clears slowly, but intraocular pressure quickly falls if surgery is successful.

• For young infants, examination under anesthesia may be required frequently in the first 3 to 4 years of life to ensure adequate control of intraocular pressure.

• Contact with social services for blind and visually handicapped individuals must be made for children even if they are only suspected of being visually impaired. Encourage families to make the contact even when the child may be too young to provide objective data on the extent of visual handicap.

PITFALLS

• Even when pressure is well controlled and amblyopia treatment is undertaken vigorously, the child is still at high risk for visual impairment.

• The child and its family must understand that glaucoma may recur at any point and that continued, long-term surveillance is essential.

• Ensure that potential systemic medicines do not raise intraocular pressure.

 Common Questions and Answers

Q: Can glaucoma be painful?
A: If the ocular pressure rises quickly (hours), pain occurs frequently. Very high intraocular pressures may be present without pain if they occur slowly (months to years).

Q: Can glaucoma occur after eye trauma?
A: Yes. This is a very common cause of glaucoma and may be asymptomatic, thus requiring follow-up ophthalmic examinations for early detection and treatment.

ICD-9-CM 743.20

BIBLIOGRAPHY

Dickens CJ, Hoskins HD. Developmental glaucoma. In: Isenberg SJ, ed. *The eye in infancy. 2nd ed.* Chicago: Yearbook Medical, 1994:318–335.

Quigley HA. Childhood glaucoma. *Ophthalmology* 1982;89:219–225.

Shields MB. Primary congenital glaucoma. In: Shields MB, ed. *Textbook of glaucoma.* Baltimore: Williams & Wilkins, 1992:220–234.

Author: Graham E. Quinn

Glomerulonephritis

 Database

DEFINITION

Glomerulonephritis (GN) presents with hematuria, oliguria, hypertension, and volume overload. Acute GN (AGN) is associated with inflammation and proliferation of the glomerular tuft. AGN may be rapidly progressive (RPGN). Chronic GN (CGN) implies that permanent damage has occurred.

PATHOPHYSIOLOGY

Causes

• Low serum complement level: systemic diseases

—Vasculitis and autoimmune disease, e.g., systemic lupus erythematosus (SLE)
—Subacute bacterial endocarditis (SBE)
—Shunt nephritis
—Cryoglobulinemia

• Low serum complement level: renal diseases

—Acute poststreptococcal GN (APSGN)
—Membranoproliferative glomerulonephritis (types 1, 2, and 3)

• Normal serum complement level: systemic diseases

—Polyarteritis nodosa group
—Wegener vasculitis
—Henoch-Schönlein purpura
—Hypersensitivity vasculitis
—Visceral abscess

• Normal serum complement level: renal diseases

—IgA nephropathy
—Idiopathic rapidly progressive glomerulonephritis
—Immune-complex disease
—Pauci-immune glomerulonephritis

PATHOLOGY

In APSGN, light microscopy reveals enlarged, swollen glomerular tufts, mesangial and epithelial cell proliferation, with polymorphonuclear cell infiltration. There is granular deposition of C3 and IgG on immunofluorescence, and electron-dense subepithelial deposits or humps on electron microscopy. The histology varies in CGN and depends on the cause. RPGN is associated with crescent formation.

EPIDEMIOLOGY

• APSGN can occur in all ages but is most frequent in males between 5 and 15 years.
• Incidence of APSGN in the United States has declined in the past two decades.

—GN occurs more often at the end of the first decade of life and in adults.

• Genetic predisposition

—Familial GN (e.g., Alports, X-linked)
—Autoimmune diseases (e.g., SLE, familial)

COMPLICATIONS

• Acute renal failure
• Hyperkalemia
• Hypertension
• Volume overload (congestive cardiac failure, pulmonary edema, hypertension)
• Chronic renal failure

PROGNOSIS

Prognosis is excellent in APSGN and variable for other causes of GN in childhood.

 Differential Diagnosis

• Acute postinfectious GN (Lancefield group A (β-hemolytic streptococci, pneumococcus, *Mycoplasma*, mumps, Epstein-Barr virus)
• Infection-related (hepatitis B and C, syphilis)
• IgA nephropathy
• Membranoproliferative GN
• Autoimmune GN (e.g., SLE)
• Familial GN
• Acute interstitial nephritis
• Hemolytic-uremic syndrome
• Pyelonephritis

 Data Gathering

HISTORY

• Macroscopic hematuria (coke-colored urine)
• Sore throat
• Impetigo
• A prior upper respiratory infection (URI) of at least 1 week or skin lesions in the preceding 3 to 4 weeks suggests APSGN.
• A URI in the proceeding few days suggests IgA nephropathy.
• Reduced urine output
• Dyspnea, fatigue, lethargy
• Headache
• Seizures (hypertensive encephalopathy)
• Symptoms of a systemic disease, such as fever, rash (especially on the buttocks and legs posteriorly), arthralgia, and weight loss

Special Questions

Establish the time relationship between a sore throat and the AGN. The onset of APSGN is usually associated with a time delay of more than 1 week.

 Physical Examination

Look for:

• Hypertension
• Pallor
• Signs of volume overload (edema, jugular venous distention, hepatomegaly, basal pulmonary crepitation, and a triple cardiac rhythm)
• Signs of vasculitis, such as rash, loss of fingertip pulp space tissue, Raynaud, and vascular thrombosis
• Signs of a systemic disorder (see vasculitis above)
• Signs of chronic renal insufficiency, such as short stature, pallor, sallowness, edema, excoriations, pericardial friction rub, pulmonary rales and effusion, uriniferous breath, asterixis, myoclonus, and neuropathy

Glomerulonephritis

 ## Laboratory Aids

TESTS

• Throat culture for β-hemolytic streptococcus (positive in 15%–20% with APSGN)
• Microscopy of the urine for crenated RBCs and RBC casts. CBC is normal in AGN; with chronic renal insufficiency, a normocytic normochromic or hypochromic microcytic anemia is found.
• Serum chemistries will reflect the degree of renal failure (raised serum urea and creatinine). The serum potassium and phosphate will be elevated and the calcium decreased.
• ASOT (antistreptolysin-O) titer: positive in 60% of patients with APSGN
• Streptozyme test: a mixed antigen test for β-hemolytic streptococcus. Together, the ASOT plus Streptozyme tests have a greater than 85% sensitivity.
• Complement C3 serum level will be low in APSGN and in other causes of GN, as detailed above.
• ECG to assess ventricular size and for hyperkalemia

Imaging

• CXR to look for pulmonary edema and cardiac size
• Renal ultrasound if presentation or course is not typical of APSGN. The ultrasound is to assess the size and parenchymal texture.

PITFALLS

• Look for and treat hyperkalemia.
• To control seizures, treat the hypertension; anticonvulsants have a secondary role.
• Monitor the degree of renal failure.
• Home testing: Blood pressure monitoring may be required.

 ## Therapy

DIET

Restricted fluid, sodium, potassium, and phosphate are initially required.

DRUGS

The following may be required:

• Loop diuretics (furosemide) for volume, blood pressure, and potassium control
• Antihypertensive agents: Vasodilators such as calcium channel blockers (nifedipine, isradipine, amlodipine) and loop diuretics are useful as first-line agents. Intravenous hydralazine, labetalol, nicardipine, or nitroprusside may be required to treat severe refractory hypertension.
• Serum potassium-lowering agents (kayexalate, furosemide, bicarbonate, insulin/glucose, salbutamol). Intravenous calcium is used to stabilize the myocardium in severe hyperkalemia.
• Phosphate binders
• Immunosuppressive agents such as prednisone, cyclophosphamide, and sometimes azathioprine are used in the treatment of vasculitis-associated GN, membranoproliferative GN, and RPGN. Plasmapheresis may be used to treat RPGN. Penicillin is used in APSGN but does not affect the course of the disease.

DURATION

APSGN is a self-limiting disease. Acute therapy is usually sufficient. The therapy of CGN depends on the underlying disease process, may include immunosupressives, and, ultimately, depends on the management of CRF.

 ## Follow-Up

Drug doses may need modification if conflicts with other treatments arise. In APSGN, improvement usually occurs within 3 to 7 days, hypertension is not sustained, and macroscopic hematuria is transient. Watch for ongoing oliguria, unresolved hypertension, increasing proteinuria, or progressive azotemia.

PITFALLS

• Not checking a serum potassium level stat
• Not recognizing fluid overload
• Not recognizing the severity and type of renal failure

 ## Common Questions and Answers

Q: When does the complement return to normal?
A: Hemolytic complement levels (C3) return to normal within a 6- to 8-week period in APSGN. Persistently low C3 levels suggest a cause other than APSGN.

Q: What are the indications for renal biopsy in AGN?
A: Patients in whom there is sustained hypertension, ongoing or progressive azotemia, or persistent proteinuria of more than 1.5 g/d should be biopsied.

ICD-9-CM 580.9

BIBLIOGRAPHY

Clark G, White RH, Glasgow EF, et al. Post-streptococcal glomerulonephritis in children: clinicopathological correlations and long-term prognosis. *Pediatr Nephrol* 1988;2:381–388.

Cole B, Salinas-Madrigal L. Acute proliferative glomerulonephritis and crescentic glomerulonephritis. In: Holliday M, Barratt TM, Avner ED, eds. *Pediatric nephrology,* 3rd ed. Baltimore: Williams & Wilkins, 1994:697–718.

Jordan S, Lemire JM. Acute glomerulonephritis. diagnosis and treatment. *Pediatr Clin North Am* 1982;29:857-873.

Madaio MP, Harrington JT. The diagnosis of acute glomerulonephritis. *N Engl J Med* 1984;309:1299–1302.

Author: Kevin E.C. Meyers

Glucose-6-Phosphate Dehydrogenase Deficiency

 Database

DEFINITION

Deficiency of the enzyme glucose-6-phosphate dehydrogenase (G6PD) in the red blood cell, which in some individuals may result in a hemolytic anemia. Children inherit abnormal G6PD genes that result either in deficient enzyme production or in production of an enzyme with diminished activity.

• Although the majority of patients with G6PD deficiency are never anemic and have mild to no hemolysis, the classic manifestation is acute hemolytic anemia.
• (AHA) World Health Organization (WHO) classification

—*Class 1: Congenital nonspherocytic hemolytic anemia:* a rare form manifesting itself as a chronic hemolysis without exposure to oxidative stressors. Patients have a mild-to-moderate anemia, although some patients are transfusion dependent. Can present as neonatal jaundice, hemolytic anemia, or a secondary manifestation of the chronic hemolysis (e.g., gallstones). Splenomegaly is present in 40% of patients. Affected individuals tend to be white males of Northern European background.
—*Class 2: Severe deficiency* (<5% detectable enzyme activity): oxidative stress-induced hemolysis only. The prototype is G6PD-Mediterranean. Because of severe deficiency, all RBCs are sensitive to stressors, and hemolysis may be severe and persistent.
—*Class 3: Mild deficiency* (approximately 10% enzyme activity): the most common type of G6PD deficiency. Acute hemolytic anemia is uncommon and occurs only with stressors. The prototype is G6PD A (African or of African descent). Because the enzyme is present and active in young RBCs, the hemolysis preferentially affects older cells and is milder and self-limited (i.e., all cells produced in response to the anemia have adequate G6PD levels).
—*Class 4: Nondeficient variant:* no symptoms, even during oxidant stressors, e.g., G6PD A (variant with normal activity); 20% to 40% alleleic frequency in Africans.

• Deficient neonates may have hyperbilirubinemia out of proportion to their anemia. In severe subtypes, this may lead to kernicterus. Elevated bilirubin is only partially due to the hemolysis; the liver plays a role as well.

PATHOPHYSIOLOGY/PATHOLOGY

• Normal G6PD activity is 7 to 10 IU/g hemoglobin.
• G6PD is necessary for the prevention of cell damage during oxidative stress.
• It is critically important in RBCs because of continuous oxidant stress (from O_2 metabolism) and because anuclear RBCs cannot synthesize more enzyme, unlike cells in other tissues.
• Also, all RBCs lose G6PD activity throughout their life span, so older cells are more prone to oxidative hemolysis.

• The normal RBC life span of approximately 120 days is unaffected in *unstressed* states, even with severe enzyme deficiency, but may be shortened during oxidant stress.
• G6PD-deficient RBCs are destroyed via *intravascular* hemolysis upon exposure to the oxidative stressor, and the acute hemolytic anemia results.
• Hemolysis usually follows stressor by 1 to 3 days.
• Hemoglobin nadir occurs 8 to 10 days postexposure. It is therefore necessary to obtain hemoglobins for over a week after the initial exposure.
• Oxidant stressors include infections (bacterial, viral, hepatitis) and drugs (mothballs, antimalarials, some sulfonamides, methylene blue, among others).
• Favism, a severe hemolytic anemia related to fava bean ingestion, is always caused by G6PD deficiency, but not all deficient patients will develop this.

GENETICS

• G6PD gene is on the X chromosome (Xq28), meaning that it is inherited primarily from mother to son (sex-linked).
• Males express the enzyme (mutant or normal) from their single X chromosome (hemizygotes). Females inheriting two deficient X chromosomes are considered homozygotes (rare) and are more severely affected than are female heterozygotes. Because of random X inactivation (the Lyon hypothesis), approximately one-half of a female's RBCs will have the deficiency and one-half will have normal G6PD activity, resulting in a milder phenotype.
• Different mutations have variable enzyme activity that in turn determines the clinical significance.
• Absolute deficiency of G6PD is not compatible with life.

EPIDEMIOLOGY

• G6PD is the most common of all clinically significant enzyme defects, as well as the most common inherited disorder of RBC defects.
• Primarily affects males
• Discovered in 1958 while studying individuals who developed hemolytic anemia when exposed to primaquine, an antimalarial drug
• Over 300 *biochemical* variants of G6PD have been identified, affecting almost 400 million people worldwide.
• The frequency of different G6PD mutations varies from population to population:

—Africans: 20% to 40% of African X-chromosomes are G6PD A (a mutant enzyme with normal activity).
—Sardinians (some regions): 30% have G6PD-Mediterranean.
—Saudi Arabians: 13% have G6PD deficiency.
—African-Americans: 10% to 15% have G6PD A- (a mutant enzyme with decreased activity; see below).
—The high incidence of mutant genes in some regions may relate to a survival advantage conferred against malarial infection (*Plasmodium falciparum*).

COMPLICATIONS

A generally asymptomatic condition with hemolysis, nausea, diarrhea, abdominal or back pain, and, frequently, low-grade fevers

PROGNOSIS

• For those with the milder forms, the prognosis is excellent.
• Can cause significant morbidity, but rarely mortality, in those with the more severe forms.

 Differential Diagnosis

Intravascular hemolysis is very rare in children, but other causes include:

• Acute hemolytic transfusion reactions (Coombs test is positive)
• Microangiopathic hemolytic disease, such as hemolytic uremic syndrome, thrombotic thrombocytopenic purpura, and prosthetic cardiac valves
• Physical trauma (e.g., March hemoglobinuria); severe burns (uncommon)
• Other inherited RBC enzyme deficiencies
• Paroxysmal nocturnal hemoglobinuria

Extravascular hemolysis can also be confused with G6PD deficiency and includes:

• Hereditary spherocytosis (spherocytes) seen on smear or detected by osmotic fragility testing
• Autoimmune hemolysis and delayed hemolytic transfusion reactions (both Coombs-positive)
• Hemoglobinopathies (e.g., sickle cell anemia; often apparent from peripheral smear). Having G6PD deficiency and a hemoglobinopathy does not worsen either disease.
• Hypersplenism or severe liver disease: Gilbert disease may present with intermittent jaundice and indirect hyperbilirubinemia after infections.
• Bleeding (which may be occult) is more common than hemolysis as a cause of acute anemia with reticulocytosis and should be ruled out.

 Data Gathering

HISTORY

• Symptoms are generally those of anemia, such as pallor, fatigue, or malaise.
• Children undergoing active hemolysis are often irritable, with nausea, diarrhea, and abdominal or back pain, and they often have low-grade fevers.
• Dark urine ("coca-cola," or tea-colored) may follow moderate-to-severe hemolysis.
• Seek information on recent drug, chemical, or food (fava bean) exposures, as well as recent or current illnesses.

Glucose-6-Phosphate Dehydrogenase Deficiency

- A detailed family history may reveal chronic anemia or intermittent jaundice or a known G6PD deficiency. Ask about a family history of splenectomy, cholecystectomy, or blood transfusion. Family ethnicity is also very important.
- Seek information on recent drug and chemical exposures, as well as recent or current illnesses.

 ## Physical Examination

- Signs include those referable to anemia, such as tachycardia, a flow murmur, or pallor.
- Significant hemolysis may cause jaundice or scleral icterus.
- Hepatosplenomegaly may occur but is unusual.

 ## Laboratory Aids

TESTS

- CBC usually reveals a normochromic normocytic anemia with an appropriate reticulocytosis. Hemoglobin can drop precipitously and should be monitored closely until stable or a trend upward is seen.
- Checking a single hemoglobin the day of exposure to the stressor is not acceptable.
- Peripheral blood smear often shows bizarre RBC morphology with marken anisocytosis and poikilocytosis.
- Can see schistocytes, hemi-ghost cells (uneven distribution of hemoglobin), bite cells, blister cells, and occasional Heinz bodies (on supravital staining)
- Hemoglobinemia can be seen in the plasma (pink-red supernatant) or may be measured as free serum hemoglobin.
- Hemoglobinuria occurs once hemoglobin-binding sites in the plasma (haptoglobin and hemopexin) are saturated and may be visible as hematuria or detected on routine urinalysis.
- Free serum haptoglobin levels decrease.
- Direct and indirect Coombs tests should be done to exclude autoimmune hemolytic anemia. They should be negative in G6PD deficiency.
- Plasma indirect bilirubin, LDH, and AST may be elevated, and hemosiderin may be found in the urine several days after hemolysis. LFTs should be normal.
- Renal functions should be obtained to rule out TTP and HUS.

Diagnostic Tests

- Rapid and relatively simple screening tests for G6PD activity in RBCs are available but are qualitative and will therefore not pick up all female heterozygotes who have a measurable but low enzyme level.

- It is necessary to confirm a deficiency or diagnose a suspected heterozygote with a test to *quantify* G6PD activity. Normal G6PD activity is 7 to 10 IU/g hemoglobin. This will accurately detect deficiency in males and homozygous females with no recent hemolysis and will be helpful with heterozygous women.

PITFALLS

- Measured enzyme levels will be higher immediately after an acute hemolytic event because younger RBCs (reticulocytes) with normal levels of G6PD will have replaced the older, more deficient population. Screening tests may be false-negative during this time. The most cost-effective approach is to defer screening until 1 to 2 weeks after the resolution of hemolysis.
- Heterozygote female detection: Two RBC populations exist because of mosaicism from random X-inactivation. On average, one-half are normal and one-half are deficient, but there may be variability. Therefore, quantitative results could be unreliable in extreme cases, which makes family counseling difficult.

 ## Therapy

- Removal of the oxidant stressor is of primary importance. Discontinue the suspected drug and/or treat the infection. In class 3 and 4 patients, essential drug therapy may be continued while monitoring for signs of severe hemolysis.
- Transfusion is rarely necessary (except in some type 1 and 2 deficiencies), but any patient who is symptomatic with anemia or has a low hemoglobin and signs of ongoing brisk hemolysis should be transfused immediately with packed RBCs. Transfused cells should not be G6PD deficient and will not undergo hemolysis.
- Supportive care, evaluation of renal function (risk of ATN with brisk hemolysis), and monitoring degree of anemia and ongoing hemolysis are important.
- Desferoxamine, xylitol, and vitamin E (strong antioxidant) have had mixed results in multiple clinical studies of their effect on severe G6PD hemolysis and are generally not warranted.
- For the affected neonate, one should monitor the bilirubin closely and start bilirubin lights early. Three-fourths of affected infants will have clinically apparent jaundice within 24 hours. If necessary, an exchange transfusion should be performed. Phenobarbital has shown some success in decreasing the bilirubin level. Early discharge is not recommended in infants with jaundice and known risk for having G6PD deficiency.

 ## Follow-Up

The majority of G6PD-deficient individuals remain asymptomatic. When hemolysis does occur, it tends to be self-limited and resolves

spontaneously, with a return to normal hemoglobin levels in 2 to 6 weeks. The development of renal failure is extremely rare in children, even with massive hemolysis and hemoglobinuria.

PREVENTION

- Avoidance of drugs and toxins known to cause hemolysis is the best prevention.
- Education regarding drug avoidance, signs and symptoms of hemolysis, and family and genetic counseling should be provided.

 ## Common Questions and Answers

Q: Do I need to follow a special diet or avoid medications if I have G6PD deficiency?
A: Though most patients will have no symptoms of their disease, certain medications may cause transient hemolytic anemia, and these should be avoided. When prescribing medications, your physician and pharmacist should know about your G6PD deficiency, but most necessary medications are safe and well tolerated. People with severe variants of the deficiency should also avoid fava beans, but otherwise, no dietary restrictions are necessary.

Q: Do I need to know which variant of G6PD deficiency I have?
A: It may be clear which variant you are likely to have based on your clinical symptoms and ethnic background.

Q: Should my family be screened if someone has G6PD deficiency?
A: In families of patients with G6PD deficiency, screening members may help provide meaningful genetic counseling to female carriers and affected but asymptomatic males.

Q: How does G6PD affect sickle cell anemia and vice versa?
A: Having sickle cell disease is somewhat protective in patients with G6PD A- deficiency, because their RBC population is young and therefore higher in enzyme activity. On the other hand, G6PD has no affect on the clinical characteristics of sickle cell disease.

ICD-9-CM 282.2

BIBLIOGRAPHY

Beutler E. G6PD deficiency. *Blood* 1994;84: 3613–3636.

Beutler E. Study of glucose-6-phosphate dehydrogenase: history and molecular biology. *Am J Hematol* 1993;42:53-58.

Mason PJ. New insights into G6PD deficiency. *Br J Haematol* 1996;94[Suppl 4]:585–591.

Author: Susan R. Rheingold

Goiter

 Database

DEFINITION

Goiter is enlargement of the thyroid gland.

PATHOPHYSIOLOGY

• Multiple causes; see Differential Diagnosis.
• The most common cause of pediatric goiter in the United States is chronic lymphocytic thyroiditis (CLT).

GENETICS

• The multinodular goiter 1 (MNG1) locus was identified on chromosome 14q by linkage analysis in one large Canadian family. This represents only one subgroup.
• Autoimmune goiters, such as CLT, occur in children with a genetic predisposition.

EPIDEMIOLOGY

Prevalence of goiter in the United States is 3% to 7%, though the incidence is much higher in regions of iodine deficiency.

COMPLICATIONS

Depending on gland size, goiters can produce a mass effect on midline neck structures. Typically, the child is euthyroid, but clinical hypothyroidism or hyperthyroidism may result from certain types of goiters.

PROGNOSIS

Depends on the cause of the goiter

 Differential Diagnosis

• Immunologic

—Chronic lymphocytic thyroiditis (often referred to as Hashimoto thyroiditis)
—Graves disease

• Infectious

—Acute suppurative thyroiditis (most often *Streptococcus pyogenes, Staphylococcus aureus,* and *Streptococcus pneumoniae*)
—Subacute thyroiditis (often viral)

• Environmental

—Goitrogens: iodide, lithium, amiodarone, oral contraceptives, perchlorate, cabbage, soybeans, cassava
—Iodine deficiency

• Neoplastic

—Thyroid adenoma/carcinoma
—TSH-secreting adenoma
—Lymphoma

• Congenital

—Ectopic gland
—Unilateral agenesis of gland
—Dyshormonogenesis
—Thyroxine resistance

• Miscellaneous

—Simple colloid goiter
—Multinodular goiter

 Data Gathering

HISTORY

• Symptoms of hypothyroidism or hyperthyroidism

—Hypothyroidism: increase in sedentary behavior, lethargy, weight gain, constipation, cold intolerance, dry skin and/or hair, hair loss
—Hyperthyroidism: hyperactivity, irritability, difficulty concentrating or focusing in school, hyperphagia, weight loss, diarrhea, heat intolerance

• Careful dietary and medication history
• History of head, neck, or chest irradiation is associated with increased risk of carcinoma.

 Physical Examination

• Inspect, palpate, and auscultate the neck.

—Neck extension aids inspection.
—Palpation is best performed standing behind the child. Determine if the thyroid is diffusely enlarged or asymmetric, evaluate gland firmness, and assess for any nodularity. Check for cervical lymphadenopathy.
—Auscultate with the stethoscope diaphragm (while patient holds his/her breath) for a bruit, which is indicative of the hyperthyroidism-associated hypervascularity.

• Pain on palpation suggests acute inflammation.
• Careful examination for signs of hypothyroidism or hyperthyroidism: pulse, linear growth and weight pattern, sexual development, deep tendon reflexes, skin

Procedure

Have patient drink water during inspection of gland. Isthmus of thyroid is just below the cricoid cartilage.

Laboratory Aids

TESTS

• Thyroid function tests: total T4 and TSH comprise the best screen for hypo- or hyperthyroidism.
• T3-RIA in cases of suspected hyperthyroidism (Note: RIA, which measures total T3, and *not* resin uptake, which indirectly assesses thyroid hormone binding capacity!)
• In cases of suspected CLT: antithyroglobulin and antimicrosomal (antiperoxidase) antibodies
• In cases of suspected Graves disease: thyroid-stimulating immunoglobulins
• Fine-needle aspiration biopsy is not a commonly used procedure in children and should be considered only in the evaluation of low-risk or purely cystic thyroid nodules.

Imaging

• Ultrasound is useful in determining the number, size, and nature (cystic, solid, or mixed) of nodules.
• I-123 thyroid scans should be done in cases of solitary nodules to establish whether or not the nodule concentrates iodide. "Cold" nodules (no I-uptake) are suggestive of neoplasia and require immediate evaluation by a pediatric endocrinologist and surgeon.
• Barium swallow studies can reveal a fistulous tract between the left piriform sinus and the left thyroid lobe in children with recurrent acute suppurative thyroiditis. Such fistulas are amenable to surgical resection.

False Positives

• Fat neck: adipose tissue, large sternocleidomastoid muscles
• Thyroglossal duct cysts
• Nonthyroidal neoplasms: lymphoma, teratoma, hygroma

Therapy

Therapy is dictated by the cause of the goiter. Surgery solely to decrease the size of a goiter is indicated only if adjacent structures are compressed.

DRUGS

L-thyroxine is indicated for the treatment of goiters with hypothyroidism. In cases of goiter with hyperthyroidism, initial treatment consists of antithyroid drugs (propylthiouracil or methimazole). Please see sections on hypothyroidism and Graves disease for further details.

DURATION

• Depends on the cause of the goiter

DIET

Depends on the cause of the goiter. The incidence of iodine deficiency (endemic) goiter has greatly declined since the addition of potassium iodide to table salt. Iodide can also be added to communal drinking water or administered as an iodized oil in isolated rural areas.

POSSIBLE CONFLICTS

In the case of manic-depressive patients on lithium and cardiac patients on amiodarone, medication-induced thyroid abnormalities can be a significant problem that should be addressed by the endocrinologist and appropriate subspecialist.

Follow-Up

• The potential for goiter regression depends on its cause. Goiters associated with CLT and Graves disease may or may not decrease in size with treatment.
• A goiter patient who is clinically and biochemically euthyroid still requires careful follow-up for the detection of the early signs of developing thyroid dysfunction.

PITFALLS

Failure to work up solitary thyroid nodules aggressively; remember, incidence of malignancy in these nodules in children is 15% to 40% (less in adults).

Common Questions and Answers

Q: Does a bigger thyroid gland mean increased thyroid functioning?
A: Goiters can be euthyroid, hypothyroid, or hyperthyroid, depending on cause.

Q: Will the goiter decrease in size with treatment?
A: This again depends on the cause of the goiter. For example, correction of an elevated TSH in CLT with treatment can result in goiter shrinkage. In iodine-deficient states, treatment will cause the *early* hyperplastic goiter to regress.

ICD-9-CM 240.9

BIBLIOGRAPHY

Aghini-Lombardi F, Antonangeli Z, Martino E, Vitti P, Maccherini D, Leoli F, Rafo T, et al. The spectrum of thyroid disorders in an iodine-deficient community: The Pescopagamo survey. *J. Clin Endocrinol Metab* 1999;84:561–566.

Alter CA, Moshang T. Diagnostic dilemma: the goiter. *Pediatr Clin North Am* 1991;38:567–578.

Bignell GR, Canzian F, Shayeghi M, et al. Familial nontoxic multinodular goiter locus maps to chromosome 14q but does not account for familial nonmedullary thyroid cancer. *Am J Hum Genet* 1997;61:1123–1130.

Hopwood NJ, Kelch RP. Thyroid masses: approach to diagnosis and management in childhood and adolescence. *Pediatr Rev* 1993;14:481–487.

Ladenson PW. Optimal laboratory testing for diagnosis and monitoring of thyroid nodules, goiter, and thyroid cancer. *Clin Chem* 1996;42:183–187.

Wang C, Crapo LM. The epidemiology of thyroid disease and implications for screening. *Endocrinol Metab Clin North Am* 1997;26:189–218.

Authors: Adda Grimberg and Marta Satin-Smith

Gonococcal Infections

 Database

DEFINITION

Gonococcal infections include all diseases caused by *Neisseria gonorrhoeae*; an aerobic gram-negative diplococci, typically appearing as pairs with flattened adjacent sides.

PATHOPHYSIOLOGY

• Gonococcal infections are included in the category of sexually transmitted diseases (i.e., their major method of transmission in adolescents and adults is through sexual contact). In neonates, gonorrheal infections can also be acquired during passage through an infected birth canal.
• Incubation period is 2 to 7 days.
• Route of spread includes exposure to any infected mucous membrane or to infectious discharge.

ASSOCIATED DISEASES

• Pediatric gonococcal infections can be categorized by age group: the neonate, prepubertal children, and sexually active adolescents.
• Neonatal gonococcal diseases include gonococcal ophthalmia neonatorum, neonatal scalp abscess (complication after fetal scalp monitoring), and, rarely, vaginitis or systemic disease with bacteremia, arthritis, meningitis, or endocarditis.
• Gonococcal disease in the pre-pubertal age group usually occurs in the genital tract with vaginitis as the most common presenting manifestation. Pelvic inflammatory disease (PID), perihepatitis, and urethritis are rare. Anorectal and pharyngotonsillar involvement can also occur. As discussed in "Pitfalls," child sexual abuse must be considered in all cases of gonococcal infection in prepubertal children outside the neonatal period and in any non-sexually active adolescent.
• Gonococcal disease in sexually active adolescents is similar to that in adults. In females, it is most frequently asymptomatic infection of the genital tract or symptomatic infection including endocervicitis, vaginitis, and urethritis, any of which can extend to cause PID, perihepatitis, or bartholinitis. In males, it most frequently occurs as symptomatic urethritis; extension can include epididymitis or proctitis. Asymptomatic or symptomatic infection of the urethra, rectum, pharynx, or conjunctivae can occur in both sexes. Hematogenous spread can cause arthritis-dermatitis syndrome, or rarely meningitis or endocarditis.
• Arthritis can occur at any age after bacteremia, most commnly in wrists, ankles, and knees, but any joint may be affected.

EPIDEMIOLOGY

• *N. gonorrhoeae* occurs only in human hosts. Approximately 1,000,000 new cases are reported each year in the United States.
• The highest incidence of infection is reported in males aged 20 to 24 years old and then in those 15 to 19 years old. The highest rates in females are from age 15 to 19 years.

COMPLICATIONS

• Gonoccal infection during pregnancy

—Both mother and infant at risk
—Gonococcal acute salpingitis or PID in first trimester has been associated with high incidence of fetal loss.
—Complications during labor and delivery include premature rupture of membranes, premature delivery, and chorioamnionitis.

• Salpingitis and PID

—Both salpingitis and PID can occur after the progression of untreated vaginal disease.
—Scarring that results from salpingitis has been estimated to cause sterility in up to 20% of women with a single infection and up to 50% of women after three episodes of infection.
—Partial obstruction of fallopian tube patency by scarring is a cause of ectopic pregnancy.
—There is an increased risk of progression of vaginal disease to salpingitis and PID in adolescents (approximately 15% of adolescents infected progress to PID).

• Disseminated disease

—Most common manifestation of disseminated gonococcal disease in children is gonococcal arthritis of the newborn; most cases involve multiple joints.
—Acute arthritis-dermatitis syndrome typically includes multiple joint tenosynovitis (with potential progression to arthritis) and papular/pustular lesions of the extremities.
—Gonococcal meningitis, endocarditis, myocarditis, and hepatitis are very rare in children.

• Ophthalmia neonatorum

—Gonococcal ophthalmia neonatorum can have a rapidly destructive course with corneal ulceration, scarring, and blindness if not treated early and aggressively.

PROGNOSIS

• Good prognosis is dependent on early diagnosis and effective irradication of infection prior to its progression and accompanying complications.
• Prognosis has been additionally improved by the recommendation to begin treatment of all forms of infection with an extended spectrum third-generation cephalosporin due to the increased prevalence of penicillin-resistant *N. gonorrhoeae*.

 Differential Diagnosis

• Neonatal ophthalmia: other organisms that can cause neonatal conjunctivitis, including staphylococcal, streptococcal, and hemophilus species.
• Vaginitis in prepubertal child, other causes include: chemical or environmental irritants; pinworms; foreign body; infection by streptococci, trichomonas, diphtheroids, and other bacteria; and in cases of sexual abuse, chlamydia, or syphilis.
• Genitourinary tract infection in adolescents: other causes include chlamydia, syphilis, or trichomonas.
• Scalp infection: other causes include other bacteria/viruses, (*see* Pitfalls).

 Data Gathering

HISTORY

Question: Vaginal itching and crusting discharge?
Significance: Pre-pubertal gonorrhea vaginitis is typically a mild disease that rarely causes ascending or disseminated infection. Most children present with vaginal itching and a minor crusting discharge that may discolor underwear. Dysuria and white cells in the urine may also occur with gonorrhea vaginitis.

Question: Dysuria and discharge?
Significance: Urethritis presents with dysuria and a history of yellow-green mucopurulent discharge.

Question: Evidence of vaginal infection?
Significance: Post-pubescent vaginitis presents acutely with vulvar discomfort, dysuria, frequency, inflamed vulvar and vaginal mucosa, and a thick, yellow purulent discharge.

Question: Problem with walking or abdominal pain?
Significance: Ascending infection is characterized by difficulty walking, fever, emesis, and abdominal pain that is diffuse in the lower quadrants, or in perihepatitis, in the right upper quadrant with possible radiation to right scapula.

Gonococcal Infections

 Physical Examination

Finding: Neonatal ophthalmia
Significance: Usually presents 2 to 5 days after delivery as a bilateral discharge that is initially watery but quickly becomes mucopurulent with or without streaks of blood (incubation can be less than 3 days and up to 2 or 3 weeks postpartum). Conjunctivae are usually edematous with advanced disease showing edema or ulceration of the cornea. Lid edema is common.

Finding: Neonatal scalp abscess
Significance: Frequent complication of fetal scalp monitoring; determination of causative agent can be difficult.

Finding: Cervical motion tenderness
Significance: Characteristic on pelvic examination in patients with ascending cervical infection.

Finding: Purulent discharge
Significance: Common in both cervicitis and urethritis.

 Laboratory Aids

Test: Typical gram stain
Significance: Intracellular gram-negative diplococci. Confirmation is dependent of culture of *N. gonorrhoeae.*

Test: *N. gonorrhoeae* is cultured in a CO_2-enriched atmosphere on chocolate agar or Thayer-Martin medium.
Significance: Culture and Gram stain are taken of the area of suspected infection by swabbing secretions (vagina, endocervix, male urethra, pharynx, rectum, conjunctivae) or by collecting the body fluid (such as cerebrospinal fluid, blood, or abscess or synovial).

Test: Cultures
Significance: In suspected sexual abuse, genital, rectal, and pharyngeal cultures should be collected prior to administration of antibiotics.

Test: STD panel
Significance: Test for other sexually transmitted diseases in the child in whom sexual abuse is suspected or when evaluating the sexually active adolescent. This includes testing for *Chlamydia,* syphilis, *Trichomonas,* and HIV.

Test: Non-culture methods for rapid identification are available.
Significance: Enzyme immunoassay, immunofluorescence, and DNA probes (they should not be used without culture in investigations of possible sexual abuse).

 Therapy

- Recommended therapy for all gonococcal infections in any age group is third-generation cephalosporin because of the increasing appearance of penicillin-resistant *N. gonorrhoeae.*
- Neonate: hospitalize after appropriate cultures (blood, cerebrospinal fluid, eye, or other site of infection) and initiation of treatment

—Non-disseminated dz: single dose of ceftriaxone, 25 to 50 mg/kg IV or IM (up to maximum dose of 125 mg); alternate for infant with hyperbilirubinemia is cefotaxime 100 mg/kg single dose.
—Disseminated dz: ceftriaxone 25 to 50 mg/kg IV or IM daily for 7 days, or cefotaxime 50 to 100 mg/kg/day IV or IM in two divided doses for 7 days; continue treatment for 10 to 14 days for meningitis.

- Neonates with gonococcal ophthalmia should have their eyes irrigated with sterile saline at presentation and at frequent intervals until the mucopurulent drainage has ceased.
- For patients outside the neonatal period, treatment and dosing charts from the *1997 Red Book.*

 Follow-Up

INFECTION CONTROL

- Neonatal ophthalmia: Routine use of prophylactic ophthalmic ointment is mandatory in the United States. Instillation in both eyes of ointment occurs immediately after birth; choice of drugs includes 1% silver nitrate, 1% tetracycline, and 0.5% erythromycin ophthalmic ointments.

ISOLATION OF HOSPITALIZED PATIENT

Contact isolation precautions for all patients with gonococcal disease in the neonatal and pre-pubescent age groups is recommended; no special policies are recommended for other patients.

CONTROL MEASURES

- Infants of mothers with active gonococcal infections at birth should receive 25 to 50 mg/kg (maximum, 125 mg) ceftriaxone IM or IV for one dose only.
- Sexual contacts of persons with known gonorrhea should be examined, cultured, and treated as if they are infected with gonococcus.
- Any patient with a sexually transmitted disease should be evaluated for other common sexually transmitted diseases, including gonorrhea, *Chlamydia,* syphilis, and HIV. Consider hepatitis vaccination.
- Routine screening cultures of endocervix of all pregnant women at first prenatal visit; repeated at term if high risk.
- All cases of gonorrhea must be reported.

PITFALLS

- The diagnosis of suspected child sexual abuse must be considered in any child with a gonococcal infection outside the neonatal period. Cases of transmission via non-sexual contact have been reported (contact with freshly infected bedding, towels, toilet seat, or other fomite, or by digital transmission from an infected caregiver) but cannot be assumed without first ruling out sexual abuse. The source of infection should be determined in all cases, if possible.
- Scalp abscesses caused by gonorrhea are sometimes difficult to differentiate from staphylococcal species, Group B strep, *H. influenzae,* gram-negative enteric flora, or herpes simplex. For this reason, hospitalization of infants with scalp abscesses is recommended for appropriate differential work-up.
- Concurrent infection with other sexually transmitted diseases, including syphilis, *Chlamydia, Trichomonas,* and possibly HIV, should be considered and tested for; presumptive treatment for *Chlamydia trachomatis* is standard of care, as discussed, for gonococcal urethritis infections in children older than 9 years.
- Treatment of partners or source contact should be initiated in all cases.
- Careful differentiation by culture from other *Neisseria* species is necessary, especially in prepubertal children, due to the underlying question of child sexual abuse.

ICD-9-CM 098.0

BIBLIOGRAPHY

American Academy of Pediatrics. Gonococcal infections. In: Peter G, ed. *1997 Red book: report of the Committee on Infectious Diseases,* 24th ed. Elk Grove Village, IL: American Academy of Pediatrics, 1997:212–219.

American Academy of Pediatrics. Prevention of neonatal ophthalmia. In: Peter G, ed. *1997 Red book: report of the Committee on Infectious Diseases,* 24th ed. Elk Grove Village, IL: American Academy of Pediatrics, 1997:601–603.

American Academy of Pediatrics. Pelvic inflammatory disease. In: Peter G, ed. *1997 Red book: report of the Committee on Infectious Diseases,* 24th ed. Elk Grove Village, IL: American Academy of Pediatrics, 1997:390–394.

Feigin RD, Cherry JD, eds. *Textbook of pediatric infectious diseases,* 2nd ed. Philadelphia: WB Saunders, 1987:562–563, 566–568, 595–606.

Sung L. MacDonald NE. Gonorrhea: a pediatric perspective. *Pediatr Rev* 1998;19(1):13–16.

Author: Molly (Martha) W. Stevens

Graft Versus Host Disease

 Database

DEFINITION

Graft versus host disease (GVHD) is a multiorgan inflammatory process that develops when immunologically competent T lymphocytes from a histoincompatible donor are infused into an immunocompromised host who is unable to reject the donor T cells. It is divided into acute and chronic forms and is caused by:

- Bone marrow transplantation (BMT)
- Transfusion of non-irradiated blood products (e.g., products containing viable T lymphocytes) to congenitally immunodeficient hosts
- Transfusion of non-irradiated blood products from a donor who is homozygous for one of the recipient's human leukocyte antigen (HLA) haplotypes
- Intrauterine materno-fetal transfusions and exchange transfusions in neonates
- Solid organ grafts that contain viable T cells (e.g., small bowel transplants)

PATHOPHYSIOLOGY

- Acute GVHD: epithelial cell necrosis involving the regenerative compartment of the three affected organ systems (e.g., the basal layer of the skin, the crypts of the large and small bowel, and the biliary epithelium of the portal triad).
- Chronic GVHD: the clinicopathologic findings are similar to those seen in autoimmune disorders such as scleroderma, systemic lupus erythematosus, and primary biliary cirrhosis (i.e., epithelial cell damage, a mononuclear inflammatory cell infiltrate, and fibrosis are prominent features).

GENETICS

- The major HLA gene complex is found on chromosome 6 and is inherited as a group or haplotype.
- Two full siblings have a 25% chance of being HLA identical.
- Minor histocompatibility antigen differences likely account for GVHD in the HLA identical sibling bone marrow transplant setting.

EPIDEMIOLOGY

- The major risk factor is HLA disparity. GVHD is most common in unrelated donor marrow transplants and absent in identical twin transplants.
- Other risk factors include:

—Prior pregnancies in the marrow donor (which give rise to allosensitization)
—Older donor or recipient age
—Gender mismatch

COMPLICATIONS

- Mortality from GVHD after BMT is usually related to infection.
- Rarely, patients die of hepatic failure or abdominal catastrophe.
- In transfusion-associated GVHD, the major cause of death is bone marrow aplasia due to destruction of the host's marrow by donor lymphocytes.

PROGNOSIS

- Acute GVHD is graded on a scale from I to IV with percent of total body surface involved (skin), volume of diarrhea (gut), and/or elevation of serum bilirubin (liver).
- Patients with grade I GVHD do not have a survival different from those without GVHD.
- Patients with grade IV GVHD have a survival of only 10% to 15% as do patients with progressive chronic GVHD (defined as acute GVHD, which does not resolve followed by chronic GVHD).

 Differential Diagnosis

ACUTE GVHD

- Skin: dermal changes from chemoradiotherapy, drug reaction, viral exanthem
- Liver: hepatic venoocclusive disease (VOD), elevations of liver function tests due to total parenteral nutrition, drug toxicity or infection, especially bacterial sepsis and cytomegalovirus
- Gastrointestinal: diarrhea secondary to the BMT preparative regimen and infectious causes, especially *Clostridium difficile* and cytomegalovirus

 Data Gathering

HISTORY

Acute GVHD

Question: Rash? Itching?
Significance: Pruritus can precede the rash, which in BMT appears as the patient's blood counts are beginning to rise. In transfusion-induced GVHD, symptoms usually start 1 week after the transfusion.

Question: Jaundice? Diarrhea?
Significance: Unusual for involvement to precede skin disease

Chronic GVHD

Question: Dry eyes? Dry mouth?
Significance: Be sure to ask if the patient forms saliva or tears because sicca syndrome can develop.

Question: Dysphagia?
Significance: Complaints of difficulty swallowing or retrosternal pain may be due to esophageal strictures.

 Physical Examination

Acute GVHD

Finding: Skin
Significance: Often begins as erythema of the palms, soles, and ears. The rash can become confluent erythroderma, and in the most severe cases can lead to bulla formation and even denudation reminscent of burn injuries.

Finding: Liver
Significance: Jaundice can be seen but painful hepatomegaly, ascites, and rapid weight gain are atypical and are more often seen in VOD.

Finding: Gastrointestinal
Significance: Stool is often watery, green, and bloody (although it may only be guaiac positive).

Chronic GVHD

Characterized as limited (localized skin involvement or hepatic dysfunction) or extensive.

Finding: Skin
Significance: Hyper- or hypopigmentation, patchy erythema, scaling, and sclerodermatous changes can be seen. The skin is involved in almost every patient.

Finding: Joints
Significance: Swelling can be seen: a detailed range of motion examination is crucial because contractures can be found in the absence of joint swelling.

Laboratory Aids

The diagnosis of GVHD is often made on clinical grounds.

Test: Laboratory
Significance: In hepatic GVHD isolated elevations of transaminases can be seen without hyperbilirubinemia. In more severe cases, a cholestatic picture is seen. Howell-Jolly bodies can be seen on peripheral blood smear in the functional asplenia of chronic GVHD.

Test: Radiological
Significance: Although total body irradiation and busulfan used in BMT can lead to pulmonary fibrosis, the picture of bronchiolitis obliterans on CT scan is considered a manifestation of chronic GVHD.

Test: Biopsy
Significance: Of note, during the first 3 weeks post-BMT, skin and gastrointestinal histological changes from chemoradiotherapy are indistinguishable from GVHD.

Therapy

The best therapy is prevention and includes irradiation of all cellular blood products for patient at risk. Also important in the BMT setting are:

• Selection of a histocompatible donor
• Immunosuppressive therapy with the combination of cyclosporine and methotrexate is the gold standard.
• Steroids, usually in combination with cyclosporine, have been used for those patients who cannot tolerate methotrexate.
• When using an unrelated donor or partially matched family member, other options include *ex vivo* depletion of T lymphocytes from the donor marrow and *in vivo* administration of anti-T cell antibodies to the recipient.
• Monoclonal antibody therapy aimed at cytokine blockade is under investigation.

Treatment of established acute GVHD includes:

• Steroids at a dose of 2 mg/kg/d for 2 weeks followed by a taper over several months
• Cyclosporine or FK506 in those patients who did not receive it as prophylaxis
• Antithymocyte globulin (ATG) for steroid-resistant patients
• Mycophenolate mofetil is presently under investigation

Options in treatment of chronic GVHD include:

• Steroids either alone or in combination with cyclosporine or FK506. Because many patients require treatment for months, the goal is alternate day therapy (e.g., steroids alternating with cyclosporine).
• Psoralen plus ultraviolet A (PUVA) is of some benefit in skin GVHD.
• Oral beclomethasone has been used for treatment of gastrointestinal GVHD.
• Ursodeoxycholic acid may be of benefit for hepatic GVHD.
• Thalidomide, clofazamine, etretinate, and, most recently, mycophenolate mofetil have shown some promise.
• Studies of azathioprine suggested a high infection rate when it was given with steroids.

Follow-Up

• Acute GVHD: The institution of steroid therapy should lead to improvement within days in those patients who are destined to respond. However, gastrointestinal symptoms are notoriously slow to respond.
• Chronic GVHD: Acute GVHD, which merges directly into chronic GVHD, is termed progressive and has an extremely poor prognosis (approximately 10% survival at 5 years post-BMT). Thrombocytopenia is another poor prognostic factor. Such patients usually die of infection.
• Of note, patients with limited chronic GVHD have a decreased rate of relapse of leukemia and an increased survival rate.

PITFALLS

• Do not immunize a patient with a live vaccine if they have chronic GVHD. This may result in symptomatic infection.
• Take sudden high fevers seriously in a patient with GVHD. Overwhelming bacterial sepsis is not infrequent. Patients with chronic GVHD are often functionally asplenic (even if Howell-Jolly bodies are not seen on peripheral blood smear). Many transplant centers place these children on prophylactic penicillin.

Common Questions and Answers

Q: If a child gets acute GVHD does that mean they will get chronic GVHD?
A: No. Approximately 30% of patients less than 10 years of age who receive an HLA identical sibling BMT will get acute GVHD, whereas only 13% will develop chronic GVHD. Of note, chronic GVHD can develop in a patient who did not have acute GVHD. This is termed *de novo* and is much more favorable than progressive chronic GVHD.

Q: Do patients with severe chronic GVHD all die?
A: No. Occasionally the GVHD will "burn out." This is rare, and the process by which it happens is not understood.

BIBLIOGRAPHY

Greenbaum BH. Transfusion associated graft versus host disease: historical perspectives, incidence and current use of irradiated blood products. *J Clin Oncol* 1991;328(9):1889–1902.

Klingebiel T, Schlegel PG. GVHD: overview on pathophysiology, incidence, clinical and biological features. *Bone Marrow Transplant* 1998;21[Suppl 2]:S45–S49.

Sullivan KM, Agura E, Anasetti C, et al. Chronic graft-versus-host disease and other late complications of bone marrow transplantation. *Semin Hematol* 1991;28(3):250–259.

Vogelsang GB, Hess AD. Graft-versus-host disease: new directions for a persistent problem. *Blood* 1994;84:2061–2067.

Author: Ann Marie Leahey

Graves Disease

 Database

DEFINITION

Multisystem autoimmune disorder that presents with the classic triad of:

- Hyperthyroidism (goiter)
- Exophthalmos
- Dermopathy (rare in children)

PATHOPHYSIOLOGY

- Autoimmune process that includes production of immunoglobulins against antigens in the thyroid, orbital tissue, and dermis.
- IgG_1 anti-TSH receptor-autoantibody (thyroid stimulating immunoglobulin; TSI) activates the receptor, resulting in constitutive stimulation; thyroid follicular cells hyperfunction, leading to increased production and release of thyroid hormone.

GENETICS

- No simple hereditary pattern (genetic susceptibility plus environmental factors).

—Up to 60% of patients have a familial history of autoimmune thyroid disease (hyper- or hypothyroidism).
—Concordance rates of Graves disease: 30% to 60% in monozygotic twins; 3% to 9% in dizygotic twins.

- Associated with increased frequency of haplotype HLA-DR3.
- Linkage studies identified CTLA-4 locus on chromosome 14q as a susceptibility gene.

EPIDEMIOLOGY

- 10% to 15% of all childhood thyroid disorders.
- Incidence increases with age, peaking in adolescence and the third to fourth decade.
- Male/female ratio: 1:4–5

COMPLICATIONS

- Endocrine disturbances: delayed/early puberty, menstrual irregularity, hypercalcemia
- Ophthalmological: 3% to 5% of patients develop severe ophthalmopathy, including eye muscle dysfunction and optic neuropathy, requiring specific treatment by an ophthalmologist. Pediatric ophthalmological findings are more common but usually less severe than in adults.

PROGNOSIS

- Good, if compliant with treatment.
- Mortality in severe thyrotoxicosis is possible from cardiac arrhythmias or cardiac failure.
- Spontaneous remission occurs in up to 25% of children after 2 years and 50% by 4.5 years. Relapse is not uncommon (3–40%).

 Differential Diagnosis

(For other causes of hyperthyroidism; *see* Goiter.)

INFECTIOUS

- Acute suppurative thyroiditis (transient thyroxine elevations).
- Subacute thyroiditis after viral illness (also transient hyperthyroidism).

ENVIRONMENTAL

- Thyroid hormone ingestion
- Ingestion of excess iodine (escape from Wolff-Chaikoff effect due to impaired autoregulation)

TUMORS (ALL RARE IN CHILDHOOD)

- TSH-producing pituitary adenoma
- Thyroid adenoma/hyperfunctioning autonomous thyroid nodule (most pediatric cases are euthyroid; incidence of nodule hyperfunctioning rises with increasing patient age).
- Thyroid carcinoma (rarely presents with hyperthyroidism)

CONGENITAL

- Neonatal Graves disease (transplacental antibody transfer from mothers with Graves disease or chronic thyroiditis)

GENETIC AND DEVELOPMENTAL

- Pituitary resistance to thyroid hormones (dominant negative thyroid-receptor gene mutations causing loss of the usual pituitary negative feedback loop and hence, inappropriately elevated TSH; pituitary resistance can be isolated, with clinical hyperthyroidism, or associated with peripheral thyroid resistance as well, leading to clinical euthyroidism or hypothyroidism).
- TSH-receptor gene mutations (rare; germline activating TSH-receptor mutations cause autosomal dominant nonautoimmune hereditary hyperthyroidism).
- McCune-Albright syndrome (activating G-protein mutation can lead to indolent hyperthyroidism in addition to the classic features of this syndrome).
- Ectopic thyroid tissue

 Data Gathering

HISTORY

Question: Growth acceleration? May also be associated with precocious puberty
Significance: Hyperthyroidism can accelerate the bone age (developmental tempo).

Question: Declining school performance?
Significance: Mind racing, difficulty concentrating; may be mistaken for attention deficit/hyperactivity disorder.

Question: Any symptoms of hyperthyroidism and their duration?

- Restlessness, emotional lability and nervousness
- Fine tremor
- Insomnia and disturbed sleep pattern; may result in daytime fatigue
- Weight loss, despite increased appetite
- Palpitations and even chest pain with minimal exertion or at rest; diminished exercise tolerance
- Heat intolerance
- Diarrhea
- Muscle weakness (proximal)
- Plummer nails (separation of nail from nail bed)
- Menstrual irregularities
- Increased urination

Significance: If child complains of these symptoms, evaluate for possible hyperthyroidism.

Question: Notice any thyroid gland enlargement? Its duration? Tenderness?
Significance: Goiter can be a presenting sign of Graves. Tenderness suggests an infectious etiology.

Question: Bulging of the eyes or change in facial appearance? Increased "staring"? Change in vision?
Significance: Expothalmus due to retro-orbital immune depositions are a hallmark of Graves disease.

Question: Familial history of thyroid disease?
Significance: Increased incidence of Graves disease in families with positive history.

 Physical Examination

Finding: Accelerated growth, or height above that expected by genetic potential
Significance: Due to bone age advancement.

Finding: Symmetrically enlarged, smooth, non-tender goiter
Significance: More than 95% of cases

Finding: Auscultate the thyroid gland for bruit while patient holds his/her breath
Significance: Due to glandular hyperperfusion associated with hyperthyroidism.

Finding: Resting tachycardia with widened pulse pressure; hyperdynamic precordium
Significance: Effects of excessive thyroid hormone cardiac.

Finding: Slightly elevated temperature
Significance: Thyroid hormone is the main controller of basal metabolic rate and a positive modulator for catecholamine-induced thermogenesis.

Finding: Lid lag/stare; exophthalmos and proptosis
Significance: Severe ophthalmopathy is rare

Finding: Fine tremor especially visible in hands and tongue
Significance: Occurs in about 60% of children with Graves disease

Finding: Proximal muscle weakness
Significance: Common but seldom severe.

Finding: Exaggerated deep tendon reflexes
Significance: Variable.

Finding: Skin warmth and moisture
Significance: Heat intolerance and excessive sweating occur in more than 30% of children with Graves.

 ## Laboratory Aids

TESTS

Test: Total or free T4
Significance: Elevated

Test: T_3 RIA
Significance: Elevated (T_3 RIA, as direct measurement of T_3, and not T_3 RU, which indirectly evaluates thyroid hormone binding capacity).

Test: TSH
Significance: Significantly suppressed or undetectable

Test: TSI titer
Significance: Positive in 90% of children

IMAGING

Test: I-123 scan
Significance: Usually not necessary to diagnose Graves disease, which would show diffuse increased uptake at 6 and 24 hours. If palpation suggests a nodule, however, a scan may be useful to reveal a "hot" nodule within a suppressed gland.

FALSE POSITIVES

• Elevated total T_4 can also be due to conditions of increased protein binding, but does not signify hyperthyroidism.

—Increased estrogen states (e.g., pregnancy and oral contraceptive use) lead to augmented hepatic thyroid binding globulin (TBG) production
—Familial dysalbuminemic hyperthyroxinemia: mutation affecting the binding affinity leads to increased protein-bound pool

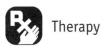 ## Therapy

DRUGS

• First line of therapy in children
• Medications block thyroid hormone synthesis but not the release of already existing hormone.
• Anti-thyroid medications (thiourea derivatives): 65% to 95% effective

—Methimazole
—Propylthiouracil (PTU)

• Propranolol or atenolol: block beta-adrenergic related symptoms; should be used in conjunction with anti-thyroid medications at the initiation of treatment and whenever cardiac symptoms are prominent.

• Duration of treatment

—Anti-thyroid medications can be weaned and potentially discontinued after 2 to 3 years of therapy, depending on the patient's course.
—Beta-blockers: used until T_4/T_3 levels are under control (approximately 6 weeks).

• Other therapies should be considered in patients who are unresponsive to drug therapy, who have significant side effects from drug therapy, or who are chronically non-compliant.

I-131 ABLATION THERAPY

• 90% to 100% effective; safe and definitive, with predictable outcome
• Results in permanent hypothyroidism requiring life-long thyroxine replacement

SUBTOTAL THYROIDECTOMY

• 80% to 100% effective; rapid and definitive
• Expensive and invasive, with risk of significant complications
• Life-long thyroxine replacement usually needed

POSSIBLE CONFLICTS

• Antihistamines and cold medications may exacerbate sympathetic nervous system symptoms.
• Treatment for severe ophthalmopathy: must refer to an ophthalmologist

—Three options: high-dose glucocorticoids, orbital radiotherapy, surgical orbital decompression
—Rehabilitative surgery involving the eye muscles or eyelids is commonly needed following ophthalmopathy treatment.

• Radioiodine ablation may exacerbate the ophthalmopathy, but this effect can be prevented with concomitant glucocorticoid administration.

 ## Follow-Up

WHEN TO EXPECT IMPROVEMENT

• Propranolol or atenolol should result in rapid relief of symptoms of sympathetic hyperactivity.
• 4 to 6 weeks of medical treatment should result in normalization of T_4/T_3 levels, though TSH may remain suppressed due to persistent underlying TSI activity.
• Duration and type of treatment depends on remission and relapse pattern.

SIGNS TO WATCH FOR

• Side effects of medications: agranulocytosis (in 0.2–0.5%), rash (the most common side effect), gastrointestinal upset, headache, transient transaminitis/hepatitis with PTU

PITFALLS

• Discontinuation of anti-thyroid drugs because of low T_4 values while TSH is still suppressed, reflecting continued TSI activity, will likely result in relapse. Anti-thyroid medication dose should be decreased or L-thyroxine should be added.
• Failure to recognize thyroid storm—an endocrinological medical emergency.

 ## Common Questions and Answers

Q: Does hyperthyroidism mean my child has thyroid cancer?
A: No. The vast majority of pediatric thyroid cancers are euthyroid because even well-differentiated carcinomas synthesize thyroid hormone much less efficiently than does normal tissue.

Q: Does Graves disease lead to thyroid cancer?
A: No. However, there is an increased incidence of benign thyroid adenoma from 0.6% to 1.9% after use of I-131 ablation.

Q: Does hyperthyroidism affect long-term growth or final adult height?
A: No. Hyperthyroidism can cause tall stature and acceleration of skeletal maturity but does not typically affect final adult height.

Q: Should routine white blood cell counts be monitored while on anti-thyroid medications due to the risk of agranulocytosis?
A: No. Routine monitoring is not cost-effective due to the acuity and rarity of agranulocytosis. However, white blood cell counts should be checked whenever a patient on anti-thyroid medication develops a fever.

Q: Will the ophthalmopathy correct with anti-thyroid treatment?
A: Not necessarily. It may require specific intervention by an ophthalmologist.

ICD-9-CM 242.0

BIBLIOGRAPHY

Bartalena L, Marcocci C, Pinchera A. Treating severe Grave's ophthalmopathy. *Baillieres Clin Endocrinol Metab* 1997;11:521–536.

Cooper DS. Antithyroid drugs for the treatment of hyperthyroidism caused by Graves' disease. *Endocrinol Metab Clin North Am* 1998;27:225–247.

Kaplan MK, Meier DA, Dworkin HJ. Treatment of hyperthyroidism with radioactive iodine. *Endocrinol Metab Clin North Am* 1998;27:205–223.

Lippe BM, Landau EM, Kaplan SA. Hyperthyroidism in children treated with long term medical therapy: twentyfive percent remission every two years. *J Clin Endocrinol Metab* 1987;64:1241.

Tomer Y, Davies TF. The genetic susceptibility to Grave's disease. *Baillieres Clin Endocrinol Metab* 1997;11:431–450.

Zimmerman D, Lteif AN. Thyrotoxicosis in children. *Endocrinol Metab Clin North Am* 1998; 27:109–126.

Authors: Adda Grimberg and Marta Satin-Smith

Growth Hormone Deficiency

 Database

DEFINITION

Growth hormone (GH) deficiency is a lack of growth hormone synthesis, release, or effect.

CAUSES

- Idiopathic (the most common form)
- Congenital

—Congenital absence of the pituitary (empty sella syndrome)
—Deletion of the GH gene in familial isolated GH deficiency
—Familial panhypopituitarism
—Growth hormone receptor defect (Laron syndrome)
—Post-growth hormone receptor defect
—Often associated with other midline defects: cleft lip, cleft palate, septo-optic dysplasia, holoprosencephaly

- Acquired

—Trauma: perinatal insult, birth trauma, surgical resection of pituitary gland, surgical damage to pituitary stalk, child abuse
—Infection: viral encephalitis, bacterial or fungal infection, tuberculosis
—Vascular: pituitary infarction, pituitary aneurysm
—Pituitary or hypothalamic irradiation
—Chemotherapy
—Tumors: craniopharyngioma, glioma, pinealoma, primitive neuroectodermal tumor (PNET; medulloblastoma)
—Histiocytosis involving the pituitary gland or sella turcica
—Sarcoidosis
—Psychosocial dwarfism

PATHOPHYSIOLOGY

Lacking GH decreases levels of insulin-like growth factor I (IGF-I) which acts on cartilage to stimulate linear growth.

GENETICS

- Autosomal recessive
- Autosomal dominant
- X-linked forms

EPIDEMIOLOGY (AGE RELATED)

- Incidence in the United States is 1 per 4,000
- Males are more commonly diagnosed than females.
- Two peak ages of diagnosis:

—Less than 1 year of age, usually because of associated hypoglycemia
—After 4 years of age, usually because of poor linear growth

COMPLICATIONS

- Short stature
- Lack of self-esteem due to the short stature
- Delay in pubertal changes (sexual characteristics and growth spurt) due to delayed bone age
- Hypoglycemia (in the newborn period)
- Osteopenia

PROGNOSIS

- Excellent

 Differential Diagnosis

- Constitutional delay of growth and adolescence
- Familial short stature
- Renal failure
- Inflammatory bowel disease
- Hypo- or achondroplasia
- Turner syndrome
- Malnutrition
- Cystic fibrosis
- Congenital heart disease
- Hyperinsulinism (in the newborn period)
- Hypothyroidism
- Hypercortisolism
- Russell-Silver syndrome
- Prader-Willi syndrome
- Sprue

 Data Gathering

HISTORY

Question: Complications during pregnancy or delivery?
Significance: Growth failure associated with congenital GH deficiency manifests by third trimester; however, you must exclude material factors causing late intrauterine growth retardation such as oligohydramnios.

Question: Birth weight?
Significance: Birth weight is usually normal and birth length below the fifth percentile; length-for-weight at birth will be low.

Question: Hypoglycemia during infancy (the first months of life)?
Significance: GH is important to maintain euglycemia in the first months of life.

Question: Plot previous lengths/heights and characterize growth pattern (velocity)?
Significance: Growth velocity will be low, but the GH-deficient infant may not drop below the third percentile for length until the end of the first year of life.

Question: Signs/symptoms of systemic illness or chronic disease?
Significance: Vomiting, polyuria, loose stools, food-provoked gastrointestinal distress, etc., may suggest a cause other than GH deficiency.

Question: Heights of family members?
Significance: Measure both parents' heights whenever the family history reveals a man below 5'4" or a woman below 4'11" tall.

Question: Family timing of pubertal development: age at menarche or pubertal growth spurt?
Significance: Constitutional delay of growth and development tends to occur in multiple close family members.

SPECIAL QUESTIONS

Question: Document patient's growth pattern and heights of family members
Significance: Measure height and weight of siblings whenever practical; always review prior growth records for the patient and siblings.

 Physical Examination

- Measure accurate weight and height with wall stadiometer
- Look for signs of syndromes, chronic disease, or malnutrition
- Evaluate Tanner stages of pubertal development
- Check males for micropenis (especially newborns)

Finding: Observe body habitus
Significance: Classic GH-deficient patient has:

- Protrusion of the frontal bones (frontal bossing)
- Midline facial defects such as poor development of nasal bridge and single central maxillary incisor
- Thin hair
- Poor nail growth
- High-pitched voice
- Truncal obesity and relative adiposity
- Cherubic facies

Finding: Observe dental development
Significance: Typically delayed

PROCEDURE

- Calculate dental age based on tooth eruption
- Quantify penile and testicular sizes:

—Small penis in GH deficiency
—Testicular size (volume using Prader beads)

- Palpate for submucosal cleft palate
- Test visual fields
- Calculate growth velocity between growth measurements

Growth Hormone Deficiency

 ## Laboratory Aids

SPECIFIC TESTS

Test: Growth factors
Significance: IGF-I and IGFBP-3 (insulin-like growth factor binding protein-3) production is regulated directly by GH

Test: GH provocative testing
Significance: A random GH level is generally useless to diagnose GH deficiency because beyond the neonatal period, GH is only secreted in brief pulses during deep sleep (at night).

NON-SPECIFIC TESTS

Growth factors and the following general tests should be used to screen for common causes of poor growth before embarking on GH provocative testing.

- CBC with differential
- Sedimentation rate: looking for inflammatory processes
- Hepatic and renal function tests
- Chromosomes in females (to exclude Turner syndrome)
- Thyroid function tests

IMAGING

- Bone age: radiography of left hand and wrist
- If proven GH deficient, head MRI to look for central nervous system tumor

REQUIREMENTS FOR TESTING

All blood tests, except GH provocative testing, do not require any form of preparation.

 ## Therapy

DRUGS

- Recombinant human growth hormone (rhGH) by subcutaneous injection daily: 0.3 mg/kg/wk
- Recombinant human GH releasing hormone (rhGHRH) by subcutaneous injection

DURATION OF THERAPY

- In children and adolescents:

—Until growth velocity drops to 0.5 cm/year
—Once puberty is complete

- In adulthood:

—GH-deficient adults may benefit from lifelong rhGH therapy due to its effects on body composition and glucose metabolism
—Patient should again undergo GH provocative testing (off rhGH therapy)

DIET

- Unrestricted

POSSIBLE CONFLICTS

Usually not given in cancer patients until one year has elapsed without recurrence

 ## Follow-Up

- Every 3 months by an endocrinologist

WHEN TO EXPECT IMPROVEMENT

- Immediate effect on hypoglycemia
- Growth velocity improves within 3 to 6 months

SIGNS TO WATCH FOR

- Pseudotumor cerebri (headache, vision problems)
- Slipped capital femoral epiphysis (SCFE)
- Theoretically, increased risk of leukemia

PITFALLS

- GH provocative testing may yield false-positive or false-negative results. 20% of normal children will fail at least one GH provocative test; obese but otherwise normal children are more likely to fail provocative GH testing.
- Malnutrition can cause low IGF-I.
- Psychosocial deprivation mimics GH deficiency. Such deprived patients may have low growth factors and respond poorly to GH provocative testing.
- rhGH therapy is associated with idiopathic intracranial hypertension (pseudotumor cerebri). This side effect is often transient, is usually reversible when the rhGH dose is decreased, and does not require cessation of therapy in all cases.
- Carefully evaluate any limp and knee or hip pain in patients on rhGH therapy because these symptoms may hail the onset of SCFE. SCFE mandates orthopedic consultation.
- There has been a slightly increased incidence of leukemia in rhGH-treated children. It is controversial whether this is due to rhGH or predisposing factors in these children (e.g., selection bias when studying children with growth failure).

 ## Common Questions and Answers

Q: Does growth hormone increase adult height in patients with familial short stature or constitutional delay of growth and adolescence?
A: Clinical studies have not shown that rhGH consistently improves final adult height for these patients.

Q: Does growth hormone cause tumors?
A: Clinical studies have not confirmed an association.

ICD-9-CM 253.3

BIBLIOGRAPHY

Chrisoulidou A, Kousta E, Beshyah SA, Robinson S, Johnston DG. How much, and by what mechanisms, does growth hormone replacement improve quality of life in GH-deficient adults? *Baillieres Clin Endocrinol Metab* 1998;12(2): 261–279.

Ghigo E, Arvat E, Aimaretti G, Broglio F, Giordano R, Camanni F. Diagnostic and therapeutic uses of growth hormone-releasing substances in adult and elderly subjects. *Baillieres Clin Endocrinol Metab* 1998;12(2):341–358.

Loder RT, Wittenberg B, DeSilva G. Slipped capital femoral epiphysis associated with endocrine disorders. *J Pediatr Orthop* 1995;15(3): 349–356.

Preece MA. Making a rational diagnosis of growth-hormone deficiency. *J Pediatr* 1997;131(1 Pt 2):S61–S64.

Romeo JH. Hyperfunction and hypofunction in the anterior pituitary. *Nurs Clin North Am* 1996;31(4):769–778.

Saggese G, Ranke MB, Saenger P, Rosenfeld RG, Tanaka T, Chaussain JL, Savage MO. Diagnosis and treatment of growth hormone deficiency in children and adolescents: Towards a consensus. *Horm Res* 1998;50(6):320–340.

Wit JM, Kamp GA, Rikken B. Spontaneous growth and response to growth hormone treatment in children with growth hormone deficiency and idiopathic short stature. *Pediatr Res* 1996;39(2):295–302.

Authors: Robert J. Ferry, Jr. and Paulo F. Collett-Solberg

Guillain-Barré Syndrome

 Database

DEFINITION

Guillain-Barré syndrome (GBS) is an autoimmune disease affecting the myelin of peripheral nerves causing weakness in the limbs, face, and respiratory muscles. Parathesias or loss of sensation in the hands and feet are often present.

CAUSES

Unknown; autoimmune attack sometimes follows viral or bacterial infection, surgery, or vaccination; often no precipitating event can be identified.

PATHOPHYSIOLOGY

Inflammatory infiltrate can be seen in areas of demyelination on nerve biopsy; lymphocytes and macrophages likely participate in myelin destruction. Both cell-mediated and humoral immune mechanisms play a role in pathogenesis.

ASSOCIATED DISEASES

• GBS is seen in a higher-than-expected rate in patients with sarcoidosis, systemic lupus erythematosis, lymphoma, HIV infection, Lyme disease, and solid tumors.
• Complications include respiratory failure, autonomic disturbances, aspiration, fluid balance and nutritional deficiencies, deep venous thrombosis, infection susceptibility, muscle atrophy, and joint contractures.

EPIDEMIOLOGY

Overall yearly incidence rate of 0.6 to 1.9 cases per 100,000. Of 95 recently reported pediatric GBS patients, 45 were age 1 to 5, 36 were age 6 to 10, and 14 were age 11 to 15.

GENETICS

Sporadic genetic factors may influence susceptibility to GBS, but there is no clear relationship between GBS and HLA-type; few cases of GBS are reported among first-order relatives.

PROGNOSIS

85% have a good recovery; ultimate functional recovery depends on the degree of axonal loss, which can be predicted from electrodiagnostic studies. Death from early respiratory failure, autonomic instability, or other complications occurs in 3% to 6% in modern series.

 Differential Diagnosis

• Myasthenia gravis
• Botulism
• Intoxication (heavy metals, organophosphates, etc.)
• Myopathy
• Poliomyelitis and other acute (viral) motor neuron dieases
• Acute cerebellar ataxia
• Transverse myelitis
• Chronic inflammatory demyelinating polyneuropathy (CIDP)
• Vasculitic neuropathy
• Diphtheric neuropathy (rare)
• Porphyric neuropathy
• Locked-in state
• Psychogenic

 Data Gathering

HISTORY

Question: Problems walking?
Significance: Most patients first note leg weakness or gait instability that progresses over days to weeks.

Question: Diminished finger and toe sensation?
Significance: Parasthesias and pain frequently appear early in the course.

Question: Respiratory problems?
Significance: Weakness may interfere with breathing.

 Physical Examination

Finding: Deep tendon reflexes are lost.
Significance: Typical sign of GBS.

Finding: Facial weakness
Significance: Occurs in many cases, and respiratory failure dictates intubation in up to 10% of patients.

Finding: "Floppy infant"
Significance: Neonates and infants may present as floppy infants.

 Laboratory Aids

Test: Lumbar puncture
Significance: Nearly all patients, particularly children, have elevated cerebrospinal fluid protein with minimal pleocytosis (<50 WBC/mm^3).

Test: Electrodiagnosis
Significance: Often helpful when clinical/cerebrospinal fluid findings are ambiguous. Evidence of demyelinating neuropathy is in clinically affected areas. Slowing of motor conduction, motor conduction block, prolonged distal motor latencies, temporal dispersion of motor responses, and abnormalities of F waves are the electrodiagnostic features of demyelinating neuropathy.

Test: In atypical cases, consider heavy metal screen, HIV titer, Lyme titer, porphyria screen, acetylcholine receptor antibodies.
Significance: See Differential Diagnosis.

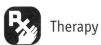 Therapy

Immunomodulatory and supportive therapies are the mainstay:

- Plasma exchange is the primary therapy for GBSA. Total plasma exchange volume of 200 to 250 mL/kg divided in three to five treatments over 7 to 14 days, beginning within 30 days of the onset of weakness significantly hastens recovery in GBS. Plasma exchange has not been studied in large trials in children, but its use in children is widespread and it is well tolerated.
- Intravenous immunoglobulin (IVIG) has been tried with success in adults and children. One large study showed it to be of equivalent efficacy to plasma exchange in adults. Many investigators have reported an increased rate of relapse in patients treated with IVIG. A trial comparing IVIG with plasma exchange in adults is nearly complete, and a similar trial in children is planned.
- Corticosteroids have not been shown to be helpful and generally not used.
- Management in an intensive care unit is usually required. Respiratory vital capacity should be frequently monitored and elective intubation performed when the vital capacity falls below 10 mL/kg. Particular attention should be given to preventing secondary pressure neuropathies.
- Pain is common in GBS and should be treated aggressively.
- Prevention measures are not known.

 Follow-Up

- First improvement typically begins 2 to 3 weeks after onset of symptoms but may not occur for 1 to 2 months in some patients.
- Improvement continues for 1 to 2 years.

PITFALLS

- Respiratory failure may occur quickly.
- Approximately 10% of patients present with a variant syndrome—pure motor GBS, pharyngeal-cervical-brachial weakness, paraparetic form, ataxic form or Fisher syndrome (ophthalmoplegia, ataxia, and arreflexia).
- Many patients appear to have psychogenic instability early in the course of GBS

 Common Questions and Answers

Q: Is GBS contagious?
A: No.

Q: Will I get GBS again?
A: Acute relapses occur in 1% to 5% of patients in large series. CIDP can rarely begin with a rapid onset of weakness indistinguishable from GBS.

ICD-9-CM 357.0

BIBLIOGRAPHY

Abd-Allah SA, Jansen PW, Ashwal S, Perkin RM. Intravenous immunoglobulin as therapy for pediatric Guillain-Barre syndrome. *J Child Neurol* 1997;12(6):376–380.

Evans OB, Vedanarayanan V. Guillain-Barre syndrome. *Pediatr Rev* 1997;18(1):10–16.

Jones HR Jr. Guillain-Barre syndrome in children. *Curr Opin Pediatr* 1995;7(6):663–668.

Author: James W. Teener

Gynecomastia

Database

DEFINITION

Any visible or palpable proliferation of breast glandular tissue, unilateral or bilateral, due to an increase in estrogen action relative to androgen action at the level of the breast.

ETIOLOGY

Physiological

• Neonatal: transient palpable breast tissue developing in newborns due to the high estrogen levels in the feto-placental unit. This condition resolves as estrogen levels decline.
• Pubertal: benign transient gynecomastia occurring in otherwise healthy adolescent males. Breast tissue in pubertal gynecomastia measuring less than 4 cm in diameter has a high likelihood of spontaneous regression.
• Involutional: breast enlargement occurring in elderly men.

Pathological

• Drug-induced

—Hormones: estrogen, androgens, gonadotropins, anabolic steroids, growth hormone, anti-androgens
—Anti-infective agents: ethionamide, isoniazid, ketoconazole, metronidazole
—Anti-ulcer drugs: cimetidine, ranitidine, omeprazole
—Chemotherapeutic agents: alkylating agents, methotrexate, vinca alkaloids
—Cardiovascular agents: amiodarone, captopril, digitoxin, diltiazem, enalapril, methyldopa, nifedipine, reserpine, spironolactone, verapamil
—Psychotropic agents: diazepam, haloperidol, phenothiazines, tricyclic antidepressants
—Drugs of abuse: alcohol, amphetamines, heroin, marijuana, methadone
—Miscellaneous: metoclopramide, phenytoin, penicillamine, theophylline

• Hypogonadism: primary or secondary
• Tumors: testicular, adrenal, ectopic hCG-producing tumors
• Chronic disease: hyperthyroidism, renal failure, liver disease, malnutrition with refeeding, HIV infection
• Congenital disorders: Klinefelter syndrome, vanishing testes syndrome (also known as anorchia, gonadal agenesis, or testicular regression), androgen resistance syndromes, true hermaphroditism, excessive peripheral tissue aromatase
• Chest wall trauma
• Intercostal nerve damage following surgery or herpes zoster
• Psychological stress
• Spinal cord injury

PATHOPHYSIOLOGY

Any situation that leads to an increase in the net effect of estrogen action relative to androgen action at the level of the breast may lead to gynecomastia. These situations could include:

• Increased estrogen concentration (endogenous or exogenous)
• Normal estrogen levels with decreased androgen concentrations
• Congenital reduction in estrogen receptors
• Pharmacological blockade of androgen receptors
• Increased breast or peripheral tissue aromatase (aromatase converts androgens to estrogens)
• Testicular dysfunction
• High serum gonadotropins or increased sex hormone binding globulin
• Elevated estrogen levels lead to proliferation of the ducts and surrounding mesenchymal tissue resulting in breast enlargement.
• Mechanism of drug-induced gynecomastia depends on drug type. Reversibility with drug withdrawal is the rule.

If gynecomastia is present for less than 1 year, tissue samples reveal prominent ductules with epithelial hyperplasia embedded in stromal connective tissue, which may spontaneously regress. If present for more than 1 year, tissue samples reveal dense collagen fibers, dilatation of the ducts with significant reduction in epithelial proliferation, which will persist despite hormonal imbalance correction.

GENETICS

Gynecomastia is occasionally familial, following X-linked or sex-limited autosomal dominant patterns.

EPIDEMIOLOGY

• Two peaks in age distribution occur in the pediatric population: in the neonatal period and in puberty.
• Neonatal gynecomastia occurs in 60% to 90% of all newborns
• 40% of boys develop transient gynecomastia (measuring >0.5 cm) during puberty
• Peak incidence at 14 years (range 10–16 years)
• No racial differences exist

COMPLICATIONS

• Physical pain, which may interfere with sports
• Psychological pain
• Embarrassment
• Skin erosion of the nipple due to rubbing against clothing
• Breast cancer: patients with Klinefelter syndrome have a 16-fold increased risk of breast cancer; other causes of gynecomastia are not associated with an increased risk of breast cancer

PROGNOSIS

• Overall, good
• Pubertal gynecomastia: 75% disappears spontaneously within 2 years, and 90% within 3 years

• Neonatal gynecomastia usually resolves within the first year of life

Differential Diagnosis

INFECTIOUS

• Breast abscess

NEOPLASTIC

• Breast neoplasm
• Neurofibroma
• Lymphangioma
• Lipoma
• Neuroblastoma metastasis

TRAUMA

• Hematoma

MISCELLANEOUS

• Pseudogynecomastia: excessive adipose tissue only; no discrete subareolar tissue
• Dermoid cyst

Data Gathering

HISTORY

Question: Time of onset relative to puberty?
Significance: Genitalia development will be present for at least 6 months before onset of breast development.

Question: Rate of progression?
Significance: Rapidly enlarging, painful gynecomastias with acute onset is more concerning than long-standing enlargement.

Question: Drug exposures, including alcohol and substance abuse?
Significance: Marijuana and heroin addiction may cause gynecomastia.

• Symptoms suggestive of hyperthyroidism? 30% of young men with hyperthyroidism develop gynecomastia.
• Symptoms suggestive of liver disease?
• Symptoms suggestive of renal failure?
• Symptoms suggestive of neoplastic disease? In patients <10 yrs of age, consider pituitary adrenal or testicular tumor.
• Symptoms suggestive of hypogonadism, such as decreased libido, decreased erectile function, and infertility suggest abnormal estrogen to androgen ratio.

Physical Examination

• Assess height, weight, growth velocity, and blood pressure.
• Assess for malnourishment. Malnourishment may result in hepatic dysfunction causing higher estrogen to androgen ratio.

Finding: Perform a complete breast examination

Significance: With patient in the supine position, grasp the breast between the thumb and forefinger and move digits toward the nipple: look for a firm, rubbery, mobile, disk-like mound of tissue arising concentrically below the nipple and areola. Measure the diameter of the disk of glandular tissue. Asymmetry and tenderness are common.

Finding: Pseudogynecomastia

Significance: If pseudogynecomastia (fatty enlargement of breasts) is present, no glandular disk will be palpable.

Finding: Check for galactorrhea

Significance: Seen with drug ingestion and pituitary tumor.

Finding: Determine if macrogynecomastia (disk diameter >5 cm with a secondary mound above the level of the breast) is present.

Significance: Macrogynecomastia may be physiological or pathological, and is unlikely to regress.

Finding: Examine the thyroid gland for the presence of a goiter

Significance: Gynecomastia seen in puberty and hyperthyroidism.

Finding: Determine the Tanner staging

Significance: Perform a careful testicular examination with measurement of size. Rule out Klinefelter syndrome if testes less than 3 cm in length or 8 mL in volume.

 ## Laboratory Aids

- None indicated for pubertal and neonatal gynecomastia.
- Renal, hepatic, and/or thyroid function tests if indicated.

Test: Karyotype

Significance: Klinefelter syndrome suspected.

Test: Luteinizing hormone (LH), follicle-stimulating hormone (FSH), estradiol, testosterone, and hCG.

Significance: To determine if hypogonadism, precocious puberty, or macrogynecomastia present.

Test: Prolactin level

Significance: To rule out a prolactin-secreting pituitary tumor: if galactorrhea present or if decreased testosterone with decreased or normal LH.

RADIOGRAPHIC STUDIES

Test: Testicular ultrasound

Significance: If elevated hCG, elevated estradiol or asymmetric testes on physical examination to rule out testicular tumor.

Test: Chest x-ray with abdominal CT

Significance: If hCG elevated and testicular ultrasound is normal to rule out extragonadal germ cell tumor or hCG-secreting nontrophoblastic neoplasm.

Test: Adrenal CT or MRI

Significance: To rule out adrenal neoplasm, if estradiol elevated, LH decreased or normal, and testicular ultrasound normal

Test: Skull x-ray, brain MRI or CT

Significance: If pituitary tumor is suspected.

 ## Therapy

- Reassurance for patients with pubertal gynecomastia measuring more than 4 cm. Treatment guidelines are variable for gynecomastia measuring 4 to 5 cm. Consultation in these patients should be considered.
- Re-examine at 3-month intervals
- Discontinue any drugs known to induce gynecomastia and follow-up in 1 month.
- Correct any underlying disorders (hyperthyroidism, malnutrition, etc.).

DRUGS

- The effectiveness of drugs in the treatment of gynecomastia has been difficult to evaluate due to the high prevalence of spontaneous regression
- Generally, drug therapy should proceed under the guidance of an endocrinologist
- Tamoxifen and testolactone have shown some benefit in adolescents with benign pubertal gynecomastia
- If gynecomastia has been present for more than 1 year, pharmacological therapy is of little benefit. After 1 year, regardless of the etiology of gynecomastia, epithelial growth becomes less prominent while periductal fibrosis and hyalinization are more evident. Because of the increase in fibrosis, gynecomastia of longer duration is less amenable to medical treatment.
- Surgery is the therapy of choice for macrogynecomastia, or persistent gynecomastia resistant to medical therapy
- Surgical options include periareolar incision with adjunctive liposuction or glandular tissue removal through two incisions in the anterior axillary regions

 ## Follow-Up

- Watch for signs of psychological stress
- Watch for symptoms of chronic disease, abnormal physical changes

PITFALLS

- Mistaking pseudogynecomastia (i.e., fatty enlargement of the breasts) from true gynecomastia
- Overlooking a potentially drug-related etiology. Drug-related gynecomastia is usually reversible if diagnosed within 1 year of onset.

 ## Common Questions and Answers

Q: When should a patient with gynecomastia be referred to a specialist?

A: If macrogynecomastia is present, if there is an abnormal hormonal work-up or an abnormal imaging study, or if there is an abnormal rate of progression

Q: For how long does neonatal gynecomastia persist?

A: Studies of healthy term infants have shown that the diameter of the breast tissue may actually increase during the first 2 weeks of life. The breast tissue then decreases to an average diameter of 10 mm until about 4 to 6 months of age. The breast tissue of female infants is generally larger and may persist longer than in males. Occasionally, the breast tissue will fail to regress and remain after the first year of life.

Q: Is it normal for a newborn baby's breasts to secrete milk?

A: In the later stages of gestation, the developing breast undergoes a small amount of secretory activity. This produces the so-called "witch's milk" that is expressed from the breasts of many full-term infants from the fifth to seventh day of life. Witch's milk may persist for 1 to 7 weeks after birth. As fetal prolactin, placental estrogen, and progesterone decline, the breast tissue regresses.

Q: How is gynecomastia distinguished from breast cancer?

A: Breast cancer usually presents as a unilateral, eccentric hard or firm mass that is fixed to underlying tissues. Associated findings can include dimpling of the skin, retraction of the nipple, nipple discharge, or axillary lymphadenopathy. The incidence of breast cancer in the pediatric population is extremely low. Less than 0.1% of all breast cancers occur in patients less than 20 years of age. Benign tumors, such as fibroadenomas, are much more common than malignant breast tumors.

ICD-9-CM 611.1

BIBLIOGRAPHY

Braunstein GD. Gynecomastia. *N Engl J Med* 1993;328(7):490–495.

Cangir A. Miscellaneous childhood tumors. In: Fernbach DJ, Vietti TJ, eds. *Clinical pediatric oncology,* 4th ed. St. Louis: Mosby Year Book, Inc., 1991:638–639.

Glass AR. Gynecomastia. *Endocrinol Metab Clin North Am* 1994;23(4)825–837.

Mahoney CP. Adolescent gynecomastia: differential diagnosis and management. *Pediatr Clin North Am* 1990;37:1389–1404.

Author: Julie A. Boom

Hand-Foot-and-Mouth Disease

 Database

DEFINITION

Hand-foot-and-mouth disease is a viral illness with the characteristic clinical features of:

- Vesiculoulcerative stomatitis
- Papular or vesicular exanthem on the hands and/or the feet
- Mild constitutional symptoms such as fever and malaise

CAUSES

Coxsackie A16 virus is the most common causative agent. Occasionally, hand-foot-and-mouth disease results from infection with:

- Coxsackie viruses A5, A7, A9, A10, A16, B1, and B3
- Enterovirus 71
- Other enteroviruses
- Herpesviruses

PATHOPHYSIOLOGY

- Enteroviruses are acquired by the oral or respiratory route.
- Lymphatic invasion leads to viremia and spread to secondary sites.
- Viremia ceases with antibody production.
- Direct inoculation of the extremities from oral lesions has been suggested in regard to hand-foot-and-mouth disease.

EPIDEMIOLOGY

- In temperate climates hand-foot-and-mouth disease is most common in the late summer and fall (a pattern common to many of the enterovirus infections).
- Spread primarily by fecal contamination and contact. Oral and respiratory secretions may also transmit the virus.
- Incubation period is 3 to 7 days.
- Highly contagious, afflicting up to one-half of those exposed.
- Close household contacts are particularly susceptible.
- May occur as an isolated case or in an epidemic distribution
- Most common in children under 5 years, but may affect adults.

COMPLICATIONS

- Hand-foot-and-mouth disease is usually self-limited and uncomplicated, resolving within 10 days.
- Dehydration is the most frequent morbid complication:

—Oral ulcerations are painful and interfere with feeding.
—Infants and children are at highest risk.

- Rare reports of other complications include:

—Neurological complications such as aseptic meningitis, encephalitis, and a polio-like paralytic disorder
—Pneumonia
—Myocarditis
—A possible association with first trimester spontaneous abortions in previously infected women

PROGNOSIS

- In the vast majority of instances hand-foot-and-mouth disease will resolve quickly requiring only supportive care.
- Young children bear the closest scrutiny because they suffer the greatest morbidity.
- Careful history and examination should distinguish those individuals with the rare, aforementioned, complications.
- Rare cases may recur at intervals for up to 1 year.

 Differential Diagnosis

Few infectious diseases have such characteristic clinical findings. Oral ulcerations followed by lesions on the distal extremities are virtually pathognomonic. The most difficult diagnostic dilemmas may be early in the disease course when isolated oral lesions predominate.

- Herpangina

—Also caused by coxsackie A viruses
—Associated with higher fever
—Usually limited to the posterior oropharynx

- Herpetic gingivostomatitis

—Most common cause of stomatitis in children
—Associated with higher fever
—More frequently associated with lymphadenopathy
—Gingival involvement severe

- Aphthous ulcers

—Generally occur without fever or upper respiratory symptoms
—Do not occur in "outbreaks"

- Stevens-Johnson syndrome

—Ulcerations frequently coalesce
—Usually affects other mucous membranes
—Often appears with separate cutaneous manifestations

- The "Boston exanthem"

—Caused by echovirus 16
—Mild febrile illness with a macular rash on the palms and soles
—Oral lesions absent

 Data Gathering

HISTORY

Question: History of cataracts?
Significance: Incubation period may be up to 1 week.

Question: Any fever, pain, or other symptoms?
Significance: A mild prodrome occasionally precedes the characteristic enanthem and exanthem by 1 or 2 days: low-grade fever (usually near 38.3°C), malaise, sore mouth, anorexia, coryza, diarrhea, abdominal pain.

Question: Bone pain?
Significance: Bone and joint aches infrequently accompany this illness.

Question: Lesions in mouth?
Significance: Oral lesions typically occur shortly before the hand and foot manifestations.

Question: Anyone in family sick?
Significance: Family members or close contacts are often similarly affected.

Question: Hydration status?
Significance: Determine quality and amount of oral intake, quality and amount of urine output, recent weight loss, duration of symptoms.

 Physical Examination

Finding: Enanthem characteristics
Significance:

- Oral lesions begin as small, red papules.
- Papules quickly evolve to small vesicles on an erythematous base.
- Lesions progress to ulcerations.
- Tongue, buccal mucosa, palate, gingiva, uvula, and/or tonsillar pillars may be involved.
- Usually 2 to 10 lesions.
- Oral lesions may persist up to 1 week.

Finding: Exanthem characteristics
Significance:

- Less consistently present than oral lesions (occur in one-fourth to two-thirds of patients)
- Maculopapular eruptions progress to vesicles
- Rarely tender or pruritic
- Most frequent on the dorsal aspects of fingers and toes
- May also occur on the palms, soles, arms, legs, buttocks, and face
- Enlarged anterior cervical, or submandibular nodes are present in one-fourth of cases.
- Attention should be given to the patient's vital signs, general appearance, and respiratory, cardiac, and neurological functioning to help identify the rare patient with a threatening complication of hand-foot-and-mouth disease.

Hand-Foot-and-Mouth Disease

Laboratory Aids

Test: None
Significance: Hand-foot-and-mouth disease has rather unique clinical features and a relatively benign course. Laboratory confirmation of the diagnosis is seldom needed or indicated.

Test: Culture
Significance: Causative viruses may be cultured from many sites:

- Oral ulcers
- Cutaneous vesicles
- Nasopharyngeal swabs
- Stool (isolation of an enterovirus from the stool does not confirm it to be the cause of disease; such a result must be paired with clinical suspicion or serological findings)
- Cerebrospinal fluid (in cases where meningoencephalitis is suspected)

Test: Electron microscopy
Significance: Can identify virus particles from similar sources.

Test: Neutralization technique
Significance: Acute and convalescent specific antibody titers may provide indirect confirmation.

Therapy

- Most cases will spontaneously resolve and require no therapy other than parental reassurance.
- Acetaminophen may relieve malaise and minor discomfort associated with the oral ulcers. It also may be used as an anti-pyretic in those children with fever.
- Dietary adjustments often improve oral intake and prevent or relieve dehydration:

—Avoid spicy or acidic foods.
—Provide cool or iced liquids in small quantities frequently.

- Symptomatic relief from particularly painful oral ulcers may be accomplished by application of a topical antihistamine or anesthetic directly to the sores (*see* Common Questions and Answers).
- Dehydration should be treated when present. Intravenous fluids may be required in the more severe cases, especially in infants and young children.
- Good supportive care is generally sufficient to treat most complications

PREVENTION

- Frequent hand washing, especially after changing diapers, and good personal hygiene are the most useful means to prevent spread of enteroviral illnesses.
- Enteric precautions should be maintained with all hospitalized patients.
- The prodromal and enanthem periods appear to be the most contagious; however, some carriers of coxsackie A16 may shed virus in the stool 3 months after infection (*see* Common Questions and Answers).

Follow-Up

- Hand-foot-and-mouth disease generally resolves spontaneously within 1 week after diagnosis.
- Small children must be followed closely for signs of dehydration.
- The extremely rare complication of myocarditis has been reported to result in at least two fatalities.
- Some patients may become asymptomatic carriers.

Common Questions and Answers

Q: What is in the "magic mouthwash" often used to relieve the pain of stomatitis?
A: Many health care providers will prescribe a "magic mouthwash" for symptomatic relief of oral ulcers, pharyngitis, and teething pain. The most common such treatment consists of an aluminum hydroxide/magnesium hydroxide gel suspension and diphenhydramine elixir (12.5 mg/5 mL) in a 1:1 formulation. It can be applied directly to the sores with a cotton swab or a small syringe before meals.

Q: Should lidocaine be used topically for symptomatic relief of oral ulcers?
A: The routine use of lidocaine in this situation is not recommended. Lidocaine is an effective topical anesthetic and comes in a 2% viscous suspension. In practice, the pain relief is short-lived, which encourages frequent administration. Lidocaine is absorbed from the mucous membranes (bypassing first-pass liver metabolism) and has been frequently reported to cause poisoning of the cardiovascular and central nervous system. Both pediatric and adult fatalities have occurred. The use of topical viscous lidocaine should be reserved for use by physicians knowledgeable regarding its proper dosage and potential side effects, and by educated, compliant parents or caretakers.

Q: When may children with hand-foot-and-mouth disease return to school?
A: This is a matter of some controversy for this highly contagious, but relatively benign, condition. However, good hygiene will greatly reduce viral transmission. And, affected patients are contagious often before the diagnosis is made. Most now suggest isolation from school or daycare contacts while febrile and/or while the enanthem persists. As mentioned, some may shed the virus in their stool for months after symptoms have resolved (again stressing the need for good personal hygiene).

ICD-9-CM 074.3

BIBLIOGRAPHY

Cherry JD. Enteroviruses: polioviruses, coxsackieviruses, echoviruses, and enteroviruses. In: Feigin RD, Cherry JD, eds. *Textbook of pediatric infectious diseases,* 3rd ed. Philadelphia: WB Saunders, 1992:1705–1753.

Gilbert GL, Dickson KE, Waters MJ, et al. Outbreak of enterovirus 71 infection in Victoria, Australia, with a high incidence of neurologic involvement. *Pediatr Infect Dis J* 1988;7: 484–488.

Robinson CR, Doane FW, Rhoades AJ. Report of an outbreak of febrile illness with pharyngeal lesions and exanthem: Toronto, 1957-isolation of coxsackie virus. *Can Med Assoc J* 1958;79: 615–621.

Slavin KA, Frieden IJ. Picture of the month: hand-foot-and-mouth disease. *Arch Pediatr Adolesc Med* 1998;152:505–506.

Thomas I, Janniger CK. Hand, foot, and mouth disease. *Cutis* 1993;52:265–266.

Wright HT, Landing BH, Lennette EH, et al. Fatal infection in an infant associated with coxsackie virus group A, type 16. *N Engl J Med* 1963;268:1041–1044.

Author: Kevin C. Osterhoudt

Hantavirus/Hantapulmonary Syndrome

 Database

DEFINITION

Hantapulmonary syndrome (HPS) is a disease in humans due to Hantavirus and acquired from certain chronically infected rodent species. When acquired by humans, it results in a syndrome characterized by rapidly progressive cardiac and respiratory failure with a high mortality.

CAUSE

Original human outbreak recognized in Southwest United States was caused by the *Sin nombre* strain of Hantavirus transmitted from chronically infected deer mice (*Peromyscus maniculatus*). Subsequent cases were recognized throughout the ubiquitous distribution of the deer mouse. Since then, additional strains of Hantavirus have been recognized each with a unique rodent host. The resulting human cases of HPS have now been identified from Canada to Argentina.

EPIDEMIOLOGY

• The host rodent develops a chronic non-fatal infection and excretes virus in urine, feces, and saliva.
• Humans acquire the infection by inhaling virus contaminated airborne particles from the dried rodent excreta. Typically, this occurs when sweeping or otherwise disturbing a rodent infested building.
• Human cases are more common in the spring and summer and also in years when the population of the rodent host has increased.
• Nosocomial transmission has only been observed with the *Andes* strain in Argentina.
• In the United States, HPS has occurred primarily in young healthy adults, although in South America a larger proportion of cases are in children.

PATHOLOGY/PATHOPHYSIOLOGY

• Pathophysiological changes of most importance are myocardial depression resulting in shock and alveolar capillary leak pulmonary edema resulting in hypoxia.
• The cardiac dysfunction is characterized by a falling cardiac output, increased systemic vascular resistance and normal or low pulmonary artery wedge pressure.
• The pulmonary alveoli are flooded with fluid devoid of red cells but with a protein content similar to serum.

 Differential Diagnosis

• Pneumonic plague
• Influenza
• Bacterial sepsis especially that caused by pneumococcus and other streptococci.

 Data Gathering

The clinical symptoms, physical findings and laboratory findings progress in sequence. Early suspicion of the syndrome allows the clinician to prepare for that phase of the illness characterized by the rapid onset of respiratory failure and shock.

HISTORY

Question: Fever and myalgia?
Significance: Usually severe, characterize the prodromal phase lasting 3 to 6 days.

Question: Gastrointestinal complaints?
Significance: Frequently prominent including combinations of nausea, vomiting, diarrhea, or abdominal pain.

Question: Headache?
Significance: Is present in over one-half of patients.

Question: Cough?
Significance: Uncommon at the onset of the prodrome but precedes the onset of dyspnea and tachypnea, which is then followed by the rapid progression of cardiorespiratory failure.

Question: Coryza and sore throat?
Significance: Not part of the prodrome.

Question: A history of activities that might expose the patient to airborne virus contaminated particles should be sought.
Significance: HPS acquired by inhalation on airborne particles.

 Physical Examination

• Tachycardia and hypotension

Finding: Fever
Significance: During the prodromal phase, fever is the only finding.

Finding: Cough
Significance: With the onset of the cardiopulmonary phase, there is cough and dyspnea associated with the production of frequently copious amounts of non-purulent material.

 Laboratory Aids

TESTS

Test: Platelet count
Significance: The platelet count falls on serial testing during the prodromal phase.

• In addition to leukocytosis, myelocytes, and immunoblasts appear in the peripheral blood.
• Liver function tests are mildly abnormal.
• Hypoxemia accompanies the onset of the cardiopulmonary phase.
• Diagnostic serology demonstrates IgM antibody present at the time of clinical presentation.

IMAGING

Test: Chest radiograph
Significance: During the prodrome, chest radiography is normal. With the onset of respiratory symptoms, chest radiography will show evidence of interstitial fluid manifested by Kerley B lines, hilar indistinctness, and peribronchial cuffing. Alveolar flooding and pleural effusions develop in severe cases. Heart size remains normal.

PITFALLS

• The diagnosis depends on serologic testing, which can take some time.
• Lacking serologic confirmation, one mostly depends on clinical history and serial hematologic tests.
• In anticipation of the rapid progression of the cardiopulmonary phase, it is preferable to have the patient closely observed in the hospital.

Therapy

Because of the rapid progression of the cardio-respiratory failure, all patients with HPS should be managed in an intensive care setting with a pulmonary artery catheter to guide therapy.

• Oxygen, intubation, and mechanical ventilation are frequently needed.
• Use fluids cautiously in view of the capillary leak.
• If the patient develops hypotension, an inotropic agent such as dobutamine should be added; if the patient continues to be hypotensive on maximal doses of dobutamine, vasopressors can be added to maintain blood pressure.
• Use empiric antibiotics because serologic tests confirming HPS are usually delayed and the differential diagnosis includes sepsis from a variety of antibiotic responsive organisms.
• Extracorporeal membrane oxygenation has been used for patients who fail to respond to maximal inotropic and ventilatory support.
• To date, antiviral agents have not been shown to be beneficial.

PREVENTION

• Universal precautions are appropriate in caring for persons with HPS; person-to-person transmission has been demonstrated only with the *Andes* strain in the southern hemisphere, not in the United States.
• Preventing infection depends on avoiding contact with airborne particles contaminated by rodent excreta.
• Eliminate rodents and seal off rodent access into the house.
• Reduce rodent shelter and food sources in the immediate vicinity of the home by cutting brush, removing trash, and storing grain and animal feed in rodent-proof containers.
• Wearing gloves, clean up rodent-contaminated areas by spraying nests and droppings with household disinfectants or dilute bleach, and sealing material in bags for burning or burial.
• Ventilate closed areas before initiating cleanup.

 Follow-Up

WHEN TO EXPECT IMPROVEMENT

• Patients who survive the shock phase typically then diurese fluid, which has been third spaced. Recovery is then generally rapid.
• Easy fatigability and mild pulmonary function abnormalities may persist.

PITFALLS

Recognizing the prodrome of HPS is difficult and requires a careful history, evaluation of the risk of exposure and rapid access to testing.

 Common Questions and Answers

Q: What should I do if I find a dead mouse indoors?
A: Identify if it is a house mouse or a species which could be infected with Hantavirus. If the latter, assume that it is infected and dispose of as described previously and then seal off rodent access to the home and eliminate any still left inside the home.

Q: What should I do if I find what look like rodent droppings?
A: Clean up with gloves and disinfectant as noted here. Then use traps to catch and identify the rodents involved and proceed as answered in the previous question.

Q: Could I have HPS without knowing it?
A: In the United States, asymptotic HPS infections would appear to be uncommon based on serum screening of household contacts of cases and other populations at high risk, which show only infrequent evidence of prior infection.

ICD-9-CM 518.89;09.81

BIBLIOGRAPHY

All About Hantavirus Web Page; http//www.cdc.gov/ncidod/diseases/hanta/hps/index.htm

Butler JC, Peters CJ. Hantaviruses and hantavirus pulmonary syndrome. *Clin Infect Dis* 1994;19:387–395.

Duchin JS, et al. Hantavirus pulmonary syndrome: a clinical description of 17 patients with a newly recognized disease. *N Engl J Med* 1994;330:949–955.

Levy H, Simpson SQ. Hantavirus pulmonary syndrome. *Am J Respir Crit Care Med* 1994;149:1710–1713.

Author: Bruce Tempest

Headache

Database

DEFINITION

Headache may be "primary" or "secondary," symptomatic of a specific oral, cranial, or cervical pathological process (e.g., trauma or tumor).

- Chronic or recurrent: recurring repeatedly over years or persisting relentlessly over days
- Acute: rapid onset or progression
- Tension headaches, also known as muscle contraction headaches, are thought due to simple traction on pain sensors during prolonged contraction of the scalp and neck.
- Migraine is a recurrent, throbbing headache of vascular origin, usually bilateral in children and unilateral in adults. The majority of primary pediatric headaches are migraine headaches.

MIGRAINE TYPES INCLUDE

- Classic migraine

—A visual aura consisting of scintillations, scotomata, or blurred vision precedes the headache followed by a unilateral or bilateral throbbing headache that intensifies over a few hours, can last several hours to a day, and is generally relieved with rest or sleep.
—Nausea, vomiting, anorexia, abdominal pain, irritability, malaise, fatigue, and photophobia are all common associated symptoms.

- Common migraine

—Is the most common form of headache in children and adolescents
—Has the characteristic throbbing headache but without the visual prodrome of classic migraine. All other symptoms noted here are frequently seen.

- Complicated migraine

—Is the association of migraine with transient neurological deficits such as ophthalmoplegic migraine, hemiplegic migraine, and migraine with aphasia
—Basilar artery migraine is the combination of occipital headache with neurological dysfunction referable to the brainstem, cerebellum, inferior temporal, and occipital lobes.
—Symptoms may include blurred vision, dizziness, vertigo, ataxia, sensory and motor abnormalities, obtundation, and loss of consciousness.
—Acute confusional migraine begins with headache and is followed by confusion, agitation, and altered sensorium and is confused with the confusional state of illicit drug use in adolescents.

- Migraine variants: include paroxysmal vertigo, paroxysmal vertigo, and cyclic vomiting or periodic syndrome.

—Are episodes of transient neurological dysfunction in a patient with known migraine, a patient who develops migraine later, or in a patient who has a family predisposition to migraine.

EPIDEMIOLOGY

- Migraine occurs in 3% to 5% of children before puberty and increases to 10% to 20% during the second decade.
- Female:male ratio is approximately equal before puberty and increases to 2:1 after puberty.
- Migraine has a strong genetic component; may be autosomal dominant in many families.

PATHOPHYSIOLOGY

Although there is a lack of consensus regarding the pathogenesis of migraine, underlying theories include involvement of the cerebral vasculature, neural hypotheses of the brainstem and cortex, involvement of bioactive amines such as serotonin and substance P.

GENETICS

Familial history of migraine headache is common (60%) and supports the diagnosis of migraine headache.

CAUSES

- Acute diffuse: trauma, infection (systemic), stress, meningitis, encephalitis, stroke (thrombotic, embolic, hemorrhagic), subarachnoid hemorrhage, toxins (e.g., lead), hypertension, hypoglycemia, post-lumbar puncture, collagen vascular disease (arteritis), drug abuse
- Acute focal: trauma, infection (otitis, sinusitis, brain abscess, encephalitis, meningitis), dental process, orbital disease, cranial neuralgias
- Subacute recurrent/progressive: migraine (common and classic), complicated migraine, migraine variants
- Chronic progressive: benign intracranial hypertension, abscess, tumor, hydrocephalus, subdural hematoma, drug abuse
- Chronic, non-progressive: chronic myositis, psychogenic or tension headache, post-concussive syndrome, depression, conversion disorder, cervical osteoarthritis, temporomandibular joint syndrome, atypical facial pain

Differential Diagnosis

- Sinusitis
- Trigeminal neuralgia
- Atypical facial pain and factitious pain disorders
- Systemic features of migraine may lead to evaluation for metabolic or cerebrovascular disorders: episodic vomiting-hyperammonemias, transient hemiparesis-stroke, acute/recurrent ataxia-amino acidopathy, mitochondrial disorders, epilepsy

Other diagnostic considerations are dictated by the temporal characteristics of headache:

- Chronic: A minority of children with chronic headache have structural brain lesions: brain tumors, hydrocephalus, abscess.
- Benign intracranial hypertension usually accompanied by papilledema, normal imaging, and cerebrospinal fluid analysis.
- Post-concussive syndrome should be considered in appropriate setting.
- Children with psychogenic or tension headaches often lack associated history of social/emotional stress.
- Occipital neuralgia from trauma, shingles, or Lyme disease
- Acute: meningitis, encephalitis, intracranial hemorrhage, sinus thrombosis, dental infection, hydrocephalus

Data Gathering

HISTORY

Question: Background?
Significance: Important features include duration of the problem, location of the headache, time of onset, mode of onset, associated symptoms, response to therapy, and familial history.

Question: Migraine?
Significance: The mode of onset is usually gradual, rarely paroxysmal. The location of the headache is typically bilateral either bifrontal, bitemporal, or bioccipital or diffuse and ill-defined. The quality of the pain may be aching/steady or throbbing.

Question: Stress?
Significance: May exacerbate either migraine or tension headache. Although many adults with migraine are depressed, the prevalence of depression in children with chronic headaches is not known.

Physical Examination

Finding: Blood pressure measurement
Significance: Hypertension

Finding: Auscultation for bruits
Significance: A-V malformations

Finding: Signs of meningeal irritation
Significance: Fundoscopy for papilledema

Finding: Examination of jaw (range of motion), teeth/oral cavity, otoscopy, and palpation of maxillary, frontal, and mastoid sinuses.
Significance: TMJ syndrome; sinusitis

Finding: Neurological examination
Significance: Should be normal in primary headache syndromes (migraine, tension), except perhaps during a migraine ictus; focal neurological deficits suggest a structural (symptomatic) basis of headache.

Laboratory Aids

Test: Sinus films
Significance: Indicated if symptoms point to sinusitis. These may not be obvious in sphenoid sinusitis, which may produce unremitting, chronic frontal headache.

Test: Chronic anemia
Significance: May be associated with headache, although it rarely presents in children as headache.

Test: Neuroimaging studies (CT/MRI)
Significance: Indicated when neurological examination indicates a focal abnormality; if the history suggests a specific diagnosis such as a brain tumor; or, if headaches are associated with persistent vomiting. Neuroimaging may also be indicated for atypical headaches, persistently unilateral headaches, and headaches that are increasing in frequency and severity, or that are refractory to treatment.

Test: EEG
Significance: Should be obtained when the headache is paroxysmal and/or focal.

Test: Lumbar puncture
Significance: Examination of cerebrospinal fluid to detect infection may occasionally be indicated. Opening pressure necessary in diagnosis of pseudotumor cerebri.

Therapy

• Evaluation and treatment is similar to that of adult migraine. Treatment may be categorized as symptomatic, abortive, or preventive. Rare to occasional migraines may be treated symptomatically with aspirin or acetaminophen.
• Abortive therapy: ergotbomine, sumatriptan
• Prophylactic therapy includes beta blockers, cyproheptadine, tricyclic antidepressants, calcium channel blockers, anti-inflammatory drugs, and occasionally anticonvulsants.
• Other treatment modalities may include behavior therapy, relaxation training including biofeedback, avoidance of specific foods or substances that may be migraine triggers. Treatment may also include appropriate psychological counseling.

PITFALLS

• Headaches with vomiting may suggest elevated intracranial pressure, not just migraine.
• Depression and migraine may be due to temporal lobe tumor.
• Arteriovenous malformation may mimic migraine and should be considered if headache is persistently on the same side of the head or if response to therapy is poor.

Common Questions and Answers

Q: When should migraine be treated?
A: Many children with migraine headaches have attacks so infrequently that prophylactic medical therapy is not warranted. Treatment should be considered when attacks occur at least once a month.

Q: What about allergy and headache?
A: Many believe that headache may represent a symptom of hypersensitivity. Headache in the setting of allergic rhinitis/asthma may be due to associated sinusitis/sinus congestion, side effect of treatment (especially theophylline), or muscle tension.

Q: At what age may migraine begin?
A: Even 2 to 3 year olds may present with headache or migraine equivalent symptoms: episodic vomiting, episodic ataxia that improves after sleep.

ICD-9-CM 346.9

BIBLIOGRAPHY

Holden EW, Levy JD, Deichmann MM, Gladstein J. Recurrent pediatric headaches: assessment and intervention. *J Dev Behav Pediatr* 1998;19(2):109–116.

Kain ZN, Rimar S. Management of chronic pain in children. *Pediatr Rev* 1995;16(6):218–222.

Lipton R, Stewart W. Migraine in the United States: a review of epidemiology and health care use. *Neurology* 1993;43(6):6–10.

Raskin N. Acute and prophylactic treatment of migraine: practical approaches and pharmacologic rationale. *Neurology* 1993;43(6):39–42.

Singh BV, Roach ES. Diagnosis and management of headache in children. *Pediatr Rev* 1998;19(4):132–135; quiz 136.

Smith MS. Comprehensive evaluation and treatment of recurrent pediatric headache. *Pediatr Ann* 1995;24(9):450, 453–457.

Author: Patricia T. Molloy

Heat Stroke and Related Illness

 Database

DEFINITION

Heat stroke results from an imbalance between heat production, absorption, and dissipation. This can result from excessive body heat generation and storage without appropriate dissipation due to high ambient temperature, low radiation or convective heat loss, decreased evaporation, medical predisposition, and inadequate sweat (water and/or salt) replacement. Heat illness actually encompasses a spectrum of heat related disease processes.

PREDISPOSING CONDITIONS

- Environmental predisposition
—Hot and humid without wind, heat wave, hot indoor environment, lack of air conditioning
—Age extremes; children have increased heat production, sweat less, and a large body surface area to weight ratio as well as inability to regulate fluid intake and environment
- Drugs/medications
—Anti-cholinergics; inhibit perspiration
—Diuretics
—Phenothiazines
—Psychiatric medications
—Drugs of abuse; hallucinogens, cocaine
—Salicylates
—Sympathomimetics
—MAO inhibitors
—Lithium
—Antihistamines
—Ethanol
- Behaviors
—Overexertion
—Athletics
—Inappropriate clothing; heavy, dark, tight-fitting, overbundling
—Lack of acclimatization and conditioning
—Inadequate fluid intake
—Children in enclosed space within motor vehicle

PATHOPHYSIOLOGY

- When environmental temperature greater than body temperature, body gains heat by conduction and radiation and can lose heat by evaporation.
- Heat production increased 10 to 20 times by strenuous exercise
- Heat dissipation (conduction to objects and air, convection, radiation, evaporation)
—If high humidity or little air movement, effectiveness of evaporative heat loss is lessened.
- Heat syncope: venous pooling (redistribution of blood volume) during strenuous or upright event, decreased central venous return, cardiac output, and cerebral perfusion pressure
- Heat exhaustion (prostration)
—Water depletion: inadequate water replacement in hot environment
—Salt depletion: salt (sweat) loss; water, but not salt replacement
—Can progress to heat stroke

- Heat stroke
—Impaired heat dissipation with extreme elevations of body temperature
—Temperature more than 42°C can uncouple oxidative phosphorylation and allow enzyme systems to cease functioning. Cell membrane integrity is lost, proteins denature, and necrosis occurs; leads to dysfunction and organ failure.
—Classic (epidemic) heat stroke
  —Sedentary, older person or young child in hot environment, medication use
  —High ambient temperature and humidity
  —Compromised homeostatic mechanisms with environmental heat stress exposure
  —Poor heat dissipation
  —Hot, dry skin (sweating usually absent)

ASSOCIATED DISEASES

- Heat cramps/spasms
—Related to physical exercise, fluid loss, poor sodium repletion (normal body temperature)
- Heat tetany
—Parasthesias, carpopedal spasm, tetany
- Heat syncope
—Alteration of consciousness (dizziness, syncope) at end of strenuous or upright event
- Heat exhaustion (prostration)
—Relatively slow onset
—Headache, nausea, vomiting, malaise, myalgias, pale skin, dizziness, visual disturbances, syncope, temperature 38 to 40°C, dehydration, electrolyte imbalance, hemoconcentration
—Can progress to heat stroke
- Heat stroke
—Central nervous system (CNS) symptoms (delirium, convulsion, coma), acute, sudden onset (80%), slower onset (minutes to hours in 20%), high fever (>40–41°C), hypotension, tachycardia, hyperventilation

COMPLICATIONS

- Heat stroke
—Electrolyte imbalance, seizures, adult respiratory distress syndrome (ARDS), acute renal, liver, cardiac failure, pulmonary edema, rhabdomyolysis (may be delayed 2–3 days), disseminated intravascular coagulation (DIC), death
—Severe dehydration if sweating occurred
—May have persistent neurological dysfunction (cerebellar, hemiparesis, dementia)

PROGNOSIS

- Heat illness (heat rash, edema, cramps, tetany, syncope, exhaustion): rapid recovery with supportive care
- Heat stroke: poor prognosis if not recognized and aggressively managed

 Differential Diagnosis

- Heat cramps
—Rhabdomyolisis
- Heat edema
—Thrombophlebitis, lymphedema, congestive heart failure

- Heat stroke
—CNS process with fever (CVA, meningitis, encephalitis), other infections, anti-cholinergic poisoning (dilated pupils), drug induced (medication, recreational), temperature rise, head injury during contact sports, severe dehydration
—Chills suggest febrile illness, not heat stroke

 Data Gathering

HISTORY

Question: Initial temperature, if taken at scene
Significance: The initial temperature can alert one to the potential for and extent of heat-related illness. If the first temperature is not obtained until after cooling interventions, extent of illness may not be fully appreciated, and appropriate therapy may be delayed.

Question: Cooling maneuvers en route to hospital
Significance: Cooling maneuvers should be instituted immediately upon consideration of heat-related illness. Interventions can avoid clinical deterioration and improve recovery. As above, however, a lower temperature may falsely reassure or mislead the definitive caretakers.

Question: History of CNS dysfunction
Significance: A history of CNS dysfunction in conjunction with an environment consistent with or predisposing conditions conducive to development of heat-related illness should lead one to a presumptive diagnosis of heat stroke. Other diagnosis leading to altered mental status, with and without fever, must also be considered.

Question: Predisposing medical, environmental or activity issues
Significance: Knowledge of environmental issues and predisposing medical or activity issues that might lead to a heat-related illness can be helpful in determining a rapid diagnosis and intervention plan. It can also enable one to predict illnesses, activities, and environments which are conducive to development of heat-related illness and potentially prevent those situations.

 Physical Examination

Finding: Heat exhaustion
Significance: Weakness, lethargy, thirst, malaise, diminished ability to work or play, headache, nausea, vomiting, myalgias, pale skin, dizziness, visual disturbances, syncope, mild CNS dysfunction, impaired judgment, cramps, vertigo, hypotension, tachycardia, hyperventilation, paresthesias, agitation, incoordination, psychosis, T less than 40°C, sweating, environmental exposure and activity

Finding: Heat stroke
Significance:

- Temperature more than 40.5°C (may be cooler due to prehospital maneuvers), with or

without hot, dry (classic), or clammy (exercise induced) skin
—Pink or ashen color
—Weakness, nausea, vomiting, anorexia, headache, dizziness, confusion, drowsiness, irritability, CNS dysfunction, euphoria, combativeness, abrupt or impending alteration of consciousness
—Obtundation, tachycardia, hypotension or normotension with wide pulse pressure, tachypnea, ataxia, posturing, incontinence, seizures, purpura, petechia
—May have muscle rigidity with tonic contractions and dystonia that mimic seizures

Finding: Temperature measurement
Significance:

• Esophageal thermometry probably the best
• Deep rectal thermometry also a good approximation of core temperature
• Tympanic temperature reasonable estimation of CNS temperature
• Oral temperature not as useful due to mouth breathing

 ## Laboratory Aids

Tests only to confirm diagnosis, evaluate extent of injury, or rule out other processes as treatment should be empiric.

• Heat cramps. Decreased serum and urine sodium and chloride; BUN normal or slightly increased
• Heat exhaustion
—May see hyponatremia (salt loss) or hypernatremia (water loss), hypochloremia, low urine sodium and chloride, hemoconcentration
—Differentiated from heat stroke by lack of significant liver function test abnormalities
• Heat stroke
—Blood chemistries: NaCl normal or high, hypokalemia, increased BUN/CR; hypophosphatemia, hypomagnesemia, hypocalcemia, lactate high; hypoglycemia
—Hematologic: CBC (hemoconcentration, leukocytosis, thrombocytosis), coagulation profile for DIC (more likely in exertional than classic heat stroke): PT/PTT, fibrin split products, fibrinogen, malaria evaluation (thick smear), hematuria
—Others: LFTs (abnormal and useful to distinguish heat stroke from heat exhaustion), CPK (rhabdomyolysis), ABG (classic heat stroke: respiratory alkalosis and hypokalemia early; lactic acidosis later; exertional heat stroke: lactic acidosis), U/A (proteinuria, microscopic hematuria, myoglobinuria), CSF, ECG, CXR.

 ## Therapy

• Rapid recognition and cooling imperative
• Specific therapy:
—Heat cramps:
    —Rest, salt and water replacement

—Heat syncope:
    —Self-limited as return to horizontal position is treatment; rest and fluids, salted liquids
—Heat exhaustion:
    —Clinical findings (HR, BP, orthostatic changes, urine output) should direct therapy
    —Most treated as outpatient with rapid recovery (older patients or those with pre-existing illnesses may require hospitalization); rest, rehydration, cooling; mild case: oral electrolyte solution (0.1% saline); if CNS/GI dysfunction (nausea, vomiting, inability to drink); IV (0.5 NSS) similar to sweat losses; avoid rapid overcorrection of hypernatremia (treat as with hypernatremic dehydration); if hyponatremic seizures, treat with 3% saline at approximately 5 mL/kg
—Heat stroke:
    —Immediate cooling
    —Remove clothing from patient and patient from hot environment; use air conditioning, open vehicle for transport if possible; esophageal or rectal temperature probe (constant temperature measurements); cooling should exceed 0.1 to 0.2°C/min; slow cooling down at 38.5 to 39°C to avoid overshoot; cooling options (ice bath, cold water bath (15–16°C) as effective as ice bath without discomfort, shivering or vasoconstriction), massage with ice, ice packs to neck, groin, axilla, wet sheet over patient, moisten skin with water spray, convection increase (fan) to increase evaporative cooling, cool water lavage (peritoneum, rectum, gastric), cold to room temperature IV fluids, alcohol sponge baths (use with caution due to potential absorption), cardiopulmonary bypass.

NON-SPECIFIC

• Heat stroke:
—Treat empirically, then rule out other causes of presentation
—ABCs
—Fluid replacement:
    —Usually only modest fluid requirements (patients often normovolemic with a distributive shock picture due to vasodilatation; cooling redistributes volume from periphery to core; aggressive fluid resuscitation can lead to fluid overload and pulmonary edema)
    —Oral hydration if alert; IV 0.5% NSS
—CNS: supportive care, seizure therapy, ICP management as indicated
—Consider antibiotics if CNS infection a possibility
—Miscellaneous therapies:
    —Nasogastric tube
    —Chlorpromazine may help with peripheral vasodilatation and prevent shivering (dose: 0.5–1.0 mg/kg [25–50 mg for adult] IV/IM; may cause hypotension);
    —Benzodiazepine for sedation;
    —Fresh frozen plasma for DIC

MEDICATIONS

• Anti-pyretics not useful because intact hypothalamus required for action

• Avoid anti-cholinergic drugs (atropine), which can inhibit sweating

PREVENTION

• Recognize and intervene for those at risk in conditions that predispose to heat illness
• Avoid enclosed spaces (children in closed cars)
• Limit physical activity, keep cool, use shaded areas
• Air conditioning all or part of hot days
• Cool or tepid baths
• Increase fluid intake: unlimited fluid replacement during strenuous activity, cool water and large volumes increase gastric emptying (high osmolality decreases gastric emptying), do not usually need glucose
• Loose, light-colored clothing, protective hat
• Acclimatization, gradual conditioning to hotter environment (7–14 days)
• Liberal dietary sodium
—Avoid sodium chloride tablets: hypernatremia and potassium depletion, gastric irritant, delayed gastric emptying
• Frequently flex leg muscles when standing and avoid prolonged standing in hot environments

 ## Common Questions and Answers

Q: How can one distinguish between heat exhaustion and heat stroke?
A: If CNS abnormalities are present, temperature is greater than 40.6°C and liver function tests are elevated, the patient is likely to have heat stroke. Remember, however, that CNS examination and temperature on arrival to medical care may not be representative of the maximal abnormalities due to preceding interventions.

Q: When should heat stroke be suspected?
A: Suspect heat stroke in a patient with or without sweating who demonstrates alterations of CNS function in environment that would be conducive to heat illness.

Q: Does the presence or absence of sweating help with the diagnosis of heat exhaustion versus heat stroke?
A: No. Sweating will be present with heat exhaustion and may or may not be present with heat stroke.

ICD-9-CM 992.0

BIBLIOGRAPHY

Heat related illnesses and deaths—United States, 1994–1995. *MMWR* 1995;44:465–468.

Kellermann AL, Todd KH. Killing heat. *N Engl J Med* 1996;335:126–127.

Simon HB. Hyperthermia. *N Engl J Med* 1993;329:483–487.

Tek D, Olshaker JS. Heat illness. *Emerg Med Clin North Am* 1992;10:299–310.

Author: George Anthony Woodward

Hemangioma (Vascular Nevi)

 Database

DEFINITION

• Hemangiomas: non-malignant neoplasms consisting of vascular endothelial cells and mast cells that enhance neoangiogenesis. Multiple cutaneous hemangiomas may be associated with other sites of hemangiomas, including the liver, lung, and gastrointestinal (GI) tract. Rarely, the meninges, brain, spinal cord, pancreas, spleen, and adrenals may be involved.
• Vascular malformations: capillaries, veins, lymphatics, or arteries that underwent errors of morphogenesis (i.e., hamartomas); includes port-wine stains (nevus flammeus) and arteriovenous malformations. Port-wine stains can signal underlying developmental defects especially of central nervous system and spine.
• Salmon patches (nevus simplex): distended dermal capillaries (nevus simplex, telangiectatic nevus).

PATHOPHYSIOLOGY

• Hemangiomas: appear in first few weeks of life, grow rapidly in first 6 to 12 months of life, followed by static period, and then involution.
• Vascular malformations: grow proportionally with the affected individual. Congenital by definition, may not become apparent until adolescence or adulthood, port-wine stain apparent at birth.
• Salmon patches: Grow proportionally with affected individual.

GENETICS

• Hemangiomas

—Usually no genetic association when isolated finding
—Seen with Klippel-Trénaunay syndrome, Parks-Weber syndrome, Maffucci syndrome, blue rubber bleb nevus syndrome (dominant inheritance), diffuse neonatal hemangiomatosis, Cobb syndrome

• Vascular malformations

—Seen with Sturge-Weber syndrome, Cobb syndrome, Wyburn-Mason (or Bonnet-Dechaume-Blanc) syndrome, Klippel-Trénaunay syndrome, Parks-Weber syndrome

• Salmon patches

—No genetic association

EPIDEMIOLOGY

• Hemangiomas

—Female:male ratio 3:1
—Increased incidence with very low birthweight (<1000 g) infants
—Present in up to 12% of infants
—80% are single lesions
—60% are found on head and neck
—25% are found on trunk

• Vascular malformations

—Port-wine stains female:male ratio 1:1

• Salmon patches

—Found in 30% to 40% of all newborns

COMPLICATIONS

• Hemangiomas

—Local ulceration, bleeding, superinfection
—Obstruction of important structures including eye, airway, GI tract
—High output cardiac failure in presence of large number of lesions
—Iron-deficiency anemia secondary to hemorrhage from GI lesions
—Kasabach-Merritt syndrome: platelet trapping, coagulopathy, thrombocytopenia; rarely cause skeletal overgrowth secondary to increased blood flow

• Vascular malformations

—Can lead to "steal" causing ischemic necrosis, pain, and increased cardiac output
—Frequently associated with skeletal abnormalities including hypertrophy (low flow) or destruction (high flow)
—Localized or disseminated intravascular coagulopathy possible, but uncommon

PROGNOSIS

• Hemangiomas: excellent except when associated with other syndromes.
• Vascular malformations: varied depending on type of malformation and associated syndromes.
• Salmon patches: excellent.

 Differential Diagnosis

INFECTION

• Bacillary angiomatosis

TUMORS

• Glomus tumor
• Angioendothelioma
• Sarcoma

CONGENITAL

• Verrucous hemangioma

MISCELLANEOUS

• Pyogenic granuloma
• Angiokeratomas
• Acquired tufted angioma

 Data Gathering

HISTORY

Question: Hemangiomas
Significance: Present in first few weeks of life, but not at birth, rapid growth noted in first year of life.

Question: Vascular malformations
Significance: Most present at birth, sometimes not noted until adolescence or adulthood.

Question: Salmon patches
Significance: Noted at birth.

Physical Examination

HEMANGIOMAS

Finding: Young lesion in superficial dermis
Significance: Raised, bright red-pink color, sharply demarcated border, stippled surface—hence term "strawberry hemangioma"

Finding: Young lesion in lower dermis or subcutaneous tissue
Significance: Bluish in color, raised with smooth overlying skin

Finding: Superficial and deep components
Significance: Can be combined in a single lesion

Finding: Involuting lesion
Significance: Develops gray or white areas, usually centrally located, which spread toward periphery

Finding: Overlying spine
Significance: Raises concern of underlying pathology

VASCULAR MALFORMATIONS

Finding: Port-wine stains
Significance: Apparent at birth, pink-to-red sharply demarcated macule, possibly slightly raised, darkens with age, may develop papules over time

Finding: Other vascular malformations
Significance: May not be noticed until adolescence or adulthood and are usually soft, easily compressed, and emptied of blood.

SALMON PATCHES

Finding: Salmon patches
Significance: Often have more than one lesion; 80% on nape of neck, 45% on eyelids, 33% on glabella.

 ## Laboratory Aids

RADIOGRAPHIC STUDIES

• Occasionally necessary to differentiate hemangiomas from vascular malformations
• Head MRI: performed to rule out anomalies of the choroid plexus and leptomeninges (Sturge-Weber); must be performed when port-wine stains include first distribution of the trigeminal nerve. Lesions in second and third distribution of trigeminal nerve do not have this risk.

 ## Therapy

• Hemangiomas

—For bleeding: direct pressure
—For ulceration: observation or wet compresses and topical antibacterials
—For infection: intravenous antibiotics for cellulitis, topical antibiotics with dressing changes for mild involvement
—Treatment is necessary for lesions that interfere with critical structures (e.g., eye, airway, GI tract) or for serious symptoms, such as consumptive coagulopathy. No therapy indicated in 95%.
—Intralesional or systemic steroids
—Interferon-alpha-2a for steroid non-responders
—Liquid nitrogen, laser therapy occasionally beneficial
—Surgical resection utilized infrequently

• Vascular malformations

—Port-wine stain: cosmetic camouflage or laser therapy. Laser therapy is being continuously improved in terms of quality of outcome and decreased complications as different types of lasers are developed and tested. Multiple laser treatment sessions at 2- to 3-month intervals are usually necessary.

 ## Follow-Up

• Hemangiomas

—50% will spontaneously resolve by 5 years.
—70% will spontaneously resolve by 7 years.
—90% will spontaneously resolve by 9 to 12 years.

• Vascular malformations

—No spontaneous resolution of lesions.

• Salmon patches

—50% on nape of neck spontaneously resolve.
—95% of others spontaneously resolve.
—Tendency toward erythema in affected area may persist after lesions resolve.

PITFALLS

• For hemangiomas, treatment significantly increases the risk of poor cosmetic outcome.
• For vascular malformations, treatment of port-wine stains may achieve color lightening rather than complete resolution of the lesion.

 ## Common Questions and Answers

Q: What will happen to my child's hemangioma?
A: Expect it to enlarge, get a bluish hue, and then get smaller. In the first year of life, it may enlarge at a rate more rapid than the rest of the child's growth. After that time it will involute, and should resolve by 9 to 12 years of age; most resolve earlier.

Q: What are the problems of the involuting hemangioma?
A: Infection and ulceration.

Q: What happens to the "stork bite" on the back of the neck?
A: It fades but still may be seen when vessels dilate.

ICD-9-CM
Port wine stain 757.32
Hemangioma 228.0

BIBLIOGRAPHY

Brown RL, Azizkhan RG. Pediatric head and neck lesions. [Tutorial]. *Pediatr Clin North Am* 1998;45(4):889–905.

Burrows PE, Laor T, Paltiel H, Robertson RL. Diagnostic imaging in the evaluation of vascular birthmarks. *Dermatol Clin* 1998;16(3):455–488.

Fishman SJ, Mulliken JB. Hemangiomas and vascular malformations of infancy and childhood. *Pediatr Clin North Am* 1993;40(6):1177–1200.

Garden JM, Bakus AD. Laser treatment of port-wine stains and hemangiomas. *Dermatol Clin* 1997;15:373–383.

Hurwitz S. Vascular disorders of infancy and childhood. In *Clinical pediatric dermatology*. Philadelphia: WB Saunders, 1993:242–272.

Jacobs AH, Walton RG. The incidence of birthmarks in the neonate. *Pediatrics* 1976;58(2):218–222.

Author: Laura N. Sinai

Hemolytic Disease of the Newborn

 Database

DEFINITION

Hemolytic anemia occurring in the newborn due to passive transfer of maternal antibodies (IgG) against fetal red cells.

CAUSES

- Most severe disease due to Rh (D) antigen sensitization
  - A and B antigens may also be responsible
  - 1% of cases due to other antigens
  - Other antigens: Kell, Duffy, C, E, and c

PATHOPHYSIOLOGY

- Rh-negative mothers may have prior sensitization due to transfusion or previous pregnancy.
- Fetomaternal bleed from Rh-positive fetus across the placenta leading to maternal sensitization
- Anti-D IgG produced in the maternal circulation crosses the placenta, coats fetal red blood cells (RBC) that are then destroyed in fetal spleen
- May lead to severe anemia, hydrops, and hyperbilirubinemia
- Extramedullary hematopoiesis in fetal liver and spleen as a response to fetal anemia leading to severe hepatosplenomegaly
- ABO isoimmunization usually in case of type O mothers with type A or B fetus; clinically milder hemolysis

EPIDEMIOLOGY

- 15% of Caucasians are Rh-negative (dd)
- 48% are heterozygous (Dd)
- 35% are homozygous (DD)
- Prevalence of Rh-positive fetus in Rh-negative mother: 15%
- Incidence of Rh hemolytic disease: 6–7/1000 live births
- Of all Rh-sensitized pregnancies:

—50% require no treatment
—31% require treatment after a full-term delivery
—10% delivered early and require exchange transfusion
—9% require intrauterine transfusion

- Reasons for spectrum of clinical severity:

—Rh immunization rarely occurs in first pregnancy
—Many second infants may be Rh-negative
—Only fraction of women at risk develop antibodies

- 50% of cases of ABO disease occur in first pregnancy

GENETICS

See Epidemiology.

COMPLICATIONS

- Hydrops fetalis
- Still births
- Neonatal hyperbilirubinemia and kernicterus
- Fetal anemia

PROGNOSIS

Approximately one-half the infants have minimal anemia and hyperbilirubinemia and require either no treatment or only phototherapy.

- One-fourth will require exchange transfusions.
- Hydropic infants have high mortality.

 Differential Diagnosis

- Neonatal hyperbilirubinemia

—ABO incompatibility
—Galactosemia
—G6PD deficiency
—Hypothyroidism
—Pyruvate kinase deficiency
—Crigler-Najjar syndrome
—Alpha-thalassemia
—Gilbert syndrome
—Spherocytosis
—Breast milk jaundice

- Hydrops fetalis

—Hematological: alpha-thalassemia, severe G6PD deficiency, twin-to-twin transfusion
—Cardiac: hypoplastic left heart syndrome, myocarditis, endocardial fibroelastosis, heart block
—Congenital infections: parvovirus, syphilis, cytomegalovirus (CMV), rubella
—Renal: renal vein thrombosis, urinary tract obstruction, nephrosis
—Placental: umbilical vein thrombosis, true knot
—Miscellaneous: trisomy 13, 18, 21, triploidy, aneuploidy, diaphragmatic hernia

 Data Gathering

HISTORY

- Previous stillbirths, abortions?
- Neonatal hyperbilirubinemia requiring therapy in previous pregnancy?
- Exposure of mother to blood products?
- Father's ABO and Rh type?
- Rh immune globulin given after previous pregnancy or abortion?

 Physical Examination

- Pallor, tachycardia, tachypnea due to congestive heart failure (CHF) secondary to severe anemia
- Icterus developing within 12 hours of birth
- Usually no icterus at birth
- Generalized edema in cases with severe anemia and hydrops
- Massive hepatosplenomegaly in severe cases
- Milder cases manifest with neonatal hyperbilirubinemia only
- ABO incompatibility usually manifests jaundice at 24 hours

Hemolytic Disease of the Newborn

 ## Laboratory Aids

ANTENATAL

- ABO and Rh type of all mothers early in pregnancy
- Monitor antibody titer by indirect Coombs test in Rh-negative mothers starting at 20 weeks.
- Amniocentesis if maternal antibody titer more than one-eighth at any time
- Spectrophotometric assessment of bilirubin concentration in amniotic fluid
- Amniotic fluid values in Lileys zone 3 and high zone 2 indicative of severe fetal disease
- Fetal blood sampling in severe cases to assess degree of anemia

NEONATAL

- Cord blood ABO and Rh types
- Cord blood hemoglobin (Hb), hematocrit (Hct), bilirubin (direct and indirect), reticulocyte count
- Direct Coombs test on cord blood: positive in immune hemolytic disease
- Indirect Coombs test on cord blood for passively transferred antibody
- Identification of antibody after elution from RBC
- Peripheral smear: nucleated RBC (spherocytes in ABO disease)

 ## Therapy

- Neonatal resuscitation as required in severe Rh isoimmunization
- Phototherapy to start as soon as possible
- Exchange transfusion

—To correct anemia in severely anemic infants
—To prevent or correct hyperbilirubinemia
—To remove circulating antibodies

- Indications for early exchange transfusion:

—Cord blood bilirubin more than 4.5 mg/dL and cord blood Hb less than 11 g/dL
—Bilirubin rising at rate more than 1 mg/dL/h despite phototherapy
—Bilirubin more than or equal to 20 mg/dL or rising to reach that level
—Hb between 11 and 13 g/dL and bilirubin rising at rate
—More than 0.5 mg/dL/h despite phototherapy

- In hydropic infants, immediate partial exchange may be needed to correct anemia and CHF.
- Late exchanges are needed for hyperbilirubinemia.
- Exchange transfusion removes sensitized RBC and bilirubin.
- For hyperbilirubinemia double-volume exchange is indicated.
- Type of blood for exchange transfusion:

—As fresh as possible (<72 hours old), CMV negative, and irradiated
—For Rh disease (if prepared before delivery): type O Rh-negative crossmatched against mother's blood; after delivery then O negative crossmatched against infant also
—For ABO disease: type O Rh-negative or Rh-compatible crossmatched against mother and infant

- Most infants with ABO incompatibility require phototherapy only.
- Some infants with milder Rh isoimmunization may only have exaggerated physiologic anemia at 12 weeks.
- Discontinue drugs that interfere with bilirubin metabolism (Novobiocin) or its binding to albumin (sulphonamides).

ANTENATAL MANAGEMENT

- Unsensitized Rh-negative mother: Rhogam at 28 weeks
- If previous stillbirth or hydrops and fetus high risk after amniocentesis plan early delivery (30 weeks)
- Careful fetal monitoring and induction of pulmonary maturation
- If fetus too immature for delivery, then intrauterine transfusions every 10 to 14 days

 ## Follow-Up

- Watch for exaggerated physiological anemia at 12 weeks.
- Assess for neurological damage.

PREVENTION

Rh hemolytic disease can be prevented by administration of Rhogam to the Rh negative women after any exposure to Rh positive blood and prophylactically during pregnancy.

 ## Common Questions and Answers

Q: Does the condition become worse with each pregnancy?
A: Yes, if the mother is not treated with Rh immunoglobulin after each Rh-positive pregnancy or abortion.

Q: Can maternal blood be used to transfuse the affected baby?
A: It can be used as a life-saving measure in a situation when there is no other suitable blood available for the baby.

ICD-9-CM 774.6

BIBLIOGRAPHY

Bennebroek J. Diagnosis and treatment of severe alloimmunization. *Vox Sang* 1994;67(Suppl 3):235–238.

Boroman JM. Antenatal suppression of Rh alloimmunization. *Clin Obstet Gynecol* 1991;34(2): 296–303.

Nathan DG, Oski FA, eds. *Hematology of infancy and childhood*, 4th ed. Vol. I. Philadelphia: WB Saunders, 1993:44–74.

Whittle MJ. Rhesus hemolytic disease. *Arch Dis Child* 1992;67(1 Spec No):65–68.

Author: Sadhna M. Shankar

Hemolytic Uremic Syndrome

 ## Database

DEFINITION

The hemolytic uremic syndrome (HUS) is a heterogeneous group of similar entities defined by microangiopathic hemolytic anemia, thrombocytopenia, and acute renal failure. HUS is the most common cause of acute renal failure in childhood.

- Typical (shiga-toxin, diarrhea-associated) form accounts for greater than 90% of pediatric cases and is characterized by the sudden onset of hemolytic anemia, thrombocytopenia, and acute renal failure after a prodromal illness of acute gastroenteritis, usually with bloody diarrhea.
- Atypical HUS (idiopathic) is a catch-all category for several variants of HUS, including recurrent HUS, inherited HUS, and HUS associated with pregnancy, oral contraceptives, cyclosporine, antitumor drugs, malignancy, and *Streptococcus pneumoniae* infection.

PATHOPHYSIOLOGY

- Common denominator in all forms of HUS is thought to be microvascular endothelial cell injury and dysfunction.
- Typical form usually starts with an infection with a shigatoxin producing *Escherichia coli*, most commonly *E. coli* 0157:H7.
- Endothelial cell injury ultimately results in local intravascular coagulation and microthrombi formation with microangiopathic hemolytic anemia and thrombocytopenia.
- Pathogenesis of atypical, non-epidemic HUS is not understood.

GENETICS

Atypical HUS has been reported with both autosomal dominant and autosomal recessive patterns of inheritance. The pathogenesis and genetics of inherited HUS is unknown.

EPIDEMIOLOGY

HUS has been reported throughout the world.

Typical

- Typical HUS tends to occur in the summer months, and epidemics have been reported in day care centers and nursing homes.
- Typical HUS occurs mainly in older infants and young children, usually between 6 months and 4 years of age.
- The shigatoxin producing *E. coli* is found in the intestine of beef cattle. Ground beef may be contaminated throughout with shigatoxin. If the hamburger is inadequately cooked, infection may ensue.
- In reported outbreaks, the frequency of bloody diarrhea has ranged from 35 to 90%.

Atypical

Atypical HUS has no seasonal variation and may occur at any age.

COMPLICATIONS

GI

- Acute colitis is usually transient.
- Complications include rectal prolapse, toxic megacolon, bowel wall necrosis, intussusception, perforation, and stricture.
- Pancreatic involvement may result in pancreatitis or insulin-dependent diabetes mellitus.

CNS

- Most patients have mild central nervous system symptoms that include irritability, lethargy, and behavioral changes.
- Major symptoms such as stupor, coma, seizures, cortical blindness, posturing, and hallucinations occur in 20 to 40% of patients.
- Thrombotic or hemorrhagic stroke may occur.
- The risk of seizures is associated with hyponatremia.

PROGNOSIS

Typical HUS

- Improved supportive care and a better understanding of the complications of typical HUS have resulted in a decrease in mortality to an acute fatality rate of 4% to 12%.
- A substantial number of patients develop renal sequelae after typical HUS, and they should be evaluated regularly for many years.
- Persistence of proteinuria after 1 year is a poor prognostic sign and warrants additional evaluation.
- Recurrences of HUS are exceedingly uncommon.
- Chronic renal insufficiency occurs in 4% to 9%. Children who do develop end stage renal disease are good candidates for kidney transplantation.

Atypical HUS

- In general, patients with atypical HUS have a substantially worse prognosis.
- Neurological symptoms are seen more commonly.
- Hypertension is common during the initial illness and prolonged antihypertensive treatment is required.
- Recurrences have been reported both before and after renal transplantation.
- In familial HUS, relapse, end-stage renal disease, and death are common.

 ## Differential Diagnosis

- Infectious causes such as *Shigella, Salmonella, Campylobacter, Yersinia enterocolitica, C. difficile,* and *Entamoeba histolytica*
- During the gastrointestinal prodrome, it may be difficult to distinguish HUS from appendicitis, inflammatory bowel disease, diverticulosis, or intussusception.
- Thrombotic thrombocytopenic purpura (TTP) shares many features with HUS.

- Sepsis with disseminated intravascular coagulation may present with acute renal failure and a microangiopathic process.

 ## Data Gathering

HISTORY

Question: Gastrointestinal prodrome?
Significance: Affected children with typical HUS are usually healthy before the initiation of the gastrointestinal prodrome. The diarrhea is usually watery or bloody and is associated with abdominal discomfort.

Question: Duration?
Significance: The prodrome lasts from 1 to 15 days and often improves before onset of the triad of features inherent to HUS.

 ## Physical Examination

- Pallor and petechiae
- Dehydration secondary to the gastroenteritis
- May have volume overload secondary to oligoanuric renal failure
- Peripheral edema, congestive heart failure, and hypertension may be present.
- Mild neurological changes of irritability or behavioral changes

Special Questions

Finding: Recent hamburger ingestion.
Significance: Many cases of typical HUS have been associated with inadequately cooked hamburger meat. Epidemics have been reported in fast-food restaurant customers.

Finding: Consumption of unpasteurized milk, cheese, or cider.
Significance: May contain Shiga toxins.

Laboratory Aids

HEMATOLOGIC

Test: CBC
Significance: The microangiopathic hemolytic anemia may be mild or severe. Leukocytosis is often seen in typical HUS.

Test: Reticulocytes
Significance: Repeated exacerbations of the hemolysis may occur for days or weeks.

Test: Blood smear
Significance: Fragmented red blood cells or schistocytes

Test: Markers of hemolysis
Significance: Elevated lactic dehydrogenase, unconjugated bilirubin, and reticulocyte count are additional evidence of ongoing hemolysis.

Test: Platelets
Significance: The thrombocytopenia may also last for days or weeks.

Test: PT-PTT
Significance: Coagulation studies usually show increased fibrin degradation products with normal prothrombin and partial thromboplastin times.

RENAL

Test: Renal function
Significance: Elevated creatinine and BUN

Test: Electrolytes
Significance: Elevated levels of potassium, phosphorus, hydrogen ion, and uric acid; decreased concentrations of sodium, calcium, and bicarbonate

Test: Urinalysis
Significance: Microscopic hematuria; varying degrees of proteinuria; macroscopic hematuria and RBC casts may be present.

GASTROINTESTINAL

Test: Electrolytes
Significance: Decreased serum potassium

Test: Liver function tests
Significance: Albumen decreased; liver function tests are usually normal.

Test: Amylase, lipase
Significance: Pancreatic involvement may result in hyperglycemia and elevated concentrations of serum amylase and lipase. Exocrine pancreatitis is difficult to evaluate since amylase and lipase are normally cleared by the kidneys.

MICROBIOLOGY

Test: Stool
Significance: All bloody stool samples should be screened for *E. coli* 0157:H7. Since the rate of recovery of the organism may decline rapidly after the first 6 days of illness, stool cultures should be obtained as early in the course of illness as possible. The local health department should be notified of any isolates.

Test: Verotoxins
Significance: Serologic evidence of verotoxin may be diagnostic.

IMAGING

Test: Plain film of the abdomen
Significance: Often demonstrates colonic distention. Look for free air as evidence of bowel perforation.

Therapy

• Supportive therapy

—Fluid and electrolyte
—Volume resuscitation initially
—In a euvolemic patient, fluids should provide replacement of ongoing losses with meticulous attention to urine output.
—Hyponatremia is common.
—If the patient is fluid overloaded, fluid intake should be restricted accordingly.

• Dialysis

—If medical management fails to correct hypertension hyperkalemia, hyperphosphatemia, and severe metabolic acidosis, dialysis or hemofiltration may be indicated. Dialysis is required in one-half to one-third of patients.

• Anemia

—Transfusion of packed red blood cells if the hemoglobin concentration falls below 6.0 to 7.0 g/dL or if there is evidence of cardiac dysfunction. The transfusions should be given slowly since blood pressure occasionally increases during transfusions.
—Platelet transfusions should be reserved for patients with active bleeding or in preparation for an invasive procedure.
—Antibiotics are not prescribed routinely because there is evidence the antimicrobials may increase verotoxin release. Antimotility agents have also been associated with more severe disease and should be avoided.
—Nutrition must be maintained and may require total parenteral nutrition if the intestine is non-functional. The degree of renal insufficiency will dictate the need for potassium and phosphorus restriction.

• Specific therapy

—Therapies have not proven to be helpful: plasmapheresis, fresh frozen plasma, intravenous immunoglobulin, heparin, antibiotics, aspirin, vitamin E for typical HUS.
—Plasmapheresis has been advocated for atypical, or idiopathic HUS.

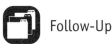

Follow-Up

WHEN TO EXPECT IMPROVEMENT

• Resolution is usually heralded by a rise in platelet count and a gradual decrease in the frequency of blood transfusions.
• During the recovery phase patients may require folic acid and iron supplementation.
• Anuria rarely lasts more than 2 weeks. In general, a longer duration of anuria is a poor prognostic feature.
• Children who sustain structural neurologic damage during the acute phase of HUS may have residual impairment, but there is tremendous potential for improvement and recovery.
• Pancreatic insufficiency may persist requiring long-term insulin therapy beyond resolution of the acute illness.

PREVENTION

Most cases of typical HUS can be avoided by thoroughly cooking all hamburger-containing foods. Other sources of contaminated foods include unpasteurized apple cider or milk.

Common Questions and Answers

Q: What are some predictors of the severity of typical HUS?
A: Predictors include an elevated white cell count, a severe gastrointestinal prodrome, anuria early in the course of illness, and age under 2 years.

Q: In a patient with atypical HUS, what is the chance other siblings will be affected?
A: If there are no other affected family members, it is not possible to determine if the patient has the familial (i.e., autosomal recessive) form of HUS. Therefore, other siblings may be at no additional risk or may have up to 25% chance of developing HUS.

Q: How many patients with gastroenteritis from *E. coli* 0157:H7 will develop HUS?
A: 10% to 20%

Q: What should the family tell the day care staff and neighbors?
A: If the patient has typical HUS, contacts should be informed that any episodes of gastroenteritis merit close follow-up for evidence of anemia, thrombocytopenia, and renal insufficiency. No prophylaxis is indicated. Exclusion of infected children from day care centers until two consecutive stool cultures are negative for *E. coli* 0157:H7 has been shown to prevent additional transmission.

ICD-9-CM 283.11

BIBLIOGRAPHY

Boyce TG, Swerdlow DL, Griffin PM. Current concepts: Escherichia coli 0157:H7 and the hemolytic-uremic syndrome. *N Engl J Med* 1995;333:364–368.

Kaplan BS, Meyers KE, Schulman SL. The pathogenesis and treatment of hemolytic uremic syndrome. *J Am Soc Nephrol* 1998;9:1126–1133.

Neuhaus TJ, Calonder S, Leumann EP. Heterogeneity of atypical haemolytic uraemic syndromes. *Arch Dis Child* 1997;518–521.

Siegler RL. The hemolytic uremic syndrome. *Pediatr Clin North Am* 1995;42:1505–1529.

Taylor CM, Monnens LA. Advances in haemolytic uraemic syndrome. *Arch Dis Child* 1998;78(2):190–193.

Author: Mary B. Leonard

Hemophilia

 Database

DEFINITION

Inherited bleeding disorder caused by the absence, severe deficiency or defective functioning of plasma coagulation factor VIII (hemophilia A) or IX (hemophilia B).

PATHOPHYSIOLOGY

• Thrombin generation via the intrinsic pathway is delayed in patients with absent or reduced (<25%) factor VIII or factor IX.
• Patients do not bleed more rapidly; instead there is delayed formation of a clot.
• The friable clot formed has a tendency to rebleed.
• In closed spaces (e.g., joint), bleeding stops by tamponade; in open spaces (e.g., iliopsoas muscle, open wounds), large amounts of blood may be lost.
• Repeated joint hemorrhages lead to synovial thickening and joint cartilage erosion. Joint space becomes narrowed and eventually fuses.

GENETICS

• X-linked recessive disorder
• Carrier status and prenatal testing available:
• Hemophilia A:

—Gene inversion in the factor VIII gene is present in 45% of severe hepatitis A. Detectable by genetic screening
—In families with unknown mutations, a coagulation assay comparing the level of factor VIII with von Willebrand factor can be used to identify carriers
—Accuracy of screening: 90%

• Hemophilia B:

—Majority of factor IX gene defects are due to missense point mutations, which can be identified in nearly all affected individuals and carriers

EPIDEMIOLOGY

• Most common severe hereditary coagulation disorder
• Distribution

—Hemophilia A: 80% to 85%
—Hemophilia B: 10% to 15%

• Incidence:

—Hemophilia A: 1 per 5,000 male births
—Hemophilia B: 1 per 25,000 male births

• No geographic or ethnic associations

COMPLICATIONS

Complications of Disease

• Hemophilic arthropathy: joint contractures, limited range of motion, and chronic pain
• Intracranial bleeding
• Compartment syndrome
• Airway compromise due to bleeds in the pharynx, tongue, or neck
• Life-threatening hemorrhage due to gastrointestinal, post-traumatic or perioperative bleeds

Complications of Therapy

• Viral transmission through pooled coagulation factor concentrates (HIV, hepatitis B, C)
• Inhibitors: Antibodies against factor VIII or IX, which can inactivate infused factor
• Anaphylaxis: Continued factor IX replacement in severe factor IX deficient patients with inhibitors may lead to anaphylaxis
• Thromboembolic disease: Use of prothrombin complex concentrates is associated with thromboembolism and myocardial infarctions in children

 Differential Diagnosis

Prolonged Coagulation Time Associated with Increased Bleeding Tendency

• von Willebrand disease
• "Acquired hemophilia" due to development of an inhibitor to factor VIII or IX
• Hereditary factor XI deficiency

Prolonged Coagulation Time But No Increased Bleeding Tendency

• Factor XII deficiency
• High molecular weight kininogen deficiency
• Prekallikrein deficiency
• Antiphospholipid antibody (lupus anticoagulant)
• Heparin artifact

 Data Gathering

HISTORY

Question: Familial history?
Significance: Familial history of hemophilia in male offspring of female blood relatives is present in 30% to 40% of cases.

Question: Excessive bleeding in male neonate?
Significance: Excessive bleeding with circumcision or of the umbilical cord may be an initial presentation of hemophilia. 1% to 2% of neonates may present with an intracranial hemorrhage.

Question: Pattern of bleeding?
Significance: Characterized by spontaneous joint and muscle hemorrhages, easy bruising and prolonged and potentially fatal hemorrhage after trauma or surgery.

Question: Age of onset of bleeding?
Significance: Bleeds generally occur with increasing frequency around the time the child begins to walk or starts teething.

Question: Location of hemarthrosis?
Significance: Large weight bearing joints are most often involved: knees, elbows, ankles, shoulders, hips.

Question: Early symptoms of a hemarthrosis?
Significance: Aura of tingling or warmth, followed by increasing pain and decreasing range of motion.

 Physical Examination

Finding: Joint examination
Significance:

• Acute hemathrosis: limitation of motion of the joint, warmth, swelling, tenderness
• Chronic joint: crepitus, decreased range of motion, proximal muscle weakness; typically occurs in knees, ankles, elbows
• Intramuscular hematomas: often little seen on exam; vague feeling of pain with motion

 Laboratory Aids

TESTS

Test: Prothrombin time (PT), partial thromboplastin time (PTT), fibrinogen or thrombin time and platelet count.
Significance: Screen for bleeding disorder.

Test: Factor VIII, IX levels
Significance:

• Less than 1%: severe hemophilia. Most common, characterized by spontaneous hemarthroses; will need frequent factor replacement therapy.
• 1% to 5%: moderate hemophilia. Spontaneous hemorrhage common; will require occasional factor replacement therapy.
• 5% to 25%: mild hemophilia. Rare bleeding; requires factor replacement therapy only with significant trauma or surgery.

PITFALLS

• Neonates have a physiological reduction in the vitamin K dependent factors, including factor IX, making a determination of the degree of factor IX deficiency difficult in the neonatal period
• Delivery-related stress and other neonatal problems may cause a transient elevation of factor VIII levels
• Poor venipuncture technique can artifactually elevate or normalize the PTT.

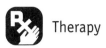 Therapy

ACUTE BLEEDING EPISODES

Factor Replacement

• Factor VIII replacement products

—Recombinant non–plasma-derived factor VIII
—Monoclonal purified plasma-derived factor VIII concentrate; heat or detergent treated for viral inactivation
—Cryoprecipitate (rarely used today)

• Factor IX replacement products

—Recombinant non–plasma-derived factor IX
—Monoclonal purified plasma-derived factor IX concentrate; heat or detergent treated for viral inactivation
—Prothrombin complex concentrate: crude plasma fraction, which contains variable amounts of factors II, VII, IX, and X viral inactivated
—Rarely used: fresh frozen plasma

• Dose

—Factor VIII dose = % desired rise in factor VIII level × body weight (kg) × 0.5
—Factor IX dose = % desired rise in factor IX level × body weight (kg)

• Target Levels:

—30% twice for most joint bleeds
—70% repeated over 12 to 48 hours for large muscle bleeds
—100% maintained over 10 to 14 days for intracranial bleeds, surgery

DDAVP

• Synthetic vasopressin analog which stimulates release of endogenous factor VIII and von Willebrand factor
• Only suitable for patients with mild or moderate factor VIII deficiency who have shown a response to DDAVP in a therapeutic trial
• Tachyphylaxis may occur with repeated dosing

Antifibrinolytic Therapy

• Antifibrinolytic agents for oral mucosal bleeding, dental extractions
• Epsilon aminocaproic acid 50 to 100 mg/kg/dose PO every 6 hours, or Tranxemic acid 25 mg/kg/dose every 6 to 8 hours

Immobilization

• Splints, casts, crutches, and/or bedrest
• Prolonged immobilization may reduce recovery of joint range of motion; initiation of physical therapy with factor coverage is recommended, particularly after joint surgery

SPECIAL BLEEDING SITUATIONS

Intracranial Hemorrhage

• Significant bleeding can occur despite the absence of external bruising

• Factor replacement to 100% should be administered immediately
• CT scan of the head is useful but may be negative early in a bleed

Major Surgery

• Factor replacement to 100% pre- and post-operatively
• Regular dosing of factor for a minimum of 1 week post-operatively, even in mild hemophilia

Compartment Syndrome

• Bleeding within the fascial compartments of muscles
• Most often occurs in the forearm and calf
• Neurovascular compromise can lead to Volkman contracture

Iliopsoas Bleed

• Lower abdominal or upper thigh pain may be first symptom
• Examination is notable for inability to extend hip with preservation of internal and external rotation (which distinguishes it from hip joint bleed)
• Diagnosis confirmed by ultrasound or CT scan
• Large volumes of blood can be lost into the retroperitoneal space. Check CBC.

Oral Bleeding/Epistaxis

• Constant pressure for 15 to 20 minutes
• Epsilon amino caproic acid or tranxemic acid
• Topical thrombin directly to the site of bleeding

Dental Care

• Significant dental procedures (e.g., tooth extraction) should be performed by a dentist with experience treating hemophiliac patients and preferably, in a hospital setting where hematology consultation is available
• Factor replacement is required pre- and post-procedures

Lacerations

• Sutures should be avoided when possible
• If sutures are required, factor replacement is necessary at time of placement and removal

Hematuria

• Increased fluid intake and bedrest as initial treatment
• If hematuria persists, factor replacement
• Prednisone in HIV negative patients

 Follow-Up

Patients should be followed regularly at a comprehensive hemophilia treatment center, in which care is coordinated by a team including the pediatric hematologist, nurse coordinator, social worker, psychologist, physical therapist, dentist, orthopedic surgeon, and financial counselor.

PREVENTION

Prophylaxis

• Primary prophylaxis: regular dosing in patients with no complications to prevent chronic joint damage
• Secondary prophylaxis: regular dosing in patients with target joints to prevent additional damage and facilitate healing and rehabilitation

Anticipatory Guidance and Prevention

• Good dental hygiene
• Immunizations: no intramuscular injections; give SC with a small gauge needle
• Rapid treatment of hemarthrosis to avoid chronic joint damage
• Avoidance of aggressive contact sports, e.g., football, basketball, lacrosse, hockey, rugby; tennis, baseball are okay, but may be prone to small joint bleeds
• Home infusion therapy as appropriate
• Self-infusion training: usually start at age 11 years

 Common Questions and Answers

Q: Are there any medications contraindicated in a child with hemophilia?
A: Aspirin should not be given as it interferes with platelet function. Non-steroidal inflammatory agents cause a milder effect on platelets, and should also be avoided when possible.

Q: Can immunizations be given to a child with hemophilia?
A: Immunizations should be given SC (instead of IM) with the smallest gauge needle; ice or cold packs should be applied to the area to minimize hematoma formation; if excessive bleeding occurs, the child should receive factor replacement.

ICD-9-CM 286.0

BIBLIOGRAPHY

DiMichele D. Hemophilia 1996. New approach to an old disease. *Pediatr Clin N Am* 1996; 43(3):709–736.

Hoyer LW. Hemophilia A. *N Engl J Med* 1994; 330(1):38–47.

Roberts HR, Eberst ME. Current management of hemophilia B. *Hematol Oncol Clin North Am* 1993;7:1269–1280.

Author: Kara M. Kelly

Hemoptysis

 Database

DEFINITION

Blood loss into the respiratory tract with amounts ranging from mild to massive which can cause hypoxia or exsanguination.

CAUSES

- Bronchiectasis
- Cavitary infections (e.g., tuberculosis, abscess, histoplasmosis)
- Tumors (lymphomas)
- Trauma (pulmonary contusion, bronchoscopy, airway manipulation)
- Congenital heart disease with large collateral vessels
- Foreign body aspiration
- Pneumonia
- Hemorrhagic diathesis including anticoagulant therapy
- H-type tracheaesophageal fistula

PATHOPHYSIOLOGY

- Related to the underlying pulmonary disease

EPIDEMIOLOGY

- Large series of pediatric patients with massive hemoptysis have not been described.
- Most instances of massive hemoptysis take place in older children.

COMPLICATIONS

- Respiratory insufficiency
- Hypovolemic shock

 Differential Diagnosis

- Infections: pneumonia, pulmonary abscess, tuberculosis
- Pulmonary disease: cystic fibrosis, bronchiectasis, foreign body, arteriovenous malformation, congenital lung malformation, pulmonary emboli, pulmonary hemosiderosis
- Cardiovascular disease
- Collagen vascular disease: lupus, vasculitis, Goodpasture disease
- Trauma
- Coagulation disorder
- Munchausen syndrome
- Complications: anemia, pneumonia

 Data Gathering

HISTORY

- Familial history of pulmonary disease or bleeding disorder?
- Exposure to environmental toxins?
- Exposure to tuberculosis?
- Drug use: cocaine, marijuana?

Question: Recurrent episodes of hemoptysis with significant spectrum production and cyst formation on chest x-ray?
Significance: Suggests a diagnosis of bronchiectasis.

Question: Acute pleuritic chest pain?
Significance: Raises the possibility of pulmonary embolism with infarction or some other pleurally based lesion. A pleural friction rub may be present.

Physical Examination

Finding: Pleural friction rub
Significance: May be associated with pulmonary embolism.

Finding: Pulmonary hypertension
Significance: Raise the diagnostic possibilities of primary pulmonary hypertension, mitral stenosis, and Eisenmenger syndrome.

Finding: Localized wheeze over a major lobar airway
Significance: Suggests an intramural lesion such as a foreign body or carcinoma.

Finding: Presence of a murmur over the lung fields
Significance: May suggest pulmonary arteriovenous malformation.

 ## Laboratory Aids

Test: Complete blood count and reticulocyte count
Significance: May reveal the volume of blood loss and chronicity.

Test: Sputum and PPD
Significance: Tuberculosis is suspected.

Test: Drug screen
Significance: If appropriate.

Test: Chest x-ray both AP and lateral
Significance: May reveal pleural effusion, bronchiectasis, foreign bodies, or consolidation.

Test: Bronchoscopy
Significance: Usually performed to localize the site of bleeding and at times may be therapeutic (e.g., in foreign body removal).

Test: CT
Significance: May identify source of bleeding.

Test: Angiogram
Significance: Used to detect bleeding from arteriovascular malformation.

 ## Therapy

- Initial management should follow the lines of Basic Life Support.
- Support intravascular volume by packed red blood cells or fresh frozen plasma.
- Methods used to stop localized bleeding include tamponade with balloon-tipped catheters, ice water lavage, catheter-directed umbilication, intravenous pitressin, and surgical resection. The last option is usually reserved for most difficult cases such as extensive collateralization of bronchial arteries or arteriovenous malformations not responsive to embolization.

PROGNOSIS

It depends on the etiology and the nature of hemoptysis. Immediate management of airway central decreases the morbidity and mortality.

ICD-9-CM 786.3

BIBLIOGRAPHY

Blumer JL. Pulmonary hemorrhage. *Practical guide to pediatric intensive care,* 3rd ed. 1991:359–361.

Cahill BC, Ingbar DH. Massive hemoptysis, assessment and management. *Clin Chest Med* 1994;15(1):147–167.

DiLeo MD, Gianoli GJ. Diagnosis and management of hemoptysis. *LA State Med Soc* 1994;146(4):115–118.

Thompson AB, Teschler H, Rennard SI. Pathogenesis, evaluation and therapy for massive hemoptysis. *Clin Chest Med* 1992;13(1):69–82.

Author: Helen Anita John-Kelly

Henoch-Schönlein Purpura

Database

DEFINITION

- Henoch-Schönlein purpura (HSP) is an immunologically mediated systemic vasculitis involving the small blood vessels of the skin, gastrointestinal (GI) tract, joints, and kidneys.
- Defined by the presence of two of the following:

—Palpable purpura
—Age of onset less than 20
—Abdominal pain
—Granulocytic infiltration of vessel walls

- In children, only palpable purpura with normal platelet count need be documented, and while most children do have purpura, colicky abdominal pain and arthritis, up to one-half may present with symptoms other than purpura.

PATHOPHYSIOLOGY

- Most cases associated with preceding upper respiratory infections, usually Group A Beta-Hemolytic Streptococci, but also reported following infections with parvovirus, adenovirus and *Mycoplasma pneumoniae*. Also reported after drug ingestion (thiazides) and insect bites.
- Capillaries, arterioles, and venules are affected in HSP as opposed to polyarteritis nodosa, Wegener and systemic lupus erythematosus (SLE), where small arteries are affected.
- Biopsy of skin lesions show leukocytoclastic vasculitis with perivascular infiltration of small vessels with polymorphonuclear and mononuclear cells. Eosinophils, granular deposits of IgA, C3, and fibrin may also be present.
- Biopsy of the involved kidneys show endocapillary proliferative glomerulonephritis involving endothelial and mesangial cells. Crescent formation may also be present. IgA, IgG, C3, and fibrin are commonly found in the mesangial regions.
- Considered to be an immune-mediated vasculitis disorder involving primarily IgA. This is indirectly suggested by the elevation of serum IgA levels, circulating IgA immune complexes, IgA rheumatoid factor, IgA—fibronectin complexes and immunoregulatory abnormalities involving IgA production.
- IgA from mucosal B cells interacts with IgG to for immune complexes which activate the alternate pathway of the complement system. Circulating IgA is deposited in the affected organs causing the inflammatory process.

GENETICS

- There is only anecdotal evidence of genetic predisposition.
- Familial history of IgA-related disorders or inherited defects in complement (C2, C4 deficiency) may predispose to HSP.

EPIDEMIOLOGY

- Incidence of 13.5 cases per 100,000 school aged children per year.
- Slightly more common in males (e.g., M:F ratio of 58:42 in one study).
- Year round occurrence, but more common in spring, winter, and fall.
- Most common in Whites, Japanese, and Native Americans. Low incidence in Black, both in Africa and North America.

COMPLICATIONS

- Persistent hypertension
- End stage kidney disease (acute or as a late sequela)
- Intussusception (most common GI complication; affecting 1% to 5% of patients)
- Protein losing enteropathy
- Pancreatitis
- Hydrops of the gallbladder
- Strictures of the esophagus and ileus
- Bowel perforations and infarctions
- Pseudomembranous colitis
- Appendicitis
- Skin necrosis
- Subarachnoid, subdural, and cortical hemorrhage and infarction
- Peripheral mono- and polyneuropathies (Guillan-Barré)
- Pulmonary hemorrhage (uncommon, but may result in death)
- Torsion of the testis and appendix epididymis

PROGNOSIS

- Generally excellent
- Better prognosis associated with younger age
- Recurrence within the first 6 weeks in up to 33%
- Most have only one to three episodes of purpura; however, a few will continue to experience symptoms for months or years. These patients have a poor prognosis and are more likely to develop severe nephritis.
- Renal involvement is the cause of the most serious long-term morbidity. Microscopic hematuria alone or with mild proteinuria generally has a good outcome. A nephritic and nephrotic combination is more guarded, and those patients with a high percentage of crescent formation do less well.

Differential Diagnosis

- Petechial and purpuric rashes seen in thrombocytopenia from:

—Idiopathic thrombocytopenic purpura (ITP)
—Sepsis/infection: meningococcemia, Rocky Mountain Spotted Fever
—Leukemia
—Hemolytic uremic syndrome (HUS)
—Coagulopathies

- Vasculitic rashes may result from primary and secondary vasculitides:

—Polyarteritis nodosa
—Wegener granulomatosis
—Infection-related
—Connective tissue diseases (e.g., SLE) Berger (IgA nephropathy): glomerulonephritis similar to HSP both clinically and immunologically, but not associated with the skin, GI, or joint manifestations of HSP
—Streptococcal glomerulonephritis
—Infantile acute hemorrhagic edema: vasculitis that presents with urticarial or maculopapular rash that then becomes purpuric. It is differentiated from HSP in that it usually affects infants from 4 months to 2 years, is more common in the winter, and is not associated with systemic symptoms. On biopsy, IgA deposits are not found.
—Rheumatoid arthritis
—Rheumatic fever

Data Gathering

HISTORY

Question: Previous disease?
Significance: Especially infections such as hepatitis, URI, and streptococcal infections.

Question: Abdominal pain?
Significance: This is the most common GI symptom. Emesis and melena are also reported.

Question: Transient, non-migratory arthritis of knees, ankles, wrists, elbows, and digits.
Significance: Frequent problem

Question: Presence of testicular pain or scrotal swelling, headache, cough, edema of the ankles or periorbital region, and hematuria?
Significance: Vasculitic lesion in GU system.

Physical Examination

Finding: Particular attention to blood pressure.
Significance: Hypertension common.

Finding: Low grade fever is present in 50% of the cases.
Significance: Hypertension common.

Finding: Rash
Significance: Petechial or purpuric in a pressure-dependent, symmetric distribution, usually around the lateral malleoli of the ankles, on the ventral surfaces of the feet and on the buttocks.

Finding: Joints should be examined for swelling and limitation of motion.
Significance: Redness and warmth are not common.

Finding: Non-pitting subcutaneous edema of the scalp, periorbital region, hands and feet is often noted.
Significance: Generalized edema is more common in children under 2 years of age.

Finding: Abdomen is often tender to palpation, but without rebound tenderness.
Significance: Hepatosplenomegaly may be found.

Finding: Affected testicle may be tender and swollen. Swelling and bruising may be noted on the scrotum.
Significance:

Laboratory Aids

There are no definitive tests to confirm the diagnosis of HSP

Test: CBC
Significance: Hemoglobin is usually normal, leukocytosis may be present, platelet count is normal or elevated

Test: ESR
Significance: normal or elevated

Test: PT and PTT
Significance: normal

Test: IgA
Significance: often elevated in the acute phase of illness, with normal or increased IgG and IgM

Test: C3
Significance: normal (decreased in post-streptococcal glomerulonephritis and SLE)

Test: Antinuclear antibody
Significance: negative (elevated in SLE)

Test: Throat swab for Group A Beta-Hemolytic Strep
Significance: positive in up to 75% of cases

Test: Elevated BUN and creatinine, decreased protein and albumin, and urinalysis with rbcs, wbcs, casts or protein are seen with renal involvement

Test: Renal biopsy
Significance: With severe renal failure, a biopsy should be performed to determine the extent of disease

RADIOGRAPHIC STUDIES

Test: Chest radiograph
Significance: May show interstitial lung disease.

Test: Barium enema
Significance: Useful in diagnosing intussusception; with HSP, often displays "thumbprinting" in jejunum and ileum, which represents submucosal edema, hemorrhage, spasm, and ulceration.

Therapy

HSP usually resolve spontaneously without specific therapy.

• Analgesics and NSAIDs may be used for control of joint pain and inflammation.
• Steroids are used for painful cutaneous edema (2 mg/kg/d of prednisone until clinical resolution).
• No consensus on management of GI and renal involvement. Oral prednisone at 2 mg/kg/d has shown faster resolution of abdominal pain, while other studies indicate the symptoms will resolve similarly without intervention.
• In nephritis, immediate treatment with steroids may prevent more serious renal disease; however, the majority will improve spontaneously. Treatment should be considered for children at high risk for chronic renal insufficiency or failure (those presenting with nephrotic syndrome or renal insufficiency).
• More than 50% crescentic glomerulonephritis on renal biopsy has a greater risk of future renal failure and should be considered for aggressive therapy with pulse or oral steroids and/or immunosuppressants (azathioprine, cyclophosphamide, cyclosporine) or plasmapheresis, IVIG, Danazol or fish oil.
• Treatment of hypertension may delay or prevent progression of renal disease in patients with glomerulonephritis.

Follow-Up

• Patients should be seen weekly during the acute illness. Visits should include history and physical, along with blood pressure measurement and urinalysis.
• All patients, even those who did not present with renal involvement, should have urine checked for blood weekly for 6 months, and then monthly for 3 years.

PREVENTION

No specific prevention is available.

ICD-9-CM 287.0

Common Questions and Answers

Q: When should I consider hospitalization?
A: Often it is not necessary. Severe complications may require admission. These include GI hemorrhage, protein losing enteropathy requiring TPN, decreased GFR or hypertension, and pulmonary hemorrhage.

Q: Is there a use for prophylactic penicillin?
A: In patients with frequent relapses, where Group A Beta-hemolytic Strep is often is the inciting agent, administration of penicillin may be helpful.

Q: Who are Henoch and Schönlein?
A: The clinical finding of joint pain associated with purpura was named, "purpura rheumatica," in 1837 by Schönlein. Henoch, a student of Schönlein, later described the association of GI and renal involvement. However, the first report was by Heberden in 1801. Of note, it has been speculated that Mozart—whose symptoms included fever, vomiting, exanthem, arthritis, anasarca and coma—died of HSP.

BIBLIOGRAPHY

Cuttica RJ. Vasculitis in children: a diagnostic challenge. *Curr Probl Pediatr* 1997;27:309–318.

Piette WW. What is Schönlein-Henoch purpura, and why should we care? *Arch Dermatol* 1997;133:515–518.

Robson WL, Leung AK. Henoch-Schönlein purpura. *Adv Pediatr* 1994;41:163–194.

Szer IS. Henoch-Schönlein purpura: when and how to treat. *J Rheumatol* 1996;23:1661–1665.

Author: Blaze Robert Gusic

Hepatic Encephalopathy

 Database

DEFINITION

Abnormal mental status in patients with severe hepatic insufficiency.

CAUSES

- Hepatic failure
- Viral hepatitis
- Drug-induced hepatotoxicity
- End-stage chronic liver disease secondary to biliary atresia, α-1-antitrypsin deficiency, Wilson disease
- Inborn errors of metabolism: urea cycle enzyme disorders, organic acidemias, and fatty acid oxidation disorders. All hypotheses depend somewhat on the accompanying features of liver failure, such as porto-systemic shunting and an increased blood-brain barrier permeability to chemical substrates.

—Appears to be of a metabolic origin because the damage is nonstructural and the manifestations are reversible with a protein-restricted diet. Treatment with lactulose, neomycin, and occasionally branched-chain amino acid supplementation may imrpove the clinical signs and symptoms.
—May be secondary to accumulation of end-stage toxic products such as ammonia, short-chain fatty acids, and methylmercaptans, which bypass the portal circulation and may exert direct toxic effects on the brain, especially with an altered blood-brain barrier
—Altered neurotransmission secondary to inhibitory effects of γ-amino benzoic acid (GABA)
—Lack of nutrients such as glucose may impair brain energy metabolism. Even with glucose infusion, the brain's demands for energy may not be met in liver failure.
—Endogenous benzodiazepine theory: Increased substances identified biochemically as benzodiazepines are found on human autopsy in liver failure patients. Whether the source is in fact endogenous or whether they may be synthesized by bacteria is unknown.
—Increased aromatic amino acids and decreased branched-chain amino acids in plasma and in the brain in liver failure. Various studies testing this hypothesis by supplying protein with a high branched-chain amino acid load have been done with conflicting results. These may act as false neurotransmitters, competing for catecholamine receptor sites.

PATHOLOGY

In patients with cerebral edema associated with hepatic encephalopathy (HE), astrocyte neuronal swelling is noted in the brain upon autopsy.

 Differential Diagnosis

- Infection: meningitis, encephalitis
- Tumors: intracranial lesions
- Trauma: cerebral hemorrhage, cerebral hematoma
- Metabolical: inborn errors of metabolism, lactic acidemias, urea cycle deficiencies
- Immunological: AIDS dementia

 Data Gathering

HISTORY

Question: Alteration in mental status and personality?
Significance: Classic feature

 Physical Examination

Finding: Neurological exam
Significance: Mainly see central nervous system and neuromuscular abnormalities

Finding: Central nervous system manifestations
Significance: Range from altered mood to frank coma. Four clinical stages of hepatic coma are described, based on changes in conscious intellectual functioning and behavior. Usually, the clinical picture starts slowly.

- Trivial lack of awareness, euphoria, or anxiety, shortened attention span. (Therefore, in a child with acute onset of combative or irrational behavior in the classroom, liver disease should always be ruled out.)
- Lethargy, apathy, disorientation, change in personality
- Somnolence, but responsive to stimuli, confused
- Coma

Finding: Neuromuscular signs
Significance: May include varying degrees of asterixis and loss of tone. Asterixis (a hand-flapping tremor) is characteristic of hepatic encephalopathy, although it may also be seen with uremia, respiratory failure, and hypokalemia. Asterixis is due to sudden inappropriate relaxation of muscle groups.

Finding: Signs of end-stage liver failure
Significance: Portal systemic shunting, varices, and ascites.

Finding: Evaluation: Check for asterixis.
Significance: Ask the patient to stand with both arms raised horizontally in front of him, palms down. Patient should dorsiflex the wrist and hold fingers far apart for at least 15 seconds. A flap will be seen when the patient has small brief intermittent movements of the individual fingers, either in flexion or laterally in the ulnar direction, with a rapid return of fingers to the original position. In more severe cases, this flap can spread more proximal including the wrist and even the shoulders.

Hepatic Encephalopathy

 Laboratory Aids

TESTS

Test: EEG
Significance: May show a decrease in wave frequency, with an increase in wave amplitude. In more advanced cases delta waves are seen. These findings are non-specific and may be seen in other disease processes.

Test: Visual evoked potentials
Significance: May become more useful than EEGs.

Test: Number connection test
Significance: Connect randomly placed numbers 1 to 25 on a sheet of paper; better used to follow a course of HE rather than in initial diagnoses.

IMAGING

Head CT scan checks for signs of increased intracranial pressure or cerebral edema. These do not help with diagnosis but may indicate severity of encephalopathy and suggest prognosis.

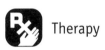 Therapy

SUPPORTIVE CARE

• Fluids and electrolyte monitoring, vital signs, paying close attention to development of infection (respiratory, urinary)

DRUGS

• Flumazenil in animal studies reverses the electrophysiological and clinical abnormalities in HE. As a benzodiazepine receptor antagonist, the agent may block the binding receptor for GABA in the brain. In some human studies, the benefits of flumazenil have also been seen but are not consistent for all patients.
• Branched-chain amino acids may reverse the altered ratio of branched-chain to aromatic amino acids, and clinical improvements have been seen. Results are not permanent and clinical deterioration resumes.
• Neomycin reduces intestinal bacterial flora responsible for ammonia synthesis.
• Lactulose: a disaccharide not able to be digested in the human intestine hydrolyzed by bacteria in the colon. Hypernatremia may result with therapy.

DURATION

These methods to improve HE are generally used as long as the acute state of HE continues.

DIET

• A low protein or even protein-free diet is recommended, to avoid increase in levels of ammonia.
• Conflicts with other treatment
• Placement of a portosystemic shunt before the onset of the acute development of neurological deterioration may suggest that the shunt is not allowing enough circulation through the liver. Suppression of the shunt, either by ballooning or by surgical ligation, may improve the clinical picture.
• Liver transplantation

 Follow-Up

WHEN TO EXPECT IMPROVEMENT

Often, improvement (a change in the level of HE by 1 or 2 stages) is seen 2 to 3 days after initiation of therapy.

SIGNS TO WATCH FOR

• Progression of mental status through deeper stages of HE

PROGNOSIS

Depends to some degree on stage of encephalopathy. In stage 4 encephalopathy, the most common cause of death is increased intracranial pressure and brain edema. Prognosis also depends on underlying cause and, therefore, methods of reversibility of liver failure. Orthotopic liver transplantation should be performed in children with severe and worsening encephalopathy before the development of radiographically apparent cerebral edema. In one study, on multiple logistic regression analysis, presence of GI hemorrhage (p = 0.005), degree of coma (p = 0.02) and serum bilirubin level (p = 0.025) were identified as independent predictors of mortality.

 Common Questions and Answers

Q: My child has chronic liver failure and has experienced two episodes of hepatic encephalopathy managed in the ICU. Is there any special diet I should be providing him?
A: Because dietary intake of protein can lead to accumulation of nitrogenous waste that can accumulate into ammonia, it is best to keep your child on a low-protein diet.

ICD-9-CM 572.2

BIBLIOGRAPHY

Alper G, Jarjour IT, Reyes JD, Towbin RB, Hirsch WL, Bergman I. Outcome of children with cerebral edema caused by fulminant hepatic failure [Review]. *Pediatr Neurol* 1998;18(4):299–304.

Basile SA, Jones EA, Skolnick P. The pathogenesis and treatment of hepatic encephalopathy: evidence for involvement of benzodiazepine receptor ligands. *Pharmacol Rev* 1991;32:27–71.

Butterworth RF. Pathogenesis and treatment of porto-systemic encephalopathy. *Digest Dis Sci* 1992;37(3):321–327.

Ferenci P. Brain dysfunction in fulminant hepatic failure. *J Hepatol* 1994;21:487–490.

Hawkins RA, Mans AM. Brain metabolism in hepatic encephalopathy and hyperammonemia. In: Felipo V, Grisola S, eds. *Cirrhosis, hyperammonemia, and hepatic encephalopathy*. New York: Plenum, 1994:13–19.

Mullen KD, Weber FL. Role of nutrition in hepatic encephalopathy. *Semin Liver Dis* 1991; 11(4):292–304.

Riegler JI, Lake JR. Fulminant hepatic failure. *Med Clin North Am* 1993;77(5):1057–1083.

Rodes J. Clinical manifestations and therapy of hepatic encephalopathy. In: Felipo V, Grisola S, eds. *Cirrhosis, hyperammonemia, and hepatic encephalopathy*. New York: Plenum, 1994:39–44.

Srivastava KL, Mittal A, Kumar A, Gupta S, Natu SM, Kumar R, Govil YC. Predictors of outcome in fulminant hepatic failure in children. *Indian J Gastroenterol* 1998;17(2):43–45.

Author: Andrew E. Mulberg

Hereditary Spherocytosis

 Database

DEFINITION

Anemia with shortened red cell survival due to selective trapping of osmotically fragile, spherocytic red blood cells in the spleen secondary to an inherent defect of the red cell membrane.

CAUSES

- Fundamental abnormality is not known and is probably in a structural protein of the red cell membrane "skeleton."
- Several intrinsic red cell defects have been identified with no single defect responsible for all the phenomena observed in this disease:

—Deficiency of one or more of the membrane proteins: spectrin, ankyrin, band 3 and protein 4.2.
—Defect in the interactions of these proteins: secondary to decreased levels of protein 4.1 or reduced phosphorylation of proteins.

PATHOPHYSIOLOGY

A membrane skeletal defect results in red cell membrane instability and loss of membrane surface. The sequelae are as follows:

- Loss of cell surface area relative to volume (spherocytosis) causing a decrease in cellular deformability.
- The spleen detains and "conditions" the non-deformable spherocytic red cells.
- Conditioning of cells involves depletion of ATP, increased glycolysis, increased influx and efflux of sodium, and loss of membrane lipid.
- Ultimately, the events lead to premature red cell destruction.

GENETICS

- Approximately three-fourths of families show autosomal-dominant inheritance pattern.
- The other one-fourth are autosomal-recessive forms, dominant disease with reduced penetrance, or new mutations.

EPIDEMIOLOGY

- Most common in people of Northern European extraction (about 1:5000)

COMPLICATIONS

- Post-splenectomy sepsis: lower risk of infection if postponed until 4 to 5 years of age, and immunized with pneumococcal vaccine (50–70% sepsis due to *Streptococcus pneumoniae*). Recurrence of hemolysis may occur due to regrowth of an accessory spleen.
- Gallstones: most common complication of hereditary sperocytosis (HS), major indication for splenectomy, pigment stones can lead to cholecystitis and/or biliary obstruction, cholelithiasis in HS manifests in second and third decades of life.
- Hemolytic crises: most frequent crises but usually not severe, develop transient increase in jaundice precipitated by infection.
- Aplastic crises: clinically more severe due to dramatic fall in hemoglobin and reticulocyte count, often caused by parvovirus B19 infection.
- Megaloblastic crises: caused by insufficient dietary intake of folic acid for increased bone marrow requirement. Folate need particularly acute during pregnancy and recovery from aplastic crises.
- Hemochromatosis (rare)
- Multiple myeloma: association of myeloma with chronic gallbladder disease.
- Other rare complications: gout, indolent leg ulcers, or chronic erythematous dermatitis on legs.

PROGNOSIS

- Severity of disease depends on classification:
- Silent carrier

—Patient can remain undetected unless thoroughly investigated due to subtle changes in lab findings

- Mild HS

—Patient may only be diagnosed late in life
—Anemia does not develop unless subjected to additional stresses (e.g., infection, exercise, pregnancy)

- Typical HS

—Patient presents in early childhood or neonatal period
—Often have baseline anemia and splenomegaly

- Severe HS

—Patient presents early in life
—Morbidity may be considerable with growth and sexual retardation

 Differential Diagnosis

- Hemolysis secondary to intracorpuscular RBC defects

—Membrane defects secondary to inherited disorders of membrane skeleton (hereditary spherocytosis and elliptocytosis) and red cell cation permeability and volume (stomatocytosis and xerocytosis)
—Enzyme defects: Embden-Meyerhof pathway (i.e., pyruvate kinase deficiency) and hexose monophosphate pathway (i.e., G6PD deficiency)
—Hemoglobin defects: heme, congenital erythropoietic porphyria; globin, qualitative (e.g., HbS, C, H, M); quantitative (e.g., thalassemias)
—Congenital dyserythropoietic anemias

- Hemolysis secondary to extracorpuscular RBC defects

—Immune-mediated (important in differential because spherocytes are present on smear): isoimmune (e.g., hemolytic disease of the newborn, blood group incompatibility) and autoimmune (e.g., cold agglutinin disease, warm auto immune hemolytic anemia)
—Non–immune-mediated: idiopathic and secondary to underlying disorder (e.g., HUS, TTP)

 Data Gathering

HISTORY

Question: Anemia, jaundice, dark urine, fatigue?
Significance: Signs of hemolysis

Question: Requiring phototherapy in newborn period (50% cases)?
Significance: Hyperbilirubinemia due to hemolysis

Question: Positive familial history (for disease, gallstones, or splenectomy)?
Significance: Autosomal dominant inheritance

Physical Examination

Finding: Splenomegaly, icterus/jaundice, pallor
Significance: All increased with hemolysis

Finding: Linear growth, weight gain and sexual development may be delayed
Significance: Delayed growth is indication for splenectomy.

 ## Laboratory Aids

Test: CBC
Significance: Mild to moderate anemia; MCV usually normal; MCHC elevated (useful screening test with high specificity); in aplastic crises, hemoglobin may drop 2 to 3 g/dL.

Test: Reticulocyte count increased
Significance: Level usually >6%; often accompanied with an elevated RDW.

Test: Indirect hyperbilirubinemia
Significance: Present in 50% to 60% of cases

Test: Peripheral smear
Significance: Microspherocytes, polychromasia

Test: Coombs test
Significance: Negative. Important differential test.

Test: Urinalysis
Significance: Hemoglobinuria, increased urobilinogen.

SPECIAL TESTS

Test: Osmotic fragility (most useful test in diagnosis)
Significance: Spherocytes are more fragile; therefore, less resistant to osmotic stress and lyse in higher concentration of saline than normal red cells.

Test: Autohemolysis test (screening test, not routinely used)
Significance: HS cells have increased autohemolysis at 24 and 48 hours, which is corrected by the addition of glucose.

Test: Bone marrow aspiration (optional)
Significance: Normoblastic hyperplasia, increased iron staining

Test: Survival of 51-Cr-labeled cells
Significance: Reduced with increased splenic sequestration

Test: Acidified glycerol lysis test, mechanical fragility test, oubain autohemolysis test
Significance: Additional test; usually not necessary

 ## Therapy

- Folic acid supplement
- Penicillin prophylaxis
- Pneumococcal and *H. influenza* B vaccines (if splenectomized)

SPLENECTOMY

- High response rate (i.e., almost sure to get increase in hemoglobin)
- Indications: moderate-to-severe anemia with significant hemolysis (reticulocyte count repeatedly >5%) resulting in transfusion dependence, decreased exercise tolerance, skeletal deformities, or delayed growth. Also, it may prevent symptomatic gallbladder disease.
- Complications: see post-splenectomy sepsis

CHOLECYSTECTOMY

- Indications: symptomatic gallbladder disease. Sometimes done concomitantly with splenectomy if gallstones evident by ultrasound.
- Complications: morbidity of surgical procedure and post-operative period.

 ## Follow-Up

- Patient monitoring
- Physical examination: splenomegaly, follow growth curves for FTT
- CBC with reticulocyte count every 2 to 6 months (dependent on clinical course)

PITFALLS

- False-negative osmotic fragility tests can occur in several situations; therefore, index of suspicion must be high to follow-up clinical course and repeat test (e.g., in neonatal period, during megaloblastic crisis, and recovery from aplastic crisis after transfusion).
- 20% to 25% HS patients have normal unincubated osmotic fragility (incubated test almost always positive; therefore, must have both).
- Autohemolysis test is sensitive but not specific. Results can be lab dependent with some labs with high false-positives in the normal population.
- Spherocytes are often present in immune-mediated hemolysis.

 ## Common Questions and Answers

Q: Will my child require blood transfusions?
A: It depends on the clinical severity of his/her disease.

Q: What are the risks and benefits of splenectomy:
A: Splenectomy is almost always successful in ameliorating anemia, but adds the risk of post-splenectomy infections.

Q: Does the age at diagnosis reflect the severity of disease?
A: Yes. In general, children diagnosed at an older age tend to be less symptomatic and have a milder form of the disease.

ICD-9-CM 282.0

BIBLIOGRAPHY

Becker PS, Lux SE. Disorders of the red cell membrane. In: Nathan DG, Oski FA, eds. *Hematology of infancy and childhood,* 4th ed. Philadelphia: WB Saunders, 1993:557–576.

Hassoun H, Palek J. Hereditary spherocytosis: a review of the clinical and molecular aspects of the disease. *Blood Rev* 1996;10:129–147.

Lanzkowsky P. Hemolytic anemia. In: Lanzkowsky P, ed. *Manual of pediatric hematology and oncology.* New York: Churchill Livingstone, 1989:91–92.

Michaels LA, Cohen AR, Huaqing Z, Raphael RI, Manno CS. Screening for hereditary spherocytosis by use of automated erythrocyte indexes. *J Pediatr* 1997;130(6):957–960.

Schroter W, Kahsnitz E. Diagnosis of hereditary spherocytosis in newborn infants. *J Pediatr* 1983;103:460–463.

Author: Deborah L. Kramer

Herpes Simplex Virus (HSV)

 Database

DEFINITION

Herpes simplex virus (HSV) is a moderately large double-stranded DNA virus. There are two serologically distinguishable subtypes: HSV-1 and HSV-2. HSV produces a wide spectrum of illness ranging from fever blisters to fatal viral encephalitis.

PATHOPHYSIOLOGY

- Initial viral replication occurs at the portal.
- Vesicular fluid contains infected epithelial cells.
- After primary HSV infection, the virus remains latent in sensory neural ganglia innervating portions of the skin or mucous membranes originally involved. The virus can be reactivated by an appropriate stimulus such as sunlight or immune suppression.
- HSV can be replicated easily in the laboratory in tissue cultures.

EPIDEMIOLOGY

- HSV-1 usually causes infections of the upper torso, head, and neck.
- HSV-2 usually causes genital infection. However, both forms can infect either oral or genital cells and thus the virus type is not a reliable indicator of the anatomic site of infection.
- Neonatal HSV infections are acquired from maternal strains and 75–85% are caused by HSV-2.
- After the neonatal period, HSV-1 infections predominate and 40–60% of children are seropositive for HSV-1 by age 5 years.
- During puberty and early adolescence, the prevalence of HSV-2 increases and 20–35% of adults are seropositive for HSV-2.
- Route of spread is usually by close bodily contact or trauma such as teething or a break in the skin.
- Incubation period is 2–12 days (average, 6 days).

ASSOCIATED DISEASES

- Neonatal infection is usually acquired from the maternal genitourinary tract and causes serious disease with high mortality and morbidity.
- Gingivostomatitis is the most common form of HSV primary infection in children.
- Encephalitis due to HSV accounts for 2–5% of all encephalitis in the United States.
- Vulvovaginitis due to primary infection with HSV-2 and sometimes HSV-1 has increased markedly in the past two years.

 Differential Diagnosis

- Neonatal HSV infection must be distinguished from viral or bacterial sepsis especially in the first 4 weeks of life.
- HSV infection should be considered in all neonates with vesicular rash, chorioretinitis, microcephaly, or hepatosplenomegaly. It must be distinguished from other congenital viral infections such as rubella or CMV.
- Herpes gingivostomatitis must be distinguished from herpangina, an enteroviral infection usually presenting as posterior pharyngeal ulcers, and sometimes as hand-foot-and-mouth disease.
- HSV encephalitis must be distinguished from other viral encephalitis and from the HSV-induced aseptic meningitis syndrome, which is a complication of primary genital infection.
- HSV vulvovaginitis must be distinguished from chancroid and syphilis. Syphilis lesions are usually nonpainful hard ulcers. Chancroid lesions are multiple purulent ulcers from which Haemophilus ducreyi can be cultured.

 Data Gathering

HISTORY

Neonatal Infection

- HSV-2, the most common cause of neonatal infection, is usually acquired from maternal labial lesions, but a history of previous or current genital HSV infection is only present in 20–30% of mothers who deliver infected infants. HSV-2 can be transmitted to the infant without rupture of the amniotic membranes or after delivery by cesarean section.
- HSV-1 can be transmitted to a neonate by any adult with active herpes labialis.
- A vesicular rash or bullae are present at birth or within a few days in almost all infants.
- Disseminated infection (32% of cases) involves the liver, lungs, adrenals, and sometimes the central nervous system (CNS).
- Localized CNS infection (33% of cases) presents with irritability, bulging fontanelle, or seizures.
- Localized skin, eye or mouth infection (35% of cases) present with rash alone, or keratitis or chorioretinitis.

Gingivostomatitis

- Fever and irritability precede the development of vesicular lesions on the lips, gingiva, and tongue. The vesicles then break down and become gray ulcers that are friable and bleed easily.
- Children refuse to drink because of the mouth pain and are at risk of dehydration.
- The child usually starts to improve in 3–5 days and has recovered in 14 days.
- Latent virus causes recurrent stomatitis or labiitis.

Encephalitis

- The illness begins with fever malaise and irritability that last 1–7 days and progress to mental status changes, seizures, and coma. Meningeal signs are not common.
- Patients can develop hemiparesis, cranial nerve palsy, and visual field defects.
- No presence of oral or genital lesions

Vulvovaginitis

- 35–50% of patients with the first episode of genital herpes will be able to give a history of genital HSV infection in their contact.
- The primary illness is characterized by fever, headache, malaise, and myalgias. Local genital symptoms include severe pain, itching, dysuria, vaginal or urethral discharge, and tender inguinal adenopathy. The genital lesions begin as vesicles and progress to ulcers before they crust over. Lesions last for 2–3 weeks.
- An aseptic meningitis syndrome occurs in 1–35% of cases. Patients will have fever, headache, meningismus, and photophobia.
- Latent virus causes recurrent episodes, which are painful but less severe than in primary infections.

 Laboratory Aids

Neonatal Infection

- Samples for viral isolation can be obtained from viral transport media.
- Serologic tests are not useful for diagnosis of maternal or neonatal herpes during the acute phase of the disease.
- PCR testing of the CSF is now recommended, and in some studies is proving to be quite useful in making the diagnosis.
- Cells from the base of freshly unroofed vesicles can be smeared on a slide for monoclonal antibody immunofluorescence.

Encephalitis

- Cerebrospinal fluid (CSF) reveals a pleocytosis with up to 2000 WBC/mm^3 and usually over 60% of the cells are lymphocytes.
- In an atraumatic lumbar puncture red blood cells, indicating hemorrhagic necrosis occur in 75 to 85 percent of cases.
- CSF protein is elevated (median, 80 mg/dL).
- HSV almost never grows from CSF.
- Electroencephalogram (EEG) can reveal a "typical pattern" of unilateral or bilateral focal spikes.
- A focal abnormality on EEG, CT, or MRI is highly suggestive of HSV encephalitis.
- The only definitive way to make the diagnosis is to perform a brain biopsy, which is essential to provide appropriate therapy.

Gingivostomatitis

Physicians usually make this diagnosis clinically since it is so common in young children.

Vulvovaginitis

- A Tzanck preparation from the base of a lesion will show multinucleate giant cells in 60% of cases.
- Viral culture obtained by unroofing a vesicle and rubbing a sterile swab over the base of the vesicle to have a sensitivity of 94% for early lesions. Sensitivity decreases to 27% for crusted lesions.
- Immunofluorescence has a sensitivity of 90%.

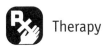 Therapy

NEONATAL INFECTION

Intravenous acyclovir (30 mg/kg/d in 3 divided doses) is the preferred drug. Some experts give higher doses (45–60 mg/kg/d). The recommended minimal duration of therapy is 14 days, and sometimes courses as long as 21 days may be indicated. Infants with ocular involvement due to HSV infection should receive a topical ophthalmic drug (1–2% trifluridine, 1% iododeoxyuridine, or 3% vidarabine) in addition to parenteral antiviral therapy.

ENCEPHALITIS

Intravenous acyclovir (30 mg/kg/d) three times a day for 14–21 days is appropriate therapy for HSV encephalitis after the neonatal period. In addition to parenteral antiviral therapy appropriate management of fluids, intracranial pressure, and seizures is essential.

GINGIVOSTOMATITIS

Most patients are managed with symptomatic therapy including antipyretics and oral fluids like popsicles. Oral anesthetics can be harmful and result in self injury when children chew on anesthetized lips. Topical acyclovir is often used in the treatment of recurrent oral herpes. It decreases the duration of HSV shedding but has minimal effect on the symptoms.

VULVOVAGINITIS

Acyclovir (Zovirax) is the appropriate therapy for genital herpes infection. Oral acyclovir is used for patients with primary genital HSV infection. Intravenous acyclovir is used for patients with severe local or systemic or complications like aseptic meningitis syndrome.

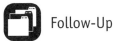 Follow-Up

PREVENTION

- Neonatal infection
- Cesarean section in a mother with active genital herpes at the time of delivery is the main way to prevent neonatal infection. The risk of HSV infection in an infant born vaginally to a mother with a first-episode primary genital infection is high (33–50%). The risk to an infant born to a mother with recurrent HSV infection at delivery is much lower (3–5%). However, this does not prevent all cases since 60–80% of mothers of infected infants are asymptomatic or have unrecognized infection.
- Postnatal infection

—Universal body substance precaution policies
—Adults with oral herpes must be particularly careful to use appropriate hygiene.
—Wrestlers with skin lesions suggestive of herpes
—Patients with genital lesions from HSV should not have intercourse until the lesions heal.
—Condoms can prevent the spread of virus.

PROGNOSIS

- Neonatal infection

—Overall mortality from untreated neonatal HSV infection is 50% and only 26% of survivors are normal.
—Combined treatment with vidarabine and acyclovir lowers mortality to 17% and increases survival.
—Infants with disseminated disease or localized CNS disease have the worst prognosis to 67%.
—The major sequelae in survivors are brain damage, seizures, and blindness.

 Common Questions and Answers

Q: What about recurrent cutaneous eruptions in a neonate? Should they be treated?
A: The need for retreatment of infants with recurrent skin lesions is undetermined and under study. Because of concerns about silent CNS recurrent infection, some experts are recommending acyclovir, 300 mg/m^2 in three doses for 6–12 months. One needs to look for neutropenia, which will occur in 25% of patients.

Q: Is prophylactic therapy for recurrent herpes genitalia helpful? When is it indicated?
A: Antiviral therapy has minimal effect on recurrent genital herpes. Oral acyclovir initiated within 2 days of onset of symptoms shortens the course. Topical acyclovir is not helpful.

Q: What steps should be taken in the nursery for an infant born to an HSV-positive mother?
A: Neonates with documented perinatal exposure to HSV may be in the incubation phase of infection and should be observed carefully. Infants of mothers with active HSV should be isolated if they have been delivered vaginally or by cesarean section after membranes were ruptured for more than 4–6 hours. The risk of HSV infection in possibly exposed infants (e.g., those born to a mother with a history of recurrent genital herpes) is low, and isolation is not necessary.

ICD-9-CM 054.9

BIBLIOGRAPHY

Corey L, Adams HG, Brown ZA, et al. Genital herpes simplex virus infections, clinical manifestations, course, and complications. *Ann Intern Med* 1983;98:958–972.

Corey L, Spear PG. Infections with herpes simplex virus. *N Engl J Med* 1986;314:686–691, 749–757.

Emans SJ, Goldstein DP. *Vulvovaginal complaints in the adolescent in pediatric and adolescent gynecology,* 3rd ed. Boston: Little, Brown, 1990:307–343.

Kohl S. Postnatal herpes simplex virus infection. In: Feigin RD, Cherry JD, eds. *Pediatric infectious diseases,* 3rd ed. Philadelphia: WB Saunders, 1992:1558–1583.

Marshall GS. Epidemiology and clinical manifestations of herpes infections in infants and children. *Semin Pediatr Infect Dis* 1997;8:151–168.

Nahmias AJ, Keyserling HL, Kevich GM. Herpes simplex. In: Remington JS, Klein JU, eds. *Infectious diseases of the fetus and newborn infant,* 2nd ed. Philadelphia: WB Saunders, 1983: 636–678.

Nahmias AJ, Whitley RJ, Herpes simplex virus encephalitis in pediatrics. *Pediatr Rev* 1981; 2:259–266.

Whitley RJ. Kimberlin DW. Treatment of viral infections during pregnancy and the neonatal period. *Clin Perinatol* 1997;24(1):267–283.

Author: Jane M. Gould

Hiccups

Database

DEFINITION

• Known medically as singultus, from the Latin "singult" (a sob or speech punctuated by sobs), hiccups are a result of involuntary spasm of the diaphragm and intercostal muscles, leading to inspiration and abrupt closure of the glottis. Hiccups affect nearly everyone at one time or another.
• Hiccup bouts may last up to 48 hours. Persistent hiccups last from 48 hours up to 1 month and intractable hiccups last for longer than 1 month.

PATHOPHYSIOLOGY

• Hiccups serve no physiological function and are often simply a benign affliction.
• A hiccup reflex arc has been postulated, although the exact anatomical mechanism remains unknown. The arc consists of:

—The afferent limb: phrenic and vagus nerves and the thoracic sympathetic chain from T6 to T12
—The efferent limb: phrenic nerve, and
—A central connection: a non-specific location incorporating the brainstem and the respiratory center, the hypothalamus, and the phrenic nerve nuclei

• Hiccups have negligible effect on ventilation and usually involve only unilateral diaphragmatic contraction, most frequently on the left

CAUSES

• Hiccup bouts may be precipitated by a number of benign causes including:

—Gastric distention: aerophagia, ingestion of excessive food, carbonated beverages or alcohol, and gastric insufflation during endoscopy
—Changes in the ambient or gastrointestinal temperature: cold showers, ingestion of hot or cold beverages
—Sudden excitement or stress
—Tobacco use

• Persistent and intractable hiccups have many causes, which can be characterized as psychogenic, organic, or idiopathic:
• Psychogenic

—Stress
—Conversion reactions
—Anorexia nervosa
—Malingering
—Personality disorders

• Organic

—Central nervous system disorders: V-P shunts, hydrocephalus, A-V malformations, stroke, temporal arteritis, CNS trauma, encephalitis, meningitis, brain abscess
—Peripheral nervous system disturbances: irritation of the phrenic or vagus nerve, from a variety of causes, including:

—Goiter, tumors or cysts of the neck, hiatal hernia, esophagitis, pneumonia, bronchitis, asthma, mediastinal lymphadenopathy, pericarditis, peptic ulcer disease, pancreatitis, inflammatory bowel disease, appendicitis, cholecystitis, and renal and hepatic disorders (stones or infections)
—Infectious etiologies: sepsis, influenza, herpes zoster, malaria and tuberculosis
—Metabolic or pharmacological causes: anesthesia, IV methylprednisolone, barbiturates, diazepam, methyldopa, uremia, hypocalcemia and hyponatremia

EPIDEMIOLOGY

• There is no male or female predominance for hiccup bouts; however, persistent and intractable hiccups have been shown to have a greater frequency in males, and are seen predominantly in adults.
• There is no racial, geographical, seasonal or socioeconomic variability.
• Fetal hiccups are common in the third trimester of pregnancy.

COMPLICATIONS

Adverse effects that have been associated with intractable hiccups include malnutrition and dehydration, weight loss, insomnia, and fatigue. Rarely, cardiac dysrhythmia and reflux esophagitis may occur.

PROGNOSIS

• Self-limited and resolves without complications

Differential Diagnosis

• Hiccups are not often mistaken for any other entity
• The differential diagnosis for persistent and intractable hiccups is outlined above (see Definition)

Data Gathering

HISTORY

• Severity, duration, and characteristics of hiccups?
• Medication and alcohol use?
• Hiccups persisting during sleep suggests an organic etiology.

Physical Examination

Finding: Head and neck examination
Significance: May reveal evidence of trauma, foreign body in the ear, nuchal rigidity, masses, cervical lymphadenopathy, or an enlarged thyroid.

Finding: Assess the chest
Significance: Evidence of pneumonia, bronchitis, pericarditis

Finding: Assess the abdomen
Significance: Evidence of appendicitis, intestinal obstruction, ruptured viscus, pancreatitis, or hepatobiliary disease

Finding:
Significance: Evidence of trauma, meningitis, encephalitis, V-P shunt malfunction or neoplasm

Laboratory Aids

SPECIFIC TEST

Test:
Significance: Chosen based on historical and physical findings

NON-SPECIFIC TEST

- CBC
- Renal function and electrolytes
- LFTs and calcium
- Toxicology screen and blood gas

RADIOGRAPHIC STUDIES

Test: Chest x-ray
Significance: May rule out phrenic, vagal, and diaphragmatic irritation by pulmonary, cardiac, and mediastinal abnormalities.

 ## Therapy

- Directed at the underlying disease.
- If etiology is unknown, empiric therapy may be necessary.

DRUGS

- Studies confined to adult populations. Pharmaceuticals rarely recommended for children.
- Chlorpromazine widely used in adults in IV preparations. Intramuscular Haloperidol has also been effective in adults.
- Anticonvulsants, including diphenylhydantoin, valproic acid, and carbamazapine reported effective.
- Combination of Cisapride, Omeprazole, and Baclofen has been reported to be effective.

NON-PHARMACOLOGICAL MODALITIES

- Interruption of respiratory function: sneezing, coughing, breath holding, hyperventilation, sudden pain or fright.
- Disruption of phrenic nerve transmission: tapping over the fifth cervical vertebra, ice applied to the skin over the area of the phrenic nerve, and even transecting the phrenic nerve.
- Behavioral modification, hypnosis, and acupuncture.
- Nasopharyngeal stimulation: traction of the tongue, stimulation of the pharynx with a cotton swab, lifting the uvula with a spoon.
- Old-fashioned home remedies such as sipping ice water, swallowing granulated sugar, drinking water from the far side of a glass, and biting on a lemon.

 ## Follow-Up

No specific follow-up is indicated unless a specific organic cause has been identified.

PREVENTION

Avoid precipitating factors.

PITFALLS

- Failure to recognize a serious underlying condition and assigning the label of idiopathic or psychogenic hiccups to an otherwise serious illness

 ## Common Questions and Answers

Q: Does breathing into a paper bag really work?
A: As a fall in pCO_2 can increase frequency of hiccups, rebreathing air will increase pCO_2 and thus terminate hiccups.

Q: Will hiccups harm my baby?
A: Hiccups alone are harmless. If they are truly persistent, intractable, or disrupt sleep, they may have the side effects as mentioned.

ICD-9-CM 786.8

BIBLIOGRAPHY

Pelig R, Shvartzman P, Hiccup. *J Fam Pract* 1996;42(4):424.

Petroiano G, Hein G, Petroiano A, Bergler W, Rufer R. Idiopathic chronic hiccup: combination therapy with cisapride, omeprazole, and baclofen. *Clin Ther* 1997;19:1031–1038.

Rousseau P. Hiccups. *South Med J* 1995;88(2):175–181.

Author: Blaze Robert Gusic

Hirschsprung Disease

 Database

DEFINITION

• Intestinal abnormality of abnormal innervation of the distal bowel beginning at the anus and extending proximately for a variable distance causing partial or complete intestinal obstruction, difficulty in passing stools and in some cases enterocolitis.
• Also known as congenital megacolon and was first reported by Harold Hirschsprung in 1886.
• Present as complete obstruction, delayed passage of meconium, "chronic constipation," or enterocolitis.

PATHOPHYSIOLOGY

• Basic histological finding is the absence of Meissner and Auerbach plexuses, hypertrophied nerve bundles between the circular and the longitudinal muscles and in the submucosa.
• Defect considered as a failure of caudal migration of the neural crest cells.

GENETICS

• Possible gene locus on the long arm of chromosome 10. Recent mouse models suggest a defect in the endothelin receptor.

EPIDEMIOLOGY

• Most common cause of lower intestinal obstruction in neonates: 1 in 5000 births
• Overall rate of male:female patients is 2.8:1; in long-segment disease, it is 2.8:1 and in total colonic aganglionosis, it is 2.2:1.
• No racial predilection
• Familial incidence in total colonic aganglionosis: 75% of cases, rectosigmoid involved, 14%, descending colon involved; 8%, colon involved; 3%, small bowel affected.

ASSOCIATED DISEASES

In 3% of the patients, there has been an association with Down syndrome, cardiac anomalies, and coexistent multiple neuroblastomas.

 Data Gathering

HISTORY

Question: Age of presentation
Significance: 80% of the time patients present in the neonatal period.

Question: Typical symptoms
Significance: Failure to pass meconium by 48 hours of life; delayed passage of meconium after 24 hours of life; history of constipation; history of chronic laxative use, abdominal distention, bilious vomiting, diarrhea in 22% of patients.

Question: Growth pattern
Significance: Neonates usually have normal weight, but growth retardation may occur when the disease is severe.

 Physical Examination

Finding: On rectal examination, the sphincter is usually normal or increased.
Significance: Removal of the finger may be followed by explosive diarrhea; transition zone is usually not felt in infants under 2 months of age.

Finding: Stool in rectum.
Significance: In most instances, especially in older children, the rectum is empty.

Finding: Anemic?
Significance: Patients are usually anemic due to chronic blood loss from the large bowel secondary to infection.

Laboratory Aids

TESTS

Test: Complete blood count
Significance: Anemia, leukocytosis in the presence of enterocolitis.

Test: Plain film of abdomen
Significance: May show distended loops of colon. Small bowel air is usually present in the bowel proximal to the obstruction.

Test: Barium enema
Significance: Useful but not diagnostic; transition zone is a funnel-shaped area of intestine with normal distal area and dilated proximal area. Barium enema reveals large mucosal pattern, prominently thickened folds and irregular margins secondary to ulceration.

Test: Anorectal manometry
Significance: Diagnostic but usually reserved for those cases causing diagnostic difficulties, as in the ultrashort segment disease.

Test: Biopsy
Significance: Suction biopsy should be done approximately 2 to 4 cm from the anal verge depending on the age of the patient. The biopsies must have adequate submucosa to demonstrate neurofibrils detected using acetylcholinesterase as a stain. With the absence of ganglion cells, biopsy is diagnostic. If the suction biopsies are not conclusive, a full-thickness biopsy is mandatory.

COMPLICATIONS

Enterocolitis is the most important complication:

- Secondary to obstruction causing an increase in intraluminal pressure and decreased intramural capillary blood flow.
- Affects the protective mucosal barrier enabling fecal breakdown products, bacteria, and toxins, to enter into the bloodstream.
- Usually present with fever, diarrhea, and frequent, bloody, bilious vomiting.

 Therapy

- Stabilizing treatment is fluid resuscitation, nasogastric decompression, broad-spectrum antibiotics, and saline enemas.
- The initial operation is a defunctionalizing colostomy or an ileostomy for total colonic aganglionosis. This is performed to avoid the hazards of enterocolitis. If the child has already developed enterocolitis, colostomy is deferred until the general condition improves.
- Definitive surgery is performed 6 months to a year after the initial colostomy. The various surgical procedures performed are:

—Endorectal pull-through: widely used. Basic principle is to strip the aganglionic rectum of its mucosa and then to bring normally innervated colon through the residual rectal muscular cuff, thereby bypassing the abnormal bowel from within. Advantages: sphincter function is preserved and minimal danger of injury to pelvis.
—Retrorectal transanal pull-through (Duhamel procedure): The normally innervated bowel is brought behind the abnormally innervated rectum approximately 1 to 2 cm above the pectinate line and an end-to-side anastomosis is performed. This procedure creates a neorectum with the anterior one-half having normal sensory receptors and a posterior one-half with normal propulsion. Advantages: reduces pelvic dissection to a minimum and retains the sensory pathway of rectal reflexes. Disadvantages: incontinence if anastomosis is too low and obstructive symptoms if anastomosis is too high or if the aganglionic segment is too long.

- Other procedures include the Soave (endorectal pull through).
- In total colonic aganglionosis, the modified Lester Martin technique is performed. It involves the anastomosis of the cecum and ascending colon as an on-lay patch graft in the more distal normal small bowel, which is then pulled through the amputated rectum that has been stripped of its mucosa and a primary anastomosis is performed.

PITFALLS

Early recognition is of utmost importance in reducing the morbidity and mortality of Hirschsprung disease.

BIBLIOGRAPHY

Abi-Hanna A, Lake AM. Constipation and encopresis in childhood. *Pediatr Rev* 1998;19(1): 23–30.

Athow AL, Filipe MI, Drake DP. Problems and advantages of acetyl cholinesterase histochemistry of rectal suction biopsies in Hirschsprung's disease. *J Pediatr Surg* 1990;25(5): 520–526.

Diseth TH, Egeland T, Emblem R. Effects of anal invasive treatment and incontinence on mental health and psychosocial functioning of adolescents with Hirschsprung's disease and low anorectal anomalies. *J Pediatr Surg* 1998;33(3): 468–475.

Fitzgerald CJ. New concepts of the etiology, diagnosis, and treatment of congenital megacolon (Hirschsprung's disease), by Orvar Swenson, MD, et al., *Pediatrics*, 1949;4:201–209. *Pediatrics* 1998;102(1 Pt 2):205–207.

Lyonnet S, Bolino A, Pelet A, et al. A gene for Hirschsprung's disease maps to the proximal long arm of chromosome 10. *Nature Genet* 1993;4(4):346–501.

Mahboubi S, Schnaufer L. The barium enema and rectal manometry in Hirschsprung's disease. *Radiology* 1979;130:643–647.

So HB, Becker JM, Schwartz DL, Kutin ND. Eighteen years' experience with neonatal Hirschsprung's disease treated by endorectal pull-through without colostomy. *J Pediatr Surg* 1998;33(5):673–675.

Author: Helen Anita John-Kelly and Andrew E. Mulberg

Histiocytic Disorders

 Database

DEFINITION

Clinical conditions resulting from or associated with proliferation of the mononuclear phagocytic system.

CLASSIFICATION

- Dendritic cell-related disorders (e.g., Langerhans cell histiocytosis)
- Macrophage-related disorders (e.g., hemophagocytic lymphohistiocytosis)
- Malignant histiocytic disorders

Langerhans Cell Histiocytosis

 Database

DEFINITION

- Reactive disorder of unknown etiology in which cells similar to Langerhans cells of the skin cause damage to organs by excessive production of cytokines and prostaglandins.
- Previously known as histiocytosis X, eosinophilic granuloma, Hand-Schüller-Christian disease and Letterer-Siwe disease

PATHOPHYSIOLOGY

- Lesions have proliferation of abnormal Langerhans cells in locations where they are not typically found; electron microscopy reveals tennis racquet-shaped inclusions (Birbeck granules)
- May arise as a result of an underlying immunodeficiency or as an abnormal response to a viral infection
- Monoclonal histiocytes have been detected in all forms of disease.

GENETICS

Generally familial. There are rare reports of recurrence within families.

COMPLICATIONS

- Single-system disease
- —Rarely progressive
- —Requires minimal treatment
- —Often remits spontaneously and completely
- Multisystem disease
- —Much more variable course
- —Spontaneous remission 10%
- —Complete remission with treatment and no recurrence 20% to 30%
- Chronic disease
- —Diabetes insipidus
- —Lung scarring 10%
- —Liver fibrosis less than 10%
- Fatal disease
- —Usually in children less than 2 years of age with organ failure (liver, bone marrow) 10% to 20%

PROGNOSIS

- Remissions and relapses
- Tendency to "burn out" eventually
- Survival curves flatten out 5 years from diagnosis

 Differential Diagnosis

- Hemophagocytic lymphohistiocytosis
- Sinus histiocytosis with massive lymphadenopathy (cervical nodes grossly enlarged)
- Malignant histiocytosis
- Bone tumors
- Craniopharyngioma
- Rhabdomyosarcoma
- Metastatic neuroblastoma

 Data Gathering

HISTORY

- Swelling? Pain? Mass effect
- Persistent otitis? Associated with histocytosis
- Early loss of teeth? Mandibular lesions
- Failure to thrive? Fever? Anorexia? Systemic sign
- Polydipsia? Polyuria? Diabetes insipidus
- Dyspnea? Cough? Pulmonary involvement; effusions

 Physical Examination

- Height, weight, and head circumference
- Reddish papules often involving the skin creases, scalp rashes, purpura, petechial rash, seborrheic dermatitis and other rashes
- Otorrhea, orbital abnormalities, gingivitis, palatal lesions, abnormal dentition with loose teeth, palpable skull lesions.
- Tachypnea, intercostal retractions
- Hepatosplenomegaly, ascites, edema, jaundice, stool with blood or mucous
- Papilledema, cranial nerve abnormalities, cerebellar dysfunction

 Laboratory Aids

MANDATORY INITIAL INVESTIGATIONS

- CBC with differential, PT, PTT, electrolytes, liver function tests.
- Chest X-ray, skeletal survey
- Early morning urine for osmolarity to assess pituitary involvement.

 Therapy

SINGLE SYSTEM

- Observation
- Local treatment
- —Surgery
- —Intralesional steroids (bone lesions)
- —Radiation therapy is not recommended unless there is compromise to vital structures (optic nerve, spinal cord)
- —Topical nitrogen mustard for refractory skin lesions
- —Indomethacin may be effective for refractory bone lesions for both its analgesic and antiprostaglandin effects

MULTISYSTEM

- Chemotherapy: usually a 6-month course; most commonly used agents: prednisone, vinblastine, etoposide, 6-mercaptopurine, methotrexate, 2-chlorodeoxyadenosine
- Immunotherapy: cyclosporin A, antithymocyte globulin
- Radiation therapy
- Bone marrow transplantation for high risk patients with organ dysfunction
- Most patients are treated at pediatric oncology centers.

 Follow-Up

LATE EFFECTS

- Poor dentition
- Deafness
- Orthopedic problems
- Small stature
- Diabetes insipidus
- Cerebellar ataxia
- Lung fibrosis
- Hepatic cirrhosis

Hemophagocytic Lymphohistiocytosis

 Database

DEFINITION

Reactive disorder characterized by an accumulation of erythrophagocytic histiocytes:

- Primary (also known as Familial Erythrophagocytic Lymphohistiocytosis)
- —Immunodysregulatory disorder
- —Classically an inherited disease
- Infection associated
- —Microorganisms implicated include: cytomegalovirus, Epstein-Barr virus (EBV), herpes simplex virus, HIV, adenovirus, tuberculosis, brucellosis, typhoid fever, leishmaniasis

PATHOPHYSIOLOGY

- Characterized by an accumulation of phagocytic histiocytes and lymphocytes in the reticuloendothelial system, skin, and central nervous system (CNS)
- Immune system dysregulation with defective T cell function, low or absent natural killer cell activity and elaboration of large amounts of inflammatory cytokines

GENETICS

- Primary
—Autosomal recessive
—Often a history of consanguinity; however, familial history is frequently negative
- Infection associated
—Sporadic

EPIDEMIOLOGY

- Primary
—Incidence is 0.12 per 100,000 children
—Males and females equally affected
—70% present in the first year of life
—Occurs in all races
- Infection associated
—Incidence variable
—Patients often have an underlying immunodeficiency disorder or are medically immunosuppressed (e.g., cancer chemotherapy)

PROGNOSIS

- Primary
—Usually fatal secondary to bleeding, infection (usually gram negative sepsis) or progressive cerebral damage from CNS involvement
—Untreated the median survival is 2 to 3 months, 12% live more than 6 months
—Allogeneic bone marrow transplantation has resulted in a few long-term survivors
- Infection associated
—Mortality rates: immunocompromised 40%, immunocompetent 20%
—Improved recovery in cases associated with bacterial infections; EBV-associated has the worst prognosis

 Differential Diagnosis

- Langerhans cell histiocytosis
- Sepsis with disseminated intravascular coagulation
- Syphilis
- Leishmaniasis
- Encephalitis
- Hepatitis
- Acute monoblastic leukemia
- Malignant histiocytosis
- Systemic juvenile rheumatoid arthritis
- Degenerative cerebral disorders
- Neurometabolic disorders
- Severe combined immunodeficiency disorder
- X-linked lympoproliferative disease
- Chédiak-Higashi syndrome

 Data Gathering

HISTORY

- Primary, rapid progression of symptoms
- Fever? Anorexia? Failure to thrive?
- Irritability, seizures, and vomiting?
- Often a viral prodrome for 2 to 6 weeks followed by constitutional symptoms, especially fever.

 Physical Examination

- Fever
- Hepatosplenomegaly
- Jaundice
- Percussion dullness from pleural effusions
- Seizure, irritability, bulging fontanel, neck stiffness, cranial nerve palsy, hypertonia or hypotonia, blindness, hemiplegia, coma, and increased intracranial pressure

 Laboratory Aids

- CBC with cytopenias
- Decreased fibrinogen
- Elevated serum triglycerides
- Bone marrow aspirate
—Early: hypercellular progressing to hypocellular, granulocytic and erythrocytic cell necroses.
—Late: diffuse benign appearing histiocytic hyperplasia with prominent hemophagocytosis of cells, especially red blood cells.
- Liver biopsy may demonstrate hemophagocytosis.
- Cerebrospinal fluid pleocytosis; (5–50 × 106/L) confirm CNS involvement.

 Therapy

- Primary
—Cytotoxic drugs: etoposide, intrathecal methotrexate, corticosteroids
—Immunosuppressive therapy: cyclosporin A, anti-thymocyte globulin
—Plasmapheresis or exchange blood transfusions
—Allogeneic bone marrow transplantation is necessary for cure
- Infection associated
—Withdrawal of immunosuppression if possible
—Anti-microbial therapy
—Corticosteroids

—Intravenous immunoglobulin
—Plasmapheresis
—For patients with uncontrolled fever, progressive pancytopenia, DIC or impending organ failure, cytotoxic therapy (as used for primary hemophagocytic lymphohistiocytosis) should be instituted

 Follow-Up

- Primary
—As most patients are diagnosed at an advanced stage, permanent neurological sequelae remain a significant problem
- Infection associated
—Few relapses are seen

MALIGNANT HISTIOCYTIC DISORDERS

- Acute monoblastic leukemia
- Malignant histiocytosis
- Histiocytic lymphoma

Common Questions and Answers

Q: How does one differentiate between the primary (inherited) and secondary (infection associated) forms of hemophagocytic lymphohistiocytosis?

A: There is no specific laboratory test that distinguishes the two entities. In general, diagnosis before age 2 years is strongly suggestive of primary hemophagocytic lymphohistiocytosis, whereas diagnosis after the age of 8 years is more in line with a diagnosis of secondary hemophagocytic lymphohistiocytosis. Clinical judgement should be used to decide on treatment for those children aged 2 to 8 years.

ICD-9-CM 277.8

BIBLIOGRAPHY

Egeler RM, D'Angio GJ. Langerhans cell histiocytosis. *J Pediatr* 1995;127:1–11.

Egeler RM, Neglia JP, Arico M, et al. The relation of Langerhans cell histiocytosis to acute leukemia, lymphomas, and other solid tumors. The LCH-Malignancy Study Group of the Histiocyte Society. *Hematol Oncol Clin North Am* 1998;12(2):369–378.

Author: Kara M. Kelly

Histoplasmosis

Database

DEFINITION

Infection of the lung caused by the fungus *Histoplasma capsulatum*.

CAUSES

- Inhalation of spores of the dimorphic fungus *Histoplasma capsulatum*
- Localized mononuclear cell infiltrate that may develop into a tuberculoid granuloma with multinucleated giant cells
- Lesions can undergo caseation necrosis, fibrosis, and, ultimately, calcification.
- Lesions usually localized to the lungs, though dissemination can occur.

GENETICS

- No genetic implications

EPIDEMIOLOGY

- The most common systemic fungal infection in the United States.
- Organism has been found in soil, blackbird and pigeon roosts, chicken houses, caves, attics, and old buildings.
- Endemic in the eastern and central United States, more specifically in the Mississippi and Ohio valleys, where 80% of the adults are skin test positive.
- No human-to-human or animal-to-human transmission.
- The symptoms depend on the immunological status of the host, as well as the size of the innoculum.
- The incubation period is between 1 to 3 weeks.
- Severe cases have been found to happen in the immunocompromised hosts as well as in children younger than 2 years of age.

COMPLICATIONS

In general, complications are rare.

- Include:

—Tracheobronchial compression
—Mediastinal granuloma formation
—Fistula formation
—Pericarditis
—Mediastinal fibrosis

- Disseminated disease involves:

—Skin
—Eyes
—Liver
—Spleen
—Bone marrow
—Heart

- Severe form of histoplasmosis is seen in patients with immunodeficiencies who live in endemic areas.

Differential Diagnosis

- Infections

—Pneumonia (viral, bacterial)
—Viral syndrome
—Tuberculosis
—Other fungal diseases: *aspergillosis, blastomycosis, coccidiomycosis*
—Sarcoidosis

Data Gathering

HISTORY

In children, severity of acute pulmonary histoplasmosis can vary:

Question: Upper respiratory symptoms, low grade fever, chest pain
Significance: Mild disease: 80% of patients affected; the course of the disease is 1 to 5 days. More than 95% of the patients are asymptomatic

Question: High fever, productive cough, chest pain, shortness of breath, hoarseness
Significance: Moderate disease: lasts approximately 15 days

Question: High fever, night sweats, weight loss, cough, chest pain, shortness of breath, hoarseness
Significance: Severe disease: lasts up to 3 weeks

Physical Examination

Finding: Flu-like signs and symptoms
Significance: Common presentations

- Fever
- Cough
- Hepatosplenomegaly
- Adenopathy
- Pneumonitis
- Skin lesions (erythema nodosum)
- Disseminated histoplasmosis

Laboratory Aids

Test: Identification of organism
Significance: Histologic identification from sputum, blood, bone marrow, biopsy specimens, and/or cerebrospinal fluid

Test: Staining methods (if granulomas are present)
Significance: Gomori methenamine silver (GMS), Wright, Giemsa, periodic acid-Schiff (PAS)

Test: Culture of the organism in tissue specimens or peripheral blood smears

Test: Serologic studies

Test: Complement fixation
Significance: A single titer 1:32 is diagnostic; a four-fold increase in titers is diagnostic. This test is more sensitive than the immunodiffusion test, which is more specific.

Test: Precipitating antibodies
Significance: H band suggests active infection, M band less specific, presence of H and M bands highly diagnostic

Test: Skin testing
Significance: A positive reaction to the histoplasmin test may become reactive 2 to 6 weeks after the infection positive when area of induration <5 mm at 48 hours. This test is not recommended for diagnostic purposes.

IMAGING

Test: Chest radiograph
Significance: Normal in 75% of the patients with histoplasmosis

- Most common radiologic changes include:

—Small 2- to 5-mm infiltrates in the lung bases
—Enlarged or calcified hilar nodes
—Buckshot calcifications seen in patients with large inoculurn
—Miliary pattern seen in patients with a high level of immunity
—Pleural effusions in 10% of adult films
—Calcified nodules in the liver and spleen

Therapy

DRUGS

• The uncomplicated cases of primary histoplasmosis of the lungs may not require medication therapy.
• Patients with severe or disseminated disease or the immunocompromised may require treatment with antifungal agents. The recommended length of treatment is 6 weeks:

—Amphotericin B, 0.5 to 1.0 mg/kg/d IV for 2 to 6 weeks
—Ketoconazole, 6 to 8 mg/kg/d PO (400 mg/d is maximum dose) for 3 to 6 months
—Other effective agents include fluconazole and itraconazole, although the latter has not been approved for the use in children, it is effective in the treatment of HIV patients with severe histoplasmosis

 Follow-Up

WHEN TO EXPECT IMPROVEMENT

• In mild-to-moderate cases not requiring drug therapy, usually 1 to 2 weeks
• In cases requiring therapy, improvement is usually noted within 2 weeks.

PROGNOSIS

• In most cases, prognosis is excellent.
• 90% mortality within 3 months in patients with acute disseminated histoplasmosis if left untreated.

PITFALLS

Can be difficult to distinguish between active disease and previous exposures in patients from endemic regions.

PREVENTION

• Isolation of the hospitalized patient

—Must isolate from patients with immunodeficiencies, otherwise standard universal precautions

CONTROL MEASURES

• None

 Common Questions and Answers

Q: How can histoplasmosis be prevented?
A: Prevention can only be achieved by controlling the environmental factors in the affected areas; there are no vaccines for the prevention of histoplasmosis.

Q: Do patients with histoplasmosis need to be isolated?
A: No isolation of infected patients is required.

ICD-9-CM 115.90

BIBLIOGRAPHY

American Academy of Pediatrics. *1997 Red book: report of the Committee on Infectious Diseases.* Evanston, IL; Academy of Pediatrics. 1997:277–278.

Bonner JR, Alexander WJ, Dismukes WE, et al. Disseminated histoplasmosis in patients with the acquired immune deficiency syndrome. *Arch Intern Med* 1984;144:2178–2181.

Davies SF. Serodiagnosis of histoplasmosis. *Semin Respir Infect* 1986;1:9–15.

Goodwin RA, Lloyd JE, Des Prez RM. Histoplasmosis in normal hosts. *Medicine* 1981;60:231–266.

Kanga J, Wilson HD. *Pediatric respiratory disease: diagnosis and treatment.* Philadelphia: WB Saunders, 1993:240–250.

Wheat J, French MLV, Kholer RB, et al. The diagnostic laboratory tests for histoplasmosis. *Ann Intern Med* 1982;97:680–685.

Author: Hector L. Flores-Arroyo

Hodgkin Lymphoma

 Database

DEFINITION

A malignant enlargement of lymph nodes characterized by a pleomorphic cellular infiltrate with multinucleated giant cells (Reed-Sternberg cells)

PATHOPHYSIOLOGY

• Exact cause unknown
• Reed-Sternberg cells are the malignant cells of Hodgkin lymphoma; however, their normal counterparts have not been definitively identified. They may originate from activated B or T lymphocytes or from an antigen-presenting cell. Histologically, Reed-Sternberg cells are dispersed among apparently normal reactive cells including lymphocytes, plasma cells, and eosinophils.
• The Rye classification histologically divides the disease into four categories: lymphocyte predominant, mixed cellularity, lymphocyte depleted, and nodular sclerosis.
• Unicentric in origin with spread mostly by contiguity from one chain of lymph nodes to another.

GENETICS

• Familial clustering suggests the role of both genetic and environmental factors in pathogenesis:

—three- to sevenfold increased risk of disease among siblings, in families where twins are concordant
—reports in parent-child pairs have been noted

EPIDEMIOLOGY

• Incidence shows bimodal age distribution:

—Early peak, before adolescence in developing countries, mid to late 20s in United States
—Second peak, late adulthood >50 years of age
—Childhood cases, rare before 5 years of age, males > females less than 10 years of age, more common in white race >15 years of age
—Infections with Epstein-Barr virus, cytomegalovirus, and herpesvirus 6 may play role in transmission of disease
—patients with history of EBV infection have a threefold increased risk of disease

COMPLICATIONS

• Acute toxicity of treatment

—Radiation effects are generally reversible and not serious. They are a function of total dose and volume irradiated and include erythema with or without hyperpigmentation of involved skin, nausea, fatigue, and possibly myelosuppression. Lhermitte syndrome, a sensation of "electric shock" radiating down the back into the extremities, may occasionally be seen.
—Chemotherapy regimens will cause nausea, vomiting, and reversible alopecia to some degree. Transfusions may be required for anemia and thrombocytopenia. Each individual agent also has a list of toxicities that must be reviewed before using alone or in combination. Most important of these include cardiac toxicity with Adriamycin, neurotoxicity with vincristine, and pulmonary toxicity with bleomycin.

• Infection

—Most common dose-limiting acute toxicity of chemotherapy is myelosuppression. Patients may have to be admitted for antibiotics if fever develops during neutropenia. Prophylactic antibiotics and vaccines have reduced the incidence of serious bacterial infections in the splenectomized host.

PROGNOSIS

• With current therapy including chemotherapy and/or radiation, five-year disease-free survival ranges from:

—88–100% in low stage disease
—54–94% in advanced stage disease

 Differential Diagnosis

• Infection is most common cause for acute lymphadenopathy.

—Bacterial (Staphylococcus aureus, β-hemolytic streptococcus, TB, atypical mycobacteria)
—Other (EBV, CMV, Cat-scratch disease, toxo, HIV, histoplasmosis)

• Malignancy is more common with chronic adenopathy.

—Non-Hodgkin lymphoma, neuroblastoma, leukemia, rhabdomyosarcoma

• Mediastinal masses divided anatomically:

—Anterior: lymphoid and thyroid tumors, bronchogenic cysts, aneurysms, lipomas
—Middle: lymphoid tumors, angiomas, pericardial cysts, teratomas, esophageal lesions, hernias
—Posterior: neurogenic tumors, cysts, thoracic meningocele, sarcomas

 Data Gathering

HISTORY

• Nonspecific clinical findings probably result from cytokine production

—Fatigue, anorexia, weight loss in one-third of patients
—"B" symptoms (part of staging classification) include one of the following:
—Unexplained fever with temp >38°C for at least 3 days
—Unexplained weight loss >10% body weight in previous 6 months
—Drenching night sweats

—"A" disease (asymptomatic)
—Pruritis or pain that worsens with ingestion of alcohol seen in some patients

 Physical Examination

• Painless lymphadenopathy most common

—Nodes are usually firmer and less mobile than inflammatory nodes
—Mediastinal mass in two-thirds of patients, may cause nonproductive cough or difficulty breathing
—Hepatosplenomegaly and bone tenderness in advanced stages
—Unusual signs and symptoms: nephrotic syndrome, dermatomyositis, and acute dysautonomia

 Laboratory Aids

• CBC, ESR
• Liver and renal function studies
• Serum copper, fibrinogen
• Baseline thyroid functions (preradiotherapy)
• Baseline echocardiogram and pulmonary function tests

PATHOLOGY

• Lymph node biopsy for definitive diagnosis

RADIOLOGIC STUDIES

• Chest x-ray (PA and lateral), looks for mediastinal mass
• CT scan (chest, abdomen, pelvis), to rule out disseminated disease
• CT or MRI of spine (if bony tenderness or symptoms of cord compression suspected)

SPECIAL TESTS

- Bone marrow biopsy
- Gallium scan (detects residual disease in the mediastinum)
- Bone scan (evaluates bone involvement, optional)
- Lymphangiogram (evaluates retroperitoneal adenopathy, optional)
- Cardiac Troponin-T levels (elevated after myocardial damage possibly due to therapy, investigational)

STAGING

- Staging laparotomy is indicated in patients with equivocal abdominal findings from clinical staging or in patients with radiotherapy treatment only.

—I: Involvement of a single lymph node region (I) or of a single extralymphatic organ or site (IE) by direct extension
—II: Involvement of two or more lymph node regions on the same side of the diaphragm (II) or localized involvement of an extralymphatic organ or site and one or more lymph node regions on the same side of the diaphragm (IIE)
—III: Involvement of lymph node regions on both sides of the diaphragm (III), which may be accompanied by involvement of the spleen (IIIS) or by localized involvement of an extralymphatic organ or site (IIIE) or both (IIISE)
—IV: Diffuse or disseminated involvement of one or more extralymphatic organs or tissues with or without associated lymph node involvement

- Staging is further subclassified "A" or "B" according to absence or presence of symptoms (listed above), respectively.

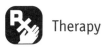

Therapy

RADIOTHERAPY (XRT)

- Exquisitely responsive to XRT
- Decisions to use XRT based on patient age, tumor burden, and potential complications
- Standard dose XRT, 3500 cGy; low dose, 2500 cGy; total dose given to all involved areas
- Doses administered in fractions, 150–200 cGy per day/five times a week

CHEMOTHERAPY

Multiple agents allow different mechanisms of action (to circumvent resistance) and nonoverlapping toxicities so that full doses can be given.

- MOPP: mechlorethamine + vincristine (Oncovin) + procarbazine + prednisone
- COPP: cyclophosphamide substituted for mechlorethamine in MOPP

- COMP: methotrexate substituted for procarbazine in COPP
- ABVD: doxorubicin (Adriamycin) + bleomycin + vinblastine + dacarbazine
- DBVE: doxorubicin + bleomycin + vincristine + etoposide
- DBVE-PC: DBVE + prednisone and cyclophosphamide
- Each cycle consists of 21–28 days, dependent on toxicity. Some regimens alternate therapy (i.e., MOPP alternating with ABVD), or use growth factor support to intensify schedule.
- Stages IA, IIA

—Attained full growth; no unfavorable signs: standard-dose XRT alone
—Still growing, bulky disease, or E lesions: (see staging) low dose XRT + two to four courses multiagent chemotherapy

- Stages IB, IIB, IIIA/B, IVA/B

—Attained full growth; no unfavorable signs: combined modality therapy with three to five courses multiagent chemotherapy + low-dose XRT
—Still growing or large mediastinal mass: low-dose XRT + chemotherapy (same as above)

Follow-Up

- Office visits monthly with CBC
- CT scan of involved areas every 3 months for first 2 years, then every 6 months for 3 years
- Special studies as needed for toxicity-related complications
- Relapse of disease usually occurs within first 3 years. Some may relapse as late as 10 years after initial diagnosis.

PITFALLS

- Late effects

—Pulmonary damage (radiation-induced and/or chemotherapy-bleomycin): pneumonitis, pulmonary fibrosis, decreased pulmonary function, pneumothorax
—Cardiac damage (XRT-induced and/or chemotherapy-Adriamycin): cardiomyopathy resulting in CHF, arrhythmias with conduction defects, pericarditis, valvular damage, coronary heart disease, and myocardial infarction
—Radiation nephritis
—Azoospermia induced by alkylating agents is almost always permanent in postpubertal boys
—Amenorrhea occurs in 20% of patients under 25 years using the MOPP regimen. Radiation-induced ovarian damage can be avoided by performing oophoropexy during laparotomy.
—Hypothyroidism results from XRT.
—Damage to soft tissue and bone growth can occur with high doses of XRT (>3500 cGy), resulting in a disproportionate alteration in sitting height versus standing height. Risk is highest during active bone growth (under 6 years of age and puberty).

—Secondary malignant neoplasms are a major concern in selecting therapy. The risk of developing leukemia (AML) is highest when both radiotherapy and alkylating agents are used. One study showed the risk of second neoplasm 15 years after diagnosis was 7%, with breast cancer as the most common solid tumor. Other secondary neoplasms associated with treatment are thyroid and skin carcinomas, brain tumor, and malignant fibrous histiocytoma.

Common Questions and Answers

Q: Is my child at risk for other cancers?
A: Yes. Although the incidence is low, children with Hodgkin disease are primarily at risk for cancers resulting from their treatment. Breast cancer is the most common solid tumor and can occur decades after therapy. Therefore, long term follow-up is essential.

Q: Will my child be infertile following treatment?
A: It depends on the therapy he/she received. Certain chemotherapy agents are associated with a higher risk of infertility (alkylating agents). Radiation to the gonads is also associated with infertility.

ICD-9-CM 201.9

BIBLIOGRAPHY

Aviles A, Soto B, Guzman R, et al. Results of a randomized study of early stage Hodgkin's disease using ABVD, EBVD, or MBVD. *Med Pediatr Oncol* 1995;24:171–175.

Bhatia S, Robinson LL, Oberlin O, et al. Breast cancer and other second neoplasms after childhood Hodgkin Disease. *N Engl J Med* 1996;334:745–751.

Lanzkowsky P. Hodgkin's disease. *Manual of pediatric hematology and oncology.* New York: Churchill Livingstone, 1989:251–269.

Leventhal BG, Donaldson SS. Hodgkin disease. In: Pizzo PA, Poplack DG, eds. *Principles and practice of pediatric oncology,* 2nd ed. Philadelphia: JB Lippincott, 1993:577–594.

Mack TM, Cozen W, Shibata DK, et al. Concordance for Hodgkin's disease in identical twins suggesting genetic susceptibility to the young-adult form of the disease. *N Engl J Med* 1995;332:413–418.

Ottlinger ME, Sallan SE, Rifai N, Sacks DB, Lipshultz SE. Myocardial damage in doxorubicin-treated children: a study of serum cardiac troponin-T. *Proc Am Soc Clin Oncol* 1995;14:345.

Author: Deborah L. Kramer

Human Immunodeficiency Virus Infection

 Database

DEFINITION

• HIV-1 and HIV-2 are the etiologic agents of HIV infection and the acquired immunodeficiency syndrome (AIDS).
• HIV infection is lifelong.
• For most infected individuals, a long clinically asymptomatic period (5–15 years in adults, frequently shorter in children), is followed by the development of generalized non-specific signs and symptoms (weight loss, adenopathy, hepatosplenomegaly) and mild clinical immunodeficiency.
• Eventually, after progressive immunologic deterioration, patients are susceptible to a wide variety of opportunistic infections and cancers, which represent the clinical syndrome known as AIDS.

PATHOLOGY

• The HIV outer envelope protein has a strong affinity for cells that express the CD4 molecule, a protein that coats the surface of various normal cells, including specific T lymphocytes and macrophages. The virus attaches to and then penetrates these cells, followed by transcription (using viral reverse transcriptase) of viral RNA into double-stranded DNA. This viral DNA is then integrated into the host cell genome and will remain there for the lifetime of the cell.
• Active viral replication continues after the primary infection. Even during the clinically latent period, more than 10^6 viral particles are produced daily. Over time, the host immune system loses the ability to contain viral replication and replace lost CD4 cells.

EPIDEMIOLOGY

• HIV infection is transmitted via:

—Sexual contact: male to female transmission more efficient than female to male; anal receptive sex more likely to transmit than vaginal sex.
—Exposure to infected blood: almost always involves parenteral exposure to infected blood (via transfusions or sharing needles). In occupational exposure, the risk of transmission from percutaneous exposure to needle contaminated with HIV-infected blood is 1/300.
—Breast milk
—Perinatally, either *in utero* or during labor and delivery. Of perinatally infected infants, 25% to 50% are believed infected *in utero;* the rest acquire the infection around the time of birth. The risk of an HIV-infected mother giving birth to an infected infant is approximately 25%, with increased rate of transmission for women with low CD4 counts, higher viral titers, and who were previously diagnosed with AIDS. In addition, vaginal delivery, especially with rupture of membranes longer than 12 hours, appears to increase the risk of infant infection.

• HIV is not believed to be transmitted by:
—Bites
—Sharing utensils, bathrooms, bathtubs
—Exposure to urine, feces, vomitus (except where these fluids may be grossly contaminated with blood, and even then transmission is rare, if at all)
—Casual contact in the home, school, or day care center

COMPLICATIONS

• *Pneumocystis carinii* pneumonia (PCP): With a peak age of 3 to 9 months, PCP is most common early fatal illness in HIV-infected children. In infancy, the mortality is 30% to 50% for the acute episode, with a median survival after first episode of less than 24 months. A high index of suspicion necessary for prompt diagnosis (by lavage) and initiation of therapy. 40% of new cases of HIV-related pediatric PCP involve infants not previously recognized as HIV-infected.
• Lymphocytic interstitial pneumonitis (LIP): Frequently asymptomatic, LIP can lead to slow onset of chronic respiratory symptoms. LIP causes a distinctive diffuse reticulonodular pattern on chest radiographs. Usually diagnosed between 2 and 4 years of age, LIP is related to dysfunctional immune response to EBV infection. Definitive diagnosis is made by lung biopsy. For symptomatic patients, prednisone is effective.
• Recurrent invasive bacterial infections: The risk of bacteremia is approximately 10%/year in HIV-infected children. Pneumococcal bacteremia is the most common invasive bacterial disease. Bacterial pneumonia, sinusitis, and otitis media are common among infected children.
• Progressive encephalopathy: Generally diagnosed between 9 and 18 months of age, the hallmark is progressive loss of developmental milestones or neurologic dysfunction. Cerebral atrophy is noted on CAT scan.
• Disseminated *Mycobacterium avium-intracellulare* (MAC): DMAC occurs in older children, usually older than 5 years of age, with severe immunodeficiency (CD4 < 100). Symptoms include prolonged fevers, abdominal pain, anorexia, and diarrhea.
• *Candida* esophagitis: As with dMAC, seen in older children with severe immunodeficiency. Patients usually present with dysphagia or chest pain. Oral thrush is noted on examination. Diagnosis suggested by findings on barium swallow. Definitive diagnosis made by biopsy.
• Disseminated CMV disease: Retinitis less common in HIV-infected children than adults. CMV may also cause pulmonary disease, colitis, and hepatitis.
• HIV-related cancers: Non-Hodgkin lymphoma most common cancer, with primary site usually located in the CNS.
• Other organ dysfunction associated with HIV-infection in children: cardiomyopathy, hepatitis, renal disease, thrombocytopenia/ITP.

PROGNOSIS

Prior to the advent of aggressive combination therapies, data suggested a bimodal survival curve, with 25% of perinatally infected infants developing early symptomatic disease, with an AIDS diagnosis by 1 to 2 years of life and frequently dying by 3 years of age. The remaining 75% have a delayed onset of symptoms, usually after 5 years of age, and the median survival of this group was to 8 to 12 years old. Since the use of three drug combinations have become standard, morbidity and mortality are both greatly decreased. The median survival is now clearly into adolescence. In addition, the incidence of new opportunistic infections has decreased greatly.

 Differential Diagnosis

• Neoplastic disease: lymphoma, leukemia, histiocytosis X
• Infectious: congenital/perinatal CMV, toxoplasmosis, congenital syphilis, acquired EBV
• Congenital immunodeficiency syndromes: Wiskott-Aldrich syndrome, chronic granulomatous disease

 Data Gathering

HISTORY

• Parental risk factors?
• Intravenous drug use?
• Non-injectable drug use?
• Sexually transmitted diseases, especially syphilis?
• Bisexuality?
• Transfusions before 1986?
• Frequent infections?
• Sinopulmonary infections?
• Recurrent pneumonia/invasive bacterial disease?
• Severe acute pneumonia (PCP)?
• Recurrent or resistant thrush, especially after 12 months of age?
• Congenital syphilis?
• Presence of sexually transmitted diseases in an adolescent?
• Acquired microcephaly?
• SProgressive encephalopathy, loss of developmental milestones?
• History of ITP/thrombocytopenia?
• Failure to thrive?
• Recurrent/chronic diarrhea?
• Recurrent/chronic enlargement of parotid gland?

Physical Examination

May be entirely normal in the first few months of life; 90% will have some physical findings by age 2. The most common findings are:

- Adenopathy, generalized
- Hepatosplenomegaly
- Failure to thrive
- Recurrent/resistant thrush, especially after 1 year of age
- Recurrent or chronic parotitis

 ## Laboratory Aids

Test: ELISA antibody screen
Significance: For children over 18 months of age, repeatedly reactive ELISA antibody screen, followed by confirmation with Western blot analysis, is diagnostic of HIV infection. Any positive test should always be repeated before a definitive diagnosis is discussed with family. In first year of life, positive HIV ELISA and Western blot antibody tests simply confirm maternal infection, because the antibody test is IgG based, and maternal anti-HIV antibodies readily cross placenta. Maternal antibodies may remain detectable until 15 months of age.

Test: HIV blood culture and/or PCR DNA testing
Significance: Most reliable way of diagnosing HIV infection in infancy. The PCR test has slightly more false-positives and false-negatives; the blood culture is more expensive, takes longer to run, and is technically more difficult. Both tests have sensitivities and specificities greater than 95% when performed after 4 weeks of age.

Test: Elevated IgG levels
Significance: First observed immune abnormality noted in HIV-infected infants, generally reaching twice the normal values by 9 months of age.

Test: CD4 counts
Significance: Obtained at diagnosis and every 1 to 3 months. Results need to be evaluated on the basis of age-adjusted normal values. Absolute CD4 counts are elevated in childhood, with normal median values greater than 3000/mm^3 in the first year of life, which then gradually decline with age, reaching values comparable with adult levels (800–1000/mm^3) by age 7.

Test: Neurological evaluation, with psychometric testing, and an initial CAT scan/MRI screening for cerebral atrophy.
Significance: Should be repeated at yearly intervals.

Test:
Significance: Post-immunization antibodies are measured to assess B cell function.

Other frequent lab abnormalities include thrombocytopenia, anemia, and elevated liver enzymes.

 ## Therapy

- Immunizations: All infected children receive standard childhood immunizations with the exception of substituting the IPV for the OPV. Infected children should receive yearly influenza A/B immunizations and the pneumococcal vaccine at age 2.
- Anti-retroviral therapy: Specific combination anti-retroviral therapy delays progression of illness, promotes improved growth and (possibly) neurological outcome. The standard of care now involves the administration of combination (usually three or more drugs) therapy. The most potent agents are those that inhibit viral protease (termed protease inhibitors). Drug regimens are complex, with as many as 9 doses of medicine a day. Adherence to prescribed schedules is critical. When patients miss even 20% to 25% of doses, the durability of response is short.
- Immune enhancement

—Passive: Recent studies suggest that monthly gammaglobulin infusions decrease, somewhat, febrile episodes and pneumococcal bacteremia. The children who benefit the most are those with CD4 counts greater than 200/mm^3 and not on antibiotic prophylaxis for PCP or otitis media.
—Active: Studies continue on reconstitution of the immune system. Intravenous interleukin-2, given for 5 days every 8 weeks, has proven efficacy in increasing CD4 counts (above that achieved with antiretroviral therapy alone).
—Prophylaxis: One of the major advances in the care of HIV-infected children and adults has been the ability to offer prophylaxis against the most common opportunistic infections. For each illness, a profile of those most at risk has been developed and drugs approved or under study.

PREVENTION

- HIV infection is almost completely preventable. Educational efforts aimed at achieving behavior change is a key component of HIV-directed work.
- It is now possible to significantly decrease the risk to newborns of HIV-infected women. Prenatal ZDV therapy, followed by continuous IV ZDV therapy during labor, and treatment of the infant for the first 6 weeks of life has been shown to decrease the risk of HIV infection in the infant from 25% to 8%. With the newer combination therapies, perinatal transmissions rates have now fallen below 5% in many parts of the country. Partly in response to these results, in 1995 both the CDC and AAP recommended that all pregnant women should receive counseling about the benefits of HIV testing, including the possibility of preventing fetal or infant infection, and should be offered HIV testing at the first prenatal visit.

 ## Follow-Up

Psychosocial support for the family is critical. For many families confronted with HIV infection, it is just one more stressor in addition to others related to urban life: inadequate finances, hard-to-access health care, inadequate housing and child care, domestic violence, and substance abuse.

PITFALLS

The result of failing to screen for HIV infection is the inability to offer anti-retroviral therapy for pregnant women, therefore, possibly preventing infant infection, and also the inability to prescribe PCP prophylaxis to infected newborns.

 ## Common Questions and Answers

Q: Once the HIV-exposed infant has seroreverted to antibody negative status, how sure are we that he/she is uninfected?
A: With today's technology, if the child has also been PCR and/or HIV blood culture negative at least twice, and is clinically well, the chance that the child still harbors HIV is very low and appears to be less than 1/5000. The child should continue to be followed by a health care provider aware of his/her past HIV antibody status. If clinical conditions warrant, retesting would be an option at a later date.

BIBLIOGRAPHY

Committe on Pediatric AIDS. Evaluation and Medical Treatment of the HIV-Exposed Infant. *Pediatrics* 1997;99:909–917.

Guideline for the use of antiretroviral agents in pediatric infection. *MMWR* 1998;47:1–38.

Recommendations of the U.S. Public Health Service Task Force on the use of Zidovudine to reduce perinatal transmission of human immunodeficiency virus. *MMWR* 1994;43:1–20.

Simonds RJ, Lindegren ML, Thomas P, et al. Prophylaxis against Pneumocystis carinii pneumonia among children with perinatally acquired human immunodeficiency virus infection in the United States. *N Engl J Med* 1995;332:786–790.

Author: Richard M. Rutstein

Hydrocephalus

 ## Database

DEFINITION

Hydrocephalus is accumulation of cerebrospinal fluid in the ventricles, leading to their enlargement.

CAUSES

- Developmental

—Chiari malformation type II (inferior displacement of medulla and cerebellum)
—Primary aqueductal stenosis
—Dandy-Walker malformation (absence of cerebellar vermis, small cerebellar hemispheres, enlarged posterior fossa, often with cystic fourth ventricle)

- Tumors of any histologic type located near foramina or the aqueduct
- Infection (meningitis) can lead to leptomeningeal adhesions and granulations.
- Hemorrhage (usually grade III to IV intraventricular hemorrhage or trauma-related) may result in a blood clot, meningeal adhesions, or granular ependymitis.

PATHOPHYSIOLOGY

- Normal pathway of CSF: choroid plexus, lateral ventricles, foramina of Monroe, third ventricle, aqueduct of Sylvius, fourth ventricle, foramina of Lushka and Magendie, subarachnoid space, arachnoid granulations, venous circulation
- Hydrocephalus often involves obstruction to CSF flow, even in the rare case of choroid plexus papilloma (overproduction of CSF).
- Noncommunicating hydrocephalus: The obstruction is in the ventricular system.
- Communicating hydrocephalus: The obstruction is outside of the ventricular system.
- Although the noncommunicating/communicating distinction has traditionally been fundamental in the literature, it has no prognostic significance; the value of the distinction concerns choice of a site for palliative drainage, and etiologic considerations.

COMPLICATIONS

- Acute hydrocephalus

—Herniation of temporal lobes may be fatal.

- Chronic hydrocephalus

—Macrocephaly
—Spastic paraparesis may lead to gait and motor problems.
—Developmental delay

 ## Differential Diagnosis

- Other causes of macrocephaly:

—Familial macrocephaly
—Pericerebral effusions
—Congenital anomalies of intra- or extracerebral veins
—Achondroplasia
—Tumors, intracranial cysts
—Neurocutaneous syndromes
—Dysmorphic syndromes
—Primary megalencephaly
—Some leukodystrophies
—GM2 gangliosidosis
—Mucopolysaccharidoses
—Head-sparing intrauterine growth retardation (relative macrocephaly)
—Rapid catch-up growth following prolonged malnutrition

- Other causes of ventriculomegaly include brain atrophy and chronic ethanol or corticosteroid exposure (reversible)
- In benign external hydrocephalus, both the ventricles and extraaxial CSF spaces are proportionately enlarged, and macrocephaly is common.

 ## Data Gathering

HISTORY

- Hydrocephalus is more common in preterm neonates in the intensive care nursery.
- Infants and children may also present to the primary pediatrician with new-onset hydrocephalus.
- Concerning complaints, especially in infants, include:

—Behavioral changes
—Enlarging head
—Nausea and vomiting

 ## Physical Examination

- Vital signs: The Cushing triad (hypertension, bradycardia, respiratory irregularities), which is characteristic of increased intracranial pressure, may be present in acute hydrocephalus.
- HEENT: Increasing head circumference in infants, sometimes with a bulging fontanelle; transillumination of the skull (using an intense light source) is seen in severe hydrocephalus; specificity of MacEwan "cracked pot" head percussion note is uncertain.
- Mental status: irritability in infants, behavioral changes in children
- Cranial nerves: Parinaud syndrome (setting sun sign, paralysis of upward gaze), papilledema or optic atrophy, visual changes
- Motor: spastic paraparesis in chronic hydrocephalus
- Reflexes: increased in chronic hydrocephalus

Laboratory Aids

TESTS

Imaging

- Head ultrasound

—Standard screening test for neonates with suspected hydrocephalus or intraventricular hemorrhage
—The anterior fontanelle must be patent for this test.
—Shows size of ventricles and presence or absence of blood

- Computed tomography (CT)

—Mainly used in infants and children whose anterior fontanelles have closed
—Advantage compared to ultrasound: better visualization of fourth ventricle/brainstem, calcifications

- Magnetic resonance imaging (MRI)

—Definitive test for analyzing brain anatomy
—Can identify developmental malformations such as Chiari and Dandy-Walker

Therapy

Neurosurgeons' use of therapeutic lumbar or ventricular puncture has decreased in recent years. These procedures must be weighed against risk of herniation (decreased when sutures are open).

VENTRICULAR SHUNT

• Indication: symptomatic progressive hydrocephalus
• Contraindications: active central nervous system infection, active intraventricular hemorrhage, and poor overall prognosis
• Components: ventricular catheter, reservoir (target of "shunt taps"), valve, distal catheter
• Distal sites: The peritoneum is the safest choice; the gall bladder, pleura, ureter, and right atrium are other choices.
• Siphon effect: drop in ventricular pressure on sitting or standing, alleviated in newer shunt systems, such as the Delta shunt, by antisiphon devices that close the valve when there is excessive negative pressure in the distal catheter
• Complications: Obstruction and infection are the main complications and often coincide, requiring replacement of the shunt system, ideally after any infection has been cleared.
• Rarely, shunting may be followed by acute decompensation, which may be due to upward transtentorial herniation of the brainstem.

THIRD VENTRICLE FENESTRATION

• Background: An old procedure that has fallen out of favor with development of modern shunt systems
• Current status: New endoscopic techniques make this procedure useful in rare cases of isolated intraventricular obstruction.

 Follow-Up

• When the etiology or need for shunt placement may not be clear, it is important to follow clinical status, head circumference, and ventricular size (by head ultrasound or CT).
• Chronic hydrocephalus is often accompanied by spastic paraparesis, visual problems, and developmental delay.
• Most important interventions are supportive, including physical therapy, occupational therapy, and orthopedic therapies for spasticity; interdisciplinary cerebral palsy clinics can be critical in providing easy access to these resources. Special education programs may be appropriate for children with severe developmental delay.

PITFALLS

• It is important for long-term patients in intensive care nurseries to have head circumferences recorded at least once a week. Macrocephaly is not always obvious on visual inspection.
• Papilledema is a sign of increased intracranial pressure, but its absence does not rule out this possibility.

—Head CT often will not show developmental malformations that may accompany hydrocephalus. MRI is the imaging procedure of choice.
—Timing of shunt placement is critical. A shunt placed too early may become infected or obstructed, while waiting too long may worsen permanent brain damage.

 Common Questions and Answers

Q: When does an infant need a head ultrasound?
A: Preterm infants below a certain gestational age or birth weight (varies from hospital to hospital) should all receive screening head ultrasounds while in the intensive care nursery, as well as any infant (inpatient or outpatient) whose head circumference crosses two percentile lines on the growth chart.

Q: When should an infant or child receive an MRI first rather than an ultrasound or CT?
A: Ordering an MRI first is reasonable in outpatients in whom the suspicion of hydrocephalus is strong and there are no obvious causes, such as infection or hemorrhage.

Q: What is the work-up for shunt obstruction and shunt infection?
A: Symptoms and signs of increased intracranial pressure should lead to a neurosurgical evaluation, head CT (to assess ventricular size and placement of ventricular catheter), and shunt series (plains films of the entire shunt system to check for disruptions). Fever is the most important indication for a shunt infection evaluation (shunt tap with CSF cell count, protein, glucose, Gram stain, and culture). Often patients will be evaluated for both complications.

ICD-9-CM 741.0

BIBLIOGRAPHY

Aicardi J. *Diseases of the nervous system in childhood.* Oxford: Blackwell Scientific, 1992.

Drake JM, Kestle J. Determining the best cerebrospinal fluid shunt valve design: the pediatric valve design trial. *Neurosurgery* 1996; 38:604–607.

Guertin SR. Cerebrospinal fluid shunts: evaluation, complications, and crisis management. *Pediatr Clin North Am* 1987;34:203–217.

Turner MS. The treatment of hydrocephalus: a brief guide to shunt selection. *Surg Neurol* 1995;43:314–323.

Wilkins RH, Rengachary SS, eds. *Neurosurgery,* 2nd ed. New York: McGraw-Hill, 1996.

Author: Peter M. Bingham

Hydronephrosis

Database

DEFINITION

Hydronephrosis is the anomalous dilatation of the upper urinary tract.

CAUSES

• Ureteropelvic junction (UPJ) obstruction: obstruction of ureter at the narrow junction with the renal pelvis, resulting in dilatation of the upper collecting system proximal to the obstruction; usually unilateral; may be due to intrinsic fibrotic narrowing of the ureter or due to extrinsic compression (i.e., accessory renal artery to the lower pole)
• Ureterovesical junction (UVJ) obstruction: usually due to a ureterocele that consists of cystic dilatations of the terminal ureter, often protruding into bladder; usually unilateral but can obstruct contralateral side as well as the bladder neck, associated with duplex anomalies of upper urinary tract (usually associated with the upper pole but may be associated with a single system)
• Vesicoureteral reflux (VUR): passage of urine from bladder to kidneys during voiding secondary to an incompetent valvular mechanism at the ureterovesical junction; may be unilateral or bilateral; usually no oligohydramnios; may be primarily due to incompetent vesicoureteral valve or secondary to bladder outlet obstruction
• Posterior urethral valves (PUVs): most common form involves mucosal folds protruding from the distal aspect of the verumontanum, which fuse to form an oval-shaped diaphragm, resulting in bladder outlet obstruction; may have primary reflux due to short intravesical tunnels or secondary reflux due to paraureteral diverticulae causing obstruction; may have renal dysplasia in severe cases; most common cause of urinary ascites or urinoma (1%–10% of infants with PUV have urinary ascites)
• Prune-belly syndrome: hypoplastic abdominal muscles associated with undescended testes and urinary tract abnormalities; associated with oligohydramnios, chronic renal failure, and pulmonary hypoplasia, VUR, and malrotation with a universal mesentery may be present
• Hydronephrosis may be associated with other congenital anomalies: urethral atresia, cloacal plate anomalies, midureteral stricture, ectopic ureter, multicystic kidney, retrocaval ureter, obstructive megaureter, hydrocolpos, pelvic tumor

EPIDEMIOLOGY

The incidence of congenital hydronephrosis is 0.17% to 0.93%. In unilateral neonatal hydronephrosis, fewer than 15% have obstruction; most resolve spontaneously, indicating either transient obstructive or nonobstructive etiology (i.e., VUR).

• UPJ obstruction: 1 in 1,500 births, 65% male, 5% bilateral, most common cause of hydronephrosis
• UVJ obstruction secondary to ureterocele: Those associated with duplex systems affect females seven times more than males; single-system ureteroceles usually affect males; 10% of cases are bilateral.
• VUR: Prevalence is unknown, but genetic factors may be involved; 33% of siblings of index cases and 66% of children of parents with VUR have VUR
• PUV: 1 in 5,000 to 8,000 males; most common cause of lower urinary tract obstruction in males
• Prune-belly syndrome: 1 in 40,000 births

Differential Diagnosis

• Renal tumors, such as Wilms tumor, may present as an abdominal mass; ultrasonography or abdominal computed tomography should distinguish a tumor.
• Multicystic dysplastic kidney, unilateral; most common renal cystic disease in infants, and second most common cause of unilateral abdominal mass; DMSA scan reveals no renal tissue, and intravenous urography shows no kidney function.

PROGNOSIS

• For congenital hydronephrosis, there is increased mortality if associated with nonrenal congenital anomalies: 52% versus 17% in isolated hydronephrosis.
• Oligohydramnios is a poor prognostic factor.
• Normal amniotic fluid volumes and unilateral hydronephrosis are associated with a better neonatal course.
• Long-term survival is related to the extent of preservation of renal function: 50% of long-term survivors of prune-belly syndrome require renal replacement therapy or transplantation.

Data Gathering

HISTORY

• In general: prenatal hydronephrosis, oligohydramnios, neonatal abdominal mass, urinary ascites, urinoma, pulmonary hypoplasia with respiratory distress, particularly if seen in full-term baby

—UPJ: abdominal, flank, or back pain; hematuria after minimal trauma; flank pain after large volume load
—Ureterocele: Sonography detects hydronephrosis, a double- or single-collecting system, and possible dysplasia.
—VUR: upper tract infection, sibling with VUR, symptoms of voiding dysfunction
—PUV: poor urinary stream or dribbling seen in approximately 30% of cases

Physical Examination

• In general: abdominal mass, signs of renal insufficiency (i.e., hypertension, failure to thrive, acidosis)
• PUV: palpable walnut-shaped bladder, hydroceles due to urinary ascites
• Prune-belly: wrinkled appearance of abdominal wall due to lack of abdominal wall musculature

—Ten percent with cardiac anomalies, 50% with anomalies of the musculoskeletal system (i.e., limb anomalies and scoliosis)
—Three percent of infants with prune-belly syndrome are female: anomalies of urethra, uterus, and vagina usually associated

Laboratory Aids

TESTS

Laboratory Tests

• Serial serum creatinine and electrolytes, especially if bilateral hydronephrosis is present—90% of infants with PUV present with some degree of renal insufficiency; children may have renal insufficiency from dysplasia or acquired damage due to VUR and infection.

—At birth, the infant's creatinine is the same as the mother's, but it should decrease to 0.4 by the end of the first week of life.
—Creatinine levels in premature babies may not decrease until 34 to 35 weeks' gestation.
—If hydronephrosis is unilateral, document normal creatinine and electrolytes.

Imaging

• Prenatal ultrasound can detect hydronephrosis and oligohydramnios; US performed later detects more anomalies.

—Neonates have transient oliguria, so the collecting system may appear falsely normal; 72 hours of life is the best time to perform US.
—UPJ obstruction: theoretically, dilated cysts communicate but can be difficult to distinguish from multicystic renal dysplasia; distal ureter should not be seen, and bladder appears normal.
—Ureterocele: cystic dilatation of distal ureter
—VUR: findings of intermittent hydronephrosis
—PUV: hypertrophied and thickened bladder and bladder neck
—Serial US is helpful. Progressive hydronephrosis indicates the presence of obstruction, while resolution of hydronephrosis indicates absence of obstruction.

• Voiding cystourethrography, in general, detects degree of VUR and dilatation or tortuosity of the lower collecting system.

—PUV thickened and trabeculated bladder wall, 50% with diverticulae, VUR in 60% of cases

• Intravenous urography, in general, evaluates excretory function of renal parenchyma.

—Ureterocele appears as a radiolucent circular shadow in bladder; if there is poor function, a duplicated upper pole may not be visualized, producing the drooping lily appearance of the lower collecting system.

• A DMSA scan, in general, identifies the presence of renal tissue which is found in the case of UPJ obstruction with communicating cysts. Multicystic renaldysplasia has noncommunicating cysts with no renal parenchyma. A DMSA scan is also important in detecting renal scarring that may be a long-term consequence of infection and reflux.

—Forty percent with VUR show scarring at baseline.

• Diuretic renography is useful in assessing renal function. Mercaptoacetyl triglycine (MAG-3) (excreted by renal tubules) is more accurate in newborns and infants than is diethylenetriamine pentaacetic acid (DTPA).

—Uptake is used to calculate differential renal function; normally each side is 50%.
—Then furosemide is administered to assess the efficiency of drainage of kidneys. This is useful only if there is brisk washout, which indicates that there is no anatomic obstruction.
—In unilateral neonatal hydronephrosis, if RUS and VCUG show no definite signs of anatomic obstruction, serial diuretic renography is useful.
—If the first study shows function greater than 40%, repeat in 3 months; if 30% to 40%, repeat in 2 months; if 20% to 30%, repeat in 1 month; if less than 20%, repeat in 2 weeks.
—If there is no deterioration in function of the involved kidney and no compensatory growth in the contralateral kidney, there is no evidence of anatomic obstruction.
—If there is any decrement in renal function, indicating obstruction, surgical intervention is indicated.
—Since less than 15% of infants will require surgery for obstruction, careful observation with serial diuretic renography is a reasonable option.

Therapy

CONSERVATIVE

Antibiotic prophylaxis at birth to prevent upper tract infection, especially if VUR is present: Use amoxicillin until 2 months of age, when trimethoprim-sulfamethoxazole or nitrofurantoin can be used.

SURGICAL

• Prenatal surgery: carries a high rate of complication; consider only if the condition is life-threatening (i.e., PUV) or if hydronephrosis is unilateral or there is normal amniotic fluid volume and pulmonary development; prenatal intervention is not indicated.
• Circumcise boys to decrease the risk of UTI.
• UPJ obstruction: Surgical excision (pyeloplasty) of obstructed portion of UPJ with re-anastomosis is 91% to 99% successful if performed as soon as diagnosis is made; perform nephrectomy if no renal function is evident.
• Ureterocele: endoscopic incision with flap to minimize VUR; nephrectomy if poor renal function; in duplicated system, if upper pole is nonfunctional, may perform upper segment nephrectomy; if upper pole functions, may anastomose upper pole ureter with the lower pole ureter
• VUR: reimplantation of ureter for high-grade reflux, persistent VUR, or associated with breakthrough upper tract infections on antibiotic prophylaxis
• PUV: Drain the bladder with a urethral catheter or vesicostomy. Definitive treatment involves transurethral ablation of valves with resectoscope or fulguration. The prognosis is better if there was a normal US at less than 24 weeks' gestation.
• Prune-belly: orchiopexy in the first year of life

ICD-9-CM 591

BIBLIOGRAPHY

Belman A. A perspective on vesicoureteral reflux. *Urol Clin North Am* 1995;22:139.

Behrman R, ed. *Nelson textbook of pediatrics*. Philadelphia: WB Saunders, 1992.

Elder JS. Antenatal hydronephrosis: fetal and neonatal management. *Pediatr Clin North Am* 1997;44(5):1299.

King L. Hydronephrosis: when is obstruction not obstruction? *Urol Clin North Am* 1995; 22:31.

Koff S. Pathophysiology of ureteropelvic junction obstruction: clinical and experimental observations. *Urol Clin North Am* 1990;17:263.

Koff SA. Neonatal management of unilateral hydronephrosis: role for delayed intervention. *Urol Clin North Am* 1998;25(2):181.

Mandell J, Peteres C, Retik A. Current concepts in the perinatal diagnosis and management of hydronephrosis. *Urol Clin North Am* 1990; 17:247.

Schulman S, Snyder H. Vesicoureteral reflux and reflux nephropathy in children. *Curr Opin Pediatr* 1993;5:191.

Author: Christina Lin Master

Hyperimmunoglobulinemia E Syndrome

 Database

DEFINITION

Hyperimmunoglobulinemia E syndrome is a rare disorder characterized by markedly elevated serum IgE levels, chronic eczematoid dermatitis, and recurrent infections.

PATHOPHYSIOLOGY

The syndrome is poorly understood; the following abnormalities have been noted in subgroups of patients:

- Phagocytic: impaired chemotaxis
- T cell: impaired proliferative response to antigens
- B cell: variable heterogeneity of ability to form antibodies to antigens

 Differential Diagnosis

- Atopic dermatitis
- Wiskott-Aldrich syndrome
- Chronic granulomatous disease

 Data Gathering

HISTORY

- Recurrent infection: otitis media, pneumonia, sinusitis, subcutaneous abscesses, pneumatoceles
- Organisms that cause infection: *Staphylococcus aureus, Candida, Haemophilus influenzae, Streptococcus pneumoniae,* group A streptococcus
- Severe eczematoid dermatitis as early as 1 week of age

 Physical Examination

- Coarse facial features, broad nasal bridge, prominent nose
- Growth retardation can occur with recurrent illnesses.
- Osteoporosis complicated by recurrent fractures

Laboratory Aids

TESTS

- Eosinophilia: peripheral eosinophils, >500 cells/mL
- Quantitative immunoglobulins: IgG, IgA, IgM usually normal, but IgE elevated, usually >5,000 IU/mL
- IgE antibodies against *S. aureus*
- Functional antibodies to diphtheria, tetanus, HIB, and pneumococcus results are variable, but there is a subgroup of patients that is unable to mount an appropriate antibody response to these antigens.
- Pulmonary function tests to evaluate extent of lung disease from infections such as pneumatoceles

 Therapy

- Supportive, based on clinical and laboratory findings
- Life-long use of antistaphylococcal therapy (i.e., dicloxacillin or augmentin at therapeutic doses)
- Surgical intervention for management of pneumatoceles for drainage or secondary to compression of nearby parenchyma
- IVIG as replacement therapy for abnormal functional antibodies is usually given at 400 g/kg on a monthly basis.

 Follow-Up

Long-term outcome is unknown; it depends on a timely diagnosis that allows for close monitoring and aggressive treatment of infections. Sequelae from recurrent infections such as pneumonias and pneumatoceles can result in a debilitating course. An increased chance of malignancy has been reported in some cases.

 Common Questions and Answers

Q: Is this disease also referred to as Job syndrome?
A: Yes, because Job suffered from difficulties with boils and other skin manifestations.

ICD-9-CM 279.3 (unspecified)

BIBLIOGRAPHY

Amman AJ. Phagocytic dysfunction diseases. In: Stites DP, Terr AI, eds. *Basic and clinical immunology*. Norwalk, CT: Appleton & Lange, 1991:356–360.

Douglas SD, Campbell DE. The hyperimmunoglobulinemia E-recurrent infection syndrome. *Clin Immunol Newsletter* 1984;5:86–87.

Lavoie A, Rottem M, Grodofsky MD, Douglas SD, et al. Anti-staphylococcus aureus IgE antibodies for diagnosis of hyperimmunoglobulinemia E-recurrent infection syndrome in infancy. *Am J Dis Child* 1989;143:38–104.

Leung DYM, Geha RS. Clinical and immunologic aspects of the hyperimmunoglobulin E syndrome. *Hematol Oncol Clin North Am* 1988; 2(1):81–97.

Sheerin KA, Buckley RH. Antibody response to protein, polysaccharide, and 0x174 antigens of the hyperimmunoglobulinemia E syndrome. *J Allergy Clin Immunol* 1991;87(4):803–811.

Author: Michelle M. Klinek

Hyperinsulinism/Hypoglycemia

Database

DEFINITION

Hyperinsulinism (HI) is a disorder of dysregulated insulin secretion characterized by excessive insulin secretion and excessive insulin action, and resulting in hypoglycemia.

CAUSES

Mutations in the sulfonylurea receptor or ATP-sensitive potassium channel or glutamate dehydrogenase result in uncoupling of insulin secretion from the glucose-sensing machinery of the pancreatic beta cell, and insulin secretion occurs regardless of blood glucose levels. Activating mutations in glucokinase lower the set point for insulin secretion from the beta cell. Transient HI may be caused by neonatal stress (maternal hypertension or precipitous delivery, hypoxia). Focal lesions may be due to loss of maternal alleles of imprinted genes specific for growth regulation.

PATHOLOGY

A variety of lesions may be found:

- Nesidioblastosis, in which beta cells are increased in number and arise from ductular epithelium
- Beta-cell adenomatosis, a diffuse abnormality of beta-cell development
- Islet-cell hyperplasia
- Focal lesions such as beta-cell adenomas
- Normal histology

GENETICS

- Autosomal recessive form: defect of sulfonylurea receptor (SUR) or K_{ATP} channel at chromosomal locus 11p14-15.1
- Autosomal dominant variant: some may have an activating mutations in the glucokinase gene
- Hyperinsulinism with hyperammonemia variant: autosomal dominant and sporadic forms, due to activating mutations of glutamate dehydrogenase (GDH) enzyme at regulatory GTP-binding site
- Sporadic focal lesions may be due to loss of maternal alleles of specific tumor suppressor gene loci in the 11p15 region

EPIDEMIOLOGY

- Most common cause of persistent hypoglycemia in children beyond the immediate neonatal period
- Annual incidence estimated at about 1:50,000 live births
- May be as high in 1:2500 in select populations (Saudi Arabians, Ashkenazi Jews)

COMPLICATIONS

- Severe refractory hypoglycemia
- Cognitive deficits, especially short-term memory, visuomotor integration, and arithmetic skills
- Seizures
- Coma
- Glucose intolerance or frank diabetes mellitus after treatment

PROGNOSIS

- Historically, over 50% patients sustained severe brain damage from hypoglycemia.
- Today the prognosis is more favorable, provided hypoglycemia is avoided.
- Glucose intolerance: Diabetes may develop later in life, especially postpancreatectomy.

Differential Diagnosis

- Sepsis
- Congenital heart disease
- Infant of diabetic mother (IDM)
- Beckwith-Wiedemann syndrome (BWS)
- Panhypopituitarism
- Respiratory distress syndrome
- Erythroblastosis fetalis
- Other inborn errors of metabolism

Data Gathering

HISTORY

Symptoms of hypoglycemia in the infant:

- Poor feeding
- Lethargy
- Cyanosis
- Tachypnea
- Jitteriness
- Seizures
- Early-morning irritability that responds to feeding

Physical Examination

Finding: Macrosomia
Significance: Suggests autosomal recessive SUR defect variant

Finding: Absence of macroglossia, umbilical hernia, visceromegaly
Significance: Signs of BWS

Finding: Normal palate genitalia
Significance: Abnormal palate or micropenis suggests hypopituitarism

Laboratory Aids

Finding: Inappropriately elevated insulin level (>2 μU/mL on newer assays) at time of hypoglycemia
Significance: Indicates uncoupling of insulin secretion from

Finding: Suppressed levels of free fatty acids and ketones at time of hypoglycemia:

- Free fatty acid level <0.5 mM
- β-Hydroxybutyrate level <1.1 mM

Significance: Indirect signs of excessive insulin action

Finding: Glycemic response to glucagon (blood sugar rise >30 mg/dL) at time of hypoglycemia
Significance: Sign of inappropriately stored glycogen at time of hypoglycemia (sign of excessive insulin action)

Finding: Suppressed insulin-like growth factor binding protein-1 (IGFBP-1) level
Significance: IGFBP-1 production is inhibited by insulin (sign of excessive insulin action)

Finding: Normal growth hormone, cortisol, and thyroxine levels
Significance: Excludes hypopituitarism

Therapy

- The major goal is prevention of brain damage by controlling blood glucose.

—Parenteral dextrose infusions to stabilize blood sugar acutely
—Supplemental oral or nasogastric feeds
—Diazoxide, a suppressant of insulin secretion, at 10 to 15 mg/kb/d divided q12h
—Octreotide, a long-acting somatostatin analog, at 5 to 20 mcg/kg/d divided q6h
—Subtotal pancreatectomy in those children refractory to medical therapy or in those with focal lesions

- Diet

—Frequent feedings and avoidance of long fasts
—Avoidance of protein loads in those with protein-sensitive hyperinsulinism

- Prognosis

—Historically, over 50% of patients sustained severe brain damage from hypoglycemia.
—Today that percentage is higher, provided hypoglycemia is avoided
—Glucose intolerance; diabetes may develop later in life, especially post-pancreatectomy.

DIET

Frequent feedings and avoidance of long fasts

Follow-Up

- Home blood glucose monitoring, especially with longer fasts or intercurrent illnesses
- Hospitalizations for intravenous glucose infusions may be necessary during illnesses with vomiting.
- After 4 to 6 years of treatment, fasting studies may be performed to evaluate disease regression.
- Close observation of linear growth is necessary, because octreotide can suppress GH secretion

Common Questions and Answers

Q: What is the chance of hyperinsulinism in the sibling of an affected child?
A: Twenty-five percent in the autosomal recessive type; as high as 50% in the autosomal dominant type.

Q: How low and for how long can glucose go before brain damage occurs?
A: Hypoglycemia is traditionally defined as glucose less than 40 mg/dL, but levels should be less than 55 to 60 mg/dL. Duration of hypoglycemia necessary for brain damage to occur is unknown.

Q: What is the chance that it will eventually resolve without surgery?
A: Only approximately 40% to 50% of cases are controlled with medication alone. The autosomal recessive form may be more likely to require surgery than will the dominant form.

ICD-9-CM 251.1

BIBLIOGRAPHY

Baker L, Thornton P, Stanley C. Management of hyperinsulinism in infants. *J Pediatr* 1991; 119(5):755–757.

De Lonlay P, Fournet J-C, Rahier J, et al. Somatic deletion of the imprinted 11p15 region in sporadic persistent hyperinsulinemic hypoglycemia of infancy is specific of focal adenomatous hyperplasia and endorses partial pancreatectomy. *J Clin Invest* 1997;100:802–807.

Glaser B, Kesavan P, Heyman M, et al. Familial hyperinsulinism caused by an activating glucokinase mutation. *NEJM* 1998;338(4):226–230.

Nestorowicz A, Inagaki N, Gonoi T, et al. A nonsense mutation in the inward rectifier potassium channel gene, Kir6.2, is associated with familial hyperinsulinism. *Diabetes* 1997;46: 1743–1748.

Stanley CA, Baker L. Hyperinsulinism in infants and children: Diagnosis and therapy. *Adv Pediatr* 1976;23:315–355.

Stanley CA. Hyperinsulinism in infants and children. *Ped Clin N Am* 1997;44:363–374.

Stanley CA, Lieu YK, Hsu BY, et al. Hyperinsulinism and hyperammonemia in infants with regulatory mutations of the glutamate dehydrogenase gene. *NEJM* 1998;338:1352–1357.

Thornton PS, Satin-Smith MS, Herold K, et al. Familial hyperinsulinism with apparent autosomal dominant inheritance: Clinical and genetic differences from the autosomal recessive variant. *J Pediatr* 1998;132:9–14.

Weinzimer SA, Stanley CA, Berry GT, Yudkoff M, Tuchman M, Thornton PS. A syndrome of congenital hyperinsulinism and hyperammonemia. *J Pediatr* 1997;130:661–664.

Author: Stuart A. Weinzimer

Hyperlipidemia

Database

DEFINITION

Hyperlipidemia refers to serum elevations of cholesterol, triglycerides, and lipoprotein. Total cholesterol consists of very low density lipoprotein (VLDL), low-density lipoprotein (LDL), and high-density lipoprotein (HDL).

• Normal serum concentrations:

—Total cholesterol: 170 mg/dL (borderline, 170–199 mg/dL)
—LDL cholesterol: 110 mg/dL (borderline, 110–129 mg/dL)
—Total triglycerides: 100 mg/dL (borderline, 100–140 mg/dL)

Primary hypercholesterolemia or hypertriglyceridemia (hyperlipidemia): elevation in serum cholesterol as a result of an inherited disorder of lipid metabolism (i.e., familial hypercholesterolemia)

Secondary hypercholesterolemia or hypertriglyceridemia: elevation in serum cholesterol as a result of another disease process (i.e., nephrotic syndrome)

PATHOPHYSIOLOGY

Primary hypercholesterolemia:

• Familial hypercholesterolemia (FH): defect of LDL receptor, resulting in the body's inability to properly utilize circulating LDL cholesterol
• Familial hypertriglyceridemia (FHTG): a severe elevation in serum triglycerides; can be associated with lipoprotein lipase deficiency or apolipoprotein C-II deficiency

GENETICS

• Familial hypertriglyceridemia (FHTG): dominantly inherited disorder
• Familial hypercholesterolemia (FH): dominantly inherited defect of LDL receptor
• Familial combined hyperlipidemia (FCHL): dominantly inherited lipid disorder

EPIDEMIOLOGY

The incidence of familial hypercholesterolemia homozygotes is 1 in 1,000,000; heterozygotes, 1 in 500, with unknown cause resulting in hypercholesterolemia and/or hypertriglyceridemia occurring in 2% of the population

COMPLICATIONS

Hypercholesterolemia has been linked to premature coronary artery disease and vascular disease. Severe hypertriglyceridemia can cause pancreatitis. The presence of significant atherosclerotic vessel disease is unusual in most children; however, it can occur in the first decade of life in children with homozygous familial hypercholesterolemia.

PROGNOSIS

• Familial hypercholesterolemia:

—Homozygotes: coronary artery disease in first or second decade of life
—Heterozygotes: Fifty percent of males develop premature heart disease by age 50 (females, age 60)

• Familial combined hyperlipidemia: occurs in 1% to 2% of population and accounts for 10% of all premature heart disease. A reduction of LDL cholesterol by 1% reduces risk by 2%.

Differential Diagnosis

• Hypercholesterolemia

—Primary hypercholesterolemia (see above)
—Hypothyroidism
—Nephrotic syndrome
—Liver disease (cholestatic)
—Renal failure
—Anorexia nervosa
—Acute porphyria
—Myelomatosis
—Medications (antihypertensives, estrogens, steroids, microsomal enzyme inducers, cyclosporine, diuretics)
—Pregnancy
—Dietary: excessive dietary intake of fat, cholesterol and/or calories

• Hypertriglyceridemia

—Primary hypertriglyceridemia (see above)
—Acute hepatitis
—Nephrotic syndrome
—Chronic renal failure
—Medications (diuretics, retinoids, oral contraceptives)
—Diabetes mellitus
—Alcohol abuse
—Lipodystrophy
—Myelomatosis
—Glycogen storage disease
—Dietary: excessive dietary intake of fat and/or calories

Data Gathering

HISTORY

Question: Is there a family history of premature heart disease?
Significance: Almost all cases of primary hyperlipidemia are of dominant inheritance; thus, questions should be asked regarding the occurrence of premature heart disease and hyperlipidemia in parents and grandparents.

Question: Does your child smoke?
Significance: Smoking reduces HDL cholesterol levels and increases the risk of vascular disease.

Question: Does your daughter use oral contraceptives?
Significance: Birth control pills have been shown to cause elevations in lipoprotein levels and, when coupled with already elevated lipid levels, can increase the risk of atherosclerosis.

Question: Does your child exercise regularly?
Significance: Lower levels of cholesterol and triglycerides are generally found in children and adolescents who are physically fit.

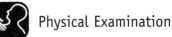

Physical Examination

• Eye examination:

—Arcus corneae: deposits of cholesterol, resulting in a thin, white circular ring located on the outer edge of the iris

• Skin examination:

—Tendon xanthomas: thickened tissue surrounding the Achilles' and extensor tendons
—Xanthelasma: yellowish deposits of cholesterol surrounding the eye
—Palmar xanthomas: pale lines in creases of palms
—Eruptive xanthomas: characteristic of hypertriglyceridemia; papular yellowish lesions with a red base that occur on the buttocks, elbows, and knees.

Laboratory Aids

TESTS

• Fasting serum lipoprotein levels: total cholesterol, HDL cholesterol, and triglycerides

—Determine the type of hyperlipidemia

• Calculated LDL cholesterol: LDL cholesterol = total cholesterol − [HDL cholesterol + triglycerides/5]

—Determines the level of LDL cholesterol
Chemistry panel (ALT, AST, Bili, BUN, creatinine, urinalysis)
—Screening test for liver and kidney disease

• Thyroid evaluation (T4, TSH)

—Determines the presence of hypothyroidism
—Three-day diet history
—Evaluates dietary intake of calories and cholesterol with 3-day diet

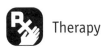

Therapy

GENERAL MEASURES

Outpatient management unless secondary hyperlipidemia caused by liver or renal failure, which would necessitate inpatient management of primary illness
NOTE: The cause of secondary hyperlipidemia should be treated with disease-specific therapy to affect a reduction in elevated lipid levels.

FOR PRIMARY HYPERLIPIDEMIA

Dietary management (recommended dietary intake):

• Total calories: age-appropriate to promote normal growth (do not limit children <3 years)
• Total fat: <20% total fat <30% of calories
• Saturated fat: 10% of calories
• Cholesterol: up to 100 mg/1,000 calories
• Protein: approximately 15% to 20% of calories
• Carbohydrates: approximately 55% of calories

NOTE: Hypertriglyceridemia almost always responds to strict dietary management (10–15 g/d of fat) and weight loss.

Risk Factors

The following are factors that contribute to heart disease:

• Smoking
• Excessive weight gain: <110% ideal body weight
• Hypertension
• Diabetes mellitus
• Low HDL cholesterol (35 mg/dL)
• Physical inactivity (bedridden)
• Family history of premature heart disease (55 years of age)

Patient education: Instruct patients on risk factors of premature heart disease, American Heart Association STEP I diet, and the need for adequate exercise and routine follow-up.

NOTE: Therapy is indicated if hyperlipidemia is caused by a dominantly inherited lipid disorder and the child is over 10 years of age and either LDL cholesterol greater than 190 mg/dL after dietary trial (6 months) or LDL cholesterol greater than 160 mg/dL after dietary trial and two or more additional risk factors exist. When drug therapy is considered, a referral to a pediatric lipid specialist is necessary.

DRUG OF CHOICE

Cholestyramine (bile acid resins) is the drug of choice for the initial treatment of primary hypercholesterolemia. It is not indicated for hypertriglyceridemia. It is contraindicated in patients with biliary obstruction or in patients with prior allergic reaction. All causes of secondary hyperlipidemia should be ruled out before starting therapy. Side effects include foul taste, constipation, nausea, and possible vitamin K deficiency. Cholestyramine may reduce or delay the absorption of concomitant oral medications secondary to drug binding.

ALTERNATIVE DRUGS

• Lovastatin (HMG-CoA reductase inhibitor) is an effective drug in adults and may prove to be beneficial in children in the future. Side effects include hepatitis and myositis.
• Niacin in megavitamin doses has been effective in the reduction of both serum LDL cholesterol and triglycerides; however, side effects occur in more than 50% of individuals, including flushing, itching, and headache.
• Experimental gene therapy has been shown to be effective in an animal model for familial hypercholesterolemia and may be the treatment of choice in the future for genetic disorders of lipid metabolism; it has been used recently in adult patients.

Follow-Up

For patients with primary hyperlipidemia who are off medication, follow-up should be performed every 1 to 2 years with lipoprotein profile evaluation. For those patients on medication, follow-up should be conducted every 3 months.

PREVENTION

• Avoid other risk factors (see above).
• Limit dietary intake of fat and cholesterol (see above).
• Increase exercise.
• Become educated about heart disease and atherosclerosis.

POSSIBLE COMPLICATIONS

• Hypercholesterolemia

—Premature heart disease
—Stroke
—Carotid artery disease

• Hypertriglyceridemia:

—Pancreatitis

CLINICAL PEARLS

Serum total cholesterol is inaccurate when serum triglycerides are greater than 400 mg/dL.

ICD-9-CM 272.4

BIBLIOGRAPHY

Cortner JA, Coates PM, Tershakovec AM. Disorders of lipoprotein metabolism and transport. In: Berman R, ed. *Nelson textbook of pediatrics,* 14th ed. Philadelphia: Saunders, 1992: 352–359.

Havel RJ. Approach to the patient with hyperlipidemia. *Med Clin North Am* 1982;66:319.

National Cholesterol Education Program. Report of the Expert Panel on Blood Cholesterol Levels in Children and Adolescents. *Pediatrics* 1992;89[Suppl]:525–584.

Newman WP, Freedman DS, Voors AW, et al. Relation of serum lipopotein levels and systolic blood pressure to early atherosclerosis: the Bogalusa Heart Study. *N Engl J Med* 1986; 314:138.

Poskitt EME, ed. *Practical paediatric nutrition.* London: Butterworths, 1988.

Author: Chris A. Liacouras

Hypertension

Database

DEFINITION

Hypertension is average systolic and/or diastolic blood pressures above the 95th percentile for age and gender as defined by the Second Task Force on Blood Pressure Control in Children. References also include norms based on the patient's height percentile. The final determination should be based on at least three measurements obtained on separate occasions. The significance of this definition with regard to morbidity and mortality is unclear.

PATHOPHYSIOLOGY

Hypertension is either primary (essential) or secondary. Secondary causes, with examples, include:

- Renal: acute glomerulonephritis, chronic renal failure, polycystic kidney disease, reflux nephropathy
- Renovascular: fibromuscular dysplasia, neurofibromatosis, vasculitis
- Cardiac: coarctation of the aorta
- Endocrine: pheochromocytoma, neuroblastoma, glucocorticoid-remediable aldosteronism
- Neurologic: increased intracranial pressure, Guillain-Barré syndrome
- Drugs: corticosteroids, oral contraceptives, sympathomimetics, illicit drugs (cocaine, phencyclidine)
- Other: obesity, burns, traction

GENETICS

Primary hypertension is more likely to develop in individuals when there is a strong family history. The genetics of secondary causes depend on the condition (e.g., polycystic kidney disease: autosomal dominant, autosomal recessive; neurofibromatosis: autosomal dominant; glucocorticoid-remediable aldosteronism: autosomal dominant).

EPIDEMIOLOGY

Primary hypertension is the most common cause of hypertension in adolescents and adults. Various rates of hypertension in children have been reported, from 1.2% to 13%, but less than 1% appear to require medication. African American adults have a greater incidence of hypertension. Differences in children, however, are not seen until after age 12. Tracking (i.e., determining the risk of hypertension based on earlier blood pressure measurements) is not reliable in children.

COMPLICATIONS

- Congestive heart failure
- Renal failure
- Encephalopathy
- Retinopathy

PROGNOSIS

The patient's prognosis depends on the underlying cause of the hypertension. It is excellent if the blood pressure is well controlled.

Differential Diagnosis

The initial objective after diagnosing hypertension in children is distinguishing primary from secondary causes. Generally, the younger the child and more elevated the blood pressure measurements, the more likely the cause of hypertension is secondary.

Data Gathering

HISTORY

Question: Is there a family history of hypertension?
Significance: Hypertension may be familial.

Question: Do you have symptoms of headache or blurry vision?
Significance: These are signes of increased intracranial pressure.

Question: Do you have chest pain?
Significance: This may indicate hypertensive heart disease or decreased coronary blood flow.

Question: Do you have epistaxis, weight gain or loss?
Significance: These are other signs of hypertension.

Question: Do you have flushing?
Significance: Flushing may be a sign of pheochromocytoma.

Question: Do you have a history of urinary tract infections?
Significance: Infections can be associated with reflux nephropathy and hypertension.

Special Questions

- Medical history: umbilical artery line, urinary tract infection
- Medications: corticosteroids, cold preparations, oral contraceptives, illicit drugs
- Family history: hypertension, phakomatosis, endocrinologic disorders
- Trauma: AV fistula, traction
- Review of symptoms: other systemic diseases

Hypertension

Physical Examination

- Body habitus: thin, obese, growth failure, virilized, stigmata of Turner or Williams syndrome
- Skin: café-au-lait spots, neurofibromas, rashes
- Head: moon facies
- Eyes: funduscopic changes, proptosis
- Lungs: rales
- Heart: rub, gallop, murmur
- Abdomen: mass, hepatosplenomegaly, bruit
- Genitalia: ambiguous, virilized
- Neurologic: Bell palsy

Laboratory Aids

TESTS

The laboratory evaluation for hypertension should proceed in a stepwise fashion.

- All patients should have:

—Urinalysis, urine culture
—Serum electrolytes, BUN, creatinine, calcium, uric acid, cholesterol
—CBC
—Echocardiogram: the most sensitive study to monitor end-organ changes
—Renal ultrasound

- Further evaluation, based on history, physical examination, and/or to prove secondary causes, includes:

—Voiding cystourethrogram
—DMSA renal scan
—Urine for catecholamines and metanephrines
—Plasma renin activity
—Aldosterone levels

- More invasive studies include:

—Renal angiogram
—Renal vein renin concentrations
—MIBG (metaiodobenzylguanidine) scan
—Renal biopsy

Therapy

- Mild primary hypertension may be managed with nonpharmacologic treatment: weight reduction, exercise, sodium restriction, avoidance of certain medications.
- Pharmacologic therapy should be directed to the cause of secondary hypertension when this is known or for severe, sustained hypertension. Medications may be needed in children with mild-to-moderate hypertension if nonpharmacologic therapy has failed or if end-organ changes are present.
- Classes of antihypertensive agents include α- and β-blockers, diuretics, vasodilators (direct and calcium channel blockers), and angiotensin converting enzyme (ACE) inhibitors.
- Other *specific therapies* include surgery (renovascular hypertension, coarctation of the aorta), percutaneous transluminal angioplasty (renovascular hypertension), and dialysis (chronic renal failure).

Follow-Up

The reduction of blood pressure with medication should be gradual to avoid side effects. The medications themselves cause adverse effects, such as exercise intolerance (β-blockers), headaches (vasodilators), renal insufficiency (ACE inhibitors), and hypokalemia (diuretics). Certain classes of medication should be avoided in patients with specific conditions, such as asthma and diabetes (β-blockers) and renal artery stenosis (ACE inhibitors).

PITFALLS

- Use the proper cuff size. The inflatable bladder should completely encircle the arm and cover approximately 75% of the upper arm. A cuff that is inappropriately small will artifactually increase the measurement.
- ACE inhibitors and β-blockers alter plasma renin activity levels.
- Several medications, such as labetolol, can affect an MIBG scan.
- Avoid multiple medications with the same mechanism of action.
- Elicit a history of adverse effects and adjust medications accordingly.
- If patients feel the medication is making them feel ill, they will discontinue it themselves.
- Attempt to wean medication intermittently.

Common Questions and Answers

Q: How does licorice cause hypertension?
A: British licorice contains glycyrrhizinic acid, a mineralocorticoid-like substance that causes sodium retention, potassium wasting, and hypertension. This substance is not found in most commercially available licorice in the United States.

Q: What percentage of children have renovascular causes for their hypertension?
A: Studies looking at the etiology of hypertension indicate that 10% to 24% of children may have a renovascular cause. Children under 5 years of age are four times more likely to have renal artery stenosis than are adolescents.

Q: What are the indications for invasive studies such as angiography?
A: This decision should be individualized and based on the severity of the hypertension, response to medication, the clinical presentation (e.g., neurofibromatosis), and results of other studies. In general, young children and all children with severe, unexplained hypertension should be completely evaluated.

Q: Can adolescents with elevated blood pressure compete in sports?
A: Adolescents with hypertension should be encouraged to participate in athletics if their blood pressures are well controlled. The use of stress testing in this population is controversial.

ICD-9-CM 401.9 (unspecified)

BIBLIOGRAPHY

Daniels SR. Hypertension in childhood. *Pediatr Rev* 1997;18:331.

Fivush B, Neu A, Firth S. Acute hypertensive crises in children: emergencies and urgencies. *Curr Opin Pediatr* 1997;9:233–236.

Rocchini AP, ed. Childhood hypertension. *Pediatr Clin North Am* 1993;40:1–212.

Rosner B, Prineas RJ, Loggie JMH, Daniels SR. Blood pressure nomograms for children and adolescents, by height, sex, and age, in the United States. *J Pediatr* 1993;123:871–876.

Sinaiko AR. Hypertension in children. *N Engl J Med* 1996;335:1968–1973.

Task Force on Blood Pressure Control in Children. Report of the Second Task Force on Blood Pressure Control in Children. *Pediatrics* 1987;79:1–25.

Author: Seth L. Schulman

Hypoparathyroidism

Database

DEFINITION

Hypoparathyroidism is decreased parathyroid hormone (PTH) effect.

PATHOPHYSIOLOGY

- Diminished or absent PTH activity results in:

—Hypocalcemia and hyperphosphatemia
—Reduced vitamin D activation to $1,25(OH)_2$ Vitamin D
—Hypocalcemia leads to increased neural excitability.

- Hypoparathyroidism

—Transient

　—Fetal parathyroid suppression: maternal hypercalcemia, diabetic mother
　—Hypomagnesemia: direct effects (suppressed PTH secretion, increased PTH resistance)
　—Alcohol intoxication

—Congenital

　—Familial: X-linked recessive, autosomal dominant, autosomal recessive
　—Sporadic and isolated
　—DiGeorge syndrome: parathyroid gland hypoplasia, thymic hypoplasia/aplasia, facial abnormalities, aortic arch and cardiac defects

—Acquired

　—Postsurgical
　—Postirradiation
　—Type 1 polyglandular autoimmune disease (Blizzard syndrome): hypoparathyroidism associated with chronic mucocutaneous candidiasis and autoimmune adrenal insufficiency; can also have diabetes mellitus, lymphocytic thyroiditis, hypogonadism, pernicious anemia, chronic hepatitis
　—Iron deposition: thalassemia, hemochromatosis
　—Copper deposition: Wilson disease
　—Metastatic carcinoma
　—Miliary tuberculosis

- Pseudohypoparathyroidism: resistance to PTH

—Albright Hereditary Osteodystrophy: G protein mutation

GENETICS

- X-linked recessive: neonatal onset
- Autosomal dominant and autosomal recessive forms

—Chromosome 3q13: mutations in the calcium-sensing receptor gene
—Chromosome 11p: mutations in the PTH gene
—Chromosome 22q11: DiGeorge syndrome
—Chromosome 21q22: Type 1 polyglandular autoimmune disease
—Chromosome 20q13: Albright hereditary osteodystrophy

- Mitochondria diseases: Kearns-Sayre syndrome (hypoparathyroidism and deafness)

EPIDEMIOLOGY

Many normal neonates can have hypocalcemia (serum calcium less than 8 mg/dL) during the first 3 weeks of life due to physiologic transient hypoparathyroidism.

- Parathyroid gland immaturity can lead to deficient PTH release and exaggerated normal fall in serum calcium concentration during the first 3 days of life.
- Relative immaturity of renal phosphorus handling and response to PTH can lead to late neonatal hypocalcemia precipitated by a high phosphate diet (cow's milk–based formulas).

COMPLICATIONS

Hypocalcemia can cause tetany, arrhythmias, seizures, and respiratory arrest.

PROGNOSIS

Fair; long-term outcome: development of nephrocalcinosis resulting in renal insufficiency

Differential Diagnosis

HYPOCALCEMIA

- Vitamin D deficiency
- Vitamin D–dependent rickets type I and II
- Hyperphosphatemia
- Prematurity
- Acute pancreatitis
- Malignancy: osteoblastic metastases, tumor-lysis syndrome
- Medication: citrated blood products, phenobarbital, dilantin, phosphate

Data Gathering

HISTORY

- In neonates: maternal calcium and magnesium abnormalities, maternal diabetes
- Family history of calcium disorders
- Medications
- Recurrent infections
- Recurrent muscle cramps
- Paresthesias

Hypoparathyroidism

Physical Examination

- Chvostek sign: Facial nerve stimulation (tapping anterior of external auditory meatus) causes contraction of orbicularis oris, producing upper lip or mouth twitch.
- Trousseau sign: Insufflation of blood pressure cuff reduces the blood flow to peripheral motor nerves and thereby can elicit carpopedal spasm in latent tetany.
- Carpopedal spasm
- Laryngeal stridor
- Mental status changes
- Irritability
- Papilledema
- Cataracts
- Bradycardia, hypotension
- Dry skin, coarse hair, brittle nails
- Albright hereditary osteodystrophy (pseudohypoparathyroidism type Ia): short stature, round face, thick neck, barrel chest, obesity, subcutaneous calcifications, brachydactyly (short 4th metacarpal bones)

Laboratory Aids

TESTS

Laboratory Tests

- Total and ionized serum calcium concentrations: low
- Serum phosphorus concentration: elevated in hypoparathyroidism; low in rickets
- Serum magnesium concentration: rule out hypomagnesemia
- Albumin: assess calcium binding (if cannot get ionized calcium)
- Intact PTH levels
- 25-OH- and 1,25(OH)$_2$-Vitamin D levels: distinguish hypoparathyroidism from rickets
- Urinary cyclic AMP response to PTH: diagnostic test if concerned about pseudohypoparathyroidism; otherwise, not routinely done

Imaging

- Chest x-ray: rachitic rosary (rickets), absence of thymus (DiGeorge syndrome)

False Positives

- Hypomagnesemia

Therapy

DRUGS

Titrate therapy to maintain serum calcium concentrations greater than 8.0 mg/dL. In cases requiring lifelong therapy, compromise for serum calciums in the 8- to 9-mg/dL range to decrease the long-term risk for developing nephrocalcinosis.

- 1,25(OH)$_2$ Vitamin D: less than 1 year: 0.04 to 0.08 μg/kg/d; 1 to 5 years: 0.25 to 0.75 μg/d; greater than 6 years and adults: 0.5 to 2.0 μg/d.
- Calcium: Dose depends on preparation and on patient needs.

DURATION

- For life

DIET

- Unrestricted

Follow-Up

Regularly with the endocrinologist

WHEN TO EXPECT IMPROVEMENT

- Immediately

SIGNS TO WATCH FOR

- Patients with acute, severe hypercalcemia should be placed on telemetry to monitor for cardiac arrhythmias (especially prolonged QTc).
- Muscle cramps
- Carpopedal spasms
- Seizures

Common Questions and Answers

Q: Is the thyroid also involved?
A: No.

Q: Are seizures common?
A: Yes, seizures are a common presentation of hypoparathyroidism in childhood, and physiologic transient hypoparathyroidism is the most common cause of neonatal seizures.

Q: Can hypoparathyroidism be associated with other abnormalities?
A: Yes. Investigate neonates at the time of diagnosis for cardiac defects and thymic aplasia (DiGeorge syndrome), and monitor patients with hypoparathyroidism for development of other autoimmune endocrinopathies and chronic mucocutaneous candidiasis (type 1 polyglandular autoimmune disease).

Q: When should IV versus oral calcium supplementation be used?
A: IV calcium supplementation provides the quickest correction of hypocalcemia and is therefore useful in severe cases (seizures, stridor, tetany, cardiac arrhythmias) or in the initiation of therapy (as you await establishment of adequate vitamin D levels, which are necessary for enteral calcium absorption). Switch to oral calcium supplementation as soon as possible to reduce the risk of potential IV calcium-mediated venous sclerosis and tissue extravasation.

ICD-9-CM 252.1

BIBLIOGRAPHY

Bassett JH, Thakker RV. Molecular genetics of disorders of calcium homeostasis. *Baillieres Clin Endocrinol Metab* 1995;9:581–608.

Betterle C, Greggio NA, Volpato M. Clinical Review 93: autoimmune polyglandular syndrome type 1. *J Clin Endocrinol Metab* 1998;83:1049–1055.

Cuneo BF, Driscoll DA, Gidding SS, Langman CB. Evolution of latent hypoparathyroidism in familial 22q11 deletion syndrome. *Am J Med Genet* 1997;69:50–55.

Eronocodelu Y, Bober E, Tunnessen W Jr. Picture of the Month: Albright hereditary osteodystrophy. *Arch Pediatr Adolesc Med* 1997;151:1263–1264.

Gertner JM. Disorders of calcium and phosphorus homeostasis. *Pediatr Clin North Am* 1990;6:1441–1465.

Guise TA, Mundy GR. Evaluation of hypocalcemia in children and adults. *J Clin Endocrinol Metab* 1995;5:1473–1478.

Authors: Adda Grimberg and Paulo F. Collett-Solberg

Hypoplastic Left Heart Syndrome

 Database

DEFINITION

Hypoplastic left heart syndrome (HLHS) is a collective term describing a group of cardiac malformations that share various degrees of hypoplasia of the structures of the left side of the heart (aorta, aortic valve, left ventricle, mitral valve, and left atrium).

PATHOPHYSIOLOGY

The etiology of HLHS appears multifactorial, most likely resulting from either an in utero reduction of left ventricular inflow or outflow. As a result, the right ventricle (RV) supplies both the pulmonary and the systemic (through the ductus arteriosus) circulations before and after birth. The reduction in pulmonary vascular resistance that occurs with lung expansion at birth reduces the proportion of RV output to the systemic circulation. If the ductus arteriosus closes, circulatory collapse may occur.

GENETICS

- Familial inheritance:

—Sibling recurrence risk (0.5%)
—Other forms of congenital heart disease (CHD) (13.5%)

- Male predominance (55%–70%)
- Definable genetic disorder (28%)

—Turner syndrome
—Noonan syndrome
—Smith-Lemli-Opitz syndrome
—Holt-Oram syndrome
—Trisomy 13, 18, 21, or other microdeletion syndromes
—Major extracardiac anomalies (diaphragmatic hernia, omphalocele, and hypospadias)

EPIDEMIOLOGY

- 0.16 to 0.36 per 1,000 live births
- Eight percent of CHD; third cause of critical CHD in the newborn
- Twenty-three percent of all neonatal mortality from CHD

COMPLICATIONS (NEONATAL PRESENTATION)

- Metabolic acidosis
- Necrotizing enterocolitis
- Multiorgan system failure (i.e., renal)

PROGNOSIS

- Fatal if untreated
- Ninety percent early survival after Stage I palliation if treated in a timely fashion at selected institutions
- Five percent mortality at hemi-Fontan (bidirectional cavopulmonary) procedure
- Ten percent to 12% mortality at Fontan operation (although significantly reduced in 1% in recent years with the addition of a fenestration to allow right-to-left shunting)

- Five-year actuarial survival:

—Seventy percent for staged palliation
—Seventy-five percent for transplantation

 Differential Diagnosis

- Neonatal sepsis (if suspicious for duct-dependent heart disease, start PGE$_1$)
- Other forms of duct-dependent CHD (critical aortic stenosis, coarctation, or interrupted aortic arch)
- Respiratory distress

 Data Gathering

HISTORY

- Respiratory distress (tachypnea, grunting, flaring, retractions)
- Cyanosis
- Cardiovascular collapse and profound metabolic acidosis when the duct closes

 Physical Examination

- Congestive heart failure (tachycardia, hepatomegaly, gallop)
- Normal S$_1$ and single S$_2$ (A$_2$ absent)

—A murmur of tricuspid regurgitation may be auscultated

- Varying degree of cyanosis
- Decreased perfusion and peripheral pulses

 Laboratory Aids

TESTS

- CXR: varying degree of cardiomegaly with increased pulmonary vascular markings (if atrial septum is intact, lungs will appear hazy with pulmonary venous obstructive pattern)
- ECG: right axis deviation (+90 to +210 degrees), RVH with qR pattern in right precordial leads, paucity of left ventricular forces with rS pattern in left precordial leads
- Echocardiogram: diagnostic procedure, demonstrating varying degrees of hypoplasia or atresia of the mitral valve, left ventricle, aortic valve, ascending aorta, and aortic arch; PDA with right-to-left shunt in systole and diastolic flow reversal; ± ASD with left-to-right flow
- Cardiac catheterization: no longer routinely performed; similar findings as with echocardiography

Therapy

MEDICAL

• The preoperative goal is to balance the systemic and pulmonary circulation provided by the right ventricle to a Qp/Qs (ratio of pulmonary to systemic blood flow) of about 1.
• Prostaglandin E1 infusion: 0.05 to 0.1 μg/kg/min
• Aggressive treatment of metabolic acidosis with fluid boluses, bicarbonate and/or THAM
• 21% FiO_2, with addition of 2% to 4% CO_2 to maintain $PaCO_2$ of 45 to 50 mmHg (thereby increasing pulmonary vascular resistance and improving systemic flow)
• Selective use of small amount of inotropic agents (in cases of sepsis or RV failure)
• Aggressive use of inotropic agents (α effect) may worsen systemic perfusion.

SURGICAL

• Palliative surgery is generally performed in three stages:

—Stage I (Norwood) palliation: performed in first few days of life; involves transection of main pulmonary artery and anastamosis of the augmented aortic arch to the pulmonary valve stump to form a neo-aortic valve and arch; placement of an aortic-to-pulmonary shunt (modified Blalock-Taussig shunt). The RV continues to provide both systemic and pulmonary blood flows.
—Hemi-Fontan procedure: involves anastamosis of the superior vena cava to the pulmonary artery, resulting in volume unloading of the RV. All prior shunts are usually removed.
—Modified-Fontan procedure: baffling the inferior vena cava to the pulmonary artery with placement of a small fenestration in the baffle, permitting a small residual right-to-left shunt

• There are many surgical modifications on these three procedures. In addition, these procedures may be performed at different ages based on an institution's experience. Our approach has been to perform the hemi-Fontan operation around 6 months of age and the Fontan operation near the age of 2 years.
• Orthotopic heart transplantation may be performed either as an initial approach or after a stage I palliation.

SUPPORTIVE

While surgical intervention has become a medical standard, some physicians still offer only supportive measures. This situation is especially true when multiple noncardiac congenital anomalies exist or when serious multiorgan system damage is present. The ultimate decision on the method of treatment must be a result of an open dialogue between parents, physicians, and other members of the care team.

 Follow-Up

Interval pediatric evaluations should include careful consideration of growth parameters, cardiovascular symptoms, and developmental milestones. Examinations should focus on the presence or absence of cyanosis, edema, effusions, and arrhythmia. Frequent echocardiograms and or cardiac catheterizations may be needed to assess:

• RV dysfunction
• AV valve regurgitation
• Aortic arch obstruction
• Branch pulmonary artery narrowing
• Collateral formation causing excessive cyanosis
• Protein-losing enteropathy
• Sinus node dysfunction
• Atrial arrhythmias

If the patient underwent heart transplantation rather than a Fontan operation, other lifelong issues need to be addressed, including:

• Graft rejection
• Infection
• Coronary vasculopathy
• Lymphoproliferative diseases

PITFALLS

During initial resuscitation and stabilization of a newly diagnosed infant:

• *Avoid using oxygen despite low pulse oximetry saturation.* Increasing FiO_2 will lower pulmonary vascular resistance and increase blood flow to the lungs, which are already "overcirculated," thereby worsening systemic perfusion.
• *Avoid overventilating the infant.* Carbon dioxide is a pulmonary vasoconstrictor and may improve systemic perfusion and cardiac output. Try to maintain normal or mildly elevated $PaCO_2$ levels.

 Common Questions and Answers

Q: What is the usual pulse oximetry reading for a child with HLHS?
A: Seventy-five percent to 85% after stage 1 palliation, 75% to 80% after a hemi-Fontan, and 92% to 95% after the Fontan.

Q: What is the usual medical therapy at various stages?
A: SBE prophylaxis at all times. Digoxin and furosemide are generally used until the hemi-Fontan. Afterload reduction (i.e., captopril) may reduce the workload. Antiplatelet (i.e., aspirin) and anticoagulant (i.e., coumadin) are used by some physicians.

ICD-9-CM 746.7

BIBLIOGRAPHY

Barber G. The hypoplastic left heart syndrome. In: Garson A, Bricker TJ, Fisher DJ, Neish SR, eds. *The science and practice of pediatric cardiology*, 2nd ed. Baltimore: Williams & Wilkins, 1998:1625–1645.

Bove EL. Current status of staged reconstruction for hypoplastic left heart syndrome. *Pediatr Cardiol* 1998;19(4):308–315.

Gentles TL, Mayer JE, Gauvreau K, et al. Fontan operation in five hundred consecutive patients: factors influencing early and late outcome. *J Thorac Cardiovasc Surg* 1997;114:376–391.

Razzouk AJ, Chinnock RE, Gundry SR, et al. Transplantation as a primary treatment for hypoplastic left heart syndrome: intermediate-term results. *Ann Thorac Surg* 1996;62(1):1–7.

Author: David M. Bush

Idiopathic Thrombocytopenia Purpura

Database

DEFINITION

Idiopathic thrombocytopenia purpura (ITP) is isolated thrombocytopenia secondary to increased destruction of platelets by circulating antiplatelet antibodies.

- Classified as *acute* when it resolves within 6 months and *chronic* if the platelet count is less than 150,000/mm³ in 6 months.

PATHOLOGY/PATHOPHYSIOLOGY

- The cause of antibody production is unknown, but it is hypothesized that antibodies generated in response to a foreign antigen or drug cross-react with the platelet membrane.
- The most frequently identified platelet antibody specificity against glycoprotein IIb/IIIa.
- Platelets are coated with antibodies, are recognized by macrophages in the spleen and other reticuloendothelial organs, and are destroyed.
- The bone marrow compensates for the platelet destruction by increasing production of platelets.

GENETICS

None described.

EPIDEMIOLOGY

- ITP is the most common acquired platelet disorder of childhood.
- Incidence is approximately 4 to 8 per 100,000 children under the age of 15 years.
- Males and females are equally affected in childhood ITP (M:F ratio is 1:3 in chronic ITP).
- The peak age for diagnosis is 2 to 5 years for acute ITP. Children younger than 1 year or older than 10 are more likely to develop chronic ITP.

COMPLICATIONS

- Intracranial hemorrhage (ICH) occurs in approximately 1 in 1,000 cases, and it is the primary cause of death in children with ITP.

—ICH occurs almost exclusively with platelet counts below 20,000/mm³ (and usually below 10,000/mm³) and may be spontaneous without preceding trauma.

—It is traditionally thought to occur more frequently early in the disease course, but recent reviews of the literature reveal that ICH can occur at any time.

- Major morbidity from hemorrhage at other sites (e.g., gastrointestinal, retinal) has been reported but is also very rare.

PROGNOSIS

- Excellent for those with acute ITP. Chronic ITP is more difficult to treat and therefore has an increased risk of bleeding complications.
- It is not possible to predict who will resolve acute ITP and who will persist with chronic ITP.
- A higher chance of chronic ITP is associated with underlying disease such as systemic lupus erythematosus, HIV, or Evan syndrome.

Differential Diagnosis

- *Thrombocytopenia from increased platelet destruction:* hemolytic uremic syndrome (HUS), thrombotic thrombocytopenic purpura (TTP), mechanical consumption from prostheses (cardiac valves or vascular grafts, catheters), DIC, sepsis, vasculitis, Kasabach-Merritt syndrome (vascular malformation with platelet consumption), hypersplenism, heparin-induced thrombocytopenia
- *Thrombocytopenia from decreased platelet production:* of bone marrow infiltration (leukemia, lymphoma, and other malignancies), drug-induced myelosuppression (e.g., chemotherapy), aplastic anemia, viral-induced suppression (e.g., EBV, HIV), type IIb von Willebrand disease, thrombocytopenia absent radii (TAR) syndrome, Fanconi anemia, Bernard-Soulier syndrome, Wiskott-Aldrich syndrome, May-Hegglin anomaly, inherited thrombocytopenia (X-linked or AD), certain metabolic and chromosomal disorders
- Clumping of platelets in the laboratory or giant platelets can artificially decrease a machine-generated platelet count. Review the smear to confirm.

Data Gathering

HISTORY

- Onset is acute in children, sometimes with overnight development of petechiae and purpura. Not associated with pallor, fatigue, weight loss, or persistent fevers.
- Half of cases are preceded by a viral infection 1 to 3 weeks before onset (particularly varicella; also EBV, CMV).
- Ask about unusual bruising, petechiae, and purpura, blood in the urine or stool, epistaxis, gum bleeding with tooth brushing, and any change in neurologic status.
- Recent immunizations, especially the MMR vaccine
- Drug history focusing on drugs with antiplatelet effects (e.g., ASA, seizure medications, heparin).
- Evidence of other autoimmune diseases (e.g., rheumatoid or collagen vascular symptoms, thyroid disease, hemolytic anemia).

- Family history is usually negative for bleeding disorders. Inquire about autoimmune disease in the family.

Special Questions

Risk factors for HIV should be elicited, because ITP-like thrombocytopenia may be a presentation of HIV in children.

Physical Examination

- Clusters of petechiae or large bruises readily apparent on skin.
- Purpura in the oropharynx and dried blood or clots in the nares.
- The physical examination should otherwise be normal.
- Consider other diagnoses if there is pallor, jaundice, adenopathy, bone pain, arthritis, or organomegaly (mild splenomegaly may occur in 5%–10%).
- A fundoscopic examination should be performed on all patients.

Laboratory Aids

TESTS

- Diagnosis based on isolated thrombocytopenia with no other laboratory or physical examination abnormality (other than bleeding)
- CBC shows thrombocytopenia with a normal WBC count and hemoglobin (mild anemia if there is ongoing bleeding).
- Peripheral blood smear should be reviewed to differentiate clumping of platelets from true thrombocytopenia. Few visible platelets are enlarged. Smear otherwise normal, with no red-cell fragmentation, no spherocytes, and no peripheral blasts.
- Platelet counts are frequently less than 20,000/mm³ (tend to be >30,000/mm³ in chronic ITP).
- PT and PTT are normal. Bleeding time would be prolonged, but testing is unnecessary.
- A direct antiglobulin test (DAT) to exclude coexisting autoimmune RBC hemolysis.
- ANA in a subset of patients, including older girls, patients with chronic ITP, and with suspicion of autoimmune disease.
- HIV testing if risk factors are identified
- Need for bone marrow aspirate is controversial. It is safe at low platelet count.

—Bone marrow test indicated if anemia, abnormal WBC count, leukemic blasts on peripheral smear, or organomegaly, jaundice, lymphadenopathy.

—Most hematologists do marrow aspirate before treating with corticosteroids.

- Marrow shows normal to increased numbers of megakaryocytes with otherwise normal morphology and cellularity.

• Assays for platelet-associated antibodies (either direct or indirect) are not established as clinically useful.

• Demonstration of platelet-associated IgG may be useful in more complicated patients in whom chronic ITP is a possible diagnosis.

Therapy

Which patients need treatment remains controversial. Guidelines put forth by the American Society of Hematology include:

—Any patient with a life-threatening bleed
—Any patient with a platelet count greater than 20,000/mm^3 and bleeding manifestations such as mucous membrane bleeding
—Any patient with a platelet count less than 10,000/mm^3

• Active toddlers or children at risk for trauma are usually treated.

• Medical treatment interferes with the antibody-mediated platelet clearance and raises platelet counts acutely, but does not alter the long-term course.

• Observation alone is acceptable for older children without serious bleeding and in whom adequate supervision and follow-up are assured.

• Avoid medications that affect platelet function, such as aspirin, ibuprofen, and cold medications with antihistamines.

• Precautions to prevent trauma: limited activity, helmet and pads around bed.

• Parental education should be for signs and symptoms of ICP.

CHOICE OF THERAPY FOR ACUTE ITP

• Corticosteroids: 80% respond with platelet counts over 20,000/mm^3 by 72 hours. Oral prednisone at 2 mg/kg/d tapered over 2 to 4 weeks is most common. Advantages: ease of dosing (oral, outpatient) and low cost. Side effects: moodiness, weight gain, more increased appetite. Disadvantage: many hematologists require a bone marrow aspirate before steroid therapy is begun to exclude leukemia. Prolonged steroid treatment has serious side effects.

• Intravenous immunoglobulin (IVIG): The usual dose is 1 g/kg/d IV and often repeated if slow or no response. Advantages: Faster time to platelet count over 20,000/mm^3 (24 hours); marrow aspirate may be deferred. Disadvantages: high cost, long infusion time of 6 to 8 hours, allergic reactions, aseptic meningitis with severe headache in 10%–30%, 50% to 75% have headache, nausea, vomiting, or fever. Premedicate with acetaminophen and diphenhydramine.

• Anti-D immunoglobulin (Win-Rho): coats RBCs with antibody to the Rh(D) antigen, which blocks the Fc receptors of the macrophages in the spleen; therefore can be used only in Rh(+) patients. Dose is 50 to 75 μg/kg IV over minutes. Anti-D is less expensive than IVIG but more costly than steroids. Lower rate of allergic side effects (10%) than IVIG and does not cause aseptic meningitis. Cause mild hemolysis with a transient hemoglobin decrease of 1 to 2 g/dL.

CHOICE OF THERAPY FOR CHRONIC ITP

• In general, children with chronic ITP have few bleeding manifestations, and observation alone is often justified.

—Splenectomy: Approximately 70% of patients will respond with complete remission. No presurgical predictors of response have been found. Disadvantages: surgical morbidity and risk of postsplenectomy sepsis with encapsulated organisms (management should include vaccination against *Haemophilus influenzae,* pneumococcus, and meningococcus, and lifelong prophylactic penicillin).
—Medical therapy: IVIG, corticosteroids, or anti-D immunoglobulin, immunosuppressives (azathioprine, cyclophosphamide, cyclosporine), vincristine, danazol, and monoclonal anti-Fc receptor have been used. Plasmapheresis and staphylococcal protein A adsorption for antibody removal have been used with limited success in refractory cases.

LIFE-THREATENING HEMORRHAGE

The goal is to stop bleeding. Transfused platelets are destroyed like native platelets but may help with hemostasis. IVIG may be given concomitantly. Multimodality therapy is frequently necessary during life-threatening hemorrhage. Emergent splenectomy is sometimes necessary. Plasmapheresis may also be beneficial.

Follow-Up

• Spontaneous recovery is the norm (60% by 3 months, 80% by 6 months, and 90% by 1 year). The incidence of significant bleeding-related morbidity and mortality is extremely low (<5%).

• Of patients with chronic ITP, 20% will ultimately have spontaneous resolution of their thrombocytopenia, as long as 10 to 20 years after diagnosis.

Common Questions and Answers

Q: Why aren't platelet transfusions used to increase the platelet count?
A: Transfused platelets are rapidly consumed and no increase in platelet count is observed.

Q: Will the ITP recur after another viral infection?
A: Only in a minority of patients.

Q: How should activities be limited until the platelet count returns to normal?
A: A common sense approach to activities for children with low platelet counts is to avoid any activity in which one foot is not on the ground at all times.

Q: How often should platelet counts be obtained?
A: Initially to follow the response to therapy. Thereafter, get counts during times of high risk of relapse (e.g., after steroid taper) and monthly until a normal platelet count is consistently seen. After resolution, platelet counts only for clinical suspicion of recurrent thrombocytopenia.

Q: Can IVIG or anti-D immunoglobulin be given repeatedly if the platelet count falls as the treatment wears off (4–5 weeks)?
A: Yes. Some patients with chronic ITP have been on monthly IVIG for years without problems. Steroids also may be resumed if there is a fall in the platelet count.

ICD-9-CM 287.3

BIBLIOGRAPHY

Albayrak D, Islek I, Kalayci AG, Gurses N. Acute immune thrombocytopenic purpura: a comparative study of very high oral doses of methylprednisolone and intravenously administered immune globulin. *J Pediatr* 1994;125(6): 1004–1007.

Bussel JB, et al. Recent advances in the treatment of idiopathic thrombocytopenic purpura. *Semin Hematol* 1998;35[Suppl 1]:1–64.

George JN, El-Harake MA, Raskob GE. Chronic idiopathic thrombocytopenic purpura. *N Engl J Med* 1994;331(18):1207–1211.

George JN, et al. Idiopathic thrombocytopenic purpura: a practice guideline developed by explicit methods for the American Society of Hematology. *Blood* 1996;88(1):3–40.

Medeiros D, Buchanan GR. Current controversies in the management of idiopathic thrombocytopenic purpura during childhood. *Pediatr Clin North Am* 1996;43(3):757–771.

Author: Susan R. Rheingold

Immune Deficiency

 Database

DEFINITION

• Immunodeficiencies can be either congenital or acquired.
• Immunodeficiencies often present as an increased susceptibility to infection as well as diarrhea, malabsorption, or failure to thrive; other manifestations can include unusual infections, including unexplained recurrent or chronic thrush.
• Consider immunodeficiencies if a child has two or more bacterial pneumonias per year, five or more episodes of otitis media per year or seven or more episodes in 2 years, recurrent or persistent sinusitis, or frequent, unusual, or unusually severe infections.

PATHOPHYSIOLOGY

• B-cell dysfunction: leads to antibody deficiency; poor opsonization of bacterial pathogens to allow for phagocytosis
• T-cell dysfunction: poor response to fungal and viral pathogens
• Complement deficiency: pyogenic infections due to poor opsonization and immune adherence of circulating white blood cells
• Granulocytopenia: poor phagocytosis of bacterial pathogens

GENETICS

• X-linked agammaglobulinemia: X-linked
• IgG subclass deficiency: autosomal recessive?
• Common variable immunodeficiency: autosomal recessive or dominant
• IgA deficiency: autosomal recessive or dominant
• Transient hypogammaglobulinemia of infancy: unknown
• Immunodeficiency with increased IgM: X-linked or autosomal recessive
• DiGeorge syndrome?
• Chronic mucocutaneous candidiasis: autosomal recessive
• Severe combined immunodeficiency: autosomal recessive or X-linked
• ADA or nucleoside phosphorylase deficiency: autosomal recessive
• Immunodeficiency with ataxia telangiectasia: autosomal recessive
• Wiskott-Aldrich syndrome: X-linked
• Natural killer-cell deficiency: unknown
• Chronic granulomatous disease: X-linked or autosomal recessive
• Hyper-IgE syndrome: autosomal dominant or unknown
• Complement deficiencies: autosomal recessive or dominant

COMPLICATIONS

• Severe invasive bacterial disease
• Recurrent respiratory tract infections
• Failure to thrive
• Unusual infection with unusual organism
• Chronic diarrhea
• Bronchiectasis, chronic or recurrent pneumonia, recurrent bronchitis

• Recurrent or resistant thrush
• Skin lesions: pyoderma or necrotic abscesses

PROGNOSIS

• X-linked agammaglobulinemia: survive to second or third decade
• IgG subclass deficiency: 50% with IgG2 or IgG4 resolve by 18 months to early childhood
• Common variable immunodeficiency: good prognosis; survive to adulthood
• IgA deficiency: earlier the onset of symptoms, guarded prognosis
• Transient hypogammaglobulinemia of infancy: self-limited with excellent prognosis
• DiGeorge syndrome: good prognosis
• Chronic mucocutaneous candidiasis: severe form: survive to third decade; mild form: survive normal lifespan
• Severe combined immunodeficiency: die by age 1 or 2 years without bone marrow transplantation
• ADA or nucleoside phosphorylase deficiency: die without bone marrow transplantation
• Ataxia telangiectasia: variable
• Wiskott-Aldrich syndrome: variable; may die from massive bleeding at a young age
• Chronic granulomatous disease: survival up to the second decade
• Hyper-IgE syndrome: may survive into adulthood
• Complement deficiencies: usually survive into adulthood

 Differential Diagnosis

CONGENITAL OR PRIMARY IMMUNODEFICIENCIES

• Antibody immunodeficiencies (B-cell–associated immunodeficiencies)

—X-linked agammaglobulinemia
—IgG subclass deficiency
—Common variable immunodeficiency
—IgA deficiency
—Transient hypogammaglobulinemia of infancy

• Cellular immunodeficiencies (T-cell–associated immunodeficiencies)

—DiGeorge syndrome: thymic aplasia or hypoplasia
—Chronic mucocutaneous candidiasis

• Combined cellular and antibody (B- and T-cell–associated immunodeficiencies)

—Severe combined immunodeficiency
—Adenosine deaminase (ADA) or nucleoside phosphorylase deficiency
—Ataxia telangiectasia
—Wiskott-Aldrich syndrome

• Natural killer-cell deficiency (adherent-cell lysis)
• Phagocytic dysfunction

—Chronic granulomatous disease
—Hyper-IgE syndrome

• Complement deficiencies

Brief Descriptions of Congenital or Primary Immunodeficiencies

• X-linked agammaglobulinemia: onset of symptoms after 6 months; infections by bacterial pathogens; respiratory system, skin, bone most commonly infected
• IgG subclass deficiency: infections with bacterial pathogens; IgG2 and IgG4 most common deficiencies in children; usually have normal or increased total IgG levels; may resolve spontaneously between 18 months and 6 years
• Common variable immunodeficiency: may appear in later childhood or adulthood; heterogeneous group of disorders
• with hypogammaglobulinemia

—B cells fail to mature into plasma cells.
—Recurrent and sinopulmonary disease is common.

• IgA deficiency: may be asymptomatic; pulmonary and GI infections are most common illnesses; difficult to establish prior to 2 years of age
• Transient hypogammaglobulinemia of infancy: occurs between 3 and 6 months of age; usually transient, although may last up to 8 years; repeated bacterial infections most common presentations
• Immunodeficiency with increased IgM: decreased IgG, IgE, IgA with increased IgM; symptoms begin in first or second year of life; recurrent bacterial infection

—May be seen as associated neutropenia

• DiGeorge syndrome: aplasia of the thymus and hypoparathyroidism, hypothyroidism, congenital heart disease, and abnormal facial features; often present with hypocalcemia
• Chronic mucocutaneous candidiasis: T-cell–deficient response to candida; 50% with endocrine abnormalities

—NLT cell response to other antigen

• Severe combined immunodeficiency: Illness begins in the first months of life; illnesses include pneumonia, sepsis, chronic diarrhea, failure to thrive, thrush *Pneumocystis carinii* pneumonia (common initial presentation and cause of pneumonia); at risk for viral and bacterial infection
• ADA deficiency: affects activity of both T- and B-cell function; associated chondro-osseus dysplasia
• Ataxia telangiectasia: progressive cerebellar ataxia; telangiectasis; sinopulmonary infections common; lymphopenia in some cases
• Wiscott-Aldrich syndrome: clinical picture of eczema, thrombocytopenia, and recurrent infections; poor antibody response to polysaccharide antigens and defective T-cell function; small platelets on peripheral blood smear; IgM low; IgG normal or slightly low; IgA and IgE elevated
• Natural killer-cell deficiency: recurrent infections, including severe herpesvirus infections; can be seen in Chediak-Higashi syndrome, leukocyte adhesion molecule deficiency, and X-linked lymphoproliferative syndrome
• Chronic granulomatous disease: granulomas in skin, lungs, and lymph nodes; impaired bac-

tericidal function of neutrophils; predisposes to infection with catalase-producing organisms; lymphadenopathy with purulent drainage and hepatosplenomegaly are common findings.
- Hyper-IgE syndrome: eczema with bacterial infections of the skin, lungs, middle ears, and sinuses; *Staphylococcus aureus* is a major cause of infection; absolute eosinophilia on peripheral smear is common.
- Complement deficiency: C2 is the most common deficiency; pyogenic infections are the most common problem; deficiencies of the terminal components of the cascade C5-C9 are associated with *Neisseria* infections.

SECONDARY IMMUNODEFICIENCIES
- HIV infection
- Malignancy
- Viral suppression
- Nephrotic syndrome

Brief Descriptions of Secondary Immunodeficiencies
- HIV infection: 18% to 20% of infants born to HIV-infected mothers will be infected; they are at risk for both viral and bacterial infections due to both B- and T-cell dysfunction.
- Malignancy: Granulocytopenia can lead to increased risk of bacterial infections.
- Viral suppression: Viral suppression of the neutrophils can occur following many viral infections; this usually does not lead to significant infections and resolves within 10 to 14 days.
- Nephrotic syndrome: increased risk of peritonitis

APPROACH TO THE PATIENT

General Goals
Screening tests should be directed to evaluate several arms of the immune system, including B-cell/antibody function, cell-mediated immunity, neutrophil/phagocytic dysfunction, and complement deficiency.

 ## Data Gathering

HISTORY
- Family history
- Number and duration of infections
- Recurrent pneumonias
- Chronic diarrhea
- Association of rashes, diarrhea, failure to thrive
- Neurologic problems
- HIV risk factors
- Endocrine disorders: hypothyroidism and hypoparathyroidism seen in DiGeorge syndrome

 ## Physical Examination

- Skin

—Telangiectasia as seen in ataxia telangiectasia

—Thrush (candidiasis) seen in T-cell deficiencies
—Eczema: seen in Wiskott-Aldrich, hyper-IgE syndromes
- Pulmonary

—Chronic lung disease seen in IgA deficiency, chronic granulomatous disease, hyper-IgE syndrome, and X-linked hypogammaglobulinemia
- Short stature

—Common presentation of immune deficiency

 ## Laboratory Aids

TESTS
- Complete blood count with differential
- Quantitative immunoglobulins
- Antibody responses to immunizations (must be certain that the child has been immunized)
- Anergy panel plus PPD: can include trichophyton, *Candida*, tetanus, mumps
- T cells: total and subsets
- Nitroblue tetrazolium test: will look at phagocytic function
- CH50: total hemolytic complement
- Complement levels: C2 to C6
- HIV ELISA and Western blot: If positive in children under 15 months of age, HIV infection should be confirmed with HIV PCR and HIV coculture.

 ## Therapy

In general, therapy should be under the guidance of a pediatric immunologist who is well trained in the treatment of these disorders.

BONE MARROW TRANSPLANTATION
- DiGeorge syndrome
- Severe combined immunodeficiency (SCID)
- SCID with ADA deficiency
- Wiskott-Aldrich syndrome
- Chronic granulomatous disease

THYMUS TRANSPLANTATION
- DiGeorge syndrome

GAMMA GLOBULIN REPLACEMENT
- X-linked agammaglobulinemia
- Immunodeficiency with elevated IgM
- Common variable immunodeficiency
- IgG subclass deficiency

PROPHYLACTIC ANTIBIOTICS/ ANTIFUNGALS
- IgG subclass deficiency
- Chronic mucocutaneous candidiasis
- Ataxia telangiectasia
- Hyper-IgE syndrome
- Complement deficiencies

Common Questions and Answers

Q: Do I have to worry about a previously well child who, on routine CBC, has neutropenia?
A: It is unlikely that a child who was previously well would have a significant immunodeficiency. The most likely diagnosis is viral suppression of the bone marrow. CBC should be repeated in approximately 2 weeks to confirm a normal neutrophil count.

Q: Does every child who has an episode of varicella-zoster need an immunologic work-up?
A: No. One isolated course of noncomplicated zoster does not require an immunologic evaluation. However, if more than one dermatome is involved or if the episodes are repeated, an immunologic evaluation is warranted.

Q: Should I be concerned about an immunodeficiency disorder in a 4-year-old child with thrush? How should such a child be evaluated?
A: There is no absolute age at which oral thrush is indicative of an underlying immunodeficiency. Obviously, one should look for predisposing factors such as antibiotic therapy or inhaled steroids as predisposing factors for oral thrush. Many authorities use 2 years as an age beyond which thrush should be evaluated. This evaluation should first include a culture from the plaque lesions to be certain that the condition is truly oral candidiasis. Immunologic work-up should include an HIV ELISA confirmed with a Western blot study when positive, T-cell subsets to include CD4 and CD8, and T-cell mitogen studies. Evaluation of these tests may require the assistance of a pediatric immunologist.

CLINICAL PEARLS

Immunodeficiency should be considered in any child with two or more bacterial pneumonias per year, five or more episodes of otitis media, chronic sinusitis or other pulmonary disease, or unusual or unusually severe infections.

BIBLIOGRAPHY

Gluckman E. Bone marrow transplantation in children with hereditary disorders. *Curr Opin Pediatr* 1996;8(1):42–44.

Hong R. Update on the immunodeficiency diseases. *Am J Dis Child* 1990;144:983–992.

Iseki M, Heiner DC. Immunodeficiency disorders. *Pediatr Rev* 1993;14(6):226–236.

Pacheco SE, Shearer WT. Laboratory aspects of immunology. *Pediatr Clin North Am* 1994;41(4):623–655.

Sorenson RU, Moore C. Immunology in the pediatrician's office. *Pediatr Clin North Am* 1994;41(4):691–714.

Author: Bret J. Rudy

Immunoglobulin A Deficiency

 Database

DEFINITION

Patients are considered IgA deficient if they have a serum IgA less than 5 mg/dL, a normal serum IgG and IgM, and they are older than 1 year.

PATHOPHYSIOLOGY

Increased incidence of the following:

- Atopy
- Sinopulmonary infections
- Gastrointestinal infections (especially *Giardia lamblia*)
- Crohn disease
- Ulcerative colitis
- Sprue
- Autoimmune illnesses

—Arthritis
—Lupus
—Immune endocrinopathies
—Autoimmune hematologic conditions

- Chronic active hepatitis

GENETICS

Most commonly autosomal dominant mode of inheritance with variable expressivity, but the following rare associations also occur:

- 18q syndrome
- Partial deletions in the long or short arm, and ring forms of chromosome 18
- Also associated with: HLA-A1, HLA-A2, B8, and Dw3.

EPIDEMIOLOGY

The prevalence is between 1 in 600 and 1 in 800 in a normal population.

COMPLICATIONS

Increased incidence of the following:

- Respiratory tract infections
- Gastrointestinal tract infections
- Atopy

PROGNOSIS

Survival into the seventh decade is common.

 Differential Diagnosis

- Toxic, environmental, drugs

—Penicillamine and anticonvulsants can induce IgA deficiency.

- Genetic/metabolic

—X-linked agammaglobulinemia (Bruton)
—Common variable immune deficiency
—Severe combined immune deficiency
—Ataxia telangiectasia
—DiGeorge syndrome
—Chronic mucocutaneous candidiasis
—Nezelof syndrome
—Selective IgG2 deficiency

- Miscellaneous

—Patients may be completely healthy and IgA deficiency may be an incidental finding.

- Common causes: may be the result of decreased synthesis or impaired differentiation of IgA B-lymphocytes into IgA plasma cells

 Data Gathering

HISTORY

Question: Does the patient have frequent sinopulmonary infections?
Significance: Patients with IgA deficiency can have frequent sinopulmonary infections.

Question: Does the patient have frequent gastrointestinal infections?
Significance: Patients with IgA deficiency can have frequent gastrointestinal infections.

Question: Does the patient have allergies?
Significance: Patients with IgA deficiency tend to be allergic.

Question: Does the patient have any autoimmune diseases?
Significance: Patients with IgA deficiency have an increased incidence of autoimmune diseases.

Question: Can healthy patients have IgA deficiency?
Significance: Approximately 30% of patients with IgA deficiency are completely healthy.

 Physical Examination

The physical examination should be geared to look for signs of recurrent infection and atopy.

Finding: Cobblestoning of the conjunctiva
Significance: Cobblestoning of the conjunctiva is caused by allergic inflammation in the eyes. Allergies are associated with IgA deficiency.

Finding: Allergic shiners
Significance: Allergic shiners are the result of allergies. Allergies are associated with IgA deficiency.

Finding: Serous otitis media
Significance: Serous otitis may be the result of recurrent ear infections. Increased ear infections can be seen in IgA deficiency. Furthermore, serous otitis media can be secondary to allergies, which is also associated with IgA deficiency.

Finding: Pain on palpation of the sinuses
Significance: Recurrent sinus infections are associated with IgA deficiency.

Finding: Pneumonia
Significance: An increased frequency of pneumonia is associated with IgA deficiency.

Finding: Swollen joints
Significance: An increased frequency of autoimmune diseases are associated with IgA deficiency.

Laboratory Aids

APPROACH TO THE PATIENT

General Goal

Decide whether the patient's complaints are consistent with IgA deficiency (frequent upper respiratory and gastrointestinal infections, or allergies).

- Measure serum IgA level.
- If the patient is IgA deficient, exclude other conditions associated with IgA deficiency.

Test: Serum IgA level
Significance: A patient is considered deficient if the serum IgA level is less than 5 mg/dL.

Test: Total immunoglobulins
Significance: If normal, this study would help rule out X-Linked agammaglobulinemia (Bruton), common variable immunodeficiency, and severe combined immunodeficiency.

Test: IgG subclasses
Significance: This study would help rule out an associated IgG2 subclass deficiency.

Test: Lymphocyte mitogens
Significance: This is a functional lymphocyte study. If normal, this study would help rule out common variable immunodeficiency, severe combined immunodeficiency, ataxia telangiectasia, DiGeorge syndrome, and Nezelof syndrome.

Test: Lymphocyte *Candida* antigen stimulation
Significance: No response to *Candida* in vivo is consistent with chronic mucocutaneous candidiasis.

Issues for Referral

Factors that may help alert you to make a referral include:

- Suggestion that IgA deficiency may be part of a more complex immune deficiency. An allergist/immunologist can assist with an appropriate immunologic evaluation.
- IgA deficiency associated with autoimmune disease. Evaluation and treatment by a rheumatologist would be indicated.
- Patient likely to need a blood transfusion. There is an increased incidence of anaphylaxis to IgA-containing blood products when administered to IgA-deficient patients. The allergist can help select appropriate blood products for these patients.

 ## Therapy

There is no specific drug therapy.

- Recurrent infections should be treated aggressively with broad-spectrum antibiotics.
- Antibiotic prophylaxis to prevent recurrent sinopulmonary infections is often indicated.
- Intravenous gamma globulin is not indicated.

CONFLICTS WITH OTHER TREATMENTS

Patients with IgA deficiency may develop antibodies against IgA in transfused blood products. These patients are at risk for anaphylactic (or anaphylactoid) transfusion reactions. To avoid these reactions, these patients may receive packed red blood cells (only if these cells have been washed three times), or they may receive plasma products from IgA deficient donors, or they may receive autologous banked blood.

 ## Follow-Up

Patients should be observed for:

- Sinopulmonary infections
- Gastrointestinal infections
- Autoimmune diseases
- Inflammatory bowel disease

NOTE: It is important to manage infectious complications aggressively, and to intervene promptly when the associated conditions present.

 ## Common Questions and Answers

Q: What is the recurrence risk for a couple with an affected child?
A: It depends on the mode of inheritance. Most commonly, the mode of inheritance is autosomal dominant and the risk would be 50%. However, the expressivity is variable and the patient's phenotype may not be that of an IgA-deficient person.

Q: Does the patient take any medications?
A: IgA deficiency can be induced by some anticonvulsants and by penicillamine.

Q: Should IgA patients wear medical alert bracelets?
A: Yes. These patients can have anaphylaxis if administered blood products containing IgA. In an emergency situation, this is important information for the caregivers to know.

BIBLIOGRAPHY

Burrows PD, Cooper MD. IgA deficiency. *Adv Immunol* 1997;65:245–276.

Middleton E, Reed CE, Ellis EF, Adkinson NF, Yunginger JW, Busse WW. *Allergy principles and practice,* 4th ed. Philadelphia: Mosby, 1993.

Rankin EC, Isenberg DA. IgA deficiency and SLE: prevalence in a clinic population and a review of the literature. *Lupus* 1997;6(4):390–394.

Sites DP, Terr AI, Parslow TG. *Basic and clinical immunology,* 8th ed. Englewood Cliffs, NJ: Prentice Hall, 1994.

Smith CA, Driscoll DA, Emanuel BS, McDonald-McGinn DM, Zackai EH, Sullivan KE. Increased prevalence of immunoglobulin A deficiency in patients with the chromosome 22q11.2 deletion syndrome (DiGeorge syndrome/velocardiofacial syndrome). *Clin Diagn Lab Immunol* 1998;5:415–417.

Author: Christopher A. Smith

Imperforate Anus

 Database

DEFINITION

Imperforate anus is a congenital abnormality whereby the bowel fails to perforate or only partially perforates the pelvic muscular floor and/or the epidermal covering.

CAUSES

- Not determined

PATHOLOGY

- The hindgut comes in contact with the cloacal membrane during the sixth week of fetal development. At this time, the hindgut is divided into a ventral urogenital and dorsal rectal component. By the eighth week, the dorsal half perforates to the exterior. In imperforate anus, the process is arrested during this critical period.
- There are many anatomic variants of imperforate anus. From the prognostic point of view, the most important is classification, distinguishing two main types: supralevator (high) and translevator (low). Separate is a group of cloacal malformations in which the urinary genital and digestive systems drain to a common channel that communicates with the perineum.
- A fistula communicating from the gut to the urogenital system or to the external opening is present in 90% of cases. In females, most commonly the fistula leads to the opening in the posterior fourchette of the vagina (in low lesions) or to the upper vagina (in high lesions). In males, the fistula leads to the raphe of the scrotum (in low lesions) or to the urethra (in high lesions).

GENETICS

- Imperforate anus can be an isolated defect or part of the syndrome or association.
- Syndromic disorders that contain imperforate anus are associated with defects on chromosomes 6, 7, 10, and 16.

EPIDEMIOLOGY

Incidence is estimated between 1 in 3,000 to 1 in 9,000. High lesions are more common in males (2:1). Low lesions occur with equal frequency in both sexes.

COMPLICATIONS

- Other anomalies are present in one-third of patients with an imperforated anus.
- Imperforate anus can be associated with vertebral and cardiac anomalies, tracheoesophageal fistula and, renal and limb anomalies (VACTERL association).
- Other anomalies associated with imperforate anus include intestinal atresia, malrotation, omphalocele, annular pancreas, urologic anomalies, spinal anomalies, duplicate uterus, septate vagina, vaginal atresia, and absence of rectal muscles.

PROGNOSIS

Continence can be attained in 90% if patients have low lesions. Less than 50% of patients with high lesions are continent before school age, but most of them continue to improve and achieve continence by adolescence.

 Differential Diagnosis

There are no disorders that can mimic imperforate anus. The task is to define the location of the termination of the bowel and the opening of the fistula.

 Data Gathering

HISTORY

- A majority of children are diagnosed in the first days of life by abnormal findings on physical examination.
- Failure to pass meconium, a history of constipation, and signs of low intestinal obstruction (abdominal distention and vomiting) should mandate reexamination of perianal area.

 Physical Examination

- Lesion presents as either no opening, an inadequate caliber of anus, or an anterior malposition of the opening.
- Physician should attempt to localize the opening of the fistula and look for associated anomalies.
- Evaluation for lumbosacral neurologic function should be done. Anal wink can usually be elicited, because a vertiginous external anal sphincter is present in a majority of the cases.

Laboratory Aids

TESTS

- Invertogram: After sufficient time for a transit of gas (>12 hours after birth), the child is placed in an upside-down position for 3 minutes, after which a lateral view of the pelvis is obtained.
- Lumbosacral films to evaluate for vertebral anomalies: An MRI of the spine should be considered to look for a tethered cord.
- Renal ultrasound, voiding cystoureterogram, and IVP can be used to evaluate for urinary tract anomalies.

 ## Therapy

- Surgery should be performed by an experienced surgeon.
- High lesions require an emergent diverting colostomy and pull-through procedure with a Pena midsagittal anorectoplasty at 3 to 9 months of age. The colostomy is closed after the anoplasty has healed and any necessary secondary dilations have been completed.
- Complications of surgery include stricture of the anocutaneous anastomosis, rectourinary fistula, mucosal prolapse, constipation, and incontinence.

 ## Common Questions and Answers

Q: Is this an isolated defect in my child?
A: Often, imperforate anus can be associated with multiple other anomalies and not necessarily isolated. Renal and vertebral anomalies must be excluded.

Q: What is the genetic basis for this defect?
A: Imperforate anus can be associated with chromosomal anomalies or can be an isolated problem.

BIBLIOGRAPHY

Bill AH, Hatch EI. Neonatal obstruction of the intestinal tract: patterns and management. In: Kelley VC, ed. *Practice of pediatrics.* Philadelphia: Harper & Row, 1987:27–32.

Javid PJ, Barnhart DC, Hirschl RB, Coran AG, Harmon CM. Immediate and long-term results of surgical management of low imperforate anus in girls. *J Pediatr Surg* 1998;33(2): 198–203.

Jona JZ. Advances in neonatal surgery. *Pediatr Clin North Am* 1998;45(3):605–617.

Raffensperger JG. *Swenson's pediatric surgery,* 4th ed. New York: Appleton-Century-Crofts, 1980:538–578.

Tempelton JN, O'Neill JA. Anorectal anomalies. In: Welsh KJ, Randolph JG, Ravitch MM, O'Neill JA, Rove MI, eds. *Pediatric surgery,* 4th ed. Chicago: Year Book, 1986:1022.

Author: Gregorz Telega

Impetigo

Database

DEFINITION

Impetigo is a superficial skin infection involving almost any part of the body. It occurs in two forms: bullous and nonbullous.

CAUSES

- Bullous: always *Staphylococcus aureus*
- Nonbullous: still predominantly *S. aureus*, but may also be group A β-hemolytic streptococcus and miscellaneous anaerobes
- Associated illnesses: varicella, tinea capitis/corporis, scabies, contact dermatitis, eczema
- Predisposing conditions: warm temperature, high humidity, prior antibiotic use (altering normal skin flora), and altered host immunity (e.g., IgA deficiency and defect in cellular immune system)
- Factors that expose fibronectin receptors in the skin, enhancing bacterial binding: underlying skin disease (atopic dermatitis, fungal skin infections), minor trauma (scratches, insect bites, burns)

PATHOPHYSIOLOGY

- Organisms colonize the skin surface and then invade superficially in areas of minor trauma (e.g., an insect bite). Bacteria are transferred from a colonized area (under the fingernails) to the another area (e.g., the nares).
- Microscopic findings: vesicle formation in the subcorneal or granular region with acantholytic cells, spongiosis, edema of the papillary dermis, infiltration of lymphocytes and neutrophils around the blood vessels (the nonbullous form will have little or no vesicle formation)

EPIDEMIOLOGY

- Most common in warm, humid areas
- Most common in warm, humid seasons
- Associated with socioeconomic disadvantage, especially crowding
- Most common bacterial skin infection in children; bacterial skin infections account for up to 17% of clinical visits.
- Rare under 2 years of age; most common between 2 and 7 years of age; seen in older groups more often as part of an epidemic

COMPLICATIONS

- Suppurative

—Cellulitis
—Lymphadenitis
—Osteomyelitis
—Pyogenic arthritis
—Pneumonia
—Sepsis

- Nonsuppurative

—Toxic shock syndrome
—Scarlet fever
—Acute poststreptococcal glomerulonephritis

PROGNOSIS

- Lesions left untreated resolve spontaneously in most cases.
- Treatment primarily prevents spread and speeds healing.
- Unless there is extension of infection beyond impetigo to cellulitis or abscess (uncommon), the infection is superficial and there is no scarring.

Differential Diagnosis

- Varicella
- Eczema herpetiformis
- Staph scalded-skin syndrome
- Tinea corporis
- Scabies
- Contact dermatitis
- Numnular eczema
- Linear IgA bullous dermatosis
- Burns (thermal and chemical)

Data Gathering

HISTORY

- Systemic symptoms are rare.
- Bullous impetigo develops in previously untraumatized skin.
- Nonbullous impetigo is frequently associated with predisposing mild trauma.

Physical Examination

- Bullous: transparent bullae that rupture easily, leaving a rim surrounding a shallow ulcer; normal surrounding skin; regional adenopathy rare
- Nonbullous: papule or vesicle progression to a honey-crusted plaque; erythema of surrounding skin; regional adenopathy common

Laboratory Aids

TESTS

- None needed in most cases: clinical diagnosis
- Gram stain and culture are indicated for recurrent or systemic illness; obtain needle aspirate from bulla or by "unroofing" crust and obtaining sample of the purulent material beneath. If positive, it may represent colonization rather than infection; it should be used to identify the organism, not to make a diagnosis.
- CBC: in the presence of systemic symptoms
- Blood culture: in the presence of systemic symptoms
- A skin biopsy may be indicated if diagnosis is in question

Therapy

SUPPORTIVE

Cleansing and debriding lesions is not necessary.

DRUGS

- Antibiotic resistance patterns in the community will guide choice of antibiotic.
- Most community-acquired cases *S. aureus* are not methicillin-resistant but may occur in households with IV drug users or in someone who works or lives in a nursing home.
- Many infections, even with organisms resistant in vitro, will still have a good clinical response.
- Topical treatment with mupirocin (Bactroban) three times per day for 7 days will not prevent nonsuppurative complications and is not appropriate when lesions are extensive, around the mouth, or there is propylene glycol hypersensitivity. Cream is preferred over the ointment unless there is so much crusting that the cream will not penetrate.
- Other topical antibacterials (bacitracin, polysporin) are *not* effective.
- Oral agents should be used when topical agents are contraindicated or when compliance with a topical agent is doubtful:

—First line: cephalexin 50 mg/kg/d in two divided doses or erythromycin ethylsuccinate 50 mg/kg/d in three to four divided doses for 7 to 10 days (compliance with cephalexin is better because of erythromycin gastrointestinal side effects)
—Second line: dicloxacillin 50 mg/kg/d (very effective, but unpalatable in liquid form), amoxicillin/clavulanic acid 40 mg/kg/d (very effective, with high cost and higher incidence of gastrointestinal side effects); clindamycin 15 mg/kg/d (very effective, but with greatest alteration of GI flora), azithromycin (very effective and fewer days [only 5 days] of dosing, but with higher cost), extended-spectrum cephalosporins (probably no more effective than first-generation, but at higher cost)

- Failed treatment: Add rifampin 20 mg/kg/d and use muciprocin in nose to decrease staph carriage

Follow-Up

- Nonbullous: If untreated, lesions progress slowly over several weeks and then heal spontaneously; occasionally ulcer forms, even when properly treated.
- Bullous: They usually rupture spontaneously (based on size and body location) and then heal over a period of several days to 1 week when properly treated.

SIGNS TO WATCH FOR

- Surrounding skin, for development of deeper infection with abscess or cellulitis
- Fever is unusual and should prompt investigation for deeper infection or another cause.
- Recurrence suggests an *S. aureus* carrier state or inadequate initial therapy.

PREVENTION

- Patient/school education (handwashing of paramount importance): very contagious; spread throughout household not unusual; easily spread via physical contact and fomites, especially on athletic teams
- Trim fingernails to prevent scratching; use gloves at night.
- Separate sleeping quarters and clothing until lesions resolved
- Treat underlying (predisposing) skin diseases and infestations.

PITFALLS

- Spread throughout a household is not uncommon, with children frequently reinfecting themselves and other family members. Children with underlying skin disease (e.g., eczema) are difficult to treat because of heavy bacterial skin colonization and mechanical trauma to skin associated with itching.
- When cultures reveal both staph and strep, there is no way to determine which is causing the infection; both must be treated empirically.

Common Questions and Answers

Q: How do you make a decision to treat topically or systemically?
A: Many factors influence this decision. It is impractical to treat a large number of lesions topically, and it is "overkill" to treat a few small lesions with a systemic course of antibiotics. Individual therapy should be tailored to the number and extent of lesions, caregivers' preference for type of therapy, and prior experience with infections in this patient.

Q: What should be done with a patient who continues to have impetigo despite repeated courses of antibiotics?
A: A search for a household source who is reinfecting the patient is probably most important. Culture with sensitivities should be performed to determine if treatment is adequate, but in most cases this is not the problem. Eliminating patient carriage of the organism (with rifampin and mupirocin) should be considered. Underlying skin diseases and irritants should be eliminated if possible. Other diagnoses should be entertained in the truly recalcitrant cases.

Q: Should the child be isolated from other family members and kept from school?
A: Until the lesions are treated, close contact of the child with other people should be discouraged through both sleeping and play.

Q: What is the difference between mupirocin cream and ointment?
A: The cream with a water base will be absorbed into the skin at a higher concentration in most cases and therefore be more effective. However, if there is significant crusting, the ointment with its oil base may penetrate better.

ICD-9-CM 684

BIBLIOGRAPHY

Bass JW, Chan DS, Creamer KM, et al. Comparison of oral cephalexin, topical mupirocin, and topical bacitracin for treatment of impetigo. *Pediatr Infect Dis J* 1997;16(7):708–710.

Dagan R. Impetigo in childhood: changing epidemiology and new treatments. *Pediatr Ann* 1993;22(4):235–240.

Sadick NS. Current aspects of bacterial infections of the skin. *Dermatol Clin* 1997; 15(2):341–349.

Scales JW, Fleischer AB, Krowchuk DP. Bullous impetigo. *Arch Pediatr Adolesc Med* 1997; 151(11):1168–1169.

Author: Jill A. Foster

Inappropriate Antidiuretic Hormone Secretion

 ## Database

DEFINITION

- Inappropriate antidiuretic hormone (ADH) or ADH-like peptide secretion in the presence of low serum sodium, low serum osmolality, and high urine osmolality, but in the absence of renal or adrenal pathology

CAUSES

- Idiopathic
- CNS pathology, causing increased secretion of ADH or ADH-like peptides: meningitis, head trauma, neurosurgical procedures, encephalitis, Guillain-Barré syndrome, brain tumor, brain abscess, hydrocephalus, hypoxia, subarachnoid hemorrhage, cerebral venous thrombosis
- Non-CNS tumor with independent secretion of ADH or ADH-like peptides: bronchogenic carcinoma, pancreatic carcinoma
- Pulmonary disease (leading to secondary elevation in ADH secretion or ADH-like peptides): tuberculosis, pneumonia, asthma, cystic fibrosis, positive-pressure ventilation
- Drugs (which mimic ADH or stimulate its release): vincristine, cyclophosphamide, carbamazepine, chlorpropamide, phenothiazines, clofibrate, nicotine, fluoxetine, sertraline

PATHOPHYSIOLOGY

- ADH is synthesized within neurons of the hypothalamus and stored in the posterior pituitary.
- ADH acts on the renal collecting ducts.
- Interaction of ADH with its receptors forms intracellular cyclic AMP (cAMP).
- cAMP increases water permeability through aquaporins (water channels) of the ducts and consequently reabsorption of free water.

The syndrome of inappropriate ADH (SIADH) results when elevated levels of ADH or ADH-like peptides cause free water retention and hypervolemia leading to hyponatremia. Three possible mechanisms include:

- Direct stimulation of the posterior pituitary (e.g., CNS disorders)
- Independent production of ADH or ADH-like substances from ectopic sources (e.g., oat-cell carcinoma, tuberculosis)
- Decreased venous return that stimulates atrial volume receptors and thereby leads to ADH release (e.g., pulmonary and intrathoracic diseases)

EPIDEMIOLOGY

SIADH can occur at any age. Its incidence depends on the various possible etiologies.

COMPLICATIONS

Severe hyponatremia can cause seizures and, rarely, brain damage. Correcting hyponatremia too quickly can lead to central pontine myelinolysis, which impairs vital functions such as breathing.

PROGNOSIS

- Based on the primary cause

 ## Differential Diagnosis

- Hyponatremic dehydration
- Congestive heart failure
- Adrenal insufficiency
- Cirrhosis
- Nephrotic syndrome
- Renal failure
- Severe potassium depletion
- Water intoxication
- Cerebral salt wasting (CSW): excess production or effects of atrial and/or brain natriuretic peptide hormones
- Hypothyroidism
- Reset hypothalamic osmostat
- Rocky Mountain spotted fever

 ## Data Gathering

HISTORY

- Unusual water intake
- Review of intake and output for inpatients
- Changes in urine output
- Anorexia, lethargy
- Weight gain or weight loss
- Renal disease
- Vomiting
- Diarrhea
- Use of diuretics
- Burns
- Heart disease
- Liver disease
- Brain injury: trauma, surgery, hypoxia, toxin

 ## Physical Examination

- No signs of dehydration
- Signs of fluid overload
- Lack of edema
- Due to hyponatremia, the patient may be lethargic or irritable with muscle cramps. In severe cases, patients may lose deep tendon reflexes, seize, or be comatose.

PITFALLS

- Failure to distinguish SIADH from various forms of salt wasting

PROCEDURE

A complete neurologic and physical examination must be performed. Classically, patients with SIADH manifest signs of hypervolemia but without increased urine output and without edema.

 ## Laboratory Aids

TESTS

Specific Tests

- Urinary osmolality and sodium with simultaneous serum osmolality, sodium, and uric acid
- Typically, serum sodium is less than 125 mEq/L, serum osmolality is less than 260 mOsm/L, and serum uric acid is less than 2.4 mg/dL, while simultaneous urinary osmolality is greater than 100 mOsm/L.
- Plasma ADH concentration: diagnostic but not helpful for rapid diagnosis

Nonspecific Tests

- Fractional renal excretion of sodium: Net sodium loss is normal or elevated.
- Urinary specific gravity

Imaging

- Head MRI if indicated

Home Testing

Timed urinary volume is helpful.

Therapy

The most important aspects of therapy for SIADH are diagnosis and treatment of the underlying cause.

DIET

- Fluid restriction

DRUGS

- For emergency use only: hypertonic saline (1.5%–3% NaCl).
- Diuretics should be avoided because they worsen hyponatremia.
- ADH antagonists: Available only through research trials now but expected to soon become standard of care
- Demeclocycline

DURATION

- Varies with different etiologies and between patients

POSSIBLE CONFLICTS

- Use of other medications that require a large volume for administration

 Follow-Up

WHEN TO EXPECT IMPROVEMENT

- Slowly, but usually during the first 48 to 72 hours

SIGNS TO WATCH FOR

- Changes in neurologic status

PREVENTION

Clinicians should have a high index of suspicion when administering certain medications, in order to serially monitor serum sodium and fluid status carefully.

 Common Questions and Answers

Q: Is the use of diuretics beneficial?
A: No. Although diuretics may relieve the effects of volume overloading, they also worsen hyponatremia. Overall, diuretics usually cause more detriment than benefit.

Q: What distinguishes SIADH from hyponatremic dehydration?
A: The history of dehydrated patients reveals excessive water loss (e.g., vomiting and diarrhea). Dehydrated patients are thirsty and have lost weight. Patients with SIADH have a history of underlying disease and weight gain. On physical examination, patients with dehydration have signs of hypovolemia in contrast to patients with SIADH who do not. Dehydrated patients have elevated blood urea nitrogen (BUN) and serum creatinine, whereas patients with SIADH have low BUN, creatinine, and albumin.

Q: What distinguishes SIADH from cerebral salt wasting (CSW)?
A: Salt wasters appear dehydrated due to decreased plasma volume, but SIADH patients do not. CSW is associated with very high urine output in contrast to SIADH, which has low urine output. Net sodium loss is very high in CSW, but SIADH has normal to slightly elevated net sodium loss. Distinguishing laboratory features of CSW include suppressed plasma aldosterone concentration, suppressed plasma ADH concentration, and normal serum uric acid concentration. Note that plasma ADH concentration is high in both SIADH and CSW.

Q: Why is it important to distinguish SIADH from CSW (and other causes of hyponatremic dehydration)?
A: Therapies differ dramatically for these conditions. Unlike the water restriction used to treat SIADH, treatment of dehydration, such as that seen in CSW, requires replacement of ongoing salt and water losses.

ICD-9-CM 253.6

BIBLIOGRAPHY

Deen PM, Knoers NV. Physiology and pathophysiology of the aquaporin-2 water channel. *Curr Opin Nephrol Hypertens* 1998;7(1):37–42.

Gross P, Wehrle R, Bussemaker E. Hyponatremia: pathophysiology, differential diagnosis and new aspects of treatment. *Clin Nephrol* 1996;46(4):273–276.

Kappy MS, Ganong CA. Cerebral salt wasting in children: the role of atrial natriuretic hormone. *Adv Pediatr* 1996;43:271–308.

Olson BR, Gumowski J, Rubino D, Oldfield EH. Pathophysiology of hyponatremia after transsphenoidal pituitary surgery. *J Neurosurg* 1997;87(4):499–507.

Soupart A, Decaux G. Therapeutic recommendations for management of severe hyponatremia: current concepts on pathogenesis and prevention of neurologic complications. *Clin Nephrol* 1996;46(3):149–169.

Authors: Robert J. Ferry, Jr. and Paulo F. Collett-Solberg

Increased Femoral Anteversion (A Cause of Intoeing)

 Database

DEFINITION

Increased femoral anteversion is an internal or medial torsion or twisting of the femur, which causes "intoeing." Lower extremity torsional problems can involve abnormal rotation of the tibia, femur, or both. In general, femoral version can be medial or internal ("ante," associated with intoeing), or lateral or external ("retro," associated with outtoeing).

CAUSES

- Heredity-family tendency
- Normal fetal development
- Intrauterine position
- Posturing (sitting position): cause or effect?
- Associated pathology (spasticity or DDH, for example)
- This condition does not, by itself, cause pain. If the child is in pain, look for another diagnosis.
- Function is usually good but may be associated with minor problems (i.e., intoeing with running).
- Increased femoral anteversion may be associated with other pathology, such as DDH, SCFE, or mild cerebral palsy.

GENETICS

There is no strong evidence to suggest that it is an inherited condition.

EPIDEMIOLOGY

Common: If "normal" is defined as being within 2 standard deviations of the mean, most children with intoeing (due to either internal tibial torsion or increased femoral anteversion) are "normal."

PROGNOSIS

- Usually excellent
- Most will correct or improve with no treatment.

 Differential Diagnosis

- DDH
- SCFE
- Mild cerebral palsy
- Fracture or osteotomy malunion
- Leg length discrepancy
- Internal tibial torsion
- Increased femoral anteversion may be associated with any of the other conditions.

 Data Gathering

HISTORY

- Intoeing is usually noticed by 2 to 3 years of age as the foot turning inward.
- Often, the family also complains of the child being clumsy, with awkward, slow running.
- Birth history (first-born common), pain, limping, family history, other "packaging" conditions (metatarsus adductus, torticollis), when first noticed, getting better or worse, functional limitations (i.e., trips and falls frequently)

 Physical Examination

- If ambulatory, watch the child walk and assess for foot-progression angle (the angle formed between the axis of the foot and the axis of forward progression of gait).
- Also assess other aspects of gait (stride, heel-toe gait, cadence, limping, other abnormalities).
- Unilateral or bilateral torsion
- Look for leg length discrepancy, hip abnormalities, contractures, spasticity.

THIGH–FOOT AXIS (TFA)

- With the child prone, the knee flexed to 90 degrees and the ankle at neutral, measure the difference between the axis of the foot and the axis of the femur.
- If the thigh–foot axis is internal, this suggests internal tibial torsion; if external, external tibial torsion.

TRANSMALLEOLAR AXIS

- With the child seated and the knee flexed to 90 degrees, assess the malleolar axis in reference to the coronal plane (less reliable than TFA).
- Look for abnormalities of the feet. Metatarsus adductus or clubfoot may be a primary cause of intoeing.
- Marked calcaneovagus may be a component of outtoeing.
- Do a careful neurologic examination to see if intoeing is related to a mild neurologic abnormality (such as mild spastic diplegic cerebral palsy).
- One can also evaluate by palpating the midpoint of the lateral greater trochanter and comparing this axis with that of the distal femoral condylar axis.
- This method is less reproducible.
- Look for increased Q-angle (angle formed by axis of pull of the quadriceps and the axis of the patellar tendon)

SPECIAL QUESTIONS

The normal torsional alignment (torsional profile) consists of the following:

- Foot-progression angle
- Medial hip rotation in extension
- Lateral hip rotation
- Thigh–foot angle
- Transmalleolar axis
- Configuration of the foot

PHYSICAL EXAMINATION TRICK

"Kissing patellae": This occurs when bilateral increased femoral anteversion causes the patellae to face one another, giving the appearance of "kissing patellae."

Increased Femoral Anteversion (A Cause of Intoeing)

 Laboratory Aids

TESTS

- Usually not helpful

Imaging

Imaging is usually not needed. Physical examination provides the information needed. If hip pathology (i.e., DDH) is suspected, then a hip x-ray may be indicated.

- X-ray: X-ray has been used, but in addition to not adding much, there are difficulties positioning the patient reproducibly, there is the factor of radiation exposure, and x-rays are not very reproducible. Complicated tables for analyzing data are available.
- CT: CT is an accurate way of measuring anteversion, but there is radiation exposure. The usual indication is the occasional patient who is being evaluated for surgery.
- Techniques for using MRI and ultrasound have also been described but, in general, are less accurate than CT.

 Therapy

- Observation and family and patient reassurance (almost always the treatment of choice)
- Devices such as casts, shoe wedges, twister cables, splints, and Denis Browne bars have no proven benefit (i.e., they will not change the natural history). They may in fact cause problems such as ligamentous damage to hip, knee, ankle, and foot.

GENERAL TREATMENT MODALITIES

- Observation (i.e., no treatment)

—Physical therapy will not change natural history, but it may help with associated patellofemoral malalignment pain.

—Devices (casts, shoe wedges, twister cables, splints, Denis Brown bars)

—Femoral osteotomy for increased femoral anteversion:
  —Very seldom needed
    —Greater than 45 degrees above normal
    —No lateral rotation of the hip
    —Major cosmetic problem with no improvement with growth

COMPLICATIONS

With surgery, there is always the creation of a surgical scar. Complications of surgery include malunion (bone may heal in the wrong position causing bowleg or knock-knee, for example), infection, second operation for hardware removal, and nonunion (while very unlikely, bone may not heal).

DRUGS

- Not helpful

 Follow-Up

WHEN TO EXPECT IMPROVEMENT

Anteversion usually decreases with age. One usually sees spontaneous correction by 8 years of age.

SIGNS TO WATCH FOR

There is no substantial evidence that increased femoral anteversion will cause arthritis of the hip or knee (chondromalacia patella).

PROGNOSIS

Overall, prognosis is good for the majority of patients.

 Common Questions and Answers

Q: How will a child with increased femoral anteversion likely sit on the floor?
A: These children often sit in a position called "w sitting," with the hips and knees flexed and the hips internally rotated such that the legs look like a "w."

Q: If a child has increased femoral anteversion but walks with the foot-progression angle close to normal, what compensatory situation likely exists?
A: The child likely also has compensatory external tibial torsion (i.e., an external rotation of the tibia that matches and in effect balances the internal rotation of the femur). This situation is sometimes a "setup" for patellofemoral subluxation and knee pain (increased Q-angle).

ICD-9-CM 755.63

BIBLIOGRAPHY

Halpern AA, Tanner J, Rinsky L. Does persistent fetal femoral anteversion contribute to osteoarthritis? *Clin Orthop* 1979;145:215.

Karol LA. Rotational deformities in the lower extremities. *Curr Opin Pediatr* 1997;9(1):77–80.

Staheli LT. Lower positional deformity in infants and children: a review. *J Pediatr Orthop* 1990;10:559.

Staheli, LT. Torsional deformities. *Pediatr Clin North Am* 1977;24:799.

Staheli LT, Corbett M, Wyss C, King H. Lower extremity rotational problems in children. Normal values to guide management. *J Bone Joint Surg* 1985;67A:39.

Tolo VT. The lower extremity. In: Morrissy RT, Weinstein SL, eds. *Lovell and Winter's pediatric orthopaedics,* 4th ed., 1996:1047–1075.

Author: John P. Dormans

Infantile Spasms

 Database

DEFINITION

Infantile spasms are myoclonic seizures, usually occurring in clusters, associated with a typical EEG pattern: high voltage, chaotic slowing, multifocal spikes, and marked asynchrony (known as hypsarrythmia). Flexor, extensor, mixed flexor/extensor, and arrest/akinetic fits occur. The combination of infantile spasms, hypsarrythmia, and mental retardation is known as West syndrome. Infantile spasms are classified as *symptomatic* if a specific etiology can be identified and *cryptogenic* if no underlying cause is found.

CAUSES

- Tuberous sclerosis (TS)
- Down syndrome
- Aicardi syndrome
- Metabolic disorders (congenital lactic acidoses, PKU)

Almost any cause of pre- or perinatal brain injury may lead to infantile spasms, including meningitis, hypoxic-ischemic injury, uremia, and congenital infection.

GENETICS

Families of probands have a higher incidence of epilepsy, suggesting multifactorial inheritance. Tuberous sclerosis may be sporadic or autosomal dominant.

EPIDEMIOLOGY

Incidence is 0.25 to 0.42 per 1,000 live births. Peak age of onset is 4 to 9 months; onset usually occurs before 1 year of age. Boys are more often affected than girls.

ASSOCIATED CONDITIONS

- Intrauterine infection
- Cerebral malformations
- Perinatal asphyxia
- Prenatal/perinatal stroke
- Lennox-Gastault syndrome
- Traumatic brain injury
- CNS infections
- Intraventricular hemorrhage
- Kernicterus
- Genetic conditions noted above
- Forty percent of infantile spasms are idiopathic

PROGNOSIS

Infantile spasms carry a poor developmental prognosis. Approximately 65% to 90% of patients are developmentally delayed at the time of initial diagnosis, and perhaps 10% of these children will achieve normal cognitive, physical, and educational development. Approximately 55% to 65% of children with infantile spasms go on to develop other seizure types, and 23% to 50% develop Lennox-Gastault syndrome. Prognosis is better in the cryptogenic group, with up to 40% having normal cognitive development and freedom from seizures on long-term follow-up.

 Differential Diagnosis

- Nonepileptic disorders: benign myoclonus, posturing related to gastroesophageal reflux, shuddering spells
- Myoclonic epilepsy of infancy

—Benign
—Severe myoclonic epilepsy (early infantile epileptic encephalopathy, or EIEE)

 Data Gathering

HISTORY

- Prenatal and perinatal history, including:

—Maternal age
—Pregnancy complications
—Perinatal difficulties

- Family history of TS or previous children with infantile spasms should be elicited.
- A detailed developmental history is needed to establish any preexisting developmental delay.
- A detailed description of spells may be useful in differentiating spasms from nonepileptic seizures, though these may be visually indistinguishable from infantile spasms.

 Physical Examination

- Check general growth parameters, specifically head circumference, because microcephaly suggests preexisting brain abnormality and a poorer prognosis.
- On general physical examination, look for dysmorphisms (Down stigmata, retinal defects as in Aicardi syndrome), suggesting genetic abnormalities, and hepatomegaly, suggesting inborn errors of metabolism or congenital infection.
- Careful skin examination, including a Wood lamp examination, should be performed for evidence of neurocutaneous disorders, specifically the hypopigmented macules associated with TS.
- On neurologic examination, particular attention should be given to level of alertness, attainment of age-appropriate developmental milestones, and motor tone.

 Laboratory Aids

TESTS

- Diagnosis depends on EEG: high voltage, chaotic slowing, multifocal spikes, marked asynchrony known as hypsarrhythmia.
- Routine blood studies should include electrolytes, calcium, and glucose but are generally unrevealing. Chromosomal analysis; metabolic screening, including blood lactate and pyruvate, serum amino acids, and urine organic acids; and TORCH titers may be helpful in identifying underlying etiology.
- If no cause is found, lumbar puncture to look for evidence of CNS infection or lactic acidosis
- Neuroimaging studies are most helpful test to determine etiology. MRI is preferred because of higher resolution for heterotopias and focal anatomic abnormalities; however, the intracranial calcifications associated with intrauterine infections and TS may be more apparent on CT.
- Infants with TS should undergo cardiologic evaluation, renal ultrasound, genetic consultation for genetic counseling, and evaluation of other family members.
- Infantile spasms can be an atypical presentation of pyridoxine-dependent seizures (see Therapy).

Therapy

DRUGS

Adrenocorticotropic hormone (ACTH) is generally considered the most effective therapy for infantile spasms. Treatment is generally initiated at 150 units/m^2/d IM for 1 to 2 weeks, and then gradually tapered over a period of 1 to 6 months. Side effects of ACTH therapy include cushingoid appearance, irritability, sleep disturbance, hyperglycemia, hypertension, electrolyte abnormalities, hypertrophic cardiomyopathy, immunosuppression, gastritis/GI bleeding, osteoporosis, and growth failure. ACTH therapy has not been proved to affect outcome in infants whose spasms are due to prenatal or perinatal brain abnormalities (symptomatic infantile spasms). Alternative therapies include topiramate (at dosages up to 20–60 mg/kg/day), clonazepam (0.1–0.15 mg/kg/d), phenobarbital (3–6 mg/kg/d), valproate (at dosages up to 100 mg/kg/d), or prednisone (2 mg/kg/d). Valproate is less frequently used as a primary agent because of the increased rate of fatal hepatotoxicity in this age group. A trial of high-dose pyridoxine (100 mg IV) should be given to all. Vigabatrin (100–150 mg/kg/day) is considered the initial treatment of choice, but is not yet available in the U.S.

 Follow-Up

Institution of ACTH therapy necessitates weekly follow-up to monitor blood pressure, glucose, electrolytes, BUN/creatinine, and signs of infection. Weight gain, cushingoid appearance, and irritability/insomnia associated with ACTH resolve as the medicine is tapered.

PITFALLS

• *Hypertension and hemorrhagic gastritis* occur in infants on ACTH therapy and must be anticipated by weekly follow-up visits.
• *Other seizure disorders* may supervene after infantile spasms have remitted and may require alternate anticonvulsant therapy.

 Common Questions and Answers

Q: Do infantile spasms ever remit spontaneously?
A: Spontaneous remission of infantile spasms has been reported but appears to be rare.

Q: What predictions can be made about prognosis of the child with idiopathic infantile spasms?
A: Periodic evaluation by a child neurologist or child developmentalist helps to detect delays in motor or cognitive development; neither the EEG nor any other laboratory test contributes prognostic information in cryptogenic infantile spasms.

ICD-9-CM 345.6

BIBLIOGRAPHY

Baram TZ, Mitchell WG, Tournay A, Snead OC, Hanson RA, Horton EJ. High-dose corticotropin (ACTH) versus prednisone for infantile spasms: a prospective, randomized, blinded study. *Pediatrics* 1996;97(3):375–379.

Chugani HT. Infantile spasms. *Curr Opin Neurol* 1995;8(2):139–144.

Kramer U, Sue WC, Mikati MA. Hypsarrhythmia: frequency of variant patterns and correlation with etiology and outcome. *Neurology* 1997;48(1):197–203.

Watanabe K. West syndrome: etiological and prognostic aspects. *Brain Dev* 1998;20(1):1–8

Author: Amy R. Brooks-Kayal

Influenza

Database

DEFINITION

Influenza is an acute febrile illness characterized by respiratory, gastrointestinal, and systemic symptoms. Due to its high global morbidity and mortality, as well as the difficulties in preventing the illness, it has been called "the last great uncontrolled plague of mankind."

CAUSES

Influenza is caused by the orthomyxoviruses influenza types A, B, and C. Influenza C virus has not been reported as a cause of influenza epidemics.

PATHOLOGY/PATHOPHYSIOLOGY

• The incubation period of influenza virus is approximately 2 to 3 days.
• Invasion of ciliated columnar epithelial cells by the influenza virus leads to necrosis of the ciliated epithelial lining of the upper and lower respiratory tracts, as well as a subsequent inflammatory response.
• Pneumonia is a result of direct invasion of the organism as well as secondary bacterial infection.

EPIDEMIOLOGY

• Although influenza affects persons of all ages, the highest morbidity and mortality occurs in infants and the elderly.
• Epidemics of influenza occur almost exclusively during winter months, peak approximately 2 weeks after the index case, and last 4 to 8 weeks. Up to 75% of schoolchildren in the epidemic region may be affected.
• Transmission of influenza virus occurs by aerosol droplets as well as by direct or indirect contact.

COMPLICATIONS

• Secondary bacterial infections (10% of children): bacterial pneumonia (pneumococcal or staphylococcal), otitis media, sinusitis
• *Primary progressive viral pneumonia:* pulmonary hemorrhage, high morbidity and mortality rates
• *Acute myositis* during convalescent period is most commonly associated with influenza B infection: rhabdomyolysis, myoglobinuria, elevated transaminase levels
• *Reye syndrome:* fatty degeneration of the liver and diffuse encephalopathy; more commonly associated with influenza B infection, although can occur after influenza A infection as well; association between aspirin use during acute illness
• *Febrile convulsions*
• *Drug toxicity:* Influenza infection may result in increased serum levels of certain medications that are metabolized by the liver (i.e., theophylline).

• *Rare sequelae* in severe cases of influenza infection include focal and diffuse myocarditis, diffuse cerebral edema, mediastinal lymph node necrosis, sudden death, and encephalitis.

ASSOCIATED ILLNESSES

• Pharyngitis
• Laryngotracheitis (croup)
• Bronchitis
• Bronchiolitis
• Pneumonia
• Gastroenteritis
• Conjunctivitis

Differential Diagnosis

INFECTION

• Viral infections, including but not limited to respiratory syncitial virus (RSV), parainfluenza, adenovirus
• *Streptococcus pyogenes* infection
• Bacterial sepsis in young infants

Data Gathering

• Infection with the influenza virus causes distinct clinical pictures based on the age of the affected individual.
• Infants and young children may suffer higher fevers and more severe respiratory symptoms.
• Many older children and adults infected with influenza are diagnosed with a "viral respiratory infection," without specific reference to the viral etiologic agent.
• The diagnosis of influenza infection is more commonly made in light of previously identified index cases or specific findings such as myositis.

HISTORY

• Abrupt onset of illness, beginning with dry cough, coryza
• Fever, headache, anorexia, malaise, myalgias, sore throat, irritability
• Respiratory complaints range from mild cough to severe respiratory distress (infants).
• Gastrointestinal complaints in younger children may include vomiting, diarrhea, and severe abdominal pain.

Physical Examination

• Cough is the predominant respiratory sign. Infants and small children may exhibit a "barky" cough (croup).
• Nasal congestion and conjunctival and pharyngeal infections are common.
• Cervical adenopathy is more common in children than in adults.

• Neonates may appear septic: apnea, circulatory collapse, petechiae.
• A generalized macular or maculopapular rash is sometimes observed.
• The myositis that accompanies the convalescent phase of influenza infection is commonly limited to or most severe in the gastrocnemius and soleus muscles. These patients may present with inability to walk or toe-walking.

SPECIAL QUESTIONS

• Patients considered to be at high risk for severe disease include those with asthma or other chronic pulmonary disease, hemodynamically significant cardiac disease, immunosuppressed children, and persons traveling to areas where an influenza outbreak is presently occurring.
• Patients considered at possible high risk for severe manifestations of influenza include those with HIV infection, sickle cell anemia, diabetes mellitus, chronic renal disease, or chronic metabolic disease.
• Patients considered likely to dangerously transmit influenza infection include hospital personnel, especially if there is contact with children or any high-risk patients; household contacts of high-risk patients, including those with HIV; and persons residing in dormitories or other institutional settings.
• Infection with the influenza virus may trigger exacerbations of asthma.

Laboratory Aids

TESTS

All specimens should include a throat swab and nasopharyngeal washing.

• Viral culture from nasopharyngeal secretions will be positive within 2 to 6 days.
• Rapid immunofluorescent tests utilizing monoclonal antibodies have variable sensitivity (70%–100%), but high specificity (100%). These are more reliable for influenza A. Polymerase chain reaction (PCR) assays are also available.
• Serologic evidence of infection involves comparison of acute and convalescent serum antibody titers (6 months). ELISA testing is now available for influenza.

IMAGING

• The chest radiographs in patients with lower airway involvement are indistinguishable from other viral lower respiratory infections.
• Chest radiographs may be normal despite significant respiratory involvement.

FALSE POSITIVES

The specificity of 100% for both the fluorescent antibody tests and culture ("gold standard") for influenza virus renders false-positive tests almost nonexistent.

Influenza

PITFALLS

- The leukocyte count in patients with influenza may be high, low, or normal.
- The differential count is too variable to be of help in diagnosis.
- Evaluation of arterial oxygenation by arterial blood gas analysis or, preferably, pulse oximetry may be required in severe cases of influenza infection. Occasional infants without roentgenographic evidence of lower respiratory tract infection have experienced apnea or rapid decrements in pulmonary function.

HOME TESTING

An ELISA kit is available for diagnosing influenza A in the office setting; however, sufficient data are not available at this time to comment upon the efficacy of this test.

REQUIREMENTS

- Diagnosis of severe viral disease
- Discovery of index cases of epidemics

 Therapy

- Most patients with influenza infection require supportive oral hydration, antipyresis, and routine decongestant therapy.
- Antitussive medications should be used cautiously, and should be appropriate to the age of the child.

IMMEDIATE

With the exception of the young infant, previously healthy children with influenza infection rarely require emergency treatment.

- Humidified air, with oxygen as needed, will be helpful to most patients with respiratory symptoms of influenza.
- Supplementary airway maneuvers, including endotracheal intubation, may be required for severe laryngotracheitis or patients with hypoxia that is unresponsive to high-flow oxygen administration.
- Hypovolemic and distributive causes of poor peripheral circulation respond well to intravascular volume repletion.

DRUGS

- Chemotherapy against influenza is recommended for patients with severe disease or children at high risk of severe illness or complications (see Special Questions).
- Amantadine hydrochloride (<9 yrs or <40 kg: 5 mg/kg/day in 1–2 divided doses; >40 kg: 200 mg/day in 1–2 divided doses) has in vitro activity against influenza A. The few pediatric studies available show some efficacy in reducing the severity of symptoms if amantadine is administered within 48 hours of symptom onset. Rimantidine, a synthetic analog of amantidine, is approved for prophylactic use only (see Prevention). Neither medication is approved for use in infants less than 1 year of age or for influenza B infection.

- Ribavirin has been used successfully as an aerosol medication in the treatment of both influenza A and influenza B; however, it is not currently approved for treatment of influenza in children.

DURATION

Therapy should be given until clinical improvement is apparent, usually between 2 and 7 days.

POSSIBLE CONFLICTS

- Amantidine dose should be reduced in patients with renal insufficiency. The side effects of amantidine include insomnia, lightheadedness, and difficulty concentrating.
- Patients with epilepsy have a higher risk of seizure activity when receiving amantidine.

PREVENTION

Vaccination

- It is necessary to provide annual vaccination to high-risk individuals and persons likely to transmit influenza infection to high-risk individuals. These groups are delineated in the list of patients under Special Questions.
- Children who are receiving chronic aspirin therapy should be considered for vaccination because of the associations between aspirin use, influenza infection, and Reye syndrome.

Chemoprophylaxis

- Prophylactic administration of amantidine is recommended for certain subgroups of patients:

—High-risk children who are exposed to influenza A infection less than 2 weeks after influenza vaccination was given (see Special Questions)
—Immunocompromised patients (poor response to vaccine)
—High-risk patients who cannot receive the vaccine (anaphylactic reaction to chicken or eggs)
—Control of outbreaks in institutions housing high-risk persons

- The dose of amantidine for prophylaxis is the same as the treatment dose. For children over 20 kg, 100 mg/d is also acceptable.

 Follow-Up

WHEN TO EXPECT IMPROVEMENT

- Fever associated with influenza infection usually lasts up to 5 days. Recrudescence of fever does not necessarily signify the onset of a secondary bacterial infection.
- Cough may last up to 2 weeks.
- Lethargy or malaise may persist for up to 2 weeks.
- Influenza A infection usually lasts longer than influenza B or influenza C infections.

SIGNS TO WATCH FOR

- Clinical signs of secondary bacterial infection (see Complications)
- Deteriorating mental status or respiratory status after initial improvement
- Myoglobinuria in the face of muscle pain

PITFALLS

The patient presenting with benign acute viral myositis might have an elevated creatinine phosphokinase (CPK). However, the presence of myoglobinuria might suggest acute viral rhabdomyolysis, which can be more damaging to the kidney. These patients should be hospitalized and monitored for adequate hydration.

 Common Questions and Answers

Q: When is it safe for a child with influenza to return to daycare or school?
A: Older children with influenza may shed the virus in nasal secretions for up to 7 days from onset of symptoms, and younger children even longer. Therefore, older children with influenza may return to school 1 week after the onset of symptoms, and infants and toddlers should remain home for 10 to 14 days.

Q: Can a child on chronic steroid therapy be immunized against influenza?
A: In general, children who require maintenance steroid therapy for their underlying illness should still receive influenza immunization. If possible, immunize while the child is on the lowest possible dose of steroids and not during a period of high-dose therapy.

Q: What are the chances of acquiring influenza despite annual vaccination?
A: Vaccination against influenza is greater than 70% effective in preventing disease and greater than 90% effective in preventing death from the infection.

ICD-9-CM 487.1

BIBLIOGRAPHY

American Academy of Pediatrics. *Influenza. Red book: report of the Committee on Infectious Diseases.* Washington, DC: American Academy of Pediatrics, 1997:307–315.

Feiste JE, Mitchell JM, Sullivan DB. After the flu: acute viral myositis. *Contemp Pediatr* 1995;(12):29–51.

Gruber WC. Influenza viruses. In Long SS, Pickering LK, Prober CG, eds. *Principles and practice of pediatric infectious diseases.* New York: Churchill Livingstone, 1997, 1267–1274.

Piedra PA. Influenza virus pneumonia: pathogenesis, treatment, and prevention. *Semin Respir Infect* 1995;10:216–223.

Prevention and control of influenza: recommendations of the Immunization Practices Advisory Committee (ACIP). *MMWR* 1991;41(RR-9):1–17.

Author: Joel A. Fein

Inguinal Hernia

 Database

DEFINITION

Hernia is a protrusion of an organ outside the compartment of the anatomic location. *Inguinal hernia* is a protrusion of a portion of the abdominal content in the area on the inguinal canal.

CAUSES

The processus vaginalis is the out-pouching of the peritoneum entering the inguinal canal during testicular migration into the scrotum. The processus vaginalis is normally obliterated after the birth but in some people remains a potential space for herniation. Local weakness of muscles and ligaments in the inguinal area and increased intraabdominal pressure predispose to this hernia.

PATHOLOGY

• The herniated contents are lined by a pouch of peritoneum and accompany the spermatic cord blood vessels and nerves in the canal.
• In girls, there may be an ovary in the hernia sac.

EPIDEMIOLOGY

Inguinal hernias are present in 1% to 3% of children; 90% of inguinal hernias are present in males. Predisposing factors:

• Prematurity
• Ascites
• Chronic lung disease
• Congenital anomalies of the pelvis and perineum
• Ehlers-Danlos syndrome

COMPLICATIONS

• Intestinal obstruction
• Incarceration
• Testicular infarction
• Bowel ischemia
• Skin ulceration
• Cryptorchidism (association)

 Differential Diagnosis

• Seminoma, teratoma, and other testicular tumors
• Scrotal trauma
• Hydrocele
• Undescended testis
• Lymphadenopathy

 Data Gathering

HISTORY

Question: Where is the location of the bulge?
Significance: Hernia presents as a swelling in the inguinal region. Hernia descending to the scrotum or labial area is known as *complete*. Hernia not entering the scrotum (labia) is known as *incomplete*.

Question: What makes the bulge larger?
Significance: The hernia can increase in size with maneuvers increasing intraabdominal pressure (coughing, crying, voiding, defecation).

Question: Is there any pain?
Significance: Uncomplicated hernias usually do not cause pain. Presence of inguinal pain in the absence of incarcerated hernia should raise the suspicion of hip disease.

Question: Are there signs of obstruction?
Significance: Question symptoms of obstruction (emesis, abdominal distention), bowel ischemia (pain, emesis, abdominal distention, fever, irritability, lethargy), reducibility, and traumatic attempts to reduce.

Physical Examination

• Ensure an empty bladder.
• Older children should be in a standing position for the examination. Ensure that your hands are warm.
• If the hernia is not present at the time of examination, maneuvers increasing intraabdominal pressure can reveal suspected hernia (Valsalva maneuver, coughing, crying, voiding, defecation).
• Translumination is achieved by shining light behind the scrotum anteriorly. Hernias as opposed to hydrocele generally do not transluminate.
• Always consider testicular torsion, epididymitis, orchitis, and trauma when examinations reveal a tender mass in the scrotum.
• Try to reduce the hernia with the child in the supine or head-down position so that gravity assists the maneuver. Use a pacifier to calm the infant. Do not force a difficult incarcerated hernia.

 Therapy

• Herniorrhaphy is the definitive treatment. Ten percent of patients will return with contralateral hernia after a unilateral repair. Surgical exploration of the contralateral inguinal canal in patients with unilateral hernia is controversial.
• The underlying cause should be addressed when present (ascites, Ehlers-Danlos syndrome).

PITFALLS

• *Richter hernia:* herniation of only part of the bowel wall, resulting in bowel ischemia without bowel obstruction; rare occurrence
• Failure to consider possibility of ovary in inguinal hernia in girls

 Common Questions and Answers

Q: Is surgery of great urgency in childhood?
A: Irreducible incarceration is common in infants less than 1 year of age, and surgery is recommended early. Surgery for uncomplicated hernia can be postponed in the premature infant or when other medical conditions need to be treated prior to surgery. An irreducible hernia requires urgent surgery.

Q: What are concerns regarding inguinal hernias in girls?
A: Of all inguinal hernias, only 10% are present in girls. The ovary is the most common organ to herniate. Detection is more difficult than in boys and is commonly mistaken for lymphadenopathy. One percent of phenotypic females with inguinal hernia have testicular feminization syndrome with a testicle present in the inguinal canal.

Author: Gregorz Telega

Insect Sting Reactions

 Database

DEFINITION

The hypersensitivity reaction that results from the sting of an insect belonging to the Hymenoptera order, including the honeybee, bumblebee, yellow jacket, hornet, and wasp

PATHOLOGY

Hypersensitivity is IgE mediated and directed against antigenic components of insect venom, including phospholipase and hyaluronidase, in addition to others.

EPIDEMIOLOGY

Incidence of insect sting allergy in the general population is 0.4% to 3.0%. Twenty-five to 40 deaths occur yearly in the United States due to insect sting anaphylaxis.

COMPLICATIONS

Reactions can span the spectrum from local to anaphylaxis and death.

PROGNOSIS

The natural history is that re-stings carry a 60% chance of producing a reaction similar to the first allegic response. There are some patients with self-limiting disease, but the majority will require immunotherapy for a cure.

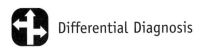 Differential Diagnosis

- Allergic mediated reaction
- Toxic reaction
- Vasovagal reflex
- Histrionic

 Data Gathering

HISTORY

Classification of Reactions

- Normal: transient pain, swelling, and erythema at sting site, which subsides within 1 hour
- Local: more extensive swelling that extends from sting site to adjacent tissue (i.e., sting on hand extending to elbow) that may peak 24 to 48 hours after sting
- Anaphylactic or systemic reaction, usually involving more than one organ system: urticaria, angioedema, bronchospasm, laryngospasm, hypotension, and shock
- Unusual: encephalitis, Guillain-Barré syndrome, serum sickness

Identification of Insect

- The honeybee is usually the only insect that leaves a stinger.
- Yellow jackets build nests in the ground.
- Hornets build large nests in trees or under branches.
- Wasp nests have a paper–honeycomb appearance and are located under eaves and roofs.

Candidates for Allergy Testing

- Children with preexisting asthma, especially poorly controlled asthmatics, are at increased risk for anaphylactic reactions.
- Re-stings usually result in a similar severity of symptoms the as initial sting reaction; therefore, testing and the use of immunotherapy are only considered in people with anaphylactic reactions.

—Multiple stings at one time may increase or broaden sensitivities.

—Children over 16 years of age with only a dermal reaction (i.e., urticaria and angioedema) are not candidates for testing because of their low risk of a worse reaction on subsequent sting.

 Laboratory Aids

TESTS

The diagnosis of insect sting allergy is made on the basis of history and the presence of specific IgE antibody detected by skin testing or RAST.

- Skin testing: gold standard; uses the six available insect venoms: honeybee, bumblebee, white-faced hornet, bald-faced hornet, yellow jacket, and wasp; need to defer skin testing 2 to 3 weeks after an anaphylactic event to avoid false negatives secondary to a refractory period. In predicting an IgE-mediated event: sensitivity 99%; specificity 80%
- RAST: radioallergosorbent test, an in vitro test that measures allergen-specific serum IgE; less sensitive and more expensive than skin testing

Insect Sting Reactions

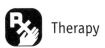 Therapy

MANAGEMENT OF ACUTE REACTIONS

• Systemic reactions: same as for anaphylaxis—SQ epinephrine (1:1000) 0.01 mL/kg up to 0.3 mL; Benadryl 1 mg/kg IV q6h; Zantac 1 mg/kg IV q6h; fluid bolus to support circulation
• Local reaction: cleansing and antibiotics if superinfection present
• Benadryl to relieve pruritus
• Topical corticosteroid to relieve local inflammation

VENOM IMMUNOTHERAPY

Candidacy is based on history, skin testing, and patient compliance. Many studies have shown 98% to 99% effectiveness in preventing systemic reactions in sting-sensitive patients. It entails a build-up phase of weekly shots for approximately 2 to 3 months and then eventually a monthly maintenance shot for 3 to 5 years. *NOTE:* For those patients with more severe reactions, such as those with cardiovascular compromise, venom immunotherapy may be continued indefinitely.

 Follow-Up

PREVENTION

• Patients with systemic reactions should carry an emergency kit for anaphylaxis:

—Epipen Sr: greater than 30 kg (0.30 mL of SQ EPI)
—Epipen Jr: less than 30 kg (0.1 mL of SQ EPI)

• Identification tag (i.e., bracelet, necklace, keychain) for patient at risk of anaphylaxis in the field

PATIENT EDUCATION

Knowledge of stinging insect habitats and their attraction by bright colors, fragrances, and sweets can help to prevent exposure to future stings. Keep in mind that things such as cotton candy, open soda cans, and flowers can attract stinging insects.

 Common Questions and Answers

Q: How many shots are involved with skin testing?
A: Between 18 and 36, depending when and if sensitivity is noted.

Q: How many Epipens should a child have?
A: It depends on with whom the child will spend time outdoors (i.e., during school recess, with school nurse, at home, at grandparents, etc.).

Q: Does the child's activity need to be restricted?
A: The child should not be in an environment that may put him or her at increased risk of bee sting without an adult supervising who has access to an Epipen.

ICD-9-CM 919.4

BIBLIOGRAPHY

Lawlor GJ, Fischer TJ, Adelman DC. Insect allergy. In: *Manual of allergy and immunology,* 3ed. Philadelphia: Lippincott Williams & Wilkens, 1995.

Li JT. Management of insect sting hypersensitivity. *Mayo Clin Proc* 1992;67:188–194.

Valentine MD, Schuberth KC, Kagey-Sobotka A, et al. The value of immunotherapy in children with allergy to insect stings. *N Engl J Med* 1990;323(23):1601–1603.

Author: Michelle M. Klinek

Intestinal Obstruction

 Database

DEFINITION

Intestinal obstruction is pathologic blockage of aboral progression of intestinal contents, which can be secondary to mechanical or paralytic etiologies.

CAUSES

Of the various etiologies that have been cited as acquired causes of intestinal obstruction, authors cite the following in decreasing order of prevalence:

- Pyloric stenosis, 25%
- Intussusception, 18%
- Atresia of the intestine, 15%
- Imperforate anus, 11%
- Hirschsprung disease, 6%
- Postoperative adhesions, 5%
- Meconium ileus, plug, 5%
- Malrotation, 5%
- Annular pancreas, 3%
- Meckel diverticulum, 3%

Generally, etiologies can be classified as:

- Intraluminal: polyp, mass, bezoar, foreign body, parasites, and tumor
- Intramural: stricture, tumor, hematoma
- Extrinsic: postoperative adhesions, adhesions from peritonitis, hernia, volvulus, and tumor

Paralytic Ileus

Caused by a failure of intestinal motor function resulting from drugs, i.e., vincristine, hypokalemia, systemic sepsis, uremia, myxedema, and diabetic ketoacidosis. Usually self-limiting and acute, characterized by an absence of bowel sounds and air throughout the intestine. Conservative therapy usually resolves the latter. *Chronic intestinal pseudo-obstruction,* a syndrome of altered intestinal and colonic motility of undefined etiology

PATHOPHYSIOLOGY

Mechanical

Mechanical obstructions can be either simple or strangulating and may be caused by congenital or acquired diseases. The latter impair intestinal blood flow and may cause intestinal necrosis, resulting in higher morbidity and mortality than caused by simple obstructions.

GENETICS

- No genetic predisposition to intestinal obstruction in general cases

EPIDEMIOLOGY

- The different causes of intestinal obstruction have their own identified epidemiologic patterns: small bowel obstruction secondary to *Ascaris lumbricoides* in Calcutta, India; colonic volvulus secondary to aerophagia and constipation in mentally retarded children; or meconium ileus equivalent in children with cystic fibrosis.
- Down syndrome with a higher prevalence of duodenal atresia

COMPLICATIONS

Perforation and peritonitis as secondary phenomena are classically the most common complications of intestinal obstruction if not corrected in the initial stages.

PROGNOSIS

- Excellent in cases of simple intestinal obstruction without strangulation

 Differential Diagnosis

Intestinal obstruction is a final common pathway for multiple etiologies, including those that lead to simple or strangulated obstruction.

- Metabolic: meconium ileus, electrolyte disturbance
- Congenital: esophageal atresia, intestinal atresia, duplication of bowel, malrotation, diaphragmatic hernia, Hirschsprung disease, imperforate anus, annular pancreas, pyloric stenosis
- Miscellaneous: adhesive bands, intussusception, meconium plug, volvulus, postoperative adhesions

 Data Gathering

HISTORY

- Pain is one of the cardinal manifestations of intestinal obstruction, resulting from distention of the intestine, producing visceral pain that is poorly localized, with nausea and vomiting.
- Pain that is well localized and associated with tenderness and rigidity results from peritonitis.
- A history of bilious emesis and feculent characteristics confirm obstruction.
- Passage of bloody stool and mucus may suggest strangulation.
- Elicit any family history of cystic fibrosis, polyps, and previous abdominal surgery, as well as recent weight loss or spinal surgery.

 Physical Examination

- Palpation may reveal the presence of hernia, a mass suggestive of feces or intussusception, and tenderness or rigidity.
- Presence of scoliosis or kyphosis should be recognized.
- Rectal examination will reveal, at times, a palpable polyp or intussusceptum.

Laboratory Aids

TESTS

Laboratory Tests

• Electrolyte balance, including sodium, chloride, bicarbonate, and potassium, are necessary for assessment of hydration and third spacing of fluids.
• No particular laboratory test will confirm the diagnosis, other than imaging techniques, as described below.

Imaging

• Plain abdominal radiographs in the supine and erect views will identify the classical features of a gasless abdomen, with air-fluid levels and distended loops of intestine.
• Paralytic ileus may present with dilation of the small and large intestines.
• Ultrasonography has been used to identify a mass (i.e., perforated appendix) as the cause of the obstruction.
• In isolated cases, contrast examinations may be helpful in making a diagnosis (e.g., barium enema to confirm intussusception or Hirschsprung disease, and upper GI series to exclude malrotation or volvulus).

 Therapy

MANAGEMENT

• Initial stages:

—Hold oral intake.
—Decompress the stomach with a nasogastric tube.
—Hydration IV and correct electrolyte imbalance
—Identify etiology of obstruction and establish definitive repair.

• Surgical:

—In cases of strangulation, immediate surgical options may be needed in cases of perforation and peritonitis. In isolated cases of distal obstruction secondary to intussusception, surgery is avoided with the institution of hydrostatic or air reduction of the mass effect.

 Common Questions and Answers

Q: Will my child need surgery for this problem?
A: Most likely; surgical treatment is necessary to correct the cause of intestinal obstruction except in a few cases, such as intussusception, pseudo-obstruction, and paralytic ileus.

Q: What is the most common cause of this problem in my 3-day-old son?
A: In an infant, the most common causes are atresias, which are absences of the normal amount of intestine in the abdomen. Other causes are defects in the large intestine, such as Hirschsprung disease.

ICD-9-CM 560.9

BIBLIOGRAPHY

Madonna MB, Boswell WC, Arensman RM. Acute abdomen. *Semin Pediatr Surg* 1997;6(2): 105–111.

Villamizar E, Mendez M, Bonilla E, Varon H, de Onatra S. Ascaris lumbricoides infestation as a cause of intestinal obstruction in children: experience with 87 cases. *J Pediatr Surg* 1996;31(1):201–206.

Wesson D. Acute intestinal obstruction. In: Walker W, Durie P, Hamilton JR, et al., eds. *Pediatric gastrointestinal disease.* Philadelphia: BC Decker, 1994:486–494.

Author: Andrew E. Mulberg

Intracranial Hemorrhage

 Database

DEFINITION

Intracranial hemorrhage is extravasation of blood from intracranial vessels to the epidural, subdural, intraparenchymal, or intraventricular space within the cranial vault.

CAUSES

- Trauma
- Prematurity
- Coagulopathies related to vitamin K deficiency, hemophilia, idiopathic thrombocytopenic purpura, protein C deficiency, hemolytic-uremic syndrome, disseminated intravascular coagulation, leukemia
- Brain tumors
- Encephalitis, especially herpes simplex infection
- Intracranial aneurysms
- Arteriovenous malformations
- Hypertension
- Cocaine use
- Cerebral infarction

PATHOPHYSIOLOGY

- Epidural hematoma (blood between the dura mater and the skull) is frequently from arterial bleeding related to skull fracture; however, approximately one-fourth of epidural hematomas in children are from venous bleeding.
- Subdural hematoma (blood between the dura mater and the arachnoid membrane) is frequently from venous bleeding resulting from trauma or a coagulopathy.
- Subarachnoid hemorrhage (blood between the arachnoid membrane and brain) is frequently from a ruptured intracranial aneurysm.
- Blood within the brain parenchyma can be the result of trauma, infections such as herpes simplex encephalitis, brain tumors, venous sinus thrombosis, or cerebral infarction.
- Subependymal germinal matrix hemorrhage occurs in newborns, more commonly in premature infants that are less than 34 weeks gestational age.
- Intraventricular hemorrhage most commonly occurs when either an intraparenchymal or subependymal germinal matrix hemorrhage extends into the ventricular system.

GENETICS

Increased frequency with hereditary disorders of coagulation, congenital heart disease, and polycystic kidney disease associated with intracranial aneurysms

COMPLICATIONS

- Death
- Increased intracranial pressure
- Hydrocephalus
- Vasospasm
- Seizures
- Motor, visual, and cognitive deficits

 Differential Diagnosis

- Stroke
- Brain tumor
- Migraine headache

POSITIVE NEUROIMAGING

- Vascular malformation
- Aneurysm
- Trauma
- Tumor
- Bleeding disorder
- Embolism
- Encephalitis
- Idiopathic

 Data Gathering

HISTORY

- Headache
- Change in consciousness
- Seizures
- Visual problems
- Epistaxis

 Physical Examination

- Onset of symptoms most frequently acute to subacute
- Change in cognitive function, including decline of consciousness, alertness, and meaningful interaction with the environment
- Seizures
- Focal motor weakness
- Signs of increased intracranial pressure, such as Cushing triad (hypertension, bradycardia, abnormal respirations), papilledema, pupils that do not constrict to light, ophthalmoparesis, decorticate or decerebrate posturing
- If associated with trauma, there may be:

—Leakage of cerebrospinal fluid from the ear or nose
—Battle sign: bruising over the mastoid process suggestive of basilar skull fracture
—Macewen sign: percussion of the skull gives a cracked pot sound suggestive of skull fracture
—Racoon eyes: periorbital ecchymosis suggestive of recent head trauma
—Retinal hemorrhages

- Herpes simplex type 1 encephalitis: frequently presents with fever, cognitive impairment, seizures
- Germinal matrix hemorrhages are frequently clinically silent but may present with apnea in the newborn.
- Intraventricular blood may present with signs of increased intracranial pressure caused by communicating hydrocephalus.
- Subarachnoid hemorrhage frequently presents as the worst headache ever experienced, subhyaloid hemorrhages, and signs of meningeal irritation.

PITFALLS

A high degree of suspicion is necessary when considering the diagnosis of an intracranial hemorrhage, especially in the context of child abuse.

Laboratory Aids

TESTS

Imaging

• Computed tomography (CT) of the head is the most important study to obtain when considering intracranial hemorrhage in the differential diagnosis because of its relative convenience, speed, and low false-negative rate. Acute blood appears as areas of increased density on head CT; however, after approximately 3 days, the blood will appear progressively less dense.

• Magnetic resonance imaging (MRI) is frequently less useful for diagnosing acute hemorrhage unless signal sequences are specifically adjusted to look for blood.

• MRI is the diagnostic study of choice for venous sinus thrombosis.

• Lumbar puncture, if not contraindicated because of increased intracranial pressure, thrombocytopenia, or skin infection, will show red blood cells and xanthochromia if the blood is contiguous with the ventricular system.

• Angiography, either with conventional dye or using magnetic resonance angiography, is helpful when looking for vasospasm and arterial venous malformations.

• Head ultrasound is the most convenient method for diagnosing subependymal germinal matrix hemorrhages in infants.

 Therapy

• Acyclovir therapy should be instituted if herpes simplex type 1 encephalitis is considered, because, if untreated, there is a high rate of mortality.

• Intracranial aneurysms are frequently amenable to neurosurgical intervention to decrease the likelihood of rebleeding; in addition, careful control of increased intracranial pressure, decreasing vasospasm with nimodipine, and prompt attention to hydrocephalus are necessary.

• Neurosurgical intervention is frequently necessary for subdural and epidural hematomas.

 Follow-Up

PREVENTION

• Using automobile seatbelts; using bicycle, skating, and skateboarding helmets; preventing child abuse; practicing diving safety; preventing falls; maintaining safe driving speeds; keeping children away from firearms

ICD-9-CM 432.9

BIBLIOGRAPHY

Golden GS. In: Swaiman KF, ed. *Pediatric neurology principles and practice,* 2nd ed. St. Louis: Mosby, 1994:791–799.

Medeiros D, Buchanan GR. Major hemorrhage in children with idiopathic thrombocytopenic purpura: immediate response to therapy and long-term outcome. *J Pediatr* 1998;133(3):334–339.

Wear WE. Index of suspicion. Case 3 presentation. Pediatr Rev 1997;18(7):248, 250–251.

Author: Douglas Hyder

Intussusception

 Database

DEFINITION

Intussusception is the telescoping of part of the bowel into an adjacent part of the bowel.

PATHOPHYSIOLOGY

- Most cases are idiopathic.
- Lead point: found in 75% of children over 5 years of age; found in 10% of children less than 2 years of age: polyp, duplication cyst, lymphoma, intestinal parasites, Meckel diverticulum, hematoma secondary to Henoch-Schönlein purpura, hypertrophied Peyer's patches, duplication cysts, intramural hematoma (hemophilia), ventriculoperitoneal shunt, hemangioma proximal to the ileocecal valve is the most common site for the lead point.
- Telescoping of the bowel causes diminished venous blood flow due to compression of the veins. This results in edema and hemorrhage, leading to decreased arterial flow and ischemia and infarction.
- Ileocolic accounts for 90% of intussusceptions.
- Ileoileal and colocolic types do occur.
- Ischemia of the bowel often does not occur in the first 24 hours of intussusception.

EPIDEMIOLOGY

- Male:female ratio: 2:1
- Most common from 6 to 12 months

COMPLICATIONS

- Bowel necrosis secondary to local ischemia
- Gastrointestinal bleeding
- Bowel perforation
- Sepsis, shock

PROGNOSIS

- Timely diagnosis results in a highly favorable prognosis.
- Hydrostatic reduction by barium enema is therapeutic in 50% to 90%.
- Risk of recurrence is approximately 10% after reduction, 1% after manual reduction, and not reported after intestinal resection.

 Differential Diagnosis

- Infection: parasites (*Enterobius*)
- Tumors: The association of lymphoma and intussusception is known.
- A series of 1,200 intussusceptions reported eleven lymphomas; all patients were over 3 years of age. Only one lymphoma was reduced, and a filling defect was noted in the cecum.
- Congenital: Hirschsprung disease
- Immunologic: Henoch-Schönlein purpura: often found at the same time
- Miscellaneous:

—Meckel diverticulum: usually painless rectal bleeding
—Incarcerated hernia
—Incarcerated malrotation
—Obstruction: adhesions, hernia, volvulus, stricture, bezoar, foreign body, fecal impaction, polyp

 Data Gathering

HISTORY

- Intermittent abdominal pain with emesis and blood and mucous stools is considered the classic presentation.
- A complete classic presentation is only found in 20% of cases.
- Colicky pain is the major symptom.
- "Currant-jelly" stools appear in about 50% of cases.

 Physical Examination

- A mass effect in the right upper quadrant may be noted.
- Absence of bowel contents in right lower quadrant (Dance sign)
- Occasionally, the intussusception can be felt on rectal examination.
- A bowel sound may be absent.

Laboratory Aids

TESTS

- CBC, electrolytes
- Plain abdominal films: obstruction, air-fluid levels, paucity of distal gas, soft tissue mass; may result in false-negative reading
- Barium enema: "cervix-like mass" or "coiled spring" on evacuation film

PITFALLS

- Some of the classic symptoms may be absent on presentation, and suspicion must be sufficient to act upon.
- Hypovolemic patients will be worsened with high osmotic contrast agents.

 Therapy

- The bowel should be decompressed by use of an NG tube.
- An intravenous line should be placed, and fluid and electrolyte losses should be corrected.
- Contraindications to reduction by BE include peritonitis, shock, and perforation.
- Caution should be used when symptoms have been present more than 5 days and when radiologic evidence of obstruction, fever, or leukocytosis are present
- A barium enema may miss a lead point.
- A surgical consultation should be obtained before the reduction attempt, because reduction may cause perforation, and failed reduction requires surgical correction.
- Perforation during reduction occurs in 1% of cases, mostly in the transverse colon.

 Follow-Up

Recurrence after nonoperative reduction has been reported in up to 10% and usually is seen within 24 hours of the reduction, so hospitalization and observation are appropriate.

 Common Questions and Answers

Q: Can my child have a recurrent intussusception?
A: Yes, the risk, though, is very low, probable below the 10% chance if the child has had a nonsurgical reduction or removal of the lead point.

Q: Can my child with constipation get this problem?
A: This is doubtful, although, in severe cases, it might be possible.

Q: What are the common ages for presentation?
A: Six months to 3 years is the age range associated with the greatest risk of intussusception, but it can occur at any age. The prevalence of pathologic conditions rises with the age of a child diagnosed with intussusception.

ICD-9-CM 560.0

BIBLIOGRAPHY

Ein SH, Stephens CA, Shandling B, Filler RM. Intussusception due to lymphoma. *J Pediatr Surg* 1986;21:786–788.

Pokorny WJ. Intussusception. In: Oski F, ed. *Principles and practice of pediatrics*, 2nd ed. Philadelphia: JB Lippincott, 1994:1856–1857.

Wesson D. Acute intestinal obstruction. In: Walker WA, Durie PR, Hamilton JR, et al., eds. *Pediatric gastrointestinal disease*. Philadelphia: BC Decker, 1991:491–492.

Author: Andrew E. Mulberg

Iron Deficiency Anemia

 Database

DEFINITION

- A decrease in hemoglobin production due to an insufficient supply of iron that results in a microcytic, hypochromic anemia.

PATHOPHYSIOLOGY

Iron is necessary for oxygen transport by hemoglobin. Most iron in the body is found in hemoglobin and liver parenchyma. Iron necessary for growth and to replace ongoing losses is supplied by the diet and is absorbed in the jejunum. Causes of iron depletion include:

- Decreased dietary intake
- Decreased iron absorption
- Rapid growth causing increased red cell production. Seen in low birth weight infants and adolescents.
- Blood loss either overt or occult. Commonly associated with cow's milk enteropathy in infants. In older children it is associated with inflammatory bowel disease, Meckel's diverticulum, and menorrhagia.

As iron stores decrease, hemoglobin synthesis becomes impaired. There is a gradual fall of red cell production in the bone marrow. Red cells formed contain less hemoglobin making them smaller and paler. Abnormal red cells cause impaired tissue oxygenation.

EPIDEMIOLOGY

Leading cause of anemia among infants and children in the United States. Most commonly seen in children ages 9 months to 3 years and in teenage girls. Prevalence is variable depending on socioeconomic status, availability of iron-fortified formulas, prevalence and duration of breast feeding, and the way that iron deficiency is defined. Prevalence is generally between 1 and 8% of children in the United States.

COMPLICATIONS

- Impaired cognitive and motor development in infants and toddlers.
- Positive correlation between cognitive and motor deficits and severity and duration of anemia.
- Impaired lymphocyte and neutrophil function leading to an increased risk of infection.
- Short term memory impairment and poor exercise performance in adolescents

PROGNOSIS

- Anemia readily corrected with iron replacement.
- Developmental delay may be long lasting or irreversible.

 Differential Diagnosis

- Recent infection
- Lead poisoning
- Thalassemia trait
- Anemia of chronic disease (JRA, IBD, renal failure)

 Data Gathering

HISTORY

- Evaluate dietary intake of iron, including breast or formula feeding and type of formula
- Age of introduction of cow's milk
- Amount of cow's milk during the day
- Blood loss from stool, urine, menorrhagia
- Birth history for prematurity or blood loss
- Pica
- Lead exposure

 Physical Examination

- Usually normal exam
- Pallor, irritability
- Tachycardia, flow murmur
- Blue sclera
- Glossitis or stomatitis
- Stool test for occult blood

 Laboratory Aids

- Low hemoglobin. Hemoglobin less than 2 standard deviations below the age specific mean. (AAP recommends screening Hgb at 9 months, 5 years, and 14 years.)
- Low MCV (red cell volume) and MCH (hemoglobin concentration) for age.
- High red cell distribution width (RDW) >14.5%. Measures the variation in red cell size. Earliest laboratory sign.
- Low serum ferritin reflects tissue iron stores. May be normal or increased with concurrent infection.
- Low serum iron
- Increased transferrin (total iron binding capacity)
- Low transferrin saturation. Measures the iron available for hemoglobin synthesis
- Increased free erythrocyte protporphyrin (FEP), a precursor molecule to hemoglobin synthesis. Also increased in lead poisoning and chronic inflammation.
- Peripheral blood smear with microcytosis, hypochromia, poikilocytosis, and anisocytosis
- Bone marrow with decreased iron stores by hemosiderin staining (rarely done)

Therapy

- Iron supplementation as ferrous sulfate orally at 4–6 mg/kg/day of elemental iron divided into two or three doses. Iron should be given on an empty stomach or with a Vitamin C-containing juice to increase absorption.
- Parenteral (IM or IV) iron dextran is rarely used. Associated with pain on injection and anaphylaxis.
- Educate family regarding age-appropriate diet including adequate iron
- May require initial inpatient observation in cases of severe anemia
- Red cell transfusion only if evidence of cardiovascular compromise (rarely indicated)

 ## Follow-Up

- Reticulocyte count should double in 1–2 weeks
- Hemoglobin concentration should be increased at least 1.0 grams per deciliter in 2–4 weeks
- Check CBC and reticulocyte count at 2 weeks to assess response
- Continue iron for 3 months to replete body stores

PREVENTION

- Maintain breast-feeding for the first five to six months of life when possible. Although the concentration of iron is lower in breast milk than in formula, iron in breast milk is much more available. For infants who are exclusively breast fed beyond six months, give iron supplementation (1 mg/kg/day).
- Give infants who are not breast fed iron-fortified formula for the first 12 months of life.
- Give low birth weight and premature infants iron supplementation after 2 months of life because of decreased iron stores and increased growth rate.
- Encourage iron-enriched cereal when infants are started on solid food.
- Avoid whole cow's milk during the first year of life.

PITFALLS

Causes of poor response to oral iron supplementation include:

- Noncompliance (most common)
- Ongoing blood loss
- Insufficient duration of therapy
- High gastric pH
- Concurrent lead intoxication
- Incorrect diagnosis (Thalassemia trait and anemia of chronic disease are not iron responsive.)

 ## Common Questions and Answers

Q: What dietary changes can help prevent the reoccurrence of iron deficiency?
A: Limit milk to not more than 24 ounces a day so that your child has a better appetite for iron-containing foods. Foods rich in iron include meats, fish, and poultry. Other foods that contain iron are raisins, dried fruit, sweet potatoes, lima beans, chili beans, green peas, peanut butter and enriched foods. Give iron on an empty stomach along with an ascorbic acid-containing juice to increase absorption of iron. Foods that decrease iron absorption include bran, vegetable fiber, tannins found in tea, and phosphates

Q: What are the side effects of iron therapy?
A: Iron can cause temporary staining of the teeth, which can be decreased by diluting the iron with a small amount of juice. Iron will also change the color of bowel movements to greenish black.

Q: What are the most important tests to do to establish the diagnosis of iron deficiency?
A: For patients with a history of dietary deficiency or known blood loss, a complete blood count that shows a low Hgb and MCV and an elevated RDW is very suggestive of iron deficiency. A therapeutic trial of iron without further laboratory testing is an appropriate next diagnostic step. An increase in the hemoglobin concentration of 1 g/dl or greater after one month of therapy confirms the diagnosis. If this does not occur, further laboratory testing is necessary and other diagnoses should be considered.

Q: How does a concurrent infection affect the diagnosis of iron deficiency?
A: Common childhood infections can be associated with a mild microcytic anemia that resembles iron deficiency. Laboratory tests to diagnose iron deficiency can be misleading while a child is acutely ill. Acute infection is associated with a shift of iron from serum to storage sites causing a decrease in serum iron and an increase in ferritin. It is therefore more helpful to screen a child for iron deficiency 3–4 weeks after an acute infection.

BIBLIOGRAPHY

Booth I, Aukett MA. Iron deficiency anaemia in infancy and early childhood. *Arch Dis Child* 1997;76:549–554.

Graham, EA. The changing face of anemia in infancy. *Ped in Rev* 1994;15:175–183.

Lozoff B, Jimenez E, Wolf, AW. Iron deficiency anemia and infant development: Effects of extended oral iron therapy. *J Pediatr* 1996; 129:382–389.

Lozoff B, Jimenez E, Wolf AW. Long-term developmental outcome of infants with iron deficiency anemia. *N Engl J Med* 1991;325: 687–694.

Nathan DG, Orkin SH, eds. *Nathan and Oski's hematology of infancy and childhood,* 5th ed. Philadelphia: WB Saunders, 1998.

Oski FA. Iron deficiency anemia in infancy and childhood. *N Engl J Med* 1993;129:190–193.

Pappas DE. Iron deficiency anemia. *Ped in Rev* 1998;19:321–322.

Author: Suzanne Shusterman

Iron Poisoning—Acute

 Database

DEFINITION

Iron poisoning (acute) is an elevation in the serum iron level secondary to an accidental or intentional ingestion of iron. Toxicity can be predicted by the amount of elemental iron ingested per kilogram of body weight. Clinical toxicity is seen with ingested doses of 20 to 60 mg/kg of elemental iron.

Stages of Iron Ingestion

• Stage 1 (0 to 6 to 12 hours postingestion)

—Direct corrosive effects of iron on gastrointestinal (GI) mucosa
—Vomiting, diarrhea, and abdominal pain
—Lethargy, hypotension, pallor possible
—Metabolic acidosis, leukocytosis, hyperglycemia possible

• Stage 2 (6 to 24 hours postingestion)

—Lasts no more than 12 to 24 hours
—A transition stage between resolving GI symptoms and the development of systemic symptoms

• Stage 3 (12 to 48 hours postingestion)

—Cerebral dysfunction, coma, myocardial depression, renal/hepatic failure
—Coagulopathies, hypoglycemia, acidosis possible

• Stage 4 (2 to 6 weeks postingestion)

—Survivors may develop GI scarring, which can lead to gastric outlet and small bowel obstructions.

PATHOPHYSIOLOGY

• Free (unbound) iron is toxic to many cellular processes. By binding this free iron to carrier/storage proteins (e.g., transferrin, ferritin), cells are protected from its harmful effects. If a cell is exposed to excessive amounts of free iron, damage occurs as free radicals attack cellular biomolecules.
• Iron has a direct corrosive effect on the intestinal mucosa, which can lead to significant GI bleeding, perforation, ischemia, necrosis, and significant fluid losses.
• Venodilation, third spacing of fluids, hepatic dysfunction, and metabolic acidosis may occur as well.
• Humans are unable to eliminate excesses in total body iron. Thus, only by limiting the absorption of dietary iron can iron balance be regulated.

EPIDEMIOLOGY

• There were more than 24,209 cases per year of exposure to iron-containing products in 1993.
• Eighty-four percent of these exposures occurred in children under 6 years of age.
• Iron exposures accounted for 2.2% of all ingestions in children under 6 years of age.

COMPLICATIONS

• GI bleeding
• GI perforation
• Renal failure
• Hepatic dysfunction
• Metabolic acidosis
• Shock
• Cerebral dysfunction
• Coma
• Myocardial depression
• Coagulopathy

PROGNOSIS

• After an iron ingestion, a majority of children remain asymptomatic or develop only minimal toxicity.
• The children remain asymptomatic 6 hours after the ingestion, they are unlikely to develop serious toxicity.
• Shock, coma, and serum iron levels greater than 500 μg/dL are poor prognostic signs.

 Differential Diagnosis

• Ingestion

—Salicylates
—Acetaminophen
—Methanol
—Ethylene glycol
—Isoniazid (INH)

• Infectious

—Sepsis
—Bacterial gastroenteritis

• Gastrointestinal

—GI hemorrhage

 Data Gathering

HISTORY

• Time since ingestion to assess staging, and degree of absorption
• Determine formulation of iron taken and calculate potential amount ingested:

—Ferrous sulfate (20% elemental iron)
—Ferrous gluconate (12%)
—Ferrous fumarate (33%)
—Ferrous chloride (28%)

• Potential milligrams of iron ingested $\times$ percentage of elemental iron = maximum potential milligrams of elemental iron ingested.
• Ask about symptoms, including vomiting, abdominal pain, and change in mental status.

 Physical Examination

• Assess vital signs.
• Assess mental status, and perform a thorough neurologic examination.
• Assess hydration status and peripheral perfusion.
• Assess abdominal examination and hematest stool.

Laboratory Aids

TESTS

Laboratory Tests

- Iron level (serum): Peak level occurs 3 to 5 hours following ingestion. Levels of greater than 350 μg/dL are often associated with serious toxicity. However, the converse is *not* true.
- CBC: helps to identify significant GI bleeding. Initial studies attempted to correlate WBC greater than 15,000 cells/L with serum iron levels greater than 300 μg/dL. However, more recent studies do not confirm this correlation.
- PT/PTT: to rule out associated coagulopathy
- Electrolytes/ABG: to rule out metabolic acidosis
- Total iron binding capacity (TIBC): total amount of iron that transferrin can bind in a particular volume of serum; no longer recommended. Previously, it was felt that toxicity occurred when the serum iron level is greater than the TIBC. Recent studies have shown fault in this theory.
- Serum glucose: Initial studies attempted to correlate serum glucose greater than 150 mg/dL with serum iron levels greater than 300 μg/dL. However, more recent studies do not confirm this correlation. Current recommendations no longer use this test as a screening tool.

Radiographic and Other Studies

- Abdominal x-ray (AXR): may identify iron tablets, which are radiopaque, in the GI tract. This study is helpful if positive, but, if negative, one cannot exclude a significant iron ingestion.
- Deferoxamine challenge test: no longer recommended because it can be falsely negative. Consists of giving an IM dose of deferoxamine, and watching for the appearance of vin rose–colored urine. A positive test suggests a significantly elevated serum iron level.

 Therapy

- Support airway, breathing, and circulation.
- Isotonic fluid rehydration for dehydration
- Ipecac: emetigenic agent; use is controversial. It is difficult to differentiate induced emesis from emesis as a result of iron toxicity.
- Gastric lavage: should be performed in patients following intentional ingestions, if AXR shows retained iron in the GI tract, or if the amount of iron ingested is greater than 20 mg/kg.
- Whole bowel irrigation: Most often, polyethylene glycol is used to flush iron out of the GI tract. This is rarely used, because no controlled studies have been done.
- Charcoal: ineffective, because it does not bind iron
- Deferoxamine: a specific ferric iron chelator. When it binds to iron, it forms ferrioxamine. This compound is excreted by the kidneys, and may turn the patient's urine a vin-rose color (red/orange). The dosage is usually 15 mg/kg/hr. It should be used in the following situations:

—Symptomatic patients with more than transient, minor symptoms
—Presence of severe symptoms: lethargy, intense abdominal pain, hypovolemia, or acidosis
—Positive AXR
—Serum iron level greater than 500 μg/dL

 Follow-Up

- Serum iron levels should be repeated until the level is normal.
- Any patient with positive AXR should have films repeated until all radiopacities have disappeared.

PREVENTION

- Education about the serious nature of iron ingestions to prevent recurrence
- Counsel families on the presence of iron in vitamins (especially prenatal vitamins), and encourage their safe storage.
- Always educate parents of young children and adolescents to keep all medications in a locked, elevated cabinet.

PITFALLS

- Relying solely on laboratory values to determine the need for therapy. Clinical symptoms alone necessitate treatment.
- Missing the diagnosis in a patient in stage 2 of iron ingestion
- Using the deferoxamine challenge test to determine if chelation therapy is indicated
- Giving prochlorperazine (Compazine) with deferoxamine. For unknown reasons, this combination of medications can lead to coma.

 Common Questions and Answers

Q: When should deferoxamine infusion be stopped?
A: Most patients will need less than 24 hours of deferoxamine. The infusion should continue until the patient has no more signs or symptoms of iron toxicity, a repeat AXR is negative (if the initial study was positive), and the urine returns to a normal color (if the patient developed vin rose–colored urine with treatment). Ideally, a serum iron level should be normal, but this may be difficult to measure in the presence of deferoxamine.

Q: Are there any major side effects of deferoxamine therapy?
A: At rapid infusion rates (>15 mg/kg/hr), hypotension has been seen. Some studies have reported the development of ARDS with prolonged infusions. Other rarer complications include *Yersinia* sepsis, ocular toxicity, ototoxicity, and acute renal failure.

Q: Can deferoxamine be given in the face of renal failure?
A: Yes. Deferoxamine offers protective effects that are independent of the renal elimination of ferrioxamine. However, the doses of deferoxamine should be adjusted accordingly.

ICD-9-CM 964.0

BIBLIOGRAPHY

Chyka P, Butler A. Assessment of acute iron poisoning by laboratory and clinical observations. *Am J Emerg Med* 1993;11(2):99–103.

Howland M. Risks of parenteral deferoxamine for acute iron poisoning. *Clin Toxicol* 1996; 34(5):491–497.

McGuigan M. Acute iron poisoning. *Pediatr Ann* 1996;25(1):33–38.

Mills K, Curry S. Acute iron poisoning. *Emerg Med Clin North Am* 1994;12(2):397–413.

Tenenbein M. Benefits of parenteral deferoxamine for acute iron poisoning. *Clin Toxicol* 1996;34(5):485–489.

Author: Debra Boyer

Irritable Bowel Syndrome

 Database

DEFINITION

• Irritable bowel syndrome (IBS) describes a cluster of symptoms that include abdominal distention and pain, improvement in the abdominal pain after a bowel movement, an increasing number of stools with the start of the pain, and looser stools with mucus associated with the onset of pain. These symptoms need to occur on a recurrent basis in order for IBS to be considered.

• Terms such as *spastic colon, nervous colon,* or *spastic colitis* have also been used to describe IBS. Spastic colitis, however, is inaccurate because these patients do not have evidence of inflammation of their colon (colitis) at colonoscopy.

PATHOPHYSIOLOGY

• Most commonly, IBS is thought to be a problem with the motility of the gastrointestinal tract.

• There are no actual histologic, microbiologic, or biochemical abnormalities noted in patients with IBS.

• A variety of investigators have hypothesized that IBS may represent an altered perception of normal gastrointestinal motility.

• A variety of other mechanisms for IBS have been proposed and include:

—Altered electric response in the colon to food

—Motility studies that in some cases demonstrated certain differences (attributed to abnormal smooth muscle function) between patients with IBS and normal controls, including poor antral contractility, high pressure/poorer contracting duodenal contractions, disrupted migrating motor complexes, and prominent duodenal contractions at inappropriate times.

—Extensive fluid intake (>2 L/d) by infants

EPIDEMIOLOGY

• IBS is thought to occur in 15% to 30% of the general population.

• In adults, IBS is the seventh most common cause of visits to primary care physicians and the most common cause of referral to a gastroenterologist.

• Fifty percent of patients present with symptoms before age 35, and 33% can trace their symptoms back into childhood.

• Female:male ratios range from 1.5 to 2.0:1.

• There is no known genetic predisposition for developing IBS.

COMPLICATIONS

• A large number of the complications that arise from IBS are psychologically based. A large number of these patients may show evidence of depression and have increased anxiety.

• Patients with IBS show a significant amount of absenteeism from both school and work.

 Differential Diagnosis

• The diagnosis of IBS is based on a clinical spectrum of symptoms and, as a result, remains a diagnosis of exclusion.

• Common disorders that need to be considered include lactose intolerance, inflammatory bowel disease, constipation, urinary tract infection, esophagitis, gastritis, duodenitis, antibiotic usage (Augmentin, erythromycin), chronic pancreatitis, chronic aspirin use, and nonsteroidal antiinflammatory drug use.

• Less common disorders that need to be considered include giardiasis, celiac disease, ureteropelvic junction obstruction, kidney stones, gallstones, cystic fibrosis, endometriosis, porphyria, duplication/mesenteric cysts, and abdominal migraines.

 Data Gathering

HISTORY

• The initial evaluation of these patients needs to include a careful and detailed history, including a description of the symptoms, with assessment if they recur on a regular basis.

• A detailed diet and travel history can be important to focus the differential.

• Careful questioning about inciting and exacerbating factors

• Clinically, patients with IBS have abdominal pain as their most common presenting complaint. This pain can be sharp, dull, crampy, or burning. It is usually periumbilical or lower abdominal in nature, but not necessarily. The pain starts after a meal and rarely awakens a patient from sleep. Patients, especially children, describe associated symptoms, such as pallor, nausea, anorexia, and fatigue with the abdominal pain.

• Another very common complaint at presentation in patients with IBS is abdominal distention and increased belching and/or flatulence.

• Patients with IBS frequently present with a change in their bowel habits. These changes appear to be progressive and at times can lead to bouts of alternating diarrhea and constipation. Patients appear to have one predominant form consistently. Most patients experience relief of pain after a bowel movement. In patients with constipation, they may go several days to a week without any stool passage.

• In some instances, mucus can be described in this group of patients. However, blood is a rare finding and is usually associated with local/anal irritation or fissure secondary to diarrhea or constipation.

• Patients with IBS rarely have other systemic complaints, such as fever, anorexia, and weight loss.

• Commonly, patients with IBS report that they can identify certain events that exacerbate or trigger an episode. These triggers may include stress, anxiety, certain foods (wheats, milk, alcohol, caffeine), and cigarette smoking.

 Physical Examination

• Findings are usually completely normal, including the abdominal and rectal examinations.

• There is usually no evidence of weight loss or growth failure.

• May have large air pockets

Laboratory Aids

TESTS

• There are no laboratory tests that are diagnostic for IBS. Since it is a diagnosis of exclusion, there are some routine laboratory tests that may be helpful in the initial evaluation. These include a CBC, ESR, urinalysis, electrolytes, and albumin. An abdominal x-ray may help to rule out an intraabdominal process, and a lactose breath test will assess lactose intolerance.

• In certain instances, further testing may include both an upper endoscopy and a colonoscopy.

 ## Therapy

• The best, but at times the most difficult, treatment for IBS is reassurance of both the parents and the child.

• The symptoms should be addressed, but the patient and/or parents should be made aware that the symptoms are not dangerous to the child.

• A variety of interventions have been attempted to decrease the severity of the symptoms.

—Fiber supplementation in the diet is a usual first step in therapy. This is an attempt to prolong stool transit time and then allow for more water absorption. Some also feel that this decreases the high pressure seen in the rectosigmoid region.

—There are a large number of medications that have been used in patients with IBS. Some that may be helpful include the anticholinergics and/or antispasmodics, such as dicyclomine (Bentyl), hyoscyamine (Levsin), Donnatal, and Mebeverine. Other agents, such as amitryptyline and lorazepam have been tried in rarer cases.

• Psychotherapy may be tried. In this therapy, patients are taught a variety of techniques and exercises to use during the episodes of pain which allow them to focus on other subjects, not on the pain.

 ## Follow-Up

There is no standard or specific follow-up needed for patients with IBS. They should continue with routine care, and one should review the clinical symptoms on a regular basis to avoid the misdiagnosis of an underlying problem.

PITFALLS

• Avoid downplaying the clinical symptoms of patients because it will make their acceptance of the treatment plan more difficult.

• Confine testing to basic screening tests so that patients are not left with the impression that there is a significant organic disease present.

 ## Common Questions and Answers

Q: Is there a genetic inheritance with IBS?
A: Although family inheritance patterns exist, no specific data are available.

Q: Are there any personality traits identified that cause certain people to be more likely to develop IBS?
A: Adult studies suggest a predilection for certain types, but no studies have been done on children.

ICD-9-CM 564.1

BIBLIOGRAPHY

Everhart JE, Renault PF. Irritable bowel syndrome in office based practice in the United States. *Gastroenterology* 1991;100:998–1015.

Friedman G. Irritable bowel syndrome: I. A practical approach. *Am J Gastroenterol* 1989;84:863–867.

Hyams JS. Recurrent abdominal pain in children. *Curr Opin Pediatr* 1995;7(5):529–532.

Hyams JS, Treem WR, Justinich CJ, Davis P, Shoup M, Burke G. Characterization of symptoms in children with recurrent abdominal pain: resemblance to irritable bowel syndrome. *J Pediatr Gastroenterol Nutr* 1995;20(2):209–214.

Mezoff AG. Irritable bowel syndrome. In: Wyllie R, Hyams JS, eds. *Pediatric gastrointestinal disease*. Philadelphia: WB Saunders, 1993:724–731.

Read NW. Irritable bowel syndrome (IBS)—definition and pathophysiology. *Scand J Gastroenterol* 1987;130[Suppl]:1–7.

Thompson WG. A strategy for management of the irritable bowel. *Am J Gastroenterol* 1986;81:95–100.

Authors: Edisio Semeao and Andrew E. Mulberg

Kawasaki Disease (Mucocutaneous Lymph Node Syndrome)

 Database

DEFINITION

• An idiopathic, multisystem disease of young children characterized by vasculitis of the small- and medium-sized blood vessels.
• Diagnosis of Kawasaki disease requires a fever for greater than 5 days and four of the following criteria:

—Non-exudative conjunctival injection
—Polymorphous, non-vesicular rash
—Mucosal involvement of the upper respiratory tract that may include erythema, fissures of the lips, crusting of the lips and mouth, or a strawberry tongue. Exudative pharyngitis and discrete oral lesions (e.g., vesicles, etc.) are rare.
—Edema or erythema of the hands and feet
—Cervical adenopathy of at least 1.5 cm in diameter, which is often unilateral.

• Atypical Kawasaki disease

—Patients may present with less than four of the five diagnostic criteria and still develop aneurysms.
—Atypical disease is more common in children less than 1 year of age.

CAUSES

• Etiology is uncertain.
• Association with recent use of rug cleaners or having had rugs shampooed has not been substantiated.

EPIDEMIOLOGY

• Median age of cases is 2.3 years with 80% of cases in children less than 4 years of age, 5% of cases in children greater than 10 years of age, and almost unheard of in children over age 15. Recurrence is low, approximately 0.8%.
• In the United States, incidence seems to be increasing, approximately 11% per year in the period 1984–1990.

GENETICS

There is no clear genetic pattern to this disease.

COMPLICATIONS

• Aneurysms usually first noted 12 to 28 days after onset of the disease. Rarely appear greater than 28 days after onset.
• Aneurysms may thrombose leading to myocardial infarction and death.
• Aneurysms may rupture rarely in patients.
• A pancarditis is often present in the first 10 days of the illness. Pericardial effusions may accompany this.

PROGNOSIS

• Without treatment with intravenous immunoglobulin (IVIG) 15% to 25% of patients develop coronary aneurysms.
• Use of IVIG decreased the incidence of coronary artery aneurysms 4–8%.

• Death occurs secondary to cardiac disease in 0.3% to 2% of cases; approximately 10% is related to early myocarditis, and the remainder due to myocardial infarctions.
• Myocardial infarction can occur several years after the initial illness.
• Patients who are younger than 1 year, older than 8 years, male, and whose fevers persist for greater than 14 days are more likely to develop aneurysms.
• Mortality rates are much higher in males and patients who develop giant coronary artery aneurysms (diameter of greater than 8 mm).

ASSOCIATED ILLNESSES

• Diarrhea and abdominal pain may be seen.
• Patients may develop arthralgias or even frank arthritis.
• Pancarditis may present as myocardial dysfunction early in the course of disease with signs of congestive heart failure.
• Infantile periarteritis nodosa (PAN) is a previously described entity in which the pathological findings of coronary artery aneurysms are indistinguishable from those seen in Kawasaki disease. Most patients with PAN do not have the other findings of Kawasaki disease.

 Differential Diagnosis

• Infections

—Measles and group A β-hemolytic streptococcal infections most closely resembled Kawasaki disease and accounted for 83% of patients referred who did not have Kawasaki disease.
—Severe staphylococcal infections with toxin release (e.g., toxic shock syndrome) may also resemble Kawasaki disease, although there is usually renal involvement (extremely rare in Kawasaki disease) and low platelets.
—Other infections that must be considered include adenovirus, Epstein-Barr virus, roseola, enterovirus, Rocky Mountain spotted fever, and leptospirosis.

• Immunological

—Juvenile rheumatoid arthritis and unusual variants of acute rheumatic fever.
—Hypersensitivity reactions and Stevens-Johnson syndrome.
—In Stevens-Johnson syndrome the conjunctivitis is more likely to be exudative, the rash is more likely to be vesicular with crusting, and there is often a history of drug ingestion.

 Data Gathering

HISTORY

Typical presentation proceeds through three recognizable phases:

• Acute phase (1–2 weeks from onset):

—Highly febrile, irritable, toxic appearing

—Fever usually greater than 40°C and may be as high as 41.6°C
—Oral changes usually quickly follow and also may last 1 to 2 weeks.
—Rash prone to occur in perineal area
—Edema and erythema of the feet are usually painful and limit ambulation.

• Subacute phase (from 2 to 8 weeks after onset)

—Without treatment gradual improvement occurs; fever decreases and there is desquamation of the perineal area, palms, soles, and/or periungual areas.
—Coronary artery aneurysms often appear during the early portion of this phase and acute myocardial infarction may be seen.
—May have persistent arthritis or arthralgias

• Convalescent phase (from months to years after)

—Resolution of remaining symptoms
—Laboratory values return to normal (see subsequent text).
—Aneurysms may resolve or patients may have persistent aneurysms, persistent cardiac dysfunction, or even myocardial infarction.

 Physical Examination

Finding: High, unremitting fevers that last 1 to 2 weeks.
Significance: Fever

Finding: Rash is polymorphous and not vesicular.
Significance: Seen in 99% of cases; predilection for perineum. Often prominent on trunk, usually maculopapular, may coalesce and may be petechial.

Finding: Conjunctivitis
Significance: Bilateral and non-exudative (96% of cases).

Finding: Oral changes may be erythema, fissures, and crusting of lips, diffuse oropharyngeal erythema, or the presence of a strawberry tongue or any combination of these findings.
Significance: Usually not exudative.

Finding: Extremity changes may include erythema of the palms and soles and/or induration of the hands and feet (99% of cases).
Significance: Desquamation, especially periungual, usually occurs in subacute phase. Transverse grooves across the fingernails (Beau lines) may be seen 2 to 3 months after onset.

Finding: Adenopathy is usually cervical and often unilateral.
Significance: Least often seen of the major criteria (75–82% of cases). May be fleeting and easily missed.

Finding: Aseptic meningitis
Significance: Is common and patients are extremely irritable and may show signs of encephalopathy or ataxia.

Kawasaki Disease (Mucocutaneous Lymph Node Syndrome)

Finding: Pancarditis during the acute phase
Significance: May present with tachycardia, gallop rhythms, muffled heart sounds, signs of congestive heart failure, and murmurs consistent with aortic or mitral insufficiency.

Finding: Abdominal exam
Significance: Patients may have a right upper quadrant mass (hydrops of gall bladder), diarrhea, hepatosplenomegaly, or jaundice.

Finding: Meatitis and vulvitis
Significance: May be seen in association with urethritis and sterile pyuria.

Finding: Arthralgias are common; frank arthritis is seen in approximately one-third of patients.
Significance: May involve large and small joints; is non-deforming. Onset may be as late as second or third week. Usually resolves in approximately 1 month.

• During acute phase, slit lamp examination may reveal anterior uveitis in approximately 80% of Kawasaki disease cases.

 Laboratory Aids

Test: White blood cell count
Significance: Usually increased with a left shift; greater than 20,000 in 50% of cases and greater than 30,000 in 15%.

Test: Increased erythrocyte sedimentation rate
Significance: Often greater than 100 mm.

Test: Platelet count
Significance: Platelets may be low, normal, or high at presentation but increase rapidly after the second week of illness; during subacute phase platelet counts may increase to 1 to 2×10^6.

Test: Other laboratory abnormalities include:

• Sterile pyuria and mild proteinuria on urinalysis
• Mild increases in hepatic transaminases
• A cerebrospinal fluid pleocytosis with a normal protein and glucose
• Mild anemia
• Mild hypoalbuminemia
• Hyponatremia
• Hypophosphatemia
• Severe hemolytic anemias

Test: ECG
Significance: During acute phase may show prolonged pr interval, decreased QRS voltage, flat T waves, and ST changes.

Test: Chest x-ray
Significance: May show dilated heart during acute phase.

Test: Echocardiogram
Significance: During acute phase can show a decreased shortening fraction and effusion. Aneurysms may be detected as early as 6 days into the illness, and peak onset is between 3 to 4 weeks.

Test: Increased BUN or creatinine
Significance: If laboratory indicators of renal involvement are present, then illnesses other than Kawasaki disease should be considered (e.g., toxic shock syndrome).

 Therapy

DRUGS

• Intravenous immunoglobulin (IVIG)

—Usual dose is 2 g/kg as a one-time dose over 10 hours.
—Efficacy of IVIG after the tenth day of illness is unclear.
—Patients who fail to respond to an initial dose of IVIG or who have a recrudescence of their symptoms should be retreated (up to two-thirds may have a good response to repeat doses).
—Side effects: Patients may develop signs of fluid overload and congestive heart failure.

• Aspirin

—High-dose aspirin was the mainstay of therapy; still used in conjunction with IVIG, although no data look at IVIG with aspirin versus IVIG alone.
—Usual initial dose is 80 to 100 mg/kg/d in divided doses. High dose required to overcome malabsorption of aspirin seen during acute phase of Kawasaki disease.

• Corticosteroids are contraindicated; may actually increase the rate of coronary artery aneurysms.

DURATION

• Aspirin is continued at high dose until day 14 of the illness or when the child has been afebrile for 48 hours.
• Aspirin dose is then decreased to 30 mg kg/d until 4 weeks after onset and additionally decreased to 3 to 10 mg/kg/d for 6 to 8 weeks or until the platelet count returns to normal.
• If there are coronary artery abnormalities dypyridamole at 3 to 5 mg/kg/d should be added to the aspirin for its vasodilatory effect. Aspirin and dypyridamole should be continued for 1 year or until coronary artery aneurysms resolve.

ACTIVITY

• Children with Kawasaki disease should be kept at bedrest until the second or third week of illness or when they have been afebrile for over 72 hours due to the possibility of myocardial involvement during the acute phase.
• Isolation of patients is not indicated.
• Even asymptomatic patients should be restricted from strenuous activities.

 Follow-Up

WHEN TO EXPECT IMPROVEMENT

• The natural course is a gradual improvement during the subacute phase.
• With IVIG children usually defervesce and show significant resolution of clinical symptoms within 2 to 3 days of treatment (70–80%).
• Two-thirds of patients who receive a repeat dose of IVIG will respond to this dose.

SIGNS TO WATCH FOR

• White blood cell count, platelet count, and ESR should be followed weekly to biweekly until they return to normal.
• Weekly echocardiograms should be done to rule out the development of coronary artery aneurysms from weeks 2 to 6 of the illness.
• If aneurysms are present, cardiology follow-up should include coronary artery catheterization and imaging at some time (usually 8–12 weeks after onset of illness).
• Symptoms of cardiac insufficiency (fatigue, chest pain, dyspnea on exertion, etc.) ECG, CXR, echocardiogram, and exercise myocardial perfusion studies should be done at regular intervals.

 Common Questions and Answers

Q: Do coronary artery aneurysms associated with Kawasaki disease ever resolve?
A: Most coronary artery aneurysms do resolve. Even some giant aneurysms (those greater than 8 mm in diameter) will resolve; there is concern, however, that even if aneurysms resolve, these patients may be at risk for the early development of atherosclerosis.

ICD-9-CD 446.1

BIBLIOGRAPHY

Melish ME. Kawasaki syndrome. *Pediatr Rev* 1996;17:153–162.

Momenah T, Sanatini S, Potts J, et al. Kawasaki disease in the older child. *Pediatrics* 1998; 102(1):e7.

Rosenfeld EA, Corydon KE, Shulman ST. Kawasaki disease in infants less than one year of age. *J Pediatr* 1995;126:524–529.

Shulman ST, DeInocencio J, Hirsch R. Kawasaki disease. *Pediatr Clin North Am* 1995;42:1205–1222.

Author: James M. Callahan

Kwashiorkor

Database

DEFINITION

• Extreme expression of protein-energy malnutrition
• Characterized by edema, growth failure, hypoalbuminemia, fatty infiltration of the liver, and specific dermatosis
• First described in West Africa by Cecily Williams. The word Kwashiorkor in Ghanian means "red or yellow boy."

CAUSES

Diet deficient in protein and a low protein-to-energy ratio are important factors in the development of Kwashiorkor. Other factors postulated include:

• Carbohydrate overloading of a severely malnourished child
• Aflatoxin poisoning
• Imbalance between the production of toxic free radical and its disposal
• Essential fatty acid deficiency
• Deficiency of trace minerals (e.g., zinc, copper, manganese, and selenium)

PATHOPHYSIOLOGY

• Hypoalbuminemia reduces colloid osmotic pressure, leading to edema.
• Reduction in renal blood flow and glomerular filtration rate due to decreased plasma volume and decreased cardiac output as a consequence of hypoalbuminemia.
• Increase in ferritin stimulates release of antidiuretic hormone and subsequent fluid retention.

EPIDEMIOLOGY

• Most common age group are children younger than 2 years of age.
• Prevalent in Third World countries; occurs in developed countries secondary to nutritional ignorance rather than food deprivation
• Other contributory factors include misconception concerning the use of foods, unstable home environment, high prevalence of alcoholism, poor sanitary conditions, and societal beliefs that prohibit the use of many nutritious foods.

COMPLICATIONS

• Fluid and electrolyte disturbances

—Hypoosmolality with moderate hyponatremia
—Mild-to-moderate metabolic acidosis
—Hypocalcemia
—Decreased body potassium without hypokalemia
—Decreased body magnesium with or without hypomagnesemia

• Infections

—Gram-positive and gram-negative organisms; the latter is more common in severe protein-energy malnutrition

• Cardiac failure

—May occur in the midst of severe anemia, during rehydration, and shortly after the introduction of high-protein and high-energy feedings

• Severe anemia

—Hemoglobin levels usually improve with proper dietary management.
—Blood transfusion should be reserved for patients with hemoglobin less than 4 g/100 mL, hypoxia, or impending cardiac failure.

• Hypothermia and hypoglycemia

—Secondary to either impaired non-regulatory mechanisms, reduced fuel substrate, or severe infection

• Severe vitamin deficiency

—Vitamin A deficiency is common

Differential Diagnosis

• Protein energy malnutrition due to the impairment in protein absorption or metabolism

Data Gathering

HISTORY

Question: Dietary history
Significance: Assess for adequacy of protein and total calories.

Question: Cultural beliefs about feeding
Significance: May contribute to low protein intake.

Question: Breastfeeding
Significance: May protect infant but expose older sibling to protein deficiency.

Question: Possible protein loss, diarrhea, renal disease
Significance: Nondietary cause of decreased serum protein.

Question: Skin rash
Significance: See Physical Examination.

Question: Growth records
Significance: Decreased growth velocity commensurate with poor protein intake.

Physical Examination

- Children appear apathetic, irritable, and sad.
- Predominant soft, pitting, painless edema of the soft tissues usually in the feet and legs, perineum, upper extremities, and face.

Finding: Dyspigmentation of the skin
Significance: Hair develops a red-brown color, loses its luster, becomes fragile and easily pluckable. Alternating bands of depigmentation and normal hair known as the "flag sign."

Finding: Characteristic dermatosis of Kwashiorkor
Significance: Also known as "flaky" dermatosis. Appears in areas of the body subject to friction or pressure, notably the flexures, groin, buttocks, behind the knees, or at the elbows. It is described as patchy areas of darkly pigmented skin with a clear margin and a slightly raised edge. As the lesions progress, these lesions peel or desquamate. In severe cases, the skin peels away in patches leaving pale, ulcerated lesions lacking pigmentation. The borders of these lesions may have new highly pigmented dark plaques. These severe peeling lesions may resemble second-degree burns, but unlike burns, the dermatosis of Kwashiorkor lacks a surrounding of erythema and is accompanied by edema.

Finding: Vesiculations of skin
Significance: Resulting in weeping lesions

Finding: Height
Significance: May be normal or retarded, depending on the chronicity of the illness.

Finding: Pale, cold, and cyanotic extremities
Significance:

Finding: Abdomen is frequently protuberant secondary to poor peristalsis
Significance: Leading to distended stomach and intestinal loops.

Laboratory Aids

Test: Common biochemical findings
Significance:

- Significant reduction in serum concentration of total protein and albumin.
- Hemoglobin and hematocrit are usually low.
- Ratio of non-essential to essential amino acids in plasma is elevated in Kwashiorkor and usually normal in marasmus.
- Increased serum elevation of free fatty acids.

Therapy

Treatment protocol is usually divided into three stages:

- Resolving life-threatening conditions

—Restoration can be achieved by oral rehydration solution. As soon as the patient improves, liquid elemental feeds can be initiated. Intravenous fluids must be used when there is persistent vomiting or abdominal distention. Electrolyte imbalances should be treated.

- Restoring nutritional status

—Nutritional status can be improved by nasogastric feeds with 6 to 12 feedings per day. High-protein, high-energy formulas are used. Initial treatment should provide average energy and protein requirements, followed by a gradual increase to 1.5 times the energy and 3 to 4 times the protein requirements by the seventh day. No change in weight or a decrease caused by loss of edema, accompanied by large diuresis, can occur.

- Ensuring nutritional rehabilitation

—Intravenous alimentation is rarely justified in primary protein-energy malnutrition and can increase mortality rates.
—Introduction of traditional home food and therapy can continue on an outpatient basis. Emotional and physical stimulation must be provided. Emphasizing nutritious use of household foods, personal and environmental hygiene, and dietary management of diarrhea and other diseases is also an aspect of management.

PROGNOSIS

Early recognition is important in treating Kwashiorkor. Treatment corrects the acute signs of the disease, but catch-up growth in height may never be achieved. A higher mortality rate is associated with severe anthropometric deficits. Mortality rate in Kwashiorkor can be as high as 40%, but adequate treatment can reduce it to less than 10%. Some of the factors that indicate poor prognosis are:

- Age of less than 6 months
- Infections
- Dehydration and electrolyte abnormalities
- Persistent tachycardia, signs of heart failure
- Total serum protein less than 3 g/100 mL
- Elevated serum bilirubin
- Severe anemia with hypoxia
- Hypoglycemia and/or hypothermia

ICD-9-CM 260

BIBLIOGRAPHY

Buno IJ, Morelli JG, Weston WL. The enamel paint sign in the dermatologic diagnosis of early-onset Kwashiorkor. *Arch Dermatol* 1998;134(1):107–108.

Chase HP, Kirmar V, Caldwell RJ, O'Brien D. Kwashiorkor in the United States. *Pediatrics* 1980;66:972–976.

Latham MC. *The dermatosis of Kwashiorkor in young children.* Ithaca, NY: Cornell University, 1991.

Rossouw JE. Kwashiorkor in North America. *Am J Clin Nutr* 1989;49:588–592.

Author: Helen Anita John-Kelly

Lacrimal Duct Obstruction

 Database

DEFINITION

• Blockage of the portion of the tear drainage system extending from the lacrimal sac to the nose

PATHOPHYSIOLOGY

• Failure of complete canalization of the naso-lacrimal duct

EPIDEMIOLOGY

• Approximately 5% of newborns

COMPLICATIONS

• Acute dacryocystitis (acute infection of the lacrimal sac)

PROGNOSIS

• Spontaneous resolution in approximately 95% of patients by 12 months of age

 Differential Diagnosis

• Causes of increased tear production: congenital glaucoma, reflex tearing secondary to dry eye, seventh nerve palsies, trichiasis, entropion.
• Other causes of decreased drainage: imperforate puncta or canaliculi, ectropion, lateral canthus dystopia, traumatic injury to the nasolacrimal duct.

 Data Gathering

HISTORY

Question: Onset of symptoms?
Significance: To determine whether the condition is congenital; symptoms include tearing, crusting of eyelashes particularly upon awaking, red eye, and discharge from eye.

 Physical Examination

Finding: Increased tear meniscus, maceration of eyelid skin, mucopurulent discharge, and conjunctival hyperemia.
Significance: Common symptoms.

Finding: Palpation
Significance: Expression of material from the puncta with pressure on the lacrimal sac.

 Laboratory Aids

Test: Dye disappearance test (DDT)
Significance: Fluorescein is applied to the conjunctival cul de sac and the patient is observed for 5 minutes. In a negative test (normal) the tear meniscus will become relatively unstained, and in a positive test the height of the stained tear meniscus will either increase or fail to decrease.

Therapy

- Initially, lacrimal sac massage and either ophthalmic antibiotic drops or ointment are applied when ocular discharge increases.
- If symptomatic at 12 months of age, probing and irrigation are performed.
- If probing and irrigation fail, then the procedure is repeated with Silastic tube intubation.
- If all else fails, a dacryocystorhinostomy (permanent surgical connection between the lacrimal sac and the nose) is performed to prevent recurrent infections (dacryocystitis) and maceration of the eyelids from tearing.

 Follow-Up

- Patients should be reevaluated at 12 months of age and referred for probing and irrigation if still symptomatic.

PITFALLS

- Referral for probing and irrigation is delayed until patient is over 12 months of age; the probing and irrigations should be performed by 13 months of age (as described previously).

 Common Questions and Answers

Q: Is my child in any danger while the nasolacrimal duct remains obstructed?
A: Occasionally, the contents of the sac can become infected and will require oral or parenteral antibiotics.

Q: Why not wait longer to do the probing and irrigation?
A: The failure rate of the initial procedure increases with age: if performed before 13 months of age 96% success rate, between 13 and 18 months of age 77% success rate, and between 18 and 24 months 54% success rate.

ICD-9-CM 375.56

BIBLIOGRAPHY

Crawford JA. Intubation of obstructions in the nasolacrimal system. *Can J Ophthalmol* 1977;12:289–293.

Crawford JA, Pashby RC. Lacrimal system disorders. *Int Ophthalmol Clin* 1984;24:39–53.

Kushner B. Congenital nasolacrimal system obstruction. *Arch Ophthalmol* 1982;100:597–600.

Author: Katrinka L. Heher

Lactose Intolerance

 Database

DEFINITION

Inability to digest the disaccharide lactose, secondary to deficiency of the enzyme lactase, resulting in symptoms of malabsorption. Two types of deficiency have been noted.

- Congenital lactase deficiency is extremely rare. It presents during the newborn period, often with the first feeding of lactose-containing formula.
- Acquired lactase deficiency can be secondary to an insult to the bowel or developmental loss of enzyme activity.

PATHOLOGY

- Disaccharide activity can be measured in biopsy specimens of the small bowel.
- Small bowel biopsy will often show no histological abnormality.

EPIDEMIOLOGY

- Deficiency is found in up to 80% of native Australians, Americans, tropical Africans, and East and Southeastern Asians. It is also highly prevalent in African Americans.
- It can be clinically evident in many African Americans by 3 years of age.

GENETICS

- Adult lactase production is a dominant trait; lactase deficiency is a recessive trait with single mendelian locus.
- The gene for lactase-phlorizin-hydrolase has been localized on chromosome 2.

PROGNOSIS

With lactose avoidance or with enzyme supplementation, the child can control and eliminate symptoms.

 Differential Diagnosis

- General

—Lactose intolerance may be secondary to a generalized small bowel mucosal dysfunction; the presence of other symptoms should prompt an evaluation.

- Infection

—Viral and bacterial infections can cause a secondary lactose intolerance.
—Parasitic infections can mimic lactose intolerance.

- Inflammatory

—Crohn disease can have an associated lactose intolerance.

- Congenital

—Other carbohydrate enzyme deficiencies can mimic lactose intolerance. This includes sucrase-isomaltase or glucose-galactose malabsorption.
—Cystic fibrosis, Shwachman syndrome, and malrotation can mimic lactose intolerance.

- Allergic/Immune

—Celiac disease often is associated with lactose intolerance.
—Protein intolerance can cause a secondary lactose intolerance.

 Data Gathering

HISTORY

Question: Symptoms?
Significance: Classic symptoms include bloating, gaseousness, colicky abdominal pain, and diarrhea.

Question: Diet history?
Significance: Provides important information.

Question: A detailed history of symptoms.
Significance: Blood in the stools, failure to thrive, fat malabsorption, or any extraintestinal symptoms strongly suggest additional etiological entities.

Question: Lactose ingestion.
Significance: Symptoms vary in severity and with dose of lactose.

Question: Milk ingestion?
Significance: Association with milk ingestion may not be evident.

 Physical Examination

Finding: Height and weight
Significance: Should be measured and plotted against age-appropriate norms; any deviation should not be evaluated as lactose intolerance alone.

Finding: Abdomen percussion
Significance: Abdomen may be distended.

Finding: Blood in the stool
Significance: Must be evaluated, because lactose intolerance does not cause bleeding.

Laboratory Aids

Test: Stool-reducing substances and fecal acidity
Significance: A positive result indicates malabsorption of carbohydrates. A pH less than 6.0 or reducing substances greater than 0.5% are interpreted as a positive result. This is a very reliable test in the presence of diarrhea; however, it is not specific for lactose alone.

Test: Lactose breath hydrogen test
Significance: Is used for lactose intolerance. It is non-invasive and highly sensitive. It is based on the fact that in the human, the only source of hydrogen is fermented unabsorbed carbohydrates. A rise of breath H_2 concentration of greater than or equal to 20 ppm over baseline appears to correlate better with subsequent symptom development than does a concentration of greater than or equal to 10 ppm. However, the frequently poor association between symptoms of lactose intolerance and breath H_2 excretion suggest caution in the interpretation of the clinical significance of the breath hydrogen test.

False-positive test results occur due to inadequate fasting before the test, rapid intestinal transit, toothpaste, smoking, and bacterial overgrowth.

False-negatives occur due to diarrhea, hyperventilation, recent antibiotics, and delayed gastric emptying. Up to 10% of the population are colonized with bacteria unable to produce hydrogen and will give a negative result.

 ## Therapy

• Removal of lactose from the diet is effective in eliminating symptoms. However, a milk-free diet may result in calcium deficiency and other nutritional issues.
• Predigestion of lactose can be done by the addition of commercially available enzyme supplementation. Multiple products are available over the counter. Liquid preparations, capsules, and chewable tablets can be obtained.
• Some acquired deficiencies, particularly those associated with infection, may resolve over time. The majority of patients with lactose intolerance will not recover the ability to digest lactose.

PITFALLS

Care must be taken to determine if the lactose intolerance is secondary to a primary pathological process (i.e., small bowel overgrowth, Crohn disease, or *Giardiasis*).

 ## Common Questions and Answers

Q: When is the usual time for presentation of lactose intolerance?
A: In whites, the age of presentation is after 5 years of age. In blacks, 2- to 3-year-old children may present. The differential diagnosis must discern between primary and secondary causes.

Q: Does lactose intolerance prevent the child from ever eating lactose?
A: No, the child or adult may have lactose in the diet if the enzyme is supplemented by tablet or caplet.

Q: Does this problem ever get better?
A: No, it is a life-long problem, but seems to become less symptomatic for adults, in light of their individual desire to tolerate symptoms.

ICD-9-CM 271.3

BIBLIOGRAPHY

Auricchio S. Genetically determined disaccharidase deficiencies. In: Walker WA, Durie PR, Hamilton JR, et al., eds. *Pediatric gastrointestinal disease.* Philadelphia: BC Decker, 1991: 657–660.

Shulman RJ. Enzyme and transport defects. In: Oski FA, DeAngelis CD, Feigin RD, et al., eds. *Principles and practice of pediatrics,* 2nd ed. Philadelphia: JB Lippincott, 1994:1895–1899.

Veligati LN, Treem WR, Sullivan B, Burke G, Hyams JS. Delta 10 ppm versus delta 20 ppm: a reappraisal of diagnostic criteria for breath hydrogen testing in children. *Am J Gastroenterol* 1994;89(5):758–761.

Author: Andrew E. Mulberg

Lead Poisoning

 ## Database

DEFINITION

- The most common pediatric environmental health problem involves a systemic intoxication by the heavy metal, lead; most commonly this is with inorganic lead.
- Children in the U.S. are predominantly exposed to lead through ingestion of paint chips and contaminated housedust and soil from deterioration of pre-1980 housing and buildings.
- The Centers for Disease Control and Prevention (CDC) considers a blood lead level of 10 μg/dL or higher to represent undue lead exposure and absorption; a level of 20 μg/dL or higher is generally considered to constitute lead poisoning.

PATHOPHYSIOLOGY

- Lead adversely effects many organ systems including the neurological (encephalopathy, peripheral neuropathy in adults, subtle neuropsychological effects), hematological (anemia due to several mechanisms), gastrointestinal (abdominal colic), renal (proximal renal tubular injury leading to Fanconi syndrome), and reproductive systems.
- Many of the toxic effects result from inhibition of enzymes involved in heme biosynthesis, as the electropositive metal binds to the negatively charged sulfhydryl groups on the active sites of delta-aminolevulinic acid dehydratase (ALA-D), ferrochelatase, porphobilinogen synthase, coproporphyrinogen oxidase, and other enzymes. Divalent lead also acts competitively with calcium in various biologic systems and lead affects nucleic acids.
- Children absorb lead more efficiently from the gastrointestinal tract and are more likely to ingest lead through hand-to-mouth activity as compared to adults.
- As the developing, immature central nervous system is susceptible to the toxic effects of lead, the neuropsychological effects of lead poisoning upon young children have been of particular concern.

EPIDEMIOLOGY

- Prevalence of elevated lead levels and geometric mean blood lead level (BLLs) have decreased significantly in the last 20 years.
- Almost 1,000,000 American children aged 1 to 5 years (4.4% of a representative national sample) are estimated to have BLLs of 10 μg/dL or higher.

- Higher prevalence occurs among children aged 1 to 3 years, African-American and Mexican-American children, those from lower income families, those living in metropolitan areas with populations of one million or greater, and those living in older housing.
- Approximately 86% of American pre-1980 publicly owned housing units and 83% of privately owned units contain some lead-based paint.

COMPLICATIONS

- Acute encephalopathy
- Seizures
- Coma
- Death (predominantly due to cerebral edema)
- Mental retardation
- Cognitive, behavioral, attentional, and neurodevelopmental impairment
- Anemia
- Fanconi syndrome

PROGNOSIS

- In general, there is an increased risk for long-term neuropsychological sequelae, which increases with lead exposure and absorption that is more intense, of longer duration, and begins at an early age when the central nervous system is still maturing.
- Recurrent episodes of symptomatic lead poisoning increase the risk for permanent sequelae.
- More subtle effects may not be detected until school entry.

 ## Differential Diagnosis

- Most lead poisoning in children is asymptomatic.
- Head encephalopathy should be considered in the differential diagnosis of a child presenting with seizures, altered mental status, and/or coma.
- Lead poisoning should also be considered in the differential diagnosis of mental retardation, behavioral disorders, and anemia.

 ## Data Gathering

HISTORY

Question: Exposure to a source of lead?
Significance: The most common sources of lead include residence in or visitation of older, deteriorated housing, a parental occupation or hobby involving lead exposure, use of remedies or cosmetics containing lead, and ingestion of contaminated water, food, or beverages.

Question: Typical symptoms?
Significance: Although many of the clinical manifestations of symptomatic lead poisoning are non-specific, a cluster of complaints including anorexia, intermittent abdominal pain, constipation, sporadic vomiting, change in mental status (such as irritability or lethargy), decreased play activity, and change in developmental status (particularly with regression of developmental milestones) may herald this condition.

Question: Lead encephalopathy?
Significance: Can present with change in consciousness, ataxia, persistent vomiting, seizures, and coma; often this presents after a prodrome of the previous symptoms.

Question: Anemia or developmental delay?
Significance: Result of lead poisoning.

 ## Physical Examination

- Not generally helpful at lower lead levels. Symptomatic and/or encephalopathic patients may have acute gastrointestinal, neurological, hematological, and systemic manifestations.
- Assess for clinical evidence of developmental delay.
- Burton gum lead line: A blue-gray discoloration at the gum-tooth interface typically along the lower incisors rarely can be seen in the setting of chronic, fairly high lead exposure and poor dental hygiene.

 ## Laboratory Aids

SPECIFIC TESTS

Test: Blood lead test, either venous or capillary.
Significance: Compare result with CDC classification system. Results may be reportable to local health authorities. Is only a measure of recent lead exposure; does not indicate total body burden of lead.

NON-SPECIFIC TESTS

Test: Complete blood count
Significance: To assess for anemia. Anemia is seen in lead poisoning starting at about 60 μg/dL from globin and heme synthesis inhibition and hemolysis. Iron deficiency anemia is often seen concomitantly. Anemia related to lead toxicity is typically normocytic and normochromic; a microcytic, hypochromic anemia may be seen with a mixed etiology. Basophilic stippling is sometimes seen on peripheral blood smear.

Test: Free erythrocyte protoporphyrin (FEP) and other blood and urine markers
Significance: Markers of lead-induced inhibition of heme synthesis. FEP can be useful clinically to follow the recovery from heme synthesis inhibition during management.

Lead Poisoning

RADIOGRAPHIC STUDIES

Test: Abdominal radiograph
Significance: Looking for radio-opaque foreign material suggestive of ingestion of lead paint chips or other lead-containing foreign body.

Test: Long bone x-rays
Significance: To look for "lead lines" or metaphysical sclerosis, characterized by increased density along transverse lines in the metaphyses of growing long bones representing increased mineralization due to interference with the metabolism of bone matrix.

Test: X-ray fluorescence for estimation of body lead burden
Significance: This has been used mainly in experimental settings.

 Therapy

- Environmental management, which includes removing children from the lead source(s), should occur when venous lead levels are recurrently 15 to 19 μg/dL (CDC Class IIB) and when levels are greater than or equal to 20 μg/dL (CDC Class III).
- Chelation therapy should complement environmental management in all children with venous levels of 45 μg/dL (CDC Class IV) or higher, using parenteral calcium disodium ethylenediamine tetraacetate (EDTA; also calcium disodium versenate) or oral agents such as meso 2,3-dimercaptosuccinic acid (DMSA, succimer, Chemet). Chelation of children with levels in the 25 to 45 μg/dL range may be considered in certain cases although it is not routinely recommended. Outpatient therapy can take place if a lead-safe environment has been identified and compliance is expected. Succimer is given at 10 mg/kg/dose (or 350 mg/m^2/dose) every 8 hours for 5 days, then every 12 hours for 14 more days. Weekly monitoring for neutropenia, platelet abnormality, and increased liver enzymes is recommended. Succimer is more lead-specific than other chelators and causes less mineral depletion.
- Children with symptomatic lead poisoning or with levels of 70 μg/dL (CDC Class V) or higher should be admitted immediately to a hospital for parenteral chelation with both intramuscular dimercaprol (BAL or British anti-Lewisite) and intravenous or intramuscular calcium disodium EDTA. As there are many issues involved with administration of both chelating agents, consultation of appropriate guidelines and pharmacological information is recommended. Children with encephalopathy constitute a medical emergency and should receive the preceding treatment in an intensive care setting with attentive neurosurgical support. Consultation with a clinician experienced in lead toxicity treatment is advised for these patients.
- Ingested lead-containing foreign bodies should be evacuated with whole bowel irrigation using a high molecular weight glycol solution.

- Nutritional support with calcium and iron supplementation should be given if intake is inadequate; deficiencies of these increase lead absorption from the gastrointestinal tract. Iron supplementation should be withheld during chelation therapy.

 Follow-Up

- Prompt environmental follow-up of current lead exposure situations and vigilance for additional exposure (with family moves, visitation of new residences, etc.) should occur.
- Follow-up of elevated venous levels from 10 to 19 μg/dL (CDC Class IIA, IIB) approximately every 3 to 4 months.
- Follow-up of venous levels of 20 μg/dL or higher at 1 to 2 month intervals until no additional lead exposure is present and levels have decreased.

PREVENTION

- Primary prevention: removal of potential environmental lead hazards.
- Secondary prevention: screening for elevated lead levels. Since 1997, CDC has recommended that state and local health departments make the determination for a universal versus targeted screening approach. Screening is recommended by use of a blood lead test for children at ages 1 and 2 and for those of 36 to 72 months of age without previous screening.

—Universal screening for communities where the risk for lead exposure is widespread and where 12% or more of children aged 12 to 36 months have lead levels of 10 μg/dL or higher and/or 27% or greater of the housing stock was built prior to 1950.
—Targeted screening for communities not meeting above criteria. Screening would be indicated for children meeting local criteria for screening such as residence in a specified geographic area, membership in a high-risk group, or a high risk status as determined by the use of a personal-risk questionnaire.

- Tertiary prevention: case management and environmental remediation for children with lead poisoning. Closer attention to the first 2 modes of prevention should obviate the need for this.

CONTROL MEASURES

- Abatement of building-based (residential) lead hazards by removal or enclosure of lead-containing structures.
- Control of environmental lead dust exposure and ingestion by good housekeeping (wet dusting and mopping of household dust) and personal hygiene (cleaning of child's hands, toys, personal items, etc.).
- Removal of any other known lead source from the child's environment.

PITFALLS

- Delay in checking a blood lead test in the presence of clinical signs or symptoms of lead poisoning or neuropsychological disorders.
- Failure to inquire about lead exposure possibilities, especially of non-urban children.

 Common Questions and Answers

Q: What is lead abatement?
A: Lead abatement is removal of a lead hazard from the environment either by replacing it (e.g., installing a new window), enclosing the area with the lead source (e.g., installing paneling), removing the lead-based paint from a surface (burning or dry sanding methods should never be used), or encapusulating the area (placement of a specific coating over the lead-containing surface, which prevents access to the lead hazard).

Q: Is lead abatement permanent?
A: Often the lead paint that is chipping or peeling is removed from a home. Any areas with intact lead-based paint may become deteriorated with aging, leading to new lead hazards.

Q: Why didn't my child's brother or sister get lead poisoned at the same age, as he/she lived in the same house?
A: Children are different; some do much more hand-to-mouth activity than others, which is the main way that children get lead into their bodies. Also, your home may not have had the same lead dangers (hazards) when the sibling was younger.

ICD-9-CM: 984.9

BIBLIOGRAPHY

American Academy of Pediatrics Committee on Drugs. Treatment guidelines for lead exposure in children. *Pediatrics* 1995;96:155–160.

American Academy of Pediatrics Committee on Environmental Health. Screening for elevated blood lead levels. *Pediatrics* 1998;101:1072–1077.

Centers for Disease Control and Prevention. Screening young children for lead poisoning: guidance for state and local public health officials. US Dept of HHS, 1997.

Centers for Disease Control and Prevention. Update: blood lead levels—United States, 1991–94. *MMWR* 1997;46:141–146.

Chisolm JJ, O'Hara DM, eds. *Lead absorption in children: management, clinical, and environmental aspects,* 1st ed. Baltimore-Munich: Urban & Schwarzenberg, 1982.

Pueschel SM, Linakis JG, Anderson AC, eds. *Lead poisoning in childhood.* Baltimore: Paul H. Brookes Publishing Co., 1996.

Author: Carla Campbell

Leprosy (Hansen Disease)

 Database

DEFINITION

• A chronic disease caused by *Mycobacterium leprae,* which affects the skin, peripheral nerves, and mucosa of upper airways

EPIDEMIOLOGY

• 90% of cases in the United States are imported, mainly refugees from Mexico and Southeast Asia. Leprosy usually spreads in overcrowded and poor hygenic conditions.
• States with indigenous disease include Texas, California, Louisiana, and Hawaii.
• Transmission is through contact with untreated or multidrug resistant cases, particularly lepromatous and "borderline" cases, and shedding from nasal secretions and skin lesions where the skin is no longer intact.
• Incubation period is 1 to 5 years (shortest for tuberculoid leprosy).
• Infectivity decreases after a couple of weeks when treatment with rifampin, and after 3 months if dapsone or clofazimine is used.

PATHOPHYSIOLOGY

• Is dependent on the cellular immune reaction to the organisms.
• Lepromatous leprosy has little cellular infiltrate, and the acid-fast bacilli (AFBs) multiply and disseminate, whereas tuberculid, the cellular reaction, is significant, forming granuloma and the AFBs are contained and few in number.
• Lepromatous leprosy usually begins with a vague skin macule, other macules form near it, and the skin thickens and becomes edematous. The lesions may coalesce leading to loss of anatomical definition. Ear lobes and cheeks are first areas affected. Lepromatous lesions are not anesthetic.
• Tuberculoid lesions are clearly defined but can disappear only to reappear later; these lesions are anesthetic, and peripheral nerves are involved secondary to granuloma around the nerve twigs that extend to the nerve plexus, destroying fibrils. Cold abscesses may develop.

ASSOCIATED DISEASES

Patients with leprosy may have other parasitic diseases common to the tropics, tuberculosis, etc.

COMPLICATIONS

• Skin nodules, plaque progression to deformation of limbs or face
• Nerve involvement leading to ulcerations, fractures, repeated trauma to affected limbs
• Infiltration and ulceration of nasal mucosa, rarely extending to larynx and trachea (lepromatous disease)
• Regional lymph nodes, may be associated with chronic sinuses (lepromatous)
• Infiltration of the testes
• Eye damage, usually secondary to the nerve anesthesia
• Rejection from familial members and or community

 Data Gathering

HISTORY

Question: Exposure history
Significance: Need to know about foreign travel at least 5 years previously.

 Physical Examination

• Skin lesions: Early skin lesions are difficult to differentiate but over a period of time become either tuberculid, lepromatous, or borderline disease (has features of both tuberculid and lepromatous). Rarely, there may be an acute presentation with fever and pain in peripheral nerves. Usually vague macules, first on the face or ear lobes, not anesthetic, which become diffusely edematous (typical leonine facies), later nodular, and may break down and ulcerate discharging many AFBs.
• Invasion of the eyes/nose. Ulceration of nasal mucosa may occur. Eye damage is secondary to nerve damage rather than invasion of AFB. Cold abscesses may form around nerve trunks. Is associated with iritis.
• Tuberculid disease: Well-demarcated raised lesions anywhere on the body, which are hairless, often depigmented, analgesic, and anesthetic. Small nerves are thickened in the vicinity of the lesion and may be palpable. Later, larger nerve trunks are thickened and palpable, with secondary signs of neuritis such as wrist or foot drop, with autonomic changes also and muscle contractures. The insensitive, atopic tissues are subject to trauma, leading to ulcers and secondary infection.

Laboratory Aids

• Skin biopsy of lesions: Organisms have not been successfully cultured. Research institutions can test for drug resistance, but results take 6 months; therefore, response to therapy is based on clinical parameters.
• Antibodies may be high in persons without disease, therefore, is not diagnostic. IgM antibody is only available in reference laboratories.
• Rheumatoid factor and Wassermann reaction are often positive and non-specific.

Therapy

• Consult with GWL Hansen's Disease Center, Carville, Louisiana, 1-800-642-2477.
• Multidrug therapy is recommended to avoid drug resistance.
• For tuberculid disease: dapsone (1 mg/kg/d); rifampin (10 mg/kg/d) for 6 months
• For lepromatous disease: dapsone (1 mg/kg/d); rifampin (10 mg/kg/d) and clofazamine (1 mg/kg/d) for 2 years and until skin biopsy smears are negative for organisms. If erythema nodosum leprum (ENL) occurs in these patients when treatment is initiated, treatment with steroids is recommended.
• Rehabilitative surgery and physical therapy are often necessary for advanced disease.

ISOLATION

• Private room for new diagnosis. Tuberculid cases are not contagious.

CONTROL MEASURES

• Handwashing for all persons in contact
• Household contacts <25 years of age of individuals with lepromatous or borderline leprosy should be treated with dapsone (1 mg/kg/d) for 3 years.
• Report to Public Health Authority.

ICD-9-CM 030.9

BIBLIOGRAPHY

Bullock ME. Mycobacterium leprae (Leprosy). In: Mandell GL, Bennett JE, Dolin R, eds. New York: Churchill Livingstone, 1994; 230:1906–1910.

Author: Barbara Watson

Lice (Pediculosis)

 Database

DEFINITION

- Infestation of the head, body, or anogenital region with one of three species of lice

CAUSES

Three species of ectoparasites (6-legged, wingless, 1- to 4-mm insects that live on humans, feeding on human blood):

- *Pediculus humanus capitus:* head louse
- *Pediculous humanus corporis:* body louse
- *Pthiris pubis:* pubic or crab louse

PATHOPHYSIOLOGY

- Head lice

—Survives for several weeks on scalp
—Typical infestation, 12 to 24 live insects per patient
—Single louse produces up to 120 eggs.
—Ova (nits) laid close to the scalp; firmly attached to hair shaft by chitinous ring (usually clustered in the parietal and occipital areas)
—Ova hatch after 8 days, leaving shell of nit on hair (readily visible to examiner).
—Transmitted by personal contact, or fomites (e.g., combs, hats, upholstery, clothing, headsets)
—Prefer to feed on scalp skin; hooks on scalp, pierces skin to feed
—Release poisonous saliva that causes pruritis, dermatitis
—Survive 1 to 2 days off human host

- Body lice

—10% to 20% larger than head lice
—Prefer to live on clothing, visiting human only to feed
—Lay eggs along seams of clothing, which hatch when warmed by wear
—Transmitted through contact with infested clothing or bedding
—Viable off of human for 10 to 21 days

- Pubic lice

—Crab-like appearance with predilection for pubic hair
—Transmitted almost exclusively by sexual contact
—Uncommonly spread by fomites (e.g., toilet seats, bedding)
—Occasionally will infest axillary hair, beard, or eyelashes
—May infest eyebrows/lashes (pediculosis palpebrum) in young children (associated with maternal infestation; but one must consider possible sexual abuse)

EPIDEMIOLOGY

- Head lice

—Common in day care setting and elementary school children
—Affects all socioeconomic groups
—Not indicative of poor hygiene
—Slightly higher incidence in girls

- Body lice

—Found on persons with poor hygiene
—More common in extreme conditions such as crowding, homelessness, wars, famine, flood, and earthquakes
—Highest incidence in the Sudan and Ethiopia

- Pubic lice

—Most common in adolescents and young adults

COMPLICATIONS

- Head lice

—Secondary dermatitis, impetigo, or furunculosis

- Body lice

—Secondary eczema, impetigo (from scratching)
—Post-inflammatory hyperpigmentation
—Known vector for disease; rickettsia prowazecki (epidemic typhus), rickettsia quintana (trench fever), borrelia recurrentis (relapsing fever).

ASSOCIATED ILLNESSES

- Pubic lice: up to 50% of patients have another sexually transmitted disease, particularly gonorrhea, or syphilis.

 Differential Diagnosis

- Seborrheic dermatitis
- Contact dermatitis
- Eczema
- Impetigo

 Data Gathering

HISTORY

Question: Pruritis?
Significance: Sign of all lice infestation

Question: Secondary skin lesion (from scratching)?
Significance: May be chief complaint

Question: Symptoms?
Significance: Review of symptoms (if body lice) to detect symptoms of rickettsial or spirochetal illness.

SPECIAL QUESTIONS

Question: Contacts?
Significance: Possible infested contacts (home, school, or sexual).

Question: Special living circumstances?
Significance: Crowding or institutionalization.

 Physical Examination

- Head lice

Finding: Lice (difficult to find) or nits on hair shaft.
Significance: Diagnostic.

Finding: Nits cluster in parietal and occipital regions.
Significance: Diagnostic.

Finding: Use of Wood light.
Significance: Live nits fluoresce under Wood light.

- Secondary skin lesions; dermatitis of the neck, shoulder area.
- Examine eyelashes, eyebrows for secondary infestation.
- Posterior occipital lymphadenapathy

- Body lice

Finding: Primary skin lesion
Significance: Pinpoint, erythematous macule, papule, or urticarial wheel

Finding: Primary lesions
Significance: Often obliterated from scratching

Finding: Parallel scratch marks in interscapular region
Significance: Often observed due to secondary infection of neck seam of clothing.

Finding: Post-inflammatory hyperpigmentation
Significance: Common

Finding: Lice in clothing or nits in clothing seams
Significance: Diagnostic

- Pubic lice

Finding: Lice or nits in pubic or perianal hair. Secondary eczema, bloody crusting common in advanced cases.
Significance: Diagnostic

Finding: Maculae cerulae (bluish/slate macules, 0.5- to 1-mm diameter)
Significance: From heavy infestation in pubic, trunk, and thigh areas.

PROCEDURES

- Head lice

—Nits only behind patient's ears in early infestation
—Nits difficult to flick away (unlike dandruff); need to be pulled along entire length of hair shaft to remove.

Lice (Pediculosis)

Laboratory Aids

Test: Rarely necessary
Significance: Can examine louse or nit under microscope to confirm characteristic appearance. Dandruff is a false positive finding.

Test: Home testing
Significance: Parents can be instructed how to examine all family members for infestation.

Test: School testing
Significance: Schools should perform examinations during epidemics.

Therapy

DRUGS

• Head lice

—Permethrin (Nix) 1% creme rinse; drug of choice
  —Acts on nerve cell membranes causing paralysis/death of insect
  —10-minute application
  —High ovicidal activity; continued activity up to 12 days after application
  —Reduced incidence of recurrence; if reapplication necessary, wait 7 to 10 days
  —Over the counter
  —Low toxicity
  —Pyrethrins (Rid, A-200)
  —Neurotoxin also
  —10-minute application
  —Low ovicidal activity; requires second application in 1 week. Available over-the-counter.
  —Some develop contact dermatitis to natural chrysanthemum base.
  —Lindane (Kwell) 1% lotion
  —4-minute application
  —Highest potential for patient neurotoxicity if used incorrectly; contraindicated in preterm infants and infants under 3 months, not recommended for children under 2 years.
  —Lindane-resistant strains of pediculosis reported in some countries
  —Malathion (Ovide) 0.5%
  —Better ovicidal activity, less toxicity than lindane and pyrethrins, but requires 8- to 10-hour application
  —Alcohol base of product causes patient to be flammable while product is on.
—Cortisone creams for secondary dermatitis; decreases pruritis
—Antibiotics for impetiginized lesions

• Pubic lice

—Same pediculicides mentioned are effective
—Second application recommended

GENERAL

• Head lice

—Treat all infested household members.

—Wash bedding, clothes, and cloth toys in hot water.
—Treat combs by washing in hot water, and soaking in pediculicide.
—Seal anything not washable in plastic bags for 10 to 14 days.
—Nit removal not necessary, especially if pediculicide reapplied 1 week later; if nit removal desired, soak hair with white vinegar for 30 to 60 minutes (breaks down chitinous adhesion, easing removal with fine-toothed comb).

• Body lice

—Pediculicide not necessary (insects live in clothing)
—Improve hygiene
—Wash clothing and bedding in hot water
—Dry cleaning is effective, as is hot ironing (particularly along seams of clothing).

• Pubic lice

—Treat sexual contact to prevent reinfestation: pediculosis palpebrum
—Petrolatum ointment applied to lashes three to four times per day for 8 to 10 days
—Removal of nits with fine-toothed comb helpful

DURATION

• As previous, single application usually effective, second application necessary in certain cases

PREVENTION

Head lice is not preventable.

Follow-Up

WHEN TO EXPECT IMPROVEMENT

Risk of transmission promptly reduced after single application, so child should be allowed to return to school or day care. Pruritis may persist for 2 weeks after therapy.

SIGNS TO WATCH FOR

Recurrence of symptoms usually represents treatment failure, most often due to not performing second application of pediculicide, failure to recognize and treat other infested contacts, failure to recognize and treat other sites of infestation, such as perianal hair, axillary hair, or sexual contacts: pediculosis pubis.

PROGNOSIS

• Excellent

PITFALLS

Pediculosis palpebrum: pediculicides are oculotoxic and must be avoided. Use lindane cautiously in patients with seizure disorder.

Common Questions and Answers

Q: Did my child get head lice because my house or my child is not clean enough?
A: No, head lice is unrelated to personal hygiene. Some experts even believe lice prefer a clean scalp.

Q: Should I cut my child's long hair to get the lice out?
A: No, meticulous application of the pediculicides to the entire scalp and pulled through all hair shafts is adequate treatment. Urgently cutting a child's hair to alleviate parental anxiety can be traumatizing to the child.

Q: Can infants become infested with pubic lice (*Phthirus pubis*)?
A: Yes. Although the primary mode of transmission of the crab louse is via sexual contact, it can be transmitted through close personal contact with an infested individual. Small children become infested on the eyebrows or lashes with crab lice.

Q: If children are infested with the head louse, how can items such as stuffed animals or other cloth toys be decontaminated?
A: Machine washable items can be washed in hot water at temperatures 128°C. An alternative method of decontamination is sealing the items in a plastic bag for 10 to 14 days.

Q: Is removal of nits necessary to prevent spread?
A: No. They can be removed from a cosmetic standpoint by using a fine-toothed comb or by soaking the hair in a solution of white vinegar followed by wrapping the head with a towel soaked in the same solution for 30 to 60 minutes.

Q: What is appropriate treatment of infestation of the eyelashes?
A: A petroleum-based ocular ointment should be applied three to four times daily for a period of 10 days. Nits should be removed mechanically from the lashes.

ICD-9-CM 132.9

BIBLIOGRAPHY

Fitzpatrick, Eisen, Wolff, et al., eds. *Dermatology in general medicine*, 4th ed, vol. II. New York: McGraw-Hill, 1993.

Harwitz S, ed. *Clinical pediatric dermatology*, 2nd ed. Philadelphia: WB Saunders, 1993.

Hogan D, Schachner L, Tanglertsaman C. Pediatric dermatology. *Pediatr Clin North Am* 1991; 38(4):953–957.

Meinking TL, Taplin D. Infestations: pediculosis. *Curr Prob Dermatol* 1996;24:157–163.

Authors: Jane Lavelle and Catherine B. Sullivan

Lupus Erythematosis

 Database

DEFINITION

Multisystem, autoimmune disease characterized by the production of antibodies to various components of the cell nucleus, in conjunction with a variety of clinical manifestations. Four of the following 11 criteria, developed by the American College of Rheumatology, must be met to classify a patient with systemic lupus erythematosis (SLE):

- Malar (butterfly) rash
- Discoid rash
- Photosensitivity
- Oral or nasal ulcers
- Arthritis
- Cytopenia: anemia, leukopenia, lymphopenia, or thrombocytopenia
- Neurological disease: seizures or psychosis
- Nephritis: >0.5 g/d proteinuria or cellular casts
- Serositis: pleuritis or pericarditis
- Immunological disorder: antibodies to dsDNA or Sm nuclear antigen, 1LE cell prep, or false-positive serologic test for syphilis
- Positive ANA

CAUSE

Although the exact etiology is unknown, lupus is an autoimmune disease, with genetic, environmental, and hormonal factors playing a role.

PATHOLOGY

- Immune complex-mediated vasculitis, which can occur in almost any organ system.
- Cutaneous lesions in SLE are very variable. They include the erythematous malar or "butterfly" rash, maculopapular rashes (which can occur anywhere on the body), periungual erythema, and mucosal membrane vasculitis.
- Arthritis in SLE can affect large and small joints and is usually symmetric and non-erosive.

- Hematological pathology in lupus includes a hemolytic anemia, anemia of chronic disease, leukopenia, lymphopenia, and thrombocytopenia.
- Neurological impairments in SLE include psychosis, depression, seizures, organic brain syndromes, and peripheral neuropathies.
- Renal pathology includes mesangial changes and glomerulonephritis (focal, diffuse, proliferative, or membraneous). The first signs of renal disease in a lupus patient are often proteinuria and an active urinary sediment. Hypertension, nephrotic syndrome, and renal failure can also occur.
- Serositis is usually seen as pericarditis or pleuritis, but peritonitis can also occur.

EPIDEMIOLOGY

- Approximately 15% of lupus patients have their onset of symptoms in childhood.
- Peak incidence of SLE is between the ages of 15 and 40.
- It has been estimated that 5,000 to 10,000 children in the United States have SLE.
- Female:male ratio is between 5:1 and 10:1.

GENETICS

- Increased frequency of lupus in first-degree family members of patients with SLE.
- Approximately 10% of patients have at least one affected relative.
- Concordance rate of 25% to 50% in monozygotic and 5% in dizygotic twins.

COMPLICATIONS

- Renal disease
- Central nervous system (CNS) involvement
- Infections secondary to the treatments used to control the disease

 Differential Diagnosis

- Systemic juvenile rheumatiod arthritis
- Other vasculitic disorders
- Dermatomyositis
- Fibromyalgia
- Drug-induced lupus

 Data Gathering

HISTORY

Question: Photosensitive?
Significance: A history of photosensitivity or a malar rash is common but not necessary in SLE.

Question: Systemic complaints?
Significance: Many patients have systemic complaints, such as fevers, fatigue, and malaise.

Question: Other complaints?
Significance: Some patients complain of joint pains, Raynaud phenonemon, or ulcers.

 Physical Examination

Finding: Rash
Significance: Vasculitis.

Finding: Oral or nasal ulcers
Significance: Usually painless and often go unnoticed by the patients.

Finding: Arthritis
Significance: Large and small joints

Finding: Pericardial friction rub
Significance: May be heard in a patient with pericarditis.

Finding: Edema
Significance: Secondary to renal disease.

Finding: CNS changes
Significance: Personality changes, psychosis, seizures.

Laboratory Aids

Test: Anti-nuclear antibodies (ANA)
Significance: Found in over 95% patients with SLE; a positive ANA can occur in many diseases.

Test: Anti–double-stranded DNA and anti-Sm.
Significance: Very specific to lupus. In many patients, the anti-DNA levels vary with the activity of disease, so it can be used as a sign for flares.

Test: CBC
Significance: For cytopenia

Test: Urinalysis
Significance: For evidence of renal dysfunction.

Test: Complement levels
Significance: Can also be useful, because they can fall very low during a lupus flare.

Test: PTT
Significance: Patients may also have a prolonged PTT, as the result of anti-phospholipid (APL) antibodies, which are often seen in SLE. Patients with APL antibodies are at an increased risk for thrombotic events, such as deep venous thromboses, strokes, and fetal losses during pregnancies.

 Therapy

• Avoid excessive sun exposure and use sunscreen liberally.
• Non-steroidal anti-inflammatory drugs may be used for the musculoskeletal and mild systemic complaints, although ibuprofen has been noted to cause an aseptic meningitis in a small number of patients with SLE.
• Hydroxychloroquine is often used to help control the cutaneous manifestations of lupus, and steroids are often necessary to control the systemic and renal problems.
• Patients with renal disease who are unresponsive to steroids often need immunosupressive agents, such as cyclophosphamide (monthly intravenous boluses or oral daily doses) or azathioprine.

PITFALLS

Overdiagnosis; a positive ANA in the absence of clinical signs or symptoms of SLE is not lupus.

PROGNOSIS

• Extremely variable. Renal disease and CNS involvement are poor prognostic signs, whereas systemic complaints and joint findings are not.
• The 10-year survival in a child presenting with SLE is over 80%.

 Common Questions and Answers

Q: If a patient has a positive ANA but no clinical signs of SLE, how often should the ANA be followed?
A: A positive ANA will usually remain positive indefinitely, but it has no real significance in the absence of clinical or other laboratory disturbances. Up to 10% of the normal population may have a positive ANA, so there is no need to repeat the test frequently.

Q: Can SLE patients take birth control pills?
A: Yes, but they should use the "mini-pill" (progesterone-only pills).

Q: Can SLE patients with end-stage renal disease obtain renal transplants?
A: Yes, and SLE usually does not recur in the new kidney.

ICD-9-CM 710.0

BIBLIOGRAPHY

Lehman TJA, McCurdy DK, Bernstein BH, et al. Systemic lupus erythematosus in the first decade of life. *Pediatrics* 1989;26:235.

Schumacher HR, ed. *Primer on the rheumatic diseases,* 10th ed. Atlanta: Arthritis Foundation, 1993.

Author: Elizabeth Candell Chalom

Lyme Disease

 Database

DEFINITION

- Multisystemic illness caused by the spirochete *Borrelia burgdorferi*

CAUSE

- The tick-borne spirochete *B. burgdorferi*

PATHOLOGY

- *Borrelia burgdorferi* are injected into the skin with the saliva of the deer tick. The spirochetes first migrate within the skin, forming the typical rash, erythema chronicum migrans. The rash starts as a red macule or papule and then expands to an annular lesion up to 30 cm in diameter with partial central clearing. The spirochetes are then spread hematogenously to other organs, including the heart, joints, and nervous system.
- Joints: Early on, the patient may experience migratory joint pain (often without frank arthritis) myalgias, and painful tendons and bursae. Months later, 60% of untreated patients will develop mono- or pauciarticular arthritis of the large joints, especially the knees. Joint fluid can have a white blood count anywhere from 500 to 110,000 cells/mm³, and the cells are mostly neutrophils.
- Neurological: 14% of untreated patients will develop neurological symptoms of Lyme disease several weeks after the initial rash. These symptoms include aseptic meningitis, cranial nerve palsies (especially facial nerve palsies), mononeuritis, plexitis, and myelitis. Months to years later, chronic neurological symptoms may occur, including a subtle encephalopathy, memory, mood, and sleep disturbances.
- Cardiac: Approximately 8% of untreated patients develop cardiac disease several weeks after the initial Lyme rash. The most common cardiac lesion is atrioventricular block (primary, secondary, or complete). Pericarditis, myocarditis, or pancarditis can also develop. Most of the cardiac manifestations will disappear with or without treatment in a short time (3–4 weeks), but they may later recur. Severe cardiac involvement rarely may be fatal.

EPIDEMIOLOGY

- Lyme disease can affect people of all ages, but one-third to one-half of all cases occur in children and adolescents.
- Male:female ratio is 1:1 to 2:1.
- Lyme disease has now become the most common tick-borne disease in the United States with over 8000 cases/year.
- Onset is most often in the summer months, and the endemic areas are in the northeast, north central, and Pacific coast states.

GENETICS

Chronic Lyme arthritis seems to be associated with an increased incidence of HLA-DR4 and less so with HLA-DR2.

COMPLICATIONS

- Chronic arthritis occurs in approximately 2% of children with the disease.
- Other complications arise from the treatment of Lyme disease, such as cholecystisis secondary to treatment with ceftriaxone, and infections from indwelling catheters used for intravenous antibiotics.

 Differential Diagnosis

- Septic arthritis
- Juvenile rheumatoid arthritis
- Post-infectious arthritis
- Primary fibromyalgia
- Systemic lupus erythematosus

 Data Gathering

HISTORY

Question: Tick bite?
Significance: History of a tick bite can only be elicited in one-third of patients with Lyme disease.

Question: Rash?
Significance: 50% to 80% will have or will recall the typical rash, which is not painful or pruritic, but does feel warm.

Question: Other symptoms?
Significance: Many patients will complain of fatigue, headaches, fevers, chills, myalgias, and arthralgias early on in the disease.

Question: Joint pain?
Significance: Many patients will complain of painful joints early on, and later will develop joint swelling.

 Physical Examination

- The rash of erythema chronicum migrans, if seen, is virtually pathognomonic for Lyme disease. If the patient does not have the rash, there is no physical finding that gives a definite diagnosis of Lyme.
- The physical examination may be completely normal early in the course of the disease.
- The patient may have arthritis, a cranial nerve palsy, or an irregular heart beat.

 Laboratory Aids

Test: ELISA
Significance: Several weeks after the tick bite, antibodies to *B. burgdorferi* can be detected by ELISA. This test, however, has a relatively high false-positive rate and occasionally false-negative results.

Test: Western blot analysis
Significance: A much more specific test. After the first few weeks of the infection, at least five of the following IgG bands must be present for the test to be positive: 18, 21, 28, 30, 34, 39, 41, 45, 58, 66, and 93 kd. During the first 2 weeks of the infection, 2 IgM bands may establish the diagnosis.

Test: A positive ELISA with a negative Western blot
Significance: Usually means the patient does not have Lyme disease and the ELISA was a false-positive.

Therapy

- Initial therapy for early Lyme disease consists of oral antibiotics. For patients over 8 years old, doxycycline or tetracycline is the drug of choice. For younger children or for people who do not tolerate tetracyclines, amoxicillin is preferred, but penicillin (PCN) V is also acceptable. For PCN-allergic patients, erythromycin may be used, but it is less effective.
- For patients with only the skin rash, 14 days of oral antibiotics is usually sufficient. If other symptoms are present, 30 days are recommended.
- For persistent arthritis unresponsive to oral medications, severe carditis, or neurological disease (other than an isolated seventh nerve palsy), intravenous antibiotics become necessary. Ceftriaxone is the drug of choice, but intravenous PCN V may also be used. Treatment should be given for 14 to 21 days.
- Lyme vaccine: Currently only approved for people 15 years and older, the Lyme vaccine is a lipoprotein from *B burgdorferi* (outer surface protein A or Osp A). The vaccine must be given in three sequential injections over the period of one year. After the third injection, the vaccine appears to be 78% effective.

PROGNOSIS

In general, the prognosis for children with Lyme disease is much better than that for adults. Only 2% of children have chronic arthritis at 6 months.

PITFALLS

Incorrect diagnosis: Many patients with vague systemic complaints (fatigue, headaches, arthralgias) are incorrectly diagnosed with Lyme disease, even though their Lyme tests are negative (or the ELISA is mildly positive and the Western blot is negative). These patients are then treated with multiple courses of oral antibiotics; if they do not respond, they are often treated with intravenous ceftriaxone, sometimes for prolonged periods of time. This delays diagnosing the true problem and subjects the patient to the unnecessary risks of long-term antibiotic use and occasionally of central venous lines.

 Common Questions and Answers

Q: What does the deer tick look like?
A: The deer tick is flat, very small (about the size of a pin head), and has eight legs. The adult male is black and the female is red and black. They can grow to 3 times their normal size when they are engorged with blood.

Q: Do all bites from infected deer ticks cause Lyme disease?
A: No. Even infected ticks will not cause Lyme disease if they are attached to the skin for a short period of time. If the tick is attached for less than 12 hours, the chances of transmitting the disease are very low. The longer the tick is attached, the higher the probability of disease transmission.

Q: Should all patients be retested for Lyme disease after a full course of treatment?
A: No. Lyme titers will remain elevated for months to years after adequate treatment for Lyme disease. If the patient's symptoms have resolved, there is no point of rechecking the titer. If the patient is still symptomatic, titers and a Western blot may be checked before starting prolonged or intravenous antibiotic therapy, to look for a rising titer and to be sure the patient truly has Lyme disease. If symptoms remain after intravenous therapy, other diagnoses should be considered.

ICD-9-CM 088.81

BIBLIOGRAPHY

Culp RW, Eichenfield AH, Davidson RS, et al. Lyme arthritis in children. *J Bone Joint Surg* 1987;69B:96.

Dressler F, Whalen JA, Reinhardt BN, et al. Western blotting in the serodiagnosis of Lyme disease. *J Infect Dis* 1993;167:392–400.

Lyme disease surveillance. *MMWR* 1991;40:417.

Pachner AR, Steere AC. The triad of neurologic manifestations of Lyme disease: meningitis, cranial neuritis, and radiculoneuritis. *Neurology* 1985;35(1):47–53.

Shapiro ED. Lyme disease. *Pediatr Rev* 1998;19(5):147–154.

Steere AC, Bartenhagen NH, Craft JE, et al. The early clinical manifestations of Lyme disease. *Ann Intern Med* 1983;99:76.

Steere AC, Bratsford WP, Weinberg M, et al. Lyme carditis: cardiac abnormalities of Lyme disease. *Ann Intern Med* 1980;93:8–16.

Steere AC, Schoen RT, Taylor E. The clinical evolution of Lyme arthritis. *Ann Intern Med* 1987;107:725–731.

Williams CL, Strobino B, Lee A, et al. Lyme disease in childhood: clinical and epidemiologic features of ninety cases. *Pediatr Infect Dis J* 1990;9:10–14.

Author: Elizabeth Candell Chalom

Lymphadenopathy

 ## Database

DEFINITION

- Enlargement of a lymph node larger than 10 mm.
- Additional differentiation should be made between lymphadenopathy, which is enlargement alone, and lymphadenitis, which is enlargement plus signs of inflammation such as erythema and tenderness.

PATHOPHYSIOLOGY

- Lymphadenitis

—Organisms enter the lymph node (either through hematogenous spread of a systemic infection or through the lymphatic drainage of an infected area) and establish a local infection with microabscess formation and suppuration.

- Etiology

—Direct invasion of node with organism regional bacterial (*Streptococcus* species, *Staphylococcus aureus*, *Haemophilus influenzae*, anaerobes).
—Systemic or locally draining pathogens
—Mycobacterium (tuberculous and nontuberculous)
—Cat-scratch disease (*Bartonella henselae*)

- Lymphadenopathy, enlargement may occur by:

—Follicular proliferation as a response to an infectious trigger or as a malignant process.
—Infiltration by metastatic tumor cells or metabolic products
—Reactive lymphadenopathy: proliferation of node in response to infectious trigger in adjacent site or systemically.
—Etiology of lymphadenopathy includes:

INFECTIOUS

- Systemic viral

—Epstein-Barr virus (EBV)
—Cytomegalovirus
—Herpes simplex
—Varicella zoster virus
—Adenovirus
—Human immunodeficiency virus

- Fungal

—Histoplasmosis
—Coccidioidomycosis
—Blastomycosis

- Bacterial

—Syphilis
—Brucellosis
—Tularemia
—Yersiniosis

- Parasitic

—Toxoplasmosis
—Leishmaniasis
—Malaria

NEOPLASTIC

- Primary lymphoid

—Hodgkin disease
—Non-Hodgkin lymphoma

- Metastatic

—Leukemia
—Neuroblastoma
—Rhabdomyosarcoma

- Immunological

—Vasculitis syndromes (systemic lupus erythematosus, rheumatoid arthritis, miscellaneous vasculitides)
—Systemic immune responses (serum sickness, autoimmune hemolytic anemias)
—Chronic granulomatous disease

METABOLIC

- Infiltrative
- Gaucher disease
- Niemann-Pick disease

DRUGS

- Phenytoin
- Isoniazid

MISCELLANEOUS

- Kawasaki syndrome
- Sarcoidosis
- Histiocytosis
- Dermatopathic lymphadenitis
- Kibuchi histiocytic necrotizing lymphadenitis

EPIDEMIOLOGY

- Adenitis is most common in children less than 5 years old.
- Age distribution for reactive adenopathy follows the pattern for each etiology.
- Hodgkin disease is rare younger than 7 years old with incidence increasing until early adulthood, more frequent in whites.

COMPLICATIONS

- Lymphadenitis

—Suppuration may progress to abscess formation and rupture through skin.
—Bacteremia may, especially in immunocompromised host.

- Lymphadenopathy

—Compression of adjacent structures, including vascular structures and airways.

PROGNOSIS

- Related to the prognosis of the underlying illness.
- In simple bacterial adenitis, most recover completely with no sequelae.
- May have scarring if drains.

 ## Differential Diagnosis

Consider the anatomy at each site and whatever variants may occur that would mimic an enlarged node (e.g., a femoral hernia may look like an enlarged inguinal node).

INFECTIOUS

- Abscess in soft tissue site near a node group
- Parotitis

ENVIRONMENTAL

- Insect bite/sting

TRAUMA

- Soft tissue swelling from blunt trauma
- Hematoma

METABOLIC

- Thyroid nodule

CONGENITAL

- Branchial cleft cyst
- Cystic hygroma
- Thyroglossal duct cyst
- Inguinal hernia

 ## Data Gathering

HISTORY

An appropriate history includes a general screening history, as well as anything that would be pertinent for diseases common to the age group (e.g., mononucleosis in an adolescent), body site (e.g., sexual history in inguinal adenopathy), or geography.

DIRECTED REVIEW OF SYSTEMS

Question: Systemic complaints?
Significance: Fever, chills, sweats, weight loss, myalgias, arthralgias, rash.

Question: Dental problems?
Significance: Tooth pain, foul taste, hot/cold sensitivity.

Question: Respiratory problems?
Significance: Upper respiratory infection symptoms, cough, dyspnea.

Question: Gastrointestinal problems?
Significance: Vomiting, diarrhea

Question: Endocrine?
Significance: Heat/cold intolerance

Question: Musculoskeletal?
Significance: Joint stiffness, pain, swelling

Question: Social?
Significance: Pets (especially kittens for cat-scratch disease); travel: especially foreign, but domestic travel for certain diseases is important (e.g., Southern California for coccidiodiomycosis); ill contacts; sexual history: unprotected intercourse, prior sexually transmitted diseases.

Physical Examination

Finding: Vital signs
Significance: Temperature, heart rate, respirations, blood pressure.

Finding: Nodes
Significance:

• Examine not just the most noticeably enlarged node, but all other regions as well to determine if this is a localized or systemic process; measure the size of each enlarged node(s) and characterize as hard or soft, fixed or mobile, and tender or non-tender. Serial measurements of nodes that are not of an obvious infectious etiology should be made weekly.
• When palpating for lymphadenopathy, gently roll the node under your fingertips to best appreciate texture and mobility.
• Have the patient in as relaxed a position as possible to appreciate nodes that are associated with large muscle groups (e.g., the neck).
• ENT: Pharyngitis commonly gives lymphadenopathy.
• Neck: Careful exam is necessary for congenital anomalies, such as skin dimples being suspicious for branchial cleft cysts.
• Chest: Adventitious sounds may indicate a systemic process such as histoplasmosis.
• Abdomen: The liver and spleen, as part of the reticuloendothelial system are usually enlarged when there is a systemic process leading to lymphadenopathy; abdominal masses may be a clue that the enlarged nodes contain metastatic disease.

Laboratory Aids

• None needed in most cases initially

Test: Complete blood count and blood culture
Significance: In cases where the patient appears systemically ill and a bacterial infection is suspected.

• In cases where the lymphadenopathy does not resolve or improve within a week, more specific testing should be guided by risk factors as assessed by the history and physical.

Test: EBV serology
Significance: In a patient with fever, pharyngitis and splenomegaly.

Test: Toxoplasmosis serology
Significance: In a patient with a cat and the appropriate clinical presentation.

Test: Lymph node biopsy
Significance: To rule out malignancy, indicated when:

• No obvious infectious etiology (e.g., lymphadenitis present or EBV serologies not suggestive of acute infection), especially if rapidly enlarging.
• Persistent supraclavicular adenopathy
• Adenopathy associated with weight loss or persistent fever and sweats

• Fixation of the lymph node to the overlying skin
• Presence of other symptoms suggesting malignancy (e.g., Horner syndrome suggestive of neuroblastoma).

RADIOGRAPHIC STUDIES

• In general, imaging techniques are not helpful in defining lymphadenopathy.
• CXR is helpful to look for hilar nodes in association with regional adenopathy.
• CT is helpful to look for hilar, other thoracic, abdominal, and pelvic adenopathy. These are indicated only if the etiology is not able to be determined through history, physical, and laboratory work-up or if malignancy is suspected.

Therapy

• Nodes with suppuration may require incision and drainage, especially if the patient is toxic appearing, there has been no response to antibiotics, or lymph node abscess is suspected.
• If there is a strong suspicion for a mycobacterial etiology, either tubercular or non-tubercular, simple aspiration often leads to fistulous tracts, so the patient should be referred to a surgeon for complete excision.

DRUG

• Lymphadenitis

—If underlying disorder is present, guide your antibiotic choice accordingly (i.e., documented staphylococcal infection distal to node group should be treated with an anti-staphylococcal agent)
—Empiric therapy: cephalexin 50 mg/kg/d in 4 divided doses or cefadroxil 30 mg/kg/d in 2 divided doses
—Penicillin-allergic patients: erythromycin 50 mg/kg/d in 4 divided doses

• Lymphadenopathy

—Treat underlying disease if treatable (e.g., penicillin for syphilis)

Follow-up

• Lymphadenitis

—Local signs of inflammation often increase within the first 24 hours of treatment, but should be improving within 24 hours
—Inflammation should be resolved within 1 week, although the node may remain enlarged for another 6 to 8 weeks

• Lymphadenopathy

—Persistence will depend on resolution of the underlying cause [e.g., lymphadenopathy from acute EBV infection will follow the intensity of the other symptoms (fever, sore throat)]. With resolution of these symptoms, lymphadenopathy may persist for several months.

SIGNS TO WATCH FOR

• Worsening of erythema, pain, or swelling on antibiotics may mean that there is an underlying abscess or that the choice of empiric antibiotics is not appropriate for the underlying organism
• Persistent fever or signs of toxicity (lethargy, tachycardia) may mean bacteremia
• Spontaneous drainage of node and formation of fistulous tract may indicate a mycobacterial infection
• "Benign" appearing node that persists beyond 2 months in absence of other symptoms or with presence of fever, chills, and weight loss may indicate malignancy.

PITFALLS

• Most episodes of lymphadenitis and lymphadenopathy are not an emergency, so a rational treatment and evaluation plan can be developed, with a minimum number of labs and interventions required in the initial stages.
• Watchful follow-up will key the physician to which nodes will require additional evaluation.
• Children in growth phases often have hypertrophy of lymphatic tissue, which can be confused for lymphadenopathy.
• Enlarged nodes may persist after trivial viral infections.

Common Questions and Answers

Q: In an otherwise well child, who presents with isolated cervical adenopathy, how extensive an initial work-up should be done?
A: Assuming that the node is soft, small, mobile, and without inflammation, the initial evaluation would be a baseline measurement and a thorough history and physical exam to uncover underlying causes. If this is unrewarding, a plan should be made for follow-up in several weeks. Acceptable alternatives other than waiting are a trial of empiric antibiotics and a complete blood count. The parent should be reassured that this may be normal and advised to return sooner if there is any worsening.

Q: How soon should I see a child with adenitis for follow-up?
A: In a child who is non-toxic appearing, but has significant inflammation, since the physical examination findings may worsen within the first 24 hours, it is best to see the child in 48 to 72 hours if the node is not improving. Parents should be instructed to return sooner if the child develops worsening systemic symptoms or appears toxic.

BIBLIOGRAPHY

Marcy S. Infections of the lymph nodes of the head and neck. *Pediatr Infect Dis J* 1983;2:397–405.

Margileth A. Sorting out the causes of lymphadenopathy. *Contemp Pediatr* 1995;12:23–40.

Suskind DL, Handler SD, Tom LH, et al. Nontubercular mycobacterial cervical adenitis. *Clin Pediatr* 1997;36(7)403–409.

Author: Jill A. Foster

Lymphedema

Database

DEFINITION

- Accumulation of interstitial fluid in part of the body (usually an extremity) secondary to malformation or malfunction of the lymphatic system.
- Divided into primary and secondary forms:

—Primary: usually an isolated finding, thought to result from abnormal development of the lymphatics. Deep tissues and muscle not affected.

—Primary lymphedema often divided into congenital lymphedema: presenting in the first few months of life.

—Lymphedema praecox: presenting from late in first year of life to early adulthood (20–35 years of age)

—Lymphedema tarda: presenting in adulthood (i.e., after 20–35 years of life).

—Secondary: the etiology of lymphatic damage has been identified, causes include surgery, neoplasm (primary or metastatic), parasitic infestation, infection, irradiation, and trauma.

PATHOPHYSIOLOGY

- Represents state of overproduction or decreased removal of lymph.
- Initially edema is pitting. Chronic edema may result in fibrosis.

GENETICS

- No increased rate of congenital anomalies of other organ systems, but may be associated with other vascular malformations.
- Many genetic disorders are associated with lymphedema: Fabry disease, Milroy (congenital familial lymphedema with ocular findings), Meige disease (familial lymphedema praecox), and Down, Turner, Noonan, yellow nail, Klippel-Tránaunay-Weber, pes cavus, and other syndromes.
- Inheritance can be autosomal dominant, recessive or sex-linked.

EPIDEMIOLOGY

- Most lymphedema in childhood is primary lymphedema.
- Congenital lymphedema comprises 10% of primary lymphedema cases; lymphedema praecox, 71%; and lymphedema tarda, 19%.
- Incidence of 1.5 per 100,000 in children less than 20 years.
- Female : male ratio in congenital lymphedema close to 1 : 1; in praecox and tarda, 2 : 1 to 9 : 1 (64–90% female).

COMPLICATIONS

- Cellulitis and lymphangitis occur in one-fourth to one-half of patients over long-term follow-up
- Lymphangiosarcoma extremely rare
- Enormous psychological burden; nearly universal
- Limitations in job-related and leisure activities
- Fibrosis

PROGNOSIS

- Edema persists throughout life.
- Natural history: plateau in severity of edema after an initial few years of progression in 50%, slow constant progression in 50%.
- Edema of contralateral extremity (usually leg) develops in up to 10% over prolonged follow-up.
- Chronic inflammation and edema ultimately lead to fibrosis and induration of the involved area.

Differential Diagnosis

INFECTION

- Cellulitis
- Lymphangitis

TUMORS

- Pelvic mass

METABOLIC

- Cushing disease

ANATOMICAL

- Venous stasis
- Deep venous thrombosis
- Hemihypertrophy
- Atrioventricular fistula

MISCELLANEOUS

- Heart failure
- Nephrosis
- Cirrhosis
- Hypoproteinemia
- Reflex sympathetic dystrophy
- Multiple enchondromatosis

Data Gathering

HISTORY

Question: Cellulitis or trauma?
Significance: Many report prior history of cellulitis or trauma of the affected limb is common.

Question: Edema?
Significance: Subacute or chronic painless swelling of one leg in an otherwise healthy pubertal female is classic for lymphedema praecox.

Question: Swelling?
Significance: Usually painless, and extremity distal to surgical or trauma site.

Physical Examination

- Subcutaneous tissue filled with fluid resulting in pitting edema
- Chronic inflammation leads to fibrosis, which corresponds to a change from pitting to non-pitting edema and induration.
- Hair loss and hyperkeratosis of the affected limb develops over time.
- Pain in affected limb uncommon.

Laboratory Aids

Test: Urine dip
Significance: Rule out nephrosis

Test: Serum total protein and albumin
Significance: Rule out hypoproteinemia

RADIOGRAPHIC STUDIES

Test: Ultrasound, CT, or MRI of pelvis
Significance: Useful to rule out obstructive pelvic lesions, which may be otherwise inapparent.

Test: Doppler ultrasound
Significance: Helpful when deep venous thrombosis is diagnostic possibility

Test: Lymphangiography or radionuclide lymphangiography
Significance: When history and physical examination yield a diagnosis of uncomplicated primary lymphedema in childhood, it is controversial as to whether or not these tests are necessary. Most feel it adds little to diagnosis and treatment.

Test: Venography and biopsy
Significance: Considered unnecessary for diagnosis.

Therapy

- Therapy should be instituted as soon as possible and before fibrosis develops.
- Goals: maintain or possibly decrease status of swelling, decrease risk of infections, minimize skin changes.
- Extremity elevation and compression (e.g., Jobst stocking, ace wrap) recommended long-term for all patients.
- Meticulous skin care.
- Pneumatic machines or manual massage: short-term recommendation to achieve greatest reduction of edema.
- Exercise (walking and swimming) thought to enhance lymphatic return.
- Cellulitis and lymphangitis treated with hospitalization and intravenous antibiotics.
- Complete decongestive physiotherapy is a comprehensive treatment program offered at few selected centers, but seems to be effective in reducing swelling and maintaining the reduction.
- Diuretics: not used in children and adolescents; efficacy debated.
- Surgery has one of two goals: removal of excess edematous tissue or attempts to restore lymph drainage; both may decrease the rate of infections but have poor cosmetic results and are recommended only for those with uncontrolled swelling with significant disability.
- Prophylactic antibiotic use is indicated for patients with recurrent cellulitis or lymphangitis.
- Compression and elevation are lifelong measures.

Follow-Up

Some edema reduction achieved with pneumatic compression or massage over short term, but persistent use of elevation and compression stockings necessary to maintain benefit.

SIGNS TO WATCH FOR

Fever, chills, red streaks on the extremity, inflamed lymph nodes all point to cellulitis or lymphangitis.

PREVENTION

- Primary disease cannot be prevented, but progression should be minimized with therapies listed here.
- Secondary disease can be prevented by altering surgical approaches to diseases that emphasize sparing of lymphatics and nodes.
- Skin care and properly fitting shoes must be emphasized to avoid skin breakdown, which can lead to cellulitis and/or lymphangitis.

PITFALLS

- Systemic reactions to lymphangiography are not uncommon.
- Compliance with compression stockings is poor because they are often hot and uncomfortable.

Common Questions and Answers

Q: Is the swelling going to go away?
A: No, this is a lifelong disorder in most cases.

Q: Could this have been prevented?
A: No, primary lymphedema is most likely due to abnormal embryological development.

Q: If the lymph channels have been abnormal since birth, why does the swelling present during adolescence?
A: No one really knows; hormones may affect lymphedema.

ICD-9-CM 457.1

BIBLIOGRAPHY

Greenlee R, Hoyme H, Witte M, et al. Developmental disorders of the lymphatic system. *Lymphology* 1993;26:156–168.

Ko DSC, Lerner R, Klose G, Cosimi AB. Effective treatment of lymphedema of the extremities. *Arch Surg* 1998;133:452–458.

Lewis JM, Wald ER. Lymphedema praecox. *J Pediatr* 1984;104:641–648.

Smeltzer DM, Stickler GB, Schirger A. Primary lymphedema in children and adolescents: a follow-up study and review. *Pediatrics* 1985; 76:206–218.

Wright NB, Carty HML. The swollen leg and primary lymphedema. *Arch Dis Child* 1994;71: 44–49.

Author: Laura N. Sinai

Malaria

 Database

DEFINITION

• Malaria is a febrile illness due to the *Plasmodium* species of protozoan parasites. *P. vivax, P. malariae, P. falciparum,* and *P. ovale* are the species that infect humans.

• Malaria was described by the earliest medical writers in China, Assyria, and India, and by the fifth century BC, Hippocrates was able to describe the characteristic fever patterns and clinical manifestations of the disease.

PATHOPHYSIOLOGY

• Two discrete stages of the *Plasmodium* life cycle: sexual stage that develops in the female Anopheles mosquito providing the sporozoites to the host, and asexual stage that occurs in the human, first in the liver producing merozoites and then in the erythrocytes as trophozoites. Trophozoites cause red cell hemolysis, therefore, releasing more merozoites to infect other erythrocytes.

• With the exception of infants with the disease, the cycle is characteristically synchronous and periodic giving the typical tertian periodicity seen in *P. falciparum, vivax,* and *ovale* and the quartan periodicity seen in *P. malariae.*

• Infection from a contaminated blood transfusion or needle can occur; congenital malaria has also been reported.

• Hemolytic anemia, the most common disease finding, can be severe, especially in *P. falciparum;* the predominant mechanism is due to intravascular hemolysis from fragile erythrocytes rather than solely rupture from infected cells.

• Cerebral malaria, the most serious consequence of malaria noted in *P. falciparum* infection, is caused by occlusion of the cerebral microvasculature from infected red cells.

• Tropical splenomegaly syndrome seen in chronic infections caused by *P. malariae* produces splenomegaly, hepatomegaly, portal hypertension, and pancytopenia. In *P. vivax* malaria, acute splenomegaly can induce rupture.

• Blackwater fever is due to acute renal failure caused by accumulation of hemoglobin in the renal tubules resulting in hemoglobinuria with dark urine. This often occurs after repeated attacks of *P. falciparum.*

• Other diseases such as pulmonary edema, distributive shock, dysentery, nephrotic syndrome have been described.

GENETICS

• Sickle cell disease and trait confers protection against malaria by two postulated mechanisms: release of a toxic form of heme from these erythrocytes that possess antimalarial properties; the hemoglobin S erythrocyte tends to lose potassium required for ATPase activation, thereby depriving the parasites of nutrients.

• Thalassemia and G6PD deficiency may also provide innate resistance to malaria.

EPIDEMIOLOGY

• High-risk areas of the world for malaria include parts of Central and South America, Africa, and Asia under tropical climates.

• Malaria is a major cause of infant death in the tropical regions of the world.

• Infection transmission is acquired through the life of the female Anopheles mosquito but can also occur through contaminated blood transfusions or needles as well as be acquired congenitally.

• The most common infecting species are *P. falciparum* and *P. vivax.*

• *P. vivax* and *P. ovale* are associated with relapsing disease because of the persistent hepatic stage of the infection.

COMPLICATIONS

• *P. falciparum* tends to cause more severe disease, and morbidity is significantly increased due to the multiorgan system involvement.

• Chronic relapses occur from *P. vivax* and ovale infections and can occur during periods ranging from every few weeks to a few months.

• In the pregnant patient, increased perinatal mortality has not been reported with malaria in stable, endemic regions. However, for semi-immune or non-immune mothers, transplacental antibodies may be lacking, and the risk of congenital infection may be higher in this subgroup.

PROGNOSIS

• The prognosis is dependent on the *Plasmodium* species, relapsing nature of the disease, chloroquine resistance, and age of the patient. The infant with *P. falciparum* infection accounts for most of the mortality due to malaria.

 Differential Diagnosis

Because there are few clearly distinctive clinical features of malaria, it can be easily overlooked if a good travel history is not obtained in any child with prolonged fever.

 Laboratory Aids

Test: Hemoglobin
Significance: Hemolytic anemia due to intravascular hemolysis as well as direct red cell infection is present initially as mild then more severe, depending on the *Plasmodium* species.

Test: WBC
Significance: Leukocyte counts are usually normal or low; there is no eosinophilia. Thrombocytopenia due to liver and splenic sequestration occurs in the more severe cases.

Test: Peripheral smear
Significance: Thick and thin peripheral blood smears are required for definitive diagnosis (thick smears enable better sensitivity if the parasitemia is low; thin smears provide for species identification). If initial smears are negative, repeat specimens should be obtained in 6 to 12 hours to confirm a truly negative result.

Test: Quantitative Buffy Coat (QBC) analysis
Significance: Available as a rapid screening test, but confirmation by blood smears is still necessary.

Test: Serologic tests
Significance: Using indirect immunofluorescent assays may be helpful but have a low sensitivity in the early phases of acute infections.

Test: PCR
Significance: Other tests using polymerase chain reaction (PCR) techniques are being studied and may be useful in the near future.

Physical Examination

- High fevers, headache, chills, sweating, and rigors are common presenting findings.
- Other features such as cough, irritability, anorexia, vomiting, abdominal pain, back pain, and arthralgias may also be present.
- Periodicity of fever is less commonly seen in young children and is dependent on the *Plasmodium* species.
- Hepatosplenomegaly may be present and is more likely observed in chronic infections due to *P. falciparum*.
- Cerebral malaria will manifest with signs of increased intracranial pressure with encephalopathy and seizures.

 ## Therapy

- For all *Plasmodium* species except chloroquine-resistant *P. falciparum,* chloroquine phosphate is recommended at a dose of 10 mg/kg PO (maximum 600 mg), then 5 mg/kg PO in 6 hours (maximum 300 mg), then 5 mg/kg PO in 24 and 48 hours (maximum 300 mg).
- If parenteral therapy is necessary, treatment with quinidine gluconate, 10 mg/kg IV initial dose (maximum 600 mg) over 2 hours followed by 0.02 mg/kg/min infusion until oral therapy can be started.
- For chloroquine-resistant *P. falciparum,* quinine sulfate, 8 mg/kg/d PO three times a day for 3 days plus tetracycline, 5 mg/kg PO four times a day for 7 days (maximum 1 g/d) is recommended.
- Alternative regimens include mefloquine, pyrimethamine-sulfadoxine (Fansidar), or clindamycin.
- Primaquine phosphate is used for the prevention of *P. vivax* and *ovale* relapses but should not be used in patients with G6PD deficiency or in pregnancy.
- Consultation with a pharmacist is recommended to identify other possible contraindications and warnings associated with these medications.

 ## Follow-Up

- Delay in the diagnosis of malaria has been shown to increase the morbidity and mortality up to 20-fold compared with diagnosis and treatment within 24 hours of presentation.
- If treated promptly, even *P. falciparum* malaria will respond well to current treatment options.

PREVENTION

- In the hospital setting, universal precautions should be followed.
- Control measures are targeted toward control of the Anopheles mosquito population, and protective measures such as remaining in well-screened areas, and wearing protective clothing should be advised. Use of insect repellents such as DEET is recommended. However, in children less than 2 years, concentration of less than 10%, and concentrations less than 35% for the older child is recommended.
- Chemoprophylaxis for travelers in endemic areas should begin 1 week before arrival, once weekly during the period of exposure, and then 4 weeks after leaving the endemic region.
- Chloroquine is the drug of choice except in resistant areas; mefloquine is then the drug of choice. Contraindications to mefloquine use include children less than 15 kg in weight, first trimester pregnancy, patients taking beta-blockers or other drugs altering cardiac conduction, patients with seizures or psychosis and patients requiring fine motor skill performance. Doxycycline or chloroquine plus proguanil are alternatives to mefloquine.
- Travelers should use pyrimethamine-sulfadoxine (Fansidar) if a febrile illness occurs while on chloroquine and access to medical care is not readily available.

PITFALLS

Failure to obtain a thorough travel history to determine exposure risk to developing malaria can delay the diagnosis and appropriate therapy.

 ## Common Questions and Answers

Q: What is the optimal drug regimen for the young infant or child or the lactating or pregnant female?
A: The only drug not contraindicated in any of these patients is chloroquine. In chloroquine-resistant areas, mefloquine has been shown to be safe in the second and third trimesters. If potential benefit justifies the potential embryotoxic and teratogenic risk to the fetus, its use in the first trimester is justified. Mefloquine is excreted in breast milk, and its safety has not been well established in young infants.

Q: Is there a vaccine available to prevent malaria?
A: Although the possibility of vaccination against malaria continues to attract interest, no adequate vaccination is available. Recent advances in the technology for introducing malarial DNA coding into bacteria may lead to an effective vaccine in the future.

Q: How can I determine if my patient is traveling to an area that has chloroquine-resistant malaria?
A: The Centers for Disease Control and Prevention has an automated traveler's hotline accessible from a touch tone phone 24 hours a day, 7 days a week at (404) 332-4559. Questions can also be faxed to (404) 332-4565. The Internet address for information is www.cdc.gov.

ICD-9-CM 084.6

BIBLIOGRAPHY

Emanuel B, Aronson N, Shulman S. Malaria in children in Chicago. *Pediatrics* 1993;92:83–85.

Fitch CD. Malaria. In: Feigin RD, Cherry JD, eds. *Pediatric infectious diseases,* 3rd ed. Philadelphia: WB Saunders, 1992:2042–2057.

Katz M. Treatment of protozoan infections: malaria. *Pediatr Infect Dis J* 1983;2:475–480.

Peter G, Halsey NA, Marcuse EK, Pickering LK. Malaria. In: *1994 Red book: report of the Committee on Infectious Diseases,* 23rd ed. Elk Grove Village, IL: American Academy of Pediatrics, 1994:301–307.

Silver HM. Malarial infection during pregnancy. *Infect Dis Clin North Am* 1997;11:99–107.

Steele RW. Malaria in children. *Adv Pediatr Infect Dis* 1997;12:325–349.

White NJ, Miller KD, Churchill FC, et al. Chloroquine treatment of severe malaria in children. *N Engl J Med* 1988;319:1493–1500.

Author: Philip V. Scribano

Mastoiditis

Database

DEFINITION

Mastoiditis is an infection of the mastoid air cells that can range from an asymptomatic illness to a severe life-threatening disease.

CAUSES

• Acute mastoiditis is caused by an extension of the inflammation of acute otitis media into the mastoid air cells.
• The bacteria causing acute mastoiditis are usually group A β-hemolytic streptococci and *Streptococcus pneumoniae* followed by *Staphylococcus aureus.*
• Chronic mastoiditis is usually caused by *Staphylococcus aureus,* anaerobic bacteria, enteric bacteria, and *Pseudomonas aeruginosa.* Chronic mastoiditis is usually a multiple organism infection.
• Unusual agents of chronic mastoiditis include *Mycobacterium tuberculosis,* atypical mycobacterium, *Nocardia asteroides,* and *Histoplasma capsulatum.*
• Cholesteatomas may contribute to the development of mastoiditis by impeding mastoid drainage of pus or erosion of underlying bone.

PATHOLOGY

• The mastoid process is the posterior portion of the temporal bone and consists of interconnecting air cells that drain superiorly into the middle ear. Because these mastoid air cells connect with the middle ear, all cases of acute otitis media are associated with some mastoid inflammation.
• Acute mastoiditis develops when the accumulation of purulent exudate in the middle ear does not drain through the Eustachian tube or through a perforated tympanic membrane but spreads to the mastoid.
• Acute mastoiditis can progress to a coalescent phase when the air cells are destroyed which may then progress to subperiosteal abscess or to chronic mastoiditis.

EPIDEMIOLOGY

• At the start of the twentieth century, about one-half the cases of otitis media developed into a coalescent mastoiditis. The routine use of antibiotics for otitis media and aggressive management of treatment failures has decreased this incidence to 0.2% to 0.4%.
• It is unusual to see mastoiditis in the very young because of incomplete pneumatization of the mastoid air cells.

COMPLICATIONS

• The mastoid's proximity to many important structures can result in serious complications from extension of infection or as a response to the inflammatory process.
• Intracranial complications include meningitis and extradural, subdural, or brain parenchymal abscesses.
• Venous sinus thrombophlebitis results from extension of disease to the sigmoid or lateral sinus. Sepsis, increased intracranial pressure, septic emboli may result.
• Facial nerve palsy is usually unilateral and can be permanent.
• Labyrinthitis or osteomyelitis may result from extension of the infection into adjacent bones. A subperiosteal abscess is an infection to the overlying mastoid periosteum.
• Hearing loss can occur from destruction of the ossicles or from labyrinthine damage.
• Bezold abscess is a deep neck abscess along medial sternocleidomastoid muscle that develops when the infection erodes through the tip of the mastoid bone and dissects down tissue planes.

PROGNOSIS

• Mastoiditis has a good prognosis if it is treated early. However, intracranial extension of mastoiditis can lead to permanent neurological deficits and death.
• Chronic mastoiditis can lead to irreversible hearing loss.

Differential Diagnosis

• Parotitis and mumps can look like mastoiditis, but the swelling is over the parotid rather than postauricular.
• Postauricular lymphadenopathy or cellulitis can be distinguished from mastoiditis with a careful physical examination.
• External otitis or a furuncle in the ear canal may produce pain or ear drainage but are not accompanied by the fever and systemic toxicity of mastoiditis.
• Leukemia, lymphoma, benign and malignant tumors of the mastoid must also be considered in the differential diagnosis of mastoiditis.

Data Gathering

HISTORY

• Symptoms include fever, ear pain, and postauricular swelling.
• Past medical history usually includes recent and often a chronic history of treatment for otitis media.
• Intracranial extension should be suspected if there is lethargy, a stiff neck, headache, focal neurological symptoms, seizures, visual changes, or persistent fevers despite appropriate antibiotic treatment.
• Labyrinthitis initially presents with tinnitus and nausea, which can progress to vomiting, vertigo, nystagmus, and loss of balance.

Physical Examination

• The ear may protrude away from the scalp. In infants, the ear protrudes out and is displaced down.
• The tympanic membrane is hyperemic with decreased mobility.
• The mastoid process is tender with soft tissue swelling and erythema. Can proceed to postauricular fluctuance.
• In chronic mastoiditis, the fever and postauricular swelling are often not present and the patient presents with ear pain, persistent drainage or hearing loss.

Laboratory Aids

Test: Middle ear aspirate obtained by myringotomy
Significance: Should be sent for Gram stain and cultures for aerobic and anaerobic bacteria. There is some correlation between middle ear bacterial cultures and mastoid cultures.

Test: Radiographs
Significance: Reveal haziness of the mastoid air cells and can show bony destruction in more advanced disease. However, radiographs are unreliable and can be falsely normal as well as falsely abnormal.

Test: CT
Significance: Helpful in the confirmation of the diagnosis, identification of coalescence or a subperiosteal abscess, and evaluation for concomitant intracranial complications. However, intracranial complications are best seen with MRI.

Test: Lumbar puncture
Significance: Must be performed in any child with symptoms of meningitis.

Test: Complete blood count with differential
Significance: May show a leukocytosis with a neutrophil predominance.

Test: Erythrocyte sedimentation rate
Significance: May be elevated in acute mastoiditis but is usually normal in the chronic stage.

Test: A purified protein derivative (PPD)
Significance: Should be placed if tuberculosis is suspected.

 Therapy

- Middle ear drainage is essential and, therefore, a myringotomy with or without tube placement should be performed early.
- Parenteral antibiotics are chosen on the basis of the most likely organisms. In acute mastoiditis, oxacillin (150 mg/kg/d in 4 doses) or cefotaxime (150–200 mg/kg/d in 4 doses) can be used. Broad-spectrum coverage such as oxacillin and gentamicin is recommended for chronic mastoiditis. If *Mycobacterium tuberculosis* is suspected, then anti-tuberculosis therapy should be started.
- Indications for surgical intervention include subperiosteal abscess, coalescence, facial nerve palsy, meningitis, intracranial abscess, venous thrombosis, or persistent symptoms despite adequate antibiotic treatment.

PREVENTION

- Appropriate early treatment of otitis media as well as timely follow up to identify treatment failures.
- Avoid factors that predispose to otitis media, including smoking and bottle feeding.
- Early recognition of mastoiditis decreases the risk of intracranial complications.

 Follow-Up

- If patients respond quickly to parenteral therapy, they can complete a 3-week course with oral antibiotics and weekly follow-up visits.
- Audiograms should be performed later to screen for hearing loss.

 Common Questions and Answers

Q: Do all children with mastoiditis need a CT scan of the head if mastoiditis is suspected?
A: No, in general if the child with mastoiditis has mild swelling, no fluctuence of the mastoid, and responds to therapy, no CT scan is needed. A patient who appears toxic, is not responding to appropriate antibiotic therapy, or one suspects is a surgical candidate should undergo additional imaging studies.

Q: Should all children with mastoiditis be admitted to the hospital?
A: Yes, in general, admission with intravenous antibiotics and ENT evaluation is warranted to rule out complications.

ICD-9-CM 383.00 (acute)
383.1 (chronic)

BIBLIOGRAPHY

Alford BR, Cohn AM. Complications of suppurative otitis media and mastoiditis. In: Paparella MM, Shumrick DA, eds. *Otolaryngology*, 2nd ed. Philadelphia: WB Saunders, 1980:1490–1509.

Bitar CN, Kluka EA, Steele RW. Mastoiditis in children. *Clin Pediatr* 1996;35:391–395.

Lewis K, Cherry JD. Mastoiditis. In: Feigin RD, Cherry JD, eds. *Textbook of pediatric infectious diseases*. Philadelphia: WB Saunders, 1992: 189–195.

Spiegel JH, Lustig LR, Lee KC, Murr AH, Schindler RA. Contemporary presentation and management of a spectrum of mastoid abscesses. *Laryngoscope* 1998;108:882–888.

Authors: Frances M. Nadel and Rosemary Casey

Measles (Rubeola—First Disease)

 Database

DEFINITION

Measles is an exanthematous disease, which has a relatively predictable course making diagnosis clinically possible. The disease involves fever, cough, conjunctivitis, or coryza with an erythematous rash, which has a characteristic progression.

CAUSES

Measles is an RNA virus classified as a morbillivirus in the *Paramyxovirus* family. It was first isolated in 1954 in human and monkey kidney tissue cultures.

PATHOPHYSIOLOGY

The infection is probably acquired by inoculation of the nose or conjunctivae.

EPIDEMIOLOGY

- Measles is a highly contagious disease in non-immune persons.
- Transmission of measles is thought to occur mainly by microaerosolized droplets of respiratory secretions.
- Hospital or clinic waiting rooms (especially pediatric emergency department waiting rooms) have been identified as a major risk accounting for up to 45% of the known exposures in this setting.
- Prior to the 1963 licensure of vaccine, approximately 500,000 cases of measles (330 cases per 100,000) population were reported annually.
- In 1983, there were only 0.7 cases per 100,000 population. However, in 1990, 27,672 cases were reported with 89 deaths.
- The reason for the 1989–1991 outbreak was failure to adequately vaccinate preschool-aged children.
- Patients are contagious from 1 to 2 days before onset of symptoms until 5 days after the appearance of the rash.
- The incubation period is generally 8 to 12 days from exposure to onset of symptoms and about 14 days until the appearance of rash.

COMPLICATIONS

- Complication rates in 1989–1990 outbreaks that occurred throughout the country was 23% and included diarrhea (9%), otitis media (7%), pneumonia (6%), and encephalitis (0.1%). Encephalitis, which can lead to permanent neurological sequelae, occur in 1 of every 1,000 cases reported in the United States.
- In 1990, approximately 18% to 20% of patients required hospitalization many for either dehydration or pneumonia.
- In patients with poor nutrition, such as found in developing countries, mortality is higher.
- Croup, pneumonia, myocarditis, pericarditis, encephalitis, and disseminated intravascular coagulation (black measles)
- Subacute sclerosis panencephalitis (SSPE) occurs in 1 per 100,000 children with naturally occurring measles. After an incubation period of several years (mean 10.8), a progressive encephalopathy develop among unvaccinated children. Patients with SSPE are not infectious.

PROGNOSIS

- Mortality in the modern outbreak of 1989–1990 occurred in 3 of every 1,000 cases in the United States.
- Case-fatality rates are increased in immunocompromised children.

ASSOCIATED DISEASES

- Typical measles
- Modified measles

—Occurs naturally in infants younger than 9 months of age because of the presence of transplacental antibody or as a result of administration of immunoglobulin to an exposed susceptible child.
—The illness is similar to typical measles but is generally mild. The patient may be afebrile and the rash may last only 1 to 2 days.

- Atypical measles

—Occurs as a result of a hypersensitivity reaction to measles infection in those who received killed virus vaccine between 1963–1967 and are, subsequently, exposed to wild virus.
—This group of young adults (second and third decade of life) become quite ill, with sudden onset of fever from 103°F to 105°F associated with headache. The rash, unlike typical measles, appears first on the distal extremities and progresses in a cephalad direction.
—Virtually all those with atypical measles have respiratory distress with clinical and radiographic signs of pneumonia often with pleural effusions.
—Diagnosis depends on recognition and on acute and convalescent measles antibody titers.
—The differential diagnoses included meningococcemia, RMSF, and toxic shock syndrome.

 Differential Diagnosis

- Steven-Johnson syndrome
- Kawasaki disease
- Viral exanthem
- With a careful history and physical examination it is almost always possible to rule in measles and rule out other possibilities.

 Data Gathering

HISTORY

- Case definition from the Centers for Disease Control and Prevention includes:

—Generalized rash lasting 3 days or longer
—A temperature of 101°F or higher and cough, coryza, or conjunctivitis

- The mean incubation period is 10 days (range: 8–21 days)
- The prodrome of measles lasts 2 to 4 days and begins with symptoms of upper respiratory infection and fever up to 104°F. General malaise, conjunctivitis with photophobia, and cough increasing in severity over this period.
- During the prodrome, Koplik spots (white spots on the buccal mucosa) appear.
- The rash appears on the face (often the nape of the neck, initially) and abdomen 14 days after exposure. The rash is erythematous and maculopapular and spreads from the head to the feet.
- After 3 to 4 days, the rash begins to clear leaving a brownish discoloration and fine scaling.
- Fever usually resolves by the fourth day of rash.
- Pharyngitis, cervical lymphadenopathy, and splenomegaly may accompany the rash.

Laboratory Aids

• The course of typical measles follows a predictable pattern and, therefore, laboratory studies to confirm infection are rarely indicated.
• At the beginning of a suspected case, confirmation of the index cases is important.
• Nasopharynx culture: Virus may be cultured from the nasopharynx if inoculated into tissue culture within 24 hours of the onset of rash.
• Monoclonal antibody immunofluorescence cells test: Rapid detection of measles virus from nasal secretions is also possible. Measles infected with epithelial cells will demonstrate fluorescence. However, after the third day of rash, detection of virus by the method becomes increasingly difficult.
• Blood sample: Measles-specific IgM titers will confirm infection but blood samples should be drawn no sooner than 5 days after the rash first appears. Prior to this IgM titers will be negative.
• Blood sample: A comparison of IgG titers obtained during the acute and convalescent stages can be done. Blood samples must be taken at least 7 to 10 days apart.

Therapy

SPECIFIC

• There is no specific therapy for this infection other than supportive care. Anti-pyretics, plenty of oral fluids, and room humidification to help reduce cough are usually all that is needed.
• In April 1993, the American Academy of Pediatrics issued a policy statement concerning vitamin A treatment of measles.

—The use of vitamin A should be considered for children 6 months to 2 years of age who are hospitalized with measles or its complications; and
—Children over 6 months of age who have an immunodeficiency, ophthalmological evidence of vitamin A deficiency, impaired intestinal absorption, or moderate to severe malnutrition or who are recent immigrants from areas of high mortality from measles.

—Children 6 months to 1 year should receive 100,000 IU of water-miscible vitamin A.
—The recommended dosage for children over 1 year of age is a single dose of 200,000 IU of water-miscible vitamin A on admission, a second dose the following day.
—The higher dose may be associated with vomiting and headache for a few hours.
—For children with ophthalmological evidence of vitamin A deficiency, a third dose at 4 weeks is indicated.
—Vitamin A is available in 50,000 IU/mL solution and may be given orally.

PREVENTION

• Vaccine recommendations

—Routine vaccination against measles, mumps, rubella (MMR) for children begins at 12 to 15 months with a second MMR vaccination at entrance to elementary school, age 4 to 6 years or middle school, age 11 to 12 years.
—With the recent resurgence of measles, aggressive employee immunization programs should be pursued for all health care workers.
—Health care workers born in 1957 or after who have no documentation of vaccination or other evidence of measles immunity should be vaccinated at the time of employment and revaccinated no sooner than one month later.

• Infection control measures

—Any patient suspected of having measles should be in a negative-pressure isolation room, in respiratory isolation.
—All health care workers involved with the patient must wear masks, gloves, and gowns.
—Isolation is required until 5 days after the first appearance of the rash, except for immunocompromised patients, who require isolation for the course of the illness.
—All suspected cases of measles should be reported immediately to the local health department.

Follow-Up

In uncomplicated measles infection the patient begins feeling better with a fading of rash on the third and fourth day.

PITFALL

Misdiagnosis is the biggest problem with measles infection. Because it is rare and may occur in outbreaks, initially cases are often misdiagnosed as Kawasaki disease or Stevens-Johnson syndrome.

Common Questions and Answers

Q: If a health care worker has had a natural measles infection or measles immunization, should one be concerned about infection following exposure?
A: Those persons born prior to 1957 who had a "wild measles virus" infection are usually immune from reinfection. However, in a report in 1993, four health care workers, who were previously vaccinated with positive pre-illness measles antibody levels, developed modified measles following exposure to infected patients. Therefore, all health care workers should observe respiratory precautions in caring for patients with measles.

Q: During an outbreak of measles, should children younger than 12 months be vaccinated?
A: In an outbreak of measles, public health officials may recommend vaccination of infants 6 months to 11 months with a single antigen measles vaccine; for children initially vaccinated before their first birthday, they should be revaccinated at 12 to 15 months of age. A second dose should be administered during the early school years.

ICD-9-CM 056.9

BIBLIOGRAPHY

American Academy of Pediatric Measles. In: Peter G, ed. *1994 red book: report on the Committee on Infectious Diseases,* 23rd ed. Elk Grove Village, IL: American Academy of Pediatrics, 1994:308–323.

Arrieta AC, Zaleska M, Stutman HR, et al. Vitamin A levels in children with measles in Long Beach, California. *J Pediatr* 1992;121:75.

Bell LM. Update on measles. *Cortlandt Forum* 1993;6:131–134.

Farizo KM, Stehr-Green PA, Simpsons DM, et al. Pediatric emergency room visits: a risk factor for acquiring measles. *Pediatrics* 1991;98:74.

Hussey GD, Klein M. A randomized controlled trial of vitamin A in children with measles. *N Engl J Med* 1990;323:169.

Author: Louis M. Bell

Meckel Diverticulum

 Database

DEFINITION

• Meckel diverticulum is a congenital anomaly that is part of the group known as the omphalomesenteric duct remnants.
• A remnant of the embryonic yolk sac remains in 1% to 3% of all infants and is the most common congenital gastrointestinal anomaly.
• Meckel diverticulum is the most common anomaly in this group and makes up more than 80% of these abnormalities.
• This diverticulum originates from the antimesenteric border of the bowel approximately 40 to 50 cm from the ileocecal valve and is between 3 and 6 cm in length.

CAUSES

• Meckel diverticulum results from a partial or complete failure or involution of the omphalomesenteric duct.
• The omphalomesenteric duct is the portion of the yolk sac that becomes incorporated into the ventral wall of the primitive gut.

PATHOLOGY

• Meckel diverticulum contains all three layers of the intestinal wall.
• The majority of these diverticuli are lined with ileal mucosa, but ectopic tissue is often present. The variety of ectopic tissue that may be present includes gastric (which is the most common), duodenal, colonic, and pancreatic.
• Of the symptomatic cases of Meckel diverticulum, 40% to 80% have some type of ectopic tissue, including gastric or pancreatic type.

EPIDEMIOLOGY

• In asymptomatic and incidentally discovered cases of Meckel diverticuli, there is no sex ratio difference. In cases in which the diverticulum is symptomatic there is a 3:1 male predominance.
• The risk of developing complications from Meckel diverticulum is approximately 4%.
• The development of symptoms seems to be age related, with the peak incidence being 2 years of age.
• 80% of all patients requiring surgery were less than 10 years of age and nearly 50% were under 2 years of age.

 Differential Diagnosis

• The differential diagnosis for Meckel diverticulum is based on its two main clinical symptoms: bleeding and obstruction.
• The causes of a lower gastrointestinal hemorrhage include milk protein colitis, gastroenteritis, intussusception, Henoch-Schönlein purpura, polyps, inflammatory bowel disease (IBD), volvulus, lymphonodular hyperplasia, hemolytic uremic syndrome, pseudomembranous colitis.
• The differential for obstruction include malrotation, volvulus, intussusception, atresias, adhesions, strictures.

 Data Gathering

HISTORY

Question: Bleeding?
Significance: The most common presentation for a Meckel diverticulum is intermittent, painless rectal bleeding secondary to peptic ulceration that arises at the junction of the ectopic gastric mucosa and the normal ileal mucosa. The bleeding can be excessive if the erosion is at the site of the remnant vitelline artery. The bleeding, even in the most severe cases, tends to be self-limiting, because of constriction of the splanchnic vessels secondary to hypovolemia.

Question: Small bowel obstruction?
Significance: A second common clinical presentation is partial or complete small bowel obstruction. The mechanism of the obstruction can be secondary to intraperitoneal bands, volvulus, intussusception (which is the most common), or an internal herniation.

Question: Similarity to appendicitis?
Significance: Meckel diverticulum may present with signs and symptoms of appendicitis with right lower quadrant pain, vomiting, and low-grade fever. This occurs when the diverticulum becomes acutely inflamed secondary to an obstruction or peptic ulceration. Approximately one-third of Meckel diverticulum may progress to perforation before exploration.

Physical Examination

Finding: None
Significance: Usually normal; may be anemic from blood loss.

 ## Laboratory Aids

Diagnosis of Meckel diverticulum depends on clinical presentation and suspicion. There are no specific laboratory evaluations that aid in the diagnosis of a Meckel diverticulum.

Test: Standard abdominal x-rays
Significance: No value in diagnosing a Meckel diverticulum.

Test: Meckel scans
Significance: An important advance in making the diagnosis, but they are only 85% sensitive and 95% specific. During the scan, the technetium-99m pertechnetate is taken up by the ectopic gastric tissue (mucous neck secreting cells). Certain substances enhance the detection of the ectopic gastric tissue including pentagastrin, glucagon, and cimetidine.

Test: Red cell tagged scans
Significance: Not specific for a Meckel diverticulum, but may be useful in localizing the site of bleeding.

Test: Superior mesenteric angiography
Significance: Have been used in making the diagnosis but are rarely indicated.

 ## Therapy

• The therapy for a Meckel diverticulum is removal, in cases in which the patient is symptomatic. The important factors in the removal are to remove all ectopic tissue during the surgery and to ensure that the closure of the bowel wall does not cause a narrowing of the lumen.
• In some cases a Meckel diverticulum is found incidentally. Some believe that if found, it should be removed secondary to the potential complications of hemorrhage, perforation, and obstruction. Others feel that the lifetime risk for developing these complications is low and, therefore, would not remove the diverticulum.
• The current favored practice is to examine the diverticulum for evidence of ectopic tissue, which includes either a thickening or a mass within the wall of the diverticulum. If present, then removal is indicated. A second feature that may lead to removal is a narrowing at the base of the diverticulum, therefore, increasing the risk for obstruction and perforation.

 ## Follow-Up

• Once the Meckel diverticulum is removed, standard post-operative care is undertaken. No specific follow-up is indicated.
• In cases in which the diverticulum is found incidentally but not removed, one should be aware of its existence. No other specific follow-up or surveillance is needed.

 ## Common Questions and Answers

Q: What are the reasons for resection of a Meckel diverticulum?
A: Narrowing at base of diverticulum or presence of ectopic tissue.

Q: What is the most common ectopic tissue present in Meckel diverticulum?
A: Gastric.

ICD-9-CM 751.0

BIBLIOGRAPHY

Anderson GF, Sfakianakis G, King DR, Boles ET. Hormonal enhancement of technectium-99m pertechnatate uptake in experimental Meckel's diverticulum. *J Pediatr Surg* 1980;15:900–905.

Connolly LP, Treves ST, Bozorgi F, O'Connor SC. Meckel's diverticulum: demonstration of heterotopic gastric mucosa with technetium-99m-pertechnetate SPECT. *J Nucl Med* 1998;39(8): 1458–1460.

Cullen JJ, Kelly KA. Current management of Meckel's diverticulum. *Adv Surg* 1996;29: 207–214.

Lobe TE. Acute abdomen. The role of laparoscopy. Semin Pediatr Surg 1997;6(2):81–87.

Ludtke FE, Mende V, Kohler H. Incidence and frequency of complications and management of Meckel's diverticulum. *Surg Gynecol Obstet* 1989;169:537–542.

Schwartz MZ, Smolens I. Meckel's diverticulum and other omphalomesenteric duct remnants. In: Wyllie R, Hyams JS, eds. *Pediatric gastrointestinal disease.* Philadelphia: WB Saunders, 1993:670–676.

Soltero MJ, Bill AJ. The natural history of Meckel's diverticulum and its relation to incidental removal. *Am J Surg* 1976;132:168–173.

Stuvil O, Brandt ML, Panic S, et al. Meckel's diverticulum in children: a 20 year review. *J Pediatr Surg* 1991;26:1289–1292.

Author: Edisio Semeao

Megaloblastic Anemia

 ## Database

DEFINITION

Anemia characterized by megaloblastic red blood cells (RBC; large cells with abundant cytoplasm) in the bone marrow and hypersegmented neutrophils on peripheral blood smears.

PATHOPHYSIOLOGY

• Abnormal DNA synthesis in hematopoietic precursors
• Anemia is due to ineffective hematopoiesis and hemolysis
• Overall causes are numerous, but the following are the most common general etiologic categories:

—Vitamin B_{12} (cobalamin) deficiency
—Folate (folic acid) deficiency
—Refractory dyserythropoietic anemias—rare in children

• Other disorders may be associated with an increased mean corpuscular volume (MCV) other than megaloblastic anemias [e.g., reticulocytes (young red blood cells)], which are increased in hemolytic anemias; liver disease; pregnancy; aplastic anemia; hypothyroidism.

EPIDEMIOLOGY

• Exact incidence and prevalence figures in American children are unknown, but overall is rare.
• In adults, pernicious anemia is a common cause.

COMPLICATIONS

• Mild congestive heart failure may develop due to anemia but this is uncommon due to the insidious onset of megaloblastic anemia in general.
• Neurological complications from vitamin B_{12} deficiency.
• Folate deficiency may complicate vitamin B_{12} deficiency.

PROGNOSIS

Prognosis depends on etiology of megaloblastic anemia; usually good if dietary deficiency. Poor prognoses may associated with inborn errors of metabolism that sometimes present with megaloblastic anemia.

 ## Differential Diagnosis

Macrocytic anemias must be differentiated from megaloblastic anemias. In macrocytic anemias, the MCV is increased but without megaloblastic bone marrow changes.

 ## Data Gathering

HISTORY

• Insidious onset of anemia and associated symptoms such as increased pallor, increased fatigue, poor appetite, irritability, etc.
• Gastrointestinal symptoms that may include:

—Malabsorption/diarrhea
—Special diets: particularly strict vegan diets
—Prior gastrointestinal surgery

• Medications such as anticonvulsants and chemotherapeutic agents that interfere with folate metabolism.
• Neurological symptoms most commonly associated with vitamin B_{12} deficiency; symptoms may include:

—Difficulty walking
—Numbness/tingling in hands and/or feet

 ## Physical Examination

• Pallor and other associated signs of anemia
• Smooth and sometimes tender tongue
• Neurological findings: Abnormal position and vibratory sensation; ataxia, muscular weakness, peripheral neuropathy, positive Babinski sign.

 ## Laboratory Aids

Complete blood count (CBC)
Significance:

• Decreased hemoglobin
• Increased MCV
• Increased red cell distribution width (RDW)
• Normal to decreased white blood count (WBC) and platelets

Test: Peripheral blood smear
Significance:

• Macroovalocytes
• Hypersegmented neutrophils
• Increased anisocytosis (variation in RBC size)
• Increased poikilocytosis (variation in RBC shape)

Test: Reticulocyte count
Significance: Low reticulocyte count

Test: B_{12}
Significance: Low serum vitamin B_{12}

Test: Folate
Significance: Low serum and RBC folate

Test: Bone marrow and biopsy examination
Significance:

• Large RBC, WBC, and platelet precursors with nuclear-to-cytoplasmic dissociation prominent in red cell line.
• Increased iron stores
• Multiple bi- and trinucleate RBC precursors and multiple mitotic figures

Test: Schilling test
Significance: B_{12} absorption

• Part 1 evaluates vitamin B_{12} absorption by measuring urine radioactivity after oral radioactive vitamin B_{12}. (Note: This test may be performed after the patient has been treated, but note that the test involves administration of vitamin B_{12} so that all other tests, particularly bone marrow examination, should be performed beforehand or shortly thereafter.)

• If the urinary excretion is lower than expected then abnormal absorption is present; this may be due to malabsorption or intrinsic factor disorders.

• Part 2 should be performed if part 1 is abnormal; this involves oral intrinsic factor. If part 2 is normal and part 1 is abnormal then pernicious anemia is highly suspected. If part 2 remains abnormal then a malabsorption syndrome is the most likely diagnosis.

Test: Barium studies
Significance: May be needed to evaluate gastric, small bowel, and large bowel anomalies.

 Therapy

• General considerations: the following three categories should be addressed for all patients:

—Adequate replacement of deficient substance, vitamin B_{12}, or folate at adequate doses for an adequate duration
—Treatment/management of underlying disorder, such as malabsorption syndromes, chronic hemolytic anemias
—Monitoring response to therapy

• Treating undiagnosed vitamin B_{12} deficiency with high doses of folate may worsen neurological complications, although a hematological response may occur.

• Folic acid deficiency: doses—folic acid at 1 to 5 mg oral daily dose for at least 2 to 3 months; parenteral preparation also available if needed.

• Vitamin B_{12} deficiency: doses acutely, daily doses of 25 to 100 mg IM; long-term, 200 to 1000 mg monthly IM. Most patients with vitamin B_{12} deficiency require lifelong treatment because most cases are due to abnormal absorption.

 Follow-Up

• The reticulocyte count should increase within the first 2 weeks of therapy, whereas the hemoglobin will take longer, in some cases months, to increase.

• If the hemoglobin fails to rise in 2 months then other causes of anemia including iron deficiency and anemia of chronic disease should be considered.

PITFALLS

• Microcytic anemias such as iron deficiency, thalassemia, and anemia of chronic disease may obscure the diagnosis of megaloblastic anemias by falsely lowering the MCV; however, hypersegmented neutrophils should be present to aid in the correct diagnoses.

• Serum B_{12} and folate rise rapidly after beginning supplements, therefore, diagnostic levels should be drawn prior to administration of supplements or normal diets.

 Common Questions and Answers

Q: What are common dietary sources of vitamin B_{12}?
A: Meat; liver contains the greatest amount of vitamin B_{12}.

Q: What are common dietary sources of folate?
A: Vegetables (primarily green, leafy vegetables), citrus fruits and berries, liver.

Q: Can food preparation destroy vitamin B_{12} and folate?
A: Food preparation cannot destroy vitamin B_{12}, but excessive heating can destroy folate.

ICD-9-CM 281.9

BIBLIOGRAPHY

Rapaport I. Introduction to hematology. *Megaloblastic anemia.* Philadelphia: JB Lippincott, 1987.

Author: Kim Smith-Whitley

Meningitis

Database

DEFINITION

Meningitis is inflammation of the membranes of the brain or spinal cord usually caused by bacteria, viruses, fungi, and rarely parasites. It is almost always a result of hematogenous spread.

CAUSES

- Bacterial

—Bacteria causing meningitis differ depending on age:
—Less than 1 month: Group B streptococcus, *Escherichia coli,* other enteric, *Listeria monocytogenes*
—4 to 6 weeks: *Haemophilus influenzae* type b, *E. coli, Streptococcus pneumoniae,* group B streptoccocus
—6 weeks to 6 years: *S. pneumoniae, Neisseria meningitides, H. influenzae* type b
—Older than 6 years: *S. pneumoniae, N. meningitis*

- Viral

—Approximately 70 different strains of enteroviruses, which include polioviruses, coxsackie A, coxsackie B, and echoviruses. Enteroviruses discovered recently are not placed in the above four groups but simply numbered (e.g., enterovirus 68) arboviruses (e.g., Eastern equine encephalitis), mumps, herpes simplex virus

- Fungal

—Fungi most commonly isolated include *Candida* spp., *Aspergillus, Cryptococcus neoformans*

- Aseptic meningitis

—Agents not easily cultured in the viral or microbiology laboratory can cause meningitis and include *Borrelia burgdorferi* (Lyme disease), *Treponema pallidum* (syphilis)
—Tuberculous meningitis

EPIDEMIOLOGY

- Bacterial meningitis

—Most bacterial meningitis (80%) occurs in patients less than 24 months of age.
—*S. pneumoniae* isolates are becoming more resistant to penicillin. Currently, approximately 20% of isolates causing invasive disease are at least relatively resistant to penicillin.

- Viral meningitis

—85% are due to enteroviruses that tend to occur in outbreaks in summer and early fall.

- Fungal meningiti

—Cryptococcus neoformans is a budding encapsulated yeast-like organism found in soil and avian excreta.

—Although associated with meningitis in immunocompromised adults (especially those with AIDS), this is rare in children with AIDS. Thirty percent of patients with cryptococcal meningitis have no underlying immunodeficiency.
—Meningitis caused by *Candida* spp. occurs in ill premature infants and other immunocompromised individuals.

- Tuberculous mening

—The incidence of disease due to *Mycobacteria tuberculosis* (TB) is on the rise throughout the world.
—TB meningitis occurs in 1 of every 300 primary TB infections.
—This is most commonly seen in children ages 6 months to 6 years.
—Meningitis will accompany miliary TB in approximately 50% of cases.
—There are increasing concerns about antimycobacterial resistant strains of TB requiring four to five antimycobacterial drugs and close follow-up for patient compliance (*see* Treatment).

COMPLICATIONS

- Bacterial meningitis

—Acute complications
—Syndrome of inappropriate ADH secretion (SIADH)
—Seizures: focal neurologic signs occur in 15–20%.
—Long-term complications
—Neurological sequelae: mental retardation
—Hearing defects

- Viral meningitis

—SIADH in 10%
—Long-term sequalae
—It is unusual to have any complication from viral meningitis. The exception to this occur in neonates (<1 month of age) or older agammaglobulinemic children with sepsis/meningitis from enterovirus infections.

- Tuberculous meningitis

—Acute complications
—The most common early on are cranial nerve findings, especially 6th cranial nerve palsy affecting the eyes.

PROGNOSIS

- Bacterial meningitis

—Approximately 500 to 1000 deaths each year
—Sequelae from the infection including hearing deficits and neurological damage may occur in up to 25% of children.

- Viral meningitis

—Prognosis for enteroviral meningitis is quite good.

- Aseptic meningitis

—Lyme disease: Prognosis with diagnosis and treatment is quite good (*see* Lyme Disease).

- Tuberculous meningitis

—The long-term prognosis in children with tuberculous meningitis depends on the stage of disease in which treatment is begun (for staging *see* Data Gathering, History, and Physical Examination).
—Complete recovery occurs in 94% of those whose treatment was started in stage 1, but only 51% and 18% for those whose treatment began in stage II or stage III, respectively.

Data Gathering

HISTORY

Bacterial Meningitis

- Children greater than 12 months of age will often complain of neck pain, headache, or back pain.
- Nausea and vomiting are commonly associated.
- Nuchal rigidity in children over 12 months. Common chief complaints by the infants' caregivers include:

—Irritable or "sleeping all the time"
—"Won't take to bottle"
—"Not acting right"
—"Cries when moved or picked up"
—"Won't stop crying"
—"Soft spot bulging out"

- Kernig and Brudzinski signs may be present. Brudzinski sign is positive: if the neck is passively flexed, flexion of legs occur. Kernig sign is positive: complete extension of the leg causes neck pain and flexion.
- In children less than 12 months symptoms are often non-specific. They may not have nuchal rigidity. Kernig and Brudzinski signs may not be present.

Other historical information that may affect your management:

Question: Is the patient immunocompromised?
Significance: This makes unusual pathogen more likely.

Question: Recurrent meningitis
Significance: Recurrent meningitis with *S. pneumoniae* or *Enterococci* may indicate a skull fracture or cubeform plate fracture with contamination of the cerebral spinal fluid (CSF) by nasopharyngeal secretions.

Viral Meningitis

Question: Early symptoms
Significance: Headache and fever may precede signs of meningitis such as stiff neck, vomiting, photophobia.

Question: Duration
Significance: The illness lasts 2 to 6 days.

Fungal Meningitis

Question: Symptoms
Significance: Cryptococcal meningitis is often indolent with complaints of worsening headaches and vomiting for days to weeks.

Question: Exposure
Significance: Exposure to pigeon droppings or other bird droppings can be a valuable clue to etiology if present.

Tuberculous Meningitis

• Symptoms often are non-specific initially with fever, nausea, and vomiting progressing to anorexia, irritability, and lethargy (stage I disease).
• Stage II disease is characterized by focal neurological signs (most often involving the cranial nerves, III, VI, VII).
• Stage III disease is characterized by coma and papilledema.

 ## Laboratory Aids

Test: Lumbar puncture with analysis of the CSF
Significance: Depending on the presentation, age, history, and physical examination, some or all of the following tests should be requested for CSF analysis.

• Opening pressure: Normal is less than 200 mm of H_2O in lateral recumbent.
• Cell count and differential
• Glucose: To be compared with the serum glucose; normal is more than 40 mg/dL or one-half to two-thirds of the serum glucose.
• Protein: Normal 5 to 40 mg/dL except in newborns who may have protein levels of 150–200 mg/dl.
• Cultures: For bacteria, fungi, viruses, and mycobacteria. Approximately 80% of blood cultures are positive in children with bacterial meningitis.

Test: PCR
Significance: TB, HSV

Test: Antibody studies
Significance: Lyme disease, HSV

Test: Other laboratory studies

• CBC: platelet count, PT/PTT, electrolytes, BUN, creatinine, glucose, arterial blood gas
• Blood culture

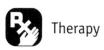 ## Therapy

• Assure adequate ventilation and cardiac function (the ABCs).
• Initiate hemodynamic monitoring and support by achieving venous access and treat shock syndrome, if present.

• Monitor serum sodium concentrations because inappropriate ADH secretion is a frequent complication during the first 3 days of treatment.
• Glucose should be given intravenously if <50 mg/dL at a dose of 0.25 to 1 g/kg.
• Acidosis should be corrected is pH if less than 7.2 with 1 to 2 mEq/kg of sodium bicarbonate.
• Coagulopathy should be treated with platelet concentrates (0.2 units per kg) if platelets are less than 50,000/mm^3 and fresh frozen plasma (10 mL/kg) if PT/PTT is prolonged
• Steroids are used commonly in the initial therapy of TB meningitis along with antibiotic drugs. Use in child with bacterial meningitis is controversial.

Bacterial Meningitis

• Antimicrobial agents: <6 weeks: ampicillin IV (200 mg/kg/d); cefotaxime IV (100–200 mg/kg/d); >6 weeks: vancomycin IV (40 mg/kg/d) in four divided doses; cefotaxime IV (180 mg/kg/d) in four divided doses.
• Note: Vancomycin and cefotaxime should be considered for presumptive therapy for bacterial meningitis until a resistant *S. pneumoniae* meningitis is ruled out; also, vancomycin and rifampin PO or IV 10 to 20 mg/kg/d in one dose is an alternative.

Fungal Meningitis

• Amphotericin B plus or minus 5-flucytosine depending on the type of fungi isolated.

Tuberculous Meningitis

• Treatment is generally with four drugs for 2 months followed by two drugs for 10 months.
• Initially, treatment can start with isoniazid, rifampin, parazinamide, and ethambutal (if <2 years) or streptomycin (if >2 years).

Viral Meningitis

• Enterovirus: no specific therapy other than supportive
• HSV: acyclovir for neonate and older child

PREVENTION

H. *influenzae* type b (HIB) vaccine has significantly reduced the incidence of meningitis and other invasive HIB infections.

 ## Follow-Up

• Most children with bacterial meningitis become afebrile by 7 to 10 days after starting therapy with gradual improvement in activity with less irritability.
• Evaluation for neurological sequelae, such as hearing and vision testing, is essential.

• Prophylaxis (for family and for patient before discharge): Rifampin should be given if the child had *H. influenzae* meningitis (20 mg/kg/dose, maximum 600 mg) once daily for 4 days or *N. meningitidis* (10 mg/kg/dose, maximum 600 mg) twice daily for 2 days.

PITFALLS

• If no etiology is discovered after the first lumbar puncture and the child is not responding to therapy, then a repeat lumbar puncturing should be performed at 36 to 48 hours.
• Remember that in tuberculous meningitis, up to 10% of children will not react to the five tuberculin unit mantoux tests. Therapy should be started if suspicious; do not rely on the skin testing.
• Be aware that the isolation of resistant strains of *S. pneumoniae* is increasing (currently it is approximately 5%); therefore, antibiotics such as vancomycin and cefotaxime should be used until antibiotic sensitivity data are available.

 ## Common Questions and Answers

Q: Is lumbar puncture required before starting antibiotics in the patient with suspected meningitis with unstable vital signs requiring resuscitation?
A: No. In the unstable patient it is contraindicated to perform a lumbar puncture. Appropriate intravenous antibiotic should be started. When resuscitated, a lumbar puncture should be performed. A latex agglutination along with routine analysis is then performed.

ICD-9-CM 322.9

BIBLIOGRAPHY

Feign RD, McGracken GH, Klein JO. Diagnosis and management of meningitis. *Pediatr Infect Dis J* 1992;11:785–814.

Lebel MH, Freij BJ, Syrogiannopoulos GA, et al. Dexamethasone therapy for bacterial meningitis: results of two double-blind, placebo-controlled trials. *N Engl J Med* 1988;319(15):964–971.

Saez-Llorens X, Ramilo O, Mustafa MM, Mertsola J, McCracken GH Jr. Molecular pathophysiology of bacterial meningitis: current concepts and therapeutic implications. *J Pediatr* 1990;116(5):671–684.

Wald ER, Kaplan SL, Mason EO Jr., et al. Dexamethasone therapy for children with bacterial meningitis. Meningitis Study Group. *Pediatrics* 1995;95:21–28.

Author: Louis M. Bell

Meningococcemia

 Database

DEFINITION

- Meningococcemia is a systemic infection with the bacterium *Neisseria meningitidis,* a gram negative diplococcus that is relatively fastidious. Despite treatment with appropriate antibiotics, this disease may have a fulminant course with a high likelihood of mortality.
- Thirteen serogroups have been described on the basis of capsular polysaccharide antigens; A, B, and C produce 90% of disease.
- Fifteen serotypes have been described on the basis of outer membrane proteins; type 2 is found in 50% of cases in United States and Canada.

PATHOPHYSIOLOGY

- Colonization and infection of the upper respiratory tract occurs after inhalation of, or direct contact with, the organism.
- Disseminated disease occurs when the organism penetrates the nasal mucosa and enters the bloodstream, where it replicates.
- Fulminant disease is signified by diffuse microvascular damage and disseminated intravascular coagulation (*see* Septic Shock).
- Death results from effects of endotoxic shock including circulatory collapse and myocardial dysfunction.
- Bacteremia without sepsis presents with fever, malaise, myalgias, and headache. Patients may clear the infection spontaneously, or it may invade meninges, joints, lungs, etc.
- Meningococcemia without meningitis occurs after initial bacteremia with systemic sepsis. A rash erupts, which may be non-specific maculopapular, morbilliform, or urticarial. Progression to petechiae or purpura signifies evolution of disease.
- Fulminant disease is signified by hypotension, oliguria, disseminated intravascular coagulation (DIC), myocardial dysfunction, and vascular collapse. Death occurs in approximately 20% of these patients.

GENETICS

Inherited deficiency of terminal complement may be found in 5% to 10% of patients during epidemics. The frequency increases to 30% in patients with recurrent disease.

EPIDEMIOLOGY

- Patients with deficiency of a terminal complement component (C5-9), asplenia or properdin deficiency are at increased risk for invasive and recurrent disease.
- Children less than age 5 are most often affected, with peak incidence between 3 and 5 months.
- During epidemics, more school-aged children may be affected.
- The disease occurs most commonly in winter and spring months.
- Increased disease activity may follow an influenza A outbreak.

COMPLICATIONS

- Complications may result directly from the infection or be classified as allergic immune complex-mediated.
- Meningococcemia may be complicated by myocarditis, arthritis, hemorrhage, and pneumonia.
- Meningococcal meningitis is most commonly complicated by deafness in 5% to 10% of survivors.
- Other complications of meningitis include seizures, subdural effusions, and cranial nerve palsies.
- Allergic complications include arthritis, vasculitis, pericarditis, and episcleritis.

PROGNOSIS

- Fatality rate of meningococcemia is 20%, even when recognized and treated.
- Fatality rate of meningococcal meningitis is 5%. The most severe cases often have a rapid progression from onset of symptoms to death over a matter of hours. At the time of hospital admission, the following signs predict poor survival:

—Lack of meningitis
—Shock
—Coma
—Purpura
—Neutropenia
—Thrombocytopenia
—DIC
—Myocarditis

 Differential Diagnosis

- Meningitis due to *N. meningitidis* is indistinguishable from that of other causes, except for one-third of children who have a petechial rash.
- Sepsis from other microbial causes may appear identically, including the petechiae or purpuric rash.

 Data Gathering

HISTORY

- Time of onset of fever, malaise, and rash?

Meningococcemia

 Physical Examination

- Recognition of abnormal vital signs and lethargy is necessary.
- Careful examination of the skin for petechiae is important.
- Nuchal rigidity, lethargy, and irritability should be carefully evaluated.

 Laboratory Aids

The organism can be cultured from blood, cerebral spinal fluid (CSF), and skin lesions.

Test: Gram stain of CSF or scraped petechia (pressed against a glass slide)
Significance: Revealing gram-negative diplococci will give a presumptive diagnosis.

Test: Rapid test for antigen detection
Significance: Best found in CSF but not sensitive for serogroup B.

 Therapy

- Patients with acute onset of petechial rash and fever should receive a prompt initial dose of antibiotics (preferably after blood culture)
- Close monitoring of vital signs and clinical status should follow, preferably in an ICU setting.
- Cefotaxime or ceftriaxone can be initiated as presumptive therapy. Once sensitivity is confirmed, penicillin is preferred.
- After isolate is proven to be sensitive to penicillin, treatment of choice is aqueous penicillin G IV at a dose of 300,000 IU/kg/d every 4 to 6 hours for 5 to 7 days.
- In penicillin-allergic patients, third-generation cephalosporins or chloramphenicol are acceptable alternatives.

 Follow-up

Patients with bacterial meningitis should have hearing test as a follow-up.

PREVENTION

- Isolation of the hospitalized patient.
- Hospitalized patients require respiratory isolation until 24 hours after appropriate antibiotic therapy.

CONTROL MEASURES

- Exposed contacts, including household, day care, and nursery school, should receive rifampin, 10 mg/kg (maximum 600 mg) every 12 hours for four doses.
- Ceftriaxone administered intramuscularly is effective prophylaxis. It's safety profile is prefered for pregnant women.
- Medical personnel should receive prophylaxis only if they had close contact with respiratory secretions.
- Vaccines for types A, C, 4, WBS are available and produce an immune response in 10 to 14 days.

PITFALLS

- Public health officials should be notified of *N. menigitidis* cases.
- Physical examination of a child with fever should include careful evaluation of the skin for petechiae and signs of early shock (tachycardia, delayed capillary refill, abnormal mental status, etc.).

 Common Questions and Answers

Q: How long should antibiotic therapy be given in a patient with septic shock?
A: 7 days.

Q: When is meningococcal vaccine indicated?
A: In asplenic, or functionally asplenic patients, in patients with terminal complement deficiency, and in epidemics in conjunction with chemoprophylaxis.

Q: When should one test for complement deficiency?
A: In patients with recurrent disease.

Q: Which hospital personnel should receive prophylaxis?
A: Only those with close contact with secretions.

ICD-9-CM 036.2

BIBLIOGRAPHY

Apicella MA. *Neisseria meningitidis.* In: Mandell GL, Douglas GR, Bennet JE, eds. *Principles and practice of infectious diseases,* 3rd ed. New York: Churchill Livingstone, 1990:1600–1613.

Baker CJ, Edwards MS. Meningococcernia. In: Oski FA, ed. *Principles and practice of pediatrics.* Philadelphia: JB Lippincott, 1990:1097–1101.

Beaty HN. Meningococcemia. In: Fauci A, Braunwald E, Isselbacher KJ, eds. *Harrison's principles of internal medicine.* New York: McGraw-Hill, 1998:574–576.

Glode MP, Smith AL. Meningococcernia. In: Feigin RD, Cherry JD, eds. *Textbook of pediatric infectious diseases.* Philadelphia: WB Saunders, 1997:1211–1224.

Peter G, ed. *1997 Red book: report of the Committee on Infectious Diseases.* Elk Grove Village, IL: American Academy of Pediatrics, 1997: 357–362.

Author: Janet H. Friday

Mental Retardation

Database

DEFINITION

• Mental retardation essentially means slow rate of learning or slow cognitive processing. By definition there are significant cognitive and adaptive delays first evident in childhood. Significant cognitive delays are defined as two standard deviations below the population mean on a standard cognitive or IQ test. This usually indicates an IQ score of less than 70 to 75. Adaptive skills are the functional skills of everyday life, including communication, social skills, daily living/self care skills, and the ability to safely move about the home and community.
• Mental retardation is typically subdivided into mild, moderate, severe, and profound categories depending on the severity of the delays. A more recent definition by the American Association on Mental Retardation (AAMR) puts more emphasis on the level of functioning and amount of supports required of an individual.

CAUSES

• The cause of the mental retardation is usually an insult to the brain or abnormal development of the central nervous system.
• Genetic
• Familial
• Metabolical
• Endocrinologic
• Infectious
• Environmental toxins
• Traumatic
• Anatomic brain malformations
• The etiology is not evident in many cases of mental retardation.

EPIDEMIOLOGY

• Prevalence of mental retardation is generally listed as 2% to 3% of the population.
• Found in both sexes and all racial and socio-economic groups.
• The mild form is the most prevalent at 85% of the mental retardation population.
• Profound mental retardation is least prevalent at about 1% of this group.
• Associated findings are more common in the more severe forms of mental retardation.

The prognosis for longevity varies with the associated findings and overall health, but individuals with mental retardation can live to adulthood and old age. An individual's level of functioning is variable depending on the level of retardation, special individual skills, and family or community supports. In general, the following applies:

• Mild mental retardation (IQ 70–55): Formerly called educable. May be in school with extra help and may achieve roughly a fourth grade level in reading and math. May be employed in an unskilled to semi-skilled job. May live in a group home or independently. Some marry.

• Moderate mental retardation (IQ 54–40): May learn to recognize basic words and learn basic skills. May work in a sheltered workshop or with supported employment in an unskilled job. May live with family or in a group home doing much of their own care.
• Severe mental retardation (IQ 39–25): May live with family or in a group home or institution. Some may be in a sheltered workshop. May be able to do some daily self care or chores with supervision.
• Profound mental retardation (IQ <25): Live with family or in a group home or institution. Usually require full care.

Mental retardation has many associated findings including, seizures, autism, cerebral palsy, communication disorders, failure to thrive, sensory impairments, and psychiatric disorders. Behavioral disorders also can be seen including attention deficit hyperactivity disorder, self injurious, and self stimulating behaviors. Families often face additional stressors when caring for a child with mental retardation.

Differential Diagnosis

The differential can include several other developmental diagnoses, including:

• Borderline cognitive abilities
• Developmental language disorder
• Autism
• Learning disability
• Cerebral palsy
• Significant visual or hearing impairment
• Degenerative disorders

Specific etiologies are too numerous to list completely but a partial list of the more common causes would include:

• Genetic/familial

—Fragile X syndrome
—Trisomy 21 (Down syndrome)
—Other chromosomal abnormalities
—Tuberous sclerosis
—Neurofibromatosis
—PKU (Phenylketonuria)
—Other inborn errors of metabolism

• Nervous system anomalies

—Hydrocephalus
—Lissencephaly
—Seizures

• Infections

—Prenatal cytomegalovirus, rubella, toxoplasmosis, HIV
—Postnatal bacterial meningitis, neonatal herpes simplex

• Endocrinologic

—Congenital hypothyroidism

• Environmental

—Heavy metal poisoning such as lead
—In utero drug or alcohol exposure, including fetal alcohol syndrome

• Trauma/injury
—Closed head trauma
—Asphyxia

Data Gathering

HISTORY

A complete and detailed history is needed including:

Question: Pregnancy history?
Significance:

• Maternal age and parity
• Maternal complications (including infections and exposures)
• Medications/drugs used
• Tobacco or alcohol used, along with quantities
• Fetal activity

Question: Birth history?
Significance:

• Gestational age
• Birth weight
• Route of delivery
• Maternal or fetal complications/distress
• Apgar scores

Question: General health?
Significance:

• Significant illnesses, hospitalizations, or surgeries
• Accidents or injuries
• Hearing and vision status
• Medications used
• Known exposures to toxins
• Any new or unusual symptoms

Question: Developmental history?
Significance:

• Current developmental achievement in each stream of development
• Age when developmental milestones were achieved
• Any loss of skills
• Where parents think their child is functioning developmentally

Question: Educational history?
Significance:

• Type of schooling and services received, if any
• Any previous educational/developmental testing

Question: Behavioral history?
Significance:

• Any perseverative or stereotypical behaviors
• Interaction skills
• Attention and activity level

Question: Family history
Significance: Anyone with developmental delays, neurological disorders, syndromes, inherited disorders, or consanguinity.

Physical Examination

A complete physical examination including growth parameters is needed looking for etiology. Key features to include are:

Finding: Observation of interactions and behavior
Significance: Any atypical behaviors and general impressions.

Finding: Head circumference
Significance: Looking for macro or microcephaly

Finding: Skin examination
Significance: Looking for neurocutaneous lesions

Finding: Major or minor dysmorphic features
Significance: Any indication of a syndrome or anatomic malformation.

Finding: Neurological examination
Significance: Looking for cranial nerve deficits, neuromuscular status, reflexes, balance and coordination and any soft signs.

DEVELOPMENTAL TESTING

When developmental delays are present and mental retardation is suspected, more formal developmental screening or testing should be done. Possible testing for the pediatrician would be the Denver Developmental Screening Test or the CAT/CLAMS. The diagnosis needs to be made on standardized tests, usually done by a clinical psychologist. Such standardized testing might involve the Stanford Binet Intelligence Scale, the Wechsler scales, the Vineland Adaptive Behavior Scales. A referral to a clinical psychologist for the formal diagnosis is indicated.

Laboratory Tests

Test: There is no specific laboratory test battery for mental retardation.
Significance: The testing needs to be tailored to the individual situation based on the history and physical examination. A high index of suspicion should be maintained for any associated findings and delays in the other streams of development. Listed here are some of the more common studies ordered for mental retardation work-up.

Test: Audiological testing
Significance: Hearing should be checked in any child with speech and language and/or cognitive delays.

Test: Genetic testing
Significance: Warranted for any dysmorphic features or a familial history of delays or genetic disorder. A karyotype and Fragile X DNA should be considered particularly for significant cognitive delays.

Test: Metabolic tests
Significance: The tests such as quantitative plasma amino acids, quantitative urine organic acids, lactate, pyruvate, or ammonia should be considered if there is any loss of skills or indication of a metabolic disorder. More specific metabolic tests may be indicated depending on symptoms.

Test: Thyroid function tests
Significance: Most infants will have had screening for hypothyroidism shortly after birth. This should be rechecked if symptoms indicate.

Test: Electroencephalogram
Significance: An EEG should be considered if there is any concern about seizures.

Test: Head MRI
Significance: Consider a head MRI for head abnormalities, significant neurological findings, loss of skills or for work up of a specific disorder such as trauma or leukodystrophy.

Test: Subspecialists
Significance: Referral to other medical specialists may also be indicated. These specialists may include developmental pediatrics, neurology, genetics, or ophthalmology.

Therapy

There is no specific cure for mental retardation. Therapy should consist of appropriate treatment for any underlying or associated medical condition. Early intervention and special education programs are available for an individualized education program based on the child's needs and abilities. Behavior management programs or selected use of medications is available for patients with severe behavioral problems. The ultimate goal of all therapies is to help the child reach his/her full potential.

Follow-Up

Children with mental retardation will need regular pediatric preventative care in addition to management of any underlying medical conditions. Ongoing monitoring of the educational programs, to assure that it is still meeting the child's needs, is important. The families will also need ongoing counseling and support in dealing with a child having special needs.

PREVENTION

There is no specific prevention for mental retardation, but prevention of some underlying causes may be possible. Immunization programs and early detection of metabolic disorders as well as education programs for head injury/asphyxia prevention may be useful in some of cases. Avoidance of alcohol and drugs during pregnancy will decrease potential injury to brain.

PITFALLS

- Children with behavioral problems may also be masking cognitive delays.
- Hearing impairment may present as a delay in development.
- Children with mild mental retardation may not be diagnosed until they are having difficulties keeping up in elementary school.

Common Questions and Answers

Q: Will my child be "normal" by adulthood?
A: Generally, mental retardation is considered a lifelong condition. Some individuals, usually with the milder form of mental retardation, can function well in the community, especially when given added supports.

Q: Can my child learn?
A: Except for the severest forms of mental retardation, children do learn. This learning may not be as rapid or as extensive as that of a typically developing child.

Q: But my child looks fine and has had appropriate motor development. How can he/she be mentally retarded?
A: Mental retardation is a slowed rate of cognitive development. Many children with mental retardation do not have obvious dysmorphic features. Other streams of development, such as gross motor skills, may be reached on time or nearly so, yet the cognitive developmental streams can be significantly delayed.

ICD-9-CM
Mild mental retardation 317
Moderate mental retardation 318.0
Severe mental retardation 318.1
Profound mental retardation 318.2
Unspecified mental retardation 319

BIBLIOGRAPHY

American Psychiatric Association. *Diagnostic and statistical manual of mental disorders*, 4th ed. Washington, DC: American Psychiatric Association, 1994.

Batshaw ML. Mental retardation. *Pediatr Clin North Am* 1993;40:507–521.

Gilbride KE. Developmental testing. *Pediatr Rev* 1995;16:338–345.

Palmer FB, Capute AJ. Mental retardation. *Pediatr Rev* 1994;15:473–479.

Author: Rita Panoscha

Mesenteric Adenitis

 Database

DEFINITION

- Inflammation of the mesenteric lymph nodes

CAUSES

- Infection

—Viral: echovirus 1 and 14, coxsackie B1 and B5
—Bacterial: streptococcus; resulting in inflammation or due to hypersensitivity reaction to a foreign protein.

PATHOPHYSIOLOGY

- Lymph nodes usually involved are those draining the ileocecal area.
- Stasis of the intestinal contents in this region; there may be absorption of toxic products or bacterial products.
- Usually nodes are enlarged, discrete, soft, and pink and with time become firm and white. Calcification and suppuration are rare.
- Reactive hyperplasia.
- Cultures of the nodes are negative.
- Probably the adenitis results from a reaction to some material absorbed from the small intestine, reaching the intestine from the blood or lymphatic system.
- Hypersensitivity reaction to a foreign protein.

EPIDEMIOLOGY

- Age related
- Most common cause of acute abdominal pain in young adults and children
- Self-limiting condition
- Can be accurately diagnosed at laparotomy
- True incidence is not known
- Probably most common cause of inflammatory adenopathy; even more common than tuberculosis.
- Can have a similar presentation to acute appendicitis.
- Most common in patients under 18 years of age.
- May have a history of recent sore throat or upper respiratory tract infection.

COMPLICATIONS

- Suppuration
- Rupture of lymph nodes
- Peritonitis
- Abscess formation

 Differential Diagnosis

- Infection:

—Acute appendicitis: 20% of patients treated for possible acute appendicitis had mesenteric adenitis.
—Infectious mononucleosis: associated lymphadenopathy more generalized than in mesenteric adenitis. Look for associated splenomegaly; can check for cold agglutinins and screen for positive mono or EBV titers.
—Tuberculosis: Look for associated intestinal involvement, positive PPD.
—Pelvic inflammatory disease: a consideration in sexually active adolescents; vaginal examination useful
—Urinary tract infections: Urine analysis is helpful.
—Abscess: related to missed acute appendicitis, IBD
—*Yersinia enterocolitica* infection: bloody diarrhea, arthropathy present; stool culture is diagnostic
—Typhlitis: Transmural inflammation of the cecum seen in patients with neutropenia and undergoing chemotherapy.

- Tumors: lymphoma: can get more generalized adenopathy; may need to get CT scan of the abdomen and even laparotomy to make or confirm the diagnosis
- Trauma: hematomas of the abdominal wall and intestines; history of trauma will be present
- Metabolic: acute intermittent porphyria; cyclical episodes of acute abdominal pain and vomiting; appropriate metabolic workup diagnostic
- Congenital: duplication cysts; may present with abdominal pain due to rupture, bleeding, intussuception, or volvulus
- Psychosocial: irritable bowel syndrome; alternating diarrhea and constipation with crampy abdominal pain
- Miscellaneous:

—Crohn disease: associated mesenteric adenitis but also intestinal involvement
—Intussuception: acute abdominal pain with currant jelly stools; barium enema is diagnostic
—Ovarian cysts: may need abdominal/pelvic ultrasound to differentiate between the two
—Volvulus: acute, severe abdominal with vomiting. No fever or prodrome. Acute surgical abdomen on physical examination.

 Data Gathering

HISTORY

Question: Abdominal pain?
Significance: Ache to severe colic; is the first symptom, due to stretch on the mesentery.

Question: Pain?
Significance: May initially be in the upper abdomen/right lower quadrant (RLQ) or generalized. If generalized, eventually becomes localized to RLQ. An important point is that the patient cannot localize the exact point of the most intense pain, unlike appendicitis.

Question: Spasms?
Significance: Between spasms the patient feels well and can walk without any difficulty. One-third of patients have nausea and vomiting.

- Anorexia and fatigue are uncommon.

 Physical Examination

- Patient flushed: Early in the attack fever may be 38°C to 38.5°C.
- May have an associated rhinorrhea or acute pharyngitis.
- Approximately 20% of patients will have cervical adenopathy.
- Abdominal examination shows tenderness of the RLQ: It may be a little higher, more medial, and less severe than acute appendicitis.
- Point of maximal tenderness may vary from one examination to the next.
- Some patients may have diffuse or periumbilical tenderness as well. There is no rigidity.
- Voluntary guarding and rebound tenderness may be seen.

Laboratory Aids

Test: CBC
Significance: One-half of the patients may have white blood cell counts over 10,000.

IMAGING

Test: Abdominal ultrasound
Significance: Will differentiate between acute appendicitis, pelvic inflammatory disease, ovarian pathology, and mesenteric adenitis.

Test: An upper GI with small bowel follow-through series
Significance: May be diagnostic for inflammatory bowel disease.

 ## Therapy

- Mainly supportive

 ## Follow-Up

WHEN TO EXPECT IMPROVEMENT

Acute symptoms may take days to resolve and generally last a few days after the associated viral symptoms have resolved.

SIGNS TO WATCH FOR

- Increasing abdominal pain
- Vomiting
- Fevers
- Toxic appearance
- Severe tenderness that is persistent
- Guarding
- Rigidity
- Decreasing bowel sounds

PROGNOSIS

- Very good. Most patients recover completely without any specific treatment.
- Death is very unusual and may only occur when secondary specific infection occurs with bacteria (i.e., hemolytic strep leading to suppuration, rupture of the nodes with resulting abscess and peritonitis).

PITFALLS

Can be frequently difficult to differentiate from acute appendicitis clinically, and many patients may have a laparotomy before the right diagnosis is made.

 ## Common Questions and Answers

Q: Can one clinically differentiate between acute appendicitis and non-specific mesenteric adenitis?
A: Patients with non-specific mesenteric adenitis cannot localize the exact point of the most intense pain, unlike appendicitis. Between spasms patients with non-specific mesenteric adenitis feel well and can walk without any difficulty. Abdominal examination shows tenderness of the RLQ that is a little higher, more medial, and less severe than in acute appendicitis. Point of maximal tenderness may vary from one examination to the next in patients with non-specific mesenteric adenitis. There is no rigidity on abdominal examination in patients with nonspecific mesenteric adenitis.

Q: What are the two investigations that can be diagnostic for RLQ pain?
A: An ultrasound of the RLQ can differentiate between acute appendicitis, ovarian pathology, and lymphadenopathy. An upper GI with small bowel follow-through series can be diagnostic for inflammatory bowel disease.

ICD-9-CM 089.2

BIBLIOGRAPHY

Adams JT. Abdominal wall, omentum, mesentery and retroperitoneum. In: Schwartz SI, Shires GT, Spencer FC, eds. *Principles of surgery*. New York: McGraw-Hill, 1989:1491–1524.

Bell TM, Steyn JH. Viruses in lymph nodes of children with mesenteric adenitis and intussusception. *Br Med J* 1962;2:700–702.

Cherry JD. Enteroviruses: poliovirus, coxsackie virus, echovirus and enterovirus. In: Feigin RD, Cherry JD, eds. *Textbook of pediatric infectious diseases*, 3rd ed., vol. II. Philadelphia: WB Saunders 1997;157:1705–1752.

Swischuk LE. Periumbilical pain and fever. *Pediatr Emerg Care* 1998 Apr;14(2):159–160.

Author: Andrew E. Mulberg and Maria R. Mascarenhas

Metabolic Disease in Newborns

 Database

DEFINITION

Inborn errors of metabolism of amino acids, carbohydrates, fats, or of energy harvesting processes within the mitochondria can present in the neonatal period. Milder forms present later with less severe manifestations. Symptoms may be incorrectly attributed to perinatal insults. Signs and symptoms suggest neonatal sepsis and may include vomiting, poor feeding, lethargy or depressed consciousness, hypo- or hypertonia, hyperreflexia, hypothermia, and the presence of odors in urine or body secretions.

PATHOPHYSIOLOGY

- Central nervous system (CNS) accumulation of lipid soluble neurotoxic metabolites
- Failure of neuronal energy production
- Severe metabolic acidosis
- Hepatic dysfunction

GENETICS

- Majority are autosomal recessive; mitochondrial disease may have a maternal inheritance pattern.

COMPLICATIONS

- Developmental delay and neurological dysfunction
- Recurrent acidosis or hyperammonemia, especially with fasting or infection
- Death
- Pancreatitis can occur in association with metabolic decompensation

 Differential Diagnosis

Metabolic disorders can mimic almost any acute disease of the neonate. Any full-term infant sick enough to warrant a blood culture, because of possible neonatal sepsis, should also have several chemical studies performed (*see* Laboratory Aids).

- Sepsis (bone marrow suppression by toxins)
- Hyperammonemia (with respiratory alkalosis)
- Encephalopathy with metabolic acidosis
- Encephalopathy without metabolic acidosis

 Data Gathering

HISTORY

Question: Have any members of your family died early in life? What was the diagnosis?
Significance: Because these disorders are genetic, a sibling or relative who died in infancy may gave been an undiagnosed case. Quite often, the stated diagnosis is sepsis or meningitis.

Question: What is the dietary intake?
Significance: Feeding history (breast feeding with lower protein content may delay presentation); lactose containing formula will increase symptoms of galactosemia. Most present in the first 2 weeks of life. Protein feeding may hasten clinical presentation but normal turnover of proteins will cause symptoms in a neonate with an inborn error of amino acid catabolism.

Question: Are there any signs of sepsis?
Significance: Septic appearing neonate with associated hepatic, renal, hematologic, or gastroenterologic abnormalities should prompt search for metabolic disorder.

SPECIAL QUESTIONS

Question: Gestational age?
Significance: Most patients are full-term.

Question: Did any sibling die in the neonatal or early infancy period?
Significance: Positive family history of previous sibling deaths, without a clear diagnosis, is an important clue.

 Physical Examination

GENERAL

Finding: Odors in urine (warm tube in hand to volatilize organic acids), cerumen, saliva
Significance: Organic acidurias

Finding: Hepatomegaly without splenomegaly
Significance: Urea cycle defects

Finding: Facial dysmorphic features
Significance: Various storage and peroxisomal diseases

Finding: Very large fontanelle
Significance: Peroxisomal diseases

NEUROLOGICAL

Finding: Level of consciousness and effect of feeding
Significance: Possible intoxication because of blocked metabolism

Finding: Seizures
Significance: CNS toxicity

Finding: Hypotonia and hypertonia
Significance: CNS toxicity

Finding: Abnormal reflexes
Significance: CNS toxicity

Laboratory Aids

Test: ABG
Significance: Acidosis

Test: Blood glucose
Significance: Hypoglycemia

Test: Blood ammonia
Significance: 1° or 2° hyperammonemia

Test: Electrolytes
Significance: Determine anion gap

Test: Urine or serum ketones
Significance: Specialized laboratory testing will probably be required and includes plasma amino acid quantitation, urinary organic acid quantitation, analysis for sulfites, very long chain fatty acids, cerebral spinal fluid examination for lactate/amino acids.

Test: Hyperammonemia without metabolic acidosis
Significance: Urea cycle defects

Test: Acidosis with ketosis
Significance: With or without secondary hyperammonemia suggests organic acidurias

Test: Ketosis with minimal acidosis
Significance: Consider MSUD

Test: Ketosis with lactic acidemia
Significance: Mitochondrial defects

Test: Hepatic dysfunction
Significance: Galactosemia, tyrosinemia, gluconeogenic defects, alpha$_1$-antitrypsin deficiency

Test: Disorders with normal routine blood chemistry
Significance: Non-ketotic hyperglycinemia, peroxisomal diseases

 ## Therapy

GENERAL

Temporizing measures while arranging transfer to a center equipped to care for a neonate with an inborn error of metabolism include:

- Caloric support: glucose 10% to 12.5% to blunt catabolism
- Restore normal acid-base balance
- Remove CNS toxins with hemofiltration or hemodialysis
- If pyruvate dehyrogenase defects suspected ketogenic diet is preferable to high glucose

SPECIFIC THERAPEUTIC MEASURES

- Consult a specialist in inherited metabolic disease
- Admit to intensive care unit pending transfer to a center expert in the care of such patients
- Pyridoxine responsive seizures respond to 100 to 300 mg IV pyridoxine
- For hyperammonemia drugs to increase waste nitrogen excretion such as Na benzoate and Na phenylbutyrate (these agents are not innocuous and should be administered by someone experienced in their use)

Follow-Up

- Prognosis depends on early diagnosis and treatment
- Recurrent episodes of metabolic decompensation occur with intercurrent illness and fasting
- Follow-up for their metabolic disorder should be at a center familiar with all aspects of these diseases

PRENATAL DIAGNOSIS

- When possible it may permit therapy at or before birth (requires close association with metabolic experts who will take care of the newborn)

PITFALLS

- Failure to consider the diagnosis of one of these rare disorders may delay appropriate therapy.
- Do not delay therapy until a definitive diagnosis is made—it may be too late.
- Failure to consult with expert in inborn errors once such a diagnosis is suspected.

 ## Common Questions and Answers

Q: If an infant dies before a diagnosis is established, what can be done to provide information for genetic counseling?
A: Explain to the family why a postmortem examination would be helpful for additional counseling. Notify the pathologist immediately that a possible inborn error was the cause of the infant's demise. Collect body fluids, skin for fibroblast culture, and tissue (to be frozen) for enzymatic assays.

Q: Does the degree of developmental disability depend on the the severity of the neonatal presentation?
A: Not entirely as the the number and severity of subsequent episodes of metabolic decompensation influence the developmental outcome.

ICD-9-CM
Hyperaminoaciduria 270.9
Hyperammonemia 270.6

BIBLIOGRAPHY

Brusilow SW, Maestri NE. Urea cycle disorders: diagnosis, pathophysiology, and therapy. *Adv Pediatr* 1996;43:127–170.

Christodoulou J, McInnes RR. Hereditary metabolic disease in early infancy: new concepts and new disorders. *Curr Opin Pediatr* 1992; 4:228–239.

Morris AAM, Leonard JV. Early recognition of metabolic decompensation. *Arch Dis Child* 1997;76:555–556.

Author: Robert M. Cohn

Metabolic Disorders with Hepatic Dysfunction

Database

DEFINITION

Some metabolic diseases present throughout the lifespan from infancy to adulthood with signs/symptoms of hepatic dysfunction including:

- Hepatomegaly
- Jaundice
- Hypoglycemia
- Elevations of hepatic enzymes
- Hyperammonemia
- Failure to thrive
- Protein/food intolerances
- Anorexia, vomiting, diarrhea

Adverse effects of hepatic dysfunction on the central nervous system (CNS) include ataxia, stupor, coma, and hypoglycemic seizures.

Examples of inborn errors with hepatic dysfunction:

- Urea cycle enzyme defects (failure to remove ammonia, a potent neurotoxin)
- Organic acidurias
- Fatty acid oxidation disorders
- Tyrosinemia type I
- Hepatic glycogen storage diseases (GSD I, III)
- Transferase deficient galactosemia
- Hereditary fructose intolerance
- Wilson disease
- Various storage diseases (*see* Metabolic Disorders with Neurologic Dysfunction)

PATHOPHYSIOLOGY

- The liver is the major organ for removal of ammonia and other toxins and carries out glucose production, glycogen storage, fat metabolism, and the synthesis of plasma proteins.
- Liver failure hampers detoxification and energy balance, adversely affecting the function of other organs.

GENETICS

Almost all of the disorders are autosomal recessive with incidences of 1:10,000 to 1:500,000.

EPIDEMIOLOGY

- Some diseases are detected by screening before any signs or symptoms are present.
- Hyperammonemic states and organic acidurias can occasionally present with hepatic more than CNS findings.

COMPLICATIONS

- Neurotoxins can cause seizures, motor and developmental delay
- Hypoglycemia
- Hepatic disease: fibrosis, cirrhosis; transplantation may have to be considered
- Pancreatitis

Differential Diagnosis

Precious time can be lost if the diagnosis of an inborn error is not considered and hepatopathy and CNS symptoms are attributed to perinatal insults:

- Infections: TORCH
- Toxins (history is key): heavy metals, acetaminophen, heterocyclic compounds, alcohol and substances of abuse
- Pancreatitis
- Congenital hepatic and bile duct malformations
- Malrotation/volvulus
- Ketotic hypoglycemia
- Reye syndrome (associated with salicylates)

Data Gathering

HISTORY

Question: Is there a family history of death in early infancy or undiagnosed severe liver disease?
Significance: Metabolic diseases involving the liver are mainly autosomal recessive.

Question: Is there any pattern to the illness?
Significance: Tipoff may be episodic nature of signs and symptoms.

- Metabolic deterioration to fasting or childhood infection.
- Association of symptoms with ingestion of protein, lactose, or sucrose (fruits).
- Avoidance of sweets (hereditary fructose intolerance, protein in urea cycle defects, anorexia.
- Salicylates and viral infection.
- Inability of patient to fast for longer than 8 to 12 hours: consider glycogenoses and fatty acid oxidation defects.
- Pancreatitis may be a presenting sign of organic acidurias.

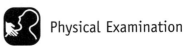

Physical Examination

Finding: Tachypnea/hyperpnea
Significance: Caused by metabolic acidosis or respiratory alkalosis (hyperammonemia)

Finding: Telltale odors on breath, in urine, saliva, cerumen
Significance: MSUD (syrup), isovaleric acidemia and glutaric aciduria type I (sweaty socks), tyrosinemia (cabbage), ketones (fruity)

Finding: Hepatomegaly
Significance: Storage diseases; urea cycle defects

Finding: Jaundice
Significance: Common in galactosemia, also in tyrosinemia and hereditary fructose intolerance

Finding: CNS findings
Significance: Lethargy after feeding, developmental delay, ataxia. In some disorders the findings are episodic.

Finding: Failure to thrive
Significance: Most inborn errors cause FTT

Laboratory Aids

ROUTINE STUDIES

Test: Blood glucose, ammonia, electrolytes, liver functions
Significance: Look for increased unconjugated bilirubin fraction

Test: Lactate; urine ketones
Significance: Organic acidemias

Test: Increased anion gap in organic acidurias.
Significance: Acid ion accumulation

Test: Reducing substances in urine
Significance: Galactosemia, hereditary fructose intolerance

Test: Amylase, lipase with findings compatible
Significance: Pancreatitis

SPECIAL

In consultation with an expert in inherited metabolic diseases the following should be considered:

Test: Plasma amino acid quantitation, copper, ceruloplasmin, urinary organic acid quantitation, urinary orotate
Significance: Amino acid, organic acid disorders, Wilson disease

Test: Enzyme studies
Significance: When glycogen storage diseases are suspected

Test: Provocative testing
Significance: Should only be performed in hospital under close observation and after consultation with expert in inborn errors. Tests like prolonged fasting and fructose challenges are best done in a center familiar with the vagaries of such protocols.

CONFIRMATION

Test: Cultured skin fibroblasts or liver biopsy
Significance: May require enzyme assays

Test: DNA analysis
Significance: May be diagnostic

SCREENING

Test: Some states screen for galactosemia and tyrosinemia
Significance: Early diagnosis but result may arrive after *E. coli* sepsis occurs

Test: Blood by blood spot card
Significance: Screening possible of acyl-carnitines

IMAGING

Test: MRI
Significance: In organic aciduria and other inborn errors which affect the CNS, MRI may shown lesions, especially in the basal ganglia.

 ## Therapy

- Acute detoxification to protect CNS—may require hemofiltration or hemodialysis
- Restore acid/base balance
- Administer intravenous glucose at 5 to 9 mg/kg/min to prevent catabolism
- Removal of ammonia: agents to shunt ammonia into minor metabolic pathways, may require dialysis
- Acute illnes may be associated with cerebral edema
- Long-term therapy requires a diet deficient in the offending dietary component (such a prescription should be developed by an expert in inborn errors). Examples of dietary measures:

—Organic acidurias: protein restriction, high carbohydrate, glycine (in isovaleric acidemia), carnitine
—Urea cycle disorders: protein restriction and agents that foster waste nitrogen removal: Na benzoate and Na phenylbutyrate
—Hypoglycemic disorders: avoidance of fasting, uncooked starch to release carbohydrate over a prolonged period, continuous night feeds by NG tube
—Hereditary fructose intolerance: avoidance of fructose and sucrose in all foods including fruits

 ## Follow-Up

- Clinical improvement in acute states may take a short time (acidosis) to days (stupor, coma)
- In galactosemia, jaundice may improve in several days
- These disorders are signified by episodic relapses

PITFALLS

Failure to consider these disorders may result in fatal outcome

 ## Common Questions and Answers

Q: Can episodic vomiting be the only symptom of an inborn error?
A: Yes, vomiting can be the only symptom in organic acid disorders, urea cycle disorders, and fatty acid oxidation disorders.

Q: What are the characteristics of ketotic hypoglycemia?
A: Hypoglycemia in a child 18 to 72 months of age, often symptomatic in the morning after overnight fast; laboratory: absence of abnormal levels of organic acids (including lactate) in urine or plasma; response to glucose alone; exclusion of other causes of hypoglycemia.

ICD-9-CM
Galactosemia 270.1
Tyrosinemia 270.2
Wilson 275.1

BIBLIOGRAPHY

Arens R, Gozal D, Williams JC, et al. Recurrent apparent life-threatening events during infancy: a manifestation of inborn errors of metabolism. *J Pediatr* 1993;123:415–418.

Clarke JTR. *A clinical guide to inherited metabolic diseases.* Cambridge, MA: Cambridge University Press, 1996.

Cohn R, Roth K. *Biochemistry and disease: bridging basic science and clinical practice.* Baltimore: Williams and Wilkins, 1996.

Author: Robert M. Cohn

Metabolic Disorders with Neurologic Dysfunction

 ## Database

DEFINITION

Neurodegenerative disorders (NDDs) may target gray matter (poliodystrophy), or white matter (leukodystrophy), or both (many inborn errors including mitochondrial encephalomyopathies). Hepatosplenomegaly or cardiomyopathy are also early findings.

PATHOLOGY

Many of these disorders are lysosomal storage diseases, which cause dysfunction or death of neurons. Some of these disorders have an unrelenting downhill course marked by inanition, respiratory failure, seizures, and worsening central nervous system (CNS) function. Biopsy of tissue outside the CNS may provide a clue to the nature of material stored.

EPIDEMIOLOGY

Different variants of these storage diseases may present at different ages. Often the disorder is not suspected until significant nervous system symptoms and signs are present.

GENETICS

- Autosomal recessive

—PKU
—Many lysosomal storage diseases
—Leukodystrophies
—Organic acidurias
—Aminoacidopathies

- Dominant

—Ataxias
—Huntington disease
—Some of the porphyrias

- X-linked

—Lesch-Nyhan
—X-linked adrenoleukodystrophy
—Ornithine transcarbamylase deficiency

- Maternal

—Several of the mitochondrial encephalomyopathies

COMPLICATIONS

- Neurological dysfunction can lead to infection
- Respiratory failure
- Decubiti

 ## Differential Diagnosis

Loss of previously acquired skills or slowdown in cognitive/motor development is the sign of these disorders: this requires a painstaking history and neurological examination. NDD must be distinguished from:

- Non-neurological disorders that may retard motor or language development:

—Hypothyroidism
—Deafness
—Osteodystrophies, Ehlers-Danlos, and other connective tissue disorders
—Rheumatoid disorders
—Prematurity or birth trauma
—Psychiatric-depression, schizophrenia, conversion

- Genetic causes of non-progressive CNS dysfunction

—Down syndrome (premature Alzheimer-type dementia occurs in adults with Down syndrome)
—Fragile X
—Duchenne or myotonic muscular dystrophy
—Tuberous sclerosis, neurofibromatosis

- Multifactorial/acquired neurological disorder

—Autism and other developmental language disorders
—Attention deficit hyperactivity disorder
—Congenital infection (TORCH)
—CNS migrational disorders: lissencephaly/pachygria (chromosome 17)

 ## Data Gathering

HISTORY

Question: Developmental history?
Significance: Decrease in development may occur rapidly or very slowly. Compounding the difficulty in recognition, many of these disorders progress very slowly until an intercurrent infection causes metabolic decompensation (e.g., organic acidurias, urea cycle defects).

Question: Is there a familial history of any other affected members?
Significance: These disorders are familial (*see* Genetics).

SPECIAL QUESTIONS

Question: Personality changes?
Significance: May be a feature

Question: Ethnic origin?
Significance: May furnish clues

Question: How has individual performed in school?
Significance: Obtain input from teachers, standardized tests to document deterioration.

FINDINGS

Question: Leukodystrophies?
Significance: Associated with dysarthria, ataxia, visual loss, spasticity (X-linked adrenoleukodystrophy, metachromatic leukodystrophy, Krabbe).

Question: Poliodystrophies?
Significance: Associated with seizures, cognitive decline, personality change (Rett syndrome, mitochondrial disease, Wilson disease, Alper disease, Lafora body disease, Huntington disease).

Question: Mitochondrial disorders?
Significance: Associated with sensorineural hearing loss, cardiac and skeletal myopathy, failure to thrive, marrow dysfunction, diabetes mellitus.

Question: Renal stones?
Significance: Lesch-Nyhan may present with renal stones.

Question: Hepatic porphyrias?
Significance: Present with abdominal pain, vomiting, weakness, sensory loss, altered mental state, seizures, liver disease.

 ## Physical Examination

Finding: Obtain height, head circumference
Significance: Also measure family members for comparison.

Finding: Microcephaly
Significance: Lactic acidoses, ceroid lipofuscinoses, Rett syndrome.

Finding: Macrocephaly
Significance: MPS, Canavan, Zellweger, glutaric aciduria type I.

Finding: Short stature
Significance: Mitochondrial disorders, storage disorders.

SKIN/HAIR

Finding: Doughy, puffy skin
Significance: Found in many storage disorders.

Finding: Hyperpigmentation
Significance: Adrenoleukodystrophy

Finding: Light complexion
Significance: In comparison to other family members: PKU

Finding: Friable hair
Significance: Menkes disease, argininosuccinic aciduria

Finding: Erythematous rash
Significance: Biotinidase deficiency, Hartnup

EYES

Finding: Retinal pigmentary changes
Significance: Ceroid lipofuscinosis, abetalipoproteinemia, MPS, Kearns-Sayre

Finding: Cherry-red macular spots
Significance: Tay-Sachs, sialidoses, Neimann-Pick, mucolipidosis I.

Finding: Nystagmus
Significance: Pelizaeus-Merzbacher, ataxias, mitochondrial disorders

FACIAL FEATURES

Finding: Coarsening
Significance: Storage diseases, except MPS III (Sanfilippo disease)

THORAX/ABDOMEN

Finding: Visceromegaly
Significance: Storage disorders, Zellweger disease

Finding: Scoliosis
Significance: Homocystinuria

EXTREMITIES

Finding: Arthropathy
Significance: Storage diseases

Finding: Arachnodactyly
Significance: Homocystinuria

NEUROLOGIC

Finding: Peripheral nervous dysfunction in some leukodystrophies
Significance:

Finding: Myopathy
Significance: Mitochondrial diseases

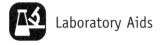 Laboratory Aids

COMMON ABNORMALITIES

Test: Blood glucose
Significance: Hypoglycemia

Test: Blood ammonia
Significance: Hyperammonemia

Test: Electrolytes
Significance: Persistent anion gap

Test: Hepatic function
Significance: Elevated liver enzymes

SPECIAL TESTS

Test: Amino acid quantitation
Significance: Amino acid disorders

Test: Urine organic acid quantitation
Significance: Organic acidemias

Test: Lysosomal enzyme studies
Significance: Storage diseases

Test: Carnitine levels
Significance: Depleted in organic acidurias, mitochondrial disorders

Test: Cholesterol and 7-deoxycholesterol
Significance: Smith-Lemli-Opitz

Test: Plasma very long chain fatty acids
Significance: Peroxisomal disorders

Test: N-acetylaspartate in urine or plasma
Significance: Canavan disease

Test: Urate elevation
Significance: Lesch-Nyhan

Test: Serum transferrin isoelectric focusing
Significance: Carbohydrate-deficient glycoprotein disease

Test: Muscle biopsy
Significance: In suspected mitochondrial disorders

Test: Porphyrins in blood, urine, stool
Significance: Various porphyrias

Test: MRI
Significance: Abnormal white matter signal in leukodystrophies

Test: MRI
Significance: Cortical atrophy in poliodystrophies

Test: MRI
Significance: Caudate atrophy in Huntington disease

Test: Basal ganglia abnormalities
Significance: Wilson, mitochondrial (Leigh's disease), organic acidurias

 Therapy

- Supportive

—Correct acidosis
—Muscle relaxants, chloral hydrate, or benzodiazepines may help relieve hypertonicity and spasticity
—Anticonvulsants for epilepsy
—Gastrostomy feeding may be required to provide adequate calories in the face of anorexia or swallowing dysfunction

- Treatment of underlying disease

—Dietary manipulation and megavitamin supplementation in vitamin dependent disorders
　　—Na benzoate and Na phenylbutyrate in hyperammonemic disorders
　　—Erucic acid (Lorenzo oil) may delay onset of symptoms in X-linked adrenoleukodystrophy.
　　—Coenzyme Q, vitamin K, vitamin C, riboflavin, electron acceptors for respiratory chain defects
　　—Biotin in holocarboxylase deficiency
　　—Pyridoxine (B6) in some cases of neonatal/infantile epilepsy
　　—Folate in folate reductase deficiency
　　—Betaine, pyridoxine, and folate in some cases of homocystinuria
　　—Vitamin E in abetalipoproteinemia
　　—Cholesterol supplementation in Smith-Lemli-Opitz
　　—Allopurinol in Lesch-Nyhan

- Treatment of porphyria

—Avoid stress triggers: certain drugs precipitate attacks
—Increase carbohydrate intake
—Protect skin from exposure to sun, use of powerful sunblocks, oral beta-carotene

 Follow-Up

- Arrange for genetic counseling and consulation with metabolic expert
- Seek out nutritional support group

PITFALLS

- Risk of recurrence requires making a specific diagnosis
- Occasionally a static encephalopathy may represent the aftermath of an unrecognized neurodegenerative process
- Lactate and pyruvate levels can be normal in individuals with lactic acidosis because compensation waxes and wanes
- Consult an expert before arranging for enzyme assays

 Common Questions and Answers

Q: Why put the patients and families through a costly and long work-up when so few of these disorders are treatable?
A: Accurate diagnosis is essential for genetic counseling for the family, will help predict the clinical course, and may identify other affected family members.

Q: Can seizure medications ever be dangerous in children with inborn errors?
A: Yes. Valproate can cause hepatotoxicity in some children with abnormal carbohydrate metabolism. Many anticonvulsants/sedatives can precipitate an acute porphyric attack.

ICD-9-CM
Lesch-Nyhan 277.2
PKU 270.1
Tay-Sachs 330.1

BIBLIOGRAPHY

Chaves-Caballo E. Detection of inherited neurometabolic disorders. *Pediatr Clin North Am* 1992;39:801—820.

Johns DR. Mitochondrial DNA and disease. *N Engl J Med* 1995;333:638—644.

Lyon G, Adams R, Kolodny EH. *Neurology of hereditary metabolic diseases of children.* New York: McGraw-Hill, 1996.

Zeviani M, Tiranti V, Piantadosi, C, Mitochondrial disorders. *Medicine* 1998;77:59—72.

Author: Robert M. Cohn

Microcytic Anemia

Database

DEFINITION

Inadequate hemoglobin synthesis leading to a decrease in hemoglobin concentration and a smaller red cell volume. Caused by either iron deficiency or the inability to utilize iron. Hemoglobin (Hgb) and mean red cell volume (MCV) are below normal for age (see the table Hematologic Values in Children).

Differential Diagnosis

METABOLIC

- Iron deficiency (most common)

ENVIRONMENTAL

- Chronic lead poisoning

CONGENITAL

- Thalassemia syndromes
—Alpha thalassemia trait
—Beta thalassemia trait

INFLAMMATORY

- Recent or chronic inflammation or infection

MISCELLANEOUS

- Sideroblastic anemia (rare in children)

APPROACH TO THE PATIENT

The child with microcytic anemia is usually diagnosed through routine laboratory screening. Most causes are chronic conditions that do not require immediate intervention. Additional laboratory work-up should be guided through careful history taking, review of red cell indices, and review of the peripheral blood smear.

- Initially identify severe anemia that requires inpatient observation and possible blood transfusion.
- Consider lead intoxication early. If history is suspicious (i.e., peeling paint, pica, etc.), draw lead level to make diagnosis.
- Iron deficiency is the most common cause of microcytic anemia. Screen by history as described below. If history is suspicious, consider therapeutic iron trial prior to additional work-up.
- If suspicious of thalassemia, send hemoglobin electrophoresis and complete blood counts from parents.

Data Gathering

HISTORY

Question: What is the child's age?
Significance: Anemia in children age 9 months to 3 years and in adolescence is most commonly due to iron deficiency. Term infants are born with adequate iron stores for 6 months. Nutritional iron deficiency, therefore, should not be responsible for anemia in term infants prior to 6 months of age.

Question: What does the child's diet include?
Significance:

- Evaluate for low dietary iron intake. Iron in breast milk is absorbed better than iron in formula or cows' milk. Formula and cereal should be iron-fortified. In preschool children and adolescents assess intake of high iron-containing foods including red meats, fish, poultry, beans, and peanut butter. Bran, vegetable fiber, and tannins found in tea can decrease iron absorption.
- Introduction of whole cows' milk before the age of 1 provides little dietary iron and can cause occult intestinal bleeding leading to iron loss. High intake of milk also causes a decreased appetite for other foods with a higher iron content.
- History of pica suggests iron deficiency or lead intoxication.

Question: Is there any history of blood loss?
Significance: Blood loss decreases iron stores. Ask about loss from stool, urine, chronic nosebleeds, and menorrhagia.

Question: Was the child born prematurely or was there history of blood loss at birth?
Significance: Premature infants have lower total body iron stores and an increased growth rate that leads to increased iron requirements.

Question: What is the child's ethnic background? Is there any familial history of anemia?
Significance: Alpha-thalassemia is most common among children of African or Asian descent. Beta-thalassemia is most common in children of Asian or Mediterranean descent.

Hematologic Values in Children

AGE	HEMOGLOBIN (g/dL)		HEMATOCRIT (%)		COUNT (10¹²/L)		MCV (L)		MCH (pg)		MCHC (g/dL)	
	MEAN	−2 SD	MEAN	−2 SD	MEAN	−2 SD	MEAN	−2 SD	MEAN	−2 SD	MEAN	−2 SD
Birth (cord blood)	16.5	13.5	51	42	4.7	3.9	108	98	34	31	33	30
1 to 3 days (capillary)	18.5	14.5	56	45	5.3	4.0	108	95	34	31	33	29
1 week	17.5	13.5	54	42	5.1	3.9	107	88	34	28	33	28
~2 weeks	16.5	12.5	51	39	4.9	3.6	105	86	34	28	33	28
1 month	14.0	10.0	43	31	4.2	3.0	104	85	34	28	33	29
~2 months	11.5	9.0	35	28	3.8	2.7	96	77	30	26	33	29
~3 to 6 months	11.5	9.5	35	29	3.8	3.1	91	74	30	25	33	30
0.5 to 2 years	12.0	10.5	36	33	4.5	3.7	78	70	27	23	33	30
2 to 6 years	12.5	11.5	37	34	4.6	3.9	81	75	27	24	34	31
5 to 12 years	13.5	11.5	40	35	4.6	4.0	86	77	29	25	34	31
12 to 18 years												
Female	14.0	12.0	41	36	4.6	4.1	90	78	30	25	34	31
Male	14.5	13.0	43	37	4.9	4.5	88	78	30	25	34	31
18 to 49 years												
Female	14.0	12.0	41	36	4.6	4.0	90	80	30	26	34	31
Male	15.5	13.5	47	41	5.2	4.5	90	80	30	26	34	31

These data have been compiled from several sources. Emphasis is given to studies employing electronic counters and to the selection of populations that are likely to exclude individuals with iron deficiency. The mean ±2 SD can be expected to include 95% of the observations in a normal population.

(From *Nathan and Oski's Hematology of Infancy and Childhood*, 5th ed. Philadelphia: WB Saunders, 1998.)

Microcytic Anemia

 Physical Examination

Finding: Child's general appearance
Significance: Most children with mild micocytic anemia are well appearing with a normal physical examination.

Finding: Irritability or pallor.
Significance: Anemia more severe than usual.

Finding: Cardiovascular examination
Significance: Check for instability including tachycardia, hypotension, and presence of a gallop. Flow murmur with chronic significant anemia.

Finding: Abnormal sclerae
Significance: Blue sclera associated with iron deficiency (very rare). Icterus with severe thalassemia syndromes.

Finding: Mouth lesions
Significance: Glossitis and stomatitis are signs of iron deficiency.

Finding: Splenic enlargement
Significance: Splenic enlargement may be seen with more severe thalassemia syndromes. The spleen is a site of extramedullary hematopoiesis and clears abnormal red cells.

 Laboratory Aids

PATIENT

Test: CBC
Significance: Low hemoglobin and low MCV (less than 2 standard deviations below age specific means) defines microcytic anemia.

Test: Red cell distribution width (RDW)
Significance: Measures the variation in red cell size. High in iron deficiency. Normal in thalassemia trait, infection, and lead poisoning.

Test: Ferretin
Significance: Serum ferritin reflects tissue iron stores. Low in iron deficiency. Normal or increased in thalassemia and infection.

Test: Serum iron
Significance: Low in iron deficiency. Normal in thalassemia (unless chronically transfused). Normal or increased in infection.

Test: Transferrin
Significance: Transferrin measures the total iron binding capacity. Increased in iron deficiency. Normal in thalassemia. Normal or increased in infection.

Test: Transferrin saturation
Significance: Transferrin saturation measures the iron available for hemoglobin synthesis. Low in iron deficiency and chronic infection. Normal in thalassemia.

Test: Free erythrocyte protoporphyrin (FEP)
Significance: Measures a precursor molecule to hemoglobin synthesis. Increased in iron deficiency, lead poisoning (very high), and chronic inflammation. Normal or increased in thalassemia.

Test: Lead level
Significance: Increase in lead intoxication.

Test: Hemoglobin electrophoresis
Significance: Increased hemoglobin A_2 in β-thalassemia trait. Normal in α-thalassemia trait and other microcytic anemia.

Test: Peripheral blood smear with microcytosis and hypochromia
Significance: In iron deficiency increased poikilocytosis and anisocytosis. Basophilic stippling in lead poisoning.

Test: Bone marrow aspirate
Significance: Bone marrow is rarely necessary. Can assess iron stores by hemosiderin staining.

FAMILY STUDIES

Test: CBC
Significance: Low or normal hemoglobin and MCV in thalassemia trait.

Test: Peripheral blood smear
Significance: May have microcytosis, poikilocytosis, and anisocytosis in thalassemia syndromes.

Test: Hemoglobin electrophoresis
Significance: Hemoglobin electrophoresis with high hemoglobin A_2 in β-thalassemia trait.

 Therapy

- May require initial inpatient observation in cases of severe anemia.
- Red cell transfusion only if evidence of cardiovascular compromise (rarely indicated).
- Removal of environmental exposure and possible chelation for lead poisoning to prevent central nervous system toxicity.
- Therapeutic trial of iron supplementation.

 Follow-Up

- In cases of mild anemia, the RDW is a helpful test to distinguish between thalassemia and iron deficiency in order to guide additional work-up. RDW is high in iron deficiency and normal in thalassemia trait.
- Lead poisoning and iron deficiency often occur together. Iron deficiency causes increased lead absorption. If history consistent, send lead levels in cases of documented iron deficiency.

 Common Questions and Answers

Q: What is a therapeutic iron trial and when is it indicated?
A: A therapeutic iron trial is a trial of oral iron therapy without additional laboratory testing in a patient with a microcytic anemia and a history of dietary deficiency or known blood loss. An increase in the hemoglobin concentration of 1 g/dL or greater after 2 to 4 weeks of therapy confirms the diagnosis of iron deficiency. If the hemoglobin does not increase, additional laboratory testing is necessary and other diagnoses should be considered.

Q: How is the diagnosis of thalassemia trait made?
A: β-Thalassemia trait, caused by decreased or absent expression of one of the β-globin genes, is diagnosed by an increase in the percentage of A_2 on hemoglobin electrophoresis. Iron deficiency can mask the diagnosis of β-thalassemia trait because it causes a decrease in hemoglobin A_2 and, therefore, hemoglobin electrophoresis should be done when iron deficiency is corrected. In α-thalassemia trait there are two abnormal α-globin genes and two normal ones. It is difficult to make an absolute diagnosis of α-thalassemia. The diagnosis can be highly suspected in patients of appropriate ethnic background who have a microcytic anemia without iron deficiency and with normal hemoglobin by A_2 electrophoresis. Familial gene analysis can be used to confirm the diagnosis if necessary.

Q: How does infection affect the diagnosis of anemia?
A: Common childhood infections can be associated with a mild microcytic anemia. Acute infection also affects some of the laboratory tests used to diagnose the cause of microcytic anemia. With infection there is a shift of iron from serum to storage sites causing a decrease in serum iron and an increase in ferritin and there is an increase in the FEP level. It is, therefore, preferable to evaluate a microcytic anemia 3 to 4 weeks after an infection resolves.

BIBLIOGRAPHY

Graham EA. The changing face of anemia in infancy. *Pediatr Rev* 1994;15:175–183.

Nathan DG, Orkin SH, eds. *Nathan and Oski's hematology of infancy and childhood,* 5th ed. Philadelphia: WB Saunders, 1998.

Oski FA. Iron deficiency anemia in infancy and childhood. *N Engl J Med* 1993;129:190–193.

Pappas DE. Iron deficiency anemia. *Pediatr Rev* 1998;19:321–322.

Segel GB. Anemia. *Pediatr Rev* 1988;10:77–88.

Walters MC, Abelson HT. Interpretation of the complete blood count. *Pediatr Clin North Am* 1996;43:599–622.

Author: Suzanne Shusterman

Milia

Database

DEFINITION

White papules that occur commonly and spontaneously on the face, and frequently elsewhere,
after healing of blisters when present on mucous membranes; referred to as Epstein pearls

PATHOPHYSIOLOGY

• Retention of keratin and sebaceous material
within the pilosebaceous duct, eccrine sweat
duct, or sebaceous collar surrounding vellus
hair.
• Lamellated keratin deposits are found in the
superficial papillary dermis.

EPIDEMIOLOGY

• Common in all age groups.
• Up to 40% of newborns have milia on the
skin
• In older patients, most often related to
trauma, site of irradiation or reepithelializing
blister.

COMPLICATIONS

• Primarily of cosmetic concern.
• Rare potential for foreign body reaction to
occur.
• If persistent milia in an unusual or widespread distribution when seen with other defects: hereditary trichodysplasia (Matie-Unna
hypotrichosis) or oral-facial-digital syndrome
type I

PROGNOSIS

• Spontaneous regression of milia occur in infants.
• In older individuals the lesions are chronic
unless treated.
• Lesions uncommonly recur.

Differential Diagnosis

• Infection

—Molluscum contagiosum
—Impetigo (pustules)
—Herpes simplex (clouded vesicles)
—Environmental (poisons)

• Tumors

—Sebaceous gland hyperplasia

• Hisllaus

—Neonatal acne
—Keratosis pilaris

Data Gathering

HISTORY

- Asymptomatic
- Recent trauma?
- History of blistering diseases?

 ## Physical Examination

- 1- to 2-mm bright white papules with smooth surface: Most often found on cheeks, nose, chin, forehead, but occasionally on dorsal surface of hands and over knees, especially if related to trauma.
- Occasionally, lesions may be seen on upper trunk, extremities, penis, or mucous membranes.
- Distinguish from pustules by palpation

 ## Laboratory Aids

Milia are firm and, when incised, reveal solid keratin rather than liquid contents.

 ## Therapy

- No need for treatment in infants because they are benign, asymptomatic, and often resolve on their own.
- Alternatively, cyst contents may be expressed by squeezing or with a comedone extractor after incision of the overlying epidermis with a needle or no. 11 scapel blade.

SPECIAL QUESTIONS

If present periocularly, ask about history of atopy/allergic conjunctivitis.

 ## Follow-Up

Without treatment, most lesions resolve in 1 to 2 weeks in infants.

 ## Common Questions and Answers

Q: Will the lesions get bigger before they go away?
A: No, there is no tendency to enlarge with time.

ICD-9-CM 706.2

BIBLIOGRAPHY

Hurwitz S. *Clinical pediatric dermatology: a textbook of skin disorders of childhood and adolescence,* 2nd ed. Philadelphia: WB Saunders, 1993.

Author: William J. Alms (revised from Carmen M. Parrott)

Milk Protein Allergy

 Database

DEFINITION

Milk protein allergy describes a group of patients in which symptoms affecting the gastrointestinal tract, skin, and respiratory tract result from ingesting cow's milk protein. This condition is usually a temporary disorder of infancy, leading to abnormalities of the intestinal mucosa while cow's milk is ingested. Predisposing factors include:

- Age (diagnosis usually before 2 years)
- Immune deficiency (low IgA, immaturity of the mucosal immune system, immaturity of mucosal barrier function)
- History or presence of atopy
- Early bottle feeding
- Allergenicity of formula supplied
- Gastrointestinal infection

PATHOPHYSIOLOGY

- Unprocessed cow's milk—80% casein and 19% whey. The whey fraction contains many types of proteins, including:

—β-lactoglobulin
—α-lactalbumin
—Bovine serum albumin
—Orosomucoid
—Folate-binding protein
—β_2-microglobulin
—Transferrin
—Lactoferrin

- Infants ingesting cow's milk appear to always develop an immune response to the proteins with the formation of circulating IgG antibodies and mucosal IgA antibodies, which is felt to be protective.
- If a children are allergic to cow's milk, they develop clinical symptoms associated with an abnormal immune response.
- Exclusively breast-fed infants may also develop milk protein allergy through exposure to allergen that has been transported from the maternal diet into the breast milk.
- Most children appear to be allergic to multiple cow's milk protein fractions; rarely are patients allergic to only one fraction. Although β-lactoglobin is suspected to be a major antigenic stimulus, no single protein fraction has been proven to be the major allergen.

EPIDEMIOLOGY

The prevalence of this entity has been estimated at between 2.0% and 7.5% of otherwise normal infants.

 Data Gathering

History and physical examination are important in raising the suspicion of cow's milk protein allergy; however, these tools have not been proven to have a positive predictive value. Additionally, no single laboratory test appears to have significant sensitivity for detecting this syndrome.

HISTORY

- The diagnosis is implied if clinical symptoms resolve upon removal of cow's milk protein–containing food products.
- Most patients will present in the first few months of life. Symptoms include:

—Failure to thrive
—Chronic diarrhea
—Vomiting
—Abdominal distention
—Occult blood loss with anemia
—Hypoproteinemia

- Infants with allergic colitis present with diarrhea associated with red blood and mucus.
- Often, the infants otherwise appear to be well.
- Rarely, infants may present with hemorrhage and shock.

 Laboratory Aids

- Occasionally, peripheral blood and stool eosinophilia may be documented.
- Certain infectious etiologies of enteropathy may mimic these histologic findings; therefore, infection should be ruled out with stool cultures and duodenal fluid cultures, if available.
- Biopsy is not routinely performed.
- Histologic changes in bowel mucosa tend to be nonspecific.
- Grossly, the mucosa appear friable and inflamed, rarely with erosions or gross ulcerations.
- Pathologic findings may include:

—Partial villous atrophy with reduction in villous height
—Moderate increase in intraepithelial lymphocytes
—Prominent eosinophilic infiltrate

Therapy

- Removal of cow's milk protein–containing products from the diet is the cornerstone of treatment.
- Because approximately 10% to 30% of children allergic to cow's milk will also be allergic to soy, hydrolyzed formulas (Pregestimil, Nutramigen, Alimentum) are the formulas of choice for infants with cow's milk protein intolerance.
- Resolution of bloody stools usually occurs within 24 to 72 hours, but guaiac-positive stools may continue for up to 2 weeks.
- Newer therapies have included the Neocate formula, which is an amino acid, simple carbohydrate and fat-based formula, which has been more effective in recalcitrant cases of allergy.

 Follow-Up

- Tolerance to cow's milk protein usually develops between the ages of 1 and 2 years, and reintroduction of a normal diet can be safely done at that time.
- Occasionally, symptoms of intolerance may persist past the third year of life, and approximately 20% will have symptoms that persist at 6 years of age.
- Cow's milk protein challenge with serologies and biopsies can help to monitor the degree of allergic response in these older children.
- If there is a history of severe anaphylactic reactions or acute urticaria, the cow's milk challenge should be performed in a hospital under medical supervision.

 Common Questions and Answers

Q: What are the newer formulas for treating milk protein allergy?
A: The newest formula is Neocate and Neocate 1+, which is for children older than 1 year. This is an amino acid–based formula that is made with single amino acids and has the least allergic potential.

Q: When does this problem usually resolve?
A: By 1 year in most infants who develop minimal symptoms, but the range can be several years.

BIBLIOGRAPHY

Justinich C. Food allergy and allergic enteropathy. In: Hyams JS, Wyllie R, eds. *Pediatric gastrointestinal disease: pathophysiology, diagnosis, and management*. Philadelphia: WB Saunders, 1998.

Savilahti E, Kuitunen M. Allergenicity of cow milk proteins. *J Pediatr* 1992;121:S12–S20.

Vinton N. Gastrointestinal bleeding in infancy and childhood. *Gastroenterol Clin North Am* 1994;23(1):93–122.

Walker-Smith JA. Cow milk-sensitive enteropathy: predisposing factors and treatment. *J Pediatr* 1992;121:S111–S1115.

Author: Donna Zeiter

Mumps/Parotitis

 Database

DEFINITION

Mumps is an acute viral disease characterized by painful enlargement of the parotids and other salivary glands.

CAUSES

• Parotitis is usually caused by mumps, a paramyxovirus.
• Other viral causes of parotitis include influenza, parainfluenza, and enteroviruses.
• Bacterial cases are usually secondary to *Staphylococcus* (suppurative parotitis).
• Recurrent parotitis is an idiopathic, rare, recurrent swelling of the parotids, without suppuration or external inflammatory changes.
• Rare childhood cases may be secondary to an obstructing calculus, foreign body (sesame seed), or various drugs (antihistamines, phenothiazines, iodine-containing drugs/contrast media).

PATHOPHYSIOLOGY

• The mumps virus enters via the respiratory tract, and a viremia ultimately ensues.
• The viremia spreads to many organs, including the salivary glands, gonads, pancreas, and meninges.

EPIDEMIOLOGY

• Humans are the only known host for mumps.
• Spread is via the respiratory route.
• Incidence of this once very common disease has declined dramatically since the advent of universal childhood immunization. Outbreaks, however, continue to occur.
• Period of communicability: 7 days before to 5 days after onset of parotid swelling
• Most communicable period: 1 to 2 days before the parotid swelling
• Incubation period: 12 to 25 days after exposure
• Mumps is most common in the late winter and spring.
• One attack of mumps (clinical or subclinical) confers lifelong immunity.

COMPLICATIONS

• Meningitis: most frequent childhood complication; this "aseptic meningitis" is usually benign.
• Encephalitis: rarely causes permanent sequelae
• Oophoritis, nephritis, thyroiditis, myocarditis, mastitis, arthritis, transient ocular involvement, deafness, and sterility (all rare)

PROGNOSIS

Complete recovery in 1 to 2 weeks is the rule.

ASSOCIATED ILLNESSES

• Salivary adenitis: This is the most common manifestation of mumps, but one-third occur subclinically.
• Epididymoorchitis: Up to 35% of adolescent and adult mumps is complicated by orchitis. It most commonly occurs in adolescents. Orchitis develops within 4 to 10 days of the onset of the parotid swelling.
• Pancreatitis: Mild inflammation is common; serious involvement is rare.

 Differential Diagnosis

• Mumps parotitis can be distinguished from the other viral causes by clinical presentation along with specialized laboratory studies (see below).
• Bacterial parotitis is usually caused by *S. aureus*, but streptococci, gram-negative bacilli, and anaerobes are also possible.
• Cases of tuberculous and nontuberculous (atypical) mycobacterial parotitis are rare, but have been reported.
• Parotid enlargement can be an initial sign in HIV-infected children.
• A salivary calculus can be diagnosed by sialogram.
• Recurrent childhood parotitis is a rare disorder in which symptoms initially manifest in children 3 to 6 years of age; it is largely a diagnosis of exclusion.
• Cervical or preauricular adenitis may simulate parotitis; close anatomic localization should be diagnostic.
• Infectious mononucleosis and cat-scratch disease are other considerations.
• Drug-induced parotid enlargement occasionally occurs.
• Malignancies of the parotid are extremely rare.
• Pneumoparotitis is seen in those with a history of playing a wind instrument, glass blowing, scuba diving, and even general anesthesia.

 Data Gathering

HISTORY

• Prodromal symptoms are uncommon in children with mumps but may include fever, anorexia, myalgia, headache, and malaise.
• Onset of mumps is usually pain and swelling in front of and below the ear.
• Swelling usually starts with one ear and then rapidly progresses to the other ear.
• Mild fever usually accompanies parotid swelling.
• Dysphagia and dysphonia are common.
• Testicular pain and swelling, along with constitutional symptoms, usually begin approximately 1 week after the parotid swelling of mumps.
• Epigastric pain and constitutional symptoms with pancreatic involvement
• Fever, headache, and stiff neck with meningitis
• Behavioral changes, seizures, and other neurologic abnormalities are rare.
• Other symptoms are analogous to the particular organ involved.

 Physical Examination

• Nonerythematous, tender parotid swelling (erythema seen with suppurative parotitis)
• Swelling ultimately obscures the mandibular ramus.
• The ear is often displaced upward and outward.
• Submaxillary and sublingual glands also may be swollen.
• Inflammation may be noted intraorally at the orifice of Stensen's duct.
• Presternal edema is occasionally noted.
• Mumps are infrequently associated with truncal rash.
• Tender, edematous testicle in mumps orchitis (usually unilateral)

SPECIAL QUESTIONS

Ask the patient if the pain (at the parotid) intensifies with the tasting of sour liquids.

PROCEDURE

Have the patient suck on a lemon drop or lemon juice, and note any discharge from Stensen's duct.

Laboratory Aids

- Uncomplicated parotitis: mild leukopenia with lymphocytosis
- Suppurative parotitis and mumps orchitis: leukocytosis
- Pancreatic involvement: hyperamylasemia and hyperlipasemia
- Salivary adenitis without pancreatic involvement: isolated hyperamylasemia
- Meningitis: CSF pleocytosis (predominately mononuclear)
- Gram stain and culture of pus expressed from Stensen's duct is diagnostic in supportive parotitis.
- Sialography is useful to evaluate for stones or strictures, but is contraindicated in acute infection.
- Serologic confirmation of mump parotitis: complement fixation, neutralization, hemagglutination inhibition, or enzyme immunoassays
- Definitive laboratory diagnosis of mumps parotitis: body fluid isolation of mumps virus in tissue culture

PITFALLS

Skin tests should not be used for tests of immunity; serologic studies are more reliable.

 ## Therapy

- Supportive therapy is all that is required in mumps parotitis.
- Antibiotics directed against *S. aureus* should be used in cases of suppurative parotitis.

 ## Follow-Up

- Most children have resolution of glandular swelling by about 1 week.
- Disappearance of testicular pain and swelling can be expected 4 to 6 days after onset.
- Testicular atrophy is common, though infertility is rare.
- Markedly elevated pancreatic enzymes should be monitored until they improve.
- Children should not return to school until at least 9 days after the onset of parotid swelling.

PREVENTION

- A single 0.5-mL subcutaneous injection of live mumps vaccine (usually given together with measles and rubella) at 12 to 15 months usually confers long-lasting immunity.
- Primary vaccine failure, as well as waning vaccine-induced immunity, have been reported.
- A second vaccination is recommended between 4 and 6 years of age.
- Vaccine should not be administered to children who are immunocompromised by disease or pharmacotherapy, or to pregnant women.
- Children with symptomatic AIDS who are to be vaccinated against measles through the MMR, however, may (and should) receive the live virus vaccine.

 ## Common Questions and Answers

Q: Should immunization be deferred in children with intercurrent illness?
A: No, children with minor illnesses, even with fever, should be vaccinated.

Q: Should vaccination be withheld in children living with immunocompromised hosts?
A: No, vaccinated children do not transmit mumps vaccine virus.

BIBLIOGRAPHY

Bakshi SS, Cooper LZ. Rubella and mumps vaccines. *Pediatr Clin North Am* 1990;37(3): 651–668.

Casella R, Leibundgut B, Lehman K, Gasser TC. Mumps orchitis: report of a mini-epidemic. *J Urol* 1997;158(6):2158–2161.

Chitre VV, Premchandra DJ. Recurrent parotitis. *Arch Dis Child* 1997;77(4):359–363.

Gold E. Almost extinct diseases: measles, mumps, rubella, and pertussis. *Pediatr Rev* 1996;17(4):120–127.

1997 Red book: report of the Committee on Infectious Diseases, 24th ed. Elk Grove Village, IL: American Academy of Pediatrics, 1997.

Quion N, DeWitt TG. Index of suspicion. Case 3. Mumps parotitis. *Pediatr Rev* 1995;16(9):349, 351.

Vetter RT, Johnson GM. Vaccination update. Diphtheria, tetanus, pertussis, mumps, rubella, measles. *Postgrad Med* 1995;98(4):133–137, 141–142, 144–145 passim.

Whitelaw CC, Kallis JM. Pediatric facial swelling. *Acad Emerg Med* 1998;5(2):146, 198–202.

Author: Nicholas Tsarouhas

Munchausen Syndrome by Proxy

 Database

DEFINITION

Munchausen syndrome by proxy (MSBP) describes an illness in a child that is fabricated by someone else (usually the parent). This results in repeated interactions with the medical care system, often leading to multiple medical procedures. The perpetrator denies the cause of the child's illnesses. Symptoms decrease when the child is separated from the perpetrator.

CAUSES

It is the parent, usually the mother, who fabricates the illnesses.

PATHOLOGY

Little is known. The mother herself may have Munchausen syndrome. She may be seeking secondary gain from the attention of medical staff.

EPIDEMIOLOGY

- Varies with presentation
- Of infants monitored in apnea programs, 0.27% are believed to be secondary to MSBP.
- Five percent of allergy patients in some clinic settings are estimated to be MSBP.
- Mortality is approximately 9%.

PROGNOSIS

If undiagnosed, mortality has been estimated at 9%. Some children go on to develop Munchausen syndrome themselves.

 Differential Diagnosis

Diagnosis depends on presentation. MSBP should be considered in unusual presentations of:

- GI bleeding
- Apnea/apparent life threatening event
- Asthma
- Seizures
- GU bleeding

PITFALLS

- Delay in making the diagnosis: The average length of time is 14 months.
- Physicians may be reluctant to suspect the parent because of their own involvement with the family.

 Data Gathering

HISTORY

- Unexplained or unusual illness, symptoms, and signs that are incongruous or present only when the perpetrator is present.
- Usual medical treatment is ineffective in treating the presenting symptom.
- The perpetrator may not be concerned about the patient, may be constantly present while the patient is in the hospital, or may form unusually close relationships with the hospital staff.

SPECIAL QUESTIONS

A history of frequent moves, other siblings who have either died or had unusual medical illnesses may suggest MSBP.

 Physical Examination

- Examination of the patient with apnea presentation may indicate evidence of intentional suffocation.
- Patients who present with unusual bleeding may have lacerations on other parts of the body.
- The perpetrator also may have lacerations.
- The patient may have evidence of old fractures.

 Laboratory Aids

TESTS

Work-up is dictated by presentation:

- Pneumogram to rule out apnea
- If bleeding is the major presentation, identify the blood as the patient's (as opposed to that of the perpetrator or an animal).
- A toxicology screen may be helpful for unusual presentations of poisoning.
- Separating the perpetrator from the patient, with resultant decrease in symptoms, may suggest the diagnosis.
- Suspect MSBP when there is blood or urine culture with many organisms.
- If GI bleeding is the presenting symptom, use endoscopy or a Meckel scan to rule out anatomic causes of bleeding.
- Video monitoring of a patient's room may demonstrate the perpetrator harming the child.
- Ensure that the perpetrator cannot tamper with testing.

Therapy

- If MSBP is documented, the patient must be separated from the perpetrator. Psychotherapy for the perpetrator is warranted.
- As long as the perpetrator is in need of intensive psychotherapy, the patient should be protected.

 Follow-Up

If the perpetrator agrees to seek help, improvement usually occurs.

SIGNS TO WATCH FOR

- Recurrence of original presentation, unusual new symptoms

 Common Questions and Answers

Q: Is it legal to use video surveillance or to separate the parent from the patient?
A: If suspicions of MSBP are high and other laboratory tests are negative, it is important to make the diagnosis. Hospital administration and/or risk management should be consulted on how to proceed.

Q: Should this be reported to child abuse authorities?
A: If documented, this should be reported to protect the child.

ICD-9-CM 301.51

BIBLIOGRAPHY

Anderson, J. McKane, JB. Munchausen syndrome by proxy. *Br J Hosp Med* 1996;56(1): 43–45.

Bools CN, Schreirer HA, Libow JA, et al. Co-morbidity associated with factitious illness (Munchausen syndrome by proxy). *Arch Dis Child* 1992;67:77–79

Light MJ, Sheridan MS. Munchausen syndrome by proxy and apnea. *Clin Pediatr* 1990;29: 162–168.

Meadow R. Munchausen syndrome by proxy: the hinterland of child abuse. *Lancet* 1977;2: 343–345.

Meadow R. Management of Munchausen syndrome by proxy. *Arch Dis Child* 1985;60: 385–393.

Schreir HA, Libow JA. Munchausen syndrome by proxy: diagnosis and prevalence. *Am J Orthopsychiatry* 1993;63:318–321.

Author: Cheryl L. Hausman

Muscular Dystrophies

 ## Database

DEFINITION

Muscular dystrophies (MDs) are hereditary diseases that cause progressive weakness and degeneration of muscle. MDs frequently involve proximal muscles and may also involve cardiac and smooth muscle. These diseases share similar electromyographic (EMG) and muscle pathologic findings and often have elevated creatine kinase (CK). Forms of MDs include:

- Duchenne muscular dystrophy (DMD)
- Becker muscular dystrophy (BMD)
- Myotonic dystrophy (MyD)
- Congenital myotonic dystrophy (CMyD)
- Emery-Dreifus muscular dystrophy (EDMD)
- Facioscapulohumeral muscular dystrophy (FMD)
- Limb-girdle muscular dystrophy (LGMD)
- Severe childhood autosomal recessive muscular dystrophy (SCARMD)
- Congenital muscular dystrophies (CMDs) (Fukuyama, merosin-deficient, others)

Classification

MDs have been classified by clinical criteria such as inheritance pattern, age of onset, pattern of muscle involvement, severity of the disease, and associated conditions. Revised classifications based on mutation analysis are evolving.

PATHOPHYSIOLOGY

Slowly, progressive weakness involves all muscle groups—some worse than others—in a symmetric fashion. Common pathologic findings:

- Loss of muscle cells and residual muscle fibers have variability in size.
- Segmental necrosis of the muscle fiber and some regenerative activity
- Accumulation of lipocytes and collagen between muscle fibers
- Smooth muscle and heart are also affected.
- In some types (MyD, EDMD, DMD, BMD), innervation of the muscle is also affected.
- Brain pathology:

—For an unknown reason, deficiency of membrane-associated cytoskeletal proteins (e.g., in DMD, merosin deficiency) interferes with brain development.
—The milder clinical course in BMD corresponds to a milder degree of dystrophin deficiency that can be measured in muscle.

GENETICS

- DMD, BMD, and EDMD are X-linked recessive; emerin, a membrane bound protein, is deficient in EDMD.
- DMD and BMD are due to mutations in the dystrophin gene. One-third of cases are sporadic and are due to new mutations in the dystrophin gene.

- MyD is autosomal dominant, caused by expansion of a normal triplet repeat sequence of a gene that codes for myotonin protein kinase. The severe congenital form, CMyD, has more than 500 repeats and is usually maternally transmitted.
- FMD is autosomal dominant, due to deletions on chromosome 4.
- LGMD: Some types are linked to deficiency of calpain-3, a muscle specific protease; the autosomal dominant form is mapped to chromosome 5. Recessive types: linked to chromosome 15; SCARMD, mutations in α-, β-, or γ-sacroglycan genes
- CMDs are autosomal recessive or sporadic: Merosin-deficient, α_2-laminin mutation; Fukuyama type (mostly in Japan), linked to chromosome 9; muscle–eye–brain disease, associated with Lissencephaly and may be synonymous with Walker-Warburg syndrome.

EPIDEMIOLOGY

- The incidence of DMD is 1 in 3,500 live male births.
- The estimated minimum incidence of MyD is 1 in 8,000, and BMD is 3 to 6 per 100,000 male births.
- Other forms of MD are less common.

COMPLICATIONS

- Patients with DMD usually die in their 20s of heart failure or pneumonia.
- MyD patients frequently die of cardiomyopathy and respiratory failure. Posterior capsular cataracts, ptosis, and ophthalmoplegia are common in adults.
- Gastrointestinal dysmotility is common in all age groups.
- Hyperinsulinemia with peripheral resistance to insulin, testicular and ovarian atrophy, and hypersomnolence also occur.
- Severe and potentially fatal cardiac arrhythmias are common in EDMD.
- CMDs are often fatal by the end of the first decade because of respiratory failure.
- The Fukuyama type has migrational abnormalities such as lissencephaly, polymicrogyria, and heterotophias.
- The Leukodystrophy type has demyelination in addition to migrational abnormalities.
- Cerebroocular muscular dystrophy has ocular anomalies and cerebral malformations (Warburg syndrome).
- Orthopedic complications, such as arthrogryposis, contractures, kyphoscoliosis, and lumbar lordosis, frequently occur in CMDs, CMyD, EDMD, DMD, and BMD.
- Retinal vascular abnormalities are common in FMD.

ASSOCIATED CONDITIONS

- Mental retardation or learning difficulty, except in LGMD, SCARMD, FMD, some cases of CMD.
- Seizures: occasional in DMD and CMD
- Hearing loss: some cases of FMD
- Malignant hyperthermia with general anesthesia may occur in MDs.

 ## Differential Diagnosis

- Nonneurologic disorders that may superficially appear to cause muscle weakness include factitious weakness and any disorder causing pain with movement.
- Electrolyte disturbance may acutely produce muscle weakness (hypercalcemia, hypokalemia).
- Weakness due to other neurologic disorders that may mimic muscular dystrophy:

—Polyneuropathy: hereditary neuropathy, such as Charcot-Marie-Tooth disease or acquired neuropathy (chronic inflammatory demyelinating polyneuropathy)
—Spinal dysraphism
—Motor neuron disease
—Myasthenia gravis
—Motor degenerative disorders or acquired structural CNS lesions (neoplastic, vascular, or demyelinating)
—Muscle diseases (electromyography usually abnormal) such as polymyositis dermatomyositis, hypothyroid or steroid myopathy, congenital or mitochondrial myopathy
—Metabolic or toxic myopathy

- Disorders causing cratine kinase isoenzyme elevation: infectious, inflammatory, and metabolic myopathies, hypothyroid myopathy, muscular trauma, and malignant hyperthermia
- Myopathy and medication: steroids, Mevacor (lovastatin), alcohol, penicillamine, antimalarials, and antiparasitic medication

 ## Data Gathering

HISTORY

- Age and rapidity of symptom onset
- Symptoms progressive or static
- Disability indicates symmetric, usually proximal, pattern of involvement.
- Pre- and perinatal history is important: Paucity of fetal movements, polyhydramnios, neonatal hypotonia, or respiratory failure could be the first signs of MD.
- Pain, fasciculations, rash, or marked fluctuation in weakness are not features of MD.
- Exposure to certain medications (diuretics, steroids, Mevacor) or toxins may suggest alternative causes of muscle weakness (see Differential Diagnosis).
- Detailed developmental and family histories are essential.
- DMD is usually apparent by the third year of life, with frequent falls, waddling gait, lumbar lordosis, difficulty climbing stairs, and difficulty arising from the floor. Most boys are wheelchair-bound by 13 years of age and die of cardiac or respiratory failure in their 20s.
- BMD appears usually beyond age 6 years. Progression is slower, and death usually occurs beyond the third decade.
- CMyD presents with generalized hypotonia, respiratory distress, facial diplegia, distal limb

weakness, and skeletal deformities at birth. The long-term prognosis poor: 50% survive into their 30s. Requirement of mechanical ventilation beyond 1 month of age is a poor indicator. Adults with MyD are often diagnosed when CMyD appears in the family, because of weakness during immobilization or during work-up for arrhythmias.

- EDMD presents between ages 5 and 15 years with weakness of upper arms and peroneal muscles. Flexion contractures are common in the elbows, neck, and calf muscles. Progression is slow, but some patients have fatal cardiac arrhythmias.
- FMD has onset between ages 5 and 25 years, with weakness of facial, shoulder, and upper arm musculature. There is an inability to close the eyes, whistle, drink through a straw, and raise the arms above the head. Progression is slow, often with periods of nearly complete arrest.
- LGMD begins in the second or third decade with complaints similar to those of DMD.
- SCARMD has a DMD phenotype in girls and boys and begins between ages 5 and 10 years.
- CMDs have neuromuscular symptoms similar to those of CMyd, but also commonly have brain or ophthalmologic disease as well. Progression is variable, but most die in the first decade.

 ## Physical Examination

- Resting tachycardia may be an early sign of cardiomyopathy in DMD and CMyD.
- The respiratory pattern may reflect hypoventilation from weakness of respiratory muscles.
- Children with decreased vital capacity may have a rapid, shallow breathing pattern.
- Check for contractures, scoliosis/lordosis, and pseudohypertrophy.
- There is frontal balding and testicular atrophy in MyD.
- Neurologic
- Cognitive developmental milestones, weakness of facial and shoulder girdle muscles. Functional testing may be most helpful in documenting extremity weakness: The ability of the child to raise the arms over the head, write, stand from a seated position, run, squat, and so on, may be more reproducible, especially when different examiners are involved in follow-up. Myotonia, seen in CMyD and MyD, is a sustained contraction of skeletal muscle in response to voluntary contraction or percussion. It is clinically apparent as an inability to release a hand grip or jaw clench. Deep tendon reflexes are diminished.
- Muscle enlargement also may be seen in motor neuron disease, glycogen storage diseases, hypothyroidism, and amyloidosis. The calf muscles in DMD feel rubbery.
- Toe walking is also seen in spastic diplegia, spinal tumors, spinal dysraphism, hereditary neuropathies, benign/developmental.
- The Gower sign (propping hands on thighs upon rising) and a waddling gait suggest pelvic

weakness. The patient stands and walks on a wide base.
- Infants with CMDs and CMyD are hypotonic, with frog-leg posture and head lag: They may be indistinguishable on examination from spinal muscular atrophy, except that MD does not cause tongue fasciculations.

 ## Laboratory Aids

TESTS

- Chemistry: creatine kinase (CK), aspartate aminotransferase (SGOT), alanine aminotransferase (SGOT), lactate dehydrogenase (LDK), and aldolase. Of these, the CK MM isoenzyme is the most sensitive and specific for primary muscle disease.
- CK measurement should be done before EMG, which might raise the level.
- DMD and the Fukuyama-type CMD have the highest CK level. CK level falls with progression of disease as muscle mass decreases. CK level is usually elevated in female carriers of DMD and BMD.
- Electrophysiologic: EMG helps to distinguish between neuropathy and myopathy. In myopathic conditions, nerve conduction velocity is normal, but motor unit action potentials have shortened duration and lower amplitude.
- Spontaneous trains of discharges by inserting the EMG needle are characteristic for myotonia.
- Electrocardiography (ECG) may reveal tall R waves and a deep Q wave in DMD and A-V block in EDMD.
- Pathologic: the gold standard (see above)
- Immunologic: proteins of DGC, α_2-laminin, merosin, calpain-3 and emerin can be identified by Western blot test, immunohistochemistry, and enzyme-linked immunosorbent assay (ELISA) in muscle biopsy. Dystrophin is measured in fetal muscle biopsies in difficult cases.
- Molecular genetics: DNA-based mutation studies are available for DMD, BMD, EDMD, LGMD, SCARMD, merosin- and Fukuyama-type CMDs, and some FMD types. Triplet repeats on chromosome 19 are identified in MyD. DNA markers can be used in prenatal diagnosis using chorionic villus cells or amniocytes, and also in the detection of carriers.

 ## Therapy

- Mainly supportive. Passive muscle stretching and night splinting delay contractures. Maintenance of upright posture delays scoliosis. Major surgery or long bedrests should be avoided while the patient is still walking. Cataract surgery is recommended in MyD. Attention to healthy diet to avoid obesity; exercise as tolerated; swimming is useful; intubation and mechanical ventilation in infantile forms; pacemakers for arrhythmias; education and support to the patient and the family.

- Vitamin therapies or specific diets have not proved beneficial.
- Dilantin (phenytoin) and Tegretol (carbamazepine) may be helpful for myotonia. Metoclopramide is useful in gastroparesis.
- Gene therapy is not currently available for any of these disorders.
- Use of genetic counseling and support groups is recommended.

PITFALLS

- Pain is usually not present in MDs, but polymyositis, dermatomyositis, and infectious myositis may be painful.
- Dermatomyositis has a typical rash not seen in MD.
- Muscle cramps, weakness, and myoglobinuria after exercise suggest metabolic muscle disease but may also be due to BMD.
- Weakness that varies during the day and involvement of bulbar and extraocular muscles suggest myasthenia gravis.

 ## Common Questions and Answers

Q: What is the recurrence risk in DMD?
A: Each time a heterozygous woman has a child, there is a 25% chance it will be an affected male. Each time a heterozygous mother has a son, the chance that she will transmit the abnormal gene is 50%. Each time a daughter is born, she will have a 50% chance of being a carrier. Affected males transmit the gene to all of their daughters.

ICD-9-CM 359.1

BIBLIOGRAPHY

Birch JG. Orthopedic management of neuromuscular disorders in children. Semin Pediatr Neurol 1998;5(2):78–91.

Fenichel FM. *Clinical pediatric neurology. A sign and symptom approach,* 3rd ed. Philadelphia: WB Saunders, 1997:151–204.

Patterson MC, Gomez MR. Muscle diseases in children: a practical approach. *Pediatr Rev* 1990;12:73–82.

Rosenberg RN, Stanley PB, DiMauro S, Barchi RL. *The molecular and genetic basis of neurological disease,* 2nd ed. Boston: Butterworth-Heinemann, 1997:867–938.

Author: Olafur Thorarenson

Myasthenia Gravis

 Database

DEFINITION

Myasthenia is a disorder caused by a disruption in signal transmission from the motor neuron to the muscle. It presents as intermittent weakness that worsens with exercise and improves with rest. The majority of patients present with ptosis and diplopia alone or in combination with swallowing difficulties and generalized weakness. There are no sensory or cognitive symptoms.

PATHOPHYSIOLOGY

In a healthy person, the motor nerve terminal lies in close proximity to the endplate, a region of the muscle cell membrane with a high concentration of acetylcholine receptors. When stimulated, the motor nerve terminal releases vesicles of acetylcholine that traverse the synaptic cleft and bind to the receptors, causing contraction of the muscle. The cleft contains acetylcholinesterase, an enzyme that breaks down acetylcholine and helps terminate the muscle contractions. In the common autoimmune form of myasthenia, an autoantibody binds to the acetylcholine receptor, and blocks its activity. The rate of receptor breakdown also increases and fewer receptors are present, resulting in decreased muscle contraction.

EPIDEMIOLOGY

There are three types of myasthenia gravis seen in childhood: neonatal transient, congenital myasthenia, and juvenile myasthenia.

• Neonatal transient: 10% to 20% of infants born to mothers with autoimmune myasthenia have maternal-fetal transmission of antibodies against the acetylcholine receptor and are born with weakness and hypotonia. The severity of maternal symptoms do not predict the likelihood of an affected infant. Occasional arthrogryposis (joint contractures) reflect in utero paralysis from transplacental transmission of the antibody. High levels of maternal antibodies against the fetal form of the acetylcholine receptor correspond to an increased risk of disease. A previous pregnancy with an affected infant places future pregnancies at much higher risk.
• Congenital myasthenia: rare; less than 10% of all childhood myasthenia. Weakness usually starts in the first year of life and is caused by an inherited disorder in neuromuscular transmission. Mutations have been described in the presynaptic nerve terminal, acetylcholinesterase, acetylcholine receptors, and postsynaptic proteins.
• Juvenile myasthenia: an autoimmune disorder caused by aberrant production of antibodies against the acetylcholine receptor. It is relatively rare, with one new diagnosis per million patients per year. The average age of onset is 10 to 13 years, with a female predominance of 2:1 or 4:1, depending on the study. Thymic pa-

thology is believed central to the pathogenesis of autoimmune myasthenia; hyperplasia is present in most children who undergo thymectomy.

PROGNOSIS

• Neonatal transient: a self-limited disorder that resolves spontaneously over the first few months of life as maternal antibodies disappear. The infant may require ventilatory and nutritional support during the first few months of life. Infants with arthrogryposis multiplex congenita (born to mothers with antibodies against the fetal form of acetylcholine receptors) may gain mobility with time.
• Congenital myasthenia: Prognosis varies, depending on the specific defect. Autosomal recessive disorders tend to be more severe than the dominant disorders. Weakness shows variable response to cholinesterase inhibitors. Immunosuppressants are not helpful. In general, these are indolent disorders.
• Juvenile myasthenia: Most patients do extremely well with treatment. Longitudinal studies suggest that the rate of spontaneous remission is approximately 2% per year and can occur throughout the lifetime of the patient. Patients with generalized weakness are slightly less likely to experience remission. The mortality rate from myasthenia is near that of the general population in patients under 50 years of age.

ASSOCIATED ILLNESSES

In juvenile myasthenia, other autoimmune disorders may occur: Hyperthyroidism is present in 3% to 9% of patients, and there is a small increase in the incidence of rheumatoid arthritis and diabetes. Some reports suggest an increased incidence of seizures in autoimmune myasthenia.

 Differential Diagnosis

• Generalized botulism, a disease of infants in specific endemic areas, may cause generalized weakness. It is caused by a *Clostridium* toxin that blocks the release of acetylcholine from the nerve terminal. The infant usually presents with generalized hypotonia and a poor suck for days (or weeks). Prominent symptoms unique to botulism are constipation and pupillary dilation. Nerve conduction studies and stool tests for the botulism toxin confirm the diagnosis.
• Guillain-Barré syndrome, or acute inflammatory demyelinating polyneuropathy, is a frequent cause of rapidly progressive generalized weakness. Unlike myasthenia, there are often sensory symptoms, and areflexia occurs even with minimal weakness.
• Acute spinal cord compression can present as generalized weakness of the extremities. If facial and extraocular muscles are not weak, then it is important to look for a sensory level, bowel or bladder dysfunction, and hyperactive reflexes.

• Organophosphate ingestion or an overdose of Mestinon (pyridostigmine bromide) can cause profound weakness. Symptoms of parasympathetic hyperactivity, such as hypersalivation, miosis, diarrhea, and bradycardia, will usually be present.
• Penicillamine is used for the treatment of autoimmune disorders and can induce autoantibodies that bind the acetylcholine receptor, causing myasthenia gravis. The weakness usually resolves when the drug is stopped.

 Data Gathering

HISTORY

• Transient neonatal: The infant is usually born to a mother with known autoimmune myasthenia or a history of weakness, ptosis, or dysphagia.
• Congenital myasthenia: The patient usually presents in the first year of life (though a later age of presentation can occur) with hypotonia and delayed motor milestones. Poor feeding and ptosis are common. There may be a family history of similar weakness. There is no response to thymectomy or immunosuppressant medications.
• Juvenile myasthenia: There is usually a gradual onset of weakness over weeks, months, or even years. The symptoms are worse after prolonged activity or late in the day. Intermittent ptosis, diplopia, dysphagia, and dysphonia are common.

 Physical Examination

• Neonatal: From birth, the infant is hypotonic, with a weak suck, a weak cry, and ptosis.
• Congenital and juvenile myasthenia:

—Weakness of neck flexion
—Ptosis and ophthalmoplegia are often the earliest findings of myasthenia.
—Generalized weakness may be asymmetric in the limbs. The weakness is more pronounced with endurance tasks.
—Shallow, rapid respirations suggest impending ventilatory failure. Vital capacity of less than 50% of predicted (in older children) indicates a danger of respiratory failure.

Laboratory Aids

Juvenile Myasthenia

• Nerve conduction and electromyography studies: Repetitive stimulation of a nerve will demonstrate a rapid decremental response. The decreased number of acetylcholine receptors limits the response to a nerve impulse. Single-fiber electromyography measures the variability in firing rates of two muscle fibers innervated by different branches of the same motor neuron. A large variability, "jitter," suggests a higher threshold for activation because of a limited number of acetylcholine receptors.

• Acetylcholine receptor antibody levels (most specific): Acetylcholine receptor antibody levels are elevated in approximately 80% of patients with generalized myasthenia. Only 50% of patients with isolated ocular myasthenia have an elevated level.

• Tensilon (edrophonium chloride) is a fast-acting acetylcholinesterase-blocking agent. A patient with myasthenia often has an immediate transient improvement in muscle strength after the IV infusion of Tensilon. A measurable weakness should be present prior to testing, and a placebo dose of saline should be given initially. Though the risk of a hyperreactive cholinergic response with muscle weakness and bradycardia is low, atropine should always be available, and the patient's vital signs should be closely monitored during a Tensilon test. A Tensilon test should not be performed if the patient has a known history of heart disease. Cranial nerve findings, such as ptosis, are often responsive to Tensilon and are easily measured.

• Children receive 20% of a 0.2-mg/kg dose of Tensilon over 1 minute; if there is no response after 45 seconds, the rest of the dose is then given, up to a maximum of 10 mg.

 ## Therapy

• The severity of disability should be used to guide the aggressiveness of therapy. Most patients benefit from Mestinon (pyridostigmine bromide) given three to four times per day. A long-acting component prior to bedtime may alleviate obstructive hypoventilation during sleep. Mestinon improves strength by blocking acetylcholinesterase activity. A normal starting dosage is approximately 7 mg/kg/d. The dosage is slowly titrated upward by following symptoms at several-day intervals. Common side effects are hypersalivation, blurry vision, and diarrhea. Most patients can take Robinul (glycopyrrholate) to decrease diarrhea.

• Medical management with immunosuppressants such as prednisone and azathioprine induces remission in 30% of patients and results in significant improvement in another 25% to 60%. Steroids may be weaned over months until weakness recurs. Calcium and every other day dosing limit the bone deterioration from chronic steroids. Azathioprine is a useful adjunctive to steroids and thymectomy. However, it takes 3 to 12 months for its suppressant effects to occur. In one long-term study of juvenile myasthenia, there was no increased risk of cancer or infection with the use of azathioprine.

• Thymectomy generally results in a 20% to 60% remission, and another 15% to 30% of patients show a marked improvement after surgery. As surgical techniques for thymectomy have improved, the complications and recovery times have decreased. Thymectomy earlier in the course of illness appears to produce a higher rate of remission. There are no studies in children, looking at CT or MRI studies of the thymus, that can predict which patients will benefit from thymectomy. On pathology, 80% to 90% of patients undergoing thymectomy have thymic hyperplasia. There are scant data about thymectomy and the risk of infection and other autoimmune disorders during childhood.

• Juvenile myasthenics with profound weakness and respiratory failure should undergo immediate therapy to decrease the number of circulating receptor antibodies. Plasmapheresis or intravenous immunoglobulin can be effective within a few days by decreasing or diluting, respectively, the acetylcholine receptor antibodies. Steroids will diminish antibody production within weeks to months. There may be a paradoxical worsening of symptoms in some patients in the weeks following an increase in steroid dosage.

 ## Follow-Up

• Penicillamine is the only drug that has been shown to induce production of antiacetylcholine receptor antibodies.

• The following medications can exacerbate myasthenia gravis and should be avoided:

—Corticosteroids may worsen symptoms, but usually only briefly, after increasing the dose.
—Aminoglycosides
—Ciprofloxacin
—β-adrenergic blocking agents, including eye drops
—Lithium
—Procainamide
—Quinidine
—Phenytoin

• Nondepolarizing neuromuscular blocking agents may cause lasting (eventually reversible) weakness.

• Always start new medications cautiously.

ICD-9-CM 358.0
Neonatal 775.2

BIBLIOGRAPHY

Gardnerova M, Eymard B, Morel E, et al. The fetal/adult acetylcholine receptor antibody ratio in mothers with myasthenia gravis as a marker for transfer of the disease to the newborn. *Neurology* 1997;48:50–54.

Lindner A, Schalke B, Toyka VK. Outcome in juvenile-onset myasthenia gravis: a retrospective study with long-term follow-up of 79 patients. *J Neurol* 1997;244:515–520.

Rodriguez M, Gomez MR, Howard F, Taylor W. Myasthenia gravis in children: long-term follow-up. *Ann Neurol* 1983;13:504–510.

Sietske R, Angela V, Beeson D, et al. Association of arthrogryposis multiplex congenita with maternal antibodies inhibiting fetal acetylcholine receptor function. *J Clin Invest* 1996; 98(10):2358–2363.

Wittbrodt ET. Drugs and myasthenia gravis: an update. *Arch Intern Med* 1997;157(4):399–408.

Author: Brenda Porter

Myocarditis

Database

DEFINITION

Myocarditis is defined as inflammation of the myocardium in association with myocellular necrosis.

PATHOLOGY

- Infective myocarditis may be caused by viral, bacterial, rickettsial, fungal, or parasitic organisms. Viruses, particularly the enteroviruses (coxsackievirus, echovirus), are the predominant causative agents. Group B coxsackieviruses are the most frequent viral agents associated with myocarditis.
- Other etiologic categories include hypersensitivity drug reactions (rare), toxic myocarditis (drug ingestion), and autoimmune or collagen vascular diseases (systemic lupus erythematosus, rheumatic fever, rheumatoid arthritis, sarcoidosis, peripartum myocarditis, and Kawasaki disease).
- "Idiopathic" myocarditis (unknown etiology) is the most common form encountered in North America.
- While some cases of myocarditis, particularly fulminant ones involving infants and children, may be the result of direct viral cytopathic effect, there is increasing evidence that most cases of myocarditis reflect immunologically mediated cellular injury in response to prior cardiotropic virus infection in genetically predisposed individuals.
- Pathologic specimens reveal lymphocytic infiltration and focal myocardial necrosis during the acute phase of myocardial inflammation. A minority of patients will have persistent lymphocytic infiltrate and ongoing focal necrosis. Rare patients will have diffuse pleomorphic infiltration and necrosis.

PATHOPHYSIOLOGY

- Seventy percent to 80% present with mild-to-moderate congestive heart failure. The vast majority of these children will fully recover in a rapid fashion. A small minority of these patients will have chronic lymphocytic infiltration and focal myocardial necrosis and progress to a dilated cardiomyopathy.
- Twenty percent to 30% present with acute left ventricular failure and shock. One-third of these patients will make a full recovery, one-third will develop dilated cardiomyopathy, and one-third will die at presentation or require cardiac transplantation.
- Left ventricular dysfunction results in pulmonary venous hypertension and pulmonary edema.

EPIDEMIOLOGY

- Enteroviruses such as coxsackievirus and echovirus are ubiquitous and very common in children.
- Enteroviral infection is most common in the summer months.
- Cardiovascular sequelae occur in less than 1% of reported enteroviral infections.
- The incidence increases to approximately 4% when coxsackievirus (Group B) is considered.

PROGNOSIS

- Seventy percent of patients with acute myocarditis will recover completely.
- Twenty percent of patients will develop dilated cardiomyopathy.
- Ten percent of patients will die during the acute phase or have cardiac transplantation.

Differential Diagnosis

- Anomalous origin of the left coronary artery from the pulmonary artery
- Critical aortic stenosis
- Critical coarctation of the aorta
- Interrupted aortic arch
- Dilated cardiomyopathy

Data Gathering

HISTORY

- Tachypnea
- Dyspnea
- Fatigability
- Malaise
- Anorexia and/or emesis (especially in children)

NOTE: Antecedent, nonspecific flulike illness or an episode of gastroenteritis?

Physical Examination

- Pulmonary

—Rales
—Tachypnea

- Cardiovascular

—Sinus tachycardia (at rest)
—Arrhythmias (atrial fibrillation, supraventricular or ventricular ectopy)
—Gallop
—Murmur (mitral and/or tricuspid insufficiency)
—Jugular venous distention (difficult to detect in infants)

- Abdomen

—Hepatomegaly

- Extremities

—Weak pulses
—Poor capillary refill
—Cool extremities

NOTE: Not all findings are present.

Laboratory Aids

TESTS

- Chest radiograph: cardiomegaly and varying amounts of pulmonary edema
- Electrocardiogram: Findings are highly variable and may include low QRS voltages, ST changes, T-wave flattening or inversion, prolongation of the QT interval, and arrhythmias, especially premature atrial or ventricular contractions.
- Echocardiogram

—Cardiac chamber enlargement
—Impaired left ventricular function
—Segmental wall abnormalities
—Global hypokinesis
—Valvar insufficiency (particularly mitral regurgitation)
—Pericardial effusion
—Left ventricular thrombi (occasionally found)

- Endomyocardial biopsy: gold standard for the diagnosis of myocarditis in both adults and children. However, the incidence of "biopsy proven" myocarditis in patients presenting with acute-onset congestive heart failure and dilated cardiomyopathy is approximately 10%. In most cases, virus is not recovered from myocardial biopsy specimens.
- Radionuclide imaging: Gallium-67 scintigraphy is a screening technique that is used routinely to detect chronic inflammatory processes. It has been shown to be sensitive, but it is limited by its low specificity and predictive accuracy in myocarditis. Similarly, indium-111 antimyosin antibody cardiac imaging has been shown to have high sensitivity for myocardial necrosis, but low specificity.
- Viral identification: Viral cultures of the blood, stool, and nasopharynx should be sent. Acute and convalescent serum should be sent for serologic titer rise.
- Laboratory tests: The erythrocyte sedimentation rates (ESR) and creatinine kinase—MB fraction (CK-MB) are variably elevated. The degree of elevation depends on the stage of disease, degree of cardiac failure, and extent of myocardial necrosis.

NOTE: One must rule out structural causes of severe left ventricular dysfunction (see Differential Diagnosis)

Therapy

- Bed rest and limited activity (during acute phase)
- Anticongestive therapy

—Diuretics
—Inotropic agents (e.g., dobutamine, dopamine, or digoxin)
—Afterload reduction (e.g., milrinone or captopril).

- High-dose gamma globulin (2 g/kg over 24 hours) therapy during the acute phase has been associated with improved recovery of left ventricular function and with a tendency to better survival during the first year after presentation.
- The role of immunosupression is unclear.
- Corticosteroids are effective in rheumatic carditis.

Follow-Up

- The patient who presents with mild-to-moderate congestive heart failure should be followed every 3 to 6 months, until full myocardial recovery is noted.
- The patient who progresses to dilated cardiomyopathy should have interval follow-up every 3 months. If myocardial function is depressed but stable, the patient may be followed expectantly. If myocardial function progressively deteriorates, cardiac transplantation may be needed.

Common Questions and Answers

Q: What can parents expect of children who have had myocarditis?
A: Most children will present with only minimal signs of heart failure and recover completely (two-thirds). Of the remaining one-third who present in shock and LV failure, one-third recover, one-third develop a cardiomyopathy, and one-third go on to transplantation.

Q: Is there a role for steroids?
A: In addition to bed rest, inotropic support, diuretics, and gamma globulin, the use of steroids is controversial and has not been prospectively studied in a large pediatric population.

ICD-9-CM
Secondary to rheumatic fever 398.0
Acute myocarditis 422.90

BIBLIOGRAPHY

Drucker NA, Newburger JW. Viral myocarditis: diagnosis and management. *Adv Pediatr* 1997; 44:141–171.

Drucker NA, Colan SD, Lewis AB, et al. Gamma-globulin treatment of acute myocarditis in the pediatric population. *Circulation* 1994;89: 252–257.

Gajarski RJ, Towbin JA. Recent advances in the etiology, diagnosis, and treatment of myocarditis and cardiomyopathies in children. *Curr Opin Pediatr* 1995;7:587–594.

Modlin JF. Update on enterovirus infections in infants and children. *Adv Pediatr Infect Dis* 1996;12:155–180.

Author: Bradley S. Marino

Near Drowning

Database

DEFINITION

Near drowning, or submersion injury, is survival, at least temporarily, after suffocation by submersion in water. Near drowning may be described by the water temperature and tonicity as "warm water" ($\geq$20°C), "cold water" (<20°C), or "very cold water" ($\leq$5°C), and as "freshwater" versus "saltwater" near drowning.

CAUSES

• "Wet drowning": aspiration of fluid into the trachea and lungs with either denaturation of surfactant by freshwater or washout of surfactant due to saltwater, which results in intrapulmonary shunting and hypoxemia.
• "Dry drowning": hypoxemia from prolonged severe laryngospasm as water enters the larynx when the near-drowning victim becomes hypercapneic and takes an involuntary gasp of air. No fluid is aspirated into the lung.

PATHOPHYSIOLOGY

• Grossly, the lungs are edematous, but not filled with aspirated fluid, with focal hemorrhages.
• Microscopically, there is thinning of the aveolar septum with emphysematous changes and frothy fluid in the airways.

EPIDEMIOLOGY

• Second only to motor vehicle accidents as the most common cause of death due to injury in childhood
• Children less than 5 years of age, especially toddlers and boys, who cannot swim and have direct access to swimming pools are at highest risk.
• Bathtub drowning and near drownings are common in babies, and child neglect or abuse should be considered.
• Adolescent near drownings usually involve substance abuse or risk-taking behavior.
• Children with seizure disorders are at higher risk of near drowning.

COMPLICATIONS

• Brain injury secondary to hypoxia
• Pulmonary injury with intrapulmonary shunting secondary to damage of the aveoli
• ARDS
• Metabolic acidosis secondary to hypoxemia
• Ischemic injury to organs such as liver, kidneys, and intestines
• Disseminated intravascular coagulation (DIC) secondary to ischemia
• Electrolyte abnormalities uncommon; may occur if a large volume of freshwater is in the stomach and not removed
• Hypothermia in cold water near drownings

PROGNOSIS

• Most children (60%–95%) recover with intact neurologic survival.
• Brain injury and death correlate with degree of hypoxia/anoxia.
• Children with warm water submersion time longer than 4 minutes, who do not receive CPR at the scene and who have absent vital signs or a Glasgow Coma Scale (GCS) score less than 5 in the emergency department, usually have a poor prognosis.
• Victims who have prolonged submersions in very cold water may have good prognosis due to "core" cooling with a concomitant decrease in metabolic rate while the brain is still being perfused.
• A good prognostic indicator is continuing improvement in the neurologic examination over the first several hours.

ASSOCIATED CONDITIONS

• C-spine injuries should be considered in older children with diving accidents.
• Signs of child abuse or neglect (burns, whip marks, bruises) should be sought in young children.
• Toxicology screens should be sent in adolescents.

Differential Diagnosis

Children with smoke inhalation or hydrocarbon ingestion may have similar presentations. However, the history and physical examination should easily determine the diagnosis.

Data Gathering

HISTORY

• Mechanism: history of diving injury, intoxication, seizure disorder, child abuse
• Prognostic indicators: length of submersion, vital signs and examination at scene, CPR done at scene, temperature of water

Physical Examination

• Vital signs with temperature
• Neurologic: pupillary response, cranial nerve findings, Glasgow Coma Score

Glasgow Coma Scale

1. Eye Opening

Spontaneous	____ 4
To voice	____ 3
To pain	____ 2
None	____ 1

2. Verbal Response

Oriented	____ 5
Confused	____ 4
Inappropriate words	____ 3
Incomprehensible words	____ 2
None	____ 1

3. Motor Response

Obeys commands	____ 6
Purposeful movement (pain)	____ 5
Withdraw (pain)	____ 4
Flexion (pain)	____ 3
Extension (pain)	____ 2
None	____ 1
Total GCS Points	____ (1 + 2 + 3)

Total GCS Score = E

14–15	= 5
11–13	= 4
8–10	= 3
5–7	= 2
3–4	= 1

• Respiratory: lower airway findings (rales, tachypnea, wheezing, retractions)
• Circulation: perfusion, strength of distal pulses, capillary refill, urine output
• GI: abdominal distention from swallowed water or ventilation

Question: Was the child apneic, cyanotic, or pulseless at the scene?
Significance: These children require admission and close observation even if they appear well at presentation to the hospital.

Question: Did the child fall through ice?
Significance: Very cold water near drownings may have good prognosis despite submersion time longer than 5 minutes.

Question: What was the estimated time of submersion, and when was CPR begun?
Significance: Shorter time periods (<2–5 minutes) for each answer correlate with better prognosis.

• Near-drowning victims may have deteriorating pulmonary involvement, despite an initially normal examination. Watch closely for signs of lower airway involvement, such as tachypnea, retractions, or rales.
• Serial neurologic examinations with pupillary response should be performed to access neurologic outcome. Children with a GCS score less than 5 after resuscitation usually have a poor neurologic outcome.

Laboratory Aids

TESTS

- Pulse oximetry is a critical aid in assessment of pulmonary involvement in the near-drowning victim. An oxygen saturation less than 97% within 4 hours after the near drowning indicates pulmonary involvement and need for admission.
- Arterial blood gases to detect and treat metabolic acidosis and hyperapnea should be done in the child with respiratory distress or apnea.
- An initial chest x-ray is indicated for endotracheal tube placement in the intubated child and as a baseline film for those with pulmonary involvement.
- Cervical spine films are indicated in the diving accident victim.
- Renal electrolytes are not indicated unless a large volume of water has been swallowed and not evacuated from the stomach.
- Anticonvulsant levels for victims with seizure disorders
- Toxicology screening when suspected
- ECG to document normal function and evaluate for prolonged QTC if indicated by history

False Positives

Initial pulse oximetry and chest x-rays may be normal in the near-drowning victim. Victims should be monitored with pulse oximetry for 4 to 6 hours for progressive respiratory distress.

Therapy

- Airway: Protect the C-spine if indicated by history. Ensure a patent airway in the arrested or comatose victim.
- Breathing: supplemental oxygen for oxygen saturations by pulse oximetry less than 95%. The near-drowning victim should be intubated and positive end-expiratory pressure (PEEP) and ventilation given if apneic or unable to maintain a PaO_2 greater than 60 or a pCO_2 less than 50 in 50% supplemental oxygen. Prophylactic antibiotics or steroids are not indicated.
- Circulation:

—For the victim with cardiopulmonary arrest, asystole protocol should be followed, using epinephrine via the ET tube or intravenously and chest compressions done.

—Since capillary leak may occur after an ischemic/anoxic episode, isotonic fluids (e.g., normal saline solution or Ringer's lactate) (10-mL/kg aliquots) should be given for signs of intravascular volume depletion (tachycardia, poor perfusion) until normalized.

—ECG monitoring should be provided with appropriate response to dysrhythmias, especially for the hypothermic, cold water near-drowning victim. For core temperature less than 29.5°C, attempts at electrical defibrillation are not likely to be successful, and "chemical defibrilla-

tion" with bretyllium or lidocaine and aggressive rewarming are tried.

- Disability: maintenance of eucapnea and adequate oxygenation to prevent further hypoxemia. There is no indication for measures to reduce ICP (hyperventilation, barbiturates, mannitol, fluid restoration, ICP monitoring, or steroids) because the brain injury and swelling is secondary to hypoxic cell injury as opposed to a traumatic lesion.
- Exposure: The near-drowning victim should be dried and warmed: for core temperatures 32°C to 35°C, active rewarming with heating blankets or radiant warmers; for less than 32°C, active internal rewarming added (heated aerosolized oxygen and intravenous fluids, gastric lavage with warm saline); for severe very cold water drowning cases and where available, peritoneal or hemodialysis, mediastinal irrigation, and cardiac bypass

DURATION

- The cold water near-drowning victim with hypothermia must be rewarmed to greater than 32°C before CPR is terminated. Remember: "The patient is not dead until he is warm and dead."
- Pulmonary treatment is provided as needed (see Breathing, above). Complications may include pneumonia; pneumothorax or pneunomediation in the ventilated patient; and ARDS.

Follow-Up

- Long-term follow-up of apparently neurologically intact survivors has shown mild coordination or gross motor deficiencies.
- The victim may be at increased risk for chronic lung disease, depending on the degree of pulmonary involvement.

PITFALLS

- Failure to observe near-drowning victim for signs of pulmonary involvement, since late deterioration can occur 24 to 48 hours postincident.
- The hypothermic patient who is a warm water near-drowning victim does not have a good prognosis or need vigorous rewarming.

PREVENTION

- Most drownings are preventable.
- Legislation to require adequate fencing and rescue equipment for public and residential pools
- Restriction of sale and consumption of alcohol in boating areas, pools, and beaches
- Parental education regarding adequate supervision during bathing and around swimming pools

Common Questions and Answers

Q: Should the near-drowning victim who arrives to the hospital with cardiopulmonary arrest be resuscitated?

A: Yes, a brief (10–15 minutes) attempt at resuscitation is indicated until circumstances of the near drowning and core temperature are known. Warm water near-drowning victims who require CPR in the emergency department may rarely (0%–25%) have good neurologic recovery but usually respond quickly (<15 minutes) to therapy.

Q: Is artificial surfactant useful in near-drowning victims?

A: Although useful in neonates, surfactant has not been well studied in near-drowning victims. In a dog model and in addicts with ARDS, it has not be beneficial. Further investigation is needed before it can be recommended for clinical use.

ICD-9-CM 994.1

BIBLIOGRAPHY

Biggarat MJ, Bohn D. Effect of hypothermia and cardiac arrest on outcome of near-drowning accidents in children. *J Pediatr* 1990; 117:179–183.

Bratton SL, Jardine DS, Morra JF. Serial neurologic examination after near drowning and outcome. *Arch Pediatr Adolesc Med* 1994;148: 167–170.

Diekma DS, Quan L, Holt VL. Epilepsy as a risk factor for submersion injury in children. *Pediatrics* 1993;91(3):512–616.

Lavelle JM, Shaw KN. Near drowning: is emergency department cardiopulmonary resuscitation or intensive care unit cerebral resuscitation indicated? *Crit Care Med* 1993;21(3): 368–373.

Lavelle JM, Shaw KN. Ten year review of pediatric bathtub near-drownings: evaluation for child abuse and neglect. *Ann Emerg Med* 1995;25:344–348.

Modell JH. Drowning: current concepts. *N Engl J Med* 1993;328(4):253–256.

O'Flaherty, JE. Prevention of pediatric drowning and near-drowning: A survey of members of the American Academy of Pediatrics. *Pediatrics* 1997;99(2):169–174.

Pearn J, Pirie PL. Pathophysiology of drowning. *Med J Aust* 1985;142:586–588.

Spack L, Rainer G, Gedeit R, et al. Failure of aggressive therapy to alter outcome in pediatric near-drowning. *Pediatr Emerg Care* 1997;13(2): 98–102.

Author: Kathy N. Shaw

Neck Masses

Database

APPROACH TO THE PATIENT

The wide range of problems causing neck masses requires a careful correlation of location, size, and tenderness with the history. The major tasks are to differentiate infections from congenital and malignant causes.

Differential Diagnosis

- Infectious

—Reactive hyperplasia: self-limited, usually viral enlargement of minimally tender nodes
—Bacterial lymphadenitis: usually staphylococcal or streptococcal infection of unilateral, tender, swollen, warm, erythematous node
—Cat-scratch disease: sometimes protracted illness caused by the gram-negative bacillus *Bartonella henselae,* which starts as a papule at a cat-scratch site and then progresses to tender, regional adenopathy

- Tuberculosis (TB): acute or insidious onset of fever and firm, nontender adenopathy in children exposed to adult infected with the acid-fast bacillus *Mycobacterium tuberculosis*
- Atypical mycobacterial disease: infection usually caused by *Mycobacterium avium* complex or *M. scrofulaceum* (ubiquitous agents found in the soil). Usually presents as a rapidly enlarging mass of firm, nontender nodes in 1- to 4-year-olds with no known exposure to TB. Nodes often with overlying skin discoloration and thinning; 25% to 50% with spontaneous drainage
- Infectious mononucleosis: Epstein-Barr viral infection most commonly seen in older children who present with fever, exudative pharyngitis, adenopathy, and hepatosplenomegaly
- Retropharyngeal abscess: suppurative adenitis of the retropharyngeal nodes that presents in children under 5 years of age with fever, toxicity, dysphagia, respiratory distress, drooling, and stridor
- Peritonsillar abscess: suppurative sequelae of a severe tonsillopharyngitis, usually caused by group A β-hemolytic *Streptococcus,* which commonly presents in older children and adolescents with trismus, "hot potato" voice, and uvular deviation from a bulging palatal abscess
- Congenital

—Thyroglossal duct cyst: remnant of the embryonic thyroglossal sinus, which presents as a nontender, mobile, anterior midline mass near the hyoid bone
—Branchial cleft cyst: remnant of the second branchial cleft, which presents as a nontender (unless infected) cyst at the anterior border of the sternocleidomastoid
—Cystic hygroma: complex, multiloculated mass of lymphatic tissue, which presents in the first year of life as a large, soft, compressible neck structure

—Dermoid cyst: small, firm, nontender mass, usually high in the midline

- Malignant
- Hodgkin lymphoma: slowly enlarging, unilateral, firm, nontender neck malignancy, which usually presents in previously well adolescents

—Non-Hodgkin lymphoma: presents in young adolescents as a painless, rapidly growing, firm collection of lymph nodes
—Neuroblastoma: most commonly presents in toddlers as a large, nontender, abdominal mass, often associated with myriad signs and symptoms as a result of its propensity for metastasis
—Rhabdomyosarcoma: head and neck malignancy that usually presents as a rapidly enlarging mass

- Thyroid

—Chronic lymphocytic thyroiditis (Hashimoto thyroiditis): autoimmune-caused childhood goiter that may be euthyroid, hypothyroid, or hyperthyroid
—Thyrotoxicosis (Graves disease): clinically hyperfunctioning thyroid caused by circulating thyroid cell-stimulating antibodies.
—Thyroiditis: painful bacterial infection of the thyroid caused by *Staphylococcus* or *Streptococcus*

- Miscellaneous

—Kawasaki disease: idiopathic vasculitis distinguished by fever, conjunctivitis, oral involvement, extremity changes, rash, and adenopathy
—Sinus histiocystosis with massive lymphadenopathy: benign form of histiocytosis that presents as massive, painless enlargement of cervical nodes
—Sternocleidomastoid tumor of infancy: benign perinatal fibromatosis, often associated with difficult deliveries or abnormal uterine positioning, that results in a hard mass in the sternocleidomastoid
—Hematoma: secondary to trauma
—Hypersensitivity reaction: secondary to bites, stings, or other allergens

Data Gathering

HISTORY

Question: Noticed at birth?
Significance: Congenital causes, especially cystic hygroma

Question: Noticed after trauma?
Significance: Hematoma

Question: Noticed with intercurrent infection?
Significance: Reactive hyperplasia, mononucleosis, adenitis, abscess

Question: Cats?
Significance: Cat-scratch disease

Question: Increasing size?
Significance: Question of malignancy

Question: Fever?
Significance: Infection, malignancy

Question: Swallowing problems?
Significance: Retropharyngeal or peritonsillar abscess, thyroglossal duct cyst

Question: Breathing problems?
Significance: Malignancy, infections

Question: Weight loss?
Significance: Malignancy, infections

Question: Cough?
Significance: Malignancy, infections

Question: Hypothyroidism/hyperthyroidism symptoms?
Significance: Thyroglossal duct cyst, thyroidal diseases

Question: Recurrence of mass?
Significance: If recurrent cervical adenitis is diagnosed in the same location, consider the possibility of an underlying congenital cyst.

Question: Recurrent infections?
Significance: Immunodeficiency

Question: Tuberculosis exposure?
Significance: Mycobacterium tuberculosis

Question: Radiation exposure?
Significance: Thyroid cancer

Question: Animal exposure/insect bites?
Significance: Cat scratch, hypersensitivity

Question: Ate undercooked meat?
Significance: Toxoplasmosis

Question: Drank unpasteurized milk?
Significance: Atypical mycobacterial infection

Physical Examination

Finding: Composed of lymph node(s)
Significance: Cervical adentitis, regional infection

Finding: Midline
Significance: Thyroglossal duct cyst, dermoid cyst, thyroidal disease

Finding: Posterior to sternocleidomastoid muscle
Significance: Consider malignancy

Finding: Painful
Significance: Infection

Finding: Indurated
Significance: Infection

Finding: Irregular
Significance: Reactive hyperplasia, malignancy

Finding: Erythematous
Significance: Adenitis

Finding: Fluctuant
Significance: Adenitis with abscess, cystic hygroma

Finding: Multiple components
Significance: Cystic hygroma

Finding: Matted down
Significance: Malignancy

Finding: Mobile
Significance: Congenital cysts, reactive hyperplasia

Finding: Moves with tongue protrusion
Significance: Thyroglossal duct cyst

Finding: Sinus opening
Significance: Branchial cleft cyst

Finding: Inferior deep cervical nodes (scalene and supraclavicular)
Significance: Malignancy

Finding: Drainage
Significance: Adenitis with abscess, atypical mycobacterial disease, infected branchial cleft cyst

Finding: Skin discoloration
Significance: Trauma, abscess, atypical mycobacterial disease

Finding: Regional adenopathy
Significance: Reactive hyperplasia, cat-scratch disease

Finding: Generalized adenopathy
Significance: Malignancy

Finding: Hepatosplenomegaly
Significance: Malignancy, infectious mononucleosis

 ## Laboratory Aids

Test: CBC
Significance: Most patients with neck malignancies present with normal CBCs.

Test: Epstein-Barr virus titers, mononucleosis spot test
Significance: Infectious mononucleosis

Test: PPD
Significance: Negative or only weakly positive in atypical mycobacterial infections

Test: Chest x-ray
Significance: TB, malignancy

Test: Lateral neck x-ray
Significance: Help detect retropharyngeal abscess

Test: Ultrasound
Significance: Often the first imaging modality for neck masses; provides immediate, noninvasive information on location, size, and composition of mass (cystic versus solid)

Test: CT scan
Significance: Useful in evaluating deep neck infections and complex or extensive neck masses

Test: MRI scan
Significance: Better than CT scan in distinguishing between soft tissue structures

Test: Thyroid scintigraphy
Significance: Useful in evaluating thyroid lesions, especially when malignancy is a concern

Test: Needle aspiration for Gram stain and culture
Significance: May help identify bacterial cause of adenitis. In the preantibiotic era, needle aspiration was avoided for fear that it might lead to chronic sinus drainage; this is not a serious concern today.

Test: Lymph node biopsy
Significance: For rapidly growing or chronic masses when malignancy is suspected

 ## Follow-Up

Close follow-up is essential for all neck masses; consider referral for biopsy in the following cases:

- Failure of antibiotics
- Toxic illness/systemic symptoms
- Clinical signs of malignancy
- Nodes that are firm, nontender, and fixed to skin/deep tissues; and nodes located posterior to the sternocleidomastoid or in the lower cervical/supraclavicular regions
- Increasing size after 2 weeks without diagnosis
- No decrease in size after 4 to 6 weeks without diagnosis
- Not back to normal size after 8 to 12 weeks

BIBLIOGRAPHY

Brodsky L, Belles W, Brody A, et al. Needle aspiration of neck abscesses in children. *Clin Pediatr* 1992;31(2):71–76.

Broughton RA. Nonsurgical management of deep neck infections in children. *Pediatr Infect Dis J* 1992;11:14–18.

Chesney PJ. Cervical adenopathy. *Pediatr Rev* 1994;15:276–285.

Connolly AA, MacKenzie K. Paediatric neck masses—a diagnostic dilemma. *J Laryngol Otol* 1997;111(6):541–545.

Cunningham MJ, Myers EN, Bluestone CD, et al. Malignant tumors of the head and neck in children: a twenty-year review. *Int J Pediatr Otorhinolaryngol* 1987;13:279–292.

DeMello DE, Liona JA, Liapis H, et al. Midline cervical cysts in children. *Arch Otolaryngol Head Neck Surg* 1987;113:418–420.

Hopwood NJ, Kelch RP. Thyroid masses: approach to diagnosis and management in childhood and adolescence. *Pediatr Rev* 1993;14:481–487.

Knight PJ, Mulne AP, Vassy LE, et al. When is lymph node biopsy indicated in children with enlarged peripheral nodes? *Pediatrics* 1982;69:391–396.

Park YW. Evaluation of neck masses in children. *Am Fam Physician* 1995;51(8):1904–1912.

1997 Red book: report of the Committee on Infectious Diseases, 24th ed. Elk Grove Village, IL: American Academy of Pediatrics, 1997.

Swischuk LE, John SD. Neck masses in infants and children. *Radiol Clin North Am* 1997;35(6):1329–1340.

Torsiglieri AJ, Tom LW, Russ AJ, et al. Pediatric neck masses: guidelines for evaluation. *Int J Pediatr Otorhinolaryngol* 1988;16:199–210.

Author: Nicholas Tsarouhas

Necrotizing Enterocolitis

 ## Database

DEFINITION

Necrotizing enterocolitis (NEC) is a necrotizing inflammatory bowel disorder affecting the premature infant; and only 10% of cases occur in term infants. NEC is the most common and most serious acquired gastrointestinal disorder among hospitalized preterm infants and is associated with significant acute and chronic morbidity and mortality.

CAUSES

NEC is a disease of unknown etiology. There are, however, several hypotheses that are believed to act in a multifactorial way to initiate the disease process.

• Hypoxia/ischemia: alterations in blood flow to mucosal surfaces secondary to hypoxic injury and other systemic factors, such as polycythemia, drug exposure, cardiac defects, and exchange transfusions
• Enteral alimentation: Since 95% of infants that develop NEC have been enterally fed, the act of initiation of feeds has been implicated as a possible cause of NEC. The composition of the formula, the rate of volume increase, and the immaturity of the mucosa have all been implicated as factors that may increase the risk of NEC.
• Infectious/inflammatory agent
• Because of the frequent report of epidemic, cluster-type episodes, a variety of microorganisms have been implicated in the development of NEC. In the majority of cases no identifiable organism is recovered, but at times certain microbes, such as *Escherichia coli, Klebsiella, Salmonella,* and *Staphylococcus epidermidis,* have been recovered. Blood cultures may be positive in 20% to 30% of cases.
• As a result of the type of injury that is seen, an endotoxin-mediated cascade has also been proposed to play a possible role in the disease process.

PATHOLOGY

• The traditional pathologic features of NEC that are most commonly seen include varying degrees of inflammation and coagulation necrosis of the colonic and intestinal mucosa.
• NEC can be transmural in nature in the most severe cases.
• The most common sites for NEC include the terminal ileum, ileocecal region, and ascending colon.
• Fifty percent of infants have both colonic and small intestine disease while the other 50% is divided fairly equally between isolated ileal or colonic involvement.

GENETICS

There is no known genetic predisposition or component in the development of NEC.

EPIDEMIOLOGY

• The prevalence for NEC is approximately 4%, and the incidence ranges from 1 in 2,000 to 4,000 live births.
• The incidence is highest in infants with birth weights between 500 and 750 g (13%–20%) and decreases to approximately 2% in infants greater than 750 g.
• NEC usually has an onset within the first 2 weeks of life and after enteral feeds have been initiated. The more premature the infant, the longer the child is at risk for developing NEC, and cases have been reported 3 months after birth.
• There is no association between NEC and sex or race.
• The overall mortality for infants with NEC is between 20% and 40%.

COMPLICATIONS

• NEC is associated with significant morbidity and mortality.
• A variety of complications may occur in infants with this disease process, including gastrointestinal perforation, acquired short bowel syndrome, DIC, sepsis and shock, intestinal strictures, enterocolic fistulae, and abscess formation.

 ## Differential Diagnosis

The clinical spectrum of signs and symptoms that can be seen in a patient with NEC leads to a variety of other disease processes that must be considered. Some processes can be related to the gastrointestinal tract, while others may be systemic in nature:

• Systemic

—Sepsis with ileus
—Pneumothorax causing a pneumoperitoneum
—Hemorrhagic disease of the newborn
—Swallowed maternal blood
—Postasphyxia bowel necrosis

• Gastrointestinal

—Volvulus
—Malrotation
—Pseudomembranous colitis
—Hirschprung colitis
—Intussusception
—Spontaneous bowel perforation
—Stress ulcer
—Meconium ileus
—Milk protein allergy
—Umbilical arterial thromboembolism

 ## Data Gathering

HISTORY

• The clinical presentation is variable in this group of patients, but the triad of abdominal distention, bloody stools, and bilious emesis is frequently seen.
• A number of more subtle, nonspecific findings may be the initial sign of NEC and include apnea and/or bradycardia, lethargy, diarrhea, acidosis, and temperature instability.
• Patients who have more advanced disease may present with more serious problems: coagulopathy and increased fluid requirements.

 ## Physical Examination

• Patients who have more advanced disease may present with more serious problems: vital sign instability (shock), ascites, and peritonitis.
• Clinical symptoms that are helpful in raising suspicion include abdominal distention, increased stool output, emesis, increased gastric residuals, decreased bowel sounds, and mottling of the extremities.

PITFALLS

The major pitfall occurs when there is a delay in making the correct diagnosis and in the institution of appropriate therapy. This leads to a rapid progression of symptoms and usually a worse outcome.

 ## Laboratory Aids

TESTS

• The diagnosis of NEC is confirmed by the presence of pneumatosis intestinalis or hepatic venous gas on x-ray. Perforation in the setting of other clinical symptoms is also indicative of NEC.
• Laboratory evaluation may be helpful in assessing the severity of the episode but is not enough to make the diagnosis.
• Laboratory abnormalities may include thrombocytopenia, disseminated intravascular coagulopathy, metabolic acidosis, anemia, neutropenia, and peripheral eosinophilia.
• Other radiologic findings may include ileus, isolated dilated intestinal loop, ascites, and free air.

Therapy

- For patients who develop NEC, therapy is based on the severity and progression of the symptoms.
- Initial management of all patients with suspected or proven NEC needs to include NPO status, intravenous fluids, NG tube placement for decompression, and intravenous antibiotics.
- Patients need to have blood and stool cultures sent and need to have frequent evaluation of CBC, fluid status, and abdominal x-ray. These should be evaluated every 6 hours to once a day, depending on the severity of the episode.
- Length of therapy and reinstitution of feeds tend to be based on the severity of the episode and on clinical, laboratory, and radiologic abnormalities.
- If the infant responds immediately to therapy and there are no laboratory or radiographic abnormalities, feeds may be started as early as 72 hours after the episode.
- If mild abnormalities arise and the patient remains only mildly ill, a 10-day course of therapy is considered.
- In cases in which laboratory and radiologic abnormalities include pneumatosis intestinalis, acidosis, and/or thrombocytopenia, a 14-day course is indicated.
- Overall, the best therapy for NEC is prevention. Although several small studies have attempted to use immunoglobulin therapy and steroid therapy as a way to decrease the incidence of NEC in premature infants, no significant change in prevalence has been reported. The best way to decrease the possibility of NEC in the premature infant is the use of slow enteral feeding protocols.

 Follow-Up

- Despite early recognition and intervention, NEC is associated with a significantly high morbidity and mortality.
- Mortality results from perforation, sepsis, shock, and DIC.
- Morbidity may be related to anemia, intravenous access difficulties, and the risk for infection. The other most common, long-term sequelae seen in 25% to 30% of infants with NEC are intestinal strictures and short gut syndrome if the patient undergoes surgical resection of bowel.

 Common Questions and Answers

Q: What is the most common complication of NEC?
A: Not recognizing the problem and the development of a short gut syndrome.

Q: Is this preventable?
A: The development of NEC is not clearly preventable, but clinicians are careful to start feeding extremely premature infants slowly with elemental diets.

ICD-9-CM 557.0

BIBLIOGRAPHY

Bell MJ, Ternberg JL, Feigin RD. Neonatal necrotizing enterocolitis: therapeutic decisions based upon clinical staging. *Ann Surg* 1978;187:1B7.

Engum SA. Grosfeld JL. Necrotizing enterocolitis. *Curr Opin Pediatr* 1998;10(2):123–130.

Kliegman RM. Neonatal necrotizing enterocolitis: bridging the basic science with clinical disease. *J Pediatr* 1990;117:833–853.

Kleigman RM. Neonatal necrotizing enterocolitis. In: Wyllie R, Hyams JS, eds. *Pediatric gastrointestinal disease*. Philadelphia: WB Saunders, 1993:788–798.

Ladd AP, Rescorla FJ, West KW, Scherer LR III, Engum SA, Grosfeld JL. Long-term follow-up after bowel resection for necrotizing enterocolitis: factors affecting outcome. *J Pediatr Surg* 1998;33(7):967–972.

Udall JN. Gastrointestinal host defense and necrotizing enterocolitis. *J Pediatr* 1990;117: 533–543.

Author: Edisio Semeao

Neonatal Apnea

Database

DEFINITION

Pathologic apnea, the cessation of respiratory airflow from the end of inspiration to the beginning of the next inspiration, is defined differently, based on patient age, gestation, and the presence of other symptoms. For term infants, it is defined as cessation of breathing for longer than 15 seconds, and for preterm infants, longer than 20 seconds. Apnea of any duration associated with cyanosis, pallor, bradycardia (heart rate less than 100 beats per minute), or hypotonia is considered to be pathologic apnea.

Types of apnea and abnormal breathing patterns:

- Central: no chest wall movement with lack of respiratory effort
- Obstructive: respiratory movement/effort with no airflow
- Mixed: combined obstructive and central apnea
- Periodic breathing: pattern of three or more respiratory pauses of greater than 3 seconds' duration separated by fewer than 20 seconds of respiration between pauses; occurs during quiet sleep; considered to be normal
- Apnea of prematurity (AOP): prolonged apnea usually associated with bradycardia in a preterm infant in whom other etiologies have been excluded
- Apnea of infancy: unexplained episode of pathologic apnea in an infant greater than 37 weeks' gestational age; reserved for those infants for whom no specific cause of an apparent life-threatening event (ALTE) can be defined
- ALTE: some combination of apnea, pallor, cyanosis, marked hypotonia, choking or gagging, and bradycardia, requiring resuscitation for its termination
- Sudden infant death syndrome (SIDS): sudden infant death unexplained by history, and with unrevealing, thorough postmortem and death scene evaluation; presumption is that death resulted from prolonged apnea

GENETICS

- No familial predisposition is noted.
- Congenital central hypoventilation syndrome is autosomal recessive when associated with Hirshsprung disease.

EPIDEMIOLOGY

- Very low birth weight (VLBW) infants most commonly experience mixed apnea and uncommonly experience obstructive or central apnea alone.
- Incidence is inversely related to gestational age: 84% of infants less than 1,000 g (28 weeks); 25% of infants less than 1,800 g (34 weeks)
- Onset by 7 days of life

- Frequency and duration decrease between 1 and 20 weeks' postnatal age; usually cease by 37 weeks' postconception

COMPLICATIONS

- Severe apnea and bradycardia, resulting in compromised cerebral blood flow
- Prolonged hypoxia and hypercarbia, resulting in derangement of central respiratory control, increased bronchomotor tone, and depressed cardiac function
- Intraventricular hemorrhage
- Necrotizing enterocolitis (NEC)
- SIDS
- ALTE

PROGNOSIS

- Apnea of prematurity: excellent prognosis with no long-term morbidity
- Obstructive apnea due to reflux: excellent prognosis
- ALTE carries a 1% to 3% mortality rate.

Differential Diagnosis

- Infection

—Systemic bacterial infection
—NEC
—Pneumonia: viral or bacterial
—Pertussis
—Meningitis
—Encephalitis

- Congenital

—Respiratory dysfunction: surfactant deficiency, bronchopulmonary dysplasia
—Congenital heart defects: patent ductus arteriosus with large left-to-right shunt, Ebstein anomaly (enlarged right atrium compressing airway)

- Environmental

—Maternal drug use: opiates, cocaine
—Maternal medications during labor: narcotics, magnesium sulfate, β-blockers
—Prostaglandins (PGE1), adenosine, opiates, barbiturates, benzodiazepines
—Hypo- or hyperthermia

- Trauma

—Intracranial hemorrhage
—Perinatal asphyxia

- Metabolic

—Hypoglycemia
—Hypocalcemia
—Hyperammonemia
—Inborn errors of metabolism

- Neurologic

—Congenital central hypoventilation syndrome
—Syringobulbia (localized syrinx of the brain stem)
—Hydrocephalus
—Arnold-Chiari II malformation
—Congenital myotonic dystrophy

—Seizures

- Anatomic

—Airway obstruction due to neck flexion in preterm (most obstructive episodes occur at the pharyngeal level)
—Structural lesions (subglottic edema/stenosis, laryngotracheomalacia, nasal secretions, choanal atresia)
—Severe micrognathia (Pierre Robin syndrome)
—Macroglossia
—Tracheoesophageal fistula

- Miscellaneous

—Impaired oxygenation: hypoxemia, anemia, hypotension
—Upper airway reflex stimulation: mechanical and chemical stimuli to nasal cavity, pharynx and larynx (gastroesophageal reflux)

Data Gathering

HISTORY

Special Questions

- Was there any maternal illness, such as diabetes or hypertension, or a history of drug use, such as cocaine or heroin?
- Were there any perinatal complications?
- Were there any risk factors for sepsis, such as maternal infection, prolonged rupture of membranes, or maternal Group B strep?
- Were any drugs given to the mother or infant?
- Postnatally, has there been any feeding intolerance or other symptoms that would raise the suspicion of gastroesophageal reflux?
- Has there been any weight loss?
- With respect to the episode of concern, how often did it occur? For how long? Was there any relationship to crying, position, sleep, or agitation?
- Were there any associated symptoms, like change in color, staring spells, or abnormal movements?
- Is there a family history of SIDS in siblings?
- Is there a family history of other disorders, including metabolic disorders and congenital central hypoventilation syndrome?

Physical Examination

- Plot growth parameters, including head circumference, weight, and length. Micro- and macrocephaly, hydrocephalus, and/or failure to thrive may indicate metabolic disorders.
- Look for dysmorphic features. Pierre Robin syndrome may be associated with apnea.
- Listen for cranial bruit to assess for a cerebral AV malformation.
- Look for pigmented or depigmented lesions of the skin. Neurocutaneous syndromes are associated with seizures, which may present as apnea.

- Assess the oropharynx, looking for malformations, including submucosal clefts, obstructed nares, and macroglossia.
- Perform a thorough neurologic examination, assessing tone, posture, head control, reflexes, and development to rule out neuromuscular disease.
- Perform a thorough cardiovascular examination. Cardiac disease may present with apnea and respiratory failure.

Laboratory Aids

TESTS

Consider the following in initial testing for a symptomatic infant:

- Polysomnogram: multichannel, simultaneous recording of various elements, typically including heart rate, chest wall impedance, nasal airflow, pulse oximetry, and pH probe for 12 to 24 hours. Indications include siblings of SIDS victims; symptomatic preterm infant; severe BPD; obstructive or mixed apnea; recurrent vomiting, choking, wheezing; and ALTE.
- Complete blood count
- Serum glucose, electrolytes, calcium, magnesium
- Chest x-ray
- Blood culture
- Spinal tap
- Arterial blood gas

If the above fails to determine the etiology of apnea, consider the following:

- Electroencephalogram (EEG)
- Electrocardiogram (ECG)
- Bronchoscopy
- Cardiology, neurology, or otolaryngology consults

Imaging

- Head ultrasound
- CT or MRI of brain
- Echocardiogram
- Lateral neck x-ray
- Barium swallow
- Upper GI

Therapy

SUPPORTIVE CARE

- Obstructive apnea secondary to anatomic problems:

—Nasopharyngeal airway
—Prone positioning (e.g., with tracheomalacia)

- Obstructive apnea secondary to reflux:

—Prone or upright positioning

- Home monitoring should be provided for all infants with any type of apnea.

DRUGS

- Apnea of prematurity and central idiopathic hypoventilation:

—Methylxanthines (e.g., theophylline, caffeine): Side effects include tachycardia, arrhythmia, vomiting, dehydration, polyuria, hyperexcitability, seizures, and hyperglycemia.
—Plasma levels for theophylline should be monitored twice per week until stable, and then weekly. Caffeine levels should be monitored weekly.

- Obstructive apnea due to reflux:

—H2-receptor antagonists (e.g., cimetidine, ranitidine): Side effects include CNS depression, renal failure, elevation of liver enzymes, vitamin B12 deficiency, and drug interaction.

- Gastrointestinal prokinetic agents (e.g., metoclopramide, and cisapride): Side effects include drowsiness, extrapyramidal reactions, seizures, and methemoglobinemia. Recent reports have raised concerns about prolongation of the QTc interval in preterm neonates treated with cisapride. Although no deaths have occurred, ECG prior to and 1 week after starting cisapride is recommended in all children, especially in neonates in whom pharmacokinetic data are lacking. If the QTc interval is greater than 0.45 seconds after treatment, reduction of the dose or discontinuation is recommended.

DIET

- Reflux activity decreases in some infants given thickened feeds (1 tablespoon rice cereal per ounce of formula). This also increases the caloric content to 30 calories per ounce.
- Small frequent feedings rather than large-volume infrequent feedings can also decrease reflux activity.

Follow-Up

- Home monitoring should continue until 2 to 3 months pass without significant alarms or apneic events and after a repeat pneumogram reveals resolution of the apnea.
- Methylxanthines should be discontinued once the infant has reached 35 to 37 weeks' postconceptional age and when no apneic spells have occurred for approximately 1 week.
- In most infants, apnea ceases by 37 weeks' postconceptional age. It may persist for up to 4 months' corrected age.

PITFALLS

- Apnea during mechanical ventilation may be a manifestation of seizure or an airway obstructive lesion.
- Cardiorespiratory monitoring cannot distinguish between central and obstructive apnea.
- There is no evidence that the pneumogram is useful in identifying risk of SIDS in premature infants, in siblings of SIDS victims, and in those with ALTEs.

- For a polysomnogram, the infant should be feeding, off H2-receptor blocking agents for at least 24 hours, and off methylxanthines for at least 5 days.

Common Questions and Answers

Q: Do I need to change the dose of methylxanthines while switching from the enteral to the parenteral route of administration, or vice versa?
A: No.

Q: Do I need to start an infant with apnea due to sepsis or RDS on methylxanthines after their initial illness is adequately treated?
A: Not unless the infant is symptomatic again.

Q: Should immunizations be delayed in infants with apnea?
A: No, routine immunization schedules should be followed.

Q: Should the pertussis portion of the DTP be avoided in infants with central apnea?
A: No, there is no reason to avoid immunizing against pertussis. Immunization with pertussis should be avoided in infants with a progressive or undiagnosed neurologic disorder.

Q: Is there a temporal association between AOP and DTP/HiB immunization?
A: Yes. About 10% of preterm neonates with a postconceptional age of less than 37 weeks experience recurrence of apnea, and another 10% have an increase in frequency of apneic episodes within 72 hours postvaccination. Cardiorespiratory monitoring should occur after immunization of these infants.

Q: Which sleeping position is recommended for preterm infants with apnea?
A: Recent data support a supine sleeping position, even for children with BPD.

ICD-9-CM 770.8

BIBLIOGRAPHY

Beckerman RC, Brouillette RT, Hunt CE. *Respiratory control disorders in infants and children*. Baltimore: Williams & Wilkins, 1992.

Marchal F, Bairam A, Vert P. Neonatal apnea and apneic syndromes. *Clin Perinatol* 1987;14:509–529.

Martin GI. Infant apnea. In: Pomerance JJ, Richardson CJ, eds. *Neonatology for the clinician*. East Norwalk, CT: Appleton-Lange, 1993:267–277.

Miller MJ, Martin RJ. Apnea of prematurity. *Clin Perinatol* 1992;19:789–808.

National Institutes of Health. Consensus development conference on infantile apnea and home monitoring, September 29 to October 1, 1986. *Pediatrics* 1987;79:292–299.

Author: Sameer Wagle

Neonatal Isoimmune Thrombocytopenia

 Database

DEFINITION

Neonatal isoimmune thrombocytopenia is thrombocytopenia caused by platelet–antigen incompatibility between a newborn and its mother. It is also called neonatal alloimmune thrombocytopenia (NATP).

PATHOPHYSIOLOGY

• Caused by maternal antibodies directed against fetal platelet antigens, inherited from the father, which cross the placenta and enter the fetal circulation
• Antibody-coated platelets in the fetus or newborn are destroyed at an increased rate.

EPIDEMIOLOGY

• Occurs in 1 in every 1,000 to 5,000 live births, including first-born offspring
• The most common antigens responsible are human platelet antigen-1a (HPA-1a, formerly PL^{A1}), HPA-5 (formerly Br^a), and HPA-3 (formerly Bak); however, many other antigens can be responsible and vary in frequency according to ethnic group.
• Less commonly, maternal antibodies directed against fetal histocompatibility antigens may cause thrombocytopenia or neutropenia.

COMPLICATIONS

• Abnormal bleeding: primarily skin and mucous membrane bleeding, including but not limited to:

—Petechiae and ecchymoses: These lesions are progressive and not confined to areas of birth trauma, such as the head and shoulders.
—Prolonged bleeding from the umbilical stump and/or phlebotomy sites
—Cephalohematomas
—Hematuria
—Gastrointestinal bleeding
—Intracranial hemorrhages: reported in 2% to 20% of cases; 50% of these occur in utero.

PROGNOSIS

• The overall prognosis is fair, as the majority of patients will experience little morbidity or mortality associated with bleeding; however, the risk of bleeding is higher than in infants of mothers with ITP, and reported mortality is 10% in some series.
• An increase in disease severity with subsequent pregnancies has been reported.

 Differential Diagnosis

• Infection: primarily related to disseminated intravascular coagulation (DIC)

—Bacterial: sepsis
—Viral: congenital rubella or cytomegalovirus
—Spirochetal: syphilis
—Protozoal: toxoplasmosis

• Tumor/malignancy

—Bone marrow disease: congenital leukemia, neuroblastoma

• Metabolic

—Methylmalonic or isovaleric acidemia

• Congenital

—Thrombocytopenia with absent radii (TAR) syndrome
—Wiskott-Aldrich syndrome
—May-Hegglin anomaly
—Hemangiomata with Kasabach-Merritt syndrome

• Immunologic

—Autoimmune neonatal thrombocytopenia: primarily seen in infants of mothers with a history of idiopathic thrombocytopenia purpura (ITP)
—Infants of mothers with systemic lupus erythematosus

• Miscellaneous

—Catheter-associated thrombosis with increased platelet consumption
—Renal vein and other large-vessel thromboses
—DIC
—Necrotizing enterocolitis

 Data Gathering

HISTORY

• Family history of bleeding disorders
• Medications used during pregnancy or in the newborn
• Infectious diseases in mother and/or newborn

Special Questions

Affirmative answers to the following questions increase the likelihood of NATP in the thrombocytopenic newborn:

• Is there no history of maternal ITP or SLE?
• Is the mother's platelet count presently normal?
• Has the mother had prior newborns with thrombocytopenia, NATP, or in utero intracranial hemorrhage?
• Has the mother ever been told that she was HPA-1a- or PL^{A1}-negative?

 Physical Examination

• Most neonates with neonatal isoimmune thrombocytopenia are well-appearing unless they have already experienced an intracranial hemorrhage
• Skin and mucous membrane bleeding, petechiae, and ecchymoses are common findings.
• Less commonly, if significant hemorrhaging occurs, the following signs may be noted: irritability, pallor, and signs of intracranial hemorrhage, including those related to increased intracranial pressure.
• If congenital anomalies, hepatosplenomegaly, or masses are present, causes of thrombocytopenia, other than immune-mediated, should be investigated.

PITFALLS

NATP is a difficult diagnosis to confirm and often requires expensive tests, the results of which are often not available to guide the acute management of the newborn; however, a complete work-up is necessary for management of future pregnancies in the affected neonate's mother.

 Laboratory Aids

TESTS

• Complete blood count (CBC) in newborn

—Low platelet count: less than 150 K, often below 50 K
—Hemoglobin and hematocrit should be normal: Infants with low values may have experienced perinatal blood loss or could have active bleeding.
—White blood cell (WBC) should be normal in uncomplicated NATP.

• Consider a PT/PTT to evaluate for DIC, particularly if the infant is ill-appearing or has a complicated pre- and perinatal history.
• Maternal platelet count: This is usually normal in NATP, but a normal maternal platelet count does not rule out autoimmune thrombocytopenia.
• Maternal serum for antiplatelet antibody analysis: In order to confirm the diagnosis of NATP, the antibody detected should be specific for a known platelet antigen.
• Maternal and paternal platelet antigen typing
• Newborn platelet antigen typing: Use only when absolutely necessary to make the diagnosis, as large amounts of blood are required for this test.
• Consider urine and stool for detection of occult blood.
• Head ultrasound to rule out intracranial hemorrhages

Therapy

• Therapy primarily involves close monitoring for severe bleeding, including intracranial hemorrhage
• Daily platelet counts at minimum during the first several days of life
• If significant bleeding occurs, the neonate should receive a platelet transfusion with the first available product, in order of preference:

—Washed, irradiated maternal platelets
—Platelets cross-matched with maternal serum
—Irradiated PL^{A1}-negative platelets
—Irradiated random donor platelets: often very limited success in increasing platelet count, as 98% of the U.S. population is PL^{A1}-positive

• Platelet transfusions, when needed, are usually required only once.
• The treatment of severely thrombocytopenic neonates without evidence of significant bleeding is controversial, because of the small but real risk of intracranial hemorrhages.
• Often transfusions are performed at platelet counts of 20 to 30 K.
• Other therapies have been reported with limited success, such as steroids, intravenous gamma globulin, and exchange transfusions.

 Follow-Up

• The thrombocytopenia of NATP usually resolves within 3 to 4 weeks but can be present for up to 12 weeks.
• Family counseling regarding management of future pregnancies after a thorough diagnostic evaluation

SIGNS TO WATCH FOR

If the thrombocytopenia persists after 3 months, other etiologies of thrombocytopenia should be investigated.

PREVENTION

Although the disease cannot be prevented, mothers of infants with NATP can be monitored during subsequent pregnancies.

ISOLATION OF HOSPITALIZED PATIENTS

Isolation of hospitalized patients is not required.

 Common Questions and Answers

Q: What is the HPA-1a- or PL^{A1}-negative mother's risk of having other affected newborns?
A: This depends on the genotype of the father:

• If the father is homozygous for HPA-1a or PL^{A1}, all offspring will be heterozygous PL^{A1}-positive and at great risk for developing NATP.
• If the father is heterozygous for HPA-1a or PL^{A1}, 50% of offspring will be at risk for developing NATP.

Q: What is the management of future pregnancies in mothers known to be HPA-1a- or PL^{A1}-negative?
A: This depends on the risk of having an affected child and the clinical course of past affected children. Unfortunately, many perinatal monitoring and therapeutic techniques have shown limited success. However, if the risk of having an affected child is 100% and the clinical course of prior affected newborns was associated with significant morbidity and/or mortality, consider the following perinatal management:

• Percutaneous umbilical blood sampling for a platelet count
• Maternal low-dose prednisone
• Maternal intravenous gamma globulin therapy
• Weekly intrauterine platelet transfusions
• Early elective cesarean section to avoid birth trauma

Q: Will the affected neonate be at increased risk for other bleeding problems later in life?
A: If the neonate has confirmed NATP, there is no increased risk for bleeding problems later in life relative to the general population.

BIBLIOGRAPHY

Bussel J, Kaplan C, MacFarland J, et al. Recommendations for the evaluation and treatment of neonatal autoimmune and alloimmune thrombocytopenia. *Thromb Haemost* 1991;65:631–634.

Glader BE, Buchanan GR. The bleeding neonate. *Pediatrics* 1976;58:548–555.

Lanzkowsky P. *Manual of pediatric hematology and oncology*. New York: Churchill Livingstone, 1995.

Pramanik AK. Bleeding disorders in neonates. *Pediatr Rev* 1992;13:163–173.

Author: Kim Smith-Whitley

Nephrotic Syndrome

 Database

DEFINITION

Nephrotic syndrome (NS) applies to any glomerular disorder associated with heavy proteinuria, hypoproteinemia, edema, and hypercholesterolemia. Nephrotic-range proteinuria is found when there is 4-plus protein on the urine dipstick, which correlates with proteinuria of more than 40/mg/kg/d.

PATHOPHYSIOLOGY

Causes

• Most pediatric cases are primary; 10% are secondary to other diseases.
• The most common primary cause of NS in childhood is minimal change nephrotic syndrome (MCNS). It is characterized by minimal histologic changes on light microscopy, usually responds to steroid therapy, and follows a relapsing course.
• Other causes of primary nephrotic syndrome include focal segmental glomerulosclerosis and membranous and membranoproliferative glomerulonephritis.
• Secondary causes of NS include infections, vasculitis, diabetes, drugs, and hereditary disorders.

Immunologic Abnormalities

A number of immunologic abnormalities are seen with NS that predispose to infection. These include defective opsonization, decreased serum levels of complement factors D and B, abnormal humoral immunity, decreased delayed hypersensitivity and proliferative responses, and increased suppressor-cell activity and suppressor lymphokine levels.

Pathology (in MCNS)

• The glomerular tuft and size are normal. Mesangial expansion is absent or minimal.
• Immunofluorescence is usually negative, although scanty staining for C3, IgM, and IgA may occasionally be found; these patients are usually steroid dependent.
• Electron microscopy reveals widening and effacement of the visceral epithelial foot processes, which are reversible, occur in association with proteinuria, and are not specific for MCNS.

EPIDEMIOLOGY

• The peak age of onset is 3 years.
• The incidence of new cases is 2 to 7 per 100,000 in children less than 16 years of age.
• The prevalence is 16 per 100,000 in children less than 16 years of age.
• Boys are more commonly affected than girls (3:2).
• A positive family history is present in 3.5% of patients.
• Atopy and MCNS have an association.
• The most common MHC haplotype associated with MCNS is HLA DR7.
• African American children have a higher incidence of focal glomerulosclerosis (FSGS) than do Caucasian and Asian children.
• Examples of congenital NS are Finnish, mesangiosclerotic, and syphilitic nephrosis.

COMPLICATIONS

• Most complications are secondary to steroid therapy and include growth retardation, glaucoma, posterior lens cataracts, obesity, mood changes, hirsutism, osteoporosis, and infection.
• Primary peritonitis and cellulitis may occur de novo or with steroid therapy.
• Diarrhea and vomiting may result in rapid severe hypovolemia.
• Vascular thromboses are found with NS in relapse, especially if hypovolemia is present.
• Acute reversible renal failure is an uncommon complication of NS of childhood.
• MCNS does not result in chronic renal failure.

PROGNOSIS

The prognosis for MCNS is excellent, with a mortality rate of less than 1%.

 Differential Diagnosis

• Edema

—Congestive cardiac failure
—Liver failure
—Protein-losing enteropathy
—Protein energy malnutrition (Kwashiorkor)

• Nephrotic syndrome

—Focal glomerulosclerosis (FSGS)
—Membranous GN
—Membranoproliferative GN
—Diffuse mesangial proliferation

 Data Gathering

HISTORY

• Fatigue and general malaise
• Reduced appetite
• Weight gain and facial swelling
• Abdominal swelling or pain
• Urine that is foamy
• Atopy

 Physical Examination

• Pitting-dependent edema
• Fluid accumulation in body spaces (ascites, pleural effusions, scrotal swelling)
• White nails, lusterless hair, soft ear cartilage
• Hepatomegaly
• Mild hypertension

SPECIAL QUESTIONS

• Inquire about known atopy or food intolerance.
• Inquire about drug exposure (especially nonsteroidal antiinflammatory agents).
• Inquire about any infections or hernias.

PROCEDURE

Look for edema in the most dependent area of the child.

Laboratory Aids

TESTS

Laboratory Tests

- The urine dipstick usually shows 2,000 mg/dL (4+) of protein.
- Timed or spot urine protein collection: The 24-hour urine shows more than 40 mg/kg/d, and the spot urine protein:creatinine ratio is above 1.

Imaging

In complicated cases, renal ultrasound to look at the kidney size and parenchymal architecture

PITFALLS

- In small children with NS, the urine dipstick may be less than 4+.
- Failure to monitor complications of glucocorticoid therapy. Growth failure, especially, must be monitored for.

HOME TESTING

The first morning urine is dipped for protein.

REQUIREMENTS

Educate the family about urine testing, complications, diet, and therapy.

 ## Therapy

DRUGS

- Corticosteroids used as first-line agents
- Alkylating agents (cyclophosphamide, chlorambucil)
- Cyclosporine
- Diuretics
- Albumin

DURATION

There are a number of similar regimens.

- On presentation: daily corticosteroids for 4 weeks, followed by alternate-day therapy for 4 weeks
- On relapse: daily corticosteroids until in remission, followed by alternate-day therapy for 8 to 12 weeks

DIET

Restrict salt intake while in relapse or on daily corticosteroids.

POSSIBLE CONFLICTS

- Live vaccines are contraindicated while daily corticosteroids or alkylating agents are being given.
- Children in relapse, on corticosteroids, or on alkylating agents and who are nonimmune and exposed to varicella should receive VZIG.
- Albumin and or Lasix must be used cautiously to prevent fluid overload or intravascular dehydration.

 ## Follow-Up

WHEN TO EXPECT IMPROVEMENT

Remission occurs 2 to 4 weeks after starting corticosteroids in MCNS.

SIGNS TO WATCH FOR

- Fever, abdominal pain, oliguria

PITFALLS

Recognize situations in which hypovolemia may occur.

 ## Common Questions and Answers

Q: Will the MCNS recur?
A: The clinical course tends to be one of multiple remissions and relapses. Relapses usually stop about the time of puberty.

Q: Can the NS return in adult life?
A: Although uncommon, this does occur.

Q: Is macroscopic hematuria ever found with MCNS?
A: Gross hematuria suggests a renovascular event or a diagnosis other than MCNS. Microscopic hematuria occurs in approximately 25% of cases.

Q: What other agents are used to treat NS?
A: Cyclosporine A is used in children with steroid-dependent or -resistant NS.

ICD-9-CM 581.9

BIBLIOGRAPHY

Barratt TM, Clark G. Minimal change nephrotic syndrome and focal segmental glomerulosclerosis. In: Holliday M, Barratt TM, Avner ED, eds. *Pediatric nephrology*, 3rd ed. Baltimore: Williams & Wilkins, 1994:767–787.

McEnery PT, Strife CF. Nephrotic syndrome in childhood. *Pediatr Clin North Am* 1982;89(4): 875–885.

Meyers KEC, Kujubu DA, Kaplan BS. Minimal-change nephrotic syndrome. In: Neilson EG, Couser WG, eds. *Immunologic renal diseases*. Philadelphia: Lippincott-Raven, 1997:975–992.

Robson WLM, Leung AKC. Nephrotic syndrome in childhood. *Adv Pediatr* 1993:40:287–323.

Author: Kevin E.C. Meyers

Neural Tube Defects

Database

DEFINITION

Neural tube defects (NTDs) include a range of defects, including some subclinical defects, resulting from failure of neural tube closure between the third and fourth week of gestation. NTDs include anencephaly, encephalocele, myelomeningocele, and occult spinal dysraphism.

PATHOPHYSIOLOGY

• Neural tube closure begins midway along the neural axis, spreads like a zipper in both rostral and caudal directions, and is completed in a few days. Failure of neural tube closure most often occurs in the lumbosacral region.
• The defect itself may be only the "tip of the iceberg," since the total extent of the malformation may involve the entire central nervous system. This includes disorganized brainstem nuclei or brainstem herniation (Chiari II malformation).

GENETICS

Most cases are due to a combination of genetic, environmental, and dietary factors. Five percent of patients are born to a couple with a family history of NTD. After one NTD, the recurrence rate is 2% to 4% for subsequent pregnancies.

EPIDEMIOLOGY

• One per 1,000 live births in the United States (not including occult defects, for which no accurate epidemiologic data are available)
• Anencephaly: 0.2 per 1,000
• Myelomeningocele: 0.2 to 0.4 per 1,000

COMPLICATIONS

• Encephalocele: hydrocephalus (50%), intellectual deficits (40%), motor and cognitive deficits, seizures likely due to dysplastic cortex surrounding the encephalocele
• Myelomeningocele: hydrocephalus (80%); Chiari II malformation (80%), with some exhibiting feeding difficulties, stridor, and apnea due to lower cranial nerve dysfunction; neurogenic bladder (80%) with risk of renal damage; orthopedic deformities; seizures (25%); below average intelligence (15%–20%); and tethered spinal cord later in childhood
• Occult dysraphism: progressive lower extremity motor or sensory deficit, gait dysfunction, sphincter dysfunction, foot deformities, scoliosis

PROGNOSIS

• Anencephaly is uniformly fatal.
• Encephalocele: Prognosis is largely dependent on the size of the defect, the amount of brain tissue contained within the sac, and any associated brain malformations.
• Myelomeningocele: Prognosis for ambulation depends on the location of the lesion. The lower the lesion, the more likely the patient will ambulate. Cognitive outcome depends in part on associated brain malformations and treatment of hydrocephalus.

Differential Diagnosis

Diagnosis reflects the embryogenesis and anatomy of each defect.

• *Anencephaly* results from failure of anterior neural tube closure. The diagnosis is obvious at birth. The cerebral hemispheres, basal ganglia, and variable amounts of the upper brainstem are absent; 75% are stillborn and the remainder die in the neonatal period.
• *Encephalocele* is a more limited failure of anterior neural tube closure. Abnormal brain tissue protrudes through a skull defect usually covered by skin. Seventy percent to 80% are occipital, 20% are frontal. Ten percent to 20% of occipital defects are meningoceles and contain no brain tissue. Frontal encephaloceles, unless accompanied by craniofacial abnormalities, may not be identified unless a neuroimaging study is performed for an associated symptom (such as developmental delay or seizures).
• *Myelomeningocele* is a failure of posterior neural tube closure. Abnormal neural tissue protrudes through a vertebral column defect. Eighty percent are thoracolumbar, lumbar, or lumbosacral. By definition, this is an open defect, and the diagnosis is obvious at birth.
• *Occult spinal dysraphism* includes a variety of lesions, all with intact skin over the defect. The wide spectrum of defects includes dermal sinus tracts, cysts, lipomas, other tumors, diastematomyelia (bifid spinal cord), tethered spinal cord, and sacral agenesis (caudal regression syndrome).
• A *syndromic basis* for dysraphism should be considered when nonneural congenital defects are present (e.g., telecanthus-Waardenburg syndrome; conotruncal defect [chromosome 22q11 deletion]).

Data Gathering

HISTORY

• NTDs are associated with maternal folic acid deficiency, gestational diabetes, maternal hyperthermia during days 20 to 28 of gestation, and use of valproic acid, carbamazepine, and alcohol during pregnancy.
• Occult frontal encephaloceles may come to attention because of a history of developmental delay, seizures, or focal neurologic signs.
• Occult spinal dysraphism presents with lower extremity weakness or sensory loss, gait abnormalities, bowel and bladder dysfunction, foot deformities, and, rarely, recurrent meningitis.

Physical Examination

• Plot head circumference as a marker of developing hydrocephalus.
• Note other dysmorphic features because NTDs are found in various syndromes and chromosomal abnormalities.
• Assess the integrity of the skin covering the defect, because this affects the timing of surgical intervention. A bony defect or sinus may be palpable in occult cases.
• Neurologic exam of the lower extremities in a myelomeningocele outlines the functional level of the lesion and provides an estimate of future ambulatory potential. Intact hip flexion (L1-L2) and knee extension (L3-L4) are favorable signs for future ambulation.
• Flaccid paralysis is present below the level of the lesion, and ultimate limb growth may be asymmetric. Sensory level may not correspond to motor level. Cranial neuropathies, such as strabismus, laryngeal paresis, and stridor, may be present at birth or may develop in the first months of life.
• Local signs of occult spinal dysraphism include a dimple, sinus, lipoma, skin pigment change, or tuft of hair in the lumbosacral area. Examination may show foot deformities, tight heel cords, unequal leg or foot length, decreased sphincter tone, lower extremity weakness, or sensory changes.

Laboratory Aids

TESTS

• Maternal serum alpha-fetoprotein (MSAFP) testing, done at 16 to 18 weeks' gestation, can identify 88% of cases of anencephaly and 79% of cases of myelomeningocele.
• Ultrasonography can diagnose more than 99% of cases of anencephaly and 90% of cases of myelomeningocele. Since most encephaloceles are skin covered, they are more likely to be diagnosed by ultrasound than by MSAFP testing.
• After delivery, serial cranial ultrasounds or CT scans can evaluate hydrocephalus, which can occur without rapid head growth in patients with NTDs.
• MRI can outline other brain anomalies, including areas of cortical dysplasia, found in 92% of patients in one neuropathologic study.
• EEG is useful in apparent or suspected seizures.
• Urodynamic evaluation of the newborn can identify infants with high-pressure bladders and sphincter dyssynergia, who are at risk for renal damage.
• Suspected occult spinal dysraphism can be initially evaluated with spine x-rays and ultrasound (in the newborn period). CT scan provides more detail of bony anatomy, and MRI more detail of spinal cord anatomy.

Therapy

- Route of delivery: One study concluded that women with known NTD pregnancies should have a scheduled cesarean-section before the onset of labor, since infants delivered in this fashion may have improved neurologic outcome compared with infants delivered vaginally or by cesarean-section after onset of labor. Other studies have not confirmed this finding.
- Neurosurgical closure of a myelomeningocele is done within the first few days of life to prevent infection and for cosmetic reasons. Prophylactic antibiotics given while awaiting surgery decrease the incidence of meningitis and ventriculitis. Closure of the defect in the first hours of life is no longer felt to be necessary, as long as the defect can be kept clean and moist.
- An encephalocele with adequate skin covering can be repaired less urgently.
- V-P shunts should probably be placed in infants with NTDs with any degree of hydrocephalus, because early treatment of hydrocephalus may improve cognitive outcome.
- Infants with high bladder pressure typically are treated initially with anticholinergics and clean intermittent catheterization.
- Occult spinal dysraphism should be referred to neurosurgery for evaluation.

Follow-Up

- Children with NTDs benefit from a multidisciplinary approach, involving a primary pediatrician, neurosurgeon, urologist, orthopedist, neurologist, physiatrist, and others.
- Prognosis for ambulation is dependent on the location of the myelomeningocele. Virtually all children with sacral lesions are able to ambulate; 95% of adolescents and 40% of younger children with low lumbar lesions will ambulate; 30% of adolescents with high lumbar or thoracic lesions will ambulate.
- Approximately 80% of children with myelomeningocele will have a neurogenic bladder, which can be characterized by urodynamic testing. The goal of therapy is urinary continence and control of high bladder pressure.
- Many children can ultimately achieve bowel control with bowel programs involving high-fiber, low-fat foods; enemas; stool softeners; and biofeedback.
- Approximately 60% of children with encephalocele and 80% to 85% with myelomeningocele are of normal intelligence.
- Risk of epilepsy generally corresponds to the degree of mental retardation and is particularly high with frontal encephaloceles. Routine EEG cannot substitute for directed history to identify possible seizure activity.
- Anticipation of skin breakdown, decubitus ulcers, and leg injuries are important, since sensory deficits impair protective reflexes.

- In an older child with a myelomeningocele, loss of motor function in the legs, increased spasticity, gait difficulties, pain, bladder dysfunction, and scoliosis may be signs of a tethered cord.

PREVENTION

- Folic acid supplementation in early pregnancy can reduce the incidence of NTDs by 50% in the general population, and by 70% in women with a history of NTD in a previous pregnancy.
- Since many pregnancies are not discovered until after the fourth week of gestation, when neural tube closure occurs, the CDC recommends that all women of childbearing age receive a minimum of 0.4 mg of folic acid daily.
- The American Academy of Pediatrics recommends women with a history of NTD in a previous pregnancy receive 4 mg of folic acid daily, starting 1 month before and through the first 3 months of pregnancy.
- Women who are taking anticonvulsants and other medications linked to NTDs may also benefit from receiving 4 mg of folic acid daily.

PITFALLS

- The neurologic status of a patient with a repaired neural tube defect should not deteriorate with time, unless something else is wrong. Have a high index of suspicion for worsening hydrocephalus, syringomyelia, and tethered spinal cord—all treatable conditions which may develop over time.
- *Tethered cord* may accompany occult dysraphism and is a surgically treatable cause of acquired neurogenic bladder/cauda equina syndrome in young children.
- *Vocal cord paralysis* may appear episodically, resembling croup, in children with myelomeningocele.
- *Shunt blockage or infection* must be diagnosed early and may be heralded by subtle symptoms of irritability, increased sleep, or low-grade fever.

Common Questions and Answers

Q: Will my child have learning problems?
A: At least 50% of those with myelomeningocele have normal intelligence. Cognitive outcome appears improved with the advent of early shunting of hydrocephalus.

Q: Could my baby have other problems besides neurologic problems?
A: Infants with NTDs need to be checked periodically for signs of bladder problems. Some develop problems with control of eye movements (strabismus), but this is often correctable.

Q: Do the child's uncles or aunts have an increased risk of having a child with a birth defect?
A: Though some families do seem to carry an increased risk for NTDs, the increase is small and seems to affect the immediate, not the extended, family.

Q: Should I stop taking anticonvulsants during pregnancy to reduce my risk of NTDs?
A: Not unless your doctor recommends doing so. In general, continuing the lowest dose of the medicine which best controls your seizures is recommended during pregnancy. There are risks to the fetus from poorly controlled seizures during pregnancy. The overall risks and benefits of medications must be weighed. Any woman of childbearing age who is taking anticonvulsants should receive at least 0.4 mg of folic acid daily (and taking 4 mg daily is often recommended).

ICD-9-CM
Myelomenigocele 741.9
Anancephaly 740.0

BIBLIOGRAPHY

American Academy of Pediatrics, Committee on Genetics. Folic acid for the prevention of neural tube defects. Pediatrics 1993;92:493–494.

Blum RW, Pfaffinger K. Myelodysplasia in childhood and adolescence. *Pediatr Rev* 1994;15:480–484.

Fernandes ET, Reinberg Y, Vernier R, et al. Neurogenic bladder dysfunction in children: review of pathophysiology and current management. *J Pediatr* 1994;124:1–7.

Marks JD, Khoshnood B. Epidemiology of common neurosurgical diseases in the neonate. *Neurosurg Clin North Am* 1998;9:63–72.

McComb JG. Spinal and cranial neural tube defects. *Semin Pediatr Neurol* 1997;4:156–166.

Volpe JJ. *Neurology of the newborn,* 3rd ed. Philadelphia: WB Saunders, 1995:4–21.

Author: Dennis J. Dlugos

Neuroblastoma

Database

DEFINITION

Neuroblastoma is tumor derived from neural crest cells that form the sympathetic ganglia and adrenal medulla.

PATHOPHYSIOLOGY

• Etiology unknown
• Neuroblastoma should be distinguished from ganglioneuroma and ganglioneuroblastoma, which, in general, show features of differentiation or maturation.
• Included in the category of small, round blue-cell tumors of childhood
• Metastatic spread by lymphatic and hematogenous routes

GENETICS

• Familial neuroblastoma has been reported but is rare (autosomal dominant with variable penetrance, 1% of patients)
• Neuroblastoma cells may acquire specific genetic alterations, which are of prognostic importance (i.e., amplification of the N-*myc* gene).

EPIDEMIOLOGY

• Most common extracranial solid tumor of children; 7% to 10% of all childhood cancers
• Prevalence: 1 in 7,000 live births in the United States; 600 new cases a year
• Majority of children are less than 4 years of age and have disseminated disease at diagnosis
• Fifty percent of tumors arise from the adrenal gland.
• Eighty percent of tumors occur below the diaphragm; 20% occur in cervical and thoracic sites.

COMPLICATIONS

• Common sites of metastases include:

—Liver
—Bone marrow
—Skin: nontender subcutaneous nodules with a bluish hue
—Lymph nodes
—Bone, particularly the skull and facial bones as well as long bones

• Mass effect at the site of the primary lesion (i.e., spinal cord compression, Horner syndrome)
• Paraneoplastic syndromes

—VIP syndrome: due to VIP (vasoactive intestinal peptide) production by tumor; watery diarrhea, abdominal distention, and electrolyte imbalances usually resolve with treatment.
—Opsoclonus-myoclonus: etiology unknown but thought to be due to an autoimmune process; associated with chaotic eye movements ("dancing eyes") and myoclonic jerks ("dancing feet") with or without cerebellar ataxia; may

not resolve with treatment of tumor. Specific therapy includes high-dose steroids and IVIG.
—Catecholamine excess: flushing, sweating, tachycardia, headache, hypertension (hypertension more commonly of renal origin than catecholamine excess)

PROGNOSIS

• Most important adverse prognostic factors are N-*myc* amplification, metastatic disease, and age over 1 year
• The following biologic properties have prognostic significance:

—Histology: "favorable" versus "unfavorable"
—N-*myc* amplification: Amplification is associated with more aggressive, higher stage tumors (22% of patients).
—Serum ferritin: High levels are associated with more aggressive tumor.
—DNA index (ploidy): Hyperdiploid tumors are associated with less aggressive tumors than diploid tumors (in infants).
—Chromosome analysis: chromosome 1 deletions associated with more advanced stage tumors.
—Lactate dehydrogenase (LDH): High levels associated with more aggressive tumors.
—Neuron-specific enolase (NSE): may be elevated in pediatric tumors other than neuroblastoma

• Children with low-risk disease, such as age younger than 1 year with low-stage tumors, have an overall cure rate of greater than 90%.
• Older children with advanced-stage tumors have significantly lower cure rates of 15% to 30%, even with intensive multimodal therapies.

Differential Diagnosis

• Depends on the presentation of the patient and the site of the primary tumor
• Included in the differential diagnosis of abdominal or thoracic mass:

—Abdominal primaries include Wilms' tumor, Burkitt lymphoma, and germ-cell tumor.
—Thoracic primaries include lymphoma (usually non-Hodgkin), leukemia with bulky disease, and germ-cell tumors.

• The differential diagnosis of a "small, round, blue-cell tumor" should include neuroblastoma, lymphoma, Ewing sarcoma, and rhabdomyosarcoma.

Data Gathering

HISTORY

Presenting signs and symptoms of neuroblastoma depend on the primary site of the tumor and the degree of dissemination.

• General well-being: Ask about activity level, change in appetite, irritability, specific areas of discomfort, and so forth. This may give some indication of the extent of disease. Patients with neuroblastoma may present appearing either well or sick, though those with disseminated disease generally appear both chronically and acutely ill.

Physical Examination

ABDOMINAL MASS

• Abdominal mass is usually firm, fixed, irregular, and frequently crosses the midline.
• Abdominal distention with or without tenderness
• Mass effect

—Signs of bowel obstruction: anorexia, vomiting, low stool output
—Hypertension
—Genital and lower extremity edema from obstruction of venous and lymphatic drainage

CERVICAL/THORACIC MASS (POSTERIOR MEDIASTINAL)

• Respiratory distress or stridor with thoracic masses
• Horner syndrome with cervical or high thoracic masses: ptosis, myosis, and anhydrosis
• Anisocoria
• Superior vena cava syndrome with large mediastinal tumors

PARASPINAL MASS

• Vertebral body involvement and nerve root compression
• Bladder and bowel dysfunction, paraplegia, and back pain due to spinal cord compression

METASTATIC DISEASE

• Liver: hepatomegaly
• Bone: with or without bony pain, periorbital ecchymoses and/or proptosis
• Bone marrow: cytopenias, pain from marrow expansion
• Lymph nodes: adenopathy
• General: fever, irritability, failure to thrive
• Periocular ecchymosis

Laboratory Aids

TESTS

• Office evaluation should include a complete blood count, a basic chemistry panel to assess electrolyte imbalance, and a radiographic study of the suspected primary tumor site (generally an ultrasound or CT scan).
• Further studies should be obtained at the referral center where the patient will receive treatment; this will avoid repeating expensive tests.

Laboratory Tests

- Complete blood count (CBC): decreased hemoglobin, platelets, and/or white blood cell counts may indicate bone marrow involvement.
- Urine catecholamines: homovanillic acid (HVA); vanillylmandelic acid (VMA): secreted by some neuroblastomas
- Liver function tests: may indicate liver involvement when elevated
- Lactate dehydrogenase (LDH): may have prognostic value
- Serum ferritin: may have prognostic value
- Bone marrow aspirate and biopsy: to evaluate bone marrow involvement

Imaging

- Plain films of the primary site (calcification suggests neuroblastoma)
- US, CT, and/or MRI of the primary site and possible metastatic sites
- Skeletal survey or bone scan to rule out bone lesions
- MIBG scan: can detect both bone and soft tissues that are involved

Staging

- The International Neuroblastoma Staging System (INSS) is the commonly used, current staging system.
- Low-risk groups usually have localized disease.
- High-risk groups have disseminated disease often involving the bones, bone marrow, liver, and/or skin. Biologic characteristics of the tumor can also help stratify risk (i.e., N-*myc* amplification).
- Stage 4S (IVS or D) are patients less than 12 months of age who have a localized primary mass (stage 1 or 2) with disseminated disease involving the liver, skin, or (minimal) bone marrow but sparing the bones.

PITFALLS

Do not use the spot VMA or HVA to screen for neuroblastoma. False positives (excretion due to other sources) and false negatives (nonsecreting tumors) are both possible.

 Therapy

Treatment protocols are based on prognostic categories:

- Patients with low-risk disease, such as stage 4S or stage 1, may only require surgery alone, particularly if surgical resection is complete and the biologic characteristics of the tumor are favorable.
- Patients with advanced-stage disease, such as stage 4 (extensive metastases), usually require a combination of surgery, chemotherapy, and radiation therapy with or without high-dose therapy and stem-cell rescue (HDT/SCR).

SURGERY

- Total surgical resection is attempted but not aggressively; if gross total resection is risky, partial resection or biopsy alone is indicated.
- After a histologic diagnosis has been established, chemotherapy and radiation therapy can be instituted to obtain tumor shrinkage for a later attempt at total gross resection.

CHEMOTHERAPY

- Multiagent chemotherapy is often used in patients that are not low risk.
- Common chemotherapeutic agents for neuroblastoma include cyclophosphamide (Cytoxan), doxorubicin (Adriamycin), etoposide (VP-16), vincristine, ifosfamide, cisplatin, and carboplatin.

RADIATION

- Radiation therapy is used for control of local disease and/or for palliation.
- Total body radiation may be a component of preparative regimens for bone marrow transplantation (BMT).

BIOLOGIC THERAPY

- 13-Cis-retinoic acid: cellular differentiating agent that has shown improved survival when used posttransplant

BONE MARROW TRANSPLANTATION

Autologous bone marrow transplantation (ABMT) or peripheral stem-cell rescue (SCR) after intensive chemotherapy is used in high-risk protocols. Use of tandem transplants is currently being explored.

DURATION

Depends on stage of disease, response, and complications: generally under 12 months. Prolonged maintenance chemotherapy does not play a role in therapy, although biologic response modification therapy may be given in the second year after diagnosis.

 Follow-Up

SIGNS TO WATCH FOR

- Patients are often followed by radiographic studies of the primary site and sites of metastases as well as laboratory tests and bone marrow studies, depending on the presentation and staging of the patient—for example, urine catecholamines, serum ferritin, and abdominal CT for a patient with an adrenal primary without metastases.
- Complications depend on the primary site of the tumor and the therapy received; acute and late effects of chemotherapy and radiation therapy require close monitoring.

ISOLATION OF HOSPITALIZED PATIENTS

- Patients with neuroblastoma should take measures to avoid contact with persons known to have active varicella.
- Neutropenic patients do not require special isolation precautions except in the transplant setting.

 Common Questions and Answers

Q: Are siblings of children with neuroblastoma at increased risk for neuroblastoma compared with the general population?
A: No, except in rare families with a known history of neuroblastoma ($<1\%$).

Q: Can neuroblastoma spontaneously regress?
A: Yes; however, this is usually seen only in children under 1 year of age with lower stage disease.

Q: What are the biggest risks during therapy?
A: The risk of infection is quite high due to the presence of an indwelling catheter and severe neutropenia secondary to aggressive chemotherapy. Platinum-containing regimens can cause significant hearing loss that may worsen the higher the cumulative dose.

Q: What therapy is available to patients who either fail to go into remission or relapse following aggressive therapy?
A: There is no standard approach to a refractory or relapsed patient with neuroblastoma. Generally, phase I or II therapies may be offered, although the outcome for these patients is generally very poor.

ICD-9-CM 194.0

BIBLIOGRAPHY

Brodeur AE, Brodeur GM. Abdominal masses in children: neuroblastoma, Wilms tumor, and other considerations. *Pediatr Rev* 1991;12(7): 196–206.

Castleberry, R.P. Biology and treatment of neuroblastoma. *Pediatr Clin North Am* 1997;44: 919–937.

Caty MG, Shamberger RC. Abdominal tumors in infancy and childhood. *Pediatr Surg* 1993; 40(6):1253–1271.

Finklestein JZ. Neuroblastoma: the challenge and the frustration. *Hematol Oncol Clin North Am* 1987;1(4):675–694.

Reynolds CP, Villablanca JG, Stram DO, Harris R, Seeger RC, Matthay KK: 13-cis-retinoic acid after intensive consolidation therapy for neuroblastoma improves event-free survival: a randomized Children's Cancer Group (CCG) study. *Proc Am Soc Clin Oncol* 1998.

Authors: Julie W. Stern
Kim Smith-Whitley (first edition)

Neurofibromatosis

 Database

DEFINITION

Neurofibromatosis (NF) is a neurocutaneous syndrome in which tumors grow along various types of nerves, both internal and external. Neurologic features include cognitive disability, intra- and extracranial tumors of the nervous system, and stroke (rare). The diagnosis is based on the presence of any two of the following physical/familial criteria:

- Two or more cutaneous neurofibroma(ta)
- Lisch nodule
- Inguinal or axillary freckling
- Six or more (smooth-edged) café-au-lait spots, at least 1-cm diameter over 6 years or 0.5 cm under 6 years
- Optic nerve glioma
- Osseous lesions, including sphenoid wing dysplasia, pseudarthrosis
- Immediate family member with NF

Tumors may be cosmetically disfiguring and physically limiting; they rarely undergo sarcomatous transformation.

GENETICS

- Neurofibromatosis type 1 (NF1) is an autosomal dominant disorder; 50% of the cases are inherited, while the other half occur as a sporadic mutation.
- Located on chromosome 17, NF1 is the most commonly inherited autosomal dominant disorder (approximately 1 in 4,000), with no known gender or ethnic predisposition.
- Expression of NF1 varies widely within and among families, from mildly affected to severely impaired.
- The course of NF1 is impossible to predict; even a relative's disease will not be an indication of progression.
- NF2 has been located on chromosome 22.

EPIDEMIOLOGY

- The frequency is 1 in every 3,000 to 4,000 live births.
- NF1 affects 100,000 Americans.
- Occurrence appears to be independent of sex, race, or environmental factors.
- NF2 affects approximately 1 in every 50,000 live births.

COMPLICATIONS

- Oncologic

—Neurofibromas are benign tumors of Schwann cells, nerve fibers, and fibroblasts that arise along the nerves.
—Plexiform neurofibromas occur in approximately 15% of patients with NF1; these are extensive tumors that grow along the nerve root and may invade adjacent structures, threatening vital structures (especially in the neck and throat) or cause gross disfigurement. Approximately 10% of these tumors undergo sarcomatous degeneration.

—CNS tumors include optic nerve/pathway gliomas or gliomas elsewhere in the brain. Meningiomas and acoustic neuromas are more characteristic of the much rarer type 2 NF.

- Neurologic: learning disability, language disorders, autism, seizures, retardation, and attention deficit occur with higher than background frequency in NF.
- Renal: hypertension
- Circulatory: moya-moya, stroke
- Endocrine: pheochromocytoma
- Hematologic: leukemia

ASSOCIATED CONDITIONS

- Head circumference greater than the 98% percentile
- Developmental speech delay
- Gross and fine motor incoordination
- Headaches, scoliosis
- Abnormalities in growth development and learning disorders, including attention deficit disorder

 Differential Diagnosis

- Café-au-lait spots are most often benign findings unrelated to NF.
- NF2, McCune-Albright syndrome, and Sturge-Weber syndrome may resemble NF1.

—NF1 versus NF2: NF2 is also known as central bilateral acoustic NF, a rare disorder characterized by multiple tumors on the cranial and spinal nerves, and by other lesions of the brain and spinal cord.
—Diagnosis of NF2 is based on bilateral acoustic neuromas, family history of NF2, and any one of the following: neurofibroma, schwannoma, meningioma, or glioma.

- Sotos syndrome features macrosomia, hypertelorism, ventriculomegaly, and cognitive difficulties.
- Tuberous sclerosis (TS) may share autosomal dominant transmission, CAL, and hypopigmented lesions in common with NF; features distinctive for TS include adenomal sebaceum, cardiac and renal tumors, and prominent epilepsy. Genetic testing for TS may soon be available.

 Data Gathering

HISTORY

- A family history is from a first-degree relative, mother, or father of the proband. The disorder shows 100% penetrance.
- Vision: Optic path tumors generally occur between the ages of 2 and 6 years.
- Development: Learning problems and ADHD are common.
- Seizures: also more common in NF
- Joint/extremity pain: neuropathic pain or abrasion due to neurofibroma

- Back pain: could signal potentially serious cord or root compression
- Headache: (hydrocephalus); migraine also common in NF
- Respiratory problems: Neurofibromas may encroach upon the airway; sexual development; abnormalities due to hypothalamic disease; psychiatric concerns; and depression are common.

 Physical Examination

- Café-au-lait spots are noted at birth or within the first year of life; the macules are generally flush and circular, although they may have jagged edges or areas of hypertrichosis. Café-au-lait spots result from collection of heavily pigmented melanocytes of neural crest origin in the epidermis. The macules will appear for the first 5 years of life and then slow or stop, although they will grow with the child.
- Axillary and inguinal freckling are generally seen by puberty. The freckling is a cluster often seen in the skin folds.
- Lisch nodules are best assessed by slit-lamp examination. The Lisch nodules are small bumps on the iris that do not interfere with vision. They are uncommon during infancy, but by age 20, 99% of NF1 patients will have Lisch nodules.
- Optic pathway tumors (OPT) are present in 20% of patients with NF1, though only approximately 20% of those will require intervention. Treatment should be limited to those patients who have uncorrectable visual acuity, a change in visual fields, and/or endocrine abnormalities, or to those lesions that extend to the hypothalamus.
- Bony dysplasias occur in approximately 3% of patients with NF1. Dysplasias frequently occur in the tibia or the sphenoid wing. A pseudarthrosis will occur due to thinning of the long bone and its inability to heal after it breaks.

GENERAL

- Blood pressure
- Review of palpable tumors for extension or "stoney" feel that could signal cancerous change
- Abdominal examination for masses
- Funduscopy and acuity check for evidence of optic pathway tumor
- Neck and spine palpation/mobility
- Reflexes for evidence of nerve root tumor
- Growth parameters (including head circumference) for evidence of hydrocephalus, hypothalamic disturbance
- Scoliosis screen

Laboratory Aids

TESTS

Laboratory Tests

- In some families, the mutation causing NF1 can be detected by DNA testing.
- Renal studies may be indicated for persistent hypertension or difficulty with urine flow.

Imaging

- X-ray of the lower legs for pseudarthrosis in infants who are not yet walking. No particular blood tests are routinely indicated. Neuroimaging of the brain may be done as signs or symptoms indicate.
- Tibial films are indicated for infants known or strongly suspected to have NF, particularly if they are not yet walking, because of the possibility of surgically remediable tibial pseudarthrosis.
- Bright areas in cerebral white matter on T2-weighted MR images are common in NF1. Indications for neuroimaging depend on findings that may warrant it, such as progressive macrocrania, sensory deficits (especially visual), new-onset seizure, and chronic headaches. Some clinicians obtain a scan as a baseline on all new cases.

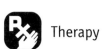 ## Therapy

- Presently, there is no treatment for tumor growth, except surgical interventions; tumors cannot be predicted based on their occurrence in another member of the family with NF. Interventions are palliative and supportive.
- Surgical intervention is performed on those tumors that are medically compromising, painful, or cosmetically disfiguring. Subcutaneous nodules are flesh-colored, raised, "pealike" nodules that may be present during childhood; these commonly appear and grow during puberty or pregnancy and do not grow into plexiform tumors.
- Family counseling regarding genetic implications, possible genetic testing using linkage, or, in some cases, mutation testing of the gene neurofibromin.
- Vigilance/anticipatory care regarding common psychological and developmental issues, such as speech delay, incoordination, hyperactivity/attention deficit, and learning disabilities. Early educational assessment and interventions may improve developmental outcome.

 ## Follow-Up

- Anticipatory care issues (see Data Gathering) are all pertinent to follow-up: monitoring for the development of tumors, hypertension, and psychological and developmental disabilities.
- Continuous yearly ophthalmologic examinations: Goldman visual field perimetry is suggested in those with any question of an optic nerve tumor. Some practitioners use yearly visual field testing (by an ophthalmologist) in lieu of MRI scanning.
- Orthopedic, oncologic, endocrine, surgery, and plastic surgery consultants may be helpful, depending on individual issues.
- Blood pressure checks are increasingly important in adolescents and adults with NF.
- Deaths have been associated with cancer, heart disease, and strokes, similar to the general population.
- Optimism: Natural history studies indicate that people with NF1 can live long, full lives.

PITFALLS

- Macrocrania is a common feature of NF, but growth curve for the head is necessary to determine whether it signifies a concern.
- Regrowth of plexiform neurofibromas: Even after apparent total resection, regrowth is common, and should be discussed before surgery.
- The possibility of nerve injury after surgery on plexiform neurofibromas should also be considered with the family/individual before surgery.

 ## Common Questions and Answers

Q: Can neurofibromatosis develop into cancer?
A: Most tumors caused by NF are benign and remain benign (even large tumors). In rare cases, they may become malignant.

Q: My child has NF1. What specialists must he see?
A: Your child should have yearly checkups with a physician familiar with the issues of NF (could be a family physician, pediatrician, child neurologist, or geneticist) who will know when to refer to other specialists. Otherwise, periodic visits to an ophthalmologist with experience in NF is the only routine recommendation.

ICD-9-CM 237.70

BIBLIOGRAPHY

Curless RG, Siatkowski M, Glaser JS, Shatz NJ. MRI diagnosis of NF-1 in children without cafe-au-lait skin lesions. *Pediatr Neurol* 1998;18(3): 269–271.

Gabriel KR. Neurofibromatosis. *Curr Opin Pediatr* 1997;9(1):89–93.

Goldberg Y, Dibbern K, Klein J, Riccardi VM, Graham JM Jr. Neurofibromatosis type 1—an update and review for the primary pediatrician. *Clin Pediatr* 1996;35(11):545–561.

Riccardi, VM. *Neurofibromatosis: phenotype, natural history, and pathogenesis,* 2nd ed. Baltimore: Johns Hopkins University, 1992.

Author: Sheila Vaughan

Neutropenia

 Database

DEFINITION

A decrease in the number of circulating neutrophils (both segmented and band forms), strictly defined as an absolute total neutrophil count (ANC) of less than 1,500/mm³. To calculate ANC, multiply the total WBC count by the percentage of segmented neutrophils and band forms. For example: WBC count 5,200 with 15% segs/polys, 4% bands, 76% lymphocytes, 5% monocytes: ANC = 5,200 × [0.15 + 0.04] = 988).

PATHOPHYSIOLOGY

Causes include:

• Decreased production in the bone marrow (congenital and acquired)
• Immune-mediated destruction
• Increased utilization (usually with overwhelming infection)
• Sequestration in the spleen

GENETICS

Some neutropenia syndromes can be inherited (i.e., Kostmann syndrome: autosomal recessive).

EPIDEMIOLOGY

• Total WBC counts and ANCs vary with age and race.
• African American children have lower total WBC counts and lower ANCs than do Caucasian children.
• Infants have a higher total WBC count and a higher percentage of lymphocytes in their differential counts.

COMPLICATIONS

• Systemic bacterial infection or localized infections such as cellulitis, labial abscesses, perirectal abscesses, oral mucosal ulceration, thrush

PROGNOSIS

• Varies
• Death from overwhelming infection does occur.
• Neutropenia resulting from infection or drug use is usually short-lived, but the congenital neutropenia syndromes may result in chronic lifelong neutropenia.
• Immune-mediated neutropenia frequently improves with age.

 Differential Diagnosis

• Neutropenia associated with infection

—Bacterial: Group B streptococcal disease, tuberculosis, brucellosis, tularemia, typhoid, paratyphoid
—Viral: hepatitis A and B, parvovirus, respiratory syncytial virus (RSV), influenza A and B, rubeola, rubella, varicella, cytomegalovirus (CMV), Epstein-Barr virus (EBV), human immunodeficiency virus (HIV)
—Other: malaria, visceral leishmaniasis, scrub typhus, sandfly fever

• Drug-induced

—Antibiotics: sulfonamides (trimethoprim-sulfamethoxazole is a common offender), penicillin, chloramphenicol (may be irreversible)
—Chemotherapy agents: alkylating agents, antimetabolites, anthracyclines
—Antipyretics: aspirin, acetaminophen (uncommon)
—Sedatives: barbiturates, benzodiazepines
—Phenothiazines: chlorpromazine, promethazine
—Antirheumatic agents: gold, penicillamine, phenylbutazone

• Tumors

—Leukemia
—Solid tumors that invade bone marrow

• Metabolic

—Nutritional: malnutrition, copper deficiency, megaloblastic anemia secondary to folate or vitamin B12 deficiency
—Inborn errors of metabolism: hyperglycinemia, isovaleric acidemia, propionic acidemia, methylmalonic acidemia

• Congenital

—Kostmann syndrome (severe congenital neutropenia)
—Cyclic neutropenia (regular oscillations in the number of circulating neutrophils: periodicity every 7–36 days; duration of neutropenia, 3–10 days)
—Chronic benign neutropenia of childhood (diagnosis of exclusion)
—Schwachman-Diamond syndrome (neutropenia and exocrine pancreatic insufficiency)
—Cartilage–hair hypoplasia (neutropenia, dwarfism, abnormal cellular immunity)
—Reticular dysgenesis

• Immunologic

—Neutropenia associated with primary immunodeficiencies (abnormalities in T- and B-lymphocytes)
—Autoimmune neutropenia: idiopathic (common in childhood; onset usually before age 2 years; diagnosis established by demonstrating antineutrophil antibodies; typically a benign course with resolution within several years; steroids may help in severe cases); Felty syndrome (neutropenia, splenomegaly, and rheumatoid arthritis); secondary to drugs, infection, or rheumatologic process
—Isoimmune neonatal neutropenia

• Miscellaneous

—Hypersplenism
—As part of evolving aplastic anemia (idiopathic, Fanconi anemia, familial aplastic anemia, dyskeratosis congenita)
—Bone marrow infiltration (tumor, osteopetrosis, Gaucher disease)
—Radiation injury

 Data Gathering

HISTORY

• Current or recurrent history of fever, skin abscesses, infection, or oral ulceration (helps establish duration of neutropenia)
• Medication use (many medications can cause neutropenia)
• Results of prior CBC with differential (a prior normal WBC count and ANC essentially rule out Kostmann syndrome)
• Symptoms of systemic infection: fever, rash, upper respiratory symptoms, jaundice
• Diet (looking for evidence of nutritional deficiency)
• Family history of neutropenia, recurrent infection, or early death (points to an inherited condition)

 Physical Examination

• Fever (temperature should not be taken rectally), tachycardia, and hypotension may indicate systemic infection.
• Oral ulceration, gingival irritation, pharyngitis, thrush
• Cellulitis, perirectal, or labial abscesses
• Hepatomegaly or splenomegaly
• Bruises, petechiae, pallor (other cell lines may be involved)
• Phenotypic abnormalities (thumb anomalies, dwarfism, joint findings)

Laboratory Aids

TESTS

• CBC with differential count (serial testing two to three times a week for 3 to 4 weeks may be necessary to evaluate for cyclic neutropenia)
• Bone marrow aspirate and biopsy (may be normal or may reveal a decrease in the number of myeloid precursors or a maturational arrest of the myeloid line [usually in the later stages], depending on the cause of neutropenia)
• Antineutrophil antibodies (present in autoimmune and isoimmune neutropenia) both on the neutrophils (direct) and in the serum (indirect)
• Cultures

 ## Therapy

GENERAL

• Correction of underlying cause of neutropenia (discontinue drug, treat infection, correct nutritional deficiency)
• Treatment of fever and suspected infection when neutropenic. Initially, broad-spectrum antibiotics are indicated; once the diagnosis has been established, this may not be necessary (i.e., individuals with chronic benign neutropenia).
• Prophylactic antibiotics are not usually beneficial and may predispose to systemic fungal infection.
• Stool softeners may be helpful in the profoundly neutropenic patient at risk for constipation to prevent development of a perirectal abscess.

SPECIFIC

• Hematopoietic growth factors

—Granulocyte colony-stimulating factor (G-CSF): drug of choice for Kostmann syndrome
—Granulocyte-macrophage colony stimulating factor (GM-CSF)

• Granulocyte transfusions (rarely indicated)
• Corticosteroids and/or plasmapheresis (most helpful in immune-mediated neutropenia)
• No therapy may be required if neutropenia is not severe and there are no serious or recurrent infections (often the case in autoimmune neutropenia and chronic benign neutropenia).

 ## Follow-Up

• CBCs and physical examinations at regular intervals while the patient is neutropenic
• Management of febrile episodes: prompt evaluation by a physician, obtain blood culture, hospitalize, and treat with intravenous antibiotics

PREVENTION

Neutropenia syndromes are not predictable and thus are not preventable.

ISOLATION OF HOSPITALIZED PATIENT

Isolation would be prudent until the etiology of the neutropenia is identified.

PITFALLS

Factitious causes of a low WBC count:

• Long time period between when blood sample is drawn and when it is tested
• Excessive leukocyte clumping (in presence of certain paraproteins)
• Leukocyte fragility secondary to leukemia or medication use

 ## Common Questions and Answers

Q: Do all episodes of fever and neutropenia require antibiotics?
A: In severe neutropenia syndromes (i.e., Kostmann syndrome) or when the etiology of the neutropenia is unclear, it is prudent to promptly evaluate the child, draw a blood culture, and administer intravenous broad-spectrum antibiotics. Certain neutropenia syndromes are not associated with an increased risk of infection (i.e., chronic benign neutropenia of childhood); children with these syndromes should be evaluated when they have fever but probably do not require intravenous antibiotics if they look well.

Q: Should a child with neutropenia be allowed to go to school?
A: Yes.

Q: Do they need to wear a mask?
A: No.

Q: When should a hematologist be consulted?
A: With any of the following:

• Chronic or profound neutropenia
• History of recurrent skin infections
• When bone marrow examination is indicated
• When hematopoietic growth factors, plasmapheresis, or granulocyte transfusion are being considered

ICD-9-CM 288.0

BIBLIOGRAPHY

Bernini JC. Diagnosis and management of chronic neutropenia during childhood. *Pediatr Clin North Am* 1996;43:773–792.

Boxer LA. Immune neutropenias: clinical and biological implications. *Am J Pediatr Hematol Oncol* 1981;3:89–96.

Brown AE. Neutropenia, fever and infection. *Am J Med* 1984;76:421–428.

Curnutte, JT. Disorders of granulocyte function and granulopoiesis. In: Nathan DG, Oski FA, eds. *Hematology of infancy and childhood*. Philadelphia: WB Saunders, 1993.

Weetman RM, Boxer LA. Childhood neutropenia. *Pediatr Clin North Am* 1980;27:361–375.

Welte K, Gabrilove J, Bronchud MH, Platzer E, Morstyn G. Filgrastim (r-metHuG-CSF): the first 10 years. *Blood* 1996;88:1907–1929.

Author: Cynthia F. Norris

Non-Hodgkin Lymphoma

 Database

DEFINITION

Non-Hodgkin lymphoma (NHL) is a malignant proliferation of cells of lymphocytic or histiocytic lineage that spread in a pattern similar to the migration of normal lymphoid cells.

PATHOPHYSIOLOGY

The exact cause is unknown. In contrast to adult lymphomas, childhood NHL is almost never nodular alone and rarely occurs in peripheral nodal areas.

Pediatric NHL can be divided into three major categories according to the NCI Formulation:

• Small noncleaved-cell lymphomas

—40% to 50% of childhood NHL
—Subdivided into Burkitt and Burkitt-like based on the degree of pleomorphism
—A variety of B-cell markers are usually present (e.g., CALLA, CD20).
—Express surface immunoglobulins, majority bearing IgM of either kappa or lambda light-chain subtype
—Terminal deoxyribonucleotidyl transferase (TdT) is negative.
—Characteristic chromosomal translocation, usually t(8;14), rarely t(8;22) or t(2;8); all translocations involve the c-*myc* proto-oncogene.

• Lymphoblastic lymphomas

—Comprise approximately 30% of childhood NHL
—Predominantly of thymocyte (T-cell) origin: Morphologically identical to acute leukemia T-lymphoblasts
—T-cell lymphomas are positive for TdT and have a T-cell immunophenotype (e.g., CD7).
—Majority lack chromosomal translocations; seldom involve T-cell receptor genes on chromosomes 7 and 14q.

• Large-cell lymphomas

—20% of childhood NHL
—The large noncleaved or cleaved type is of B-cell origin.
—Immunoblastic types are primarily of B-cell origin except for the Ki-1 antigen-positive type (anaplastic), which is of T-cell origin.

EPIDEMIOLOGY

• Third most common childhood malignancy (approximately 10% cancers in children <20 years of age in developed countries)
• Incidence is approximately 1.0 to 1.5 per 100,000 children.

—Higher frequency of endemic Burkitt type in equatorial African countries (10–15 per 100,000 children under 5–10 years of age)
—Incidence increases steadily with age; in children, usually occurs in first two decades of life (unusual <3 years of age)

• Sex: males more than females, with ratio being 2 or 3:1
• Genetic predisposition: increased risk in patients with immunologic defects (e.g., Bruton agammaglobulinemia, ataxia-telangiectasia, Wiskott-Aldrich, severe combined immunodeficiency)
• Environmental factors

—Drugs: immunosuppressive therapy and diphenylhydantoin
—Radiation: atomic-bomb survivors and ionizing radiation
—Viruses: Epstein-Barr virus (EBV), human immunodeficiency virus (HIV); EBV present in greater than 95% of cases of endemic Burkitt's versus fewer than 20% cases of sporadic

COMPLICATIONS

• Tumor lysis syndrome

—Combination of hyperuricemia, hyperkalemia, and hyperphosphatemia with hypocalcemia, resulting in uric acid nephropathy that leads to renal failure
—Correct before starting chemotherapy.

• Gastrointestinal obstruction, perforation, bleeding, intussusception
• Inferior vena cava obstruction and venous thromboembolism
• Neurologic (e.g., paraplegia, increased intracranial pressure)
• Superior vena cava (SVC) and superior mediastinum syndrome (SMS)

—Associated with lymphoblastic lymphomas that invade the thymus and nodes surrounding the vena cava and airways

• Massive pleural effusion
• Cardiac tamponade or arrhythmia

PROGNOSIS

Important prognostic factors for outcome include tumor burden at presentation and treatment administered.

• Favorable: stages I and II with primary site being head and neck (nonparameningeal), peripheral nodes, or abdominal site (80% or greater 2-year survival).
• Unfavorable: stage III or IV, parameningeal stage II, stage IV with CNS involvement (worst); incomplete initial remission within 2 months (60%–80% 2-year survival)

 Differential Diagnosis

• Abdominal masses

—Newborns: hydronephrosis, renal cysts, Wilms' tumor, or neuroblastoma.
—Older children: constipation, full bladder, hamartoma, hemangioma, cysts, leukemic or lymphomatous involvement of the liver and/or spleen, Wilms' tumor, or neuroblastoma.

• Mediastinal masses anatomically, divided into three regions:

—Anterior: masses of thymic origin, teratomas, angiomas, lipomas, or thyroid tumors
—Middle: metastatic or infection-related lesions involving the lymph nodes, pericardial or bronchogenic cysts, esophageal lesions, or hernias
—Posterior: neurogenic tumors (e.g., neuroblastoma, ganglioneuroma, neurofibroma), enterogenous cysts, thoracic meningocele, or hernias

 Data Gathering

HISTORY

• B-cell lymphomas

—Systemic manifestation (e.g., fever, weight loss, anorexia, fatigue) if disseminated; less likely if tumor localized.
—Lump in neck that does not respond to antibiotics.
—Abdominal mass with pain, swelling, change in bowel habits, nausea, or vomiting.

• T-cell lymphomas

—Mediastinal tumor symptoms include cough, hoarseness, dyspnea, orthopnea and chest pain, anxiety, confusion, lethargy, headache, distorted vision, syncope, and a sense of fullness in the ears.
—Marrow involvement
—Bleeding and/or bruising, bone pain, pallor, fatigue

 Physical Examination

• Small noncleaved-cell lymphomas

—Intraabdominal mass (up to 90%): involving ileocecal region, appendix, ascending colon, or some combination of these sites. Lymphadenopathy may be present in inguinal or iliac region; hepatosplenomegaly. Acute abdomen with intussusception, peritonitis, ascites, and acute GI bleeding. Lymphoma is the most frequent cause of intussusception in children over age 6 years.
—In endemic Burkitt lymphoma, jaw tumors are the most frequent site of disease; orbital involvement in infants; abdominal masses in 50%.
—Other sites of involvement: testis, unilateral tonsil hypertrophy, peripheral lymph nodes, parotid gland, skin, bone, CNS, and marrow.

• Lymphoblastic lymphoma

—Mediastinal mass (50%–70%) with pleural effusion present with decreased breath sounds, rales, cough with or without SVC or SMS syndrome. Signs include swelling, plethora, and cyanosis of the face, neck, and upper extremities; diaphoresis; and stridor and wheezing.
—Lymphadenopathy (50%–80%) is primarily above the diaphragm.

—Abdominal involvement is uncommon, likely to involve only liver and spleen.
—Cranial nerve involvement is rarely seen.

 ## Laboratory Aids

TESTS

Laboratory Tests

- CBC
- Liver and renal function studies
- Serum LDH and uric acid
- Serum lactate and soluble IL-2 receptor levels (optional)
- Adequate surgical biopsy

Imaging

- Abdominal ultrasound
- Chest PA and lateral
- CT scan of chest, abdomen, and pelvis
- Gallium scan
- Bone scan (optional or if gallium scan suggests bone involvement)
- MRI (especially for bone involvement)

Special Tests

- CSF examination
- Peritoneal or pleural fluid examination
- Marrow aspiration and biopsy
- Cytogenetics and immunophenotyping of tumor

STAGING

No uniform staging system exists for childhood NHL. Below is the St. Jude Children's Research Hospital staging system:

Stage I: single-tumor (extranodal) or single-nodal area, excluding mediastinum or abdomen

Stage II: single tumor with regional nodal involvement, two or more tumors or nodal areas on one side of the diaphragm, or a primary GI tract tumor (resected) with or without regional node involvement

Stage III: tumors or lymph node areas on both sides of the diaphragm, any primary intrathoracic or extensive intraabdominal disease (unresectable), or any primary paraspinal or epidural tumors

Stage IV: bone marrow or CNS disease regardless of other sites; marrow involvement defined as 0.5% to 25% of malignant cells.

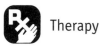 ## Therapy

A multidisciplinary approach is imperative to ensure the best therapy.

RADIOTHERAPY (XRT)

- Radiation adds no therapeutic benefit in children with limited disease.
- Increases both short- and long-term toxicity

- XRT used as emergent treatment for superior vena caval [SVC] obstruction, CNS, or testicular involvement.

SURGERY

- Performed if total resection can be achieved
- Additional indications: intussusception, intestinal perforation, suspected appendicitis, or serious GI bleeding

PRECHEMOTHERAPY MANAGEMENT

Allopurinol, hydration, and urinary alkalinization to prevent tumor lysis syndrome. Monitor uric acid, BUN, creatinine, K^+, Ca^{++}, and PO_4^-.

CHEMOTHERAPY

- Choice of a particular protocol is determined by histology and stage.
- Because of a high-conversion rate of lymphomas to leukemias, prophylactic CNS treatment is given (except in patients with totally excised intraabdominal tumor).
- Duration: 6 to 18 months (currently, as short as 9 weeks in localized nonlymphoblastic lymphomas)
- Drugs: cyclophosphamide, vincristine, methotrexate (IV + IT), prednisone, daunorubicin, asparaginase, cytarabine, thioguanine, carmustine, hydroxyurea, hydrocortisone, doxorubicin, mercaptopurine, etoposide
- Common side effects: hair loss, myelosuppression with transfusions required, nausea/vomiting

MANAGEMENT OF RELAPSE

- Relapse indicates extremely poor prognosis.
- No uniform approach to rescue therapy
- First treated to induce second remission with different/previously unused chemotherapy regimen
- Allogeneic or autologous bone marrow transplant should be considered.

 ## Follow-Up

- Patient monitoring weekly to monthly with CBC and examination.
- Radiologic imaging at intervals during and off therapy.
- Monitor for toxicity-related complications

PITFALLS

Late effects from therapy:

- Cardiac myopathy or anthracyclines
- Impaired reproductive function or infertility from alkylating agents
- Second malignant neoplasms
- Psychological consequences of life-threatening illness

 ## Common Questions and Answers

Q: Did I do something to cause this?
A: No. The majority of cases are sporadic and not associated with diet, underlying immune dysfunction, or viral illness.

Q: When will my child be "cured"?
A: For patients with small- or large-cell lymphomas, relapse most commonly occurs in the first 10 months. Therefore, a child may be considered cured if he or she remains in remission after the first year off therapy. A patient with lymphoblastic lymphoma is considered cured if he or she remains in remission after about 3 years from onset of therapy.

Q: Is this contagious?
A: No. Siblings may have slightly higher inherent risk than the general population, but they are not at risk from the affected child.

ICD-9-CM 202.8

BIBLIOGRAPHY

Kelly K, Lange B. Oncologic emergencies. *Pediatr Clin North Am* 1997;44(4):809.

Lanzkowsky P. Non-Hodgkin's lymphomas. In: Lanzkowsky P, ed. *Manual of pediatric hematology and oncology.* New York: Churchill Livingstone, 1989:271–285.

Magrath I. Lymphocyte differentiation pathways—an essential basis for the comprehension of lymphoid neoplasia. *J Natl Cancer Inst* 1981;67:501.

Magrath IT, Lee YJ, Anderson T, et al. Prognostic factors in Burkitt's lymphoma: importance of total tumor burden. *Cancer* 1980;45:1507.

Murphy SB, Fairclough DL, Hutchison RE, et al. Non-Hodgkin's lymphomas of childhood: an analysis of the histology, staging, and response to treatment of 338 cases at a single institution. *J Clin Oncol* 1989;7(2):186–193.

Shad A, Magrath I. Diagnosis and treatment of non-Hodgkin's lymphoma in childhood. In: Wernik P, Canellos G, Putcher J, eds. *Neoplastic diseases of the blood,* 3rd ed. New York: Churchill Livingstone, 1996:925.

Shad A, Magrath I. Malignant non-Hodgkin's lymphomas in children. In: Pizzo PA, Poplack DG, eds. *Principles and practice of pediatric oncology,* 3rd ed. Philadelphia: Lippincott, 1997:545–587.

Author: Deborah L. Kramer

Nosebleeds (Epistaxis)

 Database

DEFINITION

Epistaxis is bleeding from the nose. Bleeding may be evident anteriorly through the nares or posteriorly through the nasopharynx.

CAUSES

- Inflammation of, or trauma to, the nasal passages account for most nosebleeds:

—Viral upper respiratory infections, allergic rhinitis, bacterial rhinitis, childhood exanthems
—Nose picking, external trauma, foreign bodies, postsurgical bleeding, chemical or caustic agents/inhalants

- Local structural abnormalities may predispose to epistaxis:

—Rhinitis sicca, or environmental drying of the nasal mucosa, commonly promotes epistaxis (see Common Questions and Answers).
—Nasal polyps, telangiectasias, meningoceles, angiofibromas, vascular malformations

- Less commonly, nosebleeds may herald, or accompany, systemic illnesses:

—Hematologic diseases such as leukemias, thrombocytopenias, hemophilias (and von Willebrand disease), and hemoglobinopathies
—Clotting disorders due to infection, hepatic failure, or poisoning/envenomation
—Hypertension

PATHOPHYSIOLOGY

- The nasal mucosa has a rich blood supply originating from both the internal and external carotid arteries.
- Blood vessels of the nasal septum and lateral nasal walls have little anatomic support or protection. The thin mucosal surface is prone to drying.
- Blood vessels of the nose form many plexiform networks. Especially important is Kiesselbach's plexus in the anterior nasal septum, the most common site of nosebleeds in children.
- The nose is subject, by position, to traumatic injury.

EPIDEMIOLOGY

- Nosebleeds occur in all ages throughout the year.
- Children aged 2 to 10 years are most commonly affected.
- Nosebleeds are more common in the winter.

COMPLICATIONS

- Nosebleeds are most commonly uncomplicated.
- Rare complications include significant blood loss, airway obstruction, aspiration, and vomiting.

PROGNOSIS

- Uncomplicated epistaxis is most often self-limited or resolves with simple first-aid techniques.
- Refractory or recurrent epistaxis may require more specialized techniques, surgical intervention, and/or otorhinolaryngologic intervention.

ASSOCIATED ILLNESSES

Hemoptysis, hematemesis, or melena may be the presenting concerns in individuals with bleeding from the nasopharynx.

 Differential Diagnosis

Epistaxis is a common event in normal children. A careful history and physical examination should identify those children with unusual predisposing causes for nosebleeds.

 Data Gathering

HISTORY

- Frequency of occurrence
- Persistence of bleeding
- Nose-picking behavior/traumatic injury
- Nasal congestion, discharge, obstruction
- Allergies
- Medications or drugs of abuse (especially cocaine)
- Previous or concurrent bruising or bleeding
- Menstrual history
- Family history of systemic disease or hemorrhagic disorder

 Physical Examination

- Vital signs with blood pressure determination
- Inspection of nose, nasopharynx, and oropharynx
- General examination with attention to lymph nodes, liver and spleen size, rashes, icterus, pallor

PROCEDURE

- Examination of the nose may be facilitated by application of a topical vasoconstricting agent and/or anesthetic agent.
- Anxiety may interfere with examination and treatment of children. Sedation and analgesia may be beneficial in some circumstances.

 Laboratory Aids

TESTS

- Laboratory evaluation is not indicated in healthy children with readily controlled epistaxis from an anterior site.
- Recurrent or refractory nosebleeds, or suspicious findings from the history and physical examination, may warrant a directed laboratory evaluation (such as platelet count, prothrombin and partial thromboplastin times, complete blood count, and/or bleeding time) and/or consultation.

Therapy

- Elevate the head of the bed.
- Direct pressure, applied by gently squeezing the nostrils, is usually sufficient to stop most nosebleeds.
- Ice to the nasal dorsum may be combined with application of direct pressure.
- A cotton pledget beneath the upper lip may aid hemostasis by compressing the labial artery.
- Vasoconstricting agents (0.25% phenylephrine, 0.05% oxymetazoline, 1:1,000 epinephrine, or 1%–5% cocaine) will help reduce bleeding as well as improve visualization.
- Application of topical thrombin with a cotton swab may be used when direct visualization of the bleeding site is achieved.
- Once identified, an offending vessel may be cauterized with a silver nitrate stick or a swab dipped in trichloroacetic acid.
- An anterior nasal packing with oxycellulose or petroleum jelly gauze may be required to control refractory epistaxis when the site of bleeding cannot be precisely identified.
- Otorhinolaryngologic consultation may be needed for severe nosebleeds or when posterior nasal packing, fracture reduction, and/or surgery are required.
- Parental reassurance is an important, but often neglected, aspect of therapy.

PREVENTION

- Vaporizers, humidifiers, or saline sprays prevent desiccation of the nasal mucosa.
- Petroleum jelly applied to the anterior nasal septum aids healing of inflamed nasal mucosa.
- Antigen avoidance and medical therapy should be used to reduce allergic symptoms.
- Fingernails should be cut short, and nose-picking behavior should be discouraged.
- Protective athletic equipment should be worn.

 ## Follow-Up

- Nosebleeds are easily controlled and self-limited in most instances.
- Families should be given instructions in basic first aid for nosebleeds, because minor insults, such as sneezing or excessive manipulation, may cause nosebleeds to recur.
- Referral to an otorhinolaryngologist is indicated for patients with specific local abnormalities, such as polyps, tumors, or vascular malformations.
- Severe nosebleeds, recurrent nosebleeds, and/or posteriorly located nosebleeds may warrant evaluation by an otorhinolaryngologist.
- Identification of systemic illness may require referral to the appropriate specialist.
- Postsurgical nosebleeds can be particularly problematic.

PITFALLS

- Blood clots in the nasopharynx should be removed because they may obscure engorged, bleeding vessels.
- Failure to detect a posterior location within the nasal cavity as the source of bleeding may interfere with measures to control bleeding.
- After nasal packing, it is essential to examine the oropharynx to confirm adequate hemostasis.
- Absorbable-type packings should be used, if required, in patients with bleeding disorders. Standard packings are prone to rebleeding upon removal.
- Impregnation of nasal packings with antibiotic ointment reduces the risk of toxic shock syndrome.

 ## Common Questions and Answers

Q: How should the patient with nosebleeds be positioned?
A: When possible, patients with nosebleeds should be kept erect. The upright position decreases vascular congestion. Recumbent patients may appear to have less bleeding, but this is due to redirection of blood flow through the posterior pharynx.

Q: How does rhinitis sicca contribute to epistaxis, and why does it occur?
A: The nose warms, humidifies, and filters inspired air. Many modern heating systems and air-conditioning units reduce household humidity to unnaturally low levels. Rhinitis sicca is the direct result of inhaling dry air and results in friable nasal mucosa. Turbulent airflow from a septal deformity also promotes drying.

ICD-9-CM 784.7

BIBLIOGRAPHY

Alvi A, Joyner-Triplett N. Acute epistaxis: how to spot the source and stop the flow. *Postgrad Med* 1996;99:83–96.

Guarisco JL, Graham HD III. Epistaxis in children: causes, diagnosis, and treatment. *Ear Nose Throat J* 1989;68:522–538.

Mulbury PE. Recurrent epistaxis. *Pediatr Rev* 1991;12:213–217.

Author: Kevin C. Osterhoudt

Obesity

 Database

DEFINITION

Obesity is defined as excess body fat. Overweight is defined as excess body weight for height. Features:

- >120% of ideal body weight
- Triceps skinfolds greater than 85th percentile
- Body mass index (BMI) greater than or equal to 85th percentile for age, or total greater than or equal to 30

CAUSES (POSSIBLE)

- Genetic predisposition
- Positive energy balance

—Excessive caloric intake
—Decreased physical activity
—Decreased resting metabolic rate

EPIDEMIOLOGY

- Twenty-five percent prevalence in pediatric population
- Genetics: risk of childhood obesity two to three times higher in patients with family history of obesity; with one obese parent, 40% chance of obese child; with two obese parents, 70% to 80% chance of having obese child
- Ten percent to 30% of obese adults were obese as children; increasing risk with severity of childhood obesity, onset in adolescence, and family history of obesity

COMPLICATIONS

- Psychiatric: psychosocial dysfunction
- Endocrine: hyperlipidemia, diabetes mellitus type II, insulin resistance, hyperinsulinism
- Cardiovascular: hypertension, atherosclerosis, cardiac hypertrophy
- Respiratory: obstructive sleep apnea, Pickwickian syndrome
- Orthopedic: Blount disease, slipped capital femoral epiphysis, gout
- Gastrointestinal: hepatic steatosis, cholelithiasis
- Sexual development and growth: abnormal growth acceleration, earlier onset of menarche, pubertal gynecomastia

PROGNOSIS

- Poor for long-term maintenance of weight loss (with current regimens)
- Can derive significant health benefits from even modest weight reduction
- Best results:

—Family support/participation in care plan
—Treat as a chronic condition requiring long-term follow-up
—Diet restriction combined with increased physical activity
—Realistic weight goals for weight loss and maintenance

 Differential Diagnosis

- Fewer than 5% of all cases of childhood obesity are due to an underlying medical disorder.
- Endocrine

—Cushing syndrome
—Hypothyroidism, pseudohypothyroidism type I
—Hyperinsulinemia
—Growth hormone deficiency
—Hypothalamic dysfunction
—Stein-Leventhal syndrome (polycystic ovary syndrome)

- Congenital

—Muscular dystrophy
—Myelodysplasia

- Chromosomal

—Down syndrome
—Turner syndrome
—Alstrom-Hallgren syndrome
—Klinefelter syndrome
—Laurence-Moon-Biedl syndrome
—Prader-Willi syndrome
—Vasquez disease

 Data Gathering

HISTORY

- Growth and adiposity: growth chart, growth velocity chart, Tanner maturation stage
- Mental function: school performance, psychological testing
- Emotional/psychological status: concern of patient about weight, body image, self-esteem, depression
- Eating behavior: control over food intake, meal and snacking patterns, knowledge of good nutrition by patient and family
- Physical activity: exercise type and frequency, family level of activity, television viewing habits
- Family characteristics: other members with obesity, eating disorders
- Parental attitude toward weight problem: role of food in family, perception of weight problem, attempts to intervene
- Social relationships: friends, school, teasing
- Dietary intake: 3-day diet records

Physical Examination

- Anthropometric measurements: height, weight, weight for height, skinfold thickness (triceps)
- Fat distribution pattern (central or gynecoid)
- Tanner staging
- Blood pressure

Laboratory Aids

TESTS

Laboratory Tests

- Thyroid status: TSH, T$_4$ (especially if height less than 50th percentile)
- Lipoprotein profile, fasting (cholesterol, HDL, TG)
- Glucose, fasting
- Insulin level, fasting

Imaging

- Bone age

Body Composition

- Skinfolds
- Bioelectrical impedance analysis (BIA)
- Dual energy x-ray absorptiometry (DEXA)
- Underwater weighing

Therapy

DRUGS

No currently available weight-reduction drugs are indicated for use in children.

DURATION

- Lifelong, emphasizing behavioral changes and continued follow-up

DIET

- Individualized
- Reduction in total caloric intake with emphasis on decreasing fat intake
- Important to provide sufficient calories, vitamins, minerals, and protein to ensure growth
- Rarely utilize rapid weight-loss protocols (such as protein-sparing, modified fasts) unless have life-threatening complications such as pickwickian syndrome; must be monitored closely by medical staff

EXERCISE

- Incorporate exercise into the regular routine.
- Family participation
- Enjoyable activities

BEHAVIOR MODIFICATION

- Self-monitoring
- Family intervention
- Cognitive structuring

Follow-Up

- Initially should be frequent (often weekly), spacing out over time
- Referral to a multidisciplinary obesity clinic is often useful (physician, psychologist, dietitian, physical therapist).

Common Questions and Answers

Q: Is childhood obesity caused by a glandular (thyroid) problem?
A: No, only a small percentage of obesity is caused by hypothyroidism. Children with hypothyroidism are heavier and shorter compared with euthyroid children.

Q: What about the role of leptin and the genetic basis of obesity?
A: The genetics of obesity, fat-cell regulation, and body-weight set points are currently being elucidated. In the future, it may be possible to reset the body's set point for weight.

Q: What about the genetic basis of obesity and the role of leptin?
A: The genetics of obesity, fat cell regulation, and body weight set-points are currently the objects of intense scientific study. Leptin, a hormone secreted from adipose tissue, is a potential afferent signal of fat stores in humans, but its role in the pathogenesis of human obesity has yet to be determined. It is likely that in the majority of cases, obesity is due to a complex interaction between several genes and permissive environmental factors that leads to the deposition of excess calories as adipose tissue.

ICD-9-CM
Obesity 278.0
Morbid obesity 278.01

BIBLIOGRAPHY

Alemzadeh R, Lifshitz F. Childhood obesity. In Lifshitz F, ed. *Pediatric Endocrinology*, 3rd. New York: Marcel Dekker, 1996:753–774.

Behrman RE, Kliegman RN, Arvin AM, eds. *Nelson's textbook of pediatrics*, 15th ed. Philadelphia: WB Saunders, 1996.

Dietz WH. Nutrition and obesity. In: Grand RJ, Sutphen JL, Dietz WH, eds. *Pediatric nutrition: theory and practice*. Boston: Butterworth-Heinemann, 1987:525–538.

Forbes GB, Woodruff CW. *Pediatric nutrition handbook*, 2nd ed. Elk Grove Village, IL: American Academy of Pediatrics, 1985:263–273.

Krasnegjor MA, Grave GD, Kretchmer N. *Childhood obesity: a biobehavioral perspective*. Caldwell, NJ: Telford, 1988:31–44, 183–194.

National Institutes of Health Consensus Development Conference Statement. Health implications of obesity. *Ann Intern Med* 1985;103 (6):1073–1077.

Rosenbaum M, Leibel RL, Hirsch J. Obesity. *N Engl J Med* 1997;337:396–407.

Van Itallie TB, Lew EA. Assessment of morbidity and mortality risks in the overweight patient. In: Wadden TA, VanItallie TB, eds. *Treatment of the seriously obese patient*. New York: Guilford, 1992.

Author: Kathleen Graham

Osteogenesis Imperfecta

 Database

DEFINITION

Osteogenesis imperfecta (OI) is a group of genetically heterogeneous connective tissue disorders affecting bone and soft tissue, causing abnormal fragility and plasticity of bone, resulting in recurring fractures and deformity.

CAUSES

Abnormality of collagen production and organization; failure of maturation of procollagen to type 1 collagen and failure of normal collagen cross-linking

PATHOLOGY

- In general: Both enchondral and intramembranous bone formation is disturbed.

—Osteoid seams are wide and crowded by osteoblasts (woven bone).
—Osteoclasts are normal. Collagen fibrils are disorganized (by EM).

- Physis broad and irregular

—Osteopenia
—Long bones are slender and smaller.
—Fractures (recent or healed)
—Deformities
　—Spine: scoliosis, compression fractures, kyphosis
　—Skull: multiple centers of ossification, wormian bones

GENETICS

- Sillence classification:

—Type 1: autosomal dominant, blue sclera, onset preschool
　—A: teeth involved
　—B: teeth not involved
—Type II: autosomal recessive, lethal, blue sclera
—Type III: autosomal recessive, severe, normal sclera
—Type IV: autosomal dominant, normal sclera, mild form
　—A: teeth involved
　—B: teeth not involved

- Some cases of OI occur as spontaneous mutations.

EPIDEMIOLOGY

- Approximately 1 in 20,000

PROGNOSIS

- In general, the earlier the fractures occur, the more severe the disease.
- For moderate and mild types, there is a gradual tendency to improvement, with the incidence of fractures decreasing after puberty.

 Differential Diagnosis

- Severe: congenital hypophosphatasia, achondroplasia, camptomelic dwarfism
- Mild: cystinosis, pycnodysostosis, child abuse, leukemia, idiopathic juvenile osteoporosis, steroid treatment, rickets in very-low-weight infants, Menkes' kinky-hair syndrome (newborn male [X-linked recessive] with failure to thrive, metaphyseal corner fractures, and abnormal hair)

 Data Gathering

HISTORY

- Variable; family history

 Physical Examination

- Severe congenital forms: multiple fractures, limbs deformed and short, skull soft
- Mild and moderate forms

—General: short stature, hernias
—Extremities: bowing, coxa vara deformity, cubitus varus, hypermobility of joints: subluxations and dislocations
—Pelvis: trefoil pelvis, protrusio acetabuli
—Spine (cause: osteoporosis, compression fractures, and ligamentous laxity): kyphoscoliosis (30%–40%), platybasia
—Skin: thin skin, subcutaneous hemorrhages, wide surgical scars
—Eyes: blue sclera caused by thin collagen layer, Saturn's ring (white sclera immediately) hyperopia, embryotoxon or arcus juvenilis occasionally, retinal detachment occasionally
—Teeth: dentinogenesis imperfecta, enamel normal, both deciduous and permanent teeth affected, teeth easily broken, discoloration
—Deafness: either conduction or nerve type

Laboratory Aids

TESTS

Blood Tests

- Serum calcium and phosphorus is normal.
- Alkaline phosphatase may be elevated.
- There is no specific laboratory diagnostic abnormality.

Radiographs

- Osteopenia
- Fractures: new, healing, or healed; malunions
- Deformity
- Metaphyseal ends of long bones: honeycomb appearance of ends of long bones, popcorn calcifications, Erlenmeyer flask appearance, acetabular protrusio
- Spine: atlantoaxial subluxation, spondylolisthesis, scoliosis, compression fractures

 Therapy

DRUGS

None (gene therapy possibly in future). Sex hormones, fluoride, magnesium oxide, calcitonin, and special diets have all been tried; no medications have been proved to be of definite value.

ORTHOPEDIC

- Fracture treatment: Factures heal at a normal rate; splinting, orthoses, casting, operations (intramedullary rod)
- Education: fracture prevention
- Scoliosis: seen in approximately 50%; orthoses usually ineffective; spinal fusion for curves greater than 50 degrees
- Correction of deformities (e.g., shish-kebab operations)

 Follow-Up

PROGNOSIS

- Depends on severity of OI
- Spranger scoring system
- Moderate and mild types: gradual tendency to improvement, with incidence of fractures decreasing after puberty

PITFALLS

Hyperplastic callus formation may be confused with osteogenic sarcoma.

ICD-9-CM 756.51

BIBLIOGRAPHY

Minch CM, Kruse RW. Osteogenesis imperfecta: a review of basic science and diagnosis. *Orthopedics* 1998;21(5):558–567, 568–569 (quiz).

Sillence DO. Osteogenesis imperfecta: an expanded panorama of variants. *Clin Orthop* 1981;159:11.

Spanger JW, Cremin B, Beighton P. Osteogenesis imperfecta congenita. *Pediatr Radiol* 1982;12:21.

Tosi LL. Osteogenesis imperfecta. *Curr Opin Pediatr* 1997;9(1):94–99.

Zaleske DJ. Metabolic and endocrine abnormalities. In: Morrissy RT, Weinstein SL, eds. *Lovell and Winter's paediatric orthopaedics,* 4th ed. Philadelphia: Lippincott–Raven, 1996:164–170.

Author: John P. Dormans

Osteomyelitis

 Database

DEFINITION

Osteomyelitis is infection of the bone.

CAUSE

- *Staphylococcus aureus:* causes 90% of osteomyelitis in otherwise healthy children of all ages
- *Streptococcus pyogenes* or *Haemophilus influenzae* can also be the etiologic agent.
- Group B streptococci and *Escherichia coli* are often isolated in children under 1 month of age.
- *Salmonella* can be the cause in children with sickle cell anemia.
- *Pseudomonas aeruginosa* can be found in puncture wounds to the foot.

PATHOLOGY

- Usually, osteomyelitis begins as bacteremia with hematogenous spread to the bone, but direct inoculation of bacteria into the bone by trauma is also possible.
- Most bacteria that enter the bone are phagocytized, so that no infection develops. When bacteria enter areas of the bone with low blood flow, however, such as the metaphysis directly beneath the physeal plate, they may not be phagocytized, and an infection may develop.
- The first changes noted in osteomyelitis are the death of the osteoblasts in the infected area and resorption of trabeculae. Inflammation develops, which further compromises blood flow, and microabscesses are formed within the bone. Pus can spread through the bone and between the bone and the periosteum. This pus can lift the periosteum, causing point tenderness.

GENETICS

- Increased incidence in patients with sickle cell disease and other immunodeficiencies

EPIDEMIOLOGY

Incidence of 0.016% per year. The femur and tibia are most often affected.

COMPLICATIONS

- Permanent damage to the growth plate, septic arthritis, fracture in a weakened bone

 Differential Diagnosis

- Cellulitis
- Septic arthritis
- Malignancy
- Trauma
- Sickle cell crisis

 Data Gathering

HISTORY

A child with osteomyelitis usually complains of sudden onset of bone or joint pain and fever. A younger child may refuse to bear weight on or move the extremity that is involved.

 Physical Examination

- Physical examination usually reveals a febrile child with point tenderness over the area of infected bone. The child is often unwilling to move the involved extremity.
- As the infection progresses, swelling, warmth, and erythema of the skin overlying the infection may be noted.
- An infant with osteomyelitis may appear septic.

Laboratory Aids

TESTS

• Patients usually have an elevated white blood cell count and a high sedimentation rate.
• Blood cultures are positive in over 50% of patients.
• Aspiration of the infected bone, even in the absence of debridement, is useful to determine the etiologic organism.

IMAGING

• Plain films begin to show the changes of osteomyelitis 10 to 14 days into the infection, with periosteal elevation and bone destruction.
• ^{99}Tc bone scans are 80% accurate, and gallium scans are thought to be 91% accurate in diagnosing osteomyelitis.

 ## Therapy

• Antibiotic therapy for 4 to 6 weeks is usually required for osteomyelitis. Intravenous oxacillin is usually the empiric drug of choice until an organism can be isolated. Gram-negative coverage should be added for neonates, and *Salmonella* coverage is needed in sickle cell patients. If a recent foot puncture wound was experienced, coverage for *Pseudomonas* is recommended.
• Once the organism is known and sensitivities are established, the patient may be switched to oral antibiotics, as long as the serum bactericidal titer can be maintained.
• If an abscess is present in the bone, surgical debridement may also be necessary.

 ## Follow-Up

Patients should be followed to ensure adequate treatment of infection and continued growth of the extremity involved.

PITFALLS

• Delayed diagnosis, difficulty distinguishing osteomyelitis from a sickle cell crisis

 ## Common Questions and Answers

Q: Do you need to surgically debride osteomyelitis?
A: This is a very controversial topic. Many physicians feel that all osteomyelitis should be surgically debrided, while others believe that in the absence of an abscess, antibiotic therapy alone is adequate. Most agree, however, that if an abscess is present, it should be drained.

Q: Will osteomyelitis cause permanent damage in the bone?
A: If the growth plate is not damaged and the infection is adequately treated, there should be no permanent sequelae of osteomyelitis. If the growth plate is damaged, however, the affected limb may not grow evenly, or at all, even after the infection is treated.

ICD-9-CM 730.2

BIBLIOGRAPHY

Barron SA. Index of suspicion. Case 1. Diagnosis: osteomyelitis. *Pediatr Rev* 1998;19(2):51, 52.

Dirschl DR. Acute pyogenic osteomyelitis in children. *Orthop Rev* 1994;(May):305–312.

Fink CW, Nelson JD. Septic arthritis and osteomyelitis in children. *Clin Rheum Dis* 1986;12: 423.

Roy DR. Osteomyelitis. *Pediatr Rev* 1995;16(10): 380–384; 385 (quiz).

Author: Elizabeth Candell Chalom

Osteosarcoma

 Database

DEFINITION

Osteosarcoma is a tumor of the bone composed of spindle cells that produce malignant osteoid.

CAUSES

- The etiology is unknown.
- There is an association of osteosarcoma with prior radiation.
- Secondary osteosarcoma is seen in up to 5% of patients who received radiation therapy for an initial malignancy.
- Children with hereditary retinoblastoma are at increased risk of developing osteosarcoma with and without prior exposure to radiation.
- A small number of older patients with Paget disease develop osteosarcoma, but this rarely occurs in the pediatric population.

PATHOLOGY/PATHOPHYSIOLOGY

- Osteosarcoma most often involves the medullary region of bone.
- Two radiographic variants of osteosarcoma, periosteal and juxtacortical, do not involve the medullary cavity.
- Rarely, osteosarcoma occurs in soft tissue.
- Classic or conventional osteosarcoma, the largest group of osteosarcomas, is composed of connective tissue stroma containing highly malignant spindle-shaped cells as well as areas of osteoid production and calcification.
- Three common subtypes include osteoblastic, chondroblastic, and fibroblastic. Small-cell and telangiectatic variants also have been described. These variants are rare in the pediatric population, and only the conventional or classic variant is discussed in the remainder of this chapter.

EPIDEMIOLOGY

- Osteosarcoma is the most common malignant bone tumor of childhood, representing 60% of all bone tumors in the pediatric age group.
- Overall, it accounts for less than 1% of all malignant neoplasms.
- Peak incidence is in adolescence and early adulthood, with a median age of 18 at diagnosis. Osteosarcoma is felt to begin during the adolescent growth spurt.
- The most frequent site is the distal femur, followed by the proximal tibia and the proximal humerus.
- Approximately 90% of tumors will occur at the metaphyseal ends of long bones, but any portion of the skeleton may be involved.

COMPLICATIONS

Ten percent to 20% of patients have pulmonary metastases at the time of diagnosis; a smaller proportion have metastases to other bones.

PROGNOSIS

The majority of patients with osteosarcoma involving an extremity without pulmonary metastases can be cured. The following have been associated with a poorer prognosis:

- Pulmonary metastases
- Poor response of the tumor to preoperative chemotherapy
- Inability to achieve a total surgical excision of the tumor

 Differential Diagnosis

- Infection: osteomyelitis
- Tumors

—Benign: unicameral bone cyst, osteoblastoma, eosinophilic granuloma, giant-cell tumor, aneurysmal bone cyst, osteochondroma
—Malignant: Ewing sarcoma, chondrosarcoma, fibrosarcoma
—Metastatic lesions of other primary tumors

- Trauma: stress fracture

 Data Gathering

HISTORY

- Pain at the site of the tumor is the most common presentation.
- Swelling, without erythema, over the involved area is also seen on examination. The duration of symptoms varies.
- Weight loss is rare but may occur in advanced disease.
- A history of recent trauma is common, but unrelated. Trauma often brings the affected area to the patient's or parents' attention, but does not actually cause osteosarcoma.
- If fever is present, it may indicate osteomyelitis rather than osteosarcoma.

 Physical Examination

- A tender, soft-tissue mass and increased warmth may be present in the involved area.
- Regional lymphadenopathy is rare.

 Laboratory Aids

TESTS

Laboratory Tests

- Laboratory tests are not generally helpful in osteosarcoma. Serum lactate dehydrogenase (LDH) and alkaline phosphatase may be elevated.
- The prognostic significance of alkaline phosphatase is controversial.
- An elevated WBC or sedimentation rate may suggest osteomyelitis.

Imaging

- Radiographic examination should include the primary tumor site as well as areas of potential metastases, primarily the lungs and bones.
- A plain radiograph of the involved area always reveals some abnormality. Most commonly, one sees a lytic or blastic region of the bone with ill-defined borders. Other findings may include: periosteal elevation adjacent to the primary lesion; a sunburst appearance of the primary lesion caused by neoplastic spicules adjacent to the bony cortex; and a pathologic fracture.
- An MRI should be done to better evaluate the extent of the tumor. It should include the joint above and below the involved bony area. MRI can delineate the intra- and extraosseus extent of the tumor as well as evaluate the neurovascular structures involved.

Referral and Staging

- When a malignant bone tumor is suspected, the patient should be referred immediately to a pediatric tertiary care center. Any laboratory evaluation or radiographic study already performed should be sent with the patient.
- A staging work-up should include a bone scan to look for metastases or local skip lesions, as well as a chest x-ray or CT to detect macroscopic pulmonary metastases.
- The diagnosis of osteosarcoma can be confirmed only by a biopsy, which should be done by an experienced pediatric orthopedic surgeon in conjunction with a pediatric oncologist and pediatric pathologist.
- Certain surgical incisions at the time of biopsy may make patients ineligible for limb-sparing procedures.

Therapy

DRUGS

- At present, therapy incorporates preoperative chemotherapy followed by surgical resection.
- The goals of adjuvant chemotherapy are treatment of pulmonary micrometastases and shrinkage of the primary tumor mass, particularly when limb-salvage procedures are surgical options.
- The mainstays of treatment are cisplatin and doxorubicin, with many protocols also using high-dose methotrexate.
- Groups such as the Children's Cancer Group (CCG) and the Pediatric Oncology Group (POG) have developed chemotherapy protocols for osteosarcoma.

—The duration of chemotherapy varies according to the extent of the tumor at diagnosis, tumor response to therapy, and the individual protocol.

SURGERY

In the past, when osteosarcoma was managed by surgery alone, the majority of patients subsequently developed pulmonary metastases and died of progressive disease. Surgical options depend on the primary site of the tumor and the extent of tumor involvement. Complete surgical resection with wide margins is necessary for cure. Surgical options for osteosarcomas of the extremities include:

- Amputation
- Limb salvage with allograft or prosthetic reconstruction
- Rotationplasty

Macroscopic pulmonary metastases should be resected at the time of initial surgery if still visible by radiographic examination. Localized pulmonary recurrences that develop after treatment also should be resected, as this can result in long-term cure or a prolonged symptom-free period.

RADIATION

Osteosarcoma is a radiation-insensitive tumor, but radiation has been used in individual cases.

PHYSICAL THERAPY/REHABILITATION

All patients need to work with specialists to learn how to adapt to their surgically induced disability. The duration of physical therapy and rehabilitation is dependent on the disability and the individual patient's needs.

 Follow-Up

SIGNS TO WATCH FOR

- Wound infections may develop in surgical sites in the initial postoperative period. Significant pain, fever, swelling, discharge, and foul odor from the surgical site should be evaluated, preferably by the surgeon. Poor healing of the surgical site may be a problem, particularly in patients receiving chemotherapy or in those with poor nutrition. May require intravenous antibiotics, supplemental feeding or surgical revision of the wound.
- If prostheses are required, skin breakdown and fitting difficulties with prosthetic devices, such as adjustments for changes in height and weight, should be diagnosed and corrected. Scoliosis and back pain may develop in patients using improperly adjusted crutches and/or prosthetic devices after lower extremity or pelvic procedures. This requires expertise in prosthetic devices for children.
- "Phantom" pain is a normal phenomenon after amputation. Patients and their families should be reassured if this occurs. Sometimes medication can reduce the pain.

All children need to be followed by an oncologist regularly after treatment is completed to monitor for recurrence as well as long-term side effects of the chemotherapy, such as cardiac toxicity, infertility, or secondary malignancy.

 Common Questions and Answers

Q: Is there an increased risk of osteosarcoma in the contralateral limb?
A: No.

Q: Does limb salvage incur a greater risk of recurrence than does amputation?
A: Recent studies have shown that there is no increase in recurrence if wide margins are achieved at the time of surgery.

Q: How does one differentiate osteosarcoma from Ewing sarcoma, the second most common bone tumor of childhood?
A: Ultimately, only a biopsy can differentiate the two. In general, Ewing sarcoma is seen in younger children and tends to affect the axial bones, such as the pelvis. When found in the long bones, it is usually in the diaphyseal regions. Symptomatology does not differ, but Ewing sarcoma is metastaic to the bone marrow, as well as the lungs.

ICD-9-CM 170.9

BIBLIOGRAPHY

Himelstein BP, Dormans JP. Malignant bone tumors of childhood. *Pediatr Clin North Am* 1996;43(4):967–984.

Jaffe N. Osteosarcoma. *Pediatr Rev* 1991;12: 333–342.

Rougraff BT, Simon MA, Kneisl JS, Greenberg DB, Mankin HJ. Limb salvage compared with amputation for osteosarcoma of the distal end of the femur. A long-term oncologic, functional, and quality-of-life study. *J Bone Joint Surg* 1994;76(5):649–656.

Author: Susan R. Rheingold

Otitis Externa

 Database

DEFINITION

Otitis externa is inflammation of the external auditory canal. Patients with the following conditions are more at risk for otitis externa:

- Diabetes (primarily in elderly patients)
- Immunodeficiencies
- Dermatologic conditions (eczema, psoriasis)
- Foreign body
- Etiology

—Bacteria: *Pseudomonas aeruginosa, Staphylococcus aureus,* gram-negative enterics, group A streptococcus
—Viral: herpes simplex virus, varicella and herpes zoster
—Fungal: *Candida albicans, Aspergillus niger*

PATHOPHYSIOLOGY

- Disruption of the squamous epithelium of the auditory canal and alteration in the canal pH increase the susceptibility to microbial invasion, which results in inflammation.
- Excess moisture (e.g., from swimming, immersion during bathing), foreign bodies, and excessive cleaning disrupt the surface epithelium, allowing for microbial invasion.
- Cerumen is a protective substance in the ear canal, providing an acidic environment and lysozymes that provide an inhospitable environment to microbial invasion. Removal of cerumen and cleaning with soapy water disrupt the canal's acidic pH and remove antimicrobial enzymes.

EPIDEMIOLOGY

The highest incidence is during the summer months.

COMPLICATIONS

- Cellulitis of surrounding tissues
- Adenitis
- Malignant otitis externa: uncommon, seen in chronically ill or immunosuppressed children, including children with HIV; rapidly progressive severe disease that involves surrounding cartilage, bone, and nerves
- Stenosis of the auditory canal: seen with recurrent disease
- Transient conductive hearing loss

PROGNOSIS

- Excellent

 Differential Diagnosis

- Infection
—Furunculosis
—Localized abscess
—Otitis media
- Tumors
—Squamous-cell carcinoma
—Basal-cell carcinoma
—Metastatic cancer
- Trauma
—Retained foreign body

 Data Gathering

HISTORY

- Ask about predisposing risk factors.
- Symptoms may include itching, pain, a feeling of fullness, and hearing loss.
- Fever is usually absent unless there is associated cellulitis.

 Physical Examination

- Pain elicited with traction applied to pinna or tragus
- Canal erythematous, edematous
- Purulent discharge in canal
- Normal appearing tympanic membrane unless concomitant otitis media
- Procedure: Remove purulent debris from the canal with a cotton swab or gentle suction.

 Laboratory Aids

TESTS

- Obtain a bacterial culture and Gram stain in cases that do not respond to conventional topical therapy and elimination of risk factors. Also, culture immunocompromised patients.
- Fungal, viral culture in selected, refractory cases that do not respond to conventional treatment. Also, culture immunocompromised children.

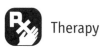 Therapy

ELIMINATION OF RISK FACTORS

• Remove foreign bodies.
• Discontinue aggravating factors, such as washing ears with water and insertion of cotton swabs.

DRUGS

• Analgesics (e.g., acetaminophen or ibuprofen) if needed
• Topical otic antibiotic/corticosteroid drops (polymixin B, neomycin, hydrocortisone) cover all major pathogens, including *Pseudomonas,* and provide some symptomatic relief via the antiinflammatory effect of the corticosteroid. Oloxacin 0.3% otic solution also covers major pathogens. It has not been approved for use in children under 1 year of age. Duration: 10 to 14 days of topical antibiotic therapy
• Acetic acid drops: useful with fungal infections and as prophylaxis in high-risk patients (e.g., swimmers)
• Antifungal drops: clotrimazole 1% solution for fungal infections
• Oral antibiotics (which cover *Streptococcus* and *Staphylococcus*) are indicated only if there is associated cellulitis, adenitis, or otitis media.
• Intravenous antibiotics are indicated for severe complications or malignant otitis externa.

 Follow-Up

Expect improvement of symptoms 24 to 48 hours after initiation of antibiotics.

SIGNS TO WATCH FOR

• Fever
• Severe local inflammation, especially in immunocompromised or chronically ill patients

PREVENTION

• Use water-impermeable ear plugs when swimming or doing other water sports.
• Blow-dry ears with the cool setting of a hair dryer.
• Use 2% acetic acid drops (or 70% ethyl alcohol) after swimming or immersion of ears; this helps to restore the acidic pH of the ear canal, decreasing the susceptibility to microbial invasion.

PITFALLS

Severe swelling may prohibit entry of antibiotic drops; placing a cotton wick in the ear for 24 hours may facilitate subsequent entry of drops into the canal.

 Common Questions and Answers

Q: For how long should one avoid swimming if diagnosed with otitis externa?
A: Until resolution of infection; then use acetic acid drops as prophylaxis.

Q: What should one consider in refractory cases of otitis externa?
A: Reevaluate for risk factors, carefully inspect the canal for a retained foreign body, and culture for routine bacterial as well as fungal pathogens.

Q: When should one refer to an otolaryngologist?
A: Refer for severe cases, when there is poor response to routine therapy, or in immunocompromised patients at risk for malignant otitis externa.

ICD-9-CM 380.10

BIBLIOGRAPHY

Bojrab D, Bruderly T, Abdulrazzak Y. Diseases of the external auditory canal: otitis externa. *Otolaryngol Clin* 1996;29(5):761–782.

Cantor R. Otitis externa and otitis media. *Emerg Med Clin* 1995;13(2):445–455.

Feigin R. Otitis externa. In: Feigin R, Cherry J, eds. *Textbook of pediatric infectious diseases*. Philadelphia: WB Saunders, 1992:172–174.

Author: Lisa M. Biggs

Otitis Media

 Database

DEFINITION

Acute otitis media (AOM) is sudden onset of infection of the middle ear. Secretory otitis media (or serous otitis media or otitis media with effusion) is persistent fluid accumulation in the middle ear without evidence of acute infection. Children with the following problems are at risk for otitis media:

- Down syndrome
- Cleft palate
- Craniofacial abnormalities
- Adenoid hypertrophy
- Oropharyngeal tumors
- Allergic rhinitis/congestion
- Immunodeficiencies
- Impaired ciliary function
- Trauma
- Upper respiratory tract infection

ETIOLOGY

- Bacterial

—*Streptococcus pneumoniae*, 30%
—*Haemophilus influenzae*, 20%
—*Moraxella catarrhalis*, 7%
—Group A streptococcus, 2%
—Enteric gram-negatives, 1%
—*Staphylococcus aureus*, 1%
—*Mycoplasma pneumoniae*

- Viral: RSV, influenza
- Fungal: rare
- Environmental: Passive smoke and "bottle propping" (bottle feeding with child in a supine position) increase risk.
- Anatomic: The normal horizontal position of the eustachian tube in infants and young children increases risk.

PATHOPHYSIOLOGY

Predilection for eustachian tube dysfunction results in fluid accumulation in the middle ear, which may be followed by proliferation of microorganisms. Infection with a microorganism results in inflammation of the mucoperiosteum.

GENETICS

- High prevalence in Eskimos and Native Americans
- May be familial predisposition

EPIDEMIOLOGY

- Highest incidence in children 6 months to 3 years
- Higher incidence in boys, Native Americans, Eskimos
- Highest incidence in winter months
- Lower incidence in breast-fed infants
- Higher incidence in children in day care
- Higher incidence in children living with smokers
- Higher incidence in children using pacifiers

COMPLICATIONS

- Perforation of tympanic membrane
- Hearing loss
- Mastoiditis
- Meningitis
- Epidural abscess
- Cholesteatoma
- Facial nerve paralysis
- Language delay
- Labyrinthitis
- Lateral sinus thrombosis
- Otitic hydrocephalus: hydrocephalus associated with decreased venous drainage secondary to venous sinus thrombosis

PROGNOSIS

- Fifty percent with middle ear effusion (MEE) at 1 month
- Ten percent with middle ear effusion (MEE) at 3 months
- Risk of recurrent otitis media higher if first episode at an early age (<12 months)

 Differential Diagnosis

- Infection

—Otitis externa: may mimic otitis media with perforated tympanic membrane (TM)

- Tumors

—Cholesteatoma

- Trauma

—Retained foreign body
—Hemotympanum: Blood behind TM may appear blue or red; look for associated signs of basilar skull fracture; traumatic perforation.

 Data Gathering

HISTORY

- Acute otitis media: Classic symptoms include acute onset, otalgia, fever, and hearing loss; nonspecific symptoms include irritability, vomiting, diarrhea, restless sleep, and "tugging" at ears.
- Serous otitis media: may be asymptomatic; nonspecific symptoms of feeling of "fullness," hearing loss

 Physical Examination

- Acute otitis media

—Pneumatic otoscopy: dull, opaque, hyperemic TM; landmarks distorted or absent; membrane may bulge; TM mobility decreased

- Serous otitis media

—Pneumatic otoscopy: TM may be dull and/or retracted; mobility is decreased; fluid level or air bubbles behind TM may be visible. Minimal erythema is present.

Special Questions

- Risk factors, previous episodes, and response to previous therapy

PROCEDURE

- Adequately restrain the child.
- Clear the canal of cerumen with curettes or irrigation.
- Ensure an adequate seal of the ear speculum in order to perform pneumatic otoscopy.
- Crying infants may have hyperemic TMs that are often confused with acute infection.

 Laboratory Aids

TESTS

- Tympanocentesis for bacterial culture and sensitivity. Indications:

—Seriously ill/toxic appearing
—Failure of antimicrobial therapy
—Patients at risk for unusual organisms: neonates, immunocompromised patients, communities with penicillin-resistant *S. pneumoniae*
—Complications (e.g., mastoiditis, facial nerve palsy)

- Tympanometry: measures middle ear pressures and TM compliance; helpful with assessment of middle ear effusion, tympanic membrane perforation, eustachian tube dysfunction, and patency of tympanostomy tubes

 Therapy

DRUGS

- Antibiotics: Duration is generally 10 to 14 days.
- Amoxicillin: first-choice antibiotic; covers most common pathogens; does not cover β-lactamase–producing organisms
- Trimethoprim/sulfamethoxazole: better coverage for β-lactamase–producing organisms
- Erythromycin/sulfisoxazole: coverage similar to that of trimethoprim/sulfamethoxazole

- Amoxicillin/clavulanate: good coverage for β-lactamase–producing bacteria; new formulation available with less diarrhea as a side effect
- Cefaclor: covers most common pathogens; serum sickness reactions reported more frequently in children than in adults
- Newer cephalosporins:

—Cefixime: once a day dosage, not ideal first-choice drug because of lower *S. pneumoniae* coverage
—Cefprozil: bid dosage
—Cefpodoxime: bid dosage
—Cefuroxime axetil: bid dosage
—Ceftibuten, cefdinir, and loracarbef

- Newer macrolides:

—Clarithromycin: bid dosing. Concurrent use with cisipride, pimozide, or terfenadine is contraindicated.
—Azithromycin: daily dosage for 5 days (days 2–5: twice the dosage of day 1). Although there are no reports of significant interactions with theophylline, terfenadine, and so on, caution is advised based on experience with other macrolides.

 Follow-Up

Expect improvement within 48 to 72 hours of treatment.

SIGNS TO WATCH FOR

- Persistent fever, pain after 3 to 5 days of therapy
- Symptoms of complications
- Seriously ill appearing

PREVENTION

- Breast feeding
- Avoidance of passive smoke
- Avoidance of pacifier use
- Avoidance of "bottle-propping" (bottle feeding with child in a supine position)
- Antibiotic prophylaxis in children meeting strict criteria for recurrent AOM

—Indicated for recurrent otitis media: three episodes in 6 months, four episodes in 12 months with one in preceding 6 months
—Drugs: Use at one-half treatment dose, and continue through the "respiratory season" (generally winter and spring) for a maximum of 6 months of therapy; amoxicillin and sulfisoxazole are the only antibiotics approved for this use.

 Common Questions and Answers

Q: Are antihistamine/decongestants recommended in the treatment of otitis media?
A: No. Antihistamine/decongestants have not been shown to be effective in the treatment of otitis media and are not recommended.

Q: Are steroids recommended in the treatment of otitis media?
A: Several studies show no difference between treatment groups and placebo groups. Steroids are generally not recommended in the treatment of AOM or serous otitis media.

Q: Are shorter courses of therapy indicated in the treatment of AOM instead of the traditional 10-day therapy?
A: There is little data supporting the traditional 10-day therapy. Recent studies indicate that shorter courses of 5 to 7 days are effective in selected patients. Until further data emerge, this practice should be restricted to children older than 2 years of age with mild AOM who are well appearing, have no underlying chronic medical conditions, have no history of recurrent AOM and on physical examination have no TM perforation.

Q: There is a lot of discussion about the emergence of antibiotic-resistant organisms. How should this affect my management of AOM?
A: The first goal of management should be the judicious use of antibiotics to prevent emergence of resistant organisms. You should educate families about the appropriate use of antibiotics. Discuss completing the course as prescribed and not sharing antibiotics with other children. Antibiotics should be reserved for use in children with documented AOM (via pneumatic otoscopy). Prophylactic antibiotic use should be restricted to children meeting the criteria for recurrent AOM and should be limited to a 6-month duration. Only amoxicillin and sulfisoxazole are approved for this use. You should generally choose amoxicillin as your first-choice antibiotic (except in cases of allergy or suspected resistant *S. pneumoniae*), because it will give adequate coverage in the majority of cases of AOM.

Q: Should I treat serous otitis media (otitis media with effusion)?
A: Clinical practice guidelines, recently published by the Agency for Health Care Policy and Research (endorsed by the American Academy of Pediatrics, the American Academy of Family Physicians, and the American Academy of Otolaryngology–Head and Neck Surgery) recommend the following:

- Middle ear effusions with no evidence of acute infection or signs of systemic infection in the previous 3 months are expected in children after a documented episode of AOM, and do not require antibiotic therapy.
- Antimicrobial therapy is indicated in children with bilateral effusions with hearing loss, effusions that persist for 3 or more months, or if new localized or systemic symptoms appear with a previously asymptomatic effusion.

ICD-9-CM 382.9

BIBLIOGRAPHY

Adderson E. Preventing otitis media: medical approaches. *Pediatr Ann* 1998;27(2):101–107.

Bluestone C. Management of otitis media in infants and children: current role of old and new antimicrobial agents. *Pediatr Infect Dis J* 1998;7:S129–S136.

Bluestone C, Stephenson J, Martin L. Ten-year review of otitis media pathogens. *Pediatr Infect Dis J* 1992;11[Suppl]:S7–S11.

Dowell S, Marcy M, Phillips W, Gerber M, Schwartz B. Otitis media–principles of judicious use of antimicrobial agents. *Pediatrics* 1998;101[Suppl 1]:165–171.

Giebink G. Progress in understanding pathophysiology of otitis media. *Pediatr Rev* 1989;11(5):133–137.

Goycoolea M, ed. Otitis media. *Otolaryngol Clin North Am* 1991;24:4.

Isaacson, G. The natural history of a treated episode of acute otitis media. *Pediatrics* 1996;98(5):968–971.

Klein J. Protecting the therapeutic advantage of antimicrobial agents used for otitis media. *Pediatr Infect Dis J* 1998;17(6):571–575.

McCracken G. Treatment of acute otitis media in an era of increasing microbial resistance. *Pediatr Infect Dis J* 1998;17(6):576–579.

Author: Lisa M. Biggs

Pancreatic Pseudocyst

 Database

DEFINITION

Pancreatic pseudocysts are cystic structures, which result as an exudative reaction to inflammation and do not communicate with the pancreatic ductular system. Pancreatic cysts come in many forms, which include:

- True cysts
- Pancreatic pseudocysts
- Pseudo-pseudocysts
- Pancreatic sequestra
- Primary cystic neoplasms
- Parasitic cysts

PATHOPHYSIOLOGY

- Pancreatic pseudocysts develop when the pancreatic ductular system has been disrupted resulting in the extravasation of pancreatic exocrine secretions including proenzymes and active enzymes such as amylase, lipase, and ribonucleases.
- These enzymes stimulate an inflammatory reaction, which ultimately leads to the formation of a fibrous capsule, which does not have a true epithelial lining.
- If these cysts remain in communication with the pancreatic ductular system, enzyme and proenzyme levels remain elevated and the cyst will persist.
- A capsule, if present, is not lined by epithelium.
- These cysts usually develop earlier in the course of acute pancreatitis and lack a fully formed fibrous capsule.
- Because there is no ductular communication, the cysts do not have persistently elevated enzyme and proenzyme concentrations.

EPIDEMIOLOGY

- Approximately 30% to 50% of patients with severe pancreatitis will develop pseudocysts.
- Pseudocysts are the most common form of pancreatic cyst, accounting for 75% of the pancreatic cystic lesions.
- In children, 60% of pseudocysts form as a result of blunt abdominal trauma.
- The second most common etiology is acute pancreatitis. The cyst fluid contains plasma concentration of electrolytes and high concentration of pancreatic enzymes. The cyst forms over a period of several weeks after ductal disruption.
- Approximately 5% to 15% of patients with acute pancreatitis will progress to developing a pseudocyst.

PROGNOSIS

The natural history of these cysts is to ultimately resolve over time.

 Differential Diagnosis

- Congenital

—Congenital cysts
—Simple cysts
—Polycystic disease
—Polycystic kidney disease
—von Hippel-Lindau

- Infections

—Parasitic
—Echinococcal (hydatid) cyst
—Taenia solium cyst

- Toxic
- Trauma
- Tumor

—Serous cystadenoma
—Cystadenocarcinoma
—Mucinous cystadenoma
—Cystic islet cell tumors
—Cystic teratoma
—Angiomatous cystic neoplasms

- Angiomas

—Lymphangiomas
—Hemangioendotheliomas

- Genetic/metabolic

—Cystic fibrosis

- Inflammatory

—Post-inflammatory cystic fluid collections
—Pancreatic sequestrum

- Miscellaneous

—Pancreatic polycystic disease
—Enterogenous cyst
—Endometriosis
—Extrapancreatic cysts
—Paraduodenal duplication cysts
—Splenic cyst
—Adrenal cyst

 Data Gathering

HISTORY

Question: When does one suspect pancreatic pseudocyst?
Significance: Pancreatic pseudocyst formation should be suspected in patients recovering from acute pancreatitis who develop recurrence or persistence of abdominal pain (a presenting symptom in 90% of pseudocyst cases).

Question: What is the patient presenting with?
Significance:

- Nausea and vomiting (70%)
- Weight loss (35%)
- Jaundice (10–15%)
- Palpable abdominal mass
- Persistently elevated amylase

Question: Other presenting complaints?
Significance:

- Sepsis from cyst infection
- Splenic or portal vein obstruction leading to esophageal varices and upper gastrointestinal tract bleeding.
- Intra-abdominal hemorrhage from pseudoaneurysms in adjacent vessels.
- Lower extremity edema from compression of the inferior vena cava.

Laboratory Aids

- Laboratory evaluations are non-specific in defining the presence of a pancreatic pseudocyst.
- Many patients will have an elevated serum amylase.
- Radiographic studies
- Computer tomography is considered to be the best means of visualizing pseudocysts because it permits a more accurate visualization of the entire pancreas in addition to providing vital information on other intra-abdominal structures and a more sensitive means of following the natural history of the pseudocyst.
- Ultrasonography will visualize pancreatic pseudocysts; however, this test is more useful in following patients for changes in cyst size.
- Endoscopic retrograde cholangiopancreatography (ERCP): Though controversial, may be important in decision making concerning additional intervention. ERCP may define whether the pseudocyst is in communication with the pancreatic ductular system which, if present, many consider is an indication for an internal drainage procedure. ERCP may also detect other abnormalities of the pancreatic duct or intrapancreatic common bile duct, which will effect the type or extent of procedure performed. ERCP may be performed safely if done within 24 hours of the definitive procedure and with broad spectrum antibiotic coverage.

Therapy

- Prior to the development of current radiological procedures, surgical treatment was recommended for clinically detected pseudocysts and a high rate of serious complications was reported. Recently, series from both Johns Hopkins and the Mayo Clinic have revealed that in patients with asymptomatic pseudocysts approximately one-half may be managed safely without any intervention (approximately 60% having complete resolution by 1 year). Factors that must be taken into account when managing patients with pseudocysts include the presence of symptoms, age and size of the pseudocyst, and presence of complications.
- In patients with acute asymptomatic pseudocysts, most surgeons recommend a 4- to 6-week period of observation to permit maturation of the pseudocyst.
- If the pseudocyst remains less than approximately 6 cm, continued observation is justified.

- If the pseudocyst is greater than 6 cm in size and increasing, an internal drainage procedure is indicated. For those patients who develop complications while being observed, an external drainage procedure should be considered. In patients with chronic pseudocysts greater than 6 cm, internal drainage or excision should be considered.
- Non-operative treatment options include:

—Percutaneous cyst aspiration (which has an overall success rate of approximately 44%)
—Percutaneous catheter drainage (which has an overall success rate of approximately 81%).

- Endoscopic treatment options include endoscopic transmural cystenterostomy and, in those patients where the pseudocyst communicates with the pancreatic duct, transpapillary stent placement. These endoscopic procedures carry the risk of bleeding (especially in patients with pseudoaneurysm formation), retroperitoneal perforation, and infection. To date, there is minimal experience with these techniques in children.

Surgical options include:

- Internal drainage

—Recurrence rate of 5%
—Mortality of less than 5%
—Cystojejunostomy
—Cystogastrostomy
—Cystoduodenostomy (usually small cysts in the head of the pancreas)

- External drainage

—Recurrence rate of 22%
—Mortality rate of 6%
—Preferred when the cyst is infected or has an immature fibrous capsule
—Development of a persistent pancreatic fistula may occur in approximately 10%

- Excision

Complications:

- Infection (incidence reported between 1–20% in the literature)

—Infected pseudocysts require immediate, surgical external drainage
—Incidence of approximately 1% to 10% in acute pancreatitis
—Mortality of 80%

- Arterial hemorrhage (incidence of approximately 7%)
- Obstruction (esophagus, stomach, duodenum, jejunum, colon, portal venous system, vena cava, urinary system, biliary tree)
- Rupture (least common, <3%)

Common Questions and Answers

Q: What is the most common cause of pancreatic pseudocyst?
A: Trauma leading to pancreatitis and the subsequent development is the most common.

Q: Which therapy has the lowest incidence of recurrence?
A: Surgical drainage and excision.

ICD-9-CM 577.2

BIBLIOGRAPHY

Grace PA, Williamson RC. Modern Management of pancreatic pseudocysts. *Br J Surg* 1993; 80(5):573–581.

Guelrud M. Endoscopic therapy of pancreatic disease in children. *Gastrointest Endosc Clin N Am* 1998;8(1):195–219.

Howell DA, Elton E, Parsons WG. Endoscopic management of pseudocysts or the pancreas. *Gastrointest Endosc Clin N Am* 1998;8(1): 143–162.

Wyllie R, Hyams J. Pediatric gastrointestinal disease: pathophysiology, diagnosis, management. Philadelphia: WB Saunders Co., 1993.

Yeo CJ, Sarr MG. Cystic and pseudocystic diseases of the pancreas. *Curr Probl Surg* 1994; 31(3):165–243.

Author: Donna Zeiter

Pancreatitis

Database

DEFINITION

Pancreatitis, which is an inflammation of the pancreas, covers a wide spectrum of inflammatory conditions of the pancreas, ranging from severe to mild and even subclinical forms. In addition, pancreatitis may be acute (where pancreatic function and morphology are restored) or chronic (where there is irreversible pancreatic insufficiency). The clinical spectrum includes abdominal pain that is aggravated by eating, nausea, and vomiting.

CAUSES

• In acute pancreatitis the most common etiological factors are trauma, multisystem disease, and drugs.
• In 25% of cases of acute pancreatitis, no cause is identified.

PATHOPHYSIOLOGY

Chronic pancreatitis is characterized by progressive and irreversible destruction of the pancreas and leads to exocrine and endocrine pancreatic insufficiency. Chronic pancreatitis leading to strictures, dilatations of the ducts, sclerosis, and destruction of pancreatic acini.

COMPLICATIONS

• The complications of pancreatitis may be divided into local and systemic complications.
• They are associated with significant risk for morbidity and mortality.

LOCAL COMPLICATIONS

• Pancreatic phlegmon/abscess/pseudocyst/hemorrhagic pancreatitis
• Pancreatic ascites

SYSTEMIC COMPLICATIONS

• Pulmonary
• Atelectasis
• Pleural effusion
• Pneumonitis
• ARDS
• Cardiovascular
• Hypotension
• Pericardial effusion
• Myocardial infarction
• Sudden death
• Circulatory
• Hematological
• Hemoconcentration
• Disseminated intravascular coagulation
• Gastrointestinal
• Paralytic ileus
• Gastritis
• Ulcer
• Upper gastrointestinal bleeding
• Portal vein thrombosis/splenic vein thrombosis/obstruction
• Renal
• Oliguria
• Azotemia
• Neurological
• Psychosis
• Stupor
• Coma
• Metabolical
• Hyperglycemia
• Hypertriglyceridemia
• Hypocalcemia

Differential Diagnosis

CAUSES

Mechanical/Structural

• Bile reflux
• Outflow obstruction (congenital or acquired, commonly gallstones)
• Trauma (abdominal/child abuse)

Multisystem Disease

• Infection/Sepsis

—Bacterial/Mycoplasma
—Viral (measles, mumps, Epstein-Barr virus, coxsackie B, rubella, influenza, echovirus, hepatitis A and B)
—Parasites (*Ascaris lumbricoides, Echinococcus granulosus, Cryptosporidium parvum, Plasmodium falciparum*)

• Shock/hypoxemia
• Hemolytic uremic syndrome
• Crohn disease
• Alagille syndrome
• Kawasaki disease
• Metabolic

—Hyperlipidemia
—Hypercalcemia
—Uremia
—α_1-Antitrypsin deficiency
—Organic acidemias

• Cystic fibrosis
• Malnutrition/refeeding/bulimia
• Diabetes mellitus
• Mitochondropathy
• Hemochromatosis
• Vasculitis

—Systemic lupus erythematosus
—Henoch-Schönlein purpura
—Kawasaki disease

• Drug

—*l*-asparaginase, azathioprine, sulfonamides, thiazides, furosemide, tetracyclines, valproic acids, estrogens, procainamide, ethacrynic acid

• Pancreatic and biliary disorders

—Cystic fibrosis
—Pancreatic divisum
—Anomalies of the pancreatic duct
—Cholelithiasis
—Choledochal cyst
—Post-endoscopic retrograde cholangiopancreatography (ERCP)

• Toxins

—Alcohol
—Organophosphates
—Yellow scorpion sting

• Unknown

—Hereditary: Recently described genetic mutation on chromosome 7, leading to recurrent acute pancreatitis and cell death. Described in family cohorts and associated with increased risk of development of insulin-dpendent diabetes mellitus and pancreatic cancer.
—Idiopathic

PROGNOSIS

• Ranson's criteria can help to assess the severity of the disease. The prognosis in the pediatric age group is good with a low mortality rate even in severe cases.
• Acute pancreatitis rarely progresses to chronic pancreatitis.
• In pediatric populations, the most common etiologies of chronic pancreatitis are hereditary pancreatitis and obstructive pancreatitis secondary to structural anomalies.
• History reveals that repeat episodes of acute pancreatitis, which may also be asymptomatic, may lead to destruction of the pancreas and diminished pancreatic function.
• Pain may exist but is not essential for diagnosis; however, most patients with chronic pancreatitis complain of chronic severe abdominal pain.
• Physical examination is remarkable for weight loss and wasting.
• Laboratory tests may indicate fat and protein malabsorption when the exocrine pancreatic capacity has decreased to approximately 10%.
• Insulin-dependent diabetes mellitus may accompany the diseases, in some cases.

Data Gathering

HISTORY

Question: Abdominal pain?
Significance: In the acute presentation, patients may present with abdominal pain radiating to the back and associated with nausea and vomiting.

Question: Febrile?
Significance: If the patient is febrile, the temperature is usually below 38.5°C. Higher temperatures are suggestive of infection. Special attention should be made to a previous history of episodes of abdominal pain.

Question:
Significance: Review of systems is important to exclude other underlying etiologies.

Question: History of abdominal trauma?
Significance: Evaluate for history of abdominal trauma and consider the possibility of child abuse.

Physical Examination

Finding: Evaluate for epigastric tenderness, decreased bowel sounds, abdominal distension, tachycardia, hypotension, hypoxemia and shock in severe cases.
Significance: Complications of pancreatitis.

Finding: Abdominal tenderness, paralytic ileus, ascites, bluish discoloration of the flanks (Grey-Turner sign) or around the umbilicus (Cullen sign).
Significance: Indicate severe necrotizing pancreatitis.

Finding: Auscultation of lungs.
Significance: Other signs include pleural effusion and adult respiratory distress syndrome (ARDS).

Finding: Palpable pancreatic mass
Significance: Suggestive of a pancreatic pseudocyst.

Laboratory Aids

• Evaluate for elevated white blood cell count (with left shift).

Test: CBC
Significance: Hemoconcentration or decreased hemoglobin in hemorrhagic pancreatitis

Test: Glucose
Significance: Transient hyperglycemia

Test: Calcium
Significance: Hypocalcemia (in 15% of patients)

Test: Liver function tests
Significance: Increased liver enzymes and bilirubin

Test: Amylase level
Significance: An elevated serum amylase is most commonly suggestive of pancreatitis; however, increased serum amylase may be associated with other etiologies. The amylase level has low sensitivity and specificity. Measuring the fractionated pancreatic amylase may help to differentiate the etiology of the elevated amylase.

CAUSES OF ELEVATED SERUM AMYLASE

• Pancreatitis
• Pancreatic tumors
• Pancreatic duct obstruction
• Pseudocyst
• Perforated ulcer
• Bowel obstruction/infarction
• ERCP–post-procedure
• Salivary/Others
• Infection (mumps)
• Trauma
• Salivary duct obstruction

• Lung carcinoma
• Ovarian tumor/cysts
• Prostate tumors
• Diabetic ketoacidosis
• Mixed (unknown)
• Cystic fibrosis
• Renal insufficiency
• Pregnancy
• Cerebral trauma
• Burns
• Macroamylasemia

IMAGING

Test: Abdominal radiographs
Significance: May identify ileus, sentinel loop, and colonic dilatation.

Test: Abdominal ultrasound
Significance: Most commonly used and can measure pancreatic size, contour, and echotexture. The measures of these parameters are not accurate and overlap with normals.

Test: Computed tomography (CT)
Significance: Procedure of choice for evaluating complications of pancreatitis such as pseudocyst and hemorrhagic pancreatitis. CT can also be helpful in providing anatomical information prior to surgery.

• Ranson's criteria are used to define the severity of pancreatitis, risk of systemic complication, and prediction of mortality. These criteria include:

—Age
—White blood cell count on presentation
—Elevated blood glucose
—Elevation of lactate dehydrogenase
—Elevated AST
—Decreased hemoglobin (hemorrhagic pancreatitis)
—Increased BUN
—Hypocalcemia
—Hypoglycemia
—Acidosis
—Hydration status

Therapy

Supportive care in an intensive care unit and anticipating complications before they occur are the major cornerstones of treatment. Management includes:

• NPO
• Placement of nasogastric tube
• Hyperalimentation (use intralipids only if triglycerides are normal)
• Antibiotic if infection suspected
• Oxygen as needed
• Pain control
• Measurement of vital signs
• Urine output and specific gravity
• Frequent labs

• Intravenous fluids (consider third spacing of intravascular fluids)
• Intravenous colloid and blood products as needed
• Treatment of disseminated intravascular coagulation
• Intravenous H_2 blockade to prevent additional gastrointestinal complications

DURATION

• Dictated by the severity of the pancreatitis and clinical improvement of the patient

Common Questions and Answers

Q: What new genetic tests are available for detecting causes of pancreatitis?
A: There have been two recently more exciting tests for detection of genetic causes of pancreatitis: cystic fibrosis gene testing and hereditary pancreatitis testing. These are available as special request testing.

Q: What is hereditary pancreatitis?
A: This has been described specifically in families with a strong history of pancreatic cancer, diabetes mellitus and recurrent pancreatitis. It is a rare diagnosis but must be considered in the right circumstances.

Q: My child has asthma, recurrent sinusitis and has chronic abdominal pain. Can she have cystic fibrosis?
A: Yes, this is definitely a concern that should be excluded by appropriate genetic and sweat testing.

ICD-9-CM 577.0

BIBLIOGRAPHY

Hirohashi S, Hirohashi R, Uchida H, et al. Pancreatitis: evaluation with MR cholangiopancreatography in children. *Radiology* 1997; 203(2):411–415.

Greenfeld JI, Harmon CM. Acute pancreatitis. *Curr Opin Pediatr* 1997;9(3):260–264.

Mader T, McHugh T. Acute pancreatitis in children. *Pediatr Emerg Care* 1992;8(3):157.

Piccoli D. Chronic pancreatitis. In: Wyllie R, Hyams JS, eds. Pediatric gastrointestinal diseases. Philadelphia: WB Saunders, 1993:880.

Tagge EP, Tarnasky PR, Chandler J, et al. Multidisciplinary approach to the treatment of pediatric pancreaticobiliary disorders. *Surgery* 1997;32(2):158–165.

Weitzman Z. Acute pancreatitis. In: Wyllie R, Hyams JS, eds. Pediatric gastrointestinal diseases. Philadelphia: WB Saunders, 1993:873.

Author: Dror Wasserman and Andrew E. Mulberg

Panhypopituitarism

Database

DEFINITION
- Deficiency of multiple pituitary hormones

CAUSES
- Idiopathic
- Congenital

—Absence of the pituitary (empty sella syndrome)
—Familial panhypopituitarism

- Acquired

—Birth trauma or perinatal insult
—Surgical resection of the gland or damage to the stalk
—Child abuse

- Infection

—Viral encephalitis
—Bacterial or fungal infection
—Tuberculosis

- Vascular

—Pituitary infarction
—Pituitary aneurysm

- Cranial irradiation
- Chemotherapy
- Tumors

—Craniopharyngioma
—Glioma
—Pinealoma
—Primitive neuroectodermal tumor (medulloblastoma)
—Histiocytosis

- Sarcoidosis

PATHOPHYSIOLOGY
Pathology is based on specific deficiency:
- Growth hormone: hypoglycemia in newborns and poor growth in other patients
- ACTH: hypocortisolism
- TSH: hypothyroidism
- LH/FSH: hypogonadism
- ADH: diabetes insipidus

GENETICS
There are rare cases of autosomal recessive, autosomal dominant, and X-linked forms.

EPIDEMIOLOGY
- Congenital forms affect both sexes equally and are diagnosed at a young age.
- The incidence of secondary forms depends on the underlying cause.

COMPLICATIONS
- Hypoglycemia in the newborn period
- Short stature
- Adrenal crisis
- Dehydration

PROGNOSIS
- Prognosis for congenital forms is excellent.
- Prognosis for secondary forms depends on the primary disease.

Differential Diagnosis

- Hyperinsulinism in newborns
- Isolated growth hormone deficiency in newborns

Data Gathering

HISTORY
Question: Birth history?
Significance: Hyperinsulinemic infants are typically large for gestational age which can be associated with shoulder dystocia; hypopituitary babies are not large.

Question: Complications during pregnancy or delivery?
Significance: Birth trauma may be associated with pituitary injury. Breech delivery or vacuum extraction have been associated.

Question: Birth weight?
Significance: Hypopituitary infants are usually normal or small for gestational age in contrast to hyperinsulinemic infants who are typically large.

Question: History of hypoglycemia during the neonatal period?
Significance: Ask about symptoms of lethargy, poor feeding, irritability, or seizures which could suggest hypoglycemia.

Question: History of surgeries and previous diseases?
Significance: Congenital hypopituitarism is often associated with midline facial defects (such as bifid uvula or cleft palate) which require repair.

Question: Growth pattern?
Significance: Plot previous heights and look for growth pattern. GH deficiency usually manifests as poor linear growth by the end of the first year of life.

Special Questions

Question: Any complaints of headache?
Significance: Headache can be a symptom of a brain tumor.

Question: Any neurological signs or symptoms?
Significance: Focal neurologic symptoms are highly suggestive of CNS pathology.

Physical Examination

Finding: Actual height and weight
Significance: Patients with panhypopituitarism have normal size in the newborn period. Patients with hyperinsulinism are typically large for gestational age.

Finding: Prolonged indirect hyperbilirubinemia
Significance: May be first sign of hypothyroidism.

Finding: Micropenis in males
Significance: Neonatal penis should be at least 2.5 cm in length; micropenis suggests gonadotropic deficiency.

PHYSICAL EXAMINATION TRICKS
Finding: Penile and testicular size
Significance: Measure stretched phallic length (from pubic ramus to glans) with patient lying supine and phallus at 90° to the body; use Prader beads to assess testicular volume.

Finding: Midline defects
Significance: Palpate for submucosal cleft palate.

Finding: Visual field testing
Significance: Visual field defects suggest a brain tumor.

ASSOCIATIONS
- Midline defects (e.g., cleft lip/palate, hypotelorism, single central maxillary incisor)
- Septo-optic dysplasia (de Morsier syndrome)
- Holoprosencephaly

Laboratory Aids

SPECIFIC TESTS
Test: Liver function tests
Significance: Typically elevated liver enzymes in the newborn period.

Test: Thyroid function tests including free thyroxine
Significance: Total T_4 and TSH may be normal, but free T_4 will be low.

Test: TRH stimulation test
Significance: Delayed, normal, or exaggerated TSH response suggests hypothalamic lesion.

Test: Serum IGF-I and IGFBP-3
Significance: May be low but normal growth factors do *not* exclude GH deficiency in children with brain tumors.

Test: Free thyroxine by equilibrium dialysis
Significance: Must measure, not calculate, the free T_4.

Test: Growth hormone stimulation tests
Significance: Should be performed by a pediatric endocrinologist.

Test: Cortrosyn stimulation test
Significance: More helpful in the diagnosis of primary adrenal insufficiency than secondary (ATCH) or tertiary (CRH) deficiency.

Test: Metyrapone or CRH stimulation test
Significance: The definitive tests for ACTH or CRH deficiency but must be performed by a pediatric endocrinologist.

Test: Water deprivation test
Significance: The definitive test for ADH deficiency but must be performed by a pediatric endocrinologist.

IMAGING

Test: Bone age
Significance: Typically delayed in GH deficiency or hypothyroidism.

Test: MRI of head
Significance: Look for tumors and presence of normal "bright spot" in posterior pituitary.

HOME TESTING

Test: Measurement of water intake and urine output
Significance: Can help diagnosis diabetes insipidus.

Test: Baseline serum tests
Significance: Can all be done in a non-fasting state.

Test: Stimulation tests
Significance: Need to be performed by a pediatric endocrinologist.

 Therapy

DRUGS

• Recombinant human growth hormone (rhGH) by subcutaneous injection daily: 0.35 mg/kg/wk
• Levo-thyroxine orally: 25 to 150 μg daily, based on weight, age, and free thyroxine levels
• Hydrocortisone

—At replacement doses if needed: 8 to 15 mg/m²/d orally, divided q8h (or three times daily)
—At stress doses for surgery, major illness, vomiting, etc.: 50 to 100 mg/m²/d IV or PO
—Intravenous doses should be divided q4h; oral stress doses should be divided q8h
—To calculate hydrocortisone dose, estimate body surface area (BSA) using a nomogram or the following formula:

$$BSA\ (m^2) = \sqrt{\frac{height(cm) \cdot weight(kg)}{3600}}$$

• DDAVP: available in oral and intranasal formulations

DURATION

• Long-term therapy: performed by a pediatric endocrinologist
• Recombinant human growth hormone (rhGH)

—In children and adolescents:
  —Until growth velocity drops to 0.5 cm/year
  —Once puberty is complete
—In adulthood:
  —GH-deficient adults may benefit from life-long rhGH therapy due to the impact of GH on body composition and glucose metabolism
  —Patient should again undergo GH provocative testing (off rhGH therapy, of course)
• Levo-thyroxine: for life
• Hydrocortisone
—Replacement dose based on individual's need
—Stress dose for life
• DDAVP: for life

DIET

• There are no restrictions; it is important to know if patient has intact thirst mechanism.

POSSIBLE CONFLICTS WITH OTHER TREATMENTS

There is a theoretical risk that growth hormone might stimulate tumor growth due to its mitogenic effect.

 Follow-Up

• Initially, every 3 months by a pediatric endocrinologist

WHEN TO EXPECT IMPROVEMENT

• Immediately, if hypoglycemic
• Growth velocity should increase within 3 to 6 months
• The growth response to thyroid hormone replacement is slow, but free T_4 levels can normalize within 4 to 6 weeks.

SIGNS TO WATCH FOR

• Headache
• Vision problems
• Seizures
• Changes in activity level
• Limp, knee, or hip pain

PITFALLS

• rhGH therapy is associated with idiopathic intracranial hypertension (pseudotumor cerebri), which typically improves whether or not medication is stopped.
• rhGH therapy is associated with slipped capital femoral epiphysis (SCFE). Carefully evaluate any limp, knee or hip pain in patients on rhGH therapy. SCFE mandates orthopedic consultation.

• Growth hormone is a mitogenic factor so there has been a theoretical potential for increasing the incidence of leukemia. Clinical studies have not confirmed this hypothesis.
• The family and the patient must understand the importance of taking stress doses of steroid appropriately (e.g., with surgery or febrile illnesses).
• You must consider the diagnosis of panhypopituitarism in patients with hypoglycemic seizures.
• Normal children can fail to respond to growth hormone provocative testing.
• Ordering a TSH level is generally not helpful when evaluating pituitary/hypothalamic causes of hypothyroidism. The unbound thyroxine level (free T4 by equilibrium dialysis) is the most useful test in these cases both to establish the diagnosis and to monitor *l*-thyroxine replacement therapy.

 Common Questions and Answers

Q: When do I give the stress dose of steroid and for how long?
A: Whenever the patient has fever, vomiting, serious illness, or surgery. Continue until 24 hours after stress resolves (e.g., the day after fever breaks or vomiting stops).

Q: What are the chances of cretinism?
A: Minimal, if medication is taken properly.

ICD-9-CM 253.2

BIBLIOGRAPHY

McGauley G, Cuneo R, Salomon F, Sonksen PH. Growth hormone deficiency and quality of life. *Horm Res* 1996;45(1-2):34–37.

Radovick S, Cohen LE, Wondisford FE. The molecular basis of hypopituitarism. *Horm Res* 1998;49(Suppl. 1):30–36.

Romeo JH. Hyperfunction and hypofunction in the anterior pituitary. *Nurs Clin North Am* 1996;31(4):769–778.

Sklar CA, Constine LS. Chronic neuroendocrinological sequelae of radiation therapy. *Int J Radiat Oncol Biol Phys* 1995;31(5):1113–1121.

Soule SG, Jacobs HS. The evaluation and management of subclinical pituitary disease. *Postgrad Med J* 1996;72(847):258–262.

Weinzimer SA, Homan SA, Ferry RJ Jr, Moshang T Jr. Serum ICF-1 and IGFBP-3 concentrations do not accurately predict growth hormone deficiency in children with brain tumors. *Clin Endocrinol* 1999;51:in press.

Authors: Robert J. Ferry, Jr. and Paulo F. Collett-Solberg

Parvovirus B19 (Erythema Infectiosum, Fifth Disease)

 Database

DEFINITION

Parvovirus B19 (B19) is a common viral infection of school-aged children that is most commonly associated with an erythematous macular rash in a patient whose appearance remains well.

CAUSES

• B19 is a single-stranded DNA virus, one of the smallest of the human viruses.
• It was first isolated from asymptomatic blood donors in 1975.

PATHOPHYSIOLOGY

• Parvovirus B19 replicates in the red blood cell precursors in the bone marrow and is associated with a number of different diseases ranging from benign to severe.
• There is no practical *in vitro* system for isolation or culture of the virus.

ASSOCIATED DISEASES

• Aplastic crisis secondary to B19 in patients with hereditary hemolytic anemias or any condition that shortens the red blood cell life span, such as sickle cell disease or spherocytosis, may cause severe anemia.
• Fifth disease or erythema infectiosum caused by B19 occurs in up to 35% of school-aged children.
• Human parvovirus arthropathy, symmetrical joint pain, and swelling especially of the hands, knees, and feet, is seen in adults much more frequently than children; among women with B19 infection, 80% to 100% develop polyarthritis.
• Hydrops fetalis may develop following maternal B19 infection and intrauterine involvement.
• Chronic bone marrow failure due to persistent B19 infection in immunocompromised patients has been reported.
• Extremity numbness and tingling, hemophagocytic syndrome, and Henoch-Schönlein purpura has recently been sporadically reported as being associated with B19 infection.

EPIDEMIOLOGY

• Most B19 infections occur in school-aged children.
• Seroprevalence of B19 IgG antibodies:

—5 years, 2% to 9%
—5 to 18 years, 15% to 35%
—Adults, 30% to 60%

• Route of spread includes exposure to:

—Nasal secretions
—Aerosolized large-droplet respiratory secretions
—Blood (1011 virions per mL or serum in patients with hereditary hemolytic anemias)

• Attack rates range from 15% to 60% of susceptibles (i.e., seronegative) will become infected on exposure.
• 40% of susceptible health care workers were infected in a Philadelphia outbreak in 1989.

COMPLICATIONS

• Parvovirus B19 during pregnancy

—Fetal loss or hydrops fetalis may occur if infected with B19 during pregnancy.
—50% of women are susceptible to B19 infection.
—The infection is not a teratogen to the fetus.
—Fetal death occurs in 3% to 9%.
—The greatest risk for B19 infection to affect the fetus exists in the first 20 weeks of gestation.
—There is no indication for elective abortion in cases of maternal infection.
—The risk of fetal death after exposure, if antibody status is unknown, is from 0.05% to 1%.

• Aplastic Crisis

—Transfusions may be necessary to treat symptoms of severe anemia.

• Arthritis/Arthropathy

—Although most cases of polyarthritis resolve within 2 weeks, persistent symptoms for months to even years (rarely) have been reported.

PROGNOSIS

The prognosis is quite good for all manifestations of B19 infections and, in general, require supportive care only until spontaneous recovery.

 Differential Diagnosis

B19 infection should be considered in all patients with arthritis or viral exanthems with a history and examination that is consistent.

 Data Gathering

HISTORY

Question: Asymptomatic infection?
Significance: May occur in approximately 20% of children and adults.

Question: Erythema infectiosum?
Significance: The most common form of infection recognized. The incubation period is 4 to 14 days; prodromal symptoms are mild and include headache, sore throat, lethargy, and low-grade fevers lasting 1 to 4 days. A facial rash that is erythematous (slapped cheeks) is noticed next, which spreads to the body and extremities. The body rash is macular erythematous and lacy appearing. It may become more intense with exercise and may be pruritic. Occasionally, it involves the palms and soles and rarely can be papular, vesicular, or purpuric. It may last for approximately 7 days but can persist more than 20 days. The child is usually unaffected and remains active and playful. Symptoms in adults are similar although often more severe. During the illness, 80% of adults have arthralgias or arthritis.

Question: Aplastic crisis
Significance: Prodromal symptoms in B19-infected children with sickle cell disease or other hereditary hemolytic anemias are non-specific and consist of fever, malaise, and headache. Laboratory testing confirms the diagnosis.

Question: Chronic marrow suppression
Significance: In immunocompromised patients, B19 infection may persist for months, leading to chronic anemia with B19 viremia. Low-grade fever and neutropenia may accompany anemia.

Parvovirus B19 (Erythema Infectiosum, Fifth Disease)

 ## Laboratory Aids

The diagnosis of B19 infection depends on recognition of typical symptoms and:

Test: Specific antibodies
Significance: Presence of specific IgM or IgG antibodies as determined by EIA and/or detection of virus. In patients with symptoms of erythema infectiosum or aplastic crisis, the presence of B19-specific IgM antibodies is diagnostic. IgM- and IgG-specific antibodies are detected in 90% of such patients by 3 to 7 days of illness. B19-specific IgG antibodies persists for years, while specific IgM antibodies begin to fall 30 to 60 days after onset of illness.

Test: Polymerase chain reaction (PCR) techniques
Significance: Immunocompromised patients with chronic marrow may be unable to produce B19-specific IgG or IgM antibodies. In such cases, B19 viral DNA can be detected using nuclear and hybridization or PCR techniques. Such techniques are also useful for detecting infection in fetuses.

Test: Hematocrit and reticulocyte count in patients with aplastic crisis
Significance: Laboratory studies reveal reticulocytopenia, usually with counts of <1%. During the illness, the patient's hematocrit may fall as low as 15%.

 ## Therapy

- There is no specific therapy for this infection other than supportive care.
- Intravenous immunoglobulin therapy has been given with some success to a few patients with chronic marrow suppression secondary to B19 infection.

PREVENTION INFECTION CONTROL

In the hospital environment, secondary attack rates approaching 40% were reported in susceptive health care workers exposed to two children with sickle cell disease and unsuspected B19 infections. In response, all patients with suspected aplastic crisis secondary to B19 should be placed in contact isolation. No measures are needed for normal hosts with rash. In addition, pregnant teachers who are at risk for infections should consider a leave of absence during community outbreaks of B19.

 ## Follow-Up

EXPECTED COURSE OF ILLNESS

- During aplastic crisis secondary to B19 the reticulocytopenia usually remains low (often <1%) for approximately 8 days before spontaneous recovery.
- The rash of erythema infectiosum in the child or adult may last up to 20 days. It may, at times, fade and/or intensify depending on sunlight exposure, exercise, or body surface temperature changes (bathing).

 ## Common Questions and Answers

Q: When may children with B19 infection return to school?
A: Children are not infectious when the rash appears. Therefore, they may return to school or daycare. The infectious period is only during the prodromal phase of illness, which is often unrecognized.

Q: What can they do to reduce risk of fetal infection?
A: Because B19 infections during pregnancy may result in fetal death, and B19 infections often occur in community outbreaks, fetal risks following maternal exposure to persons with recognized B19 infection are a frequent concern. Among pregnant women of unknown antibody status, the risk of fetal death after exposure to B19 is estimated to be <1.5%. Risk to the fetus appears to be greatest if the infection occurs prior to the 20th week of gestation. Pregnant teachers who are at risk for infection should consider a leave of absence during community outbreaks of B19.

ICD-9-CM 057.0

BIBLIOGRAPHY

Anderson LJ, Tsou C, Parker RA, et al. Detection of antibodies and antigens of human Parvovirus B19 by ELISA. *J Clin Microbiol* 1986; 24:522–526.

Bell LM. Parvovirus B19 infection: a decade of discovery. In: Long SS, Starr SE, eds. The report on pediatric infectious diseases. 1992;2:6.

Bell LM, Naides SJ, Stoffman P, Hodinka RL, Plotkin SA. Human parvovirus B19 infection among hospital staff members after contact with infected patients. *N Engl J Med* 1989; 321:485–491.

Török TJ. Parvovirus B19 and human disease. *Adv Intern Med* 1992;37:431–455.

Ware R. Human parvovirus infection. *J Pediatr* 1989;114:343–348.

Author: Louis M. Bell

Patent Ductus Arteriosus

 Database

DEFINITION

• Patent ductus arteriosus (PDA) is the persistence in postnatal life of the normal fetal vascular conduit between the central pulmonary and systemic arterial systems. Normally, the ductus arteriosus (DA) functionally closes by 18 hours of life. Structural closure is usually completed by the third week of life. If the DA remains patent beyond 3 months of life it is considered abnormal and is unlikely to close spontaneously (spontaneous closure rate 0.6% per year).
• In the infant with a normal left aortic arch, the DA connects the main pulmonary artery at the origin of the left pulmonary artery to the descending aorta, distal of the origin of the left subclavian artery.
• Many variations in the connections and the course of the DA exist. A left, right, or, rarely, bilateral ductus can persist and connect the main, proximal right or left pulmonary artery to virtually any location on the aortic arch or proximal portions of the brachiocephalic vessels.
• There are five distinct clinical conditions associated with PDA:

—Isolated cardiovascular lesion in premature infants.
—Isolated cardiovascular lesion in otherwise healthy term infants and children.
—Incidental finding associated with more significant structural cardiovascular defects.
—Compensatory structure in cases of neonatal persistent pulmonary hypertension (PPHN) without congenital heart disease.
—Critical compensatory structure in some cyanotic or left-sided obstructed lesions.

In this chapter only the issue of PDA as an isolated cardiovascular lesion will be discussed.

CAUSES

• Prematurity
• Rubella infection in the first trimester
• Genetic or familial factors
• High altitude
• Idiopathic

EPIDEMIOLOGY

• PDA, as an isolated defect is the sixth commonest congenital cardiovascular lesion.
• Incidence 1:2000 (5–10% of all types of CHD).
• Female-to-male ratio 2:1
• The incidence increases with the degree of prematurity (15–80% in preterm infants <26 weeks gestation). The incidence varies significantly depending on management style (e.g., amount of maintenance fluids prescribed, surfactant administration, use of phototherapy), coexisting diseases (e.g., RDS, hypoxemia, fluid overload, NEC, sepsis, hypocalcemia), and environmental factors (altitude).

PATHOLOGY

In premature infants and term infants with PPHN delayed closure represents impaired developmental process while in the full-term infant and older child a PDA probably reflects structural abnormality of the ductal tissue.

PHYSIOLOGY

Predominate fetal blood flow: RA⇒RV⇒MPA⇒DA⇒AO (bypasses the pulmonary vascular bed). With the first breaths after birth the pulmonary arteriolar resistance (Rp) falls abruptly, the DA constricts and pulmonary blood flow is shifted away from the DA and into the lungs. As pulmonary resistance becomes lower than the systemic, some left-to-right runoff occurs until the ductus closes. With a PDA excessive blood flow will continue from the aorta into the pulmonary artery causing pulmonary vascular flooding and volume load on the left atrium and ventricle.

COMPLICATIONS

• Pulmonary edema and congestive heart failure
• Pulmonary hemorrhage
• Pulmonary vascular obstructive disease
• Increased chronic lung disease
• Failure to thrive
• Recurrent respiratory infections
• Lobar emphysema or collapse
• Infective endarteritis
• Thromboembolism of cerebral arteries
• Aneurysm of the ductus
• Intracranial hemorrhage
• Necrotizing enterocolitis
• Renal dysfunction

 Differential Diagnosis

• Aortopulmonary window
• Systemic or pulmonary arteriovenous communications
• Ruptured sinus of Valsalva
• Coronary artery fistula
• Truncus arteriosus
• Venous hum
• Pulmonary atresia with collaterals
• Ventricular septal defect with aortic regurgitation
• Ventricular septal defect in infancy

 Data Gathering

Clinical features depend on:

• The clinical condition associated with the PDA
• The magnitude of the left-to-right shunt
• Anatomical and physiological features of the PDA in each individual
• Reaction to the increased pulmonary blood flow

HISTORY

Premature Infants

• Variable, ranging from asymptomatic to complete cardiovascular collapse.
• Tachypnea, feeding intolerance, apnea and bradycardia.

Question: Worsening lung disease?
Significance: Increase ventilator support or pulmonary hemorrhage.

Question: Respiratory and metabolic acidosis?
Significance: Low cardiac output; excessive pulmonary blood flow.

Question: Decreased urine output?
Significance: Low cardiac output.

Infants and Older Children

Question: Small PDA?
Significance: Usually asymptomatic with only an incidental finding of a heart murmur.

Question: Moderate PDA?
Significance: Can present as congestive heart failure, poor feeding, and poor weight gain.

Question: Large PDA?
Significance: Can cause, in addition to these symptoms, recurrent respiratory infections.

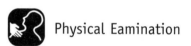 Physical Eamination

PREMATURE INFANTS

Finding: Tachypnea, rales
Significance: Increased pulmonary blood flow

Finding: Tachycardia (±S3 gallop)
Significance: Rapid ventricular filling during diastole

Finding: Hyperdynamic precordium
Significance: Large left-to-right shunt

Finding: Bounding pulses with wide pulse pressure
Significance: Reflects "run off" of the aorta

Finding: Pansystolic murmur, audible best at the left upper or mid sternal border
Significance: Typical PDA murmur

Finding: No murmur may be heard with a wide PDA
Significance: Equalization of pressure

Finding: Hepatomegaly
Significance: Increased left-to-right shunting and congestive heart failure (late sign)

INFANTS AND OLDER CHILDREN

Finding: Pansystolic murmur, heard best at second left intercostal space.
Significance: Typical PDA murmur

Finding: Murmur becomes continuous (i.e., extends into diastole) as the pulmonary vascular resistance decreases.
Significance: If heart failure occurs the murmur may lose its continuous character.

Finding: In moderate and large PDA the murmur is louder, has a harsh quality, and acquires a machinery quality and is well heard posteriorly. A systolic thrill may be felt at the left upper sternal border.
Significance: Large PDA

Finding: Tachycardia accompanied by hyperdynamic precordium.
Significance: Volume overloaded left ventricle

Finding: Bounding pulses and wide pulse pressure.
Significance: Large PDA

Finding: Apex beat may be displaced with left ventricular dilatation.
Significance: Excessive pulmonary blood flow and left-to-right shunt.

Finding: A mid-diastolic low frequency rumbling murmur may be audible at the apex.
Significance: Increased diastolic flow across the mitral valve.

Finding: With severe left ventricular failure the classic PDA signs may disappear, but there will be findings consistent with CHF (tachycardia, third sound at the apex, hepatomegaly, tachypnea, rales).
Significance: LV failure is a late finding in patients with a PDA.

• As pulmonary hypertension occurs, the murmur shortens, the diastolic component disappears and S2 becomes accentuated. A harsh diastolic blowing murmur of pulmonary regurgitation is heard in addition and the pulses become of normal or small volume. At advanced stages of irreversible pulmonary vascular disease cyanosis begins to appear with reversal of shunting, often more pronounced in the lower limbs.

 ## Laboratory Aids

Test: ECG
Significance: Usually normal in small PDA. LAE and LVH with moderate and large PDA. Biventricular hypertrophy in later stages.

Test: CXR
Significance: Usually normal with small PDA although occasionally prominence of main and peripheral pulmonary arteries may be seen. In moderate and large PDA these findings become more pronounced along with an enlarged heart and prominence of the ascending aorta. Increased pulmonary vascular markings are proportionate to the left-to-right shunt. Pulmonary edema can be seen if CHF develops. In premature infants with respiratory distress syndrome there is evidence of deteriorating lung disease with unclear cardiac borders.

Test: ECHO
Significance: 2D-echocardiogram delineates the PDA and assesses the size of dilated LA and LV. Using Doppler techniques the ductal flow pattern can be assessed and some incompetence of the foramen ovale may be discovered in cases with increased left-to-right shunt. Continuous wave Doppler examination is useful for estimating the pulmonary artery pressure.

Test: Cardiac catheterization
Significance: Not essential for diagnosis but indicated if pulmonary hypertension is suspected for assessment of the pulmonary vascular resistance and the reactivity of the pulmonary vascular bed to pulmonary vasodilators. Also can be performed for PDA closure by coil or clamshell devices.

 ## Therapy

PREMATURE INFANT

• Supportive treatment (O_2, respiratory assistance, correction of metabolic acidosis)
• Management of CHF with fluid restriction and diuretics
• If PDA persists despite above management or patient is extremely symptomatic then closure of PDA is indicated:

—Medical closure with indomethacin (or ibuprofen).

Contraindications

• Renal failure (creatinine >1.8 mg/dL), thrombocytopenia (platelets <100,000), associated conditions (NEC, IVH Grade IV)
• Surgical closure if medical treatment fails or use of indomethacin is contraindicated

INFANTS AND OLDER CHILDREN

• Medical management of CHF with digoxin and diuretics.
• Endocarditis prophylaxis with procedures.
• Closure is indicated whenever a symptomatic PDA exists. For asymptomatic PDA the procedure can be performed electively after the first year of age and is mainly performed to prevent against the potential for endocarditis.
• Closure of ductus can be achieved by:

—Surgical ligation or division
—Transcatheter closure with a coil or other occlusion device

 ## Follow-Up

PROGNOSIS

• Outcome in treated premature infants is generally good but mostly depends on the degree of prematurity and the presence of associated conditions.
• Outcome in term infants and older children is excellent if no complications have previously occurred or occurred at the time of treatment.
• PDA among adults is associated with significant mortality with or without surgery.
• Post closure of PDA no endocarditis prophylaxis is needed if complete obliteration of flow is achieved.

ICD-9-CM 747.0

BIBLIOGRAPHY

Emmanouilides GC, Riemenschneider TA, Allen HD, Gutgesell HP, eds. Moss and Adams' heart disease in infants, children and adolescents including the fetus and the young adult. Baltimore, MD: Williams & Wilkins, 1998:746–765.

Fyler DC, ed. *Nadas' pediatric cardiology*. Philadelphia: Hanley and Belfus, 1992, 525–534.

Garson A Jr., Bricker JT, McNamara DG, eds. *The science and practice of pediatric cardiology*. Malvern, PA: Lea & Febiger, 1990;1055–1069.

Author: Lazaros Kochilas

Pelvic Inflammatory Disease (PID)

Database

DEFINITION

An ascending, polymicrobial genital tract infection of sexually active females. It includes an array of inflammatory disorders, including endometritis, parametritis, salpingitis, oophoritis, tubo-ovarian abscess (TOA), peritonitis, and perihepatitis.

Centers for Disease Control and Prevention (CDC) clinical criteria:

- Minimum criteria
—Lower abdominal tenderness
—Adnexal tenderness
—Cervical motion tenderness
- Additional criteria
—Oral temperature higher than 101°F (38.3°C)
—Abnormal cervical or vaginal discharge
—Elevated erythrocyte sedimentation rate (ESR)
—Elevated C-reactive protein (CRP)
—Laboratory documented evidence of infection with *Neisseria gonorrhoeae* or *Chlamydia trachomatis*.
- Definitive criteria
—Histopathological evidence of endometritis on endometrial biopsy
—Transvaginal sonography or other imaging techniques showing thickened fluid-filled tubes with or without free pelvic fluid or TOA
—Laparoscopic abnormalities consistent with PID

ETIOLOGY

- *N. gonorrhea*
- *C. trachomatis:* tends to be associated with less fever, pain, and systemic symptoms than PID seen with gonococcus
- *Bacteroides* or *Peptostreptococcus* species

PATHOPHYSIOLOGY

- Direct spread of bacteria to ascending structures, via migration, sperm transport, refluxed menstrual blood, or intra-uterine device (IUD) string
- Direct migration may be facilitated by menstrual flow, as there is loss of protective cervical mucus
- Microbes invade epithelial cells, mucosa and serosa, causing inflammation with subsequent scarring
- An endotoxin of *N. gonorrhea* may lead to increased systemic symptomology
- Adolescents with increased susceptibility due to increased cervical ectopy (more exposed columnar epithelium), relative lack of local immunity, increased high-risk sexual behaviors, and lower compliance with barrier contraceptives.

EPIDEMIOLOGY

- Affects more than 1 million American women per year; estimated cost over $4.2 billion

- Adolescent cases account for 20% to 30%, facing a 10-fold risk compared to adults.
- Risk increases with failure to use condoms, the number of lifetime partners, new partners within 3 months, past history of STD, and the presence of IUD.
- Oral contraceptive (OCP) use decreases the risk of PID, but does not reduce the risks of vaginal or cervical infections.

COMPLICATIONS

- Chronic pelvic pain or dyspareunia
- Ectopic pregnancy: suspicion should be high in any adolescent early in pregnancy with a history of PID
- Infertility: risk increases with number of episodes of PID
- Tubo-ovarian abscess (TOA): occurs in up to one-third of all patients with PID; risk increases with time between infection and treatment; associated with higher mortality and increased rates of infertility and other sequelae
- Peritonitis
- Fitz-Hugh-Curtis syndrome (perihepatitis) results from tracking of pus along the paracolic gutters yielding inflammation of the hepatic capsule and diaphragm
- Other STDs may occur concomitantly, including HIV, syphilis, trichomaniasis, HSV, or vaginal warts

PROGNOSIS

- Overall, good
- One episode is associated with a 13% to 21% risk of infertility, two episodes with a 35% risk, and three or more episodes with a 55% to 75% risk.
- Dyspareunia or chronic pelvic pain has been reported by up to 18% of women treated for PID.
- Long-term sequelae are present in 25% of affected women, with a higher likelihood in adolescents due to later presentation, delay in diagnosis, and inadequate treatment.

Differential Diagnosis

INFECTION

- Other genital infection (e.g., *Gardnerella vaginalis,* coliforms, *Streptococcus* species, genital tract mycoplasma)
- Cervicitis
- Vaginal infection with corpus albicans, trichomonas, or *Gardnerella vaginalis:* commonly associated with malodorous discharge originating from vaginal walls
- TOA
- Pyelonephritis, urinary tract infection
- Appendicitis, appendiceal abscess
- Tuberculosis
- Viral or bacterial enteritis
- Acute cholecystitis
- Mesenteric lymphadenitis
- Pelvic thrombophlebitis

GYNECOLOGIC

- Pregnancy, intrauterine or ectopic
- Ovarian cyst or torsion
- Chronic pelvic pain secondary adhesions from prior inflammation
- Endometriosis
- Teratoma or other mass

MISCELLANEOUS

- Foreign body or pelvic trauma
- Functional pain

Data Gathering

HISTORY

Assessment begins with sensitive, private interview with a practitioner who can assure confidentiality.

Question: Review of systems.
Significance: Presentation may be "silent," with relatively few or mild symptoms.

Question: Ask about pain, fever, and synecologic symptoms.
Significance: Classic presentation of PID includes:

- Lower abdominal pain
- Abnormal vaginal discharge or bleeding
- Fever

Question: Take complete menstrual, sexual, gastrointestinal, and urinary histories.
Significance: Associated symptoms may include:

- Dysmenorrhea
- Dyspareunia
- Vomiting, diarrhea, or constipation
- Dysuria or urinary frequency

Question: Past medical, including gynecologic, history should be obtained.
Significance: Supportive historical data include:

- Recent menstruation
- Use of IUD or douche
- Inconsistent condom use
- Multiple or new sexual partners
- Prior history of PID

Physical Examination

- Perform a thorough abdominal exam, noting tenderness, rebound or guarding, and signs of perihepatitic involvement

Finding: Pelvic examination
Significance: Document the following:

- Presence of external or vaginal lesions
- Origin, quality, and quantity of discharge (e.g., "copious, mucopurulent cervical discharge," or "scant, thin vaginal discharge")
- Signs of cervical inflammation (e.g., erythema, friability)
- Cervical motion tenderness

- Adnexal tenderness or fullness
- Blot away discharge to better assess the source of new fluid accumulation

Laboratory Aids

SPECIFIC TESTS

- Urine or serum β-HCG, regardless of sexual history
- Complete blood count with differential
- ESR or CRP
- Wet prep of discharge for Trichomonads, hyphae, or Clue cells
- Gram stain of cervical discharge
- Testing for *N. gonorrhea* and *C. trachomatis*
- Culture is technique dependent, yielding an 80% sensitivity
- Antigen detection tests (e.g., DFA, ELISA) have lower sensitivities
- Genetic amplification (LCR) requires a single specimen for both organisms, has a 24-hour turnaround time, and has 90% to 95% sensitivity
- Syphilis serology (RPR) and HIV testing with appropriate counseling and follow-up
- Test of cure examination and laboratory testing should occur on all patients 6 to 8 weeks after diagnosis.

RADIOGRAPHIC STUDIES

Test: Pelvic ultrasound
Significance: To rule out TOA or other pelvic pathology

Test: Laparoscopy
Significance: Not routinely used, but considered the "gold standard" for diagnosis.

Therapy

Inpatient treatment has been the standard of care, and should occur if:

- Suspected TOA
- Patient has failed outpatient treatment
- Patient is high-risk for sequelae
- Patient with pregnancy, HIV, chronic disease

When choosing outpatient treatment:

- Re-evaluation must occur within 72 hours of initiating therapy
- Patient must be compliant with meds and follow-up
- The patient should be given a full course of doxycycline (or other oral medications) and tolerate the first dose under supervision
- All patients with PID should receive intensive education about STD prevention

DRUGS

Inpatient Management

- CDC regimen A:
—Cefotetan (2 g IV every 12 hours) or cefoxitin (2 g IV every 6 hours)

—Plus, doxycycline (100 mg PO twice a day for 14 days)
- Regimen B:
—Clindamycin (900 mg IV every 8 hours)
—Plus, gentamicin (loading dose 2 mg/kg IV or IM, followed by maintenance dose 1.5 mg/kg every 8 hours)
- Alternative parenteral regimens include:
—Ofloxacin (400 mg IV every 12 hours) plus metronidazole (500 mg IV every 8 hours), or
—Ampicillin/sulbactam (3 g IV every 6 hours) plus doxycycline (100 mg IV or PO every 12 hours), or
—Ciprofloxacin (200 mg IV every 12 hours) plus doxycycline (100 mg IV or PO every 12 hours)
—Plus metronidazole (500 mg IV very 8 hours)

The choice between parenteral regimens A or B is based on availability and the drug allergy history of the patient. Data to support the use of alternative regimens are limited.

- Regimen A should be continued for at least 48 hours after clinical improvement, and is followed by the completion of a 14-day course of doxycycline (100 mg PO twice a day).
- Regimen B should be continued for at least 24 hours after clinical improvement, and is followed by completion of a 14-day course of either doxycycline or clindamycin (450 mg PO twice a day).

Outpatient Management

- Regimen A
—Ofloxacin (400 mg PO twice a day for 14 days) (approved for ages >16 years)
—Plus, metronidazole (500 mg PO twice a day for 14 days)
- Regimen B
—Ceftriaxone (250 mg IM once) or cefoxitin (2 g IM with probenecid 1 g PO once) or other parenteral third-generation cephalosporin
—Plus, doxycycline (100 mg PO twice a day for 14 days)
- The choice between oral regimens is based on availability, cost, and patient history of drug allergy.

Emergency Care

- TOA rupture can present emergently as acute peritonitis. It requires immediate surgical or gynecologic consultation.
- If an IUD is in place, it must be removed immediately.

Follow-Up

- For inpatients, substantial clinical improvement should occur within 3 to 5 days if the patient has been properly diagnosed and treated.
- Outpatients should have significant improvement at the 48 to 72 hour follow-up.

PREVENTION

- Primary prevention involves early education and aggressive screening for STDs
- Abstinence and barrier contraceptive use should be advocated and facilitated
- Screening and treatment of sexual partners should be encouraged and facilitated

PITFALLS

- Doxycycline lowers the efficacy of oral contraceptives
- Most bacteriologic studies are technique-dependent. Therefore, the clinician should be trained in the technique for the specific method being used.
- All home pregnancy tests should be repeated
- Pelvic ultrasound requires a full urinary bladder, unlike transvaginal
- Overzealous education concerning possible sequelae or future infertility may lead to the patient "testing" fertility in the future

Common Questions and Answers

Q: A patient states she is not sexually active, should I continue to consider PID?
A: Yes, because of the risk and severity of sequelae, PID should always be considered. Continue considering alternative diagnoses.

Q: A patient does not meet the criteria for PID, however, it is still the most likely diagnosis. Should I start therapy while other studies are pending?
A: Yes, appropriate therapy for PID may be initiated while other work-ups are in progress. Delay in therapy results in increased of sequelae from PID. When considering other diagnoses, the most life-threatening processes should be considered first. These include: ectopic pregnancy, septic abortion, and appendicitis. Keep ovarian torsion high on the differential, as it must be corrected in a timely fashion to maintain function.

Q: An adolescent patient with PID has inquired about fertility. What should I tell her?
A: Many clinicians would argue that an episode of PID could serve as a "wake up" call to teenagers, inspiring them to abstain or comply with barrier contraception. However, a young woman who is told that she may have impaired fertility might try testing it through unprotected sex. Regardless, information about future sequelae must be given in a sensitive manner, taking into account the young woman's developmental status and her support network.

ICD-9-CM 614.9

BIBLIOGRAPHY

CDC. 1998 sexually transmitted disease guidelines. *MMWR* 1998;47(RR-1):79–86.

Pletcher JR, Slap GB. Pelvic inflammatory disease. *Pediatr Rev* 1998;19:361–365.

Shafer M, Sweet RL. Pelvic inflammatory disease in adolescent females. *Adolesc Med Rev* 1990;1:545–563.

Author: Jonathan R. Pletcher and Kenneth R. Ginsburg

Pericarditis

Database

DEFINITION

Inflammation of the pericardium, usually resulting in the accumulation of fluid in the pericardial space between the visceral (intimately related to the myocardium) and parietal (several layers of elastic fibers and collagen) pericardium; may be serous, fibrinous, purulent, hemorrhagic, or chylous.

CAUSES

- Infectious: viral (coxsackie B, Epstein-Barr, adenovirus, influenza, HIV), bacterial (streptococcus, pneumococcus, staphylococcus, meningococcus, mycoplasma, tularemia, *Hemophilus influenzae* type B), tuberculosis, fungal (histoplasmosis, actinomycosis), parasitic (toxoplasmosis, echinococcus).
- Rheumatologic: acute rheumatic fever, rheumatoid arthritis, systemic lupus erythematosus, systemic sclerosis, sarcoidosis, and familial Mediterranean fever.
- Metabolic/Endocrine: hypothyroidism, uremia (chemical irritation).
- Neoplastic disease: lymphoma, lymphosarcoma, leukemia, metastatic disease to the pericardium, radiotherapy induced.
- Postoperative: postpericardiotomy syndrome (after cardiac surgery), chylopericardium.
- Other: trauma, drug-induced (hydralazine, isoniazid, procainamide), aortic dissection, idiopathic.

PATHOPHYSIOLOGY

Fine deposits of fibrin develop next to the great vessels and this leads to altered function of the membranes of the pericardium, including changes in oncotic and hydrostatic pressure with subsequent accumulation of fluid in the pericardial space. In post-pericardiotomy syndrome, there appears to be a non-specific hypersensitivity reaction to the direct entrance into the pericardial space.

EPIDEMIOLOGY

- Infectious pericarditis is more frequently seen in children less than 13 years, with predominance in children less than 2 years.
- Can occur in any age group.
- Overall incidence is slightly higher in males.
- Post-pericardiotomy syndrome occurs in approximately 5% to 10% of children after uncomplicated cardiac surgery, particularly when the atrium has been entered.

COMPLICATIONS

- Cardiac tamponade: Intrapericardial pressure rises at a rapid rate secondary to decreased compliance of the pericardial membranes, resulting in restriction of ventricular filling and eventual decrease in stroke volume and cardiac output. The compliance of the pericardium is influenced by the disease process itself (i.e., the pericardium is thickened and stiff in bacterial and tuberculin pericarditis). During cardiac tamponade, ventricular end-diastolic, atrial and venous pressures are all equal. In acute pericarditis, tamponade may occur with small amounts of fluid because of rapid increase in the intrapericardial pressure. In contrast, large amounts of fluid may be tolerated if the accumulation is a chronic, slow process.
- Constrictive pericarditis: Thick, fibrotic and often calcified pericardium is seen, usually a late result of purulent or tuberculous pericarditis; it can occur months to years after the initial infection. It can also be seen in oncology patients with direct invasion of tumor into the pericardium or with significant radiation to the chest; in at least one-half the patients the etiology is unclear. Poor compliance of the pericardium leads to diminished diastolic filling of the ventricle. Patients complain of poor exercise tolerance and fatigue and they have signs of right heart failure. This entity may be difficult to distinguish from restrictive cardiomyopathy.

PROGNOSIS

Most children recover fully from pericarditis, even if it is bacterial in etiology. However, there is a small but significant morbidity and mortality associated, especially in young infants when the diagnosis is delayed and/or when *Staphylococcus aureus* is the etiologic agent. Pericarditis can also recur in as many as 15% of patients. The prognosis varies with the other causes of pericarditis, but generally is directly related to the primary disease.

Differential Diagnosis

- Acute myocarditis
- Restrictive cardiomyopathy
- Other non-specific causes of chest pain

Data Gathering

HISTORY

Question: Fever, cough, precordial chest pain, and shoulder pain (which is aggravated by changes in position)?
Significance: Most common symptoms.

Question: Respiratory distress?
Significance: Seen if there is rapid accumulation of fluid.

Question: Pain?
Significance: Often relieved if the child sits leaning forward.

Question: No symptoms?
Significance: Slow, chronic accumulation may be associated with no symptoms at all. Other symptoms are dependent on the etiology of the pericarditis.

Question: Recent upper respiratory infection or gastroenteritis?
Significance: With viral pericarditis, there may be a preceding history of a recent upper respiratory infection or gastroenteritis.

Physical Examination

Finding: On auscultation of the heart, a pericardial friction rub is the pathognomonic finding
Significance: It may be heard if only a small amount of fluid is in the pericardial space.

Finding: Quiet precordium, tachycardia and muffled heart sounds
Significance: May be heard when there is a large amount of fluid and/or tamponade.

Finding: Signs of right-sided heart failure
Significance: Tamponade, including peripheral edema, jugular venous distention, and hepatomegaly.

Finding: Pulmonary edema
Significance: Rare because the heart is underfilled and left atrial pressure, though elevated, does not exceed right atrial pressure.

Finding: Pulsus paradoxus
Significance: An exaggerated decrease in systolic blood pressure with inspiration

Finding: Kussmaul sign
Significance: Paradoxical rise in jugular venous pressure during inspiration, often considered diagnostic of tamponade.

Laboratory Aids

Test: Chest roentgenogram
Significance: Often shows enlargement of the cardiac silhouette ("water bottle") usually in association with normal pulmonary vascular markings. However, heart size may appear normal in acute pericarditis. Calcification may be seen in constrictive pericarditis.

Test: Echocardiography
Significance: Most sensitive and specific test for pericardial thickening and fluid in the pericardial space. In the presence of a large effusion, the heart may appear to swing within the pericardial cavity. In tamponade, diastolic collapse of the right atrium and ventricle may be seen as well.

Test: Electrocardiogram
Significance: Non-specific but generally demonstrates low-voltage QRS complexes secondary to dampening of the signal from the pericardial fluid. One can also see ST segment elevation throughout the leads with possible T wave inversion as well, and these findings may be secondary to inflammation of the myocardium. Electrical alternans can be seen with large effusions.

Test: Pericardiocentesis
Significance: Fluid obtained should be sent for cell count, cytology, and culture (including bacteria, viruses, *Mycobacterium tuberculosis,* and fungi).

Therapy

- Treatment depends on etiology.
- However, no matter the cause, pericardiocentesis is required if there is an effusion that causes hemodynamic compromise and it may be life saving in patients with bacterial pericarditis.
- This procedure may also be indicated for diagnostic purposes when etiology of the effusion is in question.
- Complications of pericardiocentesis include myocardial puncture, coronary artery/vein laceration, hemopericardium, and pneumothorax.
- Echocardiographic guidance is useful for this procedure but is not required if there is impending cardiovascular collapse.

THERAPY BY DIAGNOSIS

- Viral pericarditis usually resolves spontaneously in 3 to 4 weeks with bedrest and analgesics.
- Bacterial pericarditis can potentially be life threatening and requires immediate decompression of the pericardial space, most often with open drainage and possible pericardial window, intravenous antibiotic therapy for at least 4 weeks and supportive therapy (i.e., volume expansion, inotropes).

- Rheumatologic causes of pericardial inflammation usually respond to corticosteroids and/or salicylates and rarely require pericardiocentesis.
- Uremic pericarditis usually responds to dialysis but pericardiotomy (surgical removal of the pericardium) may be necessary if it becomes a chronic problem.
- In neoplastic disease, the primary disease is treated and pericardiocentesis is performed if indicated for diagnostic and/or hemodynamic reasons.
- Hemorrhagic pericarditis secondary to trauma should be drained because of the risk of developing constrictive pericarditis.
- Postpericardiotomy syndrome occurs 1 to 4 weeks after cardiac surgery and is usually treated with anti-inflammatory drugs, bedrest, and occasionally steroids. Pericardiocentesis is indicated if tamponade develops.
- Constrictive pericarditis is treated with complete stripping of the pericardium (pericardiectomy). Often, immediate clinically improvement is not seen because there has been myocardial damage as well, but full recovery is the norm.

Follow-Up

WHEN TO EXPECT IMPROVEMENT

Most forms of pericarditis resolve on their own or with anti-inflammatory medication over the course of several weeks. Follow-up is necessary to be sure that effusions have resolved and to assess for recurrence (up to 15% relapse). Patients with bacterial pericarditis require long-term therapy and close follow-up to assess for the development of constrictive pericarditis.

SIGNS TO WATCH FOR

All cardiac surgical patients need an evaluation in the first 2 to 4 weeks after their operation to assess for post-pericardiotomy syndrome, with treatment and follow-up as necessary. Signs of low cardiac output and right heart failure indicate impending cardiac tamponade. Constrictive pericarditis may present with a rapidly decreasing cardiac silhouette and calcifications seen on chest roentgenogram, as well as the onset of signs and symptoms of right heart failure.

PREVENTION

Viral and rheumatologic pericarditis cannot be prevented. The incidence of bacterial pericarditis has decreased with immunization for such bacterial infections as *Hemophilus influenza* type B.

PITFALLS

The history, physical examination, and laboratory findings of acute pericarditis can be quite similar to those found in acute myocarditis. In addition, myocarditis can be a component of pericardial disease and vice versa. Echocardiography is an excellent tool to help differentiate between these two entities.

Common Questions and Answers

Q: How does cardiac tamponade present?
A: Patients with impending tamponade appear quite ill with tachycardia, chest pain, and signs of right heart failure including jugular venous distention, hepatomegaly, and peripheral edema/ascites. They may also have signs of poor systemic perfusion secondary to low cardiac output. The chest x-ray may or may not show evidence of enlarged cardiac silhouette depending on how acutely the process occurs. It takes much less fluid to cause tamponade in an acute process than in a chronic longstanding one. Echocardiography is the standard tool to make the diagnosis and pericardiocentesis is the treatment.

Q: What is pulsus paradoxus and how does one measure it?
A: Pulsus paradoxus is an exaggerated response of the systolic blood pressure to the normal respiratory cycle. Normally with inspiration, the systolic blood pressure drops approximately 5 mm Hg secondary to the increased capacitance of the pulmonary veins from the increased systemic venous return. In tamponade, this response becomes more profound (>10 mm Hg), most likely secondary to diminished filling of the left heart. Pulsus paradoxus can also be seen in patients with severe respiratory distress such as in asthma and emphysema.

To assess for pulsus paradoxus, measure the systolic blood pressure first in expiration; then allow it to fall to the place where it is heard equally well in inspiration and expiration. The difference is the degree and paradox and greater than 10 mm Hg is considered abnormal.

ICD-9-CM 420.91, 420.90, 423.20

BIBLIOGRAPHY

Dupuis C, Gonnier P, Kachaner J, et al. Bacterial pericarditis in infancy and childhood. *Am J Cardiol* 1994;74:807–809.

Fyler DC. Pericardial disease. In: Fyler DC, ed. *Nadas' pediatric cardiology.* Philadelphia: Hanley and Belfus, Inc., 1992:1590–1599.

Pinsky WW, Friedman RA. Pericarditis. In: Garson A, Bricker JT, McNamara D, eds. The science and practice of pediatric cardiology. Kent, U.K.: Lea and Febiger, Ltd., 1990:1531–1540.

Rheuban KS. Disease of the pericardium. In: Emmanoulides GC, Allen HD, Riemenschneider TA, Gutgesell HP, eds. Heart disease in infants, children, and adolescents: including the fetus and young adult, 5th ed. Baltimore: Williams & Wilkins, 1995.

Author: Meryl S. Cohen

Periodic Breathing

Database

DEFINITION

Periodic breathing is a respiratory pattern in which 3 or more apneas lasting 3 or more seconds in duration occur separated by more than 20 seconds of respiration.

CAUSES

• Periodic breathing can be seen in healthy infants, children, and adults.
• Periodic breathing in infants is associated with:

—Apnea of prematurity or infancy
—Familial history of sudden infant death syndrome (SIDS)
—Anemia of prematurity
—Hypoxemia
—Hypochloremic alkalosis

• Periodic breathing with adults is associated with:

—Cardiac abnormalities (congestive heart failure)
—Neurological dysfunction (meningitis, encephalitis, brainstem dysfunction)
—Also referred to as Cheyne-Stokes respirations

• Abnormalities in any component of the breathing control system may result in an increased amount of periodic breathing.
• Possible etiologies for periodic breathing include:

—A delay in detecting changes in blood gas values by the chemoreceptors
—Increased chemoreceptor gain

PATHOLOGY

• There is no common pathological finding.
• Abnormalities, when they exist, are related to the underlying disorder causing the periodic breathing.

EPIDEMIOLOGY

• Usually absent in the first 48 hours of life
• More frequent during REM versus non-REM sleep
• In full term infants:

—Amount of periodic breathing usually, <4% of their sleep time
—Amount gradually decreasing through the first year of life
—By 1 year of age, the mean amount of periodic breathing, <1% of total sleep time

• In premature infants:

—Amount of periodic breathing higher than in full-term infants
—Amount correlates inversely with the gestational age

• Incidence among healthy children and adults is unknown

COMPLICATIONS

Relationship between periodic breathing and SIDS is controversial.

Differential Diagnosis

• Other forms of apnea

—Central apnea
—Obstructive apnea

• Other forms of periodic breathing

—Cheyne-Stokes respiration
—Biot breathing
—Kussmaul respiration

• Normal irregular respirations seen in infants

Data Gathering

HISTORY

• In most cases, parents notice periodicity in the respirations of the child.
• In otherwise healthy premature or term infants, there are no other symptoms.

Physical Examination

In otherwise healthy premature or term infants, the physical examination is normal.

Laboratory Aids

POLYSOMNOGRAPHY

• Assesses the extent of periodic breathing episodes.
• Determines if there is accompanying hypoxemia or bradycardia with events.
• Distinguishes between periodic breathing and obstructive and/or central apnea.
• Useful for following response to treatment (i.e., normalization of polysomnography). Variables to be monitored include:

—O_2 saturation
—End-tidal CO_2 tension
—Respiratory movements (abdomen, chest)
—Airflow
—pH probe (if gastroesophageal reflux is suspected)
—Record for a minimum of 6 hours

2-CHANNEL PNEUMOGRAM

• Variables to be monitored include:

—Heart rate
—Respiratory effort

• Gives less information than polysomnography

IMAGING

Test: Chest radiograph
Significance: Usually normal

PITFALLS

2-Channel pneumograms document periodic breathing, but can miss episodes of obstructive apnea.

Therapy

GUIDELINES

• Therapy should be directed to treating any underlying primary disease.
• If periodic breathing is associated with apnea, hypoxemia, or other sleep disturbances, treatment should be instituted.

DRUGS

Stimulants

• Caffeine

—Loading dose: 10 mg/kg
—Maintenance dose: 2.5 mg/kg daily
—Therapeutic level: 5 to 20 mg/L

• Theophylline

—Loading dose: 4 to 5 mg/kg
—Maintenance dose: 3 to 5 mg/kg/d divided tid
—Therapeutic level: 6 to 10 mg/L

Supplemental Oxygen

• Useful if periodic breathing is secondary to hypoxemia
• Nasal CPAP
• Very effective in eliminating periodic breathing

Home Monitoring

Indicated when:

• The amount of periodic breathing is significant
• There is accompanying apnea.
• There is associated hypoxia and/or bradycardia

Duration

• Dependent on the underlying cause of the periodic breathing.
• Treatment does not change the natural course of periodic breathing in otherwise healthy infants.
• Therapy should continue until the periodic breathing resolves or is no longer clinically significant.

 Follow-Up

WHEN TO EXPECT IMPROVEMENT

• Dependent on the underlying cause of the periodic breathing
• Improvement is anticipated as the infant ages.
• When treatment is started, a decrease in the amount of periodic breathing should be seen almost immediately.

PROGNOSIS

• In otherwise normal premature or term infants: excellent
• With an underlying cardiac or neurological disorder, the prognosis is governed by this primary process.

PITFALLS

• Confusing periodic breathing with obstructive or central apnea

 Common Questions and Answers

Q: What is the risk of the patient dying of SIDS?
A: The relationship between periodic breathing and SIDS is not clear, although most studies have not found a higher frequency of SIDS among patients with periodic breathing.

ICD-9-CM 786.09

BIBLIOGRAPHY

Glotzbach SF, Ariagno RL. *Respiratory control disorders in infants and children.* Baltimore: Williams & Wilkins, 1992:142.

Kelly DH, Stellwagen LM, Katz E, et al. Apnea and periodic breathing in normal full-term infants during the first twelve months. *Pediatr Pulmonol* 1985;1:215.

Lieber C, Mohsenin V. Cheyne-Stokes respiration in congestive heart failure. *Yale J Biol Med* 1992;65:39.

Shannon DC, Carley DW, Kelly DH. Periodic breathing: quantitative analyses and clinical description. *Pediatr Pulmonol* 1986;4:98.

Authors: Shmuel Goldberg and Richard Mark Kravitz

Periorbital Cellulitis

 Database

DEFINITION

Periorbital cellulitis, also called preseptal cellulitis, is an acute infection and inflammation involving the eyelid and the surrounding tissue anterior to the orbital septum without involvement of the eye or orbital contents.

PATHOPHYSIOLOGY

Infection is caused by bacteria and results from one of the following:

- Hematogenous spread/bacteremia
- Spread of focal infection due to trauma, insect bite
- Extension from paranasal sinus infection
- A pathogen is isolated in only about 30% of cases, and of those cases in which a specific bacteria is identified, two-thirds will have positive blood cultures.
- The most common bacterial pathogens are:

—*Streptococcus pneumoniae*
—*Streptococcus pyogenes* (Group A)
—*Staphylococcus aureus*
—*Haemophilus influenzae* type b (Hib)
—Anaerobes

- Staph A and Group A Strep should be strongly considered when there is a focal skin infection.
- The incidence of Hib disease has dramatically decreased since the start of routine Hib-conjugated vaccination of infants in 1990.
- *S. pneumoniae* and Hib are more likely in cases of hematogenous spread.
- Fungi should be considered if the patient is immunocompromised.

EPIDEMIOLOGY

- Periorbital cellulitis is common in young children, and the majority of children with this infection are less than 5 years old.
- Periorbital cellulitis is more common and less serious than orbital cellulitis.

COMPLICATIONS

- Orbital cellulitis or disseminated bacterial infection (e.g., sepsis, meningitis)

PROGNOSIS

Excellent in patients with uncomplicated course.

 Differential Diagnosis

- Infection

—Ethmoid, maxillary, or frontal sinusitis may cause painless swelling and redness of the eyelid related to inflammatory edema from decreased venous drainage due to obstruction of sinus ostia by swollen mucosal tissue.
—Orbital cellulitis, also called postseptal cellulitis, involves infection internal to the septum or tarsal plate, and causes pain, proptosis, ophthalmoplegia, and visual disturbance.
—Adenovirus may mimic periorbital cellulitis in young children, but should not be assumed to be the pathogen because of the drastic repercussions of not treating a bacterial source with antibiotics.

- Trauma to the soft tissues of the eyelid or surrounding structures.
- Allergy (e.g., Type I hypersensitivity reaction or blepharoconjunctivitis) or insect bite may produce a red, warm, and swollen lid.
- Miscellaneous: Cavernous venous thrombosis, rhabdomyosarcoma, and inflammatory orbital pseudotumor may initially be mistaken for infectious conditions because they may cause acute swelling, but should not be confused with periorbital cellulitis because they result in proptosis.

 Data Gathering

HISTORY

A complete immunization history should be obtained, particularly regarding the number and timing of doses of immunization against Hib. A child who has had at least two Hib vaccines, with the second dose having been given more than 1 week prior to presentation, is unlikely to have Hib disease.

Question: Was there a preceding infection?
Significance: The infection has an acute onset and is commonly associated with an upper respiratory infection with or without fever.

Question: Was there fever or headache?
Significance: Up to two-thirds of patients will have fever and headache.

Question: Any trauma?
Significance: There may be a history of local trauma in some cases.

Question: Is there itching?
Significance: The eyelid is usually tender and not pruritic, which is more suggestive of allergy-induced edema.

 Physical Examination

- The eyelid is usually swollen, red, and tender, and is unilateral in 95% of cases.
- There may be a violaceous hue of the upper and/or lower eyelids.
- Toxic-appearing or irritable child should prompt one to consider associated sepsis or meningitis.
- Other possible associated findings include upper respiratory infection, fever (75%), signs of trauma or local infection (up to 33%), otitis media (25% of patients less than 2 years), mucopurulent conjunctivitis (20%), chemosis, and difficulty opening the eye due to edema.

SPECIAL QUESTIONS

Finding: Not normal vision
Significance: Another diagnosis must be made.

Finding: Presence of pain with movement of the eyeball
Significance: The infection has extended to a postseptal (orbital) cellulitis.

Finding: Extraocular movements are not intact
Significance: Another indication of orbital involvement.

Finding: Presence of eyelid edema
Significance: Prohibits adequate evaluation of the eye to assure that extraocular movements are intact and that there is no visual disturbance, a computer tomography (CT) scan is indicated.

Finding: Presence of proptosis
Significance: By definition, periorbital cellulitis is not associated with proptosis because it is a preseptal infection; therefore, the presence of proptosis is additional evidence of orbital involvement.

PHYSICAL EXAMINATION TRICKS

- The examiner may detect proptosis by standing behind the patient and looking down at a coronal view of the patient's face from above. This allows one to see if there is any real protrusion of orbital contents when compared with the other side, because edema can make this difficult to assess.
- The examiner should retract the eyelid to rule out a foreign body. This may be accomplished by flipping the lid over a cotton swab or by fashioning a paperclip into a double-looped lid retractor.

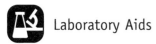 Laboratory Aids

Test: Culture purulent material
Significance: If there is a local wound infection.

Test: Complete blood count
Significance: Usually reveals a white blood cell (WBC) count between 10,000/mm³ to 15,000/mm³, and WBC greater than 15,000 is suggestive of associated bacteremia.

Test: Blood culture
Significance: Recommended but is infrequently positive because initiation of universal immunization against Hib. Streptococcal organisms are now the most common cause of bacteremia associated with periorbital cellulitis.

Test: Lumbar puncture
Significance: Indicated in cases when meningitis cannot be ruled out clinically and the patient is febrile, irritable, or appears toxic.

Test: Gram stain and culture
Significance: Needle aspiration of the leading edge of the cellulitic tissue after injecting a small amount of non-bacteriostatic sterile saline for the culture, is rarely indicated.

IMAGING

Test: CT scan
Significance: Can be useful in cases when one cannot differentiate between periorbital cellulitis and orbital cellulitis. CT scan will also reveal sinusitis, proptosis, orbital or subperiosteal abscess, or foreign body, if present.

PITFALLS

Cultures of conjunctival swabs are rarely helpful for definitive bacteriological diagnosis.

 Therapy

DRUGS

- Antibiotics selected should be β-lactamase-resistant and should cover *Streptococcus, Staphylococcus* and *H. influenzae.*
- The child should be admitted for intravenous antibiotics if appearing toxic or has evidence of disseminated disease, or if there is a purulent wound near the involved eyelid.
- If there are no signs of orbital infection or toxicity and close follow-up can be assured within 12 to 24 hours, outpatient management should be considered after giving a dose of a third-generation cephalosporin (50–75 mg of ceftriaxone per kg IM/IV).
- Oral antibiotics (e.g., amoxicillin-clavulanate or erythromycin-sulfamethoxizole) may be considered at follow-up to complete a 10-day course.

 Follow-Up

WHEN TO EXPECT IMPROVEMENT

- Ordinarily, improvement is evident within 24 to 48 hours.
- Patients should be seen daily until there are clear signs of clinical resolution and blood cultures have been negative for 48 hours.

SIGNS TO WATCH FOR

- Persistent fever
- Development of increased erythema, edema, pain, or proptosis while on antibiotics
- Evidence of other serious bacterial infection such as bacteremia/septicemia, orbital cellulitis, meningitis, arthritis, or osteomyelitis

PITFALLS

- Must rule out orbital or disseminated infection
- Must remember paranasal sinuses as possible sites of primary infection

 Common Questions and Answers

Q: Which bacteria often result in a dusky, purplish-red or "violaceous" hue of the eyelid?
A: *Haemophilus influenzae* has classically been associated with these findings, but *Streptococcus pneumoniae* may also cause this appearance.

Q: Is it safe to treat a child as an outpatient if I suspect the child of having an infection caused by Hib?
A: Any child suspected of having Hib as the etiologic agent of periorbital cellulitis, as well as any patient who appears toxic or in whom orbital infection cannot be excluded, should be hospitalized and treated with intravenous antibiotics.

BIBLIOGRAPHY

American Academy of Pediatrics. Adenovirus infections. In: *Red book: report of the Committee on Infectious Diseases,* 24th ed. Washington, DC: American Academy of Pediatrics, 1997:130.

Barone SR, Aiuto LT. Periorbital and orbital cellulitis in the Haemophilus influenzae vaccine era. *J Pediatr Ophthalmol Strabismus* 1997; 34(5):293–296.

Lessner A, Stern GA. Preseptal and orbital cellulitis. *Infect Dis Clin North Am* 1992;6(4): 933–952.

Powell KR. Orbital and periorbital cellulitis. *Pediatr Rev* 1995;16(5):163–167.

Schwartz GR, Wright SW. Changing bacteriology of periorbital cellulitis. *Ann Emerg Med* 1996; 28(6):617–620.

Author: Margaret McNamara

Perirectal Abscess

Database

DEFINITION

Abscess in the perirectal area, which may extend into surrounding soft tissues.

- Most common cause of anorectal suppuration.
- May or may not be associated with a fistula.
- Infection usually starts in the intersphincteric space, probably in one of the small anal glands.

CAUSES

- Non-specific anal gland infection
- Crohn disease
- Perforation by a foreign body
- External trauma
- Tuberculosis
- Carcinoma
- Immune deficiency (e.g., AIDS, neutropenia, diabetes mellitus)

PATHOPHYSIOLOGY

- Infection from intersphincteric space may spread vertically, horizontally, or circumferentially.
- Abscess formation is the acute phase; fistula is the chronic phase.

EPIDEMIOLOGY

- Can occur in any age group
- No racial predilection

COMPLICATIONS

- Fulminant sepsis
- Fistulas can occur if abscesses are not drained as soon as possible.

PROGNOSIS

Prognosis is good if there is early detection and drainage of abscesses.

Differential Diagnosis

- Pilonidal infection
- Hidradenitis suppurativa
- Crohn disease
- Gangrenous hemorrhoids
- Foreign body
- Tuberculosis

Data Gathering

HISTORY

- History of constipation?
- Fevers?
- Painful defecation?
- Refusing to walk?
- Rectal pain?
- Weight loss, diarrhea, abdominal pain and poor growth are symptoms associated with Crohn disease.
- Foreign body?
- Trauma?

Physical Examination

The various types of anorectal abscesses give rise to the following presentations.

Finding: Intersphincteric abscess
Significance: Is limited to the primary site. May be asymptomatic; associated with severe throbbing pain especially on defecation and continues for hours thereafter; severe enough to prevent sleep.

Finding: Perianal abscess
Significance: Result of distal vertical spread of the infection to the anal margin. Presents as tender, red swelling; often misdiagnosed as an external anal thrombosis.

Finding: Intermuscular abscess/supralevator abscess
Significance: Results of proximal vertical spread of infection. Patients usually complain of vague pelvic discomfort; rectal exam usually reveals an indurated swelling.

Finding: Ischiorectal abscess
Significance: Due to horizontal spread of infection across the external anal sphincter into the ischiorectal fossa. Sometimes infection may track across the internal anal sphincter into the anal canal. Patients may complain of pain and fever before a swelling is visible. Induration then occurs under the skin over the ischiorectal fossa and eventually a typical red fluctuant abscess is seen.

Finding: Circumferential spread
Significance: May occur from one side to the other in the intersphincteric space and can present with pain.

Laboratory Aids

- CBC
- Culture

 Therapy

- Abscesses should all be drained as soon as diagnosed.
- Pus should be sent for culture and use of antibiotics is usually reserved if infection does not respond to drainage or if gut organisms are present. The most common organism is *Escherichia coli*.
- At times, a repeat exploration of the abscess/fistula under general anesthesia may be performed to drain residual abscess.
- Sitz baths may be helpful post-procedure.

 Follow-Up

EXPECTED COURSE OF ILLNESS

- Patients usually recover well after surgical drainage of abscess.
- Fistulae may occur after aspiration of abscess.
- Additional follow-up to determine the cause of the abscess formation is crucial in attempting to prevent recurrence.

 Common Questions and Answers

Q: What are complications of this problem?
A: Fistula formation is seen in up to 25% of patients with a predilection for males.

Q: What is the most common organisms of the abscess?
A: Staphlococcus.

Q: What other disease may my child have if he has perirectal abscess?
A: Crohn disease must be excluded. If there is exposure to tuberculosis, this also must be excluded.

Q: Will the abscess recur after surgery?
A: Yes, if the disease process is secondary to a chronic disease-like inflammatory bowel disease.

Q: What treatments can be done other than surgery?
A: Antibiotics, sitz baths, and warm compresses can give symptomatic improvement.

ICD-9-CM 566

BIBLIOGRAPHY

al-Salem AH, Qaisaruddin S, Qureshi SS. Perianal abscess and fistula in ano in infancy and childhood: a clinicopathological study. *Pediatr Pathol Lab Med* 1996;16(5):755–764.

Bassford T. Treatment of common anorectal disorders. *Am Fam Physician* 1992;45(4):1787.

Festen C, van Harten H. Perianal abscess and fistula-in-ano in infants. *J Pediatr Surg* 1998;33(5):711–713.

Rosen L. Anorectal abscess-fistulae. *Surg Clin North Am* 1994;74(6):1293.

Seon-Choen F, Nicholls RJ. Anal fistula. *Br J Surg* 1993;80(12):1626.

Authors: Gregorz Telega, Helen Anita John-Kelly, and Andrew E. Mulberg

Peritonitis

Database

DEFINITION

Peritonitis is defined as inflammation of the peritoneal cavity. This inflammation may be categorized as spontaneous bacterial peritonitis (no intra-abdominal source of infection) or secondary bacterial peritonitis (intra-abdominal source of infection present).

PATHOPHYSIOLOGY

Spontaneous bacterial peritonitis (SBP) occurs when pathogenic bacteria are cultured from peritoneal fluid but no intra-abdominal surgical treatable source of infection is identified. This disease entity has gained increasing recognition as a complication in patients with ascites as a result of cirrhosis of any etiology. There have also been isolated patients reported with non-cirrhotic ascitic diseases:

- Budd-Chiari syndrome
- Congestive heart failure
- Nephrotic syndrome
- Systemic lupus erythematosis
- Rheumatoid arthritis

Secondary bacterial peritonitis results from any process leading to perforation of the gastrointestinal tract including:

- Necrotizing enterocolitis
- Volvulus with ischemia
- Intussusception with ischemia
- Trauma
- Perforation from duodenal/gastric ulcers

Translocation of organisms from the gut into the portal veins or lymphatics or, less likely, directly into the ascites may account for the source of the infection; however, other sites have been found to be infected in patients with SBP.

Therefore, the ascitic infection may be secondary to seeding from generalized bacteremia. Clearance of bacteria from the bloodstream may be impaired in patients with cirrhosis and ascites because of diminished phagocytic activity of the hepatic reticuloendothelial system (RES), which may be linked to either intrinsic cellular functional defects or shunting of blood away from the liver.

Complement, necessary for the opsonization of bacteria and ultimately clearance by phagocytes, is decreased in the ascitic fluid of patients with ascites.

EPIDEMIOLOGY

Infectious organisms include:

- Aerobic-gram negative organisms: *E. coli* (approximately 50%), *Klebsiella* (approximately 13%).
- Aerobic gram positive organisms: *Streptococcus* (approximately 19%), *Enterococcus* (5%).
- Anaerobes rarely cause SPB and polymicrobial infections occur in relatively few patients (approximately 8%).
- Urine cultures have been found to be positive for the same organism in approximately 44% of patients.
- Pneumonias and soft tissue infections have also been suggested as sources.
- In secondary bacterial peritonitis, the underlying bacterial infection tends to be a complex polymicrobial infection with an average of 2.9 to 3.9 different isolates.
- The most commonly isolated combination of organisms is *E. coli* and *Bacteroides fragilis*.
- The most common gram positive organism is non-enterococcal streptococci and enterococci.

Predisposing Factors to SBP

- Advanced liver disease
- Decreased RES activity
- Decreased serum complement levels
- Decreased ascitic protein and complement levels
- Presence of gastrointestinal hemorrhage

PROGNOSIS

- SBP is associated with a high mortality with 37% to 77% of patients dying during hospitalization.
- Retrospective studies have indicated that SBP appears to be recurrent with 51% of patients who survive the first episode going on to develop one or more recurrences.

Data Gathering

HISTORY

Clinical features depend on the stage at which peritonitis is diagnosed.

- Fever, chills?
- Generalized abdominal pain with rebound tenderness?
- Decreased bowel sounds? In SBP, approximately 10% of cases are entirely asymptomatic. Other rare findings include:
- Hypothermia?
- Hypotension?
- Diarrhea?
- Increased ascites despite diuretics?
- Encephalopathy?
- Unexplained decrease in renal function?

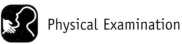

Physical Examination

- Painful palpation of abdomen
- Decreased bowel sounds

Laboratory Aids

• Diagnosis may be confirmed with paracentesis.

—To improve culture yield, culture bottles should be inoculated immediately at the bedside.

—An elevated ascitic PMN count is important in the early diagnosis of SBP and is considered the most important laboratory indicator of SBP.

• Diagnostic criteria for SBP include:

—Polymorphonuclear leukocyte counts of greater than 250/mm^3
—Ascitic fluid culture usually for a single organism.

• Diagnostic criteria for secondary bacterial peritonitis include:

—Ascitic fluid culture positive for polymicrobial infection.
—Total protein greater than 1 g/dL
—Glucose less than 50 mg/dL
—LDH greater than 225 mU/mL

 ## Therapy

• Support the patient's cardiovascular and respiratory systems.
• Control the underlying infection with antibiotics or surgery (in secondary bacterial peritonitis). Empirical antibiotic coverage should be directed primarily toward enteric gram negative aerobes and gram positive cocci.
• In SBP, Cefotaxime, a third-generation cephalosporin, has been shown to have higher resolution of infection and lower hospital mortality than the traditional Ampicillin and an aminoglycoside as empiric coverage.
• Once the organism is identified the antibiotic coverage may be optimized.
• For patients at significant risk for SBP, selective intestinal decontamination is effective in preventing bacterial infections. Antibiotics that have been studied for this use include:

—Norfloxacin
—Ciprofloxacin
—Trimethoprim-sulphamethoxazole

In SBP, surgery is the primary management tool with control of the source of the intra-abdominal infection. No particular antibiotic regimen has been shown to be superior in controlled clinical trials. Both single agents and combination regimens have been used. For mild to moderately severe infections, single drug regimens have included:

• Cefoxitin
• Cefotetan
• Cefmetazole
• Ticarcillin

Combination regimens that have been used include:

• Flagyl or Clindamycin plus aminoglycoside
• Flagyl or Clindamycin plus a third-generation cephalosporin
• Clindamycin plus aztreonam
• For severe infections, imipenem-cilastin has been used.

COMPLICATIONS

• Hypovolemia results from extra vascular extravasation and sequestration from the inflamed peritoneal membrane and the intravascular volume must be supported with crystalloids and blood products.
• Respiration may be impaired via mechanical mechanisms through diaphragmatic spasm and reflex abdominal rigidity and through increased permeability of the pulmonary vasculature in response to systemic inflammation.
• The role of surgery is to gain control of the underlying source of the abdominal infection by repairing the affected bowel through laparotomy/laparoscopy. The degree of contamination may be decreased through intraoperative peritoneal lavage, and debridement of loculations and abscesses. Adding antibiotics to lavage fluid has lost favor after the discovery that this procedure appears to impair neutrophil chemotaxis, inhibit neutrophil bacteriocidal activity, and increases the formation of adhesions. Catheters may be placed to drain well-defined abscess cavity, form a controlled fistula, or provide access for continuous postoperative peritoneal lavage.

 ## Common Questions and Answers

Q: Is peritonitis common in children with ascites?
A: Despite the frequency of ascites from many different causes, peritonitis occurs rarely.

Q: What are the most useful laboratory aids for this diagnosis?
A: Analysis of the fluid for pH, glucose content and amount of inflammatory cells provides the most useful information regarding the diagnosis of peritonitis.

ICD-9-CM 567.9

BIBLIOGRAPHY

Farber MS, Abrams JH. Antibiotics or the acute abdomen. *Surg Clin North Am* 1997;77(6):1395–1417.

Garcoa-Tsao G. Spontaneous bacterial peritonitis. *Gastroenterol Clin North Am* 1992;21(1): 257–275.

Guarner C, Soriano G. Spontaneous bacterial peritonitis. *Semin Liver Dis* 1997;17(3): 203–217.

Nathans AB, Rotstein OD. Therapeutic options in peritonitis. *Surg Clin North Am* 1994;74(3): 6577–6592.

Author: Donna Zeiter

Peritonsillar Abscess

 Database

DEFINITION

Infectious complication of tonsillitis or pharyngitis resulting in an accumulation of purulence in the tonsillar fossa.

CAUSE

- Group A beta-hemolytic *Streptococcus* (GABHS)
- *Staphylococcus aureus*
- Anaerobic bacteria

PATHOPHYSIOLOGY

- Infectious tonsillo/pharyngitis progresses from cellulitis to abscess.
- Purulence collects within one, and sometimes both, tonsillar fossa.
- Tonsillar and peritonsillar edema may lead to compromise of the upper airway.

EPIDEMIOLOGY

- Seen most commonly in adolescents, but occasionally in younger children

ASSOCIATED ILLNESS

Tonsillitis or pharyngitis usually precede its development.

COMPLICATIONS

Upper airway obstruction is the most feared complication.

PROGNOSIS

Complete, swift recovery can be expected with appropriate therapy.

 Differential Diagnosis

- Peritonsillar cellulitis: the most common diagnostic consideration; can be distinguished by its lack of peritonsillar space "fullness," uvular deviation, dysphonia, and trismus
- Retropharyngeal abscess: Minimal peritonsillar findings, along with a widened prevertebral space on lateral neck x-ray is diagnostic of this airway-compromising disease, which almost always occurs in preschool children.
- Epiglottitis: This life-threatening airway emergency presents abruptly with fever, stridor, increased work of breathing, and drooling; usually occurs in toxic-appearing children 3 to 7 years of age but becoming a rare entity advent of haemophilus influenzae type B.
- Other infectious etiologies of severe tonsillo/pharyngitis: Epstein-Barr virus (infectious mononucleosis), coxsackievirus (herpangina), *Corynebacterium diphtheriae*, *Neisseria gonorrhoeae*

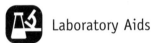 Data Gathering

HISTORY

Question: Fever and sore throat?
Significance: These are the most common initial complaints.

Question: Trouble swallowing, pain with opening the mouth (trismus), muffled ("hot-potato") voice; unilateral neck or ear pain are also common.
Significance: Classic presenting symptoms.

 Physical Examination

Finding: Unilateral peritonsillar fullness or bulging of the posterior, superior soft palate with uvular deviation.
Significance: Diagnostic

Finding: Palpable fluctuance
Significance: May be appreciated and calls for urgent aspiration.

Finding: The pharynx is erythematous and edematous, with enlarged and exudative tonsils.
Significance: Co-existing tonsillo-pharyngitis is common.

Finding: Cervical adenopathy
Significance: Common

Finding: Drooling
Significance: Often present

Finding: Torticollis
Significance: Sometimes seen

Laboratory Aids

Test: White blood cell count
Significance: Usually elevated with prominent "left shift."

Test: Rapid streptococcal throat antigen studies
Significance: Helpful to diagnose GABHS infection.

Test: Gram stain and culture of aspirate specimen
Significance: Confirms causative microorganism.

Test: CT scan or ultrasound
Significance: Differentiation of peritonsillar cellulitis from peritonsillar abscess.

Therapy

- True abscesses should be urgently/emergently drained via either needle aspiration or surgical incision and drainage.
- Antibiotic therapy can be initiated with high-dose intravenous penicillin.
- Clindamycin, nafcillin, oxacillin, or first-generation cephalosporins (e.g., cefazolin, etc.) can be used if staphylococcal and/or anaerobic bacteria are cultured or suspected.
- Surgical drainage with tonsillectomy should be considered in children not responding to parenteral antibiotics within 24 to 48 hours.
- Appropriate analgesia and adequate hydration should be ensured.

 Follow-Up

- Patients may be discharged on oral antibiotics to complete a 10- to 14-day course when afebrile and peritonsillar swelling has subsided.
- Recurrence of peritonsillar abscesses are not uncommon.
- Tonsillectomy should be considered after severe or recurrent peritonsillar abscesses.

PREVENTION

Abscess formation can often be prevented if appropriate antimicrobial therapy is initiated while the infection is still in the cellulitis stage.

PITFALLS

Treating a true abscess without incision and drainage is inadequate and can have airway-threatening implications.

 Common Questions and Answers

Q: Are radiographs necessary to make the diagnosis of peritonsillar abscess?
A: No. The physical examination is diagnostic; a lateral neck radiograph is useful only if retropharyngeal abscess or epiglottitis are diagnostic concerns.

Q: Is surgical consultation necessary in cases of peritonsillar abscess?
A: Yes. Otorhinolaryngology consultation is indicated both for acute as well as chronic management.

ICD-9-CM 475

BIBLIOGRAPHY

Fleisher GR, Ludwig S, eds. Textbook of pediatric emergency medicine, 3rd ed. Baltimore: Williams & Wilkins, 1993.

Friedman NR, Mitchell RB, Pereira KD, Younis RT, Lazar RH. Peritonsillar abscess in early childhood. Presentation and management. *Arch Otolaryngol Head Neck Surg* 1997;123(6): 630–632.

Herzon FS, Harris P. Mosher Award thesis. Peritonsillar abscess: incidence, current management practices, and a proposal for treatment guidelines. *Laryngoscope* 1995;105(8 Pt 3 Suppl. 74):1–17.

Herzon FS, Nicklaus P. Pediatric peritonsillar abscess: management guidelines. *Curr Probl Pediatr* 1996;26(8):270–278.

Passy V. Pathogenesis of peritonsillar abscess. *Laryngoscope* 1994;104(2):185–190.

Savolainen S, Jousimies-Somer HR, Makitie AA, Ylikoski JS. Peritonsillar abscess. Clinical and microbiologic aspects and treatment regimens. *Arch Otolaryngol Head Neck Surg* 1993;119: 521–524.

Strong EB, Woodward PJ, Johnson LP. Intraoral ultrasound evaluation of peritonsillar abscess. *Laryngoscope* 1995;105(8 Pt 1):779–782.

Weinberg E, Brodsky L, Stanievich J, Volk M. Needle aspiration of peritonsillar abscess in children. *Arch Otolaryngol Head Neck Surg* 1993;119:169–172.

Author: Nicholas Tsarouhas

Persistent Pulmonary Hypertension of the Newborn (PPHN)

 Database

DEFINITION

- Clinical syndrome of severe respiratory insufficiency manifesting as hypoxia in an infant with or without significant parenchymal pulmonary disease in the first few days of life in the absence of congenital heart disease.
- It is characterized by persistence of right-to-left shunting of blood through fetal channels as a result of sustained elevation of pulmonary vascular resistence following birth.
- PPHN is considered to represent a failure of adaptation of the fetal pulmonary circulation to postnatal conditions.

CAUSES

Pulmonary Venous Hypertension

- Left-sided cardiac obstructive lesions
- Left ventricular failure from severe hypoxia or congenital heart disease

Functional Obstruction

- Polycythemia

Pulmonary Arterial Vasoconstriction

- Maladaptation (abnormal vascular response)

—Developmental immaturity (idiopathic)
—Acute lung injury: sepsis, asphyxia, meconium aspiration syndrome, hyaline membrane disease, maternal lithium or dilantin therapy

- Maldevelopment (increased muscularization)

—Idiopathic or chronic intrauterine hypoxia
—Premature closure of ductus arteriosus

Pulmonary Hypoplasia

- Primary, or secondary to oligohydramnios
- Congenital diaphragmatic hernia
- Congenital chylothorax
- Neuromuscular disease
- Congenital bronchopulmonary malformations

PATHOPHYSIOLOGY

- In the fetus only 5% to 10% of the combined ventricular output flows to the lungs as a result of active pulmonary vasoconstriction (mediated by relative hypoxia) and shunting of the blood across the foramen ovale and ductus arteriosus.
- At birth, a dramatic decrease in pulmonary vascular resistance (PVR) allows 50% of the combined ventricular output to be redirected to the lungs. This process is mediated by physical tethering of capillaries by adjacent alveoli, oxygenation and lowering of CO_2 tension. It is dependent on the release of local vasodilators: nitric oxide (endothelial derived relaxing factor), bradykinin, and prostacyclin. Additional decline in PVR is associated with vascular remodeling over the next 2 weeks.

GENETICS

- Capillary alveolar dysplasia is primarily sporadic, but one familial occurrence has been documented.
- SP-B deficiency: autosomal recessive condition.

EPIDEMIOLOGY

- Incidence: 1 in 1000 newborns, and 5% of NICU admissions.
- Occurs mostly in term neonates but also occurs in preterm neonates.
- Postmature newborns with meconium-stained amniotic fluid are at an increased risk due to chronic uteroplacental insufficiency.

COMPLICATIONS

Short Term

- Pneumothorax
- Pulmonary interstitial emphysema
- Pulmonary edema
- Hypoxic ischemic encephalopathy
- Myocardial dysfunction and hypotension
- Capillary leak

Long Term

- Chronic lung disease—25%
- Reactive airway disease—25%
- Feeding difficulties and gastroesophageal reflux—20%
- Slow growth—25%
- Cerebral palsy and developmental delay—12%
- Seizure disorder
- Sensorineural deafness

PROGNOSIS

- PPHN is a self-limited disease.
- Most patients including those treated with extracorporeal membrane oxygenation (ECMO), will survive with good neurological outcome.
- Mortality rates vary with underlying etiology, the highest being associated with congenital diaphragmatic hernia and the lowest with meconium aspiration. Overall mortality is 20%.

 Differential Diagnosis

CYANOTIC CONGENITAL HEART DISEASE

- Obstruction to pulmonary venous return: total anomalous pulmonary venous return with obstruction, hypoplastic left heart, congenital mitral stenosis, cor triatrium
- Obstruction to left ventricular outflow tract: critical aortic stenosis, coarctation, interrupted aortic arch, rarely aortic thrombosis
- Ventricular dysfunction: Ebstein anomaly, endocardial fibroelastosis, myocarditis
- Obligatory left-to-right shunt: arteriovenous malformation, endocardial cushion defect, transposition of great arteries with intact ventricular septum

PULMONARY PARENCHYMAL DISEASE

- Pneumonia
- ARDS
- Hyaline membrane disease
- Aspiration syndromes (meconium, blood, amniotic fluid)

CONGENITAL BRONCHOPULMONARY MALFORMATIONS

- Alveolar capillary dysplasia: misalignment of alveolar capillary endothelium and pulmonary epithelium
- Congenital cystic adenomatoid malformation
- Surfactant protein B (SP-B) deficiency: complete absence of SP-B
- Congenital chylothorax
- Congenital diaphragmatic hernia

AIRWAY OBSTRUCTION

- Tracheomalacia
- Pierre Robin syndrome

 Data Gathering

HISTORY

Question: Details concerning the pregnancy?
Significance: Gestation, oligo/polyhydramnios, fetal anatomy on ultrasound, maternal illness and medications (e.g., NSAIDs, anticonvulsants).

Question: Details regarding labor?
Significance: Difficult, prolonged or complicated delivery, cord pH, evidence of fetal distress, meconium staining or bloody amniotic fluid.

Question: Risk factors for sepsis?
Significance: Prolonged rupture of membranes (>18 hours), maternal chorioamnionitis and urinary tract infection, positive maternal cervical culture for Group B streptococcus, intrapartum antibiotic prophylaxis.

Question: Onset of respiratory distress following birth?
Significance: Immediate (cardiac, sepsis or congenital malformations), insidious, or late in the first day.

 Physical Examination

The newborn with PPHN will nearly always display central cyanosis and respiratory distress, but these signs are common and not specific to PPHN. One must exclude other possible causes for the infant's distress. The following physical signs support a diagnosis of PPHN:

GENERAL

- Periods of central cyanosis alternating with pinkness
- Signs of intrauterine compression (Potter sequence)

Persistent Pulmonary Hypertension of the Newborn (PPHN)

RESPIRATORY DISTRESS

- Nasal flaring
- Grunting
- Tachypnea
- Intercostal and supraclavicular retractions

CHEST

- Increased anteroposterior diameter ("barrel chest") with meconium aspiration

BREATH SOUNDS

- Clear with primary idiopathic PPHN
- Coarse sounds or rales with pneumonia, aspiration, or pulmonary edema
- Diminished with diaphragmatic hernia, pulmonary hypoplasia, effusions, pneumothorax

CARDIAC

- Prominent murmur of tricuspid regurgitation

 ## Laboratory Aids

Test: Arterial blood gas
Significance: A difference of greater than 20 mm Hg between pre- and post-ductal arterial PO_2 indicates ductal right-to-left shunting and will not be seen if shunting is at the atrial level. A PaO_2 greater than 200 mm Hg in a post-ductal ABG during a hyperoxia test (100% oxygen administered for 10 minutes) rules out cyanotic congenital heart disease. A dramatic rise in PaO_2 with hyperventilation during the hyperoxia test confirms PPHN.

Test: Liver function tests
Significance: For evidence of liver injury from hypoxia and ishemia.

Test: Complete blood count
Significance: Left shift and neutropenia may be seen with sepsis.

- Blood culture
- Herpes simplex viral (HSV) cultures from eye, urine, and endotracheal aspirate if relevant.
- ECG: Abnormal axis seen in congenital heart disease.

RADIOGRAPHIC STUDIES

Test: Chest x-ray
Significance: Delineates associated parenchymal lung disease and presence/absence of pneumothorax or pneumomediostinum. Interstitial pattern of infiltrate is characteristic of idiopathic PPHN. Cardiac silhouette is often normal. Pulmonary vascular markings are normal or diminished.

Test: Echocardiography
Significance: Essential to confirm the diagnosis, and to rule out congenital heart disease. Determines the presence and degree of intracardiac shunting, estimates the pulmonary arterial pressure in presence of tricuspid or pulmonary re-

gurgitation, and estimates left ventricular function, which is necessary for determining the type of ECMO therapy used.

Test: Head ultrasound
Significance: Not mandatory, but useful to document preexisting intracranial pathology before ECMO is initiated.

 ## Therapy

- All neonates should be promptly transferred to a regional level III NICU having treatment modalities, such as high frequency ventilation, nitric oxide, and ECMO.
- Administer 100% oxygen.
- Place pre- and post-ductal pulse oximeters.
- Obtain post-ductal and pre-ductal (if saturation gradient evident) arterial blood gases.
- Obtain chest radiograph, CBC, and blood culture
- Start broad spectrum antibiotics.
- Intubate and place umbilical catheters without delay in those requiring 100% oxygen to maintain normal oxygenation and in those with elevated CO_2.
- Minimize stimulation.
- Correct metabolic acidosis.
- Start dopamine infusion if hypotensive.
- Treat underlying etiology if obvious.
- Conservatively wean therapeutic measures that have proved effective.
- Reduce pulmonary vascular resistance and eliminate intracardiac shunting.
- Maintain adequate systemic perfusion and pressure.

MODALITIES

- 100% oxygen and mechanical ventilation: conventional or high frequency oscillator, which oxygenates at less traumatic airway pressures. Maintain PO_2 between 80 to 100 mm Hg and PCO_2 within normal range.
- Paralysis and sedation: to minimize barotrauma and stress, and to prevent severe fluctuations in oxygenation during routine care.
- Maintain adequate systemic perfusion and arterial pressure with infusion of colloids and inotropes. Avoid iatrogenic hypertension.
- Vasodilator therapy:

—Metabolic alkalosis: the pulmonary vasculature is sensitive to pH rather than PCO_2. In those who respond to alkalosis as evidenced by improvement in oxygenation following a bolus of bicarbonate, pH is maintained above 7.5 by infusion of sodium bicarbonate. Hyperventilation to induce respiratory alkalosis should be avoided, and may contribute to deafness and chronic lung disease.

- Surfactant therapy: administered in those with functional (e.g., meconium aspiration syndrome) or quantitative deficiency (e.g., hyaline membrane disease).

- ECMO: used in most severely affected infants with predicted mortality of 80%. Most centers use veno-venous ECMO routinely in those with good cardiac function, and avoid cannulation of the carotid artery. Most expensive therapy, labor intensive and associated with numerous complications, such as intracranial bleed, infarction, sepsis, and metabolic disturbances. Current overall survival is 83%; and 97% for meconium aspiration.

 ## Follow-Up

All infants with PPHN should be followed at regular intervals by a developmental pediatrician for at least 2 years to look for sequelae of mechanical ventilation and monitor growth, pulmonary function, neuromotor development, and hearing.

PITFALLS

- Congenital heart disease and PPHN may coexist. Diagnosing one does not rule out the other. Infants who never attain adequate PO_2 and those who fail to improve after 5 days on ECMO should be re-evaluated for congenital heart disease.
- All modalities of treatment have potential for serious complications. Close attention to oxygenation and prompt treatment of underlying etiology is extremely important.

 ## Common Questions and Answers

Q: What are the long-term complications of ECMO therapy?
A: Intracranial bleeds and/or infarcts, and seizures are two major short-term complications; and, respectively, occur in about 10% and 20% of candidates. Long-term follow up reveals a 20% incidence of mild developmental delay, with severe handicap in 5% (all with cerebral infarcts). Eighty percent have normal developmental outcome.

ICD-9-CM 416

BIBLIOGRAPHY

Finer NN, Barrington KJ. Nitric Oxide in respiratory failure on the newborn infant. *Semin Perinatol* 1997;21:426–440.

Sahni R, Wung JT, James LS. Controversies in management of persistent pulmonary hypertension of newborn. *Pediatrics* 1994;94(3):307–309.

Steinhorn RH. Persistent pulmonary hypertension of the newborn. *Acta Anaesthsiol Scand Suppl* 1997;111:135–140.

Walsh-Sukys MC. Persistent pulmonary hypertension of the newborn: the black box re-visited. *Clin Perinatol* 1993;21:127–143.

Author: Sameer Wagle

Perthe Disease

 Database

DEFINITION

Self-limited osteonecrosis of the proximal femoral epiphysis of unknown etiology, probably related to trauma and vascular insult, that affects children.

CAUSES

Unknown; probably related to a combination of trauma and vascular insult (recent evidence suggests thrombophilia).

PATHOLOGY

• Four stages

—Initial: bone necrosis
—Fragmentation: fragmentation of necrotic bone with early revascularization
—Reossification: revascularization, resorption, and repair via creeping substitution
—Healing: remodeling

EPIDEMIOLOGY

• Seen most commonly between ages 4 to 8 years
• Boys affected more than girls, with ratio of 4.5:1
• 10% bilateral
• Majority have delayed bone age
• More common in lower socioeconomic groups

GENETICS

• No strong evidence to suggest that Perthes is an inherited condition.

COMPLICATIONS

• Osteoarthritis
• Mild limb length discrepancy
• Restriction of hip range of motion
• Pain, limping

PROGNOSIS

• Based on the following factors:

—Age of the patient at the onset of the disease; if onset older than 8 years of age, poorer prognosis than if onset at younger age
—Extent of femoral head involvement; if greater than one-half of epiphysis involved, poorer prognosis
—Subluxation of femoral head, poorer prognosis
—Growth disturbance of the physis, poorer prognosis

 Differential Diagnosis

• Toxic synovitis
• Chondrolysis
• Infection
• Juvenile rheumatoid arthritis
• Rheumatic fever
• Tuberculosis of the hip
• Tumors
• Meyer dysplasia
• Bone dysplasias

—Multiple epiphyseal dysplasia
—Trichorhinophalangeal syndrome
—Spondyloepiphyseal dysplasia

• Hypothyroidism, juvenile cretinism
• Sickle cell disease, hemophilia
• Gaucher disease

 Data Gathering

HISTORY

Question: Limping?
Significance: Weeks to months duration.

Question: Hip, thigh, or knee pain?
Significance: Insidious onset.

 Physical Examination

Finding: Limitation of range of motion
Significance: Especially internal rotation and abduction.

Finding: Irritability and tenderness of hip joint area
Significance: Early usually

Finding: Atrophy of thigh
Significance: Late finding

Finding: Slight shortening of affected limb
Significance: Due to collapse (real) or contracture (apparent)

Finding: True hip joint irritability
Significance: Early finding indicating intraarticular synovitis

Finding: Trendelenburg gait
Significance: Leaning over affected leg during stance, due to mechanical disadvantage from collapse.

SPECIAL QUESTIONS

Finding: Distribution of pain may follow the sensory distribution of the obturator nerve.
Significance: Medial thigh and knee.

PHYSICAL EXAMINATION TRICKS

The Trendelenburg test is positive when a patient stands on the affected side and the pelvis drops on the opposite side.

 Laboratory Aids

Test: Laboratory tests
Significance: Generally are not helpful, but may be necessary to rule out other conditions such as infection.

IMAGING STAGES

1. Incipient stage
2. Aseptic or avascular stage
3. Fragmentation stage
4. Residual or remodeling stage

• The first radiographic sign of Perthes is smaller size of the femoral head epiphysis and a widened articular cartilage space compared with the other side; the second sign is the subchondral fracture.

Therapy

- Most do not need treatment.
- Treatment needed generally for those with more severe involvement (Salter B).
- Two basic treatment principles.

—Restoration of range of motion.
—Containment of the femoral head epiphysis in the acetabulum.

- General treatment modalities.

—Weight relief
—Physical therapy
—Bed rest
—Traction
—Bracing
—Surgery

DRUGS

- NSAIDS for pain and inflammation

DURATION

Generally continues until patient enters the re-ossification phase.

 Follow-Up

WHEN TO EXPECT IMPROVEMENT

- The magnitude and duration of symptoms depends on the age of the patient at onset of the disease and the degree of involvement of the disease process. Most patients show improvement in symptoms by 6 months after the onset of disease.
- Patients with Perthes disease should be seen and followed by a pediatric or general orthopedic surgeon.

SIGNS TO WATCH FOR

- Stiffness
- Limping
- Pain
- Subluxation of the hip joint

PROGNOSIS

- Overall, good prognosis for the majority of patients

PITFALLS

The majority of patients with Perthes disease do not need treatment. For those who do, early recognition and appropriate early referral are key.

 Common Questions and Answers

Q: How long do you observe a patient with hip pain before ordering an X-ray?
A: It depends on the presence or absence of abnormalities on the physical examination. If any of the signs mentioned above are seen in conjunction with significant hip pain, an X-ray is indicated.

Q: Why do patients with hip pathology have knee pain?
A: This is because the nerves that innervate the hip joint also have cutaneous sensory distributions. Both the obturator and femoral nerves innervate the hip joint and both also have cutaneous sensory distribution in the region of the knee joint.

ICD-9-CM 732.1

BIBLIOGRAPHY

Harrison MH. Bassett CA. The results of a double-blind trial of pulsed electromagnetic frequency in the treatment of Perthes' disease. *J Pediatr Orthop* 1997:17(2):264–265.

Kaniklides C, Lonnerholm T, Moberg A, Sahlstedt B. Legg-Calve-Perthes disease. Comparison of conventional radiography, MR imaging, bone scintigraphy and arthrography. *Acta Radiol* 1995;36(4):434–439.

Salter RB. The present status of surgical treatment of Legg-Perthes disease: current concept review. *J Bone Joint Surg* 1984;66A:961.

Weinstein SL. Legg-Calve-Perthes disease. In: Morrissy RT, Weinstein SL, eds. Lovell and Winter's pediatric orthopaedics, 4th ed. Philadelphia: Lippincott Raven, 1996:951–992.

Author: John P. Dormans

Pertussis

Database

DEFINITION

• *Bordetella pertussis* is a small, non-motile, fastidious, gram-negative rod.
• The first description of the disease appeared in 1578 during an epidemic in Paris, France.

PATHOPHYSIOLOGY

• Replicates only in association with ciliated epithelium, causing congestion and inflammation of the bronchi; peribronchial lymphoid hyperplasia followed by a necrotizing process occurs and results in a bronchopneumonia; atelectasis can occur due to bronchiolar obstruction from accumulated secretions.
• Filamentous hemagglutinin (FHA), lymphocytosis promoting factor (LPF), and adenylate cyclase play a role in the organism's attachment and adversely affect immune cell function.
• The long incubation period (7–21 days) reflects the time necessary for *B. pertussis* to increase in numbers needed for progressive spread of infection in the respiratory tract and produce enough toxin for eliciting damage and dysfunction of the respiratory epithelium.
• Respiratory illness characterized as a bronchopneumonia.
• Apnea is a common manifestation in the young infant, <6 months of age. The characteristic "whoop" can be absent.

EPIDEMIOLOGY

• A disease of young children; the infant either nonimmunized or partially immunized is at greatest risk.
• Approximately one-third of cases reported to the Centers for Disease Control are in infants, <6 months.
• Disease in adolescents and adults is not usually recognized as pertussis despite a cough that is paroxysmal and may last for weeks. Despite improved vaccination rates in the U.S. pertussis infection rates have steadily risen since the early 1980s. This is felt to attributed to growth of a susceptible adult population and these patients are the major source of pertussis infection in children.
• Route of spread includes aerosolized respiratory droplets, direct contact with nasal secretions, and indirect contact with secretions through hand contact.

COMPLICATIONS

• Pneumonia, the most frequent complication, is responsible for more than 90% of deaths in young children with pertussis, is usually owing to secondary bacterial disease rather than *B. pertussis* itself.
• Atelectasis and interstitial or subcutaneous emphysema can also occur.
• Seizures (3%) and encephalopathy (0.9%) have been observed in infants with pertussis although these findings may be related to fever causing febrile convulsions and cerebral hypoxia due to the pulmonary complications.

PROGNOSIS

The prognosis is directly related to patient age; the highest mortality is observed in infants, <6 months of age. Infants have a 0.5% to 1% risk of death whereas, in the older child, prognosis is good.

Differential Diagnosis

• *B. parapertussis* and adenoviruses
• *B. pertussis*
• Bronchiolitis
• Bacterial pneumonia
• Cystic fibrosis
• Tuberculosis
• Foreign body aspiration should also be considered.

Data Gathering

HISTORY

Question: What are clinical stages of pertussis infection?
Significance:

• Three stages:

—Catarrhal stage (1–2 weeks) with symptoms of an upper respiratory infection
—Paroxysmal stage (2–4 weeks or longer) characterized by paroxysmal cough with increased severity and frequency producing the characteristic whoop during the sudden forceful inspiratory phase; post-tussive vomiting is also observed during this stage.
—The convalescent stage begins and lasts 1 to 2 weeks but cough can persist for several months. In the adolescent or adult, longstanding cough of 2 to 3 weeks is the hallmark symptom. Most will report a paroxysmal or staccato quality to the cough.

Physical Examination

• Rhinorrhea, lacrimation, conjunctival hyperemia and fever seen in the early stage of disease.
• Cyanosis observed during the paroxysmal stage.
• Lung auscultatory examination is usually normal unless significant atelectasis or pneumonia have occurred.

Laboratory Aids

Test: CBC
Significance: Leukocytosis with predominant lymphocytosis (77%) is commonly observed at the end of the catarrhal stage and throughout the paroxysmal stage of illness, although this phenomenon is not frequently observed in infants.

Test: Chest radiographs
Significance: May reveal perihilar infiltrates or a "shaggy right heart border" although these findings can be seen with other respiratory infections.

Test: Culture of *B. pertussis*
Significance: Achieved using calcium alginate or Dacron swabs of the nasopharynx and plated onto selective media such as Regan-Lowe or Bordet-Gengou and incubated for 7 days.

Test: Culture isolation of *B. pertussis*
Significance: Most frequently successful during the catarrhal or early paroxysmal stages and is rarely found beyond the fourth week of illness. The overall sensitivity is 60% to 70%.

Test: Direct immunofluorescent assays of nasopharyngeal specimens
Significance: Can provide a rapid and specific diagnosis but is limited by the experience of the laboratory personnel for interpretation.

Test: Polymerase chain reaction (PCR) techniques
Significance: Now available, have been shown to have a higher sensitivity than culture in the detection of *B. pertussis* from nasopharyngeal specimens.

Test: Recently developed monoclonal immunofluorescent antibody (BL-5)
Significance: Has been shown to be at least as sensitive and specific as culture but needs additional investigation.

Test: Serology
Significance: Currently, no single serologic test with adequate sensitivity and specificity is available for clinical use.

Therapy

- Patients with more severe disease manifestations (apnea, cyanosis, feeding difficulties) or other complications require hospitalization for supportive care.
- If antibiotic treatment is initiated during the catarrhal stage, it can prevent disease from progressing. Antibiotics have not been shown to shorten the course of illness if begun during the paroxysmal stage, although it will eliminate the organism from the nasopharynx within 3 to 4 days, thus shortening the potential for contagion.
- Erythromycin (50 mg/kg/d) in four doses for 14 days is recommended; an alternative dose with 40 mg/kg of erythromycin estolate twice a day for 14 days has shown equal efficacy.
- For patients not able to tolerate erythromycin, trimethoprim-sulfamethoxazole has been recommended, although its efficacy is unproved.
- Corticosteroids and β-agonist aerosols have shown anecdotal evidence in reducing the paroxysms of cough, although additional evaluation is needed.

Follow-Up

- The paroxysmal stage can last up to 4 weeks and the convalescent stage up to several months and can be quite problematic for patient and family.
- The complications of pertussis are more likely to occur in the younger infant and therefore tend to have a more serious, protracted course.

PITFALLS

The most likely source of pertussis in young infants is from the adolescent or adult with mild symptoms of pertussis. Therefore, a high index of suspicion must exist in this population before adequate control of exposure to the partially or un-immunized infant can be successful.

PREVENTION

Infection Control

- Isolation of hospitalized patient: respiratory isolation for 5 days after starting erythromycin therapy or until at least 3 weeks after the onset of the paroxysmal stage, if antibiotics were not given, is recommended.
- Control measures: exposed individuals (all household contacts, other close contacts, other children in child care) should receive erythromycin chemoprophylaxis to limit secondary transmission, regardless of immunization status.

Immunizations

- Vaccinations available in the United States include whole cell and, more recently, acellular vaccines in combination with diphtheria and tetanus toxoids. Universal immunization of the preschool child is paramount to control the rate of infection.
- The whole cell DTP should be used for the first 3 doses in infants and children and the acellular vaccine may be used for the fourth and fifth doses for children at least 15 months old.
- It seems prudent to vaccinate adults with periodic booster vaccinations given the risk they create for young infants.

Common Questions and Answers

Q: Are there any risks associated with the pertussis vaccine?
A: There are local and febrile reactions that are common to the DTP vaccine; anaphylaxis is estimated to occur in 2 cases/100,000 injections; risk of seizures occurring within 48 hours of administration is 1:1750 doses and is believed to be due to a febrile seizure; inconsolable crying for 3 or more hours is observed in 1:100 doses given; a hypertonic-hyporesponsive episode occurs in 1:1750 doses. Because of the temporal relation between administration of pertussis vaccine and severe adverse events such as death, encephalopathy, developmental delay with learning and behavioral problems or onset of seizures, much publicity has been given to this vaccine, yet causation has not been established.

Q: What are the contraindications to pertussis vaccination?
A: Contraindications to avoid initial or subsequent doses of pertussis vaccine include the following: an immediate anaphylactic reaction, encephalopathy within 7 days of a prior injection or a seizure within 3 days or persistent crying, a shock-like state or fever greater than 104.9°F within 48 hours of a prior injection. A progressive neurological disorder or history of seizure disorder are contraindications also.

ICD-9-CM 033.9

BIBLIOGRAPHY

Bass JW, Wittler RR. Return of epidemic pertussis in the United States. *Pediatr Infect Dis J* 1994;13:343.

Black S. Epidemiology of pertussis. *Pediatr Infect Dis J* 1997;16:S85–S89.

Cromer BA, Goydos J, Hackell J, et al. Unrecognized pertussis infections in adolescents. *Am J Dis Child* 1993;147:575.

Edwards KM. Pertussis in older children and adults. *Adv Pediatr Infect Dis* 1998;13:49–77

Feigin RD. Pertussis. In: Feigin RD, Cherry JD, eds. Textbook of pediatric infectious diseases, 3rd ed. Philadelphia: WB Saunders, 1990:1208.

Gordon M, Davies HD, Gold R. Clinical and microbiologic features of children presenting with pertussis to a Canadian Pediatric Hospital during and eleven-year period. *Pediatr Infect Dis J* 1994;13:617.

He Q, Mertsola J, Soini H, Viljanen MK. Sensitive and specific polymerase chain reaction assays for detection of Bordetella pertussis in nasopharyngeal specimens. *J Pediatr* 1994;124:421.

Hewlett EL. Pertussis: current concepts of pathogenesis and prevention. *Pediatr Infect Dis* 1997;16:S78–S84.

Hoppe JE. Comparison of erythromycin estolate and erythromycin ethylsuccinate for treatment of pertussis. *Pediatr Infect Dis J* 1992;11:189.

Muller FMC, Hoppe JE, Wirsing Von Konig CH. Laboratory diagnosis of pertussis: state of the art in 1997. *J Clin Microbiol* 1997;35:2435–2443.

Peter G, Halsey NA, Marcuse EK, Pickering LK. Pertussis. In: 1994 red book: report of the Committee on Infectious Diseases, 23rd ed. Elk Grove Village, IL: American Academy of Pediatrics, 1994:355.

Taranger J, Trollfors B, Lind L, et al. Environmental contamination leading to false positive polymerase chain reaction for pertussis. *Pediatr Infect Dis J* 1994;13:936.

Author: Philip V. Scribano

Pharyngitis

 Database

DEFINITION

Pharyngitis (i.e., sore throat) is inflammation of the mucous membranes and underlying structures of the pharynx and tonsils, usually secondary to viral or bacterial infection.

EPIDEMIOLOGY

• Streptococcal pharyngitis is most common in children 5 to 15 years of age; peak incidence is in the winter.
• Viral disease is more common in younger children during winter months.
• Day care attendance is a risk factor.

COMPLICATIONS

• Streptococcal pharyngitis—suppurative and non-suppurative complications.
• Infectious mononucleosis (IM) due to Epstein-Barr virus (EBV): complicated by upper airway obstruction due to tonsillar hypertrophy and splenic rupture, due to associated splenomegaly. Postanginal sepsis: can also occur in adolescents or young adults following IM.

PROGNOSIS

• Streptococcal pharyngitis: usually excellent. Morbidity associated with acute rheumatic fever (ARF) and acute post-streptococcal glomerulonephritis (APGN).
• Viral pharyngitis is usually self-limited.
• Rare mortalities from splenic rupture in IM.

 Differential Diagnosis (in approximate order of frequency)

VIRAL

• Adenovirus types 1 through 7, 7a, 9, 14, 15, and 16 are the most common cause of nasopharyngitis overall.

—Often a follicular exudative pharyngotonsillitis
—May occur in association with conjunctivitis (pharyngoconjunctival fever)

• Epstein-Barr virus (EBV)
• Influenza A, B: usually associated with more severe systemic complaints.
• Parainfluenza 1, 2, and 3.
• Enteroviruses

—Often with ulcerative lesions (herpangina or hand-foot-and-mouth disease)
—Characteristic enanthem consists of two to fourteen ulcers and vesicles (1 to 2 mm in size) in the posterior pharynx.
—May be caused by coxsackie A, B, and echoviruses.

• Measles and rubella
• Herpes simplex virus (HSV)

—Usually associated with ulcers on anterior oropharynx (gingivostomatitis) but also causes an exudative pharyngitis in adolescents which may be difficult to differentiate from streptococcal or EBV pharyngitis.

• Rhinovirus and RSV: not usually associated with pharyngeal inflammation.
• Human immunodeficiency virus (HIV): pharyngitis associated with primary HIV infection (acute retroviral syndrome), accompanied by systemic complaints simulating mononucleosis.

BACTERIAL

• *Streptococcus pyogenes* (group A β-hemolytic streptococcus)

—Most common in children 5 to 15 years old, causing at least 15% to 20% of cases of pharyngitis in this age group.
—Usually exudative with only 10% complaining of cough or rhinorrhea.

• Group C or G streptococci

—Less common, but cause outbreaks associated with contaminated foods.

• *Arcanobacterium hemolyticum*

—More commonly recognized in United Kingdom and Scandinavia.
—Exudative pharyngitis in adolescents, young adults. Can give scarletiniform rash.

• *Corynebacterium diphtheriae* (Diphtheria)

—Characterized by membrane formation that may extend from the tonsils, uvula and pharyngeal walls to the larynx and trachea. Often foul or sweet odor to breath.
—Lymphadenitis may be so severe to create "bull neck" appearance.

• *Corynebacterium hemolyticum*

—More common in adolescents and adults

• *Neisseria gonorrhea* and *N. meningitidis*
• *Mycoplasma pneumoniae*, *M. hominis*, *Chlamydia pneumoniae*
• *Francisella tularensis* (tularemia)

—Associated with undercooked meat, pet rabbits. May have membrane similar to diphtheria.
—Cervical nodes may suppurate.

• *Treponema pallidum* (syphilis)

—Usually subacute in secondary syphilis.

• Oral anaerobes (Vincent angina)

FUNGI

• *Candida* species (oral thrush)

—In infants or immunosuppressed individuals.

 Data Gathering

HISTORY

• Streptococcal pharyngitis fever is usually present. Onset is typically sudden. Headache, nausea, vomiting, and occasionally abdominal pain occur.
• Viral etiology: More likely associated with rhinorrhea, cough, hoarseness, conjunctivitis, ulcerative lesions.

Question: Has the patient been swimming in an inadequately chlorinated pool?
Significance: Consider adenoviral pharyngoconjunctival fever.

Question: Appearance of papular eruption after administration of ampicillin or amoxicillin?
Significance: Consider EBV.

Question: Travel to the former Soviet Union?
Significance: Consider diphtheria.

Question: Ingestion of undercooked meat or handling of rabbits?
Significance: Consider tularemia.

 Physical Examination

Finding: Moderate to severe pharyngeal erythema and tonsillar enlargement.
Significance: Erythema may be associated with petechiae, exudate or ulceration.

Finding: Scarletiniform rash
Significance: Strongly suggests diagnosis of GAS.

Finding: Varying degrees of cervical adenopathy.
Significance: Tender anterior lymphadenopathy is more likely associated with streptococcal disease.

Finding: Presence of an adherent membrane in pharynx extending to uvula
Significance: Suggests diphtheria.

Finding: Splenomegaly and/or generalized adenopathy
Significance: Suggests EBV.

Finding: Presence of more than six palatal petechiae
Significance: Strongly associated with streptococcal pharyngitis.

 Laboratory Aids

Because of the importance of its complications, streptococcal disease should be confirmed or excluded by laboratory testing, except in presentations suggestive of viral or other etiology of pharyngitis (e.g., a toddler with conjunctivitis and rhinorrhea, presence of gingivostomatitis, findings consistent with IM etc.).

SPECIFIC TESTS

Test: Rapid streptococcal antigen detection tests (RADTs)
Significance: Are effective as initial tests with greater than 95% specificity and 50% to 80% sensitivity. Cultures should be performed when rapid test is negative. (Hint: culture throat using two swabs initially, keeping one for culture if the rapid test is negative.) Positive rapid tests do not require culture confirmation.

Test: Throat culture
Significance: For group A β-hemolytic streptococci is still the "gold standard" with best sensitivity (>90%).

Test: Monospot (heterophile antibody) test or Epstein-Barr virus serology
Significance: For IM.

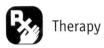 Therapy

- Usually no therapy indicated, except for streptococcal pharyngitis (and other rare cases of bacterial or fungal pharyngitis).
- May withhold treatment for GAS pharyngitis until throat culture result is available.

DRUGS

- Oral penicillin V: is the drug of choice for GAS pharyngitis except in penicillin-allergic individuals. Resistant strains have not been documented *in vitro.*

—Children: use 400,000 units (250 mg) bid or tid for 10 days.
—Adolescents/Adults: use 800,000 Units (500 mg) bid for 10 days or 400,000 units (250 mg) tid or qid for 10 days.

- Intramuscular benzathine penicillin G: assures compliance, useful in outbreaks.

—Children (<60 lbs.): 600,000 Units IM (1 dose).
—Children (>60 lbs.) and adults: 1,200,000 Units IM (1 dose). Bringing to room temperature reduces discomfort, also procaine penicillin combinations are less painful.

- Oral erythromycin: is indicated in penicillin-allergic individuals. Erythromycin ethyl succinate (40 to 50 mg/kg/d in 2–4 divided doses). Resistance is rare in the United States (<5% of isolates).
- Amoxicillin, clindamycin, and first generation oral cephalosporins (up to 15% of penicillin-allergic persons are also allergic to cephalosporins): are reasonable alternatives to penicillin in GAS pharyngitis.
- Tetracyclines and sulfonamides should *not* be used due to resistance of group A streptococci.
- Newer agents such as azithromycin, and various oral cephalosporins have also been shown to eradicate streptococci; however, because of the broad spectra of these antibiotics and the increasing incidence of antibiotic-resistant bacteria, they are not recommended.

DURATION OF THERAPY

Recent trials comparing 10 day courses of penicillin with newer oral cephalosporins or azithromycin used for 5 days have shown similar bacteriologic and clinical cure rates; but efficacy in prevention of non-suppurative sequelae is unknown, and these agents have broad spectra and greater expense.

 Follow-Up

PATIENTS WITH STREPTOCOCCAL PHARYNGITIS

- Clinical improvement is usually rapid.
- Cure rate is excellent except in non-compliant patients, *rare* co-infection with pathogens that elaborate β-lactamase (consider therapy with clindamycin) or in cases of a new infection acquired from family or classroom contact (also rare).
- No need to perform post-treatment cultures for GAS in asymptomatic patients in areas where incidence of ARF is low (e.g., United States, Canada, Western Europe).
- Watch for suppurative complications (e.g., peritonsillar abscess, cervical adenitis, mastoiditis).

PREVENTION

- Long-term penicillin prophylaxis for patients with a history of rheumatic fever.
- Immunization with diphtheria toxoid (DPT, DaPT, or dT) has dramatically decreased childhood mortality from diphtheria.

ISOLATION OF HOSPITALIZED PATIENT

- Isolation of hospitalized patients with respiratory viruses and pharyngitis.
- Droplet precautions for hospitalized children with streptococcal pharyngitis until 24 hours after initiation of therapy.

CONTROL MEASURES

- Children with GAS pharyngitis can return to school or day care 24 hours after starting antimicrobial therapy.
- Cultures of asymptomatic contacts of patients with streptococcal pharyngitis are not indicated except in outbreak situations in school or day care (where treatment of patients with positive RADT or culture is indicated) or in contacts with a history of non-suppurative complications.

PITFALLS

- Failure to use throat culture to rule out streptococcal pharyngitis when rapid test is negative.
- Failure to request identification of other organisms in the appropriate clinical setting. (e.g., *N. gonorrhea* or *A. hemolyticum*)
- Reliance on monospot test in young children (<5 years) because of a high incidence of false negatives (consider EBV serology instead).
- Positive throat culture or RADT in patients with viral pharyngitis may represent streptococcal carrier state. Diagnostic tests for GAS should be utilized in patients suspected to have streptococcal disease on clinical and epidemiologic grounds, not on all patients who complain of a "sore throat."

- Over-treatment of patients who are streptococcal carriers B asymptomatic patients (or patients with intercurrent viral infections) who have a positive test for GAS are at low, or no risk of developing suppurative or non-suppurative complications and unlikely to spread the organism to close contacts.

 Common Questions and Answers

Q: How many days after onset of GAS pharyngitis, will therapy be effective in preventing ARF?
A: Therapy started as late as 9 days after illness onset has been show to be effective in preventing ARF.

Q: Is there any benefit to starting therapy while waiting for culture results?
A: Immediate therapy probably shortens the symptomatic period, but waiting for a positive test result avoids overuse of antibiotics.

Q: Does an asymptomatic patient with a positive test for GAS from the pharynx require therapy?
A: Usually not. Between 8% and 20% of children in school or day care will have asymptomatic carriage of GAS and generally do not require therapy. Exceptions are those with a history of ARF, outbreak situations, or to achieve eradication in families with recurrent episodes of GAS pharyngitis.

Q: Is tonsillectomy indicated for recurrent GAS pharyngitis?
A: Rare patients in whom multiple symptomatic episodes of laboratory-confirmed GAS pharyngitis occur despite appropriate therapy, may be considered for tonsillectomy.

Q: Is continuous antimicrobial prophylaxis for recurrent GAS pharyngitis recommended?
A: No. There is insufficient evidence to show that it is effective, except for preventing recurrences of acute rheumatic fever.

ICD-9-CM numbers
Pharyngitis (Streptococcal) 034.0
Pharyngitis (acute, viral, infective) 462.0
Pharyngitis (influenza) 487.1
Pharyngitis (Coxsackie) 074.0, and others

BIBLIOGRAPHY

American Academy of Pediatrics. Group A streptococcal infections. In: Peter G, ed. 1997 red book: report of the Committee on Infectious Diseases, 24th ed. Elk Grove, IL: American Academy of Pediatrics. 1997:483–494.

Shulman ST. Evaluation of penicillins, cephalosporins, and macrolides for therapy of streptococcal pharyngitis. *Pediatrics* 1996; 97(Suppl):955–959.

Author: Kristine K. Macartney and Mark L. Bagarazzi

Photosensitivity

 Database

DEFINITION

• Adverse or abnormal reaction of the skin to sunlight

CAUSES

• Combination of sunlight with some abnormality in the skin such as loss of pigment, a chemical agent, a metabolic product, another skin disorder, a genetic disease, or an unknown factor, produces a cutaneous abnormality.
• Specific wavelengths of the radiant energy emitted by the sun and reaching the earth are usually responsible for each photosensitivity disorder, most commonly ultraviolet B (UVB, 290–320 nm), ultraviolet A (UVA, 320–400 nm), and visible light (400–800 nm).

PATHOLOGY

Findings are diverse for the different disorders and rarely diagnostic.

EPIDEMIOLOGY

• Variable for each disorder
• Photosensitivities with onset in childhood include albinism, hydroa aestivale, hydroa vacciniforme, the porphyrias (e.g., erythropoietic, erythropoietic protoporphyria, hepatoerythropoietic), and genetic disorders (e.g., xeroderma pigmentosa, Hartnup disease, poi kiloderma congenitale, Bloom syndrome, and Cockayne syndrome).
• Photosensitivities that occur frequently in adults but can occur in childhood are vitiligo, chemically induced photosensitivities, polymorphous light eruption, and connective tissue disease.

GENETICS

• The genetic disorders include the porphyrias and others as previously listed.
• The various porphyrias have variable inheritance patterns while most of the other genetic disorders are inherited in an autosomal recessive pattern.
• There is a positive familial history in many cases of polymorphous light eruption.

 Differential Diagnosis

• Photosensitivity resulting from pigment loss:
—Albinism
—Vitiligo
• Idiopathic photosensitivity:
—Polymorphous light eruption
—Solar urticaria
• Chemically induced reactions

—Topical agents: perfumes, plants (e.g., lemons, limes, celery, parsnips, carrots, dill, parsley, figs, meadowgrass, giant hogweed, mangos, wheat, clover, cocklebur, buttercups, Shepherd's purse, and pigweed), blankophores (e.g., optical brighteners in detergents), sunscreens
—Systemic agents: tetracyclines, sulfonamides, nalidixic acid, griseofulvin, phenothiazines, oral hypoglycemic agents, amiodarone, quinine, isoniazid, and thiazide diuretics

• Metabolic disorders:

—Porphyrias: disorders of hemoglobin synthesis producing various porphyrins that are photosensitizers

• Genetic disorders:

—(see Epidemiology)

• Cutaneous diseases aggravated by sunlight:

—Connective tissue diseases

 Data Gathering

HISTORY

• Age of onset of rash?
• Occurrence in spring and summer?
• Occurrence after sun exposure?
• How long after sun exposure?
• Occurrence after exposure to sun through glass?
• Any oral medications? May be related to oral contraceptives, sulfa drugs, iodines/bromides or phenytoin.
• Any new topical agents (e.g., perfumes, lemons, limes, sunscreens, etc.). Photosensitivity may occur on neck or places where agents were placed on skin.

 Physical Examination

Finding: Distributed lesions
Significance: The distribution of lesions is the main sign of photosensitivity reactions. Lesions are prominent on sun-exposed skin such as the face, pinnae of the ears, the V of the neck, the nuchal area, and the dorsa of the hands.

Finding: Lesion characteristics
Significance: The characteristics of individual lesions vary with the particular disease and can include papules, vesicles, and plaques (polymorphous light eruption), sunburn (chemical reaction to a systemic agent), linear areas of hyperpigmentation (chemical reaction to a topical agent), skin cancers (xeroderma pigmentosum), vesicles (porphyria).

PHYSICAL EXAMINATION TRICKS

Careful examination reveals accentuation of the rash on the nose, cheeks, and forehead with sparing of the eyelids and the submental portion of the chin. There is often a sharp cutoff in the nuchal area at the collar line.

 Laboratory Aids

Test: Phototesting
Significance: Using an artificial source of light, can confirm the presence of certain photosensitivities. Procedures are of two types. The first is exposure of skin to increasing doses of ultraviolet A and ultraviolet B to determine the erythema response (present at lower exposures than usual) and possibly reproduce lesions in certain diseases.
The second is photopatch testing in which photoallergic chemicals are applied under patches in duplicate, and one set is subsequently exposed to UVA. Patients who have photoallergic contact dermatitis develop a reaction under only the exposed patch of the agent causing the problem.

Test: Biochemical tests
Significance: Helpful for the diagnosis of the porphyrias with elevated levels of various porphyrins specific to each type in the urine, blood, or stool.

SPECIALIZED TESTS FOR GENETIC DISEASES

• Cell culture. To evaluate DNA repair for xeroderma pigmentosum, demonstration of chromosomal breaks in Bloom disease.
• Measurement of specific amino acid and indole excretion patterns in Hartnup disease.
• Measurement of antinuclear antibodies are helpful in connective tissue diseases.

Therapy

- Protection against sun exposure is necessary.

—Avoiding the sun, particularly between 10 A.M. and 2 P.M., and wearing protective clothing is important.
—Sunscreens are helpful for those sensitive to UVB.

　—They should be waterproof and reapplied every 2 hours.
　—The higher the sun protection factor (SPF—ratio of minimal erythema dose of sun-screened skin to minimal erythema dose of unprotected skin), the better.
　—Sunscreens are less effective against blocking UVA and therefore less effective in helping patients with sensitivities to longer wavelengths.
　—Shade UVA Guard offers better protection than most.
　—Opaque formulations such as zinc oxide and titanium oxide block ultraviolet and visible light but are cosmetically unacceptable.
　—Patients with severe photosensitivities may have to avoid any significant light exposure.

- Removal of the offending agent is necessary in chemically induced photosensitivities.

—Any severe and acute eruptions may require a short course of oral prednisone.
—Antimalarial agents have been used for poly-morphous light eruption, lupus erythematosus, solar urticaria, and porphyria cutanea tarda and require the experience of a specialist.

DURATION

Most patients require chronic protection against sun exposure. However, the problem is generally more acute in spring and summer months.

 Follow-Up

WHEN TO EXPECT IMPROVEMENT

- Variable, depending on the specific condition

PROGNOSIS

With the exception of chemically induced pho-tosensitivities, most of the conditions are chronic.

PITFALLS

If possible, it is important to accurately docu-ment the specific wavelength of light and the degree of photosensitivity in order to accu-rately advise the patient. This requires photo-testing by a specialist.

 Common Questions and Answers

Q: What is the best sunscreen to use?
A: It depends on your particular problem. If you are sensitive to UVB, use a sunscreen with the highest SPF. If you are sensitive to UVA, Shade UVA Guard is the best.

Q: I have heard that sunscreens with an SPF above 15 are not necessary?
A: This is definitely not true for patients with photosensitivities who have abnormal re-sponses to light and require excessive protec-tion. Even for the normal person, it is often not true. An SPF of 15 suggests that someone may receive 15 times more sun exposure with the sunscreen applied than without and not be-come sunburned. Some physicians have sug-gested that this is more than anyone should need. However, this number is calculated by testing in a controlled laboratory. Normal out-door conditions, such as wind, reflection from water and sand, perspiration, and water expo-sure, can significantly decrease the effective-ness of the sunscreen.

Q: What is "sun allergy"?
A: This is a lay term for polymorphous light eruption, one of the most common photosensi-tivities presenting with papules, vesicles, and plaques 1 to 2 days after sun exposure. It usu-ally recurs every spring and most patients learn to avoid sun exposure. However, ironically, it can improve with slow gradual sun exposure.

Q: Can I become allergic to sunscreens?
A: Certain active agents in sunscreens can pro-duce an allergic response in rare individuals. If the rash recurs with each use, switch to an-other sunscreen with different ingredients. If the problem continues, it is necessary to con-sult a specialist for evaluation.

ICD-9-CM 692.72

BIBLIOGRAPHY

Harber LC, Bickers DR. Photosensitivity dis-eases: principles of diagnosis and treatment, 2nd ed. Toronto: BC Decker, 1989.

Hurwitz S. Photosensitivity and photoreactions. In: Clinical pediatric dermatology a textbook of skin disorder of childhood and adolescence, 2nd ed. Philadelphia: WB Saunders, 1993:83.

Author: Cynthia Guzzo

Pinworms

 Database

DEFINITION

Severe perianal pruritus, usually nocturnal or early morning and associated with difficulty sleeping; caused by deposition of pinworm eggs around the anus.

ETIOLOGY

- Infection by *Enterobius vermicularis*

PATHOPHYSIOLOGY

- Adult worms inhabit the cecum and migrate to the anus, depositing eggs on the perianal skin, causing pruritus.
- Minimal inflammatory response in lower bowel mucosa correlates with few gastrointestinal symptoms.
- Ectopic locations (peritoneum, endometrium, etc.) are associated with granuloma formation.
- Pruritus in anal region may be associated with mucosal mastocytosis and histamine production.

EPIDEMIOLOGY

- Humans are the only natural host
- Spread by hand-to-mouth transmission
- Unrelated to personal hygiene
- Close contact is required for transmission
- Infection rates in the United States are 10% to 40%
- Late fall and winter infection most common
- Preschool- and school-aged children (5–10 years) predominantly

COMPLICATIONS

- Urethritis
- Vaginitis
- Salpingitis
- Pelvic peritonitis

PROGNOSIS

- Recurrence is common.
- Symptoms should resolve within a few days of treatment.

 Differential Diagnosis

INFECTION

- Other parasites
- Bacterial or fungal vulvo-vaginitis

ENVIRONMENTAL

- Irritative diaper dermatitis
- Chemical dermatitis
- Vulvitis from soaps or lotions

MISCELLANEOUS

- Habit (escalating itch-scratch cycle)
- Anal fissures (pain misinterpreted as pruritus)

 Data Gathering

HISTORY

Question: Is there a familial history of pinworms?
Significance: If yes, there may be spread between family members so treatment of one patient will not clear the problem.

Question: When is the itching greatest?
Significance: Typically pinworm infections cause perianal itching at the nocturnal or early morning times.

Question: Have you seen any evidence of tiny white worms?
Significance: It may be possible to see small, white worms in the perianal area or stool at night time.

Physical Examination

- Few physical findings present
- Excoriation from scratching around anus
- Pinworms may be visible around anus

 Laboratory Aids

Test: "Scotch-tape" slide test
Significance: Parents press sticky side of clear tape to the perianal area in the morning before child rises; apply tape to a microscope slide and examine for pinworm ova; may need to be repeated several times.

 Therapy

- Mebendazole (Vermox), 100 mg chewable tablet, once; may repeat in 2 weeks if necessary
- Second-line drugs: pyrantel pamoate (11 mg/kg, maximum 1 g) and piperazine citrate (65 mg/kg, maximum 2.5 g for 7 days)

 Follow-Up

Generally unnecessary.

PREVENTION

- Treat all affected family members.
- Decontamination of the environment (wash sheets, towels, clothing; vacuum household)

PITFALLS

Reinfection is common if all close contacts are not treated.

 Common Questions and Answers

Q: Is this caused by poor hygiene?
A: No.

Q: Is infection with pinworms usually associated with other parasitic infections?
A: No.

Q: Can they be spread at day care?
A: Yes.

ICD-9-CM 127.4

BIBLIOGRAPHY

American Academy of Pediatrics. Pinworm infestation. In: Peter G, ed. 1997 red book: report of the Committee on Infectious Diseases, 24th ed. Elk Grove, IL: American Academy of Pediatrics, 1997:407–408.

Cook GC. Enterobius vermicularis infection. *Gut* 1994 Sep;35(9):1159–1162.

Feigin RD, Cherry JD. Textbook of pediatric infectious diseases, 2nd ed. Philadelphia: WB Saunders, 1987:560.

Grencis RK, Hons BS, Cooper ES. Enterobius trichuris, Capillaria and Hookworm including Ancylostoma caninum. In: Weinstock JV ed. Gastroenterology clinics of North America. Parasitic disease of the liver and intestines, 1996 Sep; 25(3):579–597.

Russell LJ. The pinworm, enterobius vermicularis. In: Jones JE, ed. Primary care clinics in office practice: parasitic disease. 1991 Mar; 18(1):13–24.

Author: Deborah L. Silver

Plague

Database

DEFINITION

The bubonic plague is an enzootic infection that results in lymphadenitis and fever. Severe constitutional, gastrointestinal, neurological, and respiratory symptoms (pneumonic plague) can also occur. "The black death" has a secure place in history as a devastating epidemic that affected one-third of the population of Europe during the 14th century.

CAUSES

The illness commonly known as the plague is caused by *Yersinia pestis,* a gram-negative pleomorphic bacillus that is part of the Enterobacteriaceae family.

PATHOLOGY/PATHOPHYSIOLOGY

Dermatological Portal of Entry

• *Y. pestis* is most commonly transmitted from fleas to humans via the regurgitation of the organism into the skin tissue during the flea's blood meal. Rodents, as well as dogs, cats, and rabbits can thereby act as reservoirs of infection.
• Lymphatic spread of infection to the regional lymph nodes creates a localized inflammatory response. If antibody response prevents additional spread, this condition is known as *pestis minor.*
• Subsequent hematogenous spread of the organism to other organs results in the production of greater levels of bacterial endotoxin. This endotoxin is responsible for the systemic manifestations, as well as the high mortality rate, of the untreated illness.

Respiratory Portal of Entry (Pneumonic Plague)

• Acquired via contact with the saliva or respiratory droplets
• Replication of the organism within the alveolar spaces results in a fulminant localized infection and endotoxemia.

Other Organ Systems Involved

• Liver
• Spleen
• Kidney
• Meninges

EPIDEMIOLOGY (AGE RELATED)

• More than one-half of the contemporary cases of plague occur in persons under 20 years of age, possibly due to an increased tendency for children to come into contact with small animals and rodents.
• An outbreak of the pneumonic plague has been reported recently in India; however, the identification of the specific causative organism has been called into question.
• A large proportion of the cases in the United States has occurred in the southwestern part of the country.
• No cases of person to person transmissions of plague pneumonia have been reported in the United States since 1925.

ASSOCIATED ILLNESSES

• Bubonic plague: lymphadenitis (usually inguinal); systemic manifestations; 75% of plague cases worldwide.
• Pneumonic plague: pneumonia; systemic manifestations. Rapidly progressive, often fatal.
• Septicemic plague: tachycardia, hypotension, other organ involvement; either bubonic or pneumonic plague may progress to this condition.

Differential Diagnosis

• Diagnosis of plague follows a high index of suspicion and a thorough review of the patient's lifestyle, travel history, and recent activities.
• The appearance of septicemia and endotoxin-mediated shock includes a large differential diagnosis that includes sepsis due to other bacteria or viruses, as well as distributive shock resulting from toxic ingestion or anaphylaxis.

INFECTION

• Recent reports of plague-like illnesses have been associated with infections by other organisms such as *Pseudomonas pseudomallei* (melioidosis) and *Francisella tularensis* (tularemia).
• *Pestis minor,* which involves exquisitely tender lymph nodes, may be confused with bacterial adenitis, tularemia, lymphogranuloma venereum, chancroid, or cat-scratch disease.

Data Gathering

HISTORY

Question: What is the incubation period for this disease?
Significance: There is usually 2 to 6 days between exposure and first presentation of symptoms, but this period can be shorter for pneumonic plague.

Question: In the context of exposure to yersinia pestis, what are the initial symptoms of exposure?
Significance: Initial symptoms include abrupt onset of fever, weakness, malaise.

Question: What are the initial symptoms of bubonic plague?
Significance: The patient may complain of pain in the groin or axillae prior to lymph node swelling.

Physical Examination

• Patients may present initially with suppurative lymphadenitis in the groin, axillae, or neck regions.
• Patients with rapidly progressive illness are tachycardic, hypotensive, and toxic in appearance. Rashes and fever are more likely to be the initial presentation of patients with an initial pneumonic focus of infection.
• Other organ system involvement is common.

—Gastrointestinal: Abdominal pain, nausea, and diarrhea are usually due to the presence of inflammatory mediators. Hepatosplenomegaly is a common finding.
—Neurological: Weakness, delirium, and coma are due to the effects of the endotoxin of *Y. pestis.*

• Patients with septicemia can experience renal (glomerular and parenchymal damage), hematologic (disseminated intravascular coagulation), and hepatic necrosis.

SPECIAL QUESTIONS

• A thorough travel history is imperative in order to raise the index of suspicion for diagnosing plague.
• Environmental history should include the presence of rats, ground squirrels, or prairie dogs in the patient's locale.

Laboratory Aids

Test: Total white blood count
Significance: Usually 10,000 to 20,000, but may be as high as 100,000.

Test: *Yersinia pestis* culture
Significance: Can be cultured on blood agar plates from lymph node aspirate, blood, cerebrospinal fluid, or sputum from patients with pneumonic plague.

Test: Gram stain, Wayson stain, Giemsa stain, or fluorescent antibody staining of the specimen.
Significance: May reveal the bipolar organisms.

Test: Comparison of acute and convalescent sera
Significance: Taken 3 to 4 weeks apart, show at least a 4-fold increase in antibody titers by passive hemagglutination.

Therapy

DRUGS

- In the acutely ill patient suspected of *Y. pestis* infection, streptomycin (30 mg/kg/d) can be administered by the intravenous or intramuscular route.
- Tetracycline (20–30 mg/kg IV per day), or chloramphenicol (75–100 mg/kg per day IV), should be added in severe cases or if meningitis is present.
- For the patient who does not require hospitalization, streptomycin (30 mg/kg/d), tetracycline (20–30 mg/kg/d) or IV chloramphenicol (75–100 mg/kg/d) may be administered enterally after cultures are obtained.
- Drainage of affected lymph nodes or abscesses, if necessary, should wait until at least 24 hours after initiation of therapy to prevent unnecessary spread of infected drainage.

DURATION

- Therapy continued for at least 10 days. Severely ill patients may require a substantially longer course of therapy. Patients treated with streptomycin can be switched to other medications a few days after improvement is noted.

POSSIBLE CONFLICTS WITH OTHER TREATMENTS

To avoid permanent dental staining, patients less than 8 years of age should not receive tetracycline unless absolutely necessary.

PREVENTION

- General prevention: Suppression of the rodent population in endemic areas, as well as deinfestation of cats and dogs, may reduce the prevalence of disease considerably.
- Hospital isolation (negative pressure) should be continued for 3 days after initiation of therapy.

—Pneumonic plague patients require strict respiratory and secretion isolation precautions.
—Bubonic plague patients with no evidence of pneumonia require drainage and secretion precautions.

- Exposed persons: All contacts of patients thought to suffer from plague should undergo:

—Deinfestation of all clothing, pets and bedding, and homes
—Observation for fever or symptoms of disease for 7 to 10 days (inpatient or outpatient)

- Persons who have had contact with a patient with pneumonic plague require antimicrobial prophylaxis with tetracycline (15 mg/kg/d), a sulfonamide (40 mg/kg/d), or IM streptomycin (20 mg/kg/d) for a total of 7 to 10 days.
- Vaccination with a 5-vaccine regimen (3 primary and 2 boosters) of inactivated whole-cell product is indicated for:

—Persons who intend to travel to or reside in endemic regions in which the domestic rats are infested.
—Laboratory workers or other professional that will be in contact with potentially infected rodents or their fleas.
—Booster doses should continue every 1 to 2 years as long as the exposure exists.

Follow-Up

WHEN TO EXPECT IMPROVEMENT

Resolution of symptoms should begin in the first 3 days after initiation of therapy; however, the rate of clinical improvement depends on the initial severity of illness.

SIGNS TO WATCH FOR

Neurological sequelae of the plague often manifest during the course of treatment for the illness.

PITFALLS

- Certain strains of *Y. pestis* are resistant to streptomycin. In general, these organisms are sensitive to chloramphenicol.
- A high index of suspicion is needed to diagnose plague. Patients who present with fever, tachycardia, or tachypnea, rather than lymphadenitis, are at higher risk for delayed diagnosis and serious sequelae.

Emergency Care

For septicemic patients, initial attention should be given to airway management and fluid resuscitation.

Common Questions and Answers

Q: Can one determine the risks of being exposed to plague during international travel?
A: Yes. The Centers for Disease Control (CDC) provides a service that contains updated information for international travel. This automated traveler's hotline is accessible from a touch-tone telephone at all hours. The telephone number is (404) 332-4559. Similar information is available by facsimile at (404) 332-4565.

Q: Does persistent fever during treatment for plague warrant altering the antibiotic regimen?
A: No, fever can persist for up to two weeks after appropriate antibiotic therapy for plague.

ICD-9-CM 020.9

BIBLIOGRAPHY

American Academy of Pediatrics. Plague. 1997 red book: Report of the Committee on Infectious Diseases. Elk Grove IL: American Academy of Pediatrics, 1997.

Centers for Disease Control and Prevention. Update: human plague—India, 1994. *MMWR* 1994;43:722–723.

Centers for Disease Control and Prevention. Human plague—United States, 1993–1994. *MMWR* 1994;43:242–246.

Centers for Disease Control and Prevention. Fatal human plague—Arizona and Colorado, 1996. *MMWR* 1997;46:617–620.

Cleri DJ, Vernaleo JR, Lombardi LJ, et al. Plague pneumonia disease caused by *Yersinia pestis. Semin Resp Inf* 1997;12:12–23.

Crook LD, Tempest B. Plague: a clinical review of 27 cases. *Arch Intern Med* 1992;152:1253.

Gomez NF, Cleary TG. Yesinia species. In: Long SS, Pickering LK, eds. Principles and practice of pediatric infectious diseases. New York: Churchill Livingstone, 1997:935–939.

Perry RD, Featherston JD. *Yersinia pestis*—etiologic agent of plague. *Clin Microbiol Rev* 1997;10:35–66.

Author: Joel A. Fein

Pleural Effusion

 Database

DEFINITION

- Accumulation of fluid in the pleural cavity

CAUSES

- There is normally 1 to 15 mL of fluid in the pleural space.
- Alterations in the flow and/or absorption of this fluid leads to fluid accumulation.
- Mechanisms influence this flow of fluid:

—Increased capillary hydrostatic pressure (congestive heart failure, overhydration)
—Decreased pleural space hydrostatic pressure (post-thoracentesis, atelectasis)
—Decreased plasma oncotic pressure (hypoalbuminemia, nephrosis)
—Increased capillary permeability (infection, toxins, connective tissue diseases, malignancy)
—Impaired lymphatic drainage from the pleural space (disruption of the thoracic duct)
—Passage of fluid from the peritoneal cavity through the diaphragm to the pleural space (hepatic cirrhosis with ascites)

PATHOPHYSIOLOGY

- Dependent on the underlying disease; two types of pleural effusion are:

—Transudate: Mechanical forces of hydrostatic and oncotic pressures are altered favoring liquid filtration.
—Exudate: Damage to the pleural surface occurs that alters its ability to filter pleural fluid; lymphatic drainage is diminished.

- Stages associated with pleural exudate:

—Exudative: simple parapneumonic effusion; pleural fluid glucose and pH normal
—Fibropurulent: increase in fibrin, polymorphonuclear leukocytes, bacterial invasion of pleural cavity
—Fluid glucose and pH falls, LDH increases
—Organizing: fibroblasts grow; pleural peal

EPIDEMIOLOGY

- Dependent on underlying cause; most common cause is pneumonia, followed by congenital heart disease and malignancy.
- For empyema, most common organism include:

—*Staphylococcus aureus*: 28%
—*Streptococcus pneumoniae*: 20%
—*Haemophilus influenzae*: 13%

COMPLICATIONS

- Hypoxia
- Respiratory distress
- Trapped lung
- Decreased cardiac function
- Shock (secondary to blood loss in cases of hemothorax)
- Malnutrition (seen in chylothorax)

PROGNOSIS

- Dependent on underlying disease process
- Properly treated infectious etiology: excellent
- Malignancy: poor prognosis

 Differential Diagnosis

TRANSUDATE

- Cardiovascular

—Congestive heart failure
—Constrictive pericarditis

- Nephrotic syndrome with hypoalbuminemia
- Cirrhosis
- Atelectasis

EXUDATE

- Infections

—Parapneumonic effusions; *Staphylococcus aureus* is most common organism
—Tuberculous effusion
—Viral effusions: adenovirus; influenza
—Fungal effusions: most not associated with effusions; *Nocardia* and *Actinomyces* are most common
—Parasitic effusions

- Neoplasms

—Seen mostly in leukemia and lymphoma

- Connective tissue disease

—Rheumatoid arthritis
—Systemic lupus erythematosus
—Wegener granulomatosis

- Pulmonary embolus
- Intra-abdominal disease

—Subdiaphragmatic abscess
—Pancreatitis

- Others

—Sarcoidosis
—Esophageal rupture
—Hemothorax
—Chylothorax
—Drugs
—Chemical injury
—Post-irradiation effusion

 Data Gathering

HISTORY

Question: Does patient have a chronic disease?
Significance: Basic disease determines most of systemic symptoms.

Question: Are there symptoms of respiratory distress?
Significance: May be asymptomatic until amount of fluid is large enough to cause cardio-respiratory distress.

Question: Is there shortness of breath or cough?
Significance: Dyspnea and cough are associated with large effusions.

Question: Fever?
Significance: High fever and chills suggest an infectious etiologic agent.

Question: Pleuritic pain?
Significance: Pneumonia may cause irritation of the parietal pleura causing pleural pain. As the effusion increases and separates the pleural membrane, the pain may disappear.

 Physical Examination

Finding: Pleural rub during early phase
Significance: Resolves as fluid accumulates in the pleural space

Finding: Decreased thoracic wall excursion
Significance: With pleural fluid accumulation, elastic resistance to lung distention increases, limiting lung expansion.

Finding: Dull or flat percussion
Significance: On the involved side, suggests the presence of consolidation or pleural effusion.

Finding: Decreased tactile and vocal fremitus
Significance: On the involved side, suggests the presence of effusion vs. increased fremitus in consolidation.

Finding: Decreased whispering pectoriloquy
Significance: As above.

Finding: Fullness of intercostal spaces
Significance: Pleural fluid may also distort the chest wall; the chest wall may bulge outward and the ipsilateral hemidiaphragm displaced downward.

Finding: Decreased breath sounds
Significance: Suggests the presence of fluid or consolidation.

Finding: Trachea and cardiac apex displaced toward the contralateral side
Significance: A large effusion may produce a mediastinal shift, reduce venous return, and compromise cardiac output.

 Laboratory Aids

Test: Thoracentesis
Significance: Indicated whenever etiology is unclear or effusion is symptomatic.

Test: Pleural fluid analysis (see the table Pleural Fluid Analysis)
Significance: Pleural fluid glucose of less than 40 mg/dL; four possibilities: parapneumonic, malignant, tuberculous, and rheumatic.

Test: Sedimentation rate (ESR)
Significance: To follow degree of inflammation and response to therapy.

IMAGING

Test: Chest radiograph, upright films
Significance:

- Anterior-posterior projection can see 400 mL
- Lateral projection can see 200 mL

Pleural Fluid Analysis

TEST	TRANSUDATE	EXUDATE
pH	7.4	<7.3
Protein (g/100 ml)	<3.0	>3.0
Pleural/serum protein	<0.5	>0.5
Pleural/serum LDH	<0.6	>0.6
LDH (IU)	<200	>200
Pleural/serum amylase	<1	>1
Glucose (mg/DL)	>40	<40
RBC	<5000	>5000
WBC	<1000 mostly monos	>1000 mostly polys

Test: Lateral decubitus films
Significance:

• Can check for free-flowing pleural fluid
• Can see as little as 50 mL of fluid

Test: Ultrasound
Significance:

• Can diagnose small (3–5 mL) loculated collections of pleural fluid.
• Useful as a guide for thoracentesis
• Can distinguish between pleural thickening and pleural effusion

Test: CT scan
Significance:

• Defines empyema, abscess, or bronchopleural fistula
• Useful for defining extent of loculated effusions

PLEURAL BIOPSY

• If thoracentesis is non-diagnostic
• Most useful for diseases that cause extensive involvement of the pleura (i.e., tuberculosis, malignancies)
• Confirms neoplastic involvement in 40% to 70% of cases

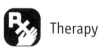 Therapy

DRAINAGE

• Thoracentesis and tube thoracostomy

—For diagnosis/relief of dyspnea or cardiorespiratory distress
—Reduce reaccumulation
—Drain empyema

• Intrapleural fibrinolytics

—Adjunct to complete drainage in complicated (i.e., multiloculated empyema) pleural effusion
—Limited studies in children, promising
—Adults, streptokinase and urokinase found to be helpful; fever most common adverse reaction reported with streptokinase

THORACOSCOPIC PLEURAL DEBRIDEMENT

• Alternative to more invasive procedures (i.e., open thoracotomy/decortication)

• Debridement through pleural visualization and adhesiolysis

OPEN THORACOTOMY WITH RIB RESECTION

• Encapsulated empyema

DECORTICATION

• Symptomatic chronic empyema
• Relief of thick fibrous peal

PLEURECTOMY

• Chylothorax
• Malignant effusions

ANTIBIOTICS

• Used if effusion secondary to infection
• Specific antibiotics dictated by organism identified

DURATION

• Drainage

—Stopped when patient is asymptomatic; drainage less than 50 mL/h
—Thick, loculated empyema requires prolonged drainage

• Antibiotics

—Clinical improvement usually occurs in 48 to 72 hours
—Dependent on organism and degree of illness:
   —*Staphylococcus aureus:* 3 to 4 weeks minimum
   —*Streptococcus pneumoniae:* 2 weeks minimum
   —*Haemophilus influenzae:* 2 weeks minimum
—Should remain on IV antibiotics until afebrile
—Complete remainder of therapy on oral antibiotics

DIET

• Chylothorax

—Medium-chain triglycerides
—Nutritional replacement
—4 to 5 weeks on this regimen

 Follow-Up

WHEN TO EXPECT IMPROVEMENT

• Clinical improvement usually within 1 to 2 weeks
• May have fever spikes up to 2 to 3 weeks

PITFALLS

• Cytologic examination

—Fresh and heparinized specimen should be refrigerated at 4°C until it can be processed.
—Fixatives should not be added.

• Malignant effusions

—Sclerosing procedures usually ineffective.

—Chest tube drainage will often create a pneumothorax because the lung is incarcerated by the tumor.

 Common Questions and Answers

Q: How sensitive/specific are the various biochemical tests of pleural fluid in children?
A: The Light criteria was developed 20 years ago for the adult. Limited information on its sensitivity or specificity in children; would advise clinical correlation with history, physical findings, and supporting laboratory tests.

Q: How long a course of antibiotics are required?
A: Dependent on the underlying organism; usually between 2 to 4 weeks total of IV/PO.

Q: When will the chest x-ray normalize?
A: May take up to 6 months to normalize.

Q: When will the pulmonary function tests normalize?
A: Dependent on extent of effusion.

ICD-9-CM 511.9

BIBLIOGRAPHY

Alrkrinawi S, Chernick V. Pleural infection in children. *Semin Respir Infect* 1996;11:148.

Bouros D, Schiza S, Patsourakis G, Chalkiadakis G, Panagou P, Siafakas N. Intrapleural streptokinase vs. urokinase in the treatment of complicated parapneumonic effusions. *Am J Resp Crit Care Med* 1997;155:291.

Chin TW, Nussbaum E, Marks M. Bacterial pneumonia. In: B. Hilman, ed. *Pediatric respiratory disease: Diagnosis and treatment.* Philadelphia: WB Saunders, 1993:271–281.

Kern J, Rodgers B. Thoracoscopy in the management of empyema in children. *J Pediatr Surg* 1993;28:1128.

Kornecki A, Sivan Y. Treatment of loculated pleural effusion with intrapleural urokinase in children. *J Pediatr Surg* 1997;32:1473.

Montgomery M. Air and liquid in the pleural space. In: V. Chernick, ed. *Kendig's disorders of the respiratory tract in children.* Philadelphia: WB Saunders, 1998:389–411.

Correa AG, Starke JK. Bacterial pneumonia. In: V. Chernick, ed. *Kendig's Disorders of the respiratory tract in children.* Philadelphia: WB Saunders, 1998;485–501.

Rosa U. Pleural effusion. *Postgrad Med* 1984; 75:252.

Sahn SA. The pleura. *Am Rev Respir Dis* 1988; 138:184.

Zeitlin PL. Pleural effusion and empyema. In: G. Loughlin, H. Eigen, eds.: Respiratory Diseases in Children, Baltimore: Williams & Wilkins, 1994:453–463.

Authors: Elizabeth C. Uong and Richard Mark Kravitz

Pneumocystis Carinii

Database

DEFINITION

Opportunistic lung infection caused by *Pneumocystis carinii* (PC). This organism is currently considered a primitive fungus. It has two developmental forms: a cyst containing sporozoites and an extracystic one named trophozoite.

- *P. carinii* pneumonia (PCP) occurs almost exclusively in the immunocompromised host. Children with congenital or acquired immune deficiency syndrome (AIDS), recipients of suppressive therapy in the treatment of malignancies or after organ transplantation are at high risk.
- Sporadic cases have been reported in patients with hematologic disorders, rheumatoid arthritis, nephrosis leading to hypoproteinemia and chronic infectious diseases.
- PCP is an AIDS-defining illness. It is the most common opportunistic life-threatening lung infection in infants with perinatally acquired HIV disease.
- PC causes a diffuse pneumonitis characterized by fever, tachypnea, hypoxemia, and bilateral diffuse infiltrates in the roentgenogram. It is a severe condition frequently leading to respiratory failure necessitating intubation and mechanical ventilation.
- Chemoprophylaxis against this microorganism has proven successful. Therefore, early identification of the HIV-infected mother becomes essential.
- Despite the advances in therapy, its infection continues to carry severe morbidity and mortality.

PATHOPHYSIOLOGY

- In the immunodeficient child the pathological changes occur predominantly in the alveoli. Cysts and trophozoites are seen adhering to the alveolar lining cells or in the cytoplasm of macrophages.
- As infection progresses, the alveolar spaces are filled with a pink, foamy exudate containing fibrin, abundant desquamative cells, and large number of organisms. Alveolar septal thickening with mononuclear cell infiltration is also seen.

EPIDEMIOLOGY

- Mode of transmission is unknown.

—Airborne person-to-person transmission is possible, but case contacts are rarely identified.
—Environmentally acquired.

- Asymptomatic infection appears early in life, more than 70% of healthy individuals have antibodies by age 4.
- Primary infection is likely to be the prominent mechanism in infants, whereas reactivation of latent disease may play a significant role later in life.

- PCP in the HIV patient can occur at any time, but usually presents during the first year of life. The higher incidence is between 3 and 6 months of age.
- In leukemic patients, the incidence of PCP has been directly related to the degree of immunodeficiency resulting from chemotherapy.
- Epidemics of PCP were reported in premature and malnourished infants during war times. This type has been termed as infantile form.

COMPLICATIONS

- High rate of respiratory failure necessitating intubation and mechanical ventilation (about 60%)

PROGNOSIS

- 10% to 40% mortality in treated patients
- Near 100% mortality if patient is untreated
- About 35% of the patients will have reoccurrence unless lifetime prophylaxis is instituted.

Differential Diagnosis

VIRAL INFECTIONS

- Common viral respiratory pathogens
- Cytomegalovirus
- Epstein-Barr virus

BACTERIAL INFECTIONS

- *Mycobaterium tuberculosis*
- *Mycobacterium avium intracellulare*

OTHER

- Lymphocytic interstitial pneumonitis

Data Gathering

HISTORY

Question: Malnourished?
Significance: Infantile form has a subacute onset with non-specific manifestations:

- Poor feeding, weight loss, and restlessness
- Chronic diarrhea
- Usually without fever
- After 1 to 2 weeks, the patient develops progressive tachypnea, respiratory distress, and cough.

Question: Sporadic or immunocompromised host?
Significance: This form has a more abrupt onset, even a fulminant one:

- Fever (>38.5°C)
- Non-productive cough
- Dyspnea at rest

These listed forms are general clinical guidelines. Symptoms may be superimposed and can be seen in infants, children, and adolescents.

Physical Examination

Finding: Fever and significant tachypnea
Significance: Are characteristic

Finding: Hypoxemia
Significance: Early in the course of disease that seems disproportionate with the auscultatory findings

Finding: Rapidly progressive respiratory distress with cyanosis
Significance: Respiratory failure early in course.

Finding: Absence of crackles
Significance: A common initial finding

Finding: Chest auscultation
Significance: Can reveal decreased breath sounds, crackles, and rhonchi

Finding: Coryza and wheezing
Significance: Have infrequently been reported

Laboratory Aids

Test: Arterial blood gas
Significance:

- pH is usually increased
- Reduced pO_2 in room air (<70 mm Hg)
- Alveolar-arterial oxygen gradient (>30 mm Hg)
- Decreased pCO_2

OTHER TESTS

- Chest radiograph

Test: Lactate dehydrogenase (LDH)
Significance: Can be elevated in patients with AIDS and PCP, but this finding is non-specific.

Test: White blood count
Significance: Is usually normal

PATHOLOGY

- Definitive diagnosis can be obtained by demonstration of the PC in pulmonary specimens:

—Induced sputum
—Bronchoalveolar lavage (90% sensitivity), usually through flexible bronchoscopy
—Open lung or transbronchial biopsy

Test: Staining
Significance:

- Cysts stain with Gomori methenamine-silver nitrate or toluidine blue-O stains
- Sporozoite and trophozoites are identified with polychrome stains (Giemsa, Wright, polychrome methylene blue)
- Immunofluorescent monoclonal antibodies (high sensitivity)

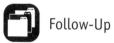

• May appear normal (4% of cases)
• Most common radiological presentation is diffuse bilateral alveolar infiltrates:

—Initially of perihilar distribution, spreads to the periphery
—Apices are the least affected
—Interstitial infiltrates and air bronchograms can be seen
—Rapid progression to whole lung consolidation

• Presence of a hilar or mediastinal adenopathy may indicate other process such as *M. tuberculosis*, Mycobacterium-avium-intracellulare, fungal infections, cytomegalovirus, or lymphoma.

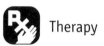

Therapy

ANTIBIOTICS

• Trimethoprim-sulfamethoxazole (TMP/SMX) is the drug of choice.

—TMP (15–20 mg/kg/d) and SMX (75–100 mg/kg/d) IV PO divided every 6 hours.
—Follow up of serum levels may be considered. Target values are 3 to 5 μg/mL TMP and 100 to 150 μg/mL SMX.
—Minimum 2 weeks, sometimes 3 weeks of therapy is required.

ALTERNATIVE THERAPY

• Pentamidine isothionate

—4 mg/kg/d IV (or IM) given in a single daily dose for minimum 2 weeks.
—Total daily dose should not exceed 300 mg.
—Used in patients who cannot tolerate TMP/SMX or unresponsive after 5 to 7 days of therapy.
—Same effectiveness as TMP/SMX, but with higher incidence of side effects. Concomitant use with didanosine increases the risk of pancreatitis.

• Atavaquone is approved for adults who cannot tolerate TMP/SMX.

—Limited pediatric experience. Suggested dose is 40 mg/kg daily divided bid.

SUPPORTIVE THERAPY

• Supply oxygen as necessary to keep PaO$_2$ above 70 mm Hg
• Mechanical ventilation must be considered if PaO$_2$ is less than 60 mm Hg on FiO$_2$ of 0.5
• Corticosteroids

—May be beneficial in HIV patients with moderate to severe PCP.
—Not systematically evaluated in children.

• Consider when PaO$_2$ is less than 70 mm Hg or the alveolar-arterial gradient is greater than 35 mm Hg.
• In patients over 13 years of age suggested dose: Prednisone 40 mg PO bid for days 1 to 5, 40 mg PO qd for days 6 to 10, 20 mg PO qd for days 11 to 21 with tappering. Younger patients may receive 2 mg/kg/d during days 7 to 10 with weaning over 10 to 14 days.

PROPHYLAXIS

• During specially high-risk periods, PCP can be effectively prevented in the immunodeficient host by chemoprophylaxis in the following groups:

—HIV-exposed: 4 to 6 weeks to 4 months.
—HIV-infected or indeterminate: 4 to 12 months.
—HIV-infected: 1 to 5 years if CD4+ T-lymphocyte count is less than 500 cells/μL or percentage less than 15%.
—HIV-infected: more than or equal to 5 years if CD4+ T-lymphocyte count is less than 200 cells/μL or percentage less than 15%.
—Severely symptomatic HIV patient or with rapidly declining CD4 count.
—High risk periods of children with congenital immunodeficiencies, cancer, or organ transplants.
—HIV patients who had previous episode of PCP.
—HIV-exposed: birth to 4 to 6 weeks require no prophylaxis.

RECOMMENDED STRATEGY

• TMP (150 mg/M^2/d) with SMX (750 mg/M^2/d) PO divided bid daily or on 3 consecutive days per week, or
• TMP (5 mg/kg/d) and SMX (25 mg/kg/d) PO divided bid daily or on 3 consecutive days per week.

ALTERNATIVE REGIMEN

• Dapsone 2 mg/kg (100 mg maximum) PO once daily
• Aerosolized pentamidine (>5 years old)

—300 mg via Respigard II inhaler once monthly

• If neither dapsone or pentamidine is tolerated, IV pentamidine 4 mg/kg administered every 2 or 4 weeks is recommended.

Follow-Up

WHEN TO EXPECT IMPROVEMENT

• After 5 to 7 days of treatment.
• If no improvement, TMP/SMX should be replaced with pentamidine.

ISOLATION OF HOSPITALIZED PATIENT

• Standard precautions required. Isolation from other immunodeficient patients is recommended.

PITFALLS

• HIV-infected patients have a higher rate of adverse reactions to TMP/SMX than in the general population, approximately in 15% of patients. One-half of them will develop rash, fever, or neutropenia.
• Prophylactic medication protects the patient as long as the drug is administered. Does not erradicate the *P. carinii*.
• Aerosolized pentamidine prophylaxis failure usually demonstrates organisms in the upper lobes. BAL of this area becomes the procedure of choice.

Common Questions and Answers

Q: Which are the most common side effects of pentamidine?
A: They include hypoglycemia, impaired renal or liver function, anemia, thrombocytopenia, neutropenia, hypotension, and skin rashes. Can be expected in 50% of the patients.

Q: How frequently is prophylaxis failure seen?
A: Adequate TMP-SMX treatment has only a 3% failure rate.

Q: Adverse reactions to TMP/SMX during PCP therapy?
A: Continuation of treatment if they are not severe is recommended.

ICD-9-CM 136.3

BIBLIOGRAPHY

American Academy of Pediatrics. 1997 red book: report of the Committee on Infectious Diseases. Elk Grove Village, IL: American Academy of Pediatrics 1997:419–424.

Hughes WT. Pneumoyctic carinair pneumonitis. In: V. Chernick, ed. *Kendig's disorders of the respiratory tract in children*, 1998;503–511.

Sanders-Laufer D, DeBruin W, Edelson PJ. Pneumocystis carinii infections in HIV-infected children. *Pediatr Clin North Am* 1991;38:69–89.

Authors: Roberto V. Nachajon

Pneumonia—Bacterial

 Database

DEFINITION

Inflammation and infection of the lung due to a bacterial pathogen: classified by anatomy such as lobar, interstitial, or broncho-pneumonia or by microbiologic pathogen.

ETIOLOGY

- *Streptococcus pneumoniae*
- Hemophilus influenzae
- Staphylococcus aureus
- Group B streptococcus (neonates)
- Anaerobic bacteria (aspiration pneumonia)
- *Legionella pneumophilia*
- Group A Streptococcus
- *Neisseria meningitidis*
- Gram-negative enteric bacilli
- *Mycoplasma pneumoniae*
- Pneumocystis carinii
- Other infections can be source of local or hematogenous spread to lungs: sinusitis, otitis media, epiglottitis, meningitis, osteomyelitis
- Predisposing conditions include: cerebral palsy, altered mental status, seizure disorder, and congenital disorders

PATHOPHYSIOLOGY

- Hematogenous spread is rare
- Acquired immunodeficiency may result in decreased host defense against infectious agents
- Impairment in any one of these areas may result in infection: Nasogastric tube, filtration in nares, epiglottal reflex (prevents aspiration), cough reflex (expulsion of infected secretions), protective epithelial lining with cilia and mucus producing cells, alveolar macrophages (bacterial killing), immune response (includes antibodies, complement, opsonins), lymphatic drainage affect host's susceptibility to infection.

GENETICS

Predisposing genetic conditions:

- Congenital anomalies (cleft palate, tracheoesophageal fistula, pulmonary sequestration, Kartegener syndrome)
- Congenital defects of immune system, sickle cell disease
- Defect in quality of secretions (cystic fibrosis)

EPIDEMIOLOGY

- Children, 2 years of age more susceptible than older children
- Male:female ratio of 2:1
- May follow epidemics of viral infections
- Human transmission via droplet spread, more rarely airborne
- All seasons; winter and spring most common

COMPLICATIONS

- Respiratory failure and cardiorespiratory collapse
- Pleural effusion
- Empyema
- Lung abscess
- Pneumothorax
- Pneumatoceles
- Pericarditis
- Bacteremia
- Sepsis

PROGNOSIS

- Excellent: 1% mortality rate in uncomplicated cases of pneumococcal pneumonia
- Longer recovery but still good outcome with other pathogens
- Uncomplicated pneumonias will recover in 1 to 5 days

 Differential Diagnosis

INFECTION

- Viral pneumonia (adenovirus, influenza, parainfluenza, respiratory syncytial virus, echovirus, and coxsackievirus)
- Fungal infections (histoplasmosis, blastomycosis, *Candida*)
- Rickettsia
- *Chlamydia*
- Tuberculosis
- Parasites

ENVIRONMENTAL

- Aspiration of foreign body
- Inhalation of toxin
- Drug reaction

TUMORS

- Metastatic (leukemia, lymphoma, solid tumors)
- Primary lung malignancy (rare in children)

TRAUMA

- Pulmonary contusion
- Traumatic airway obstruction

CONGENITAL

- Cystic fibrosis
- Pulmonary sequestration
- Congenital heart disease

IMMUNOLOGIC

- Collagen vascular disease
- Sarcoidosis

MISCELLANEOUS

- Reactive airways disease
- Pulmonary hemosiderosis
- Intra-abdominal pathology causing splinting or reactive effusion
- Atelectasis

 Data Gathering

HISTORY

- Recent upper respiratory tract is often part of the presenting history.
- Fever, headache, malaise, lethargy, chills.
- Anorexia with dehydration is common.
- Cough, shortness of breath, trouble breathing.
- Chest pain may be present.
- Nausea, vomiting, diarrhea, abdominal pain.
- Ask about underlying medical conditions.
- Inquire about duration of symptoms.
- Ask about ill contacts
- Ask about history of previous pneumonias.

 Physical Examination

- Tachypnea, dyspnea, cough, grunting, intercostal retractions, nasal flaring, splinting of affected side, abdominal distention.
- Decreased breath sounds, rales, and dullness to percussion.
- Lung examination may be normal.
- Friction rub may be heard over an effusion.
- Wheezing is rare in bacterial pneumonia (exception: *Mycoplasma pneumoniae* pneumonia)
- Observe bare-chested child in parent's arms from a distance to determine respiratory rate and work of breathing.

Laboratory Aids

• Arterial blood gas in patient with respiratory distress.

Test: CBC
Significance: White blood cell count of 15,000 frequently found; low white blood cell counts (e.g., 5000) sometimes associated with severe and overwhelming infection.

Test: Blood culture
Significance: Positive in 10% to 15% of cases of *H. influenzae, S. pneumoniae,* and *S. aureus* pneumonias.

Test: Pleural fluid studies
Significance: Gram stain, culture, cell count, glucose, protein, LDH, and pH may be helpful if effusion present.

Test: Gram stain and culture of sputum
Significance: Almost impossible to acquire in children without bronchoscopy, if obtained may identify pathogen.

Test: Pulse oximetry
Significance: Less than 92% oxygen saturation indicates significant hypoxia.

RADIOGRAPHIC IMAGING

Test: Two view (PA and lateral) chest radiograph
Significance: Lobar consolidations are common in *S. pneumoniae* and *H. influenzae;* patchy infiltrates are non-specific in infancy; hilar adenopathy is a red flag for tuberculosis; pneumatoceles suggest *S. aureus* or gram-negative organisms.

Test: Decubitus chest films
Significance: May be needed to determine the size and nature of effusions.

Test: Computed tomography scans of the chest
Significance: Allow one to differentiate parenchymal consolidation from pleural fluid when an effusion is suspected.

 ## Therapy

• ABCs (airway, breathing, circulation); life support measures including mechanical ventilation may be required.
• Supplemental humidified oxygen as needed.
• Intravenous fluid rehydration is often necessary.
• Drainage of pleural effusions (therapeutic) and chest tube placement may be necessary.
• Bronchoscopy to determine pathogen or rule out foreign body or tumor indicated when illness is protracted, recurrent, or not responding to therapy.
• Bronchodilator inhalation therapy (Albuterol) may be used if wheezing is present.

DRUGS

• Neonates

—Intravenous ampicillin
—Penicillin G
—Aminoglycoside (Gentamicin)
—Third-generation cephalosporin (Cefotaxime)

• Older children

—Inpatient—ampicillin, second- or third-generation cephalosporins
—Outpatient—penicillin V, amoxicillin, erythromycin, second- or third-generation cephalosporins, semi-synthetic macrolides. Treat for 7 to 10 days if uncomplicated. Complicated pneumonias with effusion and/or abscess formation require 14 to 21 days of IV therapy.

• Organism-specific therapy

—*Staphylococcus aureus:* Use penicillinase-resistant penicillin (Nafcillin, Oxacillin).
—Resistant *S. pneumoniae* (know prevalence in your area). If infection is life-threatening, consider Vancomycin until sensitivities are available.
—*Hemophilus influenzae* infections should be treated with cephalosporins.
—Anaerobic infections (aspiration pneumonia) should be covered with penicillin or clindamycin.
—Gram-negative pneumonia should be treated with a regimen that includes an aminoglycoside with broad activity such as amikacin or tobramycin.
—*Mycoplasma pneumoniae* requires therapy with erythromycin, macrolide or tetracycline (in children >8 years of age).

• Therapeutic procedures

—Thoracentesis (diagnostic or therapeutic) in presence of effusion
—Chest tube placement for empyema
—Surgical drainage of lung abcess may be indicated

 ## Follow-Up

• Radiograph may be abnormal for up to 6 weeks; therefore, serial x-rays are not recommended.
• Complicated pneumonias may be associated with restrictive or obstructive lung disease.
• Pulmonary function tests should be done on a case-by-case basis.

PREVENTION

• Pneumococcal vaccine should be given to immunocompromised patients and those with sickle cell disease.
• Children with sickle cell disease should take prophylactic penicillin for protection against encapsulated organisms, including pneumococcus.

PITFALLS

• Dehydration or very early detection may correspond to x-ray findings lagging behind the clinical course.
• Bacterial resistance and poor response to antimicrobial requires attention and re-evaluation.
• Hydration and nutritional status are sometimes overlooked.

 ## Common Questions and Answers

Q: When to admit?
A: Dehydration, hypoxia, significant respiratory distress, failure of outpatient management (worsening or no response in 24–72 hours), very young age (<6 months), concern for compliance with treatment, secondary complications (effusions, empyema, pneumothorax, etc.).

Q: Who should get a follow-up chest radiograph?
A: Any child with recurrent pneumonias, persistant symptoms, severe atelectasis, unusually located infiltrates, pneumothorax, or large effusions.

ICD-9-CM 482.9

BIBLIOGRAPHY

Arquedas AG, et al. Bacterial pneumonias. In: Chernick V, Kendig EL, eds. Disorders of the respiratory tract in children. 1990;371–380.

Churgay CA. The diagnosis and management of bacterial pneumonias in infants and children. In: Irons TG, Newton DA, ed. Primary care clinics in office practice: community-acquired respiratory infections in children. 1996 Dec;23(4): 821–835.

Klein JO. Bacterial pneumonias. In: Feigin RD, Cherry JD, eds. Textbook of pediatric infectious diseases. 1987:329–339.

Author: Deborah L. Silver

Pneumothorax

 Database

DEFINITION

- Air in the pleural space

PATHOPHYSIOLOGY

- Air can enter the pleural space via:

—Chest wall (i.e., penetrating trauma)
—Intrapulmonary (i.e., ruptured alveoli)

- Usually collapse of the lung on the affected side seals the leak
- If a ball valve mechanism ensues, however, air can accumulate in the thoracic cavity, causing a tension pneumothorax (a medical emergency)

CAUSES

- Spontaneous (secondary to rupture of apical blebs)
- Mechanical trauma

—Penetrating injury (i.e., knife or bullet wound)
—Blunt trauma

- Barotrauma (i.e., from mechanical ventilation)
- Iatrogenic

—Central venous catheter placement
—Bronchoscopy (especially with biopsy)

- Infection: most common organisms:

—*Staphylococcus aureus*
—Streptococcus pneumoniae
—Mycobacterium tuberculosis
—Bordetella pertussis
—Pneumocystis carinii

- Airway occlusion

—Mucus plugging (asthma)
—Foreign body
—Meconium aspiration

- Bleb formation (i.e., idiopathic spontaneous pneumothorax, cystic fibrosis)
- Malignancy

EPIDEMIOLOGY

- Dependent on the underlying lung disease
- Spontaneous pneumothorax:

—Incidence: 5 to 10/100,000
—Male:female ratio: 6:1
—Peak incidence: 16 to 24 years old

- Cystic fibrosis

—Incidence: 20% of patients more than 18 years old

COMPLICATIONS

- Pain
- Hypoxia
- Respiratory distress

- Tension pneumothorax
—Hypercarbia with acidosis
—Respiratory failure
- Pneumomediastinum with subcutaneous emphysema
- Bronchopulmonary fistula

PROGNOSIS

- Dependent on the underlying etiology of the pneumothorax
- If simple, spontaneous pneumothorax recovery is excellent

 Differential Diagnosis

PULMONARY

- Congenital lung malformations

—Cysts (i.e., bronchogenic cysts)
—Cystic adenomatoid malformation
—Congenital lobar emphysema

- Acquired emphysema
- Hyperinflation of the lung
- Bullae formation

MISCELLANEOUS

- Diaphragmatic hernia
- Infections (i.e., pulmonary abscess)
- Muscle strain
- Pleurisy
- Rib fracture

 Data Gathering

HISTORY

- May be asymptomatic
- Cough
- Shortness of breath
- Dyspnea
- Pleuritic chest pain is usually sudden in onset and especially in apices (referred pain to shoulders)
- Respiratory distress

SPECIAL QUESTIONS

Question: Does the patient have any underlying medical problems that are associated with an increased risk for pneumothoraces?
Significance: Asthma, cystic fibrosis, pneumonia, or collagen vascular disease.

Question: Did the patient do anything prior to developing symptoms that might have caused the pneumothorax?
Significance: Heavy lifting or increased coughing.

 Physical Examination

- May be normal
- Decreased breath sounds on the affected side
- Decreased vocal fremitus
- Hyperresonance to percussion on the affected side
- Tachypnea
- Tachycardia
- Shortness of breath
- Respiratory distress
- Shifting of the cardiac point of maximal impulse away from the affected side
- Shifting of the trachea away from the affected side
- Subcutaneous emphysema
- Cyanosis
- Scratch sign: listening through the stethoscope, a loud scratching sound is heard when a finger is gently stroked over the area of the pneumothorax.

Laboratory Aids

Test: Arterial blood gas
Significance:

- pO_2 can frequently be decreased
- pCO_2: elevated with respiratory compromise; decreased from hyperventilation

Test: Pulse oximetry
Significance: Useful for assessing oxygenation

Test: Electrocardiogram (ECG)
Significance:

- Diminished amplitude of the QRS voltage
- Rightward shift of the QRS axis (if left-sided pneumothorax)

IMAGING

Test: Chest radiograph
Significance:

- Radiolucency of the affected lung
- Lack of lung markings in the periphery of the affected lung
- Collapsed lung on the affected side
- Possible pneumomediastinum with subcutaneous emphysema

Test: Chest CT
Significance:

- Useful for finding small pneumothoraces
- Can help distinguish a pneumothorax from a bleb or cyst
- Helpful for locating small apical blebs associated with spontaneous pneumthoraces

Therapy

TREATMENT

- Stabilization of the patient
- Evacuation of the pleural air

—Should be done urgently if tension pneumothorax is suspected
—In small asymptomatic pneumothoraces observation of the patient indicated

- Treat the underlying condition predisposing for the pneumothorax:

—Antibiotics for infection
—Bronchodilators and anti-inflammatory agents for asthma attacks

DRUGS

- Oxygen

—Used to keep SaO_2 higher than 95%
—Breathing 100% O_2 can speed the intrapleural air's reabsorbtion into the bloodstream (useful for treating smaller pneumothoraces, especially in neonates).

SURGERY

Needle Thoracentesis

- Useful for evacuation of the pleural air in simple, uncomplicated spontaneous pneumothorax

Chest Tube Drainage

- Used for evacuation of the pleural air in recurrent pneumothoraces, complicated pneumothoraces, and cases with significant underlying lung disease.
- Thoracotomy versus video-assisted thoroscopy.

Surgical Removal of Pulmonary Blebs

- Blebs have a high rate of rupturing with resultant pneumothorax.
- In patients with established pneumothoraces, the blebs should be removed or oversewn to prevent reoccurrence of the pneumothorax.

Pleurodesis

- Used to attach the lung to the intrathoracic chest wall to prevent reoccurrence of a pneumothorax.
- Useful in cases of recurrent pneumothorax or if the pneumothorax is unresponsive to chest tube drainage (i.e., cystic fibrosis, malignancy).
- Mechanism of action: the surface of the lung becomes inflamed and adheres to the chest wall via the formation of scar tissue.

- Two commonly used methods:

—Surgical pleurodesis
  —Mechanical abrasion of part of the lung
  —Pleurectomy
  —Advantages: very effective: low reoccurrence rate; site specific (limits affected area)
  —Disadvantages: requires surgery and general anesthesia; not indicated in an unstable patient
  —Chemical pleurodesis

- Chemicals are used to cause inflammation
- Chemicals commonly used: tetracycline, minocycline, doxycycline, quinacrine, talc

—Advantages: requires no surgery or general anesthesia
—Disadvantages: less effective than surgery; generalized (rather than site-specific; makes future thoracic surgery more difficult; very painful)

DURATION

- Chest tube should be left in until:

—Majority of the air is reabsorbed
—No reaccumulation of air is seen on sealing of the chest tube

- Usually 2 to 4 days

 Follow-Up

WHEN TO EXPECT IMPROVEMENT

- Symptomatic relief within seconds of the air being evacuated

SIGNS TO WATCH FOR

- Unable to remove the chest tube without reaccumulation of air (suggestive of a bronchopulmonary fistula; requires surgical exploration if no improvement in 7–10 days)

PITFALLS

- Not considering the diagnosis in otherwise healthy patients.
- Confusing the symptoms with those of an underlying lung disease.
- Inserting a needle into a cyst or bleb (can cause a tension pneumothorax with rapid respiratory compromise).

PROGNOSIS

- Dependent on the underlying etiology of the pneumothorax
- If simple, spontaneous pneumothorax: excellent

 Common Questions and Answers

Q: Can a pneumothorax reoccur?
A: Reoccurrence is dependent on the underlying cause of the pneumothorax.

- Spontaneous pneumothorax (reoccurrence rates):

—Observation alone: 20% to 50%
—If thoracentesis performed: 25% to 50%
—If chest tube drainage performed: 32% to 38%

- Chemical pleurodesis:

—25% for tetracycline
—8% to 10% for talc

- Surgical pleurodesis:

—13% for video-assisted thoroscopy
—3% for thoracotomy

- Cystic fibrosis (reoccurrence rates):

—If no drainage attempted: 60%
—Thoracentesis alone: 79%
—Chest tube drainage alone: 63%

- Chemical pleurodesis:

—42% to 86% for tetracycline
—11% to 12.5% for quinacrine

- Surgical pleurodesis:

—0% to 4% for thoracotomy with pleurectomy

BIBLIOGRAPHY

Baumann MH, Strange C. Treatment of spontaneous pneumothorax: a more aggressive approach? *Chest* 1997;112:789–804.

Boutin C, Astoul P, Rey F, et al. Thoroscopy in the diagnosis and treatment of spontaneous pneumothorax. *Clin Chest Med* 1995;16: 497–503.

Jantz MA, Pierson DJ. Pneumothorax and barotrauma. *Clin Chest Med* 1994;15:75–91.

Kirby TJ, Ginsberg RJ. Management of the pneumothorax and barotrauma. *Clin Chest Med* 1992;13:97–112.

McLaughlin FJ, Matthews WJ, Streider DJ, et al. Pneumothorax in cystic fibrosis: management and outcome. *J Pediatr* 1982;100:863–869.

Pagtakhan RD, Chernick V. *Kendig's disorders of the respiratory tract in children*. Philadelphia: WB Saunders, 1990:545–557.

Schidlow DV, Taussig LM, Knowles MR. Cystic fibrosis foundation consensus conference report on pulmonary complications of cystic fibrosis. *Pediatr Pulmonol* 1993;15:187–198.

Tucker WY. *Pediatric respiratory disease: diagnosis and treatment*. Philadelphia: WB Saunders, 1993:839–844.

Warick WJ. *Pediatric respiratory disease: diagnosis and treatment*. Philadelphia: WB Saunders, 1993:575–578.

Author: Richard Mark Kravitz

Polyarteritis Nodosa

 Database

DEFINITION

An inflammatory process of medium and small muscular arteries resulting in dysfunction of affected organs.

CAUSES

- Idiopathic

PATHOLOGY

- Necrotizing arteritis of small- and medium-sized arteries resulting in segmental fibrinoid necrosis

EPIDEMIOLOGY

- Extremely rare in childhood
- Prevalence equal in boys and girls

GENETICS

- No specific HLA types known to be at increased risk

COMPLICATIONS

- Hypertension
- Renal failure
- Digital necrosis
- Intestinal infarction

 Differential Diagnosis

INFECTION

- Bacterial endocarditis
- Brucellosis

TUMORS

- Left atrial myxoma

METABOLICAL

- Homocystinuria

CONGENITAL

- Immunologic

—Systemic necrotizing vasculitis
—Systemic lupus erythematosus
—Kawasaki disease
—Systemic juvenile rheumatoid arthritis
—Wegener granulomatosis
—Takayasu arteritis
—Cryoglobulinemia
—Antiphospholipid antibody syndrome

PSYCHOLOGICAL

- Munchausen syndrome

MISCELLANEOUS

- Degos disease (malignant atrophic papulosis)

 Data Gathering

HISTORY

- Moderate constitutional symptoms?
- Abdominal pain?
- Weight loss?
- Unexplained fever?
- Headache?
- Arthralgia/myalgia?
- Rashes?
- Seizures?
- Weakness?

 Physical Examination

- Assess BP and pulses
- Check skin for livedo reticularis, splinter hemorrhages, and necrotic digits
- Neurological examination for findings consistent with neuropathy (mononeuritis multiplex)

PHYSICAL EXAMINATION TRICKS

Finding: The lacy network of superficial vessels of livedo reticularis
Significance: Does not blanche and is somewhat tender. Mottling of the skin seen in fair-skinned individuals will blanche and is not tender, and disappears with warming.

Laboratory Aids

Test: ESR
Significance: Usually extremely elevated, leuko-cytosis and thrombocytosis are seen.

Test: Urine analysis
Significance: Proteinuria and hematuria can be present

Test: Cr and BUN
Significance: May be elevated

Test: ANA and RF
Significance: Usually negative

Test: Anti-neutrophil cytoplasmic antibody (ANCA)
Significance: Detectable in some; usually perinu-clear (p) type, rarely cytoplasmic (c) type.

Test: Hepatitis B serologies
Significance: Hepatitis B has been associated in some series of PAN patients.

Test: Biopsy of affected tissue/organ
Significance: As indicated, usually skin, kidney, nerve, testicle.

IMAGING

Test: MRA (magnetic resonance angiography)
Significance: Can demonstrate vessel wall steno-ses and aneurysm.

FALSE-POSITIVES

Elevated ESR is seldom due to PAN. Conse-quently, a vigorous search for alternate explana-tions should be sought prior to making this di-agnosis.

PITFALLS

The detection of ANCA, previously thought to be highly specific for vasculitis, now appears to be less so. Hence, it remains important to con-firm the diagnosis of PAN with biopsy or angi-ography.

HOME TESTING

• May wish to have patients monitor blood pressure periodically if renal involvement sus-pected

 ## Therapy

DRUGS

• Corticosteroids are mainstay; usually start at dose of 1 to 2 mg/kg/d and adjusting based on response.
• Immunosuppressives such as methotrexate, azathioprine, and cyclophosphamide may be necessary.
• Hypertension should be managed aggres-sively, especially with calcium channel blockers.

DURATION

• May require long-standing therapy

DIET

• If renal system involved, low in sodium and potassium.
• Possible conflicts with other prescriptions.

 ## Follow-Up

WHEN TO EXPECT IMPROVEMENT

Initiation of steroid therapy may bring re-sponse in 1 to 2 weeks; however, management of specific organs affected during acute stage is essential.

SIGNS TO WATCH FOR

• Rising creatinine and BUN
• Abdominal pain
• Uncontrolled hypertension

PROGNOSIS

• May be extremely poor over the long term
• Risk high for renal failure, hypertension, myo-cardial infarction, bowel infarction, and death
• Due to low incidence/prevalence, precise data not available

PITFALLS

• Initiation of therapy prior to efforts to clinch the diagnosis

 ## Common Questions and Answers

Q: What is the difference between PAN and sys-temic necrotizing vasculitis?
A: PAN has a fairly strict definition. There are many children who clearly have vasculitis of the small- and medium-sized arteries who do not fit precisely into the description of PAN. In most ways the search for organ involvement and therapy is the same.

Q: Who should manage the patient with PAN?
A: Usually one discipline provides comprehen-sive management plan (either the pediatrician or rheumatologist). Subspecialist(s) of the af-fected organ systems provide management guidelines for specific organ issues.

ICD-9-CM 446.0

BIBLIOGRAPHY

Cassidy JT, Petty RE. *Textbook of pediatric rheu-matology,* 3rd ed. Philadelphia: WB Saunders, 1995.

Cuttica RJ. Vasculitis in children: a diagnostic challenge. *Curr Probl Pediatr* 1997;27(8): 309–318.

Author: Gregory F. Keenan

Polycystic Kidney Disease

 Database

DEFINITION

Polycystic kidney disease (PKD) is an heritable disorder with diffuse cystic involvement of both kidneys without other dysplastic elements.

There are two forms with considerable overlap in the pediatric population:

• Autosomal dominant polycystic kidney disease (ADPKD):

—Characterized by the presence of cysts at any point along the nephron or collecting duct
—Occasionally associated with characteristic cardiovascular and gastrointestinal manifestations
—Referred to as adult polycystic kidney disease because usually presents with clinical symptoms in the third to fifth decade
—May present in early childhood

• Autosomal recessive polycystic kidney disease (ARPKD):

—Cystic dilation of renal collecting ducts
—All cases accompanied by hepatic abnormalities such as biliary dysgenesis and periportal fibrosis (congenital hepatic fibrosis)
—Was called infantile polycystic kidney disease but can present at any time from the prenatal period through adolescence

• Diffuse cystic disease occurs in several other conditions in children and adults. Examples include tuberous sclerosis, multicystic dysplastic kidney, and a variety of malformation syndromes.

PATHOPHYSIOLOGY

• ARPKD

—In the infant and young child the kidneys are enlarged, spongy, and reniform. The cystic cortical collecting ducts are grossly visible as pinpoint dots on the capsular surface. The dilated ducts are 1 to 2 mm in diameter.
—Microscopic examination reveals medullary ductal ectasia, which is the characteristic feature of ARPKD. The glomeruli and remaining tubular structures are decreased in number.
—In older patients larger renal cysts and fibrosis develop.
—Hepatic involvement is invariably present.

• ADPKD

—Kidneys are enlarged with numerous round protuberances on their surfaces, and cysts are irregularly dispersed through the parenchyma. The cysts may measure from a few millimeters to many centimeters.

GENETICS

• ARPKD

—Sexes involved equally
—Gene recently localized to chromosome 6

• ADPKD

—Each offspring has a 50% chance of inheriting the gene.
—Expression may vary among affected individuals in terms of age of presentation, severity of involvement, and frequency of associated abnormalities.
—Causative gene is on the short arm of chromosome 16 (PKD1) in the majority.
—Second locus on chromosome 4 has been reported, which is responsible for a clinically indistinguishable form of ADPKD (PKD2).

EPIDEMIOLOGY

• Estimated incidence of ARPKD is 1:10,000 to 1:40,000.
• ADPKD is one of the most common hereditary disorders and accounts for 8% to 10% of cases of end-stage renal disease. Prevalence rates range from 1:200 to 1:1000.

COMPLICATIONS

• ARPKD

—Most patients present in infancy.
—Severely affected infants may have the oligohydramnios sequence at birth, with pulmonary hypoplasia and Potter phenotype.
—As renal function diminishes, the child may develop growth failure, anemia, and renal osteodystrophy.
—In the older child, complications of hepatic fibrosis and portal hypertension predominate. Hepatosplenomegaly, bleeding esophageal varices, and hypersplenism causing thrombocytopenia, anemia, and leukopenia may occur.

• ADPKD

—Patients may present with hypertension, urinary tract infection, abdominal pain, hematuria, or a palpable abdominal mass.
—The extrarenal complications seen in adults with ADPKD such as hepatic cysts, pancreatic cysts, colonic diverticulae, cardiac valvular abnormalities, and intracranial aneurysms are very rarely seen in pediatric patients.

PROGNOSIS

• Patients who are symptomatic at birth may die from pulmonary insufficiency.
• ADPKD

—In ARPKD, those who survive to 1 year have a much better prognosis.
—Renal insufficiency begins in early childhood and the progression is extremely variable.
—Causes of death outside of the neonatal period include renal failure, sepsis, hypertension, and complications of bacterial cholangitis and portal hypertension.
—Treatment with renal transplantation and liver transplantation may increase longevity.

• ADPKD

—Patients who present during infancy with symptomatic renal involvement may have an ominous prognosis and up to 50% die in the neonatal period.

—Presentation of ADPKD in the older child has a better prognosis.
—Control of hypertension and urinary tract infection improves the prognosis.

 Differential Diagnosis

• Multicystic dysplasia (MDK)

—Congenital condition with multiple large cysts of various sizes with no overall structural pattern to the kidney and no functional tissue, rarely bilateral renal involvement; often associated with cardiac, gastrointestinal and CNS abnormalities

• Glomerular cystic kidney disease (GCKD)

—Consists of bilateral cystic dilations of Bowman space with lack of significant tubular involvement and may have clinical and radiologic features consistent with ARPKD or ADPKD.

• Malformation syndromes
• Renal cysts occur in many hereditary syndromes in the form of peripheral cortical microcysts:

—Examples include trisomy 9, trisomy 13, Meckel syndrome, Jeune syndrome, Ivemark syndrome, Zellweger syndrome, and Bardet-Biedl syndrome.
—Acquired cystic disease may occur in patients with end-stage renal disease.

 Data Gathering

HISTORY

ARPKD?

• Patients usually present in infancy.
• Prenatal ultrasound may reveal oligohydramnios, large renal masses, or absence of urine in the bladder.
• Patients may present during the neonatal period with flank masses or respiratory distress.
• May present older children with symptoms of enlarged kidneys or hepato-splenomegaly.
• A concentrating defect may result in polydipsia and polyuria.
• Hypertension is common and may result in cardiac hypertrophy and congestive heart failure.

ADPKD?

• The most common presenting complaint in adults is pain.
• Older children may present with hypertension, abdominal pain, abdominal mass, hematuria, or urinary tract infection.
• Cerebral vessel aneurysms are rarely detected before age 20.

Physical Examination

ARPKD

- Flank mass most common.
- May also reveal evidence of portal hypertension (hematemesis, hepatosplenomegaly) or hypersplenism (pallor, petechiae).

ADPKD

- The clinical spectrum of disease is highly variable.
- Most common presentation in neonates is flank masses or palpable kidneys.
- Older children may present with hypertension, abdominal pain, abdominal mass, hematuria, urinary tract infection, or renal insufficiency.

 Laboratory Aids

Patients should undergo evaluation for renal insufficiency including BUN, creatinine, electrolytes, calcium, phosphorus, and a complete blood count (CBC).

IMAGING

ARPKD

Test: Ultrasound

- Will reveal, in patients with ARPKD, bilateral, enlarged kidneys with increased echogenicity of the parenchyma, and loss of corticomedullary differentiation.
- Occasional macrocysts may be present, >2 cm in diameter.
- The liver is enlarged and hyperechoic but usually less echogenic than the kidney. Dilated intrahepatic biliary ducts or decreased visualization of peripheral portal veins due to fibrous tissue may be seen.
- The disease may be diagnosed after 24 to 30 weeks gestation by ultrasonographic evidence of hyperechogenic enlarged kidneys, oligohydramnios, and no evidence of bladder filling.

Test: Intravenous Pyelogram (IVP)
Significance:

- Usually shows the classic finding of medullary streaking (radial striations) corresponding to accumulation of contrast in dilated collecting ducts.
- In older children with ARPKD the kidneys may be less enlarged, with evidence of macrocysts and loss of radial striations.

ADPKD

Test: Ultrasound
Significance:

- The kidneys of ADPKD may be enlarged with macrocysts of varying size. In children, renal involvement is frequently asymmetric and occasionally unilateral. However, the renal enlargement and macrocysts may not develop until adulthood. In children at risk, even single cysts in normal-sized kidneys are highly predictive of future ADPKD.
- Extrarenal cysts may also be seen in the liver, pancreas, ovary or spleen, although rarely in children.
- May not always distinguish ADPKD and ARPKD

Test: IVP
Significance:

- Will reveal enlarged, lobular kidneys
- The calyces are stretched and distorted
- Numerous cysts of various sizes are seen in the parenchyma.

False-Positives/Negatives

- The sonographic features of ADPKD and ARPKD may be present in the second trimester but usually are not manifested until after 30 weeks. Both false-positives and false-negatives have been reported.
- Although the combination of renal collecting tubule ectasia and biliary ectasia with periportal fibrosis is unique to ARPKD, portal duct fibrosis and bile duct proliferation may be seen in a variety of renal diseases such as Jeune and Zellweger syndromes and trisomy 9 and 13.

 Therapy

- Medical management of PKD is supportive.

—Hypertension is common in ADPKD and ARPKD. Patients may require antihypertensive therapy such as calcium-channel blockers.

- Supplemental bicarbonate may be indicated for metabolic acidosis.

—Urinary tract infections or bacterial cholangitis require aggressive antibiotic therapy.
—Infection of hepatic cysts may require drainage.

- Overall, renal replacement therapy with maintenance dialysis and renal transplantation is at least as successful in PKD as in non-PKD patients.

DIET

- The degree of renal insufficiency will dictate the need for a low potassium or low phosphorus diet.

 Follow-Up

SIGNS TO WATCH FOR

- Asymptomatic children in families with ADPKD are at risk and should be followed closely for hypertension, hematuria, and the development of an abdominal mass and the extrarenal manifestations
- Routine screening with cerebral arteriography for evidence of possible intracranial aneurysms in pediatric ADPKD patients is not recommended.

ICD-9-CM 753.1

 Common Questions and Answers

Q: What can be done to slow the progression of renal insufficiency in ADPKD?
A: Well-controlled blood pressure and rapid treatment of urinary tract infections may decrease the progression of renal failure.

Q: Should asymptomatic, older siblings of an infant with ARPKD be evaluated?
A: Yes. An older child may have congenital hepatic fibrosis with minimal renal involvement.

Q: Should one screen ADPKD-affected family members for the presence of cerebral vessel aneurysms if other family members have berry aneurysms?
A: Although routine screening is not recommended, intrafamilial clustering of aneurysms has been reported and it may be advisable to screen children with magnetic resonance imaging or cranial computer tomography in a family with aneurysms.

BIBLIOGRAPHY

Gabow PA. Medical progress: autosomal dominant polycystic kidney disease. *N Engl J Med* 1993;329(5):332.

Grantham JJ. The etiology, pathogenesis, and treatment of autosomal dominant polycystic kidney disease: recent advances. *Am J Kidney Dis* 1996;28:788–803.

Kaplan BS, Kaplan P, Rosenberg HK, et al. Polycystic kidney disease in childhood. *J Pediatr* 1989;115(6):867.

Author: Mary B. Leonard

Polycystic Ovarian Syndrome

 Database

DEFINITION

Polycystic ovarian syndrome (PCOS) is an endocrinologic disorder characterized by chronic anovulation, excessive androgen production, and noncyclical gonadotropin secretion. It begins perimenarcheally, and its clinical manifestations include hirsutism, amenorrhea or oligomenorrhea, and obesity.

CAUSES

• The characteristic polycystic ovary emerges when a state of anovulation persists for any length of time.
• Although the ovaries of these women produce excessive amounts of androgens, there is no inherent endocrinologic abnormality in the ovaries.
• The tonically elevated levels of luteinizing hormone (LH) cause the ovarian stromal tissue to produce more androgens, which in turn produce premature follicular atresia.
• Because there are many causes of anovulation, there are many causes of polycystic ovaries.
• It has been suggested that heredity, central catecholamine abnormalities, psychological stress, insulin resistance, and obesity may be involved.
• At least one group of patients with this condition inherits the disorder, possibly by means of an X-linked-dominant transmission.

PATHOPHYSIOLOGY

• The ovaries of most women with PCOS are enlarged as much as 5 cm in diameter, and the ovarian capsule is smooth, white, and thickened.
• Beneath the capsule are numerous small follicular cysts.
• For years it was erroneously believed that the thick sclerotic capsule acted as a mechanical barrier to ovulation.
• Instead of the characteristic picture of fluctuating hormone levels in the normal menstrual cycle, a steady state of gonadotropin and sex steroids are produced in association with persistent anovulation.
• There is an increased pulse amplitude of gonadotropin-releasing hormone (GnRH) and tonically elevated levels of LH.
• The polycystic ovary is a sign of these underlying endocrinologic abnormalities, not a disease intrinsic to the ovary.

EPIDEMIOLOGY

PCOS is relatively common and usually begins soon after menarche.

COMPLICATIONS

• The elevated levels of androgens that are produced are associated with hirsutism.
• The lack of a normal menstrual cycle leads to irregular bleeding, amenorrhea, and infertility.
• Because of the increased levels of unopposed estrogens, there is a threefold increased risk of endometrial cancer, and a 34-fold greater risk of breast cancer appearing in the postmenopausal years.

 Differential Diagnosis

• Congenital adrenal hyperplasia
• Cushing syndrome
• Adrenal androgen-producing tumors
• Ovarian- androgen-producing tumors
• Extragonadal sources of androgens

 Data Gathering

HISTORY

• Complete menstrual history
• Amenorrhea or irregular vaginal bleeding
• Infertility

 Physical Examination

HIRSUTISM

• Most patients with this syndrome are obese.
• Obesity probably enhances the syndrome because of the decrease in sex hormone-binding globulin, but is probably not important in its pathogenesis, because the syndrome occurs in some thin women and because many obese women do not have PCOS.

Laboratory Aids

- Because FSH levels are normal or low, an LH/FSH ratio greater than 3 (provided the LH level is not lower than 8 mIU/mL) may be used to suggest the diagnosis in women with clinical features of PCOS.
- Androgen levels are elevated. Serum testosterone levels are usually between 70 and 120 ng/dL, and androstenedione levels are usually between 3 and 5 ng/mL.

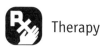

Therapy

- The best treatment for PCOS is oral contraceptives, unless pregnancy is desired, because these agents inhibit LH, decrease circulating testosterone levels, and increase levels of sex hormone-binding globulin, which binds and inactivates more of the testosterone in the circulation.
- Use oral contraceptives that contain less than 50 μg estrogen and a progestin other than norgestrel, which is the most androgenic progestin in current use.
- Patients who desire fertility should be treated with ovulation-inducing agents, starting with clomiphene citrate and proceeding to human menopausal gonadotropin or GnRH agonists if unresponsive.

- If adrenal androgens (DHEAs) are elevated, dexamethasone (0.25-0.5 mg at bedtime) should be given along with the oral contraceptive to reduce adrenal androgens to normal.
- Patients with amenorrhea or irregular bleeding should be treated with monthly progestins, such as oral medroxyprogesterone acetate 10 mg daily for the first 10 days of the month, to prevent the effects of unopposed estrogens.
- Spironolactone 50 to 100 mg twice daily causes regression of the hirsutism in women with PCOS by decreasing androgenic action in the target organs.
- Ovarian wedge resection was advocated in the past for treatment of androgen excess, but the decrease in circulating androgens occurred for only a short time, and this therapy should no longer be used.

Follow-Up

In the patient who has long-standing anovulation, an endometrial biopsy, with extensive sampling, should be done because of the link between unopposed estrogen and endometrial cancer.

Common Questions and Answers

Q: Can I still get pregnant if I have this syndrome?
A: Yes. Although the best treatment for this syndrome is oral contraceptives, those patients who desire to become pregnant can be treated with ovulation-inducing agents.

Q: I've noticed increased facial hair recently. Is there anything I can do about this?
A: Yes. In most cases, the oral contraceptives will decrease circulating androgen levels sufficiently so that this will regress, but if increased body hair (hirsutism) persists, another drug, called spironolactone, which blocks the action of androgens, can be added to more effectively treat this.

ICD-9-CM 256.4

BIBLIOGRAPHY

DeVane GW, Czckala NM, Judd HL, et al. Circulating gonadotrophins, estrogens, and androgens in polycystic ovarian disease. *Am J Obstet Gynecol* 1975;121:496.

Givens JR, Andersen RN, Wiser WI, et al. The effectiveness of two oral contraceptives in suppressing plasma androstanedione, testosterone, LH and FSH and stimulating plasma testosterone binding capacity in hirsute women. *Am J Obstet Gynecol* 1976;124:333.

Goldzicher JW. Polycystic ovarian syndrome. *Fertil Steril* 1981;35:371.

Kazar AR, Kessel B, Yen SSC. Circulating luteinizing hormone pulse frequency in women with polycystic ovary syndrome. *J Clin Endocrinol Metab* 1987;65:233.

Lobo RA, Goebelsmann U. Effect of androgen excess on inappropriate gonadotropin secretion as found in polycystic ovary syndrome. *Am J Obstet Gynecol* 1982;142:394.

Author: Ernest M. Graham

Polycythemia

 Database

DEFINITION

• Polycythemia is elevated hemoglobin and hematocrit owing to an absolute increase in red-cell mass. Polycythemia can be divided into subcategories, as follows:
• *Primary polycythemia:* primary defect of bone marrow erythropoiesis, resulting in overproduction of red cells
• *Secondary polycythemia:* stimulation of red-cell production by increased levels of erythropoietin (EPO), which may be appropriately secreted in response to tissue hypoxia, or may be inappropriately secreted because of renal disease or from a tumor
• *Relative polycythemia:* increased hematocrit without true increase in red-cell mass

PATHOPHYSIOLOGY

Primary Polycythemias

• Polycythemia vera (PCV): myeloproliferative disease with abnormal multipotent progenitor cells with abnormally high sensitivity to EPO; EPO levels are normal.
• Familial erythrocytosis: Usually idiopathic; some families have mutations in the EPO receptor (EPOR), which make red-cell precursors highly sensitive to EPO

Secondary Polycythemias

Relative tissue hypoxia resulting from deficiency of oxygen delivery, due to:

• Chronic lung disease and inadequate oxygenation due to a defect in gas exchange
• Cyanotic heart disease: desaturation of arterial blood because of admixture of oxygen-poor venous blood due to right-to-left shunt
• Circulatory: right-to-left shunting outside the heart
• Hemoglobinopathy: abnormal oxygen transport to tissues because of a mutant hemoglobin with higher than normal oxygen affinity.

—At the partial pressure of oxygen of the tissues, high oxygen-affinity hemoglobins release less oxygen than normal, resulting in hypoxia.
—Tissue hypoxia leads to supernormal secretion of EPO by the kidney, and increased production of red cells from the marrow.

• 2,3 DPG deficiency: increased oxygen affinity of hemoglobin because of reduced level of red-cell 2,3 DPG
• Inappropriate EPO secretion associated with kidney disease (not end-stage, where EPO is usually deficient)
• Malignant tumor, which secretes EPO

GENETICS

• High oxygen-affinity hemoglobins: autosomal dominant
• Familial erythrocytosis: may be autosomal dominant or recessive; Finnish and Chuvash clusters described
• 2,3-Diphosphoglycerate mutase deficiency: autosomal recessive

EPIDEMIOLOGY

• Uncorrected cyanotic congenital heart disease: most common cause of polycythemia
• PCV: Fewer than 50 reported childhood cases; 0.1% of cases of PCV are in children.
• High oxygen-affinity hemoglobins; 2,3-DPG dismutase deficiency; EPOR mutations; familial erythrocytosis: all rare

COMPLICATIONS

• Hyperviscosity: Blood viscosity increases dramatically when hematocrit >65%. Decreased exercise tolerance, dyspnea, and mental status changes are due to slowed microcirculation in the CNS.
• Thrombosis: Budd-Chiari syndrome from hepatic vein thrombosis, deep vein thrombosis, pulmonary embolus; seen especially in PCV
• Stroke: Cerebral thrombosis due to hyperviscosity
• Malignant transformation of PCV

PROGNOSIS

• Depends on underlying condition:

—High oxygen-affinity hemoglobinopathies: very good for normal life
—PCV: guarded, as may progress to myelodysplastic syndrome
—Eisenmenger syndrome: poor; progressive pulmonary hypertension and cor pulmonale

 Differential Diagnosis

PRIMARY POLYCYTHEMIA

• PCV

—Myeloproliferative disease
—May have thrombocytosis or leukocytosis

• Familial erythrocytosis

SECONDARY POLYCYTHEMIA

• Cyanotic congenital heart disease
• Eisenmenger syndrome

—Pulmonary hypertension from long-standing uncorrected congenital heart disease with left-to-right shunting (acyanotic) leads to elevated right-sided pressures and reversal of shunt to flow right to left, leading to cyanosis

• Extreme high altitude

—Compensation for low O_2 pressure includes an increase in red-cell mass.

• Alveolar hypoventilation: neuromuscular

—Muscular dystrophy
—Poliomyelitis
—Pickwickian syndrome
—Central hypoventilation

• End-stage lung disease
• Abnormal hemoglobins with high O_2 affinity
• 2,3-Diphosphoglycerate mutase deficiency
• Inappropriate EPO secretion may occur in:

—Renal disease

• Iatrogenic

—Excessive red-cell transfusion, possible in trauma, neonatal blood exchange
—Excessive exogenous dosing of EPO

• Neonatal polycythemia

—Twin-to-twin or placental transfusion

• Cobalt poisoning

RELATIVE POLYCYTHEMIA

• May be seen in smokers
• Dehydration or diuretic use

 Data Gathering

HISTORY

• Diagnosis of congenital heart disease, uncorrected or partially corrected
• History of cyanosis
• Delivery history

—Baby held below placenta
—Delayed clamping of cord
—Twins of disparate size

• Transfusion history
• Headache, paresthesias, dizziness, syncope
• Transient blindness
• Decreased exercise tolerance, respiratory distress, dyspnea on exertion, oxygen requirement
• Pruritis
• Lethargy
• Cigarette smoking
• Family history of cyanosis, high hematocrit, need for phlebotomy
• Cobalt poisoning: Homemade beer and magnets may contain cobalt.

Physical Examination

- Central and acral cyanosis
- Signs of dehydration: dry mucous membranes, no tears, poor skin turgor
- Heart murmur
- Clubbing
- Plethora: conjunctival, mucous membranes, nailbeds
- Splenomegaly: present in 75% of PCV

Laboratory Aids

TESTS

Laboratory Tests

Initial

- Complete blood count (CBC).
- Serum EPO: Distinguish 1° from 2° polycythemia.
- Pulse oximetry: to determine percent saturation of hemoglobin
- Arterial blood gas: pO_2 low in lung disease or right-to-left shunt

To Investigate High Oxygen-Affinity Hemoglobin

- Hemoglobin electrophoresis
- Whole-blood P_{50} and red-cell 2,3-DPG level
- Met-hemoglobin level: apparent cyanosis

To Investigate PCV

- Total red-cell mass measurement by ^{51}Chromium-tagged red cells: top normal range (adults) is less than 36 mL/kg in male, less than 32 mL/kg in female; gold standard test for true polycythemia
- Bone marrow aspirate with chromosomes: morphologic evidence of myelodysplastic syndrome; abnormal clone by karyotype
- Serum B_{12}, unsaturated B_{12}-binding capacity ($UB_{12}BC$): markedly elevated in PCV

Other Testing

- Total blood viscosity: rarely measured
- Iron studies: serum Fe, TIBC, ferritin
- BUN, creatinine, urinalysis: underlying renal disease

Imaging

- Echocardiography: to evaluate shunting
- Chest radiograph: to evaluate chronic lung disease, lung malignancies
- Abdominal ultrasound: to evaluate renal disease, spleen size, abdominal tumors
- Sleep study: looking for nighttime airway obstruction and desaturation

Therapy

OBSERVATION ONLY

Many patients require no therapy.

THERAPEUTIC PHLEBOTOMY

- Removal of red cells every 3 to 4 weeks to maintain hematocrit below threshold for symptoms; usually below 50% to 55%
- Patients with Eisenmenger syndrome and symptoms of hyperviscosity may not tolerate intravascular volume reduction if a large volume of blood is removed at one time.
- Patients on a chronic phlebotomy program may require iron supplementation.

DRUGS

- Hydroxyurea, alkylating agents, ^{32}P (in adults) to suppress red-cell production in PCV

SUPPLEMENTAL OXYGEN

- Helpful for secondary polycythemia due to underlying lung disease; may not help in right-to-left shunt

SURGERY

- Correction of underlying cardiac disease

DIET

- No specific recommendation
- Dietary restriction of water and salt intake may be required for underlying renal disease.

Follow-Up

SIGNS TO WATCH FOR

- Insufficient phlebotomy

—Headache
—Dizziness
—Syncope
—Decreased exercise tolerance between phlebotomies

- Progression of myelodysplastic disease

—Thrombocytopenia
—Bleeding

- Thrombosis

—Stroke
—Severe headache
—Jaundice
—Ascites

PREVENTION

- There are no preventive measures for primary conditions such as PCV, hemoglobinopathies, or familial erythrocytosis.
- Treatment of the underlying condition, such as correction of a cyanotic heart lesion, will prevent the development of secondary polycythemia.

PITFALLS

- Fingerstick CBC: Squeezing the finger to collect a specimen may give a falsely elevated hematocrit.
- Arterial blood gas: cannot interpret low pO_2 if specimen is mixture of venous and arterial blood
- Relative polycythemia: red-cell mass normal

—Decreased plasma volume with normal red-cell mass; seen in adult cigarette smokers
—Dehydration; elevated hematocrit due to hemoconcentration

- Hemoglobin electrophoresis does not identify all high-affinity hemoglobins.

—Many comigrate with normal hemoglobins
—Hemoglobin electrophoresis cannot be interpreted if the patient has been transfused within the past 3 months.

- Whole blood P_{50}

—Fresh specimen required; normals different from red cell lysates, purified hemoglobin

Common Questions and Answers

Q: Can a child with uncorrected cyanotic congenital heart disease be supported indefinitely with phlebotomy?
A: No. Phlebotomy will relieve the symptoms of hyperviscosity, but does not stop the progression of pulmonary hypertension.

Q: When should a child with polycythemia be referred to a pediatric hematologist?
A: If the high hematocrit is persistent and not clearly related to dehydration or neonatal causes (i.e., placental transfusion) then the child should be referred to a pediatric hematologist. Unexplained cyanosis is also a reason for referral. In the case of congenital heart disease, the pediatric cardiologist may be comfortable managing polycythemia without consultation with a hematologist.

ICD-9-CM 238.4

BIBLIOGRAPHY

Danish EH, Rasch CA, Harris JW. Polycythemia vera in childhood: case report and review of the literature. *Am J Hematol* 1980;9:421.

Nathan DG, Oski FA, eds. *Hematology of infancy and childhood,* 4th ed. Philadelphia: WB Saunders, 1993.

Pearson TC, Messinezy M. Investigation of patients with polycythemia. *Postgrad Med J* 1996:519–524.

Prchal JT, Sokol L. "Benign erythrocytosis" and other familial and congenital polycythemias. *Eur J Haematol* 1996:57:263–268.

Author: David F. Friedman

Porencephaly Cortical Dysplasia/Neuronal Migration Disorders

 Database

DEFINITION

Cortical dysplasia (CD) or neuronal migration disorders (NMDs) are a heterogeneous group of central nervous system developmental disorders in which there is disruption of normal cytoarchitecture in the cerebral cortex. Normal cerebral cortex has six layers, but in CD there may be a reduction to only three to four layers. CD may be classified as diffuse, in which the entire brain is affected, or focal, in which restricted regions are affected. Most CD/NMDs manifest clinically as epilepsy, mental retardation, focal neurologic deficits, or global neurologic dysfunction. Other tip-offs include intrauterine growth retardation, failure to thrive, and hypotonia. In general, the more extensive the brain area affected, the more severely compromised is the neurologic function.

Diffuse CD

• Etiologic agent likely before 20 weeks' gestation
• *Lissencephaly* (smooth brain): loss of cerebral cortical convolutions (sulci) and cortical laminations; may occur in combination with agyria-pachygyria (see below).
• *Agyria-pachygyria:* a more heterogeneous pathologic classification in which there are broad regions of cortex without gyri (similar to lissencephaly), but, in addition, focal areas of thickened cortical gyri also may be present.
• *Hemimegalencephaly:* a rare condition in which one cerebral hemisphere is enlarged and may exhibit concomitant agyric-pachygyric features. The normal-sized hemisphere may also contain subtle, focal abnormalities.

Focal CD

• Etiologic agent likely after 20 weeks' gestation
• *Dysplastic cortical architecture:* focal regions of disorganized cortical architecture and abnormally shaped neurons
• *Heterotopia:* clusters of neurons found within the white matter (where neurons are not typically found); may be nodular and confined to small region in cortex or adjacent to the ependyma (nodular forms); may extend across portions of a hemisphere (laminar heterotopia)
• *Schizencephaly:* large cleft in one or both hemispheres
• *Porencephaly:* nonloculated cavities in the brain that communicate with the ventricular system and/or subarachnoid space

CAUSES

CD/NMDs result from a variety of causes, including infectious, toxic-metabolic, ischemic, and genetic etiologies, which are all in utero insults.

• Genetic

—*Lissencephaly* may occur as a sporadic syndrome but has been associated with a 17p13.3 deletion in the Miller-Dieker lissencephaly syndrome.
—Other lissencephaly-associated syndromes, including the Norman-Roberts, Neu-Laxova, Walker-Warburg, and Fukuyama types of muscular dystrophy syndromes, are believed to have an autosomal recessive pattern of inheritance.
—The HARD syndrome (hydrocephalus, agyria, retinal dysplasia, and encephalocele) is autosomal recessive.
—*Cortical tubers* are regions of CD in tuberous sclerosis (TSC), which is associated with mutations on chromosomes 9q34 and 16p13.
—Subtle CD may be identified in neurofibromatosis (NF).
—Cortical cytoarchitectural abnormalities may also occur in trisomy 13, 18, and 21.

• Infectious

—*Polymicrogyria, pachygyria-agyria,* and *heterotopias* may occur in the setting of toxoplasmosis, other agents, rubella, cytomegalovirus, and herpes virus (TORCH) infections of the central nervous system during early development.

• Ischemic

—*Polymicrogyria* and *heterotopia* may occur in the setting of in utero hypoxic-ischemic injury.
—*Schizencephaly* may reflect intrauterine infarction and is characterized by a large cleft in one or both hemispheres. Whether schizencephaly is truly an NMD remains to be shown.
—*Porencephaly* (porencephalic cysts) are intraparencymal cavities that communicate with the ventricular system, which also result from intrauterine hypoxic-ischemic injury.

• Toxins

—Ethanol
—Ionizing radiation
—Carbon monoxide
—Isoretinoin
—Methyl mercury

• Metabolic

—CD/NMDs have been reported in association with Zellweger cerebrohepatorenal syndrome, neonatal adrenoleukodystrophy, Menkes disease, and GM2 gangliosidoses.

• Miscellaneous

—CD/NMDs may occur in syndromes characterized by numerous other congenital anomalies, such as the Smith-Lemli-Opitz, Potter, and Meckel syndromes.

PATHOLOGY

The most characteristic feature is disruption of normal cerebral cortical architecture. In lissencephaly, there are few cerebral convolutions (sulci and gyri) in the entire brain, and the normal layering of cortex is abnormal. Neurons are often abnormally shaped and are oriented incorrectly within the cortex. In heterotopias, cells are located inappropriately in the white matter. Disruption of the synaptic connections between various brain regions likely accounts for epilepsy and other neurologic problems. (See above definitions.)

GENETICS

See Causes.

EPIDEMIOLOGY

• Incidence varies according to syndrome.
• Many children die at birth or in early childhood, owing to global devastation.
• Approximate estimates are that from 20% to 40% of specimens resected during epilepsy surgery contain CD.

PROGNOSIS

Most patients with CD/NMDs will continue to suffer from seizures and cognitive impairment.

 Differential Diagnosis

In patients presenting with either overt or subtle neurologic symptoms or signs, consider a developmental central nervous system abnormality. Seizures and/or developmental delay are especially common manifestations of CD/NMDs. Epilepsy in pediatric patients may be a manifestation of a neurocutaneous disorder such as TSC. Tumors, vascular malformations, and in utero ischemic insults also should be considered.

Porencephaly Cortical Dysplasia/Neuronal Migration Disorders

 Data Gathering

HISTORY

• Important questions include family history of genetic or chromosomal syndromes, family members with mental retardation, neurologic dysfunction or seizures, and infant deaths associated with profound neurologic impairment.
• Ask about parental consanguinity.
• Subtle manifestations of neurocutaneous syndromes may be identified in family members with skin lesions or, in more overt cases, as individuals with CNS or other cancers, as in TSC or NF. Inquire about head or truncal flexion movements suggestive of infantile spasms.

 Physical Examination

• Many children with CD/NMDs have no overt signs of dysfunction, while others have global neurologic impairment.
• Developmental delay, seizures (especially infantile spasms), and focal neurologic signs may be observed.
• Microcephaly or macrocephaly also may be identified.
• Some children will have dysmorphic facies characterized by hypotelorism, malformed skull, and midline deformities.
• Characteristic facies of the Miller-Dieker lissencephaly syndrome include a thin upper lip, high forehead, anteverted nares, micrognathia, and microcephaly.
• Cutaneous manifestations such as café-au-lait or ash leaf spots, adenoma sebaceum, shagreen patches, or other regions of hyper/hypopigmentation may identify patients with neurocutaneous disorders such as TSC or NF.
• Funduscopic examination may reveal retinal hamartomas in TSC.

PHYSICAL EXAMINATION TRICKS

• Cutaneous examination with a Wood lamp may be useful in identifying ash leaf or café-au-lait spots.
• A linear sebaceous nevus on the forehead is associated with hemimegalencephaly.
• Tooth enamel pits may be identified in TSC.

 Laboratory Aids

TESTS

• Most routine blood tests and cerebrospinal fluid will be normal.
• Metabolic derangements characteristic of disorders such as gangliosidoses may be identified with specific blood tests.
• Chromosomal karyotyping analysis (genetic screening) for NF Miller-Dieker syndrome, and various trisomies can be performed to aid in both diagnosis and further genetic counseling.
• Screening for TSC will soon be available.
• Electroencephalography (EEG) is critical in diagnosing seizures and assessing the degree of underlying brain dysfunction. Characteristic findings may be sharp waves, spikes, hypsarrhythmia (in infantile spasms), and slow spike-wave discharges (Lennox-Gastaut syndrome). In children with developmental delay, formal neuropsychiatric assessment may be useful.

IMAGING

• *Magnetic resonance imaging* (MRI) with and without gadolinium contrast is essential in confirming CD/NMDs and in ruling out a CNS tumor, which may present in similar fashion.
• *Computed tomography* (CT) may be useful but has lower resolution than does MRI.
• Functional brain imaging with *single-photon emission tomography* (SPECT) and *positron-emission tomography* (PET) is gaining popularity in assessing regional changes in glucose or oxygen metabolisms within regions of dysplasia.
• A *serial brain MRI* will be necessary to monitor the appearance of CNS malignancies characteristic of NF and TSC. In addition, renal ultrasonography is necessary to monitor renal tumors, which appear in TSC.

 Therapy

DRUGS

Many children will require anticonvulsants such as phenytoin, phenobarbital, or valproate for seizure control. Children with infantile spasms may need ACTH therapy.

 Follow-Up

WHEN TO EXPECT IMPROVEMENT

Adequate seizure control may be difficult in CD/NMD patients. Cognitive and other neurologic deficits may benefit somewhat from neuropsychological intervention, education, and physical therapy. In children with a documented CD/NMD and refractory seizures, resective epilepsy surgery provides a safe and often successful alternative to conventional anticonvulsant medications.

SIGNS TO WATCH FOR

Most worrisome would be a persistent change in mental status, which could indicate status epilepticus. Other worrisome signs include development of new neurologic symptoms in patients with NF or TSC, suggesting a CNS neoplasm.

ICD-9-CM
Lissencephaly 742.2

BIBLIOGRAPHY

Barth P. Disorders of neuronal migration. *Can J Neurol Sci 1987;14:1.*

Debus O, Koch HG, Kurlemann G, et al. Factor V Leiden and genetic defects of thrombophilia in childhood porencephaly. *Arch Dis Child Fetal Neonatal Ed* 1998;78(2):F121–F124.

Eller KM, Kuller JA. Fetal porencephaly: a review of etiology, diagnosis, and prognosis. *Obstet Gynecol Surv* 1995;50(9):684–687.

Ho SS, Kuzniecky RI, Gilliam F, Faught E, Bebin M, Morawetz R. Congenital porencephaly: MR features and relationship to hippocampal sclerosis. *Am J Neuroradiol* 1998;19(1):135–141.

Author: Peter B. Crino

Portal Hypertension

Database

DEFINITION

Portal hypertension (HTN) is elevation of portal blood pressure above 10 to 12 mm Hg (normal, approximately 7 mm Hg).

PATHOPHYSIOLOGY

• Portal HTN is the result of a combination of increased portal blood flow and increased portal resistance.
• The portal vein carries blood from the stomach, spleen, pancreas, gall bladder, small intestine, and large intestine.
• Since no valves exist in the portal venous system, direction of flow reflects the pressure gradient and patency.
• All the major sequelae result from decompression of the venous pressure through portosystemic collaterals.
• The collaterals that develop are areas of decreased vascular resistance that become congested and lead to splenomegaly, esophageal varices, rectal varices, and caput medusae (periumbilical varices).

COMPLICATIONS

• The clinical manifestations of engorged collateral vessels include:

—Hemorrhage from esophageal varices
—Malabsorption due to congestion of the intestinal mucosa
—Ascites due to increased venous congestion with weeping of the mesentery
—Hypersplenism from splenic engorgement.

• Hemorrhage from esophageal varices is the most common presenting symptom (70%).

Differential Diagnosis

Portal HTN can be seen in many different diseases. Conceptually, it is easiest to divide the causes of increased portal pressure by location of the underlying lesion.

• Suprahepatic (6% of cases)

—Budd-Chiari (associated with congenital web, tumor, trauma, clotting disorder, contraceptives)
—Congestive heart failure
—Veno-occlusive disease

• Intrahepatic (60% of cases)

—Cirrhosis from any disorder (biliary atresia, cystic fibrosis liver disease, autoimmune hepatitis, chronic hepatitis, tyrosinemia, Wilson disease, α_1-antitrypsin
—Schistosomiasis (parasitic eggs located in the hepatic venule)
—Peliosis hepatitis (associated with androgens)
—Vitamin A toxicity (Ito-cell hyperplasia)
—Congenital hepatic fibrosis

• Subhepatic (34% of cases)

—Splenic vein thrombosis
—Portal vein thrombosis

Data Gathering

HISTORY

• History of umbilical catheterization
• History of hepatitis, abdominal trauma, clotting disorder, contraceptive pills, underlying medical problem such as cystic fibrosis, tyrosinemia, Wilson disease
• Ingestion of vitamin A
• Hematemesis

—Upper GI bleed from varices may be the first sign of long-standing silent liver disease or previously undiagnosed portal vein thrombosis.
—In patients with a stoma and portal HTN, life-threatening stomal variceal bleeds can develop.

Physical Examination

• Splenomegaly (although size of spleen does not correlate with pressure)
• Hemorrhoids
• Prominent vascular pattern on the abdomen
• The direction of flow through these veins can be indicative of the site of obstruction.

—For example, with inferior vena cava obstruction, the blood flow of the abdominal surface vessels is cephalad.
—Another clue may be the lack of a caput medusae. This typically occurs with portal vein obstruction due to obliteration of the umbilical vein. Physical examination of the liver may also provide information about the etiology.

• Hepatomegaly is commonly present with suprahepatic processes and may or may not be present for intrahepatic disease; for example, Budd-Chiari is associated with a large, tender liver; chronic intrahepatic liver disease may have a shrinking liver and an enlarging spleen.
• Prehepatic processes may have either a normal or atrophied liver, depending on the adequacy of blood flow.

Laboratory Aids

TESTS

• CBC and smear (will detect hypersplenism, GI blood loss, and chronic liver disease)
• PT, PTT
• Liver function tests
• Ultrasound with Doppler: used to identify whether the portal HTN results from a prerahepatic, intrahepatic, or subhepatic process

—Can investigate liver echogenicity, biliary tree, spleen size, renal abnormalities associated with cystic disease of the liver, vessel diameter, and direction of blood flow
—Hepatofugal flow in the left gastric, paraduodenal, or paraumbilical veins is consistent with portal HTN.
—Sonographically engorged collateral vessels can be identified; can see if there are esophageal varices

- Esophagogastroduodenoscopy (EGD): used for definitive determination of the presence of esophageal varices and identification of bleeding source in the patient who presents with bleeding
- Barium swallow: rarely useful because it is an insensitive measure of varices (only 70% detection in adults)
- Liver biopsy and/or appropriate serologic tests: may be needed to identify the underlying cause of the portal hypertension
- Hepatic venous wedge pressure gradient is used in adults because of the correlation of pressure with bleeding risk. However, it is not used in pediatrics because of a lack of well-documented pediatric measurements.

Therapy

ACUTE MANAGEMENT OF VARICEAL BLEED

- Lavage

—Use room temperature saline until clear.

- Blood products

—Replace blood products as needed
—Coagulopathy should be corrected with parenteral vitamin K and FFP.

- Medications

—Vasopressin: increases splanchnic vascular tone
—Somatostatin
—Nitroglycerin

- Endoscopy

—Sclerotherapy
—Ligation

- Direct tamponade

—Sengstaken-Blakemore tube

- Surgical intervention

—Portosystemic shunt
—Esophageal devascularization and/or transsection
—Liver transplantation
—TIPS (transjugular intrahepatic portosystemic shunting)

CHRONIC MANAGEMENT

- Beta-blockade: Nonselective blockers lower portal pressure by a combination of two mechanisms. β_2-blockade will increase splanchnic tone and subsequently decrease portal perfusion, and β_1-blockade will lower cardiac output and portal perfusion. Propranolol may have a specific effect in decreasing collateral circulation. Beta-blockade has been shown to be effective in preventing both initial and recurrent bleeds. It is unclear if its administration changes survival. In pediatrics it is rarely used in patients prior to adolescence for fear of lack of adaptive response if the patient should bleed.
- Sclerotherapy: not used prophylactically because of the lack of consistent data demonstrating a benefit. However, it has been successfully used to prevent recurrence of bleeding.
- Shunt: infrequently used in pediatrics. Portosystemic shunting has not been shown to improve long-term survival in patients with intrahepatic disease.
- Liver transplantation: A number of studies have established that long-term survival is better for transplanted patients than for patients treated with any other mode of therapy for bleeding. Therefore, the current approach at most institutions is liver transplantation for those patients with life-threatening bleeds not amenable to beta-blockade or sclerotherapy.

Follow-Up

- Depends on the etiology of the disease
- Most patients are followed closely for hepatic compensation.
- Growth failure, poor quality of life, and life-threatening bleeds not controllable with prophylactic intervention are indications for transplantation.

PITFALLS

- The site of bleeding needs to be identified and managed appropriately.
- Not all GI bleeding in a patient with portal HTN is upper.
- NG tube lavage, as well as being therapeutic, will help determine if the problem is from the upper tract. In some cases, the GI bleeding is from hemorrhoids or another area of the GI tract.
- The second most common pitfall is to overestimate the hemoglobin, because equilibration may not have taken place at the time of presentation with an acute bleed.

Common Questions and Answers

Q: What is my child's long-term prognosis?
A: The prognosis depends on the underlying etiology. Upper GI bleeding associated with portal vein thrombosis typically becomes less problematic as the child ages. Therefore, this group of patients will most likely not require a shunt and may be easily managed with sclerotherapy. Similarly, the group of patients with congenital hepatic fibrosis also does very well, because the underlying disease is nonprogressive and bleeding may be easily managed with sclerotherapy. In contrast, progressive liver disease and uncorrectable suprahepatic problems have a worse prognosis, and discussion needs to be tailored to the underlying pathology.

Q: Should I restrict my child's activities?
A: Limit contact sports if splenomegaly is present or use a spleen guard. Avoid aspirin and NSAID-containing products.

ICD-9-CM 306.2

BIBLIOGRAPHY

Gitnick G, LaBrecque DR, Moody FG. *Diseases of the liver and biliary tract*. St. Louis: Mosby-Year Book, 1992.

Mowat AP. *Liver disorders in childhood*. Boston: Butterworth-Heinemann, 1987.

Suchy F. *Liver disease in children*. St. Louis: Mosby, 1994.

Wyllie R, Hyams JS, eds. *Pediatric gastrointestinal disease*. Philadelphia: WB Saunders, 1993.

Author: Barbara Haber

Posterior Urethral Valves

Database

DEFINITION

• Valvular obstruction of the posterior urethra that results in variable dysfunction of all segments of the urinary tract, including the bladder, ureters, and renal parenchyma

PATHOPHYSIOLOGY

• The embryogenesis of posterior urethral valves (PUVs) is unclear.
• PUVs may arise from abnormal insertion and persistence of the distal end of the mesonephric duct.
• The valve is a fold of mucosa and fibrous tissue that usually forms a diaphragm with a slit-like orifice
• Children with PUVs commonly have renal parenchymal dysplasia.
• With flow of urine from the bladder in patients with PUVs, the valves balloon into the urethra, causing obstruction. As a result of the increased work of voiding, the bladder hypertrophies, with trabeculation and diverticulum formation. The bladder develops poor compliance, decreased capacity, increased pressure, and spastic hyperreflexia.
• The segment of the urethra proximal to the obstruction dilates and elongates.
• Obstructive uropathy produced by PUVs is the result of transmission of high bladder pressures to the ureters and kidneys.
• Hydroureteronephrosis, vesicoureteral reflux, perirenal urinoma, or urinary ascites may occur.
• Renal parenchymal damage may result.

GENETICS

• The genetic basis of PUVs remains unclear.
• The majority of cases are sporadic, although rare cases in siblings have been reported.

EPIDEMIOLOGY

• PUVs is the most common cause of lower urinary tract obstruction in male infants.
• There are rare reports of obstructive valves in the female urethra; however, they differ embryologically from PUVs seen in males.
• The majority of boys with PUVs present in the first year of life.

COMPLICATIONS

• Severe cases may suffer the effects of intrauterine oligohydramnios, including Potter syndrome and pulmonary hypoplasia.
• The renal parenchymal damage results in the sequelae of progressive renal failure, such as anemia, acidosis, fluid and electrolyte abnormalities, and failure to thrive.
• Urinary tract infections and vesicoureteral reflux are common complications.
• Urinary incontinence may result from uninhibited bladder contractions, bladder noncompliance, and polyuria.

PROGNOSIS

• The prognosis for infants with severe PUVs has improved due to earlier recognition and improved management of pulmonary hypoplasia and fluid and metabolic derangements. Pulmonary hypoplasia and renal dysplasia account for most causes of death in infants with PUVs.
• Measures of renal function at the time of presentation may not correlate with ultimate outcome. Rather, the rate of improvement following relief of obstruction is more indicative of prognosis. An early nadir creatinine below 1.0 mg/dL does not preclude renal failure, as the child attains greater body mass.
• During the course of many years, many children who seem to do well initially will suffer progressive renal failure and require renal transplantation.
• Patients with an abnormal serum creatinine at 2 years of age often develop end-stage renal disease by adolescence or young adulthood.
• Children with significant bilateral reflux, renal dysplasia, and/or bladder dysfunction are more likely to eventually develop renal insufficiency and hypertension.

Differential Diagnosis

• Nonobstructive urinary tract dilation may occur secondary to:

—Vesicoureteral reflux
—Prune-belly syndrome
—Detrusor-sphincter dyssynergia
—Polyuria
—Urinary tract infection

• Other entities that may mimic PUVs include:

—Urethral strictures
—Primary vesical neck contractures
—Anterior urethral valves

Data Gathering

HISTORY

• The clinical presentation depends on the age of presentation and the severity of the obstruction.
• Many severe cases are diagnosed postnatally as the result of evaluation of hydronephrosis detected antenatally on maternal ultrasound.
• Severely affected infants may present with respiratory distress and other sequelae of oligohydramnios, azotemia, sepsis, dehydration, acidosis, and electrolyte disorders.
• Patients may present with palpable bladder, urinary tract infection, abnormal urinary stream, or failure to thrive as a result of renal failure.
• Toddlers may present with urinary tract infection or voiding symptoms such as dysuria and a weak urinary stream.
• Older boys may present with daytime incontinence, nocturnal enuresis, or urinary frequency as a result of bladder hypertrophy coupled with polyuria secondary to a renal concentrating defect.
• A strong urinary stream does not exclude the diagnosis of PUVs because an adequate flow may be generated by the hypertrophied bladder.

Physical Examination

Palpably enlarged bladder and kidneys are the most common physical finding.

 ## Laboratory Aids

Infants with severe PUVs may have urinary tract infections and/or azotemia and fluid and electrolyte abnormalities such as dehydration, acidosis, hyperkalemia, and hyponatremia.

IMAGING

- The *voiding cystourethrogram* (VCUG) is the most important study in the diagnosis of PUVs. VCUG will reveal a sharply defined lucency in the posterior urethra and bladder hypertrophy. Bladder trabeculation, diverticuli, and vesicoureteral reflux may also be demonstrated.
- *Abdominal ultrasound* may demonstrate hydroureteronephrosis, evidence of renal dysplasia, dilation of the posterior urethra, a thickened bladder, and urinary ascites.
- Hydronephrosis is present in 90% of infants with PUVs.
- Definitive diagnosis requires *endoscopic examination*.

 ## Therapy

SUPPORTIVE

- Initial management in the neonate consists of inserting a fine urethral catheter into the bladder and treating any fluid and electrolyte disturbances and/or urinary tract infection.
- A large postobstructive diuresis may occur, requiring ongoing management of fluids and electrolytes.

SPECIFIC

- Valve ablation (destruction of the obstructive valve leaflet) is the definitive treatment of the primary lesion. The most common approach is to incise the valves transurethrally through an endoscope.
- In utero drainage of the fetal bladder, with unclear benefits, has been attempted at a few medical centers.
- Unless the patient has renal insufficiency that does not improve after fluid resuscitation and catheter drainage, the next step is endoscopic ablation of the valves.
- If the infant's urethra is too small for the endoscope, cutaneous vesicostomy may be necessary.
- If rapid recovery does not occur following placement of the catheter or after valve ablation, vesicostomy or supravesical urinary diversion (such as ureterostomy or nephrostomy) may be required. The optimal anatomic level of urinary diversion remains controversial.
- Following valve ablation, the posterior urethra will appear less dilated on VCUG. However, improvement in hydroureteronephrosis and vesicoureteral reflux occurs more slowly, over years.

 ## Follow-Up

- Growth problems, renal insufficiency, and end-stage renal disease can occur at any time during childhood, puberty, or beyond.
- Patients who require extensive urinary diversion, such as vesicostomy, pyelostomy, or ureterostomy, will require long-term reconstruction, including possible bladder reconstruction.
- Delayed obstruction may occur owing to urethral stricture.
- Patients with persistent incontinence require urodynamic evaluation to determine the case and individualized therapy.
- All children with PUVs should have careful follow-up through childhood and puberty. Each visit should include imaging for renal function and upper tract dilation and drainage, urodynamic studies of bladder function, assessment of growth, blood pressure, urinary protein, and serum creatinine.

PITFALLS

When a catheter is passed into the bladder, the valves flatten and are nonobstructive. This may give the misleading impression that there is no obstruction.

 ## Common Questions and Answers

Q: What can be done for children with long-term bladder dysfunction and incontinence?
A: Voiding dysfunction may occur as the result of myogenic failure, detrusor hyperreflexia, and bladder hypertonia. Patients may require a combination of clean intermittent catheterization (CIC), pharmacologic therapy, and bladder augmentation. Approximately 20% of patients with PUVs have secondary bladder pathology that is not reversible by primary therapy of the valves.

Q: Are patients with PUVs good candidates for renal transplantation?
A: Patients with valves have a 5-year graft survival rate of only 50%, compared with 75% for patients with other diagnoses. The main adverse factor is poor bladder function. Better results may follow more aggressive correction of the bladder anomalies. Transplantation has been successful in patients with bladder augmentation and in patients using clean intermittent catheterization.

Q: Do patients with PUVs have impaired sexual and reproductive function?
A: In a small study, patients had good sexual function and some were fertile. Ninety-five percent had normal erections and were able to achieve penetration. Thirty-four percent and 50% had normal or slow ejaculation, respectively. Approximately one-half had normal semen.

BIBLIOGRAPHY

Churchill BM, Jayanthi RV, McLorie GA, Khoury AE. Pediatric renal transplantation into the abnormal urinary tract. *Pediatr Nephrol* 1996;10:113–120.

Churchill BM, McLorie GA, Khoury AE, et al. Emergency treatment and long-term follow-up of posterior urethral valves. *Urol Clin North Am* 1990;17:343.

Parkhouse HF, Woodhouse CRL. Long-term status of patients with posterior urethral valves. *Urol Clin North Am* 1990;17:373.

Radhakrishnan J. Obstructive uropathy in the newborn. *Clin Perinatol* 1990;17:215–239.

Author: Mary B. Leonard

Premature Adrenarche

Database

DEFINITION

Premature adrenarche is characterized by appearance of small amounts of pubic hair, before age 8 in girls and age 9 in boys. Axillary hair development and apocrine sweat gland secretion are not always present. There are no other signs of sexual development.

PATHOPHYSIOLOGY

• Dehydroepiandrosterone (DHEA) and dehydroepiandrosterone sulfate (DHEAS) from the adrenal glands rise earlier than typically seen in normal puberty.
• Zona reticularis of the adrenals normally begins to increase androgen secretion at age 7 to 8 years.

GENETICS

• A familial pattern suggesting either recessive or dominant inheritance has been described.
• Occurs more frequently in African Americans

COMPLICATIONS

Can be the first sign of true precocious puberty (i.e., development of breast tissue and advancement of bone age) and thus warrants careful observation

PROGNOSIS

• Undergo puberty appropriately with normal fertility
• Ovarian hyperandrogenism is more common in some girls with premature adrenarche.
• Final adult height is normal.

Differential Diagnosis

• Tumors
—Androgen-secreting tumors can arise in the gonads or adrenal glands.
• Congenital
—Nonclassic congenital adrenal hyperplasia (CAH)
• Miscellaneous
—Central precocious puberty
—Familial male precocious puberty (testotoxicosis)

Data Gathering

HISTORY

• Careful attention to presence of any other signs of sexual precocity as well as temporal nature of the adrenarche (i.e., rate of progression)
• Family history of pubertal development

Physical Examination

• The presence of pigmented, curly hairs in the pubic area is consistent with the androgen effect.
• In girls, clitoromegaly suggests CAH or androgen-secreting tumors.

PITFALLS

Failure to differentiate between true pubic hair (curly and short) and dark lanugo hair (straight and long)

Laboratory Aids

TESTS

Specific Tests

• Adrenal steroids: DHEA and DHEAS are often in the early pubertal range, but testosterone and 17α-hydroxyprogesterone (17-OHP) should be at prepubertal levels.
• GnRH stimulation test: not recommended but would have a normal prepubertal response
• Children with systemic signs of virilization (such as a significantly advanced bone age) or elevated adrenal steroids (17-OHP or DHEA) should have CRH or ACTH stimulation testing to exclude CAH and other hyperandrogen syndromes.

Imaging

• Bone age usually is normal (not significantly advanced).
• CT scan or MRI should be considered if there are other signs of significant virilization; look for intracranial or intraabdominal masses, especially if androgens are markedly elevated.

 Therapy

• No treatment
• Reassure parents and children that this is a benign process.
• Reassess every 6 months to look for signs of virilization or pubertal progression.

 Follow-Up

WHEN TO EXPECT IMPROVEMENT

Regression does not occur.

SIGNS TO WATCH FOR

• Watch for other signs of puberty, such as breast development or testicular enlargement (≥4 mL), that suggest true precocious puberty.
• Further signs of virilization, especially postpuberty, suggest nonclassic CAH or early polycystic ovarian syndrome.

 Common Questions and Answers

Q: Is there a dietary cause for excess adrenal hormones?
A: No.

Q: Does premature adrenarche mean puberty will be early?
A: The onset of puberty in these children is within the normal range and should follow the familial pattern.

Q: Can anything be done to reverse the changes?
A: This is a benign process that does not have long-term sequelae. Antiandrogen drugs are available but are not recommended.

ICD-9-CM 255.3

BIBLIOGRAPHY

Karth-Schutz S, Levine LS, New MI. Serum androgens in normal prepubertal and pubertal children and in precocious adrenarche. *J Clin Endocrinol Metab* 1976;42:117.

Kornreich L, Horev G, Blaser S, et al. Central precocious puberty: evaluation by neuroimaging. *Pediatr Radiol* 1995;25(1):7–11.

Morris AH, Reiter EO, Geffner ME, et al. Absence of non-classical congenital adrenal hyperplasia in patients with precocious adrenarche. *J Clin Endocrinol Metab* 1989;69:709.

Pere A, Perheentupa J, Peter M, Voutilainen R. Follow up of growth and steroids in premature adrenarche. *Eur J Pediatr* 1995;154(5): 346–352.

Styne DM. New aspects in diagnosis and treatment of pubertal disorders. *Pediatr Clin North Am* 1997;44(2):505–529.

Authors: Robert J. Ferry, Jr. and Marta Satin-Smith

Premature Thelarche

 Database

DEFINITION

Premature thelarche is breast development before age 8 years with no other signs of pubertal development.

CAUSE

• Intermittent estrogen secretion by ovarian cysts

PATHOPHYSIOLOGY

• Low levels of estrogen secretion by normal follicular cysts
• Increased sensitivity of breast tissue to low levels of estrogen (surmised to be environmental)
• Ovarian response to transient increases in FSH levels and possibly to variations in ovarian sensitivity to FSH

EPIDEMIOLOGY

• Sixty percent noted between 6 months to 2 years of age

COMPLICATIONS

• May be the first sign of precocious puberty

PROGNOSIS

• No known effects on growth or fertility
• Onset after age 2 years may be associated with increased risk of progression to precocious puberty.

 Differential Diagnosis

• Environmental
—Exposure to exogenous estrogens in form of creams or birth control pills
—Intake of food with high estrogen levels (e.g., chicken liver)
• Tumors
—Benign lipomas
• Congenital
—Neonatal breast hyperplasia (*ICD-9-CM 778.7*) is benign breast enlargement in newborn boys or girls that is apparent shortly after birth and is due to gestational hormones. This kind of breast development usually regresses.
• True precocious puberty

 Data Gathering

HISTORY

• Careful assessment of onset and progression of breast tissue
• Family history of early puberty
• Exposure to estrogens

Special Questions

• Ingestion of foods with high estrogen levels

 Physical Examination

• Areolar enlargement is usually not present.
• Galactorrhea is not present.
• Look carefully for other signs of puberty:
—Menstrual blood
—Dull, gray-pink, or rugated vaginal mucosa (versus prepubertal appearance: shiny, bright red, and smooth)
—Pubic or axillary hair
• Inspect skin for birthmarks suggestive of McCune-Albright syndrome (café-au-lait spots in a "coast of Maine" pattern)

PROCEDURE

Palpate carefully to distinguish fat from true breast tissue.

 Laboratory Aids

TESTS

No test is specific. Serum FSH and estradiol may be slightly higher than age-matched controls but are not consistently elevated.

IMAGING

• Bone age is not significantly or very mildly advanced (<1 year ahead of chronologic age). Useful in guiding the need for more intensive evaluation of true precocious puberty
• Pelvic sonography: may demonstrate presence and regression of small ovarian cysts (1–15 mm)

Therapy

- Observation
- Reassurance that this is a benign process

 Follow-Up

WHEN TO EXPECT IMPROVEMENT

Regression may occur up to 6 years after onset.

SIGNS TO WATCH FOR

Evidence of pubertal progression should prompt additional evaluation by an endocrinologist:

- Rapid increase in size of breast tissue
- Vaginal bleeding
- Growth spurt
- Development of pubic and axillary hair

PITFALLS

- Must distinguish fat from breast tissue in obese girls
- Removal of a breast bud will result in failure of that breast to develop during adolescence.

 Common Questions and Answers

Q: Does premature thelarche predispose the child to abnormalities in pubertal development?
A: If onset occurs after age 2 years, the girl may be more likely to enter puberty earlier. However, the majority of girls with premature thelarche will have normal pubertal development and fertility.

Q: Is my child susceptible to breast cancer?
A: There are no data to suggest that premature thelarche increases the risk of breast neoplasia.

Q: Can it happen in boys?
A: Many newborn male and female infants have breast buds as a result of exposure to maternal estrogen in utero. This neonatal gynecomastia usually resolves quickly.

Q: My daughter has breast development on only one side. Is this a tumor?
A: Asymmetric breast development is quite common in the early stages of normal pubertal development. Malignant tumors of the breast during childhood are extremely rare. As mentioned earlier, any removal of breast tissue prior to or during puberty must be avoided if possible.

ICD-9-CM 259.1

BIBLIOGRAPHY

Haber HP, Wollmann HA, Ranke MB. Pelvic ultrasonography: early differentiation between isolated premature thelarche and central precocious puberty [see comment in Eur J Pediatr 1997;156(1):78–79]. Eur J Pediatr 1997; 154(3):182–186.

Klein Ko, Mericq V, Brown-Dawson JM, Larmore KA, Cabezas P, Cortinez A. Estrogen levels in girls with premature thelarche compared with normal prepubertal girls as determined by an ultrasensitive recombinant cell bioassay. J Pediatr 1999;134(2):190–192.

Mills JL, Stolley PD, Davies J, Moshang T Jr. Premature thelarche. Natural history and etiologic investigation. J Dis Child 1981; 135(8):743–745.

Pasquino AM, Pucarelli I, Passeri F, Segni M, Mancini MA, Municchi G. Progression of premature thelarche to central precocious puberty [see comment in J Pediatr 1995;127(2):336–337]. J Pediatr 1995;126(1):11–14.

Salardi S, Cacciari E, Mainetti B, Mazzanti L, Pirazzoli P. Outcome of premature thelarche: relation to puberty and final height. Arch Dis Child 1998;79(2):173–174.

Styne DM. New aspects in the diagnosis and treatment of pubertal disorders. Pediatr Clin North Am 1997;44(2):505–529.

Authors: Robert J. Ferry, Jr. and Marta Satin-Smith

Premenstrual Syndrome (PMS)

 Database

DEFINITION

Premenstrual syndrome (PMS) is a recurrent luteal-phase syndrome characterized by physical, psychological, and/or behavioral changes of sufficient severity to result in deterioration of interpersonal relationships and/or interference with normal activities.

CAUSES

Causes are related to the hormonal fluctuations of the menstrual cycle. Women with PMS symptoms are believed to have an abnormal response to normal hormonal changes.

PATHOPHYSIOLOGY

Currently, the preferred theories explaining PMS symptomatology involve alterations in serotonin and other neurotransmitters in response to changes in the ovarian steroid hormone levels. Other theories include:

- Estrogen excess
- Progesterone deficiency
- Pyridoxine (vitamin B6) deficiency
- Alterations in glucose metabolism
- Fluid-electrolyte imbalance
- Increased endorphins
- Hyperprolactinemia
- Serotonin deficiency
- Abnormalities in norepinephrine system

GENETICS

PMS may be found by family history in female relatives.

EPIDEMIOLOGY

- Thirty percent of all women are affected, with 10% severely affected.
- Three percent to 5% of women meet the criteria for premenstrual dysphoric disorder (PDD).

COMPLICATIONS

No permanent sequelae

PROGNOSIS

- High relapse rate after medications discontinued
- Symptoms may improve with age.

 Differential Diagnosis

- PDD is a severe form of PMS, consisting of more depressive, anxiety, and mood-swing symptoms.
- Dysmenorrhea
- Exacerbations of:

—Migraine headaches
—Epilepsy
—Asthma
—Allergies

 Data Gathering

HISTORY

- Description of cyclic symptoms occurring before the menstrual period
- Resolution at the onset of menses
- Emotional symptoms

—Irritability
—Depression
—Fatigue/lethargy
—Tearfulness
—Anxiety
—Impaired concentration

- Physical complaints

—Headaches
—Mastalgia
—Edema of legs, abdomen, or breasts
—Backache
—Clumsiness
—Increased appetite and food cravings
—Weight gain
—Decreased libido

- To establish diagnosis, use daily prospective charting of symptoms for two cycles. This will demonstrate clustering of symptoms around the luteal phase, with resolution when menses begins.
- Use a numeric scoring system for symptoms (1 = mild, 2 = moderate, 3 = severe) when recording symptoms.

 Physical Examination

No physical examination findings have proved to be helpful.

SPECIAL QUESTIONS

- Does the patient have severe behavioral symptoms and significant dysfunction?
- Does the patient meet DSM-IV criteria for PDD?

 Laboratory Aids

- None

 Therapy

DRUGS

No single treatment has been found to be universally effective, and conflicting results have been shown in studies with all therapies.

For Physical Symptoms

- Pyridoxine (vitamin B6): 50 to 100 mg/d throughout the cycle
- Natural progesterone: 200 to 400 mg vaginal suppositories taken daily from mid-cycle to menses. However, recent studies have shown progesterone to be equivalent to placebo in treating premenstrual symptoms.
- Oral contraceptives
- Gonadotropin-releasing hormone agents: suppress LH and FSH secretion, leading to a hypoestrogenic state. Available in subcutaneous and depot injections, as well as a nasal spray. Side effects include vaginal dryness, hot flashes, urinary discomfort, and osteoporosis.
- Danazol: 200 to 400 mg/d; decreases mastalgia, anxiety, irritability, and lethargy. Side effects include weight gain and androgenic activity, which limit its use.
- Nonsteroidal antiinflammatory drugs (NSAIDs): helpful in relieving dysmenorrhea, headaches, mastalgia, dizziness, and weakness
- Diuretics: Spironolactone, an aldosterone antagonist, has been effective in decreasing weight fluctuations and affective symptoms. Dosage: 25 mg orally four times daily, 2 to 3 days prior to the onset of symptoms. Do not use in adolescents at risk for pregnancy.
- Bromocriptine: helpful in the treatment of severe mastalgia not responsive to NSAIDs.

For Emotional Symptoms

• Antidepressants: the serotonergic antidepressants, fluoxetine (Prozac) and sertraline (Zoloft) are the first-line drugs for severe emotional symptoms. They work best when taken throughout the month and not solely during the luteal phase. Clomipramine (Anafranil) in doses of 25 to 75 mg daily, given for the full cycle or half-cycle, has been efficacious in treatment of emotional symptoms. Nefazodone, an antidepressant that blocks serotonergic and noradrenergic uptake, has recently been shown to be efficacious in relieving symptoms.
• Antianxiety agents: Alprozolam (Xanax) and buspirone (BuSpar) have helped patients with PDD in relief of anxiety and irritability symptoms. These are taken during the luteal phase.
• Oral contraceptives: have long been used to treat the emotional symptoms of PMS, yet recent studies show that they are less efficacious than previously thought.

DIET

• Avoidance of salt, caffeine, alcohol, and simple carbohydrates can improve symptoms.
• Regular aerobic exercise has also been shown to decrease symptoms in some women.

PREVENTION

No effective means of prevention are known.

Follow-Up

• After menses begins, the patient may see improvement.
• Following medication, the patient may see improvement within the first two menstrual cycles. If there is no improvement after 6 months, an alternate drug should be considered.

SIGNS TO WATCH FOR

• Worsening of premenstrual symptoms
• Sensory neuropathy: seen with pyridoxine (vitamin B6) use in doses as low as 200 mg/d for several months
• Psychotic behavior may necessitate psychiatric evaluation.

Common Questions and Answers

Q: What is the best way to monitor patient improvement during treatment?
A: Using a calendar and symptom rating scale may help to determine whether the chosen therapy is effective.

Q: Are there any nonpharmacologic therapies for premenstrual syndrome?
A: Yes, proper diet, rest, and exercise. Some investigators have used progressive relaxation exercises to help women manage their symptoms. Recently, reflexology therapy (manual pressure to reflex points on the ears, hands, and feet) was shown to reduce the somatic and psychological PMS symptoms in the women studied. Also, evening light therapy reduced depressive symptoms in one study of women with PDD.

Q: How do I manage the patient with mild PMS symptoms?
A: The patient should keep a symptom diary. For the physical complaints, use diet and exercise. For the emotional complaints, use relaxation and behavior modification therapy.

Q: How do I manage the patient with severe PMS symptoms?
A: The patient should keep a symptom diary. For the physical complaints, use NSAIDs, hormones, or diuretics. For the emotional symptoms, use antidepressants and/or anxiolytics.

ICD-9-CM 625.4

BIBLIOGRAPHY

Barnhart KT, Freeman EW, Sondheimer SJ. A clinician's guide to the premenstrual syndrome. *Med Clin North Am* 1995;79(6):1457–1472.

Camera EG. Premenstrual syndrome: a guide for the clinician. *Hawaii Med J* 1994;53:254–255, 259.

Coupey SM, Ahlstrom P. Common menstrual disorders. *Pediatr Clin North Am* 1989;36(3): 567–571.

Daugherty JE. Treatment strategies for premenstrual syndrome. *Am Fam Physician* 1998;58(1): 183–192, 197–198.

DeMonico SO, Brown CS, Ling FW. Premenstrual syndrome. *Curr Opin Obstet Gynecol* 1994;6: 499–502.

Emans SJ, Laufer MR, Goldstein DP. *Pediatric and adolescent gynecology,* 4th ed. Philadelphia: Lippincott-Raven, 1998:399–404.

Freeman EW. Premenstrual syndrome: current perspectives on treatment and etiology. *Curr Opin Obstet Gynecol* 1997;9(3):147–153.

Freeman EW, Rickels K, Sondheimer SJ, Polansky M. A double-blind trial of oral progesterone, alprazolam, and placebo in treatment of severe premenstrual syndrome. *JAMA* 1995; 274(1):51–57.

Johnson SR. Premenstrual syndrome therapy. *Clin Obstet Gynecol* 1998;41(2):405–421.

Mortola JF. A risk-benefit appraisal of drugs used in the management of premenstrual syndrome. *Drug Saf* 1994;10(2):160–169.

Pearlstein TB. Hormones and depression: what are the facts about premenstrual syndrome, menopause, and hormonal replacement therapy? *Am J Obstet Gynecol* 1995;173(2): 646–653.

Schmidt PJ, Neiman LK, Danaceau MA, Adams LF, Rubinow DR. Differential behavioral effects of gonadal steroids in women with and those without premenstrual syndrome. *N Engl J Med* 1998;338(4):209–216.

Steiner M, Steinberg S, Stewart D, et al. Fluoxetine in the treatment of premenstrual dysphoria. *N Engl J Med* 1995;332(23):1529–1534.

Yonkers KA, Halbreich U, Freeman E, et al. Symptomatic improvement of premenstrual dysphoric disorder with sertraline treatment. *JAMA* 1997;278(12):983–988.

Author: Liana R. Clark

Primary Adrenal Insufficiency

 Database

DEFINITION

Primary adrenal insufficiency is a deficiency in the secretion of cortisol by the adrenal glands, which may also be associated with deficiencies of other hormones, including aldosterone and adrenal androgens.

PATHOPHYSIOLOGY

- Addison disease: primary hypoadrenalism due to bilateral destruction of the adrenal cortices; autoimmune destruction (isolated or part of polyendocrine autoimmune syndromes), tuberculosis, hemorrhage, fungus, neoplastic infiltration, AIDS
- Adrenoleukodystrophy: inherited disorders of impaired peroxisomal degradation of very long chain fatty acids, resulting in adrenal insufficiency and progressive neurologic deterioration
- ACTH unresponsiveness: an inherited defect in the ACTH receptor, resulting in isolated glucocorticoid deficiency with hypoglycemia in infancy and hyperpigmentation

GENETICS

- Addison disease: Autoimmune adrenal insufficiency may be isolated or part of polyendocrine autoimmune syndromes. Familial and sporadic cases have been reported. An association exists between idiopathic Addison disease and HLA138 and Dw3.
- Adrenoleukodystrophy: X-linked recessive disorder of very long chain fatty acid metabolism. An autosomal recessive form of the disease exists, with presentation during infancy.
- ACTH unresponsiveness: autosomal recessive ACTH receptor defect

EPIDEMIOLOGY

Age

- Addison disease is uncommon in children and usually presents between ages 20 and 50 years. In the pediatric population, it is most often seen in late childhood and adolescence.
- Adrenoleukodystrophy typically presents late in the first decade of life with neurologic symptoms. Signs and symptoms of adrenal insufficiency may present at any age.
- ACTH unresponsiveness presents in late infancy or the toddler period.

Sex

- Addison disease is more common in females.
- Adrenoleukodystrophy, an X-linked disorder, predominantly affects males.
- ACTH unresponsiveness affects both sexes equally.

COMPLICATIONS

- If not diagnosed and/or treated properly, a significant physical stress such as surgery or illness may result in a life-threatening adrenal crisis.
- Adrenoleukodystrophy results in severe neurologic impairment and death.
- Unrecognized ACTH unresponsiveness is associated with recurrent hypoglycemia, seizures, mental retardation, and death.

PROGNOSIS

- The long-term prognosis of isolated adrenal insufficiency is good, provided adequate hydrocortisone is provided, particularly in times of illness.
- The diagnosis of adrenoleukodystrophy carries a poor prognosis.

 Differential Diagnosis

- Autoimmune adrenal cortical destruction
- Infectious adrenal cortical destruction

—Tuberculous
—Fungal
—AIDS

- Adrenal hemorrhage
- Neoplastic adrenal infiltration
- Adrenoleukodystrophy
- ACTH unresponsiveness

 Data Gathering

HISTORY

- Weakness and fatigue
- Anorexia, weight loss
- Headache
- Nausea, vomiting, diarrhea, abdominal pain
- Postural dizziness
- Muscle or joint pains
- Emotional lability
- Salt craving
- Hyperpigmentation, especially on lip borders, buccal mucosa, nipples, and over creases
- Decreased axillary or pubic hair in females due to lack of adrenal androgens
- Amenorrhea in females

 Physical Examination

- Hyperpigmentation
- Weight loss
- Hypotension
- Evaluate for other signs of autoimmune disease (e.g., thyromegaly, vitiligo).

Laboratory Aids

TESTS

Specific Tests

• Cortrosyn stimulation test: Administer cosyntropin (synthetic ACTH) 250 μg IV and measure cortisol at 30 and 60 minutes. A normal rise is a final cortisol exceeding 18 μg/dL. An insufficient cortisol response is diagnostic of adrenal insufficiency.
• A baseline ACTH greater than 200 pg/mL with inadequate cortisol is seen in primary adrenal insufficiency
• Serum adrenal antibodies may be positive in autoimmune Addison disease.
• Very long chain fatty acids are elevated in adrenoleukodystrophy.

Nonspecific Tests

Electrolytes

• Hyponatremia: result of the mineralocorticoid defect and glucocorticoid deficiency; combination sodium loss from kidneys and the inability to excrete a water load
• Hyperkalemia and acidosis: chronic mineralocorticoid deficiency with the inability to excrete potassium and acid
• Hypercalcemia: probably through increased calcium absorption due to the lack of glucocorticoid effect on the gut
• Hypoglycemia: Glucocorticoids have permissive effects on gluconeogenesis.
• Renin levels are elevated when a mineralocorticoid deficiency is present.

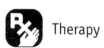

Therapy

ACUTE ADRENAL CRISIS

An intercurrent illness or surgical procedure may provoke an episode of hypotension and tachycardia, possibly leading to shock. Electrolytes reveal a decreased serum sodium, increased potassium, acidosis, and a decreased or normal glucose. Serum should be drawn and saved, but treatment should not be delayed for a diagnostic Cortrosyn stimulation test.

Treatment

• D5NS for volume repletion
• Stress dosage of hydrocortisone: 100 mg/m² followed by 100 mg/m²/24 h of hydrocortisone divided q4h. Taper steroids over the next 1 to 2 days to a physiologic replacement dosage.
• Mineralocorticoid replacement: Florinef 0.1 mg daily when able to take PO.

CHRONIC ADRENAL INSUFFICIENCY

Treatment

• Hydrocortisone 10 to 12 mg/m²/day PO divided as tid triple dose for stress of fever, illness, vomiting. For major stress (surgery, significant illness), give hydrocortisone 50 to 100 mg/m² followed by 50 to 100 mg/M²/24 h IV divided q4h. Injectable hydrocortisone is recommended for emergency home use.
• Florinef 0.1 mg PO per day
• Patient education

—Stress dosing
—Seek medical attention for significant illness, persistent vomiting, or the inability to take fluids by mouth.
—Medic-Alert bracelet

Follow-Up

An acute adrenal crisis usually improves rapidly with the administration of fluids and glucocorticoids. Steroids can usually be tapered in 12 days.

LONG-TERM MONITORING

• Clinical: reduction in hyperpigmentation
• Electrolytes, ACTH, renin
• Screen for polyautoimmune disorders.
• Growth
• Very long chain fatty acid levels and neurologic function in adrenoleukodystrophy

PREVENTION

• N/A

PITFALLS

• The symptoms of primary adrenal insufficiency are nonspecific and are similar to those found in many disease processes. The electrolyte picture of adrenal insufficiency can be seen in renal disorders, obstructive uropathy, and isolated aldosterone deficiency.
• Cosyntropin testing should definitively separate out those with true adrenal insufficiency.

Common Questions and Answers

Q: What are the indications for stress dosing and how rapidly can the stress hydrocortisone dose be tapered?
A: Patients will require stress dosing of hydrocortisone for surgical procedures, fever (>100°F), vomiting, diarrhea, and particularly vigorous exercise. The stress dose is typically given for 24 hours, after which the usual dose is resumed. Should it be necessary to administer the stress dosage for a more prolonged period, the dosage can usually be tapered to a physiologic dosage over 12 days, once the patient's clinical condition has improved.

ICD-9-CM 255.4

BIBLIOGRAPHY

Grinspoon SK, Biller BMK. Clinical review: laboratory assessment of adrenal insufficiency. *J Clin Endocrinol Metab* 1994;79(4):923–931.

Listenberg MJL, Kemp S, Sarde CO. Spectrum of mutations in the gene encoding the adrenoleukodystrophy protein. *Am J Hum Genet* 1995;56: 44–50.

Moser HW, Moser AE, Singh I, O'Neill B. Adrenoleukodystrophy: survey of 303 cases: biochemistry, diagnosis, and therapy. *Ann Neurol* 1984; 16:628–641.

New MI, del Balzo P, Crawford C, Speiser P. The adrenal cortex. In: Kaplan S, ed. *Clinical pediatric endocrinology*. Philadelphia: WB Saunders, 1990;181–234.

Tsigos C, Arai K, Hung W, Chrousos GP. Hereditary glucocorticoid deficiency is associated with abnormalities of the adrenocorticotropin gene. *J Clin Invest* 1993;92:2458–2461.

Author: Lorraine Katz

Prolonged QT Interval Syndrome

 Database

DEFINITION

Prolonged QT interval syndrome, also known as congenital long QT syndrome (LQTS), is characterized by prolongation of the surface ECG QT interval, syncope, and sudden death as a result of malignant ventricular tachyarrhythmias. This electrical instability is due to an abnormality in ventricular repolarization.

PATHOPHYSIOLOGY

There are two hypotheses to explain the pathogenesis of congenital LQTS:

• An abnormality or imbalance in the sympathetic innervation to the heart, which would explain the sinus bradycardia, abnormal repolarization, adrenergic dependence of arrhythmias, and response to antiadrenergic medications associated with the syndrome
• An intrinsic abnormality in the mechanisms responsible for cardiac repolarization. Because three of the identified gene mutations resulting in congenital LQTS occur at loci that also encode a cardiac ion protein, ion channels have been proposed as the intrinsic abnormality that is responsible for abnormal repolarization.

GENETICS

• Autosomal dominant (Romano-Ward syndrome)
• Autosomal recessive (associated congenital nerve deafness [Jervell and Lange-Nielsen syndrome])
• Genetic linkage analysis studies have attributed the autosomal dominant LQTS to at least four known gene loci (chromosomes 11, 3, 7, and 4).

	LQT1	LQT2	LQT3	LQT4
Chromosome	11	7	3	4
Gene	KVLQT1	HERG	SCN5A	

EPIDEMIOLOGY

• Exact prevalence of LQTS is not known, but it may be a common cause of syncope and sudden unexplained death in children and young adults.
• Extrapolation from sudden death data suggests that the frequency may be as high as 1 in 5,000.

COMPLICATIONS

• Complications, especially in untreated patients, include:

—Ventricular tachyarrhythmias, specifically torsades de pointes
—Syncope
—Sudden death

• In patients with the inherited form of the condition, as opposed to those with a new mutation, asymptomatic family members may be affected.

PROGNOSIS

• Children have a higher incidence of sudden death than do adults, which may reflect a bias that adult patients have already survived childhood.
• Pediatric patients with greatest risk for sudden death are believed to be those with QT$_c$ greater than 600 msec. β-Blocker therapy has been shown to reduce the incidence of sudden death.

 Differential Diagnosis

Congenital LQTS is most commonly misdiagnosed as vasovagal syncope or a seizure disorder. All patients who have a syncopal event or who are diagnosed with epilepsy should have a baseline screening ECG. Sudden infant death syndrome (SIDS) may be related to congenital LQTS (controversial). QT interval prolongation may be subtle, such that up to 10% of affected individuals may have a normal screening ECG and up to 40% may have borderline prolongation of the QT interval.

• Electrolyte abnormalities: hypokalemia, hypocalcemia, hypomagnesemia, and metabolic acidosis
• Toxins: organophosphates
• CNS trauma
• Malnutrition: anorexia
• Primary myocardial disease: myocarditis, ischemia
• Medications

—Cardiac medications: quinidine, procainamide, disopyramide, sotalol, amiodarone
—Antibiotics/antifungals: erythromycin, trimethoprim/sulfa, pentamidine, ketoconazole, fluconazole
—Psychotropic medications: tricyclics, phenothiazines, haloperidol
—Antihistamines: Seldane, Hismanal, Benadryl
—Gastrointestinal: cisapride.

 Data Gathering

HISTORY

• The history may be notable for:

—Palpitations
—Symptoms of presyncope
—Syncope

• These symptoms may be related to provocative stimuli, especially emotional or physical stress. The use of medications known to prolong the QT$_c$ interval should be established.
• Most importantly, a thorough family history for arrhythmia, syncope, epilepsy, or sudden unexplained death should be obtained.

 Physical Examination

• Usually normal, may have bradycardia

 Laboratory Aids

Bazett's formula: QT$_c$ = QT/(square root of RR interval). Generally, a QT$_c$ greater than 600 msec is considered abnormal, although some clinicians allow a slightly longer QT$_c$ for infants less than 6 months of age. In addition, some clinicians argue that the QT$_c$ should not be corrected at heart rates less than 60 bpm. The measurement should be taken in lead II without significant sinus arrhythmia. Children frequently have a prominent U wave, and it should generally be included in the measurement of the QT$_c$ if it is greater than half the amplitude of the T wave. A single measured prolonged QT$_c$ interval does not make the diagnosis of LQTS, and there is currently no single diagnostic test to confirm the diagnosis. Scoring systems may help stratify patients into high, moderate, and low probability of having the syndrome. See the table Diagnostic Criteria for Long QT Syndrome.

Diagnostic Criteria for Long QT Syndrome

Family History

Family members with definite LQTS	1
Unexplained sudden cardiac death <age 30 among immediate family members	0.5

Symptoms

Syncope*

With stress	2
Without stress	1
Congenital deafness	0.5

Electrocardiographic findings

QT_c

>480 msec	3
460–470 msec	2
450 msec (in males)	1
Torsades de pointes*	2
T-wave alternans	1
Notched T wave in 3 leads	1
Low heart rate for age	0.5
Prominent U waves	1
Miscellaneous	1

*Mutually exclusive

Total score: 0-2 = unaffected; 2.5-4.0 = intermediate; >4.5 = affected

Atrioventricular block can be seen in infants with relatively rapid heart rates and P waves that occur during the prolonged repolarization period and ventricular refractoriness. Other tests that may help confirm the diagnosis include 24-hour ambulatory Holter monitoring. This recording may disclose asymptomatic ventricular ectopy or arrhythmias, T-wave alternans, or variability in the QT_c interval during different periods of the day. Exercise stress testing may also be helpful in identifying ventricular arrhythmias or prolongation of the QT_c interval, particularly during the early recovery phase. The echocardiogram should demonstrate normal cardiac structure and function.

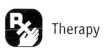

Therapy

Many clinicians argue to medically treat asymptomatic children because of a high incidence of sudden death occurring as the first symptom.

• Patients are usually treated based on symptoms and the clinical severity of their disease. The primary mode of therapy is (β-blockade, most commonly with propranolol, atenolol, or nadolol. The class Ib antiarrhythmic medications, such as mexiletine, are also used in patients with congenital LQTS. Medications do not generally help treat patients with acquired LQTS.

• Occasionally, implantation of a permanent pacemaker is indicated based on the theory that long pauses may help to promote the induction of tachyarrhythmias, such as torsades de pointes.

• Left stellate ganglionectomy is a controversial therapy performed to eliminate the hyperactive left sympathetic ganglion output.

• Automatic implantable cardioverter-defibrillators (AICDs) are usually reserved for older children and adolescents who have significant symptoms and documented ventricular arrhythmias. Recent identification of disease genes in congenital LQTS may lead to the development of therapy specific to the ion channel defect.

Follow-Up

Follow-up outpatient appointments should include the review of new or recurrent symptoms, including palpitations, near-syncope or syncope, and the efficacy and adverse effects of medical therapy. The ECG may demonstrate a normal or prolonged QT_c. Follow-up 24-hour ambulatory Holter monitor recordings and exercise stress tests may help in the assessment of adequate β-blocker therapy and the identification of ventricular arrhythmias.

PREVENTION

Preventive measures should focus on the avoidance of exposure to medications or situations that may provoke prolongation of the QT_c interval or the induction of torsades de pointes, such as certain antihistamines and antibiotics, sympathomimetics, caffeine, electrolyte abnormalities, and highly stressful environments.

PITFALLS

As reviewed in the Differential Diagnosis section, the primary pitfall is missed recognition of the syndrome. This may occur when an affected patient has a normal screening ECG (up to 10% of patients) or when a wrong diagnosis is made (epilepsy, for example). Once a diagnosis is made, family members should be thoroughly screened.

Common Questions and Answers

Q: Should activity be restricted in patients with congenital LQTS?
A: Because sudden rises in serum catecholamine levels may precipitate symptoms, it is appropriate to restrict competitive and vigorous athletics. Symptomatic patients may require greater restrictions. Documentation of appropriate β-blockade, by a lower maximal heart rate at peak exercise, on follow-up exercise stress test may be helpful.

Q: If someone is identified as having LQTS, should family members be evaluated?
A: Yes, with a high degree of suspicion. Most cases of congenital LQTS are inherited in an autosomal dominant pattern, so that each child of an affected parent has a 50% chance of having the gene. This does not predict the severity of symptoms, but parents, all siblings, and children of patients should have ECGs. Holter monitoring and exercise stress testing may be helpful in provoking an abnormal QT_c interval in suspected family members.

ICD-9-CM 426.8

BIBLIOGRAPHY

Ackerman MJ. The long QT syndrome. *Pediatr Rev* 1998;19(7):232–238.

Garson A Jr, Dick M II, Fournier A, et al. The long QT syndrome in children: an international study of 287 patients. *Circulation* 1993;87: 1866–1872.

Roden DM, Lazzara R, Rosen M, et al. Multiple mechanisms in the long QT syndrome: current knowledge, gaps, and future directions. *Circulation* 1996;94:1996–2012.

Schwartz PJ, Moss AJ, Vincent GM, et al. Diagnostic criteria for the long QT syndrome: an update. *Circulation* 1993;88:782.

Author: Ronn E. Tanel

Prune-Belly Syndrome

 Database

DEFINITION

The prune-belly syndrome is a rare congenital disorder characterized by the triad of:

- Deficiency of the abdominal musculature
- Bilateral cryptorchidism
- Dilated, anomalous development of the bladder and upper urinary tract

It presents in a broad spectrum of severity, from severe renal dysplasia and pulmonary hypoplasia to mild uropathy with stable renal function.

CAUSES

The etiology of the prune-belly syndrome remains unclear. Two theories have been proposed:

- The triad of congenital defects may be the result of a primary mesodermal defect in development with congenital deficiency of smooth muscle in the bladders, ureters, and renal pelvis.
- Outflow obstruction of the bladder in utero may result in dilation of the bladder and upper urinary tract with subsequent renal injury. The expanded bladder may block the route of the descending testicles and may cause abdominal distension and abdominal wall muscle atrophy.

PATHOPHYSIOLOGY

- Prune-belly bladder is large, irregular in shape, and thick walled. Many patients have poor urinary flow and high residual volumes.
- Ureters are usually markedly dilated, tortuous, and elongated. Peristalsis is ineffective and the distal ureters are most severely affected.
- Renal involvement is variable; the most severe dysplasia occurs in patients with worse dilation of the urinary tract. The dysplastic changes are usually symmetric.
- Usually, the bladder neck is wide and the prosthetic urethra is dilated and triangular. Most patients do not have anatomic obstruction at this point.

GENETICS

- The genetic basis of prune-belly syndrome remains unclear.
- A majority of patients have normal karyotypes.
- A majority of cases are sporadic, although rare cases in siblings have been reported.

EPIDEMIOLOGY

- Most patients are detected during the neonatal period or prenatally during maternal ultrasound.
- Prune-belly syndrome is much more common in males.

COMPLICATIONS

Many patients have other associated anomalies:

- *Gastrointestinal anomalies* include imperforate anus and increased risk of volvulus.
- *Lower extremity musculoskeletal anomalies* include talipes equinovarus and congenital hip dislocation.

Complications of the syndrome include:

- Pulmonary hypoplasia
- Vulnerability to recurrent pulmonary infections and postoperative atelectasis secondary to chest wall instability and ineffective cough because of abdominal wall deficiency
- Frequent urinary tract infections (UTIs) secondary to upper urinary stasis, vesicoureteral reflux, and bacteriuria
- Sequelae of progressive renal insufficiency

PROGNOSIS

- Patients with the most severe renal dysplasia die in the neonatal period.
- Those with a mild form do not require surgical treatment of the urinary tract; renal function is usually stable and the prognosis is excellent.
- For patients with moderate involvement, the degree of renal dysplasia and insufficiency determines outcome. In addition, upper urinary tract stasis, poor bladder emptying, vesicoureteral reflux, and bacteriuria are factors that may combine to result in a worse long-term prognosis.

 Differential Diagnosis

- The distinctly abnormal physical examination of the affected infant results in an early, accurate diagnosis in most cases.
- Pseudoprune-belly syndrome (prune-belly syndrome uropathy, normal abdominal wall examination, and incomplete or absent cryptorchidism)

 Data Gathering

HISTORY

In patients with mild involvement of the abdominal wall that are not detected in the neonatal period, evaluation of UTIs may reveal the dilated urinary tract.

 Physical Examination

- In most cases, the abdominal wall is characterized by multiple wrinkles and redundant skin.
- A large, distended bladder creates a suprapubic mass.
- Ureters and kidneys are readily palpable.
- Intestinal loops and peristalsis may be observed.
- Testes are undescended.
- Myopathy results in difficulty in sitting up from a supine position.

Laboratory Aids

TESTS

Laboratory Tests

• The initial evaluation should include assessment of renal function.
• May see elevated serum levels of creatinine and BUN
• Renal failure may result in anemia and elevated levels of potassium, phosphorus, hydrogen ion, and uric acid, and decreased concentrations of sodium, calcium, and bicarbonate.

Imaging

• An ultrasound will demonstrate the dilatation and redundancy of the upper urinary tract.
• When considering a voiding cystourethrogram, consider the risk of introducing infection into the dilated, poorly draining urinary tract.
• Renal function and drainage of the dilated tract can be assessed by radioisotope renal scan or an excretory urogram.

Therapy

SUPPORTIVE

• The basic principles of supportive care and management of renal failure apply.
• Antibiotics in the neonatal period and antibiotic prophylactic of indefinite duration are indicated to prevent infection.

SPECIFIC

• The dilated, tortuous urinary tract is managed by urologists. The optimal approach to patients with severe uropathy who survive the newborn period is very controversial.
• Some advocate minimal surgical intervention, based on the observation that there is no functional obstruction and the dilated system has a low pressure owing to the deficient smooth musculature. If renal function deteriorates, the urinary tract dilation progresses or the patient develops a urinary tract infection despite antibiotic prophylaxis; cutaneous vesicostomy is recommended to facilitate drainage.
• Others advocate extensive surgical remodeling. Possible procedures include, as indicated:

—Internal urethrotomy, reduction cystoplasty
—Excision of the redundant ureter with reimplantation of the remaining segment
—Cutaneous ureterostomy
—Pyelostomy

• Reconstruction of the abdominal wall has yielded good cosmetic results with questionable improvements in function.
• Bilateral orchiopexy is indicated.

Follow-Up

Regardless of how an individual patient might be managed, he or she will require long-term follow-up. These patients require meticulous attention to renal function, pulmonary function, and urine bacteriology.

Common Questions and Answers

Q: Are patients with prune-belly syndrome candidates for renal transplantation?
A: Yes. However, special pretransplant consideration should be given to the dilated urinary tract in order to optimize function.

Q: How does the urinary tract function in older children?
A: A tendency for bladder tone and ureteral peristalsis to improve with age has been noted.

Q: Are these patients infertile?
A: Normal sexual activity has been described. However, there are no reports of fertility, and the patients usually have azospermia.

Q: What is the usual cause of morbidity in the newborn period?
A: Respiratory failure.

ICD-9-CM 756.7

BIBLIOGRAPHY

Coplen DE, Snow BW, Duchett JW. Prune-Belly syndrome. In: Gilwater JY, Grayhack JT, Howards SS, Duchett JW, eds. Adult and pediatric urology, 3rd ed. St. Louis: Mosby, 1996;2297–2310.

Greskovich FJ III, Nyberg LM Jr. The prune belly syndrome: a review of its etiology, defects, treatment and prognosis. J Urol 1988;140:707–712.

Loder RT, Guiboux JP, Bloom DA, Hensinger RN. Musculoskeletal aspects of prune-belly syndrome. Description and pathogenesis. Am J Dis Child 1992;146:1224–1229.

Pagon RA, Smith DW, Shepard TH. Urethral obstruction malformation complex: a cause of abdominal deficiency and the "prune-belly." J Pediatr 1979;94:900.

Sutherland RS, Mevorach RA, Kogan BA. The prune-belly syndrome: current insights. Pediatr Nephrol 1995;9(6):770–778.

Wheatley JM, Stephens FD, Hutson JM. Prune-belly syndrome: ongoing controversies regarding pathogenesis and management. Semin Pediatr Surg 1996;5(2):95–106.

Woodard JR. Lessons learned in 3 decades of managing the prune-belly syndrome. J Urol 1988;159(5):1680.

Woodard JR, Zucker I. Current management of the dilated urinary tract in prune-belly syndrome. Urol Clin North Am 1990;17:407.

Author: Mary B. Leonard

Pseudotumor Cerebri

 Database

DEFINITION

Diagnostic criteria of pseudotumor cerebri include:

- Increased intracranial pressure with normal CSF
- Normal neurologic examination except for papilledema (occasional abducens nerve palsy and, rarely, meningismus)
- Normal neuroimaging study

CAUSES

- Pathogenesis is unknown but may involve abnormalities in neuroendocrine regulation of CSF circulation.
- Chronic hypercapnia due to respiratory hypoventilation may play a role in some cases.

Numerous precipitants of pseudotumor have been reported. It is clearly associated with obesity and weight gain, but weaker associations may be chance. Pseudotumor is often linked to tetracycline, sulfonamides, use of and withdrawal from corticosteroids, isotretinoin, thyroid replacements, and nalidixic acid; it is also linked to vitamin A deficiency or intoxication, chronic anemia, and hypothyroidism.

GENETICS

Sporadic, no clear genetic predisposition, unless related to an underlying hormonal, toxic, or inflammatory condition; no data are available in children.

EPIDEMIOLOGY

- Incidence in children is unknown.
- Males and females are affected equally, unlike adults.
- Pseudotumor has been reported as early as 4 months of age, with a median age of 9 years.

ASSOCIATED CONDITIONS

- Visual loss due to optic nerve pressure
- Endocrinopathies, exogenous steroids, lead exposure, tetracycline, and several other antibiotics may be associated with pseudotumor.

 Differential Diagnosis

The following may all be confused with pseudotumor, but the clinical picture and CSF analysis usually permit their distinction.

- Chronic meningitis (such as CNS Lyme disease), encephalitis, or cerebral edema (may show minimal changes on neuroimaging with elevated CSF protein and little pleocytosis)
- Cerebral venous sinus thrombosis (as in otitic hydrocephalus)

 Data Gathering

HISTORY

- Headache is the most common presenting complaint.
- Blurred vision, diplopia, transient visual obscurations, and dizziness may be present.
- Infants and young children may present with irritability, somnolence, or ataxia.
- Directed history for signs of associated endocrinopathy, antibiotic or steroid exposure, sleep disturbance, sinus infection, connective tissue, tendency for thrombosis

 Physical Examination

- Papilledema is almost always present in older children.
- Most infants have some degree of papilledema, even with open fontanelles and split sutures.
- Sixth cranial nerve palsies are common in children with pseudotumor; they were found in 29 of 68 patients in one series.
- Other cranial nerve deficits are rarely seen.
- Recording baseline visual acuity and visual fields in older children is essential.

 Laboratory Aids

TESTS

- Cranial *CT* or *MRI* should be normal. MRI is preferred because of superior imaging of brainstem, posterior fossa, and sinuses. MRA/MRV is useful in evaluating dural venous sinus thrombosis.
- *Lumbar puncture manometry* with the patient in a relaxed position should show an opening pressure of greater than 200 mm H_2O, but otherwise normal CSF composition.
- *Goldmann perimeter visual field testing* is useful in children over 5 years of age to document field deficits and monitor response to therapy.
- CBC and TFTs should be obtained because anemia, hypothyroidism, and hyperthyroidism have rarely been associated with pseudotumor.

The following may be useful in selected cases:

- ANA
- ESR
- Urine cortisol
- Serum lead level.

Some authors have reported pseudotumor in association with Lyme disease.

Therapy

• Removal of possible causative agents is the first intervention, along with treatment of associated conditions (obesity, anemia, thyroid disease).
• Acetazolamide (Diamox), a carbonic anhydrase inhibitor that decreases CSF production, is the drug of choice.

—The pediatric dosage is 60 mg/kg/d divided qid for the standard form and bid for the long-acting form (Diamox sequels).
—The adult dose is 250 mg qid or 500 mg bid, increased to 500 mg qid or 1,000 mg bid if tolerated.

• Prednisone for 10 to 14 days, followed by a 14-day taper, can be used if acetazolamide is ineffective or has intolerable side effects.
• Serial lumbar punctures are not recommended as standard therapy, although one or two LPs can be useful to relieve symptoms acutely.
• Surgical therapy, optic nerve sheath fenestration, or lumboperitoneal shunt is indicated for progressive visual loss despite medical therapy or for severe visual loss at presentation.

 ## Follow-Up

• Patients should have visual acuity, visual fields, and fundi evaluated at least monthly for 3 to 6 months.
• More frequent follow-up is required for any signs of progressive visual loss.
• Follow-up and tapering of acetazolamide should be done in conjunction with a neurologist or neuroophthalmologist.
• If visual loss resolves, acetazolamide can be tapered after 2 months of therapy.

PITFALLS

• Children are *not* exempt from permanent visual loss as a sequelae of pseudotumor.
• Ophthalmologic follow-up is important.
• Pseudotumor may be diagnosed erroneously if:

—Pseudopapilledema is mistaken for papilledema
—CSF abnormalities (i.e., isolated increase in protein) are overlooked
—Neuroimaging fails to identify a cerebral venous sinus thrombosis

 ## Common Questions and Answers

Q: What are the side effects of acetazolamide?
A: Side effects of acetazolamide include GI upset, parasthesias, loss of appetite, drowsiness, metabolic acidosis, and renal stones. An alternative is furosemide.

Q: If pseudotumor occurs on tetracycline, can the child take penicillin?
A: Penicillins/cephalosporins have not been reported as a significant cause of pseudotumor.

Q: Are there any limitations on physical activity?
A: Activity can be graded entirely according to the child's symptoms

ICD-9-CM 348.2

BIBLIOGRAPHY

Baker RS, Baumann RJ, Buncie JR, et al. Idiopathic intracranial hypertension (pseudotumor cerebri) in pediatric patients. *Pediatr Neurol* 1989;5:5.

Cox T, Bullock P, Calver DM, Robinson RO. Diagnosis and management of benign intracranial hypertension [Review]. *Arch Dis Child* 1998; 78(1):89–94.

Eggenberger ER, Miller NR, Vitale S. Lumboperitoneal shunt for the treatment of pseudotumor cerebri. *Neurology* 1996;46(6):1524–1530.

Radhakrishnan K, Ahlskog JE, Garrity JA, Kurland CT, et al. Idiopathic intracranial hypertension. *Mayo Clin Proc* 1994;69:169.

Soler D, Lessell S. Pediatric pseudotumor cerebri (idiopathic intracranial hypertension). *Surv Ophthalmol* 1992;37:155.

Author: Dennis J. Dlugos

Psittacosis/Ornithosis (Parrot Fever)

 Database

DEFINITION

Psittacosis/ornithosis (parrot fever) is an acute febrile disease characterized by pneumonitis and other systemic symptoms.

CAUSE

- *Chlamydia psittaci* (an obligate intracellular parasitic bacterium)

PATHOPHYSIOLOGY

- Inhalation of aerosolized organisms into the respiratory tract
- Incubation period of 5 to 21 days
- Spreads via bloodstream to lungs, liver, and spleen
- Lymphocytic inflammatory alveolar response

EPIDEMIOLOGY

- Birds are the major reservoir (pigeons, parrots, parakeets, turkeys, chickens, ducks).
- Infecting agent present in bird nasal secretions, urine, feces, feathers, viscera, carcasses
- While inhalation is the most common route of infection, bird bites and mouth-to-beak contact also spread infection.
- Birds may be healthy or sick.
- Most reported cases (70%) are the result of exposure to pet caged birds (especially parrots, parakeets).
- Occupational hazard of workers in poultry plants, pet shops, zoos, farms.
- Rarely transmitted person to person.
- Only 100 to 200 total cases reported in United States each year.
- Very rare disease in young children.

COMPLICATIONS

- Hepatitis, anemia
- Thrombophlebitis, pulmonary embolus
- Arthritis, keratoconjunctivitis
- Endocarditis, myocarditis, pericarditis
- Encephalitis: agitation, delirium, confusion, stupor

PROGNOSIS

Complete recovery is expected in all but a few rare cases (even without antibiotic use).

ASSOCIATED ILLNESS

Pneumonitis, along with severe headache, is the most common presentation.

 Differential Diagnosis

- Psittacosis should be considered in all fevers of unknown origin or atypical pneumonitis.
- *Mycoplasma* and *Chlamydia pneumoniae, Legionella* spp., Coxiella burnetii (Q fever), tuberculosis, viral and fungal pneumonitis, as well as pneumoccal pneumonia

 Data Gathering

HISTORY

- Abrupt onset of symptoms is usual.
- Fever, headache, cough, weakness, chills, muscle aches, and joint pain are common.
- A nonproductive cough is usual.
- Vomiting, confusion, and photophobia are less common.

PITFALLS

Failure to question parents as to the exposure of the patient to any type of bird—wild or domestic

 Physical Examination

- Ill appearance, tachypnea, rales, and splenomegaly are common.
- A relative bradycardia is a unique finding in some cases.
- Rash, meningismus, pharyngeal injection, cervical adenopathy, hepatomegaly, and mental status changes less common.

Laboratory Aids

TESTS

- Chest x-ray demonstrates diffuse interstitial infiltrates.
- Routine laboratory studies are not helpful.
- Complement fixation titers (see Common Questions and Answers)
- Isolation of the organism is diagnostic.

PITFALLS

Note that the complement fixation titers do not distinguish between the various chlamydial infections (*C. psittaci, C. pneumoniae,* and *C. trachomatis*)

 Therapy

- Tetracycline (40 mg/kg/d) or doxycycline (100 mg bid) for at least 10 to 14 days in children older than 8 years
- Erythromycin (40 mg/kg/d) in children 8 years and younger
- Chloramphenicol also an option.
- Oxygen and other supportive care (especially respiratory) as needed

 Follow-Up

- Resolution of fever and most other systemic symptoms can be expected within 48 hours of antibiotic therapy.
- Untreated patients may have severe pulmonary symptoms for 1 to 3 weeks.

PREVENTION

- Epidemiologic investigation is indicated in all possible cases.
- Birds suspected to be infected should be sacrificed, transported, and analyzed by appropriate experts.
- Potentially contaminated bird areas should be disinfected and aired.

 Common Questions and Answers

Q: In children with pneumonia and a pet bird, how is the diagnosis confirmed?
A: A fourfold rise in antibody titers by complement fixation or microimmunofluorescence (acute and convalescent specimens; 2–3 weeks apart); a single titer of 1:32 or higher (highly suggestive); culture (done through the Centers for Disease Control and Prevention).

Q: Does the source bird usually exhibit signs of infection or illness?
A: No. While the bird may show signs like anorexia, ruffled feathers, depression, or watery green droppings, often the bird is totally asymptomatic.

ICD-9-CM 073.9

BIBLIOGRAPHY

Centers for Disease Control and Prevention. Compendium of psittacosis (chlamydiosis) control, 1997. *MMWR* 1997;46(RR-13):1–13.

Gregory DW, Schaffner W. Psittacosis. *Semin Respir Infect* 1997;12(1):7–11.

Hammerschlag MR. Atypical pneumonias in children. *Adv Pediatr Infect Dis* 1995;10:1–39.

Kirchner JT. Psittacosis. Is contact with birds causing your patient's pneumonia? *Postgrad Med* 1997;102(2):181–182, 187–188, 193–194.

Peter G, ed. *1997 Red book: report of the Committee on Infectious Diseases,* 24th ed. Elk Grove Village, IL: American Academy of Pediatrics, 1997.

Schlossberg D, Delgado J, Moore MM, Wisher A, Mohn J, et al. An epidemic of avian and human psittacosis. *Arch Intern Med* 1993;153:2594.

Author: Nicholas Tsarouhas

Psoriasis

Database

DEFINITION

Psoriasis is a skin disease characterized by a chronic relapsing nature and, most commonly, clinical features of scaly, erythematous papules and plaques with thick white scale usually involving elbows, knees, and scalp (psoriasis vulgaris). Other variants include guttate, erythrodermic, and pustular psoriasis (see Physical Examination for details).

CAUSES

The pathogenesis is unknown. Trigger factors are well defined and include:

- Trauma to normal skin, producing psoriasis in the area (Koebner phenomenon)
- Infections (upper respiratory infections, *Streptococcus pyogenes*, human immunodeficiency virus)
- Stress
- Winter
- Certain drugs (systemic corticosteroids, lithium, (β-adrenergic blockers, nonsteroidal anti-inflammatory drugs, and antimalarials)

PATHOPHYSIOLOGY

- Plaque-type psoriasis is characterized by a thickened, parakeratotic epidermis with an absent granular layer above dermal papillae containing dilated tortuous capillaries.
- Collections of polymorphonuclear leukocytes extend from the dermal papillae into the epidermis (Munro microabscesses).
- A mixed perivascular infiltrate is confined to the papillary dermis.

GENETICS

- Psoriasis has a strong genetic influence.
- The mode of genetic transmission is not defined. It is likely multifactorial with more than one gene involved and modified by environmental influence.

—One-third of patients with psoriasis report a relative with the disease.
—8.1% of offspring develop psoriasis in family studies, when one parent is affected.
—When both parents have psoriasis, the percentage increases to 41%.
—In twin studies, 65% of monozygotic twins are concordant for the disease, while only 30% of dizogotic twins are concordant.

EPIDEMIOLOGY

- Psoriasis is universal in occurrence, but the prevalence varies in different populations. The average prevalence in the United States is estimated at 1%.
- Males and females are equally affected.
- Onset of psoriasis is bimodal, commonly presenting in the third decade with a smaller second peak of onset in the sixth decade; however, it can present at any age, with a mean age of onset in children of 8.1 years.
- Earlier onset is associated with more severe disease.

PROGNOSIS

- Once psoriasis appears, it generally persists throughout life.
- Spontaneous remissions of variable length and frequency occur but are unpredictable.

Differential Diagnosis

Classic plaque psoriasis is easily diagnosed. Variants of psoriasis, including guttate, erythrodermic, and pustular disease, are more difficult to recognize. The differential varies with the type of psoriasis and includes:

- Nummular eczema
- Cutaneous T-cell lymphoma
- Tinea corporis
- Pityriasis rosea
- Pityriasis lichenoides et varioliformis acuta
- Secondary syphilis
- Atopic dermatitis
- Drug eruption
- Candidiasis
- Seborrheic dermatitis

Data Gathering

HISTORY

- When the eruption first appeared
- Area involved
- Recent illness, particularly sore throat
- Recent medications, particularly systemic steroids
- Any appearance of lesions with trauma to skin
- Joint pain
- Previous treatments and response
- Improvement with sun exposure
- Family history of psoriasis

Physical Examination

- A complete cutaneous examination is necessary.
- In psoriasis vulgaris, sharply demarcated erythematous plaques with white scale are located most commonly on the elbows, knees, scalp, lumbar area, and umbilicus, but they can cover any surface and large areas of the body. Intertriginous regions are often involved, but scale is absent.
- Guttate psoriasis presents often in children and young adults as small papules (0.5–1.5 cm), with limited scale over the trunk and proximal extremities, and is frequently associated with streptococcal infection.
- Erythema with variable scale involving the majority of the body accompanied by chills is characteristic of erythrodermic psoriasis.
- Generalized pustular psoriasis is the most serious variant, with 23-mm sterile pustules arising on erythematous skin over large areas of the body and accompanied by high fevers.
- A chronic and localized variant of pustular disease involves only the palms and soles.

PHYSICAL EXAMINATION TRICKS

Classic plaque psoriasis is easily diagnosed, but variants and mild cases require careful examination for physical clues.

- Nails are frequently involved, with pinpoint pits, hyperkeratosis, and oil spots.
- Areas of hidden disease are the retroauricular portion of the scalp and the perianal region.
- Removal of scale on plaques results in bleeding points, a feature known as the Auspitz sign.
- The Koebner phenomenon may produce linear or geometric lesions corresponding to areas of trauma.
- Swollen or deformed joints suggest associated psoriatic arthritis.

Laboratory Aids

TESTS

- An elevated uric acid level is a common finding.
- *Streptococcus pyogenes* infection is frequent in guttate disease, and throat culture is appropriate.
- Other laboratory values are generally within normal limits. However, in more severe variants, anemia, elevated erythrocyte sedimentation rate, and decreased albumin levels can be seen.
- In pustular psoriasis, leukocytosis and hypocalcemia are associated.

Therapy

- Therapy is delivered by topical medications, phototherapy, or systemic medications.
- Localized disease is treated with topical therapy and more diffuse disease with phototherapy.
- Systemic medications are reserved for resistant cases.
- Except in the most severe cases, therapy for children should be limited to topical medication and ultraviolet B phototherapy (UVB).
- General skin care should include gentle washing, soaking to remove scale, and application of emollients, preferably ointments and creams.

DRUGS

Topical Medications

Topical Corticosteroids

- Mid- to high-potency topical corticosteroid ointments are applied twice daily.
- Midpotency preparations (0.1% triamcinolone acetonide) are preferred in children.
- Low-potency corticosteroids (1.0% and 2.5% hydrocortisone) are used on the face and intertriginous regions to prevent atrophy.

Anthralin

- Anthralin is applied to plaques for a 30-minute application, and is washed off carefully.
- Lower concentrations are used initially (0.1%, 0.25%) and are increased gradually as tolerated (0.5%, 1.0%).
- Irritation and staining are common, and the face and intertriginous regions cannot be treated.

Calcipotriene

- Calcipotriene ointment is a vitamin D_3 derivative recently approved for treatment of adults.
- It is applied twice daily, with avoidance of the face and intertriginous regions.
- Maximum use in adults is 100 g/wk.
- Rare cases of hypercalcemia have been reported.
- Although effective in children, safety guidelines have not been established.

Coal Tar

- A weak therapeutic agent when employed as monotherapy
- More effective when combined with UVB phototherapy
- Used in multiple shampoo preparations

PHOTOTHERAPY

UVB

- Administered between three and seven times weekly in a booth with bulbs that emit the appropriate wavelength of ultraviolet radiation
- Very effective for guttate and plaque psoriasis
- Average treatment time: 3 months
- In the summer, natural sunlight may be substituted, beginning with a 5-minute exposure to noonday sun and gradually increasing the time. Sunscreen should be used on the face.

PUVA (Psoralen and Ultraviolet B)

- PUVA and oral medications (methotrexate and etretinate) should be reserved for severe cases and carefully monitored by a dermatologist.

Possible Conflicts with Other Drugs

Photosensitizing medication (tetracyclines, sulfa derivatives, phenothiazines, and others) should be avoided with phototherapy.

DURATION

- Topical therapy is administered chronically.
- Remissions occur in summer with sun exposure, and medications may often be discontinued.
- The average treatment course with UVB therapy is 3 months; if the patient clears, treatment may be followed by an average remission period of 5 months.

Follow-Up

WHEN TO EXPECT IMPROVEMENT

- Response will depend on the potency of medication and frequency of treatment.
- Improvement with topical medication is obvious at 2 weeks and usually maximum at 2 months.
- One month of UVB therapy produces a decrease in disease.

SIGNS TO WATCH FOR

Pustules, a significant increase in degree or extent of erythema, or fever suggest progression of the disease to more serious variants and may require hospitalization and systemic therapy.

PITFALLS

- If therapy is too aggressive, disease may become irritated and worsen.
- Scrubbing by the patient to remove scale also irritates the disease.
- Psychological aspects of the disease, particularly in children, should be addressed.

Common Questions and Answers

Q: Will my disease get worse?
A: It is impossible to predict the course of an individual's disease, since it is influenced by both heredity and everyday factors in the environment. While there is no cure, with treatment the disease can be kept under control. Remissions do occur and may be for prolonged periods of time.

Q: When my disease is in remission, what can I do to prevent it from returning?
A: Avoidance of trauma and frequent moisturization of the skin is important. In the summer, controlled sun exposure is helpful. You may have to continue other treatments at less frequent intervals. Any sore throats should be cultured and treated if streptococcal disease is present. However, frequently it is impossible to prevent recurrence of the disease.

Q: Will my other children get psoriasis?
A: If neither parent has psoriasis, the chances are <10% that another child will develop the disease; if one parent is affected, the chances increase to 15%; if both parents are affected, the chances are 50%. Therefore, unless both parents are affected, it is more likely that other children will not have psoriasis.

Q: Does stress make psoriasis worse?
A: Some studies have suggested that flare-ups of psoriasis are associated with increased stress. It is difficult to evaluate whether stress is the cause or the result of the disease. Do all you can to reasonably relieve stress, but do not focus on this as the cause of your psoriasis.

ICD-9-CM 696.1

BIBLIOGRAPHY

Christophers E, Sterry W. Psoriasis. In: Fitzpatrick TB, Eisen AZ, Wolff K, et al., eds. *Dermatology in general medicine,* 4th ed. New York, McGraw-Hill, 1993:489.

de Jong EM. The course of psoriasis. *Clin Dermatol* 1997;15(5):687–692.

Farber EM. Juvenile psoriasis. Early interventions can reduce risks for problems later. *Postgrad Med* 1998;103(4):89–92, 95–96, 99–100 passim.

Stern RS. Epidemiology of psoriasis. *Dermatol Clin* 1995;13(4):717–722.

Author: Cynthia Guzzo

Pubertal Delay

 Database

DEFINITION

Pubertal delay is delay in age of onset of puberty or rate of progression of pubertal development that is greater than two standard deviations from the mean (2.5% of the population).

Constitutional or Physiologic Delay of Puberty

- Late onset of puberty as a normal variant.
- Patients grow slowly through childhood, enter puberty late, and then progress through it at a normal rate.

Male pubertal development is considered delayed if:

- Genital stage 1 persists beyond 13.7 years
- Pubic hair stage 1 persists beyond 15.1 years
- More than 5 years pass before completion of genital growth
- Pubertal development begins but progression stalls, such that the duration of a given sexual maturity rating is longer than expected:

—Genital 2: 2.2 years
—Genital 3: 1.6 years
—Genital 4: 1.9 years
—Pubic hair 2: 1.0 years
—Pubic hair 3: 0.5 years
—Pubic hair 4: 1.5 years

Female pubertal development is considered delayed if

- Breast stage 1 persists beyond 13.4 years
- Pubic hair stage 1 persists beyond 14.1 years
- No menarche beyond age 16
- More than 5 years pass between initiation of breast stage 2 and menarche
- Pubertal development begins but progression stalls, such that the duration of a given sexual maturity rating is longer than expected:

—Breast 2: 1.0 years
—Breast 3: 2.2 years
—Breast 4: 6.8 years
—Pubic hair 2: 1.3 years
—Pubic hair 3: 0.9 years
—Pubic hair 4: 2.4 years

PATHOPHYSIOLOGY

- Constitutional delay is a normal variant that is believed to result from persistence of the prepubertal (childhood) hypogonadotropic state.
- Delayed puberty and short stature associated with chronic disease is not well explained.

GENETICS

- Patients with constitutional delay will often have a family history of late pubertal onset with subsequent normal stature and development.
- The genetic transmission of delayed puberty otherwise depends on the underlying disorder.

EPIDEMIOLOGY

- Constitutional delay of puberty explains 90% to 95% of pubertal delay.
- Constitutional delay occurs in 2.5% of adolescents of both sexes.
- More than 60% of patients with constitutional delay of puberty have a positive family history.

 Differential Diagnosis

- Infection

—Viral or tuberculosis infection resulting in acquired panhypopituarism

- Tumors (may result in panhypopituitarism)

—Craniopharyngioma
—Hypothalamic glioma
—Astrocytoma
—Pituitary adenomas

- Trauma

—Panhypopituitarism resulting from severe head trauma

- Congenital

—Congenital panhypopituitarism
—Mixed gonadal dysgenesis
—Turner syndrome, Noonan syndrome
—Prader-Willi syndrome

- Immunologic

—Juvenile rheumatoid arthritis
—Systemic lupus erythematosus

- Psychosocial

—Anorexia nervosa

- Environmental

—Postradiation
—Chemotherapy

- Miscellaneous

—Constitutional delay of puberty (majority of cases)
—Glucocorticoid excess
—Chronic disease

 Data Gathering

HISTORY

- Obtain long-term growth record. Patients with gonadotropin or gonadal disorders usually have had normal growth during childhood but no increase in growth during expected pubertal spurt (i.e., growth retardation is a new event). Most children with constitutional delay have slow growth throughout childhood.

- Obtain history of progression of secondary sex characteristics. Adolescents with complete gonadal or gonadotropin deficiencies will not enter puberty, unless initiated by exogenous or adrenal hormones, whereas those with constitutional delay will progress at a normal rate after initiation of puberty. Adolescents with partial deficiencies may reach pubarche at a normal time, but will fail to progress.
- Obtain family history of pubertal development.
- Assess nutrition and socioeconomic history to rule out chronic malnutrition or eating disorder.
- Elicit history of drug use (e.g., glucocorticoids or cytotoxins).

 Physical Examination

- Examine all patients with pubertal delay thoroughly, with particular attention to:
- Thyroid examination
- Neurologic and funduscopic examination to check for intracranial pathology
- Genital and gynecologic examination: external examination for all patients; internal gynecologic examination for females with amenorrhea may be indicated; breast, pubic hair, and genital examination to assess sexual maturity ratings
- In assessment of male genitalia, consider use of orchidometer to accurately establish testicular size.
- The first sign of puberty in males is testicular size greater than 2.5 cm. Find which one of your finger segments approximates 2.5 cm and use it as a gross measure. As a screening device, this is subtler than an orchidometer.

 Laboratory Aids

TESTS

Routine Screening

Routine screening tests for chronic or systemic disease:

- Complete blood count
- Urinalysis
- Sedimentation rate
- Chemistry profile

Special Tests

Special tests to order based on history or physical examination findings:

- Thyroid function tests
- Gonadotropin levels (low levels suggest prepuberty or hypothalamic-pituitary failure; high levels suggest gonadal failure or absence)
- Karyotype
- Growth hormone levels

—Somatomedin C (IGF-I) level as baseline
—For true growth hormone levels, need growth hormone (GH) stimulation tests. Consultation with a specialist or experienced laboratory personnel is recommended before obtaining stimulation tests.

- Dynamic tests of hypothalamic–pituitary-gonadal function are usually performed by a specialist.

Imaging

- Bone age: plain film of the epiphyseal growth centers in the hand. Epiphyses change in response to growth hormone, thyroxine, and steroids of adrenal or gonadal origin. Comparison to chronologic age can help to differentiate constitutional delay from organic disorders. A bone age is almost always indicated in the initial work-up of delayed puberty.
- Pelvic ultrasound: can be useful in localization of intraabdominal testicular structures, or in determination of the presence or absence of mullerian structures. Pelvic ultrasound is indicated when testes cannot be detected in patients with a male phenotype or when mullerian structures cannot be confirmed on physical examination in patients with a female phenotype.
- Computerized tomography (CT) or magnetic resonance imaging (MRI) of the head: is useful in assessing pituitary or hypothalamic structures, mass lesions, pathologic calcifications, or increased intracranial pressure if a central cause of delayed puberty is suspected.

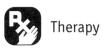 Therapy

PSYCHOSOCIAL INTERVENTIONS

Most patients with pubertal delay do not require drugs, but all need psychological and social support.

DRUGS

- In cases of presumed constitutional delay, hormones can be used to affect hypothalamic maturation, thereby initiating endogenous puberty.
- Referral to an endocrinologist or adolescent specialist is usually recommended prior to the initiation of hormonal therapy to aid in diagnosis and in monitoring response.

 Follow-Up

In cases of permanent hypogonadism, because of gonadal absence, failure, or gonadotropin deficiency, long-term hormonal therapy is necessary.

PREVENTION

- Undue stress and unneeded tests can be avoided by discussing pubertal changes with patients and their families at the outset, in late childhood.
- Even though they will not ask health care providers, teens with chronic disease may be actively worrying about slow growth and pubertal development. Open discussion with a caring provider can help allay fears and stress.

PITFALLS

- No test can make a definitive diagnosis of constitutional delay.
- Levels of sex steroids and gonadotropins vary significantly in a single patient because of pulsatile or rhythmic secretions. Consult an endocrinologist to interpret these tests.
- Sex steroid therapy in a patient with hypopituitarism can affect adult height if given before growth hormone therapy is optimized.
- Consultation with a specialist or experienced laboratory personnel is recommended before obtaining stimulation tests, as they may require special conditions.

 Common Questions and Answers

Q: Since approximately 95% of pubertal delay is constitutional or physiologic in nature, when can I avoid an expensive work-up and just observe the patient?
A: Unfortunately, only the spontaneous onset of puberty confirms the diagnosis of constitutional delay. Anxiety from delayed puberty may preclude waiting. To make a presumptive diagnosis of constitutional delay, pathology must be ruled out. Physical examination, including genital anatomy and smell sense, must be normal. There should be no signs or symptoms consistent with chronic disease. The history, including nutritional history and review of systems, must be negative. The screening blood work must be negative. Growth must progress at least 3.7 cm per year, and bone age must be delayed no more than 4.0 years compared with chronologic age. Although not always indicated, the next level of tests can be ordered. Normal prepubertal levels of LH and FSH must be present. Presumptive diagnosis is strongly supported, but not proven, by a positive family history and a height between the 3rd and 25th percentiles.

Q: When should patients with pubertal delay be seen by an endocrinologist or adolescent specialist?
A: Often, the initial work-up of pubertal delay can be completed by the primary care provider. For complex stimulation tests, or if help is needed in interpreting test results, referral to an experienced specialist is warranted. If a specific chronic disease is suspected as the underlying etiology, then referral should be made to the appropriate subspecialist

Q: Do racial differences exist concerning pubertal onset and development?
A: Several recent studies indicate that the mean ages for onset of breast development and menarche are younger for African American females than for Caucasian females. One such study reported the mean age of onset for breast development as 8.87 years for African American girls and 9.96 years for Caucasian girls. Mean age at menarche was found to be 12.16 and 12.88 years for African American and Caucasian girls, respectively.

ICD-9-CM 255.0

BIBLIOGRAPHY

Herman-Giddens ME, Slora EJ, Wasserman RL, et al. Secondary sexual characteristics and menses in young girls seen in office practice: a study from the Pediatric Research in Office Settings Network. *Pediatrics* 1997;99(4):505–512.

Hung W. Variants of male sexual development. In: *Clinical pediatric endocrinology*. Philadelphia: Mosby-Year Book, 1992.

Kulin HE. Delayed puberty. *J Clin Endocrinol Metab* 1996;81(10):3460–3464.

Lee PA, O'dea LS. Tests and variants of male sexual development. In Hung N. ed. *Clinical pediatric endocrinology*. Philadelphia: Mosby-Yearbook, 1992, 268–312.

Slap GB. Normal physiologic and psychosocial growth in the adolescent. *J Adolesc Health Care* 1986;7:13s–23s.

Styne DM. New aspects in the diagnosis and treatment of pubertal disorders. *Pediatr Clin North Am* 1997;44(2):505–529.

Authors: Jonathan R. Pletcher and Kenneth R. Ginsburg

Pulmonary Embolism

 Database

DEFINITION

Pulmonary embolism is the occlusion of a pulmonary vessel by a thrombus.

PATHOPHYSIOLOGY

- Thromboemboli may develop anywhere in the systemic venous system.
- Pulmonary embolism is characterized by the triad of hypoxemia, pulmonary hypertension, and right ventricular failure.
- Diminished pulmonary perfusion causes ventilation/perfusion (V/Q) mismatch, resulting in hypoxemia.
- Hyperventilation occurs secondary to stimulation of propriorceptors in the lung.
- Hypercapnia is seen with severe occlusion of the pulmonary artery (not often seen with smaller emboli).
- Pulmonary infarction is uncommon owing to the presence of collateral pulmonary and bronchial arteries along with the airways providing additional sources of oxygen to the tissues.

EPIDEMIOLOGY

- Pulmonary embolisms are seen more frequently in adults.
- They are underdiagnosed in children; the incidence in children is 3.7%.
- Increasing incidence is secondary to increased central catheter utilization.
- Approximately 10% of adults who present with acute pulmonary embolus die within 1 hour of onset.
- The mortality rate can be as high as 30% if delays in diagnosis are made.
- Death occurs with 85% obstruction of the pulmonary artery.
- Risk factors vary according to age groups and sex.
- In children, risk factors include:

—Presence of a central venous catheter
—Lack of mobility
—Congenital heart disease
—Ventriculoatrial shunt
—Trauma
—Solid tumors or leukemia
—Postsurgical procedures (especially scoliosis repair)
—Hypercoagulable states

- In adults, the most common risk factor is the presence of a deep vein thrombosis, usually in the legs or pelvis.

PROGNOSIS

- If treated promptly, prognosis is good.
- If treatment is delayed (especially if the patient is hemodynamically compromised prior to the event), prognosis is poor.

 Differential Diagnosis

- Cardiac

—Cardiac tamponade
—Constrictive pericarditis
—Restrictive cardiomyopathy

- Pulmonary

—Chronic cough
—Status asthmaticus
—Pneumonia with empyema
—Pneumothorax

 Data Gathering

HISTORY

- Are there any chest symptoms?
- Pulmonary embolism should be suspected in children who present with:

—Pleuritic chest pain
—Shortness of breath
—Hemoptysis
—Cough
—Acute respiratory distress
—Apprehension or anxiety
—Syncope
—Cardiovascular shock

- Symptoms may be nonspecific and indicative of other disorders.
- The clinician must have a high index of suspicion and recognize risk factors in order to establish the correct diagnosis.

 Physical Examination

Findings in physical examination are nonspecific.

- General

—Fever
—Diaphoresis
—Nervousness or apprehension (altered mental status is uncommon)

- Cardiovascular

—Increased intensity of the pulmonic component of S2
—Tachycardia
—Gallop rhythm
—New murmur

- Pulmonary

—Tachypnea
—Rales
—Cyanosis (present with 65% obstruction of the pulmonary artery)
—Pleuritic chest pain
—Dyspnea
—Cough
—Hemoptysis
—Wheezing (uncommon)

- Extremities

—Deep venous thrombosis is frequently found in the adult population.
—Phlebitis
—Edema

PITFALLS

Failure to make the diagnosis is the most common mistake. Pulmonary embolism must be suspected in the critically ill children who have a central venous catheter who develop sudden respiratory failure. Since the symptoms for severe lung disease and pulmonary embolism are similar, the diagnosis might be missed if the index of suspicion is low.

 Laboratory Aids

TESTS

Blood Tests

- In general, blood tests are nonspecific and of no significant value in the diagnosis of a pulmonary embolus.
- Arterial blood gas:

—Decreased PO_2 and PCO_2
—Increased alveolararterial (Aa) gradient

Cardiac Studies

ECG

- Useful in ruling out other conditions
- May show sinus tachycardia or nonspecific STT segment changes

Echocardiogram

- Useful for identifying:

—Abnormalities of cardiac anatomy
—Thrombi on catheter tips

Pulmonary Function Testing

Results are nonspecific.

Evaluation of the Lower Extremities

- Finding deep vein thrombosis via:

—Impedance plethysmography
—Doppler technology
—Venography

Imaging

Chest Radiograph

- May be abnormal in 70% of patients with pulmonary embolus
- Most frequent findings:

—Parenchymal infiltrates
—Atelectasis
—Pleural effusions: seen in 33% of cases, most unilateral
—Hampton hump (pyramid-shaped wedge pointing toward the hilum)

Ventilation/Perfusion (V/Q) Scan

- A V/Q scan performed to rule out a pulmonary embolus is reported in one of five categories, ranging from high probability to normal.
- An abnormal V/Q scan with normal ventilation and decreased perfusion in the appropriate clinical setting is 90% specific for a pulmonary embolus.
- A normal V/Q scan does not completely rule out pulmonary embolus, although if the patient is at low risk, a pulmonary embolus is highly unlikely.

Pulmonary Angiography

- Most sensitive and specific test
- Not done as frequently in children as in adults because of complications of the procedure
- With the introduction of newer, improved catheters and safer contrast solutions, this test is now safe to be performed in the pediatric population.
- Indicated for cases:

—Intermediate-probability V/Q scans
—High-probability scans in patients who are:
  —Poor candidates for anticoagulation
  —Hemodynamically unstable or require an embolectomy

Therapy

DRUGS

- Stabilize the patient before anticoagulation or thrombolytic therapy is begun:

—Improve oxygenation
—Correct acidosis
—Stabilize blood pressure

- The goal of therapy is anticoagulation and/or thrombolysis

Anticoagulation Therapy

- To prevent further thrombus formation

Heparin

- Bolus dose: 50 U/kg
- Maintenance dose: 10 to 25 U/kg/hr
- Keep PTT 55 to 60 seconds
- Should be given for 7 to 10 days

Coumadin

- Coumadin should be started 24 to 48 hours after heparin therapy is begun.
- Maintenance dose: 2.5 to 10.0 mg/d
- Keep PT twice normal
- Should be continued for 3 to 6 months

Thrombolytic Therapy

Agents Available

- Streptokinase: No difference in outcome has been found using streptokinase over urokinase.
- Urokinase
- rtPA (tissue plasminogen activator)

Indications

- Hemodynamically unstable
- Large embolus
- The use of low-molecular-weight heparins has been used as prophylaxis or as treatment for preexisting conditions in both adults and children.
- A synthetic, nonthrombocytopenic heparin pentasaccharide with a purely antifactor Xa activity is currently being tested.
- Ticlopidine and clopidogrel have been used successfully for the prevention of thrombotic strokes and arterial thrombotic syndromes.

Contraindications to Anticoagulant Therapy

- Active internal bleeding
- Recent cerebrovascular accident
- Major surgery
- Recent gastrointestinal bleed

EMBOLECTOMY

- Indicated when hemodynamic instability persists; is reserved for patients who have failed thrombolytic therapy or dose where medical treatment is contraindicated.
- Late results are excellent if the patient has not suffered from a perioperative cardiac arrest, which is associated with early mortality.

Follow-Up

Patients on Coumadin therapy should have the usual follow-up for those on anticoagulant.

Common Questions and Answers

Q: Is it safe for children on Coumadin to play contact sports?
A: The general recommendation is that no contact sports should be allowed while children are on coumadin therapy because of the increased risk of bleeding.

ICD-9-CM 415.1

BIBLIOGRAPHY

Buck JR, Connors RH, Coon WW, et al. Pulmonary embolism in children. *J Pediatr Surg* 1981;16:385.

Burki N. The dead space to tidal volume ratio in the diagnosis of pulmonary embolism. *Am Rev Respir Dis* 1986;133:679.

Cvitanic O, Marino PL. Improved use of arterial blood gas analysis in suspected pulmonary embolism. *Chest* 1989;95:48.

Derish MT, Smith DW, Frankel LR. Venous catheter thrombus formation and pulmonary embolism in children. *Pediatr Pulmonol* 1995;20(6):349-354.

Dobkin J, Reichel J. Pulmonary embolism: diagnosis and treatment. *Cardiol Clin* 1987;5:577.

Evans Da, Wilmott RW. Pulmonary embolism in children. *Pediatr Clin North Am* 1994;41:569.

Fulkerson WJ, Coleman RE, Ravin CE, et al. Diagnosis of pulmonary embolism. *Arch Intern Med* 1986;146:961.

Kutty K. Pulmonary embolism: how to nail down the diagnosis. *Postgrad Med* 1990;88:72.

Massicotte P, Adams M, Brooker LA, Andrew M. Low-molecular-weight heparin in pediatric patients with thrombotic disease: a dose finding study. *J Pediatr* 1996;128(3):313-318.

McCoy KS, Grossman NJ. *Pediatric respiratory diseases: diagnosis and treatment.* Philadelphia: WB Saunders, 1993:509.

Walenga JM, Fareed J. Current status on new anticoagulant and antithrombotic drugs and devices. *Curr Opin Pulm Med* 1997;3(4):291-302.

Author: Hector L. Flores-Arroyo

Pulmonary Hypertension

 Database

DEFINITION

Pulmonary hypertension is increased pulmonary vascular resistance.

CAUSES

- Hypoxemia-induced pulmonary hypertension: chronic lung disease

—Cystic fibrosis
—Bronchopulmonary dysplasia
—Interstitial lung disease

- Upper airway obstruction

—Tonsillar and/or adenoid hypertrophy
—Obesity

- Hypoventilation

—Neurologically mediated process or secondary to muscle weakness

- High pulmonary blood flow secondary to left-to-right shunting (seen in congenital heart disease)

—Atrial septal defect
—Ventricular septal defect

- Left-sided cardiac disorders that increase pulmonary venous pressure

—Left ventricular failure
—Mitral valve stenosis
—Obstructed anomalous pulmonary veins

- Occlusion of pulmonary vessels

—Sickle cell disease
—Thromboembolism
—Veno-occlusive disease

- Pulmonary vasculitis
- Persistent pulmonary hypertension of the newborn
- Idiopathic cases (primary pulmonary hypertension)

PATHOPHYSIOLOGY

- Structural alternations in pulmonary vessel architecture (remodeling)

—Smooth muscle hypertrophy
—Extension of blood vessel's smooth muscle into smaller vessels

EPIDEMIOLOGY

Incidence in children in unknown.

COMPLICATIONS

- Chronic hypoxia
- Exercise intolerance
- Right sided heart failure (cor pulmonale)
- Death

PROGNOSIS

- Dependent on the underlying disease
- In cases of primary pulmonary hypertension, improvement of pulmonary hypertension with administration of vasodilators during initial catheterization is associated with a better survival rate than if there is no response.
- Ten percent to 40% mortality in treated patients
- Near 100% mortality if patient is untreated

 Differential Diagnosis

- Pulmonary

—Asthma
—Cystic fibrosis
—Chronic obstructive pulmonary disease (COPD)
—Emphysema

- Miscellaneous

—Congestive heart failure
—Noncardiogenic pulmonary edema
—Fatigue

 Data Gathering

HISTORY

- Dyspnea (earliest complaint usually reported)
- Early on, fatigue with exercise or exertion
- At rest in later stages or if severe
- Exercise intolerance
- Feeding intolerance
- Failure to thrive
- Excessive sleeping
- Diaphoresis
- Chest pain
- Syncope
- Palpitations (late finding)

 Physical Examination

- Typically governed by the signs of the underlying lung or heart disease

COMMON FINDINGS

- Tachypnea
- Arrhythmias
- Narrowed splitting of S_2 heart sound
- Increased P_2 heart sound
- Presence of S_3 and/or S_4 heart sounds
- Murmur of pulmonary or tricuspid insufficiency (pulmonary insufficiency more common)
- Jugular venous distension
- Peripheral edema
- Hepatomegaly

SPECIAL QUESTIONS

- Consider obstructive sleep apnea as cause of pulmonary hypertension.
- Ask about snoring if suspecting pulmonary hypertension in the absence of overt cardiac or pulmonary disease.

 Laboratory Aids

TESTS

Arterial Blood Gas

Measurement of pO_2 assesses degree of hypoxia; evaluation of pCO_2 determines presence or absence of hypoventilation

Electrocardiogram (ECG)

- Can be normal if cor pulmonale has not developed; if cor pulmonale present, ECG can demonstrate:

—Right QRS axis deviation
—Right ventricular hypertrophy
—Right atrial hypertrophy

Imaging

Chest Radiograph

- Will vary according to the underlying disorder and extent of pulmonary hypertension
- Pulmonary hypertension correlates poorly with chest radiograph findings
- Cardiomegaly in primary pulmonary hypertension:

—Enlarged pulmonary artery
—Peripheral lung appears underperfused.
—"Pruning" of pulmonary vessels

Echocardiogram with Doppler Flow

- Increased pulmonary artery pressure
- Right ventricular hypertrophy
- Paradoxical movement of the intraventricular septum
- Pulmonic and tricuspid valve regurgitation
- Right-to-left shunting via an open foramen ovale

Cardiac Catheterization

- The most accurate measurement of pulmonary artery pressure is done by right heart catheterization
- Criteria for pulmonary hypertension in children:

—Mean pulmonary arterial pressure greater than >20 mm Hg; pulmonary artery systolic pressure greater than >30 mm Hg
—Pulmonary vascular resistance greater than >3 U/m_2

- Pressures should be measured before and after vasodilator to assess reversibility of pulmonary hypertension.

 Therapy

Therapy is directed toward:

- Treating the underlying disease
- Vasodilators to decrease the pulmonary hypertension and improve right heart function

DRUGS

Oxygen

Keep SaO_2 greater than 94%.

Vasodilators

- Calcium-channel blockers (PO)
- Nitroglycerin (PO)
- Hydralazine (PO)
- Prostacyclin (IV)
- Nitric oxide (NO) (inhaled)

Anticoagulation Therapy (Coumadin)

- Advocated to prevent clot formation in the narrowed pulmonary vessels
- Helpful even in the absence of thromboembolic disease

MECHANICAL VENTILATION

- Useful for correcting hypoxia and hypercarbia secondary to hypoventilation

SURGERY

- Transplantation (lung or heart-lung transplantation): reserved for patients with refractory, severe pulmonary hypertension

DURATION

Treatment can be lifelong unless the primary cause of the pulmonary hypertension can be corrected.

 Follow-Up

WHEN TO EXPECT IMPROVEMENT

- In cases of acute pulmonary hypertension, response to most of the treatment modalities will be apparent almost immediately.
- Oxygen has been shown to reverse hypoxia-related remodeling of the airways after a month of therapy.

PITFALLS

- Signs and symptoms of pulmonary hypertension are not specific and can easily be missed.
- Heart catheterization in patients with severe pulmonary hypertension is associated with increased risk of complications.
- Supplemental oxygen can cause hypercapnia in some patients by blunting their hypoxia-driven respiratory drive.
- Use of vasodilators should be done under close supervision because of their effect on systemic blood pressure (systemic hypotension can be a significant problem).

 Common Questions and Answers

Q: How many hours per day should supplemental oxygen be used?
A: Studies have shown decreased mortality in patients using oxygen 24 hours per day compared with patients using supplemental oxygen for only part of the day.

Q: Should the dosage of oxygen be adjusted during the day as per the patient's activity?
A: Increasing the supplemental oxygen should be considered for activities that require increased oxygen consumption (i.e., exercise, eating, sleeping).

ICD-9-CM 416.0

BIBLIOGRAPHY

Butt AY, Higenbottam T. New therapies for primary pulmonary hypertension. *Chest* 1994;105:21S.

Redding GJ. *Respiratory disease in children: diagnosis and management.* Baltimore: Williams & Wilkins, 1994:639.

Redding GJ. *Pediatric respiratory disease: diagnosis and treatment.* Philadelphia: WB Saunders, 1993:335.

Rich S. The medical treatment of primary pulmonary hypertension: proven and promising strategies. *Chest* 1994;105:17S.

Rich S, Kaufmann E, Levy PS. The effect of high doses of calcium-channel blockers on survival in primary pulmonary hypertension. *N Engl J Med* 1992;327:76.

Soifer SJ. Pulmonary hypertension: physiologic or pathologic disease? *Crit Care Med* 1993;21:S370.

Authors: Shmuel Goldberg and Richard Mark Kravitz

Pulmonary Valve Stenosis

 ## Database

DEFINITION

Pulmonary valve stenosis is right ventricular outflow tract obstruction (RVOTO) secondary to a conical pulmonary valve with fused leaflets. The valve is usually mobile. Some patients may have a dysplastic valve without fusion, but rather obstruction secondary to thickened, immobile cusps.

PATHOPHYSIOLOGY

Severity of clinical signs and symptoms are dependent on the degree of RVOTO, right ventricular function, and amount of right-to-left shunt.

GENETICS

Familial occurrence has been reported.

EPIDEMIOLOGY

Five percent to 8% of all CHD

COMPLICATIONS

- Bacterial endocarditis
- Sudden death (in severe pulmonary stenosis [PS])

PROGNOSIS

Generally good with appropriate medical and/or surgical management

 ## Data Gathering

HISTORY

- Exertional dyspnea and fatigue
- Cyanosis and tachypnea in the newborn period

 ## Physical Examination

- Ejection click at the left upper sternal border
- Systolic ejection murmur at the left upper sternal border that radiates to the back and sides
- May have a widely split S_2 with diminished P_2
- Magnitude of the obstruction is directly related to the length of the systolic murmur

 ## Laboratory Aids

TESTS

- *CXR*: normal heart size, prominent main pulmonary artery segment (poststenotic dilatation), normal pulmonary vascular markings
- *ECG*: right axis deviation, right ventricular hypertrophy, right atrial enlargement with severe PS. The ECG may be normal in mild valvar PS.

IMAGING

- Echocardiogram: Thick prominent pulmonary valve with restricted systolic motion (doming), poststenotic dilatation of the main pulmonary artery, and right-to-left shunting may be seen at the atrial level. Doppler can be used to estimate the pressure gradient across the stenotic valve.
- Cardiac catheterization: usually for definitive therapy, but can be used to determine the presence or absence of other cardiac defects and to determine the location and severity of the stenosis

Pulmonary Valve Stenosis

 ## Therapy

MEDICAL

- Restriction of activity with severe PS
- SBE prophylaxis
- Balloon valvuloplasty for significant PS (gradient >50 mm Hg)
- Prostaglandin E_1 for neonates with critical PS and ductal dependent pulmonary blood flow

SURGICAL

- Unsuccessful balloon valvuloplasty
- Typically needed for a dysplastic valve (e.g., Noonan syndrome)

 ## Follow-Up

PROGNOSIS

- Excellent results with both medical and surgical therapy
- May have pulmonary valve insufficiency and/ or remaining pulmonary valve stenosis after therapy

 ## Common Questions and Answers

Q: How long will patients with pulmonary valve stenosis require SBE prophylaxis after definitive therapy?
A: Indefinitely. Regardless of physical examination and gradient measured by echocardiography, these pulmonary valves are abnormal with turbulent flow. This subsequently is a nidus for infection.

Q: Are children with pulmonary valve stenosis ever cyanotic?
A: One can see right-to-left shunting at the atrial level in the newborn period and in children with severe pulmonary valve stenosis associated with an atrial septal defect.

ICD-9-CM 746.0

BIBLIOGRAPHY

Hayes CJ, Gersony WM, Driscoll, et al. Second natural history study of congenital heart defects: results of treatment with pulmonary valvar stenosis. *Circulation* 1993;87[Suppl I]:28–37.

Rocchini AP, Emmanouilides GC. *Moss and Adams: Heart diseases in infants, children and adolescents,* 5th ed. Baltimore: Williams & Wilkins, 1995:930–946.

Author: Pamela S. Ro

Purpura Fulminans

 Database

DEFINITION

Purpura fulminans is a congenital, acquired, or idiopathic condition of rapidly progressive microvascular hemorrhage into the skin. It is associated with an underlying acquired or congenital disorder of coagulation, and may lead to skin necrosis.

PATHOPHYSIOLOGY

• Common features of purpura fulminans

—Inflammation: Endothelial injury from bacterial endotoxin or other trigger may initiate secretion of inflammatory cytokines or activation of coagulation and complement proteins.
—Purpura: extravasation of formed elements of the blood from injured capillaries into the skin
—Dermal vascular thrombosis: formation of microthromboses in blood vessels of the skin, leading to hemorrhage in the skin (purpura), necrosis of skin, and gangrene

• Infection-associated purpura fulminans

—Overwhelming sepsis, usually bacterial; *Neisseria meningitidis* most common
—Disseminated intravascular coagulation (DIC): state of sustained activation of coagulation cascade and fibrinolytic mechanisms, leading to consumption of platelets, fibrinogen, and often formation of microthromboses

• Inherited defect of coagulation presenting as neonatal purpura fulminans

—Deficiency of protein C: leads to a loss of important inhibitory regulation of coagulation and uncontrolled clotting
—Protein C slows ("brakes") the coagulation cascade at two step: by degrading activated coagulation factor Va in the common part of the coagulation pathway, and by degrading factor VIIIa in the intrinsic pathway.
—Protein S is a cofactor for protein C.

• Idiopathic

—Postinfectious complication
—Complication of coumadin therapy
—Other unknown mechanisms

GENETICS

• Deficiencies of protein C and protein S are autosomally inherited with variable penetrance.
• Many different genetic mutations, leading to both qualitative and quantitative defects of the proteins, have been described.
• Heterozygous deficiency states usually cause a hypercoagulable condition, with increased risk of venous or arterial thrombosis throughout life.
• Homozygous or compound heterozygous states lead to severe deficiency (greater than 5% of normal factor activity) and neonatal purpura fulminans and are usually fatal.

EPIDEMIOLOGY

Depends on underlying cause:

• Neonatal purpura fulminans related to homozygous protein C deficiency: 1 in 250,000 to 1 in 500,000 births. Homozygous protein S deficiency is rarer.
• Purpura frequently seen in bacterial sepsis with meningococcus and other pathogens

COMPLICATIONS

• Skin necrosis and gangrene
• Scarring
• Acral amputations, from tips of digits to whole limbs
• Thrombosis in internal organs
• Death

PROGNOSIS

• Related to underlying cause of purpura fulminans
• Overall, poor for homozygous deficiencies of proteins C and S

 Differential Diagnosis

• Infection

—*Neisseria meningitidis,* most common infectious cause of purpura fulminans
—Streptococci
—*Haemophilus* species
—Staphylococci
—Gram-negative bacteremia: *Escherichia coli, Klebsiella, Proteus, Enterobacter*
—Rickettsia: Rocky Mountain spotted fever

• Environmental

—Coumadin-induced skin necrosis: 1 in 500 to 1 in 1,000 individuals starting coumadin therapy develop necrosis in subcutaneous fat, thought to be due to relative depletion of anticoagulant protein C (a vitamin K-dependent factor) during the initial phase of coumadin effect.

• Tumor

—Myeloid leukemia

• Congenital

—Inherited deficiencies of protein C and protein S. Only severe, homozygous (less than 5% activity) deficiencies of proteins C and S are associated with purpura fulminans. Milder, heterozygous deficiencies of protein C and protein S, as well as deficiency of antithrombin III, dysfibrinogenemias, the carrier state for Factor V Leiden, and other defects all give rise to hypercoagulable states with clotting tendencies, but not neonatal purpura fulminans.

• Immune

—Heparin-induced thrombocytopenia: Antibody to heparin-platelet complex causes platelet activation, thrombocytopenia, and microthrombosis, including dermal vessels.
—Antiphospholipid antibody syndrome: Predisposition to thrombosis can include skin necrosis.

• Miscellaneous

—Thrombotic thrombocytopenic purpura
—Paroxysmal nocturnal hemoglobinuria
—Henoch-Schönlein purpura

 Data Gathering

HISTORY

• Current bacterial sepsis: fever, weakness, dizziness, nausea, vomiting, onset of petechial rash
• Family history suggestive of hypercoagulable state: blood clots or thromboses at an early age, such as stroke, deep vein thrombosis, pulmonary embolism; family members taking coumadin or heparin
• Previous affected child with purpura fulminans or hypercoagulable state
• Prior exposure to heparin, therapeutically or via intravenous "heplock"
• Medications, including anticoagulation

 Physical Examination

• Signs of sepsis: fever, hypotension, tachycardia, poor perfusion, cool extremities, decreased pulses, shock
• Nonblanching purpura
• Acral purpura and necrosis: Check fingers, nose, toes, and penis for black areas.
• An erythematous border may surround purpuric areas.
• Bullae may form over purpuric skin.
• Oozing at sites of venipuncture
• Pain, ischemia, and edema of extremities, or internal organ dysfunction may result from deep vein thrombosis or arterial thrombosis, depending on location and severity.

PHYSICAL EXAMINATION TRICKS

Depress the purpuric area with a glass slide to determine whether it blanches.

Laboratory Aids

TESTS

Screening

- CBC: Platelet count may be low; hemoglobin may be low.
- Prothombin time (PT): prolonged as in DIC
- Partial thromboplastin time (PTT): prolonged as in DIC
- Fibrinogen: decreased with consumption and fibrinolysis
- Fibrin split products: increased fibrinolysis as in DIC

Etiologic

- Protein C activity in patient and parents
- Protein S antigen (total and free) in patient and parents
- Test for antiphospholipid antibodies: usually lupus anticoagulant or anticardiolipin antibody

Imaging

To document presence and extent of suspected thrombosis:

- Ultrasound with Doppler flow study
- Computed tomography
- Magnetic resonance images: better for visualization of vessels
- Angiography: Most invasive, requires vascular injury for access

—Imaging is potentially useful to:

- Distinguish thrombosis from other pathology
- Judge age of thrombus (based on collateralization)
- Assess clot size prior to anticoagulant or thrombolytic therapy
- Distinguish baseline old clot from new thrombosis

The most useful imaging strategy depends on location and clinical situation.

False Positives

- Protein C and S levels may decrease during a thrombotic episode that is not related to an underlying deficiency. Low measurements often need to be repeated at baseline after recovery.
- Protein C and S levels may be below adult normal ranges for the first 3 to 6 months of life in healthy infants.

PITFALLS

- Proteins C and S are vitamin K-dependent. Level may be affected if vitamin K is not administered at birth.
- Protein C determination is affected by coumadin therapy. It is difficult to confirm a deficiency state, especially mild deficiency, by repeat testing if coumadin is started empirically.

 ## Therapy

DRUGS

- Fresh frozen plasma (FFP) every 12 hours to replace proteins C and S in acute DIC of purpura fulminans
- Periodic FFP infusions for chronic replacement
- Prothrombin complex concentrates
- Protein C concentrate
- Oral coumadin

DURATION

- Protein C has half-life of 10 hours in circulation.
- Protein C replacement by periodic infusion of protein C concentrate
- Oral coumadin therapy indefinitely usually recommended for documented protein C or S deficiency

DIET

Patients on coumadin therapy may need to avoid foods with high vitamin K content, especially if there is variation in the dose of coumadin required to maintain adequate anticoagulation.

POSSIBLE CONFLICTS

- Many drugs can affect coumadin metabolism.
- Chronic infusion therapy for neonates may run into access problems.

 ## Follow-Up

WHEN TO EXPECT IMPROVEMENT

- Related to underlying cause of purpura fulminans

SIGNS TO WATCH FOR

- Spread of purpura, hypotension, gangrene

PITFALLS

- Individuals with protein C and protein S deficiency may have increased risk of coumadin-induced skin necrosis when starting coumadin. Patients should be heparinized for several days prior to the start of oral anticoagulation.
- Management of an infant on oral anticoagulation is difficult because of the practical problem of obtaining reliable measurements of PT, the increased risk associated with deeps sticks for blood samples, and difficulty in establishing a stable coumadin dose.

 ## Common Questions and Answers

Q: What is the risk of a second affected child with protein C or S deficiency?
A: If the diagnosis is confirmed by family studies that show both parents to be carriers of the deficiency and the affected child to be homozygous, then there is a 25% chance that each subsequent infant would have purpura fulminans, and 50% chance that each child would be a carrier. However, many hypercoagulable states cannot be attributed to an identifiable genetic defect.

Q: Should a child with purpura fulminans be followed by a specialist?
A: Generally yes, with a pediatric hematologist, to assist in acute management of purpura, establishment of diagnosis, and management of oral anticoagulation.

ICD-9-CM 286.6

BIBLIOGRAPHY

Adcock DM, Brozna J, Marlar RA. Proposed classification and pathologic mechanisms of purpura fulminans and skin necrosis. *Semin Thromb Hemost* 1990;16:333.

Beutler E, Lichtman MA, Coller BS, Kipps TJ, eds. *Williams* hematology, 5th ed. New York: McGraw-Hill, 1995.

Colman RW, Hirsh J, Marder VJ, Salzman EW. *Hemostasis and thrombosis: basic principles and clinical practice,* 3rd ed. Philadelphia: JB Lippincott, 1994.

Francis RB. Acquired purpura fulminans. *Semin Thromb Hemost* 1990;16:310.

Gerson WT, Dickerman JD, Boville G, Golden E. Severe acquired protein C deficiency in purpura fulminans associated with disseminated intravascular coagulation: treatment with protein C concentrate. *Pediatrics* 1993;91:418.

Marlar RA, Neumann A. Neonatal purpura fulminans due to homozygous protein C or protein S deficiencies. *Semin Thromb Hemost* 1990;16:299.

Author: David F. Friedman

Pyelonephritis

 Database

DEFINITION

Acute pyelonephritis (APN) (upper urinary tract infection) is defined clinically by fever and flank pain, and histologically by acute renal parenchymal (interstitial) inflammation secondary to bacterial invasion.

PATHOPHYSIOLOGY

Specific factors relating to the development of pyelonephritis:

- Host-related

—Anatomic abnormalities (e.g., obstruction, fistula)
—Functional abnormalities (e.g., dysfunctional voiding)

- Pathogen-related

—Adherence factors (P-fimbriae)
—Virulence factors (lipopolysaccharide, capsular antigen)

CAUSES

- Enterobacteriaceae: (*Escherichia coli*; most frequent cause [80%]; *Proteus, Klebsiella, Enterobacter*)
- Gram-positive organisms (cause 10%–15%): *Staphylococcus aureus, S. epidermidis, S. saprophiticus,* and enterococci
- Other organisms: *Pseudomonas, Haemophilus influenzae, Streptococcus* group B)

PATHOLOGY

- Patchy infiltration of the medullary parenchyma by polymorphonuclear leukocytes and lymphocytes, tubular disruption, and interstitial edema occurs.
- Parenchymal scarring may result as a consequence of the infection.

EPIDEMIOLOGY

- Five percent of girls develop urinary tract infection (UTI) during childhood.
- Urinary infections are more likely to involve the upper renal tracts in children less than 3 years of age.
- UTIs are more common in females, except in uncircumcised boys under 6 months of age.

COMPLICATIONS

- Acute: reduced concentrating ability, hyperkalemic RTA, bacteremia
- Chronic: focal renal scarring, hypertension, proteinuria, azotemia, and xanthogranulomatous pyelonephritis

 Differential Diagnosis

- Cystitis
- Sterile pyuria

—Vulva-vaginitis
—Balanitis
—Systemic viral illness
—Postvaccination
—Pregnancy
—Appendicitis
—Cystic renal disease
—Tuberculosis

- Lower lobe pneumonia
- Acute appendicitis

 Data Gathering

HISTORY

- A fever greater than 38.5°C may represent the only complaint.
- In the neonate, inquire about: vomiting, lethargy, irritability, fever, hypothermia, and jaundice.
- Older children will be able to tell the examiner about flank pain, dysuria, frequency, urgency, and incontinence.

Special Questions

The following are important factors that predispose to the development of UTIs and should be specifically inquired after:

- Constipation
- Bubble baths
- Incorrect toilet training
- Perineal skin irritation
- Antibiotic exposure
- Uncircumcised males

 Physical Examination

- Findings may be nonspecific.
- Fever, irritability, rigors, lethargy
- Flank tenderness: may be related to the underlying renal tract abnormality, such as flank mass due to obstruction with hydronephrosis or cystic kidney disease, spina bifida apparent or occult, as evidenced by a dimple, pilonidal sinus, or hemangioma

SPECIAL QUESTIONS

- Previous UTIs
- Investigations already performed
- A family history of UTIs or reflux nephropathy
- Symptoms suggestive of dysfunctional voiding, such as the bladder always feels full, infrequent use of the bathroom, and urgency incontinence
- Previous surgery or trauma to the lower back, lower motor milestones, and gait to assess the lower limb neuromuscular status and stool continence

PHYSICAL EXAMINATION TRICKS

- A gentle posterior punch test will reveal tenderness at the costovertebral angle.
- Bimanual palpation of the kidneys for tenderness and size
- Careful neuromuscular examination of the lower limbs and of the back to evaluate for a neurogenic bladder
- Assess the rectal tone to evaluate the integrity of the S2-S4 nerves, which also innervate the bladder.

Laboratory Aids

TESTS

Laboratory Tests

- Collect urine via one of the sterile methods (midstream, catheter, or suprapubic).
- Urine dip for WBC and nitrites as a rapid screen for infection
- As a screening test, an unspun clean-catch urine specimen with bacteria on stained microscopic examination correlates (80%–90%) with culture results of greater than 100,000 colonies per milliliter of urine.
- Urine for culture and sensitivity: A positive culture is defined by the growth of a single pathogenic organism of clean-catch 100,000 colonies/mL, catheter 1,000 colonies/mL, and by any growth from a suprapubic specimen.

Imaging

- *Renal ultrasound* to rule out obstruction and to assess the renal size and parenchyma
- *Voiding cystourethrogram* (VCUG) to rule out anatomic anomalies, including obstruction (e.g., posterior urethral valves) and vesicoureteric reflux
- *99mTc-dimecaptosuccinic acid* (DMSA) can be done to confirm the presence of APN and to look for renal scarring. This is a sensitive and specific test that some clinicians believe to be the imaging study of choice for diagnosing APN and renal scarring.

False Positives

- May be owing to nonsterile collection techniques, allowing the urine to stand unrefrigerated, or owing to prior antibiotic exposure

False Negatives

The rapid test for nitrites requires the urine to stay in the bladder for several hours and is therefore not good for infants who do not store urine in the bladder.

PITFALLS

- Imaging evaluation of the urinary tract following a UTI should be individualized based on the child's clinical presentation and on clinical judgment.
- All children less than 5 years of age should have an ultrasound and VCUG; an ultrasound is recommended in children over 5 years of age.
- Once the urine is sterile, a VCUG can be performed; there is no need to wait 4 weeks.
- Administer antibiotic prophylaxis prior to the VCUG.

Requirements for Testing

Educate the caregivers in the use and interpretation of the dipstick, and about the symptoms and signs of UTI.

 ## Therapy

DRUGS

- Antibiotics such as cotrimoxazole, Augmentin, and the second-generation cephalosporins
- Familiarity with local antibiotic patterns of resistance is particularly important in treating hospital-acquired infections.
- Antipyretics such as acetaminophen

Duration

- Give intravenous antibiotics until the patient is afebrile for at least 24 hours, then change to an oral formulation.
- In total, 10 to 14 days of antibiotic therapy are required.
- Patients with first-time UTIs should receive low-dose antibiotic prophylaxis until their work-up is completed.
- Children with frequent symptomatic recurrences of UTI and those with vesicoureteral reflux require long-term antibiotic prophylaxis.

DIET

Ensure adequate hydration.

 ## Follow-Up

- The fever usually defervesces in 3 to 5 days.
- Ongoing fever or persistent flank pain requires further evaluation to exclude a resistant organism and or an unrecognized urinary tract obstruction.
- The diagnosis and treatment of any underlying voiding dysfunction and constipation is required for the successful management of UTIs in children.
- The outcome of APN is usually good, but may result in parenchymal scarring.

 ## Common Questions and Answers

Q: Should a DMSA scan be used help diagnose APN?
A: Routine use of the DMSA scan to diagnose APN is controversial, as there is disagreement about the therapeutic implications of a positive test and routine testing will be costly. Children with hypertension and previous UTIs require a DMSA scan to look for renal cortical scarring.

Q: Does renal parenchymal scarring occur in the absence of reflux?
A: Yes. The causal relationship between reflux, APN, and renal parenchymal scarring is complex.

ICD-9-CM 590.10

BIBLIOGRAPHY

Hellerstein S. Urinary tract infections in children: why they occur and how to prevent them. *Am Fam Physician* 1998;57(10):2440–2446, 2452–2454.

Jodal U, Hansson S. Urinary tract infection. In: Holliday M, Barratt TM, Avner ED, eds. *Pediatric nephrology,* 3rd ed. Baltimore: Williams & Wilkins, 1994:950.

Kawashima A, Sandler CM, Goldman SM. Current roles and controversies in the imaging evaluation of acute renal infection. World J Urol 1998;16(1):9–17.

Rushton HG. Urinary tract infections in children. Epidemiology, evaluation and management. *Pediatr Clin North Am* 1997;44(5):1133–1169.

Author: Kevin E.C. Meyers

Pyloric Stenosis

 Database

DEFINITION

Pyloric stenosis is hypertrophy of the muscular layers of the pylorus, leading to obstruction.

ETIOLOGY

- Unknown
- No specific pattern of inheritance established
- Multifactorial inheritance likely

PATHOPHYSIOLOGY

- There is diffuse hypertrophy and hyperplasia of the pylorus, leading to narrowing of the gastric antrum.
- The antrum becomes thickened, elongated, and firm in consistency.
- Hypergastrinemia associated with hyperactivity elevations of prostaglandins and deficiency of nitric oxide as a smooth muscle neurotransmitter have been suggested as etiologic factors.

INCIDENCE AND EPIDEMIOLOGY

- Exceedingly rare in newborns as well as in patients greater than 6 months of age
- Occurs in approximately 1 in 950 live births
- More frequent among Caucasians

COMPLICATIONS

- Dehydration
- Electrolyte abnormalities, primarily hypochloremic alkalosis

PROGNOSIS

Morbidity and mortality are very low, and surgery is curative.

ASSOCIATED ANOMALIES

Increased occurrence of esophageal atresia and malrotation was noted in 5% of infants with pyloric stenosis.

 Differential Diagnosis

- Gastroesophageal reflux
- Gastroenteritis
- Pyloric atresia
- Antral web

 Data Gathering

HISTORY

- Nonbilious vomiting, classically projectile in an otherwise well and hungry child between 2 and 8 weeks of age
- Possible weight loss, varying degrees of dehydration and lethargy

 Physical Examination

- Visible peristalsis may be appreciated just after the infant feeds; this is seen as a waveform proceeding from the left upper quadrant toward the pylorus in the right upper quadrant.
- A palpable, hard, mobile, and nontender mass in the epigastrium to the right of the midline, referred to as an olive
- Best palpated after the infant has vomited

 Laboratory Aids

TESTS

- Hypochloremia and alkalosis
- Hyponatremia
- Hypokalemia

RADIOLOGIC FEATURES

Gastrointestinal Studies

- An upper gastrointestinal study can differentiate between antral webs and pylorospasm.
- In pyloric stenosis, it reveals vigorous gastric peristalsis with little or no gastric emptying.
- An elongated narrow pyloric anal canal can be seen as a single or sometimes a double tract of barium, commonly known as the "string sign."
- A pyloric bulge into the distal antrum, producing an umbrella appearance, also may be seen.

Ultrasound

- Ultrasonography identifies the hypertrophic pyloric musculature as a broad ring with low-echo density and an inner layer of high-echo density corresponding to the mucosa.
- To confirm the diagnosis, the muscle thickness should be greater than 4 mm or the pyloric length greater than 16 mm.

Therapy

- Correction of the metabolic abnormalities by replacing sodium, chloride, and potassium
- Pyloromyotomy (Ramstedt procedure): incision of the antropyloric muscle
- Pyloric stenosis is a medical emergency, not a surgical emergency.
- Postoperative vomiting is well recognized and is most likely caused by persistent local edema.
- Initiate feedings very slowly; most patients can be advanced to maintenance oral feedings 48 hours after surgery.

Follow-Up

Vomiting may persist for several days after surgery.

PITFALLS

- Failure to appreciate that chloride loss is the most significant electrolyte disorder when replacing fluids and electrolytes
- Failure to appreciate that this disorder does occur in girls as well as boys

Common Questions and Answers

Q: Can ultrasound help make the diagnosis?
A: Yes. Many will order this test first to avoid the possible aspiration of contrast material.

Q: Why is there so much chloride loss?
A: The chloride loss occurs with the loss of gastric acid, which contains HCl.

Q: What plan should I follow when replacing electrolytes?
A: Correct the deficiency of fluids with twice maintenance fluid volumes. Correct the chloride loss with normal saline, and correct the potassium loss with KCl.

ICD-9-CM 537.0

BIBLIOGRAPHY

Bissounette B, Sullivan PJ. Pyloric stenosis. *Can J Anesth* 1991;38(5):668.

Deluca SA. Hypertrophic pyloric stenosis. *Am Fam Physician* 1993;47(8):1771.

Mitchell LE, Risch N. The genetics of infantile hypertrophic pyloric stenosis: a reanalysis: *Am J Dis Child* 1993;147(11):1203.

Zenn MR, Redo SF. Hypertrophic pyloric stenosis in the newborn. *J Pediatr Surg* 1993;28(12):1577–1578.

Author: Helen Anita John-Kelly

Rabies

Database

DEFINITION

Rabies is a viral infection of the central nervous system (CNS) that is transmitted from animals to people.

CAUSES

Transmission of the virus, a rhabdovirus containing single-stranded RNA, occurs through animal bites and, rarely, via corneal transplants (from donors with unexplained encephalitis) or inhalation among laboratory workers.

PATHOPHYSIOLOGY

Except for rare cases, the rabies virus enters the body through a bite that causes a break in the skin and introduces infected saliva. From there, the virus gains access to muscle, where it is sequestered. The virus then enters the peripheral nerves, where it moves centripetally to the CNS at a rate of approximately 3 mm/hr. Once in the CNS, infection spreads rapidly to involve nearly all neurons. This, if untreated, leads to cardiopulmonary arrest and death shortly thereafter by poorly understood mechanisms.

EPIDEMIOLOGY

• While the current U.S. annual incidence of reported human rabies is about one to two cases per year, incidence rates elsewhere in the world are much higher. In addition, thousands of infected animals are identified each year in the United States.
• Endemic regions of the United States include the mid-Atlantic, southeast, south central, and north central areas, and California.
• Common vectors: Seven species of animals account for 98% of all reported U.S. animal rabies cases: skunks (38%-43%), raccoons (28%-31%), bats (14%), cats (4%), foxes (4%), cattle (4%), dogs (3%), and other (2%).
• Uncommon vectors: As noted, transmission rarely occurs via corneal transplants or inhalation among laboratory workers.

CLINICAL MANIFESTATIONS

• The *incubation period* can range between 10 days and 2 years! Most cases, however, present within 20 to 90 days postexposure.
• *Prodrome:* 2 to 10 days with vague and insidious symptoms such as sore throat, malaise, anxiety, depression, and, at times, fever or nausea. A fairly specific prodromal symptom is itching, pain, or tingling at the site of the bite.
• *Acute neurologic phase:* furious (80%) versus paralytic (20%) rabies

—*Furious rabies:* agitation, hyperactivity, bizarre behavior—nuchal rigidity, sore throat, and hoarseness. The pathognomonic sign is hydrophobia and, at times, aerophobia.
—*Paralytic rabies:* starts with flaccid paralysis in the limb that was bitten; subsequently spreads to other limbs. Cranial nerve involvement can give an expressionless face.
—*Coma:* follows the acute neurologic phase; May persist up to 2 weeks and is followed by death almost universally.

PROGNOSIS

• Once infected with the rabies virus, the prognosis is grim.
• Without postexposure rabies immunization, the disease is uniformly fatal.
• There are three documented instances of rabies in humans who survived after receiving postexposure immunization and intensive medical management.

Differential Diagnosis

• Other causes of encephalitis (i.e., HSV, enterovirus) can mimic rabies.
• Paralytic rabies can present much like Guillain-Barré syndrome or poliomyelitis.
• Pseudorabies is hysteria in an individual who thinks he or she has rabies, but does not. Here, though, normal blood gases and lack of variation in bizarre behavior are distinguishing.

Data Gathering

HISTORY

• Rabid animals: While signs of rabies in animals vary greatly, atypical behavior for the animal is the norm (i.e., passive animals become aggressive, nocturnal animals roam in daylight). Foaming at the mouth and lack of coordination may be present.
• A small minority of humans with rabies have no identifiable preceding animal exposure.

Physical Examination

• Although the neurologic findings can vary, cranial nerve paralysis (palate, vocal cords) is common. Therefore, hoarseness and stridor can be seen.
• Meningismus is also fairly common, along with involuntary movements. Beyond this, findings will depend on type of presentation (furious versus paralytic). (See Clinical Manifestations.)

SPECIAL QUESTIONS

• Type of animal inflicting the bite (domestic versus wild)
• Location of the animal and availability for observation
• History of previous rabies vaccination of the animal and patient

Laboratory Aids

 ## Therapy

 ## Common Questions and Answers

- There are no known methods for identification of rabies virus infection prior to the onset of clinical signs. However, once signs appear, laboratory diagnosis is now possible before death by several techniques:

—*Fluorescent antibodies (FA) stain* of corneal epithelial cell smears or a section of skin from the neck at the hairline
—*Serologic diagnosis* is possible if the patient survives beyond the acute period. A rise in virus-neutralizing antibody will be seen.
—*Viral isolation* from saliva, CSF, urine sedimentation, and brain is, at times, possible between days 4 and 24.

- Postmortem diagnosis is made by the presence of pathognomonic cytoplasmic inclusions (Negri bodies) in brain tissue (sensitivity, 80%).

LOCAL WOUND CARE

- The first step in preventing infection is washing out the virus mechanically or inactivating it before it has a chance to attach to and enter a neuron.
- The wound should be flushed with copious amounts of soap and water or saline.
- For puncture wounds, insertion of a catheter (i.e., angiocatheter) and irrigation with fluid by means of an attached syringe should be performed. If irrigation is too painful, infiltration of the area with local anesthesia can help.

PASSIVE AND ACTIVE IMMUNIZATION

Passive Immunization

- Human rabies immune globulin (HRIG) should be given to those who are bitten by any variety of wild animal known to be at high risk for rabies infection (skunk, raccoon, fox, coyote, bat) and any domestic dog or cat not in good health and in the custody of someone able to observe the animal for a 10-day period.
- The present recommendation for HRIG vaccination is 20 IU/kghalf injected locally into the tissue at the site of the bite and the other half administered IM.

Active Immunization

- Human diploid cell rabies vaccine (HDCV) is an inactivated rabies vaccine. This should be administered by the same criteria given above for passive immunization.
- Dosing: 1 mL IM in the deltoid region on days 0, 3, 7, 14, and 28 postexposure. Discontinue the vaccine series if fluorescent antibody testing of the animal is conducted and is negative.

PREVENTION

Immunoprophylaxis: Preexposure vaccines are offered to persons at high risk, such as veterinarians and animal handlers. Because wild animals are the largest source of rabies in the United States today, avoiding unnecessary contact is helpful. More importantly, attempts are being made to orally vaccinate wild animals by using vaccine-laden food in several areas of the United States. Last, it is essential that pet owners vaccinate their pets.

Q: Does a wild squirrel or rabbit bite necessitate rabies prophylaxis?
A: In general, rodents (squirrels, rats, mice, hamsters, gerbils), lagamorphs (rabbits and hares), and opossums are not known to serve as natural rabies reservoirs. They should not be considered rabid unless they exhibit unusual behavior.

Q: Is there any evidence of human-to-human spread?
A: No.

Q: Are there any nations in the world that require routine rabies vaccination?
A: Yes, in Nepal.

Q: What if a severe allergic reaction occurs during postexposure rabies prophylaxis?
A: The reaction should be treated at the time, as you would any systemic anaphylactic reaction. Subsequently, the rabies vaccine adsorbed (RVA), produced in rhesus diploid cells, can be given on the same schedule as HDCV.

ICD-9-CM 071

BIBLIOGRAPHY

Centers for Disease Control. Rabies surveillance, United States, 1987. *MMWR* 1988;37:1.

Gomez-Alonso J. Rabies: a possible explanation for the vampire legend. *Neurology* 1998;51(3):856–859.

NASPHV Compendium Committee. Compendium of animal rabies control. *MMWR* 1987;35:815.

Nicholson KG. Modern vaccines. *Lancet* 1990;335:1201.

Author: Susan Dibs

Rectal Prolapse

 Database

DEFINITION

There are three types of rectal prolapse:

- *Complete:* The full thickness of the rectum prolapses through the anus (two layers of rectum with an intervening peritoneal sac, which may contain small bowel).
- *Incomplete:* The prolapse is limited to the two layers of mucosa only.
- *Concealed:* an internal intussusception of the upper rectum into the lower rectum, which does not emerge through the anus

CAUSES

The exact etiology is uncertain, but is related to the following:

- Constipation
- Excessive straining with bowel movements
- Diarrhea; may be more of a cause in tropical countries
- Cystic fibrosis (CF)
- Malnutrition; can cause loss of the ischiorectal fat pad
- Complete prolapse more rare in children, but when occurs may be related to poor fixation of rectum to sacrum and weak pelvic and anal musculature
- May be complication of past surgery, such as imperforate anus repair
- Infections: hookworms

GENETICS

- No known inheritance pattern aside from the association with CF
- An autosomally recessive inherited disease

EPIDEMIOLOGY

- Occurs in more than 19% of children with CF
- It usually presents between 1 and 2 1/2 years of age in patients with CF. Presentation in these children after age 5 is rare.
- In older children and adults, it is six times more common in women than in men.
- It is seen more in underdeveloped countries, perhaps secondary to poor nutrition.

COMPLICATIONS

- In certain older patients who may also have an overactive external sphincter, the need to generate high rectal pressures in order to defecate, together with the rectal prolapse, may cause venous congestion; it may lead to the solitary rectal ulcer syndrome.
- The repetitive trauma to the mucosa can lead to a proctitis.

PROGNOSIS

With proper medical management, excellent prognosis; surgery not usually required

 Differential Diagnosis

- Tumors
- Prolapsing rectal tumor: very rare
- Trauma
- Sexual abuse (i.e., anal penetration)
- Metabolic
- Cystic fibrosis: Of significance is the fact that many (anywhere from 10%–50%) of the patients who are diagnosed with CF after age 4 have experienced rectal prolapse (either at the time of the diagnosis or as a past event).
- Anatomic

—Solitary rectal ulcer syndrome: an uncommon benign condition usually affecting older children (teen-agers). Rectal bleeding on defecation common. Some studies report an association between this entity and rectal prolapse.

—Prolapsing polyp
—Large hemorrhoids
—Surgical
—Colonic intussusception

 Data Gathering

HISTORY

- It is usually first noted by a parent after the child has defecated, and may be associated with painless rectal bleeding.
- It often reduces spontaneously. If not, it is usually easily reduced manually by the parent.
- Rectal prolapse may cause some discomfort during bowel movements.
- Trauma to the recurrently prolapsed mucosa may lead to ulceration and mucus discharge.

 Physical Examination

- Usually, prolapse is not seen on examination while the patient is at rest, unless it is irreducible.
- May see poor anal tone and/or large anal orifice, especially within hours after the prolapse
- In complete rectal prolapse, concentric mucosal rings can be seen, whereas incomplete prolapse reveals radial folds. If one sees more than 5 cm of rectum emerging, it is most likely a complete prolapse.

SPECIAL QUESTIONS

- Has the patient had history of wheezing, pneumonia, or failure to thrive?
- Does this patient have CF?

PHYSICAL EXAMINATION TRICKS

- Asking the patient to strain may allow the mucosa to prolapse. However, this is obviously not very helpful in the very young patient.
- A polyp is differentiated in that it is plum-colored and does not involve the entire anal circumference.
- In an intussusception, it is possible to insert the finger around the prolapsing apex of the intussusception, between it and the lining of the anal canal.

Laboratory Aids

TESTS

Laboratory Tests

• Sweat test: All children with prolapse should have a sweat test to rule out CF. This is a simple, noninvasive, inexpensive test with good specificity and sensitivity.
• Stool cultures: for bacterial and parasitic infestations, if diarrhea is present as a possible causative factor

Imaging

Evacuation proctography: A barium enema is given, and the movement of barium is observed under fluoroscopy during defecation. This may reveal an internal prolapse not easily recognizable on examination alone. This is not commonly used in children, as good cooperation is necessary.

PITFALLS

Although the history of rectal prolapse may be evident, it is often difficult to elicit on examination, and by the time the patient is seen after a prolapse at home, it may already be spontaneously reduced. Thus, the assumption of the diagnosis may have to rest primarily on the parental history for some time.

 ## Therapy

• Rectal prolapse has a tendency to spontaneously resolve over time.
• The prolapse will more successfully and quickly resolve if the patient is treated for constipation. This should include both dietary manipulations (increased fiber, water) and improved toilet regime. It also will usually necessitate the use of supplemental aids such as mineral oil and, occasionally, laxatives. A small child should try to defecate on a regular toilet and not a potty. In this way, the feet are off the floor, relieving pressure on the abdomen.
• In the rare case of stool infection with diarrhea as the underlying etiology, the appropriate therapy for that infection should be instituted.

DRUGS

In a patient with CF, the addition of pancreatic enzyme supplementation, if not already a part of the regime, has shown to cause dramatic improvement in rectal prolapse.

DURATION

The treatment of constipation should continue indefinitely, or until the child has demonstrated regular bowel habits on a high-fiber diet on his or her own without evidence of prolapse for at least several months.

SURGICAL

Numerous approaches have been attempted and advocated with varying degrees of enthusiasm, suggesting that none is perfect. These include:

• *Perianal sutures:* has poor results and high complication rate
• *Delorme procedure:* The rectal mucosa is excised and underlying rectal muscle is plicated with sutures.
• *Abdominal rectopexy:* The rectum is mobilized and attached to the sacrum by prosthetic material. Although this procedure provides good results, it has a high complication rate of constipation (greater than 50%).
• *Anterior resection rectopexy:* includes resection of the sigmoid loop and upper rectum; good results, but again, high complication rate because of the anastamosis
• *Perineal resection:* perineal rectosigmoidectomy with a coloanal anastamosis; good results

 ## Follow-Up

WHEN TO EXPECT IMPROVEMENT

• Over a period of months to years on a good dietary and behavioral regime

SIGNS TO WATCH FOR

• The child is beginning to strain in order to defecate.

PITFALLS

• Although usually a benign event, rectal prolapse is a very distressing condition to both the parents and the child.
• Although surgery seems to be a quicker and more definite solution, in most cases it is more prudent to allow time and medical management to solve the problem. The results from surgical procedures are not foolproof and may lead to further complications.

 ## Common Questions and Answers

Q: What should I do if my child has a rectal prolapse but I cannot reduce it?
A: You should wrap the prolapse in moist towels and bring your child to the emergency room. There, the physicians will try to reduce it. Rarely, if a prolapse is irreducible and left for a period of time, it can cause bowel ischemia and may require surgery.

Q: My child has rectal prolapse and now he is supposed to have a sweat test to determine whether or not he has cystic fibrosis. Is this very likely?
A: No. Although it is important to rule out this disease, the majority of patients with rectal prolapse do not have CF. On the other hand, many children with CF suffer from rectal prolapse.

Q: My child, who has rectal prolapse, is in day care. How will I know if he is having the prolapse?
A: You should inform someone in the school (a teacher or guardian) of his condition and he or she should check the child for prolapse after a movement. Although, if present, it usually spontaneously resolves, the caretaker should inform you so you can do a manual reduction, if necessary.

ICD-9-CM 569.1

BIBLIOGRPAHY

Andrews NJ, Jones DJ. Rectal prolapse and associated conditions. *BMJ* 1992;305:242.

Bartolo DC, Kamm MA, et al. Working party report: defecation disorders. *Am J Gastroenterol* 1994;89(8):S154.

Du Boulay DF, Fairbrother J, et al. Mucosal prolapse syndrome: a unifying concept for solitary ulcer syndrome and related disorders. *J Clin Pathol* 1983;36:1264.

Kuijpers HC. Treatment of complete rectal prolapse: to narrow, to wrap, to suspend, to fix, to encircle, to plicate, or to resect? *World J Surg* 1992;16:S26.

Author: Andrew E. Mulberg

Renal Artery Stenosis

 Database

DEFINITION

Renal artery stenosis is narrowing of one or both renal arteries or their more distal branches, resulting in decreased perfusion, increased renin release, increased vascular resistance, and systemic hypertension.

PATHOPHYSIOLOGY

- The most common cause is fibromuscular dysplasia (FMD).
- Other causes include hypoplasia of the renal artery, partial obstruction from a thromboembolism, severe dehydration, extrinsic compression of the artery, vasculitis, neurofibromatosis (NF), and following renal artery surgery (e.g., renal transplantation).
- Arterial narrowing by atheroma is very common in adults but rarely is seen in childhood.

PATHOLOGY

- FMD is a segmental sclerotic process involving smooth muscle hyperplasia. In 75% of patients it is unilateral. Stenosis is usually distal in the renal artery and sometimes involves intrarenal branches. FMD frequently gives a beaded appearance on angiography.
- In NF, the arterial narrowing is proximal, often at the vessel ostium.

GENETICS

- FMD is sporadic.
- NF is autosomal dominant.

EPIDEMIOLOGY

The majority of children with elevated blood pressure have primary or idiopathic hypertension. Of those with secondary hypertension, the majority have intrinsic renal disease (e.g., glomerulonephritis or renal scarring). Only 5% to 10% will have renal artery stenosis. Its importance, therefore, is not its frequency, but the fact that it is potentially curable.

COMPLICATIONS

- Renal artery stenosis often causes severe blood pressure elevation and may be associated with encephalopathy, seizures, or stroke.
- Chronic hypertension may cause damage to end-organs, including the heart and kidney.

PROGNOSIS

- Long-term outcome of percutaneous transluminal angioplasty (PTA) in FMD is excellent, and most children require no medications.
- Restenosis of the vessel is very infrequent.

ASSOCIATED ILLNESSES

- FMD is not associated with other conditions.
- Renal artery stenosis may occur in many other conditions, including NF, vasculitis including polyarteritis nodosa and Takayasu arteritis, moya-moya syndrome, William syndrome, Marfan syndrome, tuberous sclerosis, congenital rubella, and following trauma.
- In neonates, renal artery stenosis is usually the result of a thromboembolus, which is a complication of an umbilical artery catheter.

 Differential Diagnosis

- Renal artery stenosis should be suspected and investigated in children with sudden, severe, progressive, and/or difficult-to-manage hypertension.
- The differential diagnosis consists of other causes of significant hypertension, including coarctation of the aorta, rapidly progressive glomerulonephritis, and renal failure and pheochromocytoma.

 Data Gathering

HISTORY

- Symptoms in infants may include irritability, vomiting, and poor feeding.
- In children, symptoms may include headaches, vomiting, dizziness, and seizures.
- Many children are asymptomatic.

Special Question

Has the child ingested any medication that can increase blood pressure, such as sympathomimetic drugs, steroids, amphetamines, oral contraceptives, and so on?

 Physical Examination

- Accurate determination of blood pressure with appropriate-size cuff; done in the upper and lower extremities
- Blood pressure should be repeated until the patient is judged to be relaxed.
- Pulses should be checked in all four extremities.
- The skin must be examined for signs of neurofibromatosis (i.e., café-au-lait spots and neurofibromas) and vasculitis.
- The optic fundi must be checked for hypertensive vascular changes. Often, an ophthalmologist's examination is necessary.
- Auscultation of the lower back and abdomen should be checked for the presence of bruits.
- In infancy, signs of congestive heart failure may be present.

PHYSICAL EXAMINATION TRICKS

- The resting, relaxed blood pressure is likely to be obtained when the pulse rate has reached a basal resting level.
- Listen for an abdominal bruit just to the left of and superior to the umbilicus.
- Listen over the flanks with a bell stethoscope for a bruit.

Laboratory Aids

TESTS

- *BUN* and *creatinine* to exclude intrinsic renal disease
- *Electrolytes:* A hyperrenin state leads to hyperaldosteronism and may produce hypokalemia and mild metabolic alkalosis.
- *Selective renal vein renin determinations* are suggestive of unilateral stenosis if one side is less than one and a half times the contralateral (normal). Random venous renin concentrations have little value and may be misleading.
- *Electrocardiogram* and/or *echocardiogram* to investigate the presence of ventricular strain or hypertrophy

IMAGING

- Although a variety of imaging studies are available that may suggest renal artery stenosis, the only definitive tests are *selective* renal arteriography, and, if indicated, transluminal angioplasty.
- Renal ultrasonography may demonstrate a smaller kidney on the suspected side, but this study cannot make or exclude the diagnosis. Recently, special applications of *Doppler ultrasonography* and color-coded duplex sonography have shown promise, especially in the postoperative transplant period when immediate information regarding the renal artery is essential.
- Other *more invasive studies,* such as captopril-enhanced nuclear medicine scans, digital subtraction angiography, CT scans, and MRI, have not proved to be confirmatory for all patients, but they may be useful when used in selective children with a high likelihood of renal artery stenosis.

 ## Therapy

DRUGS

- Hypertension that accompanies renal artery stenosis is often difficult to control with antihypertensive medications. In small infants, however, long-term medical therapy may be necessary until the child is large enough for definitive correction.
- Because renal artery stenosis results in a high renin state, the angiotensin-converting enzyme (ACE) inhibitors, captopril and enalopril, are most effective. When used in conjunction with renal scintigraphy or selective renin measurements, ACE inhibitors may improve diagnosis of renal artery stenosis.
- ACE inhibitors may significantly decrease renal perfusion and function and should not be used in cases of known or suspected bilateral renal artery stenosis.
- Thrombolytic therapy with urokinase should be considered in instances of bilateral renal artery thrombosis.

DEFINITIVE CORRECTION

- PTA dilatation of the stenosis, using an intravascular balloon catheter during arteriography, is the treatment of choice. This therapy is very effective in FMD but less effective in the proximal stenosis associated with NF. Stent implantation is occasionally used as an adjunct to angioplasty.
- Surgery is indicated in cases in which PTA is not possible or successful. Autotransplantation may be effective, especially in children with bilateral renal artery and aortic narrowing.

DURATION

- Effective medical therapy should be monitored closely and continued until the renal artery stenosis can be corrected.
- Medication is generally discontinued prior to the angioplasty and used postprocedure only if the blood pressure remains elevated.

 ## Follow-Up

- If effective, response to antihypertensive therapy with ACE inhibitors should occur within 12 days.
- Response to dilation of the renal artery stenosis is often immediate, although transient vessel spasm may occur postprocedure and temporarily be associated with hypertension significant enough to require treatment.

PITFALLS

- Excessive investigation for renal artery stenosis or other secondary causes of hypertension in the majority of children identified with elevated blood pressure
- Failure to proceed rapidly to an arteriogram in a child appropriately suspected of having renal artery stenosis

ICD-9-CM 440.1

BIBLIOGRAPHY

Deal JE, Shell MF, Barratt TM, Dillon MJ. Renovascular disease in childhood. *J Pediatr* 1992;121:378.

Ellis D, Shapiro R, Scantlebury VP, Simmons R, Towbin R. Evaluation and management of bilateral renal artery stenosis in children: a case series and review. *Pediatr Nephrol* 1995;9:259.

Guzzetta PC, Davis CF, Ruley EJ. Experience with bilateral renal artery stenosis as a cause of hypertension in childhood. *J Pediatr Surg* 1991;26:532.

Author: Thomas L. Kennedy III

Renal Failure—Acute

 Database

DEFINITION

Acute renal failure is a rapidly progressive, and potentially reversible, cessation of renal function that results in the inability of the kidney to control body homeostasis. It manifests in retention of nitrogenous waste products and fluid and electrolyte imbalances.

- Oliguria: urine output less than 0.5 mL/kg/hr in infants or less than 500 mL/1.73 m² per day in older children
- Anuria: total cessation of urinary output

PATHOPHYSIOLOGY

Acute renal failure has many causes, which can be categorized into three subgroups.

- Prerenal

—Decreased perfusion of the kidney secondary either to decreased extracellular volume or diminished cardiac output
—It is the most common form of acute renal failure in children.

- Postrenal

—An obstructive process (either structural or functional)
—The obstruction can reside in the lower tract or bilaterally in the upper tracts unless the patient has a single kidney.
—This form of renal failure is more common in newborns.

- Intrinsic
- Disorders that directly affect the kidney. This form can be subcategorized:

—*Acute tubular necrosis* is the most common form of intrinsic renal failure and usually follows hypoxic or nephrotoxic injury.
—*Glomerular disorders* include the various forms of acute glomerulonephritis (AGN) such as postinfectious AGN and rapidly progressive (crescentic) AGN.
—*Vascular lesions* compromise glomerular blood flow. Hemolytic-uremic syndrome is the most common disease that causes intrinsic acute renal failure in children.
—*Interstitial nephritis* can be idiopathic or caused by reactions to drugs or infections.

- Acute renal failure is commonly precipitated by an ischemic or nephrotoxic event. Initial vasodilatation is followed by intense vasoconstriction, with blood redistributed from the cortex to the juxtamedullary nephrons. The delivery of oxygen to the kidney is impaired, leading to acute tubular necrosis. Intratubular debris and cast formation develop. Tubular fluid leaks backward across the injured tubular membrane, which, in addition to tubular obstruction, causes further hemodynamic changes.

EPIDEMIOLOGY

Acute renal failure secondary to acute tubular necrosis is commonly seen in the hospitalized patient. The combination of ischemia plus nephrotoxic agents such as aminoglycosides, amphotericin B, contrast, or chemotherapeutic agents place these individuals at increased risk.

COMPLICATIONS

- Fluid overload, resulting in congestive heart failure and hypertension
- Hyperkalemia, affecting cardiac function by causing arrhythmias
- Uremia, manifest by mental status changes, increased risk of bleeding, and infection
- Metabolic acidosis
- Hypocalcemia, causing tetany

PROGNOSIS

- Generally, patients with nonoliguric renal failure have a lower mortality rate than patients with oliguria or anuria.
- The mortality rate increases in patients with multisystem organ failure, despite good supportive care

 Differential Diagnosis

- Chronic renal failure: insidious, associated with poor growth, polyuria, and anemia
- Azotemia: caused by corticosteroid therapy, upper gastrointestinal bleeding, hypercatabolic state
- Elevated creatinine: caused by rhabdomyolysis, drugs (trimethoprimsulfa, cimetidine)

 Data Gathering

Key: POST, obstruction; PRE, prerenal; ATN, acute tubular necrosis; AIN, acute interstitial nephritis; AGN, acute glomerulonephritis; HUS, hemolytic-uremic syndrome

HISTORY

- Symptoms: fever, rash (AIN, AGN), bloody diarrhea, pallor (HUS), severe vomiting or diarrhea (PRE), abdominal pain (POST), hemorrhage, shock (ATN), anuria (AGN, POST), polyuria (ATN, AIN)
- Medical history: previous infection (AGN), neurogenic bladder, single kidney (POST)
- Medications: exposure to various medications such as nonsteroidal antiinflammatory agents, betalactam antibiotics, acyclovir (AIN), nephrotoxic drugs such as aminoglycosides, amphotericin B, cisplatinum (ATN)
- Toxins: exposure to heavy metals, organic solvents (ATN)
- Family: history of HUS
- Trauma: crush injury (ATN)
- Review of symptoms: various systemic symptoms (AGN)

 Physical Examination

- General: dehydration, shock, septic (PRE, ATN), edema (AGN), jaundice (HUS, ATN)
- Eyes: uveitis (AIN)
- Lungs: rales (AGN)
- Heart: gallop (AGN)
- Abdomen/pelvis: mass (POST)
- Skin: rash (AIN, AGN), petechia (HUS)

Laboratory Aids

TESTS

• Urinalysis: normal sediment or eumorphic RBCs, crystalluria (POST), eosinophiluria, pyuria (AIN), granular casts (PRE, ATN), pigmenturia (ATN), RBC casts, proteinuria (HUS, AGN), U_{osm} less than 350 mosm (POST, AIN, ATN), U_{osm} greater than 500 mosm (PRE, AGN, HUS)
• Serum chemistries: hyponatremia, hyperchloremic acidosis (POST), hyperkalemia (POST, AGN, HUS), BUN:Cr greater than 20 (PRE)
• CBC: microangiopathic hemolytic anemia, thrombocytopenia (HUS), eosinophilia (AIN)
• Serologies: hypocomplimentemia (AGN), antineutrophil cytoplasmic antibodies (AGN), antinuclear antibodies (AGN)
• Renal ultrasound: hydronephrosis, trabeculated bladder (POST), increased echogenicity (ATN, AIN, AGN, HUS)
• Renal biopsy: indicated in patients with prolonged, unexplained acute renal failure

SPECIAL LABORATORY TRICKS

The *fractional excretion of sodium* (FE_{Na}) is a useful urinary index that determines tubular function.

$$FE_{Na} = \frac{U_{Na}/P_{Na}}{U_{creat}/P_{creat}} \times 100$$

The FE_{Na} should not be obtained after diuretics are administered.

FE_{Na} greater than 2 (AIN, ATN), FE_{Na} less than 1 (HUS, AGN, PRE)

 ## Therapy

Therapy is preventive, supportive, or specific.

PREVENTIVE

The use of mannitol or furosemide to prevent acute renal failure is controversial. They may be used prophylactically (amphotericin B, cisplatinum, contrast) or in cases of hemoglobinuria or myoglobinuria to augment urine flow. Some feel this may convert oliguric renal failure to nonoliguric renal failure.

SUPPORTIVE

• Establish an effective circulatory volume. If the patient is in shock, administer fluids (normal saline, lactated Ringer's) liberally, even if there is no urine output.
• Maintain a normal intravascular volume. Carefully monitor output and provide appropriate fluids accordingly. Consider fluid restriction and diuretics if the patient is volume overloaded.
• Monitor serum potassium levels frequently. Avoid potassium-containing drugs, fluids, or foods in patients with oligo/anuria. If hyperkalemia is present, consider

—Calcium gluconate (0.5-1.0 mL/kg IV) over 5–10 minutes if severe
—Glucose (0.5 g/kg) and insulin (0.1 U/kg) IV over 30 minutes
—Sodium bicarbonate (1-2 mEq/kg) IV over 10–30 minutes if acidotic
—Kayexolate (1 g/kg) PO or PR in sorbitol

• Hyponatremia is usually secondary to free water excess and should be managed with fluid restriction. Hypertonic saline should be used if only CNS symptoms are present.
• Hypocalcemia, if mild, may be treated by phosphate restriction. Severe hypocalcemia requires treatment with calcium gluconate (100 mg/kg) given slowly.
• Severe acidosis (pH <7.2) requires supplementation with bicarbonate. However, this may cause hypernatremia, fluid overload, and symptomatic hypocalcemia.
• The effect of aggressive nutritional support is controversial, with the exception of use for a significantly malnourished or hypercatabolic child.
• Hypertension should be treated aggressively if encephalopathy is present.
• Dialysis is indicated for refractory acidosis, severe hyperkalemia, volume overload, and uremic symptoms (pericarditis, lethargy), or for the removal of toxins (uric acid, salicylate).

SPECIFIC

Each cause of renal failure may have a specific treatment, such as fluid resuscitation (PRE), urologic intervention (POST), and corticosteroids (AIN, some forms of AGN).

 ## Follow-Up

Patients usually remain hospitalized until their renal function improves. Long-term follow-up to monitor sequelae is indicated in patients with prolonged anuria.

PITFALLS

The excretion of many medications is influenced by acute renal failure. Careful attention to drug dosing and levels can minimize toxicity.

 ## Common Questions and Answers

Q: What is the expected recovery time in patients with acute renal failure who present with anuria?
A: Recovery time depends on the etiology of the acute renal failure. Children with HUS may recover in days to weeks. Others with ATN recover days after treatment of the inciting cause. Finally, obstructed children usually recover as soon as the obstruction is relieved.

Q: When should renal function return to normal values?
A: Renal function may not return to normal in patients with prolonged periods of anuria. In other cases, once recovery starts, a normal serum creatinine is seen within weeks.

Q: What indices should be followed after a patient recovers from acute renal failure?
A: Patients recovering from acute renal failure should have blood pressures and urinalysis for proteinuria monitored regularly. Serum creatinine should be checked if the course of acute renal failure was prolonged.

ICD-9-CM 584.0

BIBLIOGRAPHY

Sehic A, Chesney RW. Acute renal failure: diagnosis. *Pediatr Rev* 1995;16:101–106.

Sehic A, Chesney RW. Acute renal failure: therapy. *Pediatr Rev* 1995;16:137–141.

Stewart CL, Barnett R. Acute renal failure in infants, children and adults. *Crit Care Clin* 1997;13:575–590.

Thadhani R, Pascual M, Bonventre JV. Acute renal failure. *N Engl J Med* 1996;334:1448–1460.

Author: Seth L. Schulman

Renal Failure—Chronic

Database

DEFINITION

- Chronic renal failure is a reduction in the glomerular filtration rate to <25% of normal for at least 3 months' duration.
- Chronic renal insufficiency describes a reduction in the glomerular filtration rate between 25% to 50%.

PATHOPHYSIOLOGY

- Infants younger than 2 years of age develop chronic renal failure secondary to either obstructive uropathy or renal hypodysplasia.
- Children 2 to 5 years of age develop chronic renal failure secondary to neonatal vascular accidents and hemolytic uremic syndrome, obstructive uropathy, or renal hypodysplasia.
- More common etiologies of chronic renal failure in older children and adolescents include glomerulonephritis (focal segmental glomerulosclerosis, crescentic glomerulonephritis, lupus nephritis), reflux nephropathy, or hereditary causes such as Alport syndrome.

GENETICS

Several hereditary diseases can cause chronic renal failure, including:

- Alport disease (partially X-linked dominant)
- Polycystic kidney disease (autosomal recessive or dominant)
- Familial juvenile nephronophthisis (autosomal recessive)
- Cystinosis (autosomal recessive)
- Hyperoxaluria (autosomal recessive)
- Congenital nephrotic syndrome (autosomal recessive)
- Nail patella syndrome (autosomal dominant)
- Sickle cell disease (autosomal recessive)

EPIDEMIOLOGY

- The incidence of chronic renal failure is not known.
- Approximately 3 to 8 new cases of end-stage renal failure are reported per 1 million children per year
- Prevalence of chronic renal failure has been reported to be 32.4 per 1 million children in Western Europe, with 6% younger than 3 years of age, 30% between 3 and 9 years of age, and 64% between 9 and 15 years of age.
- Among children in the United States with chronic renal insufficiency entered into the North American Pediatric Renal Transplant Cooperative Study, 65.9% are male and 63.9% are white.

COMPLICATIONS

- Growth retardation is particularly severe when chronic renal failure develops in the first year of life. The etiology of growth failure may be secondary to poor nutrition, bone disease, acidosis, or a direct effect on the growth hormone-IGF-1 axis.
- Renal osteodystrophy may be seen early in chronic renal insufficiency and manifest as growth failure, bowing of the lower extremities, and slipped epiphysis. Vitamin D deficiency and secondary hyperparathyroidism are the major factors leading to bone disease.
- Anemia develops secondary to decreased erythropoietin secretion and decreased red cell survival. The anemia is normocytic associated with a low reticulocyte count.
- Neurodevelopmental delay is increased in children with chronic renal failure. This is probably secondary to uremic effects on the developing brain.
- Hypertension may be seen in some patients with chronic renal failure secondary either to hyperreninemia or hypervolemia.
- Platelet abnormalities, protein-calorie malnutrition, and immunologic disturbances are also seen in uremic patients.

PROGNOSIS

- Depends on underlying cause, child's age, degree of renal insufficiency, and need for dialysis or transplantation

Differential Diagnosis

- Differentiate acute from chronic renal failure.
- Usually chronic renal failure is insidious and associated with poor growth, polyuria, and anemia. The kidneys may be small on renal ultrasound. A renal biopsy may be indicated to determine the cause of renal failure if genetic causes are suspected (for counseling) or if treatment is being considered.

Data Gathering

HISTORY

Question: Symptoms?
Significance:

- Malaise
- Poor appetite
- Vomiting
- Bone pain
- Headache (if hypertensive)
- Polyuria

Question: Past history?
Significance:

- Perinatal complications
- Oligohydramnios
- Recurrent urinary tract infections
- Enuresis

Question: Familial history?
Significance:

- Renal disease
- Hearing impairment

Physical Examination

Finding: General
Significance:

- Short stature
- Poor weight gain
- Pale
- Fetid breath

Finding: HEENT
Significance:

- Retinal changes
- Preauricular pits
- Hearing deficit

Finding: Chest
Significance: Rales

Finding: Heart
Significance:

- Flow Murmur
- Gallop
- Rub

Finding: Abdomen
Significance:

- Palpable kidneys
- Suprapubic mass

Finding: Extremities
Significance:

- Rachitic changes
- Edema
- Absent patella

Finding: Neurological
Significance:

- Developmental delay
- Altered mental status
- Hypotonia
- Irritability

Laboratory Aids

Test: Serum chemistries
Significance: Azotemia, hyperkalemia (if advanced), acidenia, hypocalcemia, hyperphosphatemia, elevated alkalene phosphatase

Test: CBC
Significance: Microcytic anemia with low reticulocyte count

Test: Urinalysis
Significance: Isosthenuria, mild proteinuria

Test: Intact parathyroid hormone
Significance: Elevated

Test: Chest x-ray
Significance: Fluid overload, cardiomegaly

Test: Bone films
Significance: Delayed bone age, rickets, osteitis fibrosa

Test: Renal ultrasound
Significance: Small echogenic kidneys, cystic kidneys, hydronephrosis

Test: ECG (if hyperkalemic)
Significance: Peaked T waves

SPECIAL LABORATORY TRICKS

Test: 24-hour urine collection ($=1440$ minutes)
Significance: The glomerular filtration rate can be estimated with concomitant blood sampling by calculating the creatinine clearance:

$$\frac{U_{creat} \times (\text{volume voided}/1440)}{P_{creat}} \times \frac{1.73}{\text{B.S.A.}}$$

The resultant value is expressed as mL/min/1.73 m². Normal range is 80 to 120 mL/min/1.73 m².

B.S.A. = body surface area.

A simpler calculation that is already corrected for surface area and does not require a urine collection:

$$\frac{\text{Height (cm)} \times 0.55}{P_{creat}}$$

The correction factor (0.55) is applicable to most children 1 year of age. A lower factor (0.45) is suggested for infants <1 year of age and a higher one (0.7) for adolescent males.

Plotting the reciprocal of the serum creatinine versus time can approximate the rate of decline of renal function.

This may be useful in determining when renal replacement therapy will be necessary.

Therapy

MEDICATIONS

- Phosphate binders (calcium carbonate, calcium acetate, avoid aluminum if possible).
- 1,25 dihydroxy vitamin D
- Alkali therapy (sodium bicarbonate/citrate)
- Diuretic therapy
- Recombinant erythropoietin
- Recombinant human growth hormone

DIETARY RESTRICTIONS

- Protein
- Phosphate
- Potassium
- Sodium (indicated if edematous)
- Fluid (indicated in oliguric conditions)

RENAL REPLACEMENT THERAPY

- Dialysis: Indications similar to those for acute renal failure or when glomerular filtration rate <10 mL/min/1.73 m² and patient is experiencing fatigue, poor school performance, or weight loss secondary to severe dietary restrictions.
- Transplantation: In some cases a preemptive transplant may be offered in lieu of dialysis.

Follow-Up

General pediatricians should follow patients with chronic renal failure with assistance from a pediatric nephrologist.

PITFALLS

During episodes of gastroenteritis infants with chronic renal failure may be prone to dehydration because they have obligatory polyuria secondary to a concentrating defect. Do not use urine output or specific gravity as indices for hydration.

Common Questions and Answers

Q: What over-the-counter medications should be avoided in children with chronic renal failure?
A: Non-steroidal anti-inflammatorry drugs, magnesium or aluminum-containing compounds should not be used.

Q: Can children with chronic renal failure receive immunizations?
A: Children with chronic renal failure should receive all necessary immunizations especially since after transplantation some vaccines are contraindicated. In some cases booster immunizations are necessary because of an inadequate response to the initial series (e.g., hepatitis B, MMR).

Q: When is recombinant human erythropoietin indicated?
A: Generally this medication should be considered when the hematocrit is <33%.

ICD-9-CM 585.0

BIBLIOGRAPHY

Friedman AL. Etiology, pathophysiology, diagnosis, and management of chronic renal failure in children. *Curr Opin Pediatr* 1996;8:148–151.

Hanna JD, Foreman JW, Chan JCM. Chronic renal insufficiency in infants and children. *Clin Pediatr* 1991;30:365.

Seidman A, Freidman A, Boineau F, et al. Nutritional management of the child with mild to moderate chronic renal failure. *J Pediatr* 1996;129:13–18.

Warady BA, Hebert D, Sullivan EK, et al. Renal transplantation, chronic dialysis and chronic renal insufficiency in children and adolescents: the 1995 Annual Report of the North American Pediatric Renal Transplant Cooperative Study. *Pediatr Nephrol* 1997;11:49–64.

Author: Seth L. Schulman

Renal Tubular Acidosis

 Database

DEFINITION

• Renal tubular acidosis (RTA) is a clinical syndrome of disordered renal acidification in which the kidney fails to maintain a normal plasma concentration of bicarbonate in the setting of a normal rate of acid production from diet and metabolism.

• This syndrome is characterized by a hyperchloremic metabolic acidosis, bicarbonaturia, decreased production of titratable acids and ammonium with, usually, an elevated urinary pH.

TYPES

• Distal (Type I)

—Distal RTA is a primary renal acidification defect secondary either to an inability to secrete hydrogen ions or a backleak in the collecting tubule. In some cases there may be bicarbonate wasting as well.

—These infants and children present with failure to thrive, hypokalemia, nephrolithiasis, nephrocalcinosis, or rickets. The nephrolithiasis is secondary to the persistent alkaline urine, hypercalciuria, and hypocitraturia.

—Patients with complete distal RTA can never acidify their urine and, therefore, always have a urine pH higher than 6.0.

• Proximal (Type II)

—This form of RTA is caused by a defect in the sodium-hydrogen ion exchange mechanism. These infants and children spill bicarbonate into their urine because the renal threshold for reabsorption is reduced. Because the distal mechanism is intact, acidification of the urine is possible once the serum bicarbonate falls below the threshold.

—Isolated proximal RTA is rare; most children present with this abnormality as part of the Fanconi syndrome (bicarbonaturia, amino aciduria, glycosuria, and phosphaturia).

—Hypokalemia is usually present but hypercalciuria and hypocitraturia are not. Therefore, nephrocalcinosis, nephrolithiasis, and rickets are not the presenting features of this form of RTA.

• Distal Hyperkalemic (Type IV)

—Type IV RTA is the most common form of RTA in adults and children.

—Hyperkalemia distinguishes this form from types I and II.

—There are five subtypes of type IV RTA but the predominant feature is aldosterone deficiency or unresponsiveness.

—One form in children occurs with obstructive uropathy and renal insufficiency. This causes a defect in the juxtaglomerular apparatus leading to hyporeninemia with secondary hypoaldosteronism. Children with this form of RTA may present with failure to thrive.

GENETICS

• In infants and children type I RTA is usually inherited as an autosomal dominant trait. It may occur in association with other diseases such as elliptocytosis, sickle-cell disease, and the Ehlers-Danlos syndrome.

• Type II RTA with Fanconi syndrome occurs with several disorders that are autosomal recessive, including cystinosis, Lowes syndrome, Wilson disease, tyrosinemia, hereditary fructose intolerance, and galactosemia.

• Certain subtypes of type IV RTA have been reported to be familial.

EPIDEMIOLOGY

Renal tubular acidosis is an extremely rare condition.

COMPLICATIONS

• Children with RTA may develop severe growth failure, rickets, nephrocalcinosis, and nephrolithiasis.

—During episodes of vomiting or diarrhea they may be at risk of developing profound acidosis and hypokalemia.

PROGNOSIS

• Prognosis depends on the underlying etiology.

• Growth velocity increases following treatment with alkali for isolated type I and II RTA and normal stature can be achieved.

• Isolated type I RTA is a chronic condition that requires constant monitoring to avoid nephrocalcinosis.

 Differential Diagnosis

• Renal tubular acidosis is associated with a normal anion gap ($Na^+ - [Cl^- + HCO_3^-] = 8$ to 16 mEq/L).

• Other causes of metabolic acidosis with a normal anion gap include diarrhea, acetazolamide, ileal conduits, and fistulas draining the small bowel, pancreas, or biliary tree.

 Data Gathering

HISTORY

Question: Symptoms?
Significance: Failure to thrive, renal colic, bone pain, photophobia (cystinosis)

Question: Past medical history?
Significance: Prior admissions for dehydration and acidosis not associated with significant diarrhea.

Question: Medications/drugs
Significance: Amphotericin B, lithium, tetracycline (outdated), toluene.

Question: Familial history
Significance: See Genetics.

Question: Review of symptoms
Significance: Other systemic diseases

Physical Examination

Finding: General
Significance: Failure to thrive

Finding: Head
Significance: Frontal bossing

Finding: Eyes
Significance:

- Cystine deposition
- Kayser-Fleischer ring
- Cataracts

Finding: Chest
Significance: Rachitic rosary

Finding: Abdomen
Significance:

- Hepatosplenomegaly
- Enlarged kidneys

Finding: Extremities
Significance:

- Bowing
- Widening of the epiphysis of wrists

Laboratory Aids

Test: Serum electrolytes
Significance: Identify the presence of a normal anion gap metabolic acidosis, hyper/hypo-kalemia.

Test: Urinalysis
Significance: Exclude features of the Fanconi syndrome.

Test: Urine pH
Significance: Can exclude type I RTA if, <6.0; best if performed in the face of acidosis.

Test: Serum creatinine
Significance: To exclude renal insufficiency

Test: Urine anion gap
Significance:

- Negative ($Cl^- > Na^+ + K^+$) seen in gastrointestinal losses, proximal RTA
- Positive ($Cl^- < Na^+ + K^+$) seen in distal RTA

Test: Urine
Significance: Should be measured by pH meter from a fresh specimen. If this is not possible oil should be added to cover urine and protect dissipation of CO_2.

IMAGING

Test: Abdominal flat plate
Significance: Nephrocalcinosis, nephrolithiasis

Test: Bone films
Significance: Rachitic changes, delayed bone age

Therapy

- Alkali administration is the primary therapy for children with RTA.
- Sodium/potassium citrate (Polycitra2 mEq HCO_3^-/mL) is preferable for children with types I or II RTA.
- Sodium citrate (Bicitra51 mEq HCO_3^-/mL) is used in infants with type IV RTA.
- Older children can take sodium bicarbonate tablets (7.7 mEq HCO_3^-)
- Patients with type I RTA require 1 to 4 mEq/kg of alkali therapy per day in 3 to 4 divided doses. This usually decreases the chances of complications such as nephrolithiasis, nephrocalcinosis, and rickets.
- Patients with type II RTA require considerably more alkali therapy (5 to 20 mEq/kg/d in 4 to 6 divided doses).
- The dosage of alkali in children with type IV RTA ranges from 1 to 5 mEq/kg/d, which is usually sufficient to correct the hyperkalemia.

Follow-Up

- Patients with RTA should be closely monitored with frequent serum potassium and plasma bicarbonate levels until a steady state is reached.
- Normal growth may be attained once the metabolic acidosis is corrected.

PITFALLS AND PREVENTION

- Avoid hemolyzed specimens that may artificially increase the serum potassium and reduce the plasma bicarbonate levels.
- Administer alkali over several divided doses.
- Closely monitor patients during episodes of gastroenteritis to avoid dehydration and severe metabolic acidosis.

Common Questions and Answers

Q: Do children outgrow renal tubular acidosis?
A: Types I and II RTA are chronic disorders that require life-long treatment. Some children outgrow certain subtypes of type IV RTA.

Q: Can children with renal tubular acidosis develop renal failure?
A: Untreated type I RTA can lead to renal failure by causing progressive nephrocalcinosis. Children with inherited disorders associated with Fanconi syndrome such as cystinosis can also develop renal insufficiency.

ICD-9-CM 588.8

BIBLIOGRAPHY

Battle DC, Hizon M, Cohen E, et al. The use of the urinary anion gap in the diagnosis of hyperchloremic metabolic acidosis. *N Engl J Med* 1988;318:594.

McSherry E. Renal tubular acidosis in children (nephrology forum). *Kidney Int* 1981;20:799.

Rodriguez-Soriano J, Vallo A. Renal tubular acidosis. *Pediatr Nephrol* 1990;4:268.

Zelikovic I. Renal Tubular acidosis. *Pediatr Ann* 1995;24:48–54.

Author: Seth L. Schulman

Renal Venous Thrombosis

 Database

DEFINITION

- Renal venous thrombosis (RVT) is the thrombotic process that begins in the intrarenal venous radicals and usually progresses forward toward the main renal vein.
- Rarely, the thrombosis progresses in the opposite direction.

PATHOPHYSIOLOGY

- RVT in newborns and infants is commonly associated with asphyxia, dehydration (as with diarrhea), shock, sepsis, hypertonicity, and hemoconcentration.
- Additional predisposing factors in the newborn include congenital renal anomalies and maternal diabetes.
- In older children it is associated with the nephrotic syndrome, cyanotic heart disease, and hyperosmolar states such as with the use of angiography contrast agents.
- In many children, no underlying cause is apparent.
- The slow double circulation of the kidney is especially vulnerable to thrombosis.
- Thrombus formation may be initiated by vascular endothelial cell injury in conjunction with diminished vascular flow.
- RVT usually starts in the small venous radicals with progression through the arcuate and interlobular veins toward the main renal vein.
- RVT causes renal congestion and occasionally infarction.

GENETICS

- Familial occurrence is rare.
- No hereditary factors have been described.

EPIDEMIOLOGY

- RVT is predominantly a disease of the newborn.
- The incidence and prevalence are poorly defined.
- There is a small male preponderance.
- The disease is more frequently unilateral than bilateral.

COMPLICATIONS

- Bilateral RVT may lead to chronic renal failure.
- Scarring may result in hypertension.

 Differential Diagnosis

- The differential diagnosis includes other causes of renal enlargement such as hydronephrosis, cystic renal disease, renal tumors, abscess, and hematoma.
- Hemolytic uremic syndrome should also be considered because RVT may also result in fragmented red blood cells and thrombocytopenia.

PROGNOSIS

- The degree of irreversible renal damage depends on the degree of involvement and associated conditions.
- Recovery of function in affected kidneys may occur.
- Hypertension is seen in 20%.
- The majority have residual renal structural abnormalities, such as atrophy and coarse renal scarring.

 Data Gathering

HISTORY

- The majority present in the newborn period.
- Most of the symptoms are due to an underlying disorder.
- RVT is usually heralded by the sudden onset of hematuria and unilateral or bilateral flank masses.

 Physical Examination

- 60% will have a palpably enlarged kidney.
- Associated signs and symptoms include pallor, tachypnea, abdominal distention, shock, flank pain, fever, oliguria, or anuria.
- If in the thrombosis, the lower limbs may become edematous, cyanotic, and hypothermic, inferior vena cava (IVC) is involved.

 Laboratory Aids

- Proteinuria is common.
- The majority have macroscopic hematuria.
- 90% have progressive thrombocytopenia, and the majority also have microangiopathic hemolytic anemia.
- Fibrin split products may be elevated with low-plasma fibrinogen levels.
- Azotemia and other biochemical evidence of acute renal failure may be present.
- Variations in plasma electrolytes depend on the presence of diarrhea or renal failure.

IMAGING

Test: Intravenous urograms
Significance: Almost always contraindicated because of the osmolar load of intravenous contrast material.

Test: Ultrasonography
Significance: The most useful study, and will differentiate between renal enlargement and extrarenal masses. It will also identify obstruction, cystic changes, and many congenital anomalies. Also, shows renal enlargement, increased echogenicity, and loss of corticomedullary differentiation.

Test: Doppler evaluation
Significance: Of renal arterial and renal venous flow and radioisotopic reperfusion and excretion studies may be helpful.

Therapy

GENERAL

• Treatment is supportive and includes correction of fluid and electrolyte disturbances and treatment of infection.
• Correction of underlying pathophysiologic abnormalities should be attempted.
• Management of the complications of azotemia and uremia, including metabolic acidosis, hyperphosphatemia, fluid overload, and hyperosmolality, may require dialysis, particularly in infants.

ANTICOAGULANT

• The effect of anticoagulant therapy has not been documented in controlled studies and remains controversial.
• Heparin should be considered if there is laboratory evidence of continuing disseminated intravascular coagulation.
• Because the lesions are often asynchronous and asymmetrical, prophylactic heparin has been proposed for cases of RVT that are identified early and do not appear to have bilateral involvement.

SURGERY

• A surgical approach in the acute phase is rarely indicated. Surgery, complicated by disturbed fluid balance and acid-base status, and altered coagulation is risky.
• Because the thrombosis begins deep within the kidney and spreads to the larger veins, thrombectomy should be considered only in the event of bilateral involvement with IVC involvement.
• Ultimately, if the kidney has negligible function and contributes to hypertension or recurrent infections, nephrectomy may be indicated.

Follow-Up

PROGNOSIS

• Depends on the degree of involvement and associated conditions
• Mortality in infants is approximately 30%.
• Recovery of function in affected kidneys may occur. Varying degrees of renal impairment is seen in 30%.
• Hypertension is seen in 20%.
• The majority have residual renal structural abnormalities, such as atrophy and coarse renal scarring.

SIGNS TO WATCH FOR

All patients should be followed closely for evidence of hypertension.

PREVENTION

• Infants at increased risk should be recognized. The infant of a diabetic mother should be followed for evidence of RVT. Patients with nephrotic syndrome are at increased risk of thrombosis in general when treated with diuretics. If cyanotic congenital heart disease is present, contrast agents should be used judiciously. Parents and caregivers should be educated about the importance of adequate intake and good hydration in the newborn and infant. Finally, there should be an increased index of suspicion among medical staff when faced with an infant with diarrhea or a hyperosmolar state.

Common Questions and Answers

Q: Can RVT occur in the absence of gross hematuria?
A: Most patients have hematuria that may be gross. However, the hematuria may be is often microscopic or and may be absent.

Q: Do patients with RVT usually have hypertension during the acute phase?
A: Hypertension is uncommon at presentation.

ICD-9-CM 453.3

BIBLIOGRAPHY

Adelman RD. Long-term follow-up of neonatal renovascular hypertension. *Pediatr Nephrol* 1987;1:35.

Arneil GC, MacDonald AM, Murphy AV, et al. Renal venous thrombosis. *Clin Nephrol* 1973; 1:119.

Duncan RE, Evans TA, Martin LW. Natural history and treatment of renal vein thrombosis in children. *J Pediatr Surg* 1977;12:639.

Jobin J, O'Regan S, Demay G, et al. Neonatal renal vein thrombosis—long-term follow-up after conservative management. *Clin Nephrol* 1982;17:36.

Kaplan BS, Chesney RW, Drummond KN. The nephrotic syndrome and renal vein thrombosis. *Am J Dis Child* 1978;132:367.

Markowitz GS, Brignol F, Burns ER, Koenigsberg M, Folkert VW. Renal vein thrombosis treated with thrombolytic therapy: case report and brief review. *Am J Kidney Dis* 1995;25:801–806.

Mocan H, Beattie TJ, Murphy AV. Renal venous thrombosis in infancy: long term follow-up. *Pediatr Nephrol* 1991;5:45.

Oliver WJ, Kelsch RC. Renal venous thrombosis in infancy. *Pediatr Rev* 1982;4:61.

Schmidt B, Andrew M. Neonatal thrombosis: report of a prospective Canadian and international registry. *Pediatrics* 1995;96:939–943.

Author: Mary B. Leonard

Respiratory Syncytial Virus (RSV)

 Database

DEFINITION

• A pleomorphic enveloped RNA virus of the family *Paramyxoviruses*. There are two major groups, A and B, that differ in the largest surface glycoprotein, the G protein. The fusion protein, F protein, is approximately 95% homologous between the two subgroups.
• The most common cause of bronchiolitis, a viral lower respiratory disease of infants and young children.

PATHOPHYSIOLOGY

• The F protein is responsible for fusing infected cells to adjacent cells, generating a syncytium.
• Infection is initiated in the upper respiratory tract with inoculation of the nose or eyes and may spread to the lower respiratory tract in the younger age child and in those with a primary infection.
• Obstruction of smaller airways occurs secondary to edema, necrotic tissue, and inflammatory cells.
• Virus-induced epithelial damage may expose certain receptors for environmental irritants. Receptor-irritant complexes may contribute to the signs and symptoms of reactive airway disease.

EPIDEMIOLOGY

• Incubation period is 2 to 4 days.
• Virus is detected in secretions 4 days prior to clinical symptoms and 7 days after resolution of symptoms (viral shedding demonstrated for as long as 20 days).
• Most effective mode of transmission is via person-to-person spread: by droplet or hand-to-nose contact.
• Nosocomial spread occurs from infected hospital personnel-to-patient and patient-to-patient spread.
• Peak incidence is the first 2 years of life.
• 50% of children are infected by their first birthday with similar attack rate for the uninfected child during the second year of life.
• 40% to 70% of preschool children and 20% of school-age children are reinfected with exposure.
• Worldwide distribution. Temperate climates experience an annual, midwinter epidemic while epidemics are less predictable in the tropics.
• United States epidemics may begin in November (or as late as May) and last as long as 12 weeks in urban areas.
• One antigenic strain predominates during any given epidemic.

COMPLICATIONS

• Apneic episodes in very young and premature patients
• Pneumonia, rarely bacterial
• Pneumonitis
• Croup
• Respiratory failure

• Hypoxemia
• Hypercarbia
• Acute otitis media
• Dehydration

Those at greatest risk for severe infection include:

• Age less than 1 year, especially those between the ages of 6 weeks and 6 months
• Children with compromised cardiorespiratory status (e.g., bronchopulmonary dysplasia, congenital heart disease)
• Prematurity
• Immune deficits

PROGNOSIS

• Majority will have a mild-to-moderate disease course and recovery with symptomatic support.
• Some infected children proceed to more serious illness, necessitating hospitalization. An average hospital stay for previously healthy children is 5 to 7 days; full recovery is 2 weeks.
• Infants with underlying cardiac or pulmonary disease are at increased risk for more severe and longer duration of disease; mortality as high as 30%.
• Reinfections occur throughout life.

 Differential Diagnosis

INFECTION

• Influenza virus
• Parainfluenza virus type 3
• Adenovirus
• Chlamydia

ENVIRONMENTAL

• Foreign body in airway

TUMORS

• Mass compressing upper airway

CONGENITAL

• Tracheomalacia

 Data Gathering

HISTORY

Question: Initial symptoms?
Significance: Nasal discharge, cough, and fever

Question: Cough?
Significance: Typically progresses over 1 to 2 days, with tachypnea developing.

Question: Ask about duration of symptoms.
Significance: This will help in the assessment of the typical clinical progression of illness and the anticipated time course for the child.
Significance:

• Lethargy, apnea, and possible cyanotic episodes.
• Dehydration is secondary to decreased oral intake as well as increased insensible losses.
• Increasing respiratory distress?
• Did the child stop breathing/have apnea?
• Assess oral intake and urine output to rule out dehydration.

 Physical Examination

• Nasal discharge
• Otitis media
• Pharyngeal injection
• Conjunctivitis
• Respiratory distress with nasal flaring and retractions, grunting, rales, rhonchi, and expiratory wheezing noted on auscultation.
• Risk for hypoxemia increases as the respiratory rate approaches and surpasses 60 breaths per minute.
• Chest may become barrel-shaped in appearance as respiratory distress increases.
• Hyperinflation of the lungs will push liver and spleen into palpable positions within the abdomen.

 Laboratory Aids

• Rapid tests
• Immunofluorescent techniques or ELISA for antigen detection.
• Nasopharyngeal washing with inoculation into culture media.
• Growth should be detected by the appearance of the syncytial cytopathic effect in 3 to 14 days.
• Pulse oximetry to rule out hypoxemia.

RADIOGRAPHIC STUDIES

Test: Chest radiograph
Significance: Reveals hyperexpansion, increased bronchial markings, and areas of atelectasis/infiltrate. Note: the pulmonary densities, referred to as "RSV pneumonia," are frequently areas of atelectasis but may represent bacterial infection, especially in the seriously ill patient.

Therapy

- Supportive care: hydration therapy and supplemental oxygen as needed.
- Cardiorespiratory monitoring and pulse oximetry are necessary for infants at risk for apnea and hypoxemia.
- Life-threatening apnea may require emergent ventilatory support with mechanical ventilation.

DRUGS

- Ribavirin: an antiviral agent, may have some benefit. The Committee on Infectious Disease of the American Academy of Pediatrics recommends that ribavirin be considered for children with RSV who are at high risk for serious disease or those patients with an underlying condition (i.e., cardiopulmonary disease), which places them at significant risk for complications. Teratogenicity of ribavirin in humans remains a controversial issue. Apply strict isolation precautions with the use of ribavirin to minimize health care personnel exposure.
- Corticosteroids have *NOT* been shown to be effective.
- Beta-2 adrenergic agents have not been proven to be effective, but some studies have shown that 25% to 50% of patients with bronchiolitis respond to this therapy. A trial of a bronchodilator is frequently recommended.
- Mist use is considered controversial because it may irritate the airways.

Follow-Up

- Bronchiolitis will peak in severity over 48 to 72 hours; therefore, reassess the patient if seen early in the disease course.
- Symptoms usually last 7 days but may last up to 2 to 3 weeks with the evidence of reactive airway disease persisting for months to years.
- Periodic breathing may occur 48 to 72 hours post-extubation, but recurrent apneic episodes are rare, and home monitoring is usually not indicated.
- Fever commonly resolves over 48 hours.
- Respiratory symptoms commonly improve between days 2 and 5 of illness.
- Evidence of airway hyperactivity may continue for months to years in patients who have had bronchiolitis.

SIGNS TO WATCH FOR

- Respiratory rates greater than 60 per minute and other signs of respiratory failure
- Lethargy, altered mental status
- Prolonged high fever

PREVENTION

- Nosocomial and household spread can be minimized by strict hand washing and avoidance of contact with infected individuals.
- Routine use of gowns and gloves have been shown to decrease RSV nosocomial spread.
- Patients with RSV infection should be isolated in private or RSV-cohorted rooms.
- Nursing care should be cohorted so that nurses are not caring for both RSV infected and non-infected patients.
- RSV-immune globulin intravenous (RSV-IGIV) prophylaxis is available as an intravenous medication given once monthly during the RSV season. Current AAP recommendations: RSV-IGIV should be considered for infants and children younger than 2 years of age who have bronchopulmonary dysplasia and are currently receiving or received oxygen therapy during the last 6 months prior to the onset of RSV season. Infants with a gestational age of 28 weeks or less should be considered for prophylaxis until their first birthday while infants with gestational ages of 29 to 32 weeks should be considered for prophylaxis until they are 6 months old. The globulin will interfere with some vaccine activity (MMR), therefore, vaccine administration will need to modified with the administration of RSV-IGIV. MMR can not be given to a patient who received IGIV until 10 months have elapsed.
- Palivizumab (Synagis) is a prophylaxic medication that has received FDA approval and is now available. It is a humanized monoclonal antibody produced by recombinant DNA technology, directed to an epitope in the A antigenic site of the F protein of respiratory syncytial virus. Synagis, similar to RSV-IGIV, is indicated for the prevention of serious respiratory tract disease caused by RSV in pediatric patients at high risk for severe RSV disease. It is administered as an intramuscular injection monthly beginning one month prior to the RSV season and continuing monthly throughout the RSV season.

PITFALLS

- RSV is labile at room temperature. Samples should be placed in viral transport media at the bedside and transported to the lab for immediate inoculation to cell culture.
- Instillation and aspiration of 5 mL of isotonic saline is the preferred method of viral collection as opposed to nasal swabs.

Common Questions and Answers

Q: How did my child get this illness?
A: RSV bronchiolitis is caused by a virus, respiratory syncytial virus, and is passed from one person to another by contact with nasal secretions and through airborne transmission.

Q: For how long is my child contagious?
A: Viral shedding occurs for 24 hours prior to the onset of clinical symptoms and for up 21 days from the onset of symptoms.

Q: Will my child develop asthma because of the wheezing that is occurring now?
A: Evidence of airway hyperactivity following RSV bronchiolitis may continue for months or even years in some children. It is impossible to predict future episodes of reactive airway disease, but the child should be monitored clinically over time.

Q: If a patient has severe chronic lung disease with a supplemental oxygen requirement and is less than 2 years of age at the onset of the RSV season, should RSV-IGIV or Palivizumab be recommended for this patient?
A: This question does not have a clear answer based on research data currently available. The risks and benefits of each therapy must be evaluated on a patient-by-patient basis. RSV-IGIV provides additional protection against other respiratory viral illnesses and may be preferred for some selected high risk infants.

ICD-9-CM 466.1

BIBLIOGRAPHY

AAP Committee on Infectious Diseases and Committee on Fetus and Newborn. Prevention of respiratory syncytial virus infections: indications for the use of Palivizumab and update on the use of RSV-IGIV. *Pediatrics* 1998;102(5): 1211–1215.

American Academy of Pediatrics. Respiratory syncytial virus. In: Peter G, ed. *1997 Red book: report of the committee on infectious diseases,* 24th ed. Elk Grove Village, IL: American Academy of Pediatrics; 1997:443–447.

Darville T, Yamauchi T. Respiratory syncytial virus. *Pediatr Rev* 1998;19(2):55–61.

DeVincenzo JP, Malley R, Ramilo O, et al. Viral concentration in upper and lower respiratory secretions from respiratory syncytial virus (RSV) infected children treated with RSV monoclonal antibody (MEDI-493). *Pediatr Res* 1998;43:144A (Abstract 830).

Midulla F, Villani A, Panuska JR, et al. Respiratory syncytial virus lung infection in infants: immunoregulatory role of infected alveoolar macrophages. *J Infect Dis* 1993;168(6):1515–1519.

Author: Kathy Wholey Zsolway

Retinoblastoma

Database

DEFINITION

- The most common primary intraocular tumor of childhood.
- Malignant tumor of the embryonic neural retina.

PATHOPHYSIOLOGY

- Originates in retinal cell precursor (retinoblast).
- Histology: small round blue cells with large hyperchromatic nuclei and scant cytoplasm.
- Growth of tumor may be endophytic (from inner surface of retina to vitreous) or exophytic (from outer layer of retina into subretinal space); may cause retinal detachment.
- Spread is via optic nerve (common) with potential to invade CNS, direct extension beyond the eye, and lymphatic or hematogenous spread (uncommon).
- Tumor cells may break off from primary mass and grow independently within the eye (called seeding); single tumor with seeding may be confused with multifocal disease.

GENETICS

- Tumor development depends on loss of function of both *RB1* genes (located on chromosome 13) in a retinoblast.
- Hereditary and nonhereditary (sporadic) forms exist.

HEREDITARY RB

- 45% of all retinoblastoma.
- One *RB1* gene is dysfunctional in all cells (germline mutation), mutation in remaining *RB1* gene in any retinal cell will produce a tumor.
- 90% probability of second mutation occurring in at least one (but usually more) retinal cells leading to tumor development (high penetrance).
- Therefore, multiple tumors are common (bilateral and/or multifocal).
- Mean age at diagnosis: 12 months.
- Only 8% have positive familial history; remainder are new germline mutations.
- Approximately 40% to 45% of offspring will develop RB (autosomal dominant transmission, 90% penetrance).
- *RB1* gene mutation in all cells predisposes to second (non-retinoblastoma) malignances.

NON-HEREDITARY RB

- 55% of all retinoblastoma
- No germline *RB1* mutation; two somatic *RB1* mutations must occur in a single retinal cell (a rare event)
- Always unilateral
- Rarely diagnosed before 6 months (mean, 24 months)
- No increased risk of RB in offspring
- No increased risk of second malignancy

EPIDEMIOLOGY

- 1:16,000 to 1:25,000 live births
- The most common primary intraocular tumor of childhood (ocular leukemia most common overall)
- Represents 3% of all pediatric malignancies
- No sex, race, geographic, or socioeconomic predilection
- 90% diagnosed before age 4 years
- Median age at diagnosis for unilateral disease is 24 months and 12 months for bilateral disease (*see* Genetics)

COMPLICATIONS

- Metastatic spread: local spread within orbit, through the optic nerve to brain, or to distant sites (uncommon).
- Loss of eye: surgical enucleation in advanced cases.
- Blindness: in advanced, bilateral disease. Bilateral enucleation rarely required.
- Cosmetic deformity: from enucleation, ocular prosthesis lacks normal eye movements; orbital bone hypoplasia secondary to external beam radiation therapy.
- Second malignancy: patients with hereditary RB have a predisposition to cancer; this risk is increased by exposure to radiotherapy (and possibly chemotherapy).

PROGNOSIS

- Mortality from retinoblastoma is 8% (U.S.).
- Survival depends on extent (stage) of disease
- Metastatic disease occurs 5 years or less after diagnosis and has a poor outcome (same for hereditary and non-hereditary)
- Prognosis for vision depends on size and location of tumor(s)
- Second malignancy is most common cause of death in hereditary RB

—These include osteosarcoma (most frequent), pinealblastoma, melanoma, fibrosarcoma, and others
—Rates of second malignancy in hereditary RB are 10% at 10 years and as high as 40% at 30 years in patients who received XRT (70% of second tumors occur in the field of radiation, 30% elsewhere).

Differential Diagnosis

- Coats disease: acquired anomaly, males, retinal telangiectasias.
- Persistent hyperplastic primary vitreous (PHPV).
- Inflammatory conditions: hypopion, uveitis, iritis, endophthalmitis.
- Toxoplasmosis, *Toxocara canis,* other ocular infections.
- Retinopathy of prematurity (ROP).

Data Gathering

HISTORY

Question: Familial history of retinoblastoma or any eye tumors?
Significance: Hereditary retinoblastoma; siblings may require eye exam

Question: Leukocoria (white pupil, "cats eye reflex")
Significance: Often noted in photographs of children with advanced intraocular RB (60%).

Question: Strabismus, either eso- or exotropic (20%)?
Significance: Esotropia more common in general population so exotropia more suspicious.

Question: Eye complaints?
Significance: RB is rarely painful (unless secondary glaucoma or inflammation is present); vision problems are rare complaint because tumor is usually unilateral.

Question: Inflammation, heterochromia, and glaucoma
Significance: Rare presentations (<10%)

Question: Ask about neurological signs, orbital/periorbital masses, bone pain, anorexia, signs of cytopenias.
Significance: May represent metastatic disease

Question: Associated conditions?
Significance: 13q deletion syndrome has RB, dysmorphism, mental retardation, and GU or other anomalies.

Physical Examination

- Only 3% diagnosed with routine funduscopic examination. Leukomia more common as presenting sign.

Finding: Proptosis and orbital/periorbital masses
Significance: Late sequelae of mass effect

Finding: Check for red reflex in darkened room
Significance: Screen for RB in office.

- Evaluate for Anisocoria
- Cover test to assess for strabismus (20%)
- Test vision of each eye independently isolate unilateral RB.

Laboratory Aids

Test: Ophthalmologic examination
Significance: Confirmation of diagnosis based on ophthalmologic examination by a specialist in pediatric ocular tumors (via direct and indirect ophthalmoscopy and examination under anesthesia) and by imaging modalities (MRI or CT).

Test: Biopsy
Significance: Biopsy confirmation is rarely necessary.

Test: CBC
Significance: Assess for bone marrow involvement

Test: CSF cytology
Significance: Evaluate for leptomeningeal spread

Test: Chromosome analysis
Significance: Should be performed, but even in hereditary cases only 5% have mutations detectable by this means.

IMAGING

Test: CT or MRI
Significance: Evaluate primary tumor (80% have calcification) and optic nerve extension, leptomeningeal spread, pineal blastoma (in 4% of patients with hereditary RB = "trilateral RB").

STAGING

• Intraocular and extraocular staging systems exist.
• Most RB in the United States is intraocular without metastatic disease.
• Patients with tumor extension outside the globe should have an LP and bone marrow evaluation for complete staging.

Therapy

• Primary goal

—Eradicate tumor
—Prevent metastasis

• Secondary goal

—Salvage the eye and retain useful vision.

Treatment must be individualized, depending on bilateral or unilateral disease, potential for salvageable vision, and evidence of local extension or metastatic disease. Referral to a center with oncologic and ophthalmologic specialists is essential.

• Minimal (non-bulky) intraocular disease

—Plaque radiotherapy (sewn to episcleral surface above RB): local XRT to tumor in selected solitary RBs, up to 16 mm in diameter with or without vitreous seeds.
—Photocoagulation (laser): for selected small RBs, usually less than 3 mm.
—Cryotherapy (topical freeze technique): for selected RBs less than 3 to 4 mm in diameter without vitreous seeding, which are located anteriorly in the eye.

• Bulky intraocular disease

—Current trend is toward eye salvage therapy: initial chemotherapy for tumor reduction followed by local definitive therapy (as for nonbulky disease).
—Tumor resection is not possible because of risk of tumor spillage; enucleation of involved eye (with long segment of optic nerve removal to ensure tumor-free margins) may be required for large tumors refractory to chemoreduction.
—External beam radiation therapy (EBRT): RB is extremely radiosensitive; however, increases risk of second malignancy (especially in hereditary RB). Other effects: dry eye, cataract, retinopathy, and cosmetic deformity from bone maldevelopment. EBRT is still an important modality but is avoided whenever effective alternative therapies are available.

• Metastatic disease

—Multiagent chemotherapy with or without autologous bone marrow transplantation; poor results to date
—Effective treatment requires multidisciplinary collaboration between ophthalmologists, oncologists, and radiation oncologists.

Follow-Up

• Frequent ophthalmologic examinations (including EUA) are mandatory to evaluate response to therapy and to screen for disease progression, particularly in hereditary RB.
• Therapy must include genetic counseling regarding the risk of second malignancies (with or without adjuvant XRT) as well as the risk to children of affected patients (approximately 45%) in hereditary RB.
• Primary care physicians must be aware of the risks of second malignancies (*see* Prognosis) and maintain an appropriately high index of suspicion for their development.

PREVENTION

Siblings and children of patients with RB should undergo ophthalmologic examinations under anesthesia to detect the presence of RB early.

PITFALLS

• Missed or delayed diagnosis: ophthalmologic examination by a specialist in pediatric ocular tumors required to establish diagnosis and follow regression or recurrence in treated eyes, follow for development of new tumors in hereditary cases.
• Failure to recognize the possibility that a child with RB has a genetic predisposition, especially in the frequent setting where there is no familial history of RB.
• Failure to refer for appropriate genetic counseling.

Common Questions and Answers

Q: What is the risk that a child with RB will become blind?
A: Vision is salvageable in 100% of eyes with low-stage involvement, and in 81% overall. In less than 10% of patients are both eyes affected severely enough to threaten vision (bilateral disease only occurs in hereditary RB).

Q: What is the chance that a child with RB in one eye will get it in the other?
A: Bilateral disease is seen with hereditary RB. A child with unilateral disease has a 15% chance of having hereditary RB, which would put the contralateral eye at risk; this risk is much higher if the child has multifocal involvement or is less than 1 year of age.

Q: What happens to the eye socket after an enucleation?
A: Prostheses can be made to fit the socket of the enucleated eye to give excellent cosmetic results.

Q: Is there a test to identify hereditary cases?
A: Routine chromosome analysis does not reveal the defective RB gene in the majority (95%) of hereditary cases. Specialized molecular tests may be used in research labs, but since there are many possible mutations, this is costly and time-consuming. In general, hereditary cases are determined clinically because of young presentation, family history, and/or bilateral or multifocal unilateral disease.

ICD-9-CM 190.5

BIBLIOGRAPHY

Abramson DH, Frank CM, Susman M, Whalen MP, Dunkel IJ, Boyd NW 3rd. Presenting signs of retinoblastoma. *J Pediatr* 1998;132(3 Pt 1): 505–508.

Donaldson SS, Eghert PR, Newsham I, et al. Retinoblastoma. In: Pizzo PA, Poplack DG, eds. *Principles and practice of pediatric oncology,* 3rd ed. Philadelphia/New York: Lippincott-Raven Publishers, 1997, 699–715.

Gallie BL, Dunn JM, Chan HS, Hamel PA, Phillips RA. The genetics of retinoblastoma: relevance to the patient. *Pediatr Clin North Am* 1991;38:299–315.

Magramm I. Amblyopia: etiology, detection, and treatment. *Pediatr Rev* 1992;13(1):7–14.

Shields JA, Shields CL. Current management of retinoblastoma. *Mayo Clinic Proc* 1994;69:50–56.

Author: Michael D. Hogarty

Retropharyngeal Abscess

 Database

DEFINITION

A relatively rare but potentially life-threatening infection occurring in the potential space bounded by the layers of cervical fascia posterior to the esophagus and anterior to the deep cervical fascia.

CAUSES

- Infectious: Cultures usually reveal multiple organisms, predominantly
- *Streptococcus* (group A and others)
- *Staphylococcus aureus*
- Various anaerobic species (*Bacteroides, Peptostreptococcus,* and *Fusobabacterium*).
- One pediatric study cultured *Haemophilus influenzae* type b in 20% of cases; however, the study took place before the routine use of *Haemophilus influenzae* type b conjugate vaccines.
- Many of the isolates are beta-lactamase producers.

PATHOPHYSIOLOGY

The majority of infections follow a pharyngitis or supraglottitis and occur secondary to suppuration of the retropharyngeal lymph nodes, which lie in two paramedial chains and drain various nasopharyngeal structures. Other sources of infection in this space include penetrating trauma, such as from foreign object aspiration, dental procedures, or attempts at intubation. Extension of infection into this space can arise from vertebral body osteomyelitis or petrositis.

EPIDEMIOLOGY

Most large children's hospital centers report one to three cases per year. Children less than 6 years of age are most at risk, with one-half of the cases occurring in infants less than 12 months of age.

COMPLICATIONS

- Spontaneous rupture with aspiration of infected material, with subsequent asphyxia or overwhelming pulmonary infection.
- Hemorrhage from extension into local arteries, and/or venous thrombosis from involvement of major neck vessels.
- Extension of the infection inferiorly can occur, leading to a subdiaphragmatic or psoas abscess.

PROGNOSIS

- Excellent with appropriate antibiotics, expectant care, and surgery, if needed, at optimal time

 Differential Diagnosis

- Pharyngitis
- Peritonsillar or lateral wall abscess
- Epiglottitis/supraglottitis

 Data Gathering

HISTORY

- Symptoms may be present from hours to days before correct diagnosis. Many patients will have been on oral antibiotics for presumed pharyngitis/sinusitis.
- Symptoms? Most frequent symptoms include sore throat, decreased oral intake, muffled voice, drooling, stiff or painful neck, fever, dysphagia, and stridor.
- Preceding neck trauma? Especially penetrating injuries, recent surgery (especially dental), and history consistent with aspiration of a foreign object.

Physical Examination

- Most frequent signs are:
- Fever
- Stridor (seen in up to 50% of children)
- Drooling
- A tender cervical neck region with restricted range of motion
- Classic diagnostic finding of a bulging posterior pharyngeal wall. May be absent or difficult to appreciate in an ill, apprehensive child.

 Laboratory Aids

Test: CBC
Significance: Frequently reveals an elevated total WBC, with a significant left shift.

Test: Lateral neck x-ray
Significance: Reveals widening of retropharyngeal space and at times an air fluid level.

Test: CT scan or MRI of the neck
Significance: The most definitive test, which can usually differentiate abscess from local cellulitis/adenitis.

 Therapy

- Emergent therapy requires maintaining patent airway; be wary of sudden spontaneous drainage of the abscess, with catastrophic aspiration.
- Careful inhospital monitoring of airway and fluid intake.
- Start broad-spectrum parental antibiotics, active against *Streptococcus pneumoniae, Staphylococcus aureus,* and oral anaerobic organisms. If patient does not improve, broaden coverage to include drugs active against beta-lactamase producing organisms and anaerobic organisms. Clindamycin or ampicillin/sulbactam are good initial choices.
- Immediate consultation with otolaryngology surgical team. Schedule of incision/aspiration of abscess at optimal time, with team experienced in airway management of small children. CT-guided aspiration of the abscess has aided the surgical approach at many sites.
- In selected mild, early cases (especially if the CT scan is consistent with cellulitis rather than true abscess), parenteral antibiotics may be sufficient for therapy. Recent data suggest that up to 50% of patients can be successfully managed without surgical intervention. Patients treated with antibiotics alone must be followed closely for signs of worsening clinical status.

PITFALLS

- Physicians must maintain a high index of suspicion. The presentation of a retropharyngeal abscess can be subtle, with the most frequent initial diagnostic impression usually epiglottitis or severe pharyngitis.
- Both plain films and CT scan have false-positives and false-negatives.
- Once diagnosis is made, urgent consultation with experienced surgical staff is mandatory.

ICD-9-CM 478.24

BIBLIOGRAPHY

Brook I. Microbiology of retropharyngeal abscesses in children. *Am J Dis Child* 1987;141: 202–204.

Gaglani MJ, Edwards MS. Clinical indicators of childhood retropharyngeal abscess. *Am J Emerg Med* 1995;13:333–336.

Hammerschlag PE, Hammerschlag MR. Retropharyngeal abscess. In: Feigin R, Cherry JD, eds. *Textbook of pediatric infectious diseases,* 3rd ed. Philadelphia: WB Saunders, 1992:168–171.

Morrison JE Jr, Pashley RT. Retropharyngeal abscess in children: a 10-year review. *Pediatr Emerg Care* 1988;4:9–11.

Nagy M, Pizzuto M, Backstrom J, Brodsky L. Deep neck infections in children: a new approach to diagnosis and treatment. *Laryngoscope* 1997;107:1627–1634.

Author: Richard M. Rutstein

Reye Syndrome

 Database

DEFINITION

- Acute encephalopathy and fatty degeneration of the liver

PATHOPHYSIOLOGY

- Mitochondrial injury of unknown etiology results in reduction of hepatic intramitochondrial enzymes.
- Salicylates exacerbate condition when ingested after mitochondrial injury.

EPIDEMIOLOGY

- Peak incidence age 6
- Most children range from 4 to 12 years
- More common among whites in rural and suburban communities
- Association with ingestion of aspirin-containing medicines by children with varicella or influenza B

COMPLICATIONS

- Elevated intracranial pressure secondary to cerebral edema
- Mortality greater than 40%

 Differential Diagnosis

- CNS infections (e.g., meningitis, encephalitis)
- Toxins
- Drug ingestion (e.g., salicylates, valproate)
- Metabolic diseases: In report recently by Hou and colleagues, Reye-like syndrome was secondary to hereditary organic acidaemias ($n = 13$), urea cycle defects ($n = 4$), mitochondrial disorders ($n = 3$), fulminant hepatitis ($n = 2$), tyrosinaemia ($n = 1$), and valproate-associated hepatotoxicity ($n = 1$).

 Data Gathering

HISTORY

Question: Prodromal illness?
Significance: URI-Influenza A (90%), Hepatitis A, and varicella.

Question: Abrupt onset of vomiting?
Significance: Onset within 4 to 7 days of initial illness.

Question: What is natural history?
Significance: Followed by neurological deterioration in which delirium may progress to seizures, coma, or death.

 Physical Examination

- Slight liver enlargement without jaundice
- Absence of focal neurological signs

Neurological examination varies with stage of disease:

- Stage I: vomiting with obtundation, subtle cognitive and behavioral disturbances.
- Stage II: agitated delirium and coma, may see decorticate posturing.
- Stage III: hyperventilation, tachycardia, decerebrate posturing, sluggish.
- Stage IV: respiratory failure with signs of elevated intracranial pressure.
- Stage V: respiratory arrest, loss of deep tendon reflexes, fixed dilated pupils.

Laboratory Aids

Test: Ammonia
Significance: May be normal at the onset of vomiting.

Test: Liver function test
Significance: Elevated transaminases, creatinine kinase, LDH, ammonia, and prothrombin time.

Test: CSF
Significance: Normal cerebrospinal fluid except for elevated ICP.

Test: EEG
Significance: Characteristic of metabolic encephalopathy with generalized slow wave abnormalities.

PATHOLOGY (POSTMORTEM)

Test: Liver
Significance: Grossly yellowish white in appearance secondary to increased triglycerides; foamy cytoplasm with increased microvesicular fat, decreased glycogen.

Test: Brain
Significance: Marked edema with increased intracellular fluid, and abnormal neuronal mitochondria.

 ## Therapy

• Should be tailored based on severity of presentation.
• IV glucose to counteract effects of glycogen depletion.
• Fluid restriction in patients with cerebral edema (1500 mL/m^2/d), along with mannitol to increase serum osmolality and induce cerebral dehydration.
• Vitamin K, fresh frozen plasma, and platelets as needed for treatment of secondary coagulopathy.

 ## Follow-Up

• Cerebral function at presentation is the best predictor of outcome.
• Majority have mild illness without progression.
• Patients with mild disease (stage I) recover completely.
• Patients with stage II disease may show complete recovery or subtle neurologic sequelae.
• Patients with stage III to IV disease often do not survive.

PITFALLS

• Failure to recognize early and central or prevent cerebral edema—the immediate cause of death

 ## Common Questions and Answers

Q: Is Reye syndrome fatal?
A: More than 40% of children will die secondary to cerebral edema. Mortality rates are best predicted by neurological state at the onset of presentation.

Q: How can the neurological findings of Reye syndrome be differentiated from meningitis?
A: Aside from an elevated ICP, the lumbar taps of patients with Reye syndrome are at best remarkable. Elevated white count is not seen in these cases.

ICD-9-CM 331.81

BIBLIOGRAPHY

DeVivo DC. Acute encephalopathies of childhood. In: Rudolph AM, ed. *Rudolph's pediatrics,* 19th ed. Norwalk, CT: Appleton & Lange, 1991:1713–1720.

Duerksen DR, Jewell LD, Mason AL. Bain VG. Co-existence of hepatitis A and adult Reye's syndrome. *Gut* 1997;41(1):121–124.

Green CL, Blitzer MG, Shapiro E. Inborn errors of metabolism and Reye's syndrome: differential diagnosis. *J Pediatr* 1988;113:156.

Hou JW, Chou SP, Wang TR. Metabolic function and liver histopathology in Reye-like illnesses. *Acta Paediatrica* 1996;85(9):1053–1057.

Lichtenstein PK, Heubi JE, Dougherty CC, et al. Grade I Reye's syndrome: a frequent cause of vomiting and liver dysfunction after varicella and upper respiratory tract infection. *N Engl J Med* 1983;309:133.

Reye RDK, Morgan G, Baral J. Encephalopathy and fatty degeneration of the viscera: a disease entity in childhood. *Lancet* 1963;2:749.

Author: Andrew E. Mulberg

Rhabdomyolysis

 Database

DEFINITION

• Muscle injury resulting from trauma, infection, or inadequate delivery, production, or consumption of energy or oxygen relative to demands. The release of intracellular contents may cause severe electrolyte disturbances including life-threatening hyperkalemia, myoglobinuria, and acute renal failure.

• Rhabdomyolysis is uncommon in childhood.

PATHOPHYSIOLOGY

• The most common causes include muscle trauma from crush injury, burns, or electric shock. Others include viral illnesses such as influenza and Ebstein Barr infection, heat stroke, severe exertion, status epilepticus, and vasculitis with myositis.

• Rare causes in childhood include many congenital muscle enzyme and energy substrate deficiencies, acute dystonic reactions complicating hereditary torsion dystonia, other infections, exposure to certain medications (e.g., inhalation anesthetics, propofol, and chemotherapeutic agents), toxins (e.g., snake venom, hydrocarbons), and illicit drugs, and severe electrolyte abnormalities including hypophosphatemia, hypokalemia, and hypernatremia. Copper-induced rhabdomyolysis has been reported in patients with Wilson disease.

• Rhabdomyolysis is more likely to occur following exertion in the dystrophinopathies, which include all forms of muscular dystrophy.

• The insult may lead to muscle cell destruction or failure of membrane function with release of intracellular contents including proteins and electrolytes.

GENETICS

Many of the rare causes of rhabdomyolysis, including muscle enzyme deficiencies, muscular dystrophy, and disorders of mitochondrial metabolism, are heritable disorders, and a familial history should be sought.

EPIDEMIOLOGY

Rhabdomyolysis is more common in adults, where it is seen most frequently in comatose patients resulting from heroin or cocaine abuse.

COMPLICATIONS

• Electrolyte release from muscle can lead to hyperkalemia, hyperphosphatemia, and secondarily to hypocalcemia.

• Acute renal failure may occur secondary to myoglobinuria.

ASSOCIATED ILLNESSES

In addition to the previously mentioned causes, rhabdomyolysis has also been reported associated with diverse conditions, including asthma, hemolytic uremic syndrome, and diabetes mellitus.

PROGNOSIS

The prognosis depends on the amount of permanent renal disease, delay in treatment and the response to treatment. Many cases will recover completely.

 Differential Diagnosis

• Includes any condition associated with muscle pain, tenderness, and/or weakness.

• Examples include many viral illnesses, Lyme disease, suppurative myositis, Guillain-Barré syndrome, and collagen vascular diseases.

 Data Gathering

HISTORY

Question: Has there been increased exertion, viral illness, muscle injury, or electrical shock?
Significance: These conditions are associated with muscle breakdown and rhabdomyolysis.

Question: Is there familial history of muscle disease or reaction to anesthesia?
Significance: Rhabdomyolysis is associated with muscular dystrophy and reaction to drugs such as anesthesics.

SPECIAL QUESTIONS

• Antecedent history of illness or insult associated with rhabdomyolysis? Rhabdomyolysis may follow certain illnesses (e.g., influenza) and insults (e.g., crush injury) and thus a history of these should be sought.

• Muscle pain or weakness? These may result from rhabdomyolysis and may help suggest the diagnosis if present.

• Brownish discoloration of the urine?

Physical Examination

- Palpation of muscle for tenderness
- Testing for motor strength
- Eliciting reflexes to exclude neuropathy
- Examination of skin and mucous membranes for signs of vasculitis

 ## Laboratory Aids

- Serum electrolytes (high K_1, normal or low NA_1), calcium, and phosphorus
- BUN and creatinine: creatinine is elevated out of proportion to BUN.
- Creatine phosphokinase will be elevated greater than 100 times normal in rhabdomyolysis.
- Urinalysis
- CBC

Finding: Definitive tests for myoglobinuria
Significance: Immunoelectrophoresis and radio-immunoassay, are not generally available in clinical laboratories. Ammonium sulfate solubility testing is a reasonable test to differentiate myoglobin from hemoglobin.

Finding: Muscle biopsy
Significance: To demonstrate immunohistochemical features and immunoblotting to show abnormalities of the dystrophin gene may be required to evaluate the dystrophinopathies.

Finding: False-positives
Significance: The dipstick for blood is positive, but examination of a freshly voided urinary sediment will reveal few or no erythrocytes. In this instance, the possibilities are myoglobinuria or hemoglobinuria.

Finding: Very rapid rise in serum creatinine
Significance: May occur as a result of release from muscle.

 ## Therapy

GENERAL

- Treatment is supportive. If an underlying cause is identified, it should be corrected or removed.
- Adequate hydration (e.g., 2–3 times maintenance fluids) should be sufficient to provide brisk urine flow (e.g., greater than 4 mL/kg/h). Myoglobinuric nephrotoxicity is the only entity where acute renal failure can be averted by maintaining good urine flow. Alkalinization of the urine is probably beneficial. Furosemide and/or mannitol may be helpful to maintain urine output.
- Dialysis is indicated if oliguric acute renal failure occurs and/or if severe electrolyte disturbances are present.

DRUGS

- With myoglobinuria, bicarbonate therapy should be given intravenously to maintain the urine pH above 7.
- If urine output falls in the face of adequate hydration, furosemide (1–4 mg/kg/dose IV) should be given to attempt to prevent oliguric renal failure.
- If severe hyperkalemia occurs, measures should be taken to prevent cardiac dysrhythmias (calcium, bicarbonate, glucose, and insulin) and to maximize elimination of potassium by the kidneys (furosemide) and/or gastrointestinal tract (kayexalate).
- With hypocalcemia, give calcium only if symptoms are present.

POSSIBLE CONFLICTS

- Furosemide may interfere with alkalinization of the urine.
- Use of bicarbonate may precipitate symptomatic hypocalcemia.
- Calcium therapy for severe hyperkalemia is necessary, but its use with hyperphosphatemia increases risk of metastatic calcification.
- Risk factors for acute renal failure include pre-existing renal disease, concurrent use of nephrotoxic agents, volume depletion and either hypotension or hypertension.
- Failure to discontinue intravenous fluids if oligo-anuric renal failure develops could result in iatrogenic fluid overload.

 ## Follow-Up

WHEN TO EXPECT IMPROVEMENT

- Prompt cessation of rhabdomyolysis may be expected when the inciting cause is corrected or resolves.
- With resolution of the myoglobinuria, return to normal renal function is the rule.

PITFALLS

- Failure to check for muscle breakdown in cases of child abuse

ICD-9-CM 728.89

BIBLIOGRAPHY

Brumback RA, Feeback DL, Leech RW. Rhabdomyolysis in childhood. *Pediatr Clin North Am* 1992;39:821–858.

Chamberlain MC. Rhabdomyolysis in children: a 3-year retrospective study. *Pediatr Neurol* 1991;7:226–228.

Singh U, Scheld, WM. Infectious etiologies of rhabdomyolysis: three case reports and review. *Clin Infect Dis* 1996;22:642–649.

Author: Thomas L. Kennedy III

Rhabdomyosarcoma

 Database

DEFINITION

• Malignant tumor of mesenchymal cells committed to skeletal muscle lineage. Etiology is unknown.

PATHOLOGY

• One of the "small round blue" cell tumors of childhood
• Two major subtypes:

—Alveolar (19% of cases): small round cells with dense appearance, line up along spaces resembling pulmonary alveoli, associated with translocation between chromosomes 2 and 13, or less commonly 1 and 13.
—Embryonal (60% of cases): spindle-shaped cells, less densely cellular with stroma-rich appearance, associated with a chromosomal abnormality on the short arm of chromosome 11 (chromosome 11p15).
—Undifferentiated and pleomorphic types comprise the remaining cases.

GENETICS

• Majority of cases occur sporadically.
• Li-Fraumeni syndrome (family cancer syndrome associated with germline mutations of the p53 gene) includes rhabdomyosarcoma and other soft tissue sarcomas.
• Patients with Beckwith-Wiedeman syndrome (characterized by an abnormality at chromosome 11p15) have an increased incidence of rhabdomyosarcoma.

EPIDEMIOLOGY

• Slightly more than 200 new cases are diagnosed each year in the United States.
• Third most common extracranial solid tumor of childhood
• 50% of cases are diagnosed in children less than 6 years with smaller incidence peak in mid-adolescence.
• 1.3 times more common in males than females.
• Associations: fetal alcohol syndrome, central nervous system and genitourinary anomalies, cigarette smoking in fathers, marijuana and cocaine use in mothers and fathers in the year prior to the child's birth.

COMPLICATIONS

Rhabdomyosarcoma can compromise function of surrounding organs, and/or spread to lymph nodes, lung, bone, bone marrow, liver or brain.

PROGNOSIS

• Overall, 70% of patients can be cured
• Prognosis by primary site (5-year survival):

Orbit	95%
Other head and neck	78%
Parameningeal	74%
Paratesticular/Vagina	89%
Bladder/Prostate	81%
Extremities	74%
Other sites	67%

• Although 50% of patients with distant metastatic disease can be placed into remission, only 20% can be cured.
• Tumors with alveolar histology (typically extremity lesions) tend to metastasize early.
• Recurrence can occur many years after completion of therapy but is rare after 3 years.

 Differential Diagnosis

• Malignant

—Ewing sarcoma
—Neuroblastoma
—Non-Hodgkin lymphoma
—Leukemic chloroma
—Germ cell tumor
—Rare soft tissue sarcomas

• Non-Malignant

—Trauma
—Benign tumors: lipoma, rhabdomyoma, neurofibroma
—Langerhans cell histiocytosis
—Abscess

 Data Gathering

HISTORY

Question: Growth or lump that does not hurt?
Significance: Presents most often as painless, firm swelling or mass.

Question:
Significance: Other symptoms depend on site of origin:

• Head/neck: nasal congestion or discharge, otorrhea, cranial nerve palsies, proptosis, headache, vomiting or systemic hypertension (with intracranial growth of tumor)
• Genitourinary/pelvic: urinary frequency or retention, hematuria, constipation, vaginal discharge or bleeding
• Extremity: painful or painless lumps or erythema
• Trunk: usually few symptoms until tumor widespread

 Physical Examination

Can occur in any location, even in sites in which skeletal muscle is not normally found.

Finding: Location of primary tumor

• Head and neck (38%): parameningeal (middle ear, nasal cavity, paranasal sinuses, nasopharynx, infratemporal fossa, pterygopalatine fossa, parapharyngeal area); orbit (orbit, eyelid); non-parameningeal (scalp, parotid, oral cavity, larynx, oropharynx, cheek, hypopharynx, thyroid, parathyroid, neck).
• Genitourinary tract (21%): bladder and prostate; uterus, vagina, vulva and paratesticular region.
• Extremity (18%)
• Trunk (7%)
• Retroperitoneum (7%)

Significance: Prognosis varies widely by location of primary

Finding: Special attention should be made to physical examination of lymphatic structures and surrounding tissues
Significance: Spread by local invasion and lymphatogenous spread

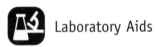 Laboratory Aids

Test: CBC
Significance: Screen for marrow invasion

Test: Electrolytes, liver and renal function tests, serum calcium, phosphorus.
Significance: Baseline values before starting chemotherapy.

IMAGING AND OTHER TESTS

Test: CT scan or preferably, MRI scan
Significance: To evaluate primary site and confirm diagnosis

Test: Biopsy
Significance: Growth of a nontender mass, especially without a history of trauma, over a 1 to 2 week period should alert examiner to consider biopsy. In addition to routine morphological and immunohistochemical stain assessments, analysis of tumor chromosomes by traditional cytogenetics, fluorescent in situ hybridization or reverse transcriptase PCR is helpful in making the diagnosis and may provide information regarding prognosis. Because of the importance of these studies, consultation with a pediatric oncologist before the biopsy is strongly encouraged.

To evaluate for evidence of distant metastases (present in 20% of patients at diagnosis)

Test: Chest radiograph and CT scan
Significance: Lung metastases, effusions

Test: 99mTc-diphosphonate bone scan
Significance: Bone metastasis

Test: Bilateral aspiration and biopsy of iliac bone marrow
Significance: Scan for marrow spread

Test: Lumbar puncture for CSF cytology (parameningeal tumors)
Significance: To determine if CNS invasion has occurred.

 ## Therapy

- Therapy is a multi-modal approach based on location and extent of disease: surgery; chemotherapy: common agents used include: vincristine, dactinomycin, doxorubicin, cyclophosphamide, etoposide and ifosphamide; radiation therapy.
- Duration of therapy depends on location and extent of disease.
- Surgical trend is towards less radical surgery with organ preservation.
- Most children are treated according to large cooperative group protocols at pediatric oncology centers.
- Treatment is characterized by significant side effects including increased susceptibility to infection, severe mucositis and poor nutritional status.
- Most patients require placement of an indwelling central venous catheter for the duration of their therapy.

 ## Follow-Up

WHEN TO EXPECT IMPROVEMENT

All patients with rhabdomyosarcoma require 1 to 2 years of chemotherapy to prevent recurrence in the original site of tumor or distant spread. However, some improvement in signs and symptoms is usually seen within the first several weeks of therapy.

ACUTE EFFECTS OF THERAPY

Therapy for rhabdomyosarcoma is intensive. Patients can expect many of the following side effects:

- Frequent admissions to the hospital for chemotherapy or complications of the therapy.
- Complications from bone marrow suppressive effects of chemotherapy or radiotherapy:

—Anemia: blood transfusions are usually necessary; erythropoietin (a stimulator of erythropoiesis) is given to many patients to reduce the number of transfusions required.
—Thrombocytopenia: platelet transfusions are often necessary to reduce the risk of serious bleeding.

—Neutropenia: increased risk of bacterial and fungal infections; G-CSF (granulocyte-colony stimulating factor) is usually administered daily following chemotherapy to shorten the duration of neutropenia.

- Complications from the gastrointestinal side effects of chemotherapy or radiotherapy:

—Nausea and vomiting; relieved with ondansetron and other anti-emetic agents.
—Malnutrition secondary to reduced appetite and mucosal ulcerations; nutritional supplements (oral, nasogastric or parenteral) may be necessary.

- Complication from radiotherapy.

—Skin erythema or breakdown.

LATE EFFECTS OF THERAPY

Therapy for rhabdomyosarcoma is intensive, and is associated with significant long-term adverse effects. Regular follow-up with a pediatric oncologist is strongly recommended.

- Cardiomyopathy

—Anthracyclines (doxorubicin) weaken cardiac muscle leading to reduced left ventricular function many years after therapy.
—Approximately 5% of patients receiving cumulative doses of doxorubicin greater than 500 mg/m^2 will develop congestive heart failure.
—Radiation to the heart can lower the cumulative dose threshold to 300 mg/m^2.
—Any patient who has received an anthracycline should be cautioned against initiating strenuous physical activity without adequate preparation.
—Pregnant women who have received anthracyclines in the past should inform their obstetrician so that appropriate cardiac assessment can be completed prior to vaginal delivery.

- Kidney and bladder damage.

—Urinalysis should be performed to detect hemorrhagic cystitis or tubular damage.
—Blood pressure should be monitored in patients who received irradiation to the kidneys; vascular damage and hypertension may develop many years after therapy.

- Infertility and delayed puberty.

—Reduced or absent gonadal function is related to high doses of alkylating agents (cyclophosphamide, ifosphamide): males are at high risk of azoospermia; females may be fertile, but are at risk for premature menopause.
—Low dose estrogen therapy with oral contraceptive medications may be necessary for amenorrheic women.
—Retrograde ejaculation may be seen following surgery for paratesticular tumors.

- Second malignant neoplasms.

—Sarcomas may occur within the radiation field.
—Myelodysplastic syndromes and acute myeloid leukemia may occur secondary to radiation or chemotherapy (cyclophosphamide, etoposide).

- Bowel obstruction and enteritis (abdominal-pelvic tumors).

—Adhesions as a consequence of surgery or radiation.
—A history of failure to gain weight or symptoms of malabsorption suggests a need for additional evaluation.

- Growth abnormalities/functional defects at the primary site.

—Radiation doses greater than 20 Gy will cause growth retardation in growing children.
—Scoliosis can occur if the vertebrae are involved in the radiation field.

- Cataracts can occur after irradiation involving the head.

 ## Questions and Answers

Q: Can a child with rhabdomyosarcoma receive immunizations during therapy?
A: Immunizations are not recommended during treatment as they are not likely to be effective since chemotherapy is immunosuppressive. The oral polio vaccine should not be administered to other household members, but they can receive the inactivated polio vaccine and all other immunizations.

Q: Can a child with rhabdomyosarcoma attend school?
A: As the chemotherapy for rhabdomyosarcoma is intensive, most children are unable to continue with school during this time, but will benefit from home-bound instruction.

Q: Is the treatment associated with infertility?
A: The present chemotherapy regimens include high cumulative doses of alkylating agents, placing males in particular, at high risk for infertility. Sperm banking is, therefore, recommended in adolescent males, prior to the initiation of chemotherapy.

ICD-9-CM 171.9

BIBLIOGRAPHY

Pappo AS, Shapiro DN, Crist WM. Rhabdomyosarcoma: biology and treatment. *Pediatr Clin N Am* 1997;44(4):953–972.

Wexler LH, Helman LJ. Pediatric soft tissue sarcomas. *CA Cancer J Clin* 1994;44:211–247.

Womer RB. Soft tissue sarcomas. *Eur J Cancer* 1997;33(13):2230–2234.

Author: Kara M. Kelly

Rheumatic Fever (ARF)

 Database

DEFINITION

• Post-infectious immune response to group A streptococcus that results in a diffuse inflammatory disease involving multiple organ systems

PATHOPHYSIOLOGY

• Immune-mediated inflammatory reaction to specific rheumatogenic strains of group A beta-hemolytic streptococci that affects connective tissue, namely the heart, joints, brain, blood vessels, and subcutaneous tissue. Streptococcal pharyngitis precedes the onset of ARF by approximately 3 weeks.
• "Antigenic mimicry" occurs in which antigen similarities between epitopes of specific rheumatogenic streptococci and host tissue cause an autoimmune cross-reaction where produced antibodies damage the host.
• "Aschoff nodules" are proliferative lesions noted in the myocardium that may persist for months to years after the initiation of disease.

GENETICS

• Increased familial incidence reported, therefore, suggesting a genetic predisposition

EPIDEMIOLOGY

• Estimated 3% of patients with untreated or inadequately treated streptococcal pharyngitis develop ARF.
• Initial episode primarily seen between 5 to 15 years of age.
• Incidence (United States) is 0.5 to 3.1/100,000 with a "resurgence" in the mid 1980s.
• No longer a disease mainly found in socially and economically disadvantaged groups in the United States, yet the incidence is higher in underdeveloped countries.
• Rheumatogenic strains of group A streptococci with specific M proteins have been associated with outbreaks of ARF.

COMPLICATIONS

Cardiac

• Pancarditis (always a component of valvulitis)

—Pericarditis (including pericardial effusion) and/or myocarditis (these entities are almost always associated with valvulitis)
—Transient arrhythmias occur infrequently.
—Carditis accounts for the greatest mortality in the acute phase and significant morbidity/mortality chronically.

• Valvulitis

—Mitral valve is most commonly affected followed by aortic (usually associated with mitral involvement). Tricuspid and pulmonary valvar involvement is rare.
—Valve inflammation leads to insufficiency.

—Prolonged immune response causes fibrosis, calcification, and valve stenosis.

Arthritis

• Two or more large joints (knees, ankles, wrists, and elbows)
• Involvement is asymmetric and migratory.
• Limitation of motion may occur.
• Unusual for the symptoms to persist beyond the acute illness.
• Symptoms improve rapidly with aspirin.

Sydenham Chorea (St. Vitus Dance)

• Involuntary, purposeless, and uncoordinated movements associated with muscle weakness and/or abnormal behavior.
• Due to inflammation of the basal ganglia/cerebellum.
• Symptoms can occur late, up to 6 months after the onset of ARF, and usually resolve within weeks but may last months to years.

PROGNOSIS

• Patients with a previous episode of ARF are at high risk for a recurrence following streptococcal pharyngitis unless secondary prophylaxis is instituted.
• Carditis can abate spontaneously or progress. The severity of the initial carditis is a major determinant to progression to rheumatic heart disease.
• Rheumatic carditis resolves in approximately 70% to 80% of patients who adhere to prophylaxis guidelines.

 Differential Diagnosis

• Carditis: viral, bacterial, rickettsial, parasitic, or myocoplasma myocarditis; Kawasaki disease
• Arthritis: poststreptococcal arthritis, serum sickness, septic arthritis (i.e., gonococcal), Lyme disease
• Collagen vascular disease: juvenile rheumatoid arthritis (small joints, not migratory, and not relieved promptly with aspirin), systemic lupus erythematosus, bacterial endocarditis
• Chorea: congenital choreoathetosis, brain tumors, Huntington chorea, Wilson disease
• Hematologic disorders with joint involvement: sickle cell anemia, leukemia
• Congenital heart defects: previously undiagnosed valvar heart disease, mitral valve prolapse with regurgitation

 Data Gathering

HISTORY

Question: How do you use the Jones criteria to make the diagnosis of ARF?
Significance: Jones criteria for diagnosis (2 major versus 1 major and 2 minor criteria with evidence of a recent streptococcal infection).

Exceptions to the Jones criteria include:
• Sydenham chorea alone.
• Indolent carditis alone (each of which may appear late and, therefore, may not be associated with supporting evidence of a recent streptococcal pharyngitis).
• Patients with a previous diagnosis of ARF who have a recurrence may not fulfill the Jones criteria due to the subtle presentation.
• Major Criteria

—Carditis: 50% of patients with ARF and always associated with a murmur of valvulitis.
—Polyarthritis: 70% of patients and manifested by a migratory arthritis of major joints.
—Sydenham chorea: 15% of patients and manifested by abnormal behavior and/or involuntary, purposeless movements.
—Erythema marginatum: 10% of patients and is an evanescent, pink rash with serpiginous borders.
—Subcutaneous nodules: 2% to 10% of patients and manifested by painless nodules over extensor surfaces of large joints, the occiput, and/or vertebral processes.

• Minor Criteria

—Arthralgia: Can only be considered in the absence of arthritis.
—Fever
—Elevated acute phase reactants (ESR, C-reactive protein).
—Prolongation of the PR interval on ECG.

 Physical Examination

CARDIAC

Finding: Murmur of valvulitis
Significance: Holosystolic mitral regurgitant murmur, Carey-Coombs apical mid-diastolic murmur, or a basal diastolic murmur of aortic insufficiency.

Finding: Murmur could be associated with a pericardial friction rub.
Significance: Pericardial effusion

MUSCULOSKELETAL

Finding: Pain, limited motion, erythema, warmth of two or more large joints.
Significance: Arthritis criterion

NEUROLOGICAL

Finding: Chorea must be differentiated from tics, athetosis, and hyperkinesis.
Significance: Sydenham's chorea criterion

SKIN

Finding: Evanescent, pink rash with pale centers and serpiginous borders on the trunk and proximal extremities.
Significance: Erythema marginatum criterion

- Firm, painless nodules over the extensor surface of large joints, occiput and/or spinous processes.

Laboratory Aids

SPECIFIC TESTS

Test: No diagnostic test is available.

NON-SPECIFIC TESTS

Test: Throat culture
Significance: May be negative in two-thirds of the patients or may be chronic carrier.

Test: Rapid streptococcal antigen test
Significance: Evidence for infection with GABHS

Test: Elevated or rising streptococcal antibody titers [antistreptolysin O (ASO), anti-Dnase B, anti-hyaluronidase]
Significance: Evidence for recent infection with GABHS

Test: Additional hematologic evaluation
Significance: Leukocytosis on complete blood count (may be normal)

Test: ESR and C-reactive protein
Significance: Minor criteria if elevated

Test: ECG
Significance: Prolonged PR interval, junctional rhythm, transient arrhythmias, ST-T wave changes.

Test: CXR
Significance: Cardiomegaly may indicate carditis or pericardial effusion.

Test: Echocardiogram
Significance: Assess valve involvement, ventricular dilatation, function, and pericardial effusions.

Therapy

- Primary prevention

—Full treatment of streptococcal pharyngitis infection

  —Penicillin V 250 mg PO tid for 10 days; or
  —Benzathine penicillin G IM (600,000 U/IM <27 kg or 1,200,000 U/IM >27 kg); or
  —Erythromycin estolate.

- Secondary prevention

—Benzathine penicillin G (1,200,000 U/IM every 3 weeks); or
—Penicillin V 250 mg PO bid; or
—Sulfadizine PO daily; or
—Erythromycin 250 mg PO daily.
—Duration depends on clinical presentation and cardiac impact of ARF
—Patients without rheumatic carditis require prophylaxis for 5 years or until age 21, whichever is longer
—Patients with a history of rheumatic carditis but with no residual cardiac disease (clinical or echo) require prophylaxis for at least 10 years and well into adulthood, whichever is longer.
—Patients with rheumatic heart disease should have prophylaxis for at least 10 years and at least until 40 years of age.

- Treatment of inflammation

—Aspirin: 100 mg/kg/d for 6 to 8 weeks (no effect on carditis)
—Prednisone: 2 mg/kg/d for 3 to 4 weeks (usually recommended for patients with severe carditis)

- Cardiac support

—Digoxin or other inotropic agents
—Afterload reducing agents such as captopril or intravenous nitroprusside
—Bedrest indicated during episode of acute carditis
—Surgical valvuloplasty or valve replacement if indicated

- Treatment of chorea

—Usually supportive
—Phenobarbital, haloperidol, chlorpromazine, diazepam, valproic acid

Follow-Up

- Patients without carditis

—Close follow-up is needed for 2 to 3 weeks to assess for development of acute carditis.
—Long-term pediatric follow-up is needed to diagnose patients with indolent carditis.
—Patients with new murmurs or clinical evidence of heart failure should be referred to a cardiologist.
—Long-term follow-up is needed to evaluate those who develop chorea.
—Prophylaxis should be stressed even in individuals without carditis.

- Patients with carditis

—Cardiology follow-up is needed to assess the development or evolution of rheumatic heart disease.
—Symptoms of worsening heart failure suggest progression of valvar or myocardial disease, recurrent ARF, or endocarditis.
—Secondary prophylaxis and bacterial endocarditis prophylaxis should be stressed.

PITFALLS

No definitive diagnostic test exists and certain clinical criteria must be present and excluded from other disease states to assure the proper diagnosis.

Common Questions and Answers

Q: Does a negative throat culture rule out ARF?
A: No. Throat cultures may be negative in as many as two-thirds of patients.

Q: Is there a vaccine available to prevent ARF?
A: Not presently; however, research efforts have been promising. Antigenic strains of group A streptococcus have been identified. Additionally, progress has been made in determining factors that cause a genetic predisposition to ARF. In the future, a vaccine may be available to those patients known to be at increased risk due to their genetic makeup.

Q: Is long-term bedrest ever indicated?
A: No. Bedrest is recommended during acute carditis. Patients who recover fully may enjoy full activity. In patients with cardiomegaly or residual valvar disease, exercise should be limited to less strenuous activities.

Q: Can echocardiographic evidence of carditis alone be used to diagnose rheumatic fever?
A: No. At the present time, carditis can only be diagnosed with a murmur consistent with valvulitis. An echocardiographic finding of valvar insufficiency without the appropriate auscultation findings cannot be used to fulfill the Jones criterion of carditis.

ICD-9-CM 398.99

BIBLIOGRAPHY

Albert DA, Harel L, Karrison T. The treatment of rheumatic carditis: a review and meta-analysis. *Medicine* 1995;74(1):1–12.

Aron AM, Freeman JM, Caters S. The natural history of Sydenham's chorea. *Am J Med* 1965; 38:83–95.

Ayoub E. Acute rheumatic fever. In: Emmanouilides GC, ed. *Moss and Adams heart disease in infants, children, and adolescents including the fetus and young adult,* 5th ed. Baltimore: Williams & Wilkins, 1995:1400–1416.

Dajani A, Taubert K, Ferrieri P, et al. Treatment of acute streptococcal pharyngitis and prevention of rheumatic fever: a statement for health professionals. *Pediatrics* 1995;96(4):758–764.

Jones TD. Diagnosis of rheumatic fever. *JAMA* 1944;126:481–484.

Kaplan MH. Rheumatic fever, rheumatic heart disease and the streptococcal connection: the role of streptococcal antigens cross reactive with heart tissue. *Rev Infect Dis* 1979;1:1988–1996.

Special Writing Group of the Committee on Rheumatic Fever, Endocarditis, and Kawasaki's Disease of the Council on Cardiovascular Disease in the Young of the American Heart Association. Guidelines for the diagnosis of rheumatic fever, Jones criteria update. *J Am Med Assoc* 1992;268(15):2069–2073.

Stollerman GH. Rheumatic fever. *Lancet* 1997; 349:935–942.

Tompkins DG, Boxerbaum B, Liebman J. Long term prognosis of rheumatic fever patients receiving regular intramuscular benzathine penicillin. *Circulation* 1972;45:543–551.

Author: Timothy M. Hoffman

Rhinitis—Allergic

 Database

DEFINITION

• Inflammation of the nasal and sinus mucosae, associated with sneezing, swelling, increased mucus production, and nasal obstruction.
• May be seasonal (periodic symptoms, most often due to pollens) or perennial (year long, may be due to multiple seasonal allergies or continual exposure to allergens, such as dust mites).

CAUSES

• Indoor allergens: house dust mite, animal dander, cigarette smoke, hair spray, paint, molds.
• Pollens: tree pollens in early spring, grass in late spring and early summer, ragweed in late summer and autumn.
• Multiple environmental factors

ASSOCIATED PROBLEMS

• Atopic dermatitis (eczema)
• Urticaria
• Asthma
• Nasal polyps
• Delayed speech and language development
• Mouth breathing
• Snoring
• Allergic conjunctivitis
• Adenoidal hypertrophy and sleep apnea

PATHOPHYSIOLOGY

Early Phase Allergic Responses to Antigen Exposure (Within First Several Hours)

• Allergen binds to specific immunoglobulin E (IgE), and then binds to receptors on mast cells and causes bridging of two or more cells.
• A cascade of enzymatic reactions occurs within the cells.
• Mediators, including histamine, leukotrienes, and prostaglandins, are released (mast cell degranulation) into the extracellular environment.
• Smooth muscle contraction, vasodilatation, edema, and secretions result, leading to narrowing and obstruction of the sinus ostia.
• Itching of the nose and sneezing occur after physical and chemical stimulation of nerve endings in the nose.
• Hypersecretion occurs as a result of parasympathetic pathways and reflex mechanisms.

Late Phase Allergic Response (Several to 8 Hours After Allergen Exposure)

• Chemotactic factors lead to eosinophil, basophil, and neutrophil infiltration, and increased numbers of lymphocytes.
• Cytotoxic proteins released by activated eosinophils may cause damage to epithelial cells.

EPIDEMIOLOGY

• Affects 8% to 20% of children and 15% to 30% of adolescents.
• Estimated that up to 75% of children with asthma also have allergic rhinitis.
• Most commonly begins during childhood and young adulthood.

GENETICS

• Increased incidence in families with atopic disease.
• If one parent has allergies, each child has a 30% chance of having an allergy; if both parents have allergies, each child has a 70% chance of having an allergy.

COMPLICATIONS

• Chronic sinusitis
• Recurrent otitis media
• Hoarseness
• Loss of smell
• Loss of hearing

 Differential Diagnosis

INFECTION

• Viral upper respiratory tract infection
• Bacterial sinusitis

ENVIRONMENTAL

• Foreign body

TUMORS

• Nasal polyps
• Dermoid cyst
• Nasal glioma

CONGENITAL

• Cystic fibrosis
• Choanal atresia
• Ciliary dyskinesia
• Septal deviation
• Meningocele/encephalocele
• Primary atrophic rhinitis

IMMUNOLOGIC

• Sarcoidosis
• Wegener granulomatosis

MISCELLANEOUS

• Vasomotor rhinitis
• Non-allergic perennial rhinitis
• Non-allergic rhinitis with eosinophilia (Mullarkey) syndrome (rare during childhood)
• Rhinitis medicamentosa
• Rhinitis associated with pregnancy
• Hypothyroidism

 Data Gathering

HISTORY

Question: What are typical symptoms?
Significance: Patient often reports stuffy nose, sneezing, itching, runny nose, noisy breathing, snoring, cough, halitosis, and repeated throat clearing may be reported. Sensation of plugged ears and wheezing may occur.

Question: Are eyes red and itching?
Significance: Suggestive of allergic conjunctivitis.

Question: Are symptoms seasonal, perennial, or episodic?
Significance: May help to identify potential allergens.

Question: Any exacerbating factors including pollen, animals, cigarette smoke, dust, molds?
Significance: Useful information to prevent symptoms from occurring.

Question: A familial history of atopic diseases?
Significance: Would suggest the diagnosis.

Question: Any related illnesses?
Significance: Include asthma, urticaria, eczema, ear infections, and delayed speech.

 Physical Examination

• Allergic shiners: Dark discoloration beneath the eyes due to obstruction of lymphatic and venous drainage, chronic nasal obstruction, and suborbital edema.
• Dennie-Morgan lines: Creases in the lower eyelid radiating outward from the inner canthus; caused by spasm in the muscles of Muller around the eye due to chronic congestion and stasis of blood.
• Check the conjunctivae for erythema and/or discharge: May suggest conjunctivitis.
• Allergic salute: A gesture characterized by rubbing the nose with the palm of the hand upwards to decrease itching and temporarily open the nasal passages.
• Allergic crease: Transverse crease near the tip of the nose, secondary to rubbing.
• Nasal mucosa: May appear pale, edematous, and mucoid or watery material may be seen in the nasal cavity; check for nasal polyps, septal deviation.

 Laboratory Aids

Test: Complete blood count
Significance: Look for eosinophilia

Test: Specimen of nasal discharge for eosinophils
Significance: Greater than 10% eosinophils is considered positive for nasal eosinophilia. (Note: use of intranasal steroids may reduce the number of eosinophils found in nasal discharge.)

Test: Sweat test
Significance: If cystic fibrosis suspected or if nasal polyps are present.

Test: Audiometry and tympanometry when indicated
Significance: Persistent fluid behind the tympani membrane may result in a hearing loss.

Test: RAST (radioallergosorbent tests)
Significance: In vitro test to measure allergen-specific IgE; very expensive; useful in patients who have diffuse atopic dermatitis

Test: Enzyme-linked immunosorbent assay
Significance: To measure allergen-specific IgE

Test: Total IgE
Significance: Elevated in allergic rhinitis.

SKIN TESTING

Test: Prick test
Significance: Qualitative test in which antigen concentrate is placed on the skin, and a needle is inserted; the skin reaction is subjectively graded from 0 to 4.

Test: Intradermal test
Significance: Qualitative test in which antigen is introduced intradermally; more sensitive than the prick test; the degree of swelling and erythema is graded from 0 to 4.

Test: Skin end-point titration (SET)
Significance: Intradermal antigen testing using differing concentrations; quantitative.

PROCEDURES

Test: Rhinoscopy
Significance: To assess the nasal turbinates and to look for nasal polyps.

Therapy

DRUGS

• Mucolytics: act to thin the mucus and thereby improve mucociliary flow; include steam inhalation, normal saline drops, bicarbonate spray, *N*-acetylcysteine: orally or inhaled, and oral guaifenesin.
• Antihistamines: competitively blocking H_1 receptors; suppresses itching, ocular symptoms, sneezing, and rhinorrhea; not very effective against nasal congestion.
—First-generation [e.g., diphenhydramine (Benadryl)]: side effects include drowsiness and paradoxical excitement; anticholinergic side effects may occur.
—Second-generation [e.g., astemizole (Hismanal)]: minimally or do not cross the blood-brain barrier and, therefore, do not have CNS side effects such as drowsiness. Zyrtec (cetirizine HCl): FDA-approved for children as young as 2 years. Dose: age 2 to 5 years: 2.5 mg = 1/2 tsp. (1 mg/mL banana-grape flavored syrup) PO daily with maximum dose of 5 mg/d. Claritin syrup or Reditabs (loratadine rapidly disintegrating tablets): approved for children as young as 6 years. Dose: 10 mg PO daily.
• Topical cromolyn (Nasalcrom): Mast-cell stabilizer; minimal side effects; does not provide immediate relief, and requires good compliance.
• Oral decongestants: Alpha$_1$- and alpha$_2$-adrenergic agonists, which act to cause vasoconstriction, decreased blood supply to the nasal mucosa, and decreased mucosal edema. Agents include ephedrine, pseudoephedrine, phenylephrine, or phenylpropanolamine.

• Topical decongestants: Sympathomimetics; side effects include drying of the mucosa and burning. Use for more than a few (3–5) days results in rebound vasodilation and congestion (rhinitis medicamentosa). Agents include phenylephrine (NeoSynephrine), which is short acting; and oxymetazoline (Afrin) which is long acting.
• Combined oral decongestants and antihistamines: examples include Extendryl (chlorpheniramine, methscopolamine, phenylephrine) and Atrohist (chlorpheniramine and pseudoephedrine).
• Topical steroids: Blunt early phase reactions and block late phase reactions; not fully effective until several days after initiation of therapy. Agents include beclomethasone (Vancenase, Beconase); flunisolide (Nasalide); fluticasone propionate (Flonase 0.05% nasal spray); budesonide (Rhinocort); triamcinolone acetonide (Nasacort); and triamcinolone (Nasacort).

IMMUNOTHERAPY

• Recommended for patients who have not responded to pharmacological therapy.
• Series of injections with specific allergens, once or twice weekly.

SURGERY

• Removal of allergic polyps.
• Inferior turbinate surgery to reduce the size of the turbinate and relieve obstruction.
• Endoscopic sinus surgery to relieve obstruction.

PREVENTION

• Minimize exposure to dust mites: consider removing carpets, upholstered furniture, and curtains; washing bedding in hot water frequently, at least every 2 weeks; using pillow and mattress covers; using solutions containing benzyl benzoate, which are mitocidal.
• Minimize exposure to animal danders: minimize exposure to all animals, consider using solutions containing tannic acid, which will denature animal allergens; shampoo pets frequently if pets cannot be removed from the household.
• Minimize exposure to pollens: keep windows closed, use air conditioning, avoid leaf-raking or lawn-mowing.
• Minimize exposure to molds: keep houseplants out of the bedroom, avoid spending time in the basement, keep humidity at 35% to 50%.

Follow-Up

• 2 to 4 weeks after initial evaluation; then every 3 to 6 months

SIGNS TO WATCH FOR

Fever, prolonged or severe headache, dizziness, pain, or purulent discharge should suggest a diagnosis other than allergic rhinitis alone.

PROGNOSIS

• Generally good. Complete recovery occurs in 5% to 10% of patients.

PITFALLS

• Skin tests may be difficult to interpret in patients with diffuse eczema and dermatographism.
• Cardiac arrhythmias have been seen with patients taking terfenadine and astemizole.

Common Questions and Answers

Q: How does one minimize exposure to dust mites?
A: Keep household temperature low; maintain humidity at approximately 40% to 50%; wash linens at hot temperatures, weekly; use a microfilter when vacuum cleaning; place mattress and boxspring in airtight plastic casing; use air conditioning; use high-efficiency particulate air filter units.

Q: How often are nasal polyps associated with cystic fibrosis?
A: In up to 40% of children, nasal polyps are associated with cystic fibrosis. Less than 0.5% of children with asthma and rhinitis have nasal polyps.

Q: When used on a daily basis, are inhaled steroids safe?
A: Yes. It is generally accepted that inhaled steroids are safe. The serious side effects seen with systemic steroids, including growth problems, hypothalamic-pituitary-adrenal suppression, and development of cataracts are not seen with daily use of inhaled steroids.

ICD-9-CM 477.9

BIBLIOGRAPHY

Cook PR, Nishioka GJ. Allergic rhinosinusitis in the pediatric population. *Otolaryn Clin North Am* 1996;29:39–56.

Meltzer EO. Treatment options for the child with allergic rhinitis. *Clin Pediatr* 1998;37:1–10.

Meltzer EO, Zeiger RS, Schatz M, Jalowayski AA. Chronic rhinitis in infants and children: etiologic, diagnostic, and therapeutic considerations. *Pediatr Clin North Am* 1983;30:847–871.

Naglerio RM. Allergic rhinitis. *N Engl J Med* 1991;325:860–869.

Simons FE. Allergic rhinitis: recent advances. *Pediatr Clin North Am* 1988;35:1053–1074.

Author: Esther K. Chung

Rickets

 Database

DEFINITION

Undermineralization of growing bone.

CAUSES

- See the table below, Causes and Management of Rickets.
- Children at high risk for rickets:

—Small premature infants
—Urban breast-fed infants who do not receive supplemental vitamin D
—Children with chronic renal insufficiency
—Children with biliary atresia or chronic liver disease
—Children with inflammatory bowel diseases

 Data Gathering

HISTORY

- Symptoms of hepatic, renal, or gastrointestinal disease?
- Calcium intake? Dairy products, legumes, green vegetables.
- Factors influencing calcium absorption? Calciferol supply, steatorrhea, antacids, anticonvulsants
- Vitamin D fortified milk?
- Exposure to sunlight?: Vitamin D metabolism

Question: Factors influencing calcium excretion?
Significance: Diuretics, polyuria, or glycosuria suggestive of renal tubular dysfunction.

- Bone pain? Fractures.
- Delayed standing, walking?
- Anorexia?
- Seizures?
- Pathological fractures?
- Tetany?
- Calcium: Familial history of rickets?

 Physical Examination

- Calcification: Slowed growth (short stature)
- Bossing deformity of the head
- Craniotabes: Soft sutures
- Premature fusion of the sutures
- Dental caries: Calcium in teeth
- Hepatic or renal enlargement: May be etiology
- Alterations in the long bones: Calcification
- Keep mass of uncalcified bone matrix
- Muscle weakness: Serum calcium
- Rachitic rosary: Enlarged costochondral junctions
- Awkward gait: Fractures and bowed leg

Causes and Management of Rickets

CAUSE	MANAGEMENT
Calcium deficiency	
Low intake	Include at least 500 mg/d of Ca
Extreme prematurity (birth weight <1500 g)	Adjust intake to 200 mg/kg/d
Steatorrhea	25-OH-D$_3$ (5–7 μg/kg/d) if serum levels are low; supplement dietary Ca
Anticonvulsants (phenobarbital or phenytoin)	Vitamin D, 1000–2000 IU/d
Renal tubular acidosis	Base supplement: 3–10 mM/kg/d as NaHCO$_3$ or citrate
Vitamin D deficiency	
Insufficient UV light	400 IU/d of vitamin D
No vitamin D supplement	400 IU/d of vitamin D
Liver disease	25-OH-D, 5–7 mg/kg/d
Renal disorders that may reduce calcitriol formation	Calcitriol, 0.25–1.0 mg/d
Hypoplasia or parenchymal damage	CaCO$_3$ to restrict P absorption and supplement dietary Ca
Specific hydroxylase deficiency	Calcitriol, 0.5–1.0 mg/d
Phosphorus deficiency	
Diet (limited to premature infants)	Adjust formula or parenteral source to give 10 mg/kg/d
Antacid excess	Alternative gastric HCl control
Excessive phosphaturia from tubular dysfunction	Supplemental P and calcitriol if low

Laboratory Aids

See the table below, Classification of Rickets and Vitamin D Metabolite Levels

- Circulating vitamin D metabolites (25-hydroxy vitamin D, 1,25-dihydroxy vitamin D)
- Circulating levels of parathyroid hormone (PTH)
- Serum Ca, P, Mg, alkaline phosphatase, and total CO_2
- Urinary Ca, P, Mg, pH, creatinine, and amino acids, exclude Fanconi syndrome and proximal renal tubular acidosis.
- Alkaline phosphatase

IMAGING

- Order one view because rickets is symmetrical.
- Knee and wrist films
- Radiographic findings: irregular cortices and bony margins, widened metaphyses, widened growth plates, osteopenia
- DEXA (dual energy x-ray absorptiometry) is The "gold standard."

 ## Therapy

See the table on the previous page.

 ## Follow-Up

- To avoid side effects of hypercalciuria and hypercalcemia, frequent monitoring (every 2–3 months) of blood and urinary calcium levels (calcium/creatinine ratio) should be done when vitamin D therapy is used.
- Should see radiographic improvement within 6 weeks.

 ## Common Questions and Answers

Q: Why are premature infants prone to rickets?
A: Premature infants have higher calcium and phosphorus requirements than full-term infants. They also tend to be sicker at birth, sometimes having feeding difficulties or malabsorption.

Q: What is the best way to diagnose rickets?
A: The most precise way to diagnose rickets is with a DEXA scan, which gives accurate measures of bone density. A routine x-ray may not show osteopenia until the disease is at a moderately severe stage.

Q: What are the sequelae of rickets?
A: The most common medical sequelae of rickets include pathological bone fractures, slowed growth (short stature), and muscle weakness.

Q: Can rickets be treated effectively?
A: Yes, rickets can be treated effectively with the right amount and combination of calcium, phosphorus, or vitamin D supplementation. Radiographic improvement can usually be seen within 6 weeks.

ICD-9-CM 268
Renal rickets 588.0

BIBLIOGRAPHY

Behrman RM, ed. Metabolic bone disease. In: *Nelson textbook of pediatrics,* 14th ed. 1997; 1748–1752.

Bergsrom WH. Twenty ways to get rickets in the 1990s. *Contemp Pediatr* 1991;8:88.

Chesney RW. Nutrition in bone disease. In: Grand RJ, Sutphen JL, Dietz WH, eds. *Pediatric nutrition: theory and practice.* Boston: Butterworth, 1987:727–742.

Author: Timothy A.S. Sentongo and Andrew E. Mulberg

Classification of Rickets and Vitamin D Metabolite Levels

	CALCIUM	PHOSPHORUS	ALKALINE PHOSPHATE	25 (0)
Deficient synthesis and supply	N or ↓	↓	↑	↓
No sunlight				
Poor diet				
Immaturity				
Malabsorption	N or ↓	↓	↑	↓
Liver disease	N or ↓	↓	↑	↓
Chronic renal failure	N or ↓	↑	↑	N
Vitamin D dependent rickets (recessively inherited)	↓	↓	↑	N
Vitamin D resistant rickets (sex-linked dominant)	N	↓	↑	N
Renal tubular disorders (defect of phosphate reabsorption)	N	↓	↑	N

N, normal; ↓, decreased; ↑, increased.

Rickettsial Disease

 Database

DEFINITION

• The rickettsial diseases are a group of illnesses caused by the *Rickettsiacceae* family of organisms. Despite some minor differences in epidemiologic, clinical, and laboratory characteristics, the illnesses caused by these organisms have similar manifestations and treatment.
• The rickettsial diseases can be divided into subgroups based on clinical presentation: the spotted fever group, the typhus group, Q fever, and ehrlichiosis.
• Because these illnesses are organized primarily by clinical similarities, the "spotted fever group" includes the tick-borne typhus classification.

CAUSES

• The rickettsial illnesses are transmitted to humans via insect vectors such as ticks, fleas, lice, or mites.
• Rickettsial diseases occur in patients of all ages. Rocky Mountain spotted fever (RMSF) has a predilection for children.
• The rickettsial diseases that occur in the United States are RMSF, murine typhus, rickettsi-alpox, epidemic typhus, Q fever, and ehrlichiosis. Note that RMSF is discussed in a separate section.

PATHOLOGY/PATHOPHYSIOLOGY

• For the spotted fever, typhus, and ehrlichiosis groups: vasculitis caused by proliferation of organisms in the endothelial lining of small blood vessels.
• Q fever: pneumonitis.

COMPLICATIONS

• Venous thrombosis
• Pneumonitis
• Pericarditis, myocarditis, heart failure
• Severe disease occurs more commonly in patients with G6PD deficiency, cardiac insufficiency, or immunocompromise.

 Differential Diagnosis

INFECTION

• Before the appearance of the rash, the constitutional symptoms associated with the spotted fevers result in a very wide differential diagnosis. After the appearance of the rash, the diagnoses are more limited: measles; meningococcemia; secondary syphilis; viral infections; coxsackievirus (hand-foot-and-mouth disease); infectious mononucleosis; enteroviral infection.
• Environmental (poisons): drug hypersensitivity reaction (toxicodermatosis)
• Tumors: leukemia with thrombocytopenia
• Immunologic: idiopathic thrombocytopenia purpura (ITP)
• Miscellaneous: leukocytoclastic angiitis; erythema multiforme/Stevens-Johnson syndrome

 Data Gathering

Differentiation between these illnesses listed, depends on the travel history, history of exposure to certain mammals or insects, and the initial clinical presentation of the patient. This clinical presentation is categorized by the grouping: spotted fever group, typhus group, Q fever, and ehrlichiosis.

HISTORY

Question: Fever, headache, and rash?
Significance: In general, rickettsial disease should be considered in a patient with these complaints. The progression of the rash can be particularly helpful in considering the diagnosis.

 Physical Examination

Differentiating clinical findings of each group are described subsequently, and the rashes associated with each illness are described in the table Characteristics of the Generalized Rashes of the Rickettsial Diseases.

• Constitutional symptoms
• Hepatosplenomegaly
• "Tache noir" (black spot): the earliest finding in the spotted fever group originates at the site of the infecting bite; becomes necrotic, forming eschar; regional lymphadenopathy related to eschar; lesion usually found on the head in children and on the legs in adults; is present in between 30% and 90% of cases.

Significance: These symptoms suggest illness caused by the spotted fever group. Tache noir is present in 30% to 90% of cases.

• Impaired level of consciousness
• Myocardial and renal involvement
• Brill-Zinsser disease (BZD) is actually a recrudescence of a previous infection with epidemic (louse-borne) typhus caused by *R. prowazekii*; BZD can occur years after the initial infection and is usually less severe than the initial episode of louse-borne typhus.

Significance: These symptoms suggest illness caused by the typhus group.

• A self-limited febrile illness characterized by headache, myalgias, and chest pain.
• Pulmonary symptoms occur in some form in over 50% of cases: mild pneumonitis/cough usually an incidental finding; radiographically confirmed pneumonia in moderately ill patients; rapidly progressive pneumonia.
• Endocarditis may occur.
• Hepatitis may range in severity.

Characteristics of the Generalized Rashes of the Rickettsial Diseases

	APPEARANCE	DISTRIBUTION	ASSOCIATED FINDINGS
Spotted fever group			*Tache noir* in 30%–90% of patients
Tick typhus	Macular → papular	Extremities → palms/ soles → trunk	
Rickettsialpox	Macular → papular → Vesicles	Extremities → palms/ soles → trunk	
Scrub typhus	Macular	Limited to trunk	Rash of shorter duration lymphadenopathy is a prominent symptom
Typhus group			No *Tache noir*
Epidemic (louse-borne) typhus	Macules → maculopapules → petechiae → hemorrhage	Trunk → extremities	
Murine typhus		Trunk → extremities	Less extensive rash of shorter duration
Miscellaneous			
Q fever	Macular or maculopapular or petechial	Trunk and extremities	No rash
Ehrlichiosis			Rash common in children; rare in adults

- Nervous system findings range from headache to meningitis and encephalitis.

Significance: These symptoms suggest illness caused by *coxiella burnetti,* the organism responsible for Q fever.

- Acute febrile illness characterized by headache, anorexia, and vomiting.
- A relative bradycardia is often noted.
- Leukopenia and thrombocytopenia.

Significance: These symptoms suggest illness caused by Ehrlicia chaffenis, the organism responsible for human ehrlichiosis.

PHYSICAL EXAM TRICKS

Rashes that involve the palms and soles present a limited differential diagnosis. This list includes rickettsial diseases, certain viral infections such as coxsackievirus (hand-foot-and-mouth), syphilis, erythema multiforme, and urticarial rash.

 ## Laboratory Aids

Test: Polymerase chain reaction (PCR)
Significance:

- Allows the identification of rickettsial-specific DNA sequences.
- *R. rickettsii, R. typhi,* and *R. prowazekii*

Test: Immunofluorescent (IgM) tests
Significance:

- Sensitive, specific, and simple.
- Can differentiate acute from past infection.
- This technique is only useful early in the course of *R. tsutsugamushi* (scrub typhus) infection.
- Biopsy of the *tache noir* may reveal rickettsial organisms of the spotted fever group by direct immunofluorescent staining. Similar testing of the generalized rash is not useful for rickettsial illnesses other than RMSF.

Test: Serologic tests

- Complement fixation tests
- Enzyme-linked immunosorbent assay (ELISA)
- Latex agglutination test
- The Weil-Felix reaction assays the patients' serologic response to rickettsiae; the highest titers occur during the second and third weeks of illness; this test will be negative in patients with rickettsialpox and Q fever.
- PCR tests in blood and tissue are available for many rickettsial diseases.

FALSE-POSITIVES

The Weil-Felix reaction may be falsely positive in testing for any of the above organisms.

PITFALLS

The headache associated with rickettsial infections can be severe. However, radiographic imaging is not necessary if there are no signs or symptoms of increased intracranial pressure.

 ## Therapy

EMERGENCY

- Fluid resuscitation for patients who appear moderately to severely ill.
- Antimicrobial therapy should be instituted as soon as the diagnosis is suspected.
- Therapy is most effective if instituted within the first week of illness. There is little benefit in waiting for confirmatory diagnostic tests.

DRUGS

- All of the rickettsial diseases respond rapidly to treatment with tetracycline; the dose is 30 to 40 mg/kg/d orally or 20 mg/kg/d IV in four divided doses (maximum dose of 2 g/d); alternatively, doxycycline may be given at dosage of 100 to 200 mg/d.
- For children under the age of 9 years, *chloramphenicol* is an acceptable alternative therapy. The dose is 100 mg/kg/d up to a maximum dose of 3 g/d.
- Erythromycin and trimethoprim-sulfamethoxizole have been used with variable success against rickettsial infections.

DURATION

The optimum duration of treatment for rickettsial infections has not been determined. In general, the more severe infections warrant 7 to 10 days of antimicrobial therapy.

POSSIBLE CONFLICTS

Prevention

- Except for *R. tsutsugamushi* (scrub typhus) and ehrlichia, all of the rickettsial diseases produce long-term immunity to the etiologic organisms within the same group.
- Fleas, ticks, and mites should be controlled in endemic areas with the appropriate insecticides.
- Clothing to cover the entire body should be worn in tick-infested areas.
- In areas where louse-borne typhus is epidemic, periodic delousing and dusting of insecticide into clothes is recommended.
- No vaccines are currently available in the United States.

 ## Follow-Up

WHEN TO EXPECT IMPROVEMENT

Improvement in the patient's clinical status usually takes place within 1 to 2 days of initiation of therapy. This improvement is delayed in severe cases, particularly if there is endocardial involvement (Q fever) or treatment is begun after the first week of illness.

PITFALLS

- Paradoxical effect of rodenticides: fleas, mites will seek alternate hosts such as humans when mice or rats are "unavailable." Therefore, rodenticides should not be the only prevention measure taken in endemic areas.

 ## Common Questions and Answers

Q: What do I do if I or my child receives a tick bite in an endemic area to rickettsial disease?
A: There is no role for prophylaxis against rickettsial diseases for patients who have suffered tick bites.

Q: Is there are difference between typhoid and typhus?
A: Typhoid, or typhoid fever, is a separate entity from typhus. Typhoid is an enteric infection caused by *Salmonella typhi* and is unrelated to the rickettsial diseases.

Q: If I contract a rickettsial illness, can I get that illness or a similar illness again?
A: With the exception of scrub typhus and ehrlichia, infection with a rickettsial organism confers immunity to other rickettsia within the same group.

ICD-9-CM 083.9

BIBLIOGRAPHY

American Academy of Pediatrics. *1997 red book: report of the committee on infectious diseases.* Elk Grove, IL: American Academy of Pediatrics, 1997.

Boyd AS. Rickettsialpox. *Dermatol Clin* 1997; 15:313–318.

Feigin RD, Snider RL, Edwards MS. Rickettsial diseases. In: Feigin RD, Cherry JD, eds. *Textbook of pediatric infectious diseases,* 3rd ed. Philadelphia: WB Saunders, 1992.

Author: Joel A. Fein

Rocky Mountain Spotted Fever

Database

DEFINITION

• Systemic illness caused by infection with *Rickettsia rickettsii*, carried by tick vectors: wood tick (*Dermacentor andersoni*) in West; dog tick (*Dermacentor variabilis*) in East; Lone star tick (*Amblyomma americanum*) in Southwest

PATHOPHYSIOLOGY

• Transmission usually from tick (reservoir) bite; can be by transfusion and aerosol route

—Usually takes more than 6 hours to be transmitted with tick bite

• Incubation period 2 to 14 days, average approximately 7 days
• After exposure, *Rickettsia* multiply in small vessel endothelium and disseminate via bloodstream, with focal areas of endothelial proliferation, thrombus, blood, and protein leakage
• Local vascular lesions account for signs and symptoms

EPIDEMIOLOGY

• Most prevalent rickettsial disease in United States
• Seasonal (April to September most common) and geographic (0%–20% prevalence in tick population reported)

—Endemic to South Atlantic and West South Central Regions
—Less often seen in Rocky Mountain states
—Also in Mexico, Central, and South America

• Two-thirds of patients less than 15 years of age (usually 5 to 9 years of age)

COMPLICATIONS

• Complications uncommon with early and appropriate treatment
• Neurological sequelae

—More common in children with severely impaired states of consciousness
—Behavioral disturbances and learning disabilities common
—Emotional lability, hyperactivity, memory loss, seizures

• Skin

—Gangrene of extremities, end organs, skin necrosis
—Skin rash usually heals without sequelae

• Hematologic

—Can progress to DIC

• Gastrointestinal

—Hepatic dysfunction
—Hypoalbuminemia from protein loss, hepatic dysfunction, protein leak from damaged vessels

• Cardiac

—Can have persistent cardiac findings, congestive heart failure, cardiovascular collapse

• Metabolic

—Hyponatremia from water shift to intracellular spaces, sodium loss in urine

• Renal

—Acute tubular necrosis

PROGNOSIS

• No known asymptomatic infection

—May be mild if treated early

• Recovery the rule if treated in 1st week
• Case fatality approximately 3% to 7%

—Higher with older age (adult >30 years of age), non-white, male, glucose-6 phosphate diesterase deficiency (G6PD), CNS involvement, renal failure, cardiovascular collapse, late rash, hepatomegaly, jaundice, thrombocytopenia, DIC, inappropriate or delayed antibiotics or diagnosis, no history of tick exposure
—Death usually between 9th and 12th day (fulminant cases with death in 5–6 days)

Differential Diagnosis

• Infection

—Sepsis, meningitis, encephalitis, rubeola, atypical measles, meningococcemia, typhoid fever, leptospirosis, toxic shock, rubella, scarlet fever, disseminated gonococcal disease, *Haemophilus influenzae*, secondary syphilis, rheumatic fever, bacterial pneumonitis, poliomyelitis, pharyngitis, mumps, hepatitis, mononucleosis, enterovirus and other virus infections, fever of unknown origin, ehrlichiosis, other rickettsial disease

• Other

—Immune thrombocytopenic purpura (ITP), thrombotic thrombocytopenic purpura (TTP), immune complex vasculitis, drug reaction, ischemic heart disease, rheumatoid arthritis, erythema multiforme, intra-abdominal process, gastroenteritis, acute surgical abdomen

Data Gathering

HISTORY

Question: Abrupt or gradual onset of fever
Significance: Often unresponsive to antipyretics or antibiotics, headache (retrobulbar, frontal), rash, confusion, myalgia, nausea, vomiting, abdominal pain.

• Classic triad of fever, headache, and rash only in approximately 50%
• Headache: characteristic; intense, persistent night and day, intractable; young child may not complain of headache
• Fever to more than 40°C with oscillations of approximately 2°C
• Onset usually 2 to 8 days post-tick bite
• Tick bite history obtained in only 50% to 70% of cases

Physical Examination

Finding: Rash
Significance: Usually appears by second or third day of illness; may be delayed until sixth day or later; small percentage (10–15%) never develop rash; absence of rash should not delay presumptive diagnosis or appropriate therapy if disease suspected.

• Usually small, irregular, erythematous macules that blanch, become maculopapular and petechial (mixed rash), and confluently hemorrhagic
• Appears first (usually) on wrists and ankles, spreads centrally within hours to extremities to trunk, neck and face; regularly occurs on palms and soles (may be spared) and scrotum; may initially appear on trunk or diffusely in some patients; can progress to necrosis of toes, ears, nose, scrotum, fingers

Finding: CNS
Significance: Meningismus, restless, irritable, apprehensive, confusion, delirium, lethargy, stupor, coma, ataxia, opisthotonos, aphasia, papilledema, seizures, cortical blindness, central deafness, ataxia, spastic paralysis, cranial nerve palsy.

Finding: Cardiac
Significance: CHF, myocarditis, arrhythmias, vascular collapse (often volume related).

Finding: Pulmonary
Significance: Pneumonitis, cough, dyspnea, pulmonary edema, hypoxemia, pleural effusions, alveolar infiltrates.

Finding: Gastrointestinal
Significance: Nausea, vomiting, abdominal pain, diarrhea, hepatomegaly, splenomegaly, anorexia, jaundice, mild pancreatitis.

Finding: Myalgias
Significance: Especially calf or thigh.

Finding: Ocular involvement
Significance: Conjunctivitis, venous engorgement, papilledema, cotton wool spots, retinal hemorrhages, retinal artery occlusion, uveitis.

Finding: Other
Significance: Edema of extremities or face; parotitis, orchitis, pharyngitis.

Laboratory Aids

Make presumptive diagnosis on signs, symptoms, and epidemiologic considerations rather than laboratory aids.

• No quick specific laboratory test; serologic data reliable by days 10 to 12; negative test does not exclude diagnosis.
• Culture impractical and potentially dangerous.

SPECIFIC TESTS

Test: Serology
Significance: Not usually useful in acute management due to time required for serology to become positive (6–10 days after clinical onset of disease).

Test: Probable confirmation
Significance: Fourfold increase in antibody titer by CF, IHA, IFA, LA, MA or single titer of at least 1:320 by Proteus OX-19 or OX-2 (Weil-Felix); 1:128 by LA, IHA, MA, 1:64 by IFA, or at least 1:16 by CF.

Test: Enzyme linked immunosorbent assay (ELISA)
Significance: Sensitive and accurate but not useful until seroconversion at approximately day 6.

Test: Direct immunofluorescence
Significance: Most sensitive and specific but observer bias; can see immunofluorescent *Rickettsia* from skin rash biopsy between days 4 to 8.

Test: Indirect fluorescent antibody (IFA)
Significance: Sensitivity 94% to 100%; specificity 100%.

Test: Indirect hemagglutination (IHA)
Significance: Sensitivity 91% to 100%; specificity 99%.

Test: Latex agglutination (LA)
Significance: Sensitivity 71% to 94%; specificity 96% to 99%; false-positive noted during pregnancy.

Test: DNA polymerase chain reaction (PCA)
Significance: Takes 48 hours but can detect the organism from lesion or blood (depends on organism load, therefore, lesion usually better than blood), specific, low sensitivity.

Test: Weil-Felix
Significance: Non-specific and insensitive, but readily available and rapid (3 to 5 minutes); sensitivity 47% to 70%, specificity 78% to 96%; positive early in course; titer greater than 1:160 suspicious. False positive with proteus infections (UTI), leptospirosis, brucellosis, typhoid fever, liver disease, pregnancy.

Test: Complement fixation (CF)
Significance: Sensitivity 0% to 63%, specificity 100%.

Test: Microagglutination (MA)
Significance: Specific, not sensitive.

NON-SPECIFIC TESTS

Test: CBC, electrolytes, BUN, CR, LFTs, DIC screen, CXR, ABG, EKG, echocardiogram
Significance: WBC normal or low for first 4 to 5 days; after that, leukocytosis (11–30,000/mm³) associated with secondary bacterial disease; elevated band count; anemia (30%); thrombocytopenia (consumptive coagulopathy); hyponatremia; hypoalbuminemia.

Test: CSF
Significance: Usually clear (WBC <10), with or without elevated protein but may see pleocytosis and increased protein in one-third of patients.

 Therapy

- Supportive care very important
- —Volume, electrolyte support as indicated
- Platelets as indicated for thrombocytopenia
- Vitamin K (IM) for prolonged clotting time
- Hyponatremia management with fluid restriction as able (avoid sodium supplements)
- Albumin if indicated

MEDICATIONS

- All rickettsiostatic, not cidal
- —Hinder replication so host can eradicate disease
- —Duration: 7 to 10 days of therapy or until afebrile 2 to 5 days
- Doxycycline (usual medication of choice in all patients, except pregnancy)
- —Dosage: child: 2.2 mg/kg/bid PO for 1 day, then 2.2 mg/kg/d PO in single dose; adult: 100 mg bid PO
- Chloramphenicol
- —Dosage: child: 75 to 100 mg/kg/d IV (initially) (modify if age <1 m), follow by 50 mg/kg/d divided qid; Adult: 500 to 1000 mg qid
- —Side effects: peripheral neuropathy, aplastic anemia, "gray baby syndrome" with high levels, possible association with leukemia, hemolytic anemia with G6PD
- Tetracycline
- —Dosage: child: 25 to 50 mg/kg/d PO divided qid or 20 to 30 mg/kg/d IV; adult: 500 mg qid PO or IV
- —Side effects: tooth discoloration if child less than 8 years of age (dose and duration related); pseudotumor cerebri, photosensitivity reaction
- Corticosteroids
- —May be helpful in severe cases, though no controlled studies
- —Not recommended for mild or moderately ill patients

 Follow-Up

- Expect improvement in 24 to 36 hours and defervescence in 2 to 3 days
- Majority improve if treated early (<1 week)

CONTROL MEASURES

- Avoidance of tick-infested areas and tick contact; pants tucked in boots, limit skin access to ticks, frequent inspection
- Tick repellants
- Early removal; ticks must attach and feed for 4 to 6 or more hours to transmit disease; avoid direct contact with tick during removal; remove tick with tweezers at point of attachment and clean wound

- Vaccine not available in United States; may not prevent disease but does prevent the deaths
- Immunity conferred after disease

PITFALLS

- Not considering diagnosis until rash present; fatal disease often without rash at initial presentation
- Not treating empirically if strong suspicion of diagnosis
- Do not exclude diagnosis even if without history or evidence of tick bite and/or negative serologic test(s)
- Disease may occur outside endemic areas and the usual summer months
- Classic descriptions of RMSF occur in second week. Initial presentations often are not classic

 Common Questions and Answers

Q: For whom should RMSF as a differential diagnosis be entertained?
A: Anyone with a fever during the spring and summer who has been in an RMSF endemic area, regardless of presence of rash or history of known tick bite.

Q: Should a child with a tick bite receive antibiotic prophylaxis when a tick is discovered?
A: To contract disease, one must be bitten by a tick that actually carries the disease (low risk), the tick must transmit the Rickettsia before it is removed (low risk), and the Rickettsia must be pathogenic if inoculated (low risk). There is no evidence that prophylaxis is necessary or efficacious in preventing disease. If considered, one must weigh risks and benefits of the therapy to be used.

ICD-9-CM 082.0

BIBLIOGRAPHY

American Academy of Pediatrics. Rocky Mountain spotted fever. In: Peter G, ed. *1997 Red book: report of the committee of infectious diseases,* 24th ed. Elk Grove Village, IL: American Academy of Pediatrics, 1997:452–454.

Raoult D, Walker DH. Rickettsia rickettsii and other spotted fever group rickettsiae (Rocky Mountain spotted fever and other spotted fevers). In: Mandell GL, Douglas RG Jr., Bennett JE, eds. *Principles and practice of infectious diseases,* 3rd ed. New York: Churchill Livingstone, 1990:1465–1471.

Shapiro ED. Tick-borne diseases. *Adv Pediatr Infect Dis* 1997;13:187–218.

Weber DJ, Walker DH. Rocky Mountain spotted fever. *Infect Dis Clin North Am* 1991;5:19–35.

Author: George Anthony Woodward

Roseola Infantum

 Database

DEFINITION

Roseola infantum is a common illness in preschool-aged children characterized by fever lasting 3 to 7 days followed by rapid defervescence and the appearance of a blanching maculopapular rash (usually on the 4th day of illness) lasting only 1 to 2 days.

CAUSES

• Roseola-like illnesses have been associated with a number of different viruses including enteroviruses (coxsackie virus A and B, echoviruses); adenoviruses (types 1, 2, 3); parainfluenza virus; measles vaccine virus.
• A major cause of roseola appears to be human herpesvirus 6 (HHV-6). HHV-6 is a herpes virus similar to Epstein-Barr virus and cytomegalovirus.
• HHV-6 was first associated with roseola infantum by Yamanishi et al. in 1988.

PATHOPHYSIOLOGY

• Unknown
• The typical pattern of rash appearing as the fever disappears may represent virus neutralization in the skin.

EPIDEMIOLOGY

• Roseola can occur throughout the year; outbreaks have occurred in all seasons of the year.
• Roseola affects children from 3 months to 4 years. The peak age was 7 to 13 months.
• 90% of cases occur in the first 2 years of life.
• Cases occur in males and females equally.
• Incubation period is 5 to 15 days.

COMPLICATIONS

• Seizures are the most common complication of roseola. Between 5% and 10% of children will have a generalized tonic-clonic seizure associated with fever.
• Aseptic meningitis with less than 200 cells with primarily mononuclear cells have been reported.
• Encephalitis
• Thrombocytopenic purpura

PROGNOSIS

The vast majority of children with roseola infantum recover without sequelae.

 Differential Diagnosis

• Roseola has a distinctive presentation but resembles other viral exanthems.
• Antibiotic-associated rash in a child taking oral antibiotics when rash develops after defervescence.
• Rubella and enteroviral infections.

 Data Gathering

HISTORY

Question: Febrile?
Significance: Period of 3 to 5 days. Commonly in the 38.9°C to 40.6°C range (102–105°F).

Question: Rash?
Significance: Appears as the fever disappears and lasts for 1 to 2 days.

Question: Mild cough and coryza?
Significance: Common symptoms.

Question: Appearance?
Significance: Usually children remain alert and are not ill appearing.

Question: Lymphadenopathy?
Significance: In the suboccipital, posterior cervical, and postauricular regions is common.

Question: Eyelid edema and a bulging fontanelle?
Significance: Has also been noted.

Laboratory Aids

Laboratory tests are not helpful in diagnosis. Commercial assays for antibody and/or antigen detection for HHV-6 are being developed.

Test: CBC
Significance: Occasionally, leukopenia with lymphocytosis is noted.

 Therapy

• Supportive care

PREVENTION

• The virus associated with roseola infantum is usually transmitted via respiratory secretions or the fecal/oral spread.
• Outbreaks in hospitals have been reported, and infection control measures, such as bedside secretion precaution, should be instituted.

PITFALLS

• Calling viral exanthems in preschool-aged children roseola even when fever is concomitant with rash

 Common Questions and Answers

Q: When can the child with roseola return to day care?
A: As soon as the child is afebrile, there is no infectious risk of spread. They may return to day care even with rash visible.

Q: Will there be long-term sequelae in the child who has a seizure associated with roseola?
A: In general, these seizures are typical febrile seizures that hold no risk for long-term neurologic sequelae, i.e., epilepsy.

ICD-9-CM 056.9

BIBLIOGRAPHY

American Academy of Pediatrics. Human herpes virus 6. In: Peter G, ed. *1994 Red book: report of the committee on infectious diseases,* 23rd ed. Elk Grove Village, IL: American Academy of Pediatrics, 1994:272–273.

Cherry JD. Roseola infantum. In: Feigin RD, Cherry JD, eds. *Textbook of pediatric infectious diseases,* 3rd ed. Philadelphia: WB Saunders, 1992:1789–1791.

Leach CT, Sumaya CV, Brown NA. Human herpes virus-6: clinical implication of a recently discovered, ubiquitous agent. *J Pediatr* 1991;121:173–181.

Author: Louis M. Bell

Salmonella Infections

Database

DEFINITION

Salmonella is responsible for a broad spectrum of pathologic states ranging from asymptomatic infection to acute gastroenteritis to enteric fever.

EPIDEMIOLOGY

• Three species are responsible for most human salmonellosis: *S. enteriditis* (over 2000 serotypes exist), *S. choleraesuis*, and *S. typhi*.
• Reservoirs

—*Salmonella* species *other* than *S. typhi*: animals and animal products (mammals, birds, reptiles, and insects); contaminated food and water; infected humans (fecal excretion may persist several months).
—Humans are the only natural reservoir for *S. typhi*: most commonly transmitted via fecally contaminated food and water; may be transmitted congenitally; chronic carriers may excrete *S. typhi* in stool for years.

• Incubation period

—*Salmonella* species *other* than *S. typhi*: 6 to 72 hours; symptoms typically begin within 24 hours

• Incubation period of invasive *Salmonella* strains and *S. typhi* is 1 to 3 weeks.
• Age distribution: children under 5 and the elderly most commonly infected with nontyphoidal *Salmonella*; *S. typhi* most common in 5 to 25 year olds.

COMPLICATIONS

• Dehydration and/or electrolyte imbalance is the most common complication arising from acute gastroenteritis.
• Invasive *Salmonella* may lead to complications of bacteremia:

—Sepsis: most common in neonates and immunosuppressed individuals
—Meningitis: vast majority of cases occur in first month of life
—Osteomyelitis: most common in patients with sickle cell anemia
—Other local infections: pneumonia, pericarditis

• Complications of enteric fever include intestinal or splenic rupture (at areas of lymphoid hypertrophy), hepatitis, pancreatitis, parotitis, orchitis, arthritis, myocarditis.
• A post-infectious form of hemolytic uremic syndrome may occur following *Salmonella* infection.

PROGNOSIS

• Most normal hosts with *Salmonella* gastroenteritis will recover spontaneously.
• Some individuals will develop a chronic carrier state, persistently shedding bacteria in the stool.

• The relapse rate of enteric fever may approach 15% of patients.

ASSOCIATED ILLNESSES

• Acute asymptomatic infection

—No clinical signs or symptoms become apparent.
—Probably most common *Salmonella* syndrome
—Patients can be identified only by recovery of organisms in stool.

• Acute gastroenteritis

—*Salmonella* is the most common type of infectious "food poisoning" in the United States.
—Symptoms begin 6–48 hours after Salmonella ingestion.
—Predominant manifestations are nausea, vomiting, crampy (often severe) abdominal pain, diarrhea (rarely, gross blood can be found).
—Other common features are malaise, myalgia, headache, fever.
—Symptoms usually resolve spontaneously in 2 to 7 days.

• Bacteremia

—*Salmonella* organisms may produce acute or intermittent bacteremia.
—Symptoms: fever/chills, diaphoresis, myalgia, anorexia
—Bacteremia may occur before clinical gastroenteritis or, in infants, present as a persistent bacteremic state with failure to thrive.
—Up to 1 in 20 patients with *Salmonella* gastroenteritis may develop bacteremia (perhaps as high as 1 in 4 in infants).

• Enteric fever (typhoid fever, paratyphoid fever)

—Caused by *S. typhi* and several other *Salmonella* serotypes
—Incubation period 1 to 3 weeks
—Insidious onset of symptoms over 2 to 7 days: fever as high as 41°C, malaise, anorexia, abdominal pain, constipation.
—Additional symptoms and signs: lethargy, myalgia, headache, cough, either diarrhea or constipation, rigors, delirium, lymphadenopathy, organomegaly, "rose spots"
—Progression of illness: when untreated, illness with high fevers may last weeks; severe morbidity or death can result from especially virulent *Salmonella* strains.

• Asymptomatic chronic carriage

—Approximately 1% of patients infected with *Salmonella* gastroenteritis or enteric fever will continue to shed *Salmonella* in the stool for more than 1 year.

Differential Diagnosis

The following illnesses may mimic *Salmonella* gastroenteritis and/or enterocolitis:

• *Shigellosis*: severe abdominal pains often are present, associated with high fevers, ulcers of

the gastrointestinal lining are common, stools are often grossly bloody with "sheets" of fecal leukocytes
• *Staphylococcal* food poisoning
• Other bacterial infections of the gastrointestinal tract.
• Viral enteritis: rotavirus, Norwalk virus, and other viruses
• Parasitic infections
• Toxic ingestion
• Non-infectious systemic illnesses marked by inflammatory colitis

Enteric fever from Salmonella infection may be confused with:

• Invasive bacterial disease
• Spirochetal infection

Data Gathering

HISTORY

• Exposure?
• Common historical features of Salmonella gastroenteritis:

—Nausea and vomiting begin 6 to 48 hours after ingestion.
—Diarrhea and abdominal pain with tenesmus follow; pain is typically periumbilical and in the right lower quadrant.
—Diarrhea lasts 2 to 4 days
—Fever seldom exceeds 39°C; occurs in one-half of affected patients.

• Common historical features of enteric fever

—Symptoms begin 3 to 60 days after exposure.
—Commonly acquired during foreign travel.
—Diarrhea uncommon early in course.
—Fever ensues, which gradually increases in magnitude.
—Malaise, anorexia, myalgia, headache, abdominal pain and vomiting may occur.

Physical Examination

Salmonella gastrointestinal disease may display certain features:

• Dehydration may be evident.
• Abdominal pain may closely mimic appendicitis and/or cholecystitis.
• Stools may be bloody, watery, or mucousy.

Finding: Important signs of enteric fever
Significance:

• Enlarged liver and spleen.
• Relative bradycardia for height of fever is a frequently distinguishing finding.
• Rose spots: 2 to 4 mm in diameter; blanching pink papules; most commonly found on anterior thorax; 5 to 20 are generally apparent at a time; fade in 3 to 4 days after appearance; characteristic of enteric fever, but not specific.

Laboratory Aids

There are several non-specific laboratory aids to diagnosis:

Test: Stool examination
Significance: May have hemoccult-positive stools; stool may be positive for fecal leukocytes in enterocolitis

Test: Complete blood cell count with differential
Significance: Normal in simple gastroenteritis; neutropenia, thrombocytopenia, and mild anemia are common in enteric fever.

Test: Serum chemistries
Significance: Metabolic acidosis and electrolyte abnormalities may occur with severe enteritis; a mild hepatitis is frequently found in enteric fever.

Test: Stool and blood culture and identification of *Salmonella* organisms
Significance: The "gold-standard" method for laboratory confirmation of infection.

Test: Bone marrow aspirate
Significance: The most sensitive source for isolation of *Salmonella* in patients with enteric fever; early in the course of invasive illness bone marrow culture may be positive even when stool samples fail to grow the bacteria; may provide positive cultures even after initial antibiotic pretreatment.

Test: Urine culture
Significance: May be a source of *Salmonella* organisms in the young or elderly and in those with enteric fever.

Test: Biopsy
Significance: Needle aspiration of purulent material may yield positive cultures; punch biopsy and culture of rose spots may confirm diagnosis of *S. typhi.*

FALSE-POSITIVES

Leukocytes in the stool are suggestive of colitis but are more typical of *Campylobacter, Shigella,* or milk allergy.

PITFALLS

Enteric fever may precede enteritis symptoms and fecal shedding of bacteria.

Therapy

• Acute asymptomatic infection

—Should not be treated with antibiotics: antibiotics do not impact duration of diarrhea and may lengthen duration of carrier state.

• Acute gastroenteritis (*see* Common Questions and Answers)

—Supportive care: maintain intravascular volume; correct electrolyte abnormalities

—Do *not* administer antidiarrheal agents, they prolong gastrointestinal transit time.
—Consider antibiotics in individuals at high risk of subsequent systemic invasive illness: children less than 3 months of age; immunocompromised hosts; patients with hemoglobinopathies; patients with chronic gastrointestinal tract disease.

• Bacteremia, enteric fever, and/or chronic carrier state:

—Supportive care.
—Antibiotics *are* indicated; initial therapy usually to be administered intravenously.
—Surgical drainage of local suppuration is indicated as in most other infections.
—Corticosteroids (3 mg/kg load, 1 mg/kg every 6 hours) may be beneficial to critically ill patients with enteric fever exhibiting neurological complications.
—Antipyretics are controversial in enteric fever syndromes because they may cause precipitous declines in temperature and shock.

• Various antibiotics may be used to treat *Salmonella* infection:

—*Salmonella* gastroenteritis at high risk of invasive disease: increasing resistance to amoxicillin, ampicillin and trimethoprim-sulfa; parenteral third-generation cephalosporins or fluoroquinolones preferred.
—Invasive *Salmonella* disease: intravenous ampicillin for 2 weeks has been first-line therapy; chloramphenicol, a third-generation cephalosporin, or a quinolone may be used for resistant organisms; cefotaxime for treatment of meningitis; meningitis or osteomyelitis may require 4 to 6 weeks of parenteral antibiotic therapy.
—Some authorities treat chronic carriers of *Salmonella* who shed more than 1 year: high-dose parenteral ampicillin; high-dose oral amoxicillin (with or without probenecid), ciprofloxacin; consider cholecystectomy for recalcitrant cases.

PREVENTION

Personal hygiene and sanitation measures are the primary means by which to prevent *Salmonella* infections:

• Carriers of *Salmonella* are a public health concern:

—Hospitalized patients: enteric precautions for length of illness.
—Outpatients: should be restricted from food preparation for others.

Follow-Up

• Acute gastrointestinal illness

—Symptoms usually resolve spontaneously within 7 days.
—Supportive care to prevent or treat dehydration may be required.
—Young children and those with underlying disease processes may be at higher risk of complications.

• Enteric fever

—Untreated, this illness will have a prolonged course over weeks.
—Life-threatening complications are most common during the second or third week of illness, often after a period of apparent clinical improvement.
—Even with appropriate treatment up to 15% of patients may suffer relapse.

• Chronic carriage

—1% to 3% of patients with *Salmonella* infection will shed bacteria in the stool for longer than 1 year.
—Chronic carriers should be identified because they represent a public health threat.

PITFALLS

• More people with *Salmonella* infestation are asymptomatic than are symptomatic.
• Antibiotic resistance is a growing problem.
• Even with appropriate therapy, patients may shed bacteria on a persistent basis or may suffer relapse.

Common Questions and Answers

Q: Should all infants with *Salmonella* gastroenteritis be treated with antibiotics?
A: Clinicians caring for children less than 1 year of life with proven, or suspected, *Salmonella* infection face many treatment dilemmas. Any toxic appearing infant, and any infant with proven *Salmonella* bacteremia, should be admitted to the hospital for parenteral antibiotics. High-risk infants (those under 3 months of age) with positive stool cultures should be treated with antibiotics after obtaining blood cultures. Well-appearing infants above the age of 3 months with *Salmonella* enterocolitis and fever can be observed off antibiotics once surveillance blood cultures are obtained.

ICD-9-CM 003.9

BIBLIOGRAPHY

Goldberg MB, Rubin RH. The spectrum of Salmonella infection. *Infect Dis Clin North Am* 1988; 2:571–598.

St. Geme JW, Hodes HL, Marcy M, et al. Consensus: management of Salmonella infection in the first year of life. *Pediatr Infect Dis J* 1988;7: 615–621.

Nataro JP. Treatment of bacterial enteritis. *Pediatr Infect Dis J* 1998;17:420–421.

Author: Kevin C. Osterhoudt

Sarcoidosis

 Database

DEFINITION

- A multisystem chronic granulomatous disease that has two distinct variations differentiated by age of onset

CAUSES

- Unknown

PATHOLOGY

- A T cell-mediated disease, resulting in non-caseating granulomas in affected organs epidemiology.
- Disease occurs before age 4 as arthritis, uveitis, fever, and rash, and in adolescence as Lofgren syndrome of erythema nodosum, periarthritis, and hilar adenopathy. Adult type disease with marked pulmonary involvement may also occur in older adolescents.

GENETICS

Blacks are more commonly affected than whites; specific genetic tendencies not identified.

COMPLICATIONS

- In children usually related to uveitis, or from hypercalciuria resulting in renal injury. In older adolescents, pulmonary problems such as restrictive lung disease can occur.

 Differential Diagnosis

- Infection: tuberculosis, bacterial sepsis, mumps, HIV, gonorrhea, Lyme disease, pulmonary mycoses
- Tumors: leukemia, neuroblastoma, lymphoma
- Immunologic: systemic JRA, SLE, dermatomyositis, Behçet syndrome

 Data Gathering

HISTORY

Question: Malaise, fever, rash, evanescent painful arthritis, swollen lymph nodes, cough, and hematuria?
Significance: May be initial complaints.

 Physical Examination

- Peripheral lymphadenopathy is most common manifestation
- Eyes may be infected
- Bilateral parotid gland enlargement and hepatosplenomegaly can be present
- The arthritis, usually in the ankles, is extremely tender
- Rash is diffuse, erythematous, and macular, or plaque-like.

SPECIAL QUESTIONS

Finding: History of papule?
Significance: Forming after needlestick (pathergy).

 Laboratory Aids

- CBC
- ESR
- Synovial effusions are typically non-inflammatory

Biopsy of peripheral lymph gland, skin, conjunctivae, or minor salivary gland demonstrating noncaseating granuloma is helpful.

Test: ACE level (angiotensin-converting enzyme)
Significance: Produced in most granulomatous diseases, but is useful where index of suspicion is high.

Test: Serum calcium and creatinine levels
Significance: Are important for baseline.

Test: Urine for blood
Significance: Seen in patients with hypercalciuria.

IMAGING

Test: CXR
Significance: May demonstrate hilar adenopathy.

Test: Gallium scan
Significance: Will demonstrate uptake diffusely in lungs (extremely sensitive test).

FALSE-POSITIVES

Test: ACE level
Significance: May be elevated in patients with miliary TB and biliary cirrhosis. Not a good single-screening test; however, can follow levels in response to treatment.

PITFALLS

Uveitis may be occult; ophthalmology evaluation is important.

Therapy

DRUGS

Non-steroidal anti-inflammatory drugs, analgesics, and steroids all have a role. In rare cases of chronic disease, immunosuppressive drugs may have a role. In cases of hypercalciuria/hypercalcemia, hydration, and lasix should be considered.

DURATION

• During times of disease activity causing clinical symptoms

DIET

Hydration is important in patients with hypercalcemia.

 Follow-Up

WHEN TO EXPECT IMPROVEMENT

Early childhood sarcoid and Lofgren syndrome typically resolve in a few months. Rarely, older children with pulmonary manifestations will develop chronic interstitial lung disease or bony infiltrates.

SIGNS TO WATCH FOR

• Climbing creatinine, shortness of breath, or persistent uveal tract inflammation

PROGNOSIS

• Generally good for most children. Lofgren disease resolves. Over 40% of older children with adult type disease have persistent pulmonary changes, but only a few will have pulmonary symptoms.

PITFALLS

• Overtreatment of asymptomatic lymphadenopathy and not detecting hypercalciuria

 Common Questions and Answers

Q: Why is the outcome better in childhood sarcoid compared with adults with sarcoid?
A: These may be two distinct granulomatous diseases. The two clearly have different patterns of organ involvement.

ICD-9-CM 135.0

BIBLIOGRAPHY

Hetherington S. Sarcoidosis in young children. *Am J Dis Child* 1982;136:13–15.

Pattishall EN, Kendig EL Jr. Sarcoidosis in children. *Pediatr Pulmonol* 1996;22(3):195–203.

Pattishall EN, Strope GL, Spinola SM, Denny FW. Childhood sarcoidosis. *J Pediatr* 1986;108: 169–177.

Author: Gregory F. Keenan

Scabies

 Database

DEFINITION

- Infestation of the stratum corneum by the human mite, *Sarcoptes scabiei* (subspecies hominis, phylum arthropoda, class arachnida, and order acarina). Etiologic agent is the gravid female mite, 0.2 to 0.4 mm in size.
- "Animal scabies," sarcoptic mange, occurs from contact with an infested canine and produces only a transient rash in humans.
- "Norwegian scabies," a variant of human scabies, occurs in institutional settings and is highly contagious, requiring isolation measures and diligent use of anti-scabetics for elimination.
- "Post-scabetic syndrome" consists of persistent pruritus, caused by hypersensitivity to mite antigen, and may persist for several days after the live mite has been eliminated.

PATHOPHYSIOGY

- The female mite burrows into the stratum corneum, rarely penetrating through the epidermis for 15 to 30 days traveling 2 to 4 mm per day and laying 1 to 3 eggs per day.
- Egg laying is completed in 4 to 5 weeks when the female dies within the burrow. Eggs, hatching within the burrow, will undergo several molts and emerge on the skin surface as nymphs. After a 2- to 3-week maturation period, mating will occur; the male will die, and the gravid female will restart the cycle with burrowing.
- 10 to 30 days after scabies infestation, perhaps the time lag necessary for the body to develop humoral or cellular hypersensitivity to the mite and/or its byproducts or the time necessary for an adequate mass of mites to exist, signs and symptoms will develop.

EPIDEMIOLOGY

- Affects all age groups
- Epidemics are reported to occur in 15-year cycles
- Sole reservoir of *Sarcoptes scabiei* is the human
- Close personal contact with an infested human (with or without clinical symptoms) is required for transmission
- Mite can live isolated from a human body for 2 to 3 days; however, the extent of fomite transmission is unclear

COMPLICATIONS

- Secondary infections, including impetigo and folliculitis
- Pruritus is often intense

PROGNOSIS

- Excellent with therapy. Resistant cases, necessitating referral to a dermatologists and consideration for oral therapy, have been reported.

 Differential Diagnosis

INFECTION

- Impetigo
- Papular viral exanthem

ENVIRONMENTAL

- Contact dermatitis

IMMUNOLOGIC

- Atopic dermatitis
- Papular urticaria

MISCELLANEOUS

- Drug eruptions
- Psoriasis
- Infantile acropustolosis

 Data Gathering

HISTORY

Question: Pruritus
Significance: Intensity worse at night when mite activity increases secondary to a rise in body temperature.

Question: Evolution of the rash
Significance: Characteristically changes over time both in appearance and distribution.

Question: Symptoms in other family members or close contacts?
Significance: Close contact is required for transmission.

 Physical Examination

- Examine the entire body surface area with particular attention to the web spaces in hands.
- Distribution of the rash is usually from the neck down in young infants and children the scalp and face may be involved.
- Lesions are typically more numerous on the hands, especially the web spaces, as well as the thenar and hypothenar eminences in older children and adults. The palms and proximal half of the foot and heel are sites of numerous lesions in infants.
- Lesions are also seen on the wrists, in the axillae, around the waistline, on the gluteal cleft, and surrounding the nipples and genitalia.
- A burrow is present in 90% to 95% of all symptomatic patients, characteristic lesion of scabies and forms a "lazy S" shape with a broad base and a punctate brown-black dot at the leading edge of the mites' path. If burrows not easily identified, washable felt tip marker can be rubbed across the web space (after the superficial ink is removed with alcohol or water, the ink will have penetrated through the stratum corneum outlining the burrow).
- Secondary lesions are more numerous and obvious than the burrows and consist of crusted papules, small vesicles, pustules, excoriated broad areas of dermatitis, and areas of secondary infection from impetigo and folliculitis.

 Laboratory Aids

Skin scrapings may be done to secure a definitive diagnosis. The burrows (most commonly found on the hands and feet) should be moistened with alcohol or mineral oil. A number 15 round-bellied blade attached to a scalpel handle should be briskly scraped across the burrows. Scraped material is placed on a slide with a drop of KOH or mineral oil with a coverslip. Under a scanning microscope the gravid female, eggs, larvae, or feces are diagnostic.

Therapy

DRUGS

- 5% Permethrin cream (Elimite): for infants older than 2 months and children. Apply to entire body surface and leave on for 8 to 12 hours and then wash off. One application is usually effective, although some recommend a second application 10 to 14 days later.
- 1% Lindane: effective for older children and nonpregnant adults; should remain on the body for 6 to 8 hours. Lindane use in young children is considered to be potentially toxic and is generally not recommended in young children.
- 10% Crotamiton cream: applied daily for 5 consecutive days (infants older than 6 months).
- 6% sulfur in a petrolatum base: applied for three consecutive 24-hour periods in older children and adults.
- Mild-to-moderate topical steroids (e.g., 1% hydrocortisone, 0.025–0.1% triamcinolone): may be beneficial in post-scabetic syndrome.
- Oral agents, such as ivermectin: used in adult patients for resistant scabies; however, referral to a dermatologist is recommended prior to the consideration of oral therapy to verify the diagnosis and to assess treatment alternatives other than oral therapy.

 Follow-Up

- Pruritus may take up to 4 weeks to resolve after effective treatment. Use of a mild-to-moderate topical steroid may improve these symptoms.
- Continued appearance of new burrows may indicate ineffective treatment (most commonly misapplication) and warrants repeat physician evaluation.

PREVENTION

- Bedding, clothing, and items of close contact should be washed and dried in hot temperatures at the time of treatment.
- All family members and close contacts should be treated concurrently regardless of clinical symptoms. Contacts may be infested without symptoms.

PITFALLS

Need to treat close contacts, symptomatic and asymptomatic, to eliminate the mite and prevent immediate reinfestation.

 Common Questions and Answers

Q: How did my child get scabies?
A: From close contact with an infested person.

Q: How long will my child continue to itch?
A: Pruritis may continue for weeks; the use of topical hydrocortisone may be helpful.

Q: Do I need to wash my child's bedding in a special detergent?
A: Simply wash all bedding in hot soapy water after your child has been treated.

ICD-9-CM 133.0

BIBLIOGRAPHY

American Academy of Pediatrics. Scabies. In: Peter G, ed. *1997 Red book: report of the committee on infectious diseases*, 24th ed. Elk Grove Village, IL: American Academy of Pediatrics; 1997:468–470.

Dourmishev AL, Serafimova DK, Dourmishev LA, et al. Crusted scabies of the scalp in dermatomyositis patients: three cases treated with oral ivermectin. *Int J Dermatol* 1998;37(3): 231–234.

Rasmussen JE. Scabies. *Pediatr Rev* 1994;15(3): 110–114.

Author: Kathy Wholey Zsolway

Scarlet Fever

 Database

DEFINITION

• A clinical syndrome consisting of fever, pharyngitis, cervical lymphadenitis, and the characteristic "sandpaper rash," which results from infection with a strain of *Streptococcus pyogenes* (group A β-hemolytic streptococcus) that elaborates streptococcal pyrogenic toxin.
• Toxins include: A, B, or C. Toxin A is associated with more virulent disease.

PATHOPHYSIOLOGY

• Susceptible individuals thought to lack toxin-specific immunity. Supported by results of "Dick test" in which a small amount of toxin introduced intradermally produces local erythema in susceptible individuals, but no reaction in those with toxin-specific immunity.
• Currently, rash and other toxic manifestations of scarlet fever have been attributed to the development of hypersensitivity to the toxin, which would, therefore, require prior exposure to the toxin.
• Toxin production is dependent on lysogeny of the infecting streptococcus by a temperate bacteriophage.
• Pharyngitis characterized by mucosal erythema and frequently by small crypt abscesses with punctate exudate in enlarged tonsils.
• Edematous papillae protrude from coated mucosa to produce "strawberry tongue."
• Histologic examination of affected skin shows dilated blood and lymphatic vessels and engorged capillaries, most prominently around hair follicles.
• Acute, edematous polymorphonuclear inflammatory reaction is seen microscopically within affected tissues.
• Epidermal inflammatory reaction is usually followed by hyperkeratosis, which accounts for scaling during defervescence.

EPIDEMIOLOGY

• Peak incidence during the first few school years.
• Rarely occurs before the age of 3 years or after the age of 15 years, possibly related to the requirement for prior sensitization and toxin-specific immunity.
• By age 10, 80% of children have developed toxin-specific antibodies.
• No sex predilection.
• All forms of streptococcal pharyngitis (i.e., with or without pyrogenic toxin) are more common in temperate and cold climates, and winter and spring months with some areas reporting an increased incidence in the fall.
• Incubation period is usually 24 to 48 hours.

COMPLICATIONS

• Acute otitis media
• Sinusitis
• Suppurative cervical lymphadenitis.
• Pneumonia with or without effusion/empyema.
• Peritonsillar cellulitis/abscess
• Retropharyngeal abscess
• Meningitis
• Brain abscess
• Thrombosis of intracranial venous sinuses
• Osteomyelitis
• Hepatitis
• Arthritis
• Acute rheumatic fever (ARF)
• Acute post-infectious glomerulonephritis (APGN)
• Erythema nodosum, possibly

PROGNOSIS

• Overall prognosis is excellent.
• Few patients suffer suppurative complications.
• Risk of developing ARF in untreated streptococcal infections is about 3% under epidemic conditions (0.3% in endemic situations).
• Risk of developing APGN depends on nephritogenicity of infecting strain. Attack rate is 10% to 15% with nephritogenic strains.

 Differential Diagnosis

• Non-scarlatinal streptococcal pharyngitis/tonsillitis
• Viral exanthems (measles, rubella, erythema infectiosum)
• Drug eruptions
• Staphylococcal scalded skin syndrome (SSSS)
• Toxic epidermal necrolysis (TEN)
• Toxic shock syndrome (streptococcal or staphylococcal)
• Kawasaki disease

UNCOMMON ENTITIES

• Infection with *Corynebacterium hemolyticum*
• Mercury poisoning (acrodynia)
• Atropine intoxication
• Boric acid poisoning
• Rifampin overdose

 Data Gathering

HISTORY

Question: Was there sudden onset of fever up to 40.5°C, sore throat, headache, nausea, vomiting and toxicity?
Significance: Classic for group A streptococcal disease.

Question: Does the rash feel like sandpaper?
Significance: Texture is more important than appearance.

Question: When did the rash start?
Significance: Characteristic rash typically occurs 12 to 48 hours after onset of fever.

Question: Any abdominal pain or muscle aches prior to rash?
Significance: May complain of abdominal pain before onset of rash, as well as aching in extremities or back.

Question: Any close contacts with streptococcal infection?
Significance: Helps in identification.

 Physical Examination

Finding: Fine maculopapular (sandpaper texture) rash on erythematous background.
Significance: Usually begins on the trunk and spreads to involve almost the entire body within hours to days.

Finding: Circumoral pallor present.
Significance: Classic finding.

Finding: Rash blanches with pressure and ultimately desquamates.
Significance: Desquamation occurs within 7 to 21 days from onset of illness.

Finding: Characteristic toxin-induced scarlet fever exanthem.
Significance: Can rarely be seen without pharyngitis in the setting of pyoderma or an infected wound (known as "surgical scarlet fever").

Finding: May see scattered petechiae.
Significance: Common finding.

Finding: Systemic toxicity.
Significance: May indicate incorrect diagnosis.

Finding: Deep red non-blanching lesions.
Significance: "Pastia lines," develop in the skin folds of joints.

Finding: Dorsum of tongue.
Significance: Has white coat early in illness with edematous red papillae. White covering desquamates and reveals swollen, red and mottled "strawberry tongue."

Other findings

• Pharynx and tonsils are beefy red and may contain exudate.
• Hemorrhagic spots on interior pillar of tonsils and soft palate.
• Large, tender anterior cervical nodes.

Laboratory Aids

Test: Rapid streptococcal antigen tests
Significance: Effective as screening tests; 50% to 80% sensitivity and greater than 95% specificity. Positive rapid tests do not require culture confirmation.

Test: Throat culture
Significance: For group A β-hemolytic streptococci is still the "gold standard" with best sensitivity (>90%). A culture should be performed when rapid test is negative.

Test: White blood cell count
Significance: Usually elevated, though may be elevated in viral pharyngitis as well. Low count would be rare with streptococcal infection.

Test: Eosinophilia (up to 30%)
Significance: Is common in the recovery phase.

Test: Dick test
Significance: Of historic interest, no longer used clinically.

Therapy

• Identical to therapy for streptococcal pharyngitis.
• Therapy started as late as 9 days after illness onset should be effective in preventing ARF.
• May withhold treatment until throat culture result is available.
• Immediate therapy probably shortens symptomatic period.

DRUGS

• Oral penicillin V: drug of choice except in penicillin-allergic individuals. Resistant strains have not been documented in the US. Dose: 25,000 – 50,000 Units/kg (1600 units = 1 mg) divided into 3 to 4 doses for 10 days. 400,000 Units (250 mg) twice daily for 10 days was shown to have comparable efficacy in a recent clinical trial, and has been recommended by the American Academy of Pediatrics.
• Intramuscular benzathine penicillin G: equally effective as oral penicillin. Dose: 600,000 Units for children less than 60 pounds. 1,200,000 Units in larger children and adults. Assures compliance. Bringing to room temperature reduces discomfort. Benzathine/Procaine penicillin combinations are less painful.

• Oral erythromycin is indicated in penicillin-allergic individuals. Dose: erythromycin ethyl succinate (40 to 50 mg/kg/d in two to four divided doses). Resistance is rare in the United States.
• Clarithromycin (10 day regimen) and azithromycin (5 day regimen) have also shown excellent clinical and bacteriologic cure rates in recent clinical trials.
• Amoxicillin, clindamycin, and first-generation oral cephalosporins (up to 15% of penicillin-allergic persons are also allergic to cephalosporins) are reasonable alternatives to penicillin.
• Tetracyclines and sulfonamides should *not* be used due to resistance.
• Recent trials comparing 10 day course of penicillin with shorter duration of therapy with newer oral cephalosporins have shown similar bacteriologic and clinical cure rates, but efficacy in prevention of nonsuppurative sequelae is unknown.
• Positive post-treatment cultures in asymptomatic patients: retreatment not recommended.

Follow-Up

• Fever and symptoms usually resolve within 24 to 48 hours of antibiotic treatment.
• Non-suppurative complications occur after unrecognized disease and when treatment is delayed for more than 9 days. ARF occurs an average of 18 days after untreated infection. APGN occurs an average of 10 days after untreated infection.

PREVENTION

• Prompt treatment leads to fewer secondary cases of streptococcal disease.
• Chemoprophylaxis with penicillin recommended by some experts in children with repeated documented episodes occurring at short intervals.

PITFALLS

• A positive throat culture may only be evidence of carriage in some cases of pharyngitis that are truly viral (e.g., Epstein Barr virus).
• Milder disease is becoming more common, and is easier to miss. Rash may only involve the bridge of the nose, face, shoulders and upper chest. Circumoral pallor and severe exudative pharyngitis are being seen less frequently.

Common Questions and Answers

Q: Should household contacts have throat cultures performed?
A: Only obtain cultures from symptomatic household contacts. Cultures should not routinely be obtained in asymptomatic contacts.

Q: Should post-treatment throat cultures be performed?
A: Only in symptomatic individuals and patients at risk for ARF and APGN.

Q: How soon can children return to school or day care?
A: When they are afebrile after at least 24 hours of therapy.

ICD-9-CM 034.1

BIBLIOGRAPHY

American Academy of Pediatrics. Group A Streptococcal infections. In: Peter G, ed. *1997 red book: report of the committee on infectious diseases*, 24th ed. Elk Grove Village, IL: American Academy of Pediatrics 1997:483–494.

Barnett BO, Frieden IJ. Streptococcal skin diseases in children. *Semin Dermatol* 1992; 11:3–10.

Bialecki C, Feder HM Jr., Grant-Kels JM. The six classic childhood exanthems: a review and update. *J Am Acad Dermatol* 1989;21:891–903.

Breese BB. Streptococcal pharyngitis and scarlet fever. *Am J Dis Child* 1978;132:612–616.

Klein JO. Management of streptococcal pharyngitis. *Pediatr Infect Dis J* 1994;13:572–575.

Pichichero ME, McLinn SE, Gooch WM, et al. Ceftibuten vs. penicillin V in group A beta-hemolytic streptococcal pharyngitis. *Pediatr Infect Dis J* 1995;14:S102–S107.

Sarkissian A, Papazian M, Azatian G, Arikiants N, Babloyan A, Leumann E. An epidemic of acute postinfectious glomerulonephritis in Armenia. *Arch Dis Child* 1997;77(4):342–344.

Shulman ST. Evaluation of penicillins, cephalosporins, and macrolides for therapy of streptococcal pharyngitis. *Pediatrics* 1996;97:955–959.

Stollerman GH. The historical role of the Dick test. *JAMA* 1983;250:3097–3099.

Wannamaker LW. Streptococcal toxins. *Rev Infect Dis* 1983;5(Suppl. 4):S723–S732.

Authors: Adam Cohen and Mark L. Bagarazzi

Scleroderma

Database

DEFINITION

Scleroderma means hard skin.

• Systemic (SSc) or progressive systemic sclerosis

—Diagnostic criteria: 1 major or 2 minor

—Major: sclerodermatous changes (tightness, thickening, induration) proximal to the MCP or MTP
—Minor: sclerodactyly-sclerodermatous changes limited to the digits: digital pitting; bibasilar pulmonary fibrosis not due to primary lung disease
—CREST (a variant form of SSc)

—Calcinosis
—Raynaud phenomenon
—Esophageal dysmotility
—Sclerodactyly
—Telangiectases
—Affects approximately one-half of patients with SSc
—Females more than males
—Earlier age of onset than SSc
—Same characteristics as SSc, but calcinosis is more severe
—Distal symptoms are more severe
—Associated with anti-centromere antibody

• Localized: fibrosis limited to the skin, subcutaneous tissue, and muscle

—Systemic features
—Rare: visceral involvement later in the disease
—Occasional: evolution into another connective tissue disease such as MCTD or SLE
—Very rarely: Raynaud

—Forms
—Morphea: one or more oval or round indurations that become hard and whitish early on, have active inflammatory border with violaceous color, forms: plaque or guttate, limited number of lesions; generalized: extensive; nodular: subcutaneous
—Linear: one or more linear areas affecting subcutaneous tissue, muscle, and bone
—Coup de sabre: involving face or scalp may be associated with seizures
—Parry-Romberg syndrome: form of linear scleroderma; congenital dysplasia of the subcutaneous tissue, neurologic changes such as TIAs.

PATHOPHYSIOLOGY

The following theories have been proposed:

• Alteration of normal glycosylation and hydroxylation of collagen
• Serum factors: endothelin
• Vasculopathy: based on high association with Raynaud
• Immune dysfunction: autoimmunity directed against connective tissue antigen such as laminin or type IV collagen

• May represent distinct early and late processes:

—Early: increase of hydrophilic glycosaminoglycan; increased T cells, macrophages, and plasma cells; mast cell hyperplasia
—Late: increase collagen content; collagen is embryonic with narrow fibrils and immature cross banding; atrophy of rete pegs

EPIDEMIOLOGY

• Systemic

—Incidence: annually 4.5 to 12 million
—Age of onset: 30 to 50 years; very rare in children
—Sex ratio: less than 8 years no difference; older than 8 years, 3:1 F:M; 15 to 44 years, 15:1 F:M
—Genetics: unknown

• Localized

—More common than SSc
—Exact incidence is unclear

COMPLICATIONS

• Systemic

—see Physical Examination

• Localized

—Skin thickening
—Joint contractures
—Leg length discrepancies

PROGNOSIS

• Natural course includes several phases: initial: inflammation; late: sclerotic, occasional regression over 3 to 5 years
• Ultimate prognosis depends on severity of skin tightness, joint contracture, and visceral involvement
• Mortality: Males more than females and non-whites more than whites
• Most common cause of death in children is secondary to cardiac, renal, and pulmonary complications

Differential Diagnosis

• Graft versus host disease
• Phenylketonuria
• *Borrelia* infection: acrodermatitis chronica atrophicans
• Porphyria cutanea tarda

Data Gathering

HISTORY

• Thickening of skin
• Tightness of joints
• Discoloration of skin
• Often insidious onset
• Morning stiffness
• Heartburn, dysphagia, reflux, cough with swallowing

Physical Examination

Finding: Skin
Significance:

• Stage 1: Edema: tense, non-pitting, perhaps warm or tender, but often asymptomatic.
• Stage 2: Sclerosis: waxy hard texture, bound to subcutaneous structures, back of digits, face (loss of forehead wrinkles, reduced mouth orifice).
• Stage 3: Atrophy: shiny appearance, hypo- or hyperpigmented, calcium deposits in subcutaneous tissue. Telangiectases: macular dilitations that fill slowly, unlike spider telangiectasias.

Finding: Raynaud
Significance:

• Subtypes:

—Phenomenon: associated with underlying disease
—Disease: no underlying disease detected
—Triple phase: blanching, cyanosis, erythema
—Present in approximately 90% of patients with systemic sclerosis
—Usually fingers, also toes, nose, ears, and tongue, often spares the thumb
—Pathophysiology: arterial vasoconstriction, venous stasis to cyanosis, reflex vasodilitation to erythema

• Calcinosis, especially over extensor joint surfaces
• Musculoskeletal
• "Creaking" of thickened tendons
• Contractures, especially PIP and elbows
• No intra-articular inflammation
• Muscle inflammation in approximately 30% of cases
• Gastrointenstinal
• Mucosal telangiectasias of mouth
• Decreased incisor distance secondary to skin thickening
• Sicca syndrome with parotitis
• Loosening of teeth secondary to periodontal membrane disease
• Esophageal disease: esophagitis, occasional ulceration or stricture
• Large bowel disease less common
• Cardiac
• Primary cause of morbidity
• Possibly due to Raynaud of coronary arteries
• Pulmonary forms

- Interstitial fibrosis with gradual obliteration of vascular bed and resulting cor pulmonale
- Parenchymal disease is almost universal, frequently assymmetric, may have hacking cough, dyspnea on exertion, pleural rub
- Combined pulmonary vascular and pulmonary parenchymal
- Primary pulmonary vascular disease with right ventricular failure
- Renal, due to decreased renal plasma flow, ominous, proteinuria, hypertension.
- CNS: Cranial nerve involvement, especially sensory branch of trigeminal N
- Sicca syndrome
- Xerostomia (dry mouth)
- Keratoconjunctivitis sicca (dry eyes)
- Diagnosis: Lip biopsy; rose bengal staining of cornea

PROCEDURES

- Schrimer test for dry eyes
- Periungual nailfold changes: capillary dropout and dilated loops; occasional redundant cuticular growth and digital pitting

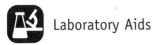 Laboratory Aids

There are no specific diagnostic tests.

NON-SPECIFIC TESTS

Systemic Form

- ANA often positive

Test: Hb
Significance: 25% have anemia due to chronic disease or vitamin B_{12} and folate deficiencies due to chronic malabsorption in sclerodermatous gut.

Test: Eosinophilia
Significance: 15%

Test: Sclero 70 (Scl-70 or Topoisomerase 1)
Significance: 26% of adults; more common with diffuse disease than peripheral vascular disease

Test: Anticentromere antibody
Significance: 22%; almost exclusively with CREST

Histologic Findings

Test: Muscle
Significance: Increased collagen and fat; negative immunofluorescence

Test: Esophageal
Significance: Atrophic muscle replaced by fibrous tissue more commonly affects smooth muscle of lower two-thirds of esophagus

ECG Findings

- ECG: first-degree block
- Right and left BBB
- PACs and PVCs: Non-specific T wave changes, ventricular hypertrophy

PFTs

Test: Restrictive lung disease
Significance: 34% of SSc

Test: Decreased DLCO
Significance: 18% SSc

Test: Acro-osteolysis
Significance: Resorption of tufts of distal phalanges, especially with severe Raynaud

- Earliest changes are decreased FVC and small airway disease.
- Bone x-ray
- Periarticular or subcutaneous calcification (15–25% patients).
- Bony erosions

CXR

- Bibasilar pulmonary fibrosis
- Rib notching
- Calcifications (in CREST)

Esophageal Studies

Test: Manometry and pH probe
Significance: Decreased or absent peristalsis of distal esophagus: distal dilatation, hiatus hernia, stricture

- Dilatation of second and third part of duodenum and proximal jejunum

LOCALIZED FORMS

- 25% to 50% eosinophilia during active disease
- 37% to 67% have positive ANA

 Therapy

- Disease modification: Many agents have been tried, however there are few controlled trials and no proven treatment. Medications include D-Penicillamine: breaks down collagen cross linkages; Colchicine: inhibit fibroproliferative process; Immunosuppressives: steroids, AZT, chlorambucil, MTX, cyclosporine.
- Supportive care: avoid cold, trauma, and excessive cold.
- Management of Raynaud: avoid cold, beta blockers, biofeedback.

 Follow-Up

- Localized forms

—Physical examination for joint mobility, muscle bulk, and growth

- Systemic forms

—Physical examination for joint mobility, muscle bulk, and growth
—Yearly PFTs
—Yearly barium swallow

PITFALLS

- Difficulty following slow disease progression, thus recommend photography of lesions every 3 to 6 months.
- Failure to appreciate limited mouth opening.
- Insufficient physical therapy resulting in permanent joint contractures.
- Excessive use of immunosupressive therapy late in disease when inflammatory component has resolved.

 Common Questions and Answers

Q: Is a biopsy necessary?
A: Biopsy is often useful to confirm diagnosis and assess degree of inflammation.

Q: Is the sclero-70 antibody useful?
A: Not for diagnosis, it is only positive in a subset of individuals with the systemic form and, therefore, useful for predicting more severe disease.

ICD-9-CM 710.1

BIBLIOGRAPHY

Cassidy JT, Petty RE. *Textbook of Pediatric Rheumatology,* 3rd ed. 1995.

Uziel Y. Miller ML. Laxer RM. Scleroderma in children. *Pediatr Clin North Am* 1995;42(5): 1171–1203.

Author: Emily von Scheven

Scoliosis/Kyphosis

Database

DEFINITION

• Lateral curvature of the spine exceeding 10 degrees (with rotation of the spine) in children older than 10 years of age. Considered idiopathic only after other causes have been excluded.

POSSIBLE CAUSES

• By definition, unknown; listed are some theories, none proven in isolation.
• Genetic

—Positive familial history for scoliosis in 30% (not predictive for severity).

• Connective tissue disorder

—Platelet calmodulin levels may be predictive of curve progression.

• Neurological (Equilibrium system)

—Most widely supported theory
—Abnormalities noted in vestibular, ocular, proprioceptive, and vibratory functions.

• Hormonal

—Lower levels of melatonin secreted from pineal body in those with AIS.
—Growth stimulating hormone: more of an influential factor than etiologic factor studies.

PATHOLOGY

• Lateral curvature of the spine with rotation

EPIDEMIOLOGY

• Prevalence

—Generally considered 1/9% to 3% for curves exceeding 10 degrees.
—0.3% for curves exceeding 20%

• Female:Male ratios

—1.4:1 for curves 11 degrees to 20 degrees
—5:1 for curves more than 20 degrees

GENETICS

• Positive familial history for idiopathic scoliosis in 30% (not predictive for severity)

COMPLICATIONS (NATURAL HISTORY)

• Reduced pulmonary function for patients with thoracic curves over 60 degrees.
• Progression of lumbar curves over 50 degrees in adult life with degenerative disc disease and pain.
• Cosmetic and emotional factors.

PROGNOSIS

• Risk of curve progression is related to patient's maturity (Risser sign, menarcheal status) and to the size of the curve.
• Curves less than 20° to 25° have a low risk of progression, even if patient is Risser 0 or Risser I
• Curves 25° to 45° have higher risk of progression, particularly in the immature
• Curves more than 45° to 50° have much higher risk of progression regardless of maturity

Differential Diagnosis

• Juvenile idiopathic scoliosis onset between 3 and 10 years of age
• Infantile idiopathic scoliosis onset younger than 3 years of age
• Congenital scoliosis
• Scoliosis associated with neurofibromatosis
• Scoliosis associated with tumors (osteoid osteoma, other)
• Neuromuscular scoliosis
• Postural scoliosis (from leg length discrepancy for example)

—No rib hump or rotation
—Disappears with forward bending
—Long curve
—No progression

Data Gathering

HISTORY

Question: Onset?
Significance: Consider when first noted, by whom, rate of worsening, previous treatment, associated signs or symptoms, familial history, etc.

Question: Pain?
Significance: Patients with idiopathic scoliosis should not have pain.

Question: Night pain?
Significance: If pain, consider tumor such as osteoid osteoma or other tumor.

Question: Other signs or symptoms?
Significance: Review of systems (especially neurological).

Physical Examination

Finding: General inspection to look for skin changes such as:

• Café au lait, pigmentation or other signs of neurofibromatosis for example, dysraphic signs (hairy patches, etc.).
• Assess for maturity, hyperelasticity, contracture, congenital anomalies.
• Assess for deformity, symmetry of spine, shoulders and trunk, including decompensation, abnormalities of thoracic kyphosis or cervical or lumbar lordosis.
• The Adam forward bending test is used to look for rib or paraspinous elevations.
• Assess for leg length discrepancy, congenital anomalies and neurological abnormalities (including abdominal reflex).

SPECIAL QUESTIONS

Finding: Crankshaft phenomenon
Significance: Progression of curve size and rotation following posterior spinal fusion, due to continued anterior spinal growth.

Finding: Patient is Risser 0, open triradiate cartilages, less than 10 years old, and is prior to the occurrence of peak height velocity (the time of maximum spinal growth).
Significance: Consider anterior fusion in addition to posterior fusion.

PHYSICAL EXAMINATION TRICKS

Finding: Scoliometer
Significance: To measure rib rotation.

Finding: Abnormal abdominal reflex
Significance: May suggest intraspinal pathology including syrinx.

Laboratory Aids

- Usually not helpful unless to rule out associated metabolic conditions.
- Pulmonary function testing are useful preoperatively.

IMAGING STAGES

- Plain standing PA and lateral scoliosis films on a long 3 foot x-ray cassette.
- Risser classification of iliac apophysis ossification is an indicator of maturity
- MRI is not routinely necessary
- 7% prevalence of abnormalities found in left thoracic curves
- Curve patterns are classified according to the King classification.
- Renal ultrasound or IVP are for evaluation of patient with congenital scoliosis.

Therapy

- Treatment
—Concepts for treatment are based on the severity of the deformity present and on the likelihood of progression
- Observation
—Curves less than 25°
  —Immature patients (Risser 0, 1, 2) should be re-evaluated in 4 to 6 months.
  —Skeletally mature patients (Risser 4 or 5) usually do not require follow up unless special circumstances
—Curves 25° to 45°
  —Risser 4 or 5 patients usually re-evaluated in 1 year

BRACE TREATMENT

- Curves 25° to 45° (Risser 0, 1): brace on initial evaluation; 30° to 45° (Risser 2 or 3): brace on initial evaluation.
- Curves 25° or greater (in Risser 0–3 patient) that have demonstrated more than 10° progression during the period of observation.
- Continue brace treatment until maturity (2 years post-menarchal and Risser 4 in females, Risser 5 in males).

OPERATIVE MANAGEMENT

- Recommended when curves exceed 45° to 50°

—Exception: Balanced thoracic and lumbar curves less than 55° may be observed for progression

- Thoracic curves and double major curves

—Posterior segmental fixation instrumentation remains current state-of-art (TSRH, Isola, CD-Horizon, etc.)
—Newer techniques of anterior spinal instrumentation for the thoracic spine
—Thorascopic technique for those who need anterior thoracic fusion to prevent the crankshaft phenomenon
—Thoracolumbar and lumbar curves

- Anterior spinal fusion using solid rod segmental constructs

GENERAL TREATMENT MODALITIES

- Brace types

—Thoracolumbosacral orthosis (TLSO): Success reported with use more than 16 hours daily.
—Milwaukee: Significantly improved outcome when compared to natural history.

DRUGS

- Post-operative continuous epidural infusion helpful for pain control

SIGNS TO WATCH FOR

- Back pain associated with idiopathic scoliosis.
- Present in 23% at time of initial evaluation (additional 9% during follow up).
- Of those with back pain, only 9% found to have identifiable cause such as spondylolysis, Scheuermann, syrinx, disc herniation, tumor, tether cord.

PROGNOSIS

- Overall, good prognosis for the majority of patients

Common Questions and Answers

Q: How long do you observe a patient with spinal asymmetry before ordering an X-ray?
A: It depends on the presence or absence of abnormalities on the physical examination. If any of the signs mentioned here are seen in conjunction with significant back pain, an X-ray or referral is indicated. The scoliometer is also a useful tool in screening patients.

Q: If a child presents with scoliosis and back pain, which occurs especially at night and is relieved with asprin, what diagnosis is suggested?
A: Scoliosis associated with osteoid osteoma.

ICD-9-CM
Scoliosis idiopathic 737.30
Scoliosis infantile progressive 737.32

BIBLIOGRAPHY

Lonstein JE. Scoliosis. In: Morrissy RT, Weinstein SL, eds. *Lovell and Winter's pediatric orthopaedics*, 4th ed. Philadelphia: Lippincott-Raven, 1996:625–685.

Lonstein JE, Carlson JM. The prediction of curve progression in untreated idiopathic scoliosis during growth. *J Bone Joint Surg* 1984;66-A:1061–1071.

Author: John P. Dormans

Seborrheic Dermatitis

 ## Database

DEFINITION

• Seborrheic dermatitis is a yellow to erythematous, scaly, greasy lesion located in areas of high concentrations of sebaceous glands (the scalp, face, postauricular and intertriginous areas).
• The term seborrhea refers to excessively oily skin.

PATHOPHYSIOLOGY

• Specific etiology is controversial.
• Does not appear to be bacterial or fungal.
• May be hormonally driven since it appears in infancy and disappears until puberty.
• Histiopathologic findings are non-specific and include evidence of low-grade inflammation, parakeratosis, acanthosis, elongation of the rete ridges, and slight intracellular edema and spongiosis.

GENETICS

• Controversial whether there is a constitutional predisposition. There is evidence that it is more common in families, but not spouses of affected patients.

EPIDEMIOLOGY

This skin disorder is first seen in infancy, and usually spontaneously resolves by the end of the first year of life. It is not usually seen again until adolescence.

COMPLICATIONS

• Usually none

PROGNOSIS

The infantile form will self-resolve by the end of the first year of life. The adolescent forms may persist through middle age as a chronic skin dermatitis.

 ## Differential Diagnosis

• Infection: Fungal infections such as *Pityrosporum ovale* and *Candida* may complicate these lesions, and on occasion may be confused with seborrhea. These can be differentiated by microscopic examination of hairs using a potassium hydroxide wet mount preparation and by fungal culture.
• Tumors: Letterer-Siwe (or Langerhans cell histiocytosis) is an uncommon disease that may present with a rash that begins with a scaly erythematous eruption on the scalp, behind the ears, in the intertriginous regions; differentiated by the presence of small reddish-brown papules or vesicles, purpuric lesions, hepatosplenomegaly, and adenopathy.
• Immunologic: Atopic dermatitis (usually affects infants at a later onset, is very pruritic, and often accompanied by a familial history of atopy). Recurrence after treatment is more indicative of atopic dermatitis. Psoriasis lacks the reddish color of seborrhea and is characterized by a micaceous scale and a tendency to locate on the flexural aspects of the extremities; it is less likely to be confined to the scalp.
• Miscellaneous: Leiner disease has severe generalized erythematous, exfoliative seborrheic dermatitis, and is accompanied by severe diarrhea, recurrent infections, and failure to thrive. It is the phenotypic appearance of a number of nutritional and immunologic disorders, such as acrodermatitis enteropathica, and complement deficiencies.

 ## Data Gathering

HISTORY

These infants usually lack a personal or familial history of atopy. The lesions are typically not pruritic and may begin early in the first few months of life.

 ## Physical Examination

• In infants, the disorder may be confined to the scalp or may spread downward to the face and back of head.
• Characteristic yellow to erythematous, scaly, greasy lesions.
• Thickened lesions of the scalp in infants is commonly referred to as cradle cap.
• Blepharitis, red eyelid margins with fine white scales.
• After adolescence, this disorder frequently manifests as dandruff, an increase of the normal desquamation of the scalp.
• Axillary involvment, the absence of pruitis, oozing, and weeping help distinguish seborrhea from atopic dermatitis.

Laboratory Aids

SPECIFIC TESTS

There are no specific test for seborrrhea.

Test: Microscopic examination of hairs
Significance: Fungal infections can be differentiated by using a potassium hydroxide wet mount preparation, and by fungal culture.

NON-SPECIFIC TESTS

Test: Skin biopsy
Significance: May help in situations that are confusing; however, findings are not necessarily diagnostic for seborrhea.

 ## Therapy

- Infantile seborrhea commonly affects the scalp and may respond to a mild shampoo. A sulfur or salicylic acid shampoo (leave on 5 minutes before rinsing off, use 2 to 3 times in the first week, then weekly afterwards) may be used if no improvement. If particularly thick, the scales can be loosened first with warm mineral oil or petrolatum, and then gently scrubbed.
- Lesions resistant to treatment may respond to a topical steroid lotion rubbed into the scalp with the fingertips.
- Adolescents should use shampoos with zinc pyrithione (e.g., Head and Shoulders), selenium sulfide (e.g., Selsun), or tar. Those with erythema and severe pruritus can consider treatment with topical corticosteroid lotions.
- Blepharitis should be treated with warm compresses, cleansing with a baby shampoo, and if necessary, sodium sulfacetamide ophthalmic ointment.
- Treatment may require long-term treatment until it resolves.

 ## Follow-Up

Some improvement should be seen with therapy by 7 to 10 days. Although this dermatitis is usually self-limited in infancy, it often takes months to resolve completely. Seborrhea may rarely be complicated by secondary bacterial or candidal infections, with erythema, tenderness, and ulceration. Seborrhea may be caused or complicated by associated underlying disorders, such as immune defects such as acquired immunodeficiency syndrome. This should be considered with seborrhea resistence to treatment.

PREVENTION

There are no known preventative measures.

PITFALLS

Treatments to infant scalp should be left on long enough to allow the scales to loosen, and then can be scrubbed off. Parents may need to be reassured that for stubborn and persistent seborrhea, scrubbing the scalp is safe and may be necessary to keep the lesions under control.

 ## Common Questions and Answers

Q: Does therapy speed resolution of the disorder?
A: Treatment does not appear to influence the underlying cause of this disorder (presumably hormonal influence on the sebaceous glands) although some suggest use of an antifungal shampoo to presumptively treat *Pityrosporum ovale.*

ICM-9-CM 690

BIBLIOGRAPHY

Hay RJ, Graham-Brown RAC. Dandruff and seborrhoeic dermatitis: causes and management. *Clin Exp Dermatol* 1997;22:3–6.

Hurwitz S. *Clinical pediatric dermatology,* 2nd ed. Philadelphia: WB Saunders, 1993.

Janniger C, Schwartz R. Seborrheic dermatitis. *Am Fam Physician* 1995;52(1):149–155.

Mimouni K, Mukamel M, Zeharia A, Mimouni M. Prognosis of infantile seborrheic dermatitis. *J Pediatr* 1995;127(5):744–746.

Author: Robert Kamei

Seizures—Febrile

Database

DEFINITION

• Single, brief (less than 15 minutes), generalized seizures occurring during rise of fever in developmentally and neurologically normal children between the ages of 6 months and 5 years without intracranial infection or other underlying cause. Febrile seizures are called complex if they last longer than 15 minutes, are focal, or recur within 1 day.

GENETICS

Febrile seizures are considered familial; may be transmitted by autosomal dominant inheritance with incomplete penetrance.

EPIDEMIOLOGY

3% to 4% of children will experience a febrile seizure.

ASSOCIATED CONDITIONS

• Associated with rapid rise in fever; familial history of febrile seizures

Differential Diagnosis

Consideration of nonepileptic causes of seizures (*see* Seizure, Major Motor). Fever may be the precipitant of seizure due to any other cause of an epileptic spell. Must exclude:

• CNS infection
• Anoxia
• Trauma
• Stroke/hemorrhage
• Intoxication
• Metabolic encephalopathy
• Neurodegenerative disorder
• Brain tumor
• Neurocutaneous syndromes (tuberous sclerosis, Sturge-Weber, neurofibromatosis)
• Previous brain injury (history of stroke, intracranial hemorrhage, birth asphyxia, cerebral palsy, head trauma, meningitis)

Data Gathering

HISTORY

Question: Previous history of seizures, febrile or afebrile, or neurologic abnormality?
Significance: One third of children with one simple febrile seizure will have another. Neurological abnormality or prior afebrile seizure increases risk of subsequent epilepsy.

Question: Precipitating factors including fever, length and symptoms of preceding illness, recent history of head trauma, possibility of ingestion?
Significance: Low fever, prolonged length of illness before seizure, ingestion, or head trauma suggest cause other than simple fever.

Question: Past medical history including gestation, birth, general health, growth and development, and current medications?
Significance: Birth complications and developmental delay may increase risk of epilepsy.

Question: Familial history?
Significance: Both febrile and afebrile seizures can be hereditary.

Question: Any recent onset of headaches, vomiting, lethargy, weakness, sensory deficits, or change in vision, behavior, balance, or gait?
Significance: Suggest underlying brain pathology and need for neuroimaging.

Physical Examination

Check vital signs for:

• Degree of fever
• Tachycardia or hypotension, suggesting possible sepsis
• Tachypnea, suggesting respiratory infection
• Head circumference

Finding: Retinal hemorrhages and evidence of intracranial hypertension such as bulging fontanelle should be noted on HEENT exam.
Significance: Signs of head trauma or possible child abuse.

Finding: Kernig and Brudzinski signs.
Significance: Possible meningitis.

Finding: Careful neurological examination. Specific attention to mental status and any focal abnormalities of motor strength, tone, or sensation should be performed.
Significance: Suggest possible meningitis or structural brain pathology.

Laboratory Aids

Test: No routine blood testing necessary
Significance: After a simple febrile seizure if the child appears clinically well.

Test: Lumbar puncture
Significance: Should be performed in any child who is thought to have a possible infection of the nervous system. This generally includes any child under 18 months of age in whom clinical signs of meningitis may be difficult to accurately assess and any older child who appears toxic or has clinical signs suggesting CNS infection.

Test: EEG
Significance: Not routinely indicated after a simple febrile seizure. EEG should be performed on children who are neurologically abnormal or experience a complex seizure.

Test: MRI
Significance: Generally reserved for children with focal seizures; focal neurologic deficits, even transitory, after a seizure; and children with focally abnormal EEGs.

Therapy

- Because only one-third of children with an initial febrile seizure have a second seizure, treatment of a single febrile seizure is not indicated.
- Anticonvulsant prophylaxis may be considered in children with an underlying neurologic abnormality and in children who have had two prolonged or more than three brief febrile seizures.
- When the initial febrile seizure is multiple, prolonged, or focal but the child recovers rapidly and completely, further investigations including EEG and possibly MRI are indicated. Decisions regarding anticonvulsant prophylaxis in these children must be individualized.

DRUGS

- Oral administration of diazepam, 0.33 mg/kg every 8 hours, during all febrile illnesses reduces the risk of recurrent febrile seizures.
- Alternatively, rectal diazepam, 0.5 mg/kg, can be administered at the onset of seizure.
- The oral route is generally simpler but has the disadvantage of significant associated sedation during every febrile illness and may not be able to be initiated early enough to be effective in children whose seizures occur immediately at the onset of fever.
- Phenobarbital (3–6 mg/kg/d) is often avoided because of possible behavioral and cognitive side effects.
- Daily valproate and primidone are considered as effective as phenobarbital but also have limiting side effects.
- Phenytoin and carbamazepine are ineffective as prophylaxis.

 Follow-Up

PROGNOSIS

- One-third of children who have a first simple febrile seizure will have a second at the time of subsequent febrile illnesses, and half of these will have a third febrile seizure.
- One-half of the recurrences occur within 6 months of the first febrile seizure, three-fourths within a year, and 90% within 2 years.
- Less than 9% of children with febrile seizures will have more than three.
- The risk of recurrence is increased if the child has a familial history of febrile seizures, first febrile seizure occurs before 12 months of age, or at a body temperature less than 40°C. Only 2% of children whose first seizure is associated with fever have nonfebrile seizures by age 7. Prolonged or focal seizures; a prior neurologic deficit; or a family history of epilepsy are associated with an increased probability of subsequent epilepsy.
- There is no evidence that occasional febrile seizures or even febrile status epilepticus causes neurologic damage, mental retardation, a decrease in IQ, cerebral palsy, or learning problems.

PITFALLS

- Diagnosis of febrile seizure in a child less than 18 months old usually entails spinal fluid examination with normal cell count, chemistry, Gram stain, and culture.
- Continued seizures with fever beyond age 6 are not compatible with diagnosis of febrile seizure.
- Infants with febrile seizures may have serious bacterial infections, bacteremia, causing fever of primary clinical significance.

 Common Questions and Answers

Q: What should be done if the child has another febrile seizure?
A: Emergency measures include placement of the child recumbent or supine with head turned to avoid aspiration, place nothing in the mouth. Antipyretic medication that can be administered PR should be kept in the home. For prolonged seizure, rectal diazepam can be given.

Q: What restrictions should be placed on general activity of a child with recurrent febrile seizures?
A: No specific restrictions are recommended.

ICD-9-CM 780.3

BIBLIOGRAPHY

Berkovic SF, Scheffer IE. Febrile seizures: genetics and relationship to other epilepsy syndromes. *Curr Opin Neurol* 1998;11(2):129–134.

Berg AT, Shinnar S, Darefsky AS, et al. Predictors of recurrent febrile seizures. A prospective cohort study. *Arch Pediatr Adolesc Med* 1997;151(4):371–378.

Freeman JM, Holmes GL. Should uncomplicated seizures be treated? Point–counterpoint. *Curr Probl Pediatr* 1994;24(4):139–148.

Freeman JM, Vining EP. Decision making and the child with febrile seizures. *Pediatr Rev* 1992;13(8):298–304.

Hirtz DG. Febrile seizures. *Pediatr Rev* 1997;18(1):5–8.

Van Esch A, Van Steensel-Moll HA, Steyerberg EW. Antipyretic efficacy of ibuprofen and acetaminophen in children with febrile seizures. *Arch Pediatr Adolesc Med* 1995;149(6):632–637.

Verity CM. Do seizures damage the brain? The epidemiological evidence. *Arch Dis Childhood* 1998;78(1):78–84.

Verity CM, Greenwood R, Golding J. Long-term intellectual and behavioral outcomes of children with febrile convulsions. *N Engl J Med* 338(24):1723–1728.

Vining EP. Gaining a perspective on childhood seizures. *N Engl J Med* 1998;338(26):1916–1918.

Author: Amy R. Brooks-Kayal

Seizures—Major Motor

Database

DEFINITION

• A transient involuntary alteration of consciousness, behavior, motor activity, sensation, or autonomic function due to an excessive rate and hypersynchrony of neuronal discharges. Seizures are classified based on the location of their onset as partial (beginning in a localized area of cerebral cortex) or primary generalized (beginning simultaneously in both hemispheres). Partial seizures are additionally divided into simple partial (consciousness not impaired), complex partial (consciousness impaired), and partial seizures evolving to generalized tonic-clonic convulsions. Primary generalized seizure types include absence, atypical absence, myoclonic, clonic, tonic, atonic, and tonic-clonic seizures.

GENETICS

• Idiopathic seizures multifactorial genetic pattern: primarily generalized epilepsies (45–55% of childhood epilepsies) may show dominant inheritance pattern.

EPIDEMIOLOGY

4% to 6% of children will have at least one seizure in the first 16 years of life; the highest incidence is in childhood, with 30% of first seizures occurring before age 4 years and nearly 80% occurring before age 20 years.

RISK FACTORS

• History of previous seizure (afebrile or febrile)
• Recent withdrawal of anticonvulsant medication
• Brain tumor
• Neurodegenerative disorder
• History of remote neurologic insult (stroke, intracranial hemorrhage, cerebral palsy, head trauma, meningitis)
• Familial history of seizures

Differential Diagnosis

• Idiopathic
• Remote symptomatic (previous history of stroke, intracranial hemorrhage, birth asphyxia, cerebral palsy, head trauma, meningitis)
• Febrile
• Acute symptomatic: CNS infection, anoxia, trauma, stroke/hemorrhage, intoxication, metabolic encephalopathy, anticonvulsant withdrawal
• Neurodegenerative disorder
• Brain tumor
• Neurocutaneous syndromes (tuberous sclerosis, Sturge-Weber, neurofibromatosis)

CAUSES OF NON-EPILEPTIC SEIZURES INCLUDE

• Syncope
• Hyperventilation
• Narcolepsy-cataplexy
• Night terrors
• Startle disease
• Breath-holding spells
• Migraine
• Shuddering spells, paroxysmal dyskinesias, tics
• Drug-induced dystonia, psychogenic seizure, movements related to GE reflux
• Segmental myoclonus

Data Gathering

HISTORY

Question: Previous history of seizures or neurologic abnormality?
Significance: Suggests child at risk of epilepsy.

Question: Precipitating factors?
Significance:

• Fever
• Preceding illness
• Recent history of head trauma
• Possibility of ingestion or recent change in antiepileptic medication
• Risk factors (*see* Database)
• Gestation, birth, general health, growth and development, and current medications, recent onset of headaches, weakness, sensory deficits, change in vision, behavior, balance, or gait.

Physical Examination

Finding: Check vital signs
Significance: Indications of fever, adequacy of air exchange and perfusion, or abnormal respiratory pattern, bradycardia, or hypertension, suggesting intracranial hypertension.

Finding: Head circumference, signs of head trauma including retinal hemorrhages and evidence of intracranial hypertension, such as bulging fontanelle
Significance: Microcephaly suggests underlying neurologic abnormality. Signs of head trauma can be a sign of child abuse. Bulging fontanelle can be a sign of meningitis, trauma, or tumor.

Finding: Signs of systemic infection
Significance: Meningismus, suggesting CNS infection.

Finding: Café-au-lait or ash leaf spots, facial hemangioma
Significance: Suggests neurocutaneous disorders.

Finding: Convulsions
Significance: If the patient is actively convulsing, neurologic examination is often limited and should be directed toward determining possibility of intracranial hypertension and any focal abnormalities (*see* Status Epilepticus).

Finding: Pupillary asymmetries, altered mental status, fixed eye deviations, and focal motor weakness (Todd paresis).
Significance: May be secondary to seizure activity or indicate underlying structural lesions.

Laboratory Aids

Test: Initial
Significance: Glucose, electrolytes, BUN, antiepileptic drug levels, complete blood count, liver function tests, toxicology screen, urinalysis. Oximetry or arterial blood gas may be indicated if child is actively seizing.

Test: Lumbar puncture (LP)
Significance: Indicated in nearly all children under 2 years of age and any older child in whom CNS infection is suspected, unless a contraindication such as intracranial hypertension, cerebral mass lesion, or obstructive hydrocephalus is present. LP should be deferred until after head CT if focal abnormalities or signs of intracranial hypertension are present on examination.

Test: EEG
Significance: Indicated immediately if convulsions continue, or the patient fails to awaken in a reasonable time period after convulsions cease. EEG also indicated in all children with first afebrile, children with complicated febrile seizure, and children with established epilepsy who have had a significant change in clinical status.

Test: Brain imaging with CT or MRI
Significance: Indicated in the initial evaluation of children with partial onset seizures, focally abnormal EEG, focal neurologic signs, history of head trauma, or difficult to control seizures. Repeat brain imaging may be indicated in children with established epilepsy who have had a significant change in clinical status. MRI is preferred because it provides more detailed images; however, CT can be obtained more rapidly and is appropriate if urgent imaging is needed or patient is medically unstable.

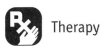

Therapy

PREVENTION

• Need for long-term antiepileptic drug (AED) therapy after a first seizure depends on the etiology, patient's age, and circumstances in which seizure occurred. Chronic AED therapy generally not indicated after a seizure resulting from a transient metabolic disturbances (hyponatremia, intoxication) or after a single unprovoked seizure in a child with normal neurologic examination and EEG. Chronic AED therapy usually indicated after first seizure symptomatic of a structural brain lesion; after two or more unprovoked seizures; and in patients with known epilepsy with recurrent seizures.

MEDICATIONS

• (*see* Status Epilepticus).
• The choice of AED for long-term management depends on the specific seizure type. Therapy should be started with a single drug, because approximately 75% of children with epilepsy will be fully controlled with monotherapy, and polytherapy increases.
• The risk of toxicity and decreases compliance. For treatment of partial onset seizures (with or without secondary generalization), carbamazepine is frequently chosen as initial therapy and is begun at 5 to 10 mg/kg/d and slowly advanced to 20 to 30 mg/kg/d divided tid. Therapeutic blood concentrations range from 8 to 12 mg/mL. LFTs and CBC must be monitored because of potential risk of aplastic anemia and hepatotoxicity.
• Phenytoin (5 to 7 mg/kg/d), valproate, and phenobarbital (3 to 5 mg/kg/d) are alternatives in children for whom carbamazepine is ineffective or poorly tolerated.
• Ethosuximide is the AED of choice for absence seizures. Initial dose is 20 mg/kg/d in two to three divided doses, increased as needed for blood levels of 40 to 100 mg/mL. For primary generalized epilepsies, refractory absence: valproate, 10 to 15 mg/kg/d increased to 20 to 60 mg/kg/d for blood levels of 50 to 100 mg/dL. Adverse effects include thrombocytopenia, pancreatitis, hyperammonemia, fatal hepatotoxicity. CBC and LFTs should be routinely monitored; phenobarbital used for partial or generalized seizures in infants. New AEDs are also available: Lamotrigine, Topiramate, Gabapentin, Tiagabine.

Follow-up

PROGNOSIS

• The reported risk of recurrence after a single unprovoked seizure in children varies from 27% to 40%.
• The risk is lowest in children with normal neurologic examinations and normal EEGs and is increased in children with abnormal examinations, focally abnormal EEGs, positive familial history of seizures, partial seizure, or postictal (Todd) paralysis.

COMPLICATIONS

No convincing evidence exists that an isolated brief seizure causes brain damage. Serious injury from a brief seizure is rare and usually related to loss of consciousness and resultant falls. Few restrictions need to be placed on patients with epilepsy, with the exceptions of driving or operating heavy machinery in adolescents or particularly dangerous sports, such as scuba diving, parachuting, and rock climbing.

• Hyponatremic seizures occur in infants with gastroenteritis usually with serum sodium well below 120 mEq/dL. Judicious correction of hyponatremia may prevent neurologic effects of rapid shifts in osmolarity: many clinicians administer normal saline to bring the sodium up to 120 mEq/dL, with slower correction thereafter.
• Apnea and hypoventilation frequently result from excessive administration of benzodiazepines to children with repetitive partial or complex partial seizures. In general, patients whose seizures do not threaten ventilation should not receive sedating doses of anticonvulsants.
• Febrile seizure is a diagnosis of exclusion in a child with first seizure associated with fever. History may suggest other possibilities; those under 18 months should undergo lumbar puncture.

Common Questions and Answers

Q: How do you know my child has epilepsy?
A: The term epilepsy is applied to children with recurrent (greater than 1) seizure not due to fever or other transient toxic/metabolic disturbance, since in general these children have a high (greater than 60%) probability of additional recurrences.

Q: Will my child always be an epileptic?
A: Depending on the circumstances, children may grow out of their seizure disorder. In many cases, anticonvulsants can be discontinued if the child has been seizure-free for 2 years.

Q: Why take an anticonvulsant(s)?
A: The purpose of anticonvulsant medication is to prevent status epilepticus and to prevent accidents and interference with normal behavior associated with brief seizures.

ICD-9-CM 345.1

BIBLIOGRAPHY

Barron TF, Hunt SL. A review of the newer antiepileptic drugs and the ketogenic diet. *Clin Pediatr* 1997;36(9):513–521.

Bourgeois BF. Temporal lobe epilepsy in infants and children. *Brain Dev* 1998;20(3):135–141.

Cantu RV. Epilepsy and athletics. *Clin Sports Med* 1998;17(1):61–69.

Scher MS. Seizures in the newborn infant. Diagnosis, treatment, and outcome. *Clin Perinatol* 1997;24(4):735–772.

Author: Amy R. Brooks-Kayal

Sepsis

Database

DEFINITION

The terms sepsis, bacteremia, sepsis syndrome, and septic shock have been used interchangeably in the medical literature, leading to confusion regarding the correct definition of each:

- Sepsis: the presence of pathogenic organisms or their toxins in the blood or tissues, and the systemic response to them.
- Bacteremia: the presence of viable bacteria in the bloodstream.
- Sepsis syndrome: sepsis accompanied by evidence of altered end-organ perfusion (e.g., changes in mental status, oliguria, elevated plasma lactate levels). This term has recently been used interchangeably with the systemic inflammatory response syndrome, which can be related to infection, trauma, burns, and other etiologies.
- Septic shock: sepsis syndrome with hypotension (systolic blood pressure <5% for age).

CAUSES

The etiology of sepsis varies with age in otherwise healthy children.

- Most common pathogens in the first 4 weeks of life: Group B *Streptococcus,* gram-negative enterics (particularly *Esherichia coli*); *Lysteria monocytogenes.*
- When there is a history of hospitalization, instrumentation, or mechanical ventilation: *Staphylococcus aureus, Staphylococcus epidermidis, Pseudomonas aeruginosa.*
- In older infants and children: *Streptococcus pneumoniae, Neisseria meningitidis,* Group A *Streptococcus, Salmonella* spp., *Haemophilus influenzae* type b (less common since vaccination available).

EPIDEMIOLOGY

- Sepsis is among the most common (10–25%) medical diagnoses on admission to pediatric intensive care units.
- Mortality rates from sepsis vary with age from 5.6 deaths per 100,000 in infants less than 1 year to 0.5 per 100,000 age 1 to 4, and 0.1 per 100,000 age 5 to 14 years.
- Although sepsis may occur in previously healthy children, it is a particular concern for children with a number of chronic underlying conditions that may render them either immunosuppressed or vulnerable to invasive infections.
- Hyposplenism, either surgical or functional (e.g., sickle cell anemia), highly prone to sepsis from encapsulated organisms—*S. pneumoniae* and *H. influenzae* type b
- Neutropenia (<1000 neutrophils/mm³ of blood), whether resulting from disease (e.g., leukemia) or from chemotherapy
- Congenital or acquired syndromes of immunodeficiency (AIDS, SCIDS)
- Organ transplant recipients
- Chronic use of high doses of steroids
- Patients with indwelling central venous catheters

COMPLICATIONS

The most common complications of sepsis are those resulting primarily from either acute hypoperfusion of vital organs, or to organ injury incurred by the uncontrolled systemic inflammatory response:

- Acute lung injury
- Acute renal failure
- Disseminated intravascular coagulation (DIC)
- Hypoglycemia
- Adult respiratory distress syndrome (ARDS)
- Refractory shock
- Multiple organ dysfunction syndrome (MODS)

PROGNOSIS

- Case fatality rates range from 10% to 50%.
- Mortality higher if shock exists on initial presentation.
- Development of ARDS or MODS associated with increased mortality.
- Survival improved in patients receiving greater than 40 mL/kg of volume resuscitation in the first hour of management.
- Presence of coagulopathy (elevated PT and PTT) associated with elevated mortality from meningococcal sepsis.

ASSOCIATED ILLNESSES

See Epidemiology for identification of subgroups of children at high risk of sepsis.

Differential Diagnosis

The differential diagnosis of the "septic-appearing" child varies somewhat with age:

- For children, <2 months:

—Viral infections (e.g., enterovirus, respiratory syncytial virus)
—Congenital heart disease (e.g., congestive heart failure due to hypoplastic left heart syndrome, coarctation of the aorta, VSD, valvular insufficiency)
—Myocarditis, pericarditis
—Cardiac arrhythmia (e.g., supraventricular tachycardia)
—Myocardial infarction secondary to anomalous coronary artery insertion
—Congenital adrenal hyperplasia
—Inborn errors of metabolism (e.g., maple syrup urine disease, methylmalonic or propionic acidemia, urea cycle disorders)
—Hypoglycemia
—Severe anemia
—Methemoglobinemia
—Gastroenteritis with dehydration
—Pyloric stenosis
—Volvulus
—Infant botulism
—Occult trauma: child abuse

- For older infants and children:

—Viral infections
—Myocarditis, pericarditis
—Cardiac arrhythmia (e.g., supraventricular tachycardia, ventricular tachycardia)
—Intussusception
—Toxic ingestion/poisoning (e.g., iron, tricyclic antidepressants, oral hypoglycemic agents, ethanol, calcium channel blockers, beta-blockers, clonidine, opioids)
—Trauma
—Infant botulism
—Diabetic ketoacidosis

Data Gathering

HISTORY

Identify children at risk of sepsis (*see* Epidemiology).

Question: Duration of illness before presentation?
Significance: Abrupt onset of symptoms more typical of invasive bacterial infection.

Question: Presence of chronic underlying illness?
Significance: Identifies children at higher risk of sepsis.

Question: Change in behavior?
Significance: May be initial sign of systemic infection.

- Exposure to known infectious agents (e.g., meningococci)?

Physical Examination

All patients with suspected sepsis should have a full set of vital signs (e.g., temperature, pulse, respiratory rate, blood pressure).

Finding: Temperature
Significance: Fever is the hallmark of an infection; however, infants in particular may demonstrate hypothermia.

Finding: Assess for signs of airway obstruction
Significance: Sterdor, stridor.

Finding: Auscultation of the chest
Significance: To assess adequacy of breathing (tachypnea, rales).

Finding: Assess circulation
Significance: Heart rate, blood pressure, skin color and temperature, capillary refill, presence of mottling.

Finding: Mental status
Significance: Level of alertness, confusion, disorientation, agitation.

Finding: Presence of petecchiae and purpura
Significance: Meningococeemia or DIC.

Finding: Thorough physical examination
Significance: Looking for focus of infection.

Sepsis

Laboratory Aids

All patients with suspected sepsis should have a thorough laboratory evaluation including:

Test: Complete blood count with WBC differential, platelet count
Significance: Elevated WBC count with increased band width.

Test: Electrolytes, glucose
Significance: Metabolic acidosis, hypoglycemia.

Test: Blood culture
Significance: Identification of causative organism.

Test: Arterial blood gas
Significance: Monitoring acid-base status.

Test: Urinalysis and urine culture
Significance: Potential source of infection.

Test: Lumbar puncture (when hemodynamically stable)
Significance: Required for diagnosis of meningitis.

Test: Chest x-ray
Significance: Potential source of infection.

Test: Prothrombin time, partial thromboplastin time
Significance: Monitor development of DIC.

Test: Fibrinogen, fibrin degradation products
Significance: Monitor development of DIC.

Test: Gram stain of petecchiae or abscess contents
Significance: May yield causative organism.

Therapy

- Ensure a patent airway (consider endotracheal intubation).
- Provide supplemental oxygen.
- Assist ventilation (e.g., bag-valve-mask device) as needed.
- Obtain intravenous access (consider placement of a femoral venous line or intraosseous line).
- Volume resuscitation: bolus 20 mL/kg of normal saline solution, repeat as needed; consider colloid solutions (5% albumin, plasma) after initial 60–80 mL/kg of crystalloid).
- Correct hypoglycemia (0.5–1 g/kg of dextrose).
- Antibiotics (depends on age, presence of meningitis, central venous catheter, immune function of patient). Generally, given IV for at least 10 days.

—Neonates, <6 weeks, no meningitis: Ampicillin and gentamicin; meningitis: ampicillin, cefotaxime
—Children, <6 weeks: cefotaxime or ceftriaxone
—Suspected infection (meningitis) with penicillin-resistant S. pneumoniae: vancomycin and cefotaxime or ceftriaxone

—Suspected Salmonella sepsis: third-generation cephalosporin or trimethoprim-sulfamethoxazole
—Nosocomially acquired infections or patients with immunosuppression, and/or central venous catheters: antistaphylococcal penicillin or vancomycin, plus aminoglycoside, and third-generation cephalosporin
—Patients with an intraabdominal focus of infection: ampicillin/sulbactam or ampicillin, gentamicin, and clindamycin

- Drainage and/or eradication of focus of infection
- Inotropic agents: dopamine (begin at 5 mg/kg/min, titrate up to 20 mg/kg/min as needed), dobutamine (begin at 5 mg/kg/min), epinephrine (begin at 1–2 mg/kg/min). To be used for persistent hemodynamic instability after adequate volume resuscitation.

PREVENTION

- Routine vaccination for *Haemophilus influenzae* type b
- Vaccination for *S. pneumoniae* in high-risk patients (e.g., sickle cell anemia, asplenia)
- Rifampin prophylaxis for household or daycare exposure to *H. influenzae* type b and *N. meningitidis*
- Prompt evaluation for fever in immunosuppressed patients

Follow-Up

- Admit all patients with suspected sepsis to the hospital; consider intensive care unit admission.
- Continuous blood pressure monitoring for the development of refractory shock
- Serial vital signs and physical examinations to monitor response to therapy
- Monitor for complications of sepsis and the development of multiple organ dysfunction syndrome (MODS).
- Chest x-ray and serial arterial blood gases for evidence of acute lung injury/ARDS
- Urine output, BUN, creatinine for acute renal failure
- Serial coagulation studies (PT/PTT) for development of disseminated intravascular coagulation (DIC)
- Serial blood glucose levels for hypoglycemia
- Serial liver function tests (glucose, albumin, ALT, AST, GGT, bilirubin) for evidence of hepatic dysfunction
- Serial neurologic examinations for evidence of central nervous system dysfunction

PITFALLS

- Recognize the patient at risk for sepsis (*see* Epidemiology).
- Initial priorities in management are the proper assessment of airway, breathing, and circulation.
- Provide adequate initial volume resuscitation; improved outcome is associated with giving greater than 40 mL/kg isotonic saline in the first hour of resuscitation.

- Eradicate the focus of infection (abscess) if present.
- Continuous monitoring and reassessment of the patient is essential.

Common Questions and Answers

Q: What are the earliest signs and symptoms of compensated shock?
A: Unexplained tachycardia and widened pulse pressure are among the earliest signs of septic shock and warrant additional observation and laboratory investigation.

Q: Are colloid solutions (e.g., 5% albumin, fresh frozen plasma) better than isotonic crystalloid (e.g., Ringer's lactate, normal saline) for volume resuscitation?
A: Both are effective for intravascular volume expansion, though less (approximately 25%) of the crystalloid volume initially given ultimately remains in the intravascular compartment. Generally, because of their ready availability and lower cost, crystalloid solutions are given for the first 60 to 80 mL/kg of resuscitation, and consideration is then given to the addition of colloid solutions for additional volume resuscitation.

ICD-9-CM 638.9

BIBLIOGRAPHY

Anderson MR, Blumer JL. Advances in the therapy for sepsis in children. *Pediatr Clin North Am* 1997;
44(1):179–205.

Beal AL, Cerra FB. Multiple organ failure syndrome in the 1990s. *J Am Med Assoc* 1994; 271:226–233.

Bone RC. Let's agree on terminology: definitions of sepsis. *Crit Care Med* 1991;19:973–976.

Bone RC. A critical evaluation of new agents for the treatment of sepsis. *J Am Med Assoc* 1991;266:1686–1691.

Carcillo JA, Davis AL, Zaritsky A. Role of early fluid resuscitation in pediatric septic shock. *J Am Med Assoc* 1991;266:1242–1245.

Martinot A, Leclerc F, Cremer R, Leteurtre S, Fourier C, Hue V. Sepsis in neonates and children: definitions, epidemiology, and outcome. *Pediatr Emerg Care* 1997;13(4):277–281.

Saez-Llorens X, McCracken GH. Sepsis syndrome and septic shock in pediatrics: current concepts of terminology, pathophysiology and management. *J Pediatr* 1993;123:497–508.

Selbst SM. Septic-appearing infant. In: Fleisher GR, Ludwig S, eds. *Textbook of pediatric emergency medicine,* 3rd ed. Baltimore: Williams & Wilkins, 1993;456–463.

Ziegler EJ, Fisher CJ, Sprung CL, et al. Treatment of gram-negative bacteremia and septic shock with HA-1A human monoclonal antibody against endotoxin. *N Engl J Med* 1991;324: 429–436.

Author: Dennis R. Durbin

Septic Arthritis

 Database

DEFINITION

Septic arthritis is an inflammatory response to the presence of infectious organisms within the joint space. See the table Types of Organisms.

CAUSES

Bacterial

- *Staphylococcus aureus*
- Streptococci
- *Haemophilus influenzae*
- *Salmonella*
- *Neisseria gonorrhoeae*
- *Neisseria meningitidis*

Aseptic Arthritis

- Rubella
- Parvovirus
- Hepatitis B or C
- Mumps
- Herpesviruses (EBV, CMV, HSV, VZV)
- Epstein-Barr virus
- Varicella
- *Candida albicans* (neonatal)

PATHOLOGY/PATHOPHYSIOLOGY

- Entry of bacteria into joint space

—Hematogenous spread
—Direct inoculation (penetrating trauma) or extension from bone infection
—Influx of inflammatory cells within the joint capsule
—Destruction of cartilaginous structures within the joint by bacterial and lysosomal enzymes
—If left untreated, can progress to necrosis of the intraarticular epiphysis

EPIDEMIOLOGY

- Predominant age: 2 to 6 years, adolescent (gonorrhea)
- Predominant sex: male:female (2:1)
- Predominantly affected joints: knee, hip, elbow, ankle

COMPLICATIONS

- Permanent limitation of range of motion can occur secondary to tissue destruction and scarring.
- Growth disturbance may occur if the epiphysis is involved.

PROGNOSIS

- Depends on duration of illness prior to institution of appropriate therapy

ASSOCIATED ILLNESSES

- *Neonatal septic arthritis* can be associated with *S. aureus*, group B streptococcus, *Escherichia coli*, and *Candida*.
- *Sickle cell disease* is associated with *Salmonella* infection, although *S. aureus* is still the most common.

- *Immunocompromise* associated with *Mycoplasma, Ureaplasma, Aspergillus* infection

 Differential Diagnosis

Infection

—Osteomyelitis with contiguous spread of infection
—Lyme arthritis
—Tuberculous arthritis
—Psoas abscess or retroperitoneal abscess with associated hip pain
—Cellulitis causing decreased range of motion of joint secondary to pain

- Tumors

—Osteogenic sarcoma (longbone pain spreading to joint space)
—Leukemia/lymphoma

- Trauma

—Occult fracture in proximity to growth plate
—Ligamentous injury (sprain)
—Foreign-body synovitis
—Traumatic knee effusion/hemarthrosis

- Immunologic

—Toxic synovitis
—Postinfectious
  —Acute rheumatic fever
  —Reactive arthritis
  —*Campylobacter, Shigella*
  —Reiter syndrome (after gastrointestinal or chlamydial infection) arthritis, uveitis, urethritis

—Collagen vascular
  —Systemic lupus erythematosus
  —Juvenile rheumatoid arthritis
  —Henoch-Schönlein purpura
  —Behçet syndrome (iridocyclitis, genital and oral ulcerations)

—Inflammatory bowel disease (Crohn disease, ulcerative colitis)
—Serum sickness
—Erythema multiforme/Stevens-Johnson syndrome

- Miscellaneous

—Knee
  —Apophysitis (i.e., Osgood-Schlatter disease)
  —Patellofemoral pain syndrome (chondromalacia patella)
  —Osteochondritis dessicans

—Hip
  —Slipped capital femoral epiphysis

 Data Gathering

HISTORY

Question: Was there trauma?
Significance: History of recent trauma does not rule out septic arthritis.

Question: Can you describe the pain?
Significance: Pain of bacterial arthritis worsens over 1 to 3 days and does not wax and wane.

Question: How many joints are involved?
Significance: Septic arthritis is rarely polyarticular.

 Physical Examination

- Fever occurs within the first few days of illness in 75% of patients, but less commonly in infants. Only 50% of children with gonococcal arthritis will have fever.
- Children with septic arthritis usually appear ill.
- The joint appears warm and swollen.
- Pseudoparalysis: decreased range of motion
- Hip effusion causes the leg to be held flexed and externally rotated.
- The child with septic arthritis will usually have pain through *any* range of motion. In contrast, most traumatic injuries will allow some painless range of motion of that joint.
- There are usually no external findings when the hip or shoulder joints are infected.
- Consider hip involvement when the patient complains of knee or thigh pain.
- In the frightened or uncooperative child, it is possible to have the parent perform an examination for tenderness and range of motion while the physician observes from a distance.

 Laboratory Aids

TESTS

Joint Fluid in Septic Arthritis

- The WBC is often greater than 100,000/mm^3, but can be as low as 50,000/mm^3 in early infections.
- The glucose level in the synovial fluid is less than 50% that of the serum.
- Culture of the joint reveals an organism in 70% to 80% of cases (except for gonorrhea).
- A Gram stain of synovial fluid reveals pathogens in 50% of cases.

Other Supportive Tests

- The ESR is elevated (>30 mm/hr) in 95% of cases.
- The C-reactive protein is increased
- Blood cultures are positive in 30% to 40% of cases.
- A high WBC count is neither sensitive nor specific for septic arthritis.

IMAGING

- Radiography is rarely helpful in diagnosis, can show widening of joint space and/or displacement of the normal fat pads in the knee or elbow, and is less often positive in the shoulder or hip.

- A Technetium-99 bone scan reveals increased uptake in the perimeter of the joint during the "blood pool" phase of the study.
- Ultrasound of the affected joint usually delineates the amount of fluid within the joint capsule. However, this test cannot differentiate between an infectious and a purely inflammatory disease.

FALSE POSITIVES

- Bone scan cannot easily differentiate septic arthritis from epiphyseal osteomyelitis.
- Evaluation of synovial fluid from patients with rheumatologic disease can mimic that of infectious arthritis; however, the clinical picture should allow differentiation of these entities.

 ## Therapy

See the table Empiric Therapy Prior to Identification of Organisms.

EMERGENCY CARE

- Drainage of infection: should occur *as soon as possible* if bacterial cause is suspected
- Indications for open surgical drainage/irrigation:

—Hip involvement
—Shoulder involvement (controversial)

—Thick, purulent, or fibrinous exudate unable to pass through 18-gauge needle
—All other joints not undergoing open drainage should undergo needle aspiration.

- Antibiotic administration as soon as possible after joint aspiration is performed
- Immobilization of extremity
- Pain management

DRUGS

Choice of antibiotics depends on age of child as outlined in the tables below.

DURATION OF THERAPY (IV + PO) FOR VARIOUS ORGANISMS

- Treat for at least 2 weeks after resolution of fever and joint effusion.
- ≥28 days: *S. aureus,* gram-negative organisms, group B streptococcus
- ≥14 days: *H. influenzae, N. meningitidis,* streptococci
- ≥7 days: *N. gonorrhoeae*

 ## Follow-Up

- Involve orthopedic surgery and physical therapy services in follow-up.
- Once the patient is receiving oral therapy, serum bactericidal titers (SBT) must be monitored

on a weekly basis if possible. Oral antibiotic titers should be kept at eight times the SBT.

WHEN TO EXPECT IMPROVEMENT

With appropriate antibacterial therapy, one should see improvement of symptoms with 2 days of initial administration.

SIGNS TO WATCH FOR

- Continued pain, fever, or lack of improvement of range of motion after 3 to 4 days of appropriate antibiotic treatment.
- Rising ESR or CRP in the face of antibiotic treatment.

PITFALLS

- Clinical examination in conjunction with the history of acute onset should raise the suspicion of septic arthritis even in the face of "negative" laboratory screening tests. The most accurate determinations can be inferred from analysis of the synovial fluid.
- Realize that some children, especially neonates and young infants, will not manifest signs of systemic disease early in the course of the illness.
- Observe failure or success of therapy, especially when the extremity is immobilized.

 ## Common Questions and Answers

Q: How can one differentiate toxic synovitis from septic arthritis on the initial visit?
A: Although this is sometimes a difficult diagnosis to make with certainty, patients with toxic synovitis usually exhibit certain characteristics that patients with septic arthritis do not:

- Almost always involves the hip joint
- History of previous viral infection
- Some painless range of motion of the involved joint is possible.
- The ESR is lower than 30 mm/hr.

BIBLIOGRAPHY

Adebajo AO. Rheumatic manifestations of infectious diseases in children. *Curr Opin Rheumatol* 1998;10:79–85.

Dagan R. Management of acute hematogenous osteomyelitis and septic arthritis in the pediatric patient. *Pediatr Infect Dis J* 1993;12:88–93.

Del Beccaro MA, Champoux AN, Bockers T, Mendelman PM. Septic arthritis versus transient synovitis of the hip: the value of screening laboratory tests. *Ann Emerg Med* 1992;21:1418–1422.

Pioro MH, Mandell BF. Septic arthritis. *Rheum Dis Clin North Am* 1997;23:239–258.

Rose CD, Eppes SC. Infection-related arthritis. *Rheu Dis Clin N Am* 1997;23:677–695

Wall EJ. Childhood osteomyelitis and septic arthritis. *Curr Opin Ped* 1998;10:73–76.

Author: Joel A. Fein

Types of Organisms

AGE	MOST COMMON ORGANISM	OTHER ORGANISMS
Newborn	Staphylococcus aureus	Candida albicans
		Group B streptococcus
		Gram-negative organisms
	(Klebsiella, Salmonella)	
Infants and children ≤5 years	S. aureus	Haemophilus influenzae *
		Streptococcus pneumoniae
Children >5 years	S. aureus	S. pneumoniae
		Neisseria meningitidis
Adolescents	Neisseria gonorrhoeae	S. aureus
		S. pneumoniae
		N. meningitidis

*Less likely in fully immunized children.

Empiric Therapy Prior to Identification of Organism

AGE	FIRST CHOICE	SECOND CHOICE	DURATION
Neonatal	Cefotaxime O/N/M	O/N/M Ampicillin Gentamicin	IV for ≥14 days PO for ≥14 days
<5 years	Cefuroxime	O/N/M Chloramphenicol Cefazolin Clindamycin	IV + PO = 28 days
>5 years	O/N/M		IV + PO = 28 days
Adolescent			
Gonococcal	Ceftriaxone	Penicillin	IV + PO = 7–10 days
Nongonococcal	O/N/M	Cefazolin	IV + PO = 28 days

O/N/M = oxicillin or nafcillin or methicillin.

Serum Sickness

Database

DEFINITION

- Serum sickness: type III hypersensitivity reaction that occurs 7 to 21 days after injection of foreign protein or serum (usually in the form of antiserums). The clinical syndrome consists of skin rash, itching, fever, malaise, proteinuria, vasculitis, and joint pain.
- Serum sickness-like reactions are characterized by fever, rash, lymphadenopathy, and arthralgia, which occurs 1 to 3 weeks after drug exposure. Immune complexes, vasculitis, and hypocomplementemia are absent. These are the types of reaction associated with cefaclor. They are commonly referred to as serum sickness.
- Serum sickness-like reactions are more common than true serum sickness since equine serum antitoxins have been replaced with human antitoxin sera. Clinically, they present identically and are treated the same.
- Common causative agents: horse antithymocyte globulins, human diploid-cell rabies vaccine, streptokinase, Hymenoptera venom, penicillins, cephalosporins, sulfonamides, hydralazine, thiouracils, metronidazole, naproxen, and dextrans.

PATHOPHYSIOLOGY

- Type III immune complex antigen-antibody complement reaction.
- Antibodies are formed 6 to 10 days after the introduction of foreign material. Antibodies interact with antigens, forming immune complexes that diffuse into vascular walls. They become fixated in tissue and activate the complement cascade. C3a and C5a are produced, resulting in increased vascular permeability and activated inflammatory cells. Polymorphonuclear cells and monocytes cause diffuse vasculitis.

GENETICS

People with a genetic predisposition to produce IgE are more susceptible.

EPIDEMIOLOGY

- Limited information is available regarding the incidence of adverse drug reactions in children; it is generally believed to occur less frequently in children than in adults.
- More than 90% of serum sickness cases are drug induced.
- Less than 5% of serum sickness cases are fatal.

COMPLICATIONS

- Shock
- Digital necrosis
- Guillain-Barré syndrome (rare)
- Generalized vasculitis (rare)
- Peripheral neuropathy (rare)
- Glomerulonephritis (rare)
- Increased risk of anaphylaxis with repeat exposure to substance
- Fatality (rare, usually due to continued administration of antigen)

PROGNOSIS

- Excellent. Most cases are mild and transient with no sequela.
- Symptoms resolve in a few days to a few weeks.

Differential Diagnosis

- Erythema multiforme
- Mononucleosis
- Systemic lupus erythematosus
- Rocky Mountain spotted fever
- Henoch-Schönlein purpura
- Hypersensitivity syndrome reaction
- Drug-induced pseudoporphyria
- Acute generalized exanthematous pustulosis
- Wegener granulomatosis

Data Gathering

HISTORY

- Suspect in any patient with an unexplained vasculitic rash who has been taking any new drug during the last 2 months

Special Questions

- Ask about presentation and evolution of rash. Typically, the rash first appears on the sides of the fingers, hands, and feet before becoming widespread.
- Is there associated pruritus? There is often pruritus.
- Fever? Often present, usually mild.
- Ask about the presence of arthritis or arthralgia. Present over half the time; usually involves the metocarpophalangeal and knee joints.
- Is there associated abdominal pain? Some cases may have visceral involvement.
- Is there a history of hematuria? There can be modest renal involvement, usually presenting as proteinuria and microscopic hematuria.
- Does the patient report any neurologic symptoms? Peripheral neuropathy, brachial plexus involvement, and Guillain-Barré syndrome have been reported associations.
- Is there a previous history of a similar rash? Was it associated with any medications in the past? The rash and symptoms of serum sickness will occur sooner on repeat exposure. Try to differentiate from simple drug rash; timing of rash after exposure is important in differentiating between the two.
- Have you had any drug or antitoxin exposure in the last month, especially to penicillins, cephalosporins, sulfonamides, hydralazine, thiouracils, streptokinase, metronidazole, naproxen, and dextrans?

Physical Examination

- Erythematous purpuric rash starts at the sides of the feet, toes, hands, and fingers and then becomes more widespread.
- Erythema multiforme, maculopapular, purpuric, or urticarial type rash
- Mild to severe fever
- Generalized lymphadenopathy; may be localized to lymph nodes that drain the injection site
- Splenomegaly, occasionally
- Edema of the face and neck.
- Joint pain

Laboratory Aids

TESTS

Tests are not extremely helpful in establishing diagnosis because no abnormality is universally present. Diagnosis is usually apparent by classic findings and history of foreign protein or drug exposure.

- Urinalysis: may show proteinuria and/or hematuria
- Complements levels variably reduced before returning to normal.
- Leukocytosis or leukopenia with or without eosinophilia
- Erythrocyte sedimentation rate may be slightly elevated.
- Direct immunofluorescent staining of rash biopsy (not routinely recommended as part of work-up) shows deposits of IgM and C3 complement in capillary walls.

Therapy

- Stop suspected medication/antigen immediately and avoid its future use.
- Topical steroids to relieve itching
- Antihistamines to inhibit the action of vasoactive mediators
- NSAIDs to relieve joint pain
- Oral corticosteroids for severe cases. The recommendation is to administer and taper over 10- to 14-day period. A shorter course may result in relapse, and recurrent symptoms are more difficult to alleviate.
- Admit if symptoms are severe or diagnosis is unclear.

Follow-Up

WHEN TO EXPECT IMPROVEMENT

- Usually self-limited illness that resolves in a few days to weeks
- If symptoms persist for more than 1 month, reconsider your diagnosis.

PREVENTION

- There is no known way to prevent a first occurrence.
- Take a careful history of previous allergic reactions.
- Skin testing prior to antiserum administration will prevent anaphylaxis but not serum sickness.
- When the need for antiserum arises, consider prophylactic antihistamines.

PITFALLS

- A history of fever, rash, and arthralgias is commonly seen with many childhood illnesses. One must always consider differential diagnoses.
- Symptoms may be so minimal that the patient does not seek medical attention.
- Often misdiagnosed as simple drug allergy

Common Questions and Answers

Q: What is the difference between serum sickness and drug allergies?
A: Drug allergies are type I IgE-mediated hypersensitivity reactions that occur very soon after drug exposure in a previously sensitized individual. Serum sickness is a type III antibody-antigen immune complex and complement amplified hypersensitivity reaction that occurs 1 to 3 weeks after an initial exposure.

Q: If my child has had serum sickness, is she at risk for getting it again?
A: Yes, if she receives the same medicine or related medicines again. The symptoms will occur more quickly, usually in 2 to 4 days, and may be more severe.

Q: Will my child have long-term effects from this illness?
A: No, this is a self-limited disease, and as long as the offending agent is stopped, your child will recover completely.

Q: Is there any way to prevent my child from getting serum sickness?
A: Unfortunately, there is no way to predict if your child will have a serum sickness-like reaction to a particular medication. It is extremely important to be aware of your child's exact allergies to medications and to inform all health care providers caring for your child.

Q: My child has had serum sickness while taking an antibiotic. Can he take other antibiotics?
A: Yes, but your child should never receive that particular antibiotic or any closely related antibiotic again. Repeat exposure will likely result in serum sickness occurring more quickly than after the first exposure. Your child can safely take antibiotics from other drug families.

Q: If one of my children has had serum sickness from an antibiotic, are my other children at risk?
A: No, there is no known genetic predisposition for serum sickness. Your other children do not need to avoid the medication that caused serum sickness.

Q: How is the Arthus reaction different from serum sickness?
A: The Arthus reaction is also a type III hypersensitivity reaction, but it causes only a local reaction. It is a local vasculitis caused by formation of antigen-antibody complexes in local vessel walls, which then activate the inflammation process. The reaction occurs within hours after an individual is injected intradermally with an antigen against which he or she has been actively immunized.

ICD-9-CM 999.5

BIBLIOGRAPHY

Erffmeyer JE. Serum sickness. *Ann Allergy* 1986;56:105–109.

Evans R, Kim K, Mahr TA. Current concepts in allergy: drug reactions. *Curr Probl Pediatr* 1991;21:185–192.

Heckbert SR, Stryker WS, Coltin ICL, Manson DE, Platt R. Serum sickness in children after antibiotic exposure: estimates of occurrence and morbidity in a health maintenance organization population. *Am J Epidemiol* 1990;132:336–342.

Knowles S, Shapiro L, Shear NH. Serious dermatologic reactions in children. *Curr Opin Pediatr* 1997;9:388–395.

Lawley TJ, Frank MM. Immune complexes and allergic disease. In: Middleton E, ed. *Allergy principles and practice,* 5th ed. St. Louis: Mosby Yearbook, 702–712.

Roujeau J, Stern RS. Severe adverse cutaneous reactions to drugs. *N Engl J Med* 1994;331: 1272–1285.

VanArsdel PP. Allergy and adverse drug reactions. *J Am Acad Dermatol* 1982;6:833–845.

Author: Denise Salerno

Severe Combined Immunodeficiency

 Database

DEFINITION

Severe combined immunodeficiency (SCID) is primary immunodeficiency characterized by onset of severe, life-threatening infections in infancy due to defective or absent T- and/or B-lymphocyte-mediated immunity.

CAUSES

• A variety of defects lead to a similar clinical presentation.
• The X-linked subset is caused by defective transcription of the gamma chain of the IL-2 receptor.
• The autosomal recessive (AR) subset is due to various defects:

—Adenosine deaminase deficiency
—Purine nucleoside phosphorylase deficiency
—Absent expression of MHC class I or II molecules
—A large percentage of AR cases have as yet unidentified defect(s).

GENETICS

• X-linked and autosomal recessive inheritance

EPIDEMIOLOGY

• Incidence: estimated to be 1 in 66,000 to 100,000 live births
• Most patients present by 6 months of age.
• The X-linked form accounts for 50% to 60% of SCID cases.
• ADA deficiency accounts for 20% to 25% of SCID cases.
• PNP deficiency accounts for 2% of SCID cases.
• Autosomal recessive forms account for most of the remainder.

COMPLICATIONS

• Untreated, most patients succumb to overwhelming infection.
• Graft versus host disease (GVHD) may result from transfusion of nonirradiated blood products.
• Clinical disease can be caused by live vaccines in previous undiagnosed SCID patients.
• Increased incidence of malignancy:

—Overall risk of malignancy is approximately 5%.
—Thirty-fold increased incidence of lymphoma

 Differential Diagnosis

• Specific diagnosis of ADA deficiency as the cause of SCID is important, because enzyme replacement therapy is available.
• Reticular dysgenesis
• Letterer-Siwe syndrome (histiocytosis)
• Omenn syndrome
• HIV infection
• Failure to thrive is the most common presenting problem.
• Recurrent and or life-threatening infections in infancy with a variety of pathogens (both common and atypical organisms)
• Chronic diarrhea
• Persistent thrush
• Skin rashes are commonly in unusual patterns or locations. They may be the presenting symptom of GVHD.

 Data Gathering

HISTORY

• Description of infections, severity, duration, response to treatment
• Family history of unexplained deaths or unusual infections

 Physical Examination

• Evaluation should focus on the presence of infection.
• Often an emaciated-appearing infant
• Marked absence of lymphoid and tonsillar tissue
• Dermatologic evaluation may reveal atypical rashes.

Laboratory Aids

TESTS

• CBC with differential to assess for degree of lymphopenia
• T- and B-lymphocyte enumeration:

—T-lymphocytes are markedly decreased or absent.
—B-lymphocytes are variable but can be normal.

• Mitogen and antigen stimulation tests are markedly decreased or absent.
• Immunoglobulin levels are usually low or absent.

—Patients can have normal IgG levels in the first few months of life due to tranplacentally derived maternal IgG.

• Appropriate cultures to identify pathogens

 Therapy

• Bone marrow transplant (BMT) is the definitive treatment in most cases. Because of the impairment of recipient immune function, conditioning for BMT may be less rigorous than in other situations requiring BMT.
• Aggressive and early specific antibiotic/antifungal/antiviral therapy for infections
• *Pneumocystis carinii* prophylaxis
• If required, patients should receive only irradiated blood products. There is a risk of GVHD due to viable donor leukocytes that may survive in nonirradiated products.
• Intravenous immunoglobulin replacement: This may be required even after BMT because of variable B-lymphocyte reconstitution.
• Enzyme replacement therapy has been used in ADA-deficient patients.

 Follow-Up

• Close monitoring of clinical status should be done before BMT. This may be every 2 to 4 weeks, depending on the patient's status.
• The posttransplant course is variable.

—The overall success rate for matched BMT in SCID is approximately 65%. Success is also being seen in partially matched BMT.
—Patients should still be followed closely for signs of infection, graft failure, and GVHD.

 Common Questions and Answers

Q: How should a child with SCID be managed before BMT?
A: Any child suspected to have SCID should be isolated from potential sources of infection. They should not attend public places such as school because of the risk of obtaining an infection. The patient should be kept away from ill siblings or relatives. This is especially true if there has been an exposure to chickenpox or other viral illnesses.

Q: Should patients with SCID receive live viral vaccines?
A: Live viral vaccines are *contraindicated* in SCID. Any patient suspected of severe immunodeficiency should not receive live viral vaccines until their immunodeficiency is defined. If the patient is receiving IVIG therapy, vaccinations are not required. In addition, siblings of patients with SCID who live in the same household should not receive live viral vaccines. This is due to the risk of viral shedding in the siblings.

Q: What is the chance of another child being affected with SCID?
A: The risk of another child being born with SCID in a family with a previously affected child will depend on the type of SCID. X-linked: 50% chance of an affected male or carrier female. Autosomal recessive causes: 25% chance of an affected child. Genetic counseling should be offered to female carriers of X-linked SCID.

Q: Can SCID be diagnosed prenatally?
A: Prenatal testing is available. Amniocentesis can be performed, and fetal cells can be tested for the presence of ADA and PNP enzymes. Fetal cord blood sampling can be done to determine the presence or absence of fetal T and/or B cells.

ICD-9-CM 279.2

BIBLIOGRAPHY

Gelfand EW, Dosch HM. Diagnosis and classification of severe combined immunodeficiency. *Birth Defects* 1983;19:65–72.

Stephan JL, Vlekova V, Le Deist F. Severe combined immunodeficiency: a retrospective single center study of clinical presentation and outcome in 117 patients. *J Pediatr* 1990;123: 564–572.

Stites DP, Terr AI, eds. *Basic and clinical immunology*, 7th ed. Norwalk, CT: Appleton & Lange 1991:341–344.

Winkelstein JA, et al., eds. *Immune Deficiency Foundation. Patient and family handbook: for the primary immune deficiency diseases*.

Author: Alex G. Yip

Sexual Abuse

 Database

DEFINITION

Sexual abuse is the involvement of a child in sexual activities that (s)he cannot understand, for which (s)he is not developmentally prepared, to which (s)he cannot give informed consent, and that violate societal taboos. It is due to a complex interaction of societal, familial, and individual factors. Associated problems are:

- Physical abuse
- Domestic violence
- Neglect
- Emotional abuse

EPIDEMIOLOGY

- Approximately 150,000 substantiated cases are identified each year in the United States. This is likely to be a significant underestimation of the actual numbers.
- Girls are victimized more than boys, who represent approximately 20% of cases reported to child protection agencies each year.
- Sexual abuse of boys is believed to be underreported.
- Children of all ages are victimized, with a peak age of vulnerability being 7 to 13 years.
- Race and socioeconomic status are not believed to play a role in the epidemiology of sexual abuse.

COMPLICATIONS

- Sexually transmitted infections, such as gonorrhea, genital warts, *Chlamydia trachomatis*, syphilis, and herpes simplex virus, are identified in only a small percentage of sexually abused children.
- Emotional problems such as posttraumatic stress disorder (PTSD), feelings of helplessness, impaired trust, low self-esteem, depression, adolescent substance abuse, and suicide attempts
- Aggressive, hypersexual, withdrawn behaviors may be consequences of having been abused.

PROGNOSIS

- Varies greatly depending on specifics of abuse sustained, available support systems
- More extensive injuries (e.g., deep lacerations, tears) may take weeks to months to heal.
- The emotional impact of abuse is very slow to resolve, and may take years to resolve.

 Differential Diagnosis

- Infection

—With genital discharge: sexually transmitted infections (*Neisseria gonorrhoeae, Chlamydia trachomatis, Trichomonas vaginalis*), group A streptococcus, *Haemophilus influenzae, Staphylococcus aureus, Corynbacterium diphtheriae, Mycoplasma hominis, Gardnerella vaginalis, Shigella* (discharge may be bloody)
—With genital bleeding: urinary tract infection, vulvovaginitis
—With genital inflammation/pruritis: sexually transmitted infections, pinworms, scabies, *Candida albicans,* group A streptococcal perianal cellulitis
—With genital bruising that may be complicated by purpura fulminans, disseminated intravascular coagulation

- Tumors

—Sarcoma botryoid: a highly malignant sarcoma, typically of the urogenital tract

- Trauma

—Accidental trauma, including straddle and impaling injuries
—Mechanical friction from tight clothing or obesity
—Accidental tourniquet of genitals by hair

- Congenital

—Variations in hymenal configuration (septated, cribriform, microperforate, imperforate hymens)
—Urethral caruncles; vestibular bands
—Ectopic ureterocele; hemangiomas
—Syndromes associated with anogenital anomalies

- Psychosocial

—Normal behaviors (masturbation, playing doctor)
—Inappropriate viewing of sexual activity (e.g., in which the child witnesses others or sees adult videos/movies)
—False allegations of sexual abuse

- Dermatologic

—Contact dermatitis
—Seborrhea
—Diaper dermatitis
—Lichen sclerosis et atrophica
—Balanitis xerotica
—Nevi

- Endocrine

—Neonatal withdrawal bleeding
—Leukorrhea

- Miscellaneous

—Nonspecific vulvovaginitis
—Rectovaginal fistula
—Labial adhesion (agglutination)
—Urethral prolapse
—Phimosis, paraphimosis
—Foreign body

 Data Gathering

HISTORY

- The physician interview should be detailed if the physician is the first professional to interview the child. Prior to the examination, however, the child may have been interviewed by the police, social service workers, or a forensic interviewer. In this case, the history does not need to include all of the following details, but should include information needed to perform an appropriate medical assessment of the child.
- The interview should be conducted with child alone in the room; diagnosis often depends on the history obtained from the child.
- Use nonleading questions.
- Use developmentally appropriate language.

Special Questions

Ask about:

- Identity of alleged perpetrator/relationship to child
- Time of last possible contact
- Method of disclosure
- Frequency of abuse (one time versus chronic)
- Specific types of sexual contact included in the abuse
- Whether the perpetrator ejaculated, if a male
- Threats made to child by alleged perpetrator
- Previous official reports of the abuse

 Physical Examination

- Varies depending on age of child
- Adolescent girls require a full pelvic examination.
- Prepubertal children require careful genital inspection only.
- A few physical findings are diagnostic of abuse. These include the finding of semen or sperm, acute genital/anal injuries without an adequate accidental explanation, gonorrhea, or syphilis (excluding perinatal infection).
- Look for acute genital injuries in the absence of an appropriate history, and marked disruptions in hymenal tissue.
- Many genital findings are unlikely to be related to abuse. These include small labial adhesions in girls who are not yet toilet trained, *Candida albicans* dermatitis, erythema of the vestibule, and small mounds or projections on an otherwise normal hymen.

PROCEDURE

- The labial traction technique (gently grabbing labia majora and pulling laterally, down and toward you) allows for the best visualization of the hymenal edges.
- A Wood lamp is useful for identification of possible semen. Note: Materials other than semen may fluoresce with a Wood lamp.

Laboratory Aids

TESTS

- Universal STD screening is not necessary.
- Vaginal cultures are obtained from within the vaginal canal. Allow 10 to 15 seconds for swabs to absorb secretions.
- Cultures for *N. gonorrhoeae* from rectum, vagina (prepubertal), cervix (adolescent), penile urethra, throat. Misidentification of *N. gonorrhoeae* can be a problem if confirmatory tests (e.g., sugar fermentation, latex agglutination) are not properly done. Know your laboratory and their methods of identification and confirmation. Cultures are the gold standard and are the only acceptable method for diagnosing sexually transmitted diseases in prepubertal children.
- *Chlamydia* cultures from rectum, vagina, cervix, penile urethra. Obtain cells for *Chlamydia* culture by gently scraping the vaginal wall with a swab (in young children). Because of the low prevalence of *Chlamydia* in the prepubertal population and normal flora that can produce false-positive results, culture remains the gold standard for *Chlamydia* testing. Rapid tests are *not* recommended for young children. PCR and LCR diagnostic techniques have not been approved for young children.
- General genital culture
- Rapid plasma reagin (RPR), hepatitis serology, HIV if indicated
- Forensic evidence collection (for an acute assault)

 Therapy

- Ensure the safety of the child.
- Report *suspected* abuse to the local child welfare agency.
- Report *suspected* sexual abuse to law enforcement.
- Consult a social worker.
- Inform the parents of the report.

DRUGS

- Prophylactic antibiotics that are effective against common STDs, such as gonorrhea, *Chlamydia*, and syphilis, are generally not used for prepubertal children, because these infections are uncommon. Prophylaxis against STDs may be considered for stranger assaults.
- Identified sexually transmitted diseases should be treated with the appropriate regimen.
- Consider pregnancy prevention (i.e., hormonal contraceptive) for adolescents.
- Tetanus booster for patients with acute, serious genital or other injuries.
- Sitz baths for comfort

 Follow-Up

- Cases will be investigated by child welfare and/or the police.
- Need for foster care placement and/or ongoing supervision is decided by investigators.
- Most children are referred for short- or long-term counseling.
- Persistent physical/genital complaints, which may indicate ongoing abuse, an STD, or psychological problems
- Patient victimizing younger child: Young perpetrators are often victims of previous abuse.
- It is important to get help for the child perpetrator so that the pattern of abuse does not continue.

PREVENTION

The efficacy of sexual abuse prevention programs is difficult to measure. Although children who are taught about personal safety learn from the experience, it is unknown whether their behavior is changed by such education.

PITFALLS

- Failing to consider sexual abuse in the differential diagnosis of nonspecific behavioral and physical complaints
- If cultures are not properly performed, the results may be uninterpretable or misleading.

 Common Questions and Answers

Q: What does an "intact hymen" mean?
A: "Intact hymen" is not a medical term and should be avoided in describing the medical examination of the genitals. The hymen is a membranous structure at the entrance to the vaginal canal. It should have an opening that varies in size depending on the child, the child's age, the position in which the child was examined, and so on. The hymen should be inspected for signs of trauma. There is a wide variation of normal hymenal appearances, and caution should be used in interpreting findings.

Q: Can there be penetration without physical findings?
A: Yes. Although full penetration of an erect penis into the prepubertal vaginal canal (through the hymen) will leave injury, the healing properties of the hymenal tissue are great, so that past injuries are sometimes difficult or impossible to identify. Furthermore, penetration may be partial (as in vulvar coitus) and may not leave any injuries to the tissue. For these reasons, physical injuries may not be identified despite a history of penetration.

Q: Are sexually transmitted diseases always transmitted sexually?
A: No. All sexually transmitted diseases may be transmitted vertically (from mother to infant). The incubation periods of different infections vary, so they are expressed at different ages accordingly. Casual transmission of sexually transmitted diseases is postulated for some organisms, but not for others. Gonorrhea and syphilis are considered diagnostic of sexual abuse outside of congenital infection. Chlamydia, herpes simplex virus 2, and trichomonas are probably due to sexual abuse and should be reported for evaluation. *Condyloma acuminata* is quite controversial at this time, is probably related to sexual abuse in preschool and older children, and should be referred for evaluation. Herpes simplex virus 1 and bacterial vaginosis are nonspecific infections that are not usually related to sexual abuse. *Candida* is unlikely to be related to sexual abuse.

Q: How often do sexually abused children have physical evidence of the abuse?
A: In the majority of cases, there are no specific physical indicators of abuse. Only a small minority of patients have physical evidence considered diagnostic of abuse. Many children have nonspecific abnormalities of the physical examination, and many have normal examinations. Classification systems for interpreting genital findings are being developed to assist in the interpretation of findings (see Physical Examination and Bibliography).

ICD-9-CM 995.5

BIBLIOGRAPHY

Adams JA, Harper K, Knudson S, et al. Examination findings in legally confirmed child sexual abuse: it's normal to be normal. *Pediatrics* 1994;94:310–317.

American Academy of Pediatrics Committee on Child Abuse and Neglect. Guidelines for the evaluation of sexual abuse of children. *Pediatrics* 1991;87:254–260.

Bays J, Chadwick D. Medical diagnosis of the sexually abused child. *Child Abuse Negl* 1993;17:91–110.

Bays J, Jenny C. Genital and anal conditions confused with child sexual abuse trauma. *Am J Dis Child* 1990;144:1319–1322.

Giardino AP, Finkel MA, Giardino ER, et al. *A practical guide to the evaluation of sexual abuse in the prepubertal child.* Newbury Park, CA: Sage Publications Inc, 1992.

Kellogg ND, Parra JM, Menard S, et al. Children with anogenital symptoms and signs referred for sexual abuse evaluations. *Arch Pediatr Adolesc Med* 1998;153:634–641.

Ludwig S. Psychosocial emergencies: child abuse. In: Fleischer GR, Ludwig S, eds. *Textbook of pediatric emergency medicine,* 3rd ed. Baltimore: Williams & Wilkins, 1993.

Author: Cindy W. Christian

Sexual Ambiguity

 ## Database

DEFINITION

Genitalia can be defined as ambiguous when it is not possible to categorize the gender of the child based on outward appearances.

PATHOPHYSIOLOGY

Gonadal Dysgenesis

- Partial dysgenesis of the gonads following differentiation into testes will result in a spectrum of abnormalities ranging from phenotypically female external genitalia with the absence of mullerian structures to micropenis or cryptorchidism.
- Mixed gonadal dysgenesis: Individuals with the mosaic genotypes XO/XY and XX/XY have gonads containing both ovarian and testicular elements and external genitalia ranging from normal female, intersex, to normal male.
- Hermaphroditism: True hermaphrodites have gonads possessing both ovarian and testicular elements. This condition includes the patients with mixed gonadal dysgenesis discussed above, in addition to those with the karyotype 46XX, and less commonly 46XY.

Disorders of Sexual Phenotype

- *Female pseudohermaphroditism:* Masculinization of the female fetus is usually caused by androgens produced by the fetus or transferred across the placenta from the mother. The most common cause is CAH.
- *Male pseudohermaphroditism:* Incomplete masculinization of the male fetus can be caused by enzyme disorders of testosterone synthesis (e.g., CAH, 5α-reductase deficiency) or unresponsiveness to testosterone action (androgen resistance syndromes).

GENETICS

- Gonadal dysgenesis is associated with chromosomal aberrations.
- The mutations causing congenital adrenal hyperplasia are autosomal recessive and display HLA linkage.
- 5_α-Reductase deficiency is an autosomal recessive disorder that manifests only in genetic males. Androgen resistance syndromes follow an X-linked recessive pattern.

EPIDEMIOLOGY

Incidence

Inherited adrenal enzymatic defects of adrenal biosynthesis are the most common cause of virilization of the newborn female. Ninety percent of these females have 21-hydroxylase deficiency.

Age

Disorders causing sexual ambiguity occur congenitally, and the time of presentation is the newborn period. Children with 5_α-reductase deficiency demonstrate virilization with puberty.

COMPLICATIONS

- 21-hydroxylase, 3_β-hydroxysteroid dehydrogenase, and cholesterol desmolase deficiencies are associated with life-threatening salt-losing adrenal crises presenting in the first 2 weeks of life.
- Dysgenetic testes and ovotestes have an increased risk of malignant degeneration and should be removed.
- An incorrect or hastily made sexual assignment can cause family members undue emotional stress.

PROGNOSIS

The cosmetic outcome from surgery is usually good. The potential for gender-appropriate sexual function is usually good with therapy. The potential for reproductive function depends on the diagnosis. Long-term studies of psychological adjustment are underway.

 ## Differential Diagnosis

- Gonadal dysgenesis

—Partial dysgenesis of the gonads
—Mixed gonadal dysgenesis
—Hermaphroditism

- Female pseudohermaphroditism

—Congenital adrenal hyperplasia: Inherited adrenal enzymatic defects, including 21-hydroxylase, 11-hydroxylase, and 3_β-hydroxysteroid dehydrogenase (3_β-HSD) deficiencies, are associated with cortisol deficiency and the production of excessive amounts of adrenal androgens, which can cause virilization. Mineralocorticoid deficiency is seen with 21-hydroxylase and 3_β-HSD deficiencies, as well.
—Maternal androgen exposure
 —Exogenous androgens or endogenous production (e.g., maternal virilizing tumor)

—Multiple congenital anomalies
 —Ambiguous genitalia can be a part of a spectrum of congenital anomalies, especially those of the urologic system and rectum.

—Idiopathic

- Male pseudohermaphroditism

—Congenital adrenal hyperplasia (CAH): Deficiencies in 3_β-HSD, 17_α-hydroxylase, and cholesterol desmolase result in insufficient androgen synthesis.
—5_α-Reductase deficiency prevents the conversion of testosterone to dihydrotestosterone (DHT), which is necessary for the development of the male external genitalia.
—Syndromes of androgen resistance are due to abnormalities in androgen receptor or postreceptor defects. Patients with incomplete forms of androgen resistance may present with sexual ambiguity.
—Multiple congenital anomalies
—Idiopathic

 ## Data Gathering

Ambiguous genitalia in the neonate should be treated as an emergency, and the diagnostic evaluation undertaken as soon as possible.

HISTORY

Obtain a careful pregnancy and family history addressing:

- Drug ingestion
- Exposure to teratogens
- Infections during the pregnancy
- Androgenic changes in the mother
- Family history suggestive of CAH

Physical Examination

Notable features include:

- Palpable gonads: imply the presence of Y-chromosome material
- Fusion of the labia
- Existence of a vagina
- Position of the urethra
- Length and diameter of the penis
- Development of the scrotum
- Other dysmorphic features
- Hypertension is seen with 17_α-hydroxylase and 11-hydroxylase deficiencies.

See the table Features of the Classical Disorders of Adrenal Steroidogenesis.

 ## Laboratory Aids

TESTS

Specific Tests

- Karyotype
- Steroid levels

—17-Hydroxyprogesterone
—17-Hydroxypregnenolone
—DHEA
—Testosterone
—Dihydrotestosterone
—11-Deoxycortisol
—Androstenedione

Imaging

- Pelvic ultrasound
- Urethrogram

Nonspecific Tests

Electrolytes: Hyponatremia, hyperkalemia, and acidosis are associated with several adrenal enzyme deficiencies.

 ## Therapy

- Gender assignment

—The results of the diagnostic evaluation should be available within 48 to 72 hours, and gender assignment made by this time. A team approach with consultations from endocrinology, urology and psychiatry is useful.

- Surgery

—Surgery may be necessary so that the sexual phenotype and gonads are consistent with the gender assignment. Dysgenetic testes and ovotestes should be removed.

- Treatment of CAH

—Acute salt-wasting adrenal crisis
  —Volume resuscitation with D5NS
  —Stress hydrocortisone 25 to 50 mg IV immediately after the serum studies are drawn. This should be followed by 100 mg/m²/24 h of hydrocortisone IV divided q4h.
  —Hydrocortisone is gradually tapered over the next few days.
  —Fludrocortisone 0.05 to 0.3 mg/d when able to take PO

—Chronic management of CAH consists of cortisol replacement 12 to 25 mg/m²/24 h divided as q8h and fludrocortisone 0.05 to 0.3 mg/d.

- Counseling of families

 ## Follow-Up

- Hormone replacement therapy at puberty may be necessary.
- Long-term follow-up may involve monitoring hormone levels, linear growth, and sexual development.

PREVENTION

- Avoid the use of androgenic steroids during pregnancy.
- Prenatal diagnosis of CAH/maternal steroid treatment is available.

PITFALLS

Girls with CAH may appear quite virilized at birth and be mistaken for boys. Nevertheless, they have good female reproductive potential with adequate control of their disease, and should be assigned a female sex.

Common Questions and Answers

Q: Should a child's sex assignment be consistent with the karyotype?
A: Karyotype should not be the major factor in gender determination because gonadal and future sexual function are more important.

Q: What clues can the physical examination give to the timing of in utero events causing sexual ambiguity?
A: In the virilized female, labioscrotal fusion results from androgen exposure prior to week 12 gestation. Thereafter, androgen exposure can only cause clitoromegaly.

ICD-9-CM 752.7

BIBLIOGRAPHY

Miller WL, Levine LS. Molecular and clinical advances in congenital adrenal hyperplasia. *J Pediatr* 1987;111:117.

Mercado AB, Wilson RC, Cheng WK, Wei J, New MI. Prenatal treatment and diagnosis of congenital adrenal hyperplasia owing to steroid 21-hydroxylase deficiency. *J Clin Endocrinol Metab* 1995;80:2014–2020.

Moshang T, Thornton PS. Endocrine disorders. In: Avery GS, ed. *Neonatology: pathophysiology and management*. Philadelphia: JB Lippincott Co., 1993.

Styne DM. The testes. In: Kaplan S, ed. *Clinical pediatric endocrinology*. Philadelphia. WB Saunders, 1990, 367–425.

Author: Lorraine Katz

Features of the Classical Disorders of Adrenal Steroidogenesis

ENZYME	CLINICAL MANIFESTATIONS	SEXUAL AMBIGUITY FEMALE	MALE	PREDOMINANT STEROIDS
Desmolase	Salt losing	No	Yes	Low levels (all steroids)
3$_\beta$-HSD	Salt losing	Yes	Yes	17-OH pregnenolone, DHEA
21-Hydroxylase	Salt losing	Yes	No	17-OH progesterone Androstenedione
11-Hydroxylase	Hypertension	Yes	No	11-Deoxycortisol
17-Hydroxylase	Hypertension	No	Yes	DOC, corticosterone

Sexual Precocity

 Database

DEFINITION

Sexual precocity is physical signs of sexual development before age 8 years in girls and age 9 years in boys.

CAUSES

• Central precocious puberty (GnRH-dependent): associated with elevated gonadotropin (LH and/or FSH) levels
• Peripheral precocious puberty (GnRH-independent): gonadotropin-independent elevation of sex steroids arising from gonads/adrenals

PATHOPHYSIOLOGY

• Central precocious puberty is associated with CNS lesions.
• Peripheral precocious puberty is associated with gonadal and adrenal lesions.
• Peripheral precocious puberty can progress to central precocious puberty, as sex steroids can mature the hypothalamic-pituitary axis.

GENETICS

• Familial male precocious puberty (testotoxicosis): sex-limited, autosomal dominant inheritance of activating mutation in the LH receptor
• McCune-Albright syndrome: sporadic, postzygotic, somatic mutation in the stimulatory subunit of G-protein receptor; more common in females

EPIDEMIOLOGY

• Precocious puberty is more common in girls.
• Precocious puberty in boys is more likely to be associated with underlying pathology.

COMPLICATIONS

• Short stature
• Psychosocial stresses of early puberty

PROGNOSIS

• With treatment, improvement in predicted height is achieved, but most do not reach target height predicted by midparental height measurements. Early treatment improves final height.
• Effect of GnRH agonists on fertility has not been fully elucidated.

 Differential Diagnosis

• Tumors
—CNS tumors
—Hypothalamic hamartoma: The CNS mass most commonly causing precocious puberty, it is a nonprogressive (benign), congenital malformation of neurons that secrete GnRH.
—Hypothalamic-chiasmatic glioma: often associated with neurofibromatosis
—Astrocytoma
—Ependymoma

—hCG-secreting tumors: may arise from pineal gland or liver
—Gonadal tumors
—Adrenal tumors

• Post-CNS trauma or damage

—Surgery
—Radiation: may occur after 18-Gy exposure

• Hydrocephalus
• Infection: brain abscess, meningitis, encephalitis, granuloma. These CNS lesions may result in abnormal stimulation or lack of inhibition of the GnRH-secreting area of the hypothalamus, resulting in early activation of the pituitary gland.
• Environmental: exogenous estrogen exposure (such as creams and oral contraceptives) and/or exogenous androgen exposure (such as anabolic steroid injections)
• Congenital adrenal hyperplasia (CAH): Poorly controlled CAH can activate the hypothalamic–pituitary–gonadal axis in either gender
• Severe acquired hypothyroidism: High levels of TSH may cross-stimulate gonadal FSH and/or LH receptors.
• McCune-Albright syndrome: triad of precocious puberty, café-au-lait spots, and polyostotic fibrous dysplasia
• Familial male precocious puberty (familial testotoxicosis)
• Refeeding after severe undernutrition during early development (such as adopted children who had kwashiorkor)
• Premature thelarche
• Premature adrenarche
• Obesity

 Data Gathering

HISTORY

• Careful chronology of physical changes, growth spurt, onset of menses
• Presence of neurologic, visual, or behavioral changes may suggest a CNS lesion.
• Family history of early puberty

Special Questions

• Family history suggestive of familial male precocious puberty

 Physical Examination

• Plot accurate height (using wall-mounted stadiometer), weight, and growth velocity.
• Carefully stage breasts, color of vaginal mucosa, and pubic hair in girls.
• Carefully stage testicular volume, penile size, and pubic hair in boys.
• Carefully evaluate for abdominal masses.
• Examine skin for acne (comedones) and café-au-lait spots.
• Perform comprehensive neurologic evaluation to assess for possible CNS pathology.

PROCEDURE

Use standard beads (Prader gonadometer) to assess testicular volumes accurately.

Laboratory Aids

TESTS

Nonspecific Tests

Bone age: If advanced, further studies are warranted, guided by history and physical examination. If not advanced, and if the patient has only mild breast or pubic hair development (but not both), premature thelarche or premature adrenarche, respectively, is the most likely diagnosis.

Specific Tests

• Sex steroids: estradiol, testosterone
• Adrenal steroids: dehydroepiandrosterone sulfate (DHEA-S)
• Gonadotropins: FSH, LH (ultrasensitive or ICMA-LH if possible)
• Prolactin: often elevated with CNS tumors
• In males, hCG levels
• Provocative tests should be done in cases in which the aforementioned tests are abnormal or equivocal:

—GnRH test for central precocious puberty; prepubertal GnRH response is predominately FSH, whereas pubertal response is predominately LH.
—ACTH stimulation test for adrenal abnormalities. Exogenous corticosteroid therapy will interfere with ACTH test but does not interfere with GnRH test of pituitary-gonadal axis.

Imaging

• MRI of head: as indicated by history, physical examination, and laboratory tests; almost always done in males because boys are much less likely than are girls to have idiopathic sexual precocity.
• Ultrasound of gonads/adrenals: as indicated by examination and studies

Therapy

• As indicated by cause of the precocious puberty, for example, removal of CNS lesions or cessation of exogenous sex steroids

DRUGS

• Central precocious puberty: GnRH agonists such as Lupron are the treatment of choice. Adjunctive therapy with recombinant human growth hormone may improve final adult height; calcium supplementation may preserve bone mass accretion in girls during GnRH agonist therapy.
• Peripheral precocious puberty: aromatase inhibitors (testolactone) and antiandrogens (spironolactone or ketoconazole)

DURATION

Until endocrinologist and family agree that pubertal progression is appropriate, guided by bone age and predicted final adult height

DIET

• No restrictions

Follow-Up

WHEN TO EXPECT IMPROVEMENT

• Depends on cause. For example, sexual changes of McCune-Albright syndrome are due to autonomously functioning ovarian cysts, which regress variably over time.
• Treatment of central precocious puberty with a GnRH agonist usually results in cessation of menses within 2 months, slowing or nonprogression of pubertal changes over 4 to 6 months, and decreased acceleration of bone age within 12 months.

SIGNS TO WATCH FOR

Typically, GnRH agonists are given in a depot form every 28 days, but some children require shortening of this time interval. Such dosing is often prompted by parental reports of moodiness, development of acne near the time of injection, or breakthrough menses (failure to suppress).

PITFALLS

• Obese children often have advanced bone age.
• Palpation of breast tissue (buds) can be difficult due to adiposity.

Common Questions and Answers

Q: If my child is treated with GnRH agonists, will he/she go through puberty when we stop the medication?
A: Yes, children on GnRH agonist treatment do proceed through normal puberty when the medication is stopped. Effects on fertility have not been fully elucidated.

Q: If a child already has some pubertal changes, can they be reversed?
A: If GnRH agonists are used, menses will cease, and breast tissue and pubic hair often regress.

ICD-9-CM 259.1

BIBLIOGRAPHY

Antoniazzi F, Bertoldo F, Lauriola S, et al. Prevention of bone demineralization by calcium supplementation in precocious puberty during gonadotropin-releasing hormone agonist treatment. *J Clin Endocrinol Metab* 1999;84(6):1992–1996.

Egli CA, Rosenthal SM, Grumbach MM, et al. Pituitary gonadotropin-independent male limited autosomal dominant sexual precocity in nine generations: familial testotoxicosis. *J Pediatr* 1985;106:33–40.

Oostdijk W, Rikken B, Schreuder S, et al. Final height in central precocious puberty after long term treatment with a slow release GnRH agonist. *Arch Dis Child* 1996;75(4):292–297.

Pasquino AM, Pucarelli I, Segni M, Matrunola M, Cerroni F. Adult height in girls with central precocious puberty treated with gonadrotropin-releasing hormone analogues and growth hormone. *J Clin Endocrinol Metab* 1999;84(2):449–452.

Shankar RR, Pescovitz OH. Precocious puberty. *Adv Endocrinol Metab* 1995;6:55–89.

Styne DM. New aspects in diagnosis and treatment of pubertal disorders. *Pediatr Clin North Am* 1997;44(2):505–529.

Authors: Robert J. Ferry, Jr., Marta Satin-Smith

Short-Bowel Syndrome

 Database

DEFINITION

Short-bowel syndrome is defined by malnutrition, malabsorption fluid, and electrolyte loss after extensive small-bowel resection.

PATHOPHYSIOLOGY

- Markedly decreased mucosal surface area due to resection
- Abnormal transit
- Malabsorption of protein, fat, carbohydrate, vitamins, electrolytes, and trace elements, depending on site of resected intestine (see the table Site of Absorption of Various Nutrients in the Intestine). The patient can lose as much as half of the intestine if the duodenum, distal ileum, and ileocecal valve (ICV) are present. If the ICV is gone, patients may not be able to tolerate even a 25% loss of intestine without the help of total parenteral nutrition (TPN).
- Normal bowel length: at 26 weeks' gestation: 150 to 200 cm; at birth in full-term infant: 200 to 300 cm; adult: 600 to 800 cm
- Infants have no intestinal reserve and do not tolerate small-bowel resection as well as adults. However, the long-term prognosis may be better because of hypertrophy and hyperplasia of the intestine.
- Gastric acid hypersection occurs soon after intestinal resection, but is transient.
- Complications include:

—Bacterial overgrowth and D-lactic acidosis due to stasis
—Renal stones due to fat malabsorption and increased oxalate absorption
—Gallstones due to disturbed enterohepatic circulation of bile salts and lithogenic bile formation

- Bowel adaptation can occur over time. Increased surface area due to bowel dilatation and villus hypertrophy and bowel lengthening can occur. Need stimulation of luminal contents for bowel growth, and factors such as glutamine, short-chain fatty acids, tropic hormones, and growth factors may be important for bowel growth.

Site of Absorption of Various Nutrients in the Intestine

SITE	NUTRIENT
Stomach	Fat
Duodenum	Calcium
	Magnesium
	Iron
	Zinc
Jejunum	Monosaccharides
	Disaccharides
	Fat-soluble vitamins A and D
	Water-soluble vitamins: thiamin, riboflavin, pyridoxine, folic acid, ascorbic acid
	Protein
Ileum	Fat
	Vitamin B12
	Bile salts
Colon	Fluid
	Electrolytes
	Short-chain fatty acids

COMPLICATIONS

- Fluid and electrolyte loss, resulting in diarrhea and dehydration and metabolic acidosis
- Calcium and magnesium deficiency, resulting in bone disease and osteoporosis
- Carbohydrate malabsorption
- Fat malabsorption
- Vitamin A deficiency: increased susceptibility to infections
- Vitamin D deficiency: bone disease (i.e., rickets)
- Vitamin E deficiency: peripheral neuropathy, hemolysis
- Vitamin K deficiency: prolonged clotting time, bruising
- Vitamin B12 and folic acid deficiency: macrocytic anemia
- Gallstones
- Renal stones
- Failure to thrive
- TPN-dependent liver disease: cholestasis, end-stage is cirrhosis and portal hypertension
- Zinc deficiency: poor growth, infections
- Carnitine deficiency: contributes to development of steatosis

PROGNOSIS

- Depends on site and amount of bowel resected
- The more of the bowel resected, the worse is the prognosis.
- Loss of ICV, worse prognosis
- Loss of jejunum and ileum worse than loss of colon
- The longer it takes to tolerate full enteral feeds, the worse is the prognosis. Most progress is made in the first year after bowel resection.
- Development of severe TPN liver disease: poor prognosis

 Differential Diagnosis

- Infants: necrotizing enterocolitis, volvulus, atresia (jejunal and ileal), gastroschisis, meconium peritonitis, congenital short-bowel syndrome
- Older children: midgut volvulus (due to malrotation), Crohn disease, adhesions causing intestinal obstruction, strictures, trauma, aganglionosis of the intestine

 Data Gathering

HISTORY

- Stooling pattern: number, size, nature (watery, bulky, foul smelling), presence of blood and mucus
- Weight loss or gain; gaining length/height
- Abdominal distention and flatulence
- Bad perianal rashes related to stool acidity and malabosrption of carbohydrates
- Bone pain
- Abdominal pain and characteristics
- Vomiting and characteristics
- Frequent infections
- Medication history
- Surgical history

 Physical Examination

- Weight, length, and head circumference measurements (if applicable); try to get previous growth chart if available.
- Look for signs of vitamin deficiencies in examination of mouth, lips, skin.
- Abdominal examination: surgical scars, ostomies, distention, hepatosplenomegaly, bowel sounds
- Rectal examination: consistency of stool, heme positivity, perianal rash

 Laboratory Aids

TESTS

Blood Tests

- CBC: Check for anemia and MCV.
- Electrolytes: sodium, potassium, chloride and bicarbonate; check for losses and adequacy of replacement.
- Minerals: calcium, phosphorus magnesium, iron; check for losses and adequacy of replacement therapy.
- Albumin and prealbumin: Check for protein stores and nutritional status.
- PT/PTT: Assess vitamin K status.
- Liver function tests: ALT, GGT, bilirubin if on parenteral nutrition (PN) to check for parenteral nutrition (PN)–associated liver disease

- Vitamin levels: vitamin A, 25-hydroxy vitamin D, vitamin E, folic acid, B12; check for adequacy
- Zinc level: Check status and adequacy of supplementation.
- Carnitine: Check status if on long-term PN and have liver disease.
- Breath tests: lactose and lactulose breath test to check for lactase deficiency and bacterial overgrowth, respectively

Stool Tests

- Stool for pH and reducing substances: Check for carbohydrate absorption.
- Stool smear for fat (Sudan stain-qualitative): Check for excessive fat loss.
- Stool for blood: Check for mucosal damage.

Tests of Absorption

- Xylose absorption test and lactose breath test to check for carbohydrate absorption
- Seventy-two-hour quantitative fecal fat collection along with concomitant diet record
- Carotene levels to check for fat absorption
- Twenty-four-hour stool collection for α_1-antitrypsin clearance to check for protein absorption

Imaging

Upper GI series with small-bowel follow-through and barium enema to evaluate length, caliber, and location of remaining bowel

Endoscopy

- Upper endoscopy: Look for presence of inflammation that may be contributing to malabsorption; get cultures for bacterial overgrowth.
- Lower endoscopy: Look for presence of colitis, especially eosinophillic colitis, as well as caliber of anastamotic site if in colon.

 Therapy

DRUGS

- Supplementation of vitamin (E, D, K, B12, folic acid) deficiencies, calcium, magnesium, iron, and zinc
- H2-receptor antagonists decrease gastric acid hypersecretion and reduce gastric secretory volume, jejunostomy volumes, as well as excessive sodium and potassium losses.
- Antidiarrheal drugs: codeine, diphenoxalate, and anticholinergic drugs (i.e., loperamide) to decrease motility
- Ion-exchange resins: Cholestyramine binds intraluminal dihydroxy bile acids to prevent bile acid–induced diarrhea.
- Octreotide: decreases gastric, pancreatic, and intestinal secretions; slows gastrointestinal motility and splanchnic blood flow
- Bacterial overgrowth: Commonly used oral antibiotics are metronidazole, trimethoprim-sulfamethoxazole, vancomycin, and gentamicin.
- Prokinetic agents: cisapride to treat bile reflux, pseudoobstruction

DURATION

Depends on amount and site of bowel resected and degree of intestinal adaptation that occurs. The more the resection, the longer is the therapy. Successful enteral feeds decrease the duration of PN. Macronutrient losses decrease with intestinal adaptation. Micronutrient supplementation may be lifelong (i.e., vitamin B12).

SURGICAL/TRANSPLANT

Surgery is useful in patients who develop strictures and partial obstruction, or in those who have very short intestine length. Intestinal interpositions (isoperistaltic or antiperistaltic) can be used to delay gastric emptying, slow intestinal transit, and increase absorption. Intestinal lengthening and tapering procedures increase absorptive surface area. In patients with extremely short intestines and PN dependency, small-bowel transplantation may be considered only as experimental and last efforts.

DIET

- Oral diet: In those patients who are able to avoid PN or tube feeds, a low-lactose diet may be well tolerated. Low-oxalate diets are helpful in preventing oxalate stones.
- Fluid and electrolyte therapy: extremely important in the acute phase immediately after bowel resection. In the chronic phase, it is important to keep up with ongoing losses, especially when enteral feeds are started.
- Enteral feeds: more successful in the patient with less extensive resection, intact ICV, and colon in continuity; no advantage of elemental formulas over intact formulas, with respect to tolerance, unless small-bowel damage is present.
- PN: important in the acute phase postoperatively when nutrition must be maintained in the face of paralytic ileus; indispensable in the chronic phase when full enteral feeds cannot be instituted and nutrition needs to be maintained. Balanced solutions of protein, glucose, and fat should be administered. Prophylactic measures to prevent PN-induced liver damage should be instituted (i.e., prevention of over feeding, early introduction of enteral feeds, cycling of PN when patient is stable). Need permanent central access to deliver concentrated PN solutions.

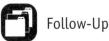 Follow-Up

WHEN TO EXPECT IMPROVEMENT

- Depends on site and extent of bowel resection

SIGNS TO WATCH FOR

- Vomiting, diarrhea, weight loss, severe fluid and electrolyte abnormalities, sepsis, bowel dilatation, intestinal obstruction

ISOLATION OF THE HOSPITALIZED PATIENT

N/A

CONTROL MEASURES

N/A

 Common Questions and Answers

Q: What are the favorable prognostic factors in short-bowel syndrome?
A: Poor prognosis is related to the greater length of the bowel resected, loss of the ileocecal valve (ICV), loss of jejunum and ileum, longer time to tolerate full enteral feeds, and development of severe TPN-liver disease. Neonates have greater chances of bowel adaptation than do adults.

Q: Are elemental formulas better than intact formulas in the management of patients with short-bowel syndrome?
A: Recent studies have shown similar rates of absorption, stomal output, and electrolyte losses between elemental and intact formulas. The disadvantages of elemental formulas include high osmolality and cost.

ICD-9-CM 579.3

BIBLIOGRAPHY

Jona JZ. Advances in neonatal surgery. *Pediatr Clin North Am* 1998;45(3):605–617.

Purdum PP, Kirky DF. Short bowel syndrome: a review of the role of nutrition support. *J Parenter Enter Nutr* 1991;15:93–101.

Scolapio JS, Fleming CR. Short bowel syndrome. *Gastroenterol Clin North Am* 1998;27(2): 467–479.

Vanderhoof JA. Invited review: short bowel syndrome. *J Pediatr Gastroenterol Nutr* 1992;14: 359–370.

Warner BW, Zeigler MM. Management of the short bowel syndrome in the pediatric population. *Pediatr Clin North Am* 1993;40;1335–1350.

Author: Maria R. Mascarenhas

Sickle Cell Disease

 Database

DEFINITION

Sickle cell disease (SCD) is a group of hemoglobin disorders in which sickle hemoglobin (HbS) predominates. SCD is characterized by hemolysis, vascular occlusion, and an increased risk of bacterial infection. Common genotypes include SCD-SS, SCD-SC, SCD-β^+thalassemia and SCD-β^0thalassemia.

GENETICS

SCD has an autosomal recessive pattern of inheritance.

PATHOPHYSIOLOGY

- The production of HbS is caused by a genetic mutation leading to a valine for glutamic acid substitution at the sixth position of the β-globin chain.
- HbS polymerizes within red cells, particularly under deoxygenated conditions, which leads to: (1) changes in red blood cell shape, (2) vascular occlusion, and (3) subsequent ischemic tissue/organ injury.

EPIDEMIOLOGY

- One in 375 African American newborns has SCD.
- One in twelve African Americans has sickle cell trait.
- The frequencies of SCD genotypes from highest to lowest are: SCD-SS (60%), SCD-SC (25%–30%), SCD-β^+thalassemia, SCD-β^0thalassemia, and other relatively infrequent variants.
- Although population data indicate that patients with SCD-SS and SCD-β^0thalassemia experience more complications than patients with other variants, disease severity varies widely among all individuals with SCD regardless of disease genotypes.

COMPLICATIONS

Acute

- Pain: can occur anywhere in the body
- Dactylitis: painful swelling of hands and feet
- Bacterial infection: Younger children are at greatest risk for sepsis/meningitis with encapsulated organisms such as *Streptococcus pneumoniae*, whereas older children and adults are at greatest risk for sepsis with gram-negative organisms. *Salmonella* infections are problematic for patients of all ages.
- Acute chest syndrome: a pneumonia-like illness defined as a new infiltrate on chest x-ray
- Neurologic: including stroke (infarctive and hemorrhagic) and transient ischemic attack (TIA)

- Acute splenic sequestration: acute enlargement of the spleen, with a decreased hemoglobin and increased reticulocyte count
- Aplastic crisis: transient decrease in RBC production characterized by a decrease in hemoglobin and reticulocyte count; parvovirus B19 is most common cause
- Cholecystitis: risk is greatest after age 10 years
- Priapism: a prolonged penile erection, which can be seen in males of all ages

Chronic

- Delayed linear growth and puberty
- Cholelithiasis
- Retinopathy: particularly in children with SCD-SC
- Neurologic: cerebral vasculopathy, silent infarction, arterial-venous malformations
- Hypersplenism: particularly in young children or patients with SCD-SC or SCD-β^+thalassemia
- Avascular necrosis: particularly of the hips
- Renal: nephrotic syndrome, acute glomerulonephritis
- Pulmonary function abnormalities
- Primary nocturnal enuresis

PROGNOSIS

Population estimates of life expectancy from 1978–1988 data range from 42 to 48 years for SCD-SS and 60 to 68 years for SCD-SC. However, many believe that early SCD diagnosis (newborn screening), penicillin prophylaxis, comprehensive medical care, and hydroxyurea therapy may increase life expectancy.

 Data Gathering

HISTORY

- SCD-phenotype
- Baseline hemoglobin and reticulocyte count
- Baseline pulse oximetry values (SpO_2)
- History of SCD complications
- Prior blood transfusions and complications

 Physical Examination

- Fever
- Pallor (may be accentuated at time of splenic sequestration or aplastic crisis)
- Scleral icterus
- Signs of respiratory distress (due to acute chest syndrome)
- A flow murmur may be present (due to anemia).
- Splenomegaly
- Warmth, tenderness, decreased range of motion at site of pain

 Laboratory Aids

TESTS

Diagnostic

- Hemoglobin electrophoresis: definitive test along with DNA analysis
- Screening test: "sickledex" or "shake" tests are not recommended to establish a diagnosis or carrier status; do not use for screening in children less than 12 months of age due to false-negative results.
- Complete blood counts: Hemoglobin values vary depending on age and SCD genotype; peripheral blood smear-sickled forms, targets, nucleated RBCs, and increased polychromasia are common RBC findings (sickle forms may be absent in transfused patients or in patients with phenotypes other than SCD-SS).
- Reticulocyte count: increased
- Quantitative hemoglobin electrophoresis
- Chemistry panel: elevated LDH, unconjugated bilirubin, AST
- Prior to the first transfusion in any sickle cell patient, draw blood for a red-cell antigen profile for future reference. (This is because of the high risk of alloimmunization in repeatedly transfused patients.)

Imaging

- Bone scan and bone marrow scan (to help differentiate osteomyelitis from bony infarction)
- Chest x-ray study (at the time of pulmonary complications): cardiomegaly
- Abdominal ultrasound (if considering cholecystitis)
- CT/MRI/arteriogram (if considering stroke)

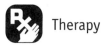 **Therapy**

GENERAL MEASURES (GENERAL WELL-PATIENT CARE)

- Children should be seen by a pediatric hematologist at least twice a year for: (1) an interim history, physical examination, and laboratory tests; (2) other ancillary studies, including transcranial Doppler ultrasound (TCD) when appropriate; (3) patient and parent education; (4) psychosocial evaluation; and (5) referrals to other specialists, such as ophthalmology, urology, and general surgery when needed.
- Infection prophylaxis with penicillin starting by 2 months of age
- Pneumococcal vaccine at 2 and 5 years
- Routine immunizations, including hepatitis B series; consider yearly influenza vaccine
- Consider folic acid supplementation.
- Parental monitoring for fever, splenomegaly, pain (including dactylitis), increased jaundice

- Encourage good oral hydration and supply family with medications to treat uncomplicated painful episodes at home.
- Transfusion therapy can prevent the development of SCD complications and decrease associated morbidity or recurrence of complications when used appropriately. When children with SCD-SS receive erythrocyte transfusions, avoid posttransfusion hemoglobin levels above 12 g/dL. Erythrocyte antigen matching for ABO as well as C, D, E, and Kell is recommended. Monitor children carefully for erythrocyte antibodies and/or delayed transfusion reactions.

MEASURES FOR SPECIFIC COMPLICATIONS

- Fever (rule out sepsis)

—History, physical examination, CBC, reticulocyte count, blood culture (urine, CSF culture, throat culture as indicated by examination)
—Parenteral antibiotics to provide 24- to 48-hour coverage until blood cultures are negative
—Close monitoring for other SCD complications

- Pain (vasoocclusive episode)

—History, physical examination; consider CBC, reticulocyte count
—Hydration
—Analgesics: Therapy should be directed toward the level of pain the child is experiencing, the medications that have been used prior to presentation, and the past experience of the child with certain interventions. Patients and their families can often tell physicians what therapies have been helpful in the past. In general, for mild pain, start with mild nonnarcotic medications (acetaminophen, ibuprofen) and mild oral narcotic analgesics (codeine, oxycodone). Consider stronger agents such as oral ketorolac, hydromorphone and morphine for initial management of moderate pain. For severe pain, use parenteral medications such as morphine, hydromorphone, and ketorolac.
—Comfort measures (massage, heating pad, warm soaks)
—Frequent reassessment for pain control and side effects of medications is mandatory.

- Acute chest syndrome

—History, physical examination, CBC, reticulocyte count, chest x-ray film (blood culture as indicated)
—Initial findings: chest pain, cough, hypoxia, fever, infiltrate on chest radiograph
—Management
  —Parenteral antibiotics
  —Pain management
  —Supplemental oxygen for hypoxia
  —Incentive spirometry or chest physiotherapy
  —Red blood cell transfusion for severe disease

- Splenic sequestration

—History, physical examination, CBC, reticulocyte count (blood culture as indicated), type and crossmatch
—Initial findings: increased spleen size, acute pallor, shock (if episode severe), anemia, and thrombocytopenia.
—A sequestration episode may have a more insidious onset or be chronic in nature.
—Management
  —Fever management (if indicated)
  —Close, frequent observation of hemoglobin level, reticulocyte count, spleen size, and cardiovascular (CV) status
  —Fluid bolus and maintenance hydration
  —Red blood cell transfusion: Avoid transfusing to hemoglobin values above 10 g/dL as hemoglobin may increase as the episode resolves and red cells are released from the spleen.
  —Repeated sequestration episodes may be an indication for splenectomy.

- Aplastic crisis

—History, physical examination, CBC, reticulocyte count (blood culture as indicated), type and crossmatch
—Initial finds: Pallor, tachycardia, *no* jaundice or splenomegaly, anemia, absent reticulocytes.
—Management
  —Fever management (if indicated)
  —Close observation of hemoglobin level, reticulocyte count, and CV status
  —Respiratory isolation (95% of cases are due to infection with parvovirus B19)
  —Red-cell transfusion for evidence of CV compromise

- Cerebral vascular accidents: *Acute care*

—History, physical examination, CBC, reticulocyte count (blood culture as indicated), type and crossmatch
—Initial findings: Syncope, weakness, numbness, limp, hemiparesis, seizure, slurred speech, aphasia, somnolence, coma.
—Imaging: head CT, MRI, MR angiography (MRA); consider arteriogram
—Management
  —Intravenous fluid bolus and maintenance hydration
  —Red blood cell transfusion (given as simple or exchange transfusion)
  —Supportive (anticonvulsives, etc.)

- Cerebral vascular accidents: *Chronic care*

—Monthly red-cell transfusions to keep HbS level below 30%

 ## Common Questions and Answers

Q: How long will my baby with SCD live?
A: No one can predict how long a child with SCD will live. When studies were done on a large number of individuals with SCD almost two decades ago, these individuals were living, on average, into their 40s if they had the SS type of SCD and into their 60s with the SC type of SCD. Most likely, new treatments such as daily penicillin, comprehensive medical care, and hydroxyurea therapy have prolonged the life expectancy of children with SCD.

Q: Is there any "cure" for sickle cell disease?
A: Bone marrow transplantation (BMT) is the only known cure for sickle cell disease in children. BMT requires destroying all the bone marrow of the child with SCD with strong drugs and/or radiation and replacing it with the bone marrow of a person without SCD. This marrow donor should be a relative, preferably a full sibling, whose bone marrow "matches" the child with SCD. Only those children with SCD who have experienced severe illness complications should be exposed to the morbidity and mortality risks of BMT at this time.

Q: What is hydroxyurea therapy?
A: Hydroxyurea is a medication that has been shown to reduce the number of painful episodes and acute chest syndrome events in adults with sickle cell disease. Individuals who receive this medication must be monitored closely for serious side effects, such as a decreased white blood count, hemoglobin, or platelets. Once these problems are detected and the drug is stopped, these problems usually resolve. The results of studies evaluating the safety of hydroxyurea therapy in children have not been published.

Q: What "triggers" or starts off a pain episode?
A: Some children say that changes in the weather (e.g., hot to cold or vice versa) will bring on painful episodes. Others say that jumping into a cold swimming pool will bring on pain. Trauma (e.g., being tackled in football), fatigue, stress, infection, and menses can also exacerbate painful episodes. However, in the majority of painful episodes, the "triggers" are unknown.

ICD-9-CM 282.6

BIBLIOGRAPHY

Nathan DG, Oski FA, eds. *Hematology of infancy and childhood*, 4th ed. Philadelphia: WB Saunders, 1993.

Reid CD, Charache S, Lubin B, eds. *Management and therapy of sickle cell disease*. National Institutes of Health, National Heart, Lung and Blood Institute. NIH Publication No. 96-2117, 1995.

Vinchinsky E, Lubin BH. Suggested guidelines for the treatment of children with sickle cell disease. *Hematol Oncol Clin North Am* 1987;1:483–501.

Author: Kim Smith-Whitley

Sinusitis

Database

DEFINITION

Sinusitis is inflammation of the mucous membranes lining the paranasal sinuses.

- Acute: persistent symptoms of nasal discharge and cough for greater than 10 but less than 30 days
- Subacute: clinical symptoms 30 to 120 days
- Chronic: symptoms lasting 3 or more months, or presumptive diagnosis based on radiographic evidence of mucosal thickening
- Recurrent: acute sinusitis with complete resolution between episodes

CAUSES

- Bacterial pathogens: *Streptococcus pneumoniae* (30%–40%); *Haemophilus influenzae,* nontypeable (approximately 20%); *Moraxella catarrhalis* (approximately 20%); group A streptococci; group C streptococci; peptostreptococci; other *Moraxella* species; *S. viridans; Eikenella corrodens; Staphylococcus aureus; Pseudomonas aeruginosa* (in patients with cystic fibrosis); anaerobic organisms
- Viral pathogens (e.g., rhinovirus, parainfluenza virus) have been recovered in respiratory isolates, but their significance is unknown; recovered organisms include respiratory syncytial virus, rhinovirus, parainfluenza virus, influenza virus, and coxsackievirus.
- Fungal pathogen: *Aspergillus*

PATHOPHYSIOLOGY

- Increased risk of sinus infection with:

—Impairment of mucociliary transport due to hypersecretion of mucus and inflammatory mediators released in response to infection or allergy
—Obstruction of the osteomeatal complex, with resultant intranasal hypoxia and increased acidity, which leads to further mucociliary dysfunction
—Immunodeficiency

- The outflow tract of the maxillary sinus is in the superior medial wall of the sinus, making gravitational drainage difficult and predisposing the sinus to infection.
- The ethmoid sinus is made up of air cells, which independently drain into 1- to 2-mm openings. These openings may become obstructed when the mucosal lining is inflamed, predisposing the sinus to infection.
- The etiology of cough is unclear and thought possibly to be due to direct contamination of the airway by nasal secretions, resulting in irritation and/or a reflex arc from the sinuses to the bronchi.

EPIDEMIOLOGY

- Complicates approximately 5% to 10% of upper respiratory tract infections

COMPLICATIONS

- Orbital subperiosteal abscess
- Periorbital cellulitis
- Orbital cellulitis/abscess
- Optic neuritis
- Meningitis
- Cavernous or sagittal sinus thrombosis
- Epidural, subdural, and brain abscesses
- Osteomyelitis of the maxilla
- Osteomyelitis of the frontal bone

PROGNOSIS

- Excellent for those who are otherwise healthy

ASSOCIATED ILLNESSES

- Recurrent viral upper respiratory infection (URI)
- Anatomic abnormalities of the sinus and nasal passages (e.g., septal deviation, unilateral choanal atresia, other craniofacial abnormalities)
- Allergies
- Cystic fibrosis with or without nasal polyps
- Immunodeficiency
- Ciliary dyskinesia
- Dental infections
- Facial trauma
- Swimming, diving

Differential Diagnosis

Infection

—Viral URI with or without mucopurulent rhinitis

Environmental

- Hayfever

Drug-induced

- Rhinitis medicamentosa

Tumors

- Nasal polyps
- Hypertrophied adenoids

Trauma

- Foreign body (e.g., bead, cotton, tissue)

Congenital

- Septal deviation
- Unilateral choanal atresia
- Ciliary dyskinesia

Data Gathering

HISTORY

- Fever; late onset may help distinguish sinusitis from viral URI.
- Recent history of an upper respiratory infection, with rhinorrhea, cough, congestion

- Nasal discharge: consistency, color. In older patients, nasal discharge may *not* be the primary complaint.
- Postnasal drip
- Sore throat may be present.
- Cough present during the day and may be worse at night, but also may not be present at night
- Malodorous breath
- Headache
- Fatigue
- Irritability
- Rarely, facial pain, which is more commonly associated with acute sinusitis
- Occasionally, painless morning eye swelling
- Check for symptoms suggestive of allergies, such as eye rubbing, tearing, sneezing.

Physical Examination

- Fever: usually high in acute sinusitis; low grade or absent in chronic sinusitis
- A nasal-sounding voice may be present.
- Malodorous breath may be noted.
- Purulent drainage in the nose and/or oropharynx may be appreciated.
- Nasal mucosa may be erythematous, pale, and boggy.
- Frontal, maxillary, and ethmoid areas may be tender to palpation/percussion.
- Headache and/or facial pain may change with position, increasing in intensity as the patient leans forward.
- Failure to transilluminate the sinuses of older children is suggestive, though not diagnostic, of sinusitis.
- Check for concurrent middle ear, tonsillar, or adenoidal disease.
- Proptosis, eye swelling, and impaired extraocular movements suggest orbital infection.
- Check for signs of meningeal irritation, focal neurologic deficits, and increased intracranial pressure.

Laboratory Aids

TESTS

- Maxillary sinus aspiration: in unresponsive/complicated cases; should be reserved for a trained otolaryngologist; cultures with 100,000 colony-forming units per milliliter or more indicate true infection

For chronic or recurrent sinusitis, consider:

- Sweat chloride test to rule out cystic fibrosis
- Immunoglobulin levels, IgG subclass levels, complement levels, and testing for human immunodeficiency virus
- Mucosal biopsy to assess ciliary function

IMAGING

• Sinus radiographs (including anteroposterior [Caldwell], lateral, and occipitomental [Waters] views): therefore, they are not felt to be reliable screens for chronic sinusitis. In acute sinusitis, however, they may be useful if air-fluid levels are seen. Abnormal findings consistent with sinusitis include opacification, air-fluid levels, and mucosal thickening of at least 4 mm. Given that empiric therapy is safe and inexpensive, these are not routinely recommended in acute sinusitis.

• CT scans of the paranasal sinuses: useful in complicated sinusitis and recurrent and chronic sinusitis

• CT scan of the head: indicated when sinusitis is accompanied by signs of increased intracranial pressure, meningeal irritation, or focal neurologic deficits

PITFALLS

• Sinus radiographs may be abnormal in asymptomatic children. Radiographs should be reserved for children in whom sinusitis is clinically suspected.

• Younger children may require sedation before CT imaging and should not have anything to eat or drink for 4 hours before the study.

 ## Therapy

If orbital or central nervous system infection is suspected by history and examination, antibiotics should be started immediately, and emergent CT studies should be performed.

DRUGS

• Amoxicillin (40 mg/kg/d divided in three doses): preferred treatment for uncomplicated cases of acute sinusitis. Side effects include hypersensitivity and diarrhea. If there is dramatic improvement of symptoms within 3 to 4 days of antibiotic therapy, a minimum of 10 days of therapy is adequate. For other patients, treat until they are symptom-free and then for an additional 7 days.

• For chronic sinusitis, use a broad-spectrum antibiotic for 3 to 4 weeks:

—Amoxicillin/clavulanate potassium (25–45 mg/kg/d of the amoxicillin component divided in two doses): may be used for recurrent or nonresponsive cases. Side effects include hypersensitivity, vomiting, and diarrhea.
—Erythromycin/sulfisoxazole (50 mg/kg/d of the erythromycin component divided in four doses), cefuroxime axetil (250–500 mg in two divided doses), or trimethoprim-sulfamethoxazole (8 mg/kg/d of the trimethoprim component divided in two doses) may also be used for cases that do not respond to amoxicillin or for recurrent cases. Erythromycin may increase levels of theophylline.

• Prophylactic amoxicillin (20 mg/kg/d) and sulfisoxazole (30 mg/kg twice per day) should be used in patients with known immunodeficiencies.

• Normal saline: squirt into each nostril daily or twice per day; removes sensitizing agents, increases humidity, and enhances mucociliary transport; vasoconstricts and improves drainage and ventilation

• Decongestants: These decrease nasal airway resistance and increase ostia patency in some studies, but the overall effect on acute sinusitis is unknown. Topical decongestants should be only for short-term therapy (5–7 days), because rebound mucosal congestion may occur. Systemic decongestants (i.e., pseudoephedrine and phenylpropanolamine) have side effects that include tachycardia, hypertension, jitteriness, and insomnia.

• Mucolytics, such as guaifenesin: may improve mucous clearance

• Topical nasal steroids: reduce and prevent mucosal swelling, which can lead to osteal occlusion; particularly useful for patients with allergic rhinitis

OTHER

• Humidifier: improves mucociliary clearance.

• Surgery: Surgery is performed as a last resort after medical therapy has been attempted; procedures include antral washout, nasal antral window, endoscopic ethmoidectomy, and middle meatus nasal antral window.

 ## Follow-Up

• Radiographic soft-tissue changes may last for up to 8 weeks; therefore, re-imaging is of limited value.

• Referral to an ear, nose, and throat (ENT) specialist when the sinusitis is chronic and not responsive to medical therapy

PITFALLS

• Diagnosis of sinusitis is being made with increasing frequency and may result in overtreatment, given that up to 45% will have spontaneous resolution.

• With widespread antibiotic use, there are increasing numbers of resistant organisms.

• Studies have shown a relatively high incidence of sinus abnormalities on CT scan in asymptomatic children, especially in infants less than 12 months of age. The significance of opacified sinuses in asymptomatic children is not well understood.

PREVENTION

• Use prophylactic amoxicillin or sulfisoxazole for refractory sinusitis.

• Avoid allergen exposure and treat allergies if present.

• Practice daily nasal hygiene through the use of normal saline drops or spray.

• Improve mucociliary clearance by increasing ambient humidity with a humidifier.

 ## Common Questions and Answers

Q: Are all of the sinuses present at birth?
A: No. The maxillary and ethmoid sinuses form during the second trimester of gestation and are present at birth. They continue to enlarge until the preteen years. The frontal sinuses are present at age 5 to 6 years and are not completely developed until late adolescence.

Q: Does the nasal discharge seen with sinusitis have to be purulent and thick?
A: No. Though the nasal discharge is often described as purulent and thick, it also may be clear or mucoid. It may be thick or thin.

Q: Are radiographs useful in the diagnosis of sinusitis?
A: There is evidence to suggest that x-rays have limited value in the diagnosis of sinusitis. Some authors feel that x-rays are useful in acute sinusitis if air-fluid levels or opacification is seen. Mucosal thickening may be seen with viral upper respiratory tract infections and allergic rhinitis. Studies have shown that x-rays do not correlate well with CT scans in the diagnosis of chronic sinusitis.

Q: Can one make the diagnosis of sinusitis based on CT scan results alone?
A: No. Up to 50% of patients who had CTs performed for other reasons had soft-tissue changes in their sinuses. Mucosal thickening and opacification on CT imaging have been seen in large numbers of asymptomatic patients. These findings seem to occur more frequently in infants less than 12 months of age. Given the poor specificity of CT imaging of the paranasal sinuses, results must be used in the context of the patient's clinical presentation.

BIBLIOGRAPHY

Aitken M, Taylor JA. Prevalence of clinical sinusitis in young children followed up by primary care pediatricians. *Arch Pediatr Adolesc Med* 1998;152:244–248.

Arjmand EM, Lusk RP. Management of recurrent and chronic sinusitis in children. *Am J Otolaryngol* 1995;16:367–382.

Isaacson G. Sinusitis in childhood. *Pediatr Clin North Am* 1996;43:1297–1318.

Kronemer KA, McAlister WH. Sinusitis and its imaging in the pediatric population. *Pediatr Radiol* 1997;27:837–846.

Manning SC. Pediatric sinusitis. *Otolaryngol Clin North Am* 1993;26:623–638.

Rosenfeld EA, Rowley AH. Infectious intracranial complications of sinusitis, other than meningitis, in children: 12-year review. *Clin Infect Dis* 1994;18:750–754.

Wald ER. Sinusitis. *Pediatr Rev* 1993;14:345–351.

Wald ER. Sinusitis in children. *N Engl J Med* 1992;326:319–323.

Author: Esther K. Chung

Sleep Apnea—Obstructive Sleep Apnea Syndrome

 Database

DEFINITION

Obstructive apnea is the cessation of airflow at the nose and mouth despite respiratory effort. Central apnea implies cessation of airflow that is not accompanied by respiratory effort.

- Many children with obstructive apnea exhibit partial airway obstruction. This is known as obstructive hypoventilation or hypopnea.
- The spectrum of abnormalities from obstructive hypoventilation to obstructive sleep apnea is known as obstructive sleep apnea syndrome (OSAS).
- Central apneas up to 20 seconds may be a normal finding in premature or newborn infants during the first months of life.
- Three or more central apneas occurring in clusters (>3 seconds, separated by <20 seconds) is known as periodic breathing.

PATHOPHYSIOLOGY

- The peak incidence of OSAS in children is between 2 and 6 years. In most cases, the cause of upper airway obstruction in these children is adenotonsillar hypertrophy.
- In infants, OSAS is uncommon; however, it may exist with craniofacial anomalies, laryngeal or tracheal malacia, as well as gastroesophageal reflux and disorders associated with hypotonia.
- Central apnea may arise from immaturity of the respiratory control system in infants. However, an underlying neurologic, cardiac, metabolic, pharmacologic, or infectious cause should be excluded.

GENETICS

- In prepubertal children, OSAS occurs equally in boys and girls. However, in adults, OSAS is more common in men.
- There is no genetic predisposition for central apneas.
- Several genetic disorders with associated craniofacial anomalies, hypotonia, and obesity may lead to OSAS. These include:

—Pierre Robin syndrome
—Treacher Collins syndrome
—Down syndrome
—Prader-Willi syndrome
—Hereditary neuromuscular disorders.

COMPLICATIONS

Complications due to chronic hypoxemia include:

- Cardiac complications
- Pulmonary hypertension and later cor pulmonale
- Systemic hypertension
- Congestive heart failure; arrhythmias are common in adults with an underlying coronary heart disease.
- Neurodevelopmental complications: daytime somnolence, poor school performance, hyperactivity, and social withdrawal
- Poor growth and failure to thrive
- Respiratory failure and death have also been reported in children with OSAS postanesthesia.
- Chronic hypercapnia/pseudotumor syndrome

ASSOCIATED CONDITIONS

- Adenotonsillar hypertrophy
- Craniofacial anomalies affecting airway patency during sleep
- Neurologic conditions causing hypotonia and upper airway obstruction, gastroesophageal reflux, central apnea of prematurity, hypoxic-ischemic encephalopathy, encephalitis
- Metabolic conditions: MCAD deficiency, OTC deficiency
- Obstructive sleep apnea: obesity, allergic rhinitis, reflux, chronic consumption of phenytoin, lymphoidal hypertrophy, acute tonsillitis/pharyngitis, velopharyngeal insufficiency, Down syndrome, neuromuscular disorders
- Central apnea: prematurity, reflux, narcotic intoxication, congenital central hypoventilation syndrome

 Differential Diagnosis

- Primary or habitual snoring: This condition is not associated with sleep-disordered breathing.
- Obesity-hypoventilation syndrome
- Central apneas: periodic breathing—Three or more central apneas occur in a repeated pattern within a 20-second period. This may be normal in newborns; if periodic breathing exceeds more than 4% of total, this is an abnormal condition. Central hypoventilation is a disorder of unknown etiology with an abnormal central chemoreceptor response.
- Metabolic disorders

Other causes of excessive daytime sleepiness include:

- Narcolepsy: onset rare before adolescence; associated cataplexy, sleep paralysis
- Epilepsy: absence spells of unresponsiveness; EEG changes
- Drug intoxication: antihistamines, anticonvulsants, nonsteroidals, methylphenidate
- Causes of obstructive apnea include any cause of lymphoidal hypertrophy in the upper airway; allergies; acute upper airway; infections (viral/bacterial tonsillitis, epiglottitis, pharyngeal abscess); chronic phenytoin exposure; excessive storage material in upper airway submucosae.
- Causes of abnormal laxity of upper airway soft tissues: Down syndrome, chronic neuromuscular disease, Prader-Willi syndrome
- Causes of abnormal control/coordination of upper airway musculature: Almost any cause of diffuse CNS disfunction may cause obstructive apnea, most commonly cerebral palsy and acquired lesions of the CNS such as stroke and head trauma.
- Causes of central apnea: beyond infancy, most commonly due to drugs suppressing ventilatory drive; in premature infants may be due to nonspecific immaturity of neural ventilatory control mechanism, sepsis, and, rarely, seizures, brainstem compression, brain tumors, Arnold Chiari type 2
- Reflux may potentiate central apnea and should be investigated (see below).
- Androgen steroid replacement has been shown to cause central apnea in adults.

 Data Gathering

HISTORY

- Children with OSAS frequently have a history of difficulty breathing when asleep, snoring, apneas during sleep, restless sleep, frequent upper respiratory infection, and mouth breathing while awake.
- Other concerns that may ultimately be attributed to or linked with sleep apnea include attention deficit, snoring, lapse in school performance, and headaches (especially morningtime/on awakening).
- Children with central apneas may have a history of cyanosis, apparent life-threatening events (ALTEs), limpness, and delayed development.

—Sleep apnea syndrome, whether obstructive or central, rarely produces these symptoms acutely, but tends to occur over weeks to months.

Physical Examination

- Assessment of the child's growth
- Obesity
- Failure to thrive
- Presence of mouth breathing, an adenoidal facies, midfacial hypoplasia, retro- and micrognathia, or other craniofacial anomalies are the key for diagnosis.
- Tongue size
- Movement of the soft palate; hard palate integrity
- Children with a history suggestive of obstructive apnea may have tonsillar enlargement or edematous nasal mucosa.
- Cardiac examination may reveal signs of pulmonary hypertension or congestive heart failure.
- A neurologic examination should be performed to evaluate muscle tone and developmental status.
- Funduscopy should be done in children with excessive sleepiness and headache to look for signs of elevated intracranial pressure from hypercapnia; a neurologic examination may show drowsiness or inattention due to sleep deficit.

Laboratory Aids

TESTS

Polysomnogram

The definitive method to establish and differentiate the type of sleep apnea is an overnight polysomnogram; variables monitored to assess sleep and respiratory states include: electroencephalogram, electrooculogram, electromyogram, arterial oxygen saturation, CO_2 tension, airflow, respiratory effort, and electrocardiogram. Normative respiratory and sleep variables have recently been published.

Other Studies

- Lateral neck x-ray to assess adenoid and tonsillar size
- CT or MRI when craniofacial anomalies are complex and assessment presurgery is required
- In severe cases, a cardiac evaluation, including ECG, chest x-ray, and Doppler echocardiogram, may be indicated.
- Diagnosis of narcolepsy depends on EEG monitoring of sleep onset to determine whether there is an abnormally shortened latency to onset of rapid eye movement (REM) sleep.
- Routine blood work is generally noncontributory.
- Evaluation of suspected reflux may include barium swallow and radionuclide studies (milk scan).
- Bronchoscopy may be done to evaluate a suspected anatomic basis of airway obstruction (laryngotracheomalacia, vocal cord polyps, papilloma).

Therapy

- Definitive treatment for children with adenotonsillar hypertrophy is adenotonsillectomy. However, some patients continue to have significant OSAS after surgery.
- Treat underlying reflux with medication, thickening the consistency of formula, and head elevation.
- Medications, such as caffeine, are intended to stimulate the respiratory drive.
- Other modalities include continuous positive airway pressure (CPAP), intraoral appliances, and weight loss.
- In extreme cases, a tracheostomy may be indicated.
- Central apneas: Apnea of prematurity may respond to stimulants such as caffeine or theophylline. If apneas are prolonged, supplemental oxygen, CPAP, or mechanical ventilation may be indicated

Follow-Up

In mild to moderate cases of OSAS, clinical improvement is expected soon after adenotonsillectomy. However, in severe cases of OSAS, or if there is an underlying craniofacial anomaly or a neurologic disorder, a repeat overnight polysomnogram is indicated 6 to 8 weeks after surgery.

- Follow-up sleep studies may help to monitor therapy.
- History of school performance should be followed, because this may be the principal indicator of how well the child is sleeping.
- Children with obstructive sleep apnea often have associated chronic middle ear disease; look for fewer episodes of otitis media after surgery.

PITFALLS

- Phenytoin may cause lymphoidal hypertrophy and potentiate sleep apnea.
- Lioresal or other muscle relaxants used to treat spasticity may also potentiate obstructive apnea, particularly in children with decreased coordination of upper airway musculature.
- Treatment of reflux in infants with obstructive apnea may be helpful even in the absence of obvious symptoms of reflux.

Common Questions and Answers

Q: What is the best sleep position for an infant with apnea?
A: A supine or lateral decubitus position in sleep is appropriate for most infants.

Q: Does apnea cause brain damage?
A: The vast majority of infants and children who are diagnosed and treated for sleep apnea have normal development. Slowed mental processing and poor attention are occasional, reversible concomitants of sleep apnea.

Q: Will my infant become addicted to caffeine?
A: Although some adults who take caffeine regularly do seem to develop signs of dependence, this reaction to caffeine has not been reported in infants.

ICD-9-CM 780.57

BIBLIOGRAPHY

Brouillette R, Hanson D, David R, et al. A diagnostic approach to suspected obstructive sleep apnea in children. *J Pediatr* 1984;105:10–14.

Gozal D, Kaufman CS. Sleep-disordered breathing and school performance in children. *Pediatrics* 1998;102(3):616–620.

Hodgman J. Apnea of prematurity and risk for SIDS. *Pediatrics* 1998;102(4):969–971.

Ponsonby AL, Dwyer T, Couper D. Sleeping position, infant apnea, and cyanosis: a population-based study. *Pediatrics* 1997;99(1):E3.

Authors: Raanan Arens and Peter M. Bingham

Slipped Capital Femoral Epiphysis

Database

DEFINITION

Slipped capital femoral epiphysis is displacement of the epiphysis; it can involve any long bone.

PATHOPHYSIOLOGY

• Unclear: abnormal stress on normal physeal plate versus a process that weakens the plate
• The femoral head slips posteriorly and inferiorly, exposing the anterior and superior aspects of the metaphysis of the femoral neck.
• Associations: endocrine dysfunction, primary hypothyroidism, pituitary dysfunction, hypogonadism, cryptorchidism, chemotherapy, pelvic radiotherapy, renal rickets

GENETICS

Five percent of cases are associated with parental disease.

EPIDEMIOLOGY

• Incidence: 1 to 3 per 100,00
• Race: Blacks more than Whites
• Sex: Males more than females (3:2)
• Age of onset: boys, 14 to 16 years; girls, 11 to 13 years (essentially never postmenarche)
• Associated with obesity, increased height, genital underdevelopment, pituitary tumors

COMPLICATIONS

• Ischemic necrosis of epiphysis: usually due to manipulative reduction of the slippage; more common in males; x-ray reveals increased density, irregularity, and ultimately collapse of epiphysis.
• Chondrolysis (acute cartilage necrosis): 1% to 40%, more common in females and Blacks; etiology unclear; x-ray reveals narrowed joint space, sclerosis of acetabular rim, and osteoporosis of femoral head.

Differential Diagnosis

• Severe sepsis
• Ischemic necrosis
• Tuberculosis of the hip; however, pain is associated with movement in all directions, and there should be other evidence of disease.
• Renal rickets
• Achondroplasia
• Schwachman syndrome: metaphyseal chondrodysplasia with pancreatic insufficiency

Data Gathering

HISTORY

• Pain in hip or knee
• Occasional history of trauma; however, usually not sufficient to explain the findings
• Three patterns:

—Chronic: most common, onset of symptoms greater than 3 weeks, lack of full internal rotation of hip
—Acute: sudden onset with inability to walk or severe pain and difficulty walking
—Acute-on-chronic: sudden exacerbation of symptoms that have been present for a while

Physical Examination

• Limp if unilateral, or waddling gait if bilateral
• Tenderness and occasional palpable thickening over hip
• Thigh atrophy
• Lack of full internal rotation of hip and decreased motion in all planes secondary to synovitis

PROCEDURE

When the hip is flexed, the thigh is forced into lateral rotation.

Laboratory Aids

TESTS

Radiographs

- Lateral view: frog leg or Lowenstein
- Measure degree of displacement:

—Minimal: alteration in plane of epiphysis relative to femoral neck; significant if angle less than 82%
—Mild: displacement less than 1 cm
—Moderate: displacement greater than 1 cm, less than two-thirds diameter of femoral neck

- Epiphyseal plate widened and irregular
- Decreased height of physis
- "Blanch sign" dense area in femoral neck
- A "Klein line" drawn along the superior femoral neck transects less of the physis than on the normal side.
- Hormonal evaluation if suspected

Pathology

Histologic findings include widening of the epiphyseal plate, large clefts, and necrotic debris in the cartilage and synovitis.

 ## Therapy

- Designed to prevent complications and further slipping
- Conservative: bed rest with traction; probably does not reduce slipping; temporizing until surgery can be scheduled
- Manipulative reduction: risk of damage to epiphyseal vessels or breakdown of callus; probably only to be considered if within 24 hours of acute slip
- Epiphyseal fixation: risk of damage to articular surface or growth plate
- Intertrochanteric osteotomy
- Salvage: hip fusion

PITFALLS

- Diagnosis is most often missed when slipped capital femoral epiphysis is not considered.
- Hip pain may be absent; there may be no pain, or only thigh or knee pain due to referred pain.

 ## Common Questions and Answers

Q: What type of x-ray should be obtained?
A: Lateral or frog lateral of hips.

Q: Is there a role for CT or MRI?
A: CT can be useful to demonstrate degree of slip. There is no role for MRI.

ICD-9-CM 732.9

BIBLIOGRAPHY

Kehn OK. Slipped capital femoral epiphysis. In: Morrissey RT, Weinstein SL, eds. *Lovell and Winter's pediatric orthopedics, Vol. 2,* 3rd ed. Philadelphia: JB Lippincott Co, 1990:885–902.

Ledwith CA, Fleisher GR. Slipped capital femoral epiphysis without hip pain leads to missed diagnosis. *Pediatrics* 1992;89(4):660–662.

Richards BS. Slipped capital femoral epiphysis. *Pediatr Rev* 1996;17(2):69–70.

Author: Emily von Scheven

Spinal Muscular Atrophy

 ## Database

DEFINITION

Spinal muscular atrophy (SMA) is a disorder of motor neurons that causes progressive weakness. The milder form (type III, Kugelberg-Welander) usually begins after age 2, while the severe, early infantile form (type I, Werdnig-Hoffman) usually starts before age 6 months. Although death due to respiratory failure is common, some individuals survive for years or decades.

PATHOPHYSIOLOGY

Theories of pathogenesis include: programmed cell death; excitotoxic amino acid; insufficiency of a trophic factor; mitochondrial injury/free radical accumulation.

GENETICS

• Most commonly autosomal recessive: A clinical DNA test is available for the most common type; rare forms of SMA are X-linked (adult-onset, male-restricted spinal and bulbar muscular atrophy).
• Juvenile amyotrophic lateral sclerosis (ALS) (see Differential Diagnosis), which also involves upper motor neurons, may be autosomal dominant.

EPIDEMIOLOGY

Worldwide incidence is approximately 1 per 4,000 live births (though areas with higher incidence have been identified), making SMA one of the most common lethal hereditary disorders in humans.

COMPLICATIONS

• Respiratory complications from hypoventilation (infection, aspiration, hypercapnia-induced stupor, hypoxia) are most prominent.
• Associated swallowing difficulty may necessitate a feeding tube.
• Contractures may occur.
• Though sphincteric function is normal, immobility may cause large-bowel stasis

ASSOCIATED CONDITIONS

• Rare forms are associated with cardiomyopathy or congenital heart disease.
• Arthrogryposis with degeneration of brainstem neurons (infantile neuronal degeneration)

 ## Differential Diagnosis

Other disorders that may resemble SMA include:

• Prader-Willi syndrome
• Down syndrome
• Metabolic disorders
• Pompe disease (glycogen excess on muscle biopsy)
• Hexosaminidase-A deficiency: organic aciduria

Neurologic disorders in the differential diagnosis of SMA include:

• Riley Day/familial dysautonomia (prominent gut/autonomic dysfunction)
• Hypomyelinating neuropathy
• Congenital myopathy/congenital muscular dystrophy
• Myasthenia gravis
• Juvenile ALS (upper motor neuron signs)
• Cervical spinal cord injury (history of birth trauma, breech)
• Polio
• Fazio-Londe disease: disproportionate bulbar dysfunction affecting swallowing
• Guillain-Barré syndrome
• Infant botulism
• Spinal cord tumor

 ## Data Gathering

HISTORY

• In some cases, onset in mid-infancy with hypotonia, poor head control, and generalized weakness may come to light during a well checkup;
• In other cases, newborns present with acute respiratory insufficiency shortly after birth and require mechanical ventilation.
• Delay or loss of motor milestones in the setting of hypotonia should always raise the possibility of SMA.
• Family history of prior floppy infants, even in the extended family, may be present.
• Occasional variation in age of onset within families, ranging from neonatal to juvenile or adolescent onset

 ## Physical Examination

Evidence supporting diagnosis of SMA includes:

• Tongue fasciculations
• Proximal pattern symmetric weakness
• Sparing of extraocular muscles and diaphragm.
• Moro and grasp reflexes are useful in the neurologic assessment of neuromuscular weakness in newborns.
• Note posture on ventral suspension and degree of head control while prone, sitting, and pulling to sit.
• The presence of deep tendon reflexes strongly weighs against the diagnosis of SMA.

Laboratory Aids

TESTS

• DNA test for "SMN" mutation is the starting point of diagnosis and can obviate further testing; if this test is normal, electromyography and muscle biopsy are done to exclude alternate diagnoses.
• Laboratory testing for alternative diagnoses is noted in Differential Diagnosis.
• Prenatal diagnosis is available when the proband is known to have a DNA abnormality.

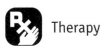 Therapy

• There is no effective therapy for motor neuron disease, though newer agents for ALS may prove useful in pediatric motor neuron disease.
• Supportive/anticipatory care directed toward respiratory complications, postural support, and genetic counseling

 Follow-Up

• Anticipatory/preventive medical issues: respiratory condition, physical therapy to prevent contractures, and so on.
• Ongoing planning and counseling regarding prognosis and appropriate medical intervention
• Follow-up genetic counseling

PITFALLS

• A seemingly minor respiratory infection in an infant or child with quadriparesis calls for close monitoring and follow-up, because it may rapidly become serious.
• Phenocopies of SMA: neonatal myasthenia, Guillain-Barré syndrome, sometimes mitochondrial disease; make laboratory confirmation of SMA important, because prognosis in these conditions may be very different from that of SMA.
• Because SMA is hereditary, genetic counseling should not be neglected once the diagnosis is established.
• Survival to the end of the first decade or later can occur in type I SMA!

 Common Questions and Answers

Q: What are prospects for specific therapy for SMA?
A: Gene therapy or use of neurotrophic factors may come to clinical trials in the next 5 years. Establishment of the sequence and function of the gene will likely accelerate this process. The Muscular Dystrophy Association and several national parents' groups have up-to-date information on therapy trials.

Q: Can routine vaccinations be given to infants with SMA?
A: Yes. In addition to routine vaccinations, yearly influenza vaccinations are recommended for older children with quadriparesis, because they are at high risk from common respiratory pathogens.

ICD-9-CM 335.10

BIBLIOGRAPHY

Crawford TO. From enigmatic to problematic: the new molecular genetics of childhood spinal muscular atrophy. *Neurology* 1996;46(2):335–340.

Matthijs G, Devriendt K, Fryns JP. The prenatal diagnosis of spinal muscular atrophy. *Prenat Diagn* 1998;18(6):607–610.

Pearn JH, Gardner-Medwin D, Wilson J. A clinical study of chronic childhood spinal muscular atrophy: a review of 141 cases. *J Neurol Sci* 37:227–248.

Russman BS, Melchreit R, Drennan JC. Spinal muscular atrophy: the natural course of disease. *Muscle Nerve* 1983;6:179.

Zerres K, Wirth B, Rudnik-Schoneborn S. Spinal muscular atrophyclinical and genetic correlations. *Neuromuscul Disord* 1997;7(3):202–207.

Author: Peter M. Bingham

Staphylococcal Scalded Skin Syndrome

 Database

DEFINITION

Staphylococcal scalded skin syndrome (SSSS) is a spectrum of generalized exfoliative skin eruptions, which resemble scalding injuries but are caused by an epidermolytic toxin produced by certain strains of *Staphylococcus aureus*. It is known as Ritter disease or pemphigus neonatorum in neonates. The spectrum of disease ranges from:

- Bullous impetigo: characterized by discrete, flaccid bullae containing clear or cloudy yellow fluid
- Staphylococcal scarlet fever: a mild generalized scarletiniform eruption with exfoliation, but without the strawberry tongue and palatal enanthem of streptococcal scarlet fever
- Classic SSSS: characterized by abrupt onset of fever, irritability, and diffuse, blanchable erythema in association with marked skin tenderness

PATHOPHYSIOLOGY

- A soluble exotoxin, referred to as epidermolytic toxin, produced by certain strains of *S. aureus* and belonging to phage group II in the United States
- Generalized desquamation with early intraepidermal bullae demonstrating a cleavage plane just beneath the granular cell layer
- Nikolsky sign develops within 12 hours to 3 days, accompanied by flaccid thin-walled bullae. Bullae spontaneously rupture within hours, separating the superficial epidermis into large sheets revealing moist red surfaces resembling burns. One to 3 days later, the denuded areas dry and the entire body surface undergoes a secondary flaky desquamation. The entire skin heals within a total of 10 to 14 days.

EPIDEMIOLOGY

- Most cases are caused by type 71 (75% of cases) or 70, with occasional cases due to types 3A, 3B, 3C, or 55.
- The vast majority of cases occur in neonates (as Ritter disease) and young children under 5 years of age.
- Rarely occurs in adults
- Most frequently occurs in association with immunosuppression or renal impairment
- No differences in incidence based on gender or socioeconomic status

COMPLICATIONS

- Occasional shedding of hair and nails
- Fungal or bacterial superinfection following desquamation
- Serious fluid and electrolyte disturbances in cases involving large surface areas that may lead to poor temperature control, hypovolemia, sepsis syndrome, and death. Neonates are particularly susceptible.

PROGNOSIS

- Exfoliated areas eventually dry, with a flaky desquamation in 3 to 5 days of initiating appropriate antibiotic therapy.
- Usually complete recovery within 10 to 14 days without scarring
- More guarded in infants and those with underlying illness
- Mortality is reported as 1% to 10% in neonates.

 Differential Diagnosis

- Toxic epidermal necrolysis (TEN)
- Kawasaki disease
- Erythema multiforme bullosum
- Erythema multiforme major (Stevens-Johnson syndrome)
- Streptococcal or staphylococcal toxic shock syndrome (TSS)
- Bullous varicella
- Burns
- Primary bullous disorders
- Chronic bullous disease of childhood
- Pemphigus vulgaris or foliaceus
- Epidermolysis bullosa

 Data Gathering

HISTORY

- Nonspecific virus-like prodrome followed by abrupt onset of fever, irritability, and extremely painful erythroderma
- Did rash begin periorally, then extend to trunk and extremities, and then finally desquamate?
- Was there any recent, seemingly trivial, localized extracutaneous infection involving the nasopharynx, middle ear, conjunctiva, pharynx, tonsils, umbilicus, or urinary tract?
- Ask about recent use of medications. A history of recent drug use suggests TEN.

 Physical Examination

- Fever
- Erythroderma and large flaccid bullae that leave behind denuded skin resembling a burn after bursting
- Bullae often appear in areas of trauma or in areas that are rubbed or even touched, including intertriginous zones.
- Lesions usually involve perineal, periumbilical, and intertriginous areas of the neonate, while the extremities are usually involved in older children.
- Crusting is seen in a radial pattern (sunburst) around the mouth, nose, and eyes without mucous membrane involvement.
- A sandpaper texture of rash and increased erythema or petechiae in skin creases (Pastia lines) are seen in the scarletiniform variant.
- Nikolsky sign: Gentle friction applied obliquely to apparently healthy skin will cause wrinkling, then sloughing.

 Laboratory Aids

TESTS

- Skin biopsy for differentiation from TEN.
- Excision of some exfoliated skin for frozen or permanent histologic section is useful, and easier to obtain than a biopsy.
- The cornified skin layer is recovered in SSSS, whereas the entire necrotic epidermis should be recognized in TEN.

Therapy

• Apply principles of good burn care in severe cases, including:

—Fluid and electrolyte management should include daily maintenance requirements as well as replacement of "third-space" fluid loss based on the percentage of affected body surface area (BSA). Fluid should be replaced as an isotonic solution calculated at 3 mL/kg of affected BSA. Most experts recommend replacement of one-half of losses over the first 8 hours and the other half over the next 16 hours.
—Children should be allowed to rest unclothed upon sterilized linens, and handling of the child should be kept to a minimum. Wound care should focus on relief of pressure on peripheral circulation by the developing eschars. This is usually followed by debridement, and affected areas are eventually dressed with silver sulfadiazine or similar agent.

• Antistaphylococcal agents: Parenteral antibiotic therapy (e.g., nafcillin, oxacillin, cephalosporins, clindamycin) should be employed for extensive skin involvement or serious systemic disease. Oral therapy (e.g., dicloxacillin, cloxacillin, amoxicillin/clavulanate, cephalexin, clindamycin) is generally sufficient for bullous impetigo. Duration of therapy is typically 7 to 10 days. Topical preparations are of no benefit.
• Corticosteroids have been shown to be detrimental both in experimental animal models as well as in clinical trials.

 Follow-Up

Patients may be followed via telephone as long as lesions are healing well and parents do not report significant complications.

PREVENTION

• Eradication of staphylococci to prevent recurrences after first attack
• Preventing skin from becoming overly moist or macerated
• Suspected or documented cases should be placed in contact isolation.

PITFALLS

• Confusion with TEN may lead to possible use of corticosteroids or simple discontinuation of antibiotics, resulting in enhanced infection from prolonged toxin production.
• Differentiation from streptococcal disease with need for penicillinase-resistant antibiotic therapy (e.g., nafcillin)
• A methicillin-resistant strain of *S. aureus* has been reported to cause SSSS.

 Common Questions and Answers

Q: Can SSSS recur?
A: Yes.

Q: Is SSSS contagious?
A: Yes, the staphylococci are primarily spread from person to person, most efficiently by someone with lesions, but asymptomatic carriers also may spread infection. However, spread of organisms does not necessarily lead to signs of toxin production in those acquiring infection.

Q: How can one distinguish TEN from SSSS?
A: TEN is frequently confused with SSSS and may be differentiated by skin biopsy showing a cleavage plane at the dermal-epidermal junction. TEN or Lyell disease is more common in adults and is usually secondary to drug hypersensitivity (e.g., sulfonamides, barbiturates, pyrazolone derivatives).

Q: Can staphylococcus be isolated from the bullae?
A: SSSS bullae are sterile, although organisms may be found in a distant focus, such as the nares or conjunctivae. In bullous impetigo, staphylococci may be isolated from the bullae.

ICD-9-CM 695.1

BIBLIOGRAPHY

Eichenfield LF, Honig PJ. Blistering disorders in childhood. *Pediatr Clin North Am* 1991;38: 959–976.

Gemmell CG. Staphylococcal scalded skin syndrome. *J Med Microbiol* 1995;43:318–327.

Ladhani S, Evans RW. Staphylococcal scalded skin syndrome. *Arch Dis Child* 1998;78:85–88.

Pollack S. Staphylococcal scalded skin syndrome. *Pediatr Rev* 1996;17:18.

Resnick SD. Staphylococcal toxin-mediated syndromes in childhood. *Semin Dermatol* 1992; 11:11–18.

Yokota S, Imagaura T, Katakura S, et al. Staphylococcal scalded skin syndrome caused by exfoliative toxin-B-producing methicillin-resistant *Staphylococcal aureus*. *Eur J Pediatr* 1996; 155:722.

Authors: Daniel H. Conway and Mark L. Bagarazzi

Status Epilepticus

 ## Database

DEFINITION

Status epilepticus (SE) is defined as more than 30 minutes of continuous seizure activity or two or more sequential seizures in 30 minutes without full recovery of consciousness between seizures. SE presents in several forms:

- Repeated generalized convulsive seizures with persistent postictal depression of neurologic function between seizures
- Nonconvulsive seizures that produce a continuous or fluctuating alteration in consciousness
- Repeated partial seizures manifested as focal motor convulsions or sensory symptoms not associated with altered consciousness (epilepsia partialis continua)

GENETICS

Some inherited conditions increase risk of SE, including neurocutaneous syndromes (tuberous sclerosis, Sturge-Weber) and familial epilepsy syndromes.

EPIDEMIOLOGY

There are 50,000 to 60,000 cases per year, and there is increased risk in young children and the elderly.

PATHOLOGY

Generalized convulsive SE is characterized by loss of consciousness and convulsive movements that may be symmetric or asymmetric. Nonconvulsive SE may be manifested only by alteration in consciousness. In epilepsia partialis continua (EPC), recurrent focal clonic activity or sensory symptoms occur without alteration of consciousness.

RISK FACTORS

- History of seizure disorder, recent withdrawal of anticonvulsant medication, brain tumor, neurodegenerative disorder, history of remote neurologic insult (stroke, cerebral palsy, head trauma, meningitis)

PROGNOSIS

The morbidity and mortality of SE are primarily a function of etiology and are lower in children than in adults. Recent mortality estimates in children range from 1% to 3%, with risk of new neurologic sequelae estimated at 9%.

 ## Differential Diagnosis

- Idiopathic
- Remote symptomatic (previous history of stroke, intracranial hemorrhage, birth asphyxia, cerebral palsy, head trauma, meningitis)
- Febrile
- Acute symptomatic (CNS infection, anoxia, trauma, stroke/hemorrhage, intoxication, metabolic encephalopathy, anticonvulsant withdrawal)
- Neurodegenerative disorder
- Brain tumor
- Neurocutaneous syndromes (tuberous sclerosis, Sturge-Weber)
- Nonepileptic seizures (including psychogenic seizures or pseudoseizures) may mimic status epilepticus.

 ## Data Gathering

HISTORY

- A history of seizures or neurologic abnormality can be clue to etiology.
- Ask specifically about precipitating factors, including:

—Fever, preceding illness
—History of head trauma
—Change in antiepileptic medication
—Family history of seizures

 ## Physical Examination

- Vital signs for indications of fever, adequacy of air exchange and perfusion, or abnormal respiratory pattern, bradycardia, or hypertension suggesting intracranial hypertension
- Signs of head trauma, including retinal hemorrhages and evidence of intracranial hypertension such as bulging fontanelle
- Look for signs of systemic infection, especially meningismus suggesting CNS infection.
- A careful skin examination, including Wood lamp examination, should be performed for evidence of neurocutaneous disorders.
- If the patient is actively convulsing, a neurologic examination is often limited and should be directed toward determining the possibility of intracranial hypertension and any focal abnormalities.
- Epileptic activity can produce transient neurologic abnormalities such as pupillary asymmetries, eye deviation, and focal motor weakness (Todd paresis), which may *not* correlate with the underlying structural lesion. Once seizure activity is controlled, conduct a neurologic examination with specific attention to mental status, abnormalities of motor strength, tone, or sensation.

 ## Laboratory Aids

TESTS

Initial

- Glucose
- Electrolytes
- BUN
- Arterial blood gas
- Antiepileptic drug levels
- Complete blood count
- Liver function tests
- Toxicology screen
- Urinalysis

Other Tests

- A lumbar puncture is indicated to rule out CNS infection unless a contraindication, such as intracranial hypertension, cerebral mass lesion, or obstructive hydrocephalus, is suspected; it may be deferred until after the head CT if suspicion of CNS infection is low.
- Brain imaging with CT or MRI is indicated in children with partial-onset seizures (including aura), focally abnormal EEG, focal neurologic signs, history of head trauma, or difficult-to-control seizures. MRI provides more detailed images; however, CT can be obtained more rapidly and is appropriate if urgent imaging is needed or the patient is medically unstable.
- An EEG is indicated immediately if convulsions continue or the patient fails to awaken in a reasonable time period after convulsions cease. An EEG also is indicated in children with first seizure and children with established epilepsy who have had a significant change in clinical status.

Therapy

- Initial management includes stabilization of airway, supporting respiration, maintaining blood pressure, and gaining intravascular access. Body temperature, blood pressure, ECG, and respiratory function should be monitored. Initially, airway control may be maintained by head positioning, and oral airway placement and oxygen supplementation provided via nasal cannula, mask, or bag-valve-mask ventilation. If the need for respiratory assistance persists, endotrachial intubation may be required. Blood glucose level should be determined promptly, and if hypoglycemia is documented, 2 to 4 mL/kg of D25 administered. Body temperature should be closely monitored and if elevated, rectal acetaminophen and a cooling blanket used.
- Antiepileptic drug administration should be initiated whenever seizure activity persists for longer than 10 to 15 minutes. Benzodiazepines are generally used in initial management of patients with active convulsions. The benzodiazepines most commonly used in SE are lorazepam (0.05–0.1 mg/kg/dose at 2 mg/min maximum, up to a total dose of 0.3–0.5 mg/kg) and diazepam (0.1–0.2 mg/kg/dose at 5 mg/min, up to a total dose of 1.0 mg/kg, not to exceed a total dose of 10 mg). Be aware that hypotension and respiratory depression can occur after benzodiazepine administration. If SE persists, administer a loading dose of 20 mg/kg phenytoin or fosphenytoin IV no faster than 1 mg/kg/min, up to maximum rate of 50 mg/min. Additional doses of 5 mg/kg may be given if needed to stop convulsion (to maximum total dose of 30 mg/kg). BP and ECG should be monitored and the rate of infusion reduced if hypotension or cardiac arrhythmias occur. Intravenous phenobarbital at a loading dose of 20 mg/kg (maximum rate, 100 mg/min) is generally a third-line drug for older children and adults but is usually given before phenytoin in infants less than 1 year of age. Additional 5- to 10-mg/kg increments (to total maximum dose of 30–40 mg/kg) may be given as necessary to stop convulsions. Sedation, respiratory depression, and hypotension are potential side effects. If intravenous access is difficult to obtain, diazepam (0.5 mg/kg to a maximum of 20 mg), paraldehyde (0.3–0.5 mL/kg diluted 1:1 in vegetable oil) and valproic acid (20 mg/kg of liquid formulation diluted 1:1 in water) can be administered.

 ## Follow-Up

PREVENTION

Need for long-term antiepileptic drug (AED) therapy after SE depends on the etiology, patient's age, and circumstances in which SE occurred. Chronic AED therapy is indicated when SE is caused by structural brain lesions or in patients with known epilepsy. Chronic AED therapy may not be needed in children who have SE solely as a result of transient metabolic disturbances such as hyponatremia, intoxication, or fever, or in neurologically normal children who experience SE as their first seizure and no cause is found.

PITFALLS

- *Anticonvulsant intoxication* may occasionally cause SE (phenytoin, carbamazepine); check levels on any patient known to take anticonvulsants.
- *Neuromuscular blockers* used in intubation may obscure ongoing electrical seizures. EEG monitoring is mandatory for all patients who have had pharmacologic paralysis for airway control during SE.
- *Psychogenic status* may be characterized by asynchronous limb movements, pelvic thrusting, and purposeful resistance to passive movement. Induction of a seizure by suggestion further supports this diagnosis.

 ## Common Questions and Answers

Q: Does SE cause brain injury?
A: Two principal determinants of outcome are hypoxic brain injury due to hypoventilation during a seizure and brain injury due to an identifiable underlying cause of SE, such as encephalitis. Outcome in children with idiopathic SE without hypoxia is usually very good.

Q: What is the toxicity of medicines used to treat SE?
A: Acute toxicity of the principal agents used to control SE includes hypotension (phenytoin), hypoventilation/respiratory arrest (barbiturates, benzodiazepines), and sedation (compounding postictal encephalopathy).

ICD-9-CM 345.3

BIBLIOGRAPHY

Mitchell WG. Status epilepticus and acute repetitive seizures in children, adolescents, and young adults: etiology, outcome, and treatment. *Epilepsia* 1996;37[Suppl 1]:S74–S80.

Perry HE, Shannon MW. Diagnosis and management of opioid- and benzodiazepine-induced comatose overdose in children. *Curr Opin Pediatr* 1996;8(3):243–247.

Author: Amy R. Brooks-Kayal

Stevens-Johnson Syndrome

 Database

DEFINITION

Stevens-Johnson syndrome (SJS) is a distinctive acute hypersensitivity syndrome marked by widespread bullous rash with mucocutaneous involvement, pronounced constitutional symptoms, and fever.

ETIOLOGY

• Hypersensitivity to viral (especially herpes simplex), bacterial, fungal, or *Mycoplasma pneumoniae* infections
• Food or drugs (especially sulfonamides, penicillins, and anticonvulsants)
• Less commonly, immunologic disorders, malignancies, and biologic products such as vaccines and immunoglobulin

PATHOPHYSIOLOGY

Acute hypersensitivity reaction, causing epidermal and dermal inflammation and destruction by invading lymphocytes and deposition of immune complexes, resulting in the following findings:

• Erythema multiforme rash and bullae diffusely involving skin
• Extensive bullae with crusting and superficial ulceration of the mucous membranes of the lips, eyes, nares, genitalia, and rectum
• Severe conjunctivitis with corneal involvement, including ulceration, keratitis, and uveitis
• Extension of oral lesions into the respiratory mucosa
• Hematuria and nephritis

EPIDEMIOLOGY

• Occurs in any age
• Highest incidence in spring and fall

COMPLICATIONS

• Severe dehydration and secondary infection (similar to burn patients)
• Sepsis
• Corneal ulceration and blindness
• Pneumonitis, pneumonia, and respiratory failure
• Nephritis and renal failure
• Stress ulcers and gastric perforation

PROGNOSIS

• Recovery can take several weeks, or longer if there are complications.
• SJS can resolve completely over time with little or no scarring.
• May have corneal scars, which may impair vision

 Differential Diagnosis

• Infection
—Varicella
—Staphylococcal or streptococcal scalded skin syndrome
—Disseminated herpes simplex virus
—Measles
• Trauma
—Burns (chemical or heat)
• Metabolic
—Drug reaction
• Congenital
—Epidermolysis bullosa
• Immunologic
—Primary immunobullous dermatoses (pemphigus, pemphigoid, linear IgA dermatosis)
—Henoch-Schönlein purpura
—Lupus erythematosus
• Miscellaneous
—Erythema multiforme minor

 Data Gathering

HISTORY

Question: Were there any exposures to drugs, especially sulfa drugs, penicillins, and anticonvulsants?
Significance: These drugs are common causes of SJS.

Question: Does the patient have another medical condition?
Significance: It is important to identify the underlying cause (infectious or toxic) and investigate underlying medical problems.

Ask about recent or current medications, vaccinations, and toxic exposures.

 Physical Examination

• Determine the surface area of skin involved.
• Examine all orifices (including anus and urethral meatus) for mucocutaneous involvement.
• Determine hydration, respiratory, gastrointestinal, and urologic status.
• Assess presence of infection or sepsis.

 Laboratory Aids

TESTS

Specific Tests

• CBC (infection); electrolytes (dehydration); BUN/creatinine (renal function); erythrocyte sedimentation rate; Tzanck smear of skin/mucosal lesions (HSV)
• Consider serologic tests, looking for specific viral etiologies and mycoplasma titers.
• Pulse oximetry

Radiographic Tests

• Chest radiograph (pneumonia)

Therapy

- Address life-threatening complications: sepsis, shock, hypovolemia, hypoxia, gastrointestinal bleeding.
- Eliminate the cause if identified.
- Admit to the intensive care unit or burn unit if indicated.
- Intravenous access is critical to provide fluid resuscitation and maintenance of large fluid requirements.
- Debridement and meticulous skin care are critical.
- Nutritional support is critical and often achieved with high-calorie nasogastric feeds or intravenous hyperalimentation.
- Ophthalmology consult
- Monitor closely for secondary infection.
- Monitor closely for airway complications.
- Skin grafts may be indicated.

DRUGS

- Cover open lesions with bacitracin ointment and gauze or Xeroform-impregnated gauze.
- Do *not* use Silvadine skin dressing because the sulfadiazene component may aggravate the condition.
- Reserve antibiotics for identified infections only. Do not use prophylactic antibiotics.
- Prevent and treat stress ulcers with antacids and H_2 blockers.
- Steroids are currently *not* indicated.

 Follow-Up

- Skin care until all areas healed
- Ophthalmology consult if corneal involvement
- Follow renal function if impaired
- Education to avoid the causative agent

PREVENTION

- None known

PITFALLS

- Discontinuation of the causative agent (e.g., anticonvulsants or antibiotics) may leave another problem untreated.
- Delay in recognition of complications

 Common Questions and Answers

Q: Why should steroids not be used?
A: Steroids are currently not indicated for SJS. A possible association with herpes simplex infection makes their use risky. Efficacy has not been shown.

Q: How do you differentiate between SJS and erythema multiforme (EM)?
A: Mucous membrane involvement is present in SJS but not in EM. SJS is more extensive and associated with more systemic symptoms.

Q: Who should be admitted to the intensive care unit?
A: Any patient with pulmonary involvement and serious infection, or if close monitoring of fluids and electrolytes or extensive skin care is not available in the regular inpatient unit.

ICD-9-CM 695.1

BIBLIOGRAPHY

Cohen B. The many faces of erythema multiforme. *Contemp Pediatr* 1994;11:19–39.

Hurwitz S. *Clinical pediatric dermatology. A textbook of skin disorders of childhood and adolescence,* 2nd ed. Philadelphia: WB Saunders, 1990.

Hurwitz S. Pediatric dermatology. *Pediatr Clin North Am* 1991;38(4):972–974.

Stewart MG, Duncan, NO III, Franklin DJ, Friedman EM, Sulek M. Head and neck manifestations of erythema multiforme in children. *Otolaryngol Head Neck Surg* 1994;111(3,1) 236–242.

Author: Deborah L. Silver

Stomatitis

Database

DEFINITION

Stomatitis is inflammation of the mucosal surfaces of the oral cavity. There are a variety of causes, but the vast majority of cases are due to viral infections (enteroviruses, herpes simplex virus I) or recurrent aphthous stomatitis.

PATHOPHYSIOLOGY

• The incubation period for enterovirus infections is 3 to 10 days. The enanthem begins as punctate macules surrounded by a ring of erythema. Vesicles develop, which eventually ulcerate, then heal without scarring. There is relative immunity to reinfection with the same serotype.
• The incubation period for HSV-I and HSV-II is 1 to 26 days. There are multiple strains of each type, with partial immunity against other strains of *both* types after infection.
• Recurrent aphthous stomatitis (canker sores) may be associated with a variety of nutritional deficiencies (B vitamins, folic acid, zinc, iron), gluten sensitivity (even in the absence of bowel symptoms), and other food sensitivities. Their occurrence may also be related to stress or oral trauma. There are three forms: the minor form (most common), the major form, and the herpetiform.

EPIDEMIOLOGY

• Viral stomatitis is spread by the fecal-oral and oral-oral routes. Asymptomatic shedding of HSV is significant.
• Enteroviral infections are more frequent during the summer and fall months.
• The prevalence of recurrent aphthous stomatitis is 5% to 66% in various studies and regions of the world, with a female predominance.

COMPLICATIONS

• Dehydration
• Extreme pain
• Secondary bacterial infection (e.g., cellulitis), uncommonly

PROGNOSIS

• Most cases are mild and self-limited, with complete resolution.
• Some less common forms (e.g., major recurrent aphthous stomatitis) can result in significant scarring and deformity.
• Recurrent aphthous stomatitis can recur at intervals of days to months, with the frequency of recurrences decreasing with increasing patient age.

Differential Diagnosis

• Infectious

—Herpangina (mostly coxsackie A, also coxsackie B and echoviruses)
—Hand-foot-mouth syndrome (coxsackie A)
—Herpes simplex virus type I and II (herpetic gingivostomatitis)
—Varicella

• Toxin

—Methotrexate, adriamycin, etoposide, 5-fluorouracil, bleomycin, cytarabine, 6-mercaptopurine, vinblastine, vincristine, dactinomycin, doxorubicin

• Trauma

—Hard foods, toothbrushes, cheek biting
—Bednar aphthae: excoriation of the hard palate in nursing infants

• Miscellaneous

—Recurrent aphthous stomatitis
—Systemic disorders: Behcet syndrome, Sweet syndrome, agranulocytosis, cyclic neutropenia, nutritional deficiencies, immunodeficiencies including HIV, inflammatory bowel disease (IBD)
—Stevens-Johnson syndrome

Data Gathering

HISTORY

Question: What is the age of the child?
Significance: Herpangina and herpetic gingivostomatitis tend to affect preschool-aged children; hand-foot-mouth syndrome typically affects toddlers and school-aged children. Recurrent aphthous stomatitis generally affects older children and young adults.

Question: How long have the oral lesions been present?
Significance: Viral stomatitis usually lasts for 1 week or less. Minor recurrent aphthous stomatitis has lesions lasting 7 to 10 days (pain usually lasts only 3–4 days); major recurrent aphthous stomatitis lesions may last weeks to months.

Question: Are the oral lesions painful?
Significance: Ulcers from hand-foot-mouth syndrome tend to be only mildly painful, whereas those in herpetic gingivostomatitis are often extremely painful. Lesions in recurrent aphthous stomatitis tend to be exquisitely painful.

Question: Are there lesions elsewhere besides the oral cavity?
Significance: With varicella, there are vesicles distributed over various skin and mucosal surfaces. In hand-foot-mouth syndrome, there are vesicles over the palms and soles and over the interdigital surfaces; there may be papules over the lower extremities and buttocks.

Question: Is there associated fever?
Significance: Sudden onset of fever often occurs with herpangina, usually low-grade but may be as high as 41°C in younger patients. Fever may occur with hand-foot-mouth syndrome (usually 38°C to 39°C), lasting 1 to 2 days. Fever is also common with herpetic gingivostomatitis, often lasting 2 to 7 days.

Question: Are there associated constitutional symptoms?
Significance: Sore throat and painful swallowing may precede the oral lesions in herpangina. Headache, vomiting, and myalgias may be early accompanying symptoms. Malaise, myalgias, and irritability may accompany herpetic gingivostomatitis (patients usually appear more ill than do those with herpangina or hand-foot-mouth syndrome). Constitutional symptoms are generally absent in recurrent aphthous stomatitis.

Question: How is the child's overall growth?
Significance: Failure to thrive/poor weight gain may be indicative of underlying disease, such as IBD or immunodeficiency states including HIV.

Question: Has the child had similar oral lesions in the past?
Significance: Think of recurrent aphthous stomatitis, immunodeficiency states, IBD, or recurrent herpes.

Question: Does the child have any chronic medical problems?
Significance: Such as HIV, cyclic or noncyclic neutropenia, IBD.

Question: Is the child taking any medications?
Significance: Chemotherapeutic agents may cause stomatitis. Stevens-Johnson syndrome may be a complication of taking certain medications (anticonvulsants, penicillins, salicylates, sulfa antibiotics).

Question: Is there a history of oral trauma? Cheek-biting?
Significance: Local trauma a common cause of stomatitis.

Physical Examination

Finding: Ulcerations or vesicles largely in posterior oral cavity (buccal mucosa, tonsils, soft palate, pharynx)
Significance: Herpangina or hand-foot-mouth syndrome

Finding: Ulcerations or vesicles largely in anterior oral cavity (buccal mucosa, gingiva, tongue)
Significance: Recurrent aphthous stomatitis, herpetic gingivostomatitis

Finding: Vesicles on lips and on skin around lips, as well as anterior oral cavity
Significance: Herpetic gingivostomatitis

Finding: Exudative pharyngitis
Significance: May occur in herpetic gingivostomatitis

Finding: Vesicles on palms, soles, and interdigital surfaces
Significance: Hand-foot-mouth syndrome

Finding: Vesicles in various stages of development over body (generally excluding palms and soles) with crusting of older lesions
Significance: Varicella

Finding: Vesicles on sucked fingers
Significance: Herpetic whitlow (from herpetic gingivostomatitis)

Finding: Target lesions and bullae on skin, ulcerations of two or more mucosal surfaces (oral, genital, conjunctival)
Significance: Stevens-Johnson syndrome

Laboratory Aids

TESTS

- In general, there is no indication for laboratory testing to make the diagnosis of stomatitis.
- Direct fluorescent antibody staining for HSV: rapid and highly specific, but less sensitive than culture.
- An office-based rapid enzyme immunoassay (EIA) for HSV-I and HSV-II has a sensitivity of 82% to 95% and a specificity of 100%.
- HSV is readily isolated for culture from skin and mucous membranes, with detection usually in 1 to 3 days.
- Enteroviruses can be isolated from stool, throat, CSF, and blood. Isolation from the throat can occur 2 days to 2 weeks after infection.

Therapy

- Soothing rinses, such as sodium bicarbonate (1 teaspoon baking soda in 32 ounces of water or normal saline), or coating agents, such as "magic mouthwash" (diphenhydramine mixed 1:1 with Maalox or Kaopectate) may provide temporary relief of pain, especially if used prior to attempting oral intake.
- Viscous lidocaine 2% may be used for severe pain, but caretakers must exercise caution in its use, as it can suppress the gag reflex and increase the risk for aspiration.
- With herpes simplex infections, oral acyclovir at a dose of 20 mg/kg q8h or 200 mg five times a day should be considered in immunocompromised patients or in patients with underlying skin disorders (e.g., eczema). Topical acyclovir has not been shown to be promising in the treatment of oral lesions.
- Treatment of recurrent aphthous stomatitis includes topical steroid gels (fluocinonide, betamethasone dipropionate, or clobetasol, applied to affected areas two to four times per day), silver nitrate cauterization, and topical analgesics.
- Chlorhexidine gluconate mouth rinse may reduce the duration of RAS lesions and decrease the rate of recurrence (taste sensation may be altered, therefore should not be used 1–2 hours before meals).

Follow-Up

Follow-up is necessary if the patient is a young infant with significant pain and poor oral intake, to ensure that the child is not becoming dehydrated.

PREVENTION

- Strict handwashing after handling an affected child is necessary in preventing spread of this disease to others (particularly other young children).
- Objects that are placed in the mouth act as fomites, and should be sterilized before being used by another child.

ISOLATION OF HOSPITALIZED PATIENT

As enteroviruses and herpes simplex virus are spread by oral-oral and fecal-oral contact, contact isolation is required for all patients with viral stomatitis.

Common Questions and Answers

Q: How can recurrent aphthous stomatitis be distinguished from recurrent intraoral herpes stomatitis?
A: Recurrent aphthous stomatitis generally affects the "movable" mucosa (lips, buccal mucosa, ventral tongue, mucobuccal fold), whereas herpes tends to involve the keratinized or "nonmovable" mucosa (hard palate, dorsum of tongue, alveolar ridge and attached gingiva).

Q: Can HSV-II (genital herpes) cause herpetic gingivostomatitis?
A: Yes, especially in sexually active patients.

Q: Do children with primary or recurrent HSV mucocutaneous infections need to be excluded from daycare or school?
A: In general, no. However, young children with primary herpetic gingivostomatitis and enteroviral stomatitis (herpangina, hand-foot-mouth syndrome) who cannot control their oral secretions should be excluded.

ICD-9-CM 528.0

BIBLIOGRAPHY

American Academy of Pediatrics. Summaries of infectious diseases. In: Peter G, ed. *1997 red book: report of the Committee on Infectious Diseases*, 24th ed. Elk Grove Village, IL: American Academy of Pediatrics; 1997:198–199, 266–276.

Amir J, Straussberg R, Harel L, Smetana Z, Varsano I. Evaluation of a rapid enzyme immunoassay for the detection of herpes simplex virus antigen in children with herpetic gingivostomatitis. *Pediatr Infect Dis J* 1996;15(7):627–629.

Annunziato PW, Gershon A. Herpes simplex virus infections. *Pediatr Rev* 1996;17(12):415–423.

Herbert AA, Berg JH. Oral mucous membrane diseases of childhood: I. Mucositis and xerostomia. II. Recurrent aphthous stomatitis. III. Herpetic stomatitis. *Semin Dermatol* 1992;11(1):80–87.

Rees TD, Binnie WH. Recurrent aphthous stomatitis. *Dermatol Clin* 1996;14(2):243–256.

Vanderhooft SL. Is the rash a drug reaction? *Contemp Pediatr* 1998;15(5):118–137.

Zaoutis T, Klein JD. Enterovirus infections. *Pediatr Rev* 1998;19(6):183–191.

Author: Bruce Oriel

Strabismus

Database

DEFINITION

From *strabos* ("to squint"), strabismus is a condition in which the visual axes of the eyes are nonparallel so that they are not directed at the same object.

- Comitant strabismus occurs when the deviation of the eyes is the same in all positions of gaze.
- Incomitant strabismus occurs when the deviation between the eyes changes with changing gaze position.
- Appearance is also classified as "esotropia" when the eyes are crossed.
- Exotropia when the eyes are divergent
- Hyper/hypotropia when an eye is up or down

PATHOPHYSIOLOGY

- Either due to a supranuclear (visual cortex) inability to use the eyes together, which usually results in comitant strabismus, or to an infranuclear disorder of the extraocular muscles or their respective cranial nerves, which results in incomitant strabismus
- Interruption of visual development in an eye (e.g., retinoblastoma tumor) also results in strabismus in infancy and childhood.

PATHOLOGY

Abnormal synaptogensis in binocular cells of the visual cortex for comitant strabismus. In incomitant strabismus, a combination of neuronal degeneration, extraocular muscle atrophy, fibrosis, or infiltration is present, depending on the etiology.

GENETICS

- Approximately 30% of children with strabismus have family members with strabismus.
- Inheritance is multifactorial, with a strabismic parent having a 12% to 17% chance of having a child with strabismus (as opposed to 4% with no family history).

EPIDEMIOLOGY

- Four percent of the population has some form of the over 100 different types of strabismus.
- Most forms of strabismus are comitant and begin in either infancy or early childhood.
- Adults with strabismus have either decompensated comitant childhood strabismus (approximately two-thirds) or acquired incomitant strabismus (approximately one-third).

COMPLICATIONS

- Approximately 50% of children under 9 years of age will develop amblyopia (see chapter on Amblyopia) in one eye if left untreated.
- Older children and adults develop constant disabling diplopia due to spatial malperception.

- Long-standing strabismus results in secondary shortening, tightening, and contracture of extraocular muscles, which limits eye excursion and binocular visual fields.
- Chronic strabismus is disfiguring and results in decreased self-esteem, poor self-image, and aberrant social interaction.

Differential Diagnosis

- Patients with increased epicanthal folds, large intercanthal distances, and other eyelid abnormalities may have the appearance of strabismus. This is called pseudostrabismus.
- Children who are developing vision in the first few months of life may appear esotropic while viewing objects at near. This is maturation of the near reflex.
- Infants and children with cicatricial retinal disease may appear to be exotropic or esotropic due to dragging of the fovea (central retinal area of vision) from its normal anatomic position.
- Orbital deformities and tumors may result in asymmetric globe position and orbital appearance without true strabismus.

Data Gathering

HISTORY

- Symmetry and direction of deviation
- Age of onset
- Amount of waking hours deviation is present
- Family history
- The presence of any trauma, prenatal, perinatal, or postnatal medical problems
- *General exposures:* contact with toxins; new climates, travel, or daycare; or recent systemic medications

Physical Examination

- Visual acuity of all patients (Snellen, HOTV) or visual behavior of each eye under 3 years old (fixation and following, with central, steady, and maintained gaze)
- The pupils should respond briskly to direct light.
- The presence of deviation can be diagnosed using corneal light reflexes (Hirschberg test).
- The light reflex should appear in the same position in each pupil while viewing a fixation light.
- A preference for one or the other eye can be noted.
- Ocular rotations should be full in each eye.
- The presence of involuntary head or ocular oscillations (nystagmus) should be noted.
- A bright, full, red-orange fundus reflex can be seen with the direct ophthalmoscope used at 2 to 4 feet.

- This is important because disruption of this reflex may herald serious ocular or systemic disease (retinoblastoma, cataract, intraocular hemorrhage).
- If any of these abnormalities are found, the infant or child will need a complete ophthalmic examination and follow-up.
- Neurologic evaluation:

—A general developmental and neurologic examination is an important part of the initial evaluation of a child with strabismus.
—Strabismus is more frequent in patients with central nervous system pathology and developmental delay (cerebral palsy, meningomyelocele, prematurity, anoxic encephalopathy, hydrocephalus, craniofacial syndromes, and intracranial tumors).

Laboratory Aids

TESTS

Hematologic

Most forms of comitant childhood strabismus do not need hematologic analysis. If incomitant strabismus (cranial nerve VI paralysis) or strabismus secondary to an inflammatory process (orbital cellulitis, myositis) is present, then hematologic studies are important.

Radiologic

CT Scans and MRI studies of the orbits and head are particularly useful in those cases of strabismus associated with trauma, craniofacial malformations, neurologic disease, or acute onset with incomitancy.

Electrophysiologic

- Visual evoked response (VER): This easily performed test represents quantification and refined measuring of the visual cortical contribution to the EEG and aids in diagnosing visual pathway abnormalities (optic nerve hypoplasia, atrophy) that contribute to strabismus pathogenesis. The VER is most useful if afferent visual pathway disease is suspected clinically.
- Electroretinogram (ERG): This test of retinal function is based on the normal electrical polarity of the retina. It is excellent for diagnosing and classifying retinal degenerations and dystrophies that may contribute to strabismus pathogenesis.
- ERG testing is most useful in patients with clinically suspected retinal abnormalities.
- Electrooculography (EOG): provides a quantitative analysis of oculomotor function and can aid in diagnosis of strabismus type (paralytic versus restrictive); the study of choice in patients with ocular oscillations (nystagmus, ocular flutter) because it provides diagnostic differentiation and pathophysiologic clues

Strabismus

Therapy

- Prompt diagnosis and treatment offers the best results, although no therapy will "cure" most forms of childhood strabismus, because we cannot yet reverse the synaptic problem serving binocular function in the visual cortex. Successful treatment includes promoting use of a cortically more primitive form of binocular cooperation. This prevents amblyopia and is characterized by intermittent recurrence of the deviation due to fatigue and sedation, or complete recurrence as an older child or adult. First medical then surgical treatments are used. All strabismus treatment includes, first, improving vision and, second, correcting alignment.
- Improve vision

—Medical: Spectacle correction of significant refractive errors is accomplished as early as 4 to 6 months of age. Spectacle treatment alone may sufficiently improve vision and binocular function. *Spectacles are medicine in children* (they impact on brain function). Penalization of the preferred eye with patching or cycloplegic drops improves vision due to amblyopia.

—Surgical: reserved for pathologic conditions that interfere with optically clear media (corneal opacification, cataract, vitreous hemorrhage) or degrade images of the work (retinal detachment, upper lid ptosis, hemangiomas).

- Correct alignment

—Medical: Spectacles with or without bifocals or optical prism alone may be sufficient in some strabismus types (accommodative esotropia, convergence insufficiency, intermittent exotropia); topical miotic drops (phospholine iodide) can manipulate accommodation and improve ocular alignment in some forms of esotropia. Visual training "exercises" have some, but limited, usefulness.

—Surgical: Extraocular muscle surgery is performed in an attempt to mechanically move the eyes into a more advantageous position for the brain (within 5%); it is successful with one operation in 75% to 80% of patients, with 20% to 25% requiring a second procedure; with new techniques, instrumentation and safe anesthesia, the incidence of any complication is rare (less than 1%).

Follow-Up

- Intermittent strabismus: Patients with deviations occurring less than half of their waking hours, with normal and equal vision in both eyes, should be evaluated every 6 months unless an increase is noticed by their caretakers.
- Constant strabismus: Amblyopia, spectacles, or necessary therapy to normalize vision is carried out immediately. If the deviation remains constant, treatment is instituted until proper alignment is achieved. Once alignment and best vision are obtained, patients are examined every 3 months if under a year of age and every 6 months up to 3 years of age, and every 6 to 12 months thereafter.
- Prognosis: Decompensation and reappearance of a new or the same deviation may occur in as many as 35% to 40% of patients into adulthood, necessitating long-term ophthalmic care.
- Contact with social services for blind and visually impaired individuals must be made for children, even if they are only suspected of being visually impaired. Encourage families to make the contact even when the child may be too young to provide objective data of the extent of disability.

PITFALLS

- Assuming that patients will "grow out" of their strabismus
- Confusing strabismus with "lazy eye" (amblyopia)
- Strabismus may be due to serious underlying ophthalmic (retinoblastoma), systemic (genetic disorders), or neurologic abnormalities (cerebral palsy).

Common Questions and Answers

Q: Does this condition interfere with learning, education, or sports?
A: No. A "learning" problem should not be blamed on the patient's eyes.

Q: Is visual training, or "eye exercises," effective treatment?
A: Although this remedy has received increased public attention, it rarely results in long-term success and requires substantial time and financial commitments.

Q: Will surgery cure this condition?
A: No. Strabismus is usually a complex neural control problem with "normal" extraocular muscles; thus, medical (glasses or drops) and surgical therapies are treatments.

ICD-9-CM 378.9

BIBLIOGRAPHY

Archer SM, Sondhi NM, Helveston EM. Strabismus in infancy. *Ophthalmology* 1989;96:133–137.

Berman N, Murphy EH. The critical period for alteration in cortical binocularity resulting from convergent and divergent strabismus. *Brain Res* 1981;254:181–202.

Foster RS, Paul TO, Jampolsky AJ. Management of infantile esotropia. *Am J Ophthalmol* 1976;82:291–299.

Graham PA. Epidemiology of strabismus. *Br J Ophthalmol* 1974;58:224–231.

Kalil RE, Spear PD, Langsetmo A. Response properties of striate cortex in cats raised with convergent or divergent strabismus. *J Neurophysiol* 1984;52:514–537.

Author: Richard W. Hertle

Stroke

Database

DEFINITION

Stroke is a neurologic deficit progressing over minutes to hours due to insufficient perfusion of the brain or spinal cord.

PATHOPHYSIOLOGY

Abnormalities of the blood, intracranial vasculature, or the heart (dysrhythmia or anatomic) lead to embolism or intravascular thrombosis.

PATHOLOGY

- Edema, neuronal swelling, cellular infiltrate, and cavitation starting from 8 hours until months after an ischemic brain injury

GENETICS

- Seen in numerous hereditary and metabolic disorders, especially coagulation disorders, hereditary AVM, and others

EPIDEMIOLOGY

Overall incidence is approximately 2.5 per 100,000, but certain groups are at higher risk (heart disease, sickle cell disease, hereditary thrombophilias).

COMPLICATIONS

- Seizures
- Respiratory insufficiency
- Intracranial hypertension
- Motor, visual, and cognitive deficits
- Autonomic disturbances
- Infection susceptibility

Differential Diagnosis

- Several disorders may mimic the presentation of stroke:

—Migraine
—Demyelinating disease
—Focal encephalitis
—Postepileptic paralysis (Todd paresis)
—Conversion disorder
—Rarely intracranial neoplasm, abscess, subdural empyema, or mitochondrial disease may present as stroke.

- Underlying causes of stroke include hematologic, circulatory, and cardiac disorders:

—*Hematologic:* factor V deficiency, lupus anticoagulant, anticardiolipin syndrome, sickle cell, hyperhomocysteinemia, dyslipidemia, proteins S or C, antithrombin III deficiency, asparaginase treatment, hyperviscosity syndromes (including leukemia), thrombocythemia, extreme dehydration; hemorrhagic stroke (see chapter on Intracranial Hemorrhage).
—*Vascular:* carotid or vertebral dissection, intracranial AVM, carotid trauma, moya-moya, cavernous angioma, vasculitis (especially due to bacterial meningitis); rarely, aneurysm, Takayusu arteritis, chronic meningitides (tuberculosis, Lyme, or sarcoidosis)
—*Cardiac:* especially rheumatic heart disease, cyanotic congenital heart disease, or heart failure due to acquired or cardiomyopathy, or perioperatively; weak association with mitral prolapse, atrial septal defects; rarely, atrial myxoma, aortic dilatation (Marfan), pulmonary AVM

Data Gathering

HISTORY

- Occurrence of stroke in specific settings may point to the diagnosis; previous migraines may point to complicated migraine (rare); details of the timing and circumstances of symptom onset may be critical in establishing diagnosis.
- Recent trauma, infection, excessive bleeding or spontaneous clotting, or history of heart disease should be established.
- Family history of premature thrombosis, hemoglobinopathy, or vascular malformations (e.g., cavernous hemangioma or hereditary hemorrhagic telangiectasia).
- Perinatal stroke may be related to a pre-, peri-, or postpartum cerebrovascular event and frequently presents with neonatal seizures.
- Complications of labor or fetal exposure to vasoactive compounds may sometimes be associated.

Physical Examination

- Vital signs, color, and respiratory pattern may disclose existing or impending respiratory failure due to loss of protective airway reflexes.
- General examination should include peripheral pulses and perfusion; palpation and auscultation of the precordium and cervical area may reveal evidence of dysrhythmia or anatomic lesions.
- Neurologic findings important to note include level of alertness, speech fluency and comprehension, confrontation visual fields, funduscopy (especially for papilledema), eye movements, facial symmetry, pattern of most severely affected limbs, and extensor response of great toe to plantar stimulation (Babinski sign).
- In the absence of sensory complaints, detailed sensory exam is often fruitless.

Laboratory Aids

TESTS

Laboratory Tests

- Blood chemistry, particularly glucose, should be tested; mild hyperglycemia may reflect stress response; marked elevation (i.e., in diabetics) should be treated, since hyperglycemia may aggravate ischemic brain injury.
- Complete blood count and PT/PTT may prompt important therapeutic decisions.

Imaging

- Individuals with stable vital signs and suspected stroke should undergo a brain imaging study promptly. Noncontrasted images are important to look for possible hemorrhage and may be followed by contrasted images for possible focal encephalitis, or to identify underlying vascular lesions.
- Many diagnostic questions can be resolved equally well by CT or MRI, though CT may be preferable in suspected subarachnoid hemorrhage; MRI is much more sensitive in the first 24 hours after symptom onset, and may identify venous or sinus thrombosis, or smaller bilateral lesions pointing to systemic embolization.

Other Tests

More extensive testing in undiagnosed cases may include:

- Tests for specific coagulopathies (see Differential Diagnosis)
- Amino acid screening
- Hemoglobin electrophoresis
- Lipid profile
- Echocardiography
- Carotid Doppler
- Specialized neuroradiologic studies (MR angiogram, standard angiography)

Therapy

- *Hospitalization:* Patients with radiologically documented or clinically suspected stroke who have stable airway, breathing, and circulation are most often hospitalized for observation and supportive therapy. Those with a diminished or fluctuating level of alertness or with radiographically extensive area(s) of infarction are often monitored in an intensive care unit for changes in respiratory status or signs of increased intracranial pressure.
- Strokes involving the posterior fossa or cerebellum are of particular concern because of the risk of tentorial herniation; a neurosurgical consult should be obtained for these cases and for those with intracranial hemorrhage above or below the tentorium.
- *Consultation* with neurology, neurosurgery, cardiology, hematology, or other pediatric subspecialists is often helpful.
- *Drugs:* In most cases, there is no contraindication to pharmacotherapy appropriate to any identified underlying condition; the decision to use antiplatelet therapy or anticoagulation is complex and depends on risk of hemorrhage or other potential side effects.
- *Rehabilitation and physical therapy* may improve outcome and should be instituted as soon as the patient's condition permits.
- *Investigational therapies* include hypervolemic hemodilution, thrombolytic agents, calcium channel antagonists, and antagonists of glutamate receptors.

Follow-Up

- The usual course in stroke of any cause is for gradual improvement after the acute onset of symptoms. Significant recovery of neurologic function may continue as long as months after the ictus, especially in infants and toddlers.
- Involvement of child developmentalists and/or ophthalmologists in follow-up depends on the etiology and residual deficits of the stroke.
- *Remote sequelae* that may not be evident for months or years after stroke include epilepsy, hydrocephalus, learning difficulties, short attention span, posture disturbances (especially cerebral palsy), sphincter disturbances, pressure sores, and susceptibility to infection if airway protective reflexes are impaired.

PITFALLS

- AVMs may not be seen on angiography immediately after a primary intracerebral hemorrhage. Some clinicians repeat angiography several weeks or months later.
- CT may be normal in the first 24 hours after nonhemorrhagic stroke. A follow-up study may be necessary.
- Diagnosis of transient ischemic attack (TIA) may depend on history; a vigorous diagnostic evaluation should be pursued.

Common Questions and Answers

Q: Will my child have another stroke?
A: Anecdotal evidence suggests that children with no identifiable underlying basis for stroke do not have recurrence. Otherwise, the chance of recurrence depends on remediation of the underlying cause.

Q: Aren't there any medicines for acute stroke?
A: Tissue plasminogen activator (TPA) appears to be useful in some cases of adult nonhemorrhagic stroke, but its usefulness in childhood stroke has not been studied.

ICD-9-CM 436

BIBLIOGRAPHY

Isaels SJ, Seshia SS. Childhood stroke associated with protein C or S deficiency. *J Pediatr* 1987;3:562–564.

Kirkham FJ. Recognition and prevention of neurological complications in pediatric cardiac surgery. *Pediatr Cardiol* 1998;19(4):331–345.

Kittner SJ, Adams RJ. Stroke in children and young adults. *Curr Opin Neurol* 1996;9(1):53–56.

Natowicz M, Kelley RI. Mendelian etiologies of stroke. *Ann Neurol* 1987;22:175–192.

Rivkin MJ, Volpe JJ. Strokes in children. *Pediatr Rev* 1996;17(8):265–278.

Author: Peter M. Bingham

Stuttering

Database

DEFINITION

Stuttering is a speech disability characterized by *abnormal dysfluency* with involuntary: repetitions of sounds, syllables, and words; prolongations; blocks; loss of control; interjections; incomplete words or phrases; revisions; word avoidance and/or substitution; tension; grimacing; loss of eye contact; and/or speech avoidance. Almost all fluent speakers have occasional dysfluencies, but without the global involvement noted in those who stutter, and occurring relatively infrequently during speech production.

PATHOPHYSIOLOGY

- Speech and language production involves a complex series of neural interactions, and precise coordination of over 100 muscles to produce speech.
- During speech production, those who stutter have neural pathways that differ from those of individuals who do not stutter (fluent individuals). Using positron-emission tomography (PET) scans, stutterers were found to have increased dopamine activity in brain regions that modulate verbalization (ventral limbic, cortical, and subcortical). Also, stutterers showed differences in glucose metabolism in Broca's area, Wernicke's area, and frontal pole areas. Metabolic differences were noted in the lower left caudate area in stutterers as well. In addition, there are apparent structural differences noted on PET scans, with right cerebral dominance, and deactivation of a left frontal and left cortex circuit felt to be involved in verbal fluency. Neurotransmitters are altered in some; certain psychopharmacologic agents (e.g., tricyclic antidepressants, phenothiazines, clozapine, selective serotonin reuptake inhibitors) can inadvertently induce stuttering in fluent individuals, and may paradoxically reduce stuttering in those who stutter (e.g., clomipramine).
- Stuttering has been described as a "central auditory processing disorder," which is an inability to differentiate, recognize, or understand sounds in individuals with normal hearing and intelligence.
- Emotional and psychological mechanisms have been implicated as well. Feelings of distress and emotional unease have no apparent contribution to the central nervous system components of stuttering, but it is well known that these feelings can contribute to increased stuttered speech.

GENETICS

- Stuttering is known to be familial, inferring a genetic or structural defect in one or more areas of the central nervous system responsible for speech and language organization and production.
- First-degree relatives of stutterers have a higher incidence of stuttering than do second- and third-degree relatives.
- Monozygotic twins have a higher incidence than do dizygotic twins. Adoption studies have demonstrated higher incidence if a biologic parent stuttered.
- Genetic studies have not clarified the exact mode of transmission, but the genetic contribution is clear.

EPIDEMIOLOGY

- Occurs in 1% to 2% of the population
- Occurs in all cultures and in all languages
- May begin as early as 2 years of age, with the majority having onset by the end of the first decade
- Male : female ratio of 3:1
- Resolves spontaneously in females more than in males

COMPLICATIONS

- Emotional distress: Those with only mild dysfluency may have emotional reactions to their stuttering far out of proportion, and this aspect may become their greatest disability.
- Social withdrawal
- Behavioral, affective, and cognitive reactions: may impact the individual more significantly than the speech disability itself. Speech avoidance and word substitutions may give the impression that the individual with stuttering is functioning at a lower intellectual level than his or her peers. Future life choices and employment may be adversely affected.

PROGNOSIS

- Spontaneous resolution in 80%.
- With appropriate speech therapy, many individuals learn to control their stuttering, or their own reactions to their stuttering.
- Some who have had appropriate speech therapy may continue to have dysfluencies, but may be able to avoid the emotional burden of their dysfluent speech in their social milieu.
- Delaying diagnosis and treatment until the child is older allows behavioral and emotional patterns to become more ingrained, with more potential disability.

Differential Diagnosis

- Developmental dysfluency

—Characterized by lack of awareness and reaction; usually occurs at 2.5 to 3.0 years of age
—Resolves spontaneously
—Sound and syllable repetitions are infrequent, but word and phrase repetitions are more common, as are substitutions.

- Cluttering

—Rapid irregular speech, which impedes intelligibility

- Spasmodic dysphonia

—Voice disorder, characterized by momentary disruption of voice caused by involuntary movements of one or more muscles of the larynx
—Usually occurs in adults

- Neurogenic stuttering

—May occur after an injury to the central nervous system, such as a stroke or serious head injury

- Tourette syndrome

—May be confused with stuttering

- Medication-induced stuttering

—May result from tricyclic antidepressants, phenothiazines, clozapine, and selective serotonin reuptake inhibitors (SSRIs)

Data Gathering

HISTORY

- Ask about the age of onset.
- Inquire into family history.
- Ask about distress with blockages and avoidance of speech.
- Ask when stuttering occurs. Stuttering usually disappears when singing, and diminishes when in a quiet, private setting and when talking alone or to pets.
- Determine if any medications may be contributing to the stuttering.
- Ask about neurologic injuries.

Physical Examination

There are no specific physical findings associated with stuttering.

- When evaluating a patient who may be stuttering, one should note what their speech sounds like most of the time.
- Tension and grimacing may be noted when speaking.
- Many children avoid speaking altogether. Some children will avoid the words and sounds that they know cause them difficulty.
- A subtle finding is use of interjections ("um," "uh"), although this may be observed in developmental dysfluency as well.
- Some will speak very slowly and in a monotone or altered speech pattern, which, to a trained speech-language pathologist, may be indicative of stuttering.
- Observation of speech may be unreliable. Review of audio or video recordings may be most helpful. Stuttering is characterized by occurrence on the initial sound or syllable, the first word of a sentence, longer words, less frequently used words, transitions from voiceless to voiced sounds, consonants more so than vowels, and content words more so than function words.
- Stuttering may be noted to be increased by talking on the telephone, saying one's name, telling jokes, time pressure, public speaking.

Laboratory Aids

There are no known laboratory tests for stuttering.

Therapy

- Evaluation and speech therapy by a speech-language pathologist knowledgeable about stuttering is necessary. Referrals for evaluation and/or therapy should be made when dysfluent speech is noted or reported, there is distress about speaking, and parental concern is expressed.
- Those who stutter have altered responses to auditory feedback of their speech, a finding that has been employed in assistive devices to eliminate stuttered speech.
- Additionally, other modalities that create diversionary central nervous system stimulation during speech production may also help eliminate stuttering to some degree.
- There are no medications that have been found to be therapeutic.
- Acupuncture, stress reduction and relaxation techniques, and hypnosis have been attempted in small studies in adults. Efficacy of these modalities is difficult to determine because spontaneous resolution occurs in a large number of stutterers.

Follow-Up

The duration and mode of speech therapy will vary with each individual. It is reasonable to expect improved speech and psychological well-being with appropriate speech therapy.

PREVENTION

Although it was once felt that inappropriate responses to developmental dysfluencies caused dysfluent speech to persist, recent evidence looking at neural involvement and genetic influences makes this seem less likely.

PITFALLS

- Missed diagnosis
- Inappropriate and/or delayed therapy

Common Questions and Answers

Q: When should a child be referred for evaluation and therapy if he or she exhibits only mild or intermittent stuttering?
A: Physicians and members of the health care team must be aware of the nature of stuttering and the natural history of the disability. The extent of the stuttering *does not* correlate with the child's emotional reaction to his or her speech disability. The focus of therapy, in addition to maximizing fluent speech, must also be to ensure the child's emotional well-being and positive self-image.

Q: What is the expected duration of speech therapy?
A: It is variable. Some individuals require only a relatively short-term course, while others require years of therapy.

Q: When should children with stuttering be referred for diagnostic PET scans?
A: The multifactorial nature of stuttering, and speech production in general, make PET and other scans useful only for research purposes at this time.

ICD-9-CM 307.0

BIBLIOGRAPHY

Ambrose N, Cox N, Yairi E. The genetic basis of persistence and recovery in stuttering. *J Speech Hear Res* 1997;40:567–580.

Brady JP. Drug-induced stuttering: a review of the literature. *J Clin Psychopharmacol* 1998;18:50–54.

Braun AR, Varga M, Stager S, et al. Altered patterns of cerebral activity during speech and language production in developmental stuttering. An $H_2(15)0$ positron emission tomography study. *Brain* 1997;120:761–784.

Fox PT, Ingham RJ, Ingham JC, et al. A PET study of the neural systems of stuttering. *Nature* 1996;382:158–162.

Perkins WH, Kent RD, Curlee RF. A theory of the neuropsycholinguistic functioning in stuttering. *J Speech Hear Res* 1991;34:734–752.

Wexler KB. Stuttering in children and adolescents. Part I. *Emerg Office Pediatr* 1996;9:73–76.

Wexler KB. Stuttering in children and adolescents. Part II: evaluation. *Emerg Office Pediatr* 1996;9:147–150.

Author: Steven C. Shapiro

Subdural Hematoma

 Database

DEFINITION

A subdural hematoma (SDH) is a collection of blood between outer pial and inner dural meningeal layers. The bleeding is usually venous in origin, although either cortical arteries or bridging veins may be torn.

PATHOPHYSIOLOGY

- SDHs may be acute or chronic. Arterial SDHs present quickly, whereas venous SDHs may accumulate slowly, not detected for weeks or months. Acute SDHs contain blood, whereas chronic SDHs contain proteinaceous exudate and blood-breakdown products.
- Significant force usually required for SDH unless there are predisposing circumstances; an SDH is only rarely due to trivial or minor trauma. However, SDH can occur with relatively minor trauma in individuals with bleeding disorders, children on chronic dialysis, and those with enlarged extracerebral spaces (cortical atrophy).
- SDHs in nonaccidental trauma may be due to the striking of the infant's head against a surface (like a mattress). The sudden deceleration associated with the impact may tear bridging veins traveling in the subdural space. The term *shaking-impact syndrome* may be more accurate than *shaken-baby syndrome*.

GENETICS

There is no clear genetic predisposition, except when hereditary coagulopathy is implicated.

EPIDEMIOLOGY

- SDHs occur in all age groups. Neonatal SDHs occur with spontaneous deliveries, but may be more frequent following deliveries with forceps or vacuum extraction.
- SDHs in infants and young children are frequently the result of nonaccidental trauma. Risk factors for nonaccidental trauma include disability or prematurity of the child, unstable family situations, parents of young age, and low socioeconomic status. One study found that fathers were the most frequent perpetrators, followed by boyfriends, female babysitters, and mothers, in descending order of frequency.
- SDHs in older children are often the result of motor vehicle accidents, and may be associated with other intracranial injuries, such as diffuse axonal injury.

COMPLICATIONS

- Traumatic SDHs are often associated with cerebral contusions. Other associated injuries include skull fractures, diffuse axonal injury, and penetrating injuries.
- SDHs may result in mass effect, focal neurologic signs, and coma.
- Increased intracranial pressure (ICP) and seizures are other serious complications.

PROGNOSIS

In general, long-term outcome is related to the condition of the child at time of presentation. Prolonged ICP or significant cerebral edema before treatment is worrisome.

 Differential Diagnosis

- SDHs are almost always traumatic, but separating accidental from nonaccidental trauma may be difficult. Falls in infants may cause linear skull fractures, rarely SDHs.
- Epidural hematomas, subarachnoid hemorrhages, and acute SDHs cannot be distinguished clinically. The lucid interval sometimes seen with epidural hematomas in adults is not a reliable sign. A head CT should differentiate.

 Data Gathering

HISTORY

- Newborn: SDHs due to birth trauma may present with lethargy, pallor, poor feeding, apnea, and seizures.
- Infants and young children: SDHs may also present with a nonspecific history of lethargy, irritability, vomiting, poor feeding, apnea, and seizures.
- Older children present with a history of trauma and alteration of consciousness.
- Chronic SDHs present with nonspecific signs, such as vomiting, irritability, failure to thrive, anemia, and seizures.

 Physical Examination

- Newborns may present with decreased responsiveness, a bulging fontanelle, hypotonia, or hypertonia. Retinal hemorrhages are not specific at this age, because they are seen in up to 40% of newborns following a vaginal delivery.
- Infants and young children may also present with nonspecific physical signs, but focal neurologic signs may be present. Retinal hemorrhages are most often associated with nonaccidental trauma, but they have been reported after accidental trauma leading to SDH. Bilateral retinal hemorrhages with retinal folds or detachments are particularly associated with nonaccidental trauma.
- Other signs of child abuse include burns, lacerations, and bruises in various stages of healing, and belt marks, choke marks, and multiple fractures of different ages.
- Older children present with signs of external head trauma, decreased responsiveness, and focal neurologic signs.

 Laboratory Aids

TESTS

Imaging

- CT scan is the imaging study of choice in acute head trauma with neurologic signs. SDH appears as an extraaxial area of increased density, crescentic in shape, and often associated with cerebral contusion or mass effect. CT also may show evidence of cerebral edema, with loss of gray matter/white matter differentiation and small ventricles.
- Subacute SDHs may be difficult to distinguish from adjacent gray matter on CT scan; loss of gray/white matter differentiation is helpful. Chronic SDHs appear as areas of low density on CT scan, often bilateral.
- MRI is helpful to clarify subacute and chronic SDHs and to identify small SDHs missed by CT.
- If child abuse is suspected, a skeletal survey or bone scan is useful to look for fractures of different ages.
- Incidental SDH is frequently found on neuroimaging studies in newborns; frequently no intervention is required other than close follow-up.

Therapy

- The treatment of choice for large, acute SDHs is surgical evacuation. Smaller SDHs may be managed conservatively, with careful monitoring for signs of neurologic deterioration.
- While awaiting surgery, attention to airway, breathing, and circulation (ABCs) is critical. Tracheal intubation should be performed if the child's Glasgow coma score is less than 8 or if airway protective reflexes are impaired.
- Isotonic fluids should be given, because hypotonic fluids may worsen cerebral edema.
- Measures to control ICP include elevating the head of the bed 30% to promote venous drainage, hyperventilation to a PCO_2 of 25 to 30 torr, and osmotic therapy with mannitol or furosemide. The efficacy of these measures in improving long-term outcome following large SDHs has not been established.
- Seizures should be treated promptly. Phenytoin is the drug of choice, with phenobarbital as a second option. Prophylactic phenytoin given for a few weeks is effective in reducing early posttraumatic seizures but does not affect long-term risk of epilepsy.
- Treatment of chronic SDHs is more controversial. If there are no signs of ICP, conservative treatment is reasonable, and most collections will resolve. Subdural taps are indicated if ICP rises. If taps are not successful, a subdural-peritoneal shunt may be placed.

 Follow-Up

- Neurologic sequelae of SDHs are more severe than epidural hematomas because of associated cerebral contusions.
- In general, long-term outcome is related to the condition of the child at the time of surgical evacuation of the hematoma. Prolonged ICP or significant cerebral edema before surgery indicates a poor prognosis.
- Children generally have a better outcome from head injury than do adults, but children less than 7 years old often do worse than older children, especially if the SDH is the result of nonaccidental trauma.
- Long-term problems include headache, seizures, hydrocephalus, vertigo, difficulty concentrating, poor school performance, fixed neurologic deficits, and neurobehavioral problems.
- Epilepsy eventually develops in approximately 10% to 15% of patients after severe head injury. This risk generally does not warrant the use of long-term prophylactic anticonvulsants.
- Children with neurologic sequelae from head injury may benefit from admission to a rehabilitation hospital.
- Social work services should be consulted in cases of known or suspected child abuse.

PREVENTION

- Parents should be counseled about appropriate methods to channel frustration and anger with infants and children. Shaking an infant when the parent is angry is never appropriate.
- Bicycle helmets, car seats, and seat belts are all valuable in preventing head injuries in children.

PITFALLS

- Be suspicious if the stated history does not fit with the pattern or severity of the injury. Physicians and other health care professionals with experience in child abuse should be consulted early if abuse is suspected.
- Chronic SDHs must be differentiated from benign external hydrocephalus, a self-limited condition characterized by increasing head size and low-density extraaxial fluid collections. MRI can differentiate benign external hydrocephalus.

 Common Questions and Answers

Q: When did the bleed occur?
A: With chronic SDHs, the time and type of injury may be difficult to establish, since no trauma may be reported and the trauma may have occurred weeks or months before. Neuroimaging can give some indication of the injury's timing.

Q: What limitations should be imposed after an acute SDH?
A: Because SDH may recur with minor trauma, it is prudent to avoid any activities that have significant risk of fall or a blow to the head.

Q: Why are anticonvulsants not used to prevent seizures following SDHs?
A: Seizure medications may be given for a few weeks to present early seizures following a SDH. After a few weeks, the risks and side effects of the medications outweigh the risk of developing seizures. If seizures begin at a time remote to the injury, then seizure medications can be re-started.

Q: My baby twisted out of my arms, fell head-first onto a tile floor, and suffered a head injury. Will I be reported for child abuse?
A: Not if the injuries fit with the stated history. In this case, the most likely injury would be a linear skull fracture. If more serious intracranial injuries do occur, they will probably not be associated with retinal hemorrhages or other injuries, such as older fractures in multiple stages of healing.

ICD-9-CM 852.2

BIBLIOGRAPHY

Duhaime AC, Christian CW, Rorke LB, Zimmerman RA. Nonaccidental head injury in infants—the "shaken-baby syndrome." *N Engl J Med* 1998;338:1822–1829.

Goldstein B, Powers KS. Head trauma in children. *Pediatr Rev* 1994;15:213–219.

Haviland J, Russell RI. Outcome after severe non-accidental head injury. *Arch Dis Child* 1997;77:504–507.

Johnston MV, Gerring JP. Head trauma and its sequelae. *Pediatr Ann* 1992;21:362–368.

Perrin RG, Rutka JT, Drake JM, et al. Management and outcomes of posterior fossa subdural hematomas in neonates. *Neurosurgery* 1997; 40:1190–1199.

Wissow LS. Child abuse and neglect. *N Engl J Med* 1995;332:1425–1431.

Author: Dennis J. Dlugos

Sudden Infant Death Syndrome

 ## Database

DEFINITION

Sudden infant death syndrome (SIDS) is sudden and unexpected death of an infant (<1 year old) that remains unexplained after a complete postmortem investigation, including autopsy, death scene evaluation, and review of the case history. Associated problems:

- Acute life-threatening event (ALTE)
- Poverty
- Low birth weight; small for gestational age (SGA)
- Prematurity
- Maternal smoking
- Maternal substance abuse

PATHOPHYSIOLOGY

- Unknown
- There are multiple theories, including central apnea, upper airway obstruction, and cardiac arrhythmias; metabolic diseases such as glycogen storage disease and medium-chain acyl-CoA dehydrogenase deficiency; and environmental factors such as hyperthermia, unsafe bedding, and prone sleeping position. Each attempts to explain SIDS, although none can adequately explain all SIDS deaths.
- "Negative" autopsy
- May see punctate petechial hemorrhages

EPIDEMIOLOGY

- Five thousand deaths per year in the United States
- 1.4 cases per 1,000 live births
- Ninety percent of cases occur before 6 months of age.
- Peak incidence: age 2 to 4 months

 ## Differential Diagnosis

- Infection
—Sepsis (bacterial, viral)
—Pneumonia
—Bronchiolitis
—Myocarditis
- Environmental
—Accidental asphyxiation
—Hyperthermia
—Hypothermia
—Toxins
—Poisonings
- Trauma
—Child abuse, including nonaccidental suffocation
—Drowning
- Metabolic
—Medium-chain acyl-CoA dehydrogenase (MCAD) deficiency
—Long-chain acyl-CoA dehydrogenase deficiency
—Pyruvate carboxylase deficiency
—Phosphoenolpyruvate carboxykinase deficiency
—Defects in glycogenolysis
—Defects in pyruvate oxidation
—Defects in oxidative phosphorylation
—Biotinidase deficiency
—3-hydroxy-3-methylglutaric aciduria
—Urea cycle defects
—Lactic acidemias
—Aminoacidopathies
—Glycogen storage disease
- Congenital
—Congenital heart disease
- Miscellaneous
—Adrenal insufficiency
—Arrhythmias

Data Gathering

HISTORY

- Previously healthy infant, with or without recent upper respiratory tract infection
- Found dead after a nap or in the morning
- No struggle or crying heard

Special Questions

- Have there been previous infant or child deaths in the family? It is unusual to have more than one SIDS death in a family. When multiple SIDS deaths occur in a family, the possibility of sequential homicide needs to be considered.
- When was the last time the baby was seen alive?
- Where was the baby found?
- In what position was the baby found?
- What was the child wearing?
- Were there blankets, stuffed toys, or bumpers at the baby's head?
- Were there any recent illnesses?
- What is the prenatal history?
- Is there a history of previous maternal miscarriages?
- What is the date of the last immunizations?
- Have there been prior medical problems?
- Is there a history of apnea?

 ## Physical Examination

- Postmortem lividity
- Pink, frothy discharge at nose and mouth
- Look for signs of injury.
- Check for dysmorphic features.

Laboratory Aids

A full autopsy must be done on all infants who die suddenly and unexpectedly.

IMAGING

A postmortem skeletal survey is indicated if there is suspicion of abuse.

 ## Therapy

Resuscitation is almost always initiated before receiving the baby at the hospital. If rigor mortis or lividity is present, resuscitation efforts should not be initiated.

 ## Follow-Up

- The medical examiner or coroner's office should be notified of all "SIDS" deaths. Remember, it's not officially SIDS until the autopsy has been completed.
- Provide support to the family.
- Refer to a SIDS center.

PITFALLS

- Not completing full postmortem examination, including autopsy, death scene review, and careful review of case and family history

PREVENTION

- Avoid a prone sleeping position for young, healthy infants.
- Provide a safe sleeping environment.
- Use apnea monitors for infants with ALTE. These monitors, although widely used, have not been shown to decrease mortality related to SIDS.

 ## Common Questions and Answers

Q: Do all infants who die suddenly and unexpectly require an autopsy?
A: Yes, it is estimated that autopsy reveals a cause of death in approximately 15% of "SIDS" deaths. The diagnosis of SIDS cannot be made without an autopsy!

Q: Does SIDS run in families?
A: Recurrence rates in families in which a sibling has died of SIDS vary greatly among studies, but large, controlled studies indicate no increased risk of SIDS in subsequent siblings. In families with recurrent SIDS death, especially after the third infant death, the possibility of serial homicide needs to be investigated.

Q: How can you tell the difference between SIDS and intentional suffocation?
A: Because the physical findings of an autopsy cannot distinguish between SIDS and intentional suffocation, other factors related to the death must be considered when attempting to distinguish the two. In comparing the features of suffocated children with the clinical features associated with SIDS, Meadow makes the following comparisons:

- The percent of suffocated children with previous apnea is approximately 90%, compared with less than 10% of SIDS infants.
- Forty-four percent of the suffocated children had a previously unexplained medical problem, whereas greater than 95% of SIDS infants were previously healthy.
- Fifty-five percent of suffocated children were older than 6 months at the time of diagnosis.
- Forty-eight percent of suffocated children had a sibling who had died, compared with 2% of SIDS deaths.

—Although these important differences may identify some children who are intentionally suffocated, differentiating fatal abuse by suffocation from SIDS is difficult.

ICD-9-CM 789.0

BIBLIOGRAPHY

American Academy of Pediatrics Task Force on Infant Positioning and SIDS. Positioning and SIDS. *Pediatrics* 1992;89:1120–1126.

Carolan PL, Moore JR, Luxenberg MG. Infant sleep position and the sudden infant death syndrome. A survey of pediatric recommendations. *Clin Pediatr* 1995;34(8):402–409.

Gilbert-Barness E, Barness L. Sudden infant death: a reappraisal. *Contemp Pediatr* 1995;12:88–107.

Keens TG, Davidson Ward SL. Apnea spells, sudden death and the role of the apnea monitor. *Pediatr Clin North Am* 1993;40:897–911.

Kohlendorfer U, Kiechl S, Sperl W. Sudden infant death syndrome: risk factor profiles for distinct subgroups. *Am J Epidemiol* 1998;147 (10):960–968.

Meadow R. Suffocation, recurrent apnea, and sudden infant death. *J Pediatr* 1990;117(3):351–357.

Peterson DR, Sabotta EE, Daling JR. Infant mortality among subsequent siblings of infants who died of sudden infant death syndrome. *J Pediatr* 1986;108:911–914.

Reece RM. Fatal child abuse and sudden infant death syndrome: a critical diagnostic decision. *Pediatrics* 1994;91:423–429.

Southall DP, Plunkett MC, Banks MW, Falkov AF, Samuels MP. Covert video recordings of life-threatening child abuse: lessons for child protection. *Pediatrics* 1997;100:735–760.

Author: Cindy W. Christian

Suicide

 ## Database

DEFINITION

Suicide is an intentional self-harming act that is meant to end life. Attempted suicide occurs when the act does not succeed, resulting in a failed (or near) suicide.

ETIOLOGY

Suicide attempts result from the interaction of a number of long-standing conditions and acute stressors:

- Mental illness (diagnosable disorder), often with psychological comorbidity (e.g., depressive disorder with personality disorder or substance use)
- Intense emotional state (e.g., hopelessness, acute interpersonal loss, conflict with parent)
- Social isolation or antisocial behavior
- Central serotonin abnormality
- A major risk factor for attempting suicide is a history of prior attempt.

PATHOPHYSIOLOGY

- A central serotonin abnormality may result in aggressive or impulsive behaviors. In suicidal patients, aggression is turned toward the self.
- An underlying psychiatric disorder, such as depression, is acutely worsened by a stressful life event.
- Feelings of isolation and lack of external support (particularly from caregivers) result in hopelessness and despair.
- Suicide may be an impulsive act designed to punish loved ones or as an act of rage.

GENETICS

- A family cluster of suicide is a risk factor for suicide. To what extent this is due to genetic factors or to behavioral influences is unknown.
- There are genetic components to depressive and many other psychiatric disorders, alcoholism, and central serotonin abnormalities.

EPIDEMIOLOGY

- Suicide is the third leading source of mortality for 15- to 24-year-olds.
- The greatest increases are occurring in African American and Caucasian teen-agers.
- Peak incidence occurs at age 20 years.
- Thirty-two deaths per 100,000 persons per year
- There are an estimated 50 to 200 attempts for every completed suicide.
- As many as 9% of young teens have reported suicidal ideation.
- Females *attempt* suicide at a rate three times that of males. Females are most likely to attempt suicide through ingestion. Many ingestions go unreported and are used as suicide "gestures."
- Males *complete* suicide at a rate three times that of females. Males are most likely to use the more lethal methods of firearm (rural) or hanging (urban) in attempting suicide.

COMPLICATIONS

- Long-term organ damage or physical disability, depending on the method used
- Long-lasting emotional scars in families of victims, resulting from frustration, anger, and guilt

PROGNOSIS

- Twenty percent to 50% of those attempting suicide will make a repeat attempt.
- Psychiatric hospitalization has not been shown to decrease risk of attempted suicide in patients with a history of mood disorder and substance abuse.

 ## Differential Diagnosis

- Central nervous system

—Brain tumors can result in disinhibitory behaviors.

- Psychiatric disorders

—Depression
—Attention deficit disorder, resulting in impulsive behaviors
—Emotional or physical abuse, with the suicide attempt being a way to gain attention, help, or a means of escape

 ## Data Gathering

HISTORY

- Patients and their families should be oriented to the evaluation process.
- Communication should be nonjudgmental and supportive.
- The provider should sensitively ascertain if the patient has a weapon or other method of self-harm.

A comprehensive history should always be obtained or reviewed by a trained mental health worker. Components of a comprehensive history include:

- Method
- Lethality of attempt (e.g., number of pills, seriousness of physical injury)
- Circumstances of attempt (e.g., remote site, public display)
- History of prior attempts
- Level of planning of attempt
- Current affect and psychological status (e.g., feelings and/or level of depression, hopelessness, impulsivity, self-esteem, etc.)
- Family consistency and dynamics
- Pharmaceuticals available at home, what is missing
- History of interpersonal conflict or personal loss
- Family history of suicide
- History of substance use
- History of psychological disorder or disease state
- History of abuse, neglect, or incest
- Social supports and coping strategies
- Willingness to make safety contract

The following historical information increases the risk for future, potentially lethal suicide attempt:

- History of potentially lethal attempt
- History of planned attempt versus impulsive attempt
- Family history of suicide or attempted suicide
- Unstable family structure
- Poor social support system, nonconnectedness

 ## Physical Examination

- Physical signs or sequelae of prior attempts
- Adolescents do not have to have the classic findings of depressed adults.
- Even without a history of ingestion, closely observe vital signs, skin, mucous membranes, and pupils for evidence of toxidrome.
- Examine the skin for signs of physical abuse or self-mutilatory behavior.
- If indicated or suspected, examine the genitalia for signs of sexual abuse.
- A complete neurologic examination is essential for the evaluation of intracranial processes, depression, and ingestions.

Laboratory Aids

TESTS

Specific Tests

- Serum and urine toxicology screens
- Urine pregnancy test, both to assess as precipitating factor and to recognize potential damage to fetus
- Acetaminophen level, as it is highly hepatotoxic and used frequently by teen-agers as a "cry for help" because of its perceived safety
- Other laboratory tests will depend on the history of method of attempt (e.g., trauma labs, metabolic screens, etc.).
- Electrocardiograms are indicated for many ingestions, including antidepressants.

Imaging

- Abdominal plain film, if history of iron or vitamin ingestion, or if severe trauma
- Other imaging studies may be indicated, depending on method of attempt.

Therapy

EMERGENCY CARE

- Trauma response as indicated
- Monitoring, both behavior and vital signs if history of ingestion
- Decontamination of GI tract and circulation as indicated (e.g., gastric lavage and/or charcoal if recent ingestion, dialysis)
- When available, a Poison Control Center can be very helpful with evaluation and treatment of most drug ingestions.
- Immediate physical protection (remove all weapons) and around-the-clock observation
- After medical evaluation and stabilization, the need for psychiatric hospitalization or outpatient follow-up can be assessed.

Psychiatric disposition should be determined by, or in conjunction with, a mental health professional. Considerations for admission include:

- Historical factors indicating high risk for repeat attempt (see Data Gathering)
- Suicidal ideation with a plan
- Male sex (increased risk of completing suicide)
- Family stability and support
- Current mental status
- Availability of alternative interventions (e.g., intensive psychiatric follow-up, day treatment program)
- Availability of insurance benefits

When discharge to a caregiver is being considered, the following minimal criteria should be in place at the time of discharge:

- The patient is not immediately suicidal.

- The patient is medically stable.
- The patient and parents agree to contact a health professional or go to the emergency department if suicidal intent recurs. The patient and family must have 24-hour access to mental health or physical health professionals.
- The patient must not have impaired mental status (e.g., severely depressed, psychoses, delirium, intoxication, etc.)
- Lethal methods of self-harm are not immediately available to the patient (e.g., guns, dangerous pharmaceuticals)
- Follow-up and treatment of underlying psychological disorders have been arranged. This should involve more than providing a phone number to psychiatric services.
- Acute precipitants and crises have been addressed.
- There is nothing to indicate to the provider that the patient and family will be non-compliant.
- Caregivers and patient are in agreement with the discharge plan.
- Insurance approval has been assured for follow-up treatment.

DRUGS

- Medications that reverse toxidromes may be indicated (flumazenil, naloxone)
- Charcoal for recent ingestions
- Tricyclic antidepressants do not exhibit the same efficacy in children and adolescents that they do in adults. Additionally, they may take a week or longer to work.
- Selective serotonin reuptake inhibitors have been shown to be effective in treating mild depressive disorders in adolescence and are much less toxic than TCAs.
- Other psychotropic medicines may be used in the acute setting for sedation or psychoses.

Follow-Up

Long-term therapy is often needed for adolescents who attempt suicide. Therefore, improvement may be slow and punctuated by frequent setbacks.

SIGNS TO WATCH FOR

- Acute life stressors
- Failure to comply with therapy or follow-up
- A sudden sense of calm or resolution may occur when a patient has decided to end life.

PREVENTION

A routine screening of all adolescents for suicide should occur and include the following:

- Change in level of functioning in school, work, or home
- Changes in mood or affect

- Direct inquiry about suicidal ideation and plans
- Exploration and discussion of coping strategies
- Discussion of social support

PITFALLS

- Adolescents often present to medical personnel before attempting suicide. The practitioner should be particularly aware of constitutional or vague complaints.
- Management must always occur in conjunction with a mental health professional.
- Minimizing attempts as "not serious" or as "just seeking attention" by parents or professionals will have serious consequences.
- Different laboratories offer different spectra and sensitivities in their toxicology screens. Providers must be familiar with what their laboratories routinely test and whether additional studies are indicated.

Common Questions and Answers

Q: Maintaining confidentiality is one of the most important aspects of the provider-patient relationship. Do I keep suicide attempts or plans confidential?
A: No. The limits of confidentiality should be clearly outlined to patients and families at the first visit or early in the patient's adolescence. These limits include anything that will directly place the patient's life in danger, such as suicidal plans, abuse, or homicidal intentions.

Q: If I directly question my patient about suicide, won't that put the idea in his or her head?
A: No. In most cases, patients will be relieved by having a professional who wants to talk about it. There is only risk in asking if nothing is done with the answer. Appropriate referral to mental health services or counseling will save your patients' lives.

ICD-9-CM 300.9

BIBLIOGRAPHY

Center for Disease Control. Suicide among children, adolescents, and young adults—United States, 1980-92. *MMWR* 1995;44:289–291.

Greenhill LL, Waslick B. Management of suicidal behavior in children and adolescents. *Psychiatr Clin North Am* 1997;20:641–665.

Press BR, Khan SA. Management of the suicidal child or adolescent in the emergency department. *Curr Opin Pediatr* 1997;9:237–241.

Authors: Jonathan R. Pletcher and Kenneth R. Ginsburg

Superior Mesenteric Artery Syndrome

 Database

DEFINITION

Superior mesenteric artery (SMA) syndrome is obstruction of the distal duodenum by the superior mesenteric artery or its branches.

CAUSES

• The mesenteric artery forms an acute downward aortomesenteric angle as it leaves the aorta. The duodenum lies within this angle and in some individuals can be compressed by the SMA anteriorly and the vertebra posteriorly, leading to symptoms of obstruction.
• Some of the conditions that predispose to narrowing of this angle are:

—Increase in lordosis of the back, as immobilization by body cast, scoliosis surgery, prolonged bed rest in a supine position
—Rapid growth in children
—Weight loss resulting in loss of mesenteric fat
—Variations of the ligament of Treitz. A short ligament lifts the third or fourth part of the duodenum into the narrower segment in the aortomesenteric angle.

PROGNOSIS

Most patients improve without need for surgery and are asymptomatic on follow-up.

 Differential Diagnosis

• Anorexia nervosa/bulimia/hysterical
• Luminal obstruction: foreign body
• Intramural obstruction: duplication cyst, web, tumor, and stricture
• Extramural obstruction: tumor, annular pancreas, bands, adhesions, volvulus, and intussusception
• Dysmotility disorder, which can be due to an intrinsic neuronal disorder, muscular weakness (holovisceral myopathy), or fibrosis (scleroderma, retroperitoneal fibrosis)

 Data Gathering

HISTORY

• Vomiting (bilious and nonbilious), nausea, postprandial nausea and vomiting, weight loss, early satiety, dehydration, bloating, abdominal pain, and failure to thrive
• The symptoms are chronic and acute, and most patients have vague abdominal pain from 18 months to 10 years in duration.
• None of the symptoms or signs for SMA syndrome are pathognomonic, but a history of weight loss, immobilization, or back surgery followed by symptoms of early satiety, bloating, and vomiting after meals would suggest the diagnosis.

 Physical Examination

• Abdominal pain
• Increased bowel gas
• Dehydration in some cases

Laboratory Aids

TESTS

Imaging

• A plain abdominal radiograph could show gas predominantly in a distended stomach with a dilated proximal duodenum with a sharp cutoff at the level where the SMA crosses the duodenum.
• An upper contrast radiography would demonstrate passage of contrast when the patient is maneuvered into a prone position, which increases the aortomesenteric angle by gravity.
• A determination of the aortomesenteric angle in severe cases may help in decision making when surgery is contemplated. In normal patients, this angle has a range of 45% to 60%, whereas in patients with SMA syndrome, it is reported to be between 10% and 22%.

 Therapy

• Refeeding to gain weight. Feeding in a prone position may help, but if this fails, a jejunal tube bypassing the obstruction or a period of parenteral feeding can be used.
• Frequent repositioning of patients in body cast
• A decrease in viscosity in feeds has a theoretical advantage.
• Reversal of back surgery may be necessary in some patients.
• Bypass surgery is unnecessary in most cases. Refractory cases in which duodenojejunostomy or derotation surgery has been tried are associated with very good results. The latter surgery consists of dividing the ligament of Treitz and the whole small intestine is passed beneath the SMA and lies in the right abdomen; the colon is separated from the retroperitoneal attachments and placed in the left abdomen.

 Common Questions and Answers

Q: When the diagnosis of SMA syndrome is suspected, what sequence do you follow?
A: The logical sequence is to see if the patient improves with refeeding and mobilization first, followed by an imaging study, such as an upper GI contrast study. CT does not improve diagnosis, and aortomesenteric angle study is almost never required.

Q: The following treatment modalities are known to be useful in treatment of SMA syndrome. Do nothing, feed with a jejunal tube, a liquid diet, prone feeding, and TPN. Which program works?
A: All of the above have been used in SMA syndrome. There is a probability that some patients have a functional disorder and do not require any of these feeding modalities. Weight gain has also been accomplished with total parenteral nutrition.

ICD-9-CM 557.1

BIBLIOGRAPHY

Atkin JT, Skandalakis JE, Gray S. The anatomic basis of vascular compression of the duodenum. *Surg Clin North Am* 1974;54:1361–1370.

Gustafsson L. Diagnosis and treatment of superior mesenteric syndrome. *Br J Surg* 1984;71: 499–501.

Marchant EA, Alvear DT, Fagelman KM. True clinical entity of vascular compression of the duodenum in adolescence. *Surg Gynecol Obstet* 1989;168:381–386.

Author: Andrew E. Mulberg

Supraventricular Tachycardia

 Database

DEFINITION

Supraventricular tachycardia (SVT) is a rapid and regular narrow complex tachycardia originating at or above the AV node. The heart rates in infants range from 220 to 320 beats/min and in older children may be slower (150–250 beats/min).

- Fifty percent of cases are idiopathic and occur in young infants and children.
- Twenty percent of cases have associated conditions such as postcardiac surgery, infection, fever, or drug exposure (i.e., cold medications).
- Ten percent to 20% of cases have Wolff-Parkinson-White (WPW) syndrome, which may be associated with congenital heart disease (Ebstein anomaly, single ventricle L-TGA) or cardiomyopathy.

PATHOPHYSIOLOGY

There are three different mechanisms for SVT:

- Reentry tachycardia: This is the most common mechanism for SVT. This involves a circuit rhythm within the atria (atrial flutter or fibrillation), AV node (AV nodal reentry tachycardia), or accessory pathway (atrioventricular reentrant tachycardia).
- Ectopic (automatic) atrial tachycardia: This is a rare mechanism for SVT and includes automatic atrial tachycardia, ectopic atrial tachycardia, and multifocal atrial tachycardia. A single focus in the atrium is responsible for rapid firing, and the heart rate may vary substantially during the day.
- Nodal tachycardia: This originates from the AV node and may resemble atrial tachycardia. The heart rates are relatively slower (120–200 beats/min).

GENETICS

SVT has been noted in several families, but no specific genetic inheritance has been described.

EPIDEMIOLOGY

- SVT is the most common arrhythmia in childhood (1/250 and 1/1,000, with a bimodal age distribution).
- Forty percent of patients present between birth and 6 months, 30% present between 4 and 9 years.

COMPLICATIONS

Complications from SVT can arise from one of three reasons:

- Persistent tachycardia can lead to congestive heart failure and cardiovascular collapse. This is especially true in the infant who may go unrecognized for 24 to 48 hours.
- Few patients with WPW syndrome (<5%) can have rapid conduction down the accessory pathway. If this occurs during atrial flutter/fibrillation, it can lead to a rapid ventricular response and ventricular fibrillation. This can especially occur in the face of receiving digoxin and/or verapamil.
- Side effects of pharmacologic agents used to treat SVT include bradycardia, other new ventricular arrhythmias due to proarrhythmic effects of antiarrhythmic agents (digoxin, procainamide, amiodarone), or noncardiac side effects (gastrointestinal, liver, pulmonary, and thyroid dysfunction).

 Differential Diagnosis

- Narrow complex SVT needs to be distinguished from normal sinus rhythm, sinus and junctional tachycardia, ventricular tachycardia, and sick-sinus syndrome with tachyarrhythmia. Structural heart disease should be excluded in all cases of newly diagnosed SVT.
- Wide complex tachycardia from aberrant SVT can be seen in a small percentage of patients with an accessory pathway and may be confused with ventricular tachycardia. As a general rule, unless there are preexisting data that the patient has aberrant SVT, *"wide complex tachycardia should always be interpreted as ventricular tachycardia until proven otherwise."*

 Data Gathering

HISTORY

- Signs and symptoms include those suggestive of low cardiac output if the tachycardia has gone unnoticed, especially in infants: tachypnea, retractions, irritability, decreased feedings, excessive sweating, hypotension, poor perfusion, and decreased urine output.
- The toddler and older child may experience palpitations, shortness of breath, chest pain, and dizziness or syncope. It is important to know what the child was doing at the time the arrhythmia started and whether the rhythm had an abrupt onset and termination.

 Physical Examination

The following need to be assessed in all patients presenting with SVT:

- Heart rate
- Respiratory rate
- Blood pressure
- Hydration
- Peripheral perfusion
- Liver size
- Mental status
- Presence gallop rhythm on auscultation
- Older children often report being able to terminate episodes of tachycardia by performing the valsalva maneuver (e.g., gagging or standing on their head).

 Laboratory Aids

TESTS

- Diagnosis can be made by a 12-lead ECG, 24-hour Holter recording, transtelephonic monitor (TTM), or a transesophageal recording.
- Patients with WPW syndrome have diagnostic ventricular preexcitation (short PR and a delta wave) on the surface ECG.
- An exercise stress test and/or electrophysiologic testing may be indicated in older patients with WPW syndrome to help prognosticate this condition.

IMAGING

- A chest x-ray may reveal cardiomegaly, suggesting congestive heart failure or underlying structural heart disease.
- Nonpharmalogic maneuvers (ice, vagal) and pharmacologic maneuvers (e.g., IV adenosine [50–300 μg/kg/dose]) may distinguish tachycardias that involve the AV node from other types of SVT.

Therapy

- Always assess the child's ABCs (airway, breathing, and circulation).
- Initial management of SVT depends on the child's hemodynamic condition.
- Presentation in cardiovascular collapse due to SVT warrants treatment with synchronized DC cardioversion (0.5–2.0 joules/kg).
- In a stable child, adenosine (bolus 50–350 mg/kg) may be used to block the AV node to achieve pharmacologic cardioversion. The half-life of the drug is less than 1 minute. Verapamil should be avoided as acute treatment of SVT in children less than 12 months of age because of its vasodilating and negative inotropic effect. Nonpharmacologic vagal maneuvers, including ice to the face, valsalva, gag, and head-stand, may be tried in older children.
- Oral digoxin is the agent of choice in hemodynamically stable SVT needing chronic therapy. Digoxin is, however, contraindicated in patients with WPW because it may potentiate faster conduction down the accessory pathway and lead to ventricular fibrillation in some patients.
- β-Blockers (propranolol or nadolol) are the treatment of choice in individuals with WPW. Procainamide and amiodarone may be used in more resistant cases. β-Blockers are usually given to patients with exercise-induced SVT.
- Radiofrequency catheter ablation is an alternative to long-term drug therapy and may be employed for the following reasons: (1) SVT refractory to medical therapy, (2) side effects from the medical regimen, (3) patient choice, (4) life-threatening arrhythmias, (5) rapid conduction properties of an accessory pathway (e.g., WPW), or (6) concomitant congenital or acquired heart disease.

Other forms of SVT, including automatic tachycardias (ectopic atrial and multifocal atrial tachycardia) and atrial flutter and fibrillation, may be responsive to antiarrhythmics such as procainamide, flecanide (should generally be avoided if the patient has structural heart disease), amiodarone or β-blockers either alone or in different combinations.

 ## Follow-Up

- As SVT may recur, neonates and infants generally should receive maintenance therapy for the first year of life and then be observed off medications, assuming that they are not having frequent breakthrough episodes of SVT.
- Individuals with recurrences in the first year of life or those requiring multiple medications should be treated for 1- to 2-year periods during which they are episode-free, and then closely followed.
- In children presenting beyond infancy, the likelihood for spontaneous resolution of the tachycardia is less likely, and treatment may need to be continued into adulthood. These patients may be considered for a radiofrequency ablation.
- Over-the-counter sympathomimetic cold medications and caffeine products should be avoided, as they may initiate SVT.

 ## Common Questions and Answers

Q: How should infants on chronic therapy be monitored?
A: Parents with infants on chronic therapy for SVT should be educated about counting the heart rate by palpation or auscultation at least one to two times daily. This method of surveillance is just as effective as HR monitors. Alarm monitors can increase anxiety level by frequent false alarms and are generally not recommended.

Q: What is the concern with verapamil?
A: Verapamil is an L-type calcium channel blocker that blocks conduction in the AV node and is very effective in treating SVT in adults. Since myocardial contractility in infants depends mostly on the trans-sarcolemmal L-type calcium channels, hypotension and cardiovascular collapse have been reported with its use in children less than 1 year of age.

Q: What are the indications and success of electrophysiology testing and radiofrequency catheter ablation?
A: Refractory arrhythmias, need for multiple medications, undesired side effects from the medications, life-threatening events (syncope, cardiac arrest), wide complex tachycardia (cannot determine whether SVT or VT), and elective ablation after 6 to 8 years of age are some of the indications. The success rate of RFA varies from 80% to 90%, depending on the location of the bypass tract or ectopic foci.

ICD-9-CM 427.89

BIBLIOGRAPHY

Brinder LS, Boeche R, Atkinson D. Evaluation and management of supraventricular tachycardia. *Ann Emerg Med* 1992;21:1499.

Fleisher G, Ludwig S. *Textbook of pediatric emergency medicine*. Baltimore: Williams & Wilkins. 1993:549–554.

Kirk CR, Gibbs JL, Thomas R, et al. Cardiovascular collapse after verapamil in supraventricular tachycardia. *Arch Dis Child* 1987;62:1265–1282.

Levin DL, Morriss FC. *Essentials of pediatric intensive care*, Vol. 1. New York: Churchill Livingstone. 1997:225–227.

Moss AJ, Adams FH. *Heart disease in infants, children, and adolescents*, Vol. 2, 5th ed. Baltimore: Williams & Wilkins. 1995:1555–1586.

Author: Venkat Ramesh

Syncope

 Database

DEFINITION

• Loss of consciousness, typically lasting no longer than 1 to 2 minutes, due to a transient drop in cerebral perfusion pressure

PATHOPHYSIOLOGY

• The most common mechanism of syncope is vasovagal, in which a variety of external stimuli (pain, emotional upset, carotid pressure) trigger increased vagal tone, leading to slowed heart rate and peripheral vasodilation and decreased cerebral perfusion pressure.
• Rarer causes include cardiac arrhythmia (heart block or tachyarrhythmia) and intracranial hypertension.

ASSOCIATED CONDITIONS

• Over one-third of syncopal spells in children are accompanied by a convulsion that may last several minutes (EEG normal); iron deficiency may accompany syncope in the setting of breath-holding spells.

 Differential Diagnosis

• Alternative causes of loss of consciousness not due to syncope include head trauma, epilepsy (temporal lobe syncope) psychogenic, stroke, hypoglycemia (rare except in certain metabolic disorders)
• Underlying causes of syncope in any age group may include congenital heart malformations, arteriovenous malformation; pulmonary hypertension; intracranial hypertension due to hydrocephalus, mass, or pseudotumor; and tachyarrhythmia or heart block (Stokes-Adams).
• Other causes of syncope by age group include the following:

—Toddlers: pallid or cyanotic breath-holding spells; these occur in response to pain, excitement, or frustration, begin with a deep inspiration or exhalation, though the precipitating gasp may not be apparent; mastocytosis (syncope preceded by dyspnea)
—Older children: prolonged QT syndrome (may be familial, with or without deafness; may occur as exercise-induced syncope ± an epileptic convulsion; adrenal insufficiency; dysautonomia

 Data Gathering

HISTORY

Question: Details of the spell?
Significance: Most important information used to distinguish syncope from seizure or head trauma.

Question: Does the child or observers recall diaphoresis, light-headedness, palpitations, visual changes lasting only seconds before loss of consciousness?
Significance: Aura of seizure.

Question: Increasing duration of unconsciousness?
Significance: Increases the probability that the event is epileptic, rather than syncopal.

Question: Generalized tonic-clonic movements?
Significance: May occur with syncope, but presyncopal signs point to the non-epileptic nature of the event.

Question: Details of body position, eye movements, and respiratory pattern?
Significance:

Physical Examination

Physical findings that could indicate the cause of syncope are usually absent.

- Vital signs
- Peripheral/central pulses
- Orthostatic pulse and blood pressure changes
- Right and left arm blood pressures
- Funduscopy (papilledema?)
- Cranial bruits
- Heart sounds

 ## Laboratory Aids

Some children may have a clear history of vaso-vagal syncope and no laboratory testing will be required.

Test: ECG and chest X-ray
Significance: Studies may be useful screening tests.

Test: Treadmill ECG, Holter monitoring, EEG/ambulatory EEG
Significance: Children with recurrent syncope may undergo more extensive testing to rule out arrhythmia or epilepsy.

Test: CBC, blood gases, echocardiogram, brain imaging, spinal tap
Significance: May be appropriate based on clinical suspicion of underlying causes (*see* Differential Diagnosis).

- Clinical intervention is primarily preventive/anticipatory: avoidance of circumstances predisposing to the most common form of syncope (vasovagal), maintaining adequate hydration during illness/exertion.
- Therapy is addressed to underlying causes, in the unusual circumstance that a specific condition is identified.

PITFALLS

- Recurrent syncope due to prolonged QT interval may be missed on routine ECG; QT interval may be prolonged only on treadmill testing.
- Carbon monoxide poisoning may cause syncopal spells; ask about potential exposure.
- Epilepsy may rarely mimic a syncopal episode or recurrent presyncopal symptoms; temporal lobe syncope seems to occur principally in adults or adolescents.
- Syncope may trigger a convulsion in an epileptic patient.

 ## Follow-Up

- A record should be kept once a child has had two or more syncopal spells within 6 months.
- Many children seem to outgrow a developmental stage when they have frequent vasovagal episodes; they may retain a tendency to syncopal spells through adulthood.
- Persistent and frequent spells may prompt more extensive laboratory testing, as described previously.

 ## Common Questions and Answers

Q: Do breath-holding spells cause brain damage?
A: Pallid breath-holding spells appear to be uniformly benign; in rare cases, older children with cyanotic breath-holding spells have had neurologic sequelae of recurrent hypoxemia.

Q: What limitations in activity are appropriate for children with recurrent syncope?
A: Precautions should be taken similar to those for children of similar age who have epilepsy: closely monitored water recreation and restrictions on climbing. Most children with recurrent syncope do not experience spells in the midst of vigorous activity.

ICD-9-CM 780.2

BIBLIOGRAPHY

Braden DS, Gaymes CH. The diagnosis and management of syncope in children and adolescents. *Pediatr Ann* 1997;26(7):422–426.

Breningstall GN. Breath-holding spells. *Pediatr Neurol* 1996;14(2):91–97.

Lerman-Sagie T, Lerman P, Mukamel M, Blieden L, Mimouni M. A prospective evaluation of pediatric patients with syncope. *Clin Pediatr* 1994;33(2):67–70.

Lombroso CT, Lerman P. Breathholding spells (cyanotic and pallid infantile syncope). *Pediatrics* 1967;39:565–581.

Prodinger RJ, Reisdorff EJ. Syncope in children. *Emerg Med Clin North Am* 1998;16(3):617–626.

Author: Peter M. Bingham

Synovitis—Transient

Database

DEFINITION

• A transient inflammatory process resulting in arthralgia and arthritis (especially affecting the hip) and occasionally rash precipitated by an exposure to an infectious agent or drug

CAUSES

• Usually viral (especially enteroviruses), post-vaccine, or drug-mediated (especially antibiotics)

PATHOLOGY

• A type III hypersensitivity reaction mediated by immune complex deposition within the skin and joint spaces

EPIDEMIOLOGY

• Any age at risk, common in ages 3–10, with males affected 1.5 times more commonly

GENETICS

• No specific associations

COMPLICATIONS

• In affected hips, rarely avascular necrosis of femoral head and coxa magna

Differential Diagnosis

• Infection: Lyme, septic, gonorrhea
• Environment: trauma (fracture, or soft tissue injury), slipped capital femoral epiphysis, avascular necrosis
• Tumors: osteoid osteoma
• Immunologic: juvenile rheumatoid arthritis
• Psychologic: psychogenic limp
• Miscellaneous: hypothyroidism

Data Gathering

HISTORY

• Exposure to individuals with viral syndromes
• Day care
• Recent use of antibiotics
• Recent vaccination, especially MMR
• Relatively rapid onset of symptoms, with refusal to bear weight, in a nontoxic appearing child

Physical Examination

Finding: General examination usually benign.
Significance: Child refuses to bear weight but may tolerate slight ranging of joint. Effusions in peripheral joints are usually small and evanescent.

PROCEDURE

• Extreme pain on passive ranging raises suspicion for septic joint

Laboratory Aids

Test: CBC
Significance: Usually mild leukocytosis

Test: ESR
Significance: Usually mid-range elevation (35–60).

IMAGING

Test: X-ray
Significance: Usually normal or demonstrates small effusion; no evidence of periosteal changes.

Test: Ultrasound
Significance: Affected hip joints may have demonstrable effusions.

Test: Joint aspirate culture
Significance: Be wary of contaminated joint aspiration cultures.

Test: Culture
Significance: Be wary of contaminated joint aspirate cultures.

PITFALLS

• Distinctions between the septic joints may be difficult.

Therapy

DRUGS

• Usually very responsive to NSAIDs such as ibuprofen (up to 10 mg/kg/dose 4 times a day).
• Rarely, a short course of oral steroids is necessary.

DURATION

Usually 1 to 3 weeks of a tapering course of NSAIDs is effective.

POSSIBLE CONFLICTS

• Avoid initiation of therapy until septic joint is not a major concern, because early use of NSAIDs
• Can mask disease progession in septic joints.

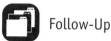 Follow-Up

WHEN TO EXPECT IMPROVEMENT

Usually significant improvement in 24 to 48 hours.

SIGNS TO WATCH FOR

• Ongoing synovitis despite therapeutic levels of NSAIDs or any bony changes indicate need to change diagnosis

PROGNOSIS

• Excellent, though on occasion, patients will experience recurrence of symptoms with subsequent viral syndrome or reexposure to a previously associated drug

PITFALLS

• Over investigation/therapy of child with features by history, physical examination, and laboratory supportive of diagnosis of serum sickness

 Common Questions and Answers

Q: Are there any chronic sequelae from serum sickness?
A: No, this is a benign disease; injury to the femoral head in affected hips is extremely rare.

Q: Is there an association with chronic arthritis?
A: No, there is no known increased risk for chronic arthritis in affected children.

ICD-9-CM 726.90

BIBLIOGRAPHY

Cassidy JT, Petty RE. *Textbook of pediatric rheumatology.* Philadelphia: WB Saunders, 1995.

Hart JJ. Transient synovitis of the hip in children. *Am Fam Physician* 1996;54(5):1587–1591, 1595–1596.

Roujeau JC, Stern RS. Severe adverse reactions to drugs. *N Engl J Med* 1994;331:1272–1285.

Author: Gregory F. Keenan

Syphilis

Database

DEFINITION

- Systemic infection caused by the spirochete, *Treponema pallidum*

Congenital Syphilis

- Transmitted from an infected mother to her unborn or newborn baby. Early congenital syphilis refers to the symptoms appearing in the first 2 years of life, and late congenital syphilis refers to those occurring later in childhood. Clinical manifestations range from asymptomatic to death or stillbirth.

Acquired Syphilis

- Sexually transmitted from an infected individual to an uninfected individual. Sexual abuse must be considered when syphilis is diagnosed in children.
- Primary stage: painless chancre(s) (indurated ulcers) at the site of inoculation; typically lasts 1 to 6 weeks
- Secondary stage: generalized rash, which is often maculopapular and involves the palms and soles; condyloma lata, hypertrophic papular lesions; fever, malaise, lymphadenopathy; follows the primary stage by 2 to 10 weeks and lasts up to 2 to 10 weeks.
- Relapse: symptoms of secondary syphilis may recur one or more times before the latent period.
- Latent period: variable, occurs after the secondary stage; first 4 years of latent period are referred to as "early latent," and subsequent years as "late latent," which lasts 1 to 40 years or more.
- Tertiary stage: many years after the primary infection; may see manifestations of neurosyphilis, aortitis, gummatous changes.

PATHOPHYSIOLOGY

- Congenital: transplacental (hematogenous) infection of the fetus at any stage of pregnancy; rarely from contact with infectious lesions during passage through the birth canal.
- Acquired: exposure to an infected genital or non-genital skin lesion.
- In late congenital syphilis, a late hypersensitivity reaction is believed to cause the findings of interstitial keratitis, deafness, and Clutton joints.

EPIDEMIOLOGY

- Occurs most frequently in urban areas.
- The incidence of congenital syphilis follows that of acquired syphilis.
- In adults, male:female ratio is 2:1.
- Acquired syphilis is spread through direct sexual contact with ulcerative lesions of the skin or mucous membranes in infected individuals.
- Syphilis enhances the transmission of HIV.
- Rate of transmission during secondary stage in pregnant women to the fetus is nearly 100%.

- Cocaine abuse during pregnancy is associated with an increased risk for maternal and congenital syphilis.
- Incubation period: 3 weeks (range: 10–90 days) following exposure for acquired primary syphilis.

COMPLICATIONS

- Stillbirth, spontaneous abortion, perinatal death: 40% of pregnancies in mothers with untreated early syphilis.
- Hydrops fetalis
- Prematurity
- Nephrosis
- Failure to thrive
- Disseminated intravascular coagulation
- Pseudoparalysis of Parrot: paralysis of one of the limbs of an infant affected by congenital syphilis; usually unilateral
- Acute syphilitic leptomeningitis
- Cranial nerve palsies
- Hearing loss (e.g., eighth nerve deafness)
- Interstitial keratitis
- Cerebral infarction
- Seizure disorder
- Mental retardation
- Rhagades: cluster of scars radiating around the mouth
- Mulberry molars: maldevelopment of the cusps in the first molars
- Clutton joints: painless arthritis of the knees and, rarely, other joints.
- Hutchinson triad: Hutchinson teeth (notched upper central incisors), interstitial keratitis, eighth nerve deafness
- Saber shins: anterior bowing of the midportion of the tibia.

PROGNOSIS

The prognosis is better the earlier syphilis is detected and treated. With late findings of syphilis, involving the nervous system and/or cardiovascular system, there may not be clinical improvement.

Differential Diagnosis

- Neonate: herpes simplex virus, toxoplasmosis, cytomegalovirus, rubella, sepsis, neonatal hepatitis, osteomyelitis.
- Primary syphilis: chancroid, granuloma inguinale, lymphogranuloma venerum, scabies, mycotic infections, herpes progenitalis.
- Secondary syphilis: infectious mononucleosis, scabies, viral exanthem.

Data Gathering

HISTORY

Newborn/Infants

Question: Always obtain a detailed prenatal history.

Significance: Inquire about all syphilis testing done on the mother; if mother has a history of syphilis, ensure documented treatment; the local department of health should have records on all cases of syphilis.

Question: Maternal history
Significance: Newborns should be evaluated for congenital syphilis if:

- Mother not adequately treated for syphilis.
- Mother treated adequately but without a four-fold decrease in antibody titers.
- Maternal syphilis treated less than 1 month before delivery.
- Maternal syphilis treated prior to pregnancy with insufficient follow-up to assess serologic response to treatment.

Older Children/Adolescents

- Possible sexual abuse in children and sexual activity in adolescents?
- History of other sexually transmitted diseases/lesions?
- Risk factors for HIV exposure?

Physical Examination

Early Congenital Syphilis

- Low birth weight
- Irritability, bulging fontanel if neurosyphilis is present.
- Loss of hair, eyebrows
- Fissures in the lips, nares, anus; mucocutaneous lesions
- Rhinitis ("snuffles") may occur at one to several weeks of age and may be blood-tinged and purulent.
- Lymphadenopathy
- Pneumonia. Check for tachypnea, respiratory distress
- Myocarditis
- Hepatosplenomegaly with or without jaundice
- Pseudoparalysis of an extremity
- Bullous ("syphilitic pemphigus") and/or maculopapular; symmetrically distributed on palms, soles, and other parts of the body.
- Condyloma lata are flat, wart-like, moist, around the anus/vagina, chancres.
- Late congenital syphilis may see:

—Boney deformities, such as short maxilla
—High arched palate
—Saddle nose
—Mulberry molars
—Higouménakis sign: enlargement of the sternoclavicular portion of the clavicle
—Protuberance of the mandible
—Saber shins
—Scaphoid scapulae

- Rhagades indicate neurologic involvement
- Acquired syphilis

—Primary syphilis
  —Chancre: painless ulcer, single, most commonly located on the genitalia

Syphilis

—Painless, inguinal adenopathy
—Secondary syphilis
—May see a flu-like illness: fever, headache, sore throat, nasal discharge, generalized arthralgias and myalgias, malaise, generalized adenopathy (painless and mobile nodes)
—Hepatosplenomegaly
—Maculopapular rash involving the palms and soles and may involve the mucous membranes
—Condyloma lata (moist, papular lesions)
—Alopecia
—Also, look for signs of meningitis, hepatitis, nephropathy, ocular involvement.

 Laboratory Aids

Test: Nontreponemal antibody tests
Significance: Measure anti-cardiolipin antibody; titers fall with syphilis therapy and may be used to follow response to treatment.

• VDRL slide test: Congenital infection if infant's titer is at least fourfold greater than the maternal titer; should be done on CSF in all neonates, when syphilis is suspected, to rule out neurosyphilis
• RPR (rapid plasma reagin): A simplified variation of the VDRL test.
• False-positive nontreponemal test: Results may occur with lab error, autoimmune disease, tuberculosis, infectious mononucleosis, endocarditis, and intravenous drug abuse. In newborns, nontreponemal testing of the cord blood may result in false-positive (e.g., from contamination with Wharton jelly) and false-negative results. Therefore, serum from the infant is preferable.
• Usually becomes nonreactive after therapy within 1 year in primary syphilis, and within 2 years in secondary and congenital syphilis.

Test: Treponemal antibody tests
Significance: Non-quantitative; used to confirm the diagnosis of syphilis; do not correlate with disease activity; positive for life once infected.

Test: FTA-ABS (fluorescent treponemal antibody) and MHA-TP (microhemagglutination assay for antibodies to *T. pallidum)* are available.
Significance: These tests connote history of infection, not only active disease. Once a patient is infected with syphilis, these tests remain positive. Positive treponemal tests may be seen in other spirochetal diseases (e.g., Lyme disease, leptospirosis).

Test: Complete blood count (CBC)
Significance: If anemia or thrombocytopenia suspected.

Test: Liver function tests
Significance: If liver disease suspected.

Test: CSF analysis
Significance: In syphilis, findings include mononuclear pleocytosis, moderately elevated protein, normal glucose; should be performed in all neonates when congenital syphilis is sus-

pected; should be performed in all patients with acquired syphilis of greater than 1 year's duration. Newborn spinal fluid protein can be as high as 200 mg/dL.

Test: Microscopy
Significance: Treponemes may be seen on darkfield microscopy of fresh exudate from skin lesions, regional lymph node, placenta, umbilical cord; or by direct fluorescent antibody staining of acetone-fixed exudate.

RADIOGRAPHIC STUDIES

Test: Long bones
Significance: To rule out metaphyseal osteochondritis and/or diaphyseal periostitis.

Test: Chest radiograph
Significance: If pneumonia is suspected (fluffy diffuse infiltrates are seen with pneumonia alba); if cardiac symptoms are present.

 Therapy

DRUGS

• Congenital syphilis: IV aqueous crystalline penicillin G (100,000–150,000 U/kg/d divided bid or tid) for 7 to 10 days is the only recommended therapy for neonates. After 4 weeks of age, use aqueous penicillin G, 200,000 to 300,000 U/kg/d divided qid.
• Acquired syphilis, less than 1 year duration: IM benzathine penicillin G 50,000 U/kg (maximum 2.4 million units) in a single dose; if penicillin-allergic, tetracycline 500 mg PO qid or doxycycline, 100 mg PO bid for 2 weeks for patients greater than 9 years old.
• Acquired syphilis, greater than 1 year duration: IM benzathine penicillin G, 50,000 U/kg, weekly for 3 consecutive weeks; if penicillin-allergic, tetracycline, 500 mg PO qid or doxycycline 100 mg PO bid for 4 weeks.
• Neurosyphilis: aqueous penicillin G 200,000 to 300,000 U/kg/d (not to exceed 24 million U/d) divided q 4 to 6 hours for 10 to 14 days. Consultation with an infectious disease specialist is therefore recommended.

 Follow-Up

• Follow-up of all infants born to positive mothers at 1, 2, 4, 6, and 12 months of age. Serologic tests should be performed 3, 6, and 12 months after therapy until they become nonreactive. If titers have not shown a decline by 3 months, retreatment should be considered.
• For patients with neurosyphilis, clinical, serologic, and CSF evaluation should occur every 6 months until the CSF is normal. A reactive CSF VDRL at 6 months is an indication for retreatment.
• Osteochondritis and periostitis in the newborn are usually self-limited and heal in the first 6 months of life.

PREVENTION

• All cases should be reported to the local department of health.
• Prenatal screening early in pregnancy is recommended in all states. In high-risk patients, screening should be repeated at 28 weeks gestation.

 Common Questions and Answers

Q: Does pregnancy cause a false-positive VDRL result?
A: There are conflicting studies regarding this issue. A positive VDRL in an otherwise healthy pregnant women should never be considered a false-positive test. A treponemal-specific test should be performed to confirm the diagnosis of syphilis, and the patient should be treated appropriately. Pregnancy can elevate a positive titer.

Q: Can an infant have congenital syphilis if his/her mother had a negative VDRL during pregnancy?
A: A mother with a negative VDRL during pregnancy may have acquired syphilis late in pregnancy and transmitted it to her fetus. If the mother was not tested at delivery, then the diagnosis may have been missed. Some recommend that VDRLs be performed at the time of delivery for mothers who are at high risk for syphilis.

Q: What is the prozone phenomenon?
A: When a nontreponemal test is falsely negative due to high concentrations of antibody to *T. pallidum.* Diluting the serum will result in positive test results.

ICD-9-CM 079.9

American Academy of Pediatrics. Syphilis. In: Peter G, ed. *1997 Red Book: report of the committee on infectious diseases,* 24th ed. Elk Grove Village, IL: American Academy of Pediatrics, 1997:504–514.

Ikeda MK, Jenson HB. Evaluation and treatment of congenital syphilis. *J Pediatr* 1990; 117:843–851.

Moyer VA, Schneider V, Yetman R, et al. Contribution of long bone radiographs to the management of congenital syphilis in the newborn infant. *Arch Pediatr Adolesc Med* 1998;152: 353–357.

Sison CG, Ostrea EM, Reyes MP, Salari V. The resurgence of congenital syphilis: a cocaine-related problem. *J Pediatr* 1997;130:289–292.

Stoll BJ. Congenital syphilis: evaluation and management of neonates born to mothers with reactive serologic tests for syphilis. *Pediatr Infect Dis J* 1994;13:845–853.

Author: Esther K. Chung

Tapeworm

 Database

DEFINITION

Tapeworms or cestodes are intestinal parasites that possess a specialized attachment organ called a scolex, which consists of sucking grooves or four circular suckers.

PATHOLOGY

• Some species have hooks to attach to the mucosa of the definitive host.
• The definitive host harbors the adult tapeworm.
• Eggs are excreted in the feces and contaminate the environment.
• If the eggs are ingested by a suitable host, eggs break down and the oncosphere is activated and penetrates the intestinal mucosa; the oncosphere travels with the lymphatics and/or blood, matures into the metacestode or mature larval stage in the tissue of the intermediate host. The definitive host consumes the metacestode.
• The adult tapeworm matures and infects the small intestine of the definitive host.

CAUSES

• *Taenia saginata:* beef tapeworm
• *Taenia solium:* pork tapeworm/cystocercosis
• *Diphyllobothrium latum:* fish tapeworm/diphyllobothriasis
• *Spirometra:* sparganosis
• *Dipylidium caninum:* dog tapeworm/dipylidiasis

PATHOPHYSIOLOGY

• Beef tapeworm

—Contamination of pastures or feed lots with human feces contaminated with eggs; ingestion by cattle (intermediate host); eggs hatch; embryo burrows through intestinal mucosa; enter bloodstream; cysticerci develop in the tissues of the intermediate host; raw or very rare meat eaten by humans; attachment of scolex of the organism to the intestinal mucosa; adult tapeworm forms

• Pork tapeworm

—Contamination of pig feeding areas; ingestion by the pig (intermediate host); invasion of the circulation through the gut mucosa; distribution to various tissues of the pig through the circulation; ingestion of the cysticercus by humans by consuming poorly cooked meat; adult worm grows in the small intestine. Humans can also act as intermediate hosts with ingestion of the eggs from food contaminated with human feces; embryos enter the bloodstream through the intestinal mucosa; most commonly involved tissues include the brain, subcutaneous tissues, muscle, and the eye; CNS symptoms develop 5 to 7 years after infection when the incysted larvae die and may include cerebral swelling with increased intracranial pressure, delirium, or hallucinations; seizures occur in the majority of patients and may be the only feature in up to 30%.

• Fish tapeworm

—Sewage contamination of fresh water lakes and streams; ingestion of plerocercoid larvae in fish, fish liver, or roe; maturation of adult tapeworm in the intestines of humans; often leads to megaloblastic anemia in individuals from certain geographic areas.

• Sparganosis

—Infection of humans occurs through placement of fish or reptile flesh to wounds leading to infection or through ingestion of copepods (small crustaceans).

• Dog tapeworm

—Larvae develop in fleas after ingestion of the eggs; humans infected through accidental ingestion of infected fleas; tapeworm develops in the human gastrointestinal (GI) tract

• Dwarf tapeworm

—Human-to-human transmission can take place; transmission is primarily through fecal-oral transmission and thus occurs more commonly in areas where hygiene is poor.

• Hydatid disease (echinococcosis)

—Humans are intermediate hosts when they ingest the eggs through contaminated dog feces; oncospheres penetrate the mesenteric vessels and they travel to various tissues in the body and commonly infect the liver and lungs; hydatid cysts develop. Within the cysts new larvae (scolices) develop associated with increase in fluid; the cysts enlarge and encroach on surrounding structures leading to echinococcocis.

ASSOCIATED DISEASES

• Abdominal pain: common manifestation due to the presence of the adult tapeworm in the GI tract; can be associated with cramping and diarrhea, vomiting, fever, and weight loss.
• Megaloblastic anemia: most commonly associated with the fish tapeworm, diphyllobothriasis; primarily found in strains from Finland; may be secondary to vitamin B_{12} absorption by the worm, interference with B_{12} absorption, low B_{12} intake, and decreased secretion of intrinsic factor.
• Encroachment of normal tissues secondary to cysts developing from larvae, especially the lungs and liver in echinococcus; fever, cough, hemoptysis; right upper quadrant pain and jaundice from intrahepatic cysts.

EPIDEMIOLOGY

• Beef tapeworm: most common in areas of the former USSR, also found in areas of Africa, such as Ethiopia and Kenya; also found in South America and Central America.
• Pork tapeworm: most common in Eastern Europe, Central and South America, Spain, Portugal, and parts of Africa, China, and India.
• Fish tapeworm: worldwide distribution but endemic areas may exist such as the Baltic countries, the lake areas of the Northern United States, Canada, and the river deltas of Alaska.
• Sparganosis: primarily found in Asia.
• Dog tapeworm: found in dogs and cats worldwide although uncommon in the United States.
• Dwarf tapeworm: children between the ages of 4 and 10 have the highest prevalence; infection is worldwide and is particularly prevalent in Algeria, Sicily, and the southern regions of the former Soviet Union.
• Echinococcocis: endemic in sheep raising areas of South America, Australia, the Mediterranean area, and areas of Africa such as Kenya and Uganda.

COMPLICATIONS

• Beef tapeworm: ectopic localization has been described including the uterus; intestinal obstruction is rare but can occur.
• Cystercosis: although man is often the definitive host, complications also occur when man becomes an accidental intermediate host. In this case the person often presents with myalgias, fever, and rarely eosinophilia; may see painless subcutaneous nodules, may see increased intracranial pressure with CNS involvement leading to papilledema, seizures, or psychotic behavior with delirium and hallucinations. The usual presentation is a new onset of seizures. Most commonly seen in the United States in those states bordering Mexico in Mexican immigrant families.
• Fish tapeworm: can cause megaloblastic anemia, fatigue, weakness, dizziness, numbness in the extremities; can rarely cause intestinal obstruction.
• Sparganosis: ocular involvement can lead to conjunctivitis, periorbital and palpebral edema, exophthalmos, chemosis, and corneal ulcerations; can see subcutaneous nodules; very rarely see CNS involvement.

- Dog tapeworm: occasionally see GI symptoms such as abdominal pain, vomiting, diarrhea.
- Dwarf tapeworm: can see restlessness, irritability, diarrhea, abdominal pain, anal and nausea pruritus, and occasionally diarrhea.
- Echinococcus: cysts develop, especially in the liver and the lung; other areas of involvement include eye, brain, spleen, heart, endocrine glands, bone, and GI tract; CNS involvement occurs more commonly in children than adults; bone involvement can lead to pathologic fractures; pulmonary lesions lead to cough and hemoptysis; CNS involvement can cause an increase in intracranial pressure and one-third have seizures.

PROGNOSIS

- Beef tapeworm: good unless there is intestinal obstruction
- Pork tapeworm: good with either surgical and/or treatment with praziquantel
- Fish tapeworm: good, including resolution of the anemia, after treatment with niclosamide; an alternative is praziquantel; B_{12} supplementation is recommended
- Sparganosis: only treatment with adequate results is surgery with complete removal of the organisms
- Dwarf tapeworm: good with treatment with niclosamide, praziquantel, or paromomycin
- Echinococcosis: variable with surgical treatment which has up to a 3% to 5% mortality

 Differential Diagnosis

Tapeworm infections can have a variable presentation depending on the site of infection and the type of infection. Tapeworm infections should be considered in all cases of diarrhea, abdominal pain, or weight loss. Larval infection should be considered in individuals with unusual end-organ disease, especially when it is cystic in nature.

 Data Gathering

HISTORY

Question: Travel recently?
Significance: Many of these infections are more prevalent in other countries.

Question: GI tract complaints?
Significance: Symptoms related to the GI tract should include weight loss, diarrhea, abdominal pain, history of intestinal obstruction, and fever. Involvement by larvae should include questions about localizing symptoms secondary to compression of normal structures. Onset of new CNS pathology, especially seizures, should include cysticercosis and echinococcosis.

 Laboratory Aids

Test: Beef tapeworm
Significance: Identification of scolex in stool; Ziehl-Neelsen stain of stool to check for eggs; cellulose tape swabs of anal and perianal skin; collection of proglottids in saline with microscopic examination; 14 or greater branches to the uterus makes the diagnosis.

Test: Pork tapeworm
Significance: ELISA test and immunoblot in combination for parenchymal cysticercosis; stool samples for intestinal worms as for beef tapeworm.

Test: Fish tapeworm
Significance: Stool samples for eggs or proglottids diagnostic.

Test: Sparganosis
Significance: CT scans helpful for cerebral sparganosis; usually diagnosed at surgery.

Test: Dog tapeworm
Significance: Diagnosis of proglottids in stool samples.

Test: Dwarf tapeworm
Significance: Saline wet mounts of stool to identify characteristic eggs.

Test: Echinococcus
Significance: Clinical presentation with or without radiographic findings is the common initial presentation and leads to the diagnosis; IgE levels may be very elevated; pulmonary lesions demonstrate a sharply demarcated smooth-bordered cyst; if it has ruptured, then there is the appearance of a crescent-shaped air level; lesions in the liver and spleen may calcify but only over many years; the Casoni skin test may be falsely positive or negative in up to 30% of infected individuals; serologic testing may be falsely negative in 10% to 50% of individuals with the disease.

 Therapy

- Beef tapeworm: niclosamide: children 25 to 75 lbs., 51.0 g; children greater than 75 lbs, 51.5 g; adults 52.0 g; administered as a single dose; contraindicated in children under 2 or in pregnancy.

—Alternative: praziquantel: 10 to 20 mg/kg in a single dose; no safety exists for children under the age of 4.
—Alternative: paromomycin: 11 mg/kg every 15 minutes for four doses (not to exceed a dose of 4 g)

- Pork tapeworm: praziquantel: 50 mg/kg body weight divided in three doses for 14 days.

—Alternative: albendazole: 15 mg/kg/d for 1 month

- Fish tapeworm: as in beef tapeworm with replacement of B_{12} in addition.
- Sparganosis: niclosamide as in beef tapeworm.
- Dwarf tapeworm: niclosamide: children 25 to 75 lbs., 51.0 g on day 1 followed by 0.5 g daily for 6 days; children 75 lbs. or greater, 51.5 g day 1 then 1.0 g per day for 6 days; adults 52.0 g per day for 7 days.

PREVENTION

Proper cooking of meat and fish can prevent transmission of beef, pork, and fish tapeworms. Also, protection measures against contamination of food and drink with human feces is essential.

 Common Questions and Answers

Q: How may one prevent tapeworm infections when traveling to other countries?
A: Obviously, proper food preparation is essential in preventing many infections. Avoiding uncooked or undercooked food products is important. In addition, avoiding drinking potentially contaminated drinking water through the use of bottled water can avoid contact with drinking water contaminated with human feces.

Q: Is treatment for cerebral cysticercosis always indicated?
A: No, for solitary calcified nodules in the brain parenchymal treatment is not needed. Seizure occurs as edema develops around the dying encysted larvae. Magnetic resonance imaging will verify if a single lesion is present. Those with multiple lesions may need therapy. An infectious disease expert familiar with these infections and the prognosis should be consulted.

ICD-9-CM 123.9

BIBLIOGRAPHY

Jones TC, Mandell GL, Dongles RG, et al. Tapeworm. In: Long SS, Pickeriny LR, Prober CG, eds. *Principles and practices of infectious diseases,* 3rd ed. Philadelphia: W.B. Saunders, 1997;2151–2156.

Rosenblatt JE. Antiparasitic agents. *Mayo Clin Proc* 1992;67:276–287.

Turner JA, Feigin RD, Cheng JD. *Textbook of pediatric infectious diseases,* vol. 2, 3rd ed. Philadelphia: W.B. Saunders, 1997;2098–2112.

Author: Bret J. Rudy

Tendonitis

 Database

DEFINITION

- Inflammation of a tendon at its insertion or along its tendon sheath

CAUSES

- Frequently associated with repetitive motion/overuse type activities

PATHOLOGY

Inflammation, microtearing, and microfracture may be present.

EPIDEMIOLOGY

- Increases with age and at time of puberty. There may be a slight increase in incidence in girls.

GENETICS

Hypermobile individuals may be prone to these injuries.

COMPLICATIONS

- Ongoing pain and predisposition for recurrence

 Differential Diagnosis

- Infection: septic arthritis, osteomyelitis
- Environmental: fracture
- Metabolic: homocystinuria
- Congenital: generalized hypermobility, Marfan syndrome, Ehler Danlos
- Immunologic: ankylosing spondylitis and the reactive spondyloarthropathies (Crohn disease, Reiter syndrome), inflammatory arthritides
- Psychological: "Touch me not" psychogenic pain

 Data Gathering

HISTORY

Question: Trauma or overuse?
Significance: Verify acute nature of injury.

 Physical Examination

Question: Any evidence of hematoma?
Significance: Palpate around and about affected areas, detecting point tenderness especially at tendon insertions as well as over bony prominences.

SPECIAL QUESTIONS

Question: Was a pop or snap felt at the time of the event?
Significance: Sometimes this is felt when tendons and ligaments are torn.

 Laboratory Aids

Test: ESR
Significance: Occasionally, an ESR will be helpful to r/o inflammatory conditions if history and/or physical examination are suggestive.

IMAGING

Test: X-ray
Significance: Affected area may be indicated to r/o a fracture or identify a bone spur.

FALSE-POSITIVES

Patients may have torn ligaments, fractures, or arthritis, not just tendinitis on examination.

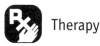 Therapy

- Rest/reduced use of the affected tendon/ muscle group is essential

PT/OT

- Either self-directed or formal help with resumption of desired activity, through gentle range of motion exercises against low resistance and advanced as tolerated

DRUGS

- Non-steroidal anti-inflammatory drugs; rarely do soft tissue steroid injections have a role in children

DURATION

- 1 to 4 weeks

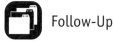 Follow-Up

WHEN TO EXPECT IMPROVEMENT

Improvement many times takes 2 to 6 weeks.

SIGNS TO WATCH FOR

If the provocative activity is resumed too soon, the irritation will recur.

PROGNOSIS

- Usually good for children; however, many will suffer recurrences if proper exercises before desired activity are not continued.

PITFALLS

Overdiagnosis in young children, in whom overuse is rare and other diagnoses should be considered. Underdiagnosis in older children in whom repetitive activities are likely to occur.

 Common Questions and Answers

Q: Which activities can result in overuse syndromes and tendonitis?
A: Virtually any repetitive activity in which children engage can cause tendonitis. For example, pain in the tendons of the thumb has occurred in children overusing video games.

ICD-9-CM 726.90

BIBLIOGRAPHY

Athreya BH, Cheh ML, Kingsland LC 3rd. Computer-assisted diagnosis of pediatric rheumatic diseases. *Pediatrics* 1998;102(4):E48.

Micheli LJ, Fehlandt AF. Overuse injuries to tendons and apophyses in children an adolescents. *Clin Sports Med* 1992;11:713–726.

Author: Gregory F. Keenan

Teratoma

 Database

DEFINITION

• An embryonal neoplasm that contains tissue derived from endoderm, mesoderm, and ectoderm, which may be benign or malignant. They are a subset of the broader class of germ cell tumors.

PATHOPHYSIOLOGY

• Abnormal migration of germ cells at about the sixth week of embryonal development, causing germ cells to come to rest outside the gonads.
• Immature teratoma: contains only immature embryonic components. Divided microscopically into four grades, 0 to 3, dependent on immature elements and mitotic activity.
• Mature teratoma: contains well-differentiated tissues such as squamous epithelium, brain, muscle, teeth, cartilage, bone, gastrointestinal, and respiratory tract linings.
• Teratoma with malignant components: foci of malignant tissue that resemble other germ cell tumors such as embryonal carcinoma, endodermal sinus tumor, and choriocarcinoma, in addition to mature or immature tissues.

EPIDEMIOLOGY

• Incidence of childhood germ cell tumors as a whole is 3.8/million in males and 4.7/million in females.
• Incidence is equal among whites and blacks.
• One suggestive epidemiologic association is with high maternal hormone levels during pregnancy.
• More controversial associations include: younger gestational age; viral infections including HSF, VZV, CMV, mumps; other congenital anomalies; maternal UTI or tuberculosis; paternal occupation in chemical industries.
• Sacrococcygeal tumors: Most prevalent in infants.
• Testicular and ovarian tumors: Most prevalent in infants and adolescents.
• Vaginal tumors: Most prevalent in girls under age 3
• Mediastinal tumors: Most prevalent in children under age 2 and in adolescents. Most common extragonadal germ cell tumor in adults.

GENETICS

• I(12p) Chromosomal abnormality is found in greater than 80% of germ cell tumors.
• No pattern of inheritance is known.

 Differential Diagnosis

• Sacrococcygeal: pilonidal cyst, meningocoele, lipomeningocoele, hemangioma, abscess, bone tumor, epidermal cyst, chondroma, lymphoma, ependymoma, neuroblastoma, glioma
• Abdominal: Wilms tumor, neuroblastoma, lymphoma, rhabdomyosarcoma, hepatoblastoma, retained twin fetus
• Vaginal: sarcoma botryoides, clear cell carcinoma
• Ovarian: cyst, appendicitis, pregnancy, pelvic infection, hematocolpos, sarcoma, lymphoma, other ovarian tumors
• Testicular: epididymitis, testicular torsion, infarct, orchitis, hernia, hydrocele, hematocoele, rhabdomyosarcoma, lymphoma, leukemia, other testicular tumors
• Mediastinal: Hodgkin and non-Hodgkin lymphoma, leukemia, thymoma

 Data Gathering

HISTORY

Question: External mass, constipation, urinary abnormalities, lower extremity weakness?
Significance: Sacrococcygnal mass may impinge on nerve structures. Anterior sacrococcygnal mass may have no external component.

Question: Cough, wheeze, dyspnea, hemoptysis, SVC syndrome?
Significance: Suggests mediastinal mass.

Question: Blood-tinged vaginal discharge?
Significance: Vaginal teratoma.

Question: Abdominal pain, nausea, vomiting, constipation, urinary tract symptoms?
Significance: Ovarian tumors present late with large mass.

Question: Painless scrotal swelling or painful testicular torsion?
Significance: Testicular mass may be teratoma.

Question: Cryptorchidism?
Significance: Associated with germ cell tumors in boys.

 Physical Examination

Finding: Palpable mass either externally or internally, signs of spinal cord compression?
Significance: Sacrococcygeal tumor.

Finding: Vaginoscopy reveals a polyploid lesion arising from the vaginal wall?
Significance: Examination under anesthesia usually necessary.

Finding: Palpable abdominal mass; peritoneal symptoms?
Significance: Ovarian mass may be large.

Finding: Palpable mass in scrotum?
Significance: Testicular origin.

Finding: Decreased breath sounds, consolidation, wheezing, SVC syndrome?
Significance: Mediastinal mass may be an emergency.

Laboratory Aids

Test: Serum alpha-fetoprotein or beta-human chorionic gonadotropin
Significance: When there are malignant components, these may be significantly elevated. Pure teratoma not associated with elevated markers.

Test: Complete blood count and chemistry profile, with electrolytes, blood urea nitrogen, creatinine, liver function tests, uric acid, and lacate dehydrogenase.
Significance: Work-up to rule out other malignancies.

IMAGING

Test: Plain x-ray
Significance: May reveal mature calcified tissues, such as bone or teeth, within the tumor.

Test: Chest x-ray
Significance: Shows mediastinal mass.

Test: Computed tomography (CT) scan
Significance: Necessary to evaluate the primary site and regional disease.

Test: Chest CT and bone scan
Significance: If malignancy is suspected or proven, these are indicated for evaluation of metastasis.

Test: Ultrasound, if CT is not readily available.
Significance: May be helpful, but it will rarely suffice as the sole imaging study of the primary site. May be first evidence of anterior sacrococcygeal mass.

 ## Therapy

• Mature teratoma: full surgical excision is curative.
• Immature teratoma: complete surgical resection is the therapy of choice. There is controversy over adjuvant chemotherapy. In cases of high alpha-fetoprotein, some support postoperative adjuvant chemotherapy.
• Teratoma with malignant components: chemotherapy with etoposide, cisplatin or carboplatin, and bleomycin, followed by surgical resection. Depends on the extent of resection, postoperative chemotherapy utilizing the same agents is often necessary. Radiation is reserved for salvage therapy.

 ## Follow-Up

• Serial exams and imaging studies of primary site
• Tumor markers (alpha-FP or beta-hCG), if initially positive
• If chemotherapy or radiation therapy utilized, need to monitor for secondary malignancies, long term. Short term, need to monitor blood counts, chemistries, renal function, and audiology.

PREVENTION

There is no known prevention for the development of teratomas and other germ cell tumors.

PITFALLS

All that appears to be a teratoma is not. Be prepared for other malignant and non-malignant histologies on biopsy.

 ## Common Questions and Answers

Q: What is the chance of cure for malignant teratomas?
A: With current chemotherapy as outlined above, disease-free survival is 85%.

Q: Can a benign tumor recur? If so, can it then be malignant?
A: Yes. If there is residual tissue left behind, the tumor can recur. If there were unrecognized areas of malignancy, the recurrence can be with a malignant teratoma. The greatest risk for the latter is with the immature teratomas.

ICD-9-CM
Benign 186.9
Sacral 653.7

BIBLIOGRAPHY

Gobel U, Calaminus G, Engert J, et al. Teratomas in infancy and childhood. *Med Pediatr Oncol* 1998;31:8–15.

Hawkins EP. Germ cell tumors. *Am J Clin Pathol* 1998;109(4):S2–S8.

Nicols CG, Fox EP. Extragonadal and pediatric germ cell tumors in children. *Hematol Oncol Clin North Am* 1991;5:1189–1209.

Rescorla FJ. Germ cell tumors. *Semin Pediatr Surg* 1997;6:29–37.

Shu XO, Nesbit ME, Buckley J, Krailo M, and Robison LL. An exploratory analysis of risk factors for childhood malignant germ cell tumors. *Cancer Causes Control* 1995;6:187–198.

Author: Debra L. Friedman

Tetanus

Database

DEFINITION

Tetanus is a disease characterized by tonic spasms of the skeletal muscles and occasionally the glottis and larynx due to intoxication with an exotoxin *tetanospasmin* produced by *Clostridium tetani*.

CAUSE

• Tetanus is caused by an anaerobic, spore-forming bacterium, *Clostridium tetani*. In anaerobic conditions, present in wounds with significant tissue damage, inoculated spores become vegetative and produce the disease-causing toxin.

• *Clostridium tetani* is a gram-positive rod found in superficial layers of soil, especially in agricultural areas throughout the world. Spores may survive in soil for months to years if not exposed to sunlight.

• *C. tetani* spores are found as part of the normal intestinal flora in many domesticated animals, rats, and humans.

PATHOPHYSIOLOGY

• *C. tetani* is found most commonly in cultivated soil in rural areas and in human and animal feces. Vegetative forms are easily killed by heat and standard disinfectants, but spores must be heated to 120°C for 15 to 20 minutes to be eradicated.

• Spores are inoculated into a variety of wounds when they are contaminated by soil or dust from houses or buildings. Under appropriate anaerobic conditions the spores become the vegetative bacillus and produce toxin. Anaerobic conditions in wounds are promoted by larger amounts of necrosis, the presence of foreign bodies, or other ongoing infections with suppuration.

• *C. tetani* produces two exotoxins, but only *tetanospasmin* is clinically important.

• *Tetanospasmin* is one of the most powerful exotoxins known, second in lethality only to *botulinum toxin*. It seems to travel from the wound site to the central nervous system (CNS) through the neurons. There may be some distribution of the toxin via the hematogenous route as well.

• The toxin may be absorbed directly into skeletal muscle adjacent to the injury and affects the motor end-plates producing sustained contractions in that area, a condition known as local tetanus.

• Once absorbed into peripheral nerves, the toxin is carried to the CNS by a yet unclear mechanism.

• The toxin has four major effects on the nervous system. At motor end-plates in skeletal muscle release of acetylcholine from neurons is inhibited. Toxin also seems to interfere with contraction and relaxation mechanisms directly. In the spinal cord action on interneurons leads to inhibition of antagonist mechanisms and uncontrolled muscle spasms result.

In the brain there is also an inhibition of antagonist mechanisms leading to uncontrolled spasms. The toxin also binds to receptors in the medullary center and can lead to direct respiratory depression. Finally, the sympathetic nervous system seems to be affected, leading to profuse sweating, vasoconstriction, labile hypertension, tachycardia, and dysrhythmias, and later hypotension.

• *Tetanospasmin* does not seem to affect cognitive processes directly. The classically described tetanic seizures are not accompanied by EEG changes consistent with seizure activity, although the EEG does show non-specific changes in many cases. "Tetanic seizures" are actually uncontrolled, generalized tetanic muscle spasms.

• The toxin binds irreversibly to neurons and resolution occurs slowly over 2 to 4 weeks.

• Pathologic changes in fatal cases are usually limited to non-specific changes in the CNS. Secondary complications may be associated with findings including pneumonia (often secondary to aspiration), pulmonary hemorrhage, CNS hemorrhage, and fractures, including vertebral body compressions related to the severe tetanic spasms.

EPIDEMIOLOGY

• Tetanus, especially neonatal tetanus, remains a major problem in developing countries but is rare in the developed world because of widespread immunization. In the United States, there are 50 to 200 cases reported annually including occasional cases of neonatal tetanus. Most cases are among the elderly but unimmunized children are also at risk.

• About two-thirds of cases in the United States occur between May and November. People from rural areas and who are involved in agriculture are more likely to have contact with the organisms, although many cases are reported among intravenous drug abusers.

COMPLICATIONS

• Most complications are related to the severe tetanic muscle contractions experienced by these patients.

• Severe spasm of the paraspinal muscles has led to compression fractures of vertebral bodies. Other bones may be broken as well, and muscle hemorrhages are not uncommon. Spasm of the chest wall as well as laryngospasm may precipitate respiratory failure and arrest. Spasms cause severe pain for patients.

• Spasms also cause dysphagia, hydrophobia, neck stiffness, and urinary retention.

• Repeated or continuous spasms may lead to elevations in body temperature.

• Cerebrovascular hemorrhages may be seen in rare cases, especially in neonatal tetanus.

• Pneumonia, including aspiration, may be a complication.

PROGNOSIS

• With advances in the ability to provide respiratory support in an intensive care setting, the prognosis has improved significantly. Overall

mortality rates have decreased from approximately 66% in the 1950s in the United States to 30% in the 1980s.

• Children and young adults have a much better prognosis than older individuals.

• In developing nations, mortality rates remain very high, reflecting an inability to provide technologically advanced tertiary care.

• A more rapid onset of disease and a more rapid progression from trismus to generalized spasms is associated with a more severe course.

• In the absence of complications, recovery is usually complete in survivors without long-term sequelae.

• Signs and symptoms usually progress for about 1 week after presentation before reaching their worst. The patient's condition then plateaus for about 1 week and then gradually improves over 2 to 6 weeks.

Differential Diagnosis

• Infections: retropharyngeal and peritonsillar abscesses, poliomyelitis, viral encephalitis, and meningoencephalitis may present with trismus or cranial nerve findings that would suggest a diagnosis of tetanus.

• Toxin: dystonic reactions to phenothiazine medications may resemble tetanus in presentation. Diphenhydramine will effectively treat these reactions.

• Metabolic: hypocalcemia due to rickets or other disorders is usually not as severe as the tetanic contractions seen with tetanus.

Data Gathering

HISTORY

Question: Incubation period?
Significance: Usually between 3 to 21 days. Cases have been reported with shorter periods, and at times it may be as long as several months. Sites of inoculation farther from the central nervous system are associated with longer incubation periods.

Question: Pain?
Significance: Local tetanus is associated with painful muscle contractions and stiffness limited to the area near the wound. This may persist for several weeks and resolve, or it may progress to generalized tetanus.

Question: Trismus?
Significance: The classic initial complaint of trismus is seen in about one-half of cases. Other early complaints include dysphagia, neck pain and stiffness, stiffness and pain in other muscle groups, urinary retention, restlessness, irritability, and headache.

Question: Progression of symptoms?
Significance: Usually occur over the first week but may progress more rapidly.

Question: Neonatal tetanus?
Significance: Usually complicates deliveries where aseptic conditions were not maintained, and the mother is either unimmunized or not up to date in her immunization status.

Physical Examination

Finding: Initial presenting sign is usually trismus.
Significance: Persistent trismus gives rise to the classic sardonic smile (wrinkling of the forehead and distortion of the eyebrows and the corners of the mouth).

Finding: Fever?
Significance: Initially, patients are usually afebrile.

Finding: As the disease progresses, other muscle groups develop tetanic contractions.
Significance: Tonic contractions of the paraspinal muscles lead to a significant opisthotonic posture. Severe spasmodic contractions, "tetanic seizures," also occur. These are extremely painful and can be associated with laryngospasm and tetany of the respiratory musculature with fatal results.

Finding: Tetanus spasms
Significance: Precipitated by a variety of stimuli including a cold draft, noise, pain, anxiety, and light touch. Because tetanus toxin does not affect the sensorium, the severe anxiety and pain associated with these spasms may precipitate additional spasms.

Finding: Tachycardia, flushing, severe and labile episodes of hypertension and tachycardia.
Significance: Autonomic nervous system involvement. Hypotension may be a late feature of the disease.

Finding: Fever
Significance: With sustained contractions, fever may develop, although it may also be a result of complications including pneumonia, infected in-dwelling catheters, or infected decubiti.

Finding: Cephalic tetanus
Significance: Involves only the cranial nerves and occurs after wounds of the face, scalp, or neck. It may also complicate chronic infections of the head and neck including chronic otitis media. Loss of airway control is a frequent and often fatal complication. Cephalic tetanus may progress to generalized tetanus.

Laboratory Aids

Test: Laboratory investigations
Significance: Yield little useful information in cases of tetanus. Anaerobic wound cultures may rarely yield *C. tetani*. The white blood cell count is usually normal or mildly elevated. CSF studies are unremarkable. EEG and EMG are non-specific. The diagnosis is made clinically.

Therapy

SPECIFIC

• Specific therapy is aimed at eradication of the vegetative organism and thereby the source of ongoing toxin production and neutralization of any toxin that has not already been irreversibly bound to neurons.
• Human tetanus immune globulin (TIG) should be administered in a dose of 500 to 3000 units in three divided doses at three separate sites. Repeat doses do not seem to be indicated. Infants with neonatal tetanus should be given a dose of 250 units.
• If TIG is not available, tetanus antitoxin (TAT) may be administered if a skin test for sensitization to this equine-derived product is negative. If the skin test is positive, desensitization must be accomplished before TAT can be administered. The dose of TAT is 50,000 to 100,000 units with one-half given intramuscularly and the remainder intravenously.
• Penicillin G, 200,000 U/kg/d should be given intravenously in four divided doses for 10 days. Oral tetracycline or intravenous vancomycin may be used in penicillin-sensitive individuals. Cephalosporins are not effective.
• Aggressive surgical debridement and removal of foreign bodies from the infected wound must be undertaken. If a wound is gangrenous, amputation may be considered.
• After resolution of the illness complete, active immunization is required in individuals who have tetanus.

SUPPORTIVE CARE

• Patients suspected of having tetanus should be rapidly transferred to a tertiary care center capable of providing sophisticated ventilatory and cardiovascular support in an intensive care setting. Transfer should occur early in the disease before these sophisticated techniques are necessary.
• Patients should be kept in a quiet, darkened room with minimum stimulus. Cardiac and respiratory status should be monitored closely.
• Tracheostomy may prevent fatal laryngospasm. It is preferable that this be done on a semiemergent rather than emergent basis.
• Parenteral nutrition is usually required to maintain adequate nutrition and hydration.

DRUGS

• Diazepam should be given to promote sedation and muscle relaxation. A dose of 0.1 to 0.2 mg/kg IV every 4 to 6 hours is an appropriate initial dose. Phenothiazines, especially chlorpromazine, may be helpful if additional sedation is needed. Sedation must be titrated to desired effect and in an attempt to avoid respiratory depression. If spasms cannot be adequately controlled or if laryngospasm or spasm of the respiratory musculature compromises ventilation, then neuromuscular blockade and mechanical ventilation should be instituted.

• Non-depolarizing neuromuscular blocking agents are usually used. Vecuronium in an initial dose of 0.1 to 0.2 mg/kg IV followed by a continuous infusion or hourly dosing intervals seems to have less cardiovascular effects than other agents.
• Beta-blockers are used as needed to manage hypertension with propranolol in a dose of 0.01 to 0.1 mg/kg every 6 to 8 hours being a popular choice.

PREVENTION

• The mainstays of prevention are good hygiene and aggressive active immunization of all individuals. All wounds should be cleaned thoroughly with soap and water, and foreign bodies should be sought aggressively and removed.
• Tetanus prophylaxis should be initiated at the time of injury in the following manner.

—If the patient has had at least three prior doses of tetanus toxoid no TIG should be given. A dose of tetanus toxoid should be given if it has been greater than 7 years since the last dose or if it has been greater than 5 years and the wound is considered to be dirty or tetanus-prone.
—If the patient has had fewer than three doses of tetanus toxoid, TIG should be given if the wound is considered tetanus-prone. The dose is 250 to 500 U IM. All of these patients should receive tetanus toxoid regardless of the nature of the wound.

Common Questions and Answers

Q: What is a tetanus-prone wound?
A: Deep puncture wounds, wounds causing a large amount of tissue necrosis including crushing wounds, large ragged lacerations, and wounds clearly contaminated with soil or feces are generally considered tetanus-prone. All wounds, including minor wounds such as corneal abrasions, insect bites, small lacerations, and burns, may be inoculated with spores and lead to the development of tetanus.

ICD-9-CM 037.0

BIBLIOGRAPHY

Loscalzo IL, Ryan J, Loscalzo J, et al. Tetanus: a clinical diagnosis. *Am J Emerg Med* 1995; 13:488–490.

Richardson JP, Knight AL. The management and prevention of tetanus. *J Emerg Med* 1993;11:737–742.

Thayaparan B, Nicoll A. Prevention and control of tetanus in childhood. *Curr Opin Pediatr* 1998;10(1):4–8.

Author: James M. Callahan

Tetralogy of Fallot

Database

DEFINITION

• Anatomical sign is anterior malalignment of infundibular septum:

—A large and unrestrictive ventricular septal defect (VSD)
—Various degrees of right ventricular outflow tract obstruction (RVOTO)
—Overriding aorta
—(Resultant) right ventricular hypertrophy (RVH)

PATHOPHYSIOLOGY

Severity of clinical signs and symptoms are dependent on the degree of RVOTO and related right-to-left shunt.

GENETICS

• Some TOF are associated with a chromosome 22q11 microdeletion.
• May be associated with other syndromes including: Down, fetal alcohol, and a variety of limb abnormality syndromes. TOF may also be associated with midline abdominal defects (e.g., omphalocele).

EPIDEMIOLOGY

• 3.5% to 8% of all CHD

COMPLICATIONS

• Paroxysmal hypoxic spells (hypercyanotic spells a.k.a. "tet spell")
• Bacterial endocarditis
• Cerebrovascular accident (CVA) secondary to cyanosis, polycythemia, and microcytic anemia
• Right ventricular dysfunction and ventricular arrhythmia
• Post-operative sudden death (ventricular arrhythmias and/or complete heart block)

PROGNOSIS

• Generally good if treated surgically in a timely manner
• More than 85% of patients with TOF are expected to survive to adulthood.

Differential Diagnosis

TOF should be considered in all infants with heart murmur and/or various degrees of cyanosis and otherwise acyanotic infants or children with history of hypercyanotic spells.

Data Gathering

HISTORY

• Heart murmur in the newborn period.
• Various degrees of progressive cyanosis.
• History of paroxysmal cyanotic especially when crying or with exercise.

Physical Examination

• Various degrees of cyanosis may be present at birth or may appear later during infancy or childhood as a result of progression of the pulmonary stenosis.
• Normal S1 and single loud S2 secondary to an aorta, which is located more anterior than normal.
• Systolic ejection murmur at left upper sternal border secondary to RVOTO

Laboratory Aids

Test: CXR
Significance: Right aortic arch (30%), decreased pulmonary vascular markings, boot-shaped heart ("Coeur en sabot") with concave main pulmonary artery segment.

Test: ECG
Significance: Right axis deviation (+90 to 180 degrees), RVH

IMAGING

Test: Echocardiogram
Significance: Anterior malalignment type VSD, presence of other VSDs, degree of infundibular stenosis, presence of valvar pulmonary stenosis and/or branch pulmonary artery stenosis, overriding aorta, arch sidedness, coronary artery anatomy.

Test: Cardiac catheterization
Significance: Presence of multiple VSDs (other than single malalignment type VSD), degree and levels of stenosis in the RVOT and pulmonary arteries, coronary artery anatomy.

Therapy

MEDICAL

- Hypercyanotic spells:

—Knee-chest position
—Oxygen
—Morphine sulfate (0.1 mg/kg IV or IM)
—Intravenous fluid bolus and/or NaHCO$_3$
—Beta-blocker (propranolol, 0.2 mg/kg IV)
—Phenylephrine (0.02 mg/kg IV)
—Polycythemia: oral Fe supplement
—SBE prophylaxis

SURGICAL

- Palliative surgery: Blalock-Taussig shunt
- Corrective surgery: VSD patch closure and RVOT reconstruction

 ## Follow-Up

PROGNOSIS

- Surgical mortality is quite low in most centers
- Residual hemodynamic abnormalities are quite common:

—Pulmonary insufficiency (with transannular patch repair)
—Residual RVOTO
—RV dysfunction
—LPA stenosis
—Residual VSD

- Conduction abnormalities (complete heart block)
- Supraventricular and ventricular arrhythmias

 ## Common Questions and Answers

Q: What is the etiology of the "tet spell"?
A: There is an increase in obstruction/vasospasm of the RVOT and/or pulmonary vascular bed that leads to a dramatic decrease in pulmonary blood flow and increased right-to-left shunt. Therefore, treatment should be aimed toward increasing pulmonary blood flow either by decreasing pulmonary vascular resistance (O$_2$, morphine) or increasing systemic vascular resistance (knee-chest position, phenylephrine).

Q: When is an optimal time for elective surgical repair of tetralogy of Fallot?
A: Still controversial. At Children's Hospital of Philadelphia, we recommend elective repair of TOF in early infancy (3–6 months).

ICD-9-CM 745.2

BIBLIOGRAPHY

Neches WH, Park SC, Ettedgui JA. Pediatric cardiology. In: *Tetralogy of Fallot and tetralogy of Fallot with pulmonary atresia.* Philadelphia: Lea & Febiger, 1990:1073–1100.

Rosenthal A. Adults with tetralogy of Fallot: repaired, yes; cured, no. *N Engl J Med* 1993;329: 355–356.

Walsh EP, Rockenmacher S, Keane JF, et al. Late results in patients with tetralogy of Fallot repaired during infancy. *Circulation* 1988;77: 1062–1067.

Zuberbuhler JR. *Moss and Adams: Heart diseases in infants, children and adolescents,* 5th ed. Baltimore: Williams & Wilkins, 1995:998–1017.

Author: Pamela S. Ro

Thalassemia

 Database

DEFINITION

• Thalassemia syndromes are hereditary anemias occurring as a result of mutations affecting the synthesis of hemoglobin.
• Normal hemoglobin is a tetramer of two alpha and two beta chains.

—Alpha thalassemia: Decrease or total lack of alpha globin synthesis. See the table Alpha Thalassemia Syndromes.
—Beta thalassemia: Decrease or lack of beta globin synthesis.

PATHOPHYSIOLOGY

• Many different mutations in alpha or beta globin genes can lead to various clinical phenotypes of alpha or beta thalassemia.
• Decrease in either alpha or beta globin synthesis leads to fewer completed $\alpha_2\beta_2$ tetramers produced per red cell leading to decrease in intracellular hemoglobin and microcytosis.
• Unpaired globin chains lead to ineffective erythropoiesis.
• Varying degrees of anemia depending on gene defect.
• Severe alpha thalassemia (HbH): Predominantly hemolytic disorder.
• Severe beta thalassemia

—Predominantly ineffective erythropoiesis and hemolysis.
—Extramedullary: Hematopoiesis leading to hepatosplenomegaly.

• Increased iron absorption from gastrointestinal tract.
• Iron overload of various organs secondary to blood transfusions and iron overload.

CLINICAL CLASSIFICATION

• Silent carrier (alpha or beta)

—Hematologically normal

• Thalassemia trait (alpha or beta)

—Mild anemia with microcytosis and hypochromia

• HbH disease (alpha thalassemia)

—Moderately severe hemolytic anemia, icterus, splenomegaly. May need transfusions.

• Hydrops fetalis (alpha thalassemia)

—Death in utero caused by severe anemia.

• Severe beta thalassemia (Cooley anemia)

—Severe anemia, growth retardation, hepatosplenomegaly bone marrow expansion and bony deformities.

• Thalassemia major

—Transfusion dependent

• Thalassemia intermedia

—No regular transfusions

GENETICS

• α thalassemia

—Each diploid cell normally has four alpha globin genes, two on each chromosome 16.
—Some mutations completely abolish the expression of an alpha globin gene (alpha 0).
—Other mutations decrease the expression of alpha globin gene (alpha +).
—The four alpha thalassemia syndromes reflect the inheritance of molecular defects affecting the output of one, two, three, or four alpha genes.

• β thalassemia

—Each diploid cell normally has two beta globin genes, one on each chromosome 11.
—Many mutations abolish the expression completely (beta 0) while others cause variable decrease in quantitative expression (beta +).
—Heterozygous state for beta globin mutation produces beta thalassemia trait.
—Homozygous state produces beta thalassemia major.
—Ability of individual patients to produce gamma globin, making fetal hemoglobin as a substitute for adult hemoglobin, modulates the clinical severity of both types of thalassemia.

EPIDEMIOLOGY

• α thalassemia

—Predominantly in Chinese subcontinent, Malaysia, Indochina, and Africa and African-American population.

• β thalassemia

—Mediterranean countries, Africa, India, Pakistan, Mideast, and China.

COMPLICATIONS

• Severe α thalassemia: Hydrops fetalis, intrauterine death.
• HbH disease: Severe hemolytic anemia, splenomegaly, hypersplenism.

• β thalassemia major: Poorly transfused patients:

—Skeletal abnormalities due to hyperplastic marrow.
—Growth retardation.
—Congestive heart failure due to severe anemia.

• Well transfused patients with iron overload:

—Endocrine disturbances: delayed puberty, growth retardation, diabetes mellitus, hypothyroidism, hypoparathyroidism.
—Cardiac abnormalities: pericarditis, arrhythmias, congestive heart failure (usually after teenage).
—Hepatic abnormalities: cirrhosis and liver failure (onset after second decade usually).

PROGNOSIS

• Life expectancy has improved over years with regular transfusions and chelation therapy.
• Bone marrow transplant from a histocompatible sibling donor may give the best long-term survival.

 Differential Diagnosis

• β thalassemia trait

—Iron deficiency anemia (Normal HbA$_2$ and HbF and decreased serum iron) and
—Increased HbA$_2$ and HbF and normal serum iron in β thalassemia trait.
—Anemia of chronic disease (Normal HbA$_2$ and HbF).

• α thalassemia trait

—Diagnosis of exclusion in older children.
—Hb Barts in neonatal hemoglobin electrophoresis.
—Familial studies helpful.

 Data Gathering

HISTORY

Question: Age of onset.
Significance: Severe α or β thalassemia. Symptomatic within first year of life.

Question: Pallor?
Significance: Sign of anemia.

Question: Failure to thrive?
Significance: Related to anemia and energy expended in ineffective erythropoiesis.

Question: Abnormal facies (frontal bossing in beta thalassemia)?
Significance: Bone marrow expansion.

Question: Abdominal distention?
Significance: Splenomegaly, hepatomegaly may be massive.

Alpha Thalassemia Syndromes

SYNDROME	CLINICAL FEATURES	ALPHA GLOBIN GENES AFFECTED
Silent carrier	No anemia, normal RBC	1
α thal trait	Mild anemia, hypochromia, microcytosis	2
HbH disease	Moderate anemia, fragmented, hypochromic and microcytic cells	3
Hydrops fetalis	Death in utero due to severe anemia	4

Question: Mediterranean, African or Asian descent?
Significance: Common ethnic background in thalassemia.

Question: Familial history of anemia or chronic transfusions?
Significance: Siblings and/or parents may be affected by a mild syndrome such as thalassemia trait.

Question: Well child with microcytosis?
Significance: Thalassemia trait is usually asymptomatic.

 ## Physical Examination

Finding: Severe pallor
Significance: Onset in first year of life. May present with signs of congestive heart failure due to severe anemia.

Finding: Variable degrees of icterus
Significance: Hemolysis is part of thalassemia.

Finding: Chipmunk facies in untransfused β thalassemia
Significance: Facial bone expansion by hypertrophic marrow.

Finding: Growth retardation
Significance: Common in thalassemia major.

Finding: Variable degrees of hepatosplenomegaly
Significance: Extramedullary hematopoiesis.

Finding: Thalassemia trait
Significance: Mild pallor only

 ## Laboratory Aids

- CBC for anemia, low MCV
- Usually Hb 9 to 10 g/dL in thalassemia trait.
- Hb usually 6 to 7 g/dL in HbH disease.
- Hb usually 7 to 8 g/dL in thalassemia intermedia.
- Hb less than 5 g/dL in thalassemia major.
- RBC indices: MCV, MCH, and MCHC decreased in both α and β thalassemia; RDW increased.
- Peripheral smear for

—Microcytosis and hypochromia.
—Mild aniso and poikilocytosis in thalassemia trait.
—Severe aniso and poikilocytosis in thalassemia major and HbH disease.
—Target cells, teardrop cells and polychromasia.

- Reticulocyte count is usually elevated in thalassemia syndromes.
- Increased indirect bilirubin in severe thalassemia.
- Serum ferritin raised in transfused β thalassemia patients.
- Hemoglobin electrophoresis is silent carrier for a thalassemia (1 abnormal gene) 1% to 2% Barts at birth, disappear in 1 to 2 months.
- α thalassemia trait (2 defective genes): 5% to 10% Hb Barts (gamma 4) at birth, remainder HbA.
- HbH disease (3 defective genes): 5% to 30% HbH (beta 4), remainder HbA.
- Hydrops fetalis (all 4 defective genes) seen mainly Hb Barts.
- β thalassemia trait: HbF 1% to 5%, HbA$_2$ 3.5% to 8%, remainder HbA.
- Thalassemia major: HbF 20% to 100%, HbA$_2$ 2% to 7%, HbA 0% to 80%. In most cases no HbA is detected.

 ## Therapy

- Silent carriers α and β thalassemia trait: Genetic counseling only.
- HbH disease

—Folic acid daily
—Transfusions whenever necessary
—Splenectomy if evidence of hypersplenism

- β thalassemia major

—Regular transfusions of red cells every 3 to 4 weeks to maintain Hb at 9 to 10 g/dL.
—Chelation therapy with Desferroxamine to avoid iron overload.
—Oral iron chelator deferiprone is still under investigation.
—Splenectomy if transfusion requirement more than 200 mL/kg/yr.
—Folic acid daily.
—Penicillin prophylaxis (125–250 mg bid) to all splectomised patients.
—*Pneumococcal* and *H. Influenzae* vaccine prior to splenectomy.
—Cholecystectomy for gallstones.
—No iron supplements.
—Genetic counseling.
—Bone marrow transplantation using histocompatible sibling donor can cure the disease and is being increasingly utilized.

 ## Follow-Up

Transfusion dependent patients need to be transfused every 3 to 4 weeks. Serum ferritin and liver function tests should be done every 3 months. Total iron binding capacity and transferrin saturation should also be measured frequently. Liver biopsy may be needed to assess the status of iron overload.

PREVENTION

Thalassemia can be prevented by identifying and counselling potential parents who can have children with thalassemia. Diagnosis can be made in early pregnancy by chorionic villus sampling.

PITFALLS

Thalassemia trait is often treated presumptively as iron deficiency anemia. Iron studies should be done to confirm the diagnosis if there is no improvement in hemoglobin level after few weeks of iron therapy.

 ## Common Questions and Answers

Q: Is prenatal testing available?
A: Yes.

Q: What would be the optimal age for bone marrow transplant?
A: Optimal age would be around five years before there is evidence of iron overload.

Q: In a transfused patient when does iron overload become a problem and when is chelation started?
A: Usually after age of five years.

ICD-9-CM 282.4

BIBLIOGRAPHY

Piomelli S. The management of patients with Cooley's anemia: transfusions and splenectomy. *Semin Hematol* 1995;32(2):262–268.

Giardina PJ, Hilgartner MW. Update on thalassemia. *Pediatr Rev* 1992;13(2):55–62.

Kazazian HH Jr. Prenatal diagnosis of beta thalassemia. *Semin Pathol* 1991;15(3 Suppl 2): 15–24.

Piomelli S, Loew T. Management of thalassemia major (Cooley's anemia). *Hematol Oncol Clin North Am* 1991;5(3):557–569.

Giardini C. Treatment of beta-thalassemia. *Curr Opin Hematol* 1997;4(2):79–87.

Author: Sadhna M. Shankar

Thyroid Cancer

 ## Database

DEFINITION

- Primary neoplasm arising in the thyroid gland

PATHOPHYSIOLOGY

- Radiation exposure is the only clearly identified causative factor in pediatric thyroid carcinogenesis.
- Etiology of most childhood thyroid carcinomas remain unknown.

GENETICS

- Usually sporadic
- Familial: medullary carcinoma can be familial (autosomal dominant), as part of Multiple Endocrine Neoplasia (MEN)-2A and 2B, or as isolated malignancy.
- Oncogenes and tumor suppressor genes implicated in thyroid cancer:

—RET protooncogene (chromosome 10q): germline mutations in MEN-2A and -2B and familial medullary carcinoma; somatic mutations in sporadic medullary carcinoma and papillary carcinoma.
—Constitutively activating mutation in the TSH receptor: follicular and papillary carcinomas.
—p53: mutations especially in poorly differentiated and anaplastic areas.

EPIDEMIOLOGY

- 0.5% to 1.5% of all malignancies in children and adolescents
- Differentiated thyroid cancer (papillary, follicular): M:F ratio 1:2, median age 12 to 13 years.
- Medullary thyroid carcinoma: M:F ratio 1:2–3, median age 10 years.

PATHOLOGY

- Follicular adenoma: benign
- Follicular, papillary, or mixed carcinoma: well differentiated; follicular 90%
- Medullary carcinoma (4–10% as part of the MEN-2 syndrome)
- In children with solitary nodules: 30% to 40% carcinoma

COMPLICATIONS

Therapy may induce hypothyroidism.

PROGNOSIS

- Course is usually indolent.
- Excellent, especially for well-differentiated follicular cell carcinoma; life expectancy is close to that of the normal population.
- Mortality is most common in medullary and undifferentiated carcinomas, which are relatively rare in children.
- Of medullary thyroid carcinomas, those associated with MEN-2B have the most aggressive coure.

 ## Differential Diagnosis

- Infections: pyogenic, viral, or granulomatous
- Tumors: lymphoma, teratoma
- Congenital: cystadenoma, cystic hygroma, dermoid cyst
- Immunologic: follicular nodules of chronic lymphocytic thyroiditis

 ## Data Gathering

HISTORY

Question: Radiation exposure?
Significance: The only identified etiologic agent of thyroid carcinogenesis in children.

Question: Rapidly enlarging neck mass?
Significance: May be the only presenting syndrome.

Question: Familial history of thyroid carcinoma or MEN syndrome?
Significance: 92% of individuals with MEN-2A or -2B develop medullary thyroid cancer.

 ## Physical Examination

Suggestive of malignancy:

Finding: Solitary nodule
Significance: Of solitary thyroid modules, the percentage that is malignant is higher in the pediatric age group than in the adult group.

Finding: Rock-hard texture
Significance: Neoplastic thyroid tissue often feels firmer on palpation than other types of goiters.

Finding: Irregular borders
Significance: Irregularity may be due to the palpable edge(s) of a thyroid neoplasm.

Finding: Associated anterior cervical adenopathy
Significance: More worrisome for thyroid malignancy with lymphatic metastases.

Laboratory Aids

• T4 and TSH are usually normal.
• Calcitonin levels are elevated in 75% of patients with medullary carcinoma, but may require pentagastrin stimulation to detect elevation in early stages of the disease.

IMAGING

Test: Ultrasound
Significance: Establishes size and presence of cystic areas.

Test: I-123 scan
Significance: Demonstrates functionality. A non-functioning nodule, i.e., does not concentrate iodine, is highly suspicious for malignancy.

FALSE-POSITIVES

• Nodules of chronic lymphocytic thyroiditis

 ## Therapy

• Surgery is recommended for a non-functioning nodule if there is a history of radiation, rapid growth of a firm nodule, satellite lymph nodes, evidence of impingement on other structures in the neck, or evidence of distant metastases.
• The affected lobe is removed and sent for frozen section; if this is suspicious, a total thyroidectomy should be done.
• Following surgery, I-131 therapy is administered if a follow-up iodine scan reveals any residual tissue or metastases.
• Suppressive doses of exogenous thyroid hormone are then given to maintain TSH levels below 0.2 mIU/mL.
• Thyroglobulin levels are useful as markers of thyroid tissue; calcitonin level serves as tumor marker for medullary carcinoma.
• Some advocate subtotal thyroidectomy, no irradiation, and suppressive T4 treatment.

 ## Follow-Up

• Palpation of tissue in the neck area after surgery: monitor for recurrent nodules.
• Elevation of thyroglobulin levels after surgery and ablation suggests residual tissue or recurrence.
• Complications of thyroid surgery include laryngeal nerve damage and hypoparathyroidism.

 ## Common Questions and Answers

Q: Does thyroid cancer usually present with hyperthyroidism?
A: No. The usual chief complaint is a solitary hard, painless nodule in a euthyroid patient.

Q: Is there an increased risk of thyroid cancer from diagnostic x-rays (chest x-rays, lateral neck films)?
A: Routine diagnostic x-rays should fall well below the levels of radiation thought to increase risk of thryoid neoplasia. During more prolonged radiologic procedures that might expose the thyroid to higher doses of radiation, a lead neck shield is used.

Q: Should prophylactic thyroidectomy be performed in children identified genetically as having familial medullary carcinoma?
A: Yes, due to the poorer prognosis associated with development of this cancer.

ICD-9-CM 193

BIBLIOGRAPHY

Feinmesser R, Lubin E, Segal K, Noyek A. Carcinoma of the thyroid in children? A review. *J Pediatr Endocrinol Metab* 1997;10:561–568.

Lafferty AR, Batch JA. Thyroid nodules in childhood and adolescence? Thirty years of experience. *J Pediatr Endocrinol Metab* 1997;10: 479–486.

Skinner MA, Wells SA Jr. Medullary carcinoma of the thyroid gland and the MEN 2 syndromes. *Semin Pediatr Surg* 1997;6:134–140.

Yeh SD, La Quaglia MP. 131I Therapy for pediatric thyroid cancer. *Semin Pediatr Surg* 1997; 6:128–133.

Zimmerman D. Thyroid neoplasia in children. *Curr Opin Pediatr* 1997;9:413–418.

Authors: Adda Grimberg and Marta Satin-Smith

Tibial Torsion

Database

DEFINITION

- Tibial torsion-twisting the tibia (can be associated with femoral torsion)
- Medial or internal tibial torsion (MTF) associated with in-toeing (most common).
- Lateral or external tibial torsion associated with out-toeing.
- Defined as within 2 standard deviations of mean.

CAUSES

- Normal fetal development
- Intrauterine position
- Heredity-familial tendency
- Posturing (sitting position)—cause or effect?
- Associated pathology (e.g., spasticity, fracture malunion or DDH)

PATHOLOGY

- Tibial torsion-twisting the tibia usually medial or internal associated with in-toeing.
- If associated with increased femoral anteversion, may be associated with patello-femoral malalignment (knee cap subluxation)

EPIDEMIOLOGY

- Common and usually normal (i.e., within 2 standard deviations of the mean)

GENETICS

No strong evidence to suggest that is an inherited condition.

COMPLICATIONS

- None proven

PROGNOSIS

- Good; usually not painful, cosmetically unattractive or dysfunctional

Differential Diagnosis

- Look for DDH, spasticity (e.g., mild cerebral palsy)

Data Gathering

HISTORY

- Familial history?

Question: Birth history?
Significance: First born common

Question: Pain, limping?
Significance: May indicate other diagnosis.

Question: Other "packaging" conditions?
Significance: Metatarsus adductus, torticollis, DDH

Question: When first noticed, getting better or worse, functional limitations (i.e., trips and falls frequently)?
Significance: Functional limitations may suggest other diagnosis such as mild cerebral palsy, especially if abnormal birth history or developmental milestones.

Physical Examination

Finding: If ambulatory, watch gait and assess for foot progression angle
Significance: The angle formed between the axis of the foot and the axis of forward progression of gait.

Finding: Also assess other aspects of gait
Significance: Stride, heel-toe gait, cadence, limping, other abnormalities. Unilateral or bilateral torsion.

Finding: Leg length discrepancy, hip abnormalities, contractures, spasticity, thigh foot axis (TFA).
Significance: With the child prone, the knee flexed to 90 degrees and the ankle at neutral measure the difference between the axis of the foot and the axis of the femur. If the thigh-foot axis is internal, this suggests internal tibial torsion; if external, external tibial torsion.

Finding: Transmalleolar axis
Significance: With the child seated and the knee flexed to 90 degrees, assess the malleolar axis in reference to the coronal plane (less reliable than TFA).

Finding: Look for abnormalities of the feet
Significance: Metatarsus adductus or clubfoot may be a primary cause of in-toeing. Significant calcaneovaigus may be a component of out-toeing.

Finding: Careful neurological examination
Significance: To see if in-toeing is related to a mild neurological abnormality, such as mild spastic diplegic cerebral palsy.

SPECIAL QUESTIONS

Physical Examination Tricks

- Normal torsional alignment
- "Torsional profile"

—1: foot-progression angle
—2: medial hip rotation in extension
—3: lateral hip rotation in extension
—4: thigh-foot angle
—5: transmalleolar axis
—6: configuration of the foot

- "Kissing patellae"

—This occurs when bilateral increased femoral anteversion causes the patellae to face one another giving the appearance of kissing patellae.

Laboratory Aids

• Usually not helpful

IMAGING STAGES

Usually not needed. Physical examination gives information needed.

Test: Hip x-ray
Significance: If hip pathology (i.e., DDH) is suspected then may be indicated.

Test: CT
Significance: CT is an accurate way of measuring tibial torsion but there is radiation exposure. An occasional indication may be a patient who is being evaluated for surgery.

Test: MRI
Significance: Techniques for using MRI and ultrasound have also been described but in general are less accurate than CT.

 Therapy

• Observation and familial and patient reassurance (almost always the treatment of choice).
• Devices such as casts, shoe wedges, twister cables, splints, Denis Brown bars have no proven benefit (i.e., they will not change the natural history). They may in fact cause problems such as ligamentous damage to hip, knee, ankle, and foot.
• Reassurance is usually enough. The condition improves spontaneously. Usually corrects enough by 8 years of age.
• Surgery seldom needed.
• Tibial osteotomy: When done is usually a distal supramaleolar osteotomy.

GENERAL TREATMENT MODALITIES

• Observation
• Physical therapy: will not change natural history (it may help with associated patellofemoral malalignment pain)
• Devices: (casts, shoe wedges, twister cables, splints, Denis Brown bars)—no proven benefit
• Tibial osteotomy is seldom, if ever, needed

DRUGS

• Not helpful

 Follow-Up

WHEN TO EXPECT IMPROVEMENT

• Usually corrects enough by 8 years of age

SIGNS TO WATCH FOR

• Should improve with growth and development. There is no substantial evidence that increased femoral anteversion will cause arthritis of the hip or knee (chondromalacia patella).

PROGNOSIS

• Overall, good prognosis for the majority of patients

 Common Questions and Answers

Q: When are special shoes or braces indicated for tibial torsion?
A: Almost never. The situation will improve without treatment in most. There is no strong evidence that any of these treatments truly alters the natural history of the condition.

Q: Why do patients with torsional pathology occasionally have knee pain?
A: Children can have increased femoral anteversion with associated external tibial torsion (i.e., an external rotation of the tibia which matches and in effect balances the internal rotation of the femur). This can be diagnosed by observing the above rotational profile and by noting increased Q-angle. This situation is sometimes a "set up" for patellofemoral pain.

ICD-9-CM 736.89

BIBLIOGRAPHY

Staheli LT. Torsional deformities. *Pediatr Clin North Am* 1977;24:799.

Staheli LT. Lower positional deformity in infants and children: a review. *J Pediatr Orthop* 1990;10:559.

Tolo VT. The lower extremity. In: Morrissy RT and Weinstein SL, eds. *Lovell and Winter's pediatric orthopaedics,* 4th ed. 1996:1047–1075.

Author: John P. Dormans

Tick Fever

Database

DEFINITION

• Relapsing fever in its endemic form is a vector-borne infection with characteristic recurrent fevers caused by several species of spirochetes of the genus *Borrelia*. In the United States the vector for endemic relapsing fever are ticks of the genus *Ornithodoros*. Epidemic relapsing fever is transmitted by the body louse and is no longer found in the United States.

• Colorado tick fever (CTF) is a febrile, usually benign, systemic illness caused by an arbovirus in the family *Reoviridae* and transmitted by ticks in the genus *Dermatocentor*.

CAUSES

• Relapsing fever is caused by several spirochetes in the genus *Borrelia* including *B. hermsii*, *B. parkerii*, and *B. turicatae*. Epidemic relapsing fever (louse-borne) is caused by *B. recurrentis*.

• Colorado tick fever is caused by an arbovirus in the family *Reoviridae*.

PATHOPHYSIOLOGY

• Endemic relapsing fever is characterized by repeated episodes of spirochetemia.

• *Borreliae* are able to undergo plasmid-mediated, antigenic variation. An antibody response against a particular strain leads to immobilization, opsonization, agglutination, and phagocytosis, and symptoms abate. The infecting organism can then again undergo antigenic variation and a recurrent episode of spirochetemia and symptoms occurs. Tick-borne disease may relapse 10 to 12 times before final resolution.

• Transmission of the infecting organism occurs when ticks of the genus *Ornithodoros* take blood meals and then detach themselves. These bites are usually painless, and the tick may remain attached for up to 15 minutes. Ticks are maintained by intermediate hosts including rodents and other small mammals.

• When a tick feeds on an infected individual, spirochetes invade all tissues including the female genital tract. Once infected, ticks remain capable of transmitting disease for many years. In addition, transovarial infection of offspring leads to increased transmission of spirochetes and increased survival.

• In the human host, organisms persist in the central nervous system (CNS), bone marrow, liver, and spleen during remissions. Pathologic findings in humans include petechial hemorrhages on visceral surfaces, hepatosplenomegaly, and a histiocytic myocarditis.

• Pneumonia, CNS hemorrhages, meningitis, disseminated intravascular coagulation (DIC), splenic rupture, hepatic coma, and dysrhythmias may result. Spirochetes may cross the placenta and lead to spontaneous abortion or severe infection in neonates.

• Colorado tick fever (CTF) is acquired when infected, adult ticks of the genus *Dermatocentor* (including *D. andersonii,* the wood tick) attach and ingest a blood meal from a human host instead of porcupines, elk, marmot, or deer (usual hosts).

• Ticks are infected while larvae as they feed on viremic, intermediate hosts such as chipmunks and ground squirrels.

• Aseptic meningitis, encephalitis, myocarditis, atypical pneumonia, epididymoorchitis, and hepatitis have been reported. Generalized hemorrhage and death have been rarely reported in children. Granulocytopenia and thrombocytopenia are often seen.

EPIDEMIOLOGY

• Endemic relapsing fever occurs in the United States among people who are exposed to the habitat of the ticks that serve as vectors. In the United States, most cases are found in the West among people who have spent time in old summer cabins in forested mountain areas. In several series, cabins that were found to be the source of cases contained large rodent nests with infected ticks in them.

• Colorado tick fever is also found among humans who travel to a location where the vector (ticks of the genus *Dermacentor*) is found. The wood tick is found in the Rocky Mountains and Western Black Hills at elevations of 4000 to 10,000 feet. Cases usually occur between April and July when adult ticks are most active. Cases have been reported as early as March and as late as November. Most cases are reported in males, and two-thirds of cases are reported in individuals between age 10 and 49 years old.

COMPLICATIONS

• Relapsing fever may be associated with hepatosplenomegaly with necrotic foci. Diffuse histiocytic interstitial myocarditis may be associated with dysrhythmias. Pneumonia, CNS hemorrhages, splenic rupture, meningitis, DIC, hepatitis, and hepatic coma may result. *In utero* infection may result in fetal loss or severe neonatal infection.

• Treatment may be associated with a marked Jarisch-Herxheimer reaction, which may require intravenous fluids and other supportive measures.

• CTF may lead to aseptic meningitis, encephalitis, myocarditis, atypical pneumonia, hepatitis, and epididymoorchitis. A prolonged convalescence with persistent lassitude, fatiguability, headache, musculoskeletal pain, and fevers may persist for weeks to months in patients who experience persistent viremia.

PROGNOSIS

• Relapsing fever generally responds rapidly to appropriate antibiotic therapy and leaves no significant sequelae. Even when untreated, the vast majority of cases are benign and self-limited. Louse-borne, epidemic relapsing fever in developing countries has been associated with mortality rates of up to 40%.

• CTF resolves without sequelae in most patients. Symptoms may persist for at least 3 weeks in a majority of the patients. Patients older than 30 years old are at a much greater risk of developing prolonged symptoms. Infection usually leads to permanent immunity.

Differential Diagnosis

• Relapsing fever and CTF resemble each other clinically, but leukopenia is more often seen with CTF. Exposure to ticks or a history of travel to an area where appropriate vectors are found is a helpful clue in diagnosing either disease.

• Relapsing fever and CTF may be misdiagnosed as influenza or enteroviral infections.

• Spirochetes may be seen on peripheral blood smears in cases of relapsing fever.

Data Gathering

HISTORY

Question: Fever?
Significance: Endemic relapsing fever has a sudden onset of high fever after an incubation period of 5 to 11 days. Patients complain of chills, headache, and myalgias. Symptoms resolve after 3 to 6 days but then recur within several days. Repeated recurrences continue with decreasing severity and lengthening periods of lack of symptoms. CTF has a usual incubation period of 4 days (range, 1–14 days). There is a history of tick exposure in 90% of patients. Patients complain of abrupt onset of fever, chills, fatigue, headache, myalgias, photophobia, and stiff neck.

Question: Headache?
Significance: Patients may complain of headache, photophobia, stiff neck, and rash, which usually begins on the trunk. There may be epistaxis.

Question: Other symptoms of CTF?
Significance: Gastrointestinal symptoms, pharyngitis, and rash may be noted by some patients.

Question: How long do symptoms of CTF last?
Significance: In about one-half of patients symptoms resolve after 2 to 4 days and then recur after 1 to 3 days. Symptoms then last for another 2 to 3 days. Some patients will have a third symptomatic period, whereas others will only have the initial symptomatic period.

Physical Examination

Finding: High fever
Significance: In relapsing fever patients have high fevers (39–41°C).

Finding: Tender hepatosplenomegaly
Significance: Is characteristic.

Finding: A macular rash
Significance: May be seen on the trunk in approximately 10% of cases, but it may fade quickly or become generalized or petechial.

Finding: Meningismus and signs of iridocyclitis
Significance: May be seen.

Finding: CTF
Significance: Patients with CTF have mostly nonspecific findings. There are often signs of CNS involvement or meningismus. Myalgias and muscle tenderness are usually seen.

Laboratory Aids

Test: Peripheral blood smear
Significance: In relapsing fever the diagnosis is often made when spirochetes are noted on a peripheral blood smear. Increased sensitivity can be obtained by examining dehemoglobinized thick smears or buffy coat preparations.

Test: Weil-Felix agglutination tests
Significance: May be positive but are nonspecific. Indirect fluorescent antibody tests are more sensitive but may be falsely positive in cases of Lyme disease.

Test: Specific test for relapsing fever
Significance: Intraperitoneal inoculation of immature laboratory mice with infected blood leads to spirochetemia in the mice and is a specific and sensitive diagnostic tool.

Test: Non-specific laboratory findings
Significance: Include thrombocytopenia, hyperbilirubinemia, and elevated hepatic transaminases.

Test: Electrocardiograms and chest roentgenogram
Significance: Should be performed to exclude the possibility of myocarditis.

Test: Diagnostic test for CTF
Significance: May be confirmed by serologic testing, immunofluorescence testing for viral antigens on the surface of red blood cells, or by viral culture.

Test: Associated laboratory findings in CTF
Significance: Include leukopenia and thrombocytopenia. Initially, both granulocytopenia and lymphopenia occur. Lymphopenia resolves first, and an atypical lymphocytosis may occur.

Test: CSF studies in CTF
Significance: Pleocytosis may be found, especially in children.

Therapy

DRUGS

• Endemic relapsing fever may be treated with oral tetracycline (in patients greater than 8 years of age) or erythromycin at doses of 40 mg/kg/d in four divided doses for 10 days.
• Patients who are symptomatic at the time treatment is begun are at significant risk of developing the Jarisch-Herxheimer reaction (severe fevers, rigors, sweating, hypotension, and prostration) related to rapid clearing of the spirochetemia. In symptomatic patients it is suggested that treatment is initiated with a single dose of oral phenoxymethyl penicillin (7.5 mg/kg) or intravenous penicillin G (10,000 U/kg given over 30 minutes). These therapies should lead to a slower clearing of the organisms and a less severe reaction.
• Close observation, intravenous fluids, and good supportive care are important in treating possible reactions.
• When the patient is afebrile, a course of tetracycline or erythromycin should be completed to prevent relapse, which has been associated with the use of penicillin alone.
• There is no specific therapy for patients with CTF. Good supportive care is usually all that is required.

PREVENTION

• Both of these diseases can be prevented by avoidance or elimination of the vector.
• Dwellings should be made of rodent-proof construction. Rodent-nesting materials should be removed from buildings where this is not possible.
• Light-colored, long-sleeved shirts, and long trousers with legs tucked inside of one's socks should be worn when infested areas cannot be avoided. Persons should inspect themselves and each other frequently for adherent ticks.
• Confirmed cases should be reported to health authorities so control measures can be instituted.

ICD-9-CM 066.1

BIBLIOGRAPHY

Boyer KM. Borrelia: relapsing fever. In: Feigin RD, Cherry JD, eds. *Textbook of pediatric infectious disease,* 3rd ed. Philadelphia: WB Saunders, 1992:1058–1062.

Doan-Wiggins L. Tick-borne diseases. *Emerg Med Clin North Am* 1991;9:303–325.

Tsai TF. Arboviral infections in the United States. *Infect Dis Clin North Am* 1991;5:73–102.

Author: James M. Callahan

Tics

Database

DEFINITION

Tics are rapid, irregular stereotyped movement (motor tics) or vocalizations (vocal tics) that are under partial voluntary control. The movements usually involve the muscles of the face, neck, and shoulder. Tics are often (but not always) brought on by stress and excitement. They typically occur in clusters, and they can be simple or complex. Simple motor tics are blinking; grimacing; neck, arm, or leg jerking; shoulder shrugging; etc. Simple vocal tics include coughing, grunting, barking, yelping, etc. Complex motor tics include jumping, smelling objects, shaking wrists, copropraxia, and echopraxia. Complex vocal tics include coprolalia, echolalia, and neologism.

- GTS is defined as a condition of chronic vocal and motor tics of more than 1 year duration.
- Typical onset in childhood with motor tics followed by vocalizations (grunts, snorts, barks) later in adolescence 50% to 60% develop coprolalia and echolalia. Obsessive-compulsive behavior, attention deficits, learning disabilities, and sleep disorders are also frequently seen.
- The natural history of GTS is exacerbation of tics in adolescence, with 80% of children improving as they reach adulthood. The lifetime prevalence in GTS has been estimated to be between 0.1 and 1.0 in 1000.

PATHOPHYSIOLOGY

- The pathophysiology of tics or Gilles de la Tourette syndrome (GTS) is not known.
- Most theories regarding GTS have implicated abnormalities in central dopaminergic transmission, but other neurotransmitters such as serotonin and norepinephrine as well as sex hormones have been implicated.

GENETICS

No single gene has been associated with tics or GTS. However, tics are frequently seen in families and GTS may be transmitted as an autosomal dominant trait.

EPIDEMIOLOGY

- Tics can occur in any age group from 2 years up.
- Simple motor tics are considered a part of normal development and occur in 10% to 20% of all school-aged children.
- There is no gender or race preference.
- The average age of onset is 7 years.

COMPLICATIONS

- Tics are usually harmless. However, in patients with complex motor tics that persist for years they may develop repetitive motion injuries with arthritic changes of the neck and spine resulting in increased risk of radiculopathy, disc herniation, and myelopathy.
- Children with tics and particularly GTS are often teased by their peers and have difficulty with social adjustments, isolation, and depression. Co-morbid learning difficulties may also contribute to these problems.

PROGNOSIS

Most children outgrow their tics within a year. If the tics last longer than 1 year they may remain as a simple tic disorder or develop into GTS.

Differential Diagnosis

- Movements resembling tics include

—Hemifacial spasm: a spastic contraction of one-half the muscles of the face. Frequency varies from occasional to constant, but the spasm usually lasts longer than a tic; results from:
  —Abnormal activity in the facial nerve
  —Aberrant regeneration after a Bell palsy
  —Arteriovenous malformation
  —Aneurysms
  —Brainstem or posterior fossa tumors
  —Idiopathic
—Myoclonus: may be difficult to differentiate as this movement can be very fast.
—Myokymia: fine repetitive, arrhythmic twitching of muscle bundles around eyes and lips; (benign and common, although severe myokymia can be seen in posterior fossa tumors, Guillain-Barré syndrome, and severe multiple sclerosis (MS).
—Paroxysmal dyskinesia: often familial, movement is more sustained and complex, may be triggered by movement.
—Partial epilepsy: may look like a tic disorder, but there is no voluntary control; EEG may show corresponding abnormalities
—Tremors: simple tics can resemble tremor; tics are more variable and lack the oscillatory appearance of tremor.
—Sleep myoclonus: tics do not occur during sleep; erratic movements during sleep are most commonly benign sleep myoclonus.

Data Gathering

HISTORY

Good tic records help to adjust medication appropriately.

- When did the first tic occur?
- What exacerbates and alleviates the tics?
- History of vocal tics (including throat-clearing, coughing, grunting, sniffing)?
- Is there some degree of voluntary control?
- Have the tics changed in character?
- Is there any other associated behavior in the child, e.g., attention deficit/hyperactivity disorder, obsessive-compulsive disorder, sleep disorders?
- Does anyone else in the family have tics?

Physical Examination

- General and neurological examinations are unrevealing. Spontaneous movements or vocalizations may be absent during the visit.
- Often the child can reproduce the tic at will.

Laboratory Aids

Because tics are generally not a symptom of an underlying brain disorder, laboratory testing is usually not indicated.

Test: MRI of the brain
Significance: Not necessarily indicated, but should be normal.

Test: EEG
Significance: May be helpful if there is a concern of partial seizures.

Test: Psychological testing
Significance: May be the most useful ancillary assessment (if any is testing is to be done) because of high incidence of associated learning disabilities, attention deficit/hyperactivity disorder, obsessive-compulsive disorder.

Therapy

Decision to treat is based on the severity of tics/vocalizations as reported by the child and parent. Medications are not needed in the majority of children with simple tics. Learning and attention difficulties associated with GTS may be the primary focus of attention.

• Haloperidol: started at 0.5 mg qhs and increased each week to effect. A usual maintenance dose is 1 to 3 mg/d divided bid. Side effects include sedation, irritability, decreased appetite, rare neuroleptic malignant syndrome, tardive dyskinesia. Risperdal has similar pharmacodynamic properties to Haloperidol and is useful in treatment of GTS but appears to have significantly fewer side effects.
• Pimozide: started at 2 mg/d divided bid, increased 2 mg q week to effect. Maintenance dose is 0.2 mg/kg/d or 10 mg (whichever is less); side effects similar to haloperidol.
• Clonidine: started at 0.05 mg/d, increased 0.05 q week. Maintenance is 0.1 to 0.6 mg/d. Sedation is the main side effect; rebound hypertension is a concern if withdrawn rapidly.
• Alternatives include fluphenazine, clonazepam (primarily used as an anticonvulsant; may cause sedation), and desipramine (primarily used as an antidepressant; potential for arrhythmia).
• Clomipramine may improve associated obsessive-compulsive behavior.
• SSRIs including fluoxetine, may be useful for tics, GTS, particularly when co-morbid obsessive-compulsive symptoms are a problem.
• CNS stimulants used for attention deficits, such as ritalin, may exacerbate tics, or be associated with onset of tics, though they do not appear to cause tic disorder per se, and are not strictly contraindicated for patients with GTS.
• Biofeedback and behavioral modification have been recommended.

 Follow-Up

The tics in GTS often become refractory to medication after prolonged use. May help to switch to another drug or to alternate between two drugs.

PREVENTION

Tics can not be prevented. However, social isolation, adjustment difficulties and depression can be prevented or minimized by informing teachers, sport coaches and other caretakers of the child's condition.

PITFALLS

Avoid exclusive focus on the tics in a child: is he or she adjusting in school, is there a learning disability, does he or she have friends, are there other stressors in the family? GTS is frequently misdiagnosed—there is an approximate 10-year interval between onset of symptoms and treatment.

 Common Questions and Answers

Q: My child just started school and now she blinks excessively. When I tell her to stop it just gets worse. What can I do?
A: Tics are considered part of normal development, they can last anywhere from a few weeks to a year, and they usually disappear if you ignore them. If they last longer than a year they are probably not a simple tic and you should contact your doctor. If there is any concern of eye irritation or a visual disturbance an ophthalmological checkup is appropriate.

Q: Our son has been diagnosed with GTS, his tics are increasing in frequency, and now he has developed vocalizations with obscenities. He has already lost his friends in school and was suspended twice last week because of his foul mouth. I tell him to stop but he does not listen. What should I do?
A: Children with GTS cannot control their vocalizations. Swearing is not intentional. Telling a child to control his vocalizations will only increase the level of anxiety and increase the tics. Once a child has been diagnosed with GTS (particularly if vocalizations are present) it may help to inform teachers, school personnel, and peers about the disease so that misunderstandings can be minimized and the child can feel comfortable at school. A review of medication with the child's physician (child psychiatrist or neurologist) is appropriate.

BIBLIOGRAPHY

Anouti A, Koller WC. Diagnostic testing in movement disorders. *Neurol Clin* 1996;14(1):169–182.

Kurlan R. Tourette syndrome. Treatment of tics. *Neurol Clin* 1997;1592:403–409.

Lumar R, Lang AE. Tourette syndrome. Secondary tic disorders. *Neurol Clin* 1997;15(2):309–331.

Author: A.G. Christina Bergqvist

Toddler's Diarrhea

 Database

DEFINITION

• Chronic diarrhea lasting at least 3 to 4 weeks in a child between 1 and 5 years of age, in a child who is normally active and growing well. Abdominal pain may be present; straining, eating and sleeping problems are not part of the syndrome. The condition is also known as chronic nonspecific diarrhea and may follow a gastroenteritis.

CAUSES

• Excess fruit juice intake usually leading to carbohydrate intolerance due to excess fructose and sorbitol.
• Motility disorder, i.e., variant of irritable bowel syndrome of infancy.
• Diet that is high in fluid but low in fat and fiber.

PATHOPHYSIOLOGY

• Chronic non-specific diarrhea is often preceded by acute gastroenteritis or other viral infection that results in dietary restrictions. Increased oral fluids, including juices are used to stay ahead of stool losses and prevent dehydration.
• Carbohydrate malabsorption

—Capacity of small intestine to absorb fructose is limited. Foods that contain equivalent amounts of fructose and glucose are more readily absorbed because of the additive effect of a glucose-dependent fructose co-transport mechanism. An excess of fructose over glucose will result in fructose malabsorption by the small intestine.
—Sorbitol is non-absorbable and inhibits fructose absorption and may cause gastrointestinal symptoms.
—Excessive intake of juices high in sorbitol and those with a high fructose to glucose ratio will result in fructose malabsorption and gastrointestinal symptoms.

• Motility disorder:

—Persistence of immature bowel motility pattern. There is failure of initiation of normal postprandial delayed gastric emptying and rapid transit due to persistence of small-bowel fasting motility pattern.
—Meals with high dietary fat delay gastric emptying. High fluid low fat meals will lack this benefit.

• Low fiber diet

—Dietary fiber (pectin) important for purpose of binding water to help form solid stools.

GENETICS

Familial members often report non-specific gastrointestinal complaints or functional bowel disorders.

EPIDEMIOLOGY

It is the most common cause of prolonged diarrhea without FTT in children.

PROGNOSIS

• Good

 Differential Diagnosis

All causes of diarrhea without malnutrition should be considered.

• Infection: Giardiasis, cryptosporidiosis, bacterial gastroenteritis, and bacterial overgrowth.
• Congenital: Cystic fibrosis, sucrase-isomaltase deficiency.
• Immunological: Celiac disease, Cow's milk-sensitive enteropathy, food allergy (multiple).
• Miscellaneous: Post-infectious enteropathy, constipation, and hormone secreting tumors like Vasoactive intestinal peptide (VIP)-oma, neuroblastoma, laxatives, Munchausen-by-proxy.

 Data gathering

HISTORY

Question: Detailed history
Significance: Essential with special attention to the "four Fs": fiber, fluid, fat, and fruit juices.

Question: Chronic diarrhea
Significance: Usually chronic diarrhea is preceded by a gastroenteritis.

Question: Stool characteristics
Significance: Typically first stool of the day is large and has better consistency than those occurring later on in the day.

Question: Timing of diarrhea
Significance: Usually no stools passed at night.

Question: Stools foul smelling and undigested food particles
Significance: Usually present due to very rapid transit.

Question: Physical appearance
Significance: Children healthy appearing, eat well, growing normally although weight might be influenced by the dietary measures.

Question: Are other children affected?
Significance: Presence of other affected family members or day care mates makes infectious etiology more likely.

Physical Examination

Finding: Normal
Significance: Although weight might be influenced by the dietary practices and measures.

 ## Laboratory Aids

Test: Stool culture
Significance: Usually normal.

Test: Infectious work-up
Significance: Negative.

Test: Stool test
Significance: Negative for WBC and blood.

Test: CBC normal
Significance:

Test: Serum electrolytes normal.
Significance:

 ## Therapy

DIET

• The child's feeding pattern should be normalized according to the "four Fs"

—Over consumption of fruit juices should be discouraged, especially those that contain sorbitol and a high fructose to glucose ratio.
—Fiber intake should be normalized by introduction of whole meal bread and fruits.
—Increase dietary fat to at least 35% to 40% of total energy intake. Substitution of low-fat milk with whole milk may be sufficient.
—Restrict fluid intake to less than 150 cc/kg/d.

• Improvement occurs within a few days to a couple of weeks after initiating the above therapy. Parental reassurance is confirmed by good response to dietary therapy.

MEDICATIONS

• Not routinely recommended and should be left to specialist's discretion. Loperamide and aspirin have been successfully used to normalize bowel patterns in cases refractory to dietary therapy but should be discouraged.

REFERRAL

• Failure of response to the above therapy
• Weight loss despite adequate intake
• Presence of other symptoms like anorexia, irritability, fever, and vomiting
• Blood and mucus in diarrhea

TESTS TO PREPARE FOR CONSULTATION

• Sweat chloride, Celiac disease panel (antigliadin and antiendomysial antibodies), serum albumin, sedimentation rate, stool Sudan III stain for fecal fat

SPECIAL INSIGHTS

• It is important to take a good history because all the illnesses in the DDx are associated with morbidity, if diagnosis is delayed.
• Consider constipation, if diarrhea alternates with normal or hard stools. KUB will show colonic fecal retention.
• Need to make follow-up phone call to parents within a few days of instituting diet. If no improvement within a week despite good compliance with dietary recommendations then rethink diagnosis and consider referral to a specialist.
• Improvement with dietary changes confirms the diagnosis and also reassures the parents.
• Excessive fruit juice consumption has been linked to decreased weight and height, and also obesity in children. It is prudent to limit its consumption to less than 12-fl oz./d.

 ## Common Questions and Answers

Q: Is growth normal in a patient with toddler's diarrhea?
A: Growth is usually normal; weight may be mildly influenced by the prior dietary practices and measures and failure to thrive has also been reported recently.

Q: What are the components of a successful treatment plan?
A: Attention to the "four F's": Decreased fruit juice intake, increased fat intake, decreased fluid, and increased fiber intake

Q: When should care by a pediatric gastroenterologist be sought?
A: If no response after 2 weeks of compliance with dietary therapy, growth delay or other gastrointestinal or systemic complaints

BIBLIOGRAPHY

Dennison BA. Fruit juice consumption by infants and children: a review. *J Am Coll Nutr* 1996;15(5 Suppl):4S–11S.

Hamdi I, Dodge JA. Toddler diarrhoea: observations on the effects of aspirin and loperamide. *J Pediatr Gastroenterol Nutr* 1985;4:362–365.

Hoekstra JH, Van den Aker JHL, Kneepkens CMF, et al. Evaluation of $^{13}CO_2$ breath tests for the detection of fructose malabsorption. *J Lab Clin Med* 1996;127(3):303–309.

Kneepkens CMF, Hoekstra JH. Chronic nonspecific diarrhea of childhood. *Pediatr Clin North Am* 1996;43:375–390.

Lifshitz F, Ament ME, Kleinman RE, et al. Role of juice carbohydrate malabsorption in chronic nonspecific diarrhea in children. *J Pediatr* 1992;120:825–829.

Author: Timothy A.S. Sentongo

Toxic Shock Syndrome (TSS)

 Database

DEFINITION

• Classic TSS is caused by TSS toxin-1 (TSST-1) producing strains of *Staphylococcus aureus*. Strains which do not produce TSST-1, coagulase-negative staphylococci, and Streptococcus pyogenes strains producing pyrogenic exotoxin A (SPE-A) have also been implicated.
• Acute febrile illness characterized by myalgia, vomiting, diarrhea, pharyngitis, diffuse desquamating macular erythroderma, mucous membrane and conjunctival erythema, multiorgan system involvement by direct inflammatory damage or ischemia, disseminated intravascular coagulopathy, and frequently hypotension.
• CDC criteria for diagnosis of staphylococcal TSS:

—Fever 38.9°C or higher
—Diffuse macular erythroderma
—Desquamation 1 to 2 weeks after onset, particularly of palms and soles
—Hypotension below fifth percentile for children, or orthostatic changes greater than 15 mm Hg or orthostatic syncope or dizziness
—Involvement of three or more organ systems: gastrointestinal, muscular, mucous membrane, renal, hepatic, hematologic or neurological

All five of these with negative blood cultures except for *S. aureus* and negative serology for RMSF, leptospirosis and measles. Four of five criteria termed "probable." Four criteria plus death prior to desquamation yields complete syndrome.

Proposed case definition of the CDC Working Group of Severe Streptococcal Infections:

• Hypotension or shock.
• Any two of the following: renal impairment, disseminated intravascular coagulopathy, thrombocytopenia, hepatic impairment, adult respiratory distress syndrome, erythematous macular rash that may desquamate, soft-tissue necrosis.
• Associated risk factors:

—Superabsorbent tampon use
—Local staphylococcal or streptococcal infection
—Surgical wounds
—Diaphragm or contraceptive sponge use
—Childbirth and abortion

PATHOPHYSIOLOGY

• TSST-1 causes extensive interstitial edema of all tissues and minimal perivascular mononuclear cellular infiltrate either directly or through cytokine (e.g., interleukin-1 and tumor necrosis factor) induction.
• Streptococcal toxins probably act similarly.
• TSST-1 acts as a superantigen, with extensive non-specific activation of lymphocytes through the T cell receptor. This activation results in an expansion of lymphocytes, the secretion of interleukin-1, tumor necrosis factor, and interleukin-2.

• These cytokines, as well as the TSST-1 toxin itself, act to decrease peripheral vascular resistance with its resultant interstitial edema. Intravascular volume becomes increasingly depleted and hypotension develops.
• An early sign of decreased intravascular volume is tachycardia out of proportion to the child's fever. This tachycardia is an attempt to increase tissue perfusion by increasing cardiac output.
• Direct toxin effects and resultant inflammatory infiltration of the myocardium may produce decreased contractility, with cardiogenic shock as the result.
• Additionally, activation of coagulation and thrombolytic enzyme systems promote a consumptive coagulopathy, requiring transfusions of blood, platelets, and fresh frozen plasma.

EPIDEMIOLOGY

• Early 1980s: over 90% of cases occurred in menstruating females; associated with "superabsorbent" tampon use. The frequency of cases occurring in menstruating females dropped in the mid-1980s because of changes to less absorbent or different composition tampons.
• Currently, 60% of cases occur in females.
• Mean age: 22 years
• Slightly higher incidence among whites
• Current incidence of menses-related disease: 1 to 5 per 100,000 women of menstrual age per year

COMPLICATIONS

Multi-system organ failure secondary to distributive shock/hypotension including:

• Pulmonary edema
• Disseminated intravascular coagulopathy (DIC)
• Renal failure (oliguric and non-oliguric); permanent renal damage extremely rare
• Hepatic failure
• Myocardial edema and decreased contractility, with or without arrhythmias
• "Stunned" myocardium demonstrating severe ventricular contractile dysfunction
• Cerebral edema with toxic or ischemic encephalopathy
• Metabolic disturbances
• Telogen effluvium; temporary hair and nail loss
• Neuropsychologic disturbances including memory loss; abnormal EEG rare

PROGNOSIS

• Recurrences are associated with inadequate treatment (parenteral antibiotics).
• Mortality approximately 7% for staphylococcal disease. Myocardial and pulmonary failure are the most common causes of death.
• Mortality higher in non-menstrual TSS due to delayed recognition.
• Death usually occurs within the first few days; may occur as late as 2 weeks following onset.

 Differential Diagnosis

• Septic shock due to *Neisseria meningitidis*
• Streptococcal and staphylococcal scarletiniform eruptions
• Leptospirosis
• Rocky Mountain Spotted Fever (RMSF) without characteristic rash
• Fulminant viral infection (e.g., adenovirus)
• Kawasaki disease although TSS may present simultaneously with Kawasaki disease. Coronary artery dilatation has been reported in cases presenting as TSS.
• Toxic epidermal necrolysis

 Data Gathering

HISTORY

• Risk factors include tampon, contraceptive sponge, and/or diaphragm use; surgical or non-surgical wounds, burns, childbirth, abortion or puerperal infections.
• Other active streptococcal or staphylococcal infections?
• Abrupt onset of high fever, chills, malaise, headache, pharyngitis, myalgias, fatigue, vomiting, diarrhea, abdominal pain, and dizziness or syncope?
• Diffuse erythroderma, severe watery diarrhea (often with fecal incontinence), decreased urine output, and altered mental status ensues 24 to 48 hours following the "influenza-like" prodrome experienced by 20% of patients.
• Review tampon package for ingredients, such as polyacrylate, polyester foam, cross-linked carboxymethylcellulose; or claim of "superabsorbency."

 Physical Examination

• Signs of soft tissue infections such as cellulitis, necrotizing fasciitis, myositis, soft-tissue abscesses, sinusitis.
• Moderately to severely ill appearance.
• Tachycardia, tachypnea, orthostasis or frank hypotension.
• Fever, erythroderma, muscle tenderness, peripheral cyanosis and edema, bulbar conjunctival hyperemia, subconjunctival hemorrhages, beefy red mucous membranes.
• Altered mental status including somnolence, agitation, disorientation, obtundation within 24 to 72 hours.
• Erythroderma may be most intense surrounding the infected focus (e.g., perineum).
• Flaky desquamation begins on trunk and extremities 5 to 7 days after symptom onset.
• Full thickness desquamation of fingers, toes, palms, and soles begins 10 to 12 days after onset.
• Vesicle or bullae formation presence of violaceous hue, are ominous findings.
• Tachycardia is the prelude to hypotension.

Laboratory Aids

Test: Antibodies to TSST-1
Significance: Will be positive several weeks after acute presentation.

Test: CBC
Significance: Usually reveals thrombocytopenia early in the course of disease, thrombocytosis during the recovery phase, anemia early in disease, normal or slightly elevated leukocyte count with left shift and absolute lymphopenia. Neutropenia is more ominous than lymphopenia.

Test: Blood cultures
Significance: Positive in 60% of streptococcal TSS; rarely positive in staphylococcal TSS.

Test: Local cultures
Significance: S. aureus may be isolated from vagina or cervix in menstrual TSS, from other infectious focus in non-menstrual cases. Isolation of group A streptococci from a sterile site is a definite case while isolation from a nonsterile site constitutes a probable case.

Test: Coagulation studies
Significance: May reveal prolonged prothrombin and partial thromboplastin times (PT/PTT) with or without evidence of DIC; low fibrinogen, elevated fibrin degradation products.

Test: Urinalysis
Significance: May reveal sterile pyuria.

Test: Lumbar puncture
Significance: May reveal CSF pleocytosis.

Test: Chemistry panel
Significance: May show elevated BUN/creatinine, abnormal liver enzymes and elevated bilirubin, hypoproteinemia, hypocalcemia, and/or hypophosphatemia.

Test: Creatinine phosphokinase
Significance: May be elevated reflecting skeletal muscle involvement.

Therapy

- Aggressive fluid resuscitation and often vasopressors in severe cases.
- Dialysis in cases with renal failure.
- Correction of coagulopathy and anemia with plasma and blood products.
- Ventilatory support in cases with adult respiratory distress syndrome.
- Removal of all foreign bodies.
- Surgical debridement with myositis and necrotizing fasciitis; abscess drainage.

- Antibiotics: parenteral administration of anti-streptococcal and staphylococcal therapy; eradicates source of the toxin, but does not affect the course of the acute illness. Continue therapy for 10 to 15 days or until causative bacteria are eradicated on follow-up cultures. Semi-synthetic anti-staphylococcal penicillins (i.e., nafcillin, oxacillin, dicloxacillin; and cefuroxime or ampicillin/sulbactam).
- Clindamycin, erythromycin if penicillin allergic (clindamycin may have theoretical advantage over penicillin for streptococcal TSS). Some advocate simultaneous use of clindamycin with semi-synthetic penicillins in face of TSS without clear etiologic agent.
- Intravenous immunoglobulin: anecdotal reports of efficacy for streptococcal TSS.
- Corticosteroids: have not been systematically studied.

Follow-Up

- Poor prognosis is often heralded by development of pulmonary edema, falling cardiac index and rising pulmonary capillary wedge pressure.
- Renal failure and cerebral edema (complication of fluid resuscitation) are other indications of complicated course.
- Temperature usually returns to normal within 2 days.
- Toxin-mediated cardiomyopathy should resolve if fatal arrhythmia does not occur during decompensated stage.
- Gastrointestinal, hepatic, and musculoskeletal changes resolve rapidly with rare permanent sequelae except for muscle weakness.
- Hair and nail loss may occur 4 to 16 weeks after illness onset; should resolve within 5 to 6 months.
- Encephalopathy is common, rarely causes seizures; both usually resolve within 4 to 5 days.

PREVENTION

- Avoidance of tampon use after first episode of TSS.
- Scrupulous wound care.
- Limitation of intravaginal foreign body use (tampon, sponge, etc.) and strict adherence to manufacturer directions.

PITFALLS

- *S. aureus* isolated from nares or vagina may represent a false positive finding because 10% to 30% of individuals are healthy carriers.
- The production of TSST-1 by isolate is only presumptive evidence unless case meets diagnostic criteria.
- Failure to meet CDC diagnostic criteria.
- Failure to identify soft-tissue or muscular site of local infection.
- Failure to identify or remove foreign body.
- Erythroderma may not be appreciated if already hypotensive.

Common Questions and Answers

Q: Can TSS recur?
A: Yes. Inadequate eradication of the nidus of infection, such as sinusitis or a foreign body, may promote TSS recurrence. Also, individuals with some immune system defects may develop recurrent TSS.

Q: Is there a test that proves TSS?
A: No, even if TSST-1 antibodies are present, they do not prove TSS unless criteria for the case definition are met.

Q: Can TSS be diagnosed in persons who have no risk factors?
A: Yes, there have been reports meeting the case definition where none of the known associated factors were present.

ICD-9-CM 040.89

BIBLIOGRAPHY

American Academy of Pediatrics. Group A Streptococcal infections. In: Peter G, ed. *1997 red book: report of the committee on infectious diseases,* 24th ed. Elk Grove Village, IL: American Academy of Pediatrics; 1997:483–494.

Ayoub EM, Ahmed S. Update on the complication of group A streptococcal infections. *Curr Probl Pediatr* 1997;27:90–101.

Bisno AL, Stevens DC. Streptococcal infection of skin and soft-tissues. *N Engl J Med* 1996; 334:240–245.

Crew JR, Harrison K, Corey RG, Steenbergen C, Bashore TM. Stunned myocardium in the toxic shock syndrome. *Ann Intern Med* 1992;117: 912–913.

Todd JK. Pathogenesis of toxic-shock syndrome: clinical bacteriologic correlates. *Surv Synth Pathol Res* 1984;3:63–72.

Todd JK. Therapy of toxic-shock syndrome. *Drugs* 1990;39:856–861.

Todd JK, Fishaut M, Kapral F, et al. Toxic-shock syndrome associated with phage-group-1 staphylococci. *Lancet* 1978;2:1116.

Authors: Daniel H. Conway and Mark L. Bagarazzi

Toxoplasmosis

 Database

DEFINITION

Toxoplasma gondii is an intracellular protozoan parasite with a complex life cycle, whose definitive host is the cat. In addition to causing asymptomatic infection and clinical disease in humans, the organism is capable of causing asymptomatic and symptomatic infections in a wide range of mammals and birds.

PATHOPHYSIOLOGY

• Toxoplasmosis is acquired by the ingestion of oocysts or intact viable tissue cysts in inadequately cooked meat.
• After ingestion, the oocysts and cysts are disrupted by the digestive process, and viable infective organisms cross the gastrointestinal lining. Hematologic spread leads to infection of multiple organs, most notably the heart, skeletal muscle, and the brain. There, slowly growing or dormant cysts remain for the patient's lifetime.
• Congenital toxoplasmosis generally occurs during a primary maternal infection. An exception may be when the pregnant woman is severely immunocompromised; congenital infection has occurred in offspring of HIV-infected women with latent toxoplasmosis infection.
• Primary infection in the first trimester is associated with a higher incidence of symptomatic congenital disease, though the majority of congenital infections occur late in pregnancy, and the neonates have subclinical infection at birth. Overall, 30% to 40% of infants born to mothers with primary infection during pregnancy will be congenitally infected.

EPIDEMIOLOGY

• The rate of acquired infection, usually asymptomatic, varies widely through the world and increases with age.
• Seroprevalence rates among pregnant women vary from 4% to 80% worldwide; in the United States rates range from 3% to 35%.
• Worldwide, the incidence of congenital infection ranges from 1 to 7/1000 live births; in the United States incidence is estimated at 0.1 to 1/1000 live births.
• 70% to 90% of children with congenital toxoplasmosis are asymptomatic at birth. Late sequelae (chorioretinitis, mental retardation, seizures, sensorineural hearing loss) occur in greater than 50% of untreated infants considered asymptomatic at birth.

COMPLICATIONS

• Congenital infection: retardation, retinitis, hydrocephalus, seizures, microcephaly, sensorineural hearing loss.
• Acquired infection (all rare): adenopathy, mononucleosis-like syndrome, myocarditis, pneumonia, meningitis/encephalitis.

PROGNOSIS

• Majority of acquired infections are asymptomatic or associated with mild short-lived symptoms.
• Majority of congenital infections are asymptomatic, though late sequelae occur in greater than 50% of untreated infants.
• Symptomatic newborns are at significant risk for sequelae, most frequently neurological (hydrocephalus, retardation) or ophthalmic (retinitis, blindness).
• Prenatal treatment appears to decrease risk to newborn; therapy of all infected infants appears to improve outcome.

 Differential Diagnosis

• Primary infection: acute disease symptoms of adenopathy, fever, rash: primary EBV, CMV, HIV infection
• For the newborn with micro/macrocephaly, hepatosplenomegaly, eye disease; other congenital infections: CMV, syphilis, rubella

 Data Gathering

HISTORY

• For acquired infection, history of contact with cats, eating raw or undercooked meat.
• For congenital infection, history of maternal exposure or positive titers (IgG and/or IgM).

 Physical Examination

• Acquired infection: Adenopathy; rash; fever, malaise; hepatosplenomegaly.
• Congenital infection: Micro- or macrocephaly, hydrocephalus, chorioretinitis, hepatosplenomegaly, petechiae, sensorineural hearing loss, intracerebral calcifications.

Laboratory Aids

- Screen all pregnant woman or their infants in high-incidence areas by use of toxoplasmosis-specific IgM or rise in IgG titer over time.
- Prenatal diagnosis by PCR on amniotic fluid appears promising, with high degree of sensitivity/specificity.
- For the at-risk neonate, diagnosis is made by demonstration of specific IgM, IgA, or IgE titers, or rise in IgG titers, and/or clinical symptoms in infant of mother with recent primary infection.
- Head CT or MRI demonstrating calcifications
- Thrombocytopenia
- Early and frequent audiologic and ophthalmic evaluations are a necessity. Many affected infants will have normal neonatal examinations.
- Elevated liver function tests

 ## Therapy

- Pyrimethamine and sulfadiazine for the first year of life for all congenitally infected infants, symptomatic or not. Folic acid is given during the course of therapy to minimize hematologic side effects.

PREVENTION

- Avoidance of undercooked meats
- Seronegative women need to exercise caution in caring for cats.
- Maternal/neonatal antibody screening is important in areas with a significant incidence of toxoplasmosis.
- Treatment of pregnant women with documented seroconversion may prevent congenital infection in many cases.
- If fetal infection is established, aggressive treatment during pregnancy with spiramycin, pyrmethamine and sulfonamide may ameliorate the severity of the disease in the infant.

 ## Follow-Up

- Continued attention to neurological development and frequent audiologic and ophthalmic evaluations throughout the first few years of life.
- For children with early symptomatic disease, careful attention to neurological condition and early intervention services to optimize outcome.

PITFALLS

- Failure to consider diagnosis in at-risk or symptomatic infant.
- Failure to consider the significant risk of late sequelae in asymptomatic exposed/infected neonate and therefore failure to offer therapy to asymptomatic infected neonate.

 ## Common Questions and Answers

Q: What is the risk of congenital infection in a mother with stable toxoplasmosis?
A: The risk of congenital infection in the offspring of a mother with long-standing toxoplasmosis infection is considered very low; the exception would be for mothers with a significant degree of immunosuppression or deficiency.

Q: What is the risk of congenital infection in offspring of a mother with documented primary infection during pregnancy?
A: Approximately 30% to 40% of infants born to mothers with primary infection during pregnancy will be infected themselves. This rate may be lower if the mother receives therapy (spiramycin or pyrimethamine/sulfadiazine) prenatally. Of the infected infants, the majority (70–90%) are normal at birth; with treatment for 12 months, it appears most will have a favorable outcome.

ICD-9-CM 130.9

BIBLIOGRAPHY

Hohlfeld P, Daffos F, Costa JM, et al. Prenatal diagnosis of congenital toxoplasmosis with a polymerase-chain-reaction test on amniotic fluid. *N Engl J Med* 1994;331:695–699.

Koppe JG, Loewer-Sieger DH, de Roever-Bonnet H. Results of 20-year follow-up of congenital toxoplasmosis. *Lancet* 1986;1:254–256.

Lappalainen M, Koskiniemi M, Hiilesmaa V, et al. Outcome of children after maternal primary toxoplasma infection during pregnancy with emphasis on avidity of specific IgG. *Pediatr Infect Dis J* 1995;14:354–361.

Lynfield R, Guerina NG. Toxoplasmosis. *Pediatr Rev* 1997;18:75–83.

Roizen N, Swisher CN, Stein MA, et al. Neurologic and developmental outcome in treated congenital toxoplasmosis. *Pediatrics* 1995;95:11–20.

Wilson CB, Remington JS, Stagno S, et al. Development of adverse sequelae in children born with subclinical congenital toxoplasma infection. *Pediatrics* 1980;66:767–774.

Author: Richard M. Rutstein

Tracheitis

Database

DEFINITION

- Acute tracheitis: potentially life-threatening bacterial infection of the trachea, which presents acutely in the otherwise normal child.
- Subacute tracheitis: infectious complication of long-term intubation or tracheostomy, predominately in children with an underlying respiratory, neurologic, or other chronic disorder.

CAUSES

- Acute

—*Staphylococcus aureus* predominately
—*Haemophilus influenza* type b (Hib), group A beta-hemolytic streptococcus (GABS), and oral anaerobes less commonly
—*Mycobacterium tuberculosis;* uncommon but known pathogen

- Subacute

—Organisms as above
—Organisms associated with nosocomial infections in a particular institution (*Pseudomonas aeruginosa,* other gram-negative enterics, *Moraxella catarrhalis,* etc.)
—Fungus (e.g., *Candida* spp.) with underlying immunodeficiency or chronic steroid use

PATHOPHYSIOLOGY

- Not clearly known; postulated disruption of the mucociliary elevator, leading to decreased clearance of bacterial pathogens
- In children with artificial airways, natural airway protective mechanisms are bypassed and pathogens inoculated directly into the trachea with suctioning.
- Viral infection may precede bacterial tracheitis; but not necessarily.
- Infection causes destruction of the tracheal wall, sloughing of mucosa, mucus, and pus production, leading to airway obstruction.

EPIDEMIOLOGY

- Infant through early adolescence
- Increased incidence during viral respiratory season
- No female/male predisposition

COMPLICATIONS

- Pneumonia
- Prolonged mechanical ventilation with associated complications (pneumothorax, pneumonia, tracheal stenosis)
- Staphylococcal toxin syndromes (Toxic shock syndrome)
- Adult respiratory distress syndrome (ARDS)
- Death

PROGNOSIS

- Acute tracheitis: outcome ranges from recovery without sequelae to tracheal stenosis (even without intubation); most patients recover fully
- Subacute tracheitis: frequent recurrences not unusual (because of altered airway mechanics and/or underlying disease)

Differential Diagnosis

INFECTIOUS

- Epiglottitis
- Pharyngitis
- Laryngitis
- Bronchitis

ENVIRONMENTAL

- Chemical or inhalation burns to airway

TUMORS

- Laryngeal tumors (rare)

TRAUMA

- Blunt trauma to neck

CONGENITAL

- Underlying airway stenosis compromised by acute viral infection, tracheal papillomatosis (human papillomavirus aspirated at birth)

Data Gathering

HISTORY

- Immunization history, especially Hib vaccine
- Upper respiratory infection prodrome?

Tracheitis Subgroups

- Acute: symptoms progress over 8- to 10-hour period; fever, lethargy, cough, dyspnea, hoarseness, stridor, noisy respirations.
- Subacute: Same as for acute with more indolent progression, increased supplemental oxygen requirement, change in pattern of breathing, stridor, noisy respirations.

Physical Examination

Finding: Acute
Significance: Toxic appearance, anxiety, and "air hunger," lethargy, fever, shortness of breath, cyanosis, labored respiration with retraction, cough, may have concomitant signs of pneumonia.

Finding: Subacute
Significance: Same as for acute with changes in secretions suctioned from trachea (thickening, change in color).

Laboratory Aids

Test: Tracheal culture
Significance: Obtain specimen directly from the trachea in controlled setting (for emergent airway management), throat swab not adequate, endotracheal tube cultures not adequate.

Test: Gram stain tracheal material
Significance: For predominant organism and white blood cells (especially polymorphonuclear leukocytes).

Test: Blood culture
Significance: Should be obtained, but bacteremia not common.

Test: CBC
Significance: Increased white count with a left shift.

Test: Erythrocyte sedimentation rate, C reactive protein
Significance: Usually elevated.

Test: Laryngoscopy or bronchoscopy
Significance: Diagnostic and therapeutic; visualize airway and suction material that obstructs airway (must be performed in setting with preparation to intubate or place tracheotomy if necessary).

RADIOGRAPHIC STUDIES

• Radiographs must be performed in controlled setting with someone prepared to intubate if necessary.
• Lateral neck and anteroposterior neck radiographs: distention of the hypopharynx, subglottic narrowing, cloudiness of the tracheal air column, irregularity of the tracheal wall, sloughing of mucosa (may mimic foreign body).

Therapy

• Control of airway essential, not all patients require intubation, but preparation must be made to perform emergent intubation or tracheotomy at any time (decline may occur gradually or suddenly if debris in airway obstructs).
• Children with pre-existing artificial airway may require increase in usual ventilatory support.

DRUGS

• Acute: (community acquired)

—If up-to-date Hib immunization: antistaphylococcal coverage with a semisynthetic penicillin (oxacillin, nafcillin); if penicillin allergy, clindamycin
—Inadequate Hib immunization: second generation cephalosporin (cefuroxime)

• Subacute: (hospital acquired, preexisting artificial airway)

—Guide therapy by known prior colonization and pathogens common in particular institution
—Mildly ill patient: empiric therapy with amoxicillin/clavulanate for 10 to 14 days
—Severely ill patient: empiric therapy with ticarcillin/clavulanate or ampicillin/sulbactam, then guide therapy by cultures (unless a predominant organism cultures, results may reflect colonizing organisms and/or mouth flora, not etiologic organism)

Follow-Up

• Acute tracheitis: because of possibility of tracheal stenosis, which may be mild and asymptomatic until the child experiences the next respiratory tract infection, the patients must be counseled to bring the child for care any time there is noisy breathing, especially stridor.
• Chronic tracheitis: no follow-up cultures should be taken; the child should be monitored the same way all children with abnormal/artificial airways would be.

SIGNS TO WATCH FOR

• Obstruction of endotracheal tube with secretions is not unusual and would be indicated by a sudden deterioration.
• Persistent fever may indicate nosocomial infection (pneumonia, urinary tract infection, etc.).
• Sudden worsening while on ventilator may indicate pneumothorax.

PREVENTION

• Routine immunization, especially for Hib in all children; immunization for influenza in children with artificial airways
• Avoid over-aggressive suctioning of children with artificial airways

PITFALLS

Patients may have rapid progression of symptoms; initial radiographic studies may be negative, close clinical observation is critical.

Common Questions and Answers

Q: Are routine surveillance cultures of patients with artificial airways helpful in prevention of tracheitis?
A: No. Children who have been hospitalized and have artificial airways rapidly become colonized with whatever organisms are common within the institution. These organisms will persist for months, are difficult to eradicate, and even if eradicated will be replaced with other, possibly more resistant flora. Routine culture is expensive and will only identify colonization.

Q: How can you differentiate a child with severe pharyngitis and tracheitis?
A: In many ways, the clinical presentation of tracheitis is similar to that of a severe pharyngitis, but in tracheitis there will be signs of respiratory compromise (e.g., stridor) and toxic appearance. The two illnesses may look very similar early in the disease course.

Q: How can you differentiate a child with tracheitis and one with tracheitis who also has systemic toxin mediated complications?
A: Children with a toxic shock syndrome presentation will usually have a diffuse erythroderma, non-purulent conjunctivitis, and inflamed oral mucosa (strawberry tongue). The hypotension and tachycardia will be out of proportion to the degree of illness and may be refractory to fluid resuscitation.

ICD-9-CM 616.0

BIBLIOGRAPHY

Britto J, Habibi P, Walters S, Levin M, Nadel S. Systemic complications associated with bacterial tracheitis. *Arch Dis Child* 1996;72:249–250.

Brook I. Aerobic and anaerobic microbiology of bacterial tracheitis in children. *Clin Infect Dis* 1995;20(S):S222–S223.

Horowitz IN. Staphylococcal tracheitis, pneumonia, and adult respiratory distress syndrome. *Pediatr Emerg Care* 1996;12(4):288–289.

Jones R, Santos J, Overall J. Bacterial tracheitis. *J Am Med Assoc* 1979;242:721–726.

Author: Jill A. Foster

Tracheoesophageal Fistula (TEF)

Database

DEFINITION

- Connection between the trachea and esophagus
- Major types are:

—Esophageal atresia (EA) with distal TEF (87%)
—Pure esophageal atresia without TEF (8%)
—"H-type" TEF without esophageal atresia (4%)
—Esophageal atresia with proximal TEF with or without distal TEF (2%)

PATHOPHYSIOLOGY

- Failure of complete separation of the primitive foregut into trachea and esophagus by tracheoesophageal septum at 4 to 8 weeks' gestation

EPIDEMIOLOGY

- Incidence: 1:3000 to 1:4000
- Slight male predominance

GENETICS

- No inheritance pattern established.
- The most likely candidate gene responsible belongs to the HOX D group.
- An increased association exists with aneuploidies specifically trisomy 13, 18, and 21.
- 50% associated with other anomalies, mostly gastrointestinal and cardiac (e.g., ventricular septal defect, right-sided aortic arch, duodenal atresia, left congenital diaphragmatic hernia, imperforate anus)
- 10% have VATER (Vertebral, Anal, Cardiac, TE fistula, Renal, Limb) syndrome
- Association with CHARGE syndrome, SCHISIS syndrome and Potter syndrome have been reported

COMPLICATIONS

- Aspiration pneumonia (usually lower lobes)
- Respiratory distress
- Respiratory failure and death
- Gastric perforation, if on positive pressure ventilation
- Esophageal dysmotility and gastroesophageal reflux
- Achalasia
- Tracheomalacia
- Chronic cough and dysphagia (foreign body impaction)
- Growth failure
- 30% associated with premature birth
- Polyhydramnios in 30% with EA + TEF; in 80% with pure EA

PROGNOSIS

- Two prognostic classifications systems exist:

—Waterston: based on birth weight, presence of pneumonia and identification of severe congenital anomalies
—Montreal: based on preoperative ventilator dependence and associated major anomalies. Appears to be more accurate in identifying infants at highest risk and is as follows:
   —Class I: No ventilator dependence and no anomalies (mortality 0%); or ventilator dependent and none or minor anomalies (mortality 9%).
   —Class II: Ventilator dependent and major anomalies (mortality 22%); or no ventilator dependence and life-threatening anomalies (mortality 88%).

Differential Diagnosis

Except for H-type, presentation is classic and usually straightforward.

TRAUMA

- Traumatic or spontaneous esophageal or pharyngeal perforation

CONGENITAL

- Pharyngeal pseudodiverticulum
- Laryngoesophageal cleft
- Esophageal stenosis
- Esophageal duplication cyst and webs
- Paraesophageal hernia

Data Gathering

HISTORY

Question: Polyhydramnios?
Significance: With or without presence of small stomach bubble

Question: Excessive salivation, coughing, emesis of undigested formula and choking with feeds in neonatal period?
Significance: Obstructional esophagus

Question: Chronic cough, recurrent aspiration pneumonia, atypical wheezing presenting after neonatal period?
Significance: May be sign of H-type TEF.

Physical Examination

- Drooling
- Cyanotic with feeding
- Associated malformations (e.g., VACTERL)
- Distended abdomen with TEF and scaphoid abdomen with pure EA
- Abnormal lung examination with rales, wheezes
- Inability to advance the NG tube into stomach, meeting resistance at approximately 10 cm; may go additional if the tube coils in the proximal esophageal pouch.

Laboratory Aids

Test: Once the diagnosis is certain, CBC, electrolytes, blood culture (as prophylactic antibiotics will likely be started), and blood type and cross, and karyotype in those with multiple anomalies and dysmorphic features consistent with trisomies.
Significance: In preparation of surgery.

RADIOGRAPHIC STUDIES

- Chest and abdominal x-ray with an 8 to 10 French NG tube in place to aid visualization of esophagus. Injecting a small amount of dilute barium or non-ionic water soluble contrast, such as Omnipaque, may help define a proximal esophageal pouch which is generally dilated and large. Bowel gas absent in isolated EA (in few cases, the distal TEF may be occluded by mucus). A narrow proximal esophageal pouch may suggest a proximal TEF. Pulmonary infiltrates are present with aspiration pneumonia.
- X-rays to rule out other anomalies (e.g., vertebrae, cardiac silhouette, limbs) should be considered.
- Contrast esophagogram: if H-type TEF suspected.
- Bronchoscopy and esophagoscopy: are indicated if esophagogram negative. Some advocate routine bronchoscopy to detect a proximal TEF, or distal TEF in an infant with a gas-less abdomen.
- Renal ultrasound: to rule out associated anomalies (post-operative: avoid abdominal pressure).
- Pre-operative echocardiogram: to rule out cardiac anomalies and evaluate position of the aortic arch to determine surgical approach.

Therapy

- Replogle sump tube or NG tube for continuous suctioning.
- Position head elevated at a 30 to 45 degree angle to minimize the risk of aspiration.
- NPO and maintenance IV fluids. Umbilical arterial and venous catheters are desirable in the neonate.
- Consult pediatric surgeon; emergent division and ligation of the TEF may be necessary as a temporizing procedure.
- Intubation of trachea in the event of respiratory distress. To minimize the escape of ventilatory gases into the stomach, it is advisable to maintain endotracheal tube tip distal to the fistula and above the carina, and with its beveled end facing forward.

SURGERY

- Primary repair: esophageal anastomosis and division of TEF via right thoracotomy in the first 1 to 2 days of life, if esophageal gap is small (usually less than 3 cm).
- Delayed repair: early gastrostomy and ligation of the TEF with delayed primary anastomosis within 30 days, performed in those with isolated esophageal atresia, long-gap atresia (more than 3 cm) and significant respiratory distress.
- Staged repair: initial gastrostomy with definitive surgery 1 month to 2 years later.
- Cervical esophagostomy (spit fistula) and esophageal replacement: for long-gap atresia (for whom primary anastomosis is considered undesirable or impossible) and repeated episodes of aspiration.
- Esophageal replacement is performed with any of the following: gastric tube, colon, jejunum, or gastric transposition.
- Post-operative care: frequent gentle suctioning of the mouth and pharynx is necessary; it is advisable to measure the suction catheters so as to avoid trauma to the repair site. Avoid aggressive suctioning and hyperextension of the neck. Endotracheal intubation should be avoided, and if necessary, must be performed by the most skilled physician available. In those with long-gap atresias with primary repair under extreme tension, prophylactic paralysis and ventilation for 5 to 7 days has been helpful in reducing stricture formation and occurrence of reflux.

DRUGS

- Prophylactic ampicillin and gentamicin. Discontinue once chest tube removed.
- H_2 antagonist to prevent stricture formation
- Antibiotics for 5 to 7 days if aspiration pneumonia is suspected.

DIET

- Pre-operative: NPO and maintenance IV fluids
- Post-operative: NPO or feed via gastrostomy/ NG tube while anastomosis heals and patency of the esophagus is demonstrated by contrast swallow (approximately 5–7 days post-op). The chest drain is left in place until barium swallow shows intact anastomosis. In those requiring mechanical ventilation, extubation is attempted cautiously since reintubation carries a risk of tracheal rupture at the repair site.

 Follow-Up

Expect improvement 5 to 10 days postoperatively.

SIGNS TO WATCH FOR

- Post-operative anastomotic leak (15%): usually closes over a period of 1 to 2 weeks.
- Stricture (30%): the higher the tension at the anastomotic site, greater the risk. High association with reflux.
- Pleural effusions or pneumothorax may accompany anastomotic leak.
- Gastroesophageal reflux (40%) and recurrent aspiration pneumonia: partial fundoplication is required in almost all with primary repair and extreme long gap atresias.
- Recurrence of fistula.
- Mortality and morbidity greater with prematurity, severe lung disease, and presence of life threatening and major associated anomalies.
- Long-term morbidity:

—Chronic cough (may be barky or croupy)
—Chronic intermittent stridor secondary to tracheomalacia
—Dysphagia and reflux in almost 50% as adults
—Increased airway resistance and rapid gastric emptying in those with gastric transposition

PITFALLS

- Prenatal diagnosis by fetal ultrasound scan has poor sensitivity (24%) and positive predictive value (56%), even in the presence of polyhydramnios when performed around 18 weeks.
- Arterial puncture in malformed extremity can compromise blood flow and cause permanent injury.
- Mechanical ventilation may result in gastric perforation before repair.

 Common Questions and Answers

Q: Could this happen to my next baby?
A: The inheritance pattern has not been established. However, there is a slight increased risk of VACTERL malformations in siblings and first-degree relatives.

ICD-9-CM 750.3

BIBLIOGRAPHY

McMullen KP, Karnes PS, Moir CR, Michels VV. Familial recurrence of tracheoesophageal fistula and associated malformations. *Am J Med Genet* 1996;63:525–528.

Nakayama DK. Esophageal atresia and tracheoesophageal stenosis. In: *Critical care of the surgical newborn*. Nakayama DK, Bose CL, Chescheir NC, et al., eds. Armonk, NY: Futura Publishing Co., Inc. 1997:227–250.

Raffensperger JG, ed. Esophageal atresia and tracheoesophageal stenosis. In: *Swenson's pediatric surgery*. Norwalk, CT: Appleton & Lange, 1990:697–734.

Stoll C, Alembik Y, Dott B, Roth MP. Evaluation of prenatal diagnosis of congenital gastrointestinal atresias. *Eur J Epidemiol* 1996; 12:611–616.

Teich S, Barton DP, Ginn-Pease ME, King DR. Prognostic classification for esophageal atresia and tracheoesophageal fistula: Waterston versus Montreal. *J Pediatr Surg* 1997;32:1075–1080.

Author: Karen D. Fairchild and Sameer Wagle

Transfusion Reaction

 Database

DEFINITION

Any acute or subacute adverse reaction that develops as a consequence of the administration of blood components. Types include:

- Acute reactions: hemolytic, febrile, allergic, hypervolemia, bacterial sepsis
- Delayed reactions: hemolytic
- Late complications of transfusion: infection, alloimmunization, iron overload, graft versus host disease (GVHD)

EPIDEMIOLOGY

5–10% of blood product recipients develop some type of transfusion reaction.

 Differential Diagnosis

CAUSE

Acute Hemolytic

- Incompatibility of donor RBC antigens and recipient RBC antibodies; usually ABO blood group incompatibility

Febrile

- Reaction between recipient antibodies to donor leukocyte or plasma protein antigens

Allergic

- Reaction between recipient antibodies and donor plasma proteins; the incidence is sporadic and donor dependent.

Hypervolemia

Administration of an excessive volume of a blood product or infusion at an excessive rate.

Bacterial Sepsis

- Contaminated blood product; most common in platelet products near the end of their shelf life

Delayed Hemolytic

- Incompatibility of donor RBC antigens and recipient RBC antibodies; usually "minor" blood group antigens

PATHOPHYSIOLOGY

Acute Hemolytic

Antigen-antibody interaction leads to complement activation on the surface of the transfused red cells, resulting in acute intravascular hemolysis and vasomotor instability

Febrile

Prior exposure to blood products may result in the formation of antibodies to leukocytes or plasma protein antigens; on reexposure the antigen-antibody interaction causes the release of pyrogens; these reactions develop only in individuals with a history of prior transfusion or pregnancy; alternatively, cytokines in the product can cause fever in the recipient.

Allergic

- Unknown

Hypervolemia

- Circulatory overload leading to heart failure

Bacterial Sepsis

Intravascular infusion of viable bacteria and endotoxins leads to acute septic shock.

Delayed Hemolytic

Previously transfused individuals who have been sensitized to a "minor" blood group antigen develop an anamnestic response on reexposure; at the time of the current transfusion, antibody titers are below detectable levels; after the transfusion is complete, titers rise (usually within 3–10 days) and extravascular hemolysis occurs.

 Data Gathering

HISTORY

Acute Hemolytic

- Fever, chills, abdominal or flank pain, pink or tea-colored urine, tachycardia, hypotension, oliguria

Febrile

- Fever, chills

Allergic

- Urticaria; sometimes bronchospasm; rarely anaphylaxis

Hypervolemia

- Hypertension, dyspnea, rales, cardiac arrhythmia

Bacterial Sepsis

- Fever, chills, hypotension

Delayed Hemolytic

- Fever, malaise, dark urine, jaundice; rarely shock, renal failure

Laboratory Aids

Acute Hemolytic

• Direct Coombs test: positive; CBC: anemia; UA: hemoglobinuria; PT/PTT/fibrinogen/FSP: disseminated intravascular coagulation (DIC)

Febrile

• Direct Coombs test, blood culture of the patient and product, and stat Gram stain of the product; all should be negative; this is a diagnosis of exclusion

Allergic

• None

Hypervolemia

• CXR: increased pulmonary vascular markings

Therapy

• Acute hemolytic: Stop transfusion immediately; hydration, pressors, and diuretics as needed to maintain circulation and urine output; treat DIC with plasma
• Febrile: Stop transfusion; antipyretics (acetaminophen); may resume transfusion if patient is stable and acute hemolytic transfusion reaction is ruled out.
• Allergic: Stop transfusion; antihistamine (diphenhydramine); steroids or epinephrine in severe reactions
• Hypervolemia: Diuretics (furosemide)

PREVENTION

• Acute hemolytic: Pre-transfusion antihistamine or administration of washed RBC products (in patients with repeated or severe allergic reactions).
• Febrile: Pre-transfusion antipyretic or administration of leukodepleted products; the latter is recommended for chronically transfused patients who have a high incidence of febrile transfusion reactions.
• Allergic: Pre-transfusion antihistamine or administration of washed RBC products (in patients with repeated or severe allergic reactions).
• Hypervolemia: Administer appropriate volumes (typically 10 mL/kg) at appropriate rate; most RBC transfusions are administered over 3 to 4 hours unless the patient is acutely hypovolemic or actively hemorrhaging; individuals with chronic anemia are frequently euvolemic and should be transfused gradually (smaller volumes over longer time period).
• Bacterial sepsis: Sterile technique in blood collection, storage and administration; careful inspection of product prior to transfusion.
• Delayed hemolytic: Appropriately performed antibody screen at time of transfusion; checking blood bank records for previously identified antibodies.

Follow-Up

LATE COMPLICATIONS

• Infection

—Posttransfusion hepatitis: caused by hepatitis B or C
—Acquired immunodeficiency syndrome (AIDS): caused by human immunodeficiency virus (HIV)
—Cytomegalovirus (CMV): problematic in individuals with inherited or acquired immunodeficiency states; these individuals should receive CMV-negative products
—Other infection: Epstein-Barr virus, syphilis, malaria, toxoplasmosis, HTLV-I, Chagas? disease, babesiosis, filariasis

• Alloimmunization

—Formation of antibodies to RBC, platelet, and leukocyte (HLA) antigens can develop in an individual who has been multiply transfused; this can cause cross-matching problems, febrile transfusion reactions, delayed hemolytic transfusion reactions, and platelet transfusion refractoriness.

• Iron Overload

—Chronically transfused individuals will accumulate iron as a byproduct of RBC breakdown; an iron-chelating drug (desferoxamine) will enhance its excretion.

• Graft Versus Host Disease

—Individuals with inherited or acquired T cell immunodeficiency states can develop GVHD from transfused immunocompetent T cells; can also occur if donor and recipient are related and share HLA types; these individuals should receive irradiated blood products.

Common Questions and Answers

Q: What is the risk of acquiring certain infections?
A:

• Hepatitis B—1:63,000 units
• Hepatitis C—1:103,000 units
• HIV—1:676,000 units

Q: Is directed donor blood safer?
A: No, there is no evidence that the infection risk is lower, and some studies suggest that the infection risk may actually be higher.

Q: Is it safe to give a transfusion to a patient with fever?
A: Yes, however, if the temperature rises during the transfusion or if symptoms such as chills or hypotension develop, the transfusion should be stopped and the patient evaluated for a transfusion reaction.

ICD-9-CM 999.8

BIBLIOGRAPHY

Busch MP. Transfusion and HIV. Curr Opin Hematol 1994;1:438.

Capon SM, Goldfinger D. Acute hemolytic transfusion reaction, a paradigm of the systemic inflammatory response: new insights into pathophysiology and treatment. Transfusion 1995;35(6):513–520.

Jones DS, Byers RH, Bush JJ, et al. Epidemiology of transfusion-associated acquired immunodeficiency syndrome in children in the United States. Pediatrics 1992;89:123.

Mollison PL, Engelfriet CP, Contreras M. Blood transfusion in clinical medicine. Oxford: Blackwell Scientific Publications, 1993.

Schreiber GB, Busch MP, Kleinman SH, et al. The risk of transfusion transmitted infection. N Engl J Med 1996;96:1685–1690.

Author: Cynthia F. Norris

Transient Erythroblastopenia of Childhood

 Database

DEFINITION

- An acquired, self-limited suppression of red cell production in an otherwise healthy child.

PATHOPHYSIOLOGY

- Unknown. Possible viral etiology is Parvovirus B19 but this remains hypothetical. A serum inhibitor, such as an IgG directed at the committed erythroid stem cell progenitor, has also been proposed but not yet proven.

GENETICS

There is no simple genetic pattern; familial TEC has been reported (rarely), suggesting a combination of environmental factors and genetic propensity.

EPIDEMIOLOGY

- Mean age at diagnosis is 26 months, less than 10% are greater than 3 years old at diagnosis.
- Slight male predominance (male : female 5.1 : 3.1)
- There is no seasonal predominance.

COMPLICATIONS

- Cardiovascular compromise secondary to severe anemia is often less than expected given the level of anemia. High output congestive heart failure is unusual.
- Neurological symptoms including confusion and transient hemiparesis have been reported but are rare.
- A significant number of patients also have neutropenia (ANC < 1500/μL) during either the acute or recovery phases of the illness.

PROGNOSIS

All children recover usually within 1 to 2 months from diagnosis (up to 8 months to recovery). Prognosis is excellent. Recurrence is rare.

 Differential Diagnosis

- Environmental: iron-deficiency anemia
- Metabolic: hypothyroidism
- Congenital: Diamond-Blackfan anemia (this diagnosis usually made within first year of life)
- Neoplasm: leukemia, myelodysplastic syndromes
- Miscellaneous: renal disease, anemia of chronic disease

 Data Gathering

HISTORY

Question: Pallor?
Significance: Typically slow in onset and, therefore, often missed by parents. Often noted by an adult who sees the child less frequently.

Question: Activity level?
Significance: Often preserved because of slow onset of anemia. An extremely anemic child may be irritable, sleepy, and/or lethargic.

SPECIAL QUESTIONS

Question: History of fever, easy bruisability, or frequent/severe infections (especially bacterial)?
Significance: Should alert the clinician to consider other diagnoses such as leukemia and bone marrow failure syndromes.

 Physical Examination

- Child is generally well appearing and not chronically ill.
- Pallor
- Tachycardia secondary to anemia
- Usually no organomegaly, ecchymosis, petechiae, or jaundice

 Laboratory Aids

Test: CBC
Significance: Low Hgb, normal MCV, normal RBC morphology. Total WBC count/morphology and platelet count should be normal, if not, think of leukemias. ANC may be decreased (rarely below 500/μL) but morphology must be normal. RDW may be elevated during recovery.

Test: Reticulocyte count
Significance: Low to zero during anemic phase, should be high during recovery.

Test: Chemistry/Blood bank
Significance: Bilirubin, LDH, ferritin, iron levels and Coombs testing should be normal to rule out iron deficiency anemia and immune hemolysis.

Test: Hemoglobin electrophoresis with quantitative HbF
Significance: Should be normal in TEC, elevated in Diamond-Blackfan anemia.

Test: Chest x-ray
Significance: To determine degree of cardiomegaly.

Test: Bone marrow aspiration
Significance: May be necessary to rule in TEC and rule out other diagnoses such as Diamond-Blackfan and the leukemias. Presence or absence of early RBC precursors may help predict time to recovery. Maturation of megakaryocytes and the myeloid cell line must be normal, especially if neutropenia is present.

Therapy

- Initial inpatient observation for complications of severe anemia. Daily CBC at least initially to gauge rate of fall of hemoglobin/rise of reticulocyte count and to estimate time to recovery.
- PRBC transfusion only if there is evidence of cardiovascular compromise. If a transfusion is needed, transfuse slowly to prevent fluid overload. A good rule of thumb is to transfuse the same number of mL/kg as the patient's hemoglobin, over 3 to 4 hours. A second transfusion is rarely required.
- Normal activity and diet for age, as tolerated.
- Instruct family on signs and symptoms of severe anemia.
- Reassurance

DRUGS

- No role for prednisone, iron supplements, anabolic steroids, or other immunosuppressive agents. Short-term folic acid may be indicated during reticulocytosis.

Follow-Up

WHEN TO EXPECT IMPROVEMENT

- Clinic visits weekly to monitor hemoglobin and reticulocytes. (These visits may need to be more frequent in the beginning of the illness and less frequent as recovery becomes evident.)
- Elevation of reticulocyte count is the first sign of recovery.

PREVENTION

There is no known way to prevent TEC.

ISOLATION

- Because of possible teratogenicity of parvovirus 19 and contagion within hospital

PITFALLS

- TEC must be an isolated normocytic, normochromic anemia. If the other cell lines are affected or if the anemia is macrocytic, think of bone marrow failure syndromes.
- Iron therapy has no place in the treatment of TEC. Be sure to check RBC indices and reticulocyte count prior to instituting iron therapy for anemia.

Common Questions and Answers

Q: Can other children in a family get this illness?
A: The cause(s) of this illness in otherwise normal children is unknown. It is very rare for other family members to be affected. It is appropriate to reassure parents with regard to this issue.

Q: Are transfusions always necessary?
A: No. Only in cases of heart failure is a transfusion necessary. Most often, children can be managed with "watchful waiting."

Q: How can you tell the difference between TEC and Diamond-Blackfan syndrome?
A: Children with Diamond-Blackfan syndrome are usually less than 1 year old and can have elevated hemoglobin F levels. If a bone marrow aspirate is obtained during the recovery phase of TEC, then the diagnosis will be clear. Often, however, only time will tell. Children with TEC always recover; those with Diamond-Blackfan syndrome do not.

ICD-9-CM 284.8

BIBLIOGRAPHY

Bhambhani K, Inoue S, Sarnaik SA. Seasonal clustering of transient erythroblastopenia of childhood. *Am J Child Dis* 1988;142:175–177.

Cherrick I, Karayalcin G, Lanzkowsky P. Transient erythroblastopenia of childhood: prospective study of fifty patients. *Am J Pediatr Hematol Oncol* 1994;16(4):320–324.

Nathan DG, Oski FA, eds. *Hematology of infancy and childhood,* 4th ed. Philadelphia: WB Saunders, 1993.

Author: Julie W. Stern
Therese B. West (first edition)

Transient Tachypnea of the Newborn (TTN)

 Database

DEFINITION

• Tachypnea (respiratory rate >60 breaths/min) in a newborn with evidence of retained fetal lung fluid and without other etiologic explanation

CAUSE

• Thought to be related to delayed maturation as a result of decreased levels of or hyporesponsiveness to catecholamines during transition.
• Not due to absence of "squeeze" of vaginal delivery

PATHOPHYSIOLOGY

• Normal term fetus has approximately 25 mL of fluid in lungs before labor; decreases to 6 mL by delivery. Through out the gestation, lung epithelium secretes chloride ion with fluid, and develops the ability to actively reabsorb sodium and fluid only late in gestation. At birth, the mature lung switches from fluid secretion to reabsorption in response to changes in oxygen tension, and levels of catecholamines, cortisol, prolactin and vasopressin. During labor, fluid is cleared from the alveoli, to the interstitium, to the pulmonary lymphatics, and to the capillaries.
• Dysfunction in catecholamine regulation, mild pulmonary capillary leak, and myocardial dysfunction with elevated filling pressures are thought to be responsible for delayed resorption of lung fluid.
• If fluid is not cleared, decreased lung compliance and increased air trapping result from compression of peripheral conducting airways by excessive interstitial fluid. Hypoxemia results from ventilation/perfusion mismatch, not from right to left shunting.

EPIDEMIOLOGY

• More common in males.
• More common in neonates born to asthmatic mothers (not related to asthma medications).
• Incidence increased with intrapartum narcotics, cesarean section without labor, maternal diabetes, and delayed clamping of the umbilical cord. Increased incidence also seen in large pre-term infants (greater than 1500 g).
• Cesarean section after normal labor does not increase the risk of TTN.
• Less common after antenatal steroid use.

COMPLICATIONS (RARE)

• Hypoxemia
• Respiratory failure necessitating mechanical ventilation
• Pneumothorax
• Persistent pulmonary hypertension of the newborn

PROGNOSIS

• Excellent: benign and a self-limited condition in all newborns.
• A single study reports an association between TTN and later development of asthma and atopy.

 Differential Diagnosis

INFECTION

• Neonatal sepsis
• Pneumonia

METABOLIC

• Metabolic acidosis
• Hypoglycemia
• Hyperammonemia
• Inborn errors of metabolism

CONGENITAL

• Cyanotic congenital heart disease
• Polycythemia
• Congenital lung malformation
• Pulmonary lymphangiectasia

MISCELLANEOUS

• Pneumothorax
• Respiratory distress syndrome
• Meconium aspiration pneumonitis
• Myocarditis
• Congestive heart failure
• CNS anomalies

 Data Gathering

HISTORY

Question: Tachypnea?
Significance: Within several hours of birth.

Question: Antenatal risk factors for sepsis?
Significance: Prematurity (less than 37 weeks), premature (before labor) or prolonged (greater than 18 hours) rupture of membranes, maternal fever, group B streptococcal colonization, recent h/o maternal genital herpes infection, rising maternal WBC count, uterine tenderness, urinary tract infection, fetal tachycardia (greater than 160 beats/min) or previous newborn with sepsis.

Question: Familial history of medical problems or deaths in the newborn period?
Significance: May suggest other diagnoses.

Transient Tachypnea of the Newborn (TTN)

 ## Physical Examination

- Respiratory rate greater than 60 and possibly up to 140 breaths/min.
- Cyanosis, nasal flaring, and/or intercostal retractions may be present. Severe retractions and air-hunger indicate a diagnosis other than TTN.
- Perfusion normal
- Barrel-shaped chest
- Breath sounds clear with occasional rales
- Cardiac and neurological examinations are normal

 ## Laboratory Aids

Test: Pulse oximetry
Significance: In the absence of prematurity, oxygen saturation should be maintained at or above 96%.

Test: Serum glucose
Significance: To rule out hypoglycemia

Test: Sequential CBC with differential count
Significance: 12 to 24 hours apart with a C-reactive protein estimation to screen for abnormalities suggestive of infection.

Test: Arterial blood gas
Significance: Frequently shows mild hypercarbia in TTN. Metabolic acidosis suggests other diagnoses, especially if persistent or severe.

Test: Blood culture
Significance: If respiratory distress does not improve in 6 hours or in those requiring mechanical ventilation.

RADIOGRAPHIC STUDIES

Test: Chest x-ray
Significance: May show hyperinflation, prominent vascular markings, interstitial edema (fluid in the fissures) and sunburst pattern of linear densities expending from the hilum and/or small pleural effusions.

 ## Therapy

- TTN is generally not an emergency.
- Rule out other more serious causes of tachypnea immediately.
- Assess and maintain airway, breathing, circulation.
- Ensure adequate hydration and obtain intravenous access if indicated.
- Oxygen as needed.
- Inpatient monitoring until full resolution of symptom.
- Use of aggressive chest percussions and suctioning in order to prevent or treat TTN should be avoided.
- Oral feedings if minimally tachypneic and without supplemental oxygen need.
- Antibiotics should be started in all those with severe and prolonged course until blood culture result is available.

 ## Follow-Up

- Usually lasts 12 to 48 hours, and almost all recover in 5 days

SIGNS TO WATCH FOR

- Worsening respiratory distress, increasing oxygen requirement, rising $PaCO_2$.
- Lethargy

PITFALLS

TTN is a diagnosis of exclusion. Infants with oxygen requirement greater than 50% probably do not have TTN.

 ## Common Questions and Answers

Q: How long will the baby need to stay in the hospital?
A: By definition, transient tachypnea of the newborn is not associated with other illnesses and is a rapidly self-resolving illness.

Q: Could this happen to my next baby?
A: There is no increased risk for the subsequent offspring.

Q: Will there be any long-lasting respiratory problems?
A: No.

Q: Did I (mother) do anything during my pregnancy to cause this?
A: No.

ICD-9-CM 770.6

BIBLIOGRAPHY

Avery ME, Gatewood OB, Brumley G. Transient tachypnea of the newborn. *Am J Dis Child* 1966;111:380–385.

Chernick V, Kendig E, eds. Respiratory disorders in the newborn. In: *Kendig's disorders of the respiratory tract in children*. Philadelphia: WB Saunders, 1990:272–353.

Demissie K, Marcella SW, Breckenridge MB, Rhoades GG. Maternal asthma and transient tachypnea of the newborn. *Pediatrics* 1998;102:84–90.

Gowen CW, Lawson EE, Gingras J, et al. Electrical potential differences and ion transport across nasal epithelium of term neonates. Correlation with mode of delivery, transient tachypnea of the newborn and respiratory rate. *J Pediatr* 1988;113:121–127.

Miller LK, Calenoff L, Boehm JJ, Riedy MJ. Respiratory distress in the newborn. *JAMA* 1980;243:1176–1179.

Rawlings JS, Smith FR. Transient tachypnea of the newborn—an analysis of neonatal and obstetric risk factors. *Am J Dis Child* 1984;138:869–871.

Authors: Karen D. Fairchild and Sameer Wagle

Tracheomalacia/Laryngomalacia

 Database

DEFINITION

• Laryngomalacia (LM)

—Inspiratory narrowing of the supraglottic structures of the larynx caused by flaccidity of its supportive cartilages. Classically presents in the first 4 to 6 weeks of life with variable degree of stridor and inspiratory effort, that gets worse with forceful breathing.
—Most common congenital anomaly of the larynx
—Most common non-infectious cause of stridor in infants

• Tracheomalacia (TM)

—Expiratory narrowing of the intrathoracic trachea. The area most frequently involved is the distal segment close to the carina. The clinical scenario most likely encountered is the so-called happy wheezer.
—The key sign on exam is monophonic wheezing.
—TM can be arbitrarily classified into primary and secondary. Primary refers to an intrinsic defect of the consistency or structure of the cartilaginous rings. It is generally idiopathic and usually a benign entity.

• Secondary TM is caused by processes that compromise in many ways the tracheal anatomy, like external compression by mediastinal tumors, vascular rings or foregut duplications. TM is often associated with tracheoesophageal fistula (TEF) and less frequently with bronchopulmonary dysplasia (BPD). Prolonged ventilation, especially in the premature newborn, is also thought to lead to this disturbance.
• The severity of the differential diagnosis involved makes TM often a diagnosis of exclusion. The combination of LT and LM is sometimes encountered.

PATHOPHYSIOLOGY

• Laryngomalacia

—It is a variable extrathoracic airway obstruction. During inspiration, due to pleural pressure changes, there is an expansion effect over the intrathoracic airways and a collapsing one over its extrathoracic portion. This physiological phenomenon becomes exaggerated in the presence of a floppy larynx. In severe cases, during inhalation, the supraglottic structures are sucked in to the point of covering completely the visualization of the vocal cords.

• Anatomically it is characterized by:

—Long, flaccid omega-shaped epiglottis that prolapses posteriorly and curves to the lumen on inspiration.
—Medial closure of the aryepiglottic folds.
—Anterior prolapse of frequently bulky arytenoid cartilage.

• Tracheomalacia

—It is a variable intrathoracic airway obstruction. During exhalation, the tracheal wall experiences a positive pressure that results in an external dynamic compression of the lumen. This mechanism is more pronounced in the presence of tracheomalacia resulting in a diminished A-P diameter.
—Sometimes is associated with main stem bronchomalacia, the left side may be more frequently affected.

 Differential Diagnosis

• Laryngomalacia

—Abnormalities of the vocal cords: vocal cord paralysis (unilateral versus bilateral, abducted versus adducted)
—Laryngeal abnormalities: laryngeal clefts, laryngeal webs, hemangiomas, papillomas
—Subglottic stenosis: congenital versus acquired

• Tracheomalacia

—Foreign body in trachea or mainstem bronchi
—Vascular abnormalities: vascular ring, vascular sling
—Tracheal stenosis: congenital versus acquired
—Asthma

 Data Gathering

HISTORY

Question: Laryngomalacia?
Significance:

• Usually mild to moderate inspiratory stridor, but may be completely asymptomatic during shallow breathing.
• Generally improves with sleep.
• Worsens with crying, agitation, feeding, and upper respiratory infections.
• Varies with positional changes: prone better than supine.

Question: Tracheomalacia
Significance:

• Audible wheezing, sometimes very persistent.
• Worsens with breathing efforts and upper respiratory infections.
• Improves during sleep.
• Usually does not affect the patient's general being and normal activities.

Physical Examination

Finding: Laryngomalacia
Significance:

- Depending on severity, stridor may be present at rest.
- Suprasternal and sometimes significant lower sternal/xyfoidal retractions may be seen.
- Positional changes noted: usually improves with neck extension and worsens with flexion.
- Stridor transmitted throughout the chest on auscultation.

Finding: Tracheomalacia
Significance:

- Coarse breath sounds with prolonged expiratory phase.
- Symmetric monotonous wheezing, best heard over the mediastinal area.
- Expiratory effort with intercostal retractions, worse during acute respiratory infections.
- Stridor may also be noted, associated laryngomalacia must be suspected.
- Normal oxyhemoglobin saturations

 ## Laboratory Aids

Test: Laryngo/bronchoscopy
Significance: Flexible fiberoptic bronchoscopy can visualize the degree and extent of laryngomalacia and/or tracheomalacia. Provides the only definitive diagnosis. Is useful in ruling out other significant pathologies in the differential diagnosis.

Test: Chest radiograph
Significance:

- Usually normal in both laryngomalacia and tracheomalacia
- It is important to rule out other abnormalities that can create external airway compression.

Test: Airway fluoroscopy
Significance:

- Lateral views are the most useful to visualize this defect.
- May be normal.
- Inspiratory collapsing larynx may be seen in laryngomalacia.
- Expiratory narrowing or collapse of the distal trachea.
- Does not confirm diagnosis.

Test: Barium swallow
Significance:

- Especially of value in patients with concomitant swallowing abnormalities.
- May see compression of esophagus from vascular malformation.

Test: Magnetic resonance imaging
Significance: Enables tipification of the vascular anomalies

 ## Therapy

- Laryngomalacia

—No definitive therapy is needed in the majority of cases.
—Observation and reassurance are frequently the only intervention indicated.
—Tracheostomy may be needed in severe cases to relieve inspiratory airway obstruction.
—In rare situations, laryngeal surgery is necessary.

- Tracheomalacia

—No specific therapy is required in most patients.
—Patients who required tracheostomy might benefit from continuous positive airway pressure (CPAP), especially younger infants.
—Humidification of secretions may help some patients, especially during respiratory infections.

 ## Follow-Up

- Periodic visits are necessary to monitor the degree of respiratory symptoms.
- Emphasis in feeding difficulties and weight gain should be done.

PROGNOSIS

- In cases of isolated laryngomalacia and/or tracheomalacia is usually excellent.
- Patients with TEF often persist with tracheal dysfunction beyond corrective surgery.

PITFALLS

- Missing other causes for presenting symptoms (*see* Differential Diagnosis).
- Not investigating lower airway in more concerning cases (14% of cases of patients with upper airway generated stridor may also have lower airway abnormalities).
- Treating the wheezing of tracheomalacia as refractory asthma, thus overmedicating the patient.
- The use of bronchodilators (β_2-agonist) may increase the tracheal wall floppiness making the symptoms worse.
- Bronchoscopy should ideally be done under conscious sedation to avoid altering vocal cord movement and airway dynamics.
- The use of rigid bronchoscopy (as opposed to flexible) may stent open the trachea, making tracheomalacia more difficult to identify. However, this scope can be of great value in patients with critical size airways (e.g., premies) as allows for ventilation through the instrument, when foreign body is suspected.

 ## Common Questions and Answers

Q: When will the symptoms improve?
A: As anatomical structures mature with age, LM symptoms have a definitive improvement by 6 months with almost always resolution by one year. TM tends to linger longer, but in both entities symptoms usually resolve completely by the second year of age.

Q: Should all patients with suspected LM have an endoscopic evaluation?
A: No. Infants with mild to moderate typical presentation deserve only careful monitoring. However, airway evaluation should be performed in all cases where a different pathology is considered. For example, significant retractions at rest, nocturnal worsening, high-pitched or persistent stridor deserve exploration. Sometimes, it is not the severity of the clinical presentation, but the parents' anxiety despite reassurance that warrants observation of the tracheobronchial tree.

Q: What should I do when symptoms worsen?
A: Calm the patient, humidification of secretions and treatment of intercurrent infection. In cases where associated bronchospasm is suspected a trial of steroids or bronchodilators may be considered.

ICD-9-CM 748.3

BIBLIOGRAPHY

Brodsky L. *Congenital stridor pediatrics in review.* 1996;17:408–410.

Handler SD, Myer CM III. *Atlas of ear, nose and throat disorders in children.* Hamilton, England: B.C. Decker Inc. 1998.

Hudak BB. *Respiratory disease in children: diagnosis and management.* Baltimore: Williams & Wilkins, 1994:501–532.

Wood RE. Spelunking in the pediatric airways: explorations with the flexible fiberoptic bronchoscope. *Pediatr Clin North Am* 1984;31:785–899.

Author: Roberto V. Nachajon

Transposition of the Great Arteries (TGA)

 Database

DEFINITION

• In TGA the aorta originates anteriorly from the right ventricle carrying desaturated blood to the body and the pulmonary artery originates posteriorly from the left ventricle carrying oxygenated blood to the lungs. There is fibrous continuity between the pulmonary and mitral valves and subaortic conus (infundibulum) is present. In the normal heart the aorta arises posteriorly from the left ventricle with fibrous continuity between the aortic and mitral valves.

• The most common type of TGA, known as D-Transposition or D-TGA is TGA (S,D,D): situs solitus of the atria and viscera (S), dextroventricular segment situs (D), aortic valve annulus to the right of the pulmonary artery (D).

• Other variations include TGA (S,D,L) where the aortic valve annulus is to the left of the pulmonary artery (L), and TGA (S,L,L) or "corrected transposition," in which there is situs solitus of the atria and the viscera (S), levoventricular segment situs (L), and the aortic valve annulus is to the left of the pulmonary artery (L).

• Associated abnormalities:

—PDA and PFO with intact ventricular septum (50%)
—Dynamic obstruction of the left ventricular outflow tract [subpulmonary obstruction, (20%)]
—Ventricular septal defect [VSD (40%)]
—VSD and left ventricular outflow tract obstruction [subaortic/aortic stenosis (10%)]
—Coarctation of the aorta or interruption of the aortic arch (10%)
—Subpulmonic/pulmonic stenosis
—Coronary branching abnormalities (33%)
—Straddling or overriding atrioventricular valve
—Juxtaposition of the atrial appendages (5%)

PATHOPHYSIOLOGY

• Systemic and pulmonary circulations are separated and function in parallel.
• Desaturated systemic venous blood passes through the right heart to the aorta, while the oxygenated pulmonary venous blood passes through the left heart and returns to the lungs.
• Survival depends on mixing (PDA, PFO/ASD, and/or VSD).

EPIDEMIOLOGY

• TGA represents 5% to 7% of all congenital heart disease
• Incidence: 20 to 30/100,000 live births
• 60% to 70% male preponderance

 Differential Diagnosis

• Cardiac (cyanosis)
—Lesions with ductal dependent pulmonary blood flow:
—Tricuspid atresia with normally related great arteries
—Tetralogy of Fallot (possible)
—Tetralogy of Fallot/Pulmonary atresia
—Critical pulmonic stenosis
—Pulmonary atresia/intact ventricular septum
—Ebstein anomaly (possible)
—Heterotaxy (most forms)
—Ductal independent mixing lesions:
—Total anomalous pulmonary venous connection without obstruction
—Truncus arteriosus
—Lesions with ductal dependent systemic blood flow:
—Hypoplastic left heart syndrome
—Interrupted aortic arch
—Critical coarctation of the aorta
—Critical aortic stenosis
• Pulmonary
—Primary lung disease
—Airway obstruction
—Extrinsic compression of the lungs
• Neurological
—CNS dysfunction
—Respiratory neuromuscular dysfunction
• Hematologic
—Methemoglobinemia
—Polycythemia

 Data Gathering

HISTORY

• Typically AGA or LGA
• Cyanosis within the first few hours or first few days of life
• Tachypnea often without retractions
• Feeding intolerance

 Physical Examination

• Cyanosis
• Tachypnea without respiratory distress (unless in heart failure from a large VSD)
• Single loud S2
• Absence of a heart murmur in infants with an intact ventricular septum
• Soft systolic murmur in infants with a VSD
• Systolic ejection murmur of valvar or subvalvar aortic or pulmonic stenosis (if present)
• Hepatomegaly if in heart failure

 Laboratory Aids

Test: Arterial blood gas
Significance: Hypoxemia (pO_2 often in low 30s) unchanged in 100% FIO_2. Infants with marginal mixing have pO_2 less than 20 with metabolic acidosis.

Test: Chest radiograph
Significance: Mild cardiomegaly with an egg-shaped heart with a narrow superior mediastinum and increased pulmonary vascular markings ("egg on a string").

Test: Electrocardiogram
Significance: Initially normal, progressing to right ventricular hypertrophy and right axis deviation.

Test: Echocardiogram
Significance: Can usually provide all the anatomic and functional information required for management of infants with D-TGA. The study should focus on the alignment of the great arteries, and other associated anomalies, specifically defects that promote intercirculatory mixing, the presence of left or right ventricular outflow tract obstruction, and the coronary anatomy.

 Therapy

DRUGS

• Correction of metabolic acidosis, hypoglycemia, and hypocalcemia improves myocardial function.
• PGE1 is used for severe cyanosis to promote mixing at the ductus arteriosus. Instituting PGE1 may increase pulmonary venous congestion if there is an inadequate interatrial communication by increasing the pulmonary blood flow. Side effects of PGE1 include apnea, fever, and hypotension.

INTERVENTIONAL CATHETERIZATION

Balloon atrial septostomy (Rashkind procedure) is used in the severely hypoxemic infant with an intact or restrictive atrial septum to promote intercirculatory mixing at the atrial level and stabilize the neonate prior to definitive or palliative surgery.

SURGERY

• Definitive surgery for D-TGA includes procedures that redirect the right- and left-sided pulmonary and systemic venous returns at the atrial, ventricular, and great artery level, and include:

—Atrial inversion: Atrial inversion procedures involve baffling the pulmonary venous blood flow to the tricuspid valve (systemic circulation), and the systemic venous blood flow to the mitral valve (pulmonary circulation). The atrial inversion operations include the Mustard procedure, in which prosthetic or pericardial baffles are used to redirect the blood, and the Senning procedure, in which the baffles are made of an atrial septal flap and the right atrial free wall. The Senning procedure, a modification of the Mustard procedure, is used in the following infants:
—Infants with D-TGA with intact ventricular septum, who have not been repaired within the first month of life.
—Neonates with D-TGA with intact ventricular septum and moderate to severe pulmonic stenosis.
—Neonates with D-TGA with "unswitchable coronaries" (<1% of cases).

—Ventricular inversion:
—D-TGA/VSD with severe pulmonic stenosis: The Rastelli operation may be used to redirect the blood at the ventricular level. In the operation the left ventricular blood flow is baffled to the aorta by creating an intraventricular tunnel between the VSD and the aortic valve. A conduit is placed from the right ventricle to the pulmonary artery to redirect the right ventricular blood flow.
—D-TGA/VSD with severe aortic stenosis: The Damus-Kaye-Stansel operation in conjunction with the Rastelli operation may be used to redirect ventricular blood flow.

—Arterial Switch: Surgical switching of the great arteries with coronary reimplantation.

PROGNOSIS

• Without treatment, 30% mortality in first week of life, 50% within first month, 70% within first 6 months and 90% within first year.
• In most centers, the mortality rate after arterial switch operation for D-TGA with intact ventricular septum or D-TGA/VSD is less than 3%. Factors that have been shown to increase the mortality include:

—An intramural course of the left coronary artery
—Retropulmonary course of the left coronary artery
—Complex arch abnormalities
—Right ventricular hypoplasia
—Multiple VSDs
—Straddling atrioventricular valves

 Follow-Up

COMPLICATIONS

• Complications of the intra-atrial surgeries include obstruction of the pulmonary venous return (<2% of the cases), obstruction of the systemic venous return (<5% of cases), residual intraatrial baffle shunt (<20% of all cases), tricuspid regurgitation (5–10%), absence of sinus rhythm (>50% of cases), frequent supraventricular arrhythmias (50%), and moderate to severely depressed RV function (10%).

—Follow-up is recommended every 6 to 12 months to detect arrhythmias, tricuspid regurgitation, and right ventricular function. Arrhythmias include sick-sinus syndrome, marked sinus bradycardia, ectopic atrial rhythm, slow junctional rhythm, and supraventricular tachycardia, especially aflutter and ectopic atrial tachycardia.
—Complications after the Rastelli operation include conduit obstruction and complete heart block (rare).

—Follow-up is recommended every 12 months to monitor for conduit obstruction, left ventricular outflow tract obstruction, and various forms of heart block.

• Complications after the arterial switch operation are much rarer relative to the atrial and ventricular inversion operations, and include supravalvar pulmonary stenosis at the anastomotic site (<5% of cases), supravalvar aortic stenosis at the anastomotic site (<5% of cases), neo-aortic regurgitation is a late finding in 25% of patients, and coronary artery obstruction, which may lead to ischemia and infarction. These complications are generally rare and hemodynamically insignificant. Mortality results from the following:

—Early mortality is usually related to kinking or obstruction of the coronary arteries during transfer to the neoaorta, an "unprepared" left ventricle, or hemorrhage from the multiple suture lines.
—Late mortality (1–2%) usually occurs from myocardial ischemia, pulmonary vascular obstructive disease, or during reoperation for supravalvular stenosis.
—Follow-up is recommended every 6 to 12 months to monitor for supravalvar aortic or pulmonic stenosis, neo-aortic valve insufficiency and coronary ischemia.

 Common Questions and Answers

Q: How do most patients with TGA present?
A: Most patients with TGA present in the newborn period with cyanosis that is not repsonsive to supplemental oxygen. A small number of patients can present later if they have good intercirculatory mixing (ASD, VSD) and possibly PS to prevent overt heart failure.

ICD-9-CM 745.10

BIBLIOGRAPHY

Blume ED, Wernovsky G. Long-term results of the arterial switch operation for transposition of the great vessels. *Semin Thorac Cardiovasc Surg* 1998;1:129–137.

Paul MH, Wernovsky G. Transposition of the great arteries. In: Emmanouilides GC, Riemenschneider TA, Allen HD, Gutgesell HP, eds. *Moss and Adams' heart disease in infants, children and adolescents including the fetus and young adult,* 5th ed. Baltimore: Williams & Wilkins, 1995:1154–1225.

Wernovsky G, Hougen TJ, Walsh EP, et al. Midterm results after the arterial switch operation for transposition of the great arteries with intact ventricular septum: clinical, hemodynamic, echocardiographic and electrophysiologic data. *Circulation* 1988;77:1333–1344.

Wernovsky G, Mayer JE Jr, Jonas RA, et al. Factors influencing early and late outcome of the arterial switch operation for transposition of the great arteries. *J Thorac Cardiovasc Surg* 1995;109:289–302.

Author: Bradley S. Marino

Transverse Myelitis

 Database

DEFINITION

- Demyelination in the spinal cord causing acute/subacute loss of motor sensory and autonomic function, often preceded by midback pain; may be postviral, associated with VZV, EBV, influenza, rubella, mumps.
- Pathophysiology suspected: analogous to that of multiple sclerosis/acute encephalomyelitis versus autoimmune versus direct viral invasion.

ASSOCIATED CONDITIONS

- Rarely, primary inflammatory disorders (e.g., lupus erythematosus, Sjögren disease) present with transverse myelitis.
- Rare metabolic causes of myelopathy include vitamin B_{12} deficiency, adrenomyeloneuropathy/leukodystrophy.

 Differential Diagnosis

- Presentation of transverse myelitis in a toddler may resemble:

—Osteomyelitis
—Arthritis
—Toxic synovitis: extreme irritability, unwillingness to bear weight
—Acute abdominal process.
—In many cases extremity weakness seen in transverse myelitis may resemble an acute neuromuscular disorder such as Guillain-Barré syndrome or polymyositis.
—Definitive myelopathic signs (spastic tone, hyperreflexia, upgoing toes, sensory level) require exclusion of alternative causes of myelopathy that are treated differently such as

- Compressive myelopathies:

—Vertebral osteomyelitis/discitis
—Intrinsic or extrinsic tumor
—Spine trauma
—Epidural abscess

- Infectious causes of myelopathy:

—Polio (raises concern of underlying immunodeficiency)
—Lyme disease (in children with possible exposure; serology is nonspecific but is sensitive unless antibiotics given early in the course)
—Syphilis: usually chronic, tertiary form (tabes dorsalis)

- Vascular:

—Cord ischemia (postcardiac surgery)
—Cord AVM

- Metabolic:

—Leukodystrophy
—Pelizaeus-Merzbacher
—Adrenoleukodystrophy (chronic presentation)
—Transverse myelitis may be part of a more generalized demyelinative disorder.
—If multiple lesions occur at different times, diagnosis of multiple sclerosis is made
—Association with demyelination of optic nerves (optic neuritis) is referred to as Devic disease.
—Multiple coincident demyelinating lesions: best seen on MRI; indicate acute disseminated encephalomyelitis

 Data Gathering

HISTORY

The most prominent symptom is often unwillingness or inability to bear weight, possibly with decreased spontaneous use of hands. History of neoplastic illness or immunodeficiency may suggest alternate causes of acute myelopathy. Details of the temporal course of the symptoms is important, since sudden onset of weakness, although not inconsistent with transverse myelitis, raise the possibility of acute structural or vascular causes of myelopathy. After 2 to 3 days, signs usually plateau and may evolve toward spasticity/hyperreflexia.

- Back pain, urinary, or fecal incontinence/retention may be suggestive of transverse myelitis.
- Episodes often preceded by respiratory illness, trauma, or surgery.

 Physical Examination

- Irritability may limit examination; extent of weakness is assessed by how vigorously the child resists examination.
- Point tenderness indicates an alternative diagnosis
- Fever, hypertension, tachycardia, meningeal signs can appear
- Neurological examination directed to visual acuity and color vision, funduscopic examination for optic nerve head pallor (optic neuritis)
- Abnormal tone, weakness is usually symmetric, legs more than arms
- Reflexes are normal or brisk
- Abnormal position sense or a sensory "level" on the trunk
- Loss of anal wink, bladder dilatation, postvoid

Laboratory Aids

- Urgent imaging of the spine must be done in acute myelopathy to rule out a surgically remediable lesion.
- MRI of spine (to lowest level that could explain level of weakness or sensory) excludes structural causes of myelopathy and can be diagnostic of transverse myelitis: cord swelling with abnormal signal within the cord.
- CSF, usually done after imaging, often shows normal or slightly increased protein, mild pleocytosis with lymphocyte predominance.
- Investigation for underlying inflammatory disorder including ESR and ANA, is appropriate.
- Investigation for granulomatous disease or spirochetal infection includes PPD/anergy panel, serum ACE (angiotensin-converting enzyme, elevated in sarcoidosis), RPR, Lyme titer.
- Viruses associated with TM include the herpesviruses (EBV, VZV, HSV), mumps, rubella, influenza, HIV.
- Investigation for underlying metabolic disorder can include VLCFA (looking for adrenoleukodystrophy), B_{12}, and urine organic acids.

 ## Therapy

- Patients with transverse myelitis whose symptoms are progressing require close monitoring, in some cases in an intensive care setting, to anticipate respiratory embarrassment or autonomic instability; mechanical ventilation may be necessary.
- Autonomic deficits may require bowel/bladder regimen, catheterization, prophylactic antibiotics, stool softeners.
- Neurosurgical consultation if imaging reveals a surgically remediable cause of myelopathy (e.g., epidural abscess, neuroblastoma)
- Intravenous glucocorticoids have been used for acute demyelinative lesion of the cord or brain to speed recovery; there is no evidence that they alter long-term outcome; alternative immunomodulatory agents have also been used
- Treatments indicated for other causes of myelopathy that may be found (e.g., emergent radiation/steroid therapy for neoplastic cord compression)

 ## Follow-Up

- 60% of individuals with transverse myelitis resolve (gradually); neurologic complications include fixed weakness, sensory, or autonomic deficits.
- In cases of suspected MS, check BAERs, VERs may provide evidence of other foci of demyelination.
- Physical and occupational therapy may help promote functional recovery and prevent contractures.

PITFALLS

- A high index of suspicion of abnormal autonomic reflexes may prevent perforated bladder.
- Use of antihypertensives requires extreme caution—iatrogenic hypotension may be refractory in this setting.
- GBS may resemble transverse myelitis, particularly when the latter presents with hyporeflexia; cytoalbuminemic dissociation (high protein, low-grade pleocytosis) in CSF from patients with GBS helps distinguish the two conditions.

 ## Common Questions and Answers

Q: What makes you think this could be MS instead?
A: History of other similar episodes that have now resolved completely, association with internuclear ophthalmoplegia, association with optic neuritis, multiple lesions in space of different ages on MRI of brain/spine.

Q: What is the usual clinical course?
A: Symptoms usually worsen for 2 to 3 days, then plateau and change to UMN before 60% resolve gradually to baseline.

Q: What causes the pain and irritability commonly seen in children with TM?
A: Pain in TM may be due to (1) neuropathic pain from nerve root inflammation, (2) nociceptive pain from dural inflammation, (3) muscle spasm from motor dyscontrol, (4) bladder distention from dysautonomia, (5) psychological distress from loss of motor control, or (6) dysesthesia from demyelination of spinothalamic tract.

ICD-9-CM 323.9

BIBLIOGRAPHY

Abele-Horn M, Franck W, Busch U, Nitschko H, Roos R, Heesemann J. Transverse myelitis associated with mycoplasma pneumoniae infection. *Clin Infect Dis* 1998;26(4):909–912.

Adams RD, Victor M. *Principles of neurology*, 5th ed. New York: McGraw Hill, 1993.

Knebusch M, Strassburg HM, Reiners K. Acute transverse myelitis in childhood: nine cases and review of the literature. *Dev Med Child Neurol* 1998;40(9):631–639.

Scott TF, Bhagavatula K, Snyder PJ, Chieffe C. Transverse myelitis. Comparison with spinal cord presentations of multiple sclerosis. *Neurology* 1998;50(2):429–433.

Authors: D. Elizabeth McNeil and Peter M. Bingham

Trichinosis

Database

DEFINITION

Disease caused by ingestion of inadequately cooked meat containing the nematode (roundworm) Trichinella spiralis larvae cysts.

• Other names trichinosis, trichinelliasis, trichinellosis

PATHOPHYSIOLOGY

• *Trichinella* larvae in poorly cooked meat eaten by patient
• Organisms released after cyst wall digestion by gastric enzymes, pass to small intestine, invade mucosa with edema, hyperemia, and ulcerations and then develop into adult worms. Fertilized females release larvae (500–5000) over approximately 2 to 6 weeks. Adult worms then expelled in feces (do not multiply in human host).
• Larvae travel via lymphatic and venules to the bloodstream and into skeletal muscle fibers to grow (10×), coil, and encyst. Muscle fibers enlarge, become edematous; may have granulomatous reactions in nonskeletal muscle, but larvae only found in skeletal muscle.
• Cysts (hyaline capsules) may calcify over several months to years.

EPIDEMIOLOGY

• Worldwide distribution, virulence varies with location and strain
• Infections occur sporadically and in epidemics (families, small communities)
• Approximately 4% of cadavers in 1970 study with evidence of previous infection (16% in 1941 study)
• Certain nationalities may be more likely to contract disease due to dietary habits
• Should be considered in patients with recent foreign travel
• Most infections involve ingestion of poorly cooked pork, wild game (bear, cougar), horse or walrus meat
• Decreasing number of cases per year in United States due to increased public awareness leading to better-cooked meat, home and commercial freezing, and laws preventing feeding of garbage to swine

COMPLICATIONS

• Myocarditis (most frequent serious complication), meningoencephalitis, CNS granulomas, pneumonitis, pericardial effusion, pleural effusion, pulmonary embolism or infarction, fatty changes of the liver, glomerulonephritis, severe enteritis, prolonged muscle aches, ocular disturbances, cardiac complaints and headaches
• Can be fatal (4–8 weeks post-infection)
• Rarely permanent damage

PROGNOSIS

• Usually resolves spontaneously over several months
• Muscle swelling and weakness may persist.
• Poorer prognosis if cardiac or CNS involvement
• Children may be more symptomatic, but fewer complications and quicker recovery than adults

Differential Diagnosis

• Infection: viral syndromes, parasitic, spirochetal, gastroenteritis, influenza, sinusitis, typhoid fever, measles, scarlet fever, meningitis, rheumatic fever, encephalitis, encephalomyelitis, poliomyelitis
• Miscellaneous: Fever of unknown origin, dermatomyositis, myocarditis, inflammatory bowel disease, angioneurotic edema, glomerulonephritis, polyneuritis, eosinophilic leukemia, polyarteritis nodosa

Data Gathering

HISTORY

Question: Most ingestions asymptomatic (subclinical).
Significance: Nonspecific signs and symptoms may mimic other nonspecific illnesses. Lack of specificity of presentation may make diagnosis less obvious in some instances.

Question: Ingestion of poorly cooked or raw meat?
Significance: Infection is transmitted by ingestion of inadequately prepared meat. History of this activity should raise suspicion of potential trichinosis infection.

Question: Ingestion of game animal?
Significance: Game animals have been associated with transmission of trichinosis. This activity may also be associated with less than ideal storage or cooking issues.

Question: Others with same diet and similar symptoms?
Significance: Because this is a dietary acquired disease, others with similar diet may be at risk of developing trichinosis. Epidemics have been reported in families and communities.

Physical Examination

• Classic presentation includes myositis, fever, periorbital edema, and eosinophilia
• Symptomatic orderly progression includes:

—GI stage (first days to week postingestion)
  —Nausea, vomiting, diarrhea (may be prolonged), abdominal pain, constipation, fever, malaise
—Dissemination (muscle invasion) stage (weeks 2–6)
  —Fever, periorbital edema, myalgias most common symptoms
  —Malaise, fatigue, facial edema and pain, tenderness, swelling, aching, weakness, or fasciculations of muscles (includes extraocular, face, tongue, larynx, neck, shoulder, chest, back, upper extremity muscles, and diaphragm)
—Convalescent (encystment) stage (weeks 3–6)
  —May have continued weakness, myalgias

Finding: Other reported signs and symptoms include cough, shortness of breath, hoarseness, headache, dysphagia, conjunctivitis, chemosis, maculopapular, urticarial or petechial rash, trunk or limb edema, conjunctival or splinter (subungual) hemorrhages, facial flushing, photophobia, blurred vision, diplopia, neck mass, cranial nerve abnormalities, meningoencephalitis, seizures, intracranial vessel thrombosis, focal neurologic findings

Laboratory Aids

SPECIFIC TESTS

- Pitfalls

—Serology takes time (3 weeks)
—No stool, body fluid (other than serology), or radiographic aid for routine specific diagnosis

- Trichinella serology (through CDC): requires several weeks to become positive; use two tests to increase sensitivity: bentonite flocculation (1:5 or fourfold increase), latex flocculation test, ELISA, immunofluorescence
- Skeletal muscle biopsy

—Most direct diagnostic tool, though usually not needed
—Best source swollen muscle, at least 2 weeks post-infection
—Encysted larvae in necrotic muscle fibers surrounded by inflammatory cells
—Granulomatous reaction in nonskeletal muscle, but not encysted larvae

- Skin test: becomes positive in 2nd to 3rd week; does not distinguish between acute or old infection as test remains positive for years after infection

NON-SPECIFIC TESTS

- CBC and differential: eosinophilia (to 70%), peaks 10 to 21 days post-infection
- Serum muscle enzymes: CPK, LDH, SGOT, SGPT often elevated; ESR may be normal or elevated
- EKG: abnormal with myocarditis
- Imaging studies: small CNS lesions, some with ring calcifications; intravenous enhancement on CT scan
- Electromyography: results resemble polymyositis and inflammatory myopathies

 ## Therapy

- No ideal or totally satisfactory therapy
- Symptomatic: bed rest, salicylates

MEDICATIONS

- Mebendazole (Vermox)

—Variable dosing recommendations (10 days)
—May be helpful during the disseminated (muscular) phase
—Successful in animal treatments
—Less toxic than thiabendazole

- Thiabendazole (Mintezol):

—Best if used within 24 hours of ingestion
—25 mg/kg PO for 7 days
—Kills some but not all established larvae
—Does not appear to alter established infection
—Better absorbed than mebendazole
—Has anti-inflammatory, antipyretic, and analgesic effects

- Pyrantel pamoate (Antiminth):

—11 mg/kg/d for 4 days
—Effective against GI worms, not encysted worms

- Systemic corticosteroids:

—May be useful, but unproven
—Should not be used alone as may prolong symptomatic disease state

 ## Follow-Up

- Expect improvement over several weeks
- Cardiac, neurologic, or pulmonary involvement indicate more severe problems
- Prognosis usually good

PREVENTION

Isolation

- Standard precautions

Control Measures

- Eat only fully cooked meat, especially pork and ground beef that may have been mixed with pork and game

—Cook until no trace of pink
—Thermal death at 55°C
—Freeze for 3 weeks at 15°C to 23°C (5–10°F)

- Smoking, salting, and drying meat are not reliable sterilization methods
- Avoid feeding swine uncooked meat scraps
- Active rat control
- Avoid breastfeeding by infected mother

PITFALLS

- Assuming only pork can transmit disease
- Not considering trichinosis in differential diagnosis

Common Questions and Answers

Q: How can I prevent infection?
A: Be sure meat fully cooked [55–77°C (170°F)] (not pink) or has been stored in a freezer at less than −15°C (5°F) for greater than 3 weeks. Trichinella larvae in game may be relatively resistant to freezing.

Q: Is trichinosis contagious from person to person?
A: No (other than through infected breastmilk).

Q: Do special precautions need to be taken when treating a patient with presumed trichinosis?
A: Only good hand washing. No isolation required.

ICD-9-CM 124

BIBLIOGRAPHY

American Academy of Pediatrics. Trichinosis (Trichinella spirallis). In: Peter G, ed. *1997 Red book: report of the committee of infectious diseases,* 24th ed. Elk Grove Village, IL: American Academy of Pediatrics, 1997:535–536.

Bia FJ, Barry M. Parasitic infections of the central nervous system. *Neurol Clin* 1986;4: 171–206.

Clausen MR, Meyer CN, Krantz T, et al. Trichinella infection and clinical disease. *QJM* 1996;89(8):631–636.

Feigin RD, Cherry JD, eds. *Textbook of pediatric infectious diseases,* 3rd ed. vol. I and II. Philadelphia: WB Saunders, 1992:361, 376, 751–752, 2088–2093.

Grove DI. Tissue nematodes (trichinosis, dracunuliasis, filariasis). In: Mandell GL, Bennet JE, Dolin R, eds. *Principles and practice of infectious diseases,* 4th ed. New York: Churchill Livingstone, 1995:2531–2533.

Kreel L, Poon WS, Nainby-Luxmoore JC. Trichinosis diagnosed by computed tomography. *Postgrad Med J* 1988;64:626–630.

McAuley JB, Michelson MK, Schantz PM. Trichinella infection in travelers. *J Infect Dis* 1991;164:1013–1016.

McAuley JB, Michelson MK, Schantz PM. Trichinosis surveillance, United States, 1987–1990. *MMWR CDC Surveill Summ* 1991;40:35–42.

MacLean JD, Viallet J, Law C, et al. Trichinosis in the Canadian Arctic: report of five outbreaks and a new clinical syndrome. *J Infect Dis* 1989;160:513–520.

Morse JW, Ridenour R, Unterseher P. Trichinosis: infrequent diagnosis or frequent misdiagnosis? *Ann Emerg Med* 1994;24:969–971.

Trichinella spiralis infection—United States, 1990. *MMWR* 1991;40:57–60.

Author: George Anthony Woodward

Tuberculosis—Pediatric

 Database

DEFINITION

Pediatric tuberculosis (TB) is the disease state caused by *Mycobacterium tuberculosis,* an acid-fast bacillus (AFB). Pediatric TB should be regarded as a spectrum of *exposure,* from *infection* to *disease,* because progression from an infected individual (exposure) to infection and subsequently disease can occur much faster in children under 2 years of age (occurring within the incubation of the disease stated below).

Progression through this spectrum is age-dependent, being 40% to 50% for 0- to 2-year-olds, approximately 20% for 2- to 4-year-olds, and 10% to 15% for those over 5 years old, the 5- to 10-year-olds being the most protected age group.

EPIDEMIOLOGY

- The most common route of infection is via the respiratory tract. TB is spread from a person with disease by droplet nuclei that are inhaled by other individuals. A child becomes infected with TB after close and prolonged contact with an adult or adolescent who has active, untreated infectious disease, usually pulmonary TB, in a poorly ventilated space. The sole risk factor is breathing air containing droplet nuclei that contain the tubercle bacillus. Thus there are individuals who develop TB without knowledge of an infectious contact.
- Congenital infection occurs, rarely, in the setting of an untreated mother in the last trimester of pregnancy.
- *Infection* with the tubercle bacillus needs to be differentiated from *disease* (i.e., tuberculosis).
- Approximately 8% (19 million) Americans have been infected with TB, 45% African Americans and 25% Whites over 70 years of age.
- The number with active contagious disease is approximately 25,000.
- The interval between onset of infection and disease is 10 to 12 weeks to many years.
- Of adults, only 10% of those infected will develop disease, and this is reduced by 60% to 90% if preventative INH is taken within the first 2 years of infection. This is the most likely time when infection replicates sufficiently to progress to a *disease* state. In most, untreated infection becomes dormant and does not progress.
- The greatest chance of disease occurring is within the first 2 years after infection (of developing a positive purified protein derivative [PPD] reaction). However, for infants and children less than 5 years old, progression through the spectrum of pediatric TB (exposure-infection-disease) is age-dependent (see Definition section).
- Postpubertal adolescents and immunosuppressed individuals, including persons with diabetes, with chronic renal failure, malnourished individuals, persons on steroids for whatever reasons (including pulse doses), have higher risks of progression of infection to disease.
- Nationwide, the past 4 years have documented an increase in TB in children under 2 years of age in the states where TB is common.

PATHOPHYSIOLOGY

- Pathology of disease includes the formation of a primary focus of infection, usually in the lung (Gohn focus), with recruitment of cell-mediated immune responses, which lead to formation of adenopathy of the hilar, cervical, mediastinal, and/or other nodes, depending on the dissemination of infection.
- Development of a PPD reaction is dependent on an adequate cell-mediated immune response, which often is not fully developed in infants less than 2 years of age and in those infected with overwhelming disease, such as miliary TB or meningitis or large pleural effusions.

COMPLICATIONS

- Missed diagnosis: Failure to consider TB in a child who is failing to thrive and whose PPD is negative.
- TB meningitis: Outcome is dependent on the stage at which anti-TB medication is begun.

—If Rx is started at stage I, complete recovery occurs in 94%, with neurologic sequelae in 6%.
—If delayed until stage II, complete recovery occurs in 51%, with neurologic sequelae in 40% and death in 7%.
—If delayed until stage III, complete recovery occurs in 18%, with neurologic sequelae in 61% and death in 20%.

- Miliary TB
- Bony TB: Most commonly spinal
- Renal TB: Presents as a fever of undetermined origin (FUO), with or without urinary symptoms
- Congenital TB manifests with hepatosplenomegaly; may have CSF abnormalities and CXR abnormalities
- Evolution of multidrug-resistant TB (MDRTB): The cost for medication alone to treat an individual with a sensitive organism is $10,000 per year; the cost of drug treatment with a resistant organism is $250,000 per year, not including any hospitalization costs.
- Drug toxicity: Pediatric patients are much more tolerant of anti-TB medications than are adults; thus regular monitoring of liver function tests is not routinely required.
- Hepatitis with INH, rifampin, and pyrazinamide (PZA); neurologic complications with INH; skin rashes with rifampin; ototoxicity with streptomycin; but ocular toxicity with EMB in the pediatric age group has not been documented, and therefore is a safe drug to use.

PROGNOSIS

- The death rate for untreated TB is 40% over 4 years.
- For miliary TB and meningeal TB, prognosis is dependent on the stage of presentation (as above).
- For outbreaks of MDRTB, death rates have ranged from 70% to 90%.

ASSOCIATED DISEASES

- Case rates for TB of all ages are highest in urban, low-income areas, in the homeless and residents of correctional facilities, and in areas with a high population of foreign-born individuals.
- The following diseases are associated with progression of infection to disease:

—CHIV infection: factor in the increase in TB, since 1 in 240 Americans is infected with HIV, and the bacillus grows better, evades detection (chest x-rays may appear normal), and is more contagious
—Lymphoma
—Diabetes
—Chronic renal failure
—Malnutrition
—Immunosuppression, including daily steroid use

 Differential Diagnosis

TB can do anything malignancy can do.

- Pulmonary infiltrate: other chronic organisms such as *Nocardia* and histoplasmosis. Infiltrates due to bacterial or viral pathogens resolve faster than TB, thus reevaluation of a suspect in 8 to 12 weeks clarifies this differential.
- Hilar adenopathy: In TB it is usually unilateral, but EBV, adenovirus, pertussis, and malignancy are possible mimickers.
- Miliary disease: pulmonary, hepatosplenomegaly with or without CNS involvement
- Gastrointestinal disease: The most common differential is Crohn disease.
- Meningitis: fungal meningitis, partially treated bacterial meningitis (rarely)

 Data Gathering

HISTORY

Inquire about the factors that are associated with tuberculosis infection:

- Exposure
- Migrant farmers
- Immigration from high-TB area such as Haiti, Southeast Asia
- Higher incidence in Native Americans
- Contact with adults who have active TB
- HIV-positive persons
- Immunosuppressed state
- Incarcerated adolescents
- Homeless persons
- Poor and medically indigent city dwellers
- Exposure to milk from untested herds
- Malnutrition
- Chronic steroid usage

Physical Examination

- May reflect underlying disease such as HIV, malnutrition, chronic steroid use
- Pulmonary rales
- Presence of sputum
- May be normal

Laboratory Aids

TESTS

Skin Testing

- The Mantoux test is 5 tuberculin units of PPD administered intradermally.
- The Centers for Disease Control does not recommend routine skin testing in low-risk groups in communities with low prevalence of TB except for one-time testing during childhood.
- Children at high risk should be tested annually.

—High-risk children include those in contact with adults from regions of world with high prevalence; adults with TB, HIV, and immunosuppressed states; those with Hodgkin disease, lymphoma, diabetes, chronic renal failure, and malnutrition; incarcerated adolescents; and those with exposure to high-risk adults.

- Skin tests become positive 3 to 6 weeks after exposure but may not turn positive for 3 months.

Other Tests

- Culture of sputum, gastric washings, pleural fluid, CSF, urine
- In children, the best source is early-morning gastric washings.
- Culture may take 2 to 3 weeks by the radiometric method.
- Positive cultures are found in fewer than 50% of children.

Imaging

Chest radiographs may show hilar adenopathy with or without atelectasis.

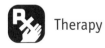

Therapy

HOSPITALIZATION

- Treatment initiated as an outpatient may not be complied with; thus hospitalization reinforces the issue of disease and allows time for education and linkage to TB control programs, which can then supervise direct observed therapy (DOT); however, in the era of managed care, direct linkage of the patient to the local TB control program through the health department and provision of DOT can avert the need to hospitalize for starting therapy; especially since the positivity rate of gastric aspirates for TB is 10% in the best hands.

- In cases of extensive disease, such as miliary or meningitis, and when an adult source case is not known, aggressive attempts should be made to obtain an organism from gastric aspirates, bronchoalveolar lavage, CSF, pleural or joint aspirate, bone aspirate, liver or tissue biopsy, and in some cases, blood cultures.

ISOLATION POLICIES

- Isolation policies are dependent on the age of the child and the manifestation of disease.
- In the past, children under 8 years of age did not require isolation for pulmonary disease, because the disease is usually a primary infection; that is, there is less organism load and more lymphatic enlargement. However, unless one knows that the parent and/or any adult visitors are *not* contagious, many infection control units require isolation of the child because the family members' state of contagion is unknown at the time of admission.
- Nonpulmonary, such as GI TB, meningitis, bone, joint, also do not require isolation.
- Children older than 8 years of age and adolescents should be isolated until they have completed 10 days of four-drug therapy (listed below)

DRUGS

- Initial treatment in areas with MDRTB of more than 4%: Until sensitivities are known, a four-drug regimen should be started: INH, 10 mg/kg/d; rifampin, 10 mg/kg/d; PZA, 30 mg/kg/d; and either streptomycin, 20 mg/kg/d (depending on whether it is meningitis or miliary TB, for which a cidal antibacterial agent is desired) or ethambutol, 25 mg/kg/d.
- If the organism is sensitive, treatment with the initial four primary drugs should continue for the first 2 months, followed by 4 months of INH and rifampin. When this regimen is adhered to, prognosis and a complete cure is achieved in 97% to 98% of patients. (*Ann Am Med* 1990;112.)

PREVENTION

- Prevention of disease by using INH, 10 mg/kg/d for 6 months orally, or if compliance is an issue, two times a week as DOT at 20 mg/kg, with a maximum dose of 900 mg, *without breaks in treatment,* is 60% to 90% effective against the development of active TB for 20 years in *nonimmunosuppressed* children. This recommendation prevents disease in the treated individual and, as a public health measure, interrupts transmission to contacts of the infected person with an efficacy of 60% to 90%.
- However, use of other regimens in cases of a contact of MDRTB are still being evaluated in children; therefore, this situation should be discussed with a specialist who has experience, one who is usually associated with the CDC or local TB control programs. Children with HIV or other immunodeficiency states require 12 months of prophylaxis. Any child (usually older children and adolescents) whose x-ray is consistent with past infection (granuloma or fibrosis) and who has not received INH prophylaxis previously requires 12 months of INH.

- BCG (bacille of Calmette and Guérin) vaccine is recommended only for infants and children who are PPD-negative, who are continually and intimately exposed to contagious adults or to adults with TB that is resistant to both INH and rifampin, and who cannot take long-term preventative medication or be removed from the contagious adult. These recommendations are currently under review.
- Follow-up and contact tracing are key to making TB a preventable disease.

Common Questions and Answers

Q: If the child has completed a course of INH and is reexposed, what are the risks of infection?
A: One course of preventive therapy is believed to confer immunity to subsequent exposure, even to MDRTB (data are preliminary).

Q: Should all children in close proximity to inner-city areas with a prevalence of TB be screened annually with PPD?
A: No. One needs to consider the risk benefit. Children under 5 years of age progress to disease more rapidly and are harder to diagnose when ill with TB; therefore, children who are under 5 years of age and live in high-risk parts of a city should be screened; otherwise, screening, according to the American Association of Pediatricians, at ages 1, 5, and 11 is sufficient.

Q: Because parents return for the PPD reading only 26% to 50% of the time, depending on which clinic they use, are there other ways to ensure that parents receive the PPD reading?
A: This is a tough question. An improved public health surveillance system, use of child care providers, or school programs requiring examination and utility are all shown to be more effective than patient education by the provider.

ICD-9-CM 011.9

BIBLIOGRAPHY

Centers for Disease Control Guidelines. *MMWR* 1990;39:1–29.

Control of tuberculosis in the United States. *Am Rev Respir Dis* 1992;142:1623–1633.

Diagnostic standards and classification of tuberculosis. *Am Rev Respir Dis* 1990;142:725–735.

Inselman LS. Tuberculosis in children: an update. *Pediatr Pulmonol* 1996;21(2):101–120.

Modern TB treatment and preventative therapy protocols. *MMWR* 1992;41.

New directions in diagnostics. *Pediatr Infect Dis J* 1997;16[Suppl 3]:S43–S48.

Author: Barbara Watson

Tuberous Sclerosis

 Database

DEFINITION

Tuberous sclerosis (TSC) is a neurocutaneous syndrome characterized by hamartomatous growths involving multiple regions of the body, such as the brain, retina, heart, kidney, and skin. First described by Bourneville (1880), the classic diagnostic triad of adenoma sebaceum, mental retardation, and seizures has been revised to include other manifestations, because many patients with TSC do not exhibit this triad.

CAUSES

TSC is either inherited in an autosomal dominant pattern or results from a spontaneous, sporadic mutation.

PATHOLOGY

Findings reflect the primary tissue in which lesions are identified (* denotes lesions that confirm the diagnosis of TSC).

- Brain

—Three characteristic lesions include *cortical tubers, *subependymal nodules, and giant-cell astrocytomas.
—In tubers, cerebral cortical architecture is disrupted, and these regions may undergo calcification, which can be visible on skull radiographs or brain computed tomography.
—Subependymal nodules consist of large abnormal astrocytes emanating from the lateral ventricular surface.
—Giant-cell astrocytomas are low-grade benign astrocytic neoplasms.

- Skin

—Adenoma sebaceum is highly suggestive of TSC and consists of pinkish-yellow plaques on the malar regions and nasolabial folds.
—Ash leaf spots are hypopigmented, hypomelanotic macules occurring anywhere on the body.
—Ungual fibromas are fleshy growths along the lateral borders of the nailbed. Shagreen patches are areas of shaggy, leathery skin typically in the lumbosacral area.
—Occasionally, café-au-lait spots also may be identified.

- Retina

—Whitish-yellow angiolipomas or *astrocytic hamartomas occur near the optic nerve head or the retinal periphery, which may calcify.

- Heart

—Rhabdomyomas in the ventricular wall occur in infancy and contain abundant nodules of large eosinophilic cells; this is the most common cardiac tumor of infancy and early childhood.

- Kidney

—Renal cysts, polycystic kidneys, *angiomyolipomas, and, rarely, renal carcinomas

- Other organ systems

—Less commonly affected are the lungs, gastrointestinal tract, spleen, vascular bed, and lymphatics.

GENETICS

Two clearly identified loci for familial and sporadic cases based on linkage analyses are 9q34 and 16p13, corresponding to *TSC1* and *TSC2* genes, respectively. The *TSC2* gene was cloned and is a 5.5-kb transcript, which encodes a 198-kd protein named tuberin. It is hypothesized that tuberin may function as a tumor suppressor. There is a loss of alleleic *TSC2* heterozygosity in TSC hamartomas, suggesting that an inactivating mutation of the *TSC2* occurring in somatic or germ-cell lines reflects a second-hit mutation.

EPIDEMIOLOGY

Current estimates suggest an incidence of 1 in 5,000 to 1 in 15,000 births. Approximately 60% to 70% of cases reflect sporadic mutation; 30% to 40% of cases are familial; it affects males and females equally.

PROGNOSIS

- Mental retardation will unfortunately not improve unless cognitive impairment results from uncontrolled seizures. Seizure control is often difficult, and many children will require epilepsy surgery to remove cortical tubers or subependymal nodules. In the rare event of neoplastic transformation of subependymal giant-cell astrocytomas, surgical intervention is necessary. Renal and cardiac tumors may require surgical intervention.

 Differential Diagnosis

Neurocutaneous syndromes in which skin lesions, mental retardation, and seizures are characteristic features should be considered:

- Neurofibromatosis
- Sturge-Weber syndrome
- von Hippel-Lindau disease
- Neurocutaneous melanosis
- Albright syndrome
- Incontinentia pigmenti
- Linear sebaceous nevus

 Data Gathering

HISTORY

- Primary symptoms include seizures, mental defect, and skin lesions.
- Seizures may begin at any time. In infancy, infantile spasms are a common presenting seizure.
- Mental retardation may manifest as developmental delay, but some patients are without cognitive defect.
- Skin lesions may appear in infancy or during early childhood.
- It is important to take a full family history, including consanguinity.
- Inquire about history of TSC, seizures, mental retardation, skin lesions, and cardiac or renal disease/cancers.

Physical Examination

- Need to maintain high level of suspicion for TSC in any patient evaluated with:

—Infantile spasms
—Seizures
—Mental retardation/developmental delay
—Peculiar skin lesions.

- Ash leaf and café-au-lait spots are small (often less than 5 mm) but may be found anywhere on skin and are often present at birth.
- Adenoma sebaceum is typically on the face around the nose and cheeks and appears similar to acne, appearing in the later childhood to adolescent years. It does not itch or suppurate.
- Ungual fibromas appear around the nailbed.
- Shagreen patches are brownish, leathery skin patches near the sacrum.
- Funduscopic examination may reveal whitish-yellow areas in epi- and peripapillary regions around the optic nerve head. They rarely cause visual impairment.
- Clinical signs of congestive heart failure in infants may be seen with cardiac TSC.
- Flank pain, nausea and vomiting, and hematuria may reflect renal involvement.

PROCEDURE

- In any suspected neurocutaneous syndrome, skin examination with a Wood lamp may be especially helpful in identifying hypo- or hyperpigmented lesions such as ash leaf or café-au-lait spots. Dilated funduscopic examination may also aid in full visualization of optic nerve head.
- One rare sign of TSC is the presence of small dental enamel pits.

 ## Laboratory Aids

TESTS

- Routine blood and cerebrospinal fluid labs are typically normal unless renal function is significantly compromised by renal cysts or renal carcinoma.
- In patients with mental retardation or seizures, electroencephalograpy is essential to evaluate cerebral activity.
- In infants, an EEG may also help diagnose infantile spasms, which are associated electrographically with a highly disorganized pattern of large-amplitude, asynchronous, sharp waves called hypsarrythmia.
- Later in childhood, children with TSC may develop the Lennox-Gastaut syndrome, which comprises of mental retardation, seizures, and a characteristic EEG pattern of slow (2.5-Hz) spike-wave complexes.

IMAGING

- Magnetic resonance imaging (MRI) of the brain with gadolinium administration performed serially every 1 to 2 years will identify tubers, subependymal nodules, and giant-cell tumors. These appear hyperintense on T-weighted images and may enhance with gadolinium. Rarely, a giant-cell astrocytoma may obstruct the foramen of Monroe, resulting in hydrocephalus, which can also be detected with MRI.
- Echocardiography can detect cardiac rhabdomyomas in infants with TSC.
- Renal ultrasound (every 1–2 years) or computed tomography (CT) will demonstrate renal lesions.

 ## Therapy

DRUGS

- Anticonvulsant therapy as needed and ACTH for infantile spasms; medical management of congestive heart failure or cardiac dysrhythmias in TSC patients with cardiac rhabdomyomas

 ## Follow-Up

SIGNS TO WATCH FOR

- A persistent change in mental status may reflect status epilepticus, an expanding mass lesion with obstructive hydrocephalus, or a new CNS neoplasm.
- Worsening renal function may reflect progressive renal involvement.

 ## Common Questions and Answers

Q: Can TSC be transmitted in subsequent pregnancies?
A: An affected individual with the TSC gene mutation has a 50% chance of transmitting the mutation to his or her offspring.

Q: Is genetic testing available?
A: The gene for TSC on chromosome 16 has been identified, but clinical use for prenatal or diagnostic testing is still in development.

Q: Will my child need brain surgery?
A: In the event of refractory seizures, removal of cortical tubers may help seizure control. If a brain tumor is detected by MRI, neurosurgical evaluation is indicated.

ICD-9-CM 759.5

BIBLIOGRAPHY

Gomez MR. *Tuberous sclerosis,* 2nd ed. New York: Raven Press, 1988.

Romanowski CA, Cavallin LI. Tuberous sclerosis, von Hippel-Lindau disease, Sturge-Weber syndrome. *Hosp Med* 1998;59(3):226–231.

Sarnat H. *Cerebral dysgenesis.* New York: Oxford University Press, 1991.

Webb DW, Osborne JP. Tuberous sclerosis. *Arch Dis Child* 1995;72(6):471–474.

Author: Peter B. Crino

Tularemia

 Database

DEFINITION

Tularemia is an infection with *Francisella tularensis,* a small, nonmotile, gram-negative coccobacillus that requires cysteine for growth. Two types have been described:

- Type A (Neartica): found in arthropods; highly virulent to rabbits and humans
- Type B (Palaeartica): found in water and aquatic animals; less virulent

Tularemia is characterized by six clinical forms, depending on the site of entry:

- Ulceroglandular tularemia constitutes 75% of all cases. A papule, which ruptures and ulcerates, occurs at the site of entry. Lymphadenopathy and hepatosplenomegaly accompany systemic symptoms of fever, chills, and headache.
- Glandular tularemia is identical to the ulceroglandular form, but without a skin lesion.
- Oculoglandular tularemia occurs when the organism gains access via the conjunctival sac, usually from rubbing the eyes with contaminated fingers. The eyelids are inflamed and the conjunctiva is infected. Yellow nodules and ulcers may appear on the palpebral conjunctiva.
- Typhoidal tularemia presents as fever of unknown origin, without localizing lymphadenopathy or skin findings. Shock, pleuropulmonary findings, odynophagia, diarrhea, and bowel necrosis are often associated.
- Oropharyngeal tularemia occurs after the ingestion of infected, improperly cooked meat. An exudative or membranous tonsillitis is seen. Lower gastrointestinal tract involvement with vomiting, diarrhea, and abdominal pain may be associated.
- Pneumonic tularemia occurs after inhalation of the organism. This presentation is seen in laboratory workers and is the most fulminant and lethal form.

PATHOPHYSIOLOGY

- Infection follows contact with rabbits or rodents.
- Ticks or deerflies are the most common vector.
- Entry into the human is via skin or mucous membranes.
- A papule or ulcer may be seen at the inoculation site.
- Bacteremia occurs after a 3- to 5-day incubation period, accompanied by fever and lymphadenopathy.
- The organism produces localized disease in reticuloendothelial organs, with areas of focal necrosis that may form granulomas.

EPIDEMIOLOGY

- *Francisella tularensis* is found in the northern hemisphere between 30° and 71° latitude.
- Wild mammals (rabbits, hares, squirrels, beavers, and deer) may be infected, as well as invertebrates (ticks, deerflies, and mosquitoes).
- Humans acquire tularemia after a bite by an infected arthropod or contact with tissues or body fluids of an infected animal.
- Most frequently affected are hunters, trappers, and farmers.

COMPLICATIONS

- Lymph node suppuration occurs in 40% of pediatric patients, regardless of treatment.
- Infection with *F. tularensis* may be complicated by necrotic and granulomatous lesions in the liver and spleen, as well as parenchymal degeneration.
- A sepsis syndrome with shock, fever, myalgias, and severe headache can be seen.
- Pneumonia and pleural involvement are frequently encountered in adults with typhoidal tularemia.

PROGNOSIS

When recognized and treated with appropriate antibiotics, the course is generally less than 1 month. Mortality is low, except in fulminant disease.

 Differential Diagnosis

Tularemia should be considered in the following differentials:

- Fever of unknown origin
- Fever with purulent conjunctivitis
- Fever with hepatosplenomegaly
- Fever with skin ulcer

Data Gathering

HISTORY

• A history of any of the following contact with affected animals should be sought: ingestion of wild animal meat, hunting or cleaning wild animals, and playing with dead wild animals.
• History of a recent tick bite is common among affected patients.
• A history of a papule that became ulcerated is classic for the ulceroglandular form.
• Fever greater than 101°F for 2 to 3 weeks is common, with associated weight loss.

 ## Physical Examination

• Skin lesions should be sought.
• Hepatosplenomegaly, purulent conjunctivitis, adenopathy, and exudative tonsillitis are other localized findings.

 ## Laboratory Aids

TESTS

• Serum agglutination titers to *F. tularensis* are positive if 1:160 or greater.
• A fourfold rise in titers after the second week of illness is characteristic and diagnostic.
• Cultures of blood, skin, ulcers, lymph nodes, gastric washings, and respiratory secretions require special media.
• Laboratory personnel should be made aware of the infection risk from specimens.

 ## Therapy

• If respiratory compromise is present, oxygen supplementation and/or assisted ventilation must be rapidly addressed.
• Recognition and prompt, aggressive treatment of shock should be a major priority.
• Intravenous antibiotic therapy should be administered. Streptomycin has been used traditionally, but gentamicin has recently been found to be equally effective.

 ## Follow-Up

PREVENTION

Isolation of the Hospitalized Patient

Infection control measures should include protection against secretions and respiratory isolation of the pneumonic form.

Control Measures

• Protective clothing and insect repellent should be used to minimize insect bites.
• Inspection for ticks (and immediate removal) should be routine after outdoor activity in endemic areas.
• Rubber gloves should be worn while cooking or handling wild rabbit meat.
• Laboratory workers should wear rubber gloves and masks when working with potentially infectious specimens.

ICD-9-CM 021.9

BIBLIOGRAPHY

Boyce JM. *Francisella tularensis*. In: Mandell GL, Douglas GR, Bennett JE, eds. *Principles and practice of infectious diseases,* 3rd ed. New York: Churchill Livingstone, 1990:1742–1746.

Cross JT, Schutze GE, Jacobs RF. Treatment of tularemia with gentamicin in pediatric patients. *Pediatr Infect Dis J* 1995;14(2): 151–152.

Kaye D. Tularemia. In: Braunwald E, ed. *Harrison's principles of internal medicine.* 14th ed. New York: McGraw-Hill, 1987:613–615.

Peter G, ed. *1997 Red Book: report of the committee on infectious disease.* Elk Grove Village, IL: American Academy of Pediatrics, 1997: 568–569.

Yow MD. Tularemia. In: Feigin RD, Cherry JD, eds. *Textbook of pediatric infectious diseases,* 2nd ed. Philadelphia: WB Saunders, 1987: 1336–1342.

Yow MD. Tularemia. In: Oski FA, ed. *Principles and practice of pediatrics.* Philadelphia: JB Lippincott Co, 1990:1132–1133.

Author: Janet H. Friday

Ulcerative Colitis

 Database

DEFINITION

Ulcerative colitis is recurrent inflammation of colonic mucosa leading to crypt abscesses. It is associated with many systemic signs and symptoms (see Complications).

CAUSES

- Unknown

PATHOLOGY

- Inflammation and ulceration of colonic mucosa with acute inflammatory cells infiltrating the villi, lamina propria, and crypts, giving rise to crypt abscesses
- In severe cases, the inflammation can infiltrate all layers of the bowel.
- Site of colon affected: rectum (100%); left side (50%–60%); pancolitis (10%); terminal ileum (backwash ileitis): radiologic, pathologic diagnosis
- Skip lesions are not seen in ulcerative colitis.

GENETICS

- HLA association: Bw52, DR2 (Japan); A2, Bw35, Bw40 (Ashkenazi Jews); A7, A11 (The Netherlands)

EPIDEMIOLOGY

- Incidence is 214 in 100,000.
- Prevalence, 50 to 75 per 100,000

COMPLICATIONS

- Bleeding
- Toxic megacolon
- Severe, acute weight loss
- Growth failure
- Anemia
- Psychosocial development
- Extraintestinal manifestations: primary sclerosing cholangitis (liver), uveitis, arthritis affecting large joints (10%), spondylitis (6%), erythema nodosum (<5%), pyoderma gangrenosum (<1%), renal calculi (5%).
- Malignancy risk is 0.51% per year after a decade of onset of disease. The risk for adenocarcinoma of the colon in children who developed disease before 14 years of age is 40% by 40 years old.
- Colonic stricture

 Differential Diagnosis

- Crohn disease
- Infectious colitis: *Salmonella, Shigella, Campylobacter, Yersinia, E. coli* (enterohemorrhagic), *Aeromonas,* ameba, *C. difficile,* CMV, herpes simplex, (lymphogranuloma inguinale, *Chlamydia*)
- Trauma due to anal sex or sexual abuse
- Congenital Hirschsprung enterocolitis
- Bleeding juvenile polyps
- Milk protein allergy
- Eosinophilic colitis
- Autoimmune enteropathy
- Irritable bowel syndrome (IBD)
- Appendicitis
- Hemolytic-uremic syndrome
- Henoch-Schönlein purpura

 Data Gathering

HISTORY

- A detailed history is important in making the diagnosis.
- Rectal bleeding (90%)
- Abdominal pain (90%)
- Diarrhea (50%)
- Weight loss (10%)
- Thirty percent present with moderate disease with cramps, bloody diarrhea, mild anemia, low-grade fever, anorexia, and weight loss.
- Ten percent present with fulminant disease defined as more than six stools a day, abdominal tenderness, fever, weight loss, anemia, leukocytosis, and hypoalbuminemia.
- Gastrointestinal symptoms: recurrent abdominal pain, diarrhea, weight loss, recent travel (enteric infections), antibiotic use (*C. difficile*), rectal bleeding, family history of IBD, appendectomy, growth failure

 Physical Examination

- Uveitis
- Signs of anemia
- Evidence of weight loss or poor growth
- Arthritis
- Mouth sores
- Abdominal tenderness
- Abdominal distention
- Rectal examination is normal except for heme positive stools.

 Laboratory Aids

TESTS

Laboratory Tests

- Complete blood count (iron deficiency)
- Iron studies: low serum iron, ferritin, elevated TIBC
- ESR (disease activity)
- Electrolytes (hydration)
- Transaminases, Aakaline phosphatase, GGT (hepatobiliary disease)
- pANCA Crohn disease (19% positive) and ulcerative colitis (80% positive)
- Stool for blood, white cells
- Stool cultures, *C. difficile* toxin A and B

Imaging

- Plain abdominal radiograph: This is important in diagnosing perforation, ileus, obstruction, and toxic megacolon. In toxic megacolon, the colon is dilated, and there are multiple air-fluid levels indicative of ileus. Serial x-rays are mandatory.
- Barium enema is useful in demonstrating strictures and mucosal disease but has the disadvantage that tissue diagnosis and direct visualization is impossible.
- An upper GI and small-bowel follow-through with extended abdominal film can demonstrate the entire gastrointestinal tract to exclude small intestinal disease.
- Ultrasound, CT, and MRI are usually not indicated in uncomplicated disease.
- Colonoscopy with biopsies are necessary to make the diagnosis of ulcerative colitis

PITFALLS

- It is often difficult to differentiate Crohn disease and ulcerative colitis. The management of both diseases is different. The combination of the pANCA and ASCA (anti-*Saccharomyces cerevisiae* antibody), for the diagnosis of ulcerative colitis, has a sensitivity of 60% to 70% and a specificity of 95% to 97%.
- Toxic megacolon is a surgical emergency. The patient has a dilated colon with breakdown of its barrier to toxins entering the systemic circulation. Signs and symptoms include peritonitis, mental status changes, and fluid and electrolyte imbalance. Plain abdominal radiograph shows a segment or total colonic dilatation. Risk factors include first attack, pancolitis, concurrent use of opiates or anticholinergics, and recent barium enema or colonoscopy.

HOME TESTING

Home testing of stool on a regular basis can alert patients and physician to alter therapy accordingly.

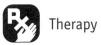 Therapy

- Mild disease and localized disease can be treated with sulfasalazine, topical corticosteroid enema or foam, and 5ASA enema or suppositories.
- Moderate disease: sulfasalazine, a short course of intravenous corticosteroid, low-residue diet
- Fulminant disease: hospitalization, complete bowel rest with total parenteral nutrition, broad-spectrum antibiotics (intravenous ampicillin, gentamicin, and metronidazole), intravenous corticosteroids, serial abdominal radiographs, frequent examinations, stool chart (frequency, amount of blood, and volume of stool output), early surgical consult

—If this treatment fails after 2 weeks, cyclosporine is started.
—After 24 weeks of failed medical treatment, subtotal colectomy is the next step. Those who respond to cyclosporine are started on oral cyclosporine; this is discontinued after 6 to 8 months. The risk of relapse may be significant after discontinuation of cyclosporine, and it is useful to start 6MP or azathioprine.

- Therapy of toxic megacolon is aimed at preventing perforation with decompression of the bowel. Management includes complete bowel rest, discontinuation of anticholinergics and narcotics, no endoscopies or contrast radiographs allowed, and broad-spectrum antibiotics; frequent examinations are required. Close communication with surgical colleagues is crucial. In the absence of improvement after 24 to 72 hours, the patient requires urgent surgery.
- Maintenance of remission: The corticosteroid dose is tapered and discontinued over a few months after initial presentation. Sulfasalazine or 5ASA is started before discharge. We recommend checking G6PD levels on patients at risk for G6PD deficiency before starting sulfasalazine.

SURGERY

- Urgently required for perforation, significant and persistent bleeding, toxic megacolon, and failure of medical treatment for fulminant colitis
- Can be electively performed for chronic incapacitating disease, growth failure, disease greater than 10 years' duration.
- Ileoanal anastomosis is the surgery of choice for most pediatric patients

DRUGS

- Methylprednisolone: 1 to 2 mg/kg/d intravenous (equivalent to prednisone 60 mg maximum)
- Prednisone 1 to 2 mg/kg/d oral (up to maximum 60 mg/d)
- Sulfasalazine 40 to 60 mg/kg/d tid (maximum, 4 g/d)
- Folic acid (to supplement sulfasalazine use) 1 mg/d
- 5ASA drugs, 4.8 g for active disease and 1.6 g for inactive disease
- Rowasa enema, 4 g at bedtime
- Rowasa suppository, 500 mg bid
- Hydrocortisone enema, 100 mg qd-bid
- Hydrocortisone foam, 80 mg qd-bid
- Cyclosporine, 4 mg/kg/d IV for 2 weeks (therapeutic levels; vary depending on the technique used in the laboratory).
- Cyclosporine PO 6 to 8 mg/kg/d for 6 to 8 months
- 6-Mercaptopurine, 1.0 to 1.5 mg/kg PO to start (keep ANC greater than 500)
- Azathioprine, 2.0 mg/kg (keep ANC greater than 500)

 Common Questions and Answers

Q: Will my child have this disease forever?
A: There are many different clinical presentations of ulcerative colitis. Some people will have only the initial attack and then be symptom-free, but usually an individual will have episodes of recurrences and remissions. Presently research is being done to identify the genetic factors in ulcerative colitis; once the genes can be identified, a cure will be possible.

Q: What is the cause of ulcerative colitis?
A: Both genetic and environmental factors are important in the development of ulcerative colitis. Possible environmental factors include aseptic environment in the first few years of life, lack of breast feeding, frequent use of antibiotics or aspirin, and diet.

Q: Where can I learn more about Crohn disease?
A: Crohn and Colitis Foundation of America (CCFA) is a nonprofit organization dedicated to the care of people with Crohn disease and ulcerative colitis.

Q: What new therapies will be used in the near future?
A: Biological agents, which is a type of therapy that uses our recently improved knowledge of the immune system, either downregulate inflammatory mediators or upregulate immunomodulatory mediators. Hopefully, this new class of therapies will greatly improve our care of people with IBD.

ICD-9-CM 556

BIBLIOGRAPHY

Grybovski JD. Crohn disease in children 10 years old or younger: comparison with ulcerative colitis. *J Pediatr Gastroenterol Nutr* 1994;18(2):174–182.

Hofley PM, Piccoli DA. Inflammatory bowel disease in children. *Med Clin North Am* 1994; 78(6):1281–1302.

Hyams J. Extraintestinal manifestations of IBD in childhood (Review). *J Pediatr Gastroenterol Nutr* 1994;19(1):7–21.

Hyams J, Davis P, Lerer T, et al. Clinical outcome of ulcerative proctitis in children. *J Pediatr Gastroenterol Nutr* 1997;25(2):149–152.

Lashner BA. Colorectal cancer in UC patients: survival curves and surveillance. *Cleve Clin J Med* 1994;62(4):272–275.

Oliva MM, Lake AM. Nutritional considerations and management of the child with inflammatory bowel disease. *Nutrition* 1996;12(3): 151–158.

Saha MT, Ruuska T, Laippala P, Lenko HL. Growth of prepubertal children with inflammatory bowel disease. *J Pediatr Gastroenterol Nutr* 1998;26(3):310–314.

Weedon DD, Shorter RG, Taylor WF, et al. Crohn disease and cancer. *N Engl J Med* 1973;289: 1099–1103.

Author: Robert N. Baldassano

Ureteropelvic Junction Obstruction

Database

DEFINITION

Ureteropelvic junction (UPJ) obstruction is obstruction of the ureter at the narrow junction with the renal pelvis, resulting in dilatation of the upper collecting system proximal to the obstruction.

CAUSES

- Intrinsic: congenital stenosis of UPJ, consisting of abnormal muscle bundles and fibrosis, producing an adynamic segment
- Extrinsic: ureteral kinks due to fibrous bands, aberrant vessels that produce a dynamic obstruction that varies, depending on the volume in the renal pelvis

PATHOPHYSIOLOGY

Obstruction may result in presentations ranging from mild dilatation of the renal pelvis with normal renal parenchyma to severe dilatation of the renal pelvis with atrophy of renal parenchyma or cystic dysplasia. It may be seen in Hirschsprung disease, esophageal atresia, imperforate anus, or adrenogenital syndrome.

GENETICS

- May be associated with other congenital anomalies: imperforate anus, contralateral multicystic kidney disease, congenital heart disease, VATER syndrome, esophageal atresia
- Ten percent of patients with UPJ obstruction have associated ipsilateral reflux significant enough to cause persistent hydronephrosis, even after relief of the obstruction.

EPIDEMIOLOGY

Most common obstructive lesion of the urinary tract in childhood

- One in 1,500 births
- Males: 65%
- Bilateral: 5%
- Forty percent of abdominal masses in neonates are due to hydronephrosis associated with UPJ obstruction.
- Fifty percent of all congenital urinary tract anomalies are UPJ obstruction.

Differential Diagnosis

- Megacalycosis: congenital dilatation without obstruction
- Vesicoureteral reflux diagnosed by a voiding cystourethrogram
- Midureteral or distal ureteral obstruction, posterior urethral valves
- Multicystic dysplasia: by ultrasound has no communicating cysts but may be difficult to distinguish; has no function on isotopic renogram
- Solid renal tumor, renal vein thrombosis

Data Gathering

HISTORY

- Antenatal: fetal hydronephrosis; oligohydramnios if bilateral involvement; polyhydramnios if intestines compressed, preventing amniotic fluid resorption; perinephric urinomas; or normal amniotic fluid volume
- Neonatal: abdominal mass
- Older childhood: intermittent abdominal, flank, or back pain; febrile urinary tract infection; hematuria after minimal trauma; flank pain after large volume load

Physical Examination

- Most newborns with UPJ have a normal physical examination.
- Neonatal: palpable abdominal mass
- Older childhood: flank mass, hypertension, failure to thrive

Laboratory Aids

TESTS

- Anemia, hematuria in older children

IMAGING

- Antenatal: ultrasonographic evaluation that shows dilatation of upper tracts with communicating calyces with nonvisualization of the lower ureter; study needs to be repeated postnatally with voiding cystography and a study to evaluate renal function, either excretory urography or an isotopic renal scan
- Diuretic renography: useful in assessing renal function; mercaptoacetyl triglycine (MAG-3) (excreted by renal tubules) is more accurate in newborns and infants than is diethylenetriamine pentaacetic acid (DTPA).

—Uptake is used to calculate differential renal function; normally each side is 50%.
—Then furosemide is administered to assess the efficiency of drainage of kidneys; this is useful only if there is brisk washout, which indicates that there is no anatomic obstruction.
—In unilateral neonatal hydronephrosis, if RUS and VCUG show no definite signs of anatomic obstruction, serial diuretic renography is useful.
—If the first study shows function greater than 40%, repeat in 3 months; if 30% to 40%, repeat in 2 months; if 20% to 30%, repeat in 1 month; if less than 20%, repeat in 2 weeks.
—If there is no deterioration in function of the involved kidney and no compensatory growth in the contralateral kidney, there is no evidence indicating anatomic obstruction.
—If there is any decrement in renal function, indicating obstruction, surgical intervention is indicated.
—Because fewer than 15% of infants will require surgery for obstruction, careful observation with serial diuretic renography is a reasonable option.

- Follow-up with postnatal ultrasound every 3 months, with a serial isotopic renogram if there is normal renal function.
- Older childhood: excretory urography with ultrasound
- Pressure-flow studies can be performed but are highly invasive.

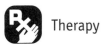

Therapy

CONSERVATIVE

- Antibiotic prophylaxis at birth to prevent upper tract infection, especially if VUR is present; use amoxicillin until 2 months of age, when trimethoprim-sulfamethoxazole or nitrofurantoin can be used.

SURGICAL

- Prenatal surgery: This carries a high rate of complication, and is to be considered only if the condition is life threatening. If hydronephrosis is unilateral or there is normal amniotic fluid volume and pulmonary development, prenatal intervention is not indicated.
- Circumcise boys to decrease the risk of UTI.

SURGERY

- Early surgical repair indicated if there is decreased function in the involved kidney, bilateral involvement, or overall decrease in renal function. Repair the better kidney to prevent decompensation.
- Surgical excision of the obstructed UPJ with reanastamosis of the ureter to the pelvis has high (91%–99%) success rates.
- Temporary preliminary urinary diversion is rarely indicated: percutaneous nephrostomy or cutaneous pyelostomy only if severe lethal anomalies make them poor risk for early surgery.
- Indications for nephrectomy: if cystic changes or infection present—isotopic scan (i.e., DMSA) shows no renal function.

Common Questions and Answers

Q: What is significance of a dilated renal pelvis seen on fetal ultrasound?
A: Frequently there is "physiologic dilatation" in the normal fetus. A renal pelvic diameter of less than 10 mm is more likely to be physiologic and not UPJ obstruction.

Q: Will the renal architecture return to normal size after the obstruction is removed?
A: Not always.

Q: Are both kidneys involved?
A: In fewer than 20% there will be bilateral UPJ.

ICD-9-CM 593.4

BIBLIOGRAPHY

Elder JS. Antenatal hydronephrosis: fetal and neonatal management. *Pediatr Clin North Am* 1997;44(5):1299.

Gloor JM, Ogburn PL Jr, Breckle RJ, Morgenstern BZ, Milliner DS. Urinary tract anomalies detected by prenatal ultrasound examination at Mayo Clinic Rochester. *Mayo Clin Proc* 1995; 70(6):526–531.

Kelalis P, King L, Belman A, eds. *Clinical pediatric urology*. Philadelphia: WB Saunders, 1992.

King L. Hydronephrosis: when is obstruction not obstruction? *Urol Clin North Am* 1995; 22:31.

Koff S. Pathophysiology of ureteropelvic junction obstruction. *Urol Clin North Am* 1990; 17:263.

Koff SA. Neonatal management of unilateral hydronephrosis: role for delayed intervention. *Urol Clin North Am* 1998;25(2):181.

Mandell J, Peters C, Retik A. Current concepts in the perinatal diagnosis and management of hydronephrosis. *Urol Clin North Am* 1990; 17:247.

Radhakrishnan J. Obstructive uropathy in the newborn. *Clin Perinatol* 1990;17:215.

Shalaby-Rana E, Lowe LH, Blask AN, Majd M. Imaging in pediatric urology. *Pediatr Clin North Am* 1997;44(5):1065.

Author: Christina Lin Master

Urethral Prolapse

 Database

DEFINITION

Urethral prolapse is circumferential eversion of urethral epithelium through the external urethral meatus, resulting in vascular congestion and possible strangulation. It may be complete or incomplete; complete is more common.

- Secondary to inadequate attachments between the smooth muscle layers of the urethra
- Exacerbated by increased intraabdominal pressure
- Possibly related to hypoestrogenic state, which causes laxity in the periurethral fascia

GENETICS

Hereditary factors may be involved, in light of increased incidence in African Americans.

EPIDEMIOLOGY

- More common in African American females than in White females
- White females comprise less than 10% of all females with urethral prolapse.
- Seen predominantly in prepubertal females, usually less than 10 to 12 years of age; age range at diagnosis, 5 days to 11 years, with average between 4 and 6 years

 Differential Diagnosis

- Sarcoma botryoides
—Hydrometrocolpos
—Condyloma accuminata
—Periurethral abscess
- Prolapsed ureterocele
—Ectopic ureter
—Urethral cysts; prolapsed urethral polyp
—Prolapsed bladder

 Data Gathering

HISTORY

- Eighty-three percent to 100% of girls present with blood on underwear from genital area, or serosanguinous discharge, a common cause of urogenital bleeding in females.
- Fifteen percent to 25% of girls present with dysuria, frequency, and even urinary retention.
- Ninety-nine percent may be asymptomatic.

 Physical Examination

- Everted doughnut-shaped, edematous mass with urethral opening in the center
- May appear as a fungating mass protruding through vulva
- May be purple or hemorrhagic in hue
- Mucosa is nontender

 Laboratory Aids

IMAGING

- If the presentation is atypical, consider pelvic ultrasound to rule out tumor, or complete renal ultrasound to rule out hydronephrosis caused by ureterocele.
- VCUG reveals an elongated urethra and a nonobstructive, doughnut-shaped mass at narrow distal urethra.

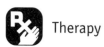

Therapy

CONSERVATIVE

- Usually cannot be reduced manually
- Sitz baths, antibiotic, and estrogen ointments to the area have been reported to be effective, especially in a premenarchal patient with mild prolapse.
- Usually resolves spontaneously or with conservative measures in approximately 2 to 3 weeks

SURGERY

- Total primary excision with reapproximation of mucosal edges if persistent or recurrent, or if complications such as urinary retention occur

Common Questions and Answers

Q: How do you manage the ureterocele?
A: By respecting the tissue and avoiding infection. Keep it moist; some use antibiotic ointment or estrogen ointment. Do not try to push the ureterocele back into the urethra.

Q: What is the most common presenting complaint?
A: Bleeding.

ICD-9-CM 599.5

BIBLIOGRAPHY

Baldwin D, Landa H. Common problems in pediatric gynecology. *Urol Clin North Am* 1995; 22:173.

Brown MR, Cartwright PC, Snow BW. Common office problems in pediatric urology and gynecology. *Pediatr Clin North Am* 1997;44(5):1091.

Kelalis P, King K, Belman A, eds. *Clinical pediatric urology*. Philadelphia: WB Saunders, 1992.

Author: Christina Master

Urinary Tract Infection

 Database

DEFINITION

Urinary tract infection (UTI) is growth of bacterial urinary tract pathogen(s) at:

- $\geq 10^2$ CFU/mL for suprapubic aspirate
- $\geq 10^4$ CFU/mL for urine obtained by catherization
- $\geq 10^5$ CFU/mL for urine obtained by clean-catch technique

PATHOLOGY

- Urinary tract pathogens include:

—Common: *E. coli, Klebsiella* spp., *Enterococcus, Proteus mirabilis*
—Less common: *Enterobacter cloacae,* group B hemolytic strep, *Citrobacter, Staphylococcus aureus,* and *Staphylococcus saprophyticus* (teenage girls)

- A specimen must be obtained sterilely, not by applying a bag to the perineum.
- Ninety percent of patients will also have pyuria (5 WBC/HPF or urine dipstick for leukocyte esterase [LE]) and bacteriuria on examination of the urine.
- Upper tract infection or pyelonephritis: infection of the renal parenchyma; vast majority of febrile babies with a positive culture have upper tract infection.
- Lower tract infection: infection limited to bladder, not involving the kidneys; occurs more in older children and adolescents; no fever.

EPIDEMIOLOGY

- Ascending infection from bladder instrumentation, perineal irritation, bacterial soilage, sexual activity
- Dysfunctional voiding
- Urinary tract abnormalities: vesiculoureteral reflux (VUR), neurogenic bladder, urethral obstruction

RISK FACTORS

- Sex/age: boys most at risk for UTI during first year of life; girls until school age and again in adolescence
- Circumcision status: Uncircumcised males have ten times the incidence of UTI compared with circumcised males.
- Race: Caucasians have a higher incidence of UTI; White females have the highest rate.
- Abnormal urinary tract: Children with VCR and obstruction are at higher risk for UTI.
- Voiding dysfunction

COMPLICATIONS

- Repeated febrile UTIs in young children may lead to renal scarring.
- Renal scarring in childhood carries a risk of hypertension, preeclampsia, and end-stage renal disease as an adult.

PROGNOSIS

Prompt treatment of febrile UTIs reduces the risk for scarring and its sequelae.

ASSOCIATED ILLNESSES

Approximately 10% of babies with febrile UTIs (pyelonephritis) are bacteremic.

 Differential Diagnosis

- Lower tract infections

—Urethral irritation for irritants such as bubble baths
—Diabetes
—Excessive drinking
—Masses adjacent to the bladder
—Normal potty training
—Dyes from ingested fluids
—Dehydration with concentrated urine

- Upper tract infections

—Gastroenteritis
—Pelvic inflammatory disease or tubo-ovarian abscess (TOA)
—Appendicitis
—Ovarian torsion

 Data Gathering

HISTORY

- Babies: Symptoms are nonspecific, such as vomiting, irritability, poor feeding, and fever.
- Older children: Classic symptoms of the lower tract include urgency, frequency, dysuria, hesitancy, suprapubic discomfort, hematuria, and malodorous urine. Classic symptoms of the upper tract include chills, nausea, flank pain, and fever.

 Physical Examination

BABIES

- Fever is the most common finding.
- Abdominal pain or distention
- Poor growth or weight gain
- Malodorous urine

OLDER CHILDREN

- Lower tract: suprapubic tenderness
- Upper tract: fever, costovertebral angle tenderness to percussion

SPECIAL QUESTION

Has the young child had a history of UTI, unexplained fevers, or urinary tract anomaly?

PROCEDURE

Suspect UTI in any febrile baby less than 1 year of age or in a preschool girl, even in the absence of signs and symptoms, especially if there is not a definite source of fever.

Urinary Tract Infection

 Laboratory Aids

TESTS

- Urinalysis: 5 WBC/HPF or bacteria on Gram stain microscopy per high-power field.
- Urine dipstick is equivalent to conventional microscopy: Trace color changes on the LE test strip indicates 5 WBC/HPF; nitrite indicates the presence of nitrate-splitting bacteria.
- Rapid filter testing for bacteriuria is equivalent to microscopic examination for bacteria; it is not as sensitive as the dipstick for detecting UTI.

—Enhanced urinalysis: 10 WBC/cm^3 or higher, or bacteria on Gram stain, may be most sensitive for detecting UTI in the neonate.

- Urine culture collected sterilely is the gold standard for diagnosis.

FALSE POSITIVES

- Contaminated urine by perineum or stool organisms

PITFALLS

- Ten percent of young babies will have a negative urinalysis despite culture or nuclear scan–documented UTI.
- Failure to culture by sterile means: unable to interpret a contaminated urine culture result

HOME TESTING

Urine dipstick for LE or nitrite with first morning void can be used to screen children at risk for repeated infections.

REQUIREMENTS

- Obtain urine sterilely to avoid false-positive results.
- The nitrite test requires urine to be in the bladder for 4 hours; therefore, the first morning specimen is best.

 Therapy

UPPER TRACT INFECTION

- Drugs: ampicillin and gentamicin intravenously until afebrile (48 hr); sterile urine, and sensitivity of the organisms to antibiotics known for neonates or infants who may have urinary tract abnormalities.
- Length of treatment: Complete a 10- to 14-day course orally.

LOWER TRACT INFECTION

- Drugs: amoxicillin, trimethoprim-sulfamethoxazole, cefprozil, nitrofurantoin orally
- Length of treatment: 7–10 days

PREVENTION

- Teaching correct wiping—front to back—to young children.
- Prophylactic antibiotics for selected children with recurrent infection, VUR, pyelonephritis
- Attention to good voiding habits

 Follow-Up

- Repeat urine culture 2 days into therapy to assess adequacy of treatment.
- Radiologic evaluation
- Renal cortical scan: all febrile children
- Ultrasound: boys, girls less than 12 years
- Voiding cystourethrogram (VCUG): all boys, all infants less than 1 year, history of voiding dysfunction, upper tract infection, or abnormal RCS or ultrasound

PITFALLS

- Not obtaining urine by a sterile method for culturing; unable to interpret contaminated results; do not know if the child should have a radiographic work-up
- Not culturing febrile babies without a documented source of fever; increased risk of long-term sequelae, untreated pyelonephritis

—Outpatient oral treatment may be satisfactory in babies older than 6 months who look well, can take oral fluids, have normal urinary tract anatomy, and have good follow-up.

 Common Questions and Answers

Q: Do all children require radiologic evaluation after their first UTI?
A: All boys, any girl with an upper tract infection, and all girls less than 3 years of age.

Q: Does a urine culture need to be sent if the dipstick or urinalysis is negative?
A: Approximately 10% of febrile infants with pyelonephritis will have a false-negative screening test (dipstick, urinalysis). A sterile urine culture should be sent.

ICD-9-CM 599.0

BIBLIOGRAPHY

Ansari BM, Jewkes F, Davies SG. Urinary tract infection in children. Part I: epidemiology, natural history, diagnosis and management. J Infect 1995;30(1):3–6.

Conway JJ, Cohn RA. Evolving role of nuclear medicine for the diagnosis and management of urinary tract infection. J Pediatr 1994;124: 87–90.

Friedman AL. Urinary tract infection. Curr Opin Pediatr 1998;10(2):197–200.

Heldrich FJ. UTI diagnosis: getting it right the first time. Contemp Pediatr 1995;12:110–133.

Hoberman A, Chao HP, Keller DM, et al. Prevalence of urinary tract infection in febrile infants. J Pediatr 1993;23(1):17–23.

Shaw KN, Gorelick M, et al. Prevalence of urinary tract infection in febrile young children in the emergency department. Pediatrics 1998; 102(2):1–5.

Shaw KN, Hexter D, McGowan KL, et al. Clinical evaluation of rapid screening test for urinary tract infection in children. J Pediatr 1991; 118(5):733–736.

Sheldon CA. Vesicoureteral reflux. Pediatr Rev 1995;16:22–27.

Author: Kathy N. Shaw

Urticaria

 Database

DEFINITION

Acute urticaria is a common, allergic skin disorder characterized by well-circumscribed localized or generalized erythematous, raised skin lesions (wheals or welts) of various sizes; it is usually intensely pruritic. Chronic urticaria is a type that recurs frequently or lasts longer than 6 weeks.

ETIOLOGY

- Ingestions (usually foods: seafood, nuts, eggs, food additives; antibiotics, especially penicillin and sulfa drugs)
- Direct contact (plants)
- Injected agents (antibiotics, blood products, insect stings and bites)
- Inhalants (pollens, danders)
- Infectious agents (viral, especially hepatitis and Epstein-Barr virus [EBV], bacterial, parasitic)
- Physical factors (cold, pressure, sun exposure, water exposure, dermatographism)
- Systemic diseases (collagen-vascular, serum sickness, malignancy, hyperthyroidism, mastocytosis)
- Associated illnesses include angioedema and anaphylaxis.

PATHOPHYSIOLOGY

- IgE or non–IgE-mediated hypersensitivity reaction causing extravasation of fluid from small blood vessels mediated by various chemicals, including histamine, kinins, prostaglandins, and serotonin

GENETICS

- Rarely hereditary (cold urticaria)

EPIDEMIOLOGY

- Nonspecific

COMPLICATIONS

- Swelling of the oropharynx or airways can be life threatening.
- Progression to anaphylaxis with wheezing and hypotension may also be life threatening.

PROGNOSIS

- Good
- Usually self-limited and benign
- Chronic urticaria: may persist intermittently for weeks to years

 Differential Diagnosis

Appearance is very distinctive and diagnosis usually straightforward.

- Infection
—Varicella
- Trauma
—Insect bites (fleas, mosquitoes, spiders)
- Immunologic
—Erythema multiforme

 Data Gathering

HISTORY

- History of urticaria
- Known exposures and ingestions
- Evanescent lesions
- Family history
- Underlying medical problems
- History of atopy
- For chronic urticaria: symptom diary including activity, diet, illnesses, sun exposure, and medications

Special Questions

- Cold/heat exposure
- Exertion or emotional stress (cholinergic urticaria)
- Water exposure (aquagenic urticaria)
- Sun exposure (solar urticaria)

 Physical Examination

- Blanching "wheal and flare" lesions
- Migratory lesions
- Examine mucous membranes and airway.
- Evaluate for wheezing (may be part of anaphylaxis).
- Check blood pressure (hypotension may be part of anaphylaxis).
- "Write" on skin with a blunt instrument; examine for wheal after a few minutes: dermatographism.
- Apply an ice cube, rewarm the area, and examine for a wheal: cold urticaria.

Laboratory Aids

TESTS

Testing is useful if a specific cause is suspected (must be individualized):

• Suspected underlying infectious agent: throat culture, titers for hepatitis or EBV, and so forth.
• Suspected underlying systemic disease: ANA, RF, ESR, CBC, thyroid studies, as indicated
• Suspected IgE-mediated urticaria: skin testing to confirm causal relationship (RAST is alternative to skin testing)

 ## Therapy

• Acute situations: epinephrine 1:1,000, 0.1 to 0.3 mL; rapid relief of itching; antihistamines relieve itching less quickly. See the Anaphylaxis chapter for further management of acute reactions.

DRUGS

• Antihistamines: diphenhydramine (Benadryl) 1.25 mg/kg/dose, or hydroxyzine (Atarax) 0.5 mg/kg/dose q4-6h, or cetrizine (Zyrtec) 5 mg for 2 to 6 years, once daily, or 5 to 10 mg/d for 6 to 12 years; cyproheptadine (Periactin) 2 to 4 mg q8-12h for cold urticaria
• Combination H1 (Benadryl, Atarax) and H2-receptor antagonists (Ranitidine, Cimetadine) for chronic urticaria
• Corticosteroids may work in chronic urticaria; high doses are often necessary, with predictable side effects.

 ## Follow-Up

SIGNS TO WATCH FOR

• Airway compromise
• Wheezing
• Hoarse voice
• Difficulty breathing or swallowing

PREVENTION

• Sun screens, protective clothing, or sun avoidance for solar urticaria
• Avoid causative agents (foods, contacts, inhalants, medications, etc.)

PITFALLS

• Discontinuation of a medication needed to treat another condition may result in problems

 ## Common Questions and Answers

Q: What duration of observation in acute urticaria is necessary to avoid missing serious sequelae?
A: In uncomplicated cases that respond rapidly to antihistamines, observation can be brief—minutes to hours. If the allergic reaction is complicated by angioedema or airway problems, or if epinephrine is administered, observation should be prolonged (several hours or overnight) to observe for worsening symptoms or anaphylaxis.

Q: Should patients with chronic urticaria be referred to a specialist?
A: If urticaria persists for more than 6 weeks and no underlying etiology is identified, the patient should be referred to an allergist or immunologist for evaluation and treatment, because it may be a sign of underlying systemic disease.

ICD-9-CM 708.9

BIBLIOGRAPHY

Greaves MW. Chronic urticaria. *N Engl J Med* 1995;332(26):1767–1771.

Hurwitz S. *Clinical pediatric dermatology: a textbook of skin disorders of childhood and adolescence,* 2nd ed. Philadelphia: WB Saunders, 1990:384–387.

Mortureux P, Leaute-Labreze C, Lamireau T, et al. Acute urticaria in infancy and childhood. *Arch Dermatol* 1998;134:319–323.

Volonakis M, Katsarov-Katsari A, Stratigos J. Etiologic factors in childhood chronic urticaria. *Ann Allergy* 1992; 69:61–65.

Author: Deborah L. Silver

Vaginal Discharge

Database

DEFINITION

Vaginal discharge is defined as secretions that come from the vagina due to hormonal influences, infection, or irritation.

• Physiologic leukorrhea is due to normal hormonal influences on the vagina and is seen in newborns and preadolescents
• Infections that cause vaginal discharge usually present in adolescence, and include:

—*Candida*
—*Gardnerella* (bacterial vaginosis)
—Gonorrhea
—*Chlamydia*
—*Trichomonas*
—*Streptococcus*

• Irritation from a vaginal foreign body will cause a discharge.
• Vaginal discharges in neonates and pubertal girls are common; however, vaginal discharges in girls over the age of 1 month and prior to puberty are usually abnormal and need to be investigated.

PATHOPHYSIOLOGY

• Physiologic leukorrhea is secondary to estrogen stimulation of the vaginal epithelium and mucous production by the paracervical glands.
• The site of the infection (vagina, endocervix, ectocervix) varies depending on the pathogen, the type of epithelium present, and other factors in the microenvironment. The squamous epithelium of the vagina and ectocervix is susceptible to *Candida* and *Trichomonas*. The columnar epithelium of the endocervix is susceptible to gonorrhea and *Chlamydia*.
• Normal vaginal flora of a postpubertal female includes lactobacilli, *Bacteroides, Gardnerella,* viridans streptococci, and *Staphylococcus epidermis.*

EPIDEMIOLOGY

• Trichomonal vaginitis is probably one of the most common causes of vaginal discharge in adolescents in an urban setting.
• Bacterial vaginosis (caused by *Gardnerella* and anaerobic bacteria) is the most common cause of vaginal discharge in postpubertal females.
• Depressed cellular immunity, antibiotic use (particularly those that are effective against lactobacilli), and perineal moisture are predisposing factors for acquiring a vaginal yeast infection.

COMPLICATIONS

• There are usually no complications with a vaginal discharge if treated promptly and appropriately.
• Sexually transmitted diseases place adolescents at risk for pelvic inflammatory disease and subsequent threat to future fertility, as well as pregnancy complications, such as ectopic pregnancies

PROGNOSIS

• Prognosis is good with appropriate treatment.
• Treating a vaginal discharge with antibiotics places the female at risk for subsequently developing a vaginal candidiasis.
• Vaginal candidiasis and bacterial vaginosis often recur despite appropriate therapy.

Differential Diagnosis

• Nonpathologic

—Physiologic discharge

• Infectious

—Enteric pathogens causing vaginitis
—Vaginitis due to sexually transmitted disease
—Urinary tract infection

• Neoplastic

—Sarcoma botryoides

• Congenital

—Ectopic ureter

• Trauma

—Foreign body
—Masturbatory behaviors
—Accidental trauma
—Sexual abuse

Data Gathering

HISTORY

• Inquire about pruritus, frequent urination, dysuria, or enuresis.
• Note the color, odor, quality, and the duration of the discharge.
• Ask about masturbation or if a foreign body was inserted into vagina.
• General health status (diabetes, HIV, etc.)
• Recent antibiotic use
• Concerns about sexual abuse in preadolescents
• Sexual activity in adolescent patients
• Contraceptive use in adolescents
• Any history of vaginal discharge: An adolescent is frequently reinfected because the partner is often untreated.

Physical Examination

• Examine in the frog-leg (supine) position or the knee-chest (prone) position.
• A speculum examination is indicated for females who are sexually active or postpubertal, whereas for prepubertal children, an otoscope can be used for illumination.
• Evaluate the color, odor, and consistency of the discharge.
• Examine the vulva for erythema, excoriations, fissures, and vesicles.
• Carefully inspect the hymen and introitus.
• Look for a foreign body in the vagina.
• A rectal examination will be helpful in detecting a firm foreign body or a mass, because the ovaries are nonpalpable in a prepubertal girl.
• The discharge from physiologic leukorrhea is clear to whitish-gray mucus with no itching, odor, or irritation.
• Chlamydia may be asymptomatic, but also may present with a mucopurulent discharge.
• Gonorrhea may remain asymptomatic, but a malodorous thick discharge that may be white, yellow, or green is often present. Labial erythema and urethral irritation are also frequently present.
• *Candida* in a prepubertal child rarely presents with the classic cottage cheese discharge. Instead, it is usually a minimally odorous, white discharge with pruritus, dysuria, dyspareunia, vaginal soreness, vulvar erythema, and edema.
• A bloody discharge can be due to tumors (such as sarcoma botryoides), trauma, vulvovaginitis, urethral prolapse, or precocious puberty.
• *Shigella* and group A β-hemolytic streptococcal vaginitis often cause a bloody discharge.

Laboratory Aids

TESTS

• There are several ways to obtain samples from the prepubertal child, all of which require care to avoid damaging the hymenal tissue:

—Use of a small cotton-tipped applicator soaked in nonbacteriostatic saline is simple, but may cause minimal discomfort.
—An eyedropper can be used to aspirate the discharge.
—A few milliliters of nonbacteriostatic saline can be instilled into the vagina and then aspirated using a syringe with a butterfly catheter with the needle removed.
—Some clinicians use the "catheter-in-a-catheter" technique. A red rubber catheter is cut to create a 4-inch distal segment, which is inserted into the vagina. A butterfly needle then has the needle removed and is cut so that the tubing is somewhat longer than the red rubber catheter. The tubing of the butterfly needle can then be inserted inside the red rubber catheter, and multiple samples can be obtained.

• Obtain a sampling of the vaginal pool for pH, wet prep (for *Trichomonas* and bacterial vaginosis), and KOH swab (for *Candida*).
• Clue cells (multiple refractile bacteria within large epithelial cells) are suggestive of bacterial vaginosis.
• A positive "whiff test" (10% KOH added to a slide with the discharge produces a fishy odor) is associated with bacterial vaginosis, but also may be seen in *Trichomonas*.
• Vaginal Gram stain and culture
• Gonorrhea and *Chlamydia* cultures are preferred over the rapid tests in prepubertal girls due to medicolegal implications of the results.
• A wet mount of a child with physiologic leukorrhea reveals numerous epithelial cells without leukocytes or pathologic bacteria.

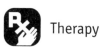 ## Therapy

• Physiologic leukorrhea: reassurance that the discharge is normal and instructions on normal vaginal hygiene. Avoid vaginal creams and antibiotics.
• Treat other etiologic agents of vaginal discharge as appropriate:

—Bacterial vaginosis can be treated with metronidazole
—For *Chlamydia,* use erythromycin or tetracycline (tetracycline should not be used in children under 8 years, given the risk of dental staining). One can also use a one-time dose of azithromycin.
—For gonorrhea, a one-time dose of ceftriaxone can be used.

• Treat yeast infections with imidazole, micanazole, or clotrimazole.

 ## Follow-Up

• Any child with a concern of sexual abuse should be evaluated by sexual abuse experts and referred for therapy as indicated.
• An adolescent with a sexually transmitted disease should be rechecked after completing the appropriate therapy. Their sexual partners also should be examined and treated.

PREVENTION

• Good perineal hygiene: Wipe front to back, wear cotton underwear, avoid tight fitting clothes, and avoid nylon tights.
• Encourage adolescent patients to use barrier contraceptives to decrease the risk of obtaining a sexually transmitted disease.
• Encourage females to eat yogurt while on antibiotics.

ISOLATION OF HOSPITALIZED PATIENT

• None required

CONTROL MEASURES

• Standard universal precautions

PITFALLS

• A sexually transmitted disease in a prepubertal girl is highly suggestive of sexual abuse. The laboratory should confirm the organism that grew in the culture for medicolegal purposes.
• *Chlamydia* may be acquired perinatally, but in rare instances is not detected until the child is 3 years old, and thus it may be difficult to differentiate between perinatally acquired *Chlamydia* and *Chlamydia* from sexual abuse in a prepubertal child.
• Gonorrhea acquired perinatally usually presents by 1 year of age; therefore, gonorrhea infections in older children are often the result of sexual abuse.

 ## Common Questions and Answers

Q: What is the best way to evaluate a prepubertal girl with a vaginal discharge?
A: It is important to perform a thorough history and physical first. If there are minimal complaints and the discharge is scant and non-odorous, then it may be physiologic leukorrhea. No treatment is needed for physiologic leukorrhea, just reassurance. If the discharge appears as anything besides the scant non-odorous discharge, then evaluation for bacteria, gonorrhea, *Chlamydia*, and yeast is indicated.

Q: What are some measures to prevent recurrence of the vaginal discharge?
A: Perineal hygiene is important to emphasize to patients to decrease the risk of fecal contamination of the vagina. Females should wipe front to back to avoid spreading fecal bacteria. Females who are sexually active should use barrier protection such as a condom.

Q: Should a patient douche?
A: No. Douching has been shown to increase the risk of pelvic inflammatory disease during an infection. It alters the normal bacterial flora of the vagina, may cause a vaginitis by introducing chemicals into the vagina, and decreases the vagina's defense mechanisms to fight infections.

ICD-9-CM 623.5

BIBLIOGRAPHY

Brown MR, Cartwright PC, Snow BW. Common office problems in pediatric urology and gynecology. *Pediatr Clin North Am* 1997;44(5):1091–115.

Emans SJ. Vulvovaginal complaints in the adolescent. In: Emans SJ, Laufer MR, Goldstein DP, eds. *Pediatric and adolescent gynecology,* 4th ed. Philadelphia: Lippincott-Raven Publishers, 1998:423–456.

Fox KK, Behets FMT. Vaginal discharge: how to pinpoint the cause. *Postgrad Med* 1995;98(3): 87–104.

Author: Philip R. Spandorfer

Vaginitis

Database

DEFINITION

Vaginitis is erythema and inflammation of the vaginal mucosa, usually associated with vaginal discharge, which varies from scant whitish to green with a foul odor. *Vaginitis, vulvitis,* and *vulvovaginitis* are terms often used interchangeably. Vaginitis can be due to poor hygiene, chemical irritation, mechanical irritation, topical allergy, trauma, or infection. Bacterial pathogens can be from normal flora, gastrointestinal flora, or respiratory flora.

- Normal flora: lactobacilli, *Staphylococcus epidermis, Streptococcus viridans,* and diptheroides
- Gastrointestinal flora: *E. coli, Klebsiella,* and *Shigella*
- Respiratory flora: group A strep, *Streptococcus pneumoniae, Staphylococcus aureus,* and *Moraxella catarrhalis*

PATHOPHYSIOLOGY

- The prepubescent vagina has a neutral pH and is lined by cuboid epithelial cells. At puberty, the pH becomes acidic and the lining changes to squamous epithelial cells.
- The bacterial colonization changes at puberty and helps fight infection.

Risk factors for vaginitis can be subdivided into the following categories:

- Anatomic

—The anatomy of a prepubertal girl may predispose her to vaginitis.
  —Absence of protective fat pad and pubic hair
  —Thin vulvar skin
  —Thin and atrophic vaginal mucosa
  —Neutral pH of the vagina

- Obesity
- Hygiene

—Inadequate cleansing of the vulva after voiding or bowel movements
—Poor handwashing
—Irritants against the vulva (chemical irritants, e.g., bubble baths and harsh soaps, and physical irritants, e.g., dirt)
—Tight, nonbreathing clothes

- Foreign body in vagina
- Trauma

—Sexual abuse
—Accidental trauma to the vulva

EPIDEMIOLOGY

- "Nonspecific vulvovaginitis" accounts for approximately 50% to 75% of vulvovaginitis seen in premenarchal girls.
- Vaginitis is the most common cause of vaginal bleeding in the pediatric age group.
- The majority of vulvovaginitis occurs during adolescence.
- One-third of women will experience vaginitis during their lifetime.

COMPLICATIONS

- Labial adhesions can develop after trauma to the labia.
- Dyspareunia
- Dysuria

PROGNOSIS

- Vaginitis is often recurrent, particularly if hygienic measures are not changed.
- Complete recovery with appropriate treatment

Differential Diagnosis

- "Nonspecific vulvovaginitis"
- Specific vulvovaginitis
- Pelvic inflammatory disease
- Cervicitis
- Vaginal or cervical polyps or tumors
- Urethral prolapse
- Systemic illnesses: e.g., scarlet fever, Kawasaki disease, Crohn disease
- Congenital anomalies: double vagina with fistula, pelvic abscess or fistula, ectopic ureter
- Dermatologic disorders: e.g., psoriasis, seborrhea, lichen sclerosis
- Trauma
- Precocious puberty
- Pinworms

Data Gathering

HISTORY

- Interview the parents and the child if she is old enough.
- The vulva is usually inflamed before the vagina.
- Common complaints are discomfort, pain, discharge, pruritus, urinary frequency, enuresis, and dysuria.
- Ask about the presence of discharge, its quantity, consistency, color, and duration.
- What home therapy has been tried?
- What other medication is the child taking, particularly antibiotics or steroids?
- Does the child use any feminine products, such as douches, feminine deodorants, soaps, or bubble baths?
- Determine if there is any concern on the caregivers part about sexual abuse (question the parents and the child separately).
- Family history of atopy
- Child's exposure to chemical and physical irritants
- Ask adolescent girls about their menstrual, sexual, and contraceptive histories (interview her in private, with the parents out of the room).
- Symptoms are often present for months in girls with nonspecific vaginitis, whereas they are often present less than a month if there is a specific cause for the vaginitis.

Physical Examination

- Examine in the frog-leg (supine) position and the knee-chest (prone) position.
- Evaluate for discharge (purulence, odor, pH).
- Examine the vulva for erythema, excoriations, fissures, and vesicles.
- Carefully inspect the hymen and introitus.
- Look for a foreign body.
- A speculum examination is indicated for females who are sexually active or post-pubertal.
- A rectal examination will be helpful in detecting a firm foreign body or a mass, because the ovaries will be nonpalpable in a prepubertal girl.
- Look for signs of dermatologic disorders.
- *Candida* will cause erythema and satellite lesions, but is usually seen in the setting of recent antibiotic use, diabetes mellitus, or diaper use. There will be intense burning, dysuria, and pruritus with *Candida.*
- *Gardnerella vaginalis* is a common cause of bacterial vaginosis. It often has a white discharge that has a fishy odor. There is usually no vulvar itching, but there is irritation.
- *Shigella* and group A β-hemolytic strep can cause bleeding of the vulva.

Vaginitis

- A foreign body (frequently toilet paper) will often cause a foul-smelling, blood-tinged purulent discharge.
- Odorless, bloody discharge can follow trauma, vulvar irritation, precocious puberty, condyloma acuminatum, urethral prolapse, or sarcoma botryoides.

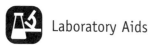 Laboratory Aids

TESTS

- If the history is benign and the physical examination reveals a scant amount of mucoid discharge with minor introital erythema, then cultures and further laboratory studies may be unnecessary.
- There are several ways to obtain samples from the prepubertal child, all of which require care to avoid damaging the hymenal tissue.

—Use of a small, cotton-tipped applicator soaked in nonbacteriostatic saline is simple, but may cause minimal discomfort.
—An eyedropper can be used to aspirate the discharge.
—A few milliliters of nonbacteriostatic saline can be instilled into the vagina and then aspirated using a syringe with a butterfly catheter with the needle removed.
—Some clinicians use the "catheter-in-a-catheter" technique. A red rubber catheter is cut to create a 4-inch distal segment, which is inserted into the vagina. A butterfly needle then has the needle removed and is cut so that the tubing is somewhat longer than the red rubber catheter. The tubing of the butterfly needle can then be inserted inside the red rubber catheter, and multiple samples can be obtained.

- Obtain a sampling of the vaginal pool for pH, wet prep (for *Trichomonas* and bacterial vaginosis), and KOH swab (for *Candida*).
- Vaginal Gram stain and culture
- Test for gonorrhea and *Chlamydia* (culture is preferred over the rapid tests in prepubertal girls).
- Urine analysis and culture

 Therapy

- Treatment for vaginitis is aimed at the particular cause of vaginitis.
- Discuss perineal hygiene, such as wiping front to back after toileting.
- Treatment of nonspecific vaginitis is aimed at improving hygiene, avoiding irritation, and techniques that promote drying the vulva (avoid tight-fitting clothes, avoid nylon tights, use cotton underwear, etc.).
- Avoidance of irritants is necessary for both chemical and physical irritants.
- Removal of a foreign body if a foreign body is the cause of the vaginitis
- Sitz baths and barrier ointments may relieve discomfort.
- If an overgrowth of bacteria is detected on vaginal culture, antibiotic therapy directed at the organism is appropriate.

—For *Gardnerella*, treat with either oral metronidazole or metronidazole vaginal suppositories. Clindamycin also can be used.
—For *Trichomonas*, use metronidazole.

- Treat vulvovaginal candidiasis with clotrimazole, miconazole, butaconazole, terconazole, or tioconazole applied topically. Oral fluconazole can be given to adolescents and adults as a one-time dose of 150 mg orally.
- Organisms associated with sexually transmitted diseases should prompt an evaluation for child abuse in the prepubertal child

 Follow-Up

- Improvement should be seen within a few days of initiating therapy.
- If symptoms recur, a thorough history and physical examination should be repeated, and alternative therapy may be indicated.

PREVENTION

Good hygiene is crucial to preventing the majority of cases of vulvovaginitis.

ISOLATION OF HOSPITALIZED PATIENT

- Not indicated

CONTROL MEASURES

Use of standard universal precautions is sufficient.

PITFALLS

- *Candida* is uncommon in prepubescent girls who are not on antibiotics; rule out diabetes mellitus.
- Avoid use of topical antifungals that contain steroids in the vulvar area.

 Common Questions and Answers

Q: What can I do to prevent my child from getting another case of vulvovaginitis?
A: The best prevention for vulvovaginitis is perineal hygiene. Girls should be instructed to wipe from front to back. They should wear cotton underwear and avoid other materials that do not promote vulvar dryness. They should avoid tight-fitting clothes. Avoidance of irritants such as dirt or harsh chemicals is beneficial.

Q: How do I know my child was not sexually abused?
A: Vulvovaginitis is a common problem in childhood. Physicians should always keep sexual abuse in their differential diagnosis so that they do not miss a case of abuse. However, a normal case of vulvovaginitis is probably just a normal case of vulvovaginitis. If there are any signs of abuse on the physical examination or if the patient reports any inappropriate sexual contact, then a further investigation is warranted.

Q: How do we treat the case of recurrent or chronic vaginitis?
A: It is crucial to emphasize the importance of appropriate hygiene to the patient. If the patient is compliant, cultures are negative, and the physical examination is nondiagnostic, a referral to a pediatric gynecologist is appropriate.

ICD-9-CM 616.10

BIBLIOGRAPHY

Brown MR, Cartwright PC, Snow BW. Common office problems in pediatric urology and gynecology. *Pediatr Clin North Am* 1997;44(5):1091–1115.

Farrington PF. Pediatric vulvo-vaginitis. *Clin Obstet Gynecol* 1997;40(1):135–140.

Vandeven AM, Emans SJ. Vulvovaginitis in the child and adolescent. *Pediatr Rev* 1993;14(4):141–147.

Author: Philip R. Spandorfer

Vein of Galen Malformations

Database

DEFINITION

Vein of Galen malformations are congenital arteriovenous malformations (AVMs). The vein of Galen connects the deep cerebral venous system with the intracranial venous sinuses. After draining the internal cerebral veins and basal veins, the vein of Galen flows into the straight sinus.

PATHOPHYSIOLOGY

Vein of Galen malformations may consist of a simple arteriovenous (AV) fistula or a more complicated AVM. Clinical symptoms develop because of high-output congestive heart failure (CHF), cerebral ischemia or hemorrhage, or hydrocephalus. Cerebral ischemia may result from the shunting of blood from the brain parenchyma to the malformation.

GENETICS

• No known genetic predisposition

EPIDEMIOLOGY

• Fifty percent of cases present as newborns, almost always with CHF.
• Older infants and children present with hydrocephalus, focal neurologic signs, headache, and subarachnoid hemorrhage.
• The incidence is unknown.

COMPLICATIONS

• High-output CHF, cerebral ischemia or hemorrhage, and hydrocephalus may result from this congenital vascular anomaly.
• Complications include mental retardation, seizures, and cerebral palsy.
• In severe cases, 80% of cardiac output may be delivered to the head because of the low vascular resistance within the malformation.

PROGNOSIS

Prognosis depends on the size of the malformation, the severity of the CHF, and the extent of cerebral injury prior to therapy. Historically, the prognosis has been poor for patients presenting as neonates with CHF. Recent advances in endovascular embolization techniques may improve prognosis.

Differential Diagnosis

• The diagnosis must be considered in any newborn with unexplained CHF (especially high-output failure), hydrocephalus, or intracranial hemorrhage.
• Other causes of high-output CHF in the newborn include anemia, hyperthyroidism, and other AVMs.
• In older infants and children, presenting symptoms may be nonspecific and raise suspicion of hydrocephalus or a mass lesion.
• Tumors that may obstruct the sylvian aqueduct include common posterior fossa tumors in children, pinealoma, hemangioblastoma, ependymoma, and hamartomas (e.g., in tuberous sclerosis).

Data Gathering

HISTORY

• Ninety-five percent of newborns with vein of Galen malformations present in CHF. Others present with hydrocephalus, subarachnoid hemorrhage, or intraventricular hemorrhage.
• Infants and older children usually present with hydrocephalus, headache, exercise-induced syncope, or subarachnoid hemorrhage.

Physical Examination

• In newborns, tachycardia, respiratory distress, hepatomegaly, a continuous cranial bruit heard over the posterior skull, and bounding carotid pulses may be present. The resting pulse may increase over time as the volume of blood shunted to the malformation increases.
• Older infants and children also may present with CHF but more often demonstrate increased head circumference, focal neurologic signs, and failure to thrive. Less common presenting signs include visual loss, proptosis, syncope, seizures, acute or progressive hemiparesis, developmental regression, epistaxis, and vertigo.

Laboratory Aids

TESTS

As with other AVMs, CBC and blood gases are often normal. Chest x-ray and ECG may reveal typical changes of high-output CHF, even in patients with resting tachycardia but no overt circulatory symptoms.

Imaging

• Neuroimaging studies are definitive.
• Prenatal diagnosis is now possible with fetal ultrasound. This allows planning for the appropriate location of delivery and postnatal management.
• In newborns, cranial ultrasound shows a large, hypoechoic structure in the region of the vein of Galen. CT shows a high-density mass that enhances with contrast. MRI shows an area of decreased signal intensity or signal void because of high flow within the malformation. CT and MRI will also show areas of cerebral ischemia or hemorrhage.
• MRI can detail the arterial supply and venous drainage of the malformation, but angiography is required before intervention.

Therapy

- Treatment of choice in all ages is endovascular embolization. A venous or arterial approach may be used, depending on the anatomy of the lesion. Direct surgical intervention has unacceptable risks and is no longer recommended.
- Refractory CHF prompts intervention (i.e., embolization of the malformation).
- The initial goal is not total obliteration of the lesion, but a reduction in blood flow to the lesion to improve cardiac function. Embolization can be completed in stages over a few months once CHF is controlled.
- Treatment in older infants and children is indicated to prevent cerebral ischemia from arterial steal or from venous infarction, and to prevent hydrocephalus and its sequelae.
- Therapy for associated conditions may include positive inotropes, diuretics, anticonvulsants, and CNS ventricular shunting.

 Follow-Up

- Survival depends largely on the severity of the CHF and the age of the patient. In the past, mortality in newborns approached 100%. Today, approximately 50% of newborns with severe CHF will survive. Critically ill infants requiring embolization in the first week of life continue to have the poorest prognosis.
- In one series of 28 children, 45% of those younger than 1 year of age had good outcomes; 61% of those ages 1 to 2 years had good outcomes, and 100% of those older than 2 years had good outcomes.
- Resting tachycardia may be an early sign of recurrent CHF in patients previously embolized.
- Patients who survive with neurologic deficits are at increased risk for the sequelae of stroke.
- Ophthalmologic complications of hydrocephalus
- A follow-up CT or MRI is indicated in evaluating patients with new neurologic signs or symptoms.

PREVENTION

There is no known prevention for these congenital malformations.

PITFALLS

- Overly rapid reduction in blood flow to the malformation can result in overperfusion of normal brain, systemic hypertension, cerebral edema, or hemorrhage.
- *Hydrocephalus* may occur in patients who have had hemorrhage from the malformation.
- *Shunt failure* may cause acute hydrocephalus, even if the malformation has not changed.

 Common Questions and Answers

Q: Can the malformation recur?
A: AVMs have a propensity to recur. Imaging studies give a good indication of the likelihood of recurrence.

Q: How does the malformation cause seizures?
A: Seizures are most often due to ischemia, acute hydrocephalus, infection, or metabolic disturbances.

ICD-9-CM 747.40

BIBLIOGRAPHY

Borthne A, et al. Vein of Galen malformations in infants: clinical, radiological and therapeutic aspects. *Eur Radiol* 1997;7:1252–1258.

Brunelle F. Arteriovenous malformation of the vein of Galen in children. *Pediatr Radiol* 1997;27:501–513.

Mickle JP, Quisling RG. Vein of Galen fistulas. *Neurosurg Clin North Am* 1994;5:529–540.

Missbach T, Davey AM. Endovascular management of vein of Galen aneurysms in neonates—two case reports and a review of the literature. *Clin Pediatr* 1997;36:663–668.

Rodesch G, et al. Prognosis of antenatally diagnosed vein of Galen malformations. *Childs Nerv Syst* 1994;10:79–83.

Volpe JJ. *Neurology of the newborn*, 3rd ed. Philadelphia: WB Saunders, 1995:802–806.

Author: Dennis J. Dlugos

Ventricular Septal Defect

Database

DEFINITION

A ventricular septal defect (VSD) is an opening in the ventricular septum.

• Seventy-five percent of all VSDs are perimembranous (located in the area adjacent to and under the aortic valve as seen from the left, and contiguous with the septal leaflet of the tricuspid valve). Malalignment defects occur from malalignment of the infundibular septum and the trabecular muscular septum. Muscular defects may be located anywhere in the muscular septum (5%–20% of all VSDs). Conoseptal defects are located under the pulmonary valve. Canal (inlet) defects are located in the atrioventricular canal beneath the AV valve.

• VSDs vary in size and number.

• In perimembranous or conoseptal defects, the right and/or noncoronary cusp of the aortic valve may herniate through the defect and cause aortic insufficiency (AI).

PATHOPHYSIOLOGY

Shunting (left-to-right or right-to-left) depends on the relative pulmonary (PVR) and systemic vascular resistances (SVR). If the defect is large, there is equilibration of right and left ventricular pressures. The larger the VSD and the lower the PVR, the greater the degree of left-to-right shunting. If the VSD is small and restrictive, the amount of left-to-right shunting depends on the size of the defect. When a large VSD is left untreated, pulmonary vascular disease (Eisenmenger syndrome) may develop.

GENETICS

Three percent of children with VSDs have a parent with a VSD.

EPIDEMIOLOGY

VSD is the most common form of congenital heart disease, occurring in approximately 1.5 to 3.5 per 1,000 live births and 4.5 to 7.0 per 1,000 premature infants.

COMPLICATIONS

• Left ventricular volume overload
• Pulmonary overcirculation
• Compromise of systemic output
• Endocarditis

PROGNOSIS

Patients with small defects have a normal lifespan, with the only risk being bacterial endocarditis. Eisenmenger syndrome may develop in children with a large VSD that is left unrepaired. Acquired right (RV muscle bundle) or left ventricular outflow tract (subaortic membrane) obstructions are associated with VSD. Aortic insufficiency may occur secondary to a poorly supported right coronary cusp.

Differential Diagnosis

• Mitral or tricuspid regurgitation
• Patent ductus arteriosus
• Atrial septal defect
• AV canal defect

Data Gathering

HISTORY

• Small VSD: The child may be asymptomatic, with normal growth and development. Most commonly, a murmur is detected at 2 to 6 weeks of age.
• Moderate VSD: There is poor weight gain, with sparing of longitudinal growth. There may be an increased incidence of respiratory infections. Sweating and fatigue with feeding may be present.
• Large VSD: The symptoms are the same as above but may be more severe.
• Children with Eisenmenger syndrome may have a history of cyanosis and fatigue.

Physical Examination

• Small VSD: The child appears healthy. A systolic thrill along the left sternal border can be palpable. Heart sounds are usually normal. A harsh, high-pitched, grade 4/6 holosystolic murmur is best heard at the left lower sternal border.
• Moderate-to-large defect: Tachycardia and tachypnea are present. There is an increased precordial impulse. The S_2 is wide, with a slight variation with respiration. The pulmonary component of S_2 may be normal or slightly accentuated. A harsh, low-pitched holosystolic murmur is heard at the left lower sternal border. A diastolic rumble represents increased flow across the mitral valve. Hepatomegaly may be present.
• In children with elevated PVR, the S_2 is loud and narrowly split. The murmur may decrease in intensity.
• A grade 1 to 3/6 early diastolic murmur of AI may be audible.

Laboratory Aids

TESTS

Electrocardiogram

- Small defect: normal
- Moderate defect: deeper than normal S wave in V1 and V2, with a larger R-wave in V5 and V6, indicating the presence of LV volume overload.
- Large defect: biventricular hypertrophy and left atrial enlargement.

Chest X-ray

- Small defect: normal
- Moderate defect: With LV volume overload, there is a prominent LV contour.
- Large defect: With increased left-to-right shunting, there may be increased pulmonary vascular markings with Kerley B lines.

Echocardiography

- Determines the anatomic location, size, and number of defects and any associated defects. Color Doppler enables one to visualize the shunt direction.

Cardiac Catheterization

- Generally reserved for children with poorly defined anatomy, associated lesions, or pulmonary hypertension with unknown reactivity

 Therapy

- Small defect: no intervention; observation and bacterial endocarditis prophylaxis for indicated procedures
- Moderate-to-large defects: If signs of congestive heart failure develop, the child should be placed on digoxin and diuretics, increased caloric intake should be provided, and the child should have regular follow-up. An early surgical repair should be undertaken during infancy.
- Perimembranous and muscular defects may become smaller or close spontaneously. Surgery can be delayed, assuming there is no evidence of heart failure or pulmonary hypertension. Because conoseptal, canal, and malalignment defects do not close spontaneously, surgical intervention is required. Repair should be undertaken for defects associated with AI.
- After 1 year of life, a significant left-to-right shunt (Qp/Qs > 2 : 1) indicates surgery.
- Children with controlled congestive heart failure but who have elevated pulmonary artery pressures (at least half-systemic) should undergo repair before the age of 2 years.
- Surgical correction may be contraindicated if the PVR is greater than 8 WU/M^2.
- The mortality of surgical repair is less than 5%.
- Complete heart block occurs in less than 2% of patients.
- A significant residual VSD may need early re-operation.

 Follow-Up

- All children with a VSD-type murmur should undergo echocardiographic evaluation to define the location, size, and number of VSDs. If the child does not demonstrate signs of congestive heart failure or pulmonary hypertension, he or she may be managed conservatively with observation. If, after the first year of life, the patient is asymptomatic and is documented to have a small defect, he or she may be followed to watch for the development of RV outflow tract obstruction and/or AI.
- Infants less than 6 months on anticongestive medications for failure to thrive should be evaluated monthly for signs of improvement. If this does not occur, the patient should be scheduled for surgery.

 Common Questions and Answers

Q: Should children with a VSD-type murmur undergo echocardiographic evaluation to define the location, size, and number of VSDs?
A: Yes.

Q: Should children with VSD have SBE prophylaxis?
A: Yes.

Q: Should asymptomatic children with VSD have restricted activity?
A: No, if there are no other problems.

ICD-9-CM 745.4

BIBLIOGRAPHY

Emmanuonilides GC, Riemenschneider TA, Allen HD, Gutgesell HP, eds. *Moss and Adams heart disease in infants, children and adolescents.* Baltimore: Williams & Wilkins, 1995:724–744.

Moe DG, Guntheroth WG. Spontaneous closure of uncomplicated ventricular septal defect. *Am J Cardiol* 1987;60:674–678.

Author: Song-Gui Yang

Ventricular Tachycardia

 Database

DEFINITION

Ventricular tachycardia (VT) is a series of three or more repetitive beats originating from the ventricle at a rate faster than 120 bpm. It usually has a wide complex rhythm but can be narrow in infants. VT may, but not always, have atrioventricular dissociation.

- *Sustained ventricular tachycardia:* lasts greater than 30 seconds or causes hemodynamic compromise
- *Nonsustained ventricular tachycardia:* lasts from 3 beats to 30 seconds but without hemodynamic compromise
- May be monomorphic or polymorphic
- *Torsade de pointes:* associated with long QT syndrome; the QRS complexes gradually change shape throughout the tachycardia.

ETIOLOGY

- Idiopathic
- Myocarditis
- Dilated cardiomyopathy
- Long QT syndrome (LQT)
- RV dysplasia
- Congenital heart disease (CHD) (e.g., tetralogy of Fallot, transposition of the great arteries, aortic stenosis, hypertrophic cardiomyopathy)
- Ventricular tumors
- Metabolic disturbances (hypoxia, acidosis, hypo/hyperkalemia)
- Drug ingestion (e.g., digitalis toxicity, antiarrhythmic agents)
- Myocardial ischemia (e.g., Kawasaki disease, congenital coronary problems)
- Trauma

PATHOPHYSIOLOGY

VT may result from a reentrant mechanism, triggered mechanism, or abnormal automaticity.

GENETICS

A long QT syndrome may be inherited as an autosomal recessive or dominant pattern. It is related to a variety of potential ion channel defects, and may be associated with hearing loss and/or a family history of sudden death.

EPIDEMIOLOGY

VT may present at any age. Premature ventricular contractions (PVCs) have been reported in 0.8% to 2.2% of otherwise healthy children (Garson 1981).

COMPLICATIONS

- Cardiovascular compromise (sudden death)
- Acquired cardiomyopathy (from long-standing VT and lack of AV synchrony)

PROGNOSIS

- Generally very good in patients with idiopathic VT and a structurally normal heart
- Suppression of ventricular ectopy with exercise has a favorable prognosis.
- In patients with heart disease (congenital or acquired) or the LQT syndrome, VT may increase the risk of presyncope, syncope, and possibly sudden death.

 Differential Diagnosis

- Supraventricular tachycardia with aberrancy
- Antidromic tachycardia (antegrade conduction down an accessory pathway, e.g., WPW)
- Atrial flutter or fibrillation with rapid conduction over an accessory pathway

 Data Gathering

HISTORY

- Mostly asymptomatic
- Palpitations
- Presyncope or syncope
- Exercise intolerance
- Dizziness
- Cardiac arrest

 Physical Examination

- Typically normal, occasional irregularity secondary to frequent PVCs
- Signs of underlying heart disease if any are present

Laboratory Aids

TESTS

• *ECG:* three or more consecutive ventricular complexes faster than 120 bpm. The bundle branch morphology (right or left) may point to the origin of the VT. Similar morphology to isolated PVCs. May have AV dissociation. Typically, repolarization (T-wave) abnormalities are present. Always measure the QTc in lead II in sinus rhythm.

• *ECHO:* Rule out congenital heart disease, tumors, and assess ventricular function.

• *Holter monitor:* Quantitative assessment of ventricular ectopy, frequency of VT, and measurement of QTc interval.

• *Exercise stress test* (5 years and up): The characteristic response is that benign PVCs are suppressed with exercise and return in the immediate recovery period. Exacerbation or worsening of ventricular arrhythmias is very concerning.

• *Cardiac catheterization:* assessment of hemodynamics and possible coronary artery imaging

• *Electrophysiologic study—Possible indications:* (1) diagnosis of a wide complex rhythm; (2) suspected VT in the setting of an abnormal heart, syncope, or cardiac arrest; (3) nonsustained VT in patients with CHD; (4) determination of appropriate medical treatment in a patient with inducible VT; (5) syncope in the setting of palpitations (SVT versus VT); and (6) characterization of the VT and consideration for radiofrequency ablation. *Note:* Electrophysiologic studies are generally not helpful in individuals with LQT syndrome.

 ## Therapy

ACUTE

• If the patient is hemodynamically compromised, prompt synchronized direct-current (1–2 joules/kg; adult, 100–400 joules) is indicated.

• CPR as necessary

• Lidocaine (1 mg/kg bolus over 1 minute, followed by an infusion at 20–50 μg/kg/min)

• If *torsade de pointes*, MgSO$_4$ may be given.

• Overdrive ventricular pacing may terminate the tachycardia. However, pacing may accelerate the VT or induce ventricular fibrillation.

• Intravenous amiodarone (may acutely depress myocardial contractility)

• Intravenous bretylium (generally reserved for ventricular fibrillation)

CHRONIC

• Medications

—Class IB (mexilitine and phenytoin)
—β-Blockers (propanolol, atenolol, nadolol): used in LQT syndrome; may be effective in exercise-induced VT and postoperative congenital heart defects
—Class III (amiodarone and sotalol): Avoid in patients with the LQT syndrome.
—Class IC (flecainide): Proarrhythmia and sudden death have been reported in patients with structural heart disease while on Class IC agents.

• Radiofrequency ablation

• Automatic implantable cardioverter defibrillators

 ## Follow-Up

• Depends on the underlying etiology
• ECG, ECHO, Holter, and exercise stress test

PITFALLS

Misdiagnosis of VT for SVT with aberrancy. Wide-complex tachycardia should always be considered to be ventricular tachycardia until proven otherwise.

 ## Common Questions and Answers

Q: Do frequent single PVCs require treatment?
A: In an otherwise healthy child with a structurally normal heart, normal QT interval, and suppressed PVCs with exercise, no treatment is indicated.

Q: Should siblings of patients with the LQT syndrome be evaluated?
A: Yes, siblings and parents (even if asymptomatic) should have an electrocardiogram, Holter monitor, and exercise stress test for definitive evaluation of the QT interval.

ICD-9-CM 427.1

BIBLIOGRAPHY

Carboni MP, Garson A Jr. Ventricular arrhythmias. In: Garson A Jr, Bricker JT, Fisher DJ, Neish SR, eds. *The science and practice of pediatric cardiology,* 2nd ed. Philadelphia: Williams & Wilkins, 1998:2121–2168.

Garson A Jr. Evaluation and treatment of chronic ventricular dysrhythmias in the young. *Cardiovasc Rev Rep* 1981;2:1164–1191.

Yabek SM. Ventricular arrhythmias in children with an apparently normal heart. *J Pediatr* 1991;119:1–11.

Author: Mitchell I. Cohen

Vesicoureteral Reflux

 Database

DEFINITION

Vesicoureteral reflux (VUR) is passage of urine from the bladder to the kidneys during voiding, secondary to an incompetent valvular mechanism at the ureterovesical junction.

CAUSES

• Primary: The ureter enters bladder through congenitally short intramuscular tunnel, which renders the flap-valve less effective.

—The normal flap-valve mechanism usually compresses the intravesical ureter against the bladder muscle during bladder filling, resulting in closure of the ureter.
—Primary VUR may be seen with other anomalies: ureteral duplication, ureterocele, ureteral ectopia, paraureteral diverticula.
—VUR is a result of abnormal development of the renal collecting system; the severity of VUR is related to the site of origin of the ureteral bud from the Wolffian duct.

• Secondary

—Due to increased intravesical pressure
—Neurogenic bladder (i.e., myelomeningocele)
—Nonneurogenic bladder dysfunction (i.e., dysfunctional voiding): related to detrusor instability and voiding dyssynergy; surgery to reimplant ureters is likely to fail in these cases.
—Bladder outlet obstruction (i.e., posterior urethral valves)
—Inflammation: bacterial cystitis, foreign body, vesical calculi

PATHOLOGY

VUR can cause hydronephrosis and increases the likelihood of renal scars because of the transmission of infectious agents into the collecting tubules in the event of urinary tract infection (UTI).

• Grade I: reflux into nondilated distal ureter
• Grade II: reflux into upper collecting system, with normal calyceal fornices and no dilatation
• Grade III: reflux into mildly dilated and tortuous ureter, with only mild blunting of calyceal fornices blunted
• Grade IV: reflux into grossly dilated ureter, with moderate dilatation and tortuosity of ureter, moderate dilatation pelvis and calyces, maintenance of papillary impressions in majority of calyces
• Grade V: massive reflux with gross ureteral dilatation and tortuosity and effacement of calyceal details, significant blunting of majority of fornices, papillary impressions no longer visible in majority of calyces
• Infection is the main cause of renal damage in VUR; reflux of sterile urine does not cause renal scarring. However, VUR is not a prerequisite for the development of pyelonephritis. In one study, 66% of children with febrile UTI had abnormal DMSA scans, but only 19% had VUR.

GENETICS

• Familial factors: VUR was found in 34% of siblings of an index case; 75% of these siblings were asymptomatic, and 13% had renal damage.
• No apparent association of grade or gender within families
• Higher incidence of VUR in sisters of female index cases
• Greater correlation between parent and child (57%–69% of children of parents with VUR are affected) than between siblings

—In 69% of the cases, the affected parent was the mother.
—In 57% of the cases, the affected parent was the father.

EPIDEMIOLOGY

There are two peaks of incidence:

• In infancy

—Primary VUR; usually males; probably secondary to higher voiding pressures
—Hydronephrosis, often with congenital renal tract anomalies
—Often diagnosed antenatally
—DMSA scans often indicate dysplasia.
—High incidence of spontaneous resolution of reflux regardless of grade: 54% of children diagnosed with Grades III–V reflux spontaneously resolve within 3 years; however, if high-grade reflux is still present beyond 2 to 3 years, spontaneous resolution is unlikely.

• In early childhood

—Three to 5 years; usually girls
—Prevalence in the general population with no history of UTI is 0.4% to 1.8%.
—Secondary VUR: may be associated with voiding dysfunction; 18% of children with reflux have symptoms of voiding dysfunction.
—Other causes of secondary VUR: 50% of children with myelomeningocele have VUR.
—Fifty percent of children with posterior urethral valves have VUR.
—Incidence of VUR in African Americans is approximately 33% less than in the White population; in those with VUR, grade distribution and rate of spontaneous resolution are similar between the two groups.

PROGNOSIS

• Spontaneous resolution of lower grades of reflux as valve mechanism becomes more efficient with growth

—Eighty-two percent grade I, 80% Grade II, 46% Grade III, and 9% Grade IV spontaneously resolve within 5 years.
—Thirty percent to 35% resolution rate per year

• Renal scarring due to UTI associated with VUR causes 15% to 29% end-stage renal disease in children and is an important cause of hypertension, although the incidence is lower now, probably due to an increased awareness of the significance of UTI in children.

—The highest risk of renal scarring is under 5 to 6 years of age.
—The presence of hypertension correlates with extent of renal scarring, especially if bilateral due to increased renin production.
—The incidence of UTI and renal damage between patients with VUR who received either medical or surgical treatment is comparable.
—Surgical correction is 95% successful for all grades of VUR if performed by an experienced pediatric urologist.

 Data Gathering

HISTORY

• Upper tract infection
• Sibling with VUR
• Renal insufficiency
• Hypertension
• Symptoms of voiding dysfunction:

—Urgency
—Dribbling
—Incontinence
—Positive curtsy sign

 Physical Examination

• Abdominal mass secondary to hydronephrosis
• Hypertension
• Signs of chronic renal insufficiency, such as hypertension or failure to thrive

Laboratory Aids

IMAGING

• Voiding cystourethrogram (VCUG) is the gold standard for diagnosis of VUR; catheterization is a necessary component.

• A standard x-ray VCUG is best for diagnosis because of better visualization of the lower urinary tract; follow-up may be conducted with isotope VCUG because of lower radiation exposure.

• A renal ultrasound is helpful for detecting hydronephrosis but can miss up to 74.2% refluxing units, including 28% with moderate-to-severe reflux.

• A DMSA cortical renal scan is the best method to detect renal scarring or renal involvement in UTI.

—Ten percent to 30% of girls with UTI and VUR will already have scarring.
—Sixty percent to 80% of girls with UTI and VUR will have a recurrence of pyelonephritis in 18 months.

• No indication for sleep cystogram

EVALUATION

• For prenatal hydronephrosis on sonogram: 18% of these infants have VUR; antibiotic prophylaxis at birth and VCUG for evaluation

• Evaluate with VCUG all children under 5 years of age who have documented UTI, any boys with UTI, and all febrile UTIs or pyelonephritis.

—Older girls with nonfebrile UTI may be evaluated by RUS and DMSA scan.

• Isotope VCUG may be used to screen family members, especially siblings less than 5 years old.

• Newborn siblings or offspring of patients with VUR should be screened at 12 months.

 ## Therapy

Based on results of the International Reflux Study

• Conservative: Most VUR resolves spontaneously over time in most patients.

• Primary VUR: Observe with antibiotic prophylaxis if less than 1 year old, even if grade IV, because of high rate of spontaneous resolution.

—Antibiotic prophylaxis prevents infection and progression to renal scarring.
—Grade I-III primary VUR or VUR associated with a duplicated ureter is also likely to resolve.
—In the United States, 25% of Grade IV resolve spontaneously, and 16% in Europe.
—Amoxicillin for 2 months and then switch to nitrofurantoin or trimethoprim-sulfamethoxazole
—Follow-up with urine cultures every 4 months or with fever.
—Change the antibiotic if breakthrough UTI occurs; do not increase the dose of the prophylactic antibiotic.
—Prophylaxis does not mask UTI.
—Obtain a VCUG and renal ultrasound every 12 to 18 mos: if negative, anitbiotics may be discontinued.
—Ninety percent of Grades I–III resolve spontaneously in 5 years.
—Reflux duration shorter if diagnosis is made when the child is less than 1 year old than if it is older.
—If VUR persists beyond 2 to 3 years of age, consider surgical intervention.
—At 6 to 8 years of age, if Grades II to III, one may attempt a trial off of prophylaxis, because risk of renal scarring decreases with age.

• Secondary to voiding dysfunction: Prevent UTI and improve urinary habits.

—May require twice-daily or two-drug prophylaxis
—Oxybutyinin hydrochloride is effective in children with detrusor instability and VUR.
—If secondary to severe cystitis: Treat the primary problem.

SURGERY

Involves reimplantation of the affected ureter to produce a competent flap-valve mechanism at the vesicoureteral junction

• Grade IV or V is unlikely to resolve spontaneously: early surgery after brief prophylaxis and confirm VUR, especially if a young infant or child is affected, because of increased risk of renal scarring higher in children less than 5 years of age

• Indicated if there are breakthrough UTIs, especially pyelonephritis on a DMSA scan; may try twice-daily or two-drug prophylaxis first

• Secondary reflux associated with diverticulum is less likely to resolve; surgery is indicated.

• Complications of surgery: increased in infancy and include persistent reflux and ureteral obstruction

• An alternative to surgery involves cystoscopic injection of material under the ureteral orifice, which appears to control reflux in the short term.

—This method is less reliable, and effective only in low-grade reflux.
—Results with collagen show a 50% recurrence rate of VUR 2 years after injection.
—Studies are ongoing with siloxane fat and acrylate polymer.

 ## Common Questions and Answers

Q: What is the significance of reflux seen after a UTI?
A: Reflux is commonly seen immediately after an infection, but this clears over the next few months in most children.

Q: Why not operate to repair the reflux when it is diagnosed?
A: Reflux tends to improve over time, especially in Grades I and II.

ICD-9-CM 593.7

BIBLIOGRAPHY

Belman A. A perspective on vesicoureteral reflux. *Urol Clin North Am* 1995;22:139.

Belman A. Vesicoureteral reflux. *Pediatr Clin North Am* 1997;44(5):1171.

Kelalis P, King L, Belman A, eds. *Clinical pediatric urology*. Philadelphia: WB Saunders, 1992.

Schulman S, Snyder H. Vesicoureteral reflux and reflux nephropathy in children. *Curr Opin Pediatr* 1993;5:191.

Author: Christina Lin Master

Viral Hepatitis

 Database

DEFINITION

Viral hepatitis is inflammation of the liver caused by hepatotropic viruses, which include hepatitis A to E, as well as other hepatotropic viruses, such as EBV, CMV, HSV, VZV, enterovirus, rubella, coxsackie B, adenovirus, parvovirus, and many others. In the United States, hepatitis B accounts for 40% of viral hepatitis cases; hepatitis A, 30%; and hepatitis C, 20%.

TYPES OF HEPATITIS

Hepatitis A

- Transmitted by the oral-fecal route
- Characterized by enteric symptoms associated with right upper quadrant pain, jaundice, diarrhea, pale stools, anorexia, nausea, hepatomegaly and splenomegaly
- The incubation period is about 15 to 40 days, and transaminases rise about 1 week after onset of symptoms; recovery is seen in over 95% of patients within 1 to 2 weeks.
- Jaundice is seen in 88% of adults, but is present in only 65% of children with hepatitis A.
- Chronic hepatitis is rarely reported in immunodeficient patients; it may represent relapsing acute hepatitis A. Fulminant liver failure occurs in less than 1% of patients.

Hepatitis B

- Hepatitis B is a DNA virus and is transmitted by body fluids.
- Hepatitis B has an incubation period of 50 to 180 days and has three phases: the prodrome, icteric, and convalescence phases. The prodrome precedes jaundice by 2 to 3 weeks, with vague symptoms of rash and arthralgia resembling serum sickness.
- Jaundice is seen less frequently in children compared with adults, and it may be accompanied by symptoms of fever, fatigue, myalgia, abdominal pain, and pruritis.
- Circulating immune complexes occasionally result in extrahepatic manifestations, which include vasculitis, nephropathy, and acrodermatitis.
- The icteric phase lasts about 4 to 6 weeks, and this is followed by clearance of antigenemia during the convalescence phase.
- The younger the age of the child with the infection, the higher the likelihood of developing chronic infection. Ninety-five percent of infected neonates, 20% of children, and 10% of adults become carriers after an acute infection.
- Only 10% to 5% lose their carrier status spontaneously.

Hepatitis C

- Hepatitis C is an RNA virus, cloned in 1990, that causes hepatitis and accounts for a significant number of what was previously called non-A non-B hepatitis.
- Hepatitis C is transmitted by blood and sexual contact.

- Clinical disease is insidious, with a long latency period before levels of ALT start to rise.
- Only about 25% of infected patients have an acute illness that is indistinguishable from other forms of hepatitis.
- It may take up to 12 months after exposure for serology to become positive. Detection is by serology or by detection of viral RNA by RT-PCR. It is not usual for HCV to cause fulminant liver failure, although it has been reported.
- After an infection, about 80% will develop viral persistence.
- After chronic HCV infection, liver functions may remain relatively normal for as long as 50 years. At present, one cannot predict the patients who will develop end-stage live failure after infection. The virus undergoes frequent mutations, which may account for the viral persistence.

Hepatitis D

- Hepatitis D is a viral parasite of the hepatitis B virus. It consists of an HDV antigen and HDV ribonucleic acid surrounded by the hepatitis B viral coat.
- Hepatitis D is transmitted by blood or sexual activity.
- Hepatitis D causes two types of acute hepatitis.

—Coinfection: Acute hepatitis B and D virus infection occurs simultaneously.
—Superinfection: Acute hepatitis D occurs in a chronic carrier of hepatitis B. Coinfection has a mortality rate of 1% to 10%, while superinfection has a mortality rate of 5% to 20%. Fulminant liver failure occurs more frequently in superinfection. Chronicity in coinfection is less than 5%, but is 75% in superinfection. Chronic HDV causes cirrhosis in 70% to 80% of patients and is a rapidly progressive disease compared with chronic hepatitis B alone.

Hepatitis E

- Hepatitis E is an RNA virus that causes epidemic hepatitis in areas where water sanitation is poor.
- Hepatitis E is transmitted via the oral-fecal route, and the disease resembles hepatitis A clinically.
- Hepatitis E has an incubation period of 6 weeks and affects young adults mainly.
- Hepatitis E has a higher mortality of 20%, which is higher than hepatitis A, and causes fulminant liver failure in pregnant women. It does not cause chronic hepatitis.

PATHOLOGY

- Acute viral hepatitis tends to affect the liver parenchyma, while chronic viral hepatitis affects portal and periportal areas. Acuteness is defined by an injury period of less than 6 months in duration. In acute hepatitis, there is spotty necrosis, panlobular disarray, increased cellularity, pleomorphism of hepatocytes, and focal parenchymal necrosis. There are multinucleated hepatocytes, indicating liver regeneration, and this leads to hepatocytes of variable sizes, staining, and shapes. Inflammatory cells line the sinusoids.

- Chronic viral hepatitis is continuing inflammation of the liver for more than 6 months. Chronic inflammation affects the portal tracts predominantly but also extends into the parenchyma. Early on, there is periportal expansion and fibrosis initially bounded by the limiting plate. Later, it extends beyond the limiting plate into the parenchyma (piecemeal necrosis). Portal bridging is the finding of extensive fibrosis that occurs between two portal tracts. When the injury is chronic and severe, attempts by the liver to regenerate lead to nodular changes and, finally, to cirrhosis.

 Differential Diagnosis

There are many disorders that give rise to elevated transaminases, and there are clues to a viral origin based on the history, serology, and histologic findings. One often invokes the diagnosis of NANB hepatitis when the cause is almost certainly viral but no virus is isolated.

 Data Gathering

- In hepatitis transmitted by blood or sexual means, the following risk factors apply:

—Positive family history of hepatitis (hepatitis B)
—Immigrants or travelers from endemic areas (E)
—Institution residents such as day care (hepatitis A), prisons (B, C)
—IV drug abusers (B, C, D)
—People with multiple sexual partners (B, C, D)
—Health care workers (B, C)
—Patients requiring multiple blood transfusions or hemodialysis (B, C)
—Dietary intake in some countries (e.g., shellfish) (A)

- Many are thought to have hepatitis A because they often present with symptoms of gastroenteritis.
- Persistence of elevated transaminases and symptoms that resemble chronic fatigue syndrome lead to repeat labs with serologic testing for viral hepatitis.
- There may be hepatomegaly and splenomegaly with or without jaundice.
- Cholestasis is sometimes seen with tea-colored urine and pale stools.
- Other common symptoms are myalgia, abdominal pain, anorexia, fever, and pale stools.

 Laboratory Aids

TESTS

- Routine liver function tests
- Prothrombin time
- Albumin
- Anti-HAV IgM: recent infection
- Anti-HAV IgG: past exposure

- HBsAg: current infection, either acute or chronic
- HBsAb IgM/IgG: resolution of disease
- HBeAg: significant infectivity, viral replication
- HBeAb: end of severe infectivity (except in precore mutants when HBV DNA is positive)
- HBcore IgM: early phase of acute infection, not present in chronic hepatitis B
- HBcore Ag: only found in liver, not serum
- HBV DNA: signifies active viral replication
- HDV Ag: active infection
- HDV Ab: exposure to hepatitis D
- HDV RNA: active replication
- HCV Ab: exposure
- HCV RNA: active replication
- Liver biopsy is useful in assessing the degree of liver damage and also to assess response to therapy. It is not indicated for diagnosis of acute viral hepatitis, although it is sometimes done inadvertently.

Hepatitis B and D

- Acute infection: HBsAg+, HBcore IgM+, HBV DNA+, HBe Ag+
- Chronic infection high risk: HBsAg+, HBe Ag+, HBsAb-, HBV DNA+
- Chronic infection low risk: HBsAg+, HBeAg-, HBeAb+, HBV DNA-
- Chronic active hepatitis: positive serology plus elevated transaminases plus hepatitis on liver biopsy (after 6 months of presenting with symptoms)
- HDV coinfection: HBcIgM+, HDV Ag+, HDV IgM-/-, HDV IgA-
- HDV superinfection: HBcIgM-, HDV Ag+, HDV IgM+, HDV IgA+
- Chronic HDV: HBcIgM-, HDV Ag-, HDV IgM+, HDV IgA+

 Therapy

HEPATITIS A

- No specific therapy is available; avoid going back to the nursery for 2 weeks after illness.
- Postexposure prophylaxis with pooled human serum globulin at dose of 0.02 mL/kg for household contacts, intimate exposure, children and staff in nursery or day care centers with outbreaks. Preexposure (short-term, 0.02 mL/kg; long-term, 0.06 mL/kg every 4–6 months) to travelers to endemic areas.
- Havrix Junior (SKB) vaccine is given by IM injection: ages 1 to 15 years: two doses of 0.5 mL; the second is given 2 to 4 weeks after the first dose; booster dose 0.5 mL, 6 to 12 months following the initial dose.
- It is sensible for children with liver disease to be vaccinated to prevent exacerbation of liver disease.

HEPATITIS B

- Postexposure prophylaxis with HBIG is indicated for neonates born to mothers who are hepatitis B carriers, after sexual contact with carriers, and after accidental exposure to infected blood products.

DRUGS

Interferon-α

- Eradication of hepatitis B is by α-interferon. Predictive factors for response are high serum ALT prior to therapy, low serum HBV DNA, nonvertically acquired hepatitis B, active hepatitis on liver biopsy, female sex, HIV−, and HDV−. The success rate based on adult studies is 33% and 37% for the loss of HBeAg and HBV DNA, respectively. In patients with cirrhosis, the use of interferon is more risky because it can cause the liver disease to become decompensated, and should only be done in centers with good access to liver transplantation.
- Interferon treatment for hepatitis C in children is not established. It is licensed for use, in adults, however, with good response—in the region of 41% improvement in ALT; 70% of patients show improved histology, but with a 50% to 70% relapse rate.
- Interferon-α (dose from published pediatric trials)

—Chronic HBV: 5 to 10 MU/m^2 given three times a week for 6 to 12 months
—Chronic HCV: 3 MU/m^2 given three times a week for 6 to 12 months
—Interferon is not licensed for use in children, and it has hematologic, infectious, autoimmune, neuropsychiatric, and systemic side effects, with myelosuppression the most common dose-dependent side effect. If platelets fall below 50,000/μL and neutrophils below 1,500/μL, the interferon dose is lowered or temporarily discontinued.

Lamivudine

There may be a role for lamivudine in the treatment of chronic hepatitis B. This is an oral nucleoside analogue that inhibits viral DNA replication. It has been shown to markedly reduce HBV DNA levels in 98% of patients during therapy, but, in general, they return to pretreatment status after the drug is discontinued. Lamivudine dosage (trial basis) is 25 to 100 mg/d for 1 year in an adult.

CURIOSITIES

- Hepatitis G was discovered a few years ago, and although so named, has not been found or proven to cause hepatitis.
- TT virus is a transfusion-transmissible virus discovered in Japan in 1997. It is a single-stranded linear DNA virus lacking an outer envelope, has similarities to parvovirus, and was found in 10% to 38% of patients with chronic liver disease. The pathogenicity of this virus in causing hepatitis is under investigation.

 Common Questions and Answers

Q: Why do patients infected at birth with HBV have a higher incidence of chronicity?
A: This is probably a dose effect, with the infecting dose being higher in vertical transmission than in other forms of transmission. In addition, early infection increases the time for the virus to integrate into the host genome.

Q: Is viral hepatitis associated with aplastic anemia?
A: There are studies that have implicated and excluded all the known hepatitis viruses (A–E) as a cause of hepatitis-associated aplastic anemia; however, parvovirus is a known hepatotropic virus and also an established cause of aplastic anemia that needs to be excluded.

Q: What is the current definition of non-A non-B (NANB) hepatitis?
A: NANB hepatitis should now be termed non-A to non-E, with all the testing available in modern hospitals. In the past, this probably included patients who are now known to have HCV.

Q: What is the best way of eradicating hepatitis B?
A: Universal vaccination in childhood has been recommended by the US Public Health Service for eradication of HBV. Vaccination is actively pursued in some Asian countries, where the disease affects about a third of the population. However, some babies born to HBsAg+ mothers develop escape mutants of hepatitis B virus.

Q: What is the relevance of genotyping of HCV?
A: Genotypes may share 65% homology based on nucleotide sequences but differ in their biologic effects, such as severity of disease and response to interferon. Western Europe; Australia type 1, 2, or 3; Far East types 1 and 2 (but Thailand type 3); Hong Kong type 6; and United States types 1a and 1b are common, while subtypes 2a, 2b, and 3a are uncommon; Africa type 4, South Africa type 5. Response to interferon is:

- Initial: 30% in type 1, 60% to 70% in types 2 and 3.
- Sustained response: 8% to 10% in type 1 and 30% in types 2 and 3.

Q: Should mothers with HCV positivity breast feed?
A: Based on the fact that viral RNA levels are very low in breast milk, it is felt that transmission of HCV via breast milk is very unlikely.

BIBLIOGRAPHY

Balistreri W. Acute and chronic viral hepatitis. In: Suchy FJ, ed. *Liver disease in children*. St. Louis: Mosby 1994:460–509.

Desmet MA, Gerber M, Hoofnagle JH, et al. Classification of chronic hepatitis: diagnosis, grading and staging. *Hepatology* 1994;19:1513–1520.

Lai CL, Chien RN, Leung NW, et al. One year trial of lamivudine for chronic hepatitis B. *N Engl J Med* 1998;339:61–68.

Niederau CN, Heingest T, Lange S, et al. Long term follow up of HBeAg-positive patients treated with interferon alpha for chronic hepatitis B. *N Engl J Med* 1996;334:1422–1427.

Popper H, Schaffner F. The vocabulary of chronic hepatitis. *N Engl J Med* 1997;284: 1154–1156.

Author: John Tung

Volvulus

 Database

DEFINITION

Volvulus is torsion of the gut upon itself or upon a narrow mesenteric pedicle. It may be acute and complete or chronic and intermittent.

CAUSES

Malrotation results in a narrow mesenteric stalk for the midgut loop and obstructing bands (Ladd bands) across the duodenum, predisposing to volvulus.

EPIDEMIOLOGY

- Malrotation with midgut volvulus is most common in neonates.
- Fifty percent to 80% of patients with abnormal rotation will be symptomatic in infancy.

COMPLICATIONS

- Intermittent or acute obstruction
- Strangulation resulting in ischemia and loss of midgut
- Protein losing enteropathy can also result from strangulation.

 Differential Diagnosis

- Perforated viscus
- Necrotizing enterocolitis
- Meconium ileus
- Hirschsprung enterocolitis
- Appendicitis
- Intussusception
- Pyelonephritis

 Data Gathering

HISTORY

- Symptoms of acute or recurrent obstruction at birth or in the first year of life
- Recurrent bilious emesis with acute abdomen
- Feeding intolerance
- Chylous ascites and/or protein-losing enteropathy due to lymphatic congestion
- In older children, recurrent abdominal pain and emesis

 Physical Examination

- Abdominal tenderness and distention
- Irritability, lethargy
- Brawny edema of abdominal wall
- Bloody stools
- Drawing up of legs
- Tachypnea and tachycardia

 Laboratory Aids

TESTS

- May see metabolic acidosis, thrombocytopenia

Imaging

- Abdominal x-ray may show dilated stomach and duodenum.
- Upper gastrointestinal tract radiography may show abnormal position of the ligament of Treitz and a "corkscrew" appearance of the midgut. The radiographic appearance, though, may be confusing because there are at least seven patterns of duodenal malrotation reported. In the absence of a *corkscrew or Z-shaped duodenum, patterns that usually indicate volvulus or obstructing Ladd bands, colon position* had greater prognostic implication, especially when the cecum is positioned in the RUQ or LUQ. In report by Long et al. (1996), these latter patterns were associated with the highest prevalence of volvulus. Barium enema shows an abnormal position of the cecum.

Therapy

- Close monitoring of fluids and electrolytes to prevent shock
- Laparotomy with resection of ischemic portions of the intestine
- Ladd procedure: volvulus is untwisted, transduodenal bands are divided, mesenteric base is broadened, and appendix is removed.
- If the entire midgut is ischemic, the volvulus may be untwisted, with reexploration in 12 to 24 hours.

Follow-Up

- Prognosis depends on extent of involvement and degree of ischemia.
- Monitor closely for feeding intolerance postoperatively.

PITFALLS

- May take hours to days to become symptomatic
- Symptoms may be mistaken for colic in infants or cyclic emesis in older children.
- Delayed diagnosis may result in strangulation and infarction, leading to short-gut syndrome.

Common Questions and Answers

Q: In what age group is volvulus most common?
A: Midgut volvulus is most common in the neonatal period.

Q: How can the signs and symptoms of volvulus be distinguished from gastroesophageal reflux?
A: Although both intermittent volvulus and gastroesophageal reflux (GER) may present with vomiting, the emesis in GER is not bilious. Bilious emesis, abdominal pain, and lethargy are signs of an abdominal obstruction, requiring further examination.

ICD-9-CM 560.9

BIBLIOGRAPHY

Gebara S, Firor HU. Congenital anomalies of the midgut. In: Wyllie R, Hyams JS, eds. *Pediatric gastrointestinal disease*. Philadelphia: WB Saunders, 1993:495–596.

Hatch EI, Sawin R. The acute abdomen. In: Wyllie R, Hyams JS, eds. *Pediatric gastrointestinal disease*. Philadelphia: WB Saunders, 1993:210–212.

Ismail A. Recurrent colonic volvulus in children. *J Pediatr Surg* 1997;32(12):1739–1742.

Kealey WD, McCallion WA, Brown S, Potts SR, Boston VE. Midgut volvulus in children. *Br J Surg* 1996;83(1):105–106.

Long FR, Kramer SS, Markowitz RI, Taylor GE. Radiographic patterns of intestinal malrotation in children. *Radiographics* 1996;16(3):547–556.

Stewart DR, Colodneg AL, Daggert WC. Malrotation of the bowel in infants and children: a 15 year review. *Surgery* 1976;79:716–720.

Author: Andrew E. Mulberg

Von Willebrand Disease

 ## Database

DEFINITION

Von Willebrand disease (vWD) is a bleeding disorder in which there is a deficiency or abnormality of the coagulation protein, von Willebrand factor (vWF), which facilitates the adherence of platelets to sites of injured endothelium as well as stabilizing factor VIII in circulation.

PATHOPHYSIOLOGY

• vWF is a large multimeric protein, found in the circulation as well as the subendothelium, which binds to collagen at sites of endothelial injury and recruits platelets to the site by binding to a specific receptor on the platelet membrane.
• When this protein is either deficient or defective, platelet "plugging" is compromised.
• vWD is an inherited bleeding disorder; however, acquired forms of vWD have been described in association with hypothyroidism, Wilms' tumor, congenital heart disease, EBV infection, and valproate therapy.
• An abnormality in the platelet receptor for vWF can lead to platelet-type pseudo-vWD.

GENETICS

• The gene for vWF is found on chromosome 12, and is autosomally inherited.
• Type I follows a dominant inheritance pattern.
• Type III follows a recessive inheritance pattern.
• Type II varies, depending on the specific type. Compound heterozygous patients have been described.

EPIDEMIOLOGY

• Incidence is estimated to be about 1 in 200 to 1 in 100. People of all races can be affected.

COMPLICATIONS

• Significant perioperative bleeding can occur, but the most common complications are recurrent epistaxis, prolonged bleeding with cuts and abrasions, and menorrhagia.
• Patients with type III (severe vWD) have a more severe bleeding disorder and can have hemarthroses and intracranial hemorrhage with trauma.

PROGNOSIS

• Type III can result in a severe bleeding disorder, but types I and II tend to be mild and often go undetected.
• With proper education and treatment, patients with the most severe forms of the disease can be expected to do well.

 ## Differential Diagnosis

• Primary hemostatic disorders

—Congenital: platelet function abnormalities
—Mild coagulation factor deficiencies
—Hemophilia (type III vWD and type IIN are similar to mild and moderate factor VIII deficiency)

• Acquired hemostatic disorders

—Mild coagulopathies, resulting in bleeding or a prolongation of the PTT or bleeding time
—Uremia
—Thrombocytopenia
—Drugs that affect platelet function

• Connective tissue disorders

—Ehlers-Danlos syndrome
—Osteogenesis Imperfecta

 ## Data Gathering

HISTORY

• A family history of vWD or bleeding tendency is an important part of the evaluation for vWD. However, be aware that variation in frequency and severity of bleeding symptoms can occur from person to person, even within an affected family.
• Mucosal bleeding is especially common in vWD.
• Gum bleeding, even with minor trauma such as brushing
• Bruising: increased number, but, more importantly, increased size (>5 cm), and often palpable rather than flat
• Recurrent epistaxis
• Menorrhagia occurs in 50% to 75% of affected women.
• Excessive or unusual posttraumatic or postsurgical bleeding
• There may be no history of bleeding manifestations.

 ## Physical Examination

• Bruises: increased number, size, and/or unusual location
• May be entirely normal

 ## Laboratory Aids

TESTS

• PTT is elevated in 25% of patients.
• Bleeding time is prolonged in 50% of patients.
• Factor VIII activity is the least sensitive of the usual screening coagulation test.
• Ristocetin cofactor is the most helpful single test for vWD.
• Factor VIII antigen (vWF)
• vWF multimeric analysis helps determine specific type:

—Type I (65%–80%): all multimers of vWF present but decreased; most common and mildest form of the disease
—Type IIA (10%–12%): absence of high-molecular-weight multimers (not uncommon for ristocetin cofactor activity to be proportionately lower than vWF antigen)
—Type IIB (3%–5%): decrease of the highest, high-molecular-weight multimers with increased low-dose, ristocetin-induced platelet aggregation
—Type IIN (1%–2%): normal multimeric analysis, factor VIII activity low due to decreased binding to vWF
—Type IIM (1%–2%): usually has normal multimeric analysis; the factor is dysfunctional due to a point mutation (not uncommon for ristocetin cofactor activity to be proportionately lower than vWF antigen).
—Type III (1%–3%): undetectable multimers of vWF; most severe form
—Platelet type (0%–1%): like type IIB

• CBC to rule out thrombocytopenia. Iron deficiency is common, and platelets can be slightly low in type IIB.
• PT to look for other coagulation abnormalities (PT is normal in vWD)

PITFALLS

• Unfortunately, a normal laboratory work-up for vWD does not necessarily indicate the absence of disease. The work-up may need to be repeated several times, preferably when the patient is well (free of infection or other stressors), before declaring that a patient does not have vWD. vWF is an acute-phase reactant.
• Another complicating problem in the laboratory diagnosis of vWD is the normal variation in vWF levels associated with different blood types.
• Conditions that alter vWF levels:

—Normal levels vary with the ABO blood group; group O can have 50% of normal levels and not have vWD.
—Increased levels: newborn period, collagen vascular disorders, postsurgical states, liver disease, intravascular clotting, hyperthyroidism, high-stress states, pregnancy, and inflammatory and infectious disease states.
—Decreased levels: hypothyroidism
—Change in the multimeric pattern of vWF: DIC, TTP, HUS, and VSDs

Von Willebrand Disease

REQUIREMENTS

- No aspirin within 7 days of bleeding time
- Avoidance of any of the many agents (antihistamines, Ca^+ channel blockers, furosemide, NSAIDs) that affect platelet function 24 hours prior to the bleeding time
- Avoid cigarette smoking and heavy exercise prior to testing for vWD.
- Steroids, oral contraceptives, and other estrogens can increase vWF levels.

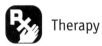 Therapy

IMMEDIATE

- Supportive measures are often enough to stop the bleeding (i.e., compression, etc.)
- Severe bleeding in a postsurgical or posttraumatic condition may require infusion with a factor concentrate known to have good levels of vWF, such as Humate-P. Severity of bleeding will be a function of the type of vWD present.

DRUGS

Knowledge of the type of vWD is required for the proper treatment of the disease.

- DDAVP (desmopressin acetate)

—Most patients with type I disease will respond to DDAVP, but because a few will not, a trial of DDAVP is recommended after the age of 1 year.
—May be administered by intravenous or intranasal routes
—May be ineffective in type IIA and type III disease
—May worsen thrombocytopenia in type IIB and platelet-type vWD
—Tachyphylaxis (failure to respond after repeated doses) can occur.

- Blood products

—Cryoprecipitate: The development of a solvent detergent-treated cryoprecipitate may reduce the risk of virus transmission. May be an appropriate product for families who wish to have a directed donor.

- vWF levels in the donor can be increased by administering DDAVP prior to collection.

—Humate P and Alphanate: Intermediate purity factor VIII concentrate product with adequate levels (especially large multimers) of vWF.

- Aminocaproic acid (Amicar): helpful for oral cavity bleeding and following tooth extraction to prevent bleeding.

PREVENTION

- Avoid heavy contact sports (football, etc.); otherwise, assume normal activity for age. Type III patients and some type II patients need to be more cautious about level of activity.
- For patients with recurrent epistaxis, measures should be taken to avoid drying of the mucosa by applying petroleum jelly and to curtail nosepicking or reduce the trauma by keeping the fingernails short.

 Follow-Up

WHEN TO EXPECT IMPROVEMENT

There is a lifelong risk of bleeding.

SIGNS TO WATCH FOR

- Pattern of bleeding
- Hepatitis, if exposed to blood products
- Some patients will become iron-deficient from chronic blood loss.

 Common Questions and Answers

Q: How can a child have a bleeding disorder if he or she went through surgery without a problem?
A: In vWD, the vWF level can change as a function of stresses in the body. Many conditions will cause the vW factor level to rise to a normal level. These conditions include infectious illnesses and pregnancy, as well as emotional stress. In surgery, the reason for the surgery itself (i.e., appendicitis, etc.) may cause enough stress to raise the factor levels to normal and prevent bleeding.

Q: Should the other family members be tested?
A: Yes, even if there is no history of bleeding in family members. Other affected family members may be unaware that they have the disease because vWD can be so mild.

Q: What sports activities can a person with vWD participate in safely?
A: People with type I vWD can participate in most activities, although it is usually advised to avoid situations in which significant trauma takes place, such as football, boxing, sky diving, and so forth. Patients with type III should try to avoid activities with even moderate trauma. For type II patients, the risk of bleeding varies.

Q: Is life expectancy lower in people with vWD?
A: For the majority of patients with vWD, their life expectancy and quality of life will be normal.

ICD-9-CM 286.4

BIBLIOGRAPHY

Blomback M, Eneroth P, Andersson OM, et al. On laboratory problems in diagnosing mild von Willebrand's disease. *Am J Hematol* 1992; 40:117–120.

Lethagen S, Harris AS, Nilsson IM. Intranasal desmopressin (DDAVP) by spray in mild hemophilia Q and von Willebrand's disease type I. *Blut* 1990;60:187–191.

Montgomery RR, Gill JC, Scott JP. Hemophilia and von Willebrand disease. In: Nathan DG, Orkin SH, eds. *Hematology of infancy and childhood,* 5th ed. Philadelphia: WB Saunders, 1993; 1644–1659.

Werner EJ, Abshire TC, Giroux DS, et al. Relative value of diagnostic studies for von Willebrand's disease. *J Pediatr* 1992;121:34–38.

Werner EJ. von Willebrand disease in children and adolescents. *Pediatr Clin North Am* 1996;43(3):683–707.

Author: J. Nathan Hagstrom

Warts

Database

DEFINITION

Warts (verrucae) are benign, proliferative, intraepithelial tumors caused by the human papillomavirus (HPV), a small double-stranded DNA virus belonging to the family Papovaviradae. To date, there have been more than 100 types of HPV isolated in vitro. The major types of warts include:

- Common warts (verruca vulgaris)
- Flat warts (verruca plana)
- Plantar warts (verruca plantaris)
- Anogenital warts (venereal warts, condyloma acuminata)
- Laryngeal warts (laryngeal papillomatosis)

PATHOPHYSIOLOGY

- Warts can potentially infect any cutaneous or mucosal membrane surface. The most likely sites include areas prone to trauma, explaining the predominance of warts on the hands and feet. Most HPV types have preferred sites of infectivity. There is a great deal of overlap, and one should not use typing to infer modes of transmission.
- The dermal papillae are thin and contain abundant blood vessels, some of which may be thrombosed. These vessels correlate clinically with the "black dots" and pinpoint bleeding seen after paring of the wart.

EPIDEMIOLOGY

- Humans are thought to be the only reservoir of HPV.
- Incubation periods range from 1 to 6 months, but latency periods of 3 or more years are suspected.
- Primary mode of transmission is thought to be by direct physical contact. Fomite spread has been postulated, and recently HPV has been spread to nasal mucosa from laser plumes.
- Once infected, individuals can spread virus to themselves (i.e., autoinoculation), primarily by manipulating warts or shaving.
- Vertical transmission, or transmission by passage through an infected birth canal, can lead to anogenital and laryngeal warts.
- Approximately 10 percent of children between 5 and 10 years of age have warts.
- Peak incidence of nongenital warts is between the ages of 12 to 16.
- Caucasians are affected more than are African Americans, for unknown reasons.
- Incidence of anogenital warts has increased dramatically in adults, but less so in children.
- Immunocompromised individuals (primarily those with impaired cell-mediated immunity), as well as individuals with preexisting skin conditions that impair skin barrier function, are at increased risk for infection.

COMPLICATIONS

Anogenital Warts

- Certain HPV types (see the table) play a prominent role in the development of squamous-cell carcinoma, particularly in the anogenital skin of men and women. Most types seen in children have low oncogenic potential.
- Bowenoid papulosis is considered a premalignant variant of anogenital warts. Clinically indistinguishable from anogenital warts, these lesions show features of dysplasia on biopsy. Despite this histology, they generally behave in a benign manner.

Laryngeal Warts

- Stridor
- Dyspnea
- Dysphonia
- Airway obstruction

Epidermodysplasia Verruciformis

- A rare autosomal recessive genodermatosis, whereby patients have impaired natural killer cell–mediated immunity. Consequently, they progressively develop widespread, refractory warts, particularly over bony prominences. The lesions in sun-exposed areas are at increased risk of cutaneous malignancy, namely invasive squamous-cell carcinomas, strongly suggesting the contribution of ultraviolet radiation to carcinogenesis.

PROGNOSIS

Spontaneous regression is seen in up to two-thirds of *untreated* common warts within 2 years. No such data on anogenital warts exist.

Differential Diagnosis

- Common warts
—Typically distinguishable on clinical grounds
- Flat warts

—Dermal nevi
—Epidermal nevi
—Molluscum contagiosum
—Milia
—Folliculitis
—Lichen planus
—Lichen nitidus
—Acrokeratosis verruciformis
- Plantar warts

—Corns
—Calluses
—Foreign bodies
- Anogenital warts

—Condyloma lata
—Molluscum contagiosum
—Skin tags
—Hemorrhoids
—Pyramidal perineal papules

Data Gathering

HISTORY

- Determine the duration of the warts, as well as the tempo of proliferation. If warts have been present for less than 6 months to 1 year, one should resist the urge to treat with aggressive modalities.
- Anogenital warts should always prompt a careful history for sexual abuse. However, the majority of children less than 3 years of age are exposed by nonsexual contact with infected parents, siblings, and caretakers. A maternal or paternal history of anogenital warts, and history of warts in individuals in close contact with the patient, should be determined.

Physical Examination

- When assessing anogenital warts, one should examine the entire patient for a potential source of infection. Presence of other warts may suggest autoinoculation. Parents and primary caretakers should likewise be checked to rule out heteroinoculation. The practitioner must check for signs of possible physical or sexual abuse. Suspicious cases should be cultured for gonorrhea and chlamydia, and serologic tests for syphilis and HIV should be performed. In cases of suspected abuse, the appropriate authorities must be notified.
- Application of 3% to 5% acetic acid to genital warts may enhance their detection.
- Paring of warts may help differentiate diagnostic possibilities by showing evidence of "black dots" or pinpoint hemorrhage at the base.
- Because of their infectious nature, warts are more likely in areas of trauma. Due to inoculation, they may be seen in a linear array.

Laboratory Aids

TESTS

- Biopsy rarely needed
- Southern blot hybridization for identification of HPV type: rarely useful in the clinical setting
- Polymerase chain reaction for identification of HPV type: rarely useful in the clinical setting

Therapy

With the likelihood for spontaneous resolution, one should never underestimate the value of benign neglect in the treatment of warts. The decision to treat must be based on the age and personality of the patient, and the number, size, and location of the warts. All therapeutic modalities work by destruction of HPV-infected epithelial cells. Treatment should include the clinically visible margins as well as immediately adjacent normal skin, as this has been shown to harbor viral DNA. Most modalities require multiple treatments and work by progressive de-bulking of virally infected cells. Painful procedures may benefit from EMLA anesthesia prior to treatment. While not all-inclusive, the following are the most well accepted modes of therapy.

READILY AVAILABLE IN MOST PEDIATRIC PRACTICES

• Surgical tape occlusion

—A benign, easy, inexpensive option with variable efficacy. Anecdotal responses have been reported, but untested. The procedure requires 24-hour occlusion, and response is slow.

• Hyperthermia

—Likewise, a benign option with anecdotal success, but untested. Treatment is time consuming, as it requires immersion in 45°C water for 30 minutes daily. Response is slow.

• Salicylic acid

—Minimally invasive, inexpensive therapy that is well tolerated and can be performed at home. Many different products are available over the counter (e.g., Duofilm, Occlusol HP, Trans-Ver-Sal, Compound W) for treatment of common warts. Plantar warts often require 40% salicylic acid in an adhesive plaster. Success rates have been reported to be as high as 84%. This procedure requires dedicated application, and response can be slow.

• Cantheridin

—Minimally invasive and usually well tolerated. Vesiculation can be unpredictable, and, therefore, it is not recommended for facial lesions. It may cause significant pigmentary changes.

• Tretinoin (Retin-A 0.1% cream)

—Primary indication is for flat warts; not effective for common warts
—Well tolerated, with the exception of mild local irritation; not for use in intertriginous sites

• Podophyllin or podophyllotoxin

—Not FDA approved for pediatric use, but has been used in children safely. Its primary indication is for anogenital warts. It should not be used in large areas due to systemic absorption. Oral ingestion can be fatal. Podophyllin requires in-office application, but podophyllotoxin (Condylox solution or gel) can be used at home.

• Immunotherapy (Imiquimod)

—Unknown mechanism of action but has been shown to upregulate interferon at sites of application. Although not FDA approved for children, it appears to be safe. It is indicated for treatment of anogenital warts. No studies with common warts exist.

• Cimetidine

—Recently, multiple anecdotal reports of success with a dosage of 30 to 50 mg/kg/d in three divided doses (maximum, 3.5-g daily dose). It is speculated to work by stimulating T-lymphocyte activity. Double-blind, placebo-controlled studies show that efficacy is no better than placebo.

TYPICALLY RESERVED FOR DERMATOLOGY PRACTICES

• Trichloroacetic/bichloroacetic acid/other keratolytics

—Work similarly to salicylic acids but are more potent medications, which can hasten response; requires in-office application

• Contact sensitization (dinitrochlorobenzene)

—Works by inducing a local allergic contact dermatitis over warts. It can be difficult to titrate and can cause severe erythema and blistering. Its application is not recommended unless by knowledgeable personnel.

• Cryotherapy

—Often very effective, and relatively rapid in comparison with topical therapies. Cryotherapy is performed with two freeze–thaw cycles of 5- to 10-second duration. Disadvantages of this procedure include pain, risk of pigmentary changes, and low risk of scarring.

• Laser ablation (CO$_2$, erbium:YAG, and flashlamp pulsed dye laser)

—An expensive but often effective option. Disadvantages of this procedure include pain, pigmentary changes, and a low risk of scarring. Laryngeal warts typically need aggressive therapy with laser ablation to prevent respiratory compromise.

• Surgery

—Should be reserved for refractory cases. Disadvantages include pain and the requirement for local anesthesia. Surgery will leave a scar.

• Electrosurgery/curettage

—Should be reserved for refractory cases. Disadvantages include pain and the requirement for local anesthesia. These procedures will leave a scar.

• Bleomycin

—Should be reserved for refractory cases. Requires multiple injections, so it is typically painful. A Raynaud-like phenomenon has been seen in a small subset of individuals when bleomycin was used in the lateral distal fingers.

 Follow-Up

• All treated warts require close follow-up, typically at 3- to 4-week intervals, to evaluate response to therapy and for possible retreatment. Prolonged intervals between treatments can delay resolution by allowing regrowth of the wart.
• Extensive, treatment-refractory HPV infection in the absence of obvious cause should prompt the practitioner to check for underlying immunodeficiency.

PREVENTION

Manipulation of warts, especially during treatment, by biting or picking should be discouraged to prevent spread.

PITFALLS

It must be emphasized that HPV typing gives no insight on actual mode of transmission of anogenital warts.

 Common Questions and Answers

Q: How likely are warts to spread?
A: Unfortunately, because we don't fully understand the mechanisms of transmission, we don't have good studies to predict infectivity. Obviously, those individuals with impaired skin integrity or immunodeficiency are at greater risk for infection with HPV. However, in the presence of normal, intact skin, infection is relatively uncommon. Good skin care (for instance, removing hangnails) can prevent potential spread to adjacent skin. Reduction of manipulation of lesions also will prevent spread. Infected children should not be prevented from going to day care or school.

Q: What can you give me to remove these warts once and for all?
A: Unfortunately, no "definitive" therapy exists. All treatments are locally destructive, and often require repetitive treatments. Despite clinical clearing, subclinical infection may persist, which can cause recurrence. Latent infections also occur. Follow-up is therefore essential, and should evidence of reinfection occur, treatment should be instituted earlier rather than later.

Q: How did my child get venereal warts? Was she or he sexually abused?
A: Although there are conflicting studies, it is generally accepted that the most common mode of transmission of anogenital warts in children under 3 years of age, is through nonsexual contact (i.e., vertical transmission, passage through the birth canal, autoinoculation, heteroinoculation [see previous discussion]). This does not negate the obligation of the physician to investigate for physical and/or sexual abuse. Should the practitioner feel uncomfortable with this type of investigation, the patient should be referred to a specialist. Development of anogenital warts in children older than 3 years of age must be investigated thoroughly for evidence of abuse.

ICD-9-CM
Verruca vulgaris 078.10
Verruca plana 078.19
Verruca plantaris 078.19
Anogenital warts 078.11

BIBLIOGRAPHY

Cohen BA. Warts and children: can they be separated? *Contemp Pediatr* 1997;14(2):128–149.

Handley J, Hanks E, Armstrong K, et al. Common association of HPV2 with anogenital warts in prepubertal children. *Pediatr Dermatol* 1997;14(5):339–343.

Siegfried EC. Warts on children: an approach to therapy. *Pediatr Ann* 1996;25(2):79–90.

Author: Ho Jin Kim

Wilms Tumor

 Database

DEFINITION

Wilms tumor is a malignant tumor of the kidney occurring in the pediatric age group. It is also called *nephroblastoma*.

CAUSES

- Not known

PATHOLOGY

- Gross: often cystic with hemorrhages and necrosis; usually no calcification (useful in differentiating from neuroblastoma, which is calcified on plain x-ray); may extend into inferior vena cava (IVC)
- Histology: Triphasic pattern blastemal, epithelial, and stromal cell. Blastemal cells aggregate into nodules like primitive glomeruli; the presence of anaplasia indicates a poor prognosis.

GENETICS

- Fifteen percent to 20% are hereditary in origin.
- Familial cases are more often bilateral and occur at an earlier age.
- A tumor-suppressor gene related to Wilms tumor (WT1) has been localized to chromosome 11p13.

EPIDEMIOLOGY

- Five percent to 6% of all childhood cancer
- Incidence: 1 in 10,000 children under 16
- Higher incidence in Black female children
- Peak age: 2 to 3 years
- May be associated with aniridia, hemihypertrophy, and cryptorchidism
- Increased incidence in children with neurofibromatosis
- Associated syndromes: WAGR (Wilms tumor, aniridia, GU abnormalities, mental retardation), Beckwith Weidman syndrome, and Denys-Drash syndrome (ambiguous genitalia, progressive renal failure, and increased risk of Wilms tumor).

COMPLICATIONS

- Extension into IVC
- Metastasis to lungs and liver
- Cardiac toxicity secondary to Adriamycin
- Liver dysfunction secondary to actinomycin D and radiation therapy (XRT)

PROGNOSIS

- Stages I and II: more than 90% cured
- Stage III: 85% cured
- Stage IV: 70% cured

 Differential Diagnosis

- Polycystic kidney
- Renal hematoma
- Renal abscess
- Neuroblastoma
- Other neoplasm of kidney: clear-cell carcinoma, rhabdoid tumor

 Data Gathering

HISTORY

- Abdominal distension
- Abdominal pain (20%–30% of cases)
- Hematuria (20%–30% of cases)
- Fever, anorexia, vomiting
- Family history of Wilms tumor
- Rapid increase in abdominal size (suggestive of hemorrhage in the tumor)

 Physical Examination

- Asymptomatic abdominal mass extending from flank toward midline (most common presentation)
- Anemia (secondary to hemorrhage in the tumor)
- Fever
- Hypertension (due to increased renin production in 25% of cases)
- Varicocele (indicates obstruction to spermatic vein due to tumor thrombus in renal vein or IVC)
- Aniridia, hemihypertrophy, cryptorchidism, hypospadias
- Signs of Beckwith Weideman and neurofibromatosis

 Laboratory Aids

TESTS

Laboratory Tests

- CBC
- Electrolytes
- Urine analysis: for microscopic hematuria
- Liver and kidney function tests

Imaging

- Ultrasound of abdomen

—Diagnostic of mass of renal origin
—Evaluate for extension of tumor into IVC

- CT scan of abdomen: useful if diagnosis doubtful
- IVP: no longer routinely used
- Chest x-ray: to evaluate for metastatic disease
- Bone scan: only if clear-cell variety on pathology
- CT of head: only for rhabdoid tumors

CLINICOPATHOLOGIC STAGING

- Stage I: Tumor is restricted to one kidney and completely resected. The renal capsule is intact.
- Stage II: Tumor extends beyond the kidney but is completely excised.
- Stage III: Residual nonhematogenous tumor is confined to the abdomen.
- Stage IV: There is hematogenous spread to lungs and liver.
- Stage V: bilateral disease

FAVORABLE PROGNOSTIC FACTORS

- Tumor weight less than 250 g
- Age at presentation less than 24 months
- Stage I disease

POOR PROGNOSTIC FACTORS

- Anaplastic pathology
- Lymph node involvement
- Distant metastasis

 Therapy

SURGERY

- Nephrectomy

—Preoperative chemotherapy in case of very large tumors with IVC extension
   —For bilateral disease nephrectomy of more affected side and partial nephrectomy of the other side, followed by chemotherapy and radiation

RADIATION THERAPY

- Not required for stage I and II patients
- Local XRT with 1,000 cGy for stages III and IV
- Whole-lung radiation (1,200 cGy) for pulmonary metastasis

CHEMOTHERAPY

- For stages I and II: vincristine (VCR) and actinomycin D (AMD) every 3 weeks for 6 months
- For stages III and IV: VCR, AMD, and doxorubicin for 6 to 15 months

SIDE EFFECTS OF THERAPY

Temporary loss of hair, peripheral neuropathy, impaired function of the remaining kidney over years following radiation, cardiac toxicity with adriamycin, second malignant neoplasms in few cases

 Follow-Up

- Every 3 months for 18 months, every 6 months for 1 year, and then yearly
- Chest x-ray, urinalysis, and abdominal ultrasound at regular intervals

PITFALLS

Rarely, Wilms tumor may present with polycythemia. It can present as fever of unknown origin without any other signs or symptoms.

 Common Questions and Answers

Q: What should be done to protect the remaining kidney during sports?
A: Children should wear a kidney guard to protect the unaffected kidney during contact sports.

Q: Can a child grow and live normally with one kidney?
A: Yes.

ICD-9-CM 189.0

BIBLIOGRAPHY

Coppes MJ, Haber DA, Grundy PE. Genetic events in development of Wilms tumor. *N Engl J Med* 1994;331(9):586–590.

Petruzzi MJ, Green DM. Wilms tumor. *Pediatr Clin North Am* 1997;44(4):939–952.

Ritchey ML, Haase GM, Shochat SJ. Current management of Wilms tumor. *Semin Surg Oncol* 1993;9(6):502–509.

Shochat SJ. Wilms tumor: diagnosis and treatment in the 1990's. *Semin Pediatr Surg* 1993;2(1):59–68.

Author: Sadhna M. Shankar

Wilson Disease

 Database

DEFINITION

Wilson disease (WD) is a treatable, recessive disorder of copper metabolism affecting brain, liver, eyes, and blood.

PATHOPHYSIOLOGY

• Primarily degenerative changes in brain, liver, and cornea, due to decreased copper excretion, and subsequent accumulation in other tissues. Copper ion is thought to inhibit pyruvate oxidase in brain and ATP in body membranes.

GENETICS

• Autosomal recessive inheritance, defect on chromosome 13. Mutations have been detected in a gene involved in copper transport.

EPIDEMIOLOGY

• Incidence of 1 in 100,000 to 500,000

ASSOCIATED CONDITIONS

• Corneal: Kayser-Fleischer rings (granular copper deposits on limbus)
• Fanconi syndrome
• Psychiatric: paranoia, delusions, schizoid-type behavior
• Pancreatitis, hepatitis
• Cardiomyopathy
• Bone disease: asymptomatic osteoporosis, osteomalacia
• Endocrinologic: gynecomastia, delayed puberty; amenorrhea due to liver disease

 Differential Diagnosis

• Liver disease resembling hepatic involvement from WD includes any cause of fulminant hepatic failure or chronic active hepatitis.
• Unexplained hemolytic anemia or thrombocytopenia may occur.
• Neurologic conditions presenting similarly to WD include Huntington disease (prominent dystonia in children), essential tremor, Sydenham chorea, hereditary dystonia, and other neurodegenerative diseases.
• Psychiatric disorders: particularly psychoses (schizophrenia, mania), may be the initial presentation of WD

 Data Gathering

HISTORY

• Children usually present with hepatic abnormalities, including fulminant hepatic failure (around 8–16 years). They can present with manifestations of subacute hepatitis followed by fulminant hepatic failure (with low ALT/AST, and low Alk Phos)
• Characteristic neurologic complications are usually not seen until puberty:

—Tremor
—Dysarthria and dystonia
—Decreased ability to perform voluntary movements
  —The most prominent symptom is the new-onset difficulty with performance of voluntary motor movements.
  —A family history of liver disease with or without associated psychiatric symptoms is helpful in the differential, though rarely present.

 Physical Examination

• Vital signs are generally normal unless anemia is present.
• Heart examination may reveal evidence of cardiomyopathy.
• GU examination may reveal delayed sexual development gynecomastia.
• Corneal abnormalities are uniformly present when there are CNS manifestations: ophthalmologic examination to evaluate for Kayser-Fleischer rings (though they can be seen on direct ophthalmologic examination in some cases).
• Examination may reveal hepatomegaly with or without splenomegaly.
• Edema and ascites can also be noted; abdominal palpation for ascites, hepatosplenomegaly
• Neurologic examination should focus on mental status, psychiatric review of systems, and motor examination: tremor, dystonia, and incoordination.

Laboratory Aids

TESTS

- Screening labs: CBC, PT/PTT, U/A
- Abdominal ultrasound for evaluation of liver size
- Liver biopsy is the definitive procedure for tissue diagnosis.
- Serum ceruloplasmin (usually low; 15% of patients have normal values)
- Elevated serum copper and urine copper
- 3x ceruloplasmin (mg/L) 5% serum Cu (mg/L) (usually 90%–95%)

 ## Therapy

- Penicillamine or Trientine (triethyl tetramine) and low-copper diet for life

—Therapy takes weeks to months to be effective.
—The amount of recovery is proportional to the amount of preexisting damage.

- Patients who present in hemolytic crisis require liver transplantation.

 ## Follow-Up

- Patients require treatment for life.
- Sudden discontinuation of therapy may precipitate fulminant hepatic failure.
- In some patients (10%–20%) with neurologic symptoms, there may be temporary exacerbation before improvement.
- Patients on penicillamine require follow-up examinations, 24-hour urine copper, serum copper, CBC, and U/A before treatment: weekly during the first month, monthly for the first year, and then yearly.
- One of the side effects of penicillamine therapy is a reversible myasthenia.
- Screen family members older than age 3 years with physical examination, LFTs, serum ceruloplasmin, and ophthalmologic examination.

PITFALLS

- Identification of Kayser-Fleischer rings may require slit-lamp examination.
- Wilson disease should be considered in patients with chronic liver disease or psychosis of unspecified etiology.
- Neurologic abnormalities in WD may be markedly asymmetrical.

 ## Common Questions and Answers

Q: Why is screening not performed in children under 3 years?
A: Normal neonatal copper excretion is similar to that of patients with WD. By the age of 3 years, the excretion rate is similar to that of adults.

Q: Can my patients with Wilson disease have children?
A: Women of reproductive age who are treated can have normal pregnancies. Both penicillamine and trientene appear safe during pregnancy in patients with WD, though the number of patients that have taken the medicine during pregnancy is few.

ICD-9-CM 275.1

BIBLIOGRAPHY

Scriver CR, Beaudet AL, Sly WS, Valle D. *Metabolic basis for inherited disease.* New York: McGraw-Hill, 1997;1416–1423.

Yarze JC, Martin P, Munoz SJ, Friedman LS. Wilson's disease: current status. *Am J Med* 1992; 92:643–654.

Author: D. Elizabeth McNeil

Wiskott-Aldrich Syndrome

Database

DEFINITION

Wiskott-Aldrich syndrome (WAS) is primary immunodeficiency with the classical clinical triad of thrombocytopenia, eczema, and recurrent infections.

CAUSES

• Mutation in a recently described novel gene, *WASP*, on the X chromosome, may lead to this syndrome.
• Abnormalities of a cell-surface glycoprotein, sialophorin, on T-lymphocytes may relate to the abnormal cell-surface cytoarchitecture seen in this syndrome.

GENETICS

• X-linked recessive disease
• Linkage analyses have localized the defective *WASP* gene to X p11.22p–11.23.
• Approximately 60% of cases will have a positive family history for WAS.

EPIDEMIOLOGY

• Incidence is rare.
• Presents in infancy with serious bleeding episodes secondary to thrombocytopenia
• Recurrent infections usually start after 6 months of age.
• Eczema is usually present by 1 year of age.

COMPLICATIONS

• Progressive decline in immunologic function with an increase in infections
• There is an increased frequency of autoimmune phenomena such as arthritis and vasculitis.
• Approximately 100-fold increased risk of malignancy compared with the general pediatric population
• Bleeding episodes can be life threatening.

Differential Diagnosis

• Other causes of thrombocytopenia
• Severe atopic disease with dermatitis and secondary skin infections
• HIV infection
• Hyper IgE syndrome

Data Gathering

HISTORY

• Persistent or severe bleeding in infancy due to thrombocytopenia
• Recurrent infections, especially by bacteria with capsular polysaccharides (e.g., *Pneumococcus*)
• Eczema can be of variable severity.
• Older patients may report recurrent viral infections.

Physical Examination

• Evaluation should focus on presence of infection.
• Dermatologic examination is significant for the extent of eczema and the presence of petechiae or ecchymoses.
• Splenomegaly

Laboratory Aids

TESTS

• CBC with differential
• Platelet count with mean platelet volume and platelet size by Coulter counter; hallmark of WAS is small platelets.
• Immunoglobulin levels typically reveal normal IgG, decreased IgM, and increased IgA and IgE.
• Functional antibody titers and isohemagglutinins; hallmark of WAS is reduced or absent responses to polysaccharide antigens and isohemagglutinins to ABO antigens.
• T- and B-lymphocyte enumeration and mitogen stimulation studies. These may progressively deteriorate with increasing age.

PROCEDURES

• Lymph node biopsy in suspected malignancy
• Bone marrow aspirate to evaluate thrombocytopenia

Therapy

- Antibiotics for acute infections and prophylactically in postsplenectomy patients
- Splenectomy may be helpful for persistent severe thrombocytopenia in select patients. However, this may greatly increase the risk of overwhelming infections with encapsulated organisms.
- Thrombocytopenia precautions: no aspirin and avoidance of situations in which trauma (especially head trauma) is likely to occur, such as contact sports.
- Platelet transfusions may be necessary for severe bleeding.
- IVIG replacement therapy is helpful in managing recurrent infections in some patients.
- Bone marrow transplant (BMT) should be considered in these patients. If a full match is available, this is the treatment of choice. The overall success rate of HLA-identical BMT is 85%. The use of haploidentical BMT is controversial because of a lower success rate.

 Follow-Up

- Signs and symptoms of malignancy should be evaluated expeditiously.
- As patients age, a progressive increase in infectious and autoimmune complications may occur.

 Common Questions and Answers

Q: What is the life expectancy for WAS patients?
A: Before currently available therapies, most affected patients died in childhood. Currently, many patients live into their third and fourth decades, even without BMT. Major morbidity and mortality are usually related to overwhelming infection or malignancy. Successfully transplanted patients may have a prolonged life expectancy.

Q: Should patients with WAS receive live viral vaccines?
A: These vaccines should be avoided because of the variable cellular immune defects associated with WAS. Any patients receiving IVIG do not require vaccinations.

Q: What is the chance of another child having WAS?
A: As with any X-linked disease, there is a 50% chance of another affected male child or asymptomatic carrier female. Genetic counseling should be offered to carrier females.

Q: Can WAS be diagnosed prenatally?
A: In families with affected males, fetal blood sampling can be performed in male fetuses to assess the size of the platelets. Small platelet size and family history of WAS suggests an affected infant.

ICD-9-CM 279.12

BIBLIOGRAPHY

Derry JMD, Ochs HD, Francke U. Isolation of novel gene mutated in Wiskott Aldrich syndrome. *Cell* 1994;78:635–644.

Litzman J, Jones A, Hann I, Chapel H, Strobel S, Morgan G. Intravenous immunoglobulin, splenectomy, and antibiotic prophylaxis in Wiskott-Aldrich syndrome. *Arch Dis Child* 1996;75(5):43–69.

Ochs HD, Skichter SJ, Harker LA, et al. The Wiskott Aldrich syndrome: studies of lymphocytes, granulocytes and platelets. *Blood* 1980;55:243–252.

Stites DP, Terr AI. *Basic and clinical immunology,* 7th ed. Norwalk, CT: Appleton-Lange, 1991:346–347.

Sullivan KS, Mullen CA, Blaise RM, Winkelstein JA. A multi-institutional survey of Wiskott Aldrich syndrome. *J Pediatr* 1994;125:876–885.

Winkelstein JA, et al., eds. *Patient and family handbook: for the primary immune deficiency diseases,* 2nd ed. Immune Deficiency Foundation, 1993.

Author: Alex G. Yip

Yersinia enterocolitica

 Database

DEFINITION

Yersinia enterocolitica is a facultative, nonlactose-fermenting, urease-positive, gram-negative coccobacillus; 34 serotypes have been recognized with serotypes 0:3, 8, and 9 the most common.

PATHOPHYSIOLOGY

- *Y. enterocolitica* adheres to epithelial cells and mucus, and heat-stable enterotoxins are produced, which play a role in the development of watery diarrhea.
- Another cytotoxin then directly injures the distal small bowel and large bowel, producing the characteristic bloody or mucous diarrhea.
- An enterocolitis develops and usually persists 5 to 14 days and is seen most commonly in the younger age groups.
- A pseudoappendicular syndrome due to mesenteric adenitis and/or terminal ileitis is seen more commonly in the older child or young adult.
- Extraintestinal manifestations include pharyngitis, suppurative lymphadenitis, pyomyositis, osteomyelitis, abscess, urinary tract infection, pneumonia, endocarditis, meningitis, peritonitis, panophthalmitis, conjunctivitis, and septic arthritis.
- If septicemia is present, mortality can be as high as 50%.

EPIDEMIOLOGY

- Most infected individuals are young children.
- *Y. enterocolitica* has been isolated from contaminated water, soil, wild and domestic animals, and unpasteurized milk products.
- Epidemics have been noted in the African American population during the winter holidays due to exposure to raw chitterlings (pork intestines) prepared for holiday meals.
- Cases due to contaminated blood transfusions from asymptomatic carriers of *Y. enterocolitica* 0:3 have been reported.
- Fecal–oral and person-to-person transmission are also possible.
- The incubation period is approximately 1 to 11 days, with symptoms persisting for 5 to 14 days. Symptoms up to several months have been reported.
- The duration of organism excretion is approximately 6 weeks after diagnosis is made.
- A clinical state of iron overload and deferoxime therapy are risk factors for developing systemic illness.

COMPLICATIONS

- Postinfectious sequelae of erythema nodosum and reactive arthritis involving weight-bearing joints (occurring 1–2 weeks after gastrointestinal symptoms) can occur, although these complications are seen most often in adults.
- Reiter syndrome, myocarditis, glomerulonephritis, erysipelas, chronic diarrhea persisting for months, and hemolytic anemia have also been reported.
- Intestinal perforation and ileocolic intussusception are possible.
- Septicemia is observed in patients with underlying medical conditions.
- Following septicemia, focal abscesses of the liver, kidney, spleen, and lungs have been reported.
- Although rare, the FDA has reported that contamination by bacterial infections of the U.S. blood is most frequently due to *Y. enterocolitica*.

PROGNOSIS

The prognosis is usually quite good, because most infections are gastrointestinal. Systemic disease (septicemia and subsequent secondary spread) have higher morbidity and mortality.

 Differential Diagnosis

Y. enterocolitica should be considered in all patients with a diarrheal illness with bloody or mucous stools with fever and abdominal pain, as well as in patients with the extraintestinal manifestations described above.

 Data Gathering

HISTORY

- Enterocolitis is the most common manifestation in young children.
- The history taking should include exposure to unpasteurized milk products and raw pork or poultry, especially the preparation of pork chitterlings.
- A history of acute onset of abdominal pain, diarrhea with blood or mucus, and mild fever suggest the diagnosis.
- Abdominal pain can be diffuse or localized to the right lower quadrant, suggestive of pseudoappendicitis due to mesenteric adenitis or terminal ileitis.

Physical Examination

Because of the wide range of clinical extraintestinal manifestations, the physical examination is nonspecific for this organism.

Laboratory Aids

TESTS

• Blood, sputum, cerebrospinal fluid, urine, and bile cultures do not require selective culture media techniques; stool samples should be plated on selective media such as cefsulodin-triclosan-novobiocin agar. If routine enteric media (MacConkey) are used, a cold enrichment technique will increase recovery of the organism.
• Serologic methods (tube agglutination assay, ELISA) are available with a rise in titers noted 1 week after onset of symptoms and peak titers observed by the second week of illness. These tests identify IgM, IgG, and IgA antibodies against *Y. enterocolitica*.
• Cross-reactivity between *Y. enterocolitica* and *Brucella abortus*, *Rickettsia* species, *Moraxella morganii*, *Salmonella* species, and thyroid tissue antigen make serodiagnosis of limited usefulness.

Therapy

• Antimicrobial therapy has been shown to benefit patients with systemic infections, focal extraintestinal infections, and enterocolitis in an immunocompromised host.
• The benefit of treatment of uncomplicated enterocolitis, mesenteric adenitis, or pseudoappendicitis has not been established.
• For most isolates, trimethoprim-sulfamethoxazole, chloramphenicol, aminoglycosides, tetracycline, quinolones, and third-generation cephalosporins are effective treatment options.

Follow-Up

• Symptoms of enterocolitis usually abate within 2 weeks from the onset of symptoms, although shedding of the organism in the stool can last at least 6 weeks after diagnosis.
• For extraintestinal manifestations, the expected course is dependent on the specific organ system involved.

PREVENTION

• Infection control: Enteric precautions are indicated for patients with enterocolitis until symptoms resolve.
• General measures: Attempts to eliminate reservoirs and reduce frequency of ingesting contaminated foods and beverages are necessary; uncooked meats, especially pork and unpasteurized milk, as well as preparation of meats near or during preparation of infant bottles for feeding, are common sources of infection.

PITFALLS

Not all bacterial colitis presents with bloody or mucus-appearing diarrhea. Therefore, suspicion should exist if the diarrhea is prolonged or environmental exposures pose a risk for developing infection.

Common Questions and Answers

Q: How long is a child considered infectious with *Y. enterocolitica*?
A: Although the typical course of enterocolitis is approximately 14 days, shedding of the organism in the stool can last at least 6 weeks. Enteric precautions should be discussed with the caretaker to ensure infection control.

Q: If there is no history of evidence of bloody or mucous stools, can you exclude *Y. enterocolitica* as the likely infectious agent in a child with diarrhea?
A: No. In fact, early in the course of illness, the diarrhea is more likely to be watery due to the enterotoxins produced (refer to the Pathophysiology section).

ICD-9-CM 027.8 (sepsis) 020.9

BIBLIOGRAPHY

Bottone EJ. *Yersinia enterocolitica*: the charisma continues. *Clin Microbiol Rev* 1997;10:257–276.

Cover TL, Aber RC. *Yersinia enterocolitica*. *N Engl J Med* 1989;321:16–24.

Kane DR, Reuman PD. Yersinia enterocolitica causing pneumonia and empyema in a child and a review of the literature. *Pediatr Infect Dis J* 1992;11:59–1593.

Krishnan LAG, Brecher ME. Transfusion-transmitted bacterial infection. *Hematol Oncol Clin North Am* 1995;9:167–185.

Lee LA, Taylor J, Carter GP, et al. *Yersinia enterocolitica* O:3: an emerging cause of pediatric gastroenteritis in the United States. *J Infect Dis* 1991;163:660–663.

Peter G, Halsey NA, Marcuse EK, et al. *Yersinia enterocolitica*. In: *1994 Red Book: report of the committee on infectious diseases*, 23rd ed. Elk Grove Village, IL: American Academy of Pediatrics, 1994:518–520.

Author: Philip V. Scribano

SECTION III

Syndromes

4p syndrome—round face, prominent nasal tip, polydactyly, scoliosis.

5p syndrome—macrocephaly, small mandible, long thin fingers, short big toes, anorectal and renal anomalies.

Aagene syndrome—hereditary recurrent intrahepatic cholestasis; with lymphedema; autosomal recessive.

abetalipoproteinemia—recessive transmission; progressive cerebellar ataxia and pigmentary degeneration of retina; starts with malabsorption of fat and progresses to ataxia; absent or reduced lipoproteins, low carotene, vitamin A, and cholesterol; acanthocytosis (spiny projections on red cells).

acanthosis nigricans—hyperpigmented lichenificated plaques in the neck and axilla; may be associated with insulin resistance (Lawrence-Seip syndrome).

acrodermatitis enteropathica—autosomal recessive; zinc deficiency; vesicobullous and eczematous skin lesions in perioral, perineal, cheeks, knees, elbows; photophobia, conjunctivitis, corneal dystrophy, chronic diarrhea, glossitis, nail dystrophy, growth retardation, superinfections, *Candida* infections.

Adie chronic pupillary syndrome—hyperreflexia involves the parasympathetic innervation of iris, resulting in large pupil with little or no reaction to light; may react to accommodation; patients have hyporeflexia.

agenesis of corpus collosum—most cases are unknown etiology; rarely as X-linked recessive; absence of major tracts that connect the right and left hemispheres; usually associated with hydrocephalus, seizures, developmental delay, abnormal head size, and hypertelorism.

Alagille syndrome—(arteriohepatic dysplasia) decreased amount of intrahepatic bile ducts with progressive destruction of bile ducts; patients have broad forehead, deep-set eyes that are widely spaced and underdeveloped, mandible, cardiac lesions, vertebral arch defects, renal changes in the tubules and interstitium.

Albers-Schönberg disease—most are autosomal dominant, few are autosomal recessive; osteopetrosis tarda or marble bone disease; increase in bony density; manifests in children, adolescents, and young adults; prone to fractures, mild anemia, craniofacial disproportion; radiologic changes include increase in density of cortical bone, longitudinal and transverse dense striations at the ends of long bones, lucent and dense bands in vertebrae-thickened base of skull.

Albright syndrome—see *McCune-Albright syndrome*.

Alexander disease—megaloencephaly in infants, dementia, spasticity, and ataxia, sometimes seizures in younger children; patients become mute, immobile, dependent; unknown pathogenesis, hyaline eosinophilic inclusions in the footplates of astrocytes in subpial and subependymal regions.

Alport syndrome—progressive hereditary nephritis; several forms of heredity male-to-male autosomal dominant, also X-linked form; neurosensory deafness, progressive renal failure.

Anderson disease—branching enzyme deficiency, amylopectinosis (glycogen storage disease type IV) accumulation of glycogen with unbranched long outer chains in various tissues; hepatomegaly and failure to thrive in first few months, progressing to liver cirrhosis and splenomegaly.

Apert syndrome—acrocephalosyndactyly; autosomal dominant, high and flat frontal bones, underdevelopment of the middle third of the face and hypertelorism and proptosis, narrow high-arched palate, short beaked nose, syndactyly of the toes and digits.

arthrogryposis multiplex congenita—fixed contractures of multiple joints, present at birth.

Bart syndrome—autosomal dominant, congenital aplasia of the skin, recurrent blisters of skin and mucous membranes, and nail defects.

Bartter syndrome—hypertrophy of juxtaglomerular apparatus; hypokalemic alkalosis, hypochloremia, and hyperaldosteronism; normal blood pressure, renin is elevated; may lead to mental retardation and small stature.

Beckwith-Wiedemann syndrome—hypoglycemia and macrosomia; visceromegaly; umbilical anomalies, renal medullary dysplasia.

Behçet syndrome—relapsing iridocyclitis and recurrent oral and genital ulcerations; 50% will have arthritis, cause unknown.

blind loop syndrome—stasis of small intestine secondary usually to incomplete bowel obstruction or problem of intestinal motility.

Bloch-Sulzberger syndrome—incontinentia pigmenti, mental retardation; one-third have seizures, ocular malformations.

Bloom syndrome—autosomal recessive; erythema and telangiectasia in a butterfly distribution, photosensitivity, and dwarfism.

Blount disease—tibia vera; disorder of growth of the medial part of the proximal tibial epiphysis; irregularity of the medial aspect of the tibial metaphysis adjacent to the epiphysis; bowing starts as angulation at the metaphysis.

blue diaper syndrome—defective tryptophan absorption.

Brill-Zinsser disease—repeat episode of typhus; a *Rickettsia* infection.

bronchiolitis obliterans—obstruction of small bronchi and bronchioles by fibrous tissue; begins with necrotizing pneumonia secondary to viral infections (adenovirus, influenza), measles, tuberculosis, fumes, talcum powder, or zinc.

Byler disease—autosomal recessive; familial cholestasis; progressive biliary cirrhosis; enlarged liver, pruritus, splenomegaly; elevated bile acids and gallstones.

Caroli disease—cystic dilatation of the intrahepatic bile ducts; autosomal recessive; recurrent bouts of cholangitis and biliary abscesses secondary to bile stasis and gallstones.

Cat's eye syndrome—autosomal dominant; ocular coloboma, downslanting eyes, congenital heart disease, and anal atresia.

Charcot-Marie-Tooth disease—peroneal muscular atrophy; most common cause of chronic peripheral neuropathy; foot drop, high-arch foot; may have stocking glove sensory loss.

Chédiak-Higashi syndrome—autosomal recessive disorder; partial oculocutaneous albinism, increased susceptibility to infection, lack of natural killer cells, large lysosome-like granules in many tissues; splenomegaly, hypersplenism, hepatomegaly, lymphadenopathy, nystagmus photophobia, peripheral neuropathy.

Coats disease—telangiectasia of retinal vessels; with subretinal exudate.

Cobb syndrome—intraspinous vascular anomaly and port wine stains.

Cockayne syndrome—autosomal recessive; dwarfism, mental retardation, birdlike facies, premature senility, photosensitivity.

Cornelia de Lange syndrome—prenatal growth retardation, microcephaly, hirsuitism, anteverted naries, downturned mouth, mental retardation, congenital heart defects.

Cri du chat syndrome—growth retardation, mental deficiency, hypotonia, microcephaly, round moon face, hypertelorism, epicanthal folds, downslanting palpebral fissures.

Crigler-Najjar disease (congenital nonhemolytic unconjugated hyperbilirubinemia)—type 1 recessive; deficiency of UDP glucoronyl transferase causing rapid rise of unconjugated bilirubin in first day of life; no hemolysis; patients have no conjugation activity; type II autosomal dominant; variable penetrance; partial activity of UDP glucoronyl transferase.

Cronkhite-Canada syndrome—diffuse intestinal polyps involving large and small intestines; alopecia, brown skin lesions, onychatrophia; patients have diarrhea and protein-losing enteropathy.

Crouzon syndrome—craniofacial dysostosis; autosomal dominant with range of expressivity; exophthalmos, hypertelorism, hypoplasia of maxilla; oral cavity anomalies; premature closure of coronal suture; bilateral atresia of external auditory meatus.

cyclic neutropenia—syndrome of fever, mouth lesions, cervical adenitis, and gastroenteritis occurring every 3 to 6 weeks; defect involves lack of granulocyte macrophage colony-stimulating factor (GMCSF); neutrophil count may be zero.

De Toni-Fanconi-Debré syndrome—fatal infantile myopathy with renal dysfunction; weak cry, poor muscle tone, poor suck; lactic acidosis; abnormal mitochondria and lipid and glycogen accumulation.

De Sanctis-Cacchione syndrome—xeroderma pigmentosum with mental retardation, dwarfism, and hypogonadism; autosomal recessive; skin unable to repair after exposure to ultraviolet light; erythema, scaling bullae, crusting telangiectasia keratoses, photophobia, corneal opacities, tumors of eyelids.

Diamond-Blackfan syndrome (congenital hypoplastic anemia)—failure of erythropoiesis, anemia, pallor, and weakness, macrocytic anemia, no hepatomegaly, elevated fetal hemoglobin; defect in abduction with retraction of the eye on adduction.

DiGeorge syndrome—thymic hypoplasia with hypocalcemia; patients have thymic hypoplasia, tetany, abnormal facies, congenital heart disease, and increased infections.

Dubin-Johnson syndrome—autosomal recessive, elevated conjugated bilirubin, large amounts of coproporphyrin I in urine deposits of melanin-like pigment in hepatocellular lysomes.

Eagle-Barrett syndrome—prune-belly syndrome; deficiency of abdominal musculature, dilatation and dysplasia of urinary tract, cryptorchidism and dilated posterior urethra; prostate hypoplastic or absent.

ectodermal dysplasia—poorly developed or absent teeth, nails, hair, sweat glands, sebaceous glands; many variations.

Ehlers-Danlos syndrome—a series of disorders of connective tissue, hyperextensible skin, hypermobile joints, and easy bruisability.

Eisenmenger syndrome—ventricular septal defect and pulmonary hypertension.

Fabry disease—X-linked, lipid storage disease; defect of ceramide trihexoside alpha-galactosidase; tingling and burning in hands and feet; small, red maculopapular lesions on the buttocks, inguinal area, fingernails, and lips. Do not sweat; proteinuria progressing to renal failure.

Farber syndrome—autosomal recessive; deficiency of acid ceramidase, hoarseness, painful swollen joints, palpable nodules over affected joints and pressure points.

fetal alcohol syndrome—small body and head size, abnormal palpebral fissures, epicanthal folds, small jaw and maxillary bone, cardiac septal defect, delayed development, and mental deficiency.

fetal hydantoin syndrome—hypoplasia of midface, low nasal bridge, ocular hypertelorism, cupid bow upper lip; slow growth, may have mental retardation, cleft lip, cardiac malformation.

Friedreich ataxia—mostly autosomal recessive, appears in late childhood or adolescence, progressive cerebellar and spinal cord dysfunction; mainly gait and arm dysfunction; high-arched foot, hammer toes, cardiac failure.

fructose intolerance, hereditary—autosomal recessive; deficiency of fructose 1-phosphate aldolase or fructose 1,6-diphosphatase, vomiting, diarrhea, hypoglycemia seizures, and jaundice.

Gardner syndrome—multiple gastrointestinal polyps with malignant transformation, skin cysts; multiple osteoma.

Gaucher disease—abnormal storage of glucosylceramide in the reticuloendothelial system; three types: type 1 (adult or chronic), type 2 (acute neuropathic or infantile), type 3 (subacute neuropathic or juvenile); splenomegaly, hepatomegaly, delayed development, strabismus, swallowing difficulties, laryngeal spasm, opisthostonos, bone pain.

Gianotti-Crosti syndrome—papular acrodermatitits and hepatitis B; usually benign and self-limited.

Gilles de la Tourette syndrome—dominant trait with partial penetrance; multiple tics: blinking, twitching, grimacing; muscles of swallowing and respiration are involved; may have swearing, can have learning disabilities.

Glanzmann disease—autosomal recessive; defective primary platelet aggregation; platelets are normal in size and survival.

Goldenhar syndrome—oculoauriculovertebral dysplasia; mandibular hypoplasia, hypoplastic zygomatic arch, and malformed displaced pinna; hearing loss.

Goltz syndrome—focal dermal hypoplasia; herniations of fat through thinned dermis, producing tan papillomas associated with other skin defects and skeletal anomalies such as syndactyly, polydactyly, and spinal defects; also colobomas, strabismus, nystagmus.

Gradenigo syndrome—acquired abducens palsy and pain in the trigeminal nerve distribution, usually after otitis media; produces diplopia; ocular and facial pain, photophobia, lacrimation.

Hand-Schüller-Christian disease—now called histiocytosis X or reticuloendotheliosis.

Hartnup disease—autosomal recessive defect in transport of monoamino monocarboxylic amino acids by intestinal mucosa and renal tubules; photosensitivity; pellagra-like skin rash; may have cerebellar ataxia.

histiocytosis X—reticuloendotheliosis; formerly was eosinophilic granuloma, Hand-Schüller-Christian, and Letterer-Siwe diseases; may be few solitary bone lesions, or seborrheic dermatitis of scalp, lymphadenopathy, hepatosplenomegaly, tooth loss, exophthalmus, pulmonary infiltrates.

Hunter syndrome—mucopolysaccharidosis II; X-linked recessive; accumulation of heparan sulfate, and dermatan sulfate; enzyme deficiency (α-L-iduronate sulfatase).

Hurler syndrome—mucopolysaccharidosis IH; autosomal recessive; accumulation of heparan sulfate, and dermatan sulfate; enzyme deficiency (α-L-iduronidase).

hyper IgE—recurrent deep-tissue and skin staphylococcal infections; eosinophilia and IgE levels that are ten times normal.

incontinentia pigmenti—see *Bloch-Sulzberger syndrome*.

Jeune thoracic dystrophy—respiratory distress, short limbs, and polydactyly; may progress to renal insufficiency.

Job syndrome—severe staphylococcal infections, chronic skin disease, and cold abscesses; may have elevated IgE.

Kallmann syndrome—isolated gonadotropin deficiency and anosmia; familial.

Kartagener syndrome—sinusitis; bronchiectasis; immotile cilia.

Kasabach-Merritt syndrome—hemangioma and consumption coagulopathy; platelet trapping and microangiopathic hemolytic anemia.

Kasai procedure—hepatoportoenterostomy; used to create drainage in patients with biliary atresia.

Kleine-Levin syndrome—unusual hunger, somnolence, and motor restlessness.

Klinefelter syndrome—seminiferous tubule dysgenesis; testicular atrophy, eunuchoid habitus, gynecomastia, XXY karyotype.

Klippel-Feil syndrome—short neck, limited neck motion, and low occipital hairline.

Krabbe leukodystrophy—cerebroside lipidosis; autosomal recessive; lack of myelin in white matter; starts in infancy, progresses to rigidity, hyperreflexia, swallowing difficulties, lack of development.

Larsen syndrome—hyperlaxicity, multiple dislocations, skin hyperlaxicity; usually autosomal dominant.

Laurence-Moon-Biedl syndrome—retinitis pigmentosa, polydactyly, obesity, hypogonadism.

Lennox-Gastaut syndrome—childhood epileptic encephalopathy; severe seizures, mental retardation, and characteristic EEG pattern; generalized bilaterally synchronous sharp-wave and slow-wave complexes; seizures start in infancy, difficult to treat; mental retardation common.

Lesch-Nyhan syndrome—X-linked recessive disorder; defect in purine metabolism; hyperuricemia results from diminished or absent HGPRT activity, choreoathetosis, compulsive self-mutilation, mental retardation, and growth failure.

Letterer-Siwe disease—part of histiocytosis X; acute disseminated histiocytosis; seborrheic-looking skin lesions; bone lesions, gingival lesions, liver and lung infiltrates.

Lowe syndrome—occulocerebral dystrophy; X-linked recessive; congenital cataracts, glaucoma, hypotonia, hyperreflexia, severe mental retardation; rickets, osteopenia, pathologic fractures, aminoaciduria, and organic aciduria.

Marfan disease—connective tissue disorder involving ectopia lentis, dilatation of aorta, long thin extremities, pectus excavatum or carinatum, scoliosis, pneumothorax.

Marfucci syndrome—multiple enchondromata and hemangioma of bone, and overlying skin; short stature, skeletal deformities, scoliosis, and limb disproportion.

McCune-Albright syndrome—polyostotic fibrous dysplasia; more common in females; prominent skin discoloration; coast of Maine (ragged edges); may have precocious puberty, hyperthyroidism, gigantism headaches, epilepsy, and mental deficiency.

MELAS syndrome—mitochondrial disorder causing neurologic problem of seizures, alternating hemiparesis, hemianopsia, or cortical blindness; has lactic acidosis, spongy degeneration of brain, sensorineural hearing loss and short stature.

Menkes syndrome—short hairs, hypopigmentation, hypothermia, growth failure, skeletal defects, arterial aneurysms, seizures, and progressive CNS failure; X-linked recessive.

Möbius syndrome—cranial nerve defects, hypoplastic tongue or digits.

Morquio syndrome—mucopolysaccharidosis; severe skeletal deformities, pectus carinatum, kyphoscoliosis, short neck hypoplasia of odontoid process C1 to C2 dislocation; neurosensory deafness, aortic insufficiency.

multiple cartilaginous exostosis—bony projections near end of tubular bones and ribs, scapula, vertebral bodies, and iliac crest; appears after age 3; exostoses become calcified; exostoses cause skeletal deformities.

nail-patella syndrome—renal proteinuria, may lead to nephrotic syndrome and renal failure; dystrophic and hypoplastic nails; hypoplastic patellae and iliac horns and malformed radial heads; autosomal dominant.

Niemann-Pick disease—storage of sphingomyelin and cholesterol; four types; normal birth followed by delayed development; hepatomegaly; 50% have cherry red spot.

Noonan syndrome—cardiac lesions (ASD or pulmonic stenosis); facial changes (palpebral slant, broad flat nose), webbed neck; short stature, high-arched palate, and malformed ears; normal karyotype.

Osler-Weber-Rendu syndrome—hereditary hemorrhagic telangiectasia; telangiectasias are present in the skin, respiratory tract mucosa, lips, nails, conjunctiva, nasal and oral mucosa.

Parinaud syndrome—weakness of upward gaze, poor convergence, and accommodation, retractive nystagmus with upward gaze and pupillary changes.

Pelizaeus-Merzbacher disease—dancing eye movements, delayed motor development and spasticity, small head, poor head control; may have optic atrophy and seizures.

Peutz-Jeghers syndrome—autosomal dominant; blueish-black macules around mouth, intestinal polyposis in small bowel.

Pickwickian syndrome—obesity, hypoventilation syndrome; may cause respiratory arrest, restless sleep.

Pierre Robin syndrome—severe micrognathia, glossoptosis, cleft palate.

Poland syndrome—unilateral hypoplastic pectoral muscle with ipsilateral upper limb deficiency, syndactyly, and defect of subclavian artery.

Prader-Willi syndrome—hypotonia, hypomentia, hypogonadism, obesity, narrow bifrontal diameter, hypotonia; may have deletion in chromosome 15.

progeria—premature aging, severe growth failure, atherosclerosis, alopecia, dystrophic nails.

prune-belly syndrome—see **Eagle-Barrett syndrome**.

Reiger syndrome—sporadic autosomal dominant; microcornea with opacity; iris hypoplasia; anterior synechiae; hypodontia, maxillary hypoplasia.

Riley-Day syndrome—familial dysautonomia, affects sensory and autonomic functions; poor feeding, aspiration, no tears, high threshold to pain, markedly decreased reflexes, smooth tongue and impaired taste, erratic blood pressure and temperature.

Rotor disease—autosomal recessive; elevated conjugated bilirubin, elevated coproporphyrin I and coproporphyrin in urine, normal liver biopsies.

Rubinstein-Taybi syndrome—broad thumbs and toes, short stature, mental retardation, beaked nose, hypoplastic mandible, congenital heart defect.

Russell-Silver dwarf syndrome—intrauterine growth retardation; subnormal growth velocity, triangular facies, clinodactyly, simian creases, GU malformations.

Sandhoff GM$_2$ gangliosidosis type II—deficient hexosaminidase activity leading to cherry red spot in macula, failure to develop motor skills, blindness, weakness, and seizures.

Sanfilippo A syndrome—mucopolysaccharidosis IIIA; autosomal recessive; accumulation of heparan sulfate, dermatan sulfate; enzyme sulfamidase.

Sanfilippo B syndrome—mucopolysaccharidosis IIIA; autosomal recessive; accumulation of heparan sulfate, dermatan sulfate; enzyme α-N-acetylglucosaminidase.

Scheie syndrome—mucopolysaccharidosis IS; autosomal recessive; accumulation of heparan sulfate, dermatan sulfate; enzyme defect α-L-iduronidase.

Scimitar syndrome—hypoplasia of right lung with systemic arterial supply, anomalous right pulmonary vein dextroposition of heart.

Seckel syndrome—intrauterine growth retardation, microcephaly, sharp facial features with underdeveloped chin, mental retardation.

Shwachman syndrome—pancreatic dysfunction, short stature, bone marrow dysfunction; skeletal abnormalities.

silo filler disease—acute pneumonitis caused by inhalation of nitrogen dioxide; chills, fever, cough, dyspnea, cyanosis, high mortality.

Smith-Lemli-Opitz syndrome—short stature, microcephaly, ptosis, anteverted nares, micrognathia, syndactyly, cryptorchidism, mental retardation.

Sotos syndrome—cerebral gigantism, large head and ears, prominent mandible, mentally retarded; poor coordination.

Stickler syndrome—autosomal dominant; high myopia, cataract formation, retinal detachment.

Sturge-Weber syndrome—port-wine stain on face in area of first branch of the trigeminal nerve; seizures and mental retardation.

Swyer-James syndrome—unilateral hyperlucent lung following bronchiolitis obliterans.

Tourette—see **Gilles de la Tourette syndrome**.

Treacher Collins syndrome—mandibulofacial dysostosis; autosomal dominant with incomplete penetration; hypoplastic mandible, hypoplastic zygomatic arches, antimongoloid slant to eyes; deformities of pinna, high-arched palate with or without cleft palate.

trisomy 9—deep set eyes, bulbous nasal tip, anxious look, cleft lip.

trisomy 13—cleft lip, microophthalmia, postaxial polydactyly.

trisomy 18—small face, high nasal bridge, short palpebral fissures, micrognathia, small mouth, overriding fingers, hypoplastic nails; mental retardation, intrauterine growth retardation.

tuberous sclerosis—epiloia; seizures, mental deficiency, adenoma sebaceum foci of intracranial calcification, hypopigmented macules, ash leaf spots, connective tissue nevi (shagreen spots) adenoma sebaceum, angiofibroma.

Turcot syndrome—adenomatous colonic polyposis associated with malignant brain tumors, especially glioblastomas.

Turner syndrome—gonadal dysplasia, short stature, sexual infantilism, streak gonads stems from XO karyotype; other features are atypical facies, low hairline, webbed neck, congenital lymphedema of extremities, coarctation aorta; increased carrying angle.

Usher syndrome—retinitis pigmentosa, cataracts, sensorineural deafness; autosomal recessive.

vanished testes syndrome—bilateral gonadal failure with normal external male genitalia, normal 46 XY karyotype, absent testes, no male puberty.

Vater syndrome—vertebral defects, anal atresia, tracheoesophageal atresia, radial dysplasia, renal dysplasia, congenital heart defect.

Vogt-Koyanagi-Harada syndrome—vitiligo, uveitis, dysacousia, and aseptic meningitis.

Von Gierke disease—type 1 glycogenosis; glucose-6-phosphate deficiency, enzyme is absent in liver, kidney, and intestinal mucosa; produces hypogylcemia under stress such as fasting; hepatomegaly, seizures.

Von Hippel-Lindau syndrome—autosomal dominant linked to chromosome 3; hemangioblastoma of cerebellum and retina; cystic cerebellar neoplasm with increased intracranial pressure.

Waardenburg syndrome—autosomal dominant; white forelock, heterochromic irides, displacement of inner canthi, broad nasal root, and confluent eyebrows.

Wegener granulomatosis—necrotizing granulomatous vasculitis of arteries and veins; involves airways, lungs, and kidneys, with resultant rhinorrhea, nasal ulceration, hemoptysis, and cough; hematuria from necrotizing vasculitis.

Werner syndrome—short stature, juvenile cataracts, hypogonadism, gray hair in second decade; autosomal recessive.

Williams syndrome—mental retardation, hypoplastic nails, periorbital fullness, supravalvular aortic stenosis, growth delay, stellate iris.

Wilson-Mikity syndrome—pulmonary immaturity; occurs in premature infants; slow onset of respiratory distress, retractions, and apnea; may clear in several weeks.

Wiskott-Aldrich syndrome—thrombocytopenia, severe eczema, and recurrent skin infections.

Wolff-Parkinson-White syndrome—short P–R interval and slow upstroke of the QRS delta wave; usually normal heart but may occur in Ebstein anomaly and cardiomyopathy.

Wolman disease—primary xanthomatosis, adrenal insufficiency, vomiting, failure to thrive, steatorrhea, hepatomegaly, and adrenal calcification; fatal.

Zellweger syndrome—cerebrohepatorenal syndrome; hepatic fibrosis and cirrhosis; seizures, mental retardation, hypotonia, glaucoma, congenital stippled epiphyses, and cysts of renal cortex.

Zollinger-Ellison syndrome—islet cell tumors producing duodenal and jejunal ulcers, high gastrin levels, and excessive acid secretion.

SECTION IV

Cardiology
Laboratory

Timothy M. Hoffman

Cardiology Laboratory

BLOOD PRESSURE MEASUREMENT

Accurate measurement of the blood pressure depends on selection of an appropriate cuff size. The recommended width of the cuff is 40% to 50% of the circumference of the measured extremity. If the cuff size is too small, then the blood pressure will be overestimated, whereas if it is too large, the blood pressure will be underestimated. Auscultation of the diastolic component of the blood pressure exhibits two endpoints: Korotkoff phases IV and V, respectively. In children, phase IV (i.e., the point of diminution or muffling of the Korotkoff sound) is generally considered a more accurate representation of the diastolic pressure. Phase V (i.e., the

disappearance of the Korotkoff sounds) should be considered the diastolic endpoint if it falls within 6 mm Hg of phase IV. Standard blood pressure measurements for children from birth to 18 years of age are shown in the figure Standard Blood Pressure Measurements in Accordance with Age and Gender, below.

Pulsus Paradoxus

Pulsus paradoxus, a decrease of more than 10 mm Hg in the systolic blood pressure during inspiration, may be associated with cardiac tamponade (e.g., as a result of pericardial effusion), constrictive pericarditis, or severe respiratory compromise (e.g., asthma exacerbation).

Hint: Pulsus paradoxus must not be confused with pulsus alternans (i.e., a decrease in the systolic pressure on alternate contractions that indicates left ventricular failure).

Using a sphygmomanometer, the clinician inflates the cuff until the pressure is 20 mm Hg above the systolic pressure. She then slowly deflates the bladder until the first Korotkoff sound is heard independent of the respiratory cycle—this is the first data point. She continues to slowly deflate the bladder until the Korotkoff phase I sound is noted in all respiratory cycles (in inspiration and expiration)—the second data point. The difference between the points is considered the reduction in systolic

A. Girls

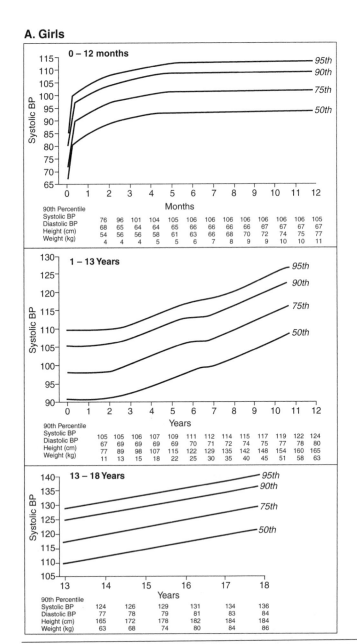

B. Boys

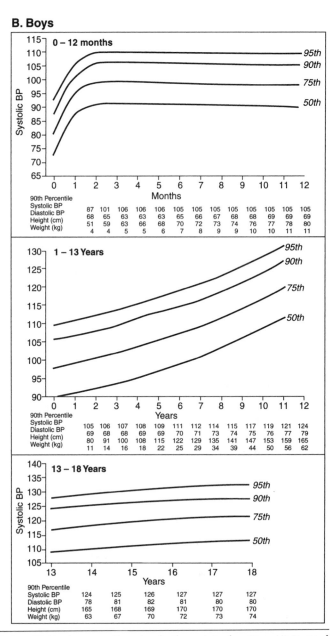

Standard blood pressure measurements in accordance with age and gender. **A:** Girls. **B:** Boys. BP, blood pressure. (Reproduced with permission from Horan MJ. Report of the Second Task Force on Blood Pressure Control in Children—1987. *Pediatrics* 1987;79:1–25.)

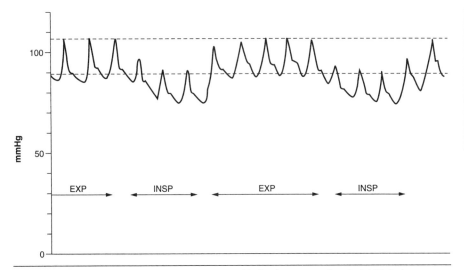

Pulsus paradoxus. EXP, expiration; INSP, inspiration. (Modified with permission from Park MK. *Pediatric cardiology for practitioners*, 3rd ed. St. Louis: Mosby–Year Book, 1996:15.)

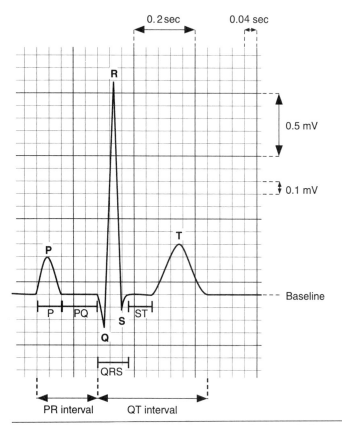

A normal electrocardiogram showing waveforms and intervals. The standard paper speed is 25 mm per second; therefore, a single 1-mm box equals 0.04 second, and a large (5-mm) box equals 0.20 second.

pressure during inspiration and is abnormal if it is greater than 10 mm Hg. The figure Pulsus Paradoxus (left) schematically depicts pulsus paradoxus.

HYPEROXITEST

The hyperoxitest can be useful for differentiating cardiac and pulmonary causes of cyanosis, and is one of the first evaluations performed when confronted with a cyanotic newborn. Cyanosis usually becomes apparent at a mean capillary concentration of 3 to 4 g/dL of reduced hemoglobin, a concentration that corresponds to an oxygen saturation of 70% to 80%.

In infants with cyanosis and hypoxemia, the arterial oxygen tension (PaO2) can range from 10 to 60 mm Hg. In an infant with a pulmonary cause for the cyanosis, administration of 100% oxygen increases the PaO2 to a level significantly greater than 150 mm Hg. In an infant with cardiac cyanosis, the PaO2 does not increase beyond 150 mm Hg in response to the administration of 100% oxygen. In patients with congenital heart disease, this phenomenon is attributable to right-to-left shunting (i.e., the mixing of unoxygenated blood and oxygenated blood within the circulatory system). Right-to-left shunting may be either intracardiac or extracardiac in nature.

ELECTROCARDIOGRAPHY

The electrocardiogram (ECG) provides data concerning the following:

- Rhythm
- Rate
- Intervals
- Axis
- Hypertrophy
- Wave changes (Q waves and ST/T waves)

Rhythm

Rhythm diagnosis is beyond the scope of this chapter.

Rate

The heart rate is determined accurately by dividing 60 by the RR interval (measured in seconds). For example, if the RR interval is 0.4 second (ten small boxes), the heart rate is 60 divided by 0.4, or 150 beats/min.

Intervals

See the figure A Normal Electrocardiogram Showing Waveforms and Intervals to the left. Interval standards include the PR, QRS, and QT intervals. The normal heart rate, PR interval, and QRS duration vary with age (see the table Heart Rate, PR Intervals and QRS Duration on the next page).

PR Interval

First-degree atrioventricular block is characterized by a PR interval that is greater than the standard range for age. A short PR interval associated with a delta wave is indicative of Wolff-Parkinson-White syndrome.

Cardiology Laboratory

Heart Rate, PR Intervals, and QRS Duration

AGE	HEART RATE (BEATS/MIN)		PR INTERVALS IN LEAD II (SECONDS)		QRS DURATION (SECONDS)	
	MEAN	RANGE	MEAN	RANGE	MEAN	RANGE
<1 day	126	95–155	0.106	0.082–0.138	0.05	0.025–0.069
1–7 days	135	100–180	0.107	0.079–0.130	0.05	0.025–0.068
8–30 days	160	120–190	0.100	0.075–0.128	0.053	0.026–0.075
<1–3 months	147	95–200	0.098	0.075–0.126	0.052	0.027–0.069
3–6 months	139	114–170	0.105	0.078–0.137	0.053	0.028–0.075
6–12 months	130	95–170	0.105	0.077–0.138	0.055	0.03 –0.070
1–3 years	121	95–150	0.113	0.090–0.140	0.056	0.032–0.070
3–5 years	98	70–130	0.119	0.092–0.150	0.058	0.03 –0.069
5–8 years	86	65–120	0.124	0.094–0.155	0.059	0.035–0.075
8–12 years	86	65–120	0.129	0.093–0.165	0.062	0.038–0.079
12–16 years	86	65–120	0.135	0.098–0.169	0.065	0.040–0.081

Adapted with permission from Liebman J, Plonsey R, Gillette PC: *Pediatric Electrocardiography*. Baltimore, Williams & Wilkins, 1982, pp 96–97 and Cassels DE, Ziegler RF: *Electrocardiography in Infants and Children*. Philadelphia, WB Saunders, 1966, p 100.

QRS Interval

The QRS duration represents the intraventricular conduction time and is normally less than 0.09 second (in children younger than 4 years) or 0.1 second (in children older than 4 years). A QRS duration greater than normal is identified as a bundle branch block:

- *Left bundle branch block* is diagnosed when there is a monophasic R wave in lead I and no Q wave in lead V_6.
- *Right bundle branch block* is diagnosed when there is a wide S wave in leads I and V_6, right axis deviation, and an M-shaped (RSR' pattern) QRS complex in lead V_1.
- *Left anterior hemiblock* can be diagnosed in the setting of left axis deviation associated with right bundle branch block.

QT Interval

The QT measurement is corrected for heart rate using the following formula:

$$QTc = \text{measured QT (seconds)} / \text{radRR interval (seconds)}$$

The QTc interval is less than 0.45 second for infants younger than 6 months, and less than 0.44 second for children.

Axis

The frontal axis should be determined for the P, QRS, and T waves from the limb leads (I, II, III, aVR, aVL, aVF). The hexaxial reference system (see the figure Hexaxial Reference System, below) is usually used. The normal axis falls between 0 and 90 degrees.

The axis is equal to the direction of the largest positive force on depolarization. A cursory way to determine the frontal axis is to note the complex that is isoelectric and locate the two planes perpendicular to it. The perpendicular plane with the greatest positive deflection is indicative of the axis.

P-Wave Axis

The location of the P-wave axis determines the origin of an atrial-derived rhythm:

- 0 to 90 degrees = a high right atrial rhythm (normal sinus rhythm)
- 90 to 180 degrees = a high left atrial rhythm
- 180 to 270 degrees = a low left atrial rhythm
- 270 to 0 degrees = a low right atrial rhythm

Hint: Classic "mirror image" dextrocardia is associated with a P-wave axis of 90 to 180 degrees in conjunction with high-amplitude forces in the right chest leads and low voltage in the left chest leads (i.e., lead V_4R has a greater amplitude than lead V_4).

QRS Axis

The QRS axis value is age-specific (see the table Age-Specific QRS Axis Values, below), but may correlate with congenital heart disease in certain clinical settings. For example, a northwest axis or left axis deviation (−30 to −120 degrees) may correlate with an endocardial cushion defect or tricuspid atresia. Left axis deviation is always abnormal in a newborn.

T-Wave Axis

The T-wave axis helps determine strain associated with ventricular hypertrophy. A T-wave axis that is 90 degrees different from the QRS axis suggests strain.

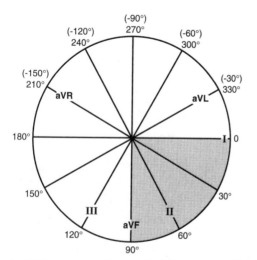

Hexaxial reference system (frontal axis). The *shaded area* represents the normal axis.

Age-Specific QRS Axis Values

AGE	MEAN (DEGREES)	RANGE (DEGREES)
<1 day	135	60–180
1–7 days	125	60–180
8–30 days	110	0–180
1–3 months	80	20–120
3–6 months	65	20–100
6–12 months	65	0–120
1–3 years	55	0–100
3–5 years	60	0–80
5–8 years	65	340–100
8–12 years	65	0–120
12–16 years	65	340–100

Adapted with permission from Liebman J, Plonsey R, Gillette PC: *Pediatric Electrocardiography*. Baltimore, Williams & Wilkins, 1982, pp 90.

Normal Range of Values (5th–95th Percentile) for R and S Waves in Leads V_1 and V_6

AGE	LEAD V_6		LEAD V_1	
	R WAVE (MM)	S WAVE (MM)	R WAVE (MM)	S WAVE (MM)
<1 day	7.0–20.0	2.5–27.0	2.3–7.0	1.6–10.3
1–7 days	9.0–27.4	4.6–18.8	2.2–13.1	0.8–9.9
8–30 days	4.2–19.8	2.5–12.8	1.7–20.5	0.6–9.0
1–3 months	3.6–17.9	2.0–17.4	3.6–12.9	0.8–5.8
3–6 months	6.1–16.7	2.1–11.8	5.0–15.8	0.6–4.9
6–12 months	4.0–16.0	1.9–14.4	5.5–17.6	0.7–3.3
1–3 years	3.6–15.0	2.2–20.5	5.0–17.5	0.6–3.4
3–5 years	2.6–15.6	5.0–24.8	5.4–20.6	0.6–2.4
5–8 years	2.6–13.5	5.3–21.0	7.9–20.5	0.6–2.9
8–12 years	3.6–11.3	4.8–22.3	8.4–19.2	0.6–2.8
12–16 years	2.1–11.1	5.5–22.3	7.9–17.4	0.7–3.1

Adapted with permission from Liebman J, Plonsey R, Gillette PC: *Pediatric Electrocardiography*. Baltimore, Williams & Wilkins, 1982, pp 84–85.

Hypertrophy

Right Atrial Hypertrophy

Diagnostic findings on ECG include a peaked P wave that exceeds 2.5 mm in any lead (often best seen in lead II).

Left Atrial Hypertrophy

A P wave with a notched contour and a duration of more than 0.08 second in lead II is diagnostic. Alternatively, a biphasic P wave in lead V1 or V_{3R} with a terminal inverted portion that measures 1×1 mm will suffice to make the diagnosis.

Right Ventricular Hypertrophy

The table Normal Range of Values for R and S Waves in Leads V_1 and V_6 (above) summarizes the normal measurements of R and S waves in leads V_1 and V_6 by age. Right ventricular hypertrophy can be diagnosed if any one of the following is seen:

- An R wave in lead V_1 that is greater than the 98th percentile for age
- An S wave in lead V_6 that is greater than the 98th percentile for age
- An upright T wave in lead V_1 in a patient older than 4 days
- Pure qR in leads V_{3R} or V_1
- A RSR' pattern in leads V_{3R} or V_1, in which the R' portion is 15 mm greater than the R wave (in a child younger than 1 year) or 10 mm greater than the R wave (in a child older than 1 year)

Left Ventricular Hypertrophy

Left ventricular hypertrophy can be diagnosed if any one of the following is seen:

- An R wave in lead V_6 that is greater than the 98th percentile for age
- A Q wave in lead V_5 or V_6 that is greater than 4 mm
- An R wave in lead V_1 that is below the 5th percentile for age
- An S wave in lead V_1 that is greater than the 98th percentile for age

Wave Changes

- *ST segment elevation* of greater than 2 mm in the precordial leads may indicate pericarditis, myocardial injury, ischemia, infarction, or digitalis effect.
- *Tall, peaked T waves* may be seen in patients with hyperkalemia.
- *Flat T waves* can occur in children with myocarditis, hypokalemia, or hypothyroidism.

CHEST ROENTGENOGRAPHY

When examining a chest radiograph, one must comment on the cardiac size, organ situs, and the pulmonary vascular markings (normal, increased, or decreased).

Cardiac Size

Cardiac size is determined by estimating the cardiothoracic ratio. The ratio is calculated by dividing the largest diameter of the heart by the largest internal diameter of the thorax. If the result is greater than 0.5, cardiomegaly is present.

Organ Situs

The normal cardiac silhouette in the anterior-posterior and lateral views is depicted in the figure Normal Cardiac Silhouette, right.

Pulmonary Vascular Markings

Pulmonary vascular markings reflect the appearance of the pulmonary arteries and veins on a chest radiograph over the lung fields. These markings can be increased in states of excessive pulmonary arterial flow [e.g., ventricular septal defect (VSD), atrial septal defect (ASD), patent ductus arteriosus (PDA)], as well as in states characterized by excessive pulmonary venous flow (e.g., congestive heart failure, conditions characterized by pulmonary edema or pulmonary venous obstruction). On the radiograph, increased pulmonary vasculature is noted when cephalization occurs and the vascular shadows extend more than two-thirds across the lung field.

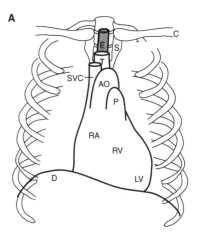

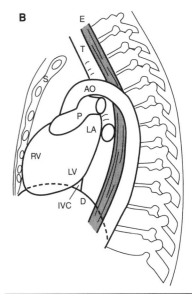

Normal cardiac silhouette. **A:** Anterior-posterior view. **B:** Lateral view. AO, aorta; C, clavicle; D, diaphragm; E, esophagus; IVC, inferior vena cava; LA, left atrium; LV, left ventricle; P, pulmonary outflow tract; RA, right atrium; RV, right ventricle; S, sternum; T, trachea; SVC, superior vena cava. (Modified with permission from Sapire DW. *Understanding and diagnosing pediatric heart disease.* East Norwalk, CT: Appleton & Lange, 1991:64.)

Decreased pulmonary vasculature markings are manifested radiographically as hyperlucency of the lung field and a paucity of pulmonary vasculature, as seen in patients with tetralogy of Fallot.

Hint: The following signs, seen on the anterior-posterior projection, offer clues to the diagnosis:

A *"boot-shaped"* heart is often seen in newborns with tetralogy of Fallot.

An *"egg on a string"* is noted in newborns with a narrow mediastinum owing to absence of a large thymus, and is associated with transposition of the great arteries.

Cardiology Laboratory

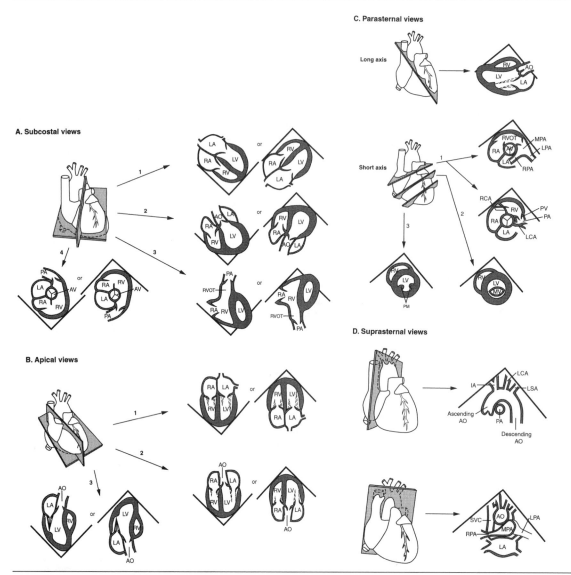

C. Parasternal views

Long axis

Short axis

A. Subcostal views

B. Apical views

D. Suprasternal views

Echocardiographic series. The *numbers* represent different planes along a sweep of the echocardiographic beam. **A:** Subcostal views. **B:** Apical views. **C:** Parasternal views. **D:** Suprasternal views. AO, aorta; AV, aortic valve; IA, innominate artery; LA, left atrium; LCA, left coronary artery; LPA, left pulmonary artery; LSA, left subclavian artery; MPA, middle pulmonary artery; MV, mitral valve; PA, pulmonary artery; PM, papillary muscle; PV, pulmonary valve; RA, right atrium; RCA, right coronary artery; RPA, right pulmonary artery; RV, right ventricle; RVOT, right ventricular outflow tract; SVC, superior vena cava. (Modified with permission from Park MK. *Pediatric cardiology for practitioners*, 3rd ed. St. Louis: Mosby–Year Book, 1996:70–73.)

A *"snowman sign"* is associated with supracardiac total anomalous pulmonary venous return. The left vertical vein, innominate vein, and the superior vena cava form the superior aspect of the snowman.

ECHOCARDIOGRAPHY

In pediatric patients, echocardiography is performed in a stepwise fashion to obtain subcostal views, apical four-chamber views, parasternal views, and suprasternal views (see the figure Echocardiographic Series, above).

M-Mode Echocardiography

A parasternal short-axis view using M-mode echocardiography reveals a cross section of the left ventricle and, therefore, can be used to estimate cardiac dimensions. Most commonly, it

is used to obtain a shortening fraction (SF), calculated in the following manner:

$$\text{SF} = 100 \times (\text{LV end-diastolic dimension} \\ - \text{LV end-systolic dimension} \\ \div \text{LV end-diastolic dimension})$$

The normal value for the SF is generally considered to be 28% to 38%, independent of age.

Doppler Echocardiography

Doppler echocardiography detects a frequency shift that reflects the direction and velocity of blood flow. Doppler echocardiography is used to detect valvular insufficiency or stenosis and abnormal vasculature flow patterns.

CARDIAC CATHETERIZATION

Cardiac catheterization allows sampling of oximetric and hemodynamic data. The normal pressures and oxygen saturations for children are depicted in the figure Normal Pressures, Mean Pressures, and Oxygen Saturations for Children on the next page. Cardiac catheterization, an invasive procedure, is often used in conjunction with angiography to confirm the diagnosis and physiology of certain acquired and congenital heart diseases. The technique also has therapeutic applications, such as patent ductus arteriosus coil embolization, coil embolization of aortopulmonary collaterals, pulmonary artery angioplasty and stent placement, and balloon valvuloplasty of semilunar valvular stenosis.

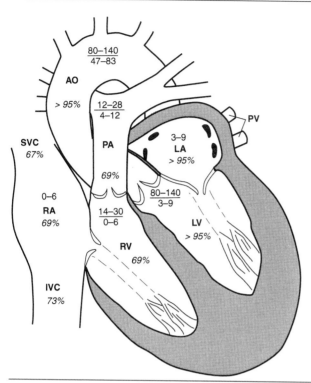

Normal pressures (systolic over diastolic, in mm Hg), mean pressures, and oxygen saturations for children. The data are based on information compiled from healthy patients between the ages of 2 months and 20 years. AO, aorta; IVC, inferior vena cava; LA, left atrium; LV, left ventricle; PA, pulmonary artery; PV, pulmonary vein; RA, right atrium; RV, right ventricle; SVC, superior vena cava.

Shunts

Data obtained from cardiac catheterization can be used to calculate the degree and direction of an intracardiac or extracardiac shunt. The calculation is based on the Fick principle, using oxygen as the indicator.

The oxygen content equals the dissolved oxygen (which is usually negligible) plus the oxygen capacity [hemoglobin (g/dL) $\times$ 1.36 mL O_2/dL $\times$ 10] multiplied by the oxygen saturation (as a percentage).

Flow (Q) is the oxygen consumption divided by the arteriovenous oxygen content difference:

$$Qp = \frac{VO_2}{PV - PA}$$

$$Qs = \frac{VO_2}{AO - MV}$$

where

Qp = pulmonary flow
Qs = systemic flow
$V.O_2$ = oxygen consumption per unit time
PV = pulmonary venous oxygen content
PA = pulmonary arterial oxygen content
MV = mixed venous oxygen content
AO = aortic oxygen content

In order to calculate the amount of a shunt, one needs to calculate the effective pulmonary blood flow (*Qp eff*):

$$Qp\ eff = \frac{VO_2}{PV - MV}$$

A left-to-right shunt is the pulmonary flow less the effective pulmonary flow ($Qp - Qp$ eff), and a right-to-left shunt is the systemic flow less the effective pulmonary flow ($Qs - Qp$ eff).

Resistance

Systemic and pulmonary vascular resistance can also be calculated using the catheterization data. This calculation is based on the Ohm law (essentially, the pressure change across the vascular bed divided by flow equals resistance):

$$Rs = \frac{AO - RA}{Qs}$$

$$Rp = \frac{PA - LA}{Qp}$$

where

Rs = systemic resistance
Rp = pulmonary resistance
AO = mean aortic pressure
RA = mean right atrial pressure
PA = mean pulmonary artery pressure
LA = mean left atrial pressure

A pulmonary resistance (Rp) of 2.5 Wood units or less is considered within the normal range; however, no vascular bed is rigid, and variations in flow can affect the result obtained.

SECTION V
Surgical Glossary

Aaron E. Carroll and
Nahush A. Mokadam

aortopexy—a procedure in which the aorta is approximated to the anterior thoracic wall; for the treatment of tracheomalacia.

Bishop-Koop procedure—resection of a dilated loop of bowel proximal to meconium obstruction, with end-to-side anastomosis between the proximal bowel and obstructed loop, combined with end ileostomy; for the treatment of meconium ileus.

bladder augmentation—a procedure in which a portion of the intra-abdominal gastrointestinal tract is used to increase the volume of the bladder.

Blalock-Taussig shunt—a procedure in which the subclavian artery is anastomosed to the pulmonary artery; for the temporary treatment of tetralogy of Fallot.

Boix-Ochoa procedure—restoration of the intra-abdominal esophageal length, repair of the esophageal hiatus, fixation of the esophagus to the hiatus, and restoration of the angle of His; for the treatment of incompetent lower esophageal sphincter.

chordee correction—a procedure in which the corpus spongiosum is moved ventrally and the corpus cavernosa are approximated dorsally; for the treatment of chordee (abnormal penile curvature associated with epispadias or hypospadias).

Clatworthy mesocaval shunt—division of the common iliac veins and side-to-end anastomosis of the inferior mesenteric vein to the left renal vein; for the treatment of portal hypertension.

Cohen procedure—trigonal reimplantation of the ureter; for the treatment of vesicoureteral reflux.

colonic conduit diversion—a procedure involving two stages: (1) a loop diversion using a colonic segment, and (2) an end-to-side anastomosis of the colonic segment to the gastrointestinal tract.

colonic interposition—replacement of the esophagus with a colonic segment; for treatment of esophageal atresia or stricture when gastric mobilization is not feasible.

diaphragmatic plication—surgical shortening of the diaphragm (abdominal, transthoracic, or bilateral); for the treatment of diaphragmatic eventration.

distal splenorenal shunt—see *Warren shunt*.

Drapanas mesocaval shunt—prosthetic graft implantation from the inferior mesenteric vein to the inferior vena cava; for the treatment of portal hypertension.

Duckett transverse preputial island flap—technique in which a flap of foreskin is used to elongate the urethra; for the treatment of hypospadias.

Duhamel procedure—resection of the aganglionic colon above the dentate line with stable anastomosis to the rectal stump, normally performed in children 6 to 12 months of age for the treatment of Hirschsprung disease (see *Martin modification*).

end-to-side portocaval shunt—procedure in which the portal vein is divided and anastomosed to the inferior vena cava; for the treatment of portal hypertension.

esophagectomy—resection of the esophagus, with gastric pull-up and anastomosis with the cervical esophagus; for the treatment of esophageal atresia or stricture.

Fontan procedure—a procedure in which a graft is created to connect the pulmonary artery to the right atrium; for the treatment of hyperplastic right heart syndrome.

Glenn shunt—a shunt from the superior vena cava to the pulmonary artery; for the treatment of tricuspid atresia or stenosis.

gridiron incision—see *McBurney incision*.

Hegman procedure—surgical release of the tarsal, metatarsal, and intertarsal ligaments; for the treatment of metatarsus adductus.

Heller myotomy—myotomy of the anterior lower esophagus (always accompanied by a Thal fundoplication); for the treatment of achalasia.

ileal loop diversion—resection and implantation of ureters into an isolated ileal segment, with an ileal stoma and primary anastomosis of ileum to cecum.

ileal ureter—ileal interposition between the renal pelvis and bladder when the ureteral length is insufficient for anastomosis; for the treatment of urinary obstruction.

ileocecal conduit diversion—bilateral ureteral diversion and anastomosis to an isolated ileocecal segment and cecostomy with primary anastomosis of ileum to the right colon.

J-pouch—creation of an ileal reservoir in the distal ileum using a "J"-shaped configuration; used following colectomy.

Jateene procedure—arterial retransposition; for the treatment of transposition of the great vessels.

Kasai procedure—resection of atretic extrahepatic bile ducts and gall bladder with Roux-en-Y anastomosis of the jejunum to the remaining common hepatic duct; for the treatment of biliary atresia or other extrahepatic obstruction.

Kimura procedure (parasitized cecal patch)—a multistep operation in which (1) a side-to-side anastomosis is made with a portion of the distal ileum and the right colon, and (2) an ileoanal pull-through is performed; for the treatment of Hirschsprung disease.

King operation—resection of the knee with placement of a Küntscher rod to fix the femur to the tibia, followed by a Syme amputation for the treatment of proximal focal femoral deficiency (PFFD).

Koch pouch diversion—a procedure involving bilateral ureteral diversion with anastomosis to a neobladder formed from an isolated ileal segment, combined with an ileal stoma and primary anastomosis of ileum to ileum.

Ladd operation—restoration of intestinal anatomy from a malrotated state; for the treatment of intestinal malrotation.

Lanz incision—an abdominal incision made in the left iliac fossa; for colostomy formation.

left hepatectomy—resection of the left hepatic lobe (medial and lateral segments).

Magpi procedure—distal advancement of the urethral meatus and granuloplasty; for the treatment of hypospadias.

Mainz pouch diversion—a procedure involving bilateral ureteral division with anastomosis to a neobladder formed from isolated cecum and terminal ileum; combined with an ileal stoma and primary anastomosis of the ileum to the right colon.

Martin modification (of Duhamel procedure)—right and transverse colectomy with ileoanal pull-through and side-to-side anastomosis of the remaining left colon to the ileum; procedure preserves some absorptive capacity of the large bowel; for the treatment of total colonic Hirschsprung disease.

McBurney (gridiron) incision—abdominal incision from the anterior superior iliac spine to the umbilicus; used for appendectomy.

Mikulicz procedure—a diverting enterostomy performed proximal to the meconium obstruction without resection; for the treatment of meconium ileus.

mini-Pena procedure—anterior sagittal anorectoplasty; for the treatment of anterior rectoperianal fistula (boys) or rectal-fourchette fistula (girls).

Mitrofanoff technique—a modification of neobladder diversion procedures, in which vascularized appendix is used to create the stoma.

Mustard technique—redirection of blood through an atrial septal defect (ASD) using a pericardial pathway; for the treatment of transposition of the great vessels; because of associated increased turbulence, this technique is not widely used today.

Mustarde procedure—correction, using simple mattress sutures, of a prominent ear with normal or absent antihelical folds.

Nissen fundoplication—a technique involving a 360-degree wrap of the gastric fundus around the gastroesophageal junction; for the treatment of incompetent lower esophageal sphincter; patient is rendered unable to vomit or belch.

Norwood procedure—a three-stage palliative procedure including (1) atrial septectomy, transection and ligation of the pulmonary artery, "neoaorta" formation using the proximal pulmonary artery, and creation of a synthetic porto-aortal shunt; (2) creation of a Glenn shunt; and (3) performance of a modified Fontan procedure; for the treatment of hypoplastic left heart syndrome.

onlay island flap—a technique in which a flap of foreskin is used to elongate the urethra; for the treatment of hypospadias.

orchidopexy—testicular pull-down and attachment; for the treatment of undescended testis.

orthoplasty—surgical correction of excessive penile curvature.

parasitized cecal patch—see **Kimura procedure**.

Pena procedure—posterior sagittal anorectoplasty performed in children 1 to 6 months of age; for the treatment of imperforate anus.

Pfannenstiel incision—an abdominal incision used to gain access to the lower abdomen and bring pelvic organs within reach without dividing muscular tissue.

pharyngoplasty—elevation of the posterior pharyngeal wall following a primary cleft palate repair (to narrow the pharyngeal space); for the treatment of velopharyngeal incompetence.

Potts shunt—anastomosis of the descending aorta to the pulmonary artery for the permanent treatment of tetralogy of Fallot.

proximal splenorenal shunt—end-to-side anastomosis of the splenic vein to the left renal vein with splenectomy; for the treatment of portal hypertension.

pyeloplasty—resection of an atretic ureter with primary anastomosis to the renal pelvis; for the treatment of ureteropelvic junction obstruction.

Ramstedt operation—relaxation of the pyloric sphincter; for the treatment of pyloric stenosis.

Rashkind procedure—balloon atrial septostomy; for the treatment of palliation of the great vessels.

Rastelli repair—a technique involving the closure of a ventricular septal defect (VSD) with a patch and the creation of a conduit from the distal pulmonary artery to the right ventricle; for the treatment of transposition of the great vessels.

Ravitch procedure—a procedure involving (1) creation of osteotomies between the manubrium and costal cartilages, (2) a greenstick fracture of the manubrium, and (3) the temporary insertion (for 6 to 12 months) of a stabilizing bar; for the treatment of pectus excavatum or pectus carinatum.

right colon pouch—a procedure involving bilateral ureteral division with anastomosis to a neobladder (formed from an isolated segment of the right colon), combined with an ileal stoma and primary anastomosis of the ileum to the transverse colon.

right hepatectomy—resection of the right hepatic lobes (anterior and posterior segments).

rooftop (bilateral subcostal) incision—an abdominal incision used to access the liver and portal structures.

Roux-en-Y anastomosis—division of the jejunum distal to the ligament of Treitz with end-to-side anastomosis of the duodenum to the distal jejunum and anastomosis of the proximal jejunum (typically) to the bile duct.

S-pouch—the creation of an ileal reservoir in the distal ileum using an "S"-shaped configuration following colectomy.

Santulli-Blanc enterostomy—a modification of the Bishop-Koop procedure that involves the resection of a distal dilated bowel segment with side-to-end anastomosis to the proximal enterostomy; for the treatment of meconium ileus.

Senning procedure (venous switch)—technique involving intra-atrial redirection of venous return so that systemic caval return is shunted through the mitral valve to the left ventricle, and pulmonary return is brought through the tricuspid valve to the right ventricle; for the treatment of transposition of the great vessels.

side-to-side portocaval shunt—a procedure in which the portal vein is anastomosed to the inferior vena cava; for the treatment of portal hypertension.

side-to-side splenorenal shunt—side-to-side anastomosis of the splenic vein to the left renal vein; for the treatment of portal hypertension.

Sistrunk operation—complete excision of a thyroglossal duct cyst.

Soave procedure—a technique involving endorectal pull-through; for the correction of rectal resection.

Stamm gastrostomy—placement of an open gastrostomy tube; the opening is designed to close spontaneously on removal of the tube.

Sting procedure—subureteric Teflon injection; for the endoscopic correction of vesicoureteral reflux.

Sugiura procedure—a technique that involves lower esophageal transection and primary anastomosis, devascularization of the lower esophagus and stomach, and splenectomy; for the treatment of esophageal varices.

Swenson procedure—resection of the posterior rectal wall to the dentate line (aganglionic region); for the treatment of Hirschsprung disease; technically difficult and rarely performed.

Syme amputation—amputation of the foot, calculated to bring the end of the stump above the opposite knee at maturity; for the treatment of proximal focal femoral deficiency (PFFD).

Thal procedure—a procedure involving a 180-degree anterior wrap of the gastric fundus around the gastroesophageal junction, preserving the patient's ability to vomit and belch; for the treatment of incompetent lower esophageal sphincter.

Thiersch operation—a procedure in which a distal rectal segment that has prolapsed is approximated to the external sphincter muscle; for the treatment of rectal prolapse.

trisegmentectomy—resection of the right hepatic lobe and the quadrate lobe of the liver (right posterior segment, right anterior segment, and medial segment).

ureteropyelostomy—partial resection and side-to-side anastomosis of a partially duplicated ureter.

uretocalycostomy—a technique for the treatment of urinary obstruction involving division of the ureter (distal to the obstruction) and intrarenal anastomosis to the most dependent renal calyx; when the renal pelvis is insufficient for anastomosis, the lower pole of the kidney is resected.

vaginal switch operation—a procedure in which the vagina is separated from the urinary tract; for treatment of duplicated vagina.

Van Ness procedure—rotational 180-degree osteotomy of the femur in which the foot and ankle are brought to the level of the opposite knee; for prosthetic attachment for the treatment of femoral deficiency.

venous switch—see **Senning procedure**.

ventricular shunt procedure—a procedure in which a Silastic catheter is positioned in a lateral ventricle and tunneled subcutaneously to drain into the central venous system or peritoneal cavity; for the treatment of hydrocephalus.

Warren (distal splenorenal) shunt—a procedure in which the splenic vein is anastomosed to the left renal vein; for the treatment of portal hypertension.

Waterston aortopulmonary anastomosis—a procedure involving anastomosis of the ascending aorta and the right pulmonary artery; for the temporary treatment of tetralogy of Fallot.

Whipple procedure—resection of the pancreatic head, duodenum, and gall bladder with gastrojejunostomy, hepatojejunostomy, and pancreaticojejunostomy.

SECTION VI
Laboratory Values

Henry R. Drott

Laboratory Values

Normal Laboratory Values

% Saturation	20%–40%	Copper	67–147 µg/dl
Absolute B₁ count	76–462/µL	Cortisol	
Absolute lymphocyte count (ALC)	1266–3022/µL	AM	10–25 µg/dl
Absolute T3	919–2419/µL	PM	2–10 µg/dl
Absolute T4	614–1447/µL	C-reactive protein (CRP), quantitative	0–1.2 mg/dl
Absolute T8	267–1133/µL	Creatine kinase	
Absolute T11	1025–2587/µL	<age 1 year	60–305 U/L
Acetaminophen	10–20 µg/ml	>age 1 year	60–365 U/L
Acid phosphatase total	2–10 U/L	Creatinine	0.6–1.2 mg/dl
Alanine aminotransferase (ALT)	5–45 U/L	Cryoglobulin	
Albumin	3.7–5.6 g/dl	C3	0.0–0.028 mg/dl
Aldolase	<6 U/L	IgA	0.0–0.026 mg/dl
Alkaline phosphatase (AP)	130–560 U/L	IgG	0.0–0.157 mg/dl
Alpha₁-antitrypsin	210–500 mg/dl	IgM	0.0–0.224 mg/dl
Alpha-fetoprotein (AFP)	0.6–5.6 ng/ml	Cyclosporin A	150–400 µg/L
Amikacin		Digoxin	0.5–2.0 ng/ml
Peak	20–30 µg/ml	DNA binding	0–149 IU/ml
Trough	0–10 µg/ml	D-Xylose, post-test	36–63 mg/dl (25-g dose)
Ammonia	9–33 µmol/L	Erythrocyte sedimentation rate (ESR)	0–20 mm/h
Amylase	30–100 U/L	Ethosuximide	25–100 µg/ml
Anion gap	7–20 mmol/L	Factor II assay	27%–108%
Antithrombin III	91%–128%	Factor V assay	50%–200%
Apolipoprotein A-I	102–215 mg/dl	Factor VII assay	50%–200%
Apolipoprotein B	45–125 mg/dl	Factor VIII assay	50%–200%
Aspartate aminotransferase		Factor IX assay	
Newborn	35–140 U/L	Newborn	14.5%–58.0%
Child	10–60 U/L	Child	50%–200%
B₁ (Total B cells)	4%–21%	Factor X assay	50%–200%
Bands	0%–4%	Factor XI assay	50%–200%
Bicarbonate	20–26 mEq/L	Ferritin	23–70 ng/ml
Bilirubin		Fibrin split products	0–10 µg/ml
δ	0.3–0.6 mg/dl	Fibrinogen	180–431 mg/dl
Neonatal	2.0–12.0 mg/dl	G6PD assay, quantitative	4.6–13.5 U/g Hb
Total	0.6–1.4 mg/dl	γ-Glutamyltransferase (GGT)	14–26 U/L
Unconjugated	0.2–1.0 mg/dl	Gentamicin	
Blasts	0%	Peak	4–10 µg/ml
Caffeine	5–20 µg/ml	Trough	0–2 µg/ml
Calcium	8.9–10.7 mg/dl	Glucose	75–110 mg/dl
Ionized	1.12–1.30 mmol/L	CSF	32–82 mg/dl
Stool	0–640 mg/24 h.	Whole blood	60–115 mg/dl
Carbon dioxide	20–26 mmol/L	Ham test	
Carboxyhemoglobin	0%–2%	Acidified	0%–1%
CD3+ and CD8+	17.4%–34.2%	Unacidified	0%–1%
CD14+	0%–10%	Haptoglobin	13–163 mg/dl
CD45+ and CD14−	90%–100%	Hematocrit	36%–46%
Ceruloplasmin	23–48 mg/dl	Spun	36%–41%
CH₅₀	104–356 U/ml	Hemoglobin	13.5–17.0 g/dl
Chloramphenicol	5–20 µg/ml	A₁C	3.8%–5.9%
Chloride	96–106 mmol/L	Total	
Sweat	0–40 mmol/L	Newborn	10–18 g/dl
Cholesterol	111–220 mg/dl	Child	12–16.0 g/dl
High-density lipoprotein (HDL)	35–82 mg/dl	HbA₂, quantitative	1.8%–3.6%
Low-density lipoprotein (LDL)	59–137 mg/dl	HbF, quantitative	0%–1.9%
Complement		Immunoglobulin A	
C3		Newborn	0–5 mg/dl
Newborn	67–161 mg/dl	Infant	27–169 mg/dl
Child	90–187 mg/dl	Child	70–486 mg/dl
C4	16–45 mg/dl		

Laboratory Values

Normal Laboratory Values (continued)

Immunoglobulin E	
Newborn	0–15 IU/ml
Child	0–200 IU/ml
Immunoglobulin G	
CSF	0.5–6 mg/dl
Child	635–1775 mg/dl
Immunoglobulin M	
Child	71–237 mg/dl
Iron	50–180 μg/dl
Urine	0–2.0 mg/24 h.
Iron-binding capacity	250–420 μg/dl
Lactate	
CSF	0–3.3 mmol/L
Plasma	0.6–2.0 mmol/L
Lactate dehydrogenase (LDH)	340–670 U/L
Latex IgE	0–20 U
Lead, blood	0–10.0 μg/dl
Lipase	25–110 U/L
Lyme antibodies (IgG/IgM)	0.00–0.79
Magnesium	1.5–2.5 mg/dl
Mean corpuscular hemoglobin (MCH)	26.0–34.0 pg
Mean corpuscular volume (MCV)	80.0–100.0 μm^3
Mean platelet volume	7.4–10.4 fl
Methemoglobin	0.0%–1.9%
Netilmicin	
Peak	5–10 μg/ml
Trough	0–2 μg/ml
Osmolality	
Urine	
Newborn	50–645 mOsm/kg
Child	50–1500 mOsm/kg
Whole blood	275–296 mOsm/kg
Partial thromboplastin time	25.0–38.0 seconds
Peroxide hemolysis	0%–20%
Phenobarbital	15–40 μg/ml
Phenytoin	10–20 μg/ml
Phosphorus	2.7–4.7 mg/dl
Platelet aggregation, 10 μm	>60.1%
Platelet count	150–400 10^3/μL
Potassium	3.8–5.4 mmol/L
Prealbumin	22.0–45.0 mg/dl
Primidone	5–12 μg/ml
Procainamide	4–10 μg/ml
Prolactin	2.7–15.2 ng/ml
Protein, 24-hour total	0–150 mg/24 h
Protein C	
Immunological	50%–122%
Functional	59%–116%
Protein S, free	40%–111%

Protein, total	6.3–8.6 g/dl
Prothrombin time	10–12 seconds
Protoporphyrin, free RBC	30–80 μmol/mol Hb
Pyruvate kinase assay	1.8–2.3 IU/ml RBC
RBC distribution width	11.5%–14.5%
Reptilase	18–22 seconds
Reticulocyte count	0.5%–1.5%
Ristocetin cofactor	48%–220%
Salicylate	<35 mg/dl
Sodium	136–145 mmol/L
Sucrose hemolysis	0%–5%
T3 (total T cells)	69%–86%
T4 (helper T cells)	39%–57%
T4–T8 ratio	0.7–2.5
T8 (suppressor T cells)	18%–45%
T11 (SRBC receptor)	75%–93%
Theophylline	10–20 μg/ml
Thrombin time	11.3–16.3 seconds
Thyroxine binding globulin	1.8–4.2 mg/dl
Thyroid stimulating hormone (thyrotropin)	0.5–5.0 μIU/ml
Thyroxine	
Newborn	3.0–14.4 μg/dl
Infant	4.6–13.4 μg/dl
Child	4.5–10.3 μg/dl
Tobramycin	
Peak	4–10 μg/ml
Trough	0–2 μg/ml
Total cell count	100
Total eosinophil count	100–300 mm^3
Total protein	
CSF	
Newborn	40–120 mg/dl
Child	15–40 mg/dl
Urine	0–20 mg/dl
Triglycerides	34–165 mg/dl
Triiodothyronine	0.9–2.25 ng/ml
Trypsin, stool	80–740 μg/g
Urea nitrogen	2–19 mg/dl
Uric acid	2.1–5.0 mg/dl
Urine specific gravity; TS meter	1.003–1.1035
Urine pH	4.8–7.8
Valproic acid	50–100 μg/ml
Vancomycin	
Peak	20–30 μg/ml
Trough	0–12 μg/ml
White blood cell count	
Newborn	9–30 10^3/μl
Child	4.5–11.0 10^3/μl
Zinc	68–94 μg/dl

SECTION VII

Herbal Treatments in Practice

Michael D. Cirigliano

Herbal Treatments in Practice

The use of herbal treatments by the public is increasing on a yearly basis, with sales exceeding $2.5 billion in 1996 (Grauds, 1997). Most clinicians have little or no basic understanding of the reported benefits and documented hazards regarding use of herbal treatments.

Many herbal treatments have great potential for treating a variety of common ailments inexpensively and with few side effects. In most cases, however, good, clinically sound data are lacking. Additionally, many herbal remedies have documented side effects and hazards, about which the public may be unaware (D'Arcy, 1991). Herbal preparations may also interact with standard pharmaceutic agents, leading to untoward effects.

Many patients obtain information about herbal treatments from friends, advertising, and other sources that may be lacking in sound scientific information. Lack of regulation and standardization in the industry also presents significant risk to the public, due to the risk of misidentification of plant species and poor quality control in manufacturing. These potential hazards are of great concern, especially in the pediatric and neonatal populations. To help advise patients who are using or wish to use herbal therapies, it is therefore imperative that physicians have some knowledge regarding herbal treatments and their potential risks.

Numerous case reports have noted that herbal treatment use is implicated in deleterious human fetal effects (Jones and Lawson, 1998; Gold and Cates, 1980). Use of a pyrrolizidine-containing herbal tea during pregnancy was felt to be the cause of a reported case of he-

patic veno-occlusive disease in an infant (Roulet et al., 1988). Use of herbal treatments should be avoided by women who are pregnant, contemplating pregnancy, or nursing (Huxtable, 1990). Much further detailed clinical study regarding safety and efficacy is required.

Herbal treatments also should be avoided in infants and young children. Adverse reactions are more likely to occur due to the tendency of infants and children to build up higher drug levels from their reduced ability to metabolize active agents (Crone and Wise, 1998).

Given the obvious potential risks and need for further study, the clinician is left with the daunting task of advising patients who wish to take herbal treatments. This is even more poignant in the pediatric realm, as the actual patient may not have an active role in considering the risk-to-benefit ratio for a particular natural product. It is imperative, therefore, that the clinician be as knowledgeable as possible regarding herbal treatments, their uses, and their potential hazards. Much has been written regarding herbal treatments, and excellent references are available for further study. With clinical trials and more regulation within the industry, herbal treatments may lead to improved treatment options for many common maladies seen in general practice.

The table Herbs Commonly Used by the Public (below) represents a compendium of the herbs more commonly used by the public (see the table Herbal Medicines on the next page for a more complete listing). This listing is by no means exhaustive, and several references have been provided.

BIBLIOGRAPHY

Crone CC, Wise TN. Use of herbal medicines among consultation-liaison populations. A review of current information regarding risks, interactions, and efficacy. *Psychosomatics* 1998;39:3–13.

D'Arcy PF. Adverse reactions and interactions with herbal medicine. *Adv Drug React Toxicol Rev* 1991;10(4):189–208.

Gold J, Cates W. Herbal abortifacients. *JAMA* 1980;243:1365–1366.

Grauds C. Botanicals: strong medicine for health and profit. The source. *Assoc Nat Med Pharm* 1997;3(1).

Huxtable RJ. The harmful potential of herbal and other plant products. *Drug Safety* 1990;5[Suppl 1]:126–136.

Jones TK, Lawson BM. Profound neonatal congestive heart failure caused by maternal consumption of blue cohosh herbal medication. *J Pediatr* 1998;132(3):550–552.

Roulet M, Laurini R, Rivier L, et al. Hepatic ven-oocclusive disease in a newborn infant of a woman drinking herbal tea. *J Pediatr* 1988;112;433–436.

FURTHER READING

The review of natural products. St. Louis: Facts and Comparisons Publishing Group.

The Complete German Commission E Monographs. *Therapeutic guide to herbal medicines.* Austin, TX: The American Botanical Council.

Alternative Medicine Alert. *A clinician's guide to alternative therapies.* Atlanta: American Health Consultants.

Herbs Commonly Used by the Public

PLANT	USE
Chamomile	Antispasmodic, antiinflammatory (GI tract)
Echinacea	Prophylaxis and treatment of cold and flu symptoms
Garlic	Antibacterial, antifungal, anithrombotic, cholesterol reduction, hypotensive, hypoglycemic, antihyperlipidemic, antiinflammatory, anticancer
Ginger	Motion sickness and nausea
	Antiinflammatory for arthritis
Goldenrod	Urinary tract inflammation
	Kidney stones
Horehound	Expectorant and cough suppressant
	Digestive aid
Kava-Kava	Sleep inducement and anxiety reduction
Milk thistle	Hepatoprotective and antioxidant
Peppermint	GI symptoms
St. John's wort	Treatment for mild-to-moderate depression
Valerian	Sleep inducement

Herbal Medicine

PLANT	_USE*_	_PRECAUTIONS & INTERACTIONS_	_TRADITIONAL DOSING**_
ALOE—Aloe vera, Aloe barbadensis, Aloe capensis (Curacao aloe, Cape aloe)—_Topical_ products (aloe vera gel) come from either the juice of the inner tissue, or the pulverized whole leaf. _Oral_ products (aloe latex) are obtained from just under the outer skin of the leaf. (6,14,15)	_Topical_ products are generally shown to be effective for promotion of wound healing and for treatment of burns and frostbite, but results are conflicting (possibly because of product variation). _Oral_ products are known to be strong cathartics and are rarely recommended for use. (6,14,22)	_Topical_ use—No side effects reported. _Oral_ use—can cause abdominal cramping, diarrhea, electrolyte imbalance, and hypokalemia. May potentiate toxicity of cardiac glycosides and thiazide diuretics. Contraindicated in pregnancy (reflex stimulation of uterine musculature). (5,14)	_Topical_ use—Apply gel as needed. Ingredients deteriorate, so use fresh product for best results. _Oral_ use—Adult daily dose is 0.05–0.2 g of powdered aloe or dry extract. May color the urine red. (5,14)
ASTRAGALUS—see Tragacanth			
BEARBERRY (Uva-Ursi)—Arctostaphylos uva-ursi (kinni-kinnik, hogberry, manzanita)—arbutin is hydrolyzed to hydroquinone in the GI. Hydroquinone is released in the urinary tract. (6,15,16)	Used as a urinary tract antibacterial and astringent. Not effective in weight loss products (used as a diuretic). (5,6,16)	May cause nausea and vomiting. Urine must be alkaline to release free hydroquinone. Bearberry is inactivated by urinary acidifiers (i.e. cranberry juice). Taking 6–8 g of sodium bicarbonate per day will alkalinize the urine, but not recommended for more than a few days. (5,6,16)	Adult mean daily dose is 10 g powdered drug (400–700 mg arbutin) macerated overnight in 150 mL of cold water.*** Maximum effect obtained 3–4 hours after ingestion. Do not use for more than 1 week. Urine may appear green. (5,6,15)
BIRCH LEAF—Betula verrucosa, Betula pubescens. (22)	Shown to be diuretic in animals. (5,22)	No side-effects reported in the literature. Contraindicated with impaired cardiac or renal function. (5)	Dose is 2–3 g in boiling water—steep for 10–15 min, strain—take several times per day. Caution pts to maintain high fluid intake. (5)
BLACK COHOSH—Cimicifuga racemosa, (baneberry, bugbane, bugwort, black snakeroot, squawroot, rattle root, Remifemin)—not the same as blue cohosh, a potentially toxic plant. (6,15,22,24,25)	Shown to decrease luteinizing hormone (LH). Decreases hot flashes. Used to treat premenstrual discomfort and dysmenorrhea. (6,22)	May affect the hypothalamus-pituitary system. Contraindicated during pregnancy and lactation. May cause GI disturbances and hypotension. (6,15)	Adult daily dose is 40–200 mg taken for no more than 6 months. Maximum effect may not be seen for up to 4 weeks. (6,22)
CAPSICUM—Capsicum frutescens, Capsicum annum (Capsaicin, Cayenne pepper, Chili pepper, Red pepper, African chilies, Tabasco pepper). (14,15,22)	Topical use depletes "substance P" and decreases the perception of pain. Shown to be effective for post-herpetic (shingles), trigeminal and diabetic neuralgia. (22)	Can cause local burning sensation. Contamination of hands can transfer to eyes and mucous membranes—wash thoroughly. (22)	Maximum effect seen after applying 4–5 times per day for at least 4 weeks, however some effect can occur within 3 days. Pain may initially increase as "substance P" is released before depletion. (15,22)
CASCARA—Rhamnus purshiana (Cascara sagrada, Bitter bark, Chittem bark, Sacred bark)—Buckthorn (Rhamnus frangula) is a different plant but with similar activities. (15)	Shown to be a stimulant laxative. (15,22)	Don't take if pregnant or lactating (passed to milk). Fresh bark can cause severe vomiting (must be stored for 1 yr or be heat treated). Misuse can cause loss of electrolytes and hypokalemia and may potentiate toxicity of cardiac glycosides and thiazide diuretics. Misuse can deposit pigment in the intestinal mucosa (melanosis coli). (5,22)	Average daily adult dose is 1 g (1/2 teaspoonful) 20 to 160 mg of cascara derivatives in 150 mL of boiling water, strain. Can be taken AM & HS. Effects are seen in 6–8 hours. Should only be taken for a few days. Tea is bitter. (5,15)
CAT'S CLAW—Uncaria tomentosa, Uncaria guianensis (Una de gato) (15)	Efficacy is anecdotal. An alkaloid constituent has been shown to be hypotensive. Other alkaloids are being studied individually. (15,19)	No reports of toxicity in the literature.	The root has less activity than the inner bark. No dose determined. (15)

Herbal Treatments in Practice

Herbal Medicine (continued)

PLANT	*USE**	*PRECAUTIONS & INTERACTIONS*	*TRADITIONAL DOSING***
CHAMOMILE—*Matricaria recutita* (German or Hungarian)—despite at least 10 names, all are the same plant. *Chamaemelum nobile* (Roman) is different but has similar constituents. (6,16,22)	Has antispasmodic, anti-inflammatory (GI tract), anti-microbial activity. Used orally to treat peptic ulcers, spasms of the GI, and inflammation of the mouth and gums. Topically used to treat mucous membrane inflammation, eczema and to promote wound-healing. (6,22)	Rarely, may cause an allergic reaction. Eating large quantities of dried flower heads can cause vomiting. (15)	Adult dose is 3 g dried flower heads (about 1 heaping Tbsp) in 250 mL hot water, steep 10–15 minutes, strain. Taken TID-QID between meals. Benefit may be cumulative. Commercial products are frequently adulterated, so best to purchase flower heads. (6,22,23)
CHASTE TREE BERRY—*Vitex agnus-castus* (6)	Inhibits prolactin release by binding dopamine receptors. Results in increase in lactation. Shown to be effective treatment for menstrual disorders (PMS, mastalgia, menopausal symptoms) by increasing progesterone in relation to estrogen. (6,15)	Rarely, causes GI disturbances, itching. May activate the pituitary, resulting in early onset of menstruation after delivery. May interfere with dopamine-receptor antagonists (animal studies). (5,15)	Adult daily dose is 20 mg of the crude fruit (as extract), or 30–40 mg of the fruits in cold water, then heated to boiling. An infusion tea (boiling water poured over drug) may have less anti-inflammatory activity. (5)
CRANBERRY—*Vaccinium macrocarpon* (6)	Used to treat UTI. Produces acid urine which prevents microorganisms from attaching to urinary tract. It also reduces urinary odor by retarding the degradation of urine by *E. coli*. (6,15,20,22)	Overuse (3–4 L per day) can cause diarrhea. (15)	Adult prophylactic dose is 90 mL (45 g fresh berries) daily. Dose to treat UTI is 360–960 mL daily. Maximum tolerated is 4 L. (6,15,22)
DONG QUAI—*Angelica polymorpha, Angelica dahurica, Angelica atropurpurea* (tang-kuei, Dang-gui, Chinese Angelica) (15)	Used to stimulate normal menstrual flow and prevent cramping. Effectiveness controversial. Still being studied for this and other uses. (15)	Contraindicated in pregnancy. Has potential to cause photodermatitis. Essential oil contains safrole, a carcinogen. (15)	Benefit not worth the risk. Not recommended for use. (15)
ECHINACEA—*Echinacea angustifolia, Echinacea pallida*—Purple cone flower (*Echinacea purpurea*) is a different species with same properties. (6,15,16,22)	Proven effective for prophylaxis and treatment of cold and flu symptoms. May work by stimulating the production of phagocytes. (6,13,15,16)	Possibly becomes immunosuppressive with continuous use (6–8 weeks). Contraindicated in patients with autoimmune diseases. Parenteral use is not recommended (can cause chills, fever, nausea, vomiting, allergies). (5,6,15)	Concentrations of chemical constituents in commercial products vary. Maximum adult daily dose is 6–9 mL of expressed fresh juice, or 1.5–7.5 mL of tincture (preferred since not all constituents are water soluble), or 2–5 g of dried root used for no more than 6–8 weeks. (5,6,15,22)
ELEUTHERA—see Siberian Ginseng			
EPHEDRA—see Ma Huang			
FEVERFEW—*Tanacetum parthenium* (6)	Shown to be effective for prophylaxis and treatment of migraine. Has spasmolytic effects on cerebral vessels. Used to treat fevers and menstrual problems. Is not effective for treating rheumatoid arthritis. (6,15,16,22)	May have GI effects. Fresh leaves can cause mouth ulceration. Do not use in pregnancy (may stimulate menstruation) or during lactation, or in children under 2 yrs. May interact with anticoagulants to increase bleeding. (6,15,16,22)	Concentrations of chemical constituents in commercial products vary. Adult dose is 125 mg dried leaves (parthenolide content no less than 0.2%) QD to BID. (6,16,22,23)
GARLIC—*Allium sativum*—when the cells of the bulb are crushed, alliin is converted to allicin (responsible for many of garlic's effects and its odor). (6,15)	Shown to be effective for reducing cholesterol, LDL, and triglycerides, and for raising HDL. May have antibacterial, antifungal, antithrombotic, hypotensive, hypoglycemic, antihyperlipidemic, antiinflammatory, and anticancer activity. (6,13,22)	Shown to inhibit platelet aggregation. May interact with anticoagulants. Reduces blood sugar so may affect glucose control. Rarely, causes allergic reactions. Heat and acid destroy ingredients responsible for cholesterol lowering, so enteric-coated products show best results. (6,15,23)	Concentrations of chemical constituents in commercial products vary. Adult daily dose is 4–12 mg of alliin (2–5 mg of allicin), or 0.4–1.2 g of dried powder, or 2–5 g of fresh bulb. Decrease in cholesterol may take 8–16 weeks, hypotensive effects 1–6 months. (6,13,23)

Herbal Medicine (continued)

PLANT	*USE**	*PRECAUTIONS & INTERACTIONS*	*TRADITIONAL DOSING***
GINGER—*Zingiber officinale* (6)	Shown to be effective for treatment of motion sickness and nausea. Shown to be an effective anti-inflammatory for treatment of arthritis. Positive inotropic effect on heat tissue being studied. (3,6,15,23)	Inhibits thromboxane synthetase (platelet aggregation inducer) and is a prostacyclin (inhibitor of platelet aggregation) agonist—may result in prolonged bleeding time. Avoid during pregnancy (controversial) and during times in chemotherapy or after surgery when bleeding is a concern. (6,22)	Adult dose is 1 g 30 min prior to travel, then 0.5–1 g q 4 hours (maximum daily dose is 2–4 g). Dose used prior to cancer chemotherapy is 1 g (3,6,23).
GINKGO—*Ginkgo biloba* (6)	Dilates arteries, capillaries and veins. Used to increase peripheral blood flow. Shown to improve intermittent claudication. Used to treat varicosity, cerebral vascular insufficiency, dementia, tinnitus, vertigo, SSRI-induced sexual dysfunction. (6,14,11)	Ginkgolide is a selective antagonist of platelet aggregation. Case report of spontaneous bleeding from the iris when given with aspirin and of a subdural hematoma with chronic use. May cause minor GI disturbances. Rarely, causes headache, dizziness, vertigo. (6,7,17,18)	Adult dose is 60–80 mg of standardized leaf extract (24% flavone glycosides and 6% terpenes) taken BID—TID. Effects can take from 1–2 months to appear. (3,6,14,22)
GINSENG—*Panax ginseng* (Korean ginseng), *Panax quinquefolium* (American ginseng)—Siberian ginseng is a different species (see separate listing). (6)	Effectiveness not adequately documented. Used prophylactically as an adaptogen to "normalize" the body and provide resistance to stress. May lower blood cholesterol and improve LDL & HDL ratios. Some ingredients raise BP and some lower BP. Not effective as an aphrodisiac. (5,6)	Nervousness and excitation can occur for first few days of intake. Over-use can cause headache, insomnia, and palpitations. Use caution in patients with hypertension. Case report of an interaction between Ginseng and furosemide (decreased diuretic effect) resulting in hospitalization (probably caused by germanium contamination). Estrogenic effects have caused vaginal bleeding, breast nodules. (3,4,9,15)	Contents of commercial products vary. Frequently mislabeled or adulterated. Roots must be a minimum of 3 yrs old to be most effective. Adult dose is 1–2 g of root daily, or 100–300 mg of extract (standardized to contain 7% ginsenosides) TID taken for 3–4 weeks. Maximum effects, if any, appear over long term (6,15,23).
GOLDENROD—*Solidago virgaurea, Solidago serotina, Solidago gigantea, Solidago canadensis* (6)	Used for prevention and treatment of urinary tract inflammation, urinary calculi and kidney stones. (6)	Rarely, causes allergies. (6)	Adult dose is 3–5 g of the herb in 240 mL boiling water, steep for 15 min, strain. Mean daily dose is 6–12 g. (5,6)
GOLDENSEAL—*Hydrastis canadensis* (6)	Efficacy not substantiated by clinical studies. Used traditionally to treat mucosal inflammation and gastritis. Does not mask urine drug screens. (6,14,22)	Contraindicated during pregnancy. High doses may cause nausea, vomiting, diarrhea, CNS stimulation and respiratory failure. (6,15)	Adult dose is 0.5–1 g of the dried root, or 2–4 mL of tincture, TID. A tea made from up to 6 g in 240 mL of water has been suggested for mouth sores. Plants take 3–4 years to grow to marketability. (6,22)
GOTU KOLA—*Centella asiatica*—Titrated extract of *C. asiatica* (TECA)—do not confuse with Kolanut, a different plant with different action. (5)	Shown topically to promote wound healing, including bladder lesions. Topical use may clear psoriasis. Being investigated for anticancer (in vitro), antihypertensive, and antifertility effects. (15)	Contact dermatitis. Large doses can be sedating. (15)	Apply topically daily. Oral adult daily dose is 600 mg powdered leaf.
GRAPESEED EXTRACT—*Vitis vinifera*—Pinebark extract (*Pinus maritima, Pinus nigra*) contains the same chemical constituents but is trademarked "pycnogenol." (6,15)	Used as an antioxidant to treat hypoxia from atherosclerosis, inflammation, cardiac or cerebral infarction. Prevention of connective tissue breakdown is not clinically proven. (6,15)	No adverse reactions reported.	Adult dose of 75–300 mg daily for 3 wks, then 40–80 mg daily maintenance dose. (6)

Herbal Treatments in Practice

Herbal Medicine (continued)

PLANT	USE*	PRECAUTIONS & INTERACTIONS	TRADITIONAL DOSING**
GUARANA—*Paullinia cupana* (Zoom)—Contains caffeine 2.5–5% (coffee seed contains 1–2%). (5,15,16)	An effective CNS stimulant. Used to treat drowsiness and to potentiate analgesics. (6,15,16)	May cause hypertension and excess stimulation. Extracts have inhibited platelet aggregation. (15)	Adult daily dose of caffeine is 100–200 mg. (7)
HAWTHORN—*Crataegus laevigata, Crataegus monogyna, Crataegus pinnatifida* (7)	Used to treat heart disease, angina, sleep disorders. Shown to dilate coronary blood vessels. (15)	High doses cause CNS depression and hypotension. May interact with blood pressure or heart medications. (15)	Minimum daily adult dose is listed as 5 mg flavone (hyperoside), 10 mg total flavonoids, or 5 mg oligomeric procyanidins (epicatechin)—or a tea of 3–4 g of dried herb taken in 1 g of doses BID-TID. (5,6)
HOPS—*Humulus lupulus*—related to marijuana. (15)	May have sedative effects, although evidence is conflicting. Active ingredients increase when herb is stored 1–2 yrs. Does not have estrogenic activity. (5,15,22)	Contact dermatitis. (15)	Tea made from .5 g (1–2 tsp) in boiling water, steeped for 5–10 min, strain. Taken BID-TID and HS. (5)
HOREHOUND—*Marrubium vulgare* (6)	Controversial use as expectorant, antitussive, cough suppressant, digestive aid, appetite stimulant. Hypoglycemic in rabbits. (6,15)	No side effects reported in humans. Large doses may produce cardiac irregularities. (22)	Adult dose is 2 g (2 heaping tsps.) of dried cut herb, in 240 mL of boiling water. Taken 3–5 times per day (up to 0.75–1 L per day). (6,22)
HORSE CHESTNUT—*Aesculus hippocastanum* (buckeye)—not the same as the sweet chestnut (*Castanea sativa*) used for cooking. (5,15)	Used traditionally to treat varicose veins and other venous insufficiencies.	Considered unsafe if not properly prepared. Misuse has resulted in death. Commercial skin cleansing products may be carcinogenic. Pollen is allergenic, and contact dermatitis has been reported. (5)	High risk/benefit ratio. Not recommended for use.
KAVA-KAVA—*Piper methylsticum* (15)	CNS depressant effects and euphoria. Used for sleep inducement and anxiety reduction. (15,21)	High doses can cause muscle weakness. Chronic ingestion causes reversible skin discoloration and eye disturbances. Potentiates alcohol and other CNS depressants. Contraindicated in pregnancy, lactation, endogenous depression. (15,21)	History of ceremonial use. Adult daily dose is 60–120 mg kava pyrones. (21)
KOLANUT—*Cola nitida* (Cola, Kola)—contains up to 3.5% caffeine (coffee seed contains 1–2%). (16,22)	Used in beverages for caffeine content. (22)	Cardiac effects (tachyphylaxis) prevent use as a diuretic. (22)	Used in commercial beverages. (16,22)
LEMON BALM—*Melissa officinalis* (sweet balm) (5,6)	Traditionally used to treat sleep disorders and nervous GI disorders. Proven effective topical treatment for early stages of herpes simplex virus lesions. (6)	No side effects reported with topical use. Decreased thyrotrophin levels in animals. (5,6)	Use topically. Tea for oral use made from 1.5–2 g (1–3 tsps) of finely chopped drug. In boiling water, steep for 5–10 min, strain. Take several times per day. (5)
LICORICE—*Glycyrrhiza glabra, Glycyrrhiza uralensis* (15)	Used to treat peptic ulcers (helps increase prostaglandins). Used as an expectorant. (6)	Considered unsafe. High doses (more than 50 g QD) can cause pseudoaldosteronism resulting in increased blood pressure, water retention, and potassium loss. Contraindicated during pregnancy and in patients with liver disorders, hypokalemia, or who are taking cardiac glycosides. Thiazide diuretics may increase potassium loss. May have estrogen-like effects. (5,6,19)	Use of deglycyrrhizinated licorice (DGL) may allow ulcer healing without major side effects, but results are inconclusive. Do not use licorice longer than 4–6 weeks. (6,15,23)

912

Herbal Medicine (continued)

PLANT	USE*	PRECAUTIONS & INTERACTIONS	TRADITIONAL DOSING**
MA HUANG—*Ephedra sinica, E intermedia, E. equisetina E. distachya* (squaw tea, Mormon tea, popotillo, sea grape)—Over 40 species, whose contents vary, some contain alkaloids including ephedrine, pseudoephedrine. (6,16,22)	Shown to be effective treatment for bronchial asthma—bronchodilator, vasoconstrictor, reduces bronchial edema. Not shown safe and effective for weight loss, although it is an ingredient in many weight loss products. (6)	Misuse has caused deaths. Can cause hypertension, CNS stimulation (nervousness, insomnia, palpitations). Can cause hyperglycemia. Ephedrine can be used to manufacture methamphetamine and methcathinone. (6,15)	Concentration of chemical constituents in commercial products varies. The North and Central American species (*Ephedra nevadensis*—Mormon Tea) contains no alkaloids. Adult dose is 2 g (1 heaping tsp—15–30 mg of ephedrine) in 240 mL boiling water, steep for 10 min. (6,22)
MILK THISTLE—*Silybum marianum* (silymarin is a mixture of derivatives found only in the fruit). (5,6)	Hepatoprotective and antioxidant. Shown to be useful in treating inflammatory liver disorders and cirrhosis (scavenges free radicals, alters outer liver cell membrane structures, blocks blinding sites, helps activate the liver's regenerative capacity). Shown to protect liver against damage from toxins. (6,22)	Few adverse effects. Mild diarrhea, allergic reactions, one report of urticaria. Do not use in decompensated cirrhosis. (6,15)	Adult dose of seeds is 12–15 g per day (200–240 mg of silymarin). Tea not an effective dosage form. (6,22)
NETTLE—*Urtica dioica* (2)	Fresh sap has shown a mild diuretic effect. Roots may relieve BPH symptoms. Root and leaves are being studied to reduce inflammation, interact with androgen transport, and stimulate the immune system. No clinical evidence for effectiveness of fruit (seed). (13,15,22)	Do not use in patients with impaired cardiac or renal function. Rarely, causes allergic reactions. (5)	Adult daily dose of root for BPH is 4–6 g. Tea is made from 4 g (3–4 tsp) herb in hot water, steep 10 min, strain. Taken TID-QID. (5)
PASSION FLOWER—*Passiflora incarnata* (Maypop) (5)	Used as a sedative, but not supported by clinical trials in humans. (15)	No adverse reactions reported. May have some MAOI activity. (15)	Adult daily dose is a tea of 4–8 g (3–6 tsp) taken in divided doses (BID-TID, HS). (5,22)
PAU D'ARCO—*Lapacho colorado, Tabebuia avellanedae* (Taheebo, Trumpet bush, lapacho) (15)	Said to be anticancer agent and antiinflammatory, but evidence is inconclusive. NCI found no significant antineoplastic effects. (15,22)	Active ingredients shown to be toxic to humans. Has anticoagulant effects. Causes nausea, vomiting, dizziness. (8,15,22)	High risk, little or no benefit. Not recommended for use.
PEPPERMINT—*Mentha × piperita* (6,15)	Shown to decrease muscle spasms of the GI tract. Used to treat abdominal pain. Oil used as a flavoring agent and a digestive aid. Enteric-coated capsules used to treat irritable bowel syndrome (IBS). (6,15)	Oil may irritate mucous membranes. Do not use in infants or children. Tea from leaves may cause laryngeal and bronchial spasms in small children. Overuse leads to heartburn and relaxation of the lower esophageal sphincter. May worsen hiatal hernia symptoms. May cause allergic reactions, contact dermatitis. (6,15)	Tea is made from 1–1.5 g (1 Tbsp) leaves in 160 mL of boiling water, steep for up to 10 min, taken TID-QID. Dose of Peppermint Spirit (10% oil and 1% leaf extract) is 1 mL (20 drops) taken with water. (6,22)
PRIMROSE, EVENING—*Oenothera biennis* (15)	Shown to lower serum cholesterol. Shown to improve atopic eczema. Used as a GLA (gamma-linoleic acid) supplement (can be converted to the prostaglandin precursor DGLA). Being studied for a variety of conditions. (15)	Studies have shown no adverse reactions or toxicity. (15)	Adult daily dose for GLA supplementation is 0.6–6 g. Adult dose for atopic eczema is 1 g BID. (6)
PSYLLIUM—*Plantago arenaria, Plantago psyllium, Plantago indica, Plantago ovata* (Plantain, Plantago) (6,16)	Shown useful as a bulk-forming laxative for constipation, irritable bowel syndrome (IBS), and for lowering cholesterol and LDL levels. (6,15)	Rarely, causes allergic reaction (anaphylaxis). May interfere with the adsorption of other drugs. Wait 30–60 minutes between dosing. Bezoars (GI blockage) may form if not taken with enough fluid. (6,15)	Dose is 7.5–10 g plus at least 150 mL water for each 5 g of drug. Take 30–60 minutes after a meal. Component in seeds may be nephrotoxic so commercial products are preferable. (6,15)

Herbal Treatments in Practice

Herbal Medicine (continued)

PLANT	USE*	PRECAUTIONS & INTERACTIONS	TRADITIONAL DOSING**
PUMPKIN SEEDS—*cucurbitae peponis* (5,13)	Used to increase urination in patients with BPH, but not substantiated by clinical trials. (5,13)	No adverse effects reported. (5)	Maximum adult dose is 15–30 g (1–2 heaping Tbsp) taken with fluid BID. Efficacy may not be seen for weeks or months. (5)
PYCNOGENOL—see Grapeseed Extract			
ST. JOHN'S WORT—*Hypericum perforatum*—the active ingredient, hypericin, has been given an IND and is being studied. (2,6,15)	Shown to be effective for the treatment of mild-to-moderate depression. May have sedative and anti-inflammatory activity. (6,10)	May have monoamine oxidase inhibitor (MAOI) activity. May cause photodermatitis. (2,5,6) Is thought to increase serotonin levels. Don't take with prozac or other antidepressants. (1)	Adult dose being studied is 300 mg TID for no more than 8 weeks. Tea made with 2–4 g (1–2 tsp) in boiling water, steep 5–10 min. Take 1–2 cups BID. (2,5)
SARSAPARILLA—*Smilax aristolochiaefolia* (Mexican), *Smilax febrifuga* (Ecuadorian), *Smilax regilii* (Honduras)—unrelated to American or Wild Sarsaparilla (*Aralia nudicaulis*). (12)	Folk use only—traditionally used to treat syphilis and as a diuretic. Being promoted erroneously for body-building. Does not contain testosterone, nor is it converted to anabolic steroids. (12,22)	Causes irritation of mucous membranes (throat, intestines). May interfere with absorption of simultaneously administered drugs. Increases absorption of digitalis and bismuth, and elimination of hypnotics. (12)	Use only as a flavoring agent. (22)
SAW PALMETTO—*Serenoa repens* (sabal, cabbage palm) (6)	Fruit extract shown to be effective for treatment of benign prostatic hyperplasia (BPH). Effects are on testosterone uptake and availability (no changes in testosterone plasma levels). Also has antiinflammatory effects. (6,2,15)	Rarely can cause upset stomach, mild headache. High doses can cause diarrhea. Do not use during pregnancy or lactation or in children. Effect on other hormone therapy not known. (15)	Adult dose is 1–2 g of ground, dried fruit daily, or 80 mg of standardized lipoidal extract (85–95% of fatty acids and sterols) BID. Teas are ineffective (aqueous extracts have little value). (6,23)
SENNA—*Cassia acutifolia, Cassia angustifolia, Senna alexandrina* (5)	Cathartic, used to treat constipation. (More drastic than cascara, but less expensive). (22)	Chronic use can result in electrolyte imbalances and potassium loss. May increase toxicity of cardiac glycosides. May turn urine red. Long term use can cause pigmentation of the colon (melanosis coli) and reversible finger clubbing. (5,6,15)	Do not take for more than 1 to 2 weeks without consulting a health care professional. Conc. of teas varies, so standardized commercial dosage forms are preferable. Tea can be made from 0.5–2 g (1/2–1 tsp) soaked in cold water 10–12 hours, or hot for 10 min. Effects can take 10 to 12 hours after ingestion to be seen. (5,6,22)
SIBERIAN GINSENG—*Eleutherococcus senticosus* (eleuthera)—same family but not the same species or composition as Panax Ginseng. (15,22)	Use not supported by adequate clinical studies. Not proven to increase endurance. Injectable form being studied to increase levels of immunocompetent cells (T-cells). (15,22)	No adverse reactions reported. (Toxicity reports have been related to adulterants). May produce aggressive behavior in animals. (22)	Frequently mislabeled or adulterated. (22)
SLIPPERY ELM—*Ulmus rubra* (6,15)	Acts as a demulcent and an emollient to treat sore throats, gastritis, colitis, gastric or duodenal ulcers. (6,15)	Pollen is allergenic. May cause contact dermatitis. (15)	Adult dose is 0.5–2 g of powdered bark steeped in 10 parts hot water (5–20 mL). (5)
TEA TREE OIL—*Melaleuca alternifolia* (Melaleuca, Australian Tea Tree) (15)	Bacteriostatic, germicidal. Used to treat boils, abscesses, cuts, abrasions and acne. Other uses not verified. (6,15)	Rarely, causes allergic reactions or skin irritation. (6)	Apply topically. Has been used in concentrations from 0.4–100%. (22)
TRAGACANTH—*Astragalus gummifera* (15)	Used as an emulsifier and thickening agent. Not proven to decrease serum lipids or blood glucose levels. (15)	Is easily contaminated. (15)	Maximum viscosity not reached for 24 hours at room temp. or 8 hrs with high heat, when mixed with water. (15)
VALERIAN—*Valeriana officinalis*—other species used for other purposes, *Valeriana edulis* (Mexican), *Valeriana wallichii* (Indian). (5,6,16)	Shown to have mild sedative/hypnotic effects. Used to promote sleep—does not decrease night awakenings. (6,15)	May cause increased morning drowsiness. Is not synergistic with alcohol, but has not been studied with opiates or other CNS depressants. (15,23)	Adult dose is 1–3 g (1–3 mL tincture) QD-TID & HS. (5,6,23)

Herbal Medicine (continued)

PLANT	USE*	PRECAUTIONS & INTERACTIONS	TRADITIONAL DOSING**
WHITE WILLOW—*Salix purpurea, Salix fragilis, Salix* daphnoides contain the most salicin, however *Salix alba* is also used. (5,6)	Used as an analgesic. Salicin is converted to salicylic acid. Probably provides a subtherapeutic source. (6,22)	May show adverse reactions similar to salicylates. However not shown to effect platelet function or to interact with anticoagulants. (5,6)	Concentrations of chemical constituents in commercial products vary. Longer to onset and longer acting than salicylic acid. Difficult to reach therapeutic dose by using plant alone. (6,22)
WITCH HAZEL—*Hamamelis virginiana* (6)	Astringent, anti-inflammatory, hemostyptic. Used to treat inflammation of skin and mucous membranes, but efficacy not supported. (6,15)	Tannins in 1 g will cause nausea, vomiting or constipation. Tannins present in oral preparations may cause liver damage. (5,15)	Apply topically. The steam distilled product does not contain tannins therefore, activity probably results from alcohol. Not recommended for oral use. (6,15,22)
YERBA MATÉ—*Ilex paraguariensis* (Maté, Paraguay tea)—contains up to 2% caffeine (similar to coffee beans). (15,16)	An effective CNS stimulant. Used to treat drowsiness and to potentiate analgesics. (6,15)	May cause hypertension, excess stimulation. Heavy use increase risk of esophageal cancer. (15)	Adult daily dose of caffeine is 100–200 mg. Tea made with 1 tsp leaves in hot water, steep for 5–10 min, strain. (5,6)
YOHIMBE—*Pausinystalia yohimbe* (Yohimbine) (16)	Used to treat impotence—has alpha-2-adrenergic blocking activity. (16)	High risk/benefit ratio. Can cause CNS stimulation, hypotension or hypertension, tachycardia, nausea, vomiting and psychoses. May have MAOI activity. (22)	Recommended for use only under the care of a physician.

*These are not FDA-approved uses. The FDA does not regulate nutritional supplements that do not claim to treat specific disease states. Therefore caution is advised before using or recommending any of these herbs for these purposes.

**In most cases, optimum doses have not been determined through adequate clinical trials. These dosages are representative of traditional use.

***Cold water maceration reduces tannins.

References: [1] American Herbal Pharmacopoeia and Therapeutic Compendium. St. John's Wort Hypericum perforatum. Herbalgram 1997;40:36. [2] Barnes J. Growing body of data for hypericum extract in depression. In Pharma 1996;No.1058:3–4, Oct 12. [3] Barnett RA. Ginkgo, Ginger, Garlic, Ginseng. Remedy 1996:33–36, 38–39, Sep/Oct. [4] Becker BN, Greene J, Evanson J, Chidsey G, Stone WU, et al. Ginseng-induced diuretic resistance. JAMA 1996;276:606–607, Aug 28. [5] Bisset NG (ed). Herbal Drugs and Phytopharmaceuticals. Boca Raton, LA: CRC Press, 1994. [6] Covington TR (ed). The Handbook of Non-Prescription Drugs. Washington, DC: APhA, 1996. [7] Foster S. Ginkgo: Ginkgo biloba, Botanical Series 304, Austin, TX: American Botanical Council: 1991:1–7. [8] Kassler WJ, Blanc P, Greenblatt R. The use of medicinal herbs by human immunodeficiency virus-infected patients. Arch Intern Med. 1991;151:2281–2288, Nov. [9] Kay MA. Healing with Plants in the American and Mexican West. Tucson, AZ: University of Arizona Press, 1996. [10] Linde K, Ramirez G, Mulrow CD, Pauls A, Weidenhammer W, Melchart D. St. John's wort for depression—an overview and meta-analysis of randomized clinical trials. BMJ 1996;313:253–8, Aug 3. [11] McCann B. Botanical could improve sex life of patients on SSRIs. Drug Topics July 7 1997:33. [12] Osborne F, Chandler F. Sarsaparilla. Canadian Pharmaceutical Journal. 1996. [13] Rawls R. Europe's strong herbal brew. C&EN. 1996:53–60, Sep 23. [14] Remington KA. A Pharmacist's guide to useful herbal remedies. Calif Pharm 1997;(suppl):1–10 April. [15] Review of Natural Products. St. Louis, MO: Facts and Comparisons, 1996. [16] Robbers JE, Speedie MK, Tyler VE. Pharmacognosy and Pharmacobiotechnology. Baltimore, MD: Williams & Wilkins, 1996. [17] Rosenblatt M, Mindel J. Spontaneous hyphema associated with ingestion of Ginkgo biloba extract. (letter). N Engl J Med 1997;336(15):1108 April 10. [18] Rowin J, Lewis SL. Spontaneous bilateral subdural hematomas associated with chronic Ginkgo biloba ingestion. Neurology 1996;46:1775–6. [19] Seligmann J, Cowley G. Sex, Lies, and Garlic. Newsweek 1995:65–68, Nov. [20] Siciliano AA. Cranberry. HerbalGram 1996;No. 38:51–54. [21] Singh YN, Blumenthal M. Kava, an overview. HerbalGram 1997;No.39:33–56. [22] Tyler VE. Herbs of Choice: The therapeutic use of phytomedicinals. New York: Haworth Press, 1994. [23] Tyler VE. What Pharmacists should know about herbal remedies. J APhA 1996;NS36 (1):29–37, Jan. [24] Vogel VJ. American Indian Medicine. Normal, OK: University of Oklahoma Press, 1970. [25] Weiner MA. Earth Medicine, Earth Food. New York: Fawcett Columbine, 1991.

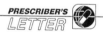

Adapted with permission from *Prescriber's Letter*, "Herbal Medicine," Document #131033. *Prescriber's Letter* is an independent advisory service providing drug therapy information to physicians by subscription. *Prescriber's Letter*, 2453 Grand Canal Blvd., Suite A, P.O.Box 8190, Stockton, CA 95208. Tel: 209-472-2240.

SECTION VIII
Tables
Monica Darby

DEVELOPMENT

Table 1   Scoring System: Draw-a-Person Test

ONE POINT ASSIGNED PER FEATURE:

Head present
Neck present
Neck, two dimensions
Eyes present
Eye detail: brows or lashes
Nose present
Nose, two dimensions
   (not round ball)
Mouth present
Lips, two dimensions
Both nose and lips in two
   dimensions
Both chin and forehead shown
Bridge of nose (straight to eyes;
   narrower than base)
Hair I (any scribble)
Hair II (more detail)
Ears present

Fingers present
Correct number of fingers shown
Opposition of thumb shown
   (must include fingers)
Hands present
Arms present
Arms at side or engaged in activity
Feet: any indication
Attachment of arms to legs I
   (to trunk or anywhere)
Attachment of arms and legs II
   (at correct point on trunk)
Trunk present
Trunk in proportion, two dimensions
   (if greater than breadth)
Clothing I (anything)
Clothing II (two articles of clothing)

MENTAL AGE (YR)	POINTS SCORED BY BOYS	POINTS SCORED BY GIRLS
3	4	5
4	7	7
5	11	11
6	13	14
7	16	17
8	18	20

Table 1—*Continued.*   Receptive Language Development

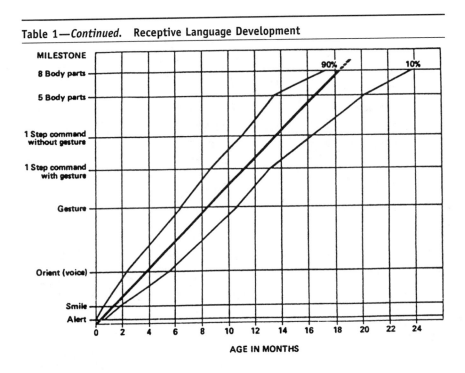

Table 1—*Continued.*   Expressive Language Development

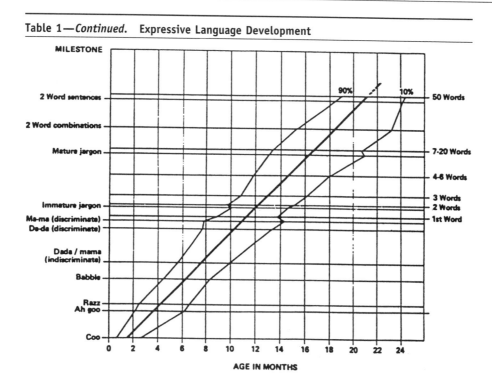

Table 2   Developmental Milestones from Birth to 5 Years

AGE (MONTHS)	ADAPTIVE/FINE MOTOR	LANGUAGE	GROSS MOTOR	PERSONAL–SOCIAL
1	Grasp reflex (hands fisted)	Facial response to sounds	Lifts head in prone position	Stares at face
2	Follows object with eyes past midline	Coos (vowel sounds)	Lifts head in prone position to 45°	Smiles in response to others
4	Hands open Brings objects to mouth	Laughs and squeals Turns toward voice	Sits: head steady Rolls to supine	Smiles spontaneously
6	Palmar grasp of objects	Babbles (consonant sounds)	Sits independently Stands, hands held	Reaches for toys Recognizes strangers
9	Pincer grasp	Says "mama," "dada" nonspecifically, comprehends "no"	Pulls to stand	Feeds self Waves bye-bye
12	Helps turn pages of book	2–4 words Follows command with gesture	Stands independently Walks, one hand held	Points to indicate wants
15	Scribbles	4–6 words Follows command no gesture	Walks independently	Drinks from cup Imitates activities
18	Turns pages of book	10–20 words Points to 4 body parts	Walks up steps	Feeds self with spoon
24	Solves single-piece puzzles	Combines 2–3 words Uses "I" and "you"	Jumps Kicks ball	Removes coat Verbalizes wants
30	Imitates horizontal and vertical lines	Names all body parts	Rides tricycle using pedals	Pulls up pants Washes, dries hands
36	Copies circle Draws person with 3 parts	Gives full name, age, and sex Names 2 colors	Throws ball overhand Walks up stairs (alternating feet)	Toilet trained Puts on shirt, knows front from back
42	Copies cross	Understands "cold," "tired," "hungry"	Stands on one foot for 2–3 sec	Engages in associative play
48	Counts 4 objects Identifies some numbers and letters	Understands prepositions (under, on, behind, in front of) Asks "how" and "why"	Hops on one foot	Dresses with little assistance Shoes on correct feet
54	Copies square Draws person with 6 parts	Understands opposites	Broad-jumps 24 inches	Bosses and criticizes Shows off
60	Prints first name Counts 10 objects	Asks meaning of words	Skips (alternating feet)	Ties shoes

---

Table 2A   Causes of Failure to Thrive

AGE AT ONSET	DIAGNOSTIC CONSIDERATIONS
Before birth (IUGR, prematurity)	Especially in "symmetric" IUGR, consider prenatal infections, congenital syndromes, teratogenic exposures (anticonvulsants, alcohol, etc.)
Neonatal	Incorrect formula preparation; failed breastfeeding; neglect; poor feeding interactions; metabolic, chromosomal, or anatomic abnormality (less common)
3–6 months	Underfeeding (possibly associated with poverty); improper formula preparation; milk protein intolerancce; oral-motor dysfunction; celiac disease; HIV infection; cystic fibrosis; congenital heart disease; GE reflux
7–12 months	Autonomy struggles; overly fastidious parent; oral-motor dysfunction; delayed introduction of solids; intolerance of new foods
After 12 months	Coercive feeding; highly distractable child; distracting environment; acquired illness; new psychosocial stressor (divorce, job loss, new sibling, death in the family, etc.)

Reproduced from Frank DA, et al., with permission from the authors.

Table 3   Primitive Reflexes

PRIMITIVE REFLEX	AGE AT DISAPPEARANCE (MONTHS)	DESCRIPTION
Palmar grasp	3–4	Pressing against the palmar surface of the infant's hand results in flexion of all fingers.
Rooting	3–4	Stroking the perioral skin at the corners of the mouth causes the mouth to open and turn to stimulated side.
Galant	2–3	Stroking along the paravertebral area causes lateral flexion of the trunk with the concavity toward the stimulated side.
Moro	4–6	Sudden movement of the head causes symmetric abduction and extension of the arms followed by gradual adduction and flexion of the arms over the body.
Asymmetric tonic neck	4–6	Turning the head to one side leads to extension of extremities on that side and flexion on the contralateral side. This puts the infant in the fencing position.
Tonic labyrinthine	2–3	In supine neck extension leads to shoulder retraction and trunk and lower extremity extension. This is reduced by neck flexion.
Positive support	2–3	Stimulation of the ball of the foot leads to cocontraction of opposing muscle groups, allowing weight to be borne.
Placing/stepping	Variable	When the dorsal surface of one foot touches the underside of a table, the infant places the foot on the table top.

Table 4 Penile and Clitoral Length in the Newborn Infant

GESTATIONAL AGE	LENGTH (MEAN ± SD) (CM)

Male Measure from pubic ramus to the tip of the glans with gentle traction applied.[a]

30 wk	2.5 ± 0.4
34 wk	3.0 ± 0.4
Term	3.5 ± 0.4

Female Measure with labia majora separated and the prepuce skin retracted.[b]

Term Infants	4.0 ± 1.24

Preterm infants—The clitoris achieves full size by 24 wk gestation and may appear more prominent relative to the labia in premature infants.

[a]Feldman KW, Smith DW. Fetal phallic growth and penile standards for newborn male infants. J Pediatr 1975;86:395.

[b]Oberfield S, Mondok A, Shanrivar F, et al. Clitoral size in full-term infants. Am J Perinatol 1989;6(4):453.

Table 5 Tanner Stages in the Female

STAGE	BREAST	PUBIC HAIR
1	Prepubertal, elevation of papilla only	Prepubertal
2	Enlargement of areola, elevation of breast and papilla ("breast bud")	Sparse, long, straight, slightly pigmented hair along labia
3	Further enlargement of breast and areola with no separation of contour	Hair is darker, curlier, and coarser with increased distribution on pubes
4	Areola and papilla form a second mount above the breast	Adult-type hair limited to pubes with no extension to medial thigh
5	Mature breast	Mature distribution of inverse triangle with spread to medial thighs

Table 6 Tanner Stages in the Male

STAGE	GENITAL DEVELOPMENT	PUBIC HAIR
1	Prepubertal	Prepubertal
2	Enlargement of testes (>4 mL volume) and scrotum with reddening of scrotal skin	Sparse, long, straight, slightly pigmented hair at base of penis
3	Growth of penis, primarily length, with further increase in size of testes and scrotum	Hair is darker and curlier with increased distribution on pubes
4	Further increase in length and breadth of penis with development of glans, increase in testes and scrotum	Adult-type hair limited to pubes with no extension to medial thigh
5	Adult size and shape	Mature distribution with spread to medial thighs and lower abdomen

Table 7 Normal Growth Rates

AGE	EXPECTED GROWTH RATE
First year	25 cm (10 inches)/y
Second year	12.5 cm (5 inches)/y
Childhood	6.25 cm (2.5 inches)/y
Adolescence, boys	15–38 cm (6–15 inches)
Adolescence, girls	15–25 cm (6–12 inches)

Table 8 Head Growth Velocity

FULL-TERM		PRETERM	
2 cm/mo	0–3 months	1 cm/wk	0–2 months
1 cm/mo	3–6 months	0.5 cm/wk	2–4 months
0.5 cm/mo	7–12 months	see full-term	>4 months

Table 9 Illustrations of the Primary and Permanent Dentition. *A* and *B,* The numbers represent the average age of eruption for the teeth, indicated in months for the primary teeth and years for the permanent dentition. *C* and *D,* The names of specific teeth in the primary and permanent dentition are shown.

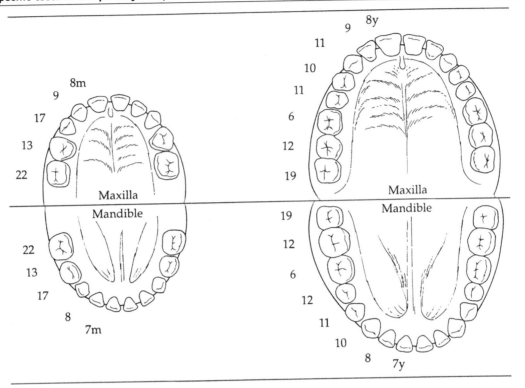

A. Primary Dentition

B. Permanent Dentition

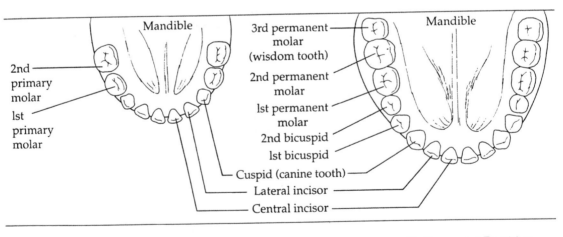

C. Primary Dentition

D. Permanent Dentition

Reproduced with permission from Nazif MM, Davis HW, McKibben DH, Roody MA. Arts of Pediatric Physical Diagnosis-3.

IMMUNIZATION

Table 10   Recommended Childhood Immunization Schedule, January–December 1998

Vaccine	Birth	1 mo	2 mos	4 mos	6 mos	12 mos	15 mos	18 mos	4–6 yrs	11–12 yrs	14–16 yrs
Hepatitis B[1,2]	Hep B-1[8]									Hep B	
			Hep B-2[8]		Hep B-3[8]						
Diphtheria-tetanus-pertussis[3]		DTaP or DTP	DTaP or DTP	DTaP or DTP			DTaP or DTP		DTaP or DTP	Td	
Haemophilus influenzae type b[4]			Hib	Hib	Hib	Hib					
Polio[5]			Polio	Polio		Polio			Polio		
Measles-mumps-rubella[6]						MMR			MMR or MMR		
Varicella[7]						Var				Var	

This schedule indicates the recommended age for the routine administration of currently licensed childhood vaccines. Some combination vaccines are available and may be used whenever administration of all components of the vaccine is indicated. Providers should consult the manufacturer's package inserts for detailed recommendations. Vaccines are listed under the routinely recommended ages. *Bars* indicate the range of acceptable ages for vaccination. *Shaded bars* indicate catch-up vaccination (i.e., at 11–12 years of age hepatitis B vaccine should be administered to children not previously vaccinated and varicella vaccine should be administered to children not previously vaccinated who lack a reliable history of chickenpox). Schedule approved by the Advisory Committee on Immunization Practices (ACIP), the American Academy of Pediatrics (AAP), and the American Academy of Family Physicians (AAFP).

[1]**Infants born to HBsAg-negative mothers** should receive 2.5 μg of Merck vaccine (Recombivax HB) or 10 μg of SmithKline Beecham (SB) vaccine (Engerix B). The second dose should be administered at least 1 month after the first dose. **Infants born to HBsAg-positive mothers** should receive 0.5 ml hepatitis B immune globulin (HBIG) within 12 hours of birth, and either 5 μg of Merck vaccine (Recombivax HB) or 10 μg of SB vaccine (Engerix-B) at a separate site. The second dose is recommended at 1–2 months of age and the third dose is recommended at 6 months of age. **Infants born to mothers whose HBsAg status is unknown** should receive either 5 μg of Merck vaccine (Recombivax HB) or 10 μg of SB vaccine (Engerix-B) within 12 hours of birth. The second dose of the vaccine is recommended at 1 month of age, and the third dose is recommended at 6 months of age. Blood should be drawn at the time of delivery to determine the mother's HBsAg status; if it is positive, the infant should receive HBIG as soon as possible (no later than 1 week of age). The dosage and timing of subsequent vaccine doses should be based on the mother's HBsAg status.

[2]Children and adolescents who have not been vaccinated against hepatitis B in infancy may begin the series during any childhood visit. Those who have not previously received three doses of hepatitis B vaccine should initiate or complete the series during the 11- to 12-year-old visit. The second dose should be administered at least 1 month after the first dose, and the third dose should be administered at least 4 months after the first dose and at least 2 months after the second dose.

[3]Diphtheria and tetanus toxoids and acellular pertussis (DTaP) vaccine is the preferred vaccine for all doses in the vaccination series, including completion of the series in children who have received at least one dose of whole-cell diphtheria-tetanus-pertussis (DTP) vaccine. Whole-cell DTP is an acceptable alternative to DTaP. The fourth dose (DtaP or DTP) may be administered as early as 12 months of age if the child is considered unlikely to return at 15–18 months of age, provided 6 months have elapsed since the third dose. Tetanus and diphtheria (Td) toxoids (absorbed, for adult use) are recommended at 11–12 years of age if at least 5 years have elapsed since the last dose of DTP, DTaP, or DT. Subsequent routine Td boosters are recommended every 10 years.

[4]Three *Haemophilus influenzae* type b (Hib) conjugate vaccines are licensed for infant use. If PRP-OMP [PedvaxHIB (Merck)] is administered at 2 and 4 months, a dose at 6 months of age is not required.

[5]Two poliovirus vaccines are currently licensed in the United States: inactivated poliovirus vaccine (IPV) and oral poliovirus vaccine (OPV). The following schedules are all acceptable by the ACIP, the AAP, and the AAFP. Parents and providers may choose among these options:
1. Two doses of IPV followed by two doses of OPV
2. Four doses of IPV recommended
3. Four doses of OPV
The ACIP recommends two doses of IPV at 2 and 4 months, followed by two doses of OPV at 12–18 months and 4–6 years. IPV is the only poliovirus vaccine recommended for immunocompromised people and their household contacts.

[6]The second dose of measles-mumps-rubella (MMR) vaccine is routinely recommended at 4–6 years of age or at 11–12 years of age, but may be administered during any visit, provided at least 1 month has elapsed since receipt of the first dose and that both doses are administered at or after 12 months of age. Those who have not previously received the second dose should complete the schedule no later than the 11- to 12-year-old visit.

[7]Susceptible children may receive varicella vaccine (Var) at any visit after the first birthday, and those who lack a reliable history of chickenpox should be immunized during the 11- to 12-year-old visit. Children older than 13 years should receive two doses, at least 1 month apart.

[8]May delay hepatitis immunization to 6 months, 7–12 months to avoid mercury until mercury-free vaccine is available.

Table 11 Recommendations for Routine Immunization of HIV-Infected Children in the United States

VACCINE	KNOWN ASYMPTOMATIC HIV INFECTION	SYMPTOMATIC HIV INFECTION
Hepatitis B	Yes	Yes
DTaP (or DTP)	Yes	Yes
IPV*	Yes	Yes†
MMR	Yes	Yes†
Hib	Yes	Yes
Pneumococcal‡	Yes	Yes
Influenza§	Yes	Yes
Varicella‖	No	No

(Adapted from the American Academy of Pediatrics. In Peter G, ed. *1997 Red Book: Report of the Committee on Infectious Diseases.* 24th ed. Elk Grove Village, IL: American Academy of Pediatrics, 1997.)

DTP = diphtheria and tetanus toxoids and pertussis vaccine; DTaP = diphtheria and tetanus toxoids acellular pertussis vaccine; IPV = inactivated poliovirus vaccine; MMR = live-virus measles, mumps, and rubella; Hib = *Haemophilus influenzae* type b conjugate.

*Only inactivated polio vaccine (IPV) should be used for HIV-infected children, HIV-exposed infants whose status is indeterminate, and household contacts of HIV-infected patients.

†Severely immunocompromised HIV-infected children should not receive MMR vaccine.

‡Pneumococcal vaccine should be administered at 2 years of age to all HIV-infected children. Children who are older than 2 years of age should receive pneumococcal vaccine at the time of diagnosis. Revaccination after 3 to 5 years is recommended in either circumstance.

§Influenza vaccine should be provided each fall and repeated annually for HIV-exposed infants 6 months of age and older, HIV-infected children and adolescents, and for household contacts of HIV-infected patients.

‖Varicella vaccine is not currently indicated for HIV-exposed or HIV-infected patients, but studies are in progress to determine safety and possible indication.

Table 12 Guide to Tetanus Prophylaxis in Routine Wound Management

HISTORY OF ABSORBED TETANUS TOXOID (DOSES)	CLEAN, MINOR WOUNDS		ALL OTHER WOUNDS*	
	Td†	TIG‡	Td†	TIG‡
Unknown or <3	Yes	No	Yes	Yes
≥3§	No‖	No	No#	No

Adapted from the American Academy of Pediatrics. In Peter G, ed. *1997 Red Book: Report of the Committee on Infectious Diseases.* 24th ed. Elk Grove Village, IL: American Academy of Pediatrics, 1997.

Td = adult-use tetanus and diphtheria toxoids; TIG = tetanus immune globulin (human).

*Such as, but not limited to, wounds contaminated with dirt, feces, soil, or saliva; puncture wounds; avulsions; and wounds resulting from missiles, crushing, burns, or frostbite.

†For children <7 years, diphtheria and tetanus toxoids and acellular pertussis (DTaP) or diphtheria-tetanus-pertussis (DTP) is recommended; if pertussis vaccine is contraindicated, diphtheria-tetanus toxoid (DT) is given. For persons ≥7 years of age, Td is recommended.

‡Equine tetanus antitoxin should be used when TIG is not available.

§If only 3 doses of fluid toxoid have been received, a fourth dose of toxoid, preferably an adsorbed toxoid, should be given.

‖Yes, if more than 10 years since the last dose.

#Yes, if more than 5 years since the last dose. (More frequent boosters are not needed and can accentuate side effects.)

Table 13   Suggested Intervals Between Immunoglobulin Administration and Measles Vaccination (MMR or Monovalent Measles Vaccine)

INDICATION FOR IMMUNOGLOBULIN	*PREPARATION*	*ROUTE*	*DOSE* U OR ML	*DOSE* MG IgG/KG	*INTERVAL (MONTHS)* *
Tetanus	TIG	IM	250 U	10	3
Hepatitis A prophylaxis	IG				
Contact prophylaxis		IM	0.02 ml/kg	3.3	3
International travel		IM	0.06 ml/kg	10	3
Hepatitis B prophylaxis	HBIG	IM	0.06 ml/kg	10	3
Rabies prophylaxis	RIG	IM	20 IU/kg	22	4
Measles prophylaxis	IG				
Standard		IM	0.25 ml/kg	40	5
Immunocompromised host		IM	0.50 ml/kg	80	6
Varicella prophylaxis	VZIG	IM	125 U/10 kg (maximum, 625 U)	20–39	5
Blood transfusion					
Washed RBCs		IV	10 ml/kg	Negligible	0
RBCs, adenine-saline added		IV	10 ml/kg	10	3
Packed RBCs		IV	10 ml/kg	20–60	5
Whole blood		IV	10 ml/kg	80–100	6
Plasma or platelet products		IV	10 ml/kg	160	7
Replacement (or therapy) of immune deficiencies	IGIV	IV	. . .	300–400	8
ITP	IGIV	IV	. . .	400	8
RSV	IGIV	IV	. . .	750	9
ITP		IV	. . .	1000	10
ITP or Kawasaki disease		IV	. . .	1600–2000	11

Adapted from the American Academy of Pediatrics. In Peter G, ed. *1997 Red Book: Report of the Committee on Infectious Diseases.* 24th ed. Elk Grove Village, IL: American Academy of Pediatrics, 1997.

IG = immune globulin; IGIV = intravenous immune globulin; IM = intramuscular; ITP = immune (idiopathic) thrombocytopenic purpura; IV = intravenous; HBIG = hepatitis B immune globulin; MMR = measles-mumps-rubella vaccine; RBCs = red blood cells; RIG = rabies immune globulin; RSV-IGIV = respiratory syncytial virus intravenous immune globulin; TIG = tetanus immune globulin; VZIG = varicella-zoster immune globulin.

*These intervals should provide sufficient time for decreases in passive antibodies in all children to allow for an adequate response to the measles vaccine. Physicians should not assume that children are fully protected against measles during these intervals. Additional doses of IG or measles vaccine may be indicated after exposure to measles.

FEEDING & NUTRITION

Table 14　Maternal Drug Use During Lactation

AVOID DURING LACTATION		*NO EFFECTS ON INFANT*
Alcohol	Meperidine	Ampicillin
Chloramphenicol	Oral contraceptives	Caffeine
Cimetidine	Paregoric	Cephalosporins
Clindamycin	Phenobarbital	Erythromycin
Codeine	Propoxyphene	Furosemide
Diazepam	Radionuclide material	Haloperidol
Ergot	Sulfonamides	Hydralazine
Iodine	Tetracycline	
Isoniazid		
LSD		
Marijuana		

Adapted from Roberts RJ. Drug therapy in infants, Philadelphia: WB Saunders, 1984.

Table 15　Commercially Available Oral Rehydration Fluids (in mEq/L)

	Na^+	K^+	Cl^-	*BASE*	*GLUCOSE*
Pedialyte	45	20	35	30	2.5
Lytren	50	25	45	30	2.0
Rehydralyte	75	20	65	30	2.5
WHO formula	90	20	80	30	2.0

Table 16　Composition of Infant Formulas (per 100 ml)

NAME (MANUFACTURER)	Kcal/oz	CHO (% of cal/type)	Fat (% of cal/type)	PRO (% of cal/type)	FE (mg)	VIT D (IU)	mg Ca/mg PO$_4$
Cow's milk–based standard formulas							
Enfamil (Mead Johnson); with/without iron	20*	44% Lactose	48% Palm olein, coconut oil, soy oil, sunflower oil	8% Cow's milk	1.22/0.34	41	52/36
Similac (Ross); with/without iron	20*	43% Lactose	48% Soy oil, coconut oil	9% Cow's milk	1.2/0.15	40	49/38
PM 60/40 (Ross)†	20	41% Lactose	50% Coconut oil, corn oil	9% Lactalbumin, casein	0.15	40	40/20
Gerber; with/without iron (Gerber)	20‡	43% Lactose	49% Corn oil, coconut oil	9% Cow's milk	1.21/0.11	40	50/39
Good Start (Carnation)†	20‡	44% Lactose, soy maltodextrin	46% Palm oil, safflower oil, coconut oil	10% Whey and whey protein	1.01	41	43/24
Soy-based standard formulas							
Isomil (Ross)	20	41% Corn syrup, sucrose	49% Coconut oil, soy oil	10% Soy protein isolate	1.2	40	70/50
Prosobee (Mead Johnson)	20	40% Corn syrup solids	48% Coconut oil, soy oil, palm oil	12% Soy protein isolate	1.3	42	63/49

Continued

Table 16 Composition of Infant Formulas (per 100 ml) (continued)

NAME (MANUFACTURER)	Kcal/oz	CHO (% of cal/type)	Fat (% of cal/type)	PRO (% of cal/type)	FE (mg)	VIT D (IU)	mg Ca/mg PO₄
Preterm formulas							
Similac Special Care (Ross)	24§	42% Lactose (50%), polycose glucose polymers (50%)	47% MCT oil (50%), soy oil (30%), coconut oil (20%)	11% Nonfat milk whey (60%), casein (40%)	1.5/0.3	122	146/81
Enfamil Premature (Mead Johnson); with/without iron	24§	44% Lactose (50%), corn syrup solids	44% MCT oil (40%), soy oil (40%), coconut oil (20%)	12% Lactalbumin (60%), casein (40%)	1.5/0.2	219	134/67
Similac Neocare (Ross)‖	22	41% Lactose (50%), glucose polymers (50%)	49% MCT oil (25%), LCT oil (75%)	10% Whey (50%), casein (50%)	1.3	59	78/46
Special formulas#							
Nutramigen (Mead Johnson)	20	54% Modified corn starch, corn syrup solids	35% Corn oil, soy oil	11% Casein hydrolysate and amino acids	1.25	42	63/42
Pregestimil (Mead Johnson)	20	41% Corn syrup solids, modified cornstarch, dextrose	48% MCT oil (60%), corn oil, soy oil, safflower oil	11% Casein hydrolysate, amino acids	1.25	50	63/42
Portagen (Mead Johnson)	20	46% Corn syrup solids, sucrose	40% MCT oil (85%), corn oil, lecithin	14% Sodium caseinate	1.25	52	63/47
Alimentum (Ross)‖	20	41% Sucrose, modified tapioca starch	48% MCT oil (50%), safflower oil (40%), soy oil (10%)	11% Casein hydrolysate, amino acids	1.2	30	70/50
Lactofree (Mead Johnson)	20	42% Corn syrup solids	49% Palm olein, soy oil, coconut oil, sunflower oil	9% Cow's milk protein isolate	1.2	40	55/37
Neocate (Scientific Hospital Supplies, Inc.)	20	47% Corn syrup solids, dextrose, maltose, maltriose, oligosaccharides	41% Hybrid safflower oil, coconut oil, soy oil	12% Synthetic free amino acids	1.2	58	83/62

CHO = carbohydrate; CF = cystic fibrosis; FE = iron; LCT = long-chain triglyceride; MCT = medium-chain triglyceride; PRO = protein.

*Also available as 24 kcal/oz and 27 kcal/oz.

†Formula with a low renal solute load.

‡Also available as 24 kcal/oz.

§Also available as 20 kcal/oz.

‖Available only as ready-to-feed.

#Indications for Special Formulas

NAME	INDICATIONS
Nutramigen	Cow's milk allergy, severe or multiple food allergies, severe or persistent diarrhea, galactosemia
Pregestimil	Malabsorption, intestinal resection, severe or persistent diarrhea, food allergies
Portagen	Steatorrhea secondary to CF, intestinal resections, pancreatic insufficiency, biliary atresia, lymphatic anomalies, celiac disease
Alimentum	Problems with digestion or absorption, severe or prolonged diarrhea, CF, steatorrhea, food allergies, intestinal resection
Lactofree	Lactose intolerance *without* cow's milk protein intolerance
Neocate	Cow's milk allergy, soy and protein hydrolysate intolerance, multiple food protein intolerance

Table 17 Uncommon Disorders Associated with Obesity

Alstrom-Hallgren syndrome
Autosomal recessive trait, obesity, retinal degeneration with blindness in childhood, sensory nerve deafness, diabetes mellitis, small testes in males, and progressive nephropathy in adults.

Carpenter syndrome
Obesity; brachycephaly with craniosynostosis; peculiar facies with lateral displacement of inner canthi and apparent exopthalmos, flat nasal bridge, low-set ears, retrognathism, and high arched palate; brachydactyly of hands with clinodactyly and partial syndactyly; preaxial polydactyly of feet with partial syndactyly; and mental retardation.

Cohen syndrome
Mild-childhood onset, truncal obesity, persistent hypotonia and muscle weakness, mild mental retardation, characteristic craniofacies with high nasal bridge, maxillary hypoplasia with mild downslant to palpebral fissures, high arched palate, short philtrum, small jaw, open mouth and prominent maxillary central incisors, mottled retina, myopia, strabismus, narrow hands and feet with shortening of metacarpals and metatarsals, simian crease, hyperextensible joints, lumbar lordosis, and mild scoliosis.

Cushing syndrome
Truncal obesity, hypertension, glucose intolerance, hirsutism, oligomenorrhea or amenorrhea, plethora, moon facies, buffalo hump, striae, ecchymoses, increased fatigability and weakness, and personality changes.

Growth hormone deficiency
Short stature, mild-to-moderate obesity.

Hyperinsulinemia (from an insulin-secreting pancreatic tumor, hypersecretion by pancreatic beta cells or a hypothalamic lesion)
Progressive obesity with hyperphagia, normal or excessive growth in stature, and signs and symptoms of hypoglycemia.

Hypothalamic dysfunction (due to tumor, trauma, or inflammation)
Hyperinsulinemia and hyperphagia may be accompanied by headache, papilledema, impaired vision, amenorrhea or impotence, diabetes insipidus, hypothyroidism, adrenal insufficiency, somnolence, temperature dysregulation, seizures, and coma.

Hypothyroidism
Short stature; delayed sexual maturation; delayed union of epiphyses; lethargy; cold intolerance; hoarse voice; menorrhagia; decreased appetite; dry skin; aching muscles and delayed relaxation phase of deep tendon reflexes; progression to dull expressionless face; sparse hair; periorbital puffiness; large tongue; pale, cool, rough-feeling skin; and presence or absence of goiter.

Laurence-Moon-Biedl (Bardet-Biedl) syndrome
Autosomal recessive trait, truncal obesity, retinal dystrophy/retinitis pigmentosa with progressively decreasing acuity, mental retardation, hypogenitalism, digital anomalies (polydactyly, syndactyly, or both), and nephropathy.

Polycystic ovary (Stein-Leventhal) syndrome
Irregular or absent menses, moderate hirsutism, weight gain shortly after menarche, increased ratio of luteinizing hormone to follicle stimulating hormone, hyperandrogenemia, and increased levels of estrone with normal levels of estradiol. May occur in association with congenital adrenal hyperplasia, Cushing syndrome, hyperprolactinemia, or insulin resistance.

Prader-Willi syndrome
Obesity, hypotonia, and feeding problems in infancy; hyperphagia in childhood and adolescence; developmental delay; mental retardation; hypogonadism; short stature; small hands and feet; and strabismus.

Pseudo-hypoparathyroidism (type I)
Short stature, round facies, short metatarsals and metacarpals, subcutaneous calcifications, moderate mental retardation, cataracts, coarse and dry skin, brittle hair and nails, hypocalcemia, and hyperphosphatemia.

Turner syndrome
Short stature, tendency to obesity, ovarian dysgenesis, broad chest with widely spaced nipples, prominent ears, narrow maxilla and small mandible, low posterior hairline, webbed posterior neck, elbow and knee anomalies, nail and skin anomalies, renal anomalies, and hearing impairment.

From Online Mendelian Inheritance in Man.

Table 18   1989 Recommended Daily Dietary Allowance[1]

AGE (YEARS) & SEX GROUP	WEIGHT* (KG)	WEIGHT* (LB)	HEIGHT* (CM)	HEIGHT* (IN)	FAT-SOLUBLE VITAMINS VITA-MIN A (μg RE)**	VITA-MIN D (μg)***	VITA-MIN E (mg TE)†	VITA-MIN K (μg)	WATER-SOLUBLE VITAMINS VITA-MIN C (mg)	THIA-MIN (mg)	RIBO-FLAVIN (mg)	NIACIN (mg NE)‡	VITA-MIN B₆ (mg)	FO-LATE (μg)	VITA-MIN B₁₂ (μg)
Infants															
0.0–0.5	6	13	60	24	375	7.5	3	5	30	0.3	0.4	5	0.3	25	0.3
0.5–1.0	9	20	71	28	375	10	4	10	35	0.4	0.5	6	0.6	35	0.5
Children															
1–3	13	29	90	35	400	10	6	15	40	0.7	0.8	9	1.0	50	0.7
4–6	20	44	112	44	500	10	7	20	45	0.9	1.1	12	1.1	75	1.0
7–10	28	62	132	52	700	10	7	30	45	1.0	1.2	13	1.4	100	1.4
Males															
11–14	45	99	157	62	1000	10	10	45	50	1.3	1.5	17	1.7	150	2.0
15–18	66	145	176	69	1000	10	10	65	60	1.5	1.8	20	2.0	200	2.0
Females															
11–14	46	101	157	62	800	10	8	45	50	1.1	1.3	15	1.4	150	2.0
15–18	55	120	163	64	800	10	8	55	60	1.1	1.3	15	1.5	180	2.0

Adapted from the National Academy of Sciences-National Research Council.

[1]The allowances, expressed as average daily intakes over time, are intended to provide for individual variations among most normal persons as they live in the United States under usual environmental stresses. Diets should be based on a variety of common foods to provide other nutrients for which human requirements have been less well defined.

*The median weights and heights of those younger than 19 years were taken from Hammill PVV, et al. Physical growth: National Center for Health Statistics percentiles. **Am J Clin Nutr.** 1979;32:607–629. The use of these figures does not imply that the height-to-weight ratios are ideal.

**RE, retinol equivalent. 1 RE = 1 μg retinol or 6 μg beta-carotene.

***As cholecalciferol. 10 μg cholecalciferol = 400 IU of vitamin D.

†TE, alpha-tocopherol equivalents. 1 TE = 1 mg d-alpha-tocopherol.

‡NE, niacin equivalent. 1 NE = 1 mg of niacin or 60 mg of dietary tryptophan.

INFECTIOUS DISEASES

Table 19   Risk Factors for Group B Streptococcal Infection

Maternal risk factors
 Prolonged rupture of membranes (>18 hours)*
 Premature rupture of membranes (<37 weeks' gestation)*
 Preterm labor (<37 weeks' gestation)*
 Fever >37.9°C (100.4°F)*
 History of previous infant with GBS sepsis*
 Clinical evidence of chorioamnionitis
 GBS bacteriuria*
 Multiple gestation
 Diabetes
Fetal/neonatal risk factors
 Prematurity
 Meconium passed *in utero*
 Low 5-minute Apgar score (<6)
 Male gender (sepsis four times more common in boys than in girls)

GBS = group B streptococci.

*Risk necessitating intrapartum antibiotic administration per 1996 Centers for Disease Control (CDC) guidelines.

Table 20   Signs and Symptoms of Sepsis in the Newborn

Respiratory distress	Tachypnea (respiratory rate >60/min), grunting, nasal flaring, retractions; sometimes present even without an oxygen requirement or abnormal chest x-ray
Temperature instability	Fever >37.9°C or hypothermia
Poor feeding	Lack of interest, abdominal distention, vomiting, diarrhea
Altered neurologic status	Lethargy, irritability, hypotonia, seizures (especially if meningitis is present)
Apnea	Especially in preterm infants
Poor perfusion	Mottled, grayish, capillary refill >3 s
Tachycardia	Often a late sign
Bulging fontanelle	Meningitis

Table 21   Neutrophil Indices

NEUTROPHIL INDICES	NORMAL VALUES
Absolute neutrophil count (ANC)*	$>1800/mm^3$
Absolute band count (ABC)†	$<2000/mm^3$
I : T ratio‡	<0.2

*ANC = % total neutrophils × WBC count

†ABC = % bands × WBC count

‡I : T = % immature (bands, metamyelocytes, myelocytes): % total (immature + segmented) neutrophils

Table 22   Clinical Features Associated with Congenital Infection

Intrauterine growth retardation
Hydrops
Hepatosplenomegaly
Microcephaly, intracranial calcifications, hydrocephalus
Anemia, thrombocytopenia, petechiae
Jaundice (especially conjugated hyperbilirubinemia)
Pneumonitis
Cardiac malformations, myocarditis
Eye abnormalities (chorioretinitis, cataracts)
Bone abnormalities (osteochondritis, periostitis)

Table 23   Clinical Findings in Congenitally Infected Infants that Suggest a Specific Diagnosis

INFECTION	SUGGESTIVE FINDINGS
Rubella	Cataracts, cloudy cornea, pigmented retina
	"Blueberry muffin" syndrome
	Vertical striation
	Malformation (PDA, pulmonary artery stenosis)
CMV	Microcephaly with periventricular calcifications
	Inguinal hernias in boys
	Petechiae with thrombocytopenia
Toxoplasmosis	Hydrocephalus with generalized calcifications
	Chorioretinitis
Syphilis	Osteochondritis and periostitis
	Eczematoid skin rash
	Mucocutaneous lesions (snuffles)
Herpes	Skin vesicles
	Keratoconjunctivitis
	Acute CNS findings

Modified with permission from Stagno S, Pass RF, Alford CA: Perinatal infections and maldevelopment. In *The Fetus and the Newborn,* Volume 17, Series 1. Edited by Bloom AD, James LS. New York: Wiley-Liss, 1981.

CMV = cytomegalovirus; CNS = central nervous system; PDA = patent ductus arteriosus.

Table 24   Interpretation of EBV Serology*

	IgG-VCA	IgM-VCA	EBV NUCLEAR ANTIGEN	EBV EARLY ANTIGENS
No evidence of infection	<10	<10	<2	<10
Acute infection	>10	≥10	<2	≥20
Convalescent infection	>10	Variable	>2	Variable
Remote past infection	≥10	<10	>2	≤20

*Values are expressed in reciprocal titers as measured by standard immunofluorescence methods.

GASTROINTESTINAL

Table 25   Classic Clinical Findings in Disorders Characterized by Abdominal Pain

DISORDER	TYPICAL CLINICAL PICTURE	DEFINITIVE DIAGNOSTIC TEST
Peptic ulcer disease	Burning or sharp midepigastric pain that occurs 1–3 hours after meals and is exacerbated by spicy food and relieved by antacids; family history of peptic ulcer disease	Endoscopy
Pancreatitis	Episodic left upper quadrant pain that occurs 5–10 minutes after meals, radiates to the back, and is exacerbated by fatty foods	Pancreatic ultrasound or CT scan Serum amylase level ($\uparrow$)
Urinary tract infection	Suprapubic pain, burning on urination, urinary frequency, urinary urgency	Urine culture Urinalysis
Renal calculi	Severe periodic cramping pain that occurs in the flank and occasionally radiates to the groin; costovertebral angle tenderness; family history of renal calculi	Urinalysis Renal ultrasound
Periappendiceal abscess	Right lower quadrant pain; rebound and direct tenderness; anorexia and vomiting; fever	Barium enema Laparoscopy WBC count ($\uparrow$)
Gallbladder disease	Right upper quadrant pain that occurs 5–10 minutes after meals and is exacerbated by fatty foods; family history of gallstones	Gallbladder ultrasound
Menstrual pain	Cramping suprapubic pain that occurs during the menses	Trial with NSAIDs
Pelvic inflammatory disease (PID)	Suprapubic pain	Cervical culture
Functional abdominal pain (irritable bowel syndrome)	Cramping periumbilical pain that is exacerbated by eating and relieved by defecation	Trial with Metamucil
Lactose intolerance	Cramping periumbilical pain that increases following ingestion of dairy products and is accompanied by flatulence and bloating	Trial with a milk-free diet Breath hydrogen study for lactose deficiency
Inflammatory bowel disease	Right lower quadrant cramping and tenderness; anemia; guaiac-positive stool	Colonoscopy Barium enema Upper gastrointestinal series ESR ($\uparrow$), platelet count ($\uparrow$), WBC count ($\uparrow$)
Esophagitis	Epigastric and substernal pain that is relieved by antacids and exacerbated by lying down; history of iron deficiency; anemia; guaiac-positive stool	Endoscopy
Lead poisoning	Abdominal pain; history of pica; microcytic anemia; basophilic stippling	Serum lead level
Pancreatic pseudocyst	Left upper quadrant pain; recurrent vomiting; history of abdominal pain	Abdominal ultrasound
Sickle cell disease (SCD)	Periumbilical pain that responds to rest and rehydration	Sickle cell preparation Hemoglobin Electrophoresis
Abdominal epilepsy	Periodic severe abdominal pain that is often associated with seizures	Trial with anticonvulsants
Abdominal migraine	Severe abdominal pain; family history of migraine; recurrent headache, fever, and vomiting; unilateral or occipital headache; somatic complaints	Trial with antimigraine medications
Depression	Social withdrawal; decreased activity; irritability; poor attention span; difficulty sleeping	Trial with antidepressant medications
School avoidance	Nonspecific abdominal pain; severe anxiety reaction; pain that is more severe on weekdays and improves on weekends	

Modified with permission from Olson AD: Abdominal pain. In *Difficult Diagnosis in Pediatrics*. Edited by Stockman JA. Philadelphia: WB Saunders, 1990, p. 283.

ESR = erythrocyte sedimentation rate; NSAIDs = nonsteroidal anti-inflammatory drugs; WBC = white blood cell; $\uparrow$ = increased.

Table 26 Abdominal Masses Commonly Associated with Calcification

Neuroblastoma
Teratoma
  Ovarian
  Sacrococcygeal
Adrenal hematoma
Hepatic hemangioma
Meconium peritonitis

Table 27 Comparison of Functional Constipation and Hirschsprung Disease

	FUNCTIONAL CONSTIPATION	*HIRSCHSPRUNG DISEASE*
Symptoms as a newborn	Rare	Almost always
Late onset (after 3 years)	Common	Rare
Difficult bowel training	Common	Rare
Stool size	Large	Small, ribbonlike
Urge to defecate	Rare	Common
Obstructive symptoms	Rare	Common
Enterocolitis	Rare	Sometimes
Failure to thrive	Rare	Common
Abdominal distention	Rare	Common
Stool in rectal ampulla	Common	None
Barium enema	Copious stool No transition zone	Delayed evacuation Transition zone
Rectal biopsy	Normal	No ganglion cells Increased anticholinesterase staining
Anorectal manometry	Distention of rectum causes relaxation of the internal sphincter	No sphincter relaxation

Table 28 Commonly Used Pediatric Medications That May Cause Cholestasis and Hepatotoxicity

Anticonvulsants
  Phenobarbital
  Diphenylhydantoin
  Carbamazepine
  Valproic acid
Antimicrobials
  Tetracycline
  Erythromycin (estolate preparations)
  Sulfonamides
  Ketoconazole
  Isoniazid
  Rifampin
  Griseofulvin

Immunosuppressants
  Cyclosporine
  Azathioprine
  Methotrexate
Steroids
  Corticosteroids
  Androgens
  Oral contraceptives
Miscellaneous drugs
  Acetaminophen
  Salicylates
  Chlorpromazine
  Cimetidine
  Iron preparations (with overdosage)

A large number of less commonly encountered agents, including antineoplastic agents, antidepressants, antipsychotics, and tranquilizers can also cause cholestasis and hepatotoxicity.

Table 29 Defects in Hepatic Bilirubin Conjugation

DISEASE	*DEFECT*	*GENETICS*
Gilbert disease	Underactivity of the transferase, defective uptake of albumin-bound bilirubin from the plasma	Autosomal recessive
Crigler-Najjar syndrome		
Type I	Complete absence of the transferase enzyme	Autosomal recessive
Type II	Partial absence of the transferase enzyme (less severe than type I)	Autosomal dominant

Table 30 Foods and Drugs Mimicking Blood in the Stool

FALSE HEMATOCHEZIA	*FALSE MELENA*	*FALSE HEME-POSITIVE STOOLS*
Foods that contain red dye	Spinach	Red meat
Juice	Blueberries	Cherries
Candy	Licorice	Tomato skin
Kool-Aid	Purple grapes	Iron supplements
Jello	Chocolate	
Tomatoes	Grape juice	
Beets	Bismuth subsalicylate	
Cranberries	Iron supplements	

Table 31   Clinical Signs of Dehydration in Children

PARAMETER	MILD	MODERATE	SEVERE
Activity	Normal	Lethargic	Lethargic to comatose
Color	Pale	Gray	Mottled
Urine output	Decreased (<2–3 ml/kg/hr)	Oliguric (<1 ml/kg/hr)	Anuric
Fontanelle	Flat	Depressed	Sunken
Mucous membranes	Dry	Very dry	Cracked
Skin turgor	Slightly decreased	Markedly decreased	Tenting
Pulse	Normal to increased	Increased	Grossly tachycardic
Blood pressure	Normal	Normal	Decreased
Weight loss	5%	10%	15%

Hypernatremic dehydration may be accompanied by moderate clinical signs. Reprinted with permission from Rogers MC: Shock. In *Handbook of Pediatric Intensive Care*, 2nd ed. Edited by Rogers MC, Helfaer MA. Baltimore: Williams & Wilkins, 1994, p. 140.

Table 32   Therapy for Hyperlipidemia

TYPE	MECHANISM	REDUCTION IN CHOLESTEROL (%)	EFFECT ON VLDL	EFFECT ON HDL	SIDE EFFECT	DOSE
Nonpharmacological therapy						
American Heart Association diet	Limits exogenous cholesterol	10–15	Decrease	Decrease		N/A
Exercise	Improves insulin resistance	Some decrease	Decrease	Increase		N/A
Weight loss	Improves insulin resistance	Some decrease	Decrease	Mild increase		N/A
Pharmacological therapy						
Bile acid resins	Accelerate LDL disposal	20–30	Mild decrease	Mild increase	Epigastric distress, constipation, bloating, interferes with some drug absorption	Up to 24 g/day cholestyramine in divided doses
Nicotinic acid or niacin	Reduces VLDL and LDL synthesis increases HDL	25	50% decrease	30%–40% increase	Flushing, headache, tachycardia, gastrointestinal distress, activation of peptic ulcer disease and inflammatory bowel disease, hepatic dysfunction	Titrate up to 1 g 3 times/day
Probucol	Increases LDL disposal; reduces HDL/LDL	5–15		Decrease	Nausea, diarrhea, flatulence, eosinophelia, hepatic dysfunction, prolongation of QT interval	0.5 g 2 times/day
Gemfibrozil	Enhances VLDL breakdown; decreases VLDL production	Decrease	40%–50% decrease	20%–30% increase	Rarely myositis; should not be used in patients with renal disease, cholelithiasis, or liver dysfunction	600 mg 2 times/day
HMG CoA reductase inhibitor (lovastatin)	Inhibits cholesterol synthesis; increases LDL disposal	30–40			Elevated liver enzymes, myositis, cataracts in animals	20–40 mg 2 times/day

HDL indicates high-density lipoprotein; HMG CoA, 3-hydroxy-3-methylglutaryl coenzyme A; LDL, low-density lipoprotein; and VLDL, very-low-density lipoprotein.

HEPATIC

Table 32A   Expected Liver Span of Infants and Children

AGE (YR)	BOYS		GIRLS	
	MEAN ESTIMATED LIVER SPAN	STANDARD ERROR OF MEAN	MEAN ESTIMATED LIVER SPAN	STANDARD ERROR OF MEAN
6 mo	2.4	2.5	2.8	2.6
1	2.8	2.0	3.1	2.1
2	3.5	1.6	3.6	1.7
3	4.0	1.6	4.0	1.7
4	4.4	1.6	4.3	1.6
5	4.8	1.5	4.5	1.6
6	5.1	1.5	4.8	1.6
8	5.6	1.5	5.1	1.6
10	6.1	1.6	5.4	1.7
12	6.5	1.8	5.6	1.8
14	6.8	2.0	5.8	2.1
16	7.1	2.2	6.0	2.3
18	7.4	2.5	6.1	2.6
20	7.7	2.8	6.3	2.9

From Lawson EE, Grand RJ, Neff RK, et al.: Am J Dis Child 1978;132:475. Used by permission.

Table 32B   Review of Liver Function Tests

I. LIVER FUNCTION TESTS

AP	AST	ALT	GGT	5 = NUC
Liver	Hepatocyte	Hepatocyte	Placenta	Biliary
Bone	Muscle	Muscle	Pancreas	
Intestine			Kidney	
Placenta			Bile Ducts	
Tumors			Choroid	

II. "TRUE" LIVER FUNCTION TESTS:
Prothrombin time
Albumin
Bile acids and salts
Factor II, V, VII, IX, X
    Vitamin k-dependent factors: II, VII, IX, X

III. LIVER FUNCTION TESTS
Clinical pearls for daily use:

	ALKALINE PHOSPHATASE	g-GGT
Low	Zinc Deficiency	Bile Acid Deficiency
	Wilson Disease	
	Cystic Fibrosis	
High	See other list	Cholestasis, ICP

IV. LIVER FUNCTION TESTS
Clinical Pearls for Daily Use: Elevated transaminases and normal bilirubin, ggt and alkaline phosphatase

Table 32C   Clinical Disease States and Age of Presentation of Hepatomegaly

AGE	CLINICAL DISEASE STATES
Newborn (Birth–2 mo)	Intrauterine and intrapartum acquired infection (TORCH, syphilis, other) Erythroblastosis fetalis Neonatal hepatitis, α_1-antitrypsin, Alagille syndrome Biliary atresia Congestive heart failure Congenital paroxysmal atrial tachycardia Sepsis
Infant (2–12 mo)	Cystic fibrosis Metabolic disease: glycogen storage, α_1-antitrypsin deficiency, galactosemia, tyrosinemia, hereditary fructose intolerance, other Neonatal hepatitis, hepatitis B HIV infection (AIDS) Histiocytosis Malnutrition Tumors (intrinsic, metastatic) Cholelithiasis Choledochal cyst
Young child (1–6 yrs)	Viral hepatitis Drug-toxic hepatitis Parasitic Tumor Leukemia, lymphoma
Older child, adolescent (7–20 yrs)	Viral hepatitis Drug-toxic hepatitis Wilson disease Chronic active hepatitis Congenital hepatic fibrosis Focal nodular hyperplasia, adenoma α_1-Antitrypsis deficiency Reye syndrome Sicle cell anemia Cholelithiasis Juvenile rheumatoid arthritis, lupus erythematous, sarcoidosis Leukemia, lymphoma Gonococcal perihepatitis Cystic fibrosis Diabetes

Adapted from Walker, WA, Mathia RK: *Pediatr Clin North Am* 1975;22:929.

ELECTROLYTES

Table 33   Assessment of Hypernatremia

UNDERLYING CAUSE	ECF VOLUME	URINE OUTPUT	URINE SODIUM	SPECIFIC GRAVITY
Sodium excess	Increased	Normal or increased	Increased	High
Water loss (DI)	Decreased	Increased	Decreased	High
Sodium and water loss (water > sodium)	Normal or decreased	Decreased	Increased	Low

DI = diabetes insipidus; ECF = extracellular fluid.

Table 34 Assessment of Hyponatremia

IF URINE OUTPUT DECREASED AND UNa <20 mEq/L	*IF URINE OUTPUT DECREASED AND UNa >20 mEq/L*	*IF URINE OUTPUT NORMAL OR INCREASED AND UNa <20 mEq/L*	*IF URINE OUTPUT NORMAL OR INCREASED AND UNa >20 mEq/L*
Effective intravascular volume, consider: CHF, nephrotic syndrome, dehydration, liver disease, third spacing conditions	Renal failure or increased ADH	Water intoxication	Renal NaCL wasting Nonoliguric renal failure, adrenal insufficiency Osmotic diuretic use or osmotic diuresis

Table 35 Conditions Associated with Increased ADH/ADH-Like Effect and Hyponatremia

Pain
Vomiting
CNS disorders: including injuries, infection, tumors
Intrathoracic disorders: including infections, mechanical ventilation
Drugs: narcotics, barbiturates, carbamazepine, NSAIDs, cyclophosphamide, vincristine, others not commonly used in pediatrics

Table 36 Determinatin of Serum Osmolality

Reliable estimate under most circumstances:
   Serum osm = 2(Na mEq/L) + 10
Estimate when there is hyperglycemia or azotemia
   Serum osm = 2(Na) + glucose/18 + BUN/2.8

Table 37 Drugs Associated with Hyperkalemia

Potassium-sparing diuretics (e.g., spironolactone, triamterene, amiloride)
Potassium supplements (e.g., potassium chloride)
Potassium-containing penicillins
Stored blood
Cyclosporine
Nonsteroidal anti-inflammatory drugs (NSAIDs)
Heparin
Angiotensin-converting enzyme (ACE) inhibitors
β-adrenergic blockers
Chemotherapeutic agents

Table 38 Treatment of Hyperkalemia

AGENT	*INDICATION*	*MECHANISM OF ACTION*	*DOSE*	*SIDE EFFECTS/POTENTIAL PROBLEMS*
10% Calcium gluconate	ECG changes	Stabilizes membranes	1 mg/kg IV over 5–10 minutes	Hypercalcemia
Sodium bicarbonate	ECG changes or very high K⁺ level	Shifts K⁺ to intracellular compartment	1 mg/kg IV over 5–10 minutes	Sodium load
Glucose plus insulin	ECG changes or very high K⁺ level	Shifts K⁺ to intracellular compartment	0.25–0.5 gm/kg glucose plus 0.3 U insulin/gm glucose over 30–60 minutes	Hyper- or hypoglycemia
Kayexalate resin	To remove K⁺ from body	K⁺ binds to resin in gut	1 gm/kg PO or PR in 50%–70% sorbitol	Constipation
Furosemide	Symptomatic hyperkalemia	Enhances urinary K⁺ excretion	1–2 mg/kg IV	May not be enough renal function to be effective
Hemo- or peritoneal dialysis	No renal function	Removes K⁺ in dialysate	. . .	Risks associated with dialysis
Exchange transfusion	ECG changes or very high K⁺ level	Donor blood has had most K⁺ removed	Double volume	Risks associated with exchange transfusion

ECG = electrocardiogram; IV = intravenous; K⁺ = potassium; PO = orally; PR = parenterally.

Table 39 Drugs Associated with Hypokalemia

Drugs associated with increased renal loss
- Aminoglycoside toxicity
- Amphotericin B
- Cisplatin
- Penicillins in high doses
- Corticosteroids
- Diuretics (except for potassium-sparing ones)

Drugs associated with increased cellular uptake of potassium
- Terbutaline
- Epinephrine
- β-adrenergic agents (e.g., albuterol)
- Theophylline toxicity
- Barium toxicity
- Insulin

Table 40 Oral Potassium Supplements

PREPARATION	FORMULATION	POTASSIUM SUPPLIED
Potassium phosphate	Tablet	1.1, 2.3, or 3.7 mEq
Potassium chloride	Extentabs	10 mEq
	Powder packet	20 mEq
	Effervescent tablets	20 mEq
	Liquid	20 mEq
Potassium citrate	Tablets, crystals, or syrup	1 mEq/ml (Polycitra) or 2 mEq/ml (Polycitra-K)
Potassium gluconate	Liquid	20 mEq/15 ml

Table 41 Commonly Used Calcium Preparations

PREPARATION	ELEMENTAL CALCIUM CONTENT	ROUTE
Calcium gluconate (10%)	1 mL = 9 mg = 0.45 mEq	IV
Calcium chloride (10%)	1 mL = 27 mg = 1.36 mEq	IV
Calcium glubionate (Neocalglucon)	1 mL = 23 mg = 1.12 mEq	PO

Table 42 Calcium Needs

Maintenance clacium (not precisely known)	20–50 mg/kg/d (elemental calcium)
Emergency calcium (for severe symptoms)	10–20 mg/kg (elemental calcium) slow IV with cardiac monitor

RENAL

Table 43 Characteristics of Renal Tubular Acidosis

	TYPE 1	TYPE 2	TYPE 4
Renal function?	Normal	Normal	Normal or decreased
Failure to thrive?	Yes	Yes	Yes
Polyuria or polydipsia?	Yes	Yes	No
Potassium level?	Normal or low	Normal or low	Elevated
Bicarbonate leak?	Usually	Significant	Small
Urine maximally acid?	No (pH > 6)	Yes	Yes
Nephrocalcinosis or nephrolithiasis?	Yes	No	No
Fanconi syndrome?	No	Often	No
Osteomalacia or rickets?	Rarely	If Fanconi syndrome is present	No

Table 44   Toxins Removed by Hemodialysis

TOXIN	MEASURED LEVEL SUGGESTIVE OF NEED FOR HEMODIALYSIS*
Acetaminophen	>100 μg/ml in conjunction with antidote
Arsenic	Only with coexistent renal failure
Bromide	>150 mg/dl and severe symptoms
Chloral hydrate	250 mg/dl
Ethanol	500 mg/dl
Ethylene glycol	50 mg/dl
Isopropanol	400 mg/dl
Lithium	4 mEq/L in acute overdose
	As needed for severe symptoms in chronic overdose
Methanol	50 mg/dl
Salicylates	100–120 mg/dl in acute overdose
	60–800 mg/dl in chronic overdose

*The decision to perform hemodialysis should be based on physical findings as well as drug levels. A repeat measure should be obtained when the drug level is elevated to ensure that a laboratory error has not occurred. In addition, units of measured should be checked before instituting hemodialysis.

Table 45   Toxins Removed by Charcoal Hemoperfusion*

TOXIN	MEASURED LEVEL SUGGESTIVE OF NEED FOR CHARCOAL HEMOPERFUSION
Amitriptyline	Based on signs and symptoms
Chloral hydrate	250 mg/dl
Digitoxin	50 ng/ml with antidotal therapy
Digoxin	15 ng/ml with antidotal therapy
Ethchlorvinyl	150 μg/ml
Glutethimide	40 mg/L
Methaqualone	40 μg/ml
Nortriptyline	Based on signs and symptoms
Pentobarbital	50 mg/L
Phenobarbital	100 mg/L
Theophylline	100 μg/ml in acute overdose
	60 μg/ml in chronic overdose

*The decision to perform hemoperfusion should be based on physical findings as well as drug levels. A repeat measure should be obtained when the drug level is elevated to ensure that a laboratory error has not occurred. In addition, units of measured should be checked before instituting hemodialysis.

Table 46   Normal Values for Fractional Excretion of Sodium (Fe$_{Na}$)

	PRERENAL ARF	INTRINSIC ARF
Adult or child	<1.0	>2.0
Infant (neonate)	<2.5	>2.5

ARF = acute renal failure.

Table 47   Causes of False-Positive Dipstick Reactions for Urinary Protein

Overlong immersion
Placing reagent strip directly in the urine
  stream
Alkaline urinary pH (pH >7.0)
Quaternary ammonium compounds and
  detergents
Pyuria
Bacteriuria
Mucoprotein

Table 48   Drugs that May Cause Hemolytic Anemia in Patients Who Have G6PD Deficiency

Acetanilid	Nitrofurantoin
Doxorubicin	Primaquine
Methylene blue	Pamaquine
Naphthalene	Sulfa drugs

PULMONARY

Table 49   Characteristics of the Three Stages of Parapneumonic Pleural Effusions

	EXUDATIVE STAGE	_FIBRINOLYTIC STAGE_	_ORGANIZING STAGE (EMPYEMA)_
Appearance	Nonpurulent, not turbid	Nonpurulent, not turbid	Purulent, turbid
Fluid consistency	Free flowing	Loculated	Organized
Gram stain and culture results	Negative	Transitional	Positive (before antibiotic treatment)
Glucose	>100 mg/dl	<50 mg/dl	<50 mg/dl
Protein	<3 g/dl	>3 g/dl	>3 g/dl
pH	>7.30	<7.30	<7.30
WBCs	Few	PMNs	PMNs

PMNs = polymorphonuclear neutrophils; WBCs = white blood cells.

Table 50   Pleural Fluid Diagnostic Studies

STUDY	_TRANSUDATE_	_EXUDATE_
Biochemical		
Pleural LDH	<200 IU	≥200 IU
Pleural fluid/serum LDH ratio[a]	<0.6	≥0.6
Pleural fluid/serum protein ratio[a]	<0.5	≥0.5
Specific gravity	<1.016	≥1.016
Protein level	<3.0 g/dl	≥3.0 g/dl
Other studies		
Glucose	_Usually_ >40 mg/dl	_Typically_ <40 mg/dl
Amylase	May be elevated in some neoplasms, GI trauma, or surgery	
Rheumatoid factor, LE prep, ANA	Are occasionally helpful if collagen vascular disorders are within the differential	
Hematologic		
WBC count	Although high counts (>100/mm³) are suggestive of an exudate, the results are quite variable	
WBC differential	May actually provide more useful information	
Lymphocyte count	May be elevated in neoplasms, tuberculosis, and some fungal infections	
Segmented neutrophils	May be elevated in bacterial infections, connective tissue disease, pancreatitis, or pulmonary infarction	
Eosinophil count	May be elevated in bacterial infections, neoplasms, and connective tissue diseases	
RBC count	If >100,000/mm³, is suggestive of trauma, neoplasms, or pulmonary infarction	
Cytology & chromosomal studies	May show evidence of malignant cells or chromosomal abnormalities	
Microbiology		
Gram stain		
Fluid culture for aerobes and anaerobes		
Acid-fast stain (if tuberculosis is in the differential)		
Fungal culture		
Viral culture		
Counterimmune electrophoresis (may aid in the detection of a bacterial infection)		

[a]These tests are more reliable in differentiating transudate from exudate than specific gravity or protein level.

Table 51 Normal Blood Gas Values from the Children's Hospital of Philadelphia Blood Gas Laboratory

PARAMETER	AGE OF PATIENT	NORMAL VALUE
pH	1 day	7.29–7.45
	3–24 months	7.34–7.46
	>7 years	7.37–7.41
Pco_2	1 day	27–40 mm Hg
	3–24 months	26–42 mm Hg
	>7 years	34–40 mm Hg
Po_2	1 day	37–97 mm Hg
	3–24 months	88–103 mm Hg
	>7 years	88–103 mm Hg
Base excess	1 day	>8–(−2)
	3–24 months	−7–0
	>7 years	−4–(+2)
HCO_3	1 day	19 mmol/L
	3–24 months	16/24 mmol/L
	>7 years	22–27 mmol/L
O_2 saturation	...	94%–99%
Venous pH	...	7.32–7.42
Venous CO_2		25–47 mm Hg
Venous O_2		25–47 mm Hg

CO_2 = carbon dioxide; HCO_3 = bicarbonate; O_2 = oxygen; Pco_2 = carbon dioxide tension; Po_2 = oxygen tension.

Table 52 Signs of Inhalation Injury

PULMONARY	CNS	SKIN
Tachypnea	Confusion	Facial burns
Stridor	Dizziness	Singed nasal hairs
Hoarseness	Headache	Cyanosis
Rales	Hallucinations	Cherry red color
Wheezing	Restlessness	
Cough	Coma	
Retractions	Seizures	
Nasal flaring		
Carbonaceous sputum		

CARDIOVASCULAR

Table 54 Common Causes of Abnormally Wide Splitting of the Second Heart Sound (S_2)

Atrial septal defect (ASD)
Mild pulmonic stenosis
Complete right bundle branch block
Left ventricular paced beats
Massive pulmonary embolus

Table 53 Pulmonary Function Test

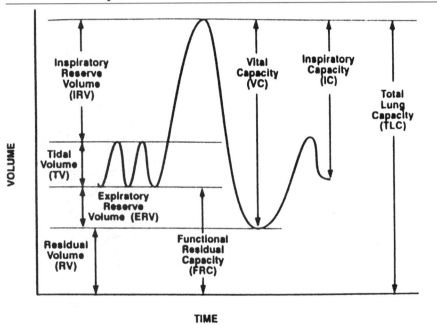

Table 55   Conditions Causing a Prominent Third Heart Sound (S_3)

Physiologic (infants and children)
Congestive heart failure (CHF)
Ventricular septal defect, with large pulmonary to systemic flow ($\dot{Q}p : \dot{Q}s$) ratio
Mitral insufficiency
Tricuspid insufficiency
Hyperdynamic ventricle with high output (e.g., anemia, thyrotoxicosis, arteriovenous fistula)

Table 56   Conditions Causing a Prominent Fourth Heart Sound (S_4)

Left ventricular outflow tract obstruction (e.g., aortic stenosis)
Right ventricular outflow tract obstruction (e.g., pulmonic stenosis)
Hypertrophic cardiomyopathy
Heart block (atrium contracting against a closed valve)

Table 57   Drugs Associated with Rapid Heart Rates

Prescription drugs
   β-adrenergic agonists (e.g., albuterol)
   Methylxanthines (e.g., theophylline)
   Tricyclic antidepressants (e.g., imipramine)
   Nonsedating histamines (e.g., terfenadine)
Over-the-counter drugs
   Decongestants (e.g., pseudoephedrine)
   Diet aids (phenylpropanolamine)
   Inhaled bronchodilators (e.g., albuterol)
   Caffeine-containing products
Drugs of abuse
   Nicotine
   Cocaine
   Amphetamines
   Alcohol
   Marijuana
   LSD
   Phencyclidine
   Amyl nitrate

Table 58   Causes of Prolonged QT Interval

Congenital
  Hereditary
    Jervell and Lange-Neilsen syndrome: long QT interval, stress-induced syncope, congenital nerve deafness, autosomal recessive inheritance
    Romano-Ward syndrome: long QT interval, stress-induced syncope, autosomal dominant inheritance (usually incomplete penetrance)
  Sporadic
Acquired
  Electrolyte abnormalities
    Hypocalcemia
    Hypomagnesemia
  Metabolic disturbances
    Malnutrition
    Liquid protein diets
  Drugs
    Phenothiazines (e.g., haloperidol)
    Tricyclic antidepressants (e.g., imipramine)
    Nonsedating antihistamines (e.g., terfenadine)
    Class Ia antiarrhythmic agents (e.g., quinidine)
    Class III antiarrhythmic agents (e.g., amiodarone)
  CNS trauma
  Cardiac abnormalities
    Ischemia
    Mitral valve prolapse
    Myocarditis
  Intraventricular conduction abnormalities
    Bundle branch blocks

Table 59 Structural Heart Disease Associated with Tachycardia

DEFECT	*TYPE OF TACHYCARDIA*
Congenital heart disease	
Mitral valve prolapse	SVT, VT
Aortic valve stenosis or regurgitation	VT
Ebstein anomaly of the tricuspid valve	SVT (WPW) commonly, VT less commonly
Tetralogy of Fallot	VT
Mustard/Senning repair of D-TGA	SVT (particularly atrial flutter)
Fontan repair of single ventricle	SVT (particularly atrial flutter)
Cardiomyopathy	
Hypertrophic cardiomyopathy	SVT, VT
Dilated cardiomyopathy	SVT, VT
Arrhythmogenic right ventricular dysplasia	VT (monomorphic, left bundle branch block)
Miscellaneous causes	
Eisenmenger complex (pulmonary vascular disease and pulmonary hypertension)	VT
Cardiac tumor (atrial myxoma, rhabdomyosarcoma)	SVT, VT (depending on tumor site)

D-TGA = D-transposition of the great arteries; SVT = supraventricular tachycardia; VT = ventricular tachycardia; WPW = Wolff-Parkinson-White syndrome.

Table 60 Poisons Causing Tachycardia

Tachycardia and hypertension
  Amphetamines
  Antihistamines
  Cocaine
  LSD/PCP
Tachycardia and hypotension
  β_2-adrenergic agonists
    Albuterol
    Terbutaline
  Carbon monoxide
  Cyclic antidepressants
  Hydralazine
  Iron
  Phenothiazines
  Theophylline
  Any agent causing vomiting, diarrhea, or hemorrhage

LSD = lysergic acid diethylamide; PCP = phencyclidine hydrochloride.

Table 61 Poisons Causing Bradycardia

Bradycardia and hypertension
  α-Adrenergic agonists
    Phenylpropanolamine
    Ephedrine
  Clonidine
  Ergotamine
Bradycardia and hypotension
  α_1-Adrenergic antagonists
    Phentolamine
    Prazosin
  α_1-Adrenergic agonists
    Clonidine
    Tetrahydrozoline
  β-adrenergic antagonists
    Propranolol
    Atenolol
    Metoprolol
  Calcium channel blockers
  Digitalis-containing drugs and plants
  Narcotics
  Organophosphate pesticides
  Sedative/hypnotics

Table 62 Poisons Causing Cardiac Arrhythmias

Atrioventricular block
  Astemizole
  β-Adrenergic antagonists
  Calcium channel blockers
  Clonidine
  Cyclic antidepressants
  Digitalis-containing drugs and plants
Ventricular tachycardia
  Amphetamines
  Carbamazepine
  Chloral hydrate
  Chlorinated hydrocarbons
  Cocaine
  Cyclic antidepressants
  Digitalis-containing drugs or plants
  Phenothiazines (especially thioridazine)
  Theophylline
  Type Ia antiarrhythmic agents
    Quinidine
    Procainamide
  Type Ic antiarrhythmic agents
    Flecainide
    Encainide
Torsades de pointes (multifocal ventricular tachycardia)
  Amantadine
  Cyclic antidepressants
  Lithium
  Nonsedating antihistamines
    Astemizole
    Terfenadine
  Quinidine
  Phenothiazines
  Sotalol

Table 63 Revised Jones Criteria for Diagnosis of Acute Rheumatic Fever

MAJOR CRITERIA	MINOR CRITERIA
Carditis	Fever
Arthritis	Arthralgia
Rash (erythema marginatum)	Elevated ESR, CRP
Chorea (Sydenham)	Prolonged PR interval on ECG
Subcutaneous nodules	History of prior attack of rheumatic fever or rheumatic heart disease

Diagnosis is likely with the presence of two major and one minor criteria, or one major and two minor criteria. Supporting evidence of a preceding streptococcal infection includes a history of recent scarlet fever, a positive throat culture for group A *Streptococcus,* and an increased antistreptolysin O (ASO) titer (or titers for other streptococcal antibodies). (Adapted from The Report of the ad hoc Committee of the American Heart Association Council on Rheumatic Fever and Congenital Heart Disease. *Circulation* 69:204A–208A, 1984.)

CRP = C-reactive protein; ECG = electrocardiogram; ESR = erythrocyte sedimentation rate.

MUSCULOSKELETAL

Table 64 Range of Motion of Major Joints

	FLEXION	EXTENSION	ABDUCTION	ADDUCTION	INTERNAL ROTATION	EXTERNAL ROTATION
Hip	120°	30°	50°	30°	35°	45°
Knee	135°	5°	0°	0°	10°	10°
Ankle	50°	20°	10°	20°	5° (eversion)	5° (inversion)
Shoulder	90°	45°	180°	45°	55°	45°
Elbow	135°	5°	0°	0°	90° (supination)	90° (pronation)
Wrist	80°	70°	20° (radial)	30° (lunar)	0°	0°

Table 65 Characteristics of Synovial Fluid

	APPEARANCE	WBC/MM²	% NEUTROPHILS	% GLUCOSE SYNOVIAL BLOOD
Normal	Clear	<2000	<40	>50
Infectious	Turbid	>75,000	>75	<50
Inflammatory (JRA, SLE)	Clear/turbid	5000–75,000	50	≥50
Traumatic	Bloody/clear	<5000	<50	>50

Table 66 Relationship Between Short Stature, Bone Age, and Growth Velocity[a]

Bone age delayed—normal growth velocity	Constitutional short stature
Bone age normal—normal growth velocity	Genetic short stature
Bone age delayed—delayed growth velocity	Organic diseases

[a]Velocity = the rate of growth during a year.

ENDOCRINOLOGY

Table 67 Clinical and Biochemical Features of Congenital Adrenal Hyperplasia (CAH)

| | SEXUAL AMBIGUITY | | | |
ENZYME DEFECT	FEMALE	MALE	ADDITIONAL CLINICAL MANIFESTATIONS	PREDOMINANT STEROIDS
Desmolase	−	+	Salt wasting	. . .
3β-Hydroxysteroid dehydrogenase	+	+	Salt wasting	17-OH-Pregnenolone, DHEA
21-Hydroxylase	+	−	Salt wasting	17-OH-Progestone, androstenedione
11-Hydroxylase	+	−	Hypertension	11-Deoxycortisol
17-Hydroxylase	−	+	Hypertension	DOC, corticosterone

DHEA = dehydroepiandrosterone; DOC = deoxycorticosterone.

Table 68 Normal Serum Adrenal Steroid Levels in Newborn Infants

| | PRETERM SICK | | PRETERM WELL | FULL TERM |
STEROID	24–28 WEEKS	31–35 WEEKS	31–35 WEEKS	
Cortisol (μg/dl)	7.5 ± 4	6 ± 2.7	6.9 ± 3.8	6.2 ± 3.9
17-OH-Preg (ng/dl)	1794 ± 1818	1395 ± 694	942 ± 739	245 ± 291
17-OH-Pro (ng/dl)	651 ± 661	373 ± 317	169 ± 95	36 ± 13*
11-deoxycortisol (ng/dl)	662 ± 548	294 ± 239	111 ± 62	87 ± 42
DHEA (ng/dl)	1872 ± 4038	675 ± 502	920 ± 1227	286 ± 238
DHEAS (μg/dl)	467 ± 312	459 ± 209	341 ± 93	162 ± 88
Androstenedione (ng/dl)	479 ± 1032	206 ± 86	215 ± 134	149 ± 67

Data based on information in Lee MM, Rajabopalan L, Berg G, et al.: Serum adrenal steroid concentrations in premature infants. *J Clin Endocrinol Metab* 69:1133–1136, 1989, and in Wiener D, Smith J, Dahlem S, et al.: Serum adrenal steroid levels in healthy term 3-day-old infants. *J Pediatr* 110(1):122–124, 1987.

17-OH-Preg = 17-OH-pregnenolone; 17-OH-Pro = 17-OH-progesterone; DHEA = dehydroepiandrosterone; DHEAS = dehydroepiandrosterone sulfate.

*17-OH-Pro values in full-term sick newborns may be double or triple the baseline values. No data are available for other steroid hormones in sick full-term infants.

Table 69 Pharmacokinetics of Common Insulin Preparations

INSULIN PREPARATION	ONSET (HOURS)	PEAK (HOURS)	DURATION OF ACTION (HOURS)
Ultra-rapid-acting (Lispro)	0.25–0.50	1–2	2–3
Short-acting (Regular, Semilente)	0.5–1.0	2–4	4–6
Long-acting (NPH, Lente)	2–4	6–12	18–24
Very long-acting (Ultralente)	6–10	18–24	24–36

NPH = neutral protein Hagedorn insulin.

Table 70 Normal Thyroid Hormone Levels

T_4	Total	7.0–15.0 μg/dL
	Free	0.8–2.3 ng/dL
T_3		100–250 ng/dL
TSH		0.5–5.0 μg/mL

Table 71   Normal Ranges for Gonadotropin and Sex Steroid Levels: Females

	LH (mIU/ml)	FSH (mIU/ml)	ESTRADIOL (ng/dl)	TESTOSTERONE (ng/dl)
0–1 year	0.02–7.0	0.24–14.2	0.5–5.0	<10
Prepubertal	0.02–0.3	1.0–4.2	<1.5	<3–10
Tanner 2	0.02–4.7	1.0–10.8	1.0–2.4	7.0–28
Tanner 3	0.10–12.0	1.5–12.8	0.7–6.0	15–35
Tanner 4	0.4–11.7	1.5–11.7	2.1–8.5	13–32
Tanner 5	0.4–11.7	1.0–9.2	3.4–17.0	20–38
Adult	. . .	. . .	. . .	10–55
Follicular phase	2.0–9.0	1.8–11.2	3.0–10.0	. . .
Mid-cycle	18.0–49	6.0–35.0	. . .	. . .
Luteal phase	2.0–11.0	1.8–11.2	7.0–30.0	. . .

FSH = follicle-stimulating hormone; LH = luteinizing hormone.

Table 72   Normal Ranges for Gonadotropin and Sex Steroid Levels: Males

	LH (mIU/ml)	FSH (mIU/ml)	ESTRADIOL (ng/dl)	TESTOSTERONE (ng/dl)
0–1 year	0.02–7.0	0.16–4.1	1.0–3.2	<10
Prepubertal	0.02–0.3	0.26–3.0	<1.5	<3–10
Tanner 2	0.2–4.9	1.8–3.2	0.5–1.6	18–150
Tanner 3	0.2–5.0	1.2–5.8	0.5–2.5	100–320
Tanner 4	0.4–7.0	2.0–9.2	1.0–3.6	200–620
Tanner 5	0.4–7.0	2.6–11.0	1.0–3.6	350–970
Adult	1.5–9.0	2.0–9.2	0.8–3.5	350–1030

FSH = follicle-stimulating hormone; LH = leuteinizing hormone.

Table 73   Classification of Total and LDL Cholesterol Levels in Children and Adolescents from Families with Hypercholesterolemia or Premature Cardiovascular Disease

CATEGORY	TOTAL CHOLESTEROL, mg/dL	LDL CHOLESTEROL, mg/dL
Acceptable	<170	<110
Borderline	170–199	110–129
High	≥200	≥130

NEUROLOGIC

Table 74   Causes of Ataxia

FORM OF ATAXIA	MAJOR CAUSES	OTHER CAUSES
Acute ataxia	Ingestion	Migraine
	Postinfectious cerebellitis	Neuroblastoma
Acute recurrent ataxia	Migraine	. . .
	Metabolic disease	
Chronic ataxia	Congenital disorders with mental deficiency	. . .
Chronic progressive ataxia	Brain tumors	Ataxia-telangiectasia
	Neuroectodermal tumors	Friedreich ataxia

Table 75   Glasgow Coma Scale

Eyes open		Best motor response	
Spontaneously	4	Obey commands	6
To speech	3	Localize pain	5
To pain	2	Withdrawal	4
None	1	Flexion to pain	3
Best verbal response		Extension to pain	2
Oriented	5	None	1
Confused	4		
Inappropriate	3		
Incomprehensible	2		
None	1		

Adapted from Fleisher G, Ludwig S, eds. *Textbook of Pediatric Emergency Medicine*, 3rd ed. Baltimore: Williams & Wilkins, 1993:272.

Table 76   Glasgow Coma Scale (GCS) for Adults and Children and Modified Score for Infants

	GLASGOW COMA SCORE (ADULTS/OLDER CHILDREN)		MODIFIED GLASGOW COMA SCORE (INFANTS)
Eye opening	Spontaneous	4	Spontaneous
	To verbal stimuli	3	To speech
	To pain	2	To pain
	None	1	None
Best verbal response	Oriented	5	Coos and babbles
	Confused speech	4	Irritable, cries
	Inappropriate words	3	Cries to pain
	Non-specific sounds	2	Moans to pain
	None	1	None
Best motor response	Follows commands	6	Normal spontaneous movements
	Localizes pain	5	Withdraws to touch
	Withdraws to pain	4	Withdraws to pain
	Flexes to pain	3	Abnormal flexion
	Extends to pain	2	Abnormal extension
	None	1	None

Table 77   Drugs that Can Cause Delirium or Coma

DRUG	PHYSICAL FINDINGS
Barbiturates	Small, reactive pupils; hypothermia; flaccidity; doll's eye reflex may be absent
Opiates	Pinpoint, reactive pupils; hypothermia; hypotension; hypoventilation; bradycardia
Psychedelics	Small, reactive pupils; hypertension; hyperventilation; dystonic posturing
Amphetamines	Dilated pupils, hyperthermia, hypertensison, tachycardia, arrhythmia
Cocaine	Dilated pupils, hyperthermia, tachycardia
Atropine-scopolamine	Dilated pupils; hyperthermia; flushing; hot, dry skin; supraventricular tachycardia
Glutethimide	Midposition, irregular fixed pupils; hypothermia; flaccidity
Tricyclic antidepressants	Hyperthermia, hypotension, supraventricular tachycardia
Phenothiazines	Hypotension, arrhythmia, dystonia
Methaqualone	Same as with barbiturates; if severe tachycardia, dystonia

Reprinted with permission from Packer RJ, Berman PH: Coma. In *Textbook of Pediatric Emergency Medicine*, 3rd ed. Edited by Fleisher GR, Ludwig S. Baltimore: Williams & Wilkins, 1993, p. 126.

Table 78   Prognostic Indicators of Poor Neurologic Outcome in Near-Drowning Victims*

At the scene
  Submersion time >4–10 minutes
  Delay in beginning CPR
  Resuscitation >25 minutes
In the emergency department
  Necessity for CPR
  Fixed, dilated pupils
  pH <7.0
  GCS score <5
After initial resuscitation
  Persistent GCS score <5
  Persistent apnea

CPR = cardiopulmonary resuscitation; GCS = Glasgow coma scale.

*Applies to victims of warm water near-drownings only. Hypothermic victims of cold water near-drownings may have a better prognosis.

Table 79   Relationship of the Lesion to the Physical Findings

LESION	*FINDINGS*
Upper motor neuron involving corticospinal tract, thalamus, centrum, semiovale, motor cortex	Altered, normal or increased reflexes, bulk normal; strength normal or decreased
Cerebellum	Uncoordinated
Spinal (upper and lower motor)	Local pain, bowel and bladder dysfunction, if anterior horn cells involved, weakness and bulk, decreased absent reflexes, fasciculations
Peripheral	Loss of distal muscles, fasciculations less than spinal lesions; sensation is affected
Muscle	Weakness, muscle atrophy, decreased reflexes, pain, cramping, stiffness
Corticospinal tract	Increased tone, clasp knife character in flexion of arms and extension of legs
Extrapyramidal (basal ganglia)	Rigidity, normal reflexes, absent Babinski, voluntary movement is preserved, may have tremor, chorea, athetosis or dystonia

Table 80   Poisons Causing Coma

Coma with miosis
    Barbiturates and other sedative/hypnotics
    Bromide
    Chloral hydrate
    Clonidine
    Ethanol
    Narcotics
    Organophosphates
    PCP
    Phenothiazines
    Tetrahydrozoline
Coma with mydriasis
    Atropine/diphenoxylate
    Carbon monoxide
    Cyanide
    Cyclic antidepressants
    Glutethimide
    LSD

LSD = lysergic acid diethylamide; PCP = phencyclidine hydrochloride.

Table 81   Poisons Causing Seizures

Amoxapine
Amphetamines
Anticonvulsants
    Phenytoin
    Carbamazepine
Antihistamines and anticholinergic drugs or plants
Camphor
Carbon monoxide
Chlorinated hydrocarbons
Cocaine
Cyanide
Cyclic antidepressants
Isoniazid
Lead
Lidocaine
Meperidine
PCP
Phenothiazines
Phenylpropanolamine
Propoxyphene
Propranolol
Theophylline

PCP = phencyclidine hydrochloride.

Table 82   Differential Diagnosis of Metabolic Neurologic Dysfunction

PROMINENT SYMPTOM	DIAGNOSES TO CONSIDER	DIAGNOSTIC TEST	METABOLIC THERAPY
Myoclonic seizures	Ceroid	DNA, tissue EM	
	Lafora body disease	Muscle biopsy	
	Prion (GSS)	DNA	
	Mitochondrial	DNA, muscle biopsy	CoQ, other vitamins
	Aminoacidopathies	Blood biochemistry	Dietary
	Biotinidase deficiency	Blood biochemistry	Biotin supplement
	Organic acidurias	Blood biochemistry	Dietary, vitamins
Stroke	Homocystinuria	Blood/urine test	B vitamins, betaine
	Mitochondrial	DNA, muscle biopsy	
Coma	Organic aciduria	Blood/urine test	
	MSUD	Blood/urine test	
	Hyperammonemias	Blood test	Dietary
Spasticity	Leukodystrophy	MRI, fibroblast analysis	Dietary
Visual loss	Leukodystrophy	MRI	
	Mitochondrial	DNA, muscle biopsy	
Psychosis	Leukodystrophy	MRI, blood biochemistry, DNA, fibroblast analysis	
	Porphyria	Blood/urine	Avoid precipitants
		Biochemistry	
	Wilson disease	Copper excretion, DNA	Penicillamine
	Homocystinuria	Blood biochemistry	(see above)
	Ceroid	DNA, tissue electron microscopy	
	Huntington disease	DNA	
Microcephaly	Ceroid	DNA, tissue EM	
	Rett syndrome	(-clinical features)	
	Krabbe disease	Blood biochemistry	
Macrocephaly	Storage disorders	DNA, blood biochemistry	
	Canavan disease	Urine biochemistry, DNA	
Neuropathy	Krabbe disease	MRI & blood biochemistry	
	Metachromatic leukodystrophy		
	Porphyria	Blood/urine biochemistry	
	Mitochondrial	DNA, muscle biopsy	
	Friedreich ataxia	(-clinical features)	
	Abetalipoproteinemia		
	Disorders/deficiency of vitamin E	Blood biochemistry	Vitamin E
	Mitochondrial	Vitamin E level	Vitamin E
	Neuroaxonal dystrophy	DNA, muscle biopsy	
		MRI, nerve biopsy	
Myopathy	Fukuyama disease	MRI	
	Mitochondrial	DNA, muscle biopsy	
	Lactic acidoses	Blood biochemistry	
Ataxia	Ataxia telangiectasia	DNA	
	Leukodystrophies	MRI, blood biochemistry	
	Friedreich		
	Mitochondrial	(clinical features)	
	Hartnup	DNA, muscle biopsy	
	Hyperammonemias	Blood biochemistry	
	Abetalipoproteinemia	Blood biochemistry	
	Sphingolipidoses	Blood biochemistry	
	Machado-Joseph, SCA-1 (hereditary ataxias)	Blood biochemistry, fibroblast analysis, DNA	

Table 83   Acquired Disorders Associated with Progressive Neurologic Dysfunction

STRUCTURAL	*HORMONAL*	*INFECTIOUS*	*ENVIRONMENTAL*	*TOXIC*	*IMMUNOLOGIC*
Hydrocephalus	Hypothyroidism	SSPE	Malnutrition/malabsorption syndromes	Lead	Demyelination/multiple sclerosis
Brain tumor	Congenital adrenal hyperplasia (visuospatia 1 deficits)	HIV	Vitamin/trace element deficiency (niacin, thiamine, folic acid, vitamin E, B12, essential fatty acids)	Organic chemicals	Opsoclonus/myoclonus or cerebellar ataxia (neuroblastoma)
Vascular anomalies		Spirochetes	Physical abuse/neglect	Carbon monoxide	Sydenham chorea
				Cocaine, hallucinogens, hypnotics	Rasmussen encephalitis
				Phenytoin (cerebellar degeneration)	

Table 84   Epidural versus Acute Subdural Hematoma

	EPIDURAL HEMATOMA	*SUBDURAL HEMATOMA*
Common mechanism	Blunt direct trauma, frequently to parietal region	Acceleration–deceleration injury
Etiology	Arterial or venous	Venous (bridging veins below dura)
Incidence	Uncommon	Common
Peak age	Usually >2 years	Usually <1 year Peak at 6 months
Location	Unilateral Commonly parietal	75% Bilateral Diffuse, over cerebral hemispheres
Skull fracture	Common	Uncommon
Associated seizures	Uncommon	Common
Retinal hemorrhages	Rare	Common
Decreased level of consciousness	Common	Almost always
Mortality	Rare	Uncommon
Morbidity in survivors	Low	High
Clinical findings	Dilated ipsilateral pupil, contralateral hemiparesis Period of lucidity prior to acute decompensation and rapid progression to herniation	Decreased level of consciousness Irritability, lethargy
Onset	Acute	Acute (within 24 hours), subacute (within 1 day–2 weeks), or chronic (after 2 weeks)
Findings on CT	Convex "lens-shaped" cerebral hemisphere	Concave, diffusely surrounding cerebral hemisphere

CT = computed tomography.

GYNECOLOGICAL

Table 85 Age-related Prevalence of Principal Laparoscopic Findings in 121 Adolescent Females 11 to 17 Years Old with Acute Pelvic Pain (The Children's Hospital, Boston, 1980–1986)

DIAGNOSIS	NUMBER OF PATIENTS		
	AGE 11–13	AGE 14–15	AGE 16–17
Ovarian cyst	12 (50%)	16 (35%)	19 (37%)
Acute pelvic inflammatory disease	4 (17%)	7 (16%)	10 (19%)
Adnexal torsion	0 (0%)	7 (16%)	2 (4%)
Endometriosis	0 (0%)	2 (4%)	4 (7%)
Ectopic pregnancy	0 (0%)	3 (7%)	1 (2%)
Appendicitis	3 (13%)	4 (9%)	6 (12%)
No pathology	5 (20%)	6 (13%)	10 (19%)
Total	24 (20%)	45 (37%)	52 (43%)

From Goldstein DP: Acute and chronic pelvic pain. *Pediatr Clin North Am* 36(3):576, 1989.

Table 86 Key Characteristics of Vaginal Discharges

	PRESENTING SYMPTOMS	DISCHARGE	NONMENSTRUAL pH	AMINE/ WHIFF TEST	VAGINAL SMEAR	TREATMENT
Nonspecific vaginitis	Foul-smelling discharge Itching	Scant to copius Brown to green in color	Variable	Negative	Leukocytes Bacteria and other debris	Improved perineal hygiene
Physiologic leukorrhea	None	Variable Scant to moderate Clear to white	<4.5	Negative	Normal epithelial cells Lactobacilli predominate	None
Bacterial vaginosis	Foul-smelling discharge	Gray-white	>4.7	Positive	Epithelial cells with bacteria ("clue cells") Gram-negative rods	Metronidazole Clindamycin
Candidiasis	Severe itching Vulvar inflammation	White, "curd-like"	<4.5	Negative	Fungal hyphae and buds	Topical or intravaginal imidazoles, triazoles Oral ketoconazole
Trichomonal vaginitis	Copious discharge Itching	Profuse Yellow to green	5.0–6.0	Occasionally present	Motile flagellated organisms	Metronidazole
Foreign body	Foul-smelling discharge	Foul-smelling Purulent Dark brown	Variable (usually >4.7)	Occasionally present	Leukocytes Epithelial cells with bacteria and debris	Remove foreign body Irrigate vagina
Contact vulvovaginitis	Vulvar inflammation Itching Edema	Scant White to yellow	Variable (usually <4.5)	Negative	Leukocytes Epithelial cells	Remove irritant Topical steroids

Table 87 Emergency Contraceptive Pills

INSTRUCTIONS FOR USE

Any of the birth control pills listed below can be used as ECPs. Use only the type of pill your health-care provider prescribed for you. Use only one type of pill.

IF YOU ARE TAKING	NUMBER OF PILLS TO SWALLOW AS SOON AS POSSIBLE (1ST DOSE)	NUMBER OF PILLS TO SWALLOW 12 HOURS LATER (2ND DOSE)
Ovral	2 white pills	2 white pills
Lo/Ovral	4 white pills	4 white pills
Levlen	4 light-orange pills	4 light-orange pills
Nordette	4 light-orange pills	4 light-orange pills
Tri-Levlen	4 yellow pills	4 yellow pills
Triphasil	4 yellow pills	4 yellow pills
Alesse	5 pink pills	5 pink pills

- To reduce the chance of nausea, take an anti-nausea medicine (like Dramamine II or Benadryl) 1 hour **before** the first ECP dose; repeat according to labeled instructions. This may make you feel tired, so don't drive or drink any alcohol.

- Take the first ECP dose as soon as convenient **WITHIN 3 DAYS (72 HOURS)** after unprotected sex. Try to time the first dose so that the timing of the second dose will be convenient.

- Take the second ECP dose **12 hours after the first dose.**

IMPORTANT: Do not take any extra ECPs. More pills will probably not make the treatment work better. More pills will increase your risk of feeling sick to your stomach.

- Use condoms, spermicides, or a diaphragm if you have sex after taking ECPs until you get your period. Talk to your health-care provider about other regular birth control methods you can use in the future.

- Your next period may be a few days early or late.

IMPORTANT: Do a home pregnancy test or see your health-care provider if your period has not started **within 3 weeks** after ECP treatment. You may be pregnant.

Source: Program for Applied Technologies (PATH): *Emergency Contraception: Resources for Providers.* Seattle, 1997. This patient handout may be reproduced without permission of the publisher.

TRAUMA

Table 88 Classification of Burns

TYPE OF BURN	AFFECTED SKIN LAYER	APPEARANCE
First degree	Epidermis	Erythema, hypersensitivity
Second degree		
Superficial	Upper (papillary) dermis	Erythema, blistering, intact hairs, exquisite pain
Deep	Deep (reticular dermis)	Skin may be white or mottled and nonblanching, or blistered and moist; pain may or may not be present; hairs easily pulled
Third degree	Entire dermis	Dry, white or charred skin; leathery appearance, painless, no hair
Fourth degree	Subcutaneous tissue	Same as third degree; may have exposed muscle and bone

Table 89 "Rule of Nines"

BODY PART	PERCENT OF BSA		
	INFANT	CHILD	ADOLESCENT/ADULT
Head	18%	13%	9%
Anterior trunk	18%	18%	18%
Posterior trunk	18%	18%	18%
Upper extremity (each)	9%	9%	9%
Lower extremity (each)	14%	16%	18%
Genitalia	1%	1%	1%

For small burns, a rough estimate of the affected BSA can be made by comparing the burn with the size of the child's palm (which represents approximately 1% of the BSA).

BSA = body surface area.

TOXICOLOGY

Table 90 Agents with Limited or Uncertain Binding to Activated Charcoal

Iron
Lithium
Heavy metals
  Arsenic
  Mercury
  Lead
  Thallium
Alcohols
  Methanol
  Ethanol
  Isopropanol
  Ethylene glycol
Hydrocarbons
  Kerosene
Gasoline
Mineral seal oil
Caustics*
  NaOH
  KOH
  HCl
  H_2SO_4
Low-molecular-weight
  compounds
Cyanide
Pesticides
  Organophosphates
  Carbamates

Administration of activated charcoal may also impede further management.

Table 91 Agents Causing Hypoglycemia in Overdosed Children

Ethanol
Salicylates
Oral hypoglycemic agents
Propranolol
Insulin

Table 92 Poisons Not Detected on the Comprehensive Drug Screen[a]

β-Adrenergic antagonists
Calcium channel blockers
Carbon monoxide
Clonidine
Cyanide
Iron
LSD
Many benzodiazepines (alprazolam, midazolam, lorazepam)
Most plants and mushrooms

[a]Partial listing of some of the most common poisons.

Table 93 Poisons Causing Respiratory Depression or Apnea[a]

Antipsychotic agents
Carbamate pesticides
Chlorinated hydrocarbons
  Trichloroethylene
  1,1,1-trichloroethane
Clonidine
Coral snake envenomation
Cyclic antidepressants
Ethanol (especially when combined with sedative/hypnotics)
Exotic snake envenomation
  Cobras
  Sea snakes
  Mambas
Mojave rattlesnake envenomation
Narcotics
Nicotine
Organophosphate pesticides
Sedative/hypnotics

[a]Partial list of representative poisons.

Table 94 Poisons Causing an Abnormal Anion Gap[a]

Increased anion gap with metabolic acidosis
Carbon monoxide[b]
Cyanide
Ethanol[b]
Ethylene glycol[b]
Iron[b]
Isoniazid
Methanol[b]
Salicylates[b]
Theophylline[b]
Decreased anion gap
Bromide
Lithium[b]
Hypermagnesemia[b]
Hypercalcemia[b]

[a]Partial list of representative poisons; anion gap = $Na^+ - (Cl^- + CO_2^-)$.

[b]Specific levels rapidly available.

Table 95 Common Poisons and Antidotes

POISON	ANTIDOTE	ADMINISTRATION
Acetaminophen	N-Acetylcysteine	Loading dose 140 mg/kg, then 17 doses at 70 mg/kg/dose. Dilute 20% solution to 5%–10% with juice or soda to improve palatability.
Anticholinergics	Physostigmine	
Benzodiazepines	Flumazenil	
β-Adrenergic antagonists	Glucagon	
Calcium channel blockers	Glucagon	0.3–0.6 ml/kg (8–16 mEq calcium/kg)
	Calcium gluconate 10%	
Carbon monoxide	Hyperbaric oxygen	
	Sodium thiosulfate 25%*	
Cyanide	Sodium nitrate 3%	Dose depends on hemoglobin (see cyanide antidote kit package insert). Do not exceed recommended dosage. Do not give to patients suffering from concomitant carbon monoxide exposure.
	Sodium thiosulfate 25%	Dose depends on hemoglobin (see cyanide antidote kit package insert).
Digitalis	Digitalis Fab fragments	Calculate dose based on level or dose ingested or 10 vials if acute overdose, 5 vials if chronic overdose.
Ethylene glycol	Ethanol	0.6 g/kg load over 1 hour followed by 100 mg/kg/hr infusion
	Pyridoxine	2 mg/kg and thiamine 0.5 mg/kg
Methanol	Folate	50–100 mg over 6 hours
	4-Methylpyrazole (investigational)	
Iron	Deferoxamine	5–15 mg/kg/hr IV infusion
Isoniazid	Pyridoxine	
Lead	Lead level 45–69 μg/dl	
	Dimercaptosuccinic acid	10 mg/kg PO three times daily for 5 days, then twice daily for 14 days (may be useful at lower levels)
	or	
	Calcium NaEDTA	50–75 mg/kg/day divided, every 6 hours either IM or by slow IV infusion (IV use not FDA-approved)
	Lead level ≥ 70 μg/dl	
	Calcium NaEDTA	Administer as described above
	and	
	British anti-lewisite (BAL)	3–5 mg/kg IM every 4 hours for 5 days
Methemoglobinemia	Methylene blue 1%	1–2 mg/kg (0.1–0.2 ml/kg)
Narcotics	Naloxone	
Organophosphates	Atropine	0.1–0.5 mg/kg initial dose with additional doses as needed to counteract bronchorrhea
	Pralidoxime	25–50 mg/kg (up to 1 g); for severe cases, consider 10–15 mg/kg/hr infusion
Phenothiazines (dystonia)	Diphenhydramine	1–2 mg/kg IM or IV
	Benztropine	1–2 mg/kg IM or IV

IM = intramuscularly; IV = intravenously; FDA = Food and Drug Administration; NaEDTA = sodium ethylenediaminetetraacetic acid; PO = orally.

*Consider for possible cyanide inhalation if the patient suffers from smoke inhalation.

Table 96 Epidemiologic Aspects of Food Poisoning

ORGANISM	PATHOGENESIS	SOURCE	PREVENTION
Salmonella	Infection	Meats, poultry, eggs, dairy products	Proper cooking and food handling, pasteurization
Staphylococcus	Preformed enterotoxin	Meats, poultry, potato salad, cream-filled pastry, cheese, sausage	Careful food handling, rapid refrigeration
Clostridium prefringens	Enterotoxin	Meats, poultry	Avoid delay in serving foods, avoid cooling and re-warming foods
Clostridium botulinum	Preformed neurotoxin	Honey, home-canned foods, un-cooked foods	Proper refrigeration (see text)
Vibrio parahaemolyticus	Infection enterotoxin	Sea fish, seawater, shellfish	Proper refrigeration
Bacillus cereus			
Diarrheal type	Sporulation enterotoxin	Many prepared foods	Proper refrigeration
Vomiting type	Preformed toxin	Cooked or fried rice, vegetables, meats, cereal, puddings	Proper refrigeration of cooked rice and other foods
Enterohemorrhagic E. coli 0157-H7	Cytotoxins	Milk, beef	Thorough cooking of beef, consumption of pasteurized milk products
Enterotoxigenic E. coli (travelers' diarrhea)	Enterotoxin	Food or water	Prognosis is not recommended for infants and young children

Table 97   Clinical Aspects of Food Poisoning

ORGANISM	INCUBATION	SYMPTOMS	DURATION	TREATMENT
Bacillus cereus	Vomiting toxin 1–6 hrs; Diarrhea toxin 6–24 hrs	Vomiting ± diarrhea; fever uncommon	8–24 hrs	None
Brucella	Several days to months; usually >30 days	Weakness, fever, headache chills, arthralgia, weight loss; splenomegaly		Bactrim, Tetracycline
Campylobacter	2–10 days; usually 2–5 days	Diarrhea (often bloody), abdominal pain, fever		Severe infection or immunocompromised: Erythromycin, Cipro, or Norfloxacin
Clostridia botulinum	2 hrs–8 days; usually 12–48 hrs	Poor feeding, weak cry, constipation, diplopia, blurred vision, resp weakness; symmetric descending paralysis		Supportive, trivalent equine antitoxin to prevent further paralysis
Clostridia perfringens	6–24 hrs	Diarrhea, abdominal cramps, vomiting and fever uncommon	<24 hrs	None
Escherichia coli	→	→		Antibiotics in systemic infections
E. coli 0157:H7	1–10 days; usually 3–4 days	Diarrhea (often bloody), abdominal cramps, little or no fever. Can cause HUS.	5–10 days	Supportive
ETEC	6–48 hrs	Diarrhea, abdominal cramps, nausea, fever, and vomiting; Uncommon	5–10 days	Supportive
Listeria monocytogenes	2–6 wks	Meningitis, neonatal sepsis, fever	Variable	Ampicillin and Gentamicin
Nontyphoidal Salmonella	6–48 hrs	Diarrhea often with fever and abdominal cramps	<7 days	None unless <3 months or immunocompromised
Salmonella typi	3–60 days; usually 7–14 days	Fever, anorexia, malaise, headache, myalgias, ± diarrhea or constipation	3–4 wks	Chloramphenicol, Ampicillin, Amoxicillin, Bactrim, Cefotaxi, Ceftriaxone
Shigella	12 hrs–6 days; usually 2–4 days	Diarrhea (often bloody), frequently fever, abdominal cramps	1 day–1 month	Bactrim, Cipro
Staphylococcus aureus	30 min–8 hrs; usually 2–4 hrs	vomiting, diarrhea	<24 hrs	None
Vibriosis	4–30 hrs	Diarrhea, cramps, nausea, vomiting	Self limited	Usually none. Treatment for patients with liver disease or immunocompromised: Cefotaxime Gentamicin, Chloramphenico Tetracycline
Yersinia enterocolitica	1–10 days; usually 4–6 days	Diarrhea, abdominal pain (often severe), mesenteric adenitis, pseudo-appendicular syndrome	1–3 wks	Septicemia or enterocolitis in immunocompromised: Cefotaxi aminoglycosides, Tetracycline, Bactrim, Chloramphenicol.

Continued

Table 98 Nomogram for Estimating Severity of Acute Poisoning

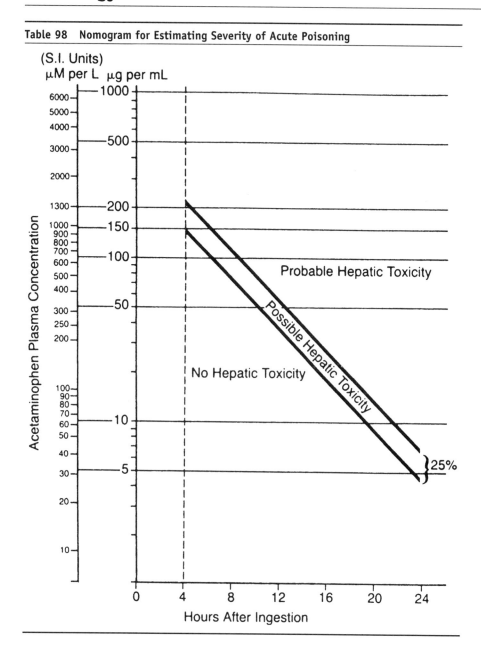

(S.I. Units)
μM per L μg per mL

Acetaminophen Plasma Concentration

Probable Hepatic Toxicity

Possible Hepatic Toxicity

No Hepatic Toxicity

25%

Hours After Ingestion

Table 99 Poisonous Plants

The following are a few common plants that are toxic:

- Azalea
- Buttercup
- Calla Lily
- Creeping Charlie—Ground Ivy
- Daffodil
- Delphinium
- Elderberry
- Holly berries
- Hyacinth bulbs
- Hydrangea
- Iris
- Ivy (Boston and English)
- Jimson Weed
- Larkspur
- Laurel
- Lily-of-the-Valley
- Mistletoe
- Morning Glory
- Nightshade
- Periwinkle
- Philodendron
- Poison Ivy
- Poison Oak
- Rhododendron
- Sweet Pea
- Tomato vines
- Tulip
- Wisteria
- Yew

GONOCOCCAL INFECTIONS

Table 100   Regimens for the Treatment of Pelvic Inflammatory Disease (PID) in Adolescents

Outpatient regimens
  Regimen A
    Ofloxacin, 400 mg PO twice daily for 14 days
                PLUS
    Metronidazole, 500 mg PO twice daily for 14 days
  Regimen B
    Ceftriaxone, 250 mg IM once
                OR
    Cefoxitin (2 mg IM) plus probenecid (1 g PO) in a single dose concurrently once
                OR
    Another parenteral third-generation cephalosporin (e.g., ceftizoxime or cefotaxime)
                PLUS
    Doxycycline, 100 mg orally twice daily for 14 days
Inpatient regimens
  Parenteral regimen A
    Cefotetan, 2 g IV every 12 hours
                OR
    Cefoxitin, 2 g IV every 6 hours
                PLUS
    Doxycycline, 100 mg IV or PO every 12 hours
  Parenteral regimen B
    Clindamycin, 900 mg IV every 8 hours
                PLUS
    Gentamicin loading dose IV or IM (2 mg/kg of body weight), followed by a maintenance dose (1.5 mg/kg) every 8 hours; single daily dosing may be substituted

The safety and effectiveness of fluoroquinolones (e.g., ciprofloxacin, ofloxacin, norfloxacin, enoxacin) in patients younger than 18 years, pregnant women, and lactating women has not been established; therefore, fluoroquinolones are presently not recommended in these patients.

IM = intramuscularly; IV = intravenously; PO = orally.

Table 101   Uncomplicated Gonococcal Infection: Treatment in Children Beyond the Newborn Period and in Adolescents. Recommended Antimicrobial Regimens Include Therapy for Presumed Concomitant Infection with *Chlamydia* trachomatis[a]

DISEASE	PREPUBERTAL CHILDREN WHO WEIGH <100 LB (45 KG)	DISEASE	PATIENTS WHO WEIGH ≥100 LB (45 KG) AND ARE 9 YEARS OR OLDER
Uncomplicated vulvovaginitis, urethritis, proctitis, or pharyngitis	Ceftriaxone, 125 mg IM,[b] in a single dose **OR** Spectinomycin[c] (max 2 g), IM, in a single dose **PLUS** Erythromycin,[e] 40 mg/kg/d in divided doses for 7 d	Uncomplicated endocervicitis, or urethritis	Ceftriaxone, 125 mg IM,[b] in a single dose **OR** Ciprofloxacin,[d] 500 mg orally, in a single dose **OR** Cefixime, 400 mg orally, in a single dose **OR** Ofloxacin,[d] 400 mg orally, in a single dose **OR** Spectinomycin,[c] 2 g IM, in a single dose **PLUS** Doxycycline, 100 mg orally, twice daily for 7 d[f] **OR** Azithromycin, 1 g orally, in a single dose

[a]Hospitalization should be considered, especially for patients who have been treated as outpatients and have failed to respond, and for those who are unlikely to adhere to treatment regimens.

[b]Some clinicians believe the discomfort of an IM injection can be reduced by using 1% lidocaine as a diluent.

[c]Spectinomycin is not recommended for treatment of pharyngeal infections; in persons who cannot take a cephalosporin, a quinolone, or spectinomycin, a 5-d oral regimen of trimethoprim-sulfamethoxazole may be given.

[d]Quinolones are contraindicated for persons younger than 18 y, pregnant women, and nursing women.

[e]Doxycycline can be given instead of erythromycin if the child is 9 y or older.

[f]Tetracycline, 500 mg, four times daily, can be substituted for doxycycline.

Reprinted with permission from American Academy of Pediatrics. In: Peter G, ed. 1994 Red book: report of the Committee on Infectious Diseases, 23rd ed. Elk Grove Village, IL: American Academy of Pediatrics, 1994:199.

Table 102   Complicated Gonococcal Infection: Treatment for Children beyond the Newborn Period and for Adolescents[a]

DISEASE	PREPUBERTAL CHILDREN WHO WEIGH <100 LB (45 KG)	DISEASE	PATIENTS WHO WEIGH ≥100 LB (45 KG) AND ARE 9 YEARS OR OLDER
Ophthalmia, peritonitis, bacteremia, or arthritis	Ceftriaxone, 50 mg/kg/d (max 1 g/d) IV or IM,[c] once daily for 7 d	Gonococcal pharyngitis Pelvic inflammatory disease	Ceftriaxone, 125 mg IM,[c] in a single dose See Table 86

[a]In all cases, in addition to the recommended treatment for gonococcal infection, doxycycline (100 mg orally, twice daily for 7 d), tetracycline (500 mg, 4 times daily for 7 d), or azithromycin (1 g orally, in a single dose) is recommended on the presumption that the patient has concomitant infection with *Chlamydia trachomatis*, for children younger than 9 y and pregnant women, erythromycin is recommended.

[b]Hospitalization is required; follow-up cultures are necessary to ensure that treatment has been effective.

[c]Some clinicians believe the discomfort of IM injection can be reduced by using 1% lidocaine as a diluent.

[d]Such as the arthritis-dermatitis syndrome.

[e]Spectinomycin is not recommended for treatment of pharyngeal gonococcal infection. For patients who cannot take a cephalosporin, spectinomycin, or a quinolone, a 5-d oral regimen of trimethoprim-sulfamethoxazole may be given.

[f]Alternatively, parenteral therapy can be discontinued 24–48 h after improvement begins and a 7-d course is completed with an appropriate oral antimicrobial. Some experts advise a 10- to 14-d course of therapy.

Reprinted with permission from American Academy of Pediatrics. In: Peter G, ed. 1994 Red book: report of the Committee on Infectious Diseases, 23rd ed. Elk Grove Village, IL: American Academy of Pediatrics, 1994:200.

MISCELLANEOUS

Table 103   Late Effects of Chemotherapy and Radiation

CHEMOTHERAPY AGENT	POSSIBLE LATE EFFECTS
Cyclophosphamide	Azoospermia, amenorrhea, hemorrhagic cystitis, secondary malignancies
Doxorubicin, daunomycin	Cardiomyopathy/pericarditis, secondary leukemia
Methotrexate, actinomycin	Avascular necrosis, hepatitis or cirrhosis, learning disabilities with intrathecal use
Vincristine	Neuropathies
Steroids	Obesity, avascular necrosis, osteoporosis, cataracts
Cisplatin	Gynecomastia, nephritis, thrombotic thrombocytopenic purpura
Etoposide	Secondary leukemia
RADIATION	
Cranium/brain	Short stature or short trunk, obesity, learning disabilities, leukoencephalopathy, cranial neuropathies, alopecia, cataracts, hypothyroidism, second malignancies (brain, thyroid)
Head and neck	Nasolacrimal duct obstruction, chronic conjunctivitis, chronic otitis media, alopecia, cataracts, dental abnormalities, voice changes, facial deformities, neuropathies, esophagitis, second malignancies (thyroid, soft-tissue sarcomas, bone tumors)
Mediastinum	Cardiomyopathy, hypothyroidism, second malignancies (thyroid, acute myeloid leukemia, breast cancer), pneumonitis/fibrosis, reduced cell-mediated immunity
Lungs	Pneumonitis or fibrosis
Spine	Short stature or short trunk, scoliosis, hypothyroidism, second malignancies (thyroid), delayed puberty
Bones	Atrophy or hypoplasia, avascular necrosis, osteoporosis, second malignancies (bone and soft-tissue sarcomas), osteochondromas
Total nodes	Reduced cell-mediated immunity, bone marrow dysfunction

Table 104   Red Eye: Common Causes by Location

CONJUNCTIVA	ADNEXA	GLOBE
infectious conjunctivitis	chalazion/hordeolum	corneal abrasion
neonatal conjunctivitis	dacryocystitis	foreign body
allergic conjunctivitis	orbital cellulitis	
periorbital cellulitis		

Table 105 Helpful Specific Drug Levels

DRUG	TIME TO PEAK BLOOD LEVEL (HOURS POSTINGESTION)	POTENTIAL INTERVENTION
Acetaminophen	4	N-Acetylcysteine administration
Carbamazepine	2–4*†	. . .
Carboxyhemoglobin	Immediate	Hyperbaric oxygen therapy
Digoxin	2–4	Fab (digoxin antibody) fragment
Ethanol	½–1†	. . .
Ethylene glycol	½–1	Ethanol infusion and hemodialysis
Iron	2–4	Deferoxamine administration
Isopropanol	½–1†	. . .
Lead	5 weeks*	Chelation and environmental abatement
Lithium	2–4	Hemodialysis
Methanol	½–1	Ethanol infusion and hemodialysis
Methemoglobinemia	Immediate	Methylene blue administration
Phenobarbital	2–4	Alkaline diuresis, multiple-dose activated charcoal
Phenytoin	1–2*	Multiple-dose activated charcoal
Salicylates	6–12*	Alkaline diuresis, multiple-dose activated charcoal, hemodialysis
Theophylline	1–36*	Multiple-dose activated charcoal, whole-bowel irrigation, charcoal hemoperfusion, hemodialysis

*Repeated measurement of levels is necessary because of significant variation in time to reach to peak level.

†The peak level is predictive of toxicity and clinical course. Adapted from Weisman RS, Howland MA, Verebey K: The toxicology laboratory. In *Goldfrank's Toxicologic Emergencies,* 5th ed. Edited by Goldfrank LR, Flomenbaum NE, Lewin NA, et al. East Norwalk, CT: Appleton & Lange, 1994, p. 105.

Table 106 Human Papilloma Viruses: Preferred Sites of Infectivity

CLINICAL TYPE	HPV TYPE
Verruca vulgaris (common warts)	1, 2, 4, 7, 26, 27, 29
Verruca plana (flat warts)	3, 10, 28, 41
Verruca plantaris (plantar warts)	1, 2, 4
Anogenital warts	1–6, 10, 11, 13, 16, 18, 31, 33, 35, 39, 41, 42
Laryngeal warts	6, 11, 13, 30, 40
Anogenital carcinoma	11, 16, 18, 31, 33, 42, 47
Bowenoid papulosis	16, 18, 30
Epidermodysplasia verruciformis	5, 8–10, 12, 14, 15, 17, 19–25, 16–38, 40

Continued

MEDICATIONS

Table 107   Medications

DRUG	DOSE	DOSAGE FORMS
Acetaminophen (Feverall, Panadol, Tempra, Tylenol)	*Orally or rectally:* Children: 10–15 mg/kg repeated every 4–6 hours, up to 5 doses daily. Adults: 325–650 mg every 4–6 hours or 1 g tid or qid. Do not exceed 4 g/day.	Drops: 100 mg/ml Suspension: 160 mg/5 ml Suppositories: 120 mg, 325 mg, 650 mg Tablets: 160 mg, 325 mg, 500 mg Tablets: chewable: 80 mg Also available in combination with codeine; see codeine monograph.
Acetazolamide (Diamox)	*Orally or IV:* Children and adults: 8–30 mg/kg/day in 4 divided doses. Do not exceed 1 g/day. *Altitude sickness (adults):* 250 mg every 8–12 hours beginning 24–48 hours before ascent and continuing for at least 48 hours after arrival.	Injection: 500 mg Tablets: 250 mg
Acetylcysteine (Mucomyst, Mucosil)	*Acetaminophen poisoning:* 140 mg/kg PO followed by 70 mg/kg for 17 doses administered every 4 hours until acetaminophen levels are nontoxic. Usually administered as a 5% solution diluted in juice or soda. *Inhalation* (administer 10% solution undiluted): Infants: 2–4 repeated tid or qid Children and adolescents: 6–10 ml repeated tid or qid	Solution for inhalation: 10% or 20% in 10-ml and 30-ml vials
Acyclovir (Zovirax)	*Oral doses for children and adults:* *Varicella zoster (chickenpox):* 80 mg/kg/day in 4 divided doses for 5 days. Do not exceed 800 mg/dose (3200 mg/day). *Herpes simplex virus:* Children: 1200 mg/m^2/day in 4–5 divided doses. Adults: 200 mg every 4 hours while awake (5 doses daily). Chronic suppressive therapy at a dose of 400 mg bid may be used for up to 1 year or longer. *IV doses for children and adults:* *Neonatal HSV encephalitis:* 30 mg/kg/day in 3 divided doses for 10–14 days. *HSV encephalitis:* 1500 mg/m^2/day in 3 divided doses for at least 10 days and up to 21 days. *Other HSV infections:* 750 mg/m^2/day in 3 divided doses for 7 days. *Varicella zoster infections:* 1500 mg/m^2/day in 3 divided doses for 7 days. *Topically:* apply ointment every 3 hours up to 6 times daily for 7 days. Use a disposable fingercot or glove when applying the ointment to avoid transmission of the virus. Dosage may need to be adjusted in patients with renal dysfunction.	Capsules: 200 mg Injection: 500-mg, 1-g vials Ointment: 5%, 15 g Suspension: 200 mg/5 ml
Adenosine (Adenocard)	*IV* (given via rapid push followed by a saline flush): Children: 0.1 mg/kg initially, followed by doses increasing in 0.05 mg/kg increments every 2 minutes to a maximum dose of 0.35 mg/kg or 12 mg/dose. Adults: 6 mg followed by 12 mg with a repeat dose of 12 mg, if needed.	Injection: 3 mg/ml (2-ml vial)
Albumin, human (Albuminar, Albutein, Plasbumin)	*IV* (as a 5% solution for hypovolemic patients or 25% for fluid- or sodium-restricted patients): Children: 0.5–1 g/kg infused over 2–4 hours. May repeat to a maximum of 6 g/kg/day. Adults: 25 g infused over 2–4 hours. Usually not to exceed 125 g/day.	Injection: 5% (50 ml, 250 ml, 500 ml); 25% (20 ml, 50 ml, 100 ml)

Continued

Table 107   Medications   (continued)

DRUG	DOSE	DOSAGE FORMS
Albuterol (Proventil, Ventolin)	*Oral:* Age 2–6: 0.3–0.6 mg/kg/day in 3 divided doses to a maximum of 12 mg/day. Age 6–12: 6–8 mg/day in 3–4 divided doses to a maximum of 24 mg/day. Over age 12: 6–16 mg/day in 3–4 divided doses to a maximum of 32 mg/day. *Inhalation:* *Metered-dose inhaler:* Under age 12: 1–2 inhalations qid. Over age 12: 1–2 inhalations up to 6 times a day. *Nebulization:* 0.01–0.05 ml/kg usually repeated every 4–6 hours, but may be administered more frequently in severely ill patients under controlled conditions.	Aerosol: 90 μg/actuation Solution for inhalation: 0.5% Syrup: 10 mg/5 ml Tablets: 2 mg, 4 mg
Allopurinol (Zyloprim)	*Orally:* Under age 6: 150 mg/day in 3 divided doses. Age 6–10: 300 mg/day in 2 or 3 divided doses. Over age 10: 600–800 mg/day in 2 or 3 divided doses. Note: The metabolism of mercaptopurine and azathioprine is decreased by allopurinol. Decrease dose of mercaptopurine or azathioprine by 75%.	Tablets: 100 mg, 300 mg
Alprostadil (Prostin VR Pediatric)	A continuous infusion beginning at a dose of 0.05–0.1 μg/kg/min. Dosage may be adjusted downward or gradually upward based on the patient's response. Usual dosage range is 0.01–0.4 μg/kg/min.	Injection: 500 μg/ml (1-ml ampule)
Aluminum acetate (Domeboro, Burow's Solution)	*Topically:* as a wet dressing or soak 2–4 times daily for 30 minutes at a time. Usual concentrations are 1:10, 1:20, or 1:40. *Ear:* 4–6 drops in the ear at first every 2–3 hours, then every 4–6 hours until itching or burning subsides.	Powder (packets): 1 packet/pint of water = 1:40 dilution Solution, otic: 1:10 dilution with 2% acetic acid
Aluminum and magnesium hydroxides (Maalox, Maalox Plus, Mylanta)	Children: 5–10 ml 4–6 times daily or more frequently. Adults: 15–30 ml 4–6 times daily or more frequently.	Suspension: aluminum hydroxide 225 mg and magnesium hydroxide 200 mg/5 ml Suspension with simethicone: as above with simethicone 25 mg/5 ml
Amikacin (Amikin)	*IV* (dose should be based on ideal body weight): Neonates: 0–4 weeks, <1200 g: 7.5 mg/kg/dose every 18–24 hours. Under 7 days of age: 1200–2000 g: 7.5 mg/kg/dose every 12–18 hours >2000 g: 10 mg/kg/dose every 12 hours. Over 7 days of age: 1200–2000 g: 7.5 mg/kg/dose every 8–12 hours. >2000 g: 10 mg/kg/dose every 8 hours. Infants and children: 15–22.5 mg/kg/day in 3 divided doses daily. The dose for the treatment of nontuberculous mycobacterial infections is 15–30 mg/kg/day in 2 divided doses, to a maximum of 1.5 g/day as part of a multiple-drug regimen. Adults: 15 mg/kg/day in 2–3 divided doses. Dosage adjustment is required in patients with renal dysfunction.	Injection: 50 mg/ml, 250 mg/ml

Continued

Table 107   Medications   (continued)

DRUG	*DOSE*	*DOSAGE FORMS*
Aminocaproic acid (Amicar)	*IV:* 　　Children: 100 mg/kg over the first hour followed by an infusion of 33.3 mg/kg/hr to a maximum daily dose of 30 g. 　　Older children and adults: 4–5 g over the first hour followed by an infusion of 1 g/hr for 8 hours or until control is achieved. *Orally:* doses are the same or alternatively, 100 mg/kg may be administered every 4–6 hours to a maximum of 5 g/dose.	Injection: 250 mg/ml (20-ml vial) Solution: 1.25 g/5 ml (16-oz bottle) Tablets: 500 mg
Amiodarone (Cordarone)	*Orally:* 　　Children (use body surface area for children age 1 year or under): loading dose of 10–15 mg/kg/day or 600–800 mg/1.73 m²/day in 1–2 divided doses for 4–14 days or until adequate control of arrhythmia is achieved or prominent adverse effects occur. Then reduce dosage to 5 mg/kg/day or 200–400 mg/1.73 m²/day as a single dose for several weeks. A further dose reduction to 2.5 mg/kg/day should be attempted if the arrhythmia does not recur. 　　Adults: loading dose of 800–1600 mg/day in 1–2 divided doses for 1–3 weeks, followed by dose of 600–800 mg/day in 1–2 divided doses for 1 month. Maintenance dose usually 400 mg/day, but may be lower for supraventricular arrhythmias. *IV:* 　　Children (only limited information is available): initial loading dose of 5 mg/kg over 1 hour followed by a continuous infusion of 5 μg/kg/min has been used. The continuous infusion dosage may be increased to 10 μg/kg/min and then to 15 μg/kg/min until the desired effect is achieved. 　　Adults: loading dose of 150 mg administered over 10 minutes (15 mg/min) followed by 360 mg over 6 hours at a rate of 1 mg/min, followed by the maintenance dose of 540 mg over 18 hours at a rate of 0.5 mg/min. If necessary, maintenance infusion of 0.5 mg/min may be continued past the initial 24 hours. Additional bolus doses of 150 mg may be administered over 10 minutes for breakthrough arrhythmias.	Injection: 50 mg/ml Tablets: 200 mg
Amitriptyline (Elavil, Endep)	*Orally:* *Chronic pain:* 0.1 mg/kg/day at bedtime initially, advancing to 0.5–2 mg/kg/day over a 2–3 week period. *Depression:* 1 mg/kg/day to start, advancing to a maximum of 5 mg/kg or 100 mg, whichever is less. 　　Adolescents and adults: 25–50 mg at bedtime or in divided doses, increasing daily doses by 25 mg to a maximum of 100 mg/day for adolescents and 300 mg for adults. Dosage should be decreased to the lowest effective dose after symptom control has been reached.	Tablets: 10 mg, 25 mg, 50 mg, 75 mg, 100 mg, 150 mg

Continued

Table 107   Medications   (continued)

DRUG	_DOSE_	_DOSAGE FORMS_
Amoxicillin (Amoxil, Polymax, Trimax, Wymox)	_Orally:_ Children ≤20 kg: 20 mg/kg/day in 3 divided doses for urinary tract infections. 40 mg/kg/day in 3 divided doses for otitis media, upper respiratory infection, or skin infections. Do not exceed adult doses recommended below. Children >20 kg and adults: 750 mg/day in 3 divided doses for urinary tract infections or 1500 mg/day in 3 divided doses for otitis media, upper respiratory infections, or skin infections. Maximum daily dose is 3 g. _Endocarditis prophylaxis:_ 50 mg/kg (up to 3 g) 1 hour before procedure and 25 mg/kg (up to 1.5 g) 6 hours later.	Capsules: 250 mg, 500 mg Drops: 50 mg/ml Suspension: 125 mg/5 ml, 250 mg/5 ml Tablets, chewable: 125 mg, 250 mg
Amoxicillin and clavulanic acid (Augmentin)	_Orally_ (based on the amoxicillin component): 20–40 mg/kg/day in 3 divided doses to a maximum of 1.5 g/day, OR 25–45 mg/kg/day in 2 divided doses to a maximum of 1.75 g/day using the BID formulation of the drug. Use the higher doses for respiratory tract infections and otitis media.	Suspension: amoxicillin 125 mg and clavulanic acid 31.25 mg/5 ml; BID formulation—amoxicillin 200 mg and clavulanic acid 28.5 mg/5 ml; amoxicillin 250 mg and clavulanic acid 62.5 mg/5 ml; BID formulation—amoxicillin 400 mg and clavulanic acid 57 mg/5 ml Tablets: amoxicillin 250 mg and clavulanic acid 125 mg; amoxicillin 500 mg and clavulanic acid 125 mg; BID formulation—amoxicillin 875 mg and clavulanic acid 125 mg Tablets, chewable: amoxicillin 125 mg and clavulanic acid 31.25 mg; BID formulation—amoxicillin 200 mg and clavulanic acid 28.5 mg; amoxicillin 250 mg and clavulanic acid 62.5 mg; BID formulation—amoxicillin 400 mg and clavulanic acid 57 mg
Amphotericin B (Fungizone)	_IV_ (infusion over 4–8 hours): _Test dose_ (infusion over 30 minutes) <10 kg: 0.1 mg in 1 ml D_5W. >10 kg: 1 mg in 10 ml D_5W. _Therapeutic dose:_ begin with 0.25–0.5 mg/kg immediately following test dose. Doses may be doubled on each subsequent day to a maximum of 1 mg/kg as the patient tolerates. Once therapy is established, alternate day doses at a maximum of 1.5 mg/kg/day may be used. Bladder irrigations of 15–50 mg daily in 1 L of sterile water instilled over 24 hours have been used to treat bladder infections.	Injection: 50-mg vial
Amphotericin B, cholesteryl (Amphotec)	_IV_ (infusion at a rate of 1 mg/kg/hr): Children and adults: 3–4 mg/kg/day as a single infusion. Doses of up to 6 mg/kg/day may be used if there is no improvement at the lower dose. Admix with 5% dextrose injection to a final concentration of about 0.6 mg/ml for administration over 3–4 hours. In patients who tolerate the longer infusion time well, the time can be shortened to 2 hours.	Injection: 50-mg vial
Amphotericin B, liposomal complex (Abelcet)	_IV_ (infusion over 2 hours): Children and adults: 5 mg/kg/day in a single infusion. Admix with 5% dextrose to a final concentration of 1 mg/ml. A final concentration of 2 mg/ml may be used for pediatric patients or patients requiring fluid restriction.	Suspension for injection: 5 mg/ml

Continued

Table 107   Medications   (continued)

DRUG	DOSE	DOSAGE FORMS

Ampicillin (Omnipen, Polycillin, Principen, Totacillin)	*IV:*
	Meningitis:
	   Neonates under age 7 days:
	      <2000 g: 100 mg/kg/day in 2 divided doses.
	      >2000 g: 150 mg/kg/day in 3 divided doses.
	   Neonates over age 7 days:
	      <1200 g: 100 mg/kg/day in 2 divided doses.
	      1200–2000 g: 150 mg/kg/day in 3 divided doses.
	      >2000 g: 200 mg/kg/day in 4 divided doses.
	   Infants and children: 150–300 mg/kg/day in 4–6 divided doses to a maximum of 12 g/day.
	   Adults: 150–200 mg/kg/day in 6–8 divided doses.
	Moderate infections:
	   Neonates under age 7 days:
	      <2000 g: 50 mg/kg/day in 2 divided doses.
	      >2000 g: 75 mg/kg/day in 3 divided doses.
	   Neonates over age 7 days:
	      <1200 g: 50 mg/kg/day in 2 divided doses.
	      1200–2000 g: 75 mg/kg/day in 3 divided doses.
	      >2000 g: 100 mg/kg/day in 4 divided doses.
	   Infants, children, and adults: 50–100 mg/kg/day in 4–6 divided doses to a maximum total dose of 12 g/day.
	Orally (mild to moderate infections):
	   Children <20 kg: 50–75 mg/kg/day in 4 divided doses. Do not exceed adult doses for the same degree of infection.
	   Children >20 kg and adults: 1–2 daily (250–500 mg/dose) in 4 divided doses.
		Capsules: 250 mg, 500 mg
		Injection: 125-mg, 250-mg, 500-mg, 1-g, 2-g vials
		Suspension: 125 mg/5 ml, 250 mg/5 ml, 500 mg/5 ml

Ampicillin and sulbactam sodium (Unasyn)	*IV:*
	   Infants and children: 150 mg/kg/day (100 mg ampicillin + 50 mg sulbactam) in 3–4 divided doses.
	   Adults: 1.5–3 g (1–2 g ampicillin + 0.5–1 g sulbactam) given every 6 hours.
		Injection: 1.5 g (1 g ampicillin + 0.5 g sulbactam), 3 g (2 g ampicillin + 1 g sulbactam)

Amrinone (Inocor)	*IV:* a bolus dose of 0.75 mg/kg administered over 2–3 minutes is followed by a maintenance infusion of 3–5 μg/kg/min for neonates or 5–10 μ/kg/min for infants, children, or adults. The bolus doses may be repeated at 30-minute intervals to a total of 3 mg/kg. Total daily dose should not exceed 10 mg/kg.	Injection: 5 mg/ml
Arginine (R-Gene)	*IV:* *Growth hormone reserve test:* 500 mg/kg to a maximum dose of 30 g (300 ml) over 30 minutes. *Metabolic alkalosis:* arginine dose (g) = weight (kg) $\times$ 0.1 [HCO$_3$ − 24] where HCO$_3$ is the patient's serum bicarbonate concentration in mEq/L. Administer one half to two thirds of the dose calculated and reevaluate.	Injection: 10% 30 g/300 ml
Ascorbic acid (vitamin C; Cecon, Cevalin, Ce-Vi-Sol)	*Orally, IV, IM:* *Scurvy:* 100–300 mg/day in 2–3 divided doses. *Supplementation:* 35–200 mg/day.	Many are available; only some examples are listed. Drops: 35 mg/0.6 ml, 100 mg/ml Injection: 100 mg/ml, 250 mg/ml, 500 mg/ml Tablets: 50 mg, 100 mg, 250 mg, 500 mg, 1 g Tablets, chewable: 100 mg, 250 mg, 500 mg, 1 g Tablets, timed release: 500 mg, 1 g, 1.5 g

Continued

Table 107   Medications   (continued)

DRUG	_DOSE_	_DOSAGE FORMS_

Aspirin (Anacin, Ascriptin, Bufferin, Easprin, Ecotrin)	_Orally or rectally:_
	Analgesic, antipyretic:
	  Children: 10–15 mg/kg every 4–6 hours.
	  Adults: 325–1000 mg every 4–6 hours, up to 4 g/day.
	Anti-inflammatory:
	  Children ≤25 kg: 60–90 mg/kg/day in 3–4 divided doses initially, with a usual range of 80–100 mg/kg/day. Monitor serum levels.
	  Children >25 kg and adults: 2.4–3.6 g/day in 4 divided doses. Maximum total daily dose usually should not exceed 5.4 g.
	Kawasaki syndrome: 100 mg/kg/day in 4 divided doses until fever resolves: then 3–8 mg/kg once daily for 6–10 weeks after onset of the disease, or longer.
		Suppositories: 60 mg, 120 mg, 300 mg, 325 mg, 600 mg, 650 mg
		Tablets: 325 mg, 500 mg, 650 mg
		Tablets, chewable: 81 mg
		Tablets, extended release: 165 mg, 325 mg, 500 mg, 650 mg, 975 mg
		Also available in buffered formulation, enteric-coated tablets, and chewing gum.

Astemizole (Hismanal)	_Orally (on an empty stomach):_
	  Under age 6: 0.2 mg/kg once daily.
	  Age 6–12: 5 mg once daily.
	  Over age 12 and adults: 10 mg once daily.
		Tablets: 10 mg

Atenolol (Tenormin)	_Orally:_
	  Children: initially 0.8–1 mg/kg/day in a single dose. Dosage may be increased to 1.5 mg/kg/day or a maximum of 2 mg/kg/day if necessary.
	  Adults: initially 25–50 mg/day, increasing to 50–100 mg/day as needed. The maximum dose for hypertension is 100 mg; for angina, 200 mg.
		Tablets: 25 mg, 50 mg, 100 mg

Atropine sulfate	_Preoperative orally or IM:_
	  Under age 6 months: 0.16 mg (NOT mg/kg!).
	  Over age 6 months: 0.02 mg/kg to a maximum dose of about 1 mg.
	Bradycardia: 0.02 mg/kg with a minimum dose of 0.1 mg and a maximum dose of 0.5 mg in children, 1 mg in adolescents, and 2 mg in adults.
	Ophthalmic: 1–2 drops of 0.5%–1% solution in the eye.
		Injection: 0.3 mg/ml, 0.4 mg/ml, 0.5 mg/ml, 0.8 mg/ml, 1 mg/ml
		Ointment, ophthalmic: 0.5%, 1%
		Solution, ophthalmic: 0.5%, 1%, 2%

Attapulgite (Kaopectate)	_Orally (dose after each loose bowel movement, up to 7 times a day):_
	  Age 3–6: 7.5 ml or 1 tablet.
	  Age 6–12: 15 ml or 2 tablets.
	  Over age 12: 30 ml or 4 tablets.
		Suspension: 600 mg/15 ml
		Tablets, chewable: 300 mg

Azathioprine (Imuran)	_IV or orally:_ Children and adults: initially 3–5 mg/kg/day as a single dose. Maintenance doses are usually 1–3 mg/kg/day. Note: Metabolism of azathioprine is decreased by allopurinol; decrease dose of azathioprine by 75%.	Injection: 100-mg vial Tablets: 50 mg

Azithromycin (Zithromax)	_Orally:_
	Otitis media (6 months of age and older): 10 mg/kg (to a maximum of 500 mg) on the first day followed by 5 mg/kg/day (to a maximum of 250 mg) for 4 days.
	Pharyngitis/tonsillitis:
	  2 yrs of age and older: 12 mg/kg/day (to a maximum of 500 mg) for 5 days.
	  Adults: 500 mg on the first day followed by 250 mg/day for 4 days.
	Uncomplicated chlamydia infection: 1 g as a single dose.
		Capsules: 250 mg
		Suspension: 100 mg/5 ml, 200 mg/5 ml, 1-g packet

Continued

Table 107   Medications   (continued)

DRUG	*DOSE*	*DOSAGE FORMS*
Aztreonam (Azactam)	*IV or IM:* Children over age 1 month: 60–100 mg/kg/day in 3–4 divided doses. Doses of up to 200 mg/kg/day have been used in severe infections. Maximum total daily dose is 8 g. Adults: 1–2 g every 6–8 hours, depending on the severity of the infection. Dose adjustment is necessary in renal impairment.	Injection: 500-mg, 1-g, 2-g vials
Bacitracin; bacitracin and polymyxin B (Polysporin); bacitracin, neomycin, and polymyxin B (Neosporin)	*Topically:* apply to affected area 1–3 times daily. *Ophthalmic:* apply to eyes every 3–4 hours.	Ointment, ophthalmic (all three): 3.5-g tube Ointment, topical (all three): 15-g, 30-g tubes
Beclomethasone dipropionate (Beclovent, Beconase, Vancenase, Vanceril)	*Intranasal:* Age 6–12: 1 inhalation in each nostril tid. Over age 12 and adults 1 inhalation in each nostril bid or qid or 2 inhalations in each nostril bid. *Oral inhalation:* Age 6–12: 1–2 inhalations tid or qid or 2–4 inhalations bid. Do not exceed 10 inhalations/day. Over age 12 and adults: 2 inhalations tid or qid not to exceed 20 inhalations/day.	Intranasal aerosol spray: 42 μg/spray Intranasal nasal suspension spray pump: 42 μg/spray Oral inhalation aerosol: 42 μg/spray
Beractant (Survanta)	*Intratracheally:* should be used only by physicians familiar with its administration. The usual dose is 4 ml/kg administered in 4 quarter doses through a #5 French endhole catheter. Patients should be ventilated and repositioned between quarter doses.	Suspension: 25 mg phospholipids/ml, 8-ml vial
Betamethasone (Diprolene, Diprosone, Maxivate, Uticort, Valisone)	Apply a thin film to the skin 1–3 times daily. Avoid application to the face, groin, or axillae.	Benzoate (Uticort): 0.025% cream, lotion, gel Diproprionate, augmented (Diprolene): 0.05% cream, lotion, gel, ointment Diproprionate (Diprosone): 0.05% cream, lotion, ointment, 0.1% aerosol Diproprionate with clotrimazole (antifungal) [Lotrisone] Valerate (Valisone): 0.01% cream, lotion, ointment
Bethanechol (Duvoid, Myotonachol, Urecholine)	*Orally:* *Gastroesophageal reflux:* Children: 0.1–0.2 mg/kg given at least 30 minutes before a meal. Up to 4 doses/day may be given. Adults: 10–50 mg up to qid. *Urinary retention:* Children: 0.6 mg/kg/day in 3–4 divided doses. Adults: 10–50 mg/dose up to qid. *SC:* 0.12–0.2 mg/kg/day in 3–4 divided doses. Usual adult dose is 2.5–5 mg tid or qid.	Injection: 5 mg/ml Tablets: 5 mg, 10 mg, 25 mg, 50 mg
Bisacodyl (Dulcolax)	*Orally* (higher doses for evacuation, lower for laxation): Age 3–12: 5–10 mg as a single dose. Over age 12: 5–15 mg as a single dose. Tablets are enteric coated and must not be chewed or crushed. *Rectally:* Under age 2: 5 mg/day as a single dose. Age 2–11: 5–10 mg/day as a single dose. Over age 12: 10 mg/day as a single dose.	Suppositories: 5 mg, 10 mg Tablets, enteric coated: 5 mg
Brompheniramine and phenylpropanolamine (Dimetapp)	*Orally:* Age 1–6 months: 1.25 ml tid or qid. Age 7–24 months: 2.5 ml tid or qid. Age 2–4: 3.75 ml tid or qid. Age 4–12: 5 ml tid or qid. Over age 12: 5–10 ml tid or qid or 1 extended-release tablet every 12 hours.	Elixir: brompheniramine maleate 2 mg, phenylpropanolamine 12.5 mg per 5 ml Tablets, extended release: brompheniramine maleate 12 mg, phenylpropanolamine 75 mg

Continued

Table 107   Medications   (continued)

DRUG	DOSE	DOSAGE FORMS
Bumetanide (Bumex)	*Orally or IV:* Neonates: 0.01–0.05 mg/kg/dose every 24–48 hours. Infants and children: 0.015–0.1 mg/kg/dose every 6–24 hours to a maximum of 10 mg/day. Adults: 0.5–1 mg/dose IV or 0.5–2 mg/dose orally once or twice daily to a maximum of 10 mg/day.	Injection: 0.25 mg/ml Tablets: 0.5 mg, 1 mg, 2 mg
Caffeine (*Note:* Not commercially available in solution or injectable form; must be compounded by the pharmacy)	*Orally or IV:* *Loading dose:* 10 mg/kg caffeine base. If theophylline has been administered within the previous 3 days, a modified dose (50%–75% of loading dose) may be given. *Maintenance:* 2.5 mg/kg caffeine base 24 hours after the loading dose. Dosage may be adjusted based on the patient's response and the results of serum level monitoring.	Do not use caffeine and sodium benzoate injection in neonates.
Calcitonin (Calcimar, Miacalcin)	*IM or SC:* *Paget disease:* initially, 100 U/day; maintenance is 50 U/day or 50–100 U every 1–3 days. *Hypercalcemia:* 4 U/kg every 12 hours; after 1–2 days may increase to 8 U/kg every 12 hours until more specific treatment is established.	Injection: 400-U vial
Calcitriol (Calcijex, Rocaltral)	Individualize to maintain normal serum calcium levels. *Orally:* *Hypocalcemia in premature infants:* 1 μg/day for 5 days. *Renal failure:* Children: 0.25–2 μg/day (hemodialysis) or 0.014–0.041 μg/kg/day (no hemodialysis). Adults: 0.25–1 μg/day. *IV:* *Hypocalcemia in premature infants:* 0.05 μg/kg/day for 4 days. *Renal failure:* Children: 0.01–0.05 μg/kg 3 times weekly (hemodialysis). Adults: 0.5–3 μg 3 times weekly (hemodialysis).	Capsules: 0.25 μg, 0.5 μg Injection: 1 μg/ml, 2 μg/ml (1-ml ampules)
Calcium salts	See dosage forms for calcium content of various salts. Dosage should be adjusted based on the desired response and serum calcium levels. *IV (gluconate or chloride salts):* *Cardiac resuscitation:* Calcium gluconate: Children: 60–100 mg/kg/dose to a maximum of 3 g. Adults: 500 mg–1 g/dose. Calcium chloride: Children: 20 mg/kg/dose to a maximum of 1 g. Adults: 2–4 mg/kg/dose to a maximum of 1 g. *Hypocalcemia* (usually the gluconate salt): Neonates: 200–800 mg/kg/day, usually as a continuous infusion. Infants and children: 200–500 mg/kg/day as a continuous infusion or in 4 divided doses. Adults: 2–15 g/day as a continuous infusion or in divided doses.	Calcium acetate = 25% Ca = 250 mg Ca per 1 g Ca acetate Calcium carbonate = 40% Ca = 400 mg Ca per 1 g Ca carbonate Calcium chloride = 27% Ca = 270 mg Ca per 1 g Ca chloride Calcium citrate = 21% Ca = 210 mg Ca per 1 g Ca citrate Calcium glubionate = 6.5% Ca = 65 mg Ca per 1 g Ca glubionate Calcium gluconate = 9% Ca = 90 mg Ca per 1 g Ca gluconate Calcium lactate = 13% Ca = 130 mg Ca per 1 g Ca lactate Injection: Chloride salt: 1 g (100 mg/ml) = 27 mg Ca/ml Gluconate salt: 1 g (100 mg/ml) = 9 mg Ca/ml Suspension: carbonate salt: 1.25 g/5 ml = 500 mg Ca/5 ml

Continued

Table 107   Medications   (continued)

DRUG	DOSE	DOSAGE FORMS
Calcium salts (*continued*)	*Orally (carbonate, glubionate, or lactate salts):* Neonates: 20–80 mg calcium/kg/day in 4–6 divided doses. Infants and children: 20–40 mg calcium/kg/day in 4–6 divided doses. Adults: 400 mg–1.2 g calcium/day or more.	Syrup: glubionate salt: 1.8 g/5 ml = 115 mg Ca/5 ml Tablets: Acetate salt: 667 mg = 169 mg Ca (PhosLo) Carbonate salt: 650 mg = 260 mg Ca; 1.25 g = 500 mg Ca; 1.5 g = 600 mg Ca Citrate salt: 950 mg = 200 mg Ca (Citracal); 2376 mg = 500 mg Ca (Citracal Liquitab) Gluconate salt: 500 mg = 45 mg Ca; 650 mg = 58.5 mg Ca; 975 mg = 87.75 mg Ca; 1 g = 90 mg Ca Lactate salt: 325 mg = 42.25 mg Ca; 650 mg = 84.5 mg Ca
Captopril (Capoten)	*Orally:* Neonates: 0.01–0.05 mg/kg up to tid, initially. Dose may be increased incrementally to a maximum of 0.5 mg/kg administered as frequently as every 6 hours (2 mg/kg/day). Infants and children: 0.15–0.3 mg/kg up to tid, initially. Dose may be increased incrementally to a maximum of 6 mg/kg/day in divided doses. Adolescents and adults: 12.5–25 mg every 8–12 hours, initially. May be titrated upward to a maximum of 6 mg/kg/day or 450 mg.	Tablets: 12.5 mg, 25 mg, 50 mg, 100 mg
Carbamazepine (Tegretol)	*Orally:* initially 5–10 mg/kg/day in 2–4 divided doses, increasing slowly to a maximum of 30 mg/kg/day (1.6–2.4 g in adults). Suspension formulation should be administered in 3–4 daily doses; tablet formulations may be administered in 2–3 divided doses.	Suspension: 100 mg/5 ml Tablets, chewable: 100 mg Tablets: 200 mg
Carbamide peroxide (Debrox, Gly-Oxide)	*Ear:* Instill up to 5–10 drops in the ear and allow to remain there for several minutes or longer. *Orally:* apply several drops to the affected area up to qid.	Drops, oral: 10% (Cank-aid, Gly-Oxide, Orajel Braceaid Rinse) Drops, otic: 6.5% (Auro Ear Drops, Debrox, Murine Ear Drops)
Carnitine (Carnitor, Vitacarn)	*Orally:* Children: 50–100 mg/kg/day in 2–3 divided doses to a maximum of 3 g/day. Adults: 660 mg–3 g/day in 2–3 divided doses. *IV:* Children and adults: a loading dose of 50 mg/kg followed by an infusion of 50 mg/kg/day. The dose may be increased if needed to a maximum of 300 mg/kg/day.	Capsules: 250 mg Injection: 200 mg/ml Solution: 100 mg/ml Tablets: 330 mg
Cefaclor (Ceclor)	*Orally:* 20–40 mg/kg/24 hr in 2–3 divided doses to a maximum of 2 g/24 hr.	Capsules: 250 mg Suspension: 125 mg/5 ml, 250 mg/5 ml
Cefadroxil (Duricef, Ultracef)	*Orally:* Children: 30 mg/kg/day in 2 divided doses to a maximum of 2 g/day. Adults: 1–2 g/day in a single or 2 divided doses.	Capsules: 500 mg Suspension: 125 mg/5 ml, 250 mg/5 ml, 500 mg/5 ml Tablets: 1 g
Cefazolin (Ancef, Kefzol)	*IV or IM:* 50–100 mg/kg/day in 3 divided doses to a maximum of 6 g/day. Usual adult doses are 500 mg–2 g/dose every 8 hours Dosing adjustment is necessary in renal impairment.	Injection: 250-mg, 500-mg, 1-g vials
Cefixime (Suprax)	*Orally:* Children: 8 mg/kg/day in 1 or 2 divided doses to a maximum of 400 mg. Adults: 400 mg/day in 1 or 2 divided doses. *Otitis media:* use suspension formula because higher serum levels are reached at the same dose when the suspension is administered.	Suspension: 100 mg/5 ml Tablets: 200 mg, 400 mg

Continued

Table 107 Medications (continued)

DRUG	DOSE	DOSAGE FORMS
Cefotaxime (Claforan)	**IV:** *Sepsis:* Infants and children: 100–120 mg/kg/day in 3–4 divided doses. Adults: 1–2 g every 6–8 hours. *Meningitis:* Neonates under age 1 week: 50 mg/kg every 12 hours. Neonates over age 1 week: 50 mg/kg every 8 hours. Infants over 4 weeks and children: 200 mg/kg/day in 4 divided doses to a maximum total daily dose of 12 g. Adults: 2 g every 4–6 hours. Dosing adjustment is necessary in renal impairment.	Injection: 1-g, 2-g vials
Cefoxitin (Mefoxin)	**IV:** Neonates: 90–100 mg/kg/day in 3 divided doses. Children: 80–160 mg/kg/day depending on the severity of the infection in 4 divided doses. Adults: 1–2 g every 6–8 hours to a maximum total daily dose of 12 g.	Injection: 1-g, 2-g vials
Cefpodaxime (Vantin)	*Orally* (with food to enhance absorption): Children: 10 mg/kg/day in 2 divided doses to a maximum of 400 mg/day (otitis media) or 200 mg/day (pharyngitis/tonsillitis). Adults: 200 mg/day in 2 divided doses for upper respiratory or uncomplicated urinary tract infection, 400 mg/day in 2 divided doses for lower respiratory tract infection (community-acquired pneumonia), 800 mg/day in 2 divided doses (skin, skin structure infection). Dosage adjustment is necessary in severe renal impairment.	Suspension: 50 mg/5 ml, 100 mg/5 ml Tablets: 100 mg, 200 mg
Cefprozil (Cefzil)	*Orally:* Children: *Otitis media:* 30 mg/kg/day in 2 divided doses to a maximum total daily dose of 1 g. *Pharyngitis, tonsillitis:* 15 mg/kg/day in 2 divided doses to a maximum total daily dose of 500 mg. Adults: *Lower respiratory tract:* 500 mg every 12 hours. *Upper respiratory tract and skin:* 500 mg every 24 hours. Dosage adjustment is necessary in renal impairment.	Suspension: 125 mg/5 ml, 250 mg/5 ml Tablets: 250 mg, 500 mg
Ceftazidime (Fortaz, Tozicef, Tazidime)	**IV:** Neonates: <2000 g: 60 mg/kg/day in 2 divided doses. >2000 g: 90 mg/kg/day in 3 divided doses. Infants and children: 90–150 mg/kg/day in 3 divided doses to a maximum total daily dose of 6 g. Adults: 3–6 g/day in 3 divided doses. Dosage adjustment is necessary in renal impairment.	Injection: 500 mg, 1 g, 2 g

Continued

Table 107   Medications   (continued)

DRUG	DOSE	DOSAGE FORMS

Ceftriaxone (Rocephin)	*IV or IM:*
	PPNG (uncomplicated pharyngeal, urethral, endocervical, rectal):
	   <45 kg: 125 mg IM as a single dose.
	   >45 kg: 250 mg IM as a single dose.
	PPNG (ophthalmia): >20 kg: 1 g IM as a single dose.
	Infants born to a mother infected with PPNG: 50 mg/kg IM to a maximum of 125 mg as a single dose.
	Other serious infections (not including meningitis):
	   Children: 50–75 mg/kg/day in 2 divided doses. Do not exceed 2 g/day.
	   Adults: usually 1–2 g as a single daily dose or in 2 divided doses.
	Meningitis:
	   Children: 100 mg/kg/day in 1–2 divided doses to a maximum total daily dose of 4 g.
		Injection: 250-mg, 500-mg, 1-g, 2-g vials

Cefuroxime (Ceftin, Kefurox, Zinacef)	*Orally (administer with food to enhance absorption):*
	Otitis media (all ages): 30 mg/kg/day in 2 divided doses to a maximum total daily dose of 1 g.
	Other infections (all ages): 20 mg/kg/day in 2 divided doses to a maximum total daily dose of 500 mg.
	IV:
	   Children: 50–100 mg/kg/day in 3–4 divided doses. A dose of 150 mg/kg/day in 3 divided doses is recommended for bone and joint infections. Do not exceed adult doses below.
	   Adults: 2.25–4.5 g/day in 3 divided doses. Higher dose is necessary for severe infections and bone and joint infections.
	Dosage adjustment is necessary in renal impairment.
		Injection: 750-mg, 1.5-g vials
		Suspension (axetil): 125 mg/5 ml
		Tablets: 125 mg, 250 mg, 500 mg

Cephalexin (Keflet, Keflex)	*Orally:*
	   Children: 50–100 mg/kg/day in 4 divided doses for otitis media and serious infections. Doses of 25–50 mg/kg/day in 2–4 divided doses may be used for less serious infections. Do not exceed adult doses.
	   Adults: 1–4 g/day in 4 divided doses.
		Capsules: 250 mg, 500 mg
		Drops: 100 mg/ml
		Suspension: 125 mg/5 ml, 250 mg/5 ml
		Tablets: 250 mg, 500 mg, 1 g

Cetirizine (Zyrtec)	*Orally:* Age 6 years–adults: 5–10 mg/day as a single dose.	Syrup: 1 mg/ml Tablets: 5 mg, 10 mg

Charcoal (Actidose-Aqua, Actidose with Sorbitol, CharcoAid, LiquiChar)	*Orally:* usually available as premixed solutions. Solutions containing sorbitol should not be used for multiple doses because diarrhea will occur. Do not administer concomitantly with ipecac because charcoal will adsorb and inactivate the ipecac. Do not administer with milk, ice cream, or sherbet because adsorptive capacity of the charcoal will be decreased.
	Single dose:
	   Children: 1–2 g/kg up to 15–30 g as soon as possible after the ingestion, preferably after emesis.
	   Adults: 30–100 g.
	   Dose should be 5 to 10 times the amount of the ingested poison.
	Multiple dose (products without sorbitol):
	   Infants: 1 g/kg every 4–6 hours.
	   Children and adults: 1–2 g/kg (up to 60 g) every 2–6 hours.
		Liquid: 25 g/120 ml, 30 g/240 ml, 50 g/240 ml
		Liquid, with sorbitol: 25 g/120 ml, 50 g/240 ml

Continued

Table 107   Medications   (continued)

DRUG	DOSE	DOSAGE FORMS
Chloral hydrate (Aquachloral, Noctec)	*Orally or rectally:* *Sedation before procedures:* 60–75 mg/kg 30 minutes to 1 hour before the procedure. May repeat with a half-dose (30–37.5 mg/kg) if the first dose is ineffective. Do not exceed 120 mg/kg or 2 g total. *Sedation for anxiety:* 25 mg/kg/day in divided doses every 6–8 hours to a maximum of the usual adult dose of 750 mg/day. Continuous therapy, especially in infants, is not recommended due to accumulation of the active metabolites.	Capsules: 250 mg, 500 mg Suppositories: 324 mg, 500 mg, 648 mg Syrup: 500 mg/5 ml
Chloramphenicol (Chloromycetin)	*IV or orally:* Neonates under age 7 days: 25 mg/kg/day in a single daily dose. Neonates age 7–21 days: 50 mg/kg/day in 2 divided doses daily. Infants and children: 50–75 mg/kg/day in 4 divided doses to a maximum total daily dose of 4 g. Adults: 50 mg/kg/day in 4 divided doses to a maximum total daily dose of 4 g. Serum levels must be monitored closely, especially in neonates and infants, and patients with renal or hepatic impairment.	Capsules: 250 mg Injection: 1-g vial
Chlorothiazide (Diuril)	*Orally:* Infants under age 6 months: 20–40 mg/kg/day in 2 divided doses. Children: 20 mg/kg/day in 2 divided doses. Adults: 0.5–1 g/day in 1 or 2 divided doses. *IV:* Infants under age 6 months: 20–40 mg/kg/day in 2 divided doses, but doses of 2–8 mg/kg/day may be sufficient in some patients. Children: 4–20 mg/kg/day in 2 divided doses. Adults: 0.5–1 g/day.	Injection: 500 mg Suspension: 250 mg/5 ml Tablets: 250 mg, 500 mg
Chlorpromazine (Thorazine)	*Nausea and vomiting or psychosis:* Over age 6 months: 0.3–0.5 mg/kg IV every 6–8 hours or 0.5–1 mg/kg PO every 4–6 hours or 1 mg/kg rectally every 6–8 hours as needed. Do not exceed adult doses. Adults: 25–50 mg IV every 6–8 hours or 10–25 mg PO every 4–6 hours or 50–100 mg rectally every 6–8 hours. Doses may be increased in the treatment of psychoses; some adults may require as much as 800 mg/day until control is achieved. Dose should then be decreased to the usual maintenance levels of 200 mg/day for adults.	Injection: 25 mg/ml Oral concentrate: 30 mg/ml, 100 mg/ml Suppositories: 25 mg, 100 mg Syrup: 10 mg/5 ml Tablets: 10 mg, 25 mg, 50 mg, 100 mg, 200 mg
Cholestyramine resin (Cholybar, Questran, Questran Light)	*Orally:* Children: 240 mg/kg/day of the resin administered in 3 divided doses. Adults: 3–4 g tid or qid. Doses should be administered mixed in liquids (4 g in 2–6 oz) or with pulpy fruits (applesauce or pineapple). Many drugs bind with cholestyramine in the GI tract. Drugs should be administered 1 hour before or 4 hours after cholestyramine. Patients should also be cautioned to ingest plenty of fluids, because constipation and fecal impaction are potential side effects of cholestyramine administration.	Bar: 4 g resin/bar (Cholybar) Powder: 4 g resin/9 g powder (Questran); 4 g resin/ 5 g powder (Questran Light, contains aspartame)

Continued

971

Table 107 Medications (continued)

DRUG	DOSE	DOSAGE FORMS

Cimetidine (Tagamet)	*Orally, IV:*
	Initial dose:
	  Neonates: 5–10 mg/kg/day in 2–3 divided doses daily.
	  Infants: 10–20 mg/kg/day in 2–4 divided doses daily.
	  Children: 20–40 mg/kg/day in 4 divided doses daily.
	  Adults: 300 mg every 6 hours. Orally, doses of 800 mg at bedtime or 400 mg bid may be used.
	  Doses may be adjusted upward, especially in hypersecretory states, as necessary to maintain the gastric pH of 5 or greater. A maximum total daily dose of 2.4 g should not be exceeded.
	  Dosage must be adjusted in renal impairment.
		Injection: 150 mg/ml
		Liquid: 300 mg/5 ml
		Tablets: 200 mg, 300 mg, 400 mg, 800 mg

Ciprofloxacin (Ciloxan, Cipro)	The drug is not approved for use in patients under age 18 due to possible adverse effects; consider risk vs benefit if for use in patients under age 18.
	Orally (on an empty stomach):
	  Children: 20–30 mg/kg/day in 2 divided doses; up to 40 mg/kg/day may be used for patients with cystic fibrosis. Do not exceed 1.5 g/day.
	  Adults: 500–1500 mg/day in 2 divided doses.
	IV (administer over 1 hour at a concentration of 1–2 mg/ml):
	  Children: 15–20 mg/kg/day in 2 divided doses; up to 30 mg/kg/day may be used in patients with cystic fibrosis. Do not exceed 800 mg/day.
	  Adults: 400–800 mg/day in 2 divided doses.
	  Dosage must be adjusted in patients with renal dysfunction.
	Ophthalmic: administer 1–2 drops every 2 hours while awake for 2 days and then every 4 hours while awake for 5 days.
		Injection: 10 mg/ml
		Solution, ophthalmic: 3.5%
		Tablets: 250 mg, 500 mg, 750 mg

Cisapride (Propulsid)	*Orally:*
	  Infants and children: 0.15–0.3 mg/kg/dose administered tid or qid. Do not exceed 10 mg/dose.
	  Adult: 10 mg/dose qid. Some patients may require a dose of 20 mg qid.
		Suspension: 1 mg/ml
		Tablets: 10 mg

Citrate and citric acid (Bicitra, Polycitra, Shohl's Solution)	*Orally (dilute in water or juice):*
	  Infants and children: 2–3 mEq/kg/day in 3–4 divided doses.
	  Adults: 15–30 ml given qid.
	  Giving doses with meals decreases the saline laxative effect.
		Content per 1 ml*

Clarithromycin (Biaxin)	*Orally:*
	  Children: 15 mg/kg/day in 2 divided doses, not to exceed 1 g/day.
	  Adults: 500 mg–1 g/day in 2 divided doses.
		Suspension: 125 mg/5 ml, 250 mg/5 ml
		Tablets: 250 mg, 500 mg

Clindamycin (Cleocin)	*IV:*
	  Neonates under age 7 days:
	    ≤2000 g: 10 mg/kg/day in 2 divided doses.
	    >2000 g: 15 mg/kg/day in 3 divided doses.
	  Neonates over age 7 days:
	    <1200 g: 10 mg/kg/day in 2 divided doses.
	    1200–2000 g: 15 mg/kg/day in 3 divided doses.
	    >2000 g: 20 mg/kg/day in 3–4 divided doses.
	  Infants and children: 25–40 mg/kg/day in 3–4 divided doses.
	  Adults: 1.2–2.7 g/day in 2–4 divided doses. Maximum total daily dose should not exceed 4.8 g and should be used for life-threatening infections only.
		Capsules: 150 mg
		Injection: 150 mg/ml
		Solution, oral: 75 mg/5 ml
		Solution, topical: 1%

Continued

Table 107   Medications   (continued)

DRUG	*DOSE*	*DOSAGE FORMS*

Clindamycin (Cleocin) (*continued*)	*Orally:*
	  Infants and children: 15–25 mg/kg/day in 4 divided doses for moderate to severe infections.
	  Adults: 150–450 mg every 6–8 hours to a maximum total daily dose of 1.8 g.
	Topically: apply to the affected area bid. Avoid the eyes, abraded skin, and mucous membranes.	

Clonazepam (Klonopin)	*Orally:*
	  Under age 10 or <30 kg: initially 0.01–0.03 mg/kg/day in 2–3 divided doses. Dose may be increased gradually (every third day) until seizures are controlled or adverse effects are seen. The usual maintenance dose range is 0.1–0.2 mg/kg/day.
	  Adults >30 kg: initially 1.5 mg/day in 3 divided doses. Dose may be increased by 0.5–1 mg every third day to a maximum total daily dose of 20 mg. Usual maintenance dose is 0.05–0.2 mg/kg/day.
		Tablets: 0.5 mg, 1 mg, 2 mg

Clorazepate dipotassium (Tranxene)	*Orally:*
	  Age 9–12: initially 3.75–7.5 mg bid. Dose may be increased by 3.75 mg at weekly intervals to a maximum total daily dose of 60 mg.
	  Over age 12 and adults: up to 7.5 mg up to tid. May be increased by 7.5 mg at weekly intervals to a maximum total daily dose of 90 mg.
		Capsules or tablets: 3.75 mg, 7.5 mg, 15 mg
		Tablets: 11.25 mg, 22.5 mg

Clotrimazole (Lotrimin, Mycelex)	*Vaginal cream:* 1 applicatorful at bedtime for 7–14 days. *Vaginal suppository:* 1 suppository intravaginally at bedtime for 7 days or 2 at bedtime for 3 days or 500 mg as a single dose. *Topically:* apply to affected areas bid.	Cream, topical: 1% (30-g tube) Cream, vaginal: 1% (45-g tube) Solution, topical: 1% (30-ml squeeze bottle) Suppositories, vaginal: 100 mg, 500 mg
Cocaine hydrochloride	*Topically:* use the lowest effective dose. Do not exceed 1 mg/kg.	Solution, topical: 4%, 10%
Codeine	*Orally:* *Analgesic:* 0.5–1 mg/kg every 3–6 hours as needed, to a maximum of 60 mg. Usual adult dose is 30 mg. *Antitussive:* 0.2–0.25 mg/kg every 4–6 hours as needed, to a maximum of 30 kg. *SC:* same doses as above may be used, although the oral route is only two thirds as effective as the SC route. It should not be used IV. If an IV analgesic is required, morphine should be used.	Injection (phosphate): 30 mg/ml, 60 mg/ml Solution, oral (phosphate): 15 mg/5 ml Tablets (sulfate): 15 mg, 30 mg, 60 mg Also available in various combinations with acetaminophen: Elixir, oral: 12 mg codeine with 120 mg acetaminophen Tablets: 7.5 mg codeine with acetaminophen 300 mg (Tylenol w/ Codeine No. 1), 15 mg codeine with acetaminophen 300 mg (Tylenol w/ Codeine No. 2), 300 mg codeine with acetaminophen 300 mg (Tylenol w/ Codeine No. 3), 60 mg codeine with acetaminophen 300 mg (Tylenol w/ Codeine No. 4)
Colfosceril palmitate (Exosurf Neonatal)	*Intratracheally:* should be used only by physicians familiar with its administration. The usual dose is 5 ml/kg divided equally between the two lungs. Second and third doses may be administered at 12-hour intervals. The infant should be suctioned before administration of colfosceril and ventilator settings should be decreased, depending on the patient's response.	Powder, lyophilized: 108 mg/10 ml

Colistin, neomycin, and hydrocortisone (Coly-Mycin S Otic)	*Otic* (shake bottle well before administering):
	  Children: 3 drops in the affected ear tid or qid.
	  Adults: 4 drops in the affected ear tid or qid.
		Suspension, OTIC: 5 ml

Continued

Table 107 Medications (continued)

DRUG	*DOSE*	*DOSAGE FORMS*
Corticotropin [ACTH (adrenocorticotropic hormone)]	*IM:* Usually 40–80 U/day as a single dose for 7–10 days, followed by a tapering schedule. Therapy should not be discontinued abruptly. Higher doses and longer therapy regimens have also been used.	Repository gel injection: 40 U/ml, 80 U/ml
Cortisone acetate (Cortone Acetate)	Depends on the use of the drug and patient response. *Orally:* *Physiologic replacement:* 0.5–0.75 mg/kg/day in 3 divided doses. *Anti-inflammatory:* 2.5–10 mg/kg/day in 3–4 divided doses. *IM:* *Physiologic replacement:* 0.25–0.35 mg/kg/day as a single dose. *Anti-inflammatory:* 1–5 mg/kg/day in 1 or 2 divided doses. In patients requiring physiologic replacement, dosage may need to be increased during periods of stress, including perioperatively and during illness.	Injection: 50 mg/ml Tablets: 5 mg, 10 mg, 25 mg
Cosyntropin (Cortrosyn)	*IV:* Under age 2: 0.125 mg. Over age 2 and adults: 0.25 mg.	Injection: 0.25 mg
Co-trimoxazole (trimethoprim and sulfamethoxazole; Bactrim, Septra)	*Orally or IV (based on trimethoprim):* Over age 2 months and adults: *Treatment doses:* *Mild to moderate infections (urinary tract or otitis media):* 8 mg trimethoprim/kg/day in 2 divided doses. Maximum dose is 320 mg trimethoprim/day. *Pneumocystis carinii pneumonitis:* 20 mg trimethoprim/kg/day in 4 divided doses. *Prophylaxis doses:* *Urinary tract infection:* 2 mg trimethoprim/kg/day as a single dose. *Pneumocystis carinii:* 10 mg trimethoprim/kg/day in 2 divided doses daily for 3 days per week. Dosage adjustment is necessary in patients with renal impairment. IV doses must be administered over 60–90 minutes and should be well diluted (1 ml injection in 25 ml infusate).	Injection: 16 mg trimethoprim and 80 mg sulfamethoxazole per 1 ml Suspension: 8 mg trimethoprim and 40 mg sulfamethoxazole per 1 ml Tablets: 80 mg trimethoprim and 400 mg sulfamethoxazole Tablets, double strength: 160 mg trimethoprim and 800 mg sulfamethoxazole
Cromolyn sodium (Intal, Nasalcrom)	Children: *Metered-dose inhaler:* 2 inhalations qid. *Spinhaler dry inhalation:* contents of 1 capsule qid. *Nebulizer solution:* 20 mg nebulized qid. *Intranasal spray:* 1 spray in each nostril 3–6 times daily.	Capsules, powder for inhalation: 20 mg Inhalation, metered dose: 800 μg/spray Solution, nasal: 5.2 mg/spray Solution, nebulizer: 20 mg/2 ml
Crotamiton (Eurax)	*Topically:* apply a thin layer to all skin surfaces from the neck to the toes and soles of the feet. Be sure to apply to all surfaces, including skin folds. Avoid the face and mucous membranes, including the urethral meatus. A second coat is applied 24 hours later. A cleansing bath should follow 48 hours after the second application. Treatment may be repeated after 7–10 days if the mites reappear. It is safe for use in infants and young children. If signs of irritation or hypersensitivity appear, remove the product immediately by bathing. Contaminated clothing and bed linens should be washed to avoid reinfestations.	Cream: 10% Lotion: 10%

Continued

Table 107   Medications   (continued)

DRUG	DOSE	DOSAGE FORMS

Cyanocobalamin (vitamin B$_{12}$; Betalin 12)	*IM:*
	Congenital pernicious anemia:
	  Children: 1000 μg/day for 2 weeks, then maintenance doses of 50 μg monthly.
	  Adults: 100 μg monthly.
	Vitamin B$_{12}$ deficiency: 100 μg for 2 weeks, then twice weekly for several months, then every other month.
	Oral dosing is not recommended due to poor absorption.
		Injection: 100 μg/ml, 1000 μg/ml

Cyclopentolate (Cyclogyl)	Instill 1 drop into each eye 5–10 minutes before exam in infants or 40–50 minutes before exam in children and adults. Finger pressure on the lacrimal duct for 1–2 minutes after instillation decreases systemic absorption. In adults, 2% solution may be necessary in patients with highly pigmented irises.	Solution, ophthalmic: 0.5%, 1%, 2%
Cyclosporine (Neoral, Sandimmune)	NOTE: The two are *not* bioequivalent. Clinical condition and serum levels must be monitored carefully when a patient's therapy is changed from one to the other, especially in patients receiving large doses (>10 mg/kg/day) of Sandimmune who are changed to Neoral therapy because significant drug toxicity may result. *Orally:* *Sandimmune:* initially 10–18 mg/kg/day (dose dependent on organ being transplanted) in 2 divided doses, tapering over several weeks with frequent monitoring to a maintenance dose usually in the range of 5–10 mg/kg/day. *Neoral:* initially about 10 mg/kg/day in 2 divided doses, tapering over several weeks based on clinical condition and serum levels. *Conversion from Sandimmune to Neoral:* start with the same dose unless the patient's Sandimmune dose is >10 mg/kg/day. Dose may then be decreased to maintain former cyclosporine serum level. Patients who require high doses of Sandimmune should have serum levels monitored daily to prevent toxicity due to higher cyclosporine levels than may be achieved with Neoral. Sandimmune liquid may be mixed with milk or juice in a glass container to improve palatability. Neoral liquid should be mixed with fruit juice because the mixture with milk may be unpalatable. In both cases, the mixture should be administered immediately and the container should be rinsed with more fluid to be sure the whole dose is administered. *IV (Sandimmune only):* 5–6 mg/kg/day in 1 or 2 divided doses. Each dose should be administered over at least 2 hours.	Capsules (Neoral): 25 mg, 100 mg Capsules (Sandimmune): 25 mg, 50 mg, 100 mg Injection (Sandimmune): 50 mg/ml Solution, oral (Neoral and Sandimmune): 100 mg/ml
Deferoxamine (Desferal)	Children: *Acute iron intoxication:* 15 mg/kg/hr IV continuous infusion; maximum 6 g/24 hr. *Chronic iron overload:* 20–25 mg/kg/day IM or 500 mg–2 g IV with each unit of blood transfused, or 20–40 mg/kg/day SC over 8–12 hours up to 1–2 g/day.	Injection: 500-mg vial

Continued

Table 107   Medications   (continued)

DRUG	_DOSE_	_DOSAGE FORMS_

Desmopressin acetate (DDAVP)	_Intranasally:_
	Nocturnal enuresis in patients under age 6: 20 μg at bedtime with half of dose in each nostril. Dose may be increased or decreased depending on the patient's response. Usual range is 10–40 μg/day.
	Diabetes insipidus in patients age 3 months–adults: initially 5 μg/day as a single dose or in 2 divided doses. Dosage should be titrated to the patient's response. The usual range is 5–40 μg/day.
	Orally:
	Diabetes insipidus:
	  Children: initially, 0.05 mg/dose with careful monitoring to prevent hyponatremia or water intoxication.
	  Over age 12 and adults: initially, 0.05 mg bid. Dosage may then be adjusted to maintain normal diurnal water turnover. The usual total daily dosage is in the range of 0.1–1.2 mg and may be administered in 2–3 divided doses.
	Nocturnal enuresis in children over age 12: 0.2–0.4 mg/day at bedtime.
	_IV:_
	To increase factor VIII levels: 0.3 μg/kg over 30 minutes.
	Diabetes insipidus: adult doses are 2–4 μg/day in 2 divided doses or approximately one tenth of the intranasal dose necessary to control the patient's symptoms, if that is known.
		Injection: 4 μg/ml
		Solution, nasal: 100 μg/ml/2.4 ml bottle with calibrated intranasal tube
		Spray, intranasal: 10 μg/actuation metered dose
		Tablets: 0.1 mg, 0.2 mg

Dexamethasone (Decadron, Hexadrol, Maxidex)	_IV or orally:_ _Bacteria meningitis:_ 0.6 mg/kg/day in 4 divided doses for the first 4 days of antibiotic therapy. It must be started at the same time or before the first dose of antibiotic. _Cerebral edema:_ 1–1.5 mg/kg/day in 4 divided doses to a maximum total daily dose of 16 mg. _Antiemetic therapy (chemotherapy-induced emesis):_ 20 mg/m²/day in 4 divided doses. _Airway edema or extubation:_ 0.5–2 mg/kg/day in 4 divided doses beginning 24 hours before and continuing for at least 24 hours after extubation. Doses should be tapered when discontinuing long-term therapy. _Ophthalmic:_ instill drops or apply ointment tid or qid.	Elixir: 0.5 mg/5 ml Injection: 4 mg/ml, 10 mg/ml, 20 mg/ml, 24 mg/ml Ointment, ophthalmic: 0.05% Solution, ophthalmic: 0.05% Solution, oral: 1 mg/ml Tablets: 0.25 mg, 0.5 mg, 0.75 mg, 1 mg, 1.5 mg, 2 mg, 4 mg, 6 mg

Dextroamphetamine sulfate (Dexedrine)	_Orally:_
	  Age 3–5: 2.5 mg/day given in the morning. Dosage may be increased 2.5 mg/day until a response is realized or side effects appear. Usual range is 0.1–0.5 mg/kg/day to a maximum of 40 mg.
	  Age 6 or older: 5 mg/day in the morning or at noon. Dosage may be increased in 5-mg increments at weekly intervals. Usual range is 0.1–0.5 mg/kg/day to a maximum of 40 mg.
		Capsules, sustained release: 5 mg, 10 mg, 15 mg
		Tablets: 5 mg, 10 mg

Dextrose (Glucose)	_IV for resuscitation:_ 1 g/kg. Usual infusion rates are 0.5–0.8 g/kg/hr.
	Orally for glucose tolerance testing:
	  Neonates to age 2: 3 g/kg (minimum dose 10 g).
	  Age 2–12: 1.75 g/kg (maximum dose 50 g).
	  Over age 12: 1.25 g/kg (maximum dose 50 g).
		Injection: 5% or 10% for infusion (available in water, half normal saline, normal saline, lactated Ringer's, etc.)
		Injection: 10%, 25%, 50%
		Solution, oral: 100 g/300 ml

Continued

Table 107   Medications   (continued)

DRUG	DOSE	DOSAGE FORMS
Diazepam (Valium)	**IV:** *Status epilepticus:* 0.05–0.3 mg/kg administered over 2–3 minutes and repeated every 15–30 minutes to a total maximum dose of 0.75 mg/kg or 30 mg, whichever is less. May be repeated in 2–4 hours, if necessary. *Sedation:* 0.04–0.2 mg/kg every 2–4 hours to a maximum of 0.6 mg/kg within an 8-hour period. *Orally for sedation or muscle relaxant:* 0.12–0.8 mg/kg/day in 3–4 divided doses to an adult dose of 6–40 mg/day. *Rectally:* 0.5 mg/kg of the injectable with a repeat dose of 0.25 mg/kg, if necessary, 10 minutes later.	Injection: 5 mg/ml Solution, oral: 5 mg/5 ml Solution, concentrated oral: 5 mg/ml Tablets: 2 mg, 5 mg, 10 mg
Diazoxide (Hyperstat IV, Proglycem)	**IV (hypertensive emergency):** 1–3 mg/kg to a maximum of 150 mg. Dose may be repeated in 5–15 minutes. **Orally (hypoglycemia due to hyperinsulinism):** Newborns and infants: initially 8 mg/kg/day in 2 or 3 divided doses. May be increased incrementally if response is inadequate to a maximum of 15 mg/kg/day. Children and adults: 3 mg/kg/day in 2 or 3 divided doses initially. May be increased to a maximum of 8 mg/kg/day.	Capsules: 50 mg Injection: 15 mg/ml Suspension, oral: 50 mg/ml
Dicloxacillin (Dycill, Dynapen, Pathocil)	**Orally:** Children <40 kg: 25–50 mg/kg/day in 4 divided doses. Doses of 50–100 mg/kg/day in 4 divided doses are necessary for follow-up oral therapy of osteomyelitis. Children >40 kg and adults: 125–500 mg/dose every 6 hours.	Capsules: 250 mg, 500 mg Suspension, oral: 62.5 mg/5 ml
Didanosine [ddl (dideoxyinisine); Videx]	**Orally:** doses must be given at 12-hour intervals on an empty stomach, but because the drug is degraded by gastric acids, each formulation contains buffers. Infants and children: 240 mg/m²/day in 2 divided doses. If the tablet formulation is used, children over age 1 should receive 2 tablets per dose to assure sufficient buffering. Children under age 1 may receive doses in a single tablet. Adults: <60 kg: 125 mg (tablets) or 167 mg (buffered powder) per dose. ≥60 kg: 200 mg (tablets) or 250 mg (buffered powder) per dose.	Powder for oral solution, buffered (single-dose packets): 100 mg, 167 mg, 250 mg, 375 mg Powder for oral solution, pediatric (mixed with an antacid at the time it is dispensed by the pharmacist): 10 mg/ml Tablets, buffered, chewable/dispersible: 25 mg, 50 mg, 100 mg, 150 mg
Digoxin (Lanoxicaps, Lanoxin)	Should be based on lean body weight. Dosage adjustment is required in patients with impaired renal function. Total digitalizing dose (TDD) is administered as follows: half TDD initially, then one fourth TDD 8–12 hours later, then one fourth TDD 8–12 hours after that. Maintenance doses are administered in 2 divided doses beginning 12 hours after the last digitalizing dose. Patients should be under continuous cardiographic monitoring during digitalization. IM doses are the same as oral doses, but that route of administration should be avoided.†	Capsules, liquid filled (Lanoxicaps): 0.05 mg, 0.1 mg, 0.2 mg (90%–100% bioavailable) Elixir: 0.05 mg/ml (75%–87% bioavailable) Injection: 0.1 mg/ml, 0.25 mg/ml (100% bioavailable IV) Tablets: 0.125 mg, 0.25 mg, 0.5 mg (60%–80% bioavailable)

Continued

Table 107 Medications (continued)

DRUG	DOSE	DOSAGE FORMS

Dimercaprol [BAL (British anti-lewisite)]	*Deep IM:*
	Lead toxicity:
	  Moderate poisoning: 2 mg/kg 6 times a day or up to 12 mg/24 hr for 2–3 days.
	  Severe poisoning: 4 mg/kg 6 times a day for 5–7 days.
	  Arsenic, mercury, or gold toxicity:
	  Mild:
	    Days 1 and 2: 3 mg/kg qid.
	    Day 3: 3 mg/kg bid.
	    Days 4–14: 3 mg/kg every day.
	  Severe:
	    Days 1 and 2: 3 mg/kg 6 times a day.
	    Day 3: 3 mg/kg qid.
	    Days 4–14: 3 mg/kg bid.
		Injection: 100 mg/ml (3-ml ampul)

Diphenhydramine (Benadryl, Benylin, Nytol, Sleep-Eze 3, Sominex Formula 2)	*IV, orally, IM:*
	  Children: 5 mg/kg/day in 3 or 4 divided doses to a maximum of 300 mg/day.
	  Adults: 10–50 mg repeated as often as every 4 hours, not to exceed 400 mg/day.
	  The drug may cause paradoxical excitement in children.
		Capsules: 25 mg, 50 mg
		Elixir (14% alcohol): 12.5 mg/5 ml
		Injection: 10 mg/ml, 50 mg/ml
		Syrup (5% alcohol): 12.5 mg/5 ml
		Tablets: 25 mg, 50 mg

Diphtheria and tetanus toxoids (Td, DT)
Diphtheria and tetanus toxoids and acellular pertussis vaccine (DaPT, DTaP, Acel-Immune, Tripedia)
	IM (0.5 ml/dose):
	  Infants age 6 weeks–1 year: 3 doses at least 4 weeks apart and a fourth dose 6–12 months after the third dose.
	  Age 1–6: 2 doses at least 4 weeks apart and a third dose 6–12 months after the second dose.
	  Over 7: 2 doses of the adult preparation (lower concentration of diphtheria taxoid) at least 4 weeks apart and a third dose 6–12 months later.
	  Booster doses: should be administered every 10 years.
	  Diphtheria and tetanus toxoids and pertussis vaccine are preferred for the initial immunization of infants.
		Injection, pediatric (DT): diphtheria 6.6–15 Lf U and tetanus 5–10 Lf U/0.5 ml
		Injection, adult (Td): diphtheria 2 Lf U and tetanus 2–10 Lf U/0.5 ml

Diphtheria and tetanus toxoids and whole-cell pertussis vaccine (DwPT, DTwP, Tri-Immunol); diphtheria and tetanus toxoids and acellular pertussis vaccine (DaPT, DTaP, Acel-Immune, Tripedia)	*IM (0.5 ml/dose):* ideally, immunization should begin at age 6–8 weeks with 3 doses at 4–8-week intervals and a fourth dose 1 year after the third dose. A booster dose is given at age 4–6. Neither should be used after the 7th birthday.	Injection: diphtheria 5–12.5 Lf U, tetanus 5–10 Lf U, and pertussis 4 U/0.5 ml Injection: diphtheria 6.7 or 7.5 Lf U, tetanus 5 Lf U, and acellular pertussis 40–46.8 μg/0.5 ml
Diphtheria and tetanus toxoids, whole-cell pertussis, and *Haemophilus influenzae* type b vaccine (Tetramune)	*IM:* 0.5 mg/dose beginning at about age 2 months at approximately 2-month intervals with a fourth dose administered at about age 15 months.	Injection: diphtheria 12.5 Lf U, tetanus toxoid 5 Lf U, pertussis ≤16 U, *Haemophilus* oligosaccharide complex 10 μg/0.5 ml
Diphtheria antitoxin	*IV by slow infusion or IM:* all patients are dosed the same. Sensitivity to horse serum should be tested before administering the dose.	Injection: 10,000-U vial, 20,000-U vial (available from the CDC)
Dobutamine hydrochloride (Dobutrex)	*IV infusion:* 2–15 μg/kg/min to a maximum of 40 μg/kg/min. Start at the lower end of the range and titrate upward based on the patient's response.	Injection: 12.5 mg/ml

Docusate sodium (dioctyl sodium sulfosuccinate; Colace, D-S-S, Doxinate)	*Orally* (in 1–4 divided doses with a glass of water):
	  Infants and children under age 3: 10–40 mg/day.
	  Age 3–6: 20–60 mg/day.
	  Age 6–12: 40–150 mg/day.
	  Over age 12 and adults: 50–500 mg. Do not administer with mineral oil because absorption of the mineral oil may be increased.
		Capsules: 50 mg, 100 mg, 240 mg, 250 mg
		Liquid: 150 mg/15 ml
		Solution: 50 mg/ml
		Syrup: 50 mg/15 ml, 60 mg/15 ml
		Also available in combination with stimulant laxatives, including senna, phenolphthalein, and casanthranol.

Continued

Table 107   Medications   (continued)

DRUG	DOSE	DOSAGE FORMS
Dopamine hydrochloride (Dopastat, Intropin)	*Continuous IV infusion:* initially 1 μg/kg/min titrated upward based on patient's response to a maximum of 20 μg/kg/min in neonates or 50 μg/kg/min in all other patients. The hemodynamic effects of dopamine occur only at doses >15 μg/kg/min.	Injection in 5% dextrose: 0.8 mg/ml, 1.6 mg/ml, 3.2 mg/ml (premixed infusions) Injection: 40 mg/ml, 80 mg/ml, 160 mg/ml
Doxycycline (Doryx, Doxy-100, Vibramycin)	*Orally or IV:* Children under age 8: should not be used unless there is no alternative. Over age 8: 2–5 mg/kg/day to a maximum of 200 mg/day in 1 or 2 divided doses. Adults: 100–200 mg/day in 1 or 2 divided doses. Inpatient treatment of PID 100 mg IV bid with cefoxitin 2 g IV every 6 hours for at least 4 days or 2 days after patient improves, whichever is longer. Doxycycline should be continued orally to complete 10–14 days of therapy.	Capsules or tablets: 50 mg, 100 mg Injection: 100 mg, 200 mg
d-Xylose (wood sugar; Xylo-Pfan)	*Orally* (prepared as a 5%–10% aqueous solution): 14.5 g/m^2 to a maximum dose of 25 g. Alternatively, a dose of 500 mg/kg may be used. Infants should fast for 4–5 hours before the dose and children should fast overnight. Blood xylose levels are then measured to determine extent of intestinal absorption.	Powder for preparing oral solutions: 25 g
Edetate calcium disodium (Calcium Disodium Versenate, Calcium EDTA)	*Mild to moderate lead poisoning:* 25–50 mg/kg. *Severe lead poisoning:* up to 75 mg/kg/24 hr not to exceed 1.5 g/day. *Usual dosage* (children): *Asymptomatic lead toxicity:* Initial: up to 1 g/m^2/24 hr in a continuous IV drip if possible or in 2–4 divided doses for 5 days. Subsequent courses: up to 50 mg/kg/24 hr in a continuous IV drip is possible or in 2–4 divided doses for 3–5 days. *Symptomatic lead toxicity or lead encephalopathy:* Initial: up to 1.5 g/m^2/24 hr in a continuous IV drip if possible or in 6 divided doses for 5–7 days; give with dimercaprol (BAL). Subsequent courses: as for asymptomatic toxicity above.	Injection: 200 mg/ml For intravenous infusion, dilute to a maximum concentration of 5 mg/ml with D$_5$W or normal saline. Infusions should be administered either continuously or over 1–2 hours if intermittent doses are used. Rapid infusion may increase intracranial pressure.
Edrophonium (Enlon, Reversol, Tensilon)	*Myasthenia gravis test:* 0.2 mg/kg as a single dose IV. Infants: Initial: 0.1 mg; if no response, follow with an additional 0.4 mg for a maximum total dose of 0.5 mg. Children: Initial: 0.04 mg/kg followed by 0.16 mg/kg if no response; maximum total dose is 10 mg. *Titration of therapy:* 0.04 mg/kg one time; if strength improves, an increase in neostigmine or pyridostigmine dose is indicated. *Reversal of nondepolarizing neuromuscular blocking agents:* 1 mg/kg/dose.	Injection: 10 mg/ml May precipitate cholinergic crisis.
Enalapril, enalaprilat (Vasotec)	*Orally:* initially 0.1 mg/kg/day in 1 or 2 divided doses to the usual adult dose of 2.5–5 mg/kg/day. Dosage may be increased as required to a maximum of 0.5 mg/kg/day or 40 mg. *IV:* 5–10 μg/kg (up to 0.625–1.25 mg) may be administered every 8–24 hours as necessary for control of hypertension.	Injection: 1.25 mg/ml Tablets: 2.5 mg, 5 mg, 10 mg, 20 mg

Continued

Table 107   Medications   (continued)

DRUG	*DOSE*	*DOSAGE FORMS*
Enalapril, enalaprilat (Vasotec) (*continued*)	Dosage must be decreased in patients with compromised renal function and also should be decreased in patients who are hyponatremic or volume depleted, in severe congestive heart failure, or in those who are receiving diuretics. The oral dosage form (enalapril) is a prodrug that is not stable in aqueous media. The injectable dosage form (enalaprilat) is the active form, but is not absorbed from the GI tract.	
Epinephrine (Adrenalin, Sus-Phrine, Vaponefrin)	*IV for bradycardia, asystole, or pulseless arrest:* Neonates: 0.01–0.03 mg/kg (0.1–0.3 ml/kg of a 1:10,000 solution) every 3–5 minutes as necessary. Infants to adults: 0.1 mg/kg to a maximum of 1 mg: may be repeated every 3–5 minutes as necessary. A continuous infusion may be started at a dose of 0.1–1 μg/kg/min and titrated to effect. *Nebulization:* 0.25–0.5 ml of a 2.25% racemic epinephrine solution diluted in 2.5–3 ml of normal saline for inhalation. *SC for allergic reactions:* 0.01 mg/kg to a maximum dose of 0.5 mg (of the 1:1000 solution). For a prolonged effect, 0.005 ml/kg/dose of the 1:200 suspension in glycerin (equivalent to 0.025 mg/kg/dose) may be given every 8–12 hours.	Aerosol: 0.2–0.3 mg/spray, depending on brand (Bronkaid Mist, Primatene Mist, AsthmaHaler Mist) Injection: 1:10,000 (0.1 mg/ml), 1:1000 (1 mg/ml) Injection pre-filled automatic syringe: 1:200 (EpiPen delivers 0.3 mg IM, EpiPen Jr. delivers 0.15 mg IM) Solution, racemic for inhalation: 2.25% (Asthma-Nefrin, S-2, Vaponefrin)
Epoetin alfa (erythropoietin; Epogen, EPO, r-HuEPO)	*IV or SC:* initially 50–100 U/kg administered 1–3 times weekly until the hematocrit reaches 30%–33%. Dosage should be lowered if the hematocrit exceeds that range or increases by more than 4 points in a 2-week period. It may be increased if the hematocrit does not reach the target range or fails to increase by 5–6 points in an 8-week period. The usual maintenance dose is 25 U/kg 3 times weekly. Hematocrit and serum iron levels should be monitored frequently. Blood pressure should also be monitored frequently, especially during initial therapy.	Injection: 2000 U/ml, 4000 U/ml, 10,000 U/ml
Ergocalciferol (vitamin D$_2$, activated ergosterol; Calciferol, Drisdol)	1 μg = 40 U. *Orally:* Healthy infants and children: 400 U/day. Infants and children with malabsorption syndromes: 1000 U/day. Children with liver disease: 4000–8000 U/day. Children with vitamin D-dependent rickets: 3000–5000 U/day. Nutritional rickets with normal absorption: 1000–5000 U/day; with malabsorption: 10,000–25,000 U/day. *IM:* should be retained for patients with rickets due to severe vitamin D deficiency. The dose for vitamin D-resistant rickets ranges from 50,000–500,000 U/day, for hypoparathyroidism from 50,000–200,000 U/day, and for familial hypophosphatemia from 10,000–80,000 U/day. The range between therapeutic and toxic doses is narrow. Patients must be closely monitored.	Capsules: 50,000 U (1.25 mg) Injection (in sesame oil): 500,000 U/ml (12.5 mg/ml) Solution, oral: 8000 U/ml (200 μg/ml)

Continued

Table 107 Medications (continued)

DRUG	*DOSE*	*DOSAGE FORMS*
Erythromycin (E-Mycin, Ery-Tab, Eryc, Erythrocin, E.E.S., Ilosone, Pediamycin)	*Orally* (do not exceed 2 g/day): Neonates: 20–30 mg/kg/day in 2 or 3 divided doses. Infants and children: Base or ethylsuccinate: 30–50 mg/kg/day in 3 or 4 divided doses. Estolate: 20–50 mg/kg/day in 3 or 4 divided doses. Adults: Base, estolate, or sterate: 250–500 mg every 6–12 hours. Ethylsuccinate: 400–800 mg every 6–12 hours. *Endocarditis prophylaxis* (penicillin-allergic patients): 20 mg/kg to a maximum of 1 g 2 hours before the procedure and 10 mg/kg to a maximum of 500 mg 6 hours later. *Bowel preparation* (erythromycin base, only): 15 mg/kg to a maximum of 1 g administered at 1:00, 2:00, and 11:00 PM on the day before surgery, usually combined with neomycin and mechanical cleansing of the bowel. *IV:* 15–20 mg/kg/day to a maximum of 4 g/day administered in 4 divided doses. *Ophthalmic ointment* for prophylaxis of neonates: apply a 0.5–1 cm ribbon of the ointment to each conjunctival sac. *Topically for acne:* apply to the affected areas bid. The skin should be washed, rinsed well, and dried before applying the erythromycin. Keep away from the eyes, nose, and mouth.	Base: Capsules, enteric-coated pellets; 250 mg Ointment, ophthalmic: 0.5% Solution, topical: 1.5%, 2% Tablets, enteric coated: 250 mg, 333 mg, 500 mg Tablets, film coated: 250 mg, 500 mg Estolate: Capsules: 250 mg Suspension: 125 mg/5 ml, 250 mg/5 ml Tablets: 500 mg Ethylsuccinate: Suspension: 200 mg/5 ml, 400 mg/5 ml Tablets: chewable: 200 mg Tablets: 400 mg Stearate: Tablets: 250 mg, 500 mg
Erythromycin and sulfisoxazole (Eryzole, Pediazole)	*Orally* (based on the erythromycin content): Up to age 2 months: 40–50 mg/kg/day in 3 or 4 divided doses to a maximum of 2 g/day. Alternatively, the following patient weights may be used: 8–15 kg: 2.5 ml every 6 hours. 16–23 kg: 5 ml every 6 hours. 24–44 kg: 7.5 ml every 6 hours. >45 kg: 10 ml every 6 hours.	Suspension: 200 mg erythromycin and 600 mg sulfisoxazole per 5 ml
Ethacrynic acid (Edecrin)	*Orally:* 1 mg/kg administered 1–2 times daily. Do not exceed the usual adult dose of 50–100 mg/day. *IV:* 0.4–1 mg/kg up to 50 mg administered 1 or 2 times daily. Serum electrolytes must be closely monitored during ethacrynic acid therapy.	Injection: 50 mg Tablets: 25 mg, 50 mg
Ethambutol (Myambutol)	*Orally* (patient should be old enough to cooperate with an eye exam; optic neuritis is an adverse effect): Children: 15 mg/kg/day in a single dose. Adolescents and adults: 15–25 mg/kg/day in a single dose. Do not exceed 2.5 g/day.	Tablets: 100 mg, 400 mg
Ethosuximide (Zarontin)	*Orally:* Under age 6: 15 mg/kg/day in 2 divided doses to a maximum of 250 mg/dose. Over age 6: 250 mg bid. Dose may be increased by 250 mg/day every 4–7 days to a maximum of 1.5 g/day or 40 mg/kg/day.	Capsules: 250 mg Syrup: 250 mg/5 ml

Continued

Table 107 Medications (continued)

DRUG	DOSE	DOSAGE FORMS
Fentanyl citrate (Sublimaze)	IV (slowly over a period of 3–5 minutes to avoid chest wall rigidity and to titrate to effect): Children: 1–2 μg/kg may be repeated at 30–60-minute intervals. For continuous therapy, after a bolus dose, a dose of 1 μg/kg/hr initially may be increased or decreased as necessary to response. Older children and adults: 0.5–1 μg/kg (25–50 μg) may be repeated at 30–60-minute intervals. The doses listed are analgesic/sedation doses. Doses used for general anesthesia may be higher.	Injection: 50 μg/ml
Ferrous sulfate (Feosol, Fer-In-Sol)	Orally (doses are expressed as elemental iron; ferrous sulfate contains 20% iron): Iron deficiency anemia: Children: 3–6 mg/kg/day depending on the severity of the deficiency. Higher doses should be administered in 3 divided doses; moderate doses may be administered in 2 divided doses to avoid GI upset. For prophylaxis, 1–2 mg/kg/day in a single dose may be used. Adults: 120–240 mg iron daily in 2–4 divided doses. For prophylaxis, 60 mg iron daily as a single dose. Administration between meals increases absorption, but may result in more GI upset. Do not administer with antacids, eggs, or milk because they may decrease absorption of the iron. Liquid preparations may stain the teeth.	Capsules: 50 mg Fe Drops: 15 mg Fe/0.6 ml Elixir: 44 mg Fe/5 ml Syrup: 18 mg Fe/5 ml Tablets: 60 mg Fe, 65 mg Fe
Fluconazole (Diflucan)	Orally or IV: Oropharyngeal or esophageal candidiasis: 6 mg/kg (up to 200 mg) on the first day; then 3 mg/kg/day (up to 100 mg). Systemic candidiasis or cryptococcal meningitis: 12 mg/kg (up to 400 mg) on the first day; then 6 mg/kg/day (up to 200 mg). Prevention of candidiasis in bone marrow transplant: 12 mg/kg/day (up to 400 mg) beginning several days before anticipated onset of neutropenia and continued until 7 days after neutrophil count is >1000/mm^3. Vaginal candidiasis: 150 mg as a single dose. Dosage should be adjusted in patients with renal dysfunction.	Injection: 2 mg/ml (ready to administer) Suspension: 10 mg/ml, 40 mg/ml Tablets: 50 mg, 100 mg, 150 mg, 200 mg
Flucytosine (Ancobon)	Orally: Children and adults: 50–150 mg/kg/day in 4 divided doses. Dosage must be adjusted in renal impairment.	Capsules: 250 mg, 500 mg
Fludrocortisone (Florinef)	Orally: Infants and children: 0.05–0.1 mg/day. Adults: 0.05–0.2 mg/day.	Tablets: 0.1 mg

Continued

Table 107 Medications (continued)

DRUG	DOSE	DOSAGE FORMS
Flumazenil (Mazicon, Romazicon)	IV: Children (little information is available on dosing in children): The following are guidelines only: 0.01 mg/kg (to a maximum of 0.2 mg) initially, followed by 0.005 mg/kg (to a maximum of 0.2 mg) every minute until a total cumulative dose of 1 mg has been reached. Adults: *Reversal of sedation:* 0.2 mg over 15 seconds; may repeat 0.2-mg dose every 60 seconds to a maximum of 1 mg. May repeat doses every 20 minutes to a maximum of 3 mg in 1 hour. *Benzodiazepine overdose:* 0.2 mg over 30 seconds, then 0.3 mg over 30 seconds if desired level of consciousness is not reached. Additional 0.5-mg doses may be given every minute until a cumulative dose of 3 mg has been reached. If a partial response is noted, further 0.5-mg doses may be given until a cumulative dose of 5 mg is reached. Resedation may occur in patients who received long-acting benzodiazepines.	Injection: 0.1 mg/ml
Flunisolide (Nasalide)	*Intranasal spray:* Age 6–14: 1 spray in each nostril tid or 2 sprays in each nostril bid initially. Maintenance dose is usually 1 spray in each nostril daily. Over age 14 and adults: 2 sprays in each nostril bid or tid initially. After symptoms are controlled, dosage should be decreased to the lowest dose that will prevent symptoms from recurring. That may be as little as 1 spray in each nostril once daily for perennial rhinitis. The maximum dose is 4 sprays to each nostril daily. Improvement in symptoms may take from several days to several weeks to occur, but therapy should not be continued for more than 3 weeks in the absence of efficacy.	Spray, intranasal: 25 μg/metered spray
Fluocinolone acetonide (Fluonid, Flurosyn, Synalar, Synemol)	*Topically:* apply a thin layer to the affected area bid to qid. Use the lowest effective potency product. Absorption is greater if the product is covered by anything that is occlusive (plastic pants, tight diapers).	Cream: 0.01%, 0.025%, 0.2% Ointment: 0.025% Shampoo: 0.01% Solution: 0.01%
Fluorescein sodium (AK-Fluor, Fluorets, Fluor-I-Strip, Ful-Glo)	Apply 1–2 drops of solution or touch conjunctiva with a moistened strip and allow 1–2 minutes for staining. Fluorescein will stain soft contact lenses permanently; allow at least 1 hour before replacing them in the eyes.	Solution, ophthalmic: 2% Strip, ophthalmic: 0.6 mg, 1 mg or 9 mg (packed in 2s)
Fluoride (Fluoritab, Karidium, Luride, Pediaflor)	*Orally:* dosage should be based on the fluoride content of the water supply. Long-term supplementation in areas with fluoridated water may result in dental fluorosis and osseous changes.* Fluoride content of drinking water <0.3 ppm: Birth–6 months: do not supplement. 6 months–3 years: 0.25 mg/day. 3–6 years: 0.5 mg/day. 6–16 years: 1 mg/day. Fluoride content of drinking water 0.3–0.6 ppm: Birth–3 years: do not supplement. 3–6 years: 0.25 mg/day. 6–16 years: 0.5 mg/day.	Most multivitamin combinations are available in formulations containing appropriate amounts of fluoride (Poly-Vi-Flor drops or chewable tablets, Tri-Vi-Flo drops, Vi-Daylin/F drops and chewable tablets). Products containing only fluoride: Drops: 0.125 mg/drop, 0.25 mg/drop, 0.5 mg/ml Solution: 0.2 mg/ml (may be used orally or as a rinse) Tablets, chewable: 0.5 mg, 1 mg

Continued

Table 107   Medications   (continued)

DRUG	DOSE	DOSAGE FORMS
Fluoride (Fluoritab, Karidium, Luride, Pediaflor) (continued)	Fluoride content of drinking water >0.6 ppm: do not supplement. *Dental gel:* usually applied by a dentist. *Rinses:* over-the-counter rinses may be used for patients over age 6 on a daily basis and contain 0.01%–0.02% fluoride.	
Folic acid (Folvite)	*Orally, parenterally:* Infants: 50 μg/day. Age 1–10: 1 mg/day initially, then 0.1–0.4 mg/day. Over age 11 and adults: 1 mg/day initially, then 0.5 mg/day.	Injection: 5 mg/ml, 10 mg/ml Tablets: 0.1 mg, 0.4 mg, 0.8 mg, 1 mg
Fosphenytoin—See phenytoin		
Furosemide (Lasix)	*Orally, IV, or IM:* Premature neonates (oral absorption may be poor): 1–2 mg/kg every 12–24 hours. Oral doses up to 4 mg/kg may be used. Children: 1–2 mg/kg every 6–12 hours but not to exceed 6 mg/kg/day. Adults: 20–80 mg/day in divided doses to a maximum of 600 mg/day. Serum electrolyte levels should be monitored closely.	Injection: 10 mg/ml Solution: 10 mg/ml, 40 mg/5 ml Tablets: 20 mg, 40 mg, 80 mg
Gabapentin (Neurontin)	*Orally (as add-on therapy):* Under age 12: no dosing recommendations are available at this time. Age 12–adults: initially, 300 mg on day 1, followed by rapid titration to 300 mg tid. The usual maintenance dosage range is 900–1800 mg/day in 3 divided doses to a maximum daily dose of 3600 mg. It is not necessary to monitor gabapentin levels or the levels of other antiepileptic drugs the patient may be taking because there are no significant drug interactions. Withdrawal of gabapentin therapy should be accomplished over a period of at least 1 week.	Capsules: 100 mg, 300 mg, 400 mg
Ganciclovir (Cytovene, DHPG)	*IV (as an infusion over 1 hour):* *Induction:* 10 mg/kg/day in 2 divided doses for 2–3 weeks. *Maintenance:* 5 mg/kg/day as a single dose for 7 days a week to 6 mg/kg/day for 5 days a week. *Orally:* *Maintenance therapy only:* in adults, a dose of 1000 mg tid with food is used. There are no guidelines for oral use in children. Dosage must be adjusted in patients with renal dysfunction.	Capsules: 250 mg Injection: 500-mg vial

Gentamicin (Garamycin)	*IV or IM (in obese patients it should be based on ideal, rather than actual, body weight):*
	Neonates under age 7 days:
	    <1000 g: 2.5 mg/kg every 24 hours.
	    <1500 g: 2.5 mg/kg every 18 hours.
	    >1500 g: 2.5 mg/kg every 12 hours.
	Neonates over age 7 days:
	    1200–2000 g: 2.5 mg/kg every 8–12 hours.
	    >2000 g: 2.5 mg/kg every 8 hours.
	ECMO patients: 2.5 mg/kg every 18 hours.
	Infants and children under age 5: 2.5 mg/kg every 8 hours.
	Age 5–10: 2 mg/kg every 8 hours.
	Over age 10 and adults: 5 mg/kg/day administered in 3 divided doses.
		Injection: 10 mg/ml, 40 mg/ml
		Ointment, ophthalmic: 0.3%
		Solution, ophthalmic: 0.3%

Continued

Table 107 Medications (continued)

DRUG	DOSE	DOSAGE FORMS
Gentamicin (Garamycin) (continued)	Cystic fibrosis patients may require doses up to 10 mg/kg/day in 4 divided doses. *Ophthalmic solution:* 1–2 drops in the affected eye every 2–4 hours. More frequent application (up to every hour) may be used initially in severe infections. *Ophthalmic ointment:* apply a ribbon of ointment to the eye bid or tid. *Intrathecal/intraventricular* (use only a preservative-free product): Neonates: 1 mg/day as a single dose. Children over age 3 months: 1–2 mg/day. Older children and adults: 4–8 mg/day. Dosage must be adjusted in renal failure. Serum levels should be monitored during therapy in all patients.	
Glucagon	*IV, IM, or SC:* *Hypoglycemia* (dose may be repeated in 20 minutes if necessary): Neonates: 0.025 mg/kg/dose. Children: 0.025–0.1 mg/kg/dose to a maximum of 1 mg. Adults: 0.5–1 mg/dose. *Infusion for the treatment of neonatal hyperinsulinemia:* 1–5 ng/kg/min to start and titrate to response. The infusion must be delivered by a pump to maintain a steady rate. Glucose levels must be monitored hourly until they are stable in an acceptable range. Rebound hypoglycemia may occur if the infusion is suddenly discontinued. *Diagnostic aid during radiography:* 0.25–2 mg 10 minutes before the procedure.	Injection: 1 mg-vial, 10 mg-vial (1 mg = 1 U)
Glycopyrrolate (Robinul)	*IM:* *Preoperatively:* Under age 2: 4.4–8.8 μg/kg 30–60 minutes before the procedure. Over age 2–adults: 4.4 μg/kg 30–60 minutes before the procedure. *Orally:* *To control respiratory secretions* (glycopyrrolate is poorly absorbed from the GI tract): 50 μg/kg administered tid or qid. *Reversal of neuromuscular blockade:* 0.2 mg for each 1 mg neostigmine or 5 mg pyridostigmine administered.	Injection: 0.2 mg/ml Tablets: 1 mg, 2 mg
Gonadorelin HCl [Factrel, LH-RH (luteinizing hormone-release hormone), GnRH (gonadotropin-releasing hormone)]	*IV:* 2–5 μg/kg to a maximum of 100 μg.	Injection: 100 μg

Griseofulvin (Microsize products: Fulvicin U/F, Grifulvin V, Grisactin; Ultramicrosize products: Fulvicin P/G, Grisactin Ultra, Gris-PEG)	Absorption of griseofulvin from the GI tract is somewhat dependent on the size of the particles of griseofulvin. The ultramicrosize is absorbed about 1.5 times as well as the microsize. Absorption is also increased by administering the dose with a fatty meal. Duration of therapy is dependent on the site of infection and ranges from 2–4 weeks for tinea corporis, to 4–8 weeks for tinea capitis and tinea pedis, to 3–6 months for tinea unguium.	Microsize:
		  Capsules: 125 mg, 250 mg
		  Suspension: 125 mg/5 ml
		  Tablets: 250 mg, 500 mg
		Ultramicrosize:
		  Tablets: 125 mg, 165 mg, 250 mg, 330 mg

Continued

Table 107 Medications (continued)

DRUG	DOSE	DOSAGE FORMS

Griseofulvin (Microsize products: Fulvicin U/F, Grifulvin V, Grisactin; Ultramicrosize products: Fulvicin P/G, Grisactin Ultra, Gris-PEG) (continued)	Children:
	  Microsize: 15–20 mg/kg/day in 1 or 2 divided doses.
	  Ultramicrosize: 10–13 mg/kg/day in 1 or 2 divided doses.
	Older children and adults:
	  Microsize: 500 mg–1 g/day in a single or 2 divided doses. Use higher dose for tinea pedis or tinea unguium.
	  Ultramicrosize: 660–750 mg/day in a single or 2 divided doses.
	During long-term therapy, renal, hepatic, and hematopoietic function should be monitored.
	Patients should also be cautioned to avoid sunlight because photosensitivity reactions have occurred.	

Haemophilus b conjugate vaccine (ActHIB, HibTITER, OmniHIB, PedvaxHIB, ProHIBIT)	Depends on the product used. If possible, the patient's immunization should be completed with the same vaccine because information on the interchangeability of the vaccines is lacking. In situations in which the brand of vaccine used previously is not known, the primary objective in infants age 2–6 months should be to assure that 3 doses of conjugate vaccine have been administered. Administer 0.5 ml of the vaccine IM in the outer aspect of the vastus lateralis or deltoid. Doses listed below are listed by age at first vaccination and by product.
	ActHIB, HibTITER, OmniHIB:
	  Age 2–6 months: 3 injections given at about 2-month intervals and a booster dose after age 15 months.
	  Age 7–11 months: 2 injections given at about 2-month intervals and a booster dose after age 15 months, but not less than 2 months after the second injection.
	  Age 12–14 months: 1 injection and a booster dose after age 15 months, but not less than 2 months after the first injection.
	  Age 15 months and older: a single injection.
	PedvaxHIB:
	  Age 2–6 months: 2 injections given at about 2-month intervals and a booster at age 12 months.
	  Age 7–11 months: 2 injections given at about 2-month intervals and a booster dose after age 15 months, but not less than 2 months after the second injection.
	  Age 12–14 months: 1 injection and a booster dose after age 15 months, but not less than 2 months after the first injection.
	  Age 15 months and older: a single injection.
	ProHIBIT:
	  Age 15 months and older: a single injection.
		ActHIB and OmniHIB: 10-μg capsular polysaccharide and 24-μg tetanus toxoid
		HibTITER: 10-μg capsular oligosaccharide and *25-μg diphtheria CRM$_{197}$ protein per 0.5-ml dose
		PedvaxHIB: 15-μg purified capsular polysaccharide and 250-μg _Neisseria meningitidis_ OMPC per 0.5-ml dose
		ProHIBIT: 25-μg purified capsular polysaccharide and 18-μg conjugated diphtheria toxoid protein per 0.5-ml dose; also available in the tetravalent vaccine (Tetramune) that includes diphtheria, tetanus, whole-cell pertussis, and _Haemophilus_ b conjugate in the same 0.5-ml dose

Haloperidol (Haldol)	_Orally:_
	Age 3–12:
	  Agitation or hyperkinesia: 0.01–0.03 mg/kg/day once daily.
	  Tourette disorder: 0.05–0.075 mg/kg/day in 2 or 3 divided doses.
	  Psychotic disorders: 0.05–0.15 mg/kg/day in 2 or 3 divided doses.
		Injection: 5 mg/ml
		Solution, concentrated oral: 2 mg/ml
		Tablets: 1 mg, 2 mg, 5 mg, 10 mg

Continued

Table 107　Medications (continued)

DRUG	DOSE	DOSAGE FORMS
Haloperidol (Haldol) (*continued*)	*IM:* 1–3 mg every 4–8 hours; maximum, 0.1 mg/kg/day. Dose should be individually adjusted to patient. Not recommended for children under age 3. Oral dosage range is 2–100 mg/24 hr.	
Heparin sodium	*IV:* *Anticoagulation:* 　Children and adults: 　　Continuous infusion: 50 U/kg then 15–25 U/kg/hr. Dose may be increased by 2–4 U/kg/hr every 6–8 hours based on the results of the APTT. 　　Intermittent infusion: 50–100 U/kg every 4 hours. This method is less desirable than continuous infusion. *Line flushing:* 　Central catheters: may be flushed as infrequently as once daily with 2–3 ml of solution containing 10 U/ml for patients under age 1 or 100 U/ml for patients age 1 or older. 　Peripheral catheters, locks: usually flushed every 6–8 hours with 10 U/ml concentration with a volume determined by the length of the catheter, but usually about 1 ml. Lines should be flushed before and after medication or blood administration or if blood is seen in the catheter. Preservative-free heparin solutions should be used for all line flushes in children under age 2 months.	Injection: 1000 U, 5000 U, 10,000 U, 20,000 U, 40,000 U/ml Injection, preservative-free: 1000 U, 5000 U, 10,000 U/ml Solution, lock flush: 10 U/ml, 100 U/ml (available preserved and preservative-free)
Hepatitis A vaccine (Havrix, VAQTA)	*IM:* Havrix: 　Children and adolescents: 360 ELISA U/0.5 ml dose with 2 doses given about 1 month apart. 　Age 18–adults: 1440 ELISA U/1 ml dose as a single dose. A booster dose is recommended to be given 6–12 months later to ensure adequate titers. VAQTA: 　Children and adolescents: 25 U/0.5 ml dose as a single dose. 　Adults: 50 U/1 ml dose as a single dose. A booster dose given 6–12 months after the initial dose ensures adequate titers.	Havrix: 　Pediatric injection: 360 ELISA U/0.5 ml 　Adult injection: 1440 ELISA U/1 ml VAQTA: 　Injection: 50 U/1 ml (0.5 ml, 1 ml)
Hepatitis B immune globulin (H-BIG, Hep-B-Gammagee, HyperHep)	*IM (anterolateral thigh in children, deltoid in adults):* If H-BIG and hepatitis B vaccine are administered at the same time, use different sites for each injection. *Neonates born to HBsAg-positive mothers:* 0.5 ml within 12 hours of birth. *Postexposure prophylaxis:* 0.06 ml/kg to a maximum of 5 ml as soon as possible, but within 7 days of exposure. A second dose should be administered 28–30 days after exposure.	Injection: 0.5-ml syringe; 1-ml, 4-ml, and 5-ml vials
Hepatitis B vaccine, recombinant (Engerix-B, Recombivax-HB)	*IM (anterolateral thigh in children, deltoid in adults):* Two different products are available. Interchangeability of the vaccines has not been documented, but Engerix-B may be used to complete a series that was initiated with Recombivax-HB.	Formulation, pediatric: 5 μg/ml in 0.5-ml and 3-ml vials Formulation, dialysis: 40 μg/ml in 1-ml vials Injection, Engerix-B: 20 μg/ml in 0.5-ml and 1-ml vials

Continued

Table 107   Medications *(continued)*

DRUG	*DOSE*	*DOSAGE FORMS*
Hepatitis B vaccine, recombinant (Engerix-B, Recombivax-HB) *(continued)*	*Engerix B:* *Infants born to HBsAg-positive mothers:* 10 μg (0.5 ml) on the first day of life, at age 1 month, and at age 6 months. Because of concern about mercury in vaccines, hepatitis may be delayed until 6 months with repeat at 7 and 12 months. *Infants born to HbsAg-negative mothers:* 10 μg (0.5 ml) on the first or second day of life, at age 1 month, and at age 6 months or at age 1–2 months, at age 4 months, and at age 6–18 months. Under age 11: 10 μg (0.5 ml) for a 3-dose series at 0, 1, and 6 months or a 4-dose series at 0, 1, 2, and 12 months. Over age 11–adults: 20 μg (1 ml) for a 3-dose series at 0, 1, and 6 months or a 4-dose series at 0, 1, 2, and 12 months. *Dialysis or immunocompromised patients:* 40 μg (2 ml) administered as two 1-ml doses at separate sites for a 4-dose series at 0, 1, 2, and 6 months. *Recombivax-HB:* Because of concern about mercury in vaccines, hepatitis may be delayed until 6 months with repeat at 7 and 12 months. *Infants born to HBsAg-positive mothers:* 5 μg (0.5 ml) on the first day of life, age 1 month, and age 6 months. *Infants born to HBsAg-negative mothers and children under age 11:* 2.5 μg (0.25 ml or 0.5 ml) at 0, 1, and 6 months. In infants, the series may be started at birth or at age 1–2 months. Age 11–19: 5 μg (0.5 ml) for a 3-dose series at 0, 1, and 6 months. Adults: 10 μg (1 ml) for a 3-dose series at 0, 1, and 6 months. *Dialysis and immunocompromised patients:* 40 μg (1 ml) of the special dialysis formula at 0, 1, and 6 months. Revaccination (booster) doses are not generally recommended except in dialysis patients whose antibody levels have fallen to <10 mIU/ml. Levels should be tested in vaccinated individuals who are exposed to HBsAb-positive blood. If levels are inadequate, a dose of H-BIG and a booster dose of vaccine should be administered at the same time in separate sites.	Injection, Recombivax-HB: 10 μg/ml in 0.5-ml, 1-ml, and 3-ml vials
Hydralazine (Apresoline)	*Orally:* Children: 0.75–1 mg/kg/day in 2–4 divided doses, but not to exceed 25 mg/dose initially. May be increased slowly over 3 or 4 weeks to a maximum of 7.5 mg/kg/day (or 200 mg). Adults: initially 10 mg qid. May be increased by 10–25 mg/dose every 2–5 days to a maximum of 300 mg/day. *IV (ratio of oral to IV dosing is about 4:1):* Children: initially 0.1–0.2 mg/kg (to a maximum of 20 mg) every 4–6 hours. May be increased to a maximum of 1.7–3.5 mg/kg/day. Adults: initially 10–20 mg every 4–6 hours. May be increased to 40 mg/dose. Dose must be adjusted in renal impairment.	Injection: 20 mg/ml Tablets: 10 mg, 25 mg, 50 mg, 100 mg

Continued

Table 107 Medications (continued)

DRUG	DOSE	DOSAGE FORMS

Hydrochlorothiazide (Esidrix, HydroDIURIL, Oretic)	*Orally* (chlorothiazide, which is available as a suspension, is usually a better choice for children requiring low doses):
	  Children over age 6 months: 2 mg/kg/day in 2 divided doses.
	  Adults: 25–100 mg/day in 1 or 2 doses.
		Tablets: 25 mg, 50 mg, 100 mg

Hydrocortisone (Cortef, Cortenema, Cortifoam, Cortril, Hydrocortone, Solu-Cortef)	*Orally:*
	Congenital adrenal hyperplasia: initially 30–36 mg/m²/day divided as one third in the morning and two thirds in the evening or one fourth in the morning, one fourth midday, and half in the evening.
	Physiologic replacement: 0.5–0.75 mg/kg/day.
	Anti-inflammatory: 2.5–10 mg/kg/day in 3 or 4 divided doses.
	IV:
	Adrenal insufficiency:
	  Infants and young children: 1–2 mg/kg bolus, then 25–150 mg/day in 3 or 4 divided doses.
	  Older children: 1–2 mg/kg bolus, then 150–250 mg/day in 3 or 4 divided doses.
	  Adults: 15–240 mg/day in 1 or 2 divided doses.
	Anti-inflammatory:
	  Infants and children: 1–5 mg/kg/day in 2–4 divided doses.
	  Adults: 15–240 mg every 12 hours.
	Shock (succinate salt):
	  Children: 50 mg/kg, then in 4 hours or every 24 hours as needed.
	  Adults: 500 mg–2 g every 2–6 hours.
	Rectal retention enemas: 1 enema nightly for 21 days. May be continued for a longer period if effective or discontinued if no effect is seen.
	Intrarectal foam: 1 applicatorful rectally nightly or bid for 2 or 3 weeks. Absorption of hydrocortisone may be greater from the foam formulation than the enema. Discontinue if not effective after 3 weeks.
	Topically (low potency corticosteroid in most formulations): apply a thin layer to the affected area tid or qid.
		Cream, topical: 0.5%, 1%, 2.5%
		Enema: 100 mg/60 ml (Cortenema)
		Foam, intrarectal: 90 mg/applicatorful (Cortifoam), rectal/anal 1% (Proctofoam-HC)
		Injection (sodium phosphate): 50 mg/ml
		Injection (sodium succinate): 100-mg, 250-mg, 500-mg, 1-g vials
		Ointment, topical: 0.5%, 1%, 2.5%
		Suspension (cypionate): 10 mg/5 ml
		Tablets: 5 mg, 10 mg, 20 mg

Hydromorphone (Dilaudid)	*IV:*
	  Young children: 0.015–0.03 mg/kg every 3–4 hours.
	  Older children and adults: 1–4 mg every 3–4 hours.
	Orally:
	  Young children: 0.04–0.07 mg/kg every 3–4 hours.
	  Older children and adults: 1–6 mg every 3–4 hours depending on size and pain severity.
	To convert a patient from oral to IV therapy: start with a ratio of 5:1. Ratios of up to 2:1 may be required in some patients on long-term chronic therapy.
	To convert a patient from IV to oral therapy: in a patient who is receiving a stable dose, use an IV to oral ratio of 1:3.
	Equianalgesic doses:
	  Oral: 7.5 mg hydromorphone = 30 mg morphine.
	  Parenteral: 1.5 mg hydromorphone = 10 mg morphine
		Injection: 1 mg/ml, 2 mg/ml, 4 mg/ml, 10 mg/ml
		Solution, oral: 1 mg/ml
		Suppositories, rectal: 3 mg
		Tablets: 2 mg, 4 mg, 8 mg

Continued

Table 107 Medications (continued)

DRUG	*DOSE*	*DOSAGE FORMS*
Hydroxyzine (Atarax, Vistaril)	*Orally:* Children: 2 mg/kg/day in 3 or 4 doses. Adults: 100–400 mg/day in 3 or 4 doses. Use lower doses for pruritus and higher doses for sedation. *Parenterally:* the use of hydroxyzine parenterally (IM, IV, SC) has been associated with severe adverse effects at the site of the injection. The reactions are characterized by local discomfort, sterile abscess, erythema, and tissue necrosis. Phlebitis and hemolysis have been reported after IV administration. The manufacturers recommend administration by deep IM injection into a well-developed large muscle. SC infiltration of the drug from an IM injection or extravasation of an IV injection must be avoided.	Capsule (pamoate): 25 mg, 50 mg, 100 mg Injection for IM use: 25 mg/ml, 50 mg/ml Solution, oral: 10 mg/5 ml Suspension, oral (pamoate): 25 mg/5 ml Tablets: 10 mg, 25 mg, 50 mg, 100 mg
Ibuprofen (Advil, Motrin, Nuprin)	*Orally:* *Antipyretic:* Age 6 months–12 years (repeat doses up to every 6 hours): Temperature <39°C (102.5°F): 5 mg/kg/dose. Temperature >39°C (102.5°F): 10 mg/kg/dose. Over age 12 and adults: 200–400 mg/dose to a maximum of 1200 mg/day. *Juvenile rheumatoid arthritis:* 30–70 mg/kg/day in 4 divided doses to a maximum of 2400 mg/day. *Adult anti-inflammatory dose:* 400–800 every 6–8 hours to a maximum of 3200 mg/day.	Suspension, oral: 100 mg/5 ml Tablets: 200 mg, 300 mg, 400 mg, 600 mg, 800 mg
Imipenem and cilastatin (Primaxin)	*IV infusion over 1 hour* (expressed as mg of imipenem): Children: 50–100 mg/kg/day in 4 divided doses to a maximum of 4 g/day. Adults: 2–4 g/day in 3 or 4 divided doses. Dosage adjustment is required in renal impairment.	Injection: imipenem 250 mg and cilastatin 50 mg, imipenem 500 mg and cilastatin 500 mg
Imipramine (Tofranil)	*Orally:* *Enuresis* in children under age 6: initially 25 mg 1 hour before bedtime nightly. Dose may be increased to 50 mg in children age 6–12 or 75 mg in children over age 12 if the initial dose is ineffective. *Depression:* Children: 1.5 mg/kg/day in 1–4 divided doses initially. May be increased in increments of about 1 mg/kg/day to a maximum of 5 mg/kg/day. Adolescents: 25–50 mg/day increased gradually to a maximum of 100 mg/day in a single or divided doses. Adults: 75–100 mg/day increased gradually to a maximum of 300 mg/day in a single or divided doses. Dosage should be decreased to the minimum effective dose after symptom control has been achieved. *Doses used to treat pain:* generally lower than those used in the treatment of depression. A starting dose of 0.2–0.4 mg/kg/day administered at bedtime may be used initially. A gradual increase to 1–3 mg/kg/day may be necessary for some patients. Administration of the total daily dose at bedtime may decrease the daytime sedative effects.	Tablets: 10 mg, 25 mg, 50 mg

Continued

Table 107   Medications   (continued)

DRUG	_DOSE_	_DOSAGE FORMS_
Immune globulin, intramuscular	IM: *Measles prophylaxis:* 0.25 ml/kg within 6 days of exposure. In immunocompromised patients, use 0.5 ml/kg (15 ml maximum). *Hepatitis A pre-exposure prophylaxis:* Risk of exposure within 3 months: 0.02 ml/kg. Risk of exposure greater than 3 months: 0.06 ml/kg. *Hepatitis A postexposure:* 0.02 ml/kg given within 2 weeks of exposure. *Immunodeficiency:* IV has largely replaced use of the IM form. An initial dose of 1.2 ml/kg is followed with doses of 0.6 ml/kg at 2–4-week intervals. The usual maximum volumes are 20–30 ml in infants and small children and 30–50 ml in adults.	Injection, IM: 165 $\pm$ 15 mg (of protein) per ml (2 ml and 10 ml)
Immune globulin, intravenous (Gamimune N, Gammagard S/D, Gammar-P IV, Iveegam, Polygam S/D, Sandoglobulin, Venoglobulin-I, Venoglobulin-S)	IV as a slow infusion: The rate of infusion varies from product to product but should always be initiated at a very slow rate and may be increased every 30 mintues to the manufacturer's maximum recommended rate or less as the patient tolerates. Infusion-related reactions usually abate if the rate of infusion is decreased. Anaphylactic hypersensitivity reactions may occur and are more likely in patients with IgA deficiency. *Immunodeficiency syndromes:* 100–400 mg/kg every 2–4 weeks. *Idiopathic thrombocytopenic purpura:* either 400 mg/kg/day for 2–5 consecutive days or 1 g/kg/day for 1 or 2 consecutive days may be used for induction. Maintenance doses are usually 400 mg/kg/dose every 4–6 weeks but may be increased to 800–1000 mg/kg if the lower dose is insufficient and are based on platelet counts and clinical response. *Kawasaki disease:* usually 2 g/kg as a single dose. Alternatively, 400 mg/kg/day for 4 days may be used.	Gamimune N: 5% or 10% solution in vials Gammagard S/D: powder with diluent to make 5% solution Gammar-P IV: powder with diluent to make 5% solution Iveegam: powder with diluent to make 5% solution Polygam S/D: powder with diluent to make 5% solution Sandoglobulin: powder with diluent to make 3%, 6%, or 12% solution Venoglobulin-I: powder with diluent to make 5% solution Venoglobulin-S: solution 5%, 10%
Indomethacin IV (Indocin IV)	IV push: Further dilution of the reconstituted injection may result in precipitation of insouble indomethacin. An initial 0.2 mg/kg/dose is followed by 2 doses based on the patient's postnatal age (PNA) *at the time of the first dose:* PNA <48 hours: 0.1 mg/kg at 12–24-hour intervals. PNA 2–7 days: 0.2 mg/kg at 12–24-hour intervals. PNA >7 days: 0.25 mg/kg at 12–24-hour intervals. The patient's renal and hepatic function should be monitored. Oral use in children is generally not recommended.	Injection (sodium trihydrate): 1 mg
Insulin	IV: *Treatment of diabetic ketoacidosis:* loading dose of 0.1 U/kg followed by a continuous infusion of 0.1 U/kg/hr (usual range 0.05–0.2 U/kg/hr) to maintain steady, but slow, decrease of serum glucose levels of 80–100 mg/dl/hr. Only regular insulin should be used by this route.	All insulins below are 100 U/ml. Regular insulin: available in beef and pork; pork; beef; human, recombinant DNA; and human, semi-synthetic Isophane (NPH) insulin: available in beef and pork; pork; beef Prompt zinc (semilente) insulin; available in beef and pork; pork; beef; and human, recombinant DNA

Continued

Table 107   Medications   (continued)

DRUG	DOSE	DOSAGE FORMS
Insulin (*continued*)	*SC:* *Maintenance:* most patients require 0.5–1 U/kg/day in 2–4 divided doses depending on how well controlled the patient's glucose levels have been. Patients should be warned not to change insulins without prior approval of their physicians. If regular insulin is to be mixed with other types of insulin, the regular insulin should always be measured first. Extemporaneously prepared doses of mixed insulins should be used as soon as possible after mixing to minimize the amount of the regular insulin that will be bound by excess protamine or zinc in the other insulin. The activity of regular insulin has a time to onset of ½ to 1 hour, peaks at 2–3 hours, and has a duration of 5–7 hours. The activity of isophane (NPH) insulin has a time to onset of about 1–2 hours, peaks at 4–12 hours, and has a duration of 18–24 hours.	Extended zinc (ultralente) insulin: available in beef and pork; beef; and human, recombinant DNA Fixed combinations: regular insulin 30 U/ml with isophane insulin 70 U/ml; available as pork; human, recombinant DNA; and human, semisynthetic isophane insulin 50 U/ml available as human, recombinant DNA
Ipecac	*Orally* (followed by 10–20 ml/kg (up to 300 ml) of water. May be repeated after 20 minutes if vomiting does not occur): Age 6–12 months: 5–10 ml. Age 1–12: 15 ml. Over age 12: 30 ml. Do not administer at the same time as activated charcoal, or with milk or carbonated beverages.	Syrup
Ipratropium bromide (Atrovent)	For patients over age 12: 2 inhalations qid. May be increased to a maximum of 12 inhalations in 24 hours.	Aerosol, metered dose: 8 μg/actuation Solution for nebulization: 0.02%, 2.5 ml
Iron dextran (INFeD)	Total replacement dosage in milliliters may be calculated using the following formula: $[0.0476 \times Wt \times (Hb_N - Hb_0)] + 1$ ml/5 kg (up to 14 ml) where: Wt = lean body weight in kilograms. Hb_N = normal hemoglobin in deciliters (12 for patients weighing ≤15 kg or 14.8 for patients weighing >15 kg). Hb_0 = patient's observed hemoglobin. This dose may be administered as an IV infusion over 1–6 hours after the successful administration of a test dose of about 25 mg of iron over 5 minutes. (Use ~10 mg iron for small children.) For IV infusion, iron dextran should be diluted in 0.9% sodium chloride rather than 5% dextrose solution, because dilution in dextrose has been associated with more adverse reactions. IM administration into a large muscle using the Z-track technique may be used, with the total dosage divided into daily doses, generally not to exceed 25 mg in infants, 50 mg in children weighing 5–10 kg, or 100 mg in heavier children and adults.	Injection: 50 mg/ml
Isoniazid (isonicotinic acid hydrozide, isonicotinyl hydrazide; INH, Nydrazid)	*Orally or IM:* *Treatment:* Children: 20 mg/kg/day in 1 or 2 divided doses (up to 300 mg/day). Adults: 5 mg/kg/day up to 300 mg; 10 mg/kg should be used for disseminated disease. *Prophylaxis:* Children: 10 mg/kg/day in a single dose up to 300 mg/day. Adults: 300 mg/day.	Injection: 100 mg/ml Solution, oral: 50 mg/5 ml (with sorbital 70%) Tablets: 100 mg, 300 mg

Continued

Table 107 Medications (continued)

DRUG	*DOSE*	*DOSAGE FORMS*
Isoniazid (isonicotinic acid hydrozide, isonicotinyl hydrazide; INH, Nydrazid) (*continued*)	Liver function should be monitored during therapy because hepatitis may occur at any time. Patients whose diets are low in milk or meat should receive pyridoxine supplements at a dose of about 10–50 mg/day.	
Isoproterenol (Isuprel)	*IV* (by continuous infusion): 0.05–3 μg/kg/min up to 2–20 μg/min. *Oral inhalation:* 1–2 metered doses up to 6 times daily. *Nebulization:* 　Age 2–9: 0.25 ml (1:200) in 2.5 ml normal saline solution up to every 4 hours. 　Over age 9: 0.5 ml (1:2000) in 2.5 ml normal saline solution up to every 4 hours.	Aerosol, metered dose inhaler: 1:400 (0.25%) Injection: 1:5000 (0.2 mg/ml, 1 mg/5 ml) Solution for inhalation: 1:200 (0.5%)
Ketoconazole (Nizoral)	*Orally* (acid must be present in the GI tract for the dissolution and absorption of ketoconazole): 　Children: 3.3–6.6 mg/kg/day in 1 or 2 divided doses to a maximum dose of 400 mg/day. 　Adults: 200–400 mg/day in a single dose. Do not administer antacids or H_2 antagonists of the same time as ketoconazole. Monitor liver function during therapy. *Topically:* apply to the affected area once or twice daily. *Shampoo for dandruff:* apply shampoo and lather, allow to remain on the scalp for at least 1 minute before rinsing. Reapply shampoo and lather again, allow to remain on the scalp for 3 minutes, and then rinse. Treatments should be done twice weekly with at least 3 days between treatments, for 4 weeks. The frequency of subsequent treatments should be determined individually.	Cream: 2% Shampoo: 2% Tablets: 200 mg
Ketorolac tromethamine (Toradol)	*IM or IV:* 　Children: limited information is available on its use in children, but doses of 0.5 mg/kg repeated every 6 hours have been recommended. Do not exceed the adult doses listed below. 　Adults: 　　<50 kg: 15 mg every 6 hours. 　　>50 kg: 30 mg every 6 hours. The duration of therapy should be held to a minimum. Because the drug may mask signs of infection post-operatively due to its anti-inflammatory and antipyretic effects, monitor the patient appropriately. *Orally:* 　Children: use of an alternative NSAID should be considered for children because there is not an appropriate dosage form and alternatives are available. 　Adults: 10 mg repeated up to qid. Ketorolac is approved for short-term therapy (5–14 days) only. Longer therapy has been associated with a higher incidence of side effects. Dosage adjustment is recommended in patients with renal impairment.	Injection: 15 mg/ml, 30 mg/ml Tablets: 10 mg
Lamivudine (Epivir)	*Orally:* 　Age 3 months–12 years: 4 mg/kg bid, to a maximum of 150 mg bid. 　Adolescents and adults: 150 mg bid. Dosage adjustment may be necessary in patients with renal dysfunction.	Solution: 10 mg/ml Tablets: 150 mg

Continued

Table 107   Medications   (continued)

DRUG	*DOSE*	*DOSAGE FORMS*
Leuprolide acetate (Lupron, Lupron Depot)	*SC:* *Anterior pituitary gonadotropic testing:* 10 μg/kg/dose. *Precocious puberty:* 50 μg/kg/day. Dosage may be titrated upward in 10 μg/kg increments if suppression of ovarian or testicular function is incomplete. *IM for precocious puberty* (higher doses may be necessary for younger children. Doses should be based on the patient's weight and age): Girls over age 8 and boys over age 9: 0.3 mg/kg (minimum 7.5 mg) repeated every 4 weeks using the depot product. Dosage may be increased in 3.75-mg increments every 4 weeks until an effective dose is achieved. Therapy should generally be discontinued at age 11 for girls or age 12 for boys.	Injection for SC use (Lupron): 5 mg/ml Injection, suspension for IM use (Lupron Depot): 3.75 mg, 7.5 mg
Levothyroxine sodium (Levothroid, Synthroid)	*Orally:* Age 0–6 months: 8–10 μg/kg or 25–50 μg/day. Age 6–12 months: 6–8 μg/kg or 50–75 μg/day. Age 1–5: 5–6 μg/kg or 75–100 μg/day. Age 6–12: 4–5 μg/kg or 100–150 μg/day. Over age 12 and adults: 2–3 μg/kg or >150 μg/day. *IV:* one half to three fourths of the oral dose for children or about half the oral dose for adults. The parenteral form of the drug is very unstable and should be used immediately after reconstitution without admixing with other solutions.	Injection: 200 μg, 500 μg Tablets: 25 μg, 50 μg, 75 μg, 88 μg, 100 μg, 112 μg, 125 μg, 175 μg, 200 μg, 300 μg
Lidocaine hydrochloride (Xylocaine)	*IV for cardiac arrythmias:* 1 mg/kg loading dose followed by a continuous infusion of 20–50 μg/kg/min. The loading dose may be repeated twice at 10–15 minute intervals, if necessary. *Infiltration for local anesthesia:* dose depends on procedure, degree, and duration of anesthesia required and the vascularity of the site. Maximum recommended dose is 4.5 mg/kg. Doses should not be repeated sooner than 2 hours. *Topical:* apply to affected area as needed. Maximum dose should not exceed 3 mg/kg or be repeated within 2 hours. Patients treated with oral lidocaine viscous should be cautioned about the hazards of biting the numbed areas and swallowing difficulties.	Aerosol, metered dose: 10% (for use before endotracheal intubation) Injection: 0.5%, 1%, 1.5%, 2%, 4%; 0.5% with epinephrine 1:200,000; 1% with epinephrine 1:100,000 or 1:200,000; 1.5% with epinephrine 1:200,000; 2% with epinephrine 1:100,000 or 1:200,000 Jelly: 2% Liquid, viscous: 2% Ointment: 2.5%, 5% Solution, topical: 2%, 4%
Lindane (gamma benzene hexachloride; Kwell)	*Topically:* *Pediculosis:* apply 15–30 ml of shampoo to the scalp and lather for 4–5 minutes, then rinse. The hair should be combed with a fine-toothed comb to remove nits. Treatment may be repeated after 1 week, if necessary. *Scabies:* apply a thin layer of the lotion to the skin from the neck to the toes (include the head in infants). The lotion should be removed by bathing after 6 hours for infants, 6–8 hours for children or 8–12 hours for adults. Treatment may be repeated after 1 week, if necessary. Percutaneous absorption may occur and cause toxicity. Do not apply to inflamed or raw skin.	Lotion: 1% Shampoo: 1%

Continued

Table 107   Medications   (continued)

DRUG	DOSE	DOSAGE FORMS

Loperamide (Imodium)	*Orally:*
	Acute diarrhea (dosage is for the initial 24 hours):
	    Age 2 up to age 6 (13–20 kg): 1 mg tid.
	    Age 6–8 (20–30 kg): 2 mg bid.
	    Age 8–12 (>30 kg): 2 mg tid.
	    Adults: 4 mg initially followed by 2 mg after each unformed stool to a maximum of 8 mg in 24 hours (16 mg/24 hr under a physician's care).
	For subsequent days, use a dose of 0.1 mg/kg for children after each loose stool, but do not exceed dosage guidelines for the first day.
	Chronic diarrhea:
	    Children: 0.08–0.24 mg/kg/day in 2 or 3 doses daily to a maximum of 2 mg/dose.
	    Adults: 4 mg followed by 2 mg after each unformed stool until symptoms are controlled, then decreased to the lowest dose that will control symptoms. Usual maintenance dose is 4–8 mg/day.
		Capsules: 2 mg
		Solution, oral: 1 mg/5 ml
		Tablets: 2 mg

Loracarbef (Lorabid)	*Orally* (administer doses on an empty stomach):
	Age 6 months–12 years:
	    Otitis media: 30 mg/kg/day in 2 divided doses. Administer only the suspension for otitis because it is absorbed more quickly and results in higher blood levels.
	    Other infections: 15 mg/kg/day in 2 divided doses.
	    Older children and adults: 200–400 mg/day in 2 divided doses.
		Capsules: 200 mg
		Suspension, oral: 100 mg/5 ml, 200 mg/5 ml

Loratadine (Claritin)	*Orally:*
	    Age 2–12: 5 mg/day in a single dose.
	    Adults >30 kg: 10 mg/day in a single dose.
		Tablets: 10 mg

Lorazepam (Ativan)	*IV:*
	Status epilepticus:
	    Neonates: 0.05 mg/kg over 2–5 minutes. Dose may be repeated in 10–15 minutes.
	    Infants and children: 0.1 mg/kg over 2–5 minutes to a maximum of 4 mg/dose. A second dose of 0.05 mg/kg may be given.
	    Adolescents: 0.07 mg/kg over 2–5 minutes to a maximum of 4 mg. Dose may be repeated in 10–15 minutes.
	    Adults: 4 mg over 2–5 minutes. Dose may be repeated in 10–15 minutes.
	Adjunct to antiemetic therapy: 0.02–0.04 mg/kg up to every 6 hours. Do not exceed a maximum of 2 mg/dose.
	Orally or IV:
	Anxiety and sedation:
	    Infants and children: 0.03–0.04 mg/kg/day, in 3–4 divided doses.
	    Adults: 2–6 mg/day, usually orally, in 2 or 3 divided doses.
		Injection: 2 mg/ml, 4 mg/ml
		Solution, oral: 2 mg/ml
		Tablets: 0.5 mg, 1 mg, 2 mg

Magnesium citrate (Citrate of Magnesia, Evac-Q-Mag)	*Orally* (chill for the better palatability):
	    Under age 6: 2–4 ml/kg.
	    Age 6–12: 100–150 ml.
	    Over age 12: 150–300 ml.
		Solution: 300 ml (carbonated; contains 3.85–4.71 mEq Mg/5 ml)

Magnesium gluconate (Almora, Magonate, Magtrate)	*Orally* (expressed in terms of mEq of magnesium):
	    Children: 0.05–0.75 mEq/kg/day in 3 or 4 divided doses.
	    Adults: 2.2–4.4 mEq administered bid or tid.
		Liquid: 1000 mg/5 ml (54 mg Mg = 4.4 mEq Mg)
		Tablets: 500 mg (27 mg Mg = 2.2 mEq Mg)

Continued

Table 107   Medications   (continued)

DRUG	*DOSE*	*DOSAGE FORMS*
Magnesium hydroxide (Milk of Magnesia)	*Orally:* Under age 2: 0.5 ml/kg/dose. Age 2–5: 5–15 ml/day. Age 6–12: 15–30 ml/day. Over age 12: 30–60 ml/day.	Suspension: contains about 13.7 mEq Mg/5 ml
Magnesium sulfate (Epsom Salts)	*IV* [expressed in terms of magnesium sulfate (and mEq Mg)]: *Hypomagnesemia* (monitor serum magnesium levels closely): Neonates: 25–50 mg/kg (0.2–0.4 mEq/kg) every 8–12 hours for 2–3 doses. Infants and children: 25–50 mg/kg (0.2–0.4 mEq/kg) every 4–6 hours for 3 or 4 doses with a maximum single dose of 2000 mg (16 mEq). Doses up to 100 mg/kg have been used in severe hypomagnesemia. Adults: 1 g (8 mEq) every 6 hours for 4 doses. Doses of 2–3 g (16–24 mEq) have been used for severe hypomagnesemia. *Maintenance dose:* 30–60 mg/kg/day (0.25–0.5 mEq/kg/day) in 3 or 4 divided doses. *Management of seizures or hypertension in children:* 25–100 mg/kg (0.2–0.8 mEq/kg) every 4–6 hours as needed. Administer the drug slowly (over 1–2 hours) in a concentration not greater than 10 mg/ml. Blood pressure should be monitored frequently during infusions because hypotension has been reported with too-fast administration.	Injection: 500 mg/ml (4 mEq magnesium = 49 mg Mg)
Mannitol (Osmitrol)	*IV:* initial dose of 2 g/kg followed by doses of 0.25–0.5 g/kg every 4–6 hours. A test dose of 0.2 g/kg (to a maximum of 12.5 g) over 3–5 minutes should produce a urine flow of about 1 ml/kg/hr for 2 or 3 hours. It should be used for patients with marked oliguria or inadequate renal function.	Injection: 5%, 10%, 15%, 20%, 25%
Measles vaccine (Attenuvax) Measles and rubella vaccine (M-R-Vax II) Measles, mumps, and rubella vaccine (M-M-R II)	*SC in the outer aspect of the upper arm:* 0.5 ml at age 15–18 months. A booster dose (principally for measles) is now recommended at age 4–6 (ACIP) or 11–12 (AAP). Federal law requires that the date of administration, manufacturer, lot number, and expiration date of the vaccine, and the name, title, and address of the person administering the dose be entered into the patient's permanent medical record. It also requires providers to distribute information on vaccines before each vaccination.	Measles 1000 $TCID_{50}$ per dose (0.5 ml) Measles 1000 $TCID_{50}$ and rubella 1000 $TCID_{50}$ per dose (0.5 ml) Measles 1000 $TCID_{50}$, rubella 1000 $TCID_{50}$, and mumps 20,000 $TCID_{50}$ per dose (0.5 ml)
Mebendazole (Vermox)	*Orally:* Over age 2 and adults: *Enterobiasis (pinworm):* 100 mg as a single dose. May be repeated at 2 weeks. *Ascariasis (roundworm), trichuriasis (whipworm), hookworm, or mixed infections:* 200 mg/day in 2 divided doses for 3 days. A second course may be administered 3–4 weeks later.	Tablets, chewable: 100 mg
Meperidine hydrochloride (Demerol)	Oral doses are about half as effective as IV doses but are generally used for less severe pain; therefore, the doses listed are for all routes of administration, but that should be kept in mind if a patient is being switched from parenteral to oral therapy. Children: 1–1.5 mg/kg every 3–4 hours. A single dose of 3 mg/kg (to a maximum of 100 mg) may be used preoperatively.	Injection: 25 mg/ml, 50 mg/ml, 75 mg/ml, 100 mg/ml Solution, oral: 50 mg/5 ml Tablets: 50 mg, 100 mg

Continued

Table 107   Medications   (continued)

DRUG	DOSE	DOSAGE FORMS
Meperidine hydrochloride (Demerol) *(continued)*	Adults: 50–150 mg every 3–4 hours. Dosage adjustment is necessary in renal impairment. Long-term or high-dose therapy may result in accumulation of normeperidine, an active metabolite that is a CNS stimulant, especially in patients with renal failure.	
Meropenem (Merrem IV)	*IV:* *Intra-abdominal infections:* Age 3 months–adults: 60 mg/kg/day in 3 divided doses to a maximum total daily dose of 3 g. *Meningitis:* Age 3 months–adults: 120 mg/kg/day in 3 divided doses to a maximum total daily dose of 6 g.	Injection: 500 mg, 1 g
Mesalamine (Asacol, Pentasa, Rowasa)	*Orally* Adults: 1 g (capsules) qid or 800 mg (tablets) tid. *Rectally:* 4 g enema administered at bed time daily. The enema should be retained overnight (8 hours) for best results.	The oral forms of the drug are formulated with an enteric coating to slowly release the drug. Capsules (Pentasa): 250 mg Suspension, rectal: 4 g/60 ml Tablets (Asacol): 400 mg
Metaproterenol (Alupent, Metaprel)	*Orally:* Under age 6: 1.3–2.6 mg/kg/day in 3 or 4 divided doses. Age 6–9 (<27 kg): 10 mg/dose tid or qid. Over age 9 (>27 kg) and adults: 20 mg/dose tid or qid. *Oral inhalation:* Over age 12 and adults: 2–3 inhalations every 3–4 hours, up to 12 inhalations daily. *Nebulizer:* Age 6–12: 0.1 ml of a 5% solution diluted in 0.9% sodium chloride solution to 3 ml, repeated up to every 4 hours. Over age 12 and adults: 0.2–0.3 ml of 5% solution (or 2.5 ml of 0.4% or 0.6% commercially available diluted solution) administered tid or qid.	Inhalation: Aerosol: 0.65 mg/inhalation spray Solution: 5%, 0.4% in normal saline solution, 0.6% in normal saline solution Solution, oral: 10 mg/5 ml Tablets: 10 mg, 20 mg
Methylene blue (Urolene Blue)	*IV for methemoglobinemia:* 1–2 mg/kg injected slowly over a period of several minutes. The dose may be repeated in 1 hour, if necessary. *Orally for adults with chronic methemoglobinemia:* 100–300 mg/day.	Injection: 10 mg/ml Tablets: 65 mg
Methylphenidate (Ritalin)	*Orally:* Over age 6: initially 0.3 mg/kg/day (2.5–5 mg/dose) before breakfast and lunch. That may be increased to the usual dosage range of 0.5–1 mg/kg/day or a maximum of 2 mg/kg/day or 60 mg. The sustained-release form may be given as a single dose at breakfast.	Tablets: 5 mg, 10 mg, 20 mg Tablets, extended release: 20 mg
Methylprednisolone (A-methaPred, Depo-Medrol, Medrol, Solu-Medrol)	*IV:* *Status asthmaticus:* 1 mg/kg every 6 hours. *Acute spinal cord injury:* 30 mg/kg over 15 minutes followed in 45 minutes by an infusion of 5.4 mg/kg/hr for 23 hours. *Shock:* 30 mg/kg and may be repeated every 4–12 hours, but not to continue for longer than 48–72 hours. *"Pulse" therapy for lupus nephritis in older children and adults:* 1 g/day for 3 days. A dose of 30 mg/kg every other day for 6 doses has been used for children. *Orally:* Children: 0.117–1.6 mg/kg/day in 4 divided doses. Adults: 2–60 mg/day in 4 divided doses.	Injection (acetate; Depo-Medrol): 20 mg/ml, 40 mg/ml, 80 mg/ml Injection (sodium succinate): 40-mg, 125-mg, 500-mg 1-g, 2-g vials Tablets: 2 mg, 4 mg, 8 mg, 16 mg, 24 mg, 32 mg

Continued

Table 107   Medications   (continued)

DRUG	DOSE	DOSAGE FORMS
Methylprednisolone (A-methaPred, Depo-Medrol, Medrol, Solu-Medrol) (*continued*)	*Intra-articular, intralesional doses (acetate):* 4–40 mg or up to 80 mg for large joints every 1–5 weeks.	
Metoclopramide (Maxolon, Octamide, Reglan)	*Orally or IV:* *Gastroesophageal reflux:* Children: initially 0.1–0.5 mg/kg/day in 4 divided doses before meals. Dosage may be increased to a maximum of 0.8 mg/kg/day. Adults: 10–15 mg 30 minutes before meals and at bedtime. *IV:* *Intubation of GI tract or radiographic exam:* Under age 6: 0.1 mg/kg. Age 6–14: 2.5–5 mg. Adults: 10 mg. *Antiemetic in chemotherapy-induced nausea:* 1–2 mg/kg administered 30 minutes before the chemotherapy and every 2–4 hours as necessary thereafter to a maximum of 3 doses. Extrapyramidal reactions are common at this dose and may be treated with diphenhydramine IV (1 mg/kg up to 50 mg) every 6 hours.	Injection: 5 mg/ml Solution, oral: 5 mg/5 ml, 10 mg/5 ml Tablets: 5 mg, 10 mg
Metolazone (Zaroxolyn)	*Orally:* Infants and children: 0.2–0.4 mg/kg/day in 1–2 divided doses. Adults: 2.5–5 mg/day for the treatment of hypertension. Edema due to cardiac or renal disease may require doses of 5–20 mg/day.	Tablets: 2.5 mg, 5 mg, 10 mg
Metronidazole (Flagyl, Protostat)	*Orally or IV:* *Anerobic bacterial infections* (IV initially, then orally): Infants other than neonates to adults: 30 mg/kg/day in 4 divided doses, not to exceed 4 g/day. *Amebiasis* (usually orally): Infants and children: 35–50 mg/kg/day in 3 divided doses. Adults: 500–750 mg every 8 hours. *Other parasitic infections* (usually orally): Infants and children: 15–30 mg/kg/day in 3 divided doses. Adults: 250 mg every 8 hours or a single 2-g dose. *Antibiotic-associated pseudomembranous colitis:* Infants and children: 20 mg/kg/day in 4 divided doses. Adults: 250–500 mg tid or qid. Oral doses may be taken with food to minimize stomach upset.	Injection: available 5 mg/ml ready to infuse solution or 500-mg vial Tablets: 250 mg, 500 mg
Midazolam (Versed)	*IV* (titrate dose slowly to avoid excessive dosing): *Conscious sedation:* Children: 0.05 mg/kg just before the procedure to a maximum dose of 2 mg. Dose may be repeated every 3 or 4 minutes up to 4 times. Adults: 0.5–2 mg over 2 minutes. Titrate to effect by repeating doses every 2–3 minutes to a usual dose of 2.5–5 mg. *Infusion for sedation during mechanical ventilation:* administer a loading dose of 0.05–0.2 mg/kg followed by a continuous infusion of 1–2 μg/kg/min and titrate to effect. *Orally:* 0.5 mg/kg to a maximum dose of 15 mg. *Intranasally:* 0.2–0.3 mg/kg/dose. The oral and intranasal routes of administration are not FDA approved.	Injection: 1 mg/ml, 5 mg/ml

Continued

Table 107   Medications   (continued)

DRUG	*DOSE*	*DOSAGE FORMS*
Mineral oil	*Orally* (do not administer concomitantly with docusate): Children: 5–20 ml/day. Adults: 15–45 ml/day. *Rectally* (as a retention enema): Children: 30–60 ml. Adults: 60–150 ml.	Enema: 133 ml Liquid
Morphine sulfate (Astramorph PF, Duramorph, MSIR, MS Contin, Roxanol)	*IV or IM:* Neonates and infants under age 6 months: these patients are particularly sensitive to the respiratory depressant effects of opiates; therefore, the doses recommended are lower: 0.03 mg/kg every 3 or 4 hours. Infusions have been used in neonatal patients at a dose of 0.01 mg/kg/hr. The dose may be increased if necessary but should not exceed 0.015–0.02 mg/kg/hr. Infants over 6 months and children: 0.1 mg/kg every 3 or 4 hours. The usual maximum dose is 10 mg. Adults: 2.5–10 mg every 2–6 hours. *Epidurally:* 0.5–5 mg in the lumbar region. Dose may be repeated every 24 hours. Maximum dose is 10 mg/24 hr. *Intrathecally:* one tenth of epidural dose or about 0.2–1 mg/dose. Repeat doses are not recommended. *Orally:* prompt-release preparations are administered every 3 or 4 hours; controlled-release preparations are administered every 8–12 hours. Oral doses are about one third as effective as IV doses. Infants over 6 months and children: 0.3 mg/kg every 3 or 4 hours (prompt release) or 0.3–0.6 mg/kg every 8–12 hours (extended release). Adults: 10–30 mg every 3–4 hours (prompt release) or 15–30 mg every 8–12 hours (extended release).	Injection: 0.5 mg/ml, 1 mg/ml, 2 mg/ml, 3 mg/ml, 4 mg/ml, 5 mg/ml, 8 mg/ml, 10 mg/ml, 15 mg/ml Solution: 10 mg/5 ml, 20 mg/5 ml, 20 mg/ml Suppositories: 5 mg, 10 mg, 20 mg, 30 mg Tablets: 15 mg, 30 mg Tablets, controlled release: 15 mg, 30 mg, 60 mg, 100 mg
Mumps virus vaccine (Mumpsvax)	*SC into the outer aspect of the upper arm:* 0.5 ml at age 15 months or older. Trivalent MMR vaccine is preferred for most vaccinations. Federal law requires that the date of administration, manufacturer, lot number, and expiration date of the vaccine, and the name, title, and address of the person administering the dose be entered into the patient's permanent medical record. It also requires providers to distribute information on vaccines before each vaccination.	Injection: $\geq$20,000 TCID$_{50}$/0.5 ml
Mupirocin (pseudomonic acid A; Bactroban)	*Topically:* apply a small amount to the affected area tid, usually for 3–5 days. Re-evaluate the patient if there has not been improvement after 5 days.	Ointment: 2%
Nafcillin (See oxacillin)	Neonates: 60 mg/kg/24 hr in 4–6 divided doses. Children: 100–200 mg/kg/24 hr in 4–6 divided doses.	Injection: 500 mg, 1 g, 2 g
Nalbuphine (Nubain)	*Parenterally:* *Reversal of morphine infusion side effects:* 0.025–0.05 mg/kg repeated every 6 hours as necessary. *Analgesia:* Children over age 10 months: 0.1–0.14 mg/kg every 3–6 hours as necessary to a maximum dose of 10 mg. Adults: 10–20 mg every 3–6 hours. Its use in narcotic-dependent patients may cause symptoms of withdrawal.	Injection: 10 mg/ml, 20 mg/ml

Continued

Table 107   Medications   (continued)

DRUG	DOSE	DOSAGE FORMS
Naloxone (Narcan)	*IV (preferred), IM, or SC:* *Neonatal opiate depression:* 0.01 mg/kg every 2 or 3 minutes until the desired response is obtained. Additional doses may be necessary at 1–2-hour intervals. *Opiate overdosage:* 0.1 mg/kg to a dose of 2 mg administered every 2 or 3 minutes until 5 doses (up to 10 mg) have been given. If the depressive condition is not reversed, causes other than opiate ingestion should be considered. Additional doses may be necessary because the duration of effect of the opiate is generally longer than that of naloxone. The drug may also be administered via continuous infusion, especially if higher doses are necessary. *Postoperative narcotic reversal (partial reversal):* 0.005–0.01 mg/kg every 2–3 minutes until the desired degree of reversal is achieved. Care should be taken to avoid excessive dosage because that might result in a decrease in analgesia and an increase in blood pressure.	Injection (neonatal): 0.02 mg/ml Injection: 0.4 mg/ml, 1 mg/ml
Naproxen (Aleve, Naprosyn)	*Orally:* 5–10 mg/kg every 8–12 hours to a maximum daily dose of 1 g.	Suspension: 125 mg/5 ml Tablets: 250 mg, 375 mg, 500 mg
Nelfinavir (Viracept)	*Orally* (to be used in combination with nucleoside analogs): Age 2–13: 60–90 mg/kg/day in 3 divided doses with food. Adolescents and adults: 750 mg/dose tid.	Powder: 50 mg/g (1 g scoop provided to measure doses) Tablets: 250 mg
Neomycin, polymyxin B, and dexamethasone (AK-Trol, Dexacidin, Maxitrol)	*Topically to the eye:* apply 1–2 drops or a small amount of the ointment to the affected eye every 4–6 hours. Finger pressure should be applied to the lacrimal sac for about 1 minute after the administration of the drops.	Ointment, ophthalmic; neomycin 3.5 mg, polymyxin B sulfate 10,000 U, and dexamethasone 0.1% per gram Suspension, ophthalmic: neomycin 3.5 mg, polymyxin B sulfate 10,000 U, and dexamethasone 0.1% per ml
Neomycin, polymyxin B, and hydrocortisone (Cortisporin)	*Ophthalmic:* Solution: 1–2 drops to the affected eye every 4–6 hours; apply finger pressure to the lacrimal sac for 1 minute after instillation. Ointment: apply about ½″ ribbon of ointment to the eye tid or qid. *Otic* (both a suspension and a solution formulation are available. The solution form may sting when instilled, but allows the ear canal to be examined easily): instill 3–4 drops into the affected ear tid or qid.	Ointment, ophthalmic: neomycin 0.35%, bacitracin 400 U, polymyxin B 10,000 U, and hydrocortisone 1% Solution or suspension, otic: neomycin 5 mg/ml, polymyxin B 10,000 U/ml, and hydrocortisone 1% Suspension, ophthalmic: neomycin 0.35%, polymyxin B 10,000 U, and hydrocortisone 1%
Neomycin sulfate (Mycifradin)	*Orally:* *Bowel preparation:* 15 mg/kg (up to 1 g) at 1 PM, 2 PM, and 11 PM on the day before surgery (with erythromycin, cleansing enemas). *Hepatic coma:* 50–100 mg/kg/day in 3 or 4 divided doses up to 12 g/day.	Solution, oral: 125 mg/5 ml Tablets: 500 mg
Neostigmine (Prostigmin)	*IM:* *Myasthenia gravis test:* 0.04 mg/kg single dose	Injection: 0.25 mg/ml, 0.5 mg/ml, 1 mg/ml

Continued

Table 107   Medications   (continued)

DRUG	DOSE	DOSAGE FORMS
Neostigmine (Prostigmin) (*continued*)	*IV:* *Reversal of non-depolarizing neuromuscular blockade after surgery in conjunction with atropine or glyco-pyrrolate:* Infants: 0.025–0.1 mg/kg/dose. Children: 0.025–0.08 mg/kg/dose. Adults: 0.5–2.5 mg, total dose not to exceed 5 mg.	
Netilmicin (Netromycin)	*IV (monitor levels carefully):* Neonates under age 7 days: <1500 g: 2.5 mg/kg every 24 hours. 1500–2000 g: 2.5 mg/kg every 18 hours. >2000 g: 2.5 mg/kg every 12 hours. Neonates age 7–21 days: <1500 g: 2.5 mg/kg every 12 hours. >1500 g: 2.5 mg/kg every 8 hours. Age 4 weeks–12 years: 2.5 mg/kg every 8 hours. Over age 12: 1.5–2 mg/kg every 8 hours. Maximum dose until serum levels are known: 100 mg/dose. Dose adjustment is required in patients with renal impairment.	Injection: 100 mg/ml
Nitrofurantoin (Furadantin, Macro-dantin)	*Orally:* *Active infection:* Children: 5–7 mg/kg/day in 4 divided doses to a maximum of 400 mg/day. Adults: 200–400 mg/day in 4 divided doses. *Chronic suppression therapy:* Children: 1–2 mg/kg/day in 1 or 2 divided doses. Adults: 50–100 mg at bedtime daily. Administer with food or milk to decrease rate of absorption because high peak levels are associated with increased GI upset.	Capsules (macrocrystals): 25 mg, 50 mg, 100 mg Suspension: 25 mg/5 ml
Nitroprusside sodium (Nipride, Nitropress)	*IV as a continuous infusion:* 0.3–0.5 μg/kg/min initially, then titrate to effect. Usual dose is 3 μg/kg/min. The maximum dose is 10 μg/kg/min. Cyanide toxicity may occur during prolonged therapy or in patients with hepatic dysfunction. Administration of sodium thiosulfate may decrease blood cyanide levels. Thiocyanate may accumulate in patients with renal impairment.	Injection: 50 mg Protect solutions from light. Do not use if highly colored (blue, green, or red).
Norepinephrine (Levarterenol, Levophed, Noradrenalin)	*IV as a continuous infusion:* initially 0.05–0.1 μg/kg/min, titrated to response. Maximum dose: 1–2 μg/kg/min.	Injection: 1 mg/ml
Nystatin (Mycostatin, Nilstat)	*Orally:* Neonates: 100,000 U administered qid. Infants: 200,000 U administered qid. Children and adults: 400,000–1 million U administered qid. *Topically:* apply ointment or cream to the affected area tid or qid.	Cream: 100,000 U/g [also available with triamcinolone, a topical steroid (Mycolog)] Ointment: 100,000 U/g [also available with triamcinolone, a topical steroid (Mycolog)] Suspension: 100,000 U/ml Tablets: 500,000 U (intestinal infections only) Troches: 200,000 U
Octreotide (somatostatin analog; Sandostatin)	*IV or SC:* the subcutaneous route is generally preferred because absorption is not immediate and the activity is somewhat prolonged. The drug may also be administered as a continuous infusion. Pediatric experience is limited, but initial doses of 1–10 μg/kg with total daily doses of 2–50 μg/kg in 2–4 divided doses. Usual adult doses are 50 μg 1 or 2 times daily initially, then titrate dose to the patient's response. The long-term effects of octreotide on growth hormone release have not been determined.	Injection: 50 μg/ml, 100 μg/ml, 200 μg/ml, 500 μg/ml, 1000 μg/ml

Continued

Table 107   Medications   (continued)

DRUG	DOSE	DOSAGE FORMS
Oxacillin (Bactocill)	**IV:** Neonates under age 7 days: <2000 g: 50 mg/kg/day in 2 divided doses. >2000 g: 100 mg/kg/day in 2 divided doses. Neonates over age 7 days: <1200 g: 50 mg/kg/day in 2 divided doses. 1200–2000 g: 75 mg/kg/day in 3 divided doses. >2000 g: 100 mg/kg/day in 4 divided doses. Infants and children (depends on severity and site of infection): *Mild to moderate infections:* 50 mg/kg/day in 4 divided doses. *Severe infections, including osteomyelitis:* 100–200 mg/kg/day in 4–6 divided doses. Total maximum dose is 12 g/day. Adults: *Mild to moderate infections:* 250–500 mg every 6 hours. *Severe infections:* 1–2 g every 4–6 hours. *Orally:* Infants and children: 50–100 mg/kg/day in 4 divided doses. Adults: 500 mg–1 g every 4–6 hours.	Capsules: 250 mg, 500 mg Injection: 250 mg, 500 mg, 1 g, 2 g, 4 g, 10 g Solution, oral: 250 mg/5 ml
Oxybutymin (Ditropan)	*Orally:* Children over age 5: 5 mg administered bid or tid. Adults: 5 mg bid or tid, to a maximum of qid.	Solution, oral: 5 mg/5 ml Tablets: 5 mg
Pancrelipase (Cotazym, Cotazym-S, Creon, Pancrease MT, Ultrase, Zymase)	*Orally:* depends on the condition being treated and the dietary content of the patient. Dosage is usually determined by the fat content of the diet. The usual starting dose is 4000–8000 U of lipase activity before or with each meal or snack for children age 1–7, 4000–12,000 U for children age 7–12, or 4000–33,000 U for adults. Further dosage adjustments may be made based on the patient's symptoms. The newer, enteric-coated products are designed to release the enzymes at pH >6 and are therefore more resistant to destruction by gastric acids.	Capsules, delayed release, containing enteric-coated spheres, microspheres, or microtablets‡
Paregoric	*Analgesic:* 0.25–0.5 ml/kg from once daily to qid. *Antidiarrheal:* 0.1 ml/kg after each loose stool up to qid. Contains 0.4 mg/ml morphine.	Tincture: 16-oz bottle
Pemoline (Cylert)	*Orally:* Children over age 6: initially 37.5 mg/day in the morning. Dose may be gradually increased in 18.75-mg increments weekly to a maximum of 112.5 mg/day. Improvement in the patient's condition is gradual and may not be significant until the third or fourth week of therapy.	Tablets: 18.75 mg, 37.5 mg, 75 mg Tablets, chewable: 37.5 mg
Penicillamine (Cuprimine, Depen)	Do not exceed a dose of 30 mg/kg/day. *Rheumatoid arthritis:* Children: Initial: 3 mg/kg/day (≤250 mg/day) for 3 months, then 6 mg/kg/day (≤500 mg/day) in divided doses bid for 3 months. Maximum: 10 mg/kg/day in 3 or 4 divided doses. *Wilson disease:* Children: 20 mg/kg/day in 4 divided doses.	Capsules: 125 mg, 250 mg Tablets: 250 mg

Continued

Table 107 Medications (continued)

DRUG	DOSE	DOSAGE FORMS

Penicillin G, aqueous (potassium and sodium salts)	*IV:*
	 Neonates under age 7 days:
	  <2000 g: 25,000 U/kg every 12 hours. For meningitis, use 50,000 U/kg every 12 hours.
	  >2000 g: 20,000 U/kg every 8 hours. For meningitis, 50,000 U/kg every 8 hours.
	 Neonates over age 7 days:
	  <2000 g: 25,000 U/kg every 8 hours. For meningitis, 50,000 U/kg every 8 hours.
	  >2000 g: 25,000 U/kg every 6 hours. For meningitis, 50,000 U/kg every 6 hours.
	 Infants and children: 100,000–250,000 U/kg/day in 6 divided doses. Up to 500,000 U/kg/day may be used for severe infections to a maximum of 20 million U/day.
	 Adults: 2–20 million U/day in 6 divided doses.
	The potassium salt contains 1.7 mEq of potassium and 0.3 mEq of sodium per 1 million U.
	The sodium salt contains 2 mEq of sodium per 1 million U.
	The potassium salt must be administered slowly at high doses due to the effect of the potassium.
		Injection, potassium salt: 1 million U, 5 million U, 10 million U
		Injection, sodium salt: 5 million U

Penicillin G procaine, benzathine	*Deep IM:* results in low but prolonged serum levels. May be given as a single daily dose. A dose of penicillin G benzathine will result in low serum levels for up to 4 weeks. Newborns: avoid use in these patients because sterile abscess and procaine toxicity are of greater concern. Infants: 50,000 U/kg up to 600,000 U. Children and adults: 600,000–1.2 million U/day. Maximum dose is 4.8 million U.	Injection, benzathine: 600,000 U/ml Injection, benzathine and procaine: combined equal parts of each in 300,000 U, 600,000 U, 1.2 million U, 2.4 million U; 900/300 (900,000 U benzathine, 300,000 U procaine) Injection, procaine: 600,000 U/ml
Penicillin V potassium (phenoxy-methylpenicillin; Pen Vee K, V-Cillin K, Veetids)	*Orally:* Children: 25–50 mg/kg/day in 4 divided doses. Adults: 125–500 mg/dose every 6 hours. *Prophylaxis:* Under age 5: 125 mg bid. Over age 5 and adults: 250 mg bid.	Liquid, oral: 250 mg/5 ml Tablets: 125 mg, 250 mg, 500 mg
Pentobarbital (Nembutal)	*Orally, IM:* *Sedation before surgery:* Children: 2–6 mg/kg/day to a maximum of 100 mg. *IV:* *For sedation before procedures:* dose should be administered slowly and incrementally to avoid oversedation. Patients must be closely observed. Dosing is very patient-specific. The rate of injection should not exceed 1 mg/kg/min (50 mg/min in adults). Allow at least 1 minute to reach full effect. Children: initially 2 mg/kg to a maximum of 100 mg. Incremental doses of 1–2 mg/kg may be used to a maximum total dose of 200 mg. Adults: initially 100 mg. Incremental doses of 100–200 mg may be given to a maximum dose of 500 mg for healthy adults. *Barbiturate coma:* 10–15 mg/kg administered over 1–2 hours, followed by a maintenance infusion of 1 mg/kg/hr. Dosage may be increased to 2–3 mg/kg/hr to maintain burst suppression on EEG. Hypothermia may necessitate a decrease in dosage.	Capsules: 50 mg, 100 mg Elixir: 20 mg/5 ml Injection: 50 mg/ml Suppositories: 30 mg, 60 mg, 120 mg, 200 mg

Continued

Table 107   Medications   (continued)

DRUG	*DOSE*	*DOSAGE FORMS*
Pentobarbital (Nembutal) (*continued*)	*Rectally* (do not divide suppositories): 4.5–9 kg: 30 mg. 9–18 kg: 30–60 mg. 19–36 kg: 60 mg. 36–50 kg: 60–120 mg. >50 kg: 120–200 mg.	
Phenobarbital	*IV or orally:* *Loading doses:* Neonates: 20 mg/kg/day in 2 divided doses for 1 day. Infants and children: 10 mg/kg/day in 2 divided doses for 2 days. Adolescents and adults: 10 mg/kg/day in 2 divided doses for 1 day. *Maintenance doses:* Neonates: 5 mg/kg/day in 2 divided doses. Infants: 5–6 mg/kg/day in 2 divided doses. Age 1–5: 6 mg/kg/day in 2 divided doses. Age 5–12: 4 mg/kg/day in 1 or 2 divided doses. Over age 12 and adults: 1–2 mg/kg/day in 1 or 2 divided doses. *IV for status epilepticus:* 15–20 mg/kg in incremental doses. Allow at least 15–30 minutes for the drug to distribute into the CNS and for the seizures to stop.	Elixir: 15 mg/5 ml, 20 mg/5 ml Injection (sodium): 30 mg/ml, 60 mg/ml, 65 mg/ml, 130 mg/ml Tablets: 15 mg, 30 mg, 60 mg, 100 mg
Phentolamine mesylate	*Test dose (pheochromocytoma):* 1 mg IM or IV.	Injection: 5-mg ampul
Phenylephrine (Neo-Synephrine, Mydfrin Ophthalmic)	*Intranasally* (do not use for longer than 3–5 days): Under age 6: 0.125% solution 2–3 drops every 4 hours as needed. Age 6–12: 0.25% solution 2–3 drops or 1–2 sprays every 4 hours as needed. Over age 12 and adults: 0.5% solution 2–3 drops or 1–2 sprays every 4 hours as needed. 1% solution may be used in adults with extreme congestion. *Ophthalmic:* Infants: 1 drop of 2.5% solution 15–30 minutes before procedure. Children and adults: 1 drop of 2.5% or 10% solution; may repeat in 15–30 minutes. *IV for severe hypotension or shock:* a bolus dose of 5–20 μg/kg (2–5 mg in adults) may be repeated every 10–15 minutes. For infusion, initial doses of 0.1–0.5 μg/kg/min are titrated to effect.	Drops only: 0.125% Injection: 10 mg/ml Solution, nasal drops or spray: 0.25%, 0.5%, 1% Solution, ophthalmic: 2.5%, 10%
Phenytoin (Dilantin) and fosphenytoin (Cerebyx)	Care must be taken when changing from one dosage form of the drug to another because some contain phenytoin sodium and some contain the free acid form of the drug. The free acid form is used for the Infatabs and the suspension. Phenytoin sodium is used for the injection and capsules. Phenytoin sodium contains 92% phenytoin. Injection labelled as 50 mg/ml phenytoin sodium contains 46 mg of phenytoin and capsules labelled 100 mg contain 92 mg phenytoin. Fosphenytoin should be ordered in terms of phenytoin equivalents.	Capsule, phenytoin sodium, extended: 30 mg, 100 mg Injection, fosphenytoin: 75 mg/1 ml (equivalent to 50 mg phenytoin sodium) Injection, phenytoin sodium: 50 mg/ml Suspension, phenytoin: 125 mg/5 ml Tablet, chewable, phenytoin: 50 mg

Continued

Table 107   Medications   (continued)

DRUG	DOSE	DOSAGE FORMS
Phenytoin (Dilantin) and fos-phenytoin (Cerebyx) (*continued*)	The patient's serum levels should be monitored whenever the dosage form is changed. In addition, the different brands of phenytoin capsules have different dissolution characteristics. Dilantin capsules are considered extended and may be dosed in adults as a single daily dose. The serum level range usually associated with clinical effectiveness is 10–20 μg/ml; that associated with mild to moderate toxicity may be as low as 25–30 μg/ml. *Loading dose (IV or PO):* 15–20 mg/kg in a single or divided doses. *Maintenance dose (IV or PO):* 5 mg/kg/day in 2 or 3 divided doses initially and then adjusted to response and serum levels. Usual ranges based on age (divided into 2 or 3 doses daily): Neonates: 5–8 mg/kg/day. Age 6 months–3 years: 8–10 mg/kg/day. Age 4–6: 7.5–9 mg/kg/day. Age 7–9: 7–8 mg/kg/day. Age 10–16: 6–7 mg/kg/day. Adults: 5–6 mg/kg/day may be given as a single dose if extended-capsule preparation is used. Higher doses are required in infants and young children due to lower absorption of the drug from the GI tract. IV doses of phenytoin should be administered at a maximum rate of about 1 mg/kg/min (50 mg/min in adults) to avoid cardiovascular side effects. The injection is not compatible with many solutions or medications. The line must be flushed well with saline before administration to avoid precipitation of phenytoin in the line. Extravasation of the drug must also be avoided because it is very alkaline and may cause severe tissue necrosis. Thorough flushing of the vessel after phenytoin administration will also decrease the incidence of local tissue inflammation that may occur even in the absence of extravasation. Fosphenytoin injection should be diluted with either 5% dextrose or normal saline to a concentration of 1.5–25 mg of phenytoin equivalents (2.3–37.5 mg fosphenytoin) per ml of diluent and may be administered at a rate of 2–3 mg phenytoin equivalents/kg/min (100–150 mg phenytoin equivalents/min in adults).	
Phosphate (potassium and/or sodium)	Should be guided by the patient's serum phosphorus and potassium levels. Severe deficits should be replaced by the IV route because the oral route may result in diarrhea and oral absorption is unreliable. In general, the deficit should be made up by incorporating it into the patient's maintenance fluids. Intermittent infusions should follow the guidelines outlined below for potassium infusions because the IV form is potassium phosphate and each 3 mmol of phosphate will also deliver 4.4 mEq of potassium. The guidelines below are meant for use in patients with severe hypophosphatemia (<1 mg/dl in adults):	Injection (potassium phosphate): 3 mmol (94 mg) phosphorus and 4.4 mEq potassium per milliliter Packets or capsules (Neutra-Phos): 250 mg (8 mmol) phosphorus, 7 mEq potassium, and 7 mEq sodium Packets or capsules (Neutra-Phos K): 250 mg (8 mmol) phosphorus, 14.25 mEq potassium Tablets (K-Phos Neutral): 250 mg (8 mmol) phosphorus, 1.1 mEq potassium, and 13 mEq sodium Tablets (Uro-KP-Neutral): 250 mg (8 mmol) phosphorus, 1.27 mEq potassium, and 10.9 mEq sodium

Continued

Table 107   Medications   (continued)

DRUG	DOSE	DOSAGE FORMS
Phosphate (potassium and/or sodium) (continued)	Neonates: 0.5 mmol/kg up to 1–2 mmol/kg/day. Children: 0.15–0.3 mmol/kg with subsequent doses only after serum levels are checked and if the patient is symptomatic. Adults: 0.08 mmol/kg (uncomplicated hypophosphatemia) or 0.16 mmol/kg for prolonged deficits. Do not exceed 0.24 mmol/kg/day (serum phosphorus ≥0.5 mg/dl) or 0.5 mmol/kg/day (serum phosphorus <0.5 mg/dl). IV doses should be administered over a 6-hour period. *Maintenance doses:* Children: 0.5–1.5 mmol/kg/day. Adults: 15–30 mmol/day. *Orally:* should be taken with food to increase GI tolerance. Each packet or capsule should be mixed in 75 ml of water. Tablets should be taken with a full glass of water. *Maintenance doses:* Children: 2–3 mmol/kg/day in 4 divided doses. Adults: 32–64 mmol/day (4–8 packets) in 4 divided doses. Do not administer at the same time as aluminum- and/or magnesium-containing antacids, sucralfate, or calcium because they may act to bind phosphorus.	
Phytonadione (vitamin K; Aqua-MEPHYTON, Konakion, Mephyton)	*IM or SC:* *Hemorrhagic disease of the newborn, prophylaxis:* 0.5–1 mg within 1 hour of birth and again 6–8 hours later, if needed. *Treatment:* 1–2 mg/day. *Treatment of deficiency caused by malabsorption or decreased synthesis or due to drugs (administer IV cautiously and slowly):* Children: 1–2 mg/day. Adults: 10 mg/day. *Treatment of oral anticoagulant overdose:* Infants: 1–2 mg repeated every 4–8 hours. Children and adults: 2.5–10 mg repeated in 6–8 hours. *Orally:* *Prevention of deficiency in malabsorption:* Children: 2.5–5 mg every other day or daily. Adults: 5–25 mg/day.	Injection: 2 mg/ml, 10 mg/ml Tablets: 5 mg
Piperacillin (Piperacil)	*IV:* Neonates: 150 mg/kg/day in 3 divided doses. Infants and children: 300 mg/kg/day in 4–6 divided doses. Doses of 300–500 mg/kg/day in 6 divided doses have been used in the treatment of children with cystic fibrosis. Adults: 2–4 g every 4–8 hours. Do not exceed 18 g/day.	Injection: 2-g, 3-g, 4-g, 40-g bulk package
Piroxicam (Feldene)	*Orally:* Children: 0.2–0.3 mg/kg/day in a single daily dose to a maximum of 15 mg/day. Adults: 10–20 mg/day in a single dose.	Capsules: 10 mg, 20 mg

Continued

Table 107   Medications   (continued)

DRUG	DOSE	DOSAGE FORMS
Pneumococcal vaccine, polyvalent (Pneumovax 23, Pnu-Imune 23)	*SC or IM:* Over age 2 and adults: 0.5 ml. The manufacturers presently do not recommend a booster dose due to the increased incidence and severity of adverse effects. The AAP and ACIP presently recommend revaccination in those patients at greatest risk (asplenia, sickle cell, and organ transplant). Revaccination should be considered in children after age 3–5 if they will be older than age 10 at the time of revaccination and in adults, after 6 or more years since the last vaccination.	Injection: 25 μg of each of 23 polysaccharide isolates per 0.5 ml
Poliovirus vaccine, live, oral, trivalent (sabin, TOPV, OPV, Orimune) Poliovirus vaccine, inactivated (Salk, IPV, Ipol)	*IPV regimen (SC):* two 0.5-ml doses are administered at least 4 weeks apart, but preferably 8 weeks apart starting at 2 months of age. A third dose is administered at 12–18 months of age and a fourth dose should be given at school entry or about 4–6 years of age. *IPV/OPV regimen (SC and orally):* two 0.5-ml doses of IPV are administered at 2 and 4 months of age with DTP or DTaP and Hib vaccines, followed by OPV doses at 12–18 months of age and again at 4–6 years of age. *OPV regimen (orally):* a total of four 0.5-ml doses of the oral vaccine are administered at 2 and 4 months of age, 12–18 months of age, and 4–6 years of age. Inactivated vaccine must be used for immunocompromised individuals and their household contacts or in patients who are inpatients in the hospital setting. Live polio virus will be excreted from the GI tract of infants given the oral polio vaccine.	Injection: 0.5 ml Solution, oral pipettes: 0.5 ml
Polyethylene glycolelectrolyte solution (Colovage, Colyte, Go-LYTELY, OCL)	*Orally after a 3–4-hour fast:* Children: 25–40 mg/kg/hr. Adults: 240 ml every 10 minutes. The patient should continue to drink the solution until the rectal effluent is clear. Rapid drinking of each portion is more effective than slow consumption. The first bowel movement should occur about an hour after starting. The solution is more palatable if chilled, but must not be poured over ice. Nothing, including other flavorings, should be added to the solution. *Nasogastric tube administration:* Adults: 240 ml every 10 minutes.	Powder for oral solution to make 4 L: PEG3350 236 g, sodium sulfate 22.74 g, sodium bicarbonate 6.74 g, sodium chloride 5.86 g, and potassium chloride 2.97 g
Potassium chloride	*Orally:* liquid doses must be well diluted before administration to avoid GI adverse effects. Capsules or tablets should be taken with a full glass of water. Capsules may be opened and emptied onto a soft food, but the beads should not be crushed or chewed. Total daily dose may be given in 1 or 2 divided doses if tolerated, or may be given in 3 or 4 divided doses to decrease GI upset. Dose is usually based on each patient's requirements and may depend on concurrent medications or medical conditions that result in potassium losses. The following may be used as general guidelines: *Normal daily requirement for either PO or IV replacement:* Newborn: 2–6 mEq/kg/day. Children: 2–3 mEq/kg/day. Adults: 40–80 mEq/day.	Capsules, controlled release: 8 mEq (600 mg), 10 mEq (750 mg) Injection, concentrated: 2 mEq/ml, 3 mEq/ml Liquids: 20 mEq/15 ml (10%), 30 mEq/15 ml (15%), 40 mEq/15 ml (20%) Powders, effervescent packets: 15 mEq, 20 mEq, 25 mEq Tablets, effervescent: 20 mEq, 25 mEq, 50 mEq Tablets, extended release: 6.7 mEq (500 mg), 8 mEq (600 mg), 10 mEq (750 mg) Other potassium salts are also available and may be desirable in patients who are acidotic. They include bicarbonate, citrate, acetate, and gluconate salts.

Continued

Table 107   Medications   (continued)

DRUG	*DOSE*	*DOSAGE FORMS*
Potassium chloride (*continued*)	*During diuretic therapy:* 　Children: 1–2 mEq/kg/day. 　Adults: 20–40 mEq/day. *For treatment of hypokalemia:* 　Children: 2–5 mEq/kg/day. 　Adults: 40–100 mEq/day. *IV:* doses should be well diluted. Usually they are incorporated into the patient's daily fluid requirement. The maximum desirable concentration is 80 mEq/L. Greater concentrations should be used cautiously and only in patients with documented hypokalemia with a serum potassium level <2.5 mEq/L. In the case of a patient in whom a shorter infusion of potassium is necessary, the following guidelines may be used: Maximum concentration of the solution must not exceed 30 mEq/100 ml (1 mEq/3 ml) and rate of infusion should not exceed 1 mEq/kg/hr in children or 40 mEq/hr in adults. The solutions should be infused using a pump to control the infusion rate. Infusion over 2–3 hours (0.3–0.5 mEq/kg/hr) is more desirable. Administration of doses greater than 0.3 mEq/kg/hr should be done only if the patient has an ECG monitor in place. Solutions should be mixed well to prevent layering of the potassium chloride, which may result in inadvertent rapid administration.	
Prednisolone and prednisone	*Orally:* depends on the condition being treated and the patient's response. The lowest dose possible should be used. Withdrawal of long-term therapy must be accomplished slowly by gradually tapering the dose. The guidelines below may be used for initial dosing. Children: 　*Anti-inflammatory or immunosuppressive:* 1–2 mg/kg/day in 1–4 divided doses. 　*Acute asthma:* 1–2 mg/kg/day in 1 or 2 divided doses for up to 5 days. 　*Inflammatory bowel disease:* 1–3 mg/kg/day in 1–2 divided doses. 　*Nephrotic syndrome:* 2 mg/kg/day in 3 or 4 divided doses. 　*Organ transplants:* 1 mg/kg/day in 2 divided doses, tapering gradually to 0.15 mg/kg/day or lowest effective dose.	Prednisolone: 　Liquid, as sodium phosphate (Pediapred): 5 mg/5 ml 　Syrup (Prelone): 15 mg/5 ml 　Tablets: 5 mg Prednisone: 　Solution: 5 mg/5 ml 　Syrup (Liquid Pred): 5 mg/5 ml 　Tablets: 1 mg, 2.5 mg, 5 mg, 10 mg, 20 mg, 50 mg
Primidone (Mysoline)	*Orally:* 　Under age 8: initially 50–125 mg/day at bedtime or in 2 divided doses. Increase dose by 50–125 mg/day at weekly intervals to the normal range of 125–250 mg tid or 10–25 mg/kg/day. 　Over age 8 and adults: initially 125–250 mg/day at bedtime or in 2 divided doses. Increase dose by 125–250 mg/day at weekly intervals to the usual maintenance dose of 250 mg tid or qid. Do not exceed 500 mg qid (2 g). Primidone is metabolized to phenobarbital and phenylethylmalonamide (PEMA). Phenobarbital levels should be monitored in addition to primidone levels.	Suspension: 250 mg/5 ml Tablets: 50 mg/ 250 mg

Continued

Table 107   Medications   (continued)

DRUG	*DOSE*	*DOSAGE FORMS*
Probenecid (Benemid)	*Uricosuric:* 　Children under age 2: not recommended. 　Age 2–14: 　　*Initial:* 25 mg/kg for 1 dose. 　　Maintenance: 40 mg/kg/24 hr in 4 divided 　　　doses.	Tablets: 500 mg
Procainamide (Procanbid, Pronestyl)	*IV:* 　Children: loading dose of 3–6 mg/kg to a maxi- 　　mum of 100 mg over 5 minutes. This may be re- 　　peated every 5–10 minutes to a maximum of 　　15 mg/kg. Follow with a maintenance infusion 　　at a dose of 20–80 μg/kg/min. 　Adults: loading dose of 50–100 mg, repeated every 　　5–10 minutes to a maximum of 15–18 mg/kg or 　　1–1.5 g. Follow with a maintenance infusion at 　　a usual dose of 3–4 mg/min (range 1–6 mg/ 　　min). *Orally* (immediate-release products must be adminis- 　tered every 3 hours; controlled-release products 　must be administered every 6 hours or every 　12 hours depending on the formulation used): 　Children: 15–50 mg/kg/day to a maximum dose of 　　4 g/day. 　Adults: usual range is 1–4 g/day in divided doses 　　as above.	Capsules, immediate release: 250 mg, 375 mg, 　500 mg Injection: 100 mg/ml, 500 mg/ml Tablets, immediate release: 250 mg, 375 mg, 500 mg Tablets, sustained release: 250 mg, 500 mg, 750 mg, 　1000 mg Tablets, sustained release, 12-hour duration (Procan- 　bid): 500 mg, 1000 mg
Prochlorperazine (Compazine)	*Orally or rectally as an antiemetic:* 0.4 mg/kg/day in 3 　or 4 divided doses or alternatively by the patient's 　weight: 　9–14 kg: 2.5 mg every 12–24 hours as needed, to 　　a maximum of 7.5 mg/day. 　14–18 kg: 2.5 mg every 8–12 hours as needed, to 　　a maximum of 10 mg/day. 　18–39 kg: 2.5 mg every 8 hours or 5 mg every 　　12 hours as needed, to a maximum of 15 mg/ 　　day. 　>40 kg: 　　Rectally: 25 mg every 12 hours. 　　Orally: 5–10 mg tid or qid. *IM* (IV is not recommended in children): 0.13 mg/kg; 　may be repeated if necessary up to tid or qid. 　Usual adult dose is 5–10 mg every 4 hours to a 　maximum of 40 mg/day.	Capsules, sustained release: 10 mg, 15 mg, 30 mg Injection: 5 mg/ml Suppositories: 2.5 mg, 5 mg, 25 mg Syrup: 5 mg/5 ml Tablets: 5 mg, 10 mg, 25 mg
Promethazine (Phenergan)	*Antihistamine* (usually orally): 　Children: 0.1 mg/kg every 6 hours during the day. 　　A dose of 0.5 mg/kg may be used at bedtime. 　Adults: 12.5 mg every 6 hours during the day with 　　a 25-mg dose at bedtime. *Antiemetic* (orally, IV, IM, or rectally): 　Children: 0.5 mg/kg up to every 4 hours. 　Adults: 12.5–25 mg every 4 hours as needed. *Motion sickness* (orally): 　Children: 0.5 mg/kg 30 minutes to 1 hour before 　　traveling; then every 12 hours as needed. 　Adults: 25 mg 30 minutes to 1 hour before travel- 　　ing; then every 12 hours as needed. *Sedation* (all routes): 　Children: 0.5–1 mg/kg every 6 hours as needed. 　Adults: 25–50 mg every 6 hours as needed.	Injection: 25 mg/ml, 50 mg/ml Suppositories: 12.5 mg, 25 mg, 50 mg Syrup: 6.25 mg/5 ml, 25 mg/5 ml Tablets: 12.5 mg, 25 mg, 50 mg

Continued

Table 107   Medications   (continued)

DRUG	DOSE	DOSAGE FORMS
Propranolol (Inderal)	*Orally:* *Arrhythmias:* Children: 0.5–1 mg/kg/day in 3 or 4 divided doses. Dosage may be titrated upward at 3–7-day intervals to the usual range of 2–4 mg/kg/day. If higher doses are necessary, up to 16 mg/kg/day (up to 640 mg) may be used. Adults: usually 10–30 mg every 6–8 hours. *Hypertension:* Children: 0.5–1 mg/kg/day in 2–4 divided doses, increasing at 3–7-day intervals to the usual range of 1–5 mg/kg/day. Adults: 40 mg bid, increasing at 3–7-day intervals to a maximum dose of 640 mg/day. *Migraine prophylaxis:* Children: 0.6–1.5 mg/kg/day in 3 divided doses. Adults: 80 mg/day in 3 or 4 divided doses. Dose may be increased to a maximum of 240 mg/day in divided doses. *Tetralogy spells:* Children: 1–2 mg/kg every 6 hours. *Thyrotoxicosis:* Neonates: 2 mg/kg/day in 2–4 divided doses. Children: 1 mg/kg/day qid. Adolescents and adults: 10–40 mg every 6 hours. *IV:* reserve for life-threatening arrhythmias. To be administered as an IV bolus *slowly* under ECG monitoring. The IV dose is much smaller than the oral dose. Children: 0.01–0.1 mg/kg to a maximum of 1 mg for arrhythmias. For tetralogy spells, 0.15–0.25 mg/kg, which may be repeated once after 15 minutes. Adults: 1–3 mg. A second dose may be given, if necessary, after 2 minutes.	Capsules, sustained release: 60 mg, 80 mg, 120 mg, 160 mg Injection: 1 mg/ml Solution: 4 mg/ml, 8 mg/ml Tablets: 10 mg, 20 mg, 40 mg, 60 mg, 80 mg, 90 mg
Propylthiouracil	*Orally:* Initially: Neonates: 5–10 mg/kg/day in 3 divided doses. Under age 10: 5–7 mg/kg/day in 3 divided doses. Over age 10: 150–300 mg/day in 3 divided doses. Adults: 300 mg/day in 3 divided doses. After control of symptoms has been achieved, the dose may be decreased to the lowest dose possible, usually one third to two thirds of the initial dose, administered in 3 doses daily.	Tablets: 50 mg
Protamine sulfate	*IV:* 1 mg of protamine sulfate neutralizes 90 mg of lung-derived heparin or 115 U of intestinal mucosa-derived heparin. Because heparin disappears rapidly from the circulation, the dose of protamine decreased rapidly with time elapsed since the heparin infusion. The dose of protamine necessary after 30 minutes is half the dose above and that necessary after 2 hours is one fourth the dose above. Because protamine itself is an anticoagulant, avoid overdosing. Protamine should be administered slowly, over a 1-minute period, and the dose should not exceed 50 mg.	Injection: 10 mg/ml
Protirelin (Thyrel TRH)	*IV* (as a bolus over 15–30 seconds with the patient remaining supine for an additional 15 minutes): Children: 7 μg/kg to a maximum of 500 μg. Adults: 500 μg.	Injection: 500 μg/ml

Continued

Table 107 Medications (continued)

DRUG	DOSE	DOSAGE FORMS
Pseudoephedrine (Dorcol, Pedia-Care Infant's Decongestant, Sudafed)	*Orally* (duration of use should usually not exceed 5 days): Under age 2: 4 mg/kg/day in 4 divided doses. Age 2–5: 15 mg every 6 hours to a maximum of 60 mg/day. Age 6–12: 30 mg every 6 hours to a maximum of 120 mg/day. Over age 12 and adults: 60 mg every 6 hours to a maximum of 240 mg/day. (Prolonged-release products for adults may be taken in 2 divided doses daily.)	Capsule: 60 mg Capsules, timed release: 120 mg Drops: 7.5 mg/0.8 ml Liquid: 15 mg/5 ml, 30 mg/5 ml Tablets: 30 mg, 60 mg Tablets, extended release: 120 mg
Psyllium (Fiberall, Hydrocil, Konsyl, Metamucil, Perdiem Fiber, Serutan)	*Orally* (each dose should be accompanied by a full glass of water or other liquid): Children: half the adult dose (½ to 1 packet or 1.7–3.4 g of psyllium) once daily to tid. Adults: 1–2 packets or 3.4–6.8 g of psyllium once daily to tid.	Powder: ~3.4 g/dose Powder, effervescent
Pyrantel pamoate (Antiminth)	*Orally* (may be taken with juice or milk and without regard to the ingestion of food): 11 mg/kg to a maximum of 1 g.	Suspension: 50 mg/ml
Pyridoxine (vitamin B_6)	*IV:* *Treatment of pyridoxine-dependent seizures in infants:* 10–100 mg. *Orally:* *Pyridoxine deficiency:* Children: 5–25 mg/day for 3 weeks. Adults: 10–20 mg/day for 3 weeks. *Drug-induced (isoniazid) neuritis:* Children: 1–2 mg/kg 24 hr (prophylaxis) or 10–50 mg/day (treatment). Adults: 25–100 mg/day (prophylaxis) or 100–200 mg/day (treatment). *Pyridoxine-dependent seizures:* 2–100 mg/day or more, probably for life.	Injection: 100 mg/ml Tablets: 25 mg, 50 mg, 100 mg Tablets, timed release: 100 mg
Rabies immune globulin (Hyperab, Imogam)	*IM:* 20 U/kg as soon as possible after exposure, but may be given as much as 8 days after exposure. Up to one half of the volume should be used to infiltrate the wound. The remaining dose should be administered at a different site and in a different extremity from the vaccine.	Injection: 150 IU/ml
Rabies virus vaccine, human diploid cell cultures (Imovax)	*IM:* *Post-exposure:* 1 ml on days 0, 3, 7, 14, and 28. *Pre-exposure:* 1 ml on days 0, 7, and 21 or 28. A booster dose or serum antibody titer measurement should be done every 2 years for those with continuing exposure.	Injection: 2.5 IU rabies antigen per 1 ml
Ranitidine (Zantac)	*Orally:* Children: 2–4 mg/kg/day in 2 divided doses initially. Dose may be higher in hypersecretory conditions. Adults: 150 mg bid or 300 mg at bedtime. Dose may be higher or more frequently administered. Up to 6 g/day has been used. *IV:* Children: 1–2 mg/kg/day in 3 or 4 divided doses. Do not exceed 6 mg/kg/day or 300 mg/day. Adults: 50 mg every 6–8 hours. Do not exceed 400 mg/day.	Injection: 25 mg/ml Syrup: 15 mg/ml Tablets: 75 mg, 150 mg, 300 mg

Continued

Table 107   Medications   (continued)

DRUG	*DOSE*	*DOSAGE FORMS*
Ribavirin (Virazole)	Aersol administered via the manufacturer's small particle aerosol generator (SPAG). 6 g of the drug are solubilized in sterile water and aerosolized over 12–18 hours daily for 3–7 days. Therapy must be started within the first 3 days of lower respiratory tract infection due to RSV. The manufacturer recommends against using the drug for patients who require assisted ventilation. Precipitation of the drug in respiratory equipment has occurred, as has accumulation of fluid in tubing. Either condition may compromise the patient.	Powder for reconstitution for aerosol: 6 g
Rifampin (Rifadin, Rimactane)	*Orally* (on an empty stomach): *Tuberculosis:* Children: 10–20 mg/kg/day as a single daily dose to a maximum of 600 mg. Adults: 600 mg/day. *Meningococcal carriers:* Under age 1 month: 10 mg/kg/day in 2 divided doses for 2 days. Infants and children: 20 mg/kg/day in 2 divided doses for 2 days, to a maximum dose of 1200 mg/day. Adults: 600 mg/dose bid for 2 days. *Hemophilus influenza type b prophylaxis:* Under age 1 month: 10 mg/kg/day as a single dose for 4 days. Over age 1 month and children: 20 mg/kg/day as a single dose for 4 days. Adults: 600 mg/day for 4 days. *IV* (over 30 minutes to 3 hours): same doses as for the oral route. Rifampin may cause a red–orange discoloration of the sweat, urine, tears, and other body fluids; soft contact lenses may be permanently stained.	Capsules 150 mg, 300 mg Injection: 600 mg Suspension: not commercially available, but may be made by mixing the powder from the capsules with simple syrup to form a 10 mg/ml suspension. Such suspensions are stable for 4 weeks at room temperature or refrigerated.
Rimantadine (Flumadine)	*Orally:* Under age 10: 5 mg/kg once daily to a maximum dose of 150 mg. Over age 10 and adults: 100 mg bid. Therapy may be continued for up to 6 weeks. Rimantadine does not completely prevent an immune response to influenza vaccine; therefore, vaccination is not contraindicated. Rimantadine should be continued for 2–4 weeks after vaccination to allow for antibody production.	Syrup: 50 mg/5 ml Tablets: 100 mg
Rubella virus vaccine (Meruvax II, German measles vaccine)	*SC:* 0.5 mg. For most patients, the combination vaccine containing measles, mumps, and rubella is the preferred vaccine.	Injection: 0.5-ml vials
Scopolamine (hyoscine; Isopto Hyoscine)	*IM, SC, or IV:* Children: 0.006 mg/kg to a maximum dose of 0.3 mg. Adults: 0.3–0.65 mg. *Ophthalmic:* Children: 1 drop (up to qid for uveitis). Adults: 1–2 drops (up to qid for uveitis).	Injection: 0.3 mg/ml, 0.4 mg/ml, 0.86 mg/ml, 1 mg/ml Solution, ophthalmic: 0.25%

Continued

Table 107   Medications   (continued)

DRUG	DOSE	DOSAGE FORMS
Senna (Fletcher's Castoria, Senokot, X-Prep)	*Orally:* *Laxative:* Age 1 month–1 year: 54.5–109 mg (1.25–2.5 ml Senokot syrup) up to bid, but usually once daily at bedtime. Age 1–5: 109–218 mg (2.5–5 ml Senokot syrup, 5–7.5 ml Fletcher's) up to bid, but usually once daily at bedtime. Age 5–15: 218–436 mg (5–10 ml Senokot syrup, 10–15 ml Fletcher's) up to bid, but usually once daily at bedtime. Alternatively, 1 tablet (187 mg senna) may be given. Adults: 2 tablets or 10–15 ml Senokot syrup up to 30 ml or 8 tablets daily. *Bowel evacuation* (usually X-Prep; given the day before the procedure): Age 2–5: 30–45 ml. Age 6–10: 60 ml. Over age 10: 75 ml.	Liquid (Fletcher's Castoria): 33.3 mg/ml Syrup (Senokot, X-Prep): 218 mg/5 ml Tablets (Senokot): 187 mg
Sermorelin acetate (growth hormone-releasing hormone; Geref)	*IV* (in the morning after an overnight fast): 1 μg/kg IV push followed by a 3 ml saline flush.	Injection: 50-μg vials
Silver sulfadiazine (Silvadene, SSD, Thermazene)	*Topically:* applied to a thickness of $\frac{1}{16}$ inch under sterile conditions (using a sterile glove) once or bid to a clean, debrided wound. Wound should always be covered with cream; reapply if it rubs off.	Cream: 10 mg/g
Sodium bicarbonate (baking soda, $NaHCO_3$)	*IV:* *Cardiac arrest* (only after adequate ventilation has been established): 1 mEq/kg IV push initially; may repeat with a dose of 0.5 mEq/kg. Further doses should not be given until the patient's acid–base status has been determined. For instants, the concentration should not exceed 4.2% (0.5 mEq/ml). *Metabolic acidosis* (after measurement of blood gases and pH): Children: mEq HCO_3 = 0.3 × weight (kg) × base deficit (mEq/L) *OR* mEq HCO_3 = 0.5 × weight (kg) × [24-serum HCO_3 (mEq/L)]. Adults: mEq HCO_3 = 0.2 × weight (kg) × base deficit (mEq/L) *OR* mEq HCO_3 = 0.5 × weight (kg) × [24-serum HCO_3 (mEq/L)]. Doses should be administered slowly with frequent monitoring of acid–base balance. *Orally:* *Urine alkalinization* (titrate dose to desired pH): Children: 1–10 mEq/kg/day in divided doses. Adults: 48 mEq initially followed by 12–24 mEq every 4 hours. Doses up to 192 mEq/day have been used.	Injection: 4.2% (0.5 mEq/ml), 7.5% (0.9 mEq/ml), 8.4% (1 mEq/ml) Tablets: 325 mg, 650 mg
Sodium chloride (NaCl; Adsorbonac, AK-NaCl, Muro 128)	*IV:* *Sodium depletion:* repletion rate should be based on the urgency of the patient's condition and as slowly as possible: Na (mEq) = 0.6 × weight (kg) × [desired Na − actual Na]. Use of hypertonic sodium chloride solutions (3%, 5%) should be reserved for emergency use only. *Maintenance sodium requirements:* Children: 3–4 mEq/kg/day. Adults: 154 mEq/day.	Injection: 0.45% (½ normal), 0.9% (normal saline), 3%, 5% Injection, concentrated (must be diluted before use): 14.6% (2.5 mEq/ml), 23.4% (4 mEq/ml) Ointment, ophthalmic: 5% Solution, nasal: 0.65% Solution, ophthalmic: 5%

Continued

Table 107   Medications   (continued)

DRUG	DOSE	DOSAGE FORMS
Sodium chloride (NaCl; Adsorbonac, AK-NaCl, Muro 128) (continued)	*Ophthalmic:* apply 1–2 drops or ¼ inch ribbon of the ointment to the affected eye every 3–4 hours. *Nasal:* use as necessary.	
Sodium polystyrene sulfonate (Kayexalate)	*Orally:* Children: base the dose on the exchange rate of 1 mEq K^+/g of resin in smaller children. Alternatively, a dose of 1 g/kg every 6 hours may be used. Adults: 15 g administered once daily to qid. *Rectally as a retention enema:* Children: 1 g/kg every 2–6 hours. Adults: 30–50 g every 6 hours. Enemas should be retained for as long as possible to increase ion exchange. Evacuation of the enema should be followed by a non-sodium-containing cleansing enema. Sorbital is frequently used for making solutions because it helps to prevent constipation. Administer cautiously to patients who may be at risk of serum sodium level increases. It is not totally selective for potassium; small amounts of calcium and magnesium may also be lost.	Powder Suspension: 15 g/60 ml (with sorbitol)
Sodium sulfacetamide (Ak-Sulf, Bleph-10, Cetamide, Sodium Sulamyd)	*Topically to the eye:* Solutions: apply 1–2 drops in the affected eye up to every 2 or 3 hours while awake. Ointment: apply to the eye once daily to qid. Drops will cause burning or stinging sensation. Ointment will cause blurred vision.	Ointment, ophthalmic: 10% Ointment, ophthalmic: 10% with prednisolone 0.2%, 0.25%, or 0.5% Suspension, ophthalmic: 10%, 15%, 30% Suspension, ophthalmic: 15% with phenylephrine 0.125% (Vasosulf) Suspension, ophthalmic: 10% with prednisolone 0.2%, 0.25%, or 0.5%
Spironolactone (Adlactone)	*Orally:* *Edema* (response may not be evident for up to 5 days): Children: 1.5–4 mg/kg/day in 1 or 2 divided doses. Adults: 100 mg/day with a range of 25–200 mg/day. *Primary aldosteronism:* Children: 125–375 mg/m^2/day in divided doses. Adults: 400 mg/day in 1 or 2 divided doses.	Tablets: 25 mg, 50 mg, 100 mg (A stable suspension may be made by crushing tablets and suspending the powder in simple syrup or cherry syrup.)
Stavudine (Zerit)	*Orally:* Age 6 months–15 years: dose has not been established, but doses of 1–2 mg/kg/day have been well tolerated. Adults: <60 kg: 30 mg bid. ≥60 kg: 40 mg bid. Dosage must be adjusted in patients with renal dysfunction.	Capsules: 15 mg, 20 mg, 30 mg, 40 mg
Streptomycin	*IM:* Newborn: 20–30 mg/kg/24 hr in 2 divided doses for 10 days. Children: 20–40 mg/kg/24 hr in 2 divided doses for 10 days. Adults: 1–2 g in 1 or 2 doses daily. Maximum dose 2 g/24 hr.	Injection: 400 mg/ml
Sucralfate (Carafate)	Sucralfate is not absorbed from the GI tract. It may bind with other drugs administered at the same time, lowering their effectiveness; therefore, it should be administered at least 2 hours before or after other drugs.	Suspension: 1 g/10 ml Tablets: 1 g

Continued

Table 107 Medications (continued)

DRUG	DOSE	DOSAGE FORMS
Sucralfate (Carafate) (continued)	*Orally:* Children: dosage has not been established, but 40–80 mg/kg/day in 4 divided doses has been used. Adults: 1 g qid. The dose for stomatitis or mucositis is about 500 mg–1 g of suspension swished around the mouth and then spit out or swallowed, repeated qid.	
Sulfasalazine (Azulfidine)	*Orally:* Over age 2: initially 40–60 mg/kg/day in 3–6 divided doses (not to exceed 6 g/day), then decreasing to a maintenance dose of 20–40 mg/kg/day in 4 divided doses to a maximum dose of 2 g/day. Adults: initially 3–4 g/day in equally divided doses. Although doses as high as 12 g/day have been used, they are generally accompanied by an increased incidence of adverse effects. Maintenance doses are usually 2 g/day in 4 divided doses. The drug may cause a yellow discoloration of urine and skin.	Tablets: 500 mg Tablets, enteric coated: 500 mg
Sulfisoxazole (Gantrisin)	*Orally:* Over age 2 months: 150 mg/kg/day in 4 or 6 divided doses to a maximum daily dose of 6 g. An initial dose of 75 mg/kg may be given. Adults: 2–4 g initially followed by 4–8 g/day in 4–6 divided doses.	Solution or suspension: 500 mg/5 ml Tablets: 500 mg
Tacrolimus (FK-506, Prograf)	Patients are usually treated concurrently with an adrenal corticosteroid. *Orally:* Children: 0.3 mg/kg/day in 2 divided doses. Adults: 0.15–0.3 mg/kg/day in 2 divided doses. Doses may be decreased to a lower maintenance dose. *IV (as a continuous infusion):* Children: 0.1 mg/kg/day. Adults: 0.05–0.1 mg/kg/day. Conversion to oral therapy should take place as soon as the patient is able to tolerate oral medication.	Capsules: 1 mg, 5 mg Injection: 5 mg/ml
Terbutaline (Brethine, Bricanyl)	*Orally:* Under age 12: initially 0.05 mg/kg tid, increased gradually as required to a maximum of 0.15 mg/kg tid or total of 5 mg/24 hr. Over age 12: initially 2.5 mg tid. Maintenance: usually 5 mg or 0.075 mg/kg tid. *Parenteral, SC:* Under age 12: 0.01 mg/kg to a maximum of 0.3 mg every 15–20 minutes for 3 doses. Over age 12: 0.25 mg, repeated in 15–30 minutes if needed once only; a total dose of 0.5 mg should not be exceeded within a 4-hour period. *Inhalation:* 2 puffs every 4–6 hours.	Aerosol, oral: 0.2 mg/activation Injection: 1 mg/ml (1-ml ampul) Tablets: 2.5 mg, 5 mg
Tetanus immune globulin (Hyper-Tet)	*IM:* 250 U as a single dose for postexposure prophylaxis. For treatment of tetanus, doses of 3000–6000 U in children or adults are recommended. The immune globulin will not block the effectiveness of tetanus toxoid, but they should be administered at different sites.	Injection: 250 U/ml

Continued

Table 107   Medications   (continued)

DRUG	*DOSE*	*DOSAGE FORMS*
Tetanus toxoid, absorbed	*IM:* 0.5 ml. Primary immunization consists of 3 doses; the second dose is administered 4–8 weeks after the first dose, and the third dose is given 6–12 months after the second dose. Alternatively, the ACIP and AAP recommend 4 doses for primary immunization, with the first 3 administered at 4–8 week intervals and the fourth dose 6–12 months after the third dose. A fifth dose is usually administered before school entry at age 4–6. Subsequent boosters should be administered at 10-year intervals throughout life.	Injection: 5 Lf or 10 Lf units/0.5 ml
Tetracycline (Acromysin, Panmycin, Robitet, Sumycin)	*Orally* (should be given on an empty stomach): Over age 8: 25–50 mg/kg/day in 4 divided doses. Adults: 1–2 g/day in 2–4 divided doses.	Capsules: 250 mg, 500 mg Suspension: 125 mg/5 ml Tablets: 250 mg, 500 mg
Theophylline	*IV or orally for apnea in infants:* Premature neonates (postconceptional age under 40 weeks): 2 mg/kg/day in 2 divided doses. Term neonates under age 4 weeks: 5 mg/kg loading dose followed by 2–4 mg/kg/day in 2 or 3 divided doses. Term neonates over age 4 weeks: 5–7.5 mg/kg loading dose followed by 3–6 mg/kg/day in 3 divided doses. *Acute bronchospasm* (all dosing should be based on lean body weight): Loading dose: 1 mg/kg will increase serum theophylline concentration by 2 μg/ml. Patients who have received no theophylline in the previous 24 hours may be given 6 mg/kg. Patients who have received theophylline within the previous 24 hours may receive 3 mg/kg. Serum theophylline level should be monitored 30 minutes after the end of a bolus infusion. Loading dose should be administered IV over 30 minutes or PO using an immediate-release product. For patients requiring a continuous IV infusion of theophylline, it should be started at the completion of the bolus dose at the following rate for children: Age 6 months–1 year: 0.5 mg/kg/hr. Age 1–9: 0.9 mg/kg/hr. Age 9–12 and adolescent smokers: 0.8 mg/kg/hr. Age 12–16 (nonsmokers): 0.7 mg/kg/hr. Theophylline levels should be monitored 12–24 hours after beginning the infusion and daily while therapy continues. *Oral therapy for chronic bronchospasm:* Age 6 months–1 year: 12–18 mg/kg/day. Age 1–9: 20–24 mg/kg/day. Age 9–12 and adolescent smokers: 20 mg/kg/day. Age 12–16 (nonsmokers): 18 mg/kg/day. Over age 16 (nonsmokers): 13 mg/kg/day (not to exceed 900 mg/day).	*Immediate release:* Capsules: 100 mg, 200 mg Injection in D_5W: 0.4 mg/ml, 0.8 mg/ml, 1.6 mg/ml, 2 mg/ml, 3.2 mg/ml, 4 mg/ml Solution: 27 mg/5 ml, 50 mg/5 ml, 90 mg/5 ml (provided by 105 mg/5 ml of aminophylline) Tablets: 100 mg, 125 mg, 200 mg, 250 mg, 300 mg *Controlled release:* Capsules: 50 mg (Slo-Bid q 8–12 h), 60 mg (Slo-Phyllin q 8–12 h), 65 mg (Aerolate III q 8–12 h), 75 mg (Slo-Bid q 8–12 h), 100 mg (Slo-Bid q 8–12 h, Theo-24 q 24 h), 125 mg (Theovent q 12 h, Slo-Bid and Slo-Phyllin q 8–12 h), 130 mg (Theoclear L.A.-130 and Theospan-SR, q 12 h, Aerolate Jr. q 8–12 h), 200 mg (Slo-Bid q 8–12 h, Theo-24 q 24 h), 250 mg (Slo-Phyllin q 8–12 h, Theovent q 24 h), 260 mg (Theoclear L.A.-260, Theobid, and Theospan-SR q 12 h, Aerolate-SR q 8–12 h), 300 mg (Slo-Bid q 8–12 h, Theo-24 q 24 h) Tablets: 100 mg (Theochron q 12 h, Theo-Dur, Theo-Sav, and Theo-X q 12–24 h), 200 mg (Theochron q 12 h, Theo-Dur, Theo-Sav, and Theo-X q 12–24 h, Theolair-SR q 8–12 h), 250 mg (Respbid q 12 h, Theolair-SR q 8–12 h), 300 mg (Quibron-T/SR and Theochron q 12 h, Theo-Dur, Theo-Sav, and Theo-X q 12–24 h, Theolair-SR q 8–12 h), 400 mg (Uniphyl and Unicontin q 12–24 h), 450 mg (Theo-Dur q 12–24 h), 500 mg (Respbid q 12 h, Theolair-SR q 8–12 h)

Continued

Table 107   Medications   (continued)

DRUG	*DOSE*	*DOSAGE FORMS*
Theophylline (*continued*)	Frequency of dosing must be based on the characteristics of the product chosen. Immediate-release products must be administered every 6 hours. Extended-release products may be administered every 8–12 hours or even every 24 hours in adolescents using products designed for daily administration. Serum levels should be monitored frequently during early therapy to maintain serum levels between 10–20 μg/ml. After a stable dose is achieved, monitoring should be done at least every 6–12 months.	

Thiamine (vitamin B$_1$; Betalin S)	*Orally, IM, or IV:*
	Thiamine deficiency (beriberi):
	  Children: 10–25 mg IM or IV daily for critically ill children or 10–50 mg PO daily in divided doses.
	  Adults: 5–30 mg/day in 3 divided doses.
	Metabolic disorders: 10–20 mg/day, but doses up to 4 g/day in divided doses have been used.
		Injection: 100 mg/ml, 200 mg/ml
		Tablets: 5 mg, 10 mg, 25 mg, 50 mg, 100 mg, 250 mg, 500 mg

Ticarcillin (Ticar)	*IV (for the treatment of severe infections):*
	  Neonates under age 1 week:
	    <2 kg: 75 mg/kg every 12 hours.
	    >2 kg: 75 mg/kg every 8 hours.
	  Neonates from age 1–4 weeks:
	    <2 kg: 75 mg/kg every 8 hours.
	    >2 kg: 100 mg/kg every 8 hours.
	  Infants over age 4 weeks and children: 200–300 mg/kg/day in 4–6 divided doses.
	  Children weighing over 40 kg and adults: 200–300 mg/kg/day in 4–6 divided doses to a maximum daily dose of 24 g.
	Dosage must be adjusted in patients with renal or hepatic dysfunction.
		Injection: 1 g, 3 g, 6 g (20-g and 30-g pharmacy bulk packages)

Ticarcillin and clavulanate potassium (Timentin)	*IV (may be expressed in terms of ticarcillin content alone or in terms of the fixed ratio (30 : 1) of the commercially available combination product):*
	  Children:
	    <60 kg: 200–300 mg/kg/day of ticarcillin (207–310 mg of ticarcillin/clavulanic acid) in 4–6 divided doses.
	    >60 kg: 3 g ticarcillin + 0.1 g clavulanic acid (3.1 g of combination) every 4–6 hours to a maximum of 24 g of ticarcillin daily.
	Dosage must be adjusted in patients with renal or hepatic dysfunction.
		Injection: 3 g ticarcillin + 0.1 g clavulanic acid labelled as a combined total potency of 3.1 g (pharmacy bulk package containing 30 g ticarcillin + 1 g clavulanic acid)

Tobramycin (Nebcin, TobraDex, Tobrex)	*IV:*
	  Infants and children: 7.5 mg/kg/day in 3 divided doses to a maximum daily dose of 300 mg.
	  Older children and adults: 5 mg/kg/day in 3 divided doses to a maximum daily dose of 300 mg.
	Patients with cystic fibrosis may require higher doses and more frequent administration (10 mg/kg/day in 4 divided doses).
	Dosage may be increased based on the results of serum level monitoring.
	Dosage must be adjusted in patients with renal dysfunction.
	Ophthalmic:
	  Ointment: apply a 1-cm ribbon of ointment to the eye bid or tid.
	  Solution: apply 1–2 drops into the eye up to every 30–60 minutes in severe infections or every 3–4 hours for moderate infections.
		Injection: 10 mg/ml, 40 mg/ml
		Ointment, ophthalmic: 0.3%
		Ointment, ophthalmic: 0.3% with dexamethasone 0.1%
		Solution, ophthalmic: 0.3%
		Solution, ophthalmic: 0.3% with dexamethasone 0.1%

Continued

Table 107 Medications (continued)

DRUG	DOSE	DOSAGE FORMS
Tolmetin (Tolectin)	*Orally for rheumatoid arthritis:* Over age 2: initially 20 mg/kg/day in 3 or 4 divided doses, adjusted to the patient's response. Usual maintenance dosage range is 15–30 mg/kg/day. Adults: 600 mg–1.8 g/day in 3 divided doses.	Capsules: 400 mg Tablets: 200 mg, 600 mg
Tretinoin (retinoic acid; Retin-A)	*Topically:* apply to the affected area once daily after cleaning, generally at bedtime. Avoid application to areas not being treated. Use should be discontinued if severe reddening, swelling, or peeling occurs. After healing, therapy may be restarted with the same or a different formulation administered less frequently.	Cream: 0.025%, 0.05%, 0.1% Gel: 0.01%, 0.025% Solution: 0.05%
Trifluride (Viroptic)	*Topically to the eye:* apply 1 drop every 2 hours while awake until re-epithelialization has occurred. Maximum daily dose of 9 drops should not be exceeded. After re-epithelialization has occurred, dosage should be reduced to 1 drop every 4 hours for an additional 7 days to prevent recurrence, but the total length of therapy should not exceed 21 days.	Solution, ophthalmic: 1%
Trimethobenzamide (Tigan)	*IM* (not for infants or young children): 200 mg tid or qid. *Rectally* (not for neonates or infants): <13.6 kg: 100 mg tid or qid. 13.6–45 kg: 100–200 mg tid or qid. >45 kg: 200 mg tid or qid. *Orally:* 13.6–45 kg: 100–200 mg tid or qid. >45 kg: 250 mg tid or qid. Alternatively, a dose of 5 mg/kg administered tid or qid rectally or orally may be used.	Capsules: 100 mg, 250 mg Injection: 100 mg/ml Suppositories: 100 mg, 200 mg
Tropicamide (Mydriacyl, Ocu-Tropic, Tropicacyl)	*Topically to the eye:* 1 to 2 drops into the eye(s) 15–20 minutes before exam. 0.5% solution is usually sufficient for exam. If cycloplegia for refraction is necessary, 1% solution must be used and repeated in 5 minutes. Exam must take place within 30 minutes because its effect is short.	Solution, ophthalmic: 0.5%, 1%
Tuberculin, purified protein derivative	*Mantoux method* (intradermal injection): generally considered the most accurate and reliable skin test method available and should be used for surveillance of individuals likely to be exposed to clinical tuberculosis or to evaluate suspected cases or their contacts. The test solution recommended is 5 TU/0.1 ml. It should be injected intradermally using a tuberculin syringe with a short (¼″ to ½″) 26- or 27-gauge needle. The test site should be examined 48–72 hours later for a reaction. Interpretation of the skin test results depends somewhat on the type of individual being tested. In general, reactions that measure 5 mm or less in diameter may be considered negative. Induration reactions measuring >5 mm should be considered significant in individuals who have HIV infection. Induration reactions >10 mm should be considered significant in individuals who are at increased risk of tuberculosis but are otherwise normal. Induration reactions >15 mm should be considered significant in normal individuals at low risk.	Injection: 1 TU/0.1 ml, 5 TU/0.1 ml, 250 TU/0.1 ml Multiple puncture device

Continued

Table 107   Medications   (continued)

DRUG	_DOSE_	_DOSAGE FORMS_
Tuberculin, purified protein derivative (_continued_)	_Multiple puncture devices:_ should not be used if tuberculosis is suspected because the dose of tuberculin administered cannot be precisely controlled. They may be useful in initial screening of populations at low risk who are asymptomatic. The lest should be administered to the cleaned forearm with moderate pressure without twisting for at least 1 second. A clear imprint of the 4 lines and the base of the device should be visible. The site should be inspected 48–72 hours later. Vesiculation and/or induration >2 mm should be considered positive.	
Urokinase (Abbokinase Open-Cath)	An appropriate volume of urokinase 5000 IU/ml solution should be slowly and gently instilled into the catheter. After at least 5 minutes, a 5-ml syringe should be used to gently aspirate the solution and clot. Aspiration should be attempted every 5 minutes for 30 minutes. If unsuccessful, the catheter may be capped and allowed to sit for 30–60 minutes before attempting aspiration again. When patency is restored, 4–5 ml of blood should be aspirated from the catheter to ensure removal of all of the residual drug. The catheter should then be gently flushed with 10 ml of normal saline. Excessive pressure should be avoided to prevent expelling the clot into the circulation or rupture of the catheter.	Injection: 5000 IU, 9000 IU
Valproic acid, valproate sodium, and divalproex sodium (Depacon, Depakene, Depakote)	_Orally_ (expressed in terms of valproic acid): Initially 15 mg/kg/day increasing by 5–10 mg/kg/day at weekly intervals until seizures are controlled or side effects occur. Usual maximum total daily dose is 60 mg/kg. Frequency of administration in part depends on dosage form, but dosage is usually divided. To prevent adverse GI effects, capsules (valproic acid) and solution are usually administered in 2 or 3 divided doses. Divalproex usually may be administered in 2 divided doses. The usual therapeutic serum concentration range is 50–100 μg/ml. The oral solution has been administered rectally in patients who are NPO by diluting it 1:1 with tap water and administering it as a retention enema. _IV_ (over 1 hour): for patients who are not on valproic acid therapy, use the dosing and frequency of administration guidelines outlined above for oral dosing. For patients already on valproic acid therapy, use the patient's total oral daily dose and frequency of dosing for the IV route. The use of the injectable form for periods of more than 14 days has not been studied.	Capsules (divalproex sodium): 125 mg valproic acid Capsules (valproic acid): 250 mg Injection: 100 mg/ml Solution (valproate sodium): 250 mg valproic acid/ 5 ml Tablets (divalproex sodium): 125 mg, 250 mg, 500 mg valproic acid

Vancomycin (Lyphocin, Vancocin, Vancoled)	_IV_ (over at least 1 hour):
	Neonates under age 7 days:
	    <1000 g: 10 mg/kg every 24 hours.
	    >1000–2000 g: 10 mg/kg every 18 hours.
	    >2000 g: 10 mg/kg every 12 hours.
	Neonates age 7–30 days:
	    <1000 g: 10 mg/kg every 18 hours.
	    1000–2000 g: 10 mg/kg every 12 hours.
	    >2000 g: 10 mg/kg every 8 hours.
		Capsules: 125 mg, 250 mg
		Injection: 500 mg, 1 g (5-g, 10-g pharmacy bulk packages)
		Solution, oral: 1 g, 10 g

Continued

Table 107   Medications   (continued)

DRUG	DOSE	DOSAGE FORMS

Vancomycin (Lyphocin, Vancocin, Vancoled) (continued)	Infants age 31–60 days: 10 mg/kg every 8 hours.
	  Infants over age 2 months and children: 40 mg/kg/day in 4 divided doses to a maximum dose of 2 g/day.
	  Adults: 0.5 g every 6 hours or 1 g every 12 hours. Dosage adjustment is necessary in renal impairment.
	Higher doses, up to 60 mg/kg/day, may be required in children with staphylococcal central nervous system infections.
	Intrathecal:
	  Neonates: 5–10 mg/day.
	  Children: 5–20 mg/day.
	  Adults: 20 mg/day.
	Orally (not absorbed; do not use for systemic infections):
	  Children: 40 mg/kg/day in 4 divided doses to a maximum daily dose of 2 g.
	  Adults: 0.5–2 g/day in 3 or 4 divided doses.	

Varicella virus vaccine (Varivax)	SC (in the outer aspect of the upper arm):
	  Age 1–12: 0.5 ml single dose.
	  Adolescents and adults: 0.5 ml/dose for 2 doses separated by 4–8 weeks.
		Injection: 1350 PFU of Oka/Merck varicella virus (live). Keep frozen. Reconstituted vaccine must be used within 30 minutes and may be stored at room temperature.

Verapamil (Calan, Isoptin, Verelan)	*IV* (push over 2 to 3 minutes):
	  Under age 1: 0.1–0.2 mg/kg (usually 0.75–2 mg).
	  Age 1–16: 0.1–0.3 mg/kg to a maximum of 10 mg. May be repeated once in 30 minutes if not effective.
	  Over age 16: 0.075–0.15 mg/kg (5–10 mg) with a repeat dose in 30 minutes if necessary.
	Orally (not well established in children):
	  Age 1–5: 4–8 mg/kg/day in 3 divided doses or about 40–80 mg every 8 hours.
	  Over age 5: 80 mg every 6–8 hours.
	  Adults: 240–480 mg/day in 3 or 4 divided doses (1–2 doses daily using extended-release products for the treatment of hypertension).
		Capsules, extended release: 120 mg, 180 mg, 240 mg
		Injection: 2.5 mg/ml
		Tablets: 40 mg, 80 mg, 120 mg
		Tablets, extended release: 120 mg, 180 mg, 240 mg

Vitamin A (Aquasol A)	*Orally:*
	For malabsorption syndromes (water miscible product):
	  Under age 8: 5000–15,000 U/day.
	  Over age 8 and adults: 10,000–50,000 U/day.
	For severe deficiency with xerophthalmia:
	  Age 1–8: 5000 U/kg/day for 5 days or until recovery.
	  Over age 8 and adults: 500,000 U/day for 3 days, then 50,000 U/day for 14 days, then 10,000–20,000 U/day for 2 months.
	Deficiency (without corneal change):
	  Under age 1: 10,000 U/kg/day for 5 days, then 7500–15,000 U/day for 10 days.
	  Age 1–8: 5000–10,000 U/kg/day for 5 days, then 17,000–35,000 U/day for 10 days.
	  Over age 8 and adults: 100,000 U/day for 3 days then 50,000 U/day for 14 days.
	Dietary supplementation:
	  Infants up to age 6 months: 1500 U/day.
	  Age 6 months–3 years: 1500–2000 U/day.
	  Age 4–6: 2500 U/day.
	  Age 7–10: 3300–3500 U/day.
	  Over age 10 and adults: 4000–5000 U/day.
		Capsules: 10,000 U, 25,000 U, 50,000 U
		Solution: 50,000 U/ml

Continued

Table 107   Medications   (continued)

DRUG	DOSE	DOSAGE FORMS
Vitamin E [alpha tocopherol, alpha tocopheryl acetate, to-copherol polyethylene glycol succinate (TPGS), Aquasol E]	*Orally* (water miscible or water soluble TPGS products are recommended, especially for patients with mal-absorption): *Deficiency:* Infants: 25–50 U/day. *Children with malabsorption:* 15–25 U/kg/day to raise and maintain plasma tocopherol levels. Patients with cystic fibrosis, thalassemia, or sickle-cell disease may require larger daily doses (400–800 U/day). Adults: 60–75 U/day.	Capsules: 100 U, 200 U, 400 U, 600 U, 1000 U Capsules, water miscible: 100 U, 200 U, 400 U Solution, water miscible: 50 U/ml Solution (TPGS): 400 U/15 ml
Vitamins, multiple	*Orally:* 1 ml or 1 tablet daily. Drops are formulated for children under age 2; chewable tablets for children over age 2. *IV:* pediatric formulation for infants and children usually administered over 24 hours in TPN or IV solutions. Adult formulation is used for older children and adults.	Many formulations are available. Specialized references should be consulted.
Warfarin sodium (Coumadin)	Infants and children: Loading dose 0.2 mg/kg (max 10 mg) on day 1. Maintenance dose 0.1 mg/kg/day with a range of 0.05–0.34 mg/kg/d; infant <12 months may require doses near high end of this range; may be difficult to maintain in children <5 years. Adults: 5–15 mg/day initially for 2–5 days until desired PT is reached. Usual maintenance dosage range is 2–10 mg/day.	Tablets: 1 mg, 2 mg, 2.5 mg, 4 mg, 5 mg, 7.5 mg, 10 mg
Zalcitabine (ddC, Hivid)	*Orally:* Under age 13: not approved for use in these patients. Adolescents age 13–adults: 0.75 mg every 8 hours on an empty stomach. Adjust dose in patients with renal dysfunction.	Tablets: 0.375 mg, 0.75 mg
Zidovudine (Retrovir)	*Orally:* Age 3 months–12 years: 180 mg/m² every 6 hours to a maximum of 200 mg every 6 hours. Dosage may be decreased in patients who develop anemia and/or granulocytopenia. Adults: *Asymptomatic:* 100 mg every 4 hours while awake (500 mg/day). *Symptomatic:* 100 mg every 4 hours (600 mg/day). *IV:* Age 3 months–13 years: 0.5–1.8 mg/kg/hr as a continuous infusion or 100 mg/m² by infusion over 1 hour every 6 hours. Adults: 1–2 mg/kg every 4 hours 6 times daily. *Maternal–fetal HIV transmission prevention:* Maternal (>14 weeks of pregnancy): 100 mg every 4 hours while awake (500 mg/day) until the onset of labor. During labor and delivery, 2 mg/kg over 1 hour followed by a continuous IV infusion of 1 mg/kg/hr until the umbilical cord is clamped. Infant: 2 mg/kg orally every 6 hours starting within 12 hours of birth and continuing for 6 weeks. For infants unable to tolerate oral drugs, 6 mg/kg/day IV in 4 evenly divided doses may be used. Dosage adjustment is necessary in severe renal impairment.	Capsules: 100 mg Injection: 10 mg/ml Solution: 50 mg/5 ml

Continued

Table 107   Medications   (continued)

DRUG	DOSE	DOSAGE FORMS

Zinc	Response may not occur for 6–8 weeks
	Orally:
	    Infants and children: 0.5–1 mg/kg/day of elemental zinc in 1–3 divided doses.
	    Adults: 25–50 mg elemental zinc tid.
	Acrodermatitis enteropathica: 10–45 mg/day elemental zinc
	Zinc sulfate 4.4 mg = 1 mg elemental zinc (220 mg = 50 mg).
		Zinc sulfate (23% zinc):
		    Capsules: 220 mg (50 mg zinc)
		    Injection: 1 mg/ml, 5 mg/ml (zinc)
		    Tablets: 66 mg (15 mg zinc), 110 mg (25 mg zinc), 220 mg (45 mg zinc)
		Zinc gluconate (14.3% zinc):
		    Tablets: 10 mg (1.4 mg zinc), 15 mg (2 mg zinc), 50 mg (7 mg zinc), 78 mg (11 mg zinc)

Table 108   Citric Acid and Citrate Dosage Forms (Content per 1 ml)

PRODUCT	SODIUM CITRATE	POTASSIUM CITRATE	CITRIC ACID	BICARBONATE EQUIVALENT
Bicitra solution	100 mg (1 mEq Na)	. . .	66.8 mg	1 mEq
Oracit solution	98 mg (1 mEq Na)	. . .	128 mg	1 mEq
Polycitra K solution	. . .	220 mg (2 mEq K)	66.8 mg	2 mEq
Polycitra-LC solution	100 mg (1 mEq Na)	110 mg (1 mEq K)	66.8 mg	2 mEq

Table 109   Digoxin Dosing

	TOTAL DIGITALIZING DOSE (µg/kg)		DAILY MAINTENANCE DOSE (µg/kg DIVIDED IN 2 DOSES)	
AGE	PO	IV	PO	IV
Preterm infant	20–30	15–25	5–7.5	4–6
Full-term infant	25–40	20–30	6–10	5–8
1 month to 2 years	35–60	30–50	10–15	7.5–12
2 years to adult	30–40	25–35	7.5–15	6–9
Maximum dose	0.75–1.5 mg	0.5–1 mg	0.125–0.5 mg	0.1–0.4 mg

IV = intravenously; PO = orally.

Table 110   Pancrelipase Dosage Forms

	LIPASE (USP UNITS)	AMYLASE (USP UNITS)	PROTEASE (USP UNITS)
Capsules (enteric coated or delayed-release microspheres)			
Cotazym-S	5000	20,000	20,000
Creon	8000	30,000	13,000
Creon-10	10,000	33,200	37,500
Creon-20	20,000	66,400	75,000
Pancrease	4500	20,000	25,000
Pancrease MT-4	4500	12,000	12,000
Pancrease MT-10	10,000	30,000	30,000
Pancrease MT-16	16,000	48,000	48,000
Pancrease MT-20	20,000	56,000	44,000
Ultrase MT-12	12,000	39,000	39,000
Ultrase MT-20	20,000	65,000	65,000
Zymase	12,000	24,000	24,000
Capsules (filled with non–enteric coated powder)			
Cotazym, Ku-Zyme HP	8000	30,000	30,000
Powder (not enteric-coated)			
Viokase (per 0.7 g)	16,800	70,000	70,000
Tablets (not enteric-coated)			
Ilozyme	11,000	30,000	30,000
Viokase	8000	30,000	30,000

Index

Page numbers in boldface indicate major discussion; page numbers in italics denote figures; those followed by "t" denote tables.

Index

Index

Index

Index

Index

Index

Index

Index

Index

Index

Index

Index

Index

Index

Index

Index